Neonatal and Pediatric Pharmacology

Therapeutic Principles in Practice

FOURTH EDITION

Neonatal and Pediatric Pharmacology

Therapeutic Principles in Practice

Sumner J. Yaffe, MD

Consulting Professor
Stanford University School of Medicine
Palo Alto, California

Jacob V. Aranda, MD, PhD, FRCP(C), FAAP

Professor of Pediatrics
Director of Neonatology
Department of Pediatrics
State University of New York Downstate Medical Center
Brooklyn, New York
Professor
Departments of Pediatrics, Pharmacology, and Pharmaceutical Sciences
Pediatric Pharmacology Research Unit Network (PPRU)
Wayne State University
Children's Hospital of Michigan
Detroit, Michigan

Wolters Kluwer | Lippincott Williams & Wilkins
Health
Philadelphia • Baltimore • New York • London
Buenos Aires • Hong Kong • Sydney • Tokyo

Acquisitions Editor: Sonya Seigafuse
Product Manager: Kerry Barrett/Nicole Walz
Vendor Manager: Alicia Jackson
Senior Manufacturing Manager: Benjamin Rivera
Marketing Manager: Lisa Lawrence
Design Coordinator: Holly Reid McLaughlin
Production Services: Aptara, Inc.

Two Commerce Square, 2001 Market Street
Philadelphia, PA 19103
LWW.com

Printed in China

Library of Congress Cataloging-in-Publication Data
Neonatal and pediatric pharmacology : therapeutic principles in practice / [edited by] Sumner J. Yaffe, Jacob V. Aranda. — 4th ed.
p. ; cm.
Includes bibliographical references and index.
Summary: "Neonatal and Pediatric Pharmacology offers guidelines for safe, effective, and rational drug therapy in newborns, children and adolescents. The book provides relevant and useful data on the molecular, physiologic, biochemical, and pharmacologic mechanisms of drug action and therapy in this population. The authors identify areas of innovative basic and translational research necessary for the continuing evaluation and development of drugs for the fetus, newborns, children and adolescents. Neonatal and Pediatric Pharmacology is a valuable reference for all health care professionals who treat the fetus, newborns, children, and adolescents, including neonatologists, nurses, pediatricians, general practitioners, students, obstetricians, perinatologists, surgeons and allied health professionals. It will be useful anytime during the day and especially in the middle of the night when knowledge of appropriate indications, safe and effective use, dosage, and therapeutic regimen for a certain drug or molecular entity is immediately needed. The book is also directed to those involved in basic, clinical, and other academic pharmacological research, the pharmaceutical industry, and regulatory agencies dealing with drug and therapeutic developments for this population. Those teaching pharmacology and therapeutics will find this compilation of information extremely useful in preparing teaching materials"—Provided by publisher.
ISBN-13: 978-0-7817-9538-8 (hardback : alk. paper)
ISBN-10: 0-7817-9538-9 (hardback : alk. paper)
1. Pediatric pharmacology. 2. Children—Diseases—Chemotherapy.
I. Yaffe, Sumner J., 1923– II. Aranda, Jacob V.
[DNLM: 1. Drug Therapy. 2. Child. 3. Infant. 4. Pharmaceutical Preparations—administration & dosage. 5. Pharmacological Phenomena.
WS 366 N4381 2010]
RJ560.P4 2010
615′.1083—dc22

2010024217

Care has been taken to confirm the accuracy of the information presented and to describe generally accepted practices. However, the authors, editors, and publisher are not responsible for errors or omissions or for any consequences from application of the information in this book and make no warranty, expressed or implied, with respect to the currency, completeness, or accuracy of the contents of the publication. Application of the information in a particular situation remains the professional responsibility of the practitioner.

The authors, editors, and publisher have exerted every effort to ensure that drug selection and dosage set forth in this text are in accordance with current recommendations and practice at the time of publication. However, in view of ongoing research, changes in government regulations, and the constant flow of information relating to drug therapy and drug reactions, the reader is urged to check the package insert for each drug for any change in indications and dosage and for added warnings and precautions. This is particularly important when the recommended agent is a new or infrequently employed drug.

Some drugs and medical devices presented in the publication have Food and Drug Administration (FDA) clearance for limited use in restricted research settings. It is the responsibility of the health care providers to ascertain the FDA status of each drug or device planned for use in their clinical practice.

To purchase additional copies of this book, call our customer service department at (800) 638-3030 or fax orders to (301) 223-2320. International customers should call (301) 223-2300.

Visit Lippincott Williams & Wilkins on the Internet: at LWW.com. Lippincott Williams & Wilkins customer service representatives are available from 8:30 am to 6 pm, EST.

10 9 8 7 6 5 4 3 2 1

To our loved ones

Kenneth Frederic and Christopher James Aranda

And

Suzie, Steve, Kristine, Jason, Noah, Ian, and Zachary Yaffe

For their unending love and unconditional support

Special thanks to Susanne Goldstein

For her editorial assistance

And to Kerry Barrett and Nicole Walz

For their dedicated enthusiasm and invaluable assistance in the preparation of the text

Nahed M. Abdel-Haq, M.D.
Associate Professor of Pediatrics
School of Medicine, Department of Pediatrics
Wayne State University;
Faculty Member, Division of Infectious Diseases
Department of Pediatrics
Children's Hospital of Michigan
Detroit, Michigan

Edward Paul Acosta, Pharm.D.
Professor
Division of Clinical Pharmacology
University of Alabama at Birmingham
Birmingham, Alabama

Mahmoud S. Ahmed, Ph.D.
Professor and Director, Maternal Fetal Pharmacology and Bio-Development Laboratories
OB/GYN, Graduate Programs in Pharmacology & Toxicology and Biochemistry & Molecular Biology
University of Texas Medical Branch
Galveston, Texas

Karel Allegaert, M.D., Ph.D.
Associate Professor
Department of Woman and Child
Katholieke Universiteit, Leuven;
Consultant
Neonatal Intensive Care Unit
University Hospitals, Leuven
Leuven, Belgium

Brian J. Anderson, Ph.D.
Departments of Anesthesia and Intensive Care
Auckland Children's Hospital
Grafton, Auckland, New Zealand

Jocelyn Y. Ang, M.D.
Associate Professor
Department of Pediatrics
Wayne State University;
Staff Physician
Department of Pediatrics
Children's Hospital of Michigan
Detroit, Michigan

John N. van den Anker, M.D., Ph.D.
Professor
Departments of Pediatrics, Pharmacology & Physiology
George Washington University School of Medicine and Health Sciences;
Vice Chairman of Pediatrics for Experimental Therapeutics and Chief Pediatric Clinical Pharmacology
Departments of Pediatrics
Children's National Medical Center
Washington, District of Colombia

Jacob V. Aranda, M.D., Ph.D., F.R.C.P.C., F.A.A.P.
Professor and Director of Neonatology
Pediatric Pharmacology Research Unit Network (NIH PPRU)
The Children's Hospital of Brooklyn
State University of New York Downstate Medical Center
Brooklyn, New York

Alana Arnold, Pharm.D.
Department of Pharmacy
Children's Hospital of Boston
Boston, Massachusetts

Basim I. Asmar, M.D.
Professor of Pediatrics
School of Medicine, Department of Pediatrics
Wayne State University;
Director, Division of Infectious Diseases
Department of Pediatrics
Children's Hospital of Michigan
Detroit, Michigan

Henrietta Bada, M.D.
Mary Florence Jones Professor of Pediatrics
Chief, Division of Neonatology
Department of Pediatrics
College of Medicine, University of Kentucky
Lexington, Kentucky

Sami L. Bahna, M.D., Dr., Ph.D.
Professor and Chief of Allergy & Immunology Section
Pediatrics
Louisiane State University Health Sciences Center
Shreveport, Louisiana

Daniel K. Benjamin Jr., M.D., Ph.D., M.P.H.
Professor of Pediatrics
Department of Pediatrics
Division of Infectious Diseases
Duke University School of Medicine
Duke University Medical Center
Durham, North Carolina

Stacey L. Berg, M.D.
Professor
Department of Pediatrics
Baylor College of Medicine;
Texas Children's Cancer Center
Texas Children's Hospital
Houston, Texas

Cheston M. Berlin Jr., M.D.
Department of Pediatrics
Pennsylvania State University College of Medicine and Penn State Children's Hospital
Hershey, Pennsylvania

Brookie M. Best, Pharm.D., M.A.S.
Assistant Clinical Professor of Pharmacy and Pediatrics
Skaggs School of Pharmacy and Pharmaceutical Sciences, and Department of Pediatrics, School of Medicine/Rady Children's Hospital San Diego
University of California, San Diego
La Jolla, California

Jeffrey L. Blumer, M.D., Ph.D.
Departments of Pediatrics and Pharmacology
School of Medicine, Case Western Reserve University
Division of Pediatric Pharmacology and Critical Care
Rainbow Babies and Children's Hospital
Cleveland, Ohio

Lisa R. Bomgaars, M.D., M.S.
Associate Professor
Pediatrics
Baylor College of Medicine;
Texas Children's Cancer Center
Texas Children's Hospital
Houston, Texas

Rada Boskovic, M.D.
The Motherisk Program
Division of Clinical Pharmacology and Toxicology
Toronto, Ontario, Canada

Mirjana Lulic Botica, B.Sc., R.Ph., B.C.P.S.
Neonatal Clinical Pharmacy specialist
Department of Pharmacy
Hutzel women's Hosptial
Detroit, Michigan

Tania S. Burgert, M.D.
Assistant Professor Pediatrics
Section of Pediatric Endocrinology
Yale University School of Medicine
New Haven, Connecticut

Edmund V. Capparelli, Pharm.D.
Clinical Professor, Pediatrics and Pharmacy
Pediatric Pharmacology and Drug Discovery
Pediatrics and Skaggs School of Pharmacy and Pharmaceutical Sciences
University of California
San Diego, California

Bruce Carleton, B.Sc., Pharm.D.
Professor
Departments of Paediatrics and Pharmaceutical Sciences
University of British Columbia;
Director
Pharmaceutical Outcomes and Policy Innovations Programme
Woman's and Children's Health Centre of British Columbia
Vancouver, British Columbia, Canada

Eda Cengiz, M.D., F.A.A.P.
Associate Research Scientist
Division of Pediatric Endocrinology
Yale School of Medicine
New Haven, Connecticut

Evangelia Charmandari, M.D., Ph.D.
Associate Professor in Pediatric and Adolescent Endocrinology
First Department of Pediatrics
University of Athens Medical School
'Aghia Sophia' Children's Hospital
Athens, Greece

Sylvain Chemtob, M.D., Ph.D., F.R.C.P.C., F.C.A.H.S.
Professor
Pediatrics, Pharmacology
University of Montreal;
Neonatologist
Pediatrics
Centre Hospitalier Universitaire Sainte-Justine
Montreal, Canada

Russell W. Chesney, M.D.
Le Bonheur Professor and Chair
Department of Pediatrics
University of Tennessee Health Science Center;
Chief of Pediatrics
Department of Pediatrics
Le Bonheur Children's Hospital
Memphis, Tennessee

John Chou, M.D., M.S.
Associate Professor of Pediatrics
Pediatrics
University of Pennsylvania;
Neonatal Quality Officer
Neonatology
Children's Hospital of Philadelphia
Philadelphia, Pennsylvania

George P. Chrousos, M.D., M.A.C.P., M.A.C.E.
Professor of Pediatrics
First Department of Pediatrics
University of Athens Medical School
'Aghia Sophia' Children's Hospital
Athens, Greece

Harry T. Chugani, M.D.
Pediatric Neurology
Children's Hospital of Michigan, and Department of Pediatrics
Wayne State University School of Medicine
Detroit, Michigan

Sanford N. Cohen, M.D.
Department of Pediatrics
Wayne State University;
Department of Pediatrics
Children's Hospital of Michigan
Detroit, Michigan

Michael Cohen-Wolkowiez, M.D.
Assistant Professor of Pediatrics
Division of Infectious Diseases
Department of Pediatrics
Duke University School of Medicine
Duke University Medical Center
Durham, North Carolina

Charles J. Coté, M.D., F.A.A.P.
Professor of Anaesthesia
Harvard Medical School;
Senior Anesthetist
Division of Pediatric Anesthesia
MassGeneral Hospital for Children
Department of Anesthesia and Critical Care
Massachusetts General Hospital
Boston, Massachusetts

Erika Crane, M.D.
Pediatric Clinical Pharmacology Fellow
Pediatrics
Children's Hospital of Michigan
Detroit, Michigan

Virginia Delaney-Black, M.D., M.P.H.
Department of Pediatrics
Wayne State University;
Department of Pediatrics
Children's Hospital of Michigan and Child Research Center of Michigan
Detroit, Michigan

David J. Diemert, M.D., F.R.C.P.(C)
Assistant Professor
Microbiology, Immunology & Tropical Medicine
The George Washington University
Washington, District of Colombia

Maria Delivoria-Papadopoulos, M.D.
Department of Pediatrics
St. Christopher's Hospital for Children
Drexel University College of Medicine
Philadelphia, Pennsylvania

Nada Djokanovic, M.D., M.Sc.
The Motherisk Program
Division of Clinical Pharmacology and Toxicology
The Hospital for Sick Children and University of Toronto
Toronto, Ontario, Canada

Véronique G. Dorval, M.D.
Neonatal Fellow
Department of Pediatrics
University of Montreal;
Neonatal Fellow
Department of Pediatrics
CHU Sainte-Justine
Montreal, Canada

Hakan Ergün, M.D.
Ankara University
Faculty of Medicine
Department of Pharmacology and Clinical Pharmacology
Sihhiye-Ankara, Turkey

Henry C. Farrar, M.D.
Professor
Department of Pediatrics & Pharmacology
University of Arkansas for Medical Sciences;
Clinical Pharmacologist
Section of Clinical Pharmacology & Toxicology
Arkansas Children's Hospital
Little Rock, Arkansas

Evridiki Vicky Fera, M.B.Ch.B.
The Children's Hospital of Buffalo
Department of Pediatrics
Buffalo, New York

Delbert A. Fisher, M.D.
Academic Associate
Quest Diagnostics Nichols Institute
San Juan Capistrano, California

Daniel A.C. Frattarelli, M.D., F.A.A.P.
Chair, AAP Committee on Drugs
Program Director and Chair, Pediatrics
Oakwood Hospital and Medical
Center
Dearborn, Michigan

Rafael Gorodischer, M.D.
Professor Emeritus
Department of Pediatrics
Ben-Gurion University of the Negev;
Patient Safety & Risk Management Unit
Hospital Administration
Soroka Medical Center
Beer-Sheva, Israel

Scott A. Gruber, M.D.
Professor and Chief, Section of Transplant Surgery
Department of Surgery
Wayne State University School of Medicine;
Director, Organ Transplant Program
Department of Surgery
Harper University Hospital
Detroit, Michigan

Jean-Pierre Guignard, M.D.
Division of Nephrology
Department of Pediatrics
University Medical Center (CHUV)
Lausanne, Switzerland

Harvey Guyda, M.D.
Chairman
Department of Pediatrics
McGill University;
Pediatrician in Chief
Department of Pediatrics
Montreal Children's Hospital
McGill University Health Centre
Montreal, Quebec, Canada

Susan R. Hintz, M.D., M.S.
Department of Pediatrics
Division of Neonatal and Developmental Medicine
Stanford University School of Medicine
Stanford, California

Matthijs de Hoog, M.D., Ph.D.
Associate professor of pediatrics
Department of Pediatrics
Erasmus MC;
Deputy director
Intensive Care
Erasmus MC—Sophia Children's Hospital
Rotterdam, The Netherlands

Mohammad Ilyas, M.D.
Associate Professor
Department of Pediatrics
University of Arkansas for Medical Sciences (UAMS);
Pediatric Nephrologist
Department of Pediatrics
Arkansas Children Hospital
Little Rock, Arkansas

Amrish Jain, M.D.
Assistant Professor
The Carman and Ann Adams
Department of Pediatrics
Wayne State University;
Clinical Educator
Division of Pediatric Nephrology and Hypertension
Children's Hospital of Michigan
Detroit, Michigan

Laura P. James, M.D.
Professor
Pediatrics & Pharmacology
University of Arkansas for Medical Science;
Section Chief
Section of Clinical Pharmacology & Toxicology
Arkansas Children's Hospital
Little Rock, Arkansas

Alan H. Jobe, M.D. Ph.D.
Professor of Pediatrics
Cincinnati Children's Hospital
University of Cincinnati School of Medicine
Cincinnati, Ohio

Deborah P. Jones, M.D.
Professor
Department of Pediatrics
University of Tennessee, Health Science Center;
Pediatric Nephrologist
LeBonheur Children's Hospital
Memphis, Tennessee

Sandra E. Juul, M.D., Ph.D.
Professor
Department of Pediatrics
University of Washington;
Associate Division Head for Scholarship and Research
Pediatrics
University of Washington
Seattle, Washington

Ralph E. Kauffman, M.D.
Department of Pediatrics
University of Missouri–Kansas City, and Children's Mercy Hospital
Kansas City, Missouri

H. William Kelly, Pharm.D.
Professor Emeritus
Department of Pediatrics
University of New Mexico Health Sciences Center
Albuquerque, New Mexico

Gregory L. Kearns, Pharm.D., Ph.D.
Associate Chairman
Pediatrics
University of Missouri Kansas City;
Director Pediatric Pharmacology Res. Unit
Division of Pediatric Pharmacology
Children's Mercy Hospitals
Kansas City, Missouri

David W. Kimberlin, M.D.
Professor of Pediatrics
Department of Pediatrics
University of Alabama at Birmingham
Birmingham, Alabama

Tomoshige Kino, M.D., Ph.D.
Division of Endocrinology and Metabolism (E.C., G.P.C.)
Clinical Research Center
Biomedical Research Foundation of the Academy of Athens
Athens, Greece;
Section on Pediatric Endocrinology (E.C., T.K., G.P.C.)
Program in Reproductive and Adult Endocrinology
Eunice Kennedy Shriver National Institute of Child Health & Human Development
Bethesda, Maryland

Gideon Koren, M.D., F.R.C.P.(C.), F.A.C.M.T.
The Motherisk Program
Division of Clinical Pharmacology and Toxicology
The Hospital for Sick Children
University of Toronto
Toronto, Ontario, Canada

J. Steven Leeder, Pharm.D., Ph.D.
Professor of Pediatric and Pharmacology
Schools of Medicine and Pharmacy
University of Missouri-Kansas City;
Marion Merrell Dow/Missouri Endowed Chair in Pediatric Clinical Pharmacology,
Chief, Division of Clinical Pharmacology and Medical Toxicology
Department of Pediatrics
Children's Mercy Hospitals and Clinics
Kansas City, Missouri

George Lambert, M.D.
Associate Professor,
Pediatric Pharmacology and Toxicology,
Department of Pediatrics;
Attending Neonatologist
Pediatrics
Robert Wood Johnson University Hospital
New Brunswick, New Jersey

Agustin Legido, M.D., Ph.D.
Department of Pediatrics
St. Christopher's Hospital for Children
Drexel University College of Medicine
Philadelphia, Pennsylvania

Mary W. Lieh-Lai, M.D.
Associate Professor of Pediatrics
Co-Chief, Critical Care Medicine
Children's Hospital of Michigan
Wayne State University School of Medicine
Detroit, Michigan

Jose Maria Lopes, M.D., Ph.D.
Department of Neonatology
Institute Fernandes Figueira
Rio de Janerio, Brazil

Victoria Tutag Lehr, R.Ph., Pharm.D.
Associate Professor
Department of Pharmacy Practice
Eugene Applebaum College of Pharmacy and Health Sciences, Wayne State University;
Associate Professor
Division of Clinical Pharmacology and Toxicology
Children's Hospital of Michigan
Detroit, Michigan

Richard L. Levine, M.D.
Professor
Department of Pediatrics and Psychiatry
Penn State College of Medicine;
Chief, Adolescent Medicine and Eating Disorders
Department of Pediatrics
Penn State Hershey
Hershey, Pennsylvania

Jennifer A. Lowry, M.D.
Assistant Professor
Department of Pediatrics
University of Missouri—Kansas City School of Medicine;
Clinical Pharmacologist and Medical Toxicologist
Clinical Pharmacology and Medical Toxicology
Children's Mercy Hospital
Kansas City, Missouri

Sanna Mahmoud, M.D., Ph.D.
Director
Allergy & Immunology
Lake Cumberland Regional Hospital
Somerset, Kentucky

Shannon F. Manzi, Pharm.D.
Department of Pharmacy
Children's Hospital of Boston and Northeastern University
Boston, Massachusetts

Cecilia C. Maramba-Lazarte, M.D., M.Sc.ID
Associate Professor
Department of Pharmacology and Toxicology
College of Medicine, University of the Philippines Manila;
Consultant, Pediatric Infectious Diseases and Tropical Medicine
Department of Pediatrics
Philippine General Hospital
Manila, Philippines

Merene Mathew, M.D.
Fellow
Clinical Pharmacology & Toxicology
Children's Hospital of Michigan
Detroit, Michigan

Doreen Matsui, M.D., F.R.C.P.C.
Children's Hospital
London Health Sciences Centre
London, ON, Canada

Tej K. Mattoo, M.D., D.C.H., F.R.C.P. (U.K.), F.A.A.P.
Professor
Department of Pediatrics
Wayne State University School of Medicine;
Chief, Pediatric Nephrology and Hypertension
Department of Pediatrics
Children's Hospital of Michigan
Detroit, Michigan

Donald R. Mattison, M.D., CAPT., U.S.P.H.S.
Eunice Kennedy Shriver
National Institute of Child Health and Human Development
National Institutes of Health, Department of Health and Human Services
Bethesda, Maryland

Paola J. Maurtua-Neumann, M.D.
Fellow
Pediatric Infectious Diseases
Tulane University Medical Center
New Orleans, Los Angeles

Mark Mirochnick, M.D.
Professor
Department of Pediatrics
Boston University School of Medicine;
Chief
Division of Neonatology
Boston Medical Center
Boston, Massachusetts

Allen A. Mitchell, M.D.
Professor of Pediatrics & Epidemiology
Boston University Schools of Medicine & Public Health;
Director
Slone Epidemiology Center at Boston University
Boston, Massachusetts

Al Patterson, Pharm.D.
Department of Pharmacy
Children's Hospital of Boston
Boston, Massachusetts

Om Prakash Mishra, M.D.
Department of Pediatrics
St. Christopher's Hospital for Children
Drexel University College of Medicine
Philadelphia, Pennsylvania

Milap C. Nahata, M.S., Pharm.D.
College of Pharmacy and Department of Pediatrics
College of Medicine, Ohio State University
Columbus, Ohio

Sumathi Nambiar, M.D., M.P.H.
Division of Anti-Infective and Ophthalmology Products
US Food and Drug Administration
Silver Spring, Maryland

Tatiana Nanovskaya, D.D.S., Ph.D.
Assistant Professor
OB/GYN
University of Texas Medical Branch
Galveston, Texas

Girija Natarajan, M.D.
Assistant Professor
Department of Pediatrics
Wayne State University;
Medical Director
NICU, Department of Pediatrics
Children's Hospital of Michigan
Detroit, Michigan

John P. Newnham, M.B.B.S., M.D., FRANZCOG, C.M.F.M.
Winthrop Professor of Obstetrics, Head of School
School of Women's and Infants' Health
The University of Western Australia;
Maternal Fetal Medicine Subspecialist
Obstetrics and Gynaecology
King Edward memorial Hospital
Perth, Western Australia

Annie Nguyen-Vermillion, M.D.
Neonatal Fellow
Department of Pediatrics, Division of Neonatology
University of Washington
Seattle, Washington

Catherine E. O'Brien, Pharm.D.
Assistant Professor
Pharmacy Practice
University of Arkansas for Medical Sciences;
Clinical Pharmacist
Section of Clinical Pharmacology & Toxicology
Arkansas Children's
Little Rock, Arkansas

Pearay L. Ogra, M.D.
Emeritus Professor
School of Medicine and Biomedical Sciences
University at Buffalo
State University of New York
Buffalo, New York;
Former John Sealy Distinguished Chair
Professor and Chairman
Department of Pediatrics
University of Texas Medical Branch at Galveston
Galveston, Texas

Kristine G. Palmer, M.D.
Assistant Professor
Department of Pediatrics
University of Arkansas for Medical Sciences;
Medical Co-Director, NICU
Department of Pediatrics
University of Arkansas for Medical Sciences
Little Rock, Arkansas

Ian M. Paul, M.D., M.Sc.
Associate Professor
Pediatrics and Public Health Sciences
Penn State College of Medicine;
Penn State Milton S. Hershey Medical Center
Hershey, Pennsylvania

Mary Frances Picciano, Ph.D.
Office of Dietary Supplements
National Institutes of Health
Bethesda, Maryland
Email: PiccianoMF@od.nih.gov

David G. Poplack, M.D.
Elise C. Young Professor of Pediatric Oncology
Head, Hematology–Oncology Section
Department of Pediatrics
Baylor College of Medicine;
Director, Texas Children's Cancer Center
Texas Children's Hospital
Houston, Texas

Hengameh H. Raissy, Pharm.D., Ph.C.
Research Associate Professor
Department of Pediatrics
University of New Mexico;
Pharmacist Clinician
Department of Pediatrics
University of New Mexico Hospital
Albuquerque, New Mexico

Anders Rane, M.D., Ph.D.
Professor
Department of Clinical Pharmacology
Karolinska Institutet
Stockholm, Sweden

Michael D. Reed, Pharm.D., F.C.P.
Department of Pediatrics
School of Medicine, Case Western Reserve University
Division of Pediatric Pharmacology and Critical Care
Rainbow Babies and Children's Hospital
Cleveland, Ohio

Michael Rieder, M.D., Ph.D., F.R.C.P.C., F.A.A.P., F.R.P.C. (Glasgow)
CIHR-GSK Chair in Paediatric Clinical Pharmacology
Departments of Paediatrics, Physiology & Pharmacology and Medicine
Schulich School of Medicine & Dentistry, University of Western Ontario;
Chief
Section of Paediatric Clinical Pharmacology
Department of Paediatrics
Children's Hospital
London Health Sciences Centre
London, Ontario, Canada

John Denis Roarty, M.D., M.P.H.
Associate Professor
Department of Ophthalmology
Wayne State University;
Chief of Ophthalmology
Department of Ophthalmology
Children's Hospital of Michigan
Detroit, Michigan

Celia Rodd, M.D.
Associate Professor
Department of Pediatrics
McGill University
Montreal, Canada

William J. Rodriguez, M.D., Ph.D.
Professor Emeritus
Department of Pediatrics
The George Washington University School of Medicine
Washington, District of Colombia;
Science Director
Office of Pediatric Therapeutics/Office of the Commissioner
US Food and Drug Administration
Rockville, Maryland

Chokechai Rongkavilit, M.D.
Associate Professor
Department of Pediatrics
Wayne State University;
Staff Physician
Department of Pediatrics
Children's Hospital of Michigan
Detroit, Michigan

Bruce A. Russell, B.A., M.A., Ph.D.
Department of Philosophy
Wayne State University
Detroit, Michigan

Ashok P. Sarnaik, M.D.
Professor of Pediatrics
Co-Chief, Critical Care Medicine
Children's Hospital of Michigan
Wayne State University School of Medicine
Detroit, Michigan

Urs B. Schaad, M.D.
Professor of Pediatrics and Pediatric Infectious Diseases
University of Basel;
Chairman of Pediatrics and Medical Director
University Children's Hospital UKBB
Basel, Switzerland

Michael W. Shannon, M.D., M.P.H.
Division of Emergency Medicine
Children's Hospital of Boston
Department of Pediatrics, Harvard Medical School
Boston, Massachusetts

Bernard H. Shapiro, Ph.D.
Professor of Biochemistry
University of Pennsylvania
School of Veterinary Medicine
Philadephia, Pennsylvania

Kelly P. Shaw, Pharm.D.
President
Kirby-Shaw Consulting
Toronto, Ontario

David W. Scheifele, M.D.
Professor
Department of Pediatrics
University of British Columbia;
Director
Vaccine Evaluation Center
BC Children's Hospital
Vancouver, BC, Canada

Sinno H.P. Simons, M.D., Ph.D.
Department of Pediatrics, VU Medical center
Amsterdam, The Netherlands

Susan C. Smolinske, Pharm.D., D.A.B.A.T., B.C.P.S.
Professor, Clinician–Educator
College of Medicine, Pediatrics
Wayne State University
Detroit, Michigan

Wayne R. Snodgrass, M.D., Ph.D.
Professor
Pediatrics, Pharmacology–Toxicology, and Obstetrics–Gynecology
Head, Clinical Pharmacology–Toxicology Unit
Medical Director, Texas Poison Center—Houston/Galveston
University of Texas Medical Branch
Galveston, Texas

Margaret Ann Springer, M.D.
Section on Clinical Pharmacology
Departments of Pediatrics and Psychiatry
Louisiana State University Health Sciences Center
Shreveport, Louisiana

William J. Steinbach, M.D.
Associate Professor
Pediatrics, Molecular Genetics & Microbiology
Duke University;
Associate Professor
Pediatrics
Duke University Medical Center
Durham, North Carolina

David K. Stevenson, M.D.
Department of Pediatrics
Division of Neonatal and Developmental Medicine
Stanford University School of Medicine
Stanford, California

Santhanam Suresh, M.D., F.A.A.P.
Attending Anesthesiologist
Professor of Anesthesiology & Pediatrics
Children's Memorial Hospital
Northwestern University's Feinberg School of Medicine
Chicago, Illinois

Stanley J. Szefler, M.D.
Professor
Department of Pediatrics and Pharmacology
University of Colorado
School of Medicine;
Head, Pediatric Clinical Pharmacology
Department of Pediatrics
National Jewish Health
Denver, Colorado

William Tamborlane, M.D.
Professor and Chief of Endocrinology
Department of Pediatrics
Yale School of Medicine;
Attending Physician
Department of Pediatric Endocrinology
Yale-New Haven Children's Hospital
New Haven, Connecticut

Alexander O. Tuazon, M.D.
Associate Professor
Department of Pediatrics
College of Medicine, University of the Philippines Manila;
Head, Section of Pediatric Pulmonology
Department of Pediatrics
Philippine General Hospital
Manila, Philippines

Dick Tibboel, M.D., Ph.D.
Professor of Research Intensive Care in Childhood
Pediatric Surgery
Erasmus University Rotterdam;
Head ICU
Pediatric Intensive Care
Erasmus MC—Sophia Children's Hospital
Rotterdam, The Netherlands

Alexander O. Tuazon, M.D.
Associate Professor
Department of Pediatrics
College of Medicine, University of the Philippines Manila;
Head, Section of Pediatric Pulmonology
Department of Pediatrics
Philippine General Hospital
Manila, Philippines

Ignacio Valencia, M.D.
Department of Pediatrics
St. Christopher's Hospital for Children
Drexel University College of Medicine
Philadelphia, Pennsylvania

Louis Vernacchio, M.D., M.Sc.
Assistant Clinical Professor
Department of Pediatrics
Harvard Medical School;
Division of General Pediatrics
Children's Hospital Boston
Boston, Massachusetts

Alexander A. Vinks, Pharm.D., Ph.D.
Professor and Director
Division of Clinical Pharmacology
Cincinnati Children's Hospital Medical Center
Cincinnati, Ohio

Hendrik J. Vreman, Ph.D.
Department of Pediatrics
Division of Neonatal and Developmental Medicine
Stanford University School of Medicine
Stanford, California

Philip D. Walson, M.D.
Visiting Professor
Department of Laboratory Medicine
Georg-August-Universitat Medical School
Goettingen, Germany

Thomas G. Wells, M.D.
Professor
Department of Pediatrics
University of Arkansas for Medical Sciences
Little Rock, Arkansas

Suzanne R. White, M.D., F.A.C.E.P., F.A.C.M.T.
Dayanandan Professor and Chair
Departments of Emergency Medicine and Pediatrics
Wayne State University School of Medicine;
Emergency Physician-In-Chief
Detroit Medical Center
Detroit, Michigan

Richard J. Whitley, M.D.
Distinguished Professor
Department of Pediatrics
University of Alabama at Birmingham;
Division Director Pediatric Infectious Diseases
Department of Pediatrics
The Children's Hospital of Alabama
Birmingham, Alabama

John T. Wilson, M.D.
Section on Clinical Pharmacology
Departments of Pediatrics and Psychiatry
Louisiana State University Health Sciences Center
Shreveport, Louisiana

Ronald J. Wong, M.D.
Department of Pediatrics
Division of Neonatal and Developmental Medicine
Stanford University School of Medicine
Stanford, California

Sumner J. Yaffe, M.D.
Consulting Professor
Stanford University School of Medicine
Palo Alto, California

Yesim Yilmaz-Demirdag, M.D.
Assistant Professor
Department of Pediatrics
West Virginia University
Morgantown, West Virginia

Eli Zalzstein, M.D.
Associate Professor
Pediatric Cardiology Unit
Ben Gurion University;
Head, Pediatric Cardiology Unit
Soroka University Medical Center
Beer-Sheva, Israel

O.L. Zharikova, M.D., Ph.D.
Postdoctoral Fellow
Department of OB/GYN
University of Texas Medical Branch
Galveston, Texas

Members of the pediatric community who depend on this book to provide the most up-to-date information and guidance in neonatal and pediatric pharmacology are fortunate in that they have had to wait just 5 years since the publication of the Third Edition in 2005 for this revised updated version, rather than the 12 years between the second and third editions. This shorter interval is important since the gain of new knowledge and the appearance of new problems and challenges have continued to accelerate, as they had for the Third Edition. This update is equal to the task of currency, describing advances in knowledge such as further improvements in preventing mother-to-child transmission of HIV by improved pharmaceutical regimens in both developed and developing countries, and new challenges posed by the need for rapid treatments tested in children for bioterrorism agents that need emergency care as new forms of poisonings.

As is customary, Drs. Yaffe and Aranda have again recruited leading experts to contribute chapters on key topics that cover the full breadth of the field. With encouraging signs of international cooperation and collaboration in testing and approval requirements, even to the extent of funding common protocols for drug testing for approval among Europe, the United States, and Canada, there is new optimism for bringing new pharmaceutical agents to market faster and more economically than in the past, and it is important for pediatrics to be at the forefront of this movement. Much of the content of this volume provides important considerations as that process develops, including searching for commonality in ethical and methodological issues.

The many chapters on individual classes of drugs provide the most recent information on the full spectrum of drugs used for newborns, infants, and children that alone would make having this book of great value.

Altogether, this book maintains and enhances the reputation and value of its previous editions. All those who prescribe drugs for children are indebted to Drs. Yaffe and Aranda for compiling yet another edition of this standard text.

Duane Alexander, MD, FAAP

Preface to the Third Edition

This third edition of the senior and standard textbook in the field of pediatric pharmacology comes none too soon. There have been enormous changes and advances in pediatrics and pediatric pharmacology in the 12 years since publication of the second edition of this text in 1991. Much has been learned about treating then-new diseases, such as pediatric AIDS and Lyme disease, and diseases entirely new to the Western hemisphere (West Nile Fever) have arrived and require informed treatment. The expansion of pediatric emergency and intensive care, and the growing numbers of extremely low-birth-weight infants being treated in Neonatal Intensive Care Units, provide new patient groups and new settings for drug treatment. Many new drugs have been added to the therapeutic armamentarium in the last 12 years, some as new molecular entities, many as variations on a theme, and others as new combination or extended action formulations. Growth in antivirals, cancer drugs, and psychoactive drugs has been particularly striking. To complicate the picture, a rapidly growing use of herbals and alternative medicines given to children by parents, often without physician awareness, requires knowledge of both their actions and their interactions with physician-prescribed regimens. In addition to drugs, numerous new vaccines and combinations thereof have also entered (and sometimes departed) use since 1991.

Accompanying these changes have been major changes in the drug testing scene that have markedly expanded our knowledge of dosage, safety, and efficacy of pharmaceutical use in children. Realization that children may metabolize and respond to drugs differently at one age than another, as well as differently from adults, has spread beyond the pediatric profession to be recognized by parents, the FDA, and Congress, and has significantly expanded and legitimized drug testing and evaluation in children. Much of this advance was made possible by the leadership of one of the authors of this text, Sumner Yaffe, in conceptualizing and establishing the Pediatric Pharmacology Research Unit (PPRU) Network of the NICHD. Initially funded in 1994, this Network quickly demonstrated that drug testing could be done safely, effectively, and ethically in children, and that reliable data for FDA submission could be obtained quickly at reasonable cost using common protocols at multiple sites. The success of the PPRU Network rapidly destroyed any legitimacy of the excuses offered for not doing drug testing in children, and made possible both the Pediatric Rule adopted by the FDA in 1998 to require testing in children for new drugs expected to have significant use in children, and the Better Pharmaceuticals for Children Act, passed by Congress in 1997, that provided a six-month extension of market exclusivity for on-patent drugs in return for the drug company testing the drug in children. That combination markedly increased industry-sponsored drug testing in children, led to pediatric labeling for a number of these drugs, and provided valuable information to guide practitioners prescribing drugs for children. While not an unqualified success, and not without controversy, the benefits of this legislation were sufficient that Congress extended it in the Best Pharmaceuticals for Children Act of 2002, adding a new provision to cover testing off-patent drugs with government funding. The expanded knowledge gained from this research is incorporated into this third edition.

Another change since the previous edition is a huge gain in scientific knowledge, represented in large part by the new fields of pharmacogenetics, pharmacogenomics, and pharmacoproteomics. Recognizing the importance of discoveries of genetic differences in drug metabolism, the ability to screen for them, and the increasing role this knowledge will play in drug prescribing practices to improve patient safety (and protect the physician), a whole new chapter is devoted to this topic.

Covering all these topics are chapters authored by leading authorities in the field. With the prestige of this text, the editors obviously had no trouble attracting the top experts as contributors. This combination of comprehensive coverage of this field by the foremost scientists is sure to continue the unquestioned position of this book as the standard text and source of information in pediatric pharmacology. Physicians and children once again will benefit from this updated authoritative source of knowledge.

Duane Alexander, MD, FAAP

Preface to the Fourth Edition

Neonatal and pediatric pharmacology and drug therapy may be viewed as corrective and manipulative physiology and biochemistry for the fetus, newborn infant, and growing child using drugs, biologicals and molecular entities. Drugs are used to correct physiological, molecular, and biochemical as well as disease-related abnormalities that occur during pre- and postnatal periods, extrauterine adaptation, and growth and development to adulthood.

As advances in the knowledge of diseases and their diagnoses are made, the complexities of treatment, particularly by drugs, increase in tandem. Therapeutic drug exposure and administration in the newborn and children has increased over the years. Moreover, the number of drugs available to physicians and health care givers continues to increase. There is an increasing variety of antimicrobials, cardiovascular drugs, diuretics, immunosuppressants and immunomodulators, antivirals, biologicals, and other drugs for the management of sick newborn and children. Safe and effective use of these agents in infants and children requires adequate knowledge of their pharmacologic properties, including drug action, metabolism, and disposition.

The fourth edition of *Neonatal and Pediatric Pharmacology: Therapeutic Principles in Practice* has been substantially revised to meet the current needs of clinicians, pharmacologists, pharmacists, and other health care givers. The book has expanded to 66 chapters in this edition, plus drug formularies for newborns and children. This edition is designed to provide relevant information on drugs and their uses in newborn infants, older infants, children, and adolescents. It was proposed as a quick reference for busy clinicians, house staff, students, nurses, pharmacists, and health care providers. It may also serve as a general and basic reference for teaching neonatal and pediatric pharmacology. It is also hoped that researchers also will find it useful to understand the unique characteristics and dynamic changes in drug requirements and action during a period of intense growth and development. The mechanisms of drug actions, the evidence of drug efficacy in certain disease states, dose, therapeutic guidelines, and drug toxicities are emphasized. The book was organized to parallel the distinct periods of early human development. Special sections useful in drug therapy such as therapeutic drug monitoring, adverse drug reactions, and epidemiologic considerations are also included. The unraveling of some of the secrets of the human genome has resulted in major progress and challenges in the understanding of drug disposition and pharmacologic effects in humans and personalized drug therapies. A chapter is devoted to this issue in this book. The importance of pharmacogenetics and pharmacogenomics in clinical therapeutics in children and in pediatric drug trials and drug development can no longer be ignored. Developmental changes in receptors, drug-metabolizing enzymes, transporters, and ion channels may have impact on the efficacy and safety of drugs in children. The determinants of drug action, metabolism, and disposition are multifaceted, and the impact of the variations in the human genome, the environment demographics, and other factors will remain a major challenge in the immediate future.

Drugs are double-edged swords; although they can cure illnesses and restore health and well-being, they can also produce unwanted and, at times, unanticipated toxicities. The rational, intelligent, and safe use of drugs springs mainly from understanding their actions, uses, problems, and limitations. This understanding, in turn, will permit selection of the appropriate drug and prescription of the optimal dosage. It is our utmost desire that this textbook can help those providers of care to newborns and children to maximize the benefits of pharmacologic agents while averting their adverse effects. Identified areas of ignorance or concern should stimulate further research in order to minimize the unknowns in neonatal and pediatric drug therapy. Thus, this book will advance and promote the health and wellness in newborns and children.

Sumner J. Yaffe
Jacob V. Aranda

Contents

SECTION III: **Drugs in Special Populations and Settings**

SECTION IV: Specific Drugs

CHAPTER

1

Sumner J. Yaffe
Jacob V. Aranda

Introduction and Historical Perspectives

The following is an excerpt from the second edition of this book:

> The past several decades have witnessed a revolution in the practice of therapeutics. It has long been recognized that the nature, duration, and intensity of drug action depend not only on the intrinsic properties of the drug, but also on its interaction with the host to whom the drug has been administered for the treatment of disease. Advances in drug development have led to the introduction of highly specific and extremely potent therapeutic agents in the marketplace.
>
> Prompted perhaps by the synthesis of these highly specific and potent chemical entities, there has developed an ever-increasing understanding of the mechanisms of drug disposition—especially those concerned with the biotransformation of xenobiotics. This has led to a burgeoning new discipline: clinical pharmacology. Awareness of host factors as major determinants of drug concentration (and hence drug effect) within the organism also has led to an enlightened efficiency in the selection of drug entities and their dosage.
>
> While these advances have been proceeding at a rapid pace in adult medicine, it is evident that pediatric pharmacology has not kept pace and, until very recently, has lagged far behind the research and attention paid to the proper use of therapeutic and diagnostic drugs in adults. Thus, a large percentage of the drugs used in sick infants and children are prescribed on empirical grounds. This information gap in pediatric practice was recognized as a crisis by Dr. Charles C. Edwards, former commissioner of the Food and Drug Administration (FDA), when he addressed the 1972 Annual Meeting of the American Academy of Pediatrics.

The two decades since the foregoing material was written has witnessed remarkable progress in drug studies in infants and children. The introductions to the first three editions of this book detailed the historical perspectives related to pediatric pharmacology and lamented the lack of studies in infants and children, which led to inadequate labeling of drugs for use in this special, vulnerable population. As a consequence, infants and children were considered therapeutic orphans. The situation changed dramatically around the time of the publication of the second edition in 1992. The following paragraphs describe the changes that have occurred, the rationale for the changes, and a glimpse into the future as well as a description of the regulatory environment in the United States and Europe.

During the last several decades, many individuals and organizations within the pediatric community, including academia and the American Academy of Pediatrics (AAP), working with the National Institutes of Health (NIH), the Food and Drug Administration (FDA), and the pharmaceutical industry, have sought to find ways to increase pediatric drug research and, consequently, labeling for children. These efforts culminated in a 1990 workshop titled Drug Development and Pediatric Populations, which was jointly sponsored by the Institute of Medicine of the National Academy of Sciences, the National Institute of Child Health and Human Development (NICHD), the FDA, the pharmaceutical industry, and the AAP. The workshop made recommendations regarding impediments to drug development for the pediatric population and their solutions. In retrospect, this was a watershed meeting. Recommendations from the workshop included (a) that the FDA explore ways to facilitate the approval of drugs for children and inclusion of pediatric information in drug labeling, (b) that economic incentives to drug development for children be addressed by granting extended patent exclusivity to sponsors for drugs that are studied in children and for which data are submitted to the FDA in support of pediatric labeling, (c) that the pharmaceutical industry take a more proactive stance with respect to drug development for children, and (d) that the National Institutes of Health establish a network of pediatric centers to facilitate the conduct of pediatric clinical studies. During the last decade, each of these recommendations has been implemented. In 1997, the FDA Modernization Act (FDAMA) was passed by Congress, giving extended patent exclusivity to companies for performing pediatric studies; in 1994 and 1998, the FDA implemented new regulations to facilitate and require pediatric studies of drugs; and in 1994, NICHD funded the first group of pediatric centers to inaugurate the Pediatric Pharmacology Research Unit (PPRU) network.

The FDA's regulatory position was first articulated in 1970, when the agency stated that "drugs used for children must be tested in children"; the Committee on Drugs (COD) of the American Academy of Pediatrics supported this view in a position paper that appeared in the journal *Pediatrics* in 1995. The COD pointed out that every time a physician prescribes an unlabeled drug for a child, he or she is performing an uncontrolled experiment with an enrollment of one with no protocol or outside overview. The COD further stated that it is unethical not to study drugs in children.

One of the Institute of Medicine's recommendations asked the FDA to take a more positive role in solving the problem of the therapeutic orphan. Several recent actions by the FDA in this regard are cited in what follows.

The FDA has taken a more proactive role in recent years in ensuring that inclusion of pediatric use information in drug labels, derived from information from clinical studies, is standard. The pediatric regulatory initiatives issued in recent years have provided an economic incentive for pharmaceutical manufacturers to conduct studies in children and have set standards and requirements for pediatric studies that the industry must meet.

A description of the regulations and law provide an understanding of the incentive for manufacturers to conduct pediatric studies as well as the current requirements for pediatric studies that the pharmaceutical industry must meet. A brief history of the regulatory efforts made to address the lack of information for children in prescription drug labeling will allow the reader to realize what a sea change has taken place both at the FDA, the academic community, and the European Medication Evaluation Agency over the last 15 years. The process by which new drugs are developed and approved for marketing in the United States and in Europe is not well understood by most observers, and the process by which drugs are developed for use in children is probably even less clear.

In the United States, the FDA is responsible for assuring that new drugs and biologics are safe and effective for their proposed uses before they are approved for marketing. The FDA's role as a regulatory agency is not to develop therapeutic agents or to conduct clinical trials to determine the safety and efficacy of the product. New drug development is the responsibility of pharmaceutical manufacturers and government or private research institutions. The FDA's responsibility is to ensure that the rights and safety of human subjects are protected during the clinical testing of investigational drugs, to review and evaluate the safety and efficacy of proposed new therapeutics on the basis of data submitted by the sponsor, and to determine whether the balance between the benefits and the risks associated with a new drug is sufficiently favorable to justify approval for marketing.

After preclinical testing of a potential new drug is completed and before clinical trials in humans can begin, the sponsor of the new drug must file an Investigational New Drug (IND) application with the FDA. Requirements for this submission are outlined in the regulations and include the results of the preclinical testing describing the pharmacologic and toxicity profile of the drug and the chemistry; the manufacturing controls; and the purity, potency, and stability of the agent. In addition, a proposed protocol for the initial phase 1 and phase 2 clinical trial in humans is included. This initial protocol may not be initiated until the FDA notifies the sponsor that based on a complete evaluation by a multidisciplinary review team the study is safe to proceed. The FDA has 30 days to complete this review and notify the sponsor of its decision.

Following this, studies to define a safe and tolerable dose and to determine the activity of the agent are undertaken in phase 1 and phase 2 studies. The sponsor may initiate these studies as soon as the protocols are approved. However, any study deemed to represent an undue risk to participants may be put on hold for safety concerns at any time information sufficient to make this assessment is obtained.

When there are data adequate to support the continuation of the new drug development process, the sponsors meet with the FDA to review the data obtained from the phase 1 and phase 2 studies and to plan for the phase 3 studies. The phase 2 and phase 3 studies should be designed with the intent to demonstrate substantial evidence of efficacy and safety. Studies likely to provide such data are described in the Code of Federal Regulations as adequate and well controlled. As such, these studies should include clear objective criteria for assessing positive and negative effects, an appropriate control group to allow valid comparison with the group receiving the investigational drug, a well-defined patient population that is randomized to assure comparability among the treatment groups, and measures to eliminate bias, such as blinding or randomization.

The completed and analyzed results of the clinical trials are submitted along with proposed labeling and technical information as a New Drug Application (NDA) by the applicant for FDA review. The FDA must determine whether the data submitted satisfy the statutory requirements for safety and effectiveness, that is, "adequate tests by all methods reasonably applicable to show whether or not such drug is safe for use under the conditions prescribed," and "substantial evidence [of efficacy] consisting of adequate and well controlled investigations." The standard time to review and take an action (i.e., approval or nonapproval) on an application is approximately 10 months. Priority applications are reviewed and have an action taken in 6 months.

Once an NDA is approved, new information about the drug's safety profile is monitored by periodic safety updates submitted by the applicant as well as reports received from the MedWatch program. MedWatch is a reporting system designed to detect rare and serious adverse events after approval of a therapeutic agent. Premarketing clinical trials do not reflect the actual use of the drug after approval. In clinical trials, the populations studied are likely to be narrow, only patients with those indications for which efficacy is being studied are included in the trials, the drug is frequently used for shorter time periods than may be the case in actual use, and most NDAs usually include between 3,000 and 4,000 patients, so that rare adverse events would be very difficult to detect.

In addition, at the time of approval, the applicant may agree to conduct further clinical trials during phase 4 (which is the time after approval), to provide additional important information regarding appropriate use of the drug. These studies are usually intended to answer questions raised during the review of the clinical data that are not substantial enough to delay approval, but are sufficiently important to warrant a request for further investigation.

Prior to 1979, it was considered unethical to enroll children in "experiments," that is, clinical trials. They were considered to be "protected." In 1977, the American Academy of Pediatrics, reacting to the paucity of information for children in drug labels, asserted that it was unethical to adhere to a system that forced physicians to use drugs in what was basically an uncontrolled experiment whenever they wrote prescriptions for children. The Academy stated that it was imperative that new drugs that were to be used in children should be studied in children under controlled circumstances so that the benefits of therapeutic advances would become available to all who would need them. This was a powerful, yet simple statement: Children deserve the same standard as adults. If adequate and well-controlled studies were required to determine the efficacy of the products used in adults, then the same should be true for products used to treat children. It was now considered unethical *not* to study children. Following this unprecedented statement, in 1979, the FDA confirmed the need to have information on how best to use a product in the pediatric population. Thereafter, a number of milestones in Pediatric Drug Development in the United States and in Europe occurred (see Table 1.1) The FDA issued a regulation in 1994 that required that statements on pediatric use of a drug for an indication approved for adults must be based on substantial evidence derived from adequate and well-controlled studies conducted in children, unless the requirement was waived.

The intent of the initial regulation (1994 rule) was to encourage manufacturers to conduct the necessary trials so that adequate prescribing information would be available to physicians. Unfortunately, it did not generate the response intended. Few clinical trials were initiated in the pediatric population. Manufacturers cited financial, medicolegal, and methodological disincentives, especially for products already approved for adults. These products were available to physicians for prescription use outside of labeled indications through the practice of medicine. The FDA could encourage but not require that a sponsor conduct the appropriate trials to support pediatric labeling.

At the time this rule was issued, approximately 80% of drugs listed in the *Physicians' Desk Reference* did not have directions for use in the pediatric population based on clinical trials. This disturbing situation was heightened by the AIDS epidemic, which served to contrast the disparity between the pace of drug development between adults and children. In 1994, the FDA issued a final, slightly modified rule requiring drug manufacturers to survey the existing data and determine whether those data were sufficient to support additional pediatric use information in a drug's labeling. In addition, the rule explicitly stated that controlled clinical studies need not be carried out in pediatric patients when the course of the disease and the response to treatment were similar in adults and children. Extrapolation from adult efficacy data to pediatric patients was permitted. Therefore, controlled clinical studies in adults, together with other information, such as pharmacokinetic and adverse reaction data in pediatric patients, could be found to be sufficient to establish pediatric safety and efficacy. Under the 1994 rule, the manufacturer could determine that existing data permitted modification of the label's pediatric use. The manufacturer, however, had to submit a supplemental new drug application to the FDA, seeking approval of the labeling change.

It is important to recognize that the 1994 rule did not require that manufacturers conduct pediatric studies if existing information was not adequate to support a labeling change. Instead, where there was insufficient information to support a pediatric indication or pediatric use statement, the 1994 rule allowed the manufacturer to

TABLE 1.1 Milestones in Pediatric Drug Development

1977—AAP Statement concerning the need to conduct clinical trials in children

1979—The US Food and Drug Administration (FDA) establishes a section for drug labels and requires trials in children parallel to adult process

1994—FDA requirement for sponsors or drug manufacturers to update drug labels, to evaluate existing data, and to determine whether these data are sufficient to support information for pediatric drug labeling. The FDA also implements a voluntary collection of data on pediatric use before and after a drug is approved. FDA introduces the "extrapolation concept"

1997—US Congress passes FDAMA (FDA Modernization Act) and prolongs patent exclusivity for 6 months to pharmaceuticals who voluntarily perform studies on the drug in children

1998—The FDA publishes the Pediatric Rule which requires manufacturers to assess the safety and efficacy of drugs and biologic products in children in specified circumstances

2002—The Best Pharmaceuticals for Children Act (BPCA) was signed into law by President G. W. Bush. BPCA renewed exclusivity or patent protection for additional 6 months. Provides additional mechanisms, such as studies funded by the National Institutes of Health to obtain drug data from "off-patent" or patented drugs (which manufacturers decline to study in children). BPCA provides process for "off-patent" drug development, public posting of results, and reporting of all AEs for 1 year after exclusivity is granted

2003—Pediatric Research Equity Act (PREA) is passed which requires the study of drugs and biologics for pediatric population except in defined situations and also creates a Pediatric Advisory Committee

2006—European Parliament passes the Best Medicines for Children Act in December 12, 2006, which became law in January 2007. The law requires studies of drug in newborns and children and a pediatric investigation plan (PIP) for all drugs being developed. It creates a pediatric committee to decide priority drugs to study and to review protocol proposals and study plans for drug development in children. It also provides procedures to study drugs for newborns and children and funding mechanisms. EMEA (European Medication Evaluation Agency) reviews data for approval and marketing licensure

2007—US Congress, reauthorized BPCA

AAP, American Academy of Pediatrics; AEs, Adverse events.

include in the drug's labeling the statement, "safety and effectiveness in pediatric patients have not been established."

The FDA was hopeful and enthusiastic about this regulation. Unfortunately, well over half of the responses to the rule concluded that there was insufficient data, and the resulting labeling change consisted of inclusion of the statement just given. Only 23% of the responses resulted in improved labeling for pediatrics.

Clearly, if the goal of ensuring the safe and effective use of therapeutic agents in children was to be met, additional steps had to be taken. Two pieces of legislation underscore the commitment of the FDA to the safe and effective use of therapeutic agents in children. The first of these is Section 111 of the FDAMA. Congress passed this act in November 1997 (see Table 1.1). Section 111 of this act created a financial incentive (called "pediatric exclusivity") consisting of an additional 6 months of marketing exclusivity for conducting pediatric studies on new drugs and drugs already on the market and under patent. The second recent advance is the 1998 Final Pediatric Rule, which was to become effective in 1999 (see later discussion). This regulation requires that pediatric studies be conducted for certain new as well as marketed drugs and biologic products. Requiring studies in the pediatric population represents a significant departure from the previous regulations, which are voluntary. Both the final rule and the pediatric exclusivity provision are critical to ensuring that necessary and timely pediatric drug development occurs and that improved pediatric labeling will be the result. The financial incentive of an additional 6 months of marketing exclusivity can apply to both new drugs and marketed drugs as defined by FDAMA. If the 6 months of additional marketing exclusivity is granted, all the sponsor's products that contain the drug ("active moiety" formulations of the drug) may receive this extension. Because of this wide application, this is seen as a significant "carrot" in getting manufacturers to conduct pediatric studies. To qualify for pediatric exclusivity, the drug manufacturer must receive a written request for pediatric studies from the FDA. This written request outlines the studies that the drug manufacturer must conduct and complete, and which complete study reports must be submitted by an agreed-on date. New and approved drugs that this law applies to are those that have been determined as likely to produce health benefits in the pediatric population. For any given drug, the FDA evaluates every indication under development or that has been previously approved and requests that the appropriate studies be performed. Conducting pediatric studies in response to a written request is voluntary. To obtain pediatric exclusivity, final reports of the submitted studies must meet the terms of the written request and the drug must have existing patent protection or exclusivity.

Because voluntary efforts such as the 1994 Pediatric Rule did not substantially increase the number of products entering the market with adequate pediatric labeling, the FDA concluded that additional steps were necessary to ensue the safety and effectiveness of drugs and biologic products for pediatric patients. In addition, even though the pediatric exclusivity offered by FDAMA is expected to provide a substantial incentive for sponsors to conduct pediatric studies, that provision does not apply to drugs that no longer have existing patent protection or exclusivity or to biologics or "old" antibiotics. It is a voluntary program, making it likely that manufacturers may elect not to conduct studies in products with smaller markets, even though there may be a great medical need for the product in pediatric patients. Therefore, it was felt that there were still many situations where there was a need to require the collection of data in children.

The 1998 Pediatric Rule requires the manufacturers of new and marketed drugs and biologic products to evaluate the safety and effectiveness of their products in pediatric patients. It is designed to ensure that new drugs and biologic products contain adequate pediatric labeling for the claimed indication at the time of, or soon after, approval. This rule establishes a presumption that all new drugs and biologics will be studied in pediatric patients, but allows manufacturers to obtain a waiver of the requirement in some circumstances (e.g., if the indication is not applicable to the pediatric population). This rule applies to new chemical entities, new indications, new dosage forms, new dosing regimens, and new routes of administration.

This rule also authorizes the FDA to require pediatric studies of marketed drugs and biologic products where there is a compelling need for studies (defined as situations in which the product is used in a substantial number of pediatric patients) and the absence of adequate labeling could pose significant risks for pediatric patients, or the product would provide a meaningful therapeutic benefit over existing treatments. Thus, this rule is mandatory and gives the FDA additional power to require studies in children. While this rule was being implemented the rule was considered by the Federal courts to be illegal and not within the FDA's authority.

The second approach to the solution of the therapeutic orphan dilemma occurred at the National Institutes of Health with the development of the Pediatric Pharmacology Research Unit (PPRU) network. This network was established in 1994 following a conference of the Forum of Drug Development of the Institute of Medicine of the National Academy of Sciences. This conference strongly recommended that steps be taken to eliminate the therapeutic orphan situation. In response to the need for appropriate therapy for pediatric patients, the NICHD established the PPRU network with the mission of facilitating and promoting pediatric labeling of new drugs or drugs already in the market. In this process, the network strives to foster cooperative and complementary research efforts among the academy, industry, and health professionals. The overall goal of the network is to provide data for the safe and effective use of drugs in children.

In 1994, after the announcement of the intent to establish a network, the NICHD received a large number of applications from children's hospitals and universities. From these applications, seven sites were selected to join with the NICHD in cooperatively dealing with the problem of the therapeutic orphan. The network had the following three functions: (a) to conduct studies on the pharmacokinetics and pharmacodynamics of drugs in infants and children, (b) to provide a focus for pre-and postmarketing clinical trials in children conducted by clinical pediatric pharmacologists in collaboration with the pharmaceutical industry and contract research organizations, and (c) to serve as an advisory body to the pharmaceutical industry, regulatory agencies, health professionals, and the public on the appropriate use of drugs in children.

The principal investigators in the PPRU network are pioneers in the field of pediatric pharmacology. Their combined contributions in this specialized area exceed 1,500 publications. The research expertise of network investigators is varied and all-encompassing within the field of pediatrics. In January 1999, the network of 7 sites was expanded to 13 sites. With this expansion in the number of sites, the network has access to a large, all-inclusive pediatric population with more than 2 million outpatient visits per year and more than 100,000 pediatric in-patient admissions. The network serves as a major resource for the training of health professionals in pediatric pharmacology and clinical trial methodology as well as the study of drugs in infants and children. The Pharmaceutical Research Manufacturer's Association has also endorsed and supported a research fellow at each PPRU site.

The involvement of children in clinical trials requires study designs that minimize discomfort in patients and do not disturb family life. The PPRU pediatric pharmacologists use their combined experience and skills, and access large numbers of children to shorten the length of the study period. The PPRU network strives to develop child-friendly protocols with minimal risk for all pediatric patients regardless of their condition. Pediatric patients involved in drug studies include those with common disorders, such as allergies, asthma, and upper respiratory infections, as well as those with less common disorders such as cystic fibrosis, severe infections, HIV (human immunodeficiency virus) infection and AIDS, sickle cell anemia, cancer, and childhood depression. The combined patient capabilities of the network are available to ensure appropriate and objective evaluation of drugs including, but not limited to, antipyretics, analgesics, antibiotics, decongestants, antihypertensives, diuretics, and bronchodilators. The network is also committed to developing safe and effective drug therapy for children in intensive care and in life-threatening situations. Studies of drugs in patients in the pediatric and neonatal intensive care units and in patients on extracorporeal membrane oxygenation, hemodialysis, and after organ transplantation put the PPRU at the forefront of pharmaceutical development. An overriding consideration for the PPRU pediatric pharmacologists who are in the network is to delineate the effects of development during infancy and childhood on the pharmacokinetics of drugs; the influence of age-specific changes in drug disposition and pharmacodynamics; and the interplay among disease states, stage of development, and response to drugs. The overall expertise of the network and its members permits achievement of these studies in a superlative and authoritative manner. In addition, studies of translational research involving molecular mechanisms of action and pharmacogenetics and pharmacogenomics are encouraged in the network.

The NICHD supports each unit by underwriting the costs of the principal investigator, who is responsible for developing and maintaining the PPRU for conducting research. In addition, NICHD supports a nurse coordinator and a core analytical and biomedical laboratory, which provides state-of-the-art study design, computer modeling of drug disposition and drug response, and data management and analysis. The latter function is subsumed by a separately funded data center, which is funded under a contract mechanism. Because the network site is located within children's hospitals and university departments of pediatrics, each site has access to clinical investigators with sufficient numbers of patients to allow appropriate studies representing all the subspecialties of pediatrics.

The organization of the PPRU network is via a cooperative agreement. The network is governed by a Steering Committee, which consists of the principal investigators of each of the 13 units and a representative from the NICHD. The Steering Committee is chaired by an independent, non-PPRU investigator. An FDA member functions in a liaison capacity and serves as a consultant to advise members of regulatory issues. The Steering Committee has several subcommittees concerned with (a) evaluation of protocols, (b) refinement of operating procedures, (c) ethics of conducting research in children, and (d) publication policy. The Steering Committee as a whole evaluates protocols for scientific merit and serves as an advisory board for issues concerning pediatric drug labeling and appropriate use of drugs in children. By the end of the decade in 2010, substantial evolution of the PPRU network is expected but its mission will continue to include the development of safe and effective medications for newborns and children.

The passage and implementation of the pediatric exclusivity section of the FDAMA had the most dramatic impact on drug research for children and on the activity within the PPRU during the last 5 years. Section 111 of the FDAMA provides 6 months of additional exclusivity for a drug if the company performs pediatric studies in compliance with a request from the FDA. The industry responded to this incentive to an unprecedented extent. More than 500 studies have been requested to the FDA, leading to more than 200 studies; more than 100 drugs have been granted additional exclusivity, and pediatric labeling has been added to more than 30 drugs, with many more pediatric labels to come. The increase in sponsored pediatric studies created an exponential increase in PPRU activity, which would not have occurred without this legislation. As non-PPRU pediatric study sites evolved in response to FDAMA, the PPRU found itself increasingly playing more of a specialty role in being a resource primarily for phase 1 and phase 2 and pharmacokinetic/pharmacodynamic studies, whereas non-PPRU study sites played an increasingly greater role in phase 3 and phase 4 studies. The PPRU might not have had this opportunity, at least not in the short time frame, had the FDAMA stimulus not been present.

The initiation of PPRU network drug trials in young children uncovered the need to expand current knowledge of pediatric clinical trial methodology and pediatric pharmacology. The explosion in the number of drug studies that occurred after implementation of the pediatric provisions of the FDAMA brings to light the problem of finding enough children with which to conduct efficacy and safety trials for drugs used in chronic childhood conditions, due mostly to the lack of adequate biomarkers to establish disease severity, recurrence, and response to therapy. The NIH Ad Hoc Committee on Surrogate Markers identified a biomarker as "a characteristic that is measured and an indicator of normal biological processes, pathogenic, or response to a therapeutic intervention" (e.g., use of clonal markers to quantify leukemic cells, CD4 counts, or measurement of viral load to estimate response to therapy in AIDS). To address these research issues, the NICHD had programs to stimulate research on clinical outcome, biomarkers, and surrogate end point development and validation.

The most challenging area of performing drug clinical trials in children is conducting efficacy and safety studies in preterm and sick newborn infants. Only a few of the 170 drugs used in newborn intensive care nurseries have been demonstrated to be effective. This population is most vulnerable to adverse drug effects because of the immaturity of their drug-metabolizing enzymes and the pathophysiologic changes that affect drug disposition and action. Studies in the sick newborn, especially the low-birth-weight infant, are difficult to conduct because of the need to distinguish between the pharmacologic effect and its toxicity and the underlying pathologic process.

A further and most significant stimulus to the solution of the therapeutic orphan problem occurred in 1999 with the convening of a conference titled Rational Therapeutics for Infants and Children under the auspices of the Institute of Medicine of the National Academy of Sciences. This conference, published in 2000, underscored the need for further studies of drugs in infants and children and emphasized support for long-term studies of safety in this population. Mention was made of studies in other vulnerable populations such as pregnant women and the elderly. The support of the Institute of Medicine was very helpful in persuading Congress to take up and enact the Best Pharmaceuticals for Children Act (BPCA).

The FDAMA was authorized for 5 years. At its termination in 2002, because of its unprecedented success, it was reauthorized for 5 to 7 additional years. In doing so, Congress incorporated the pediatric exclusivity provisions of FDAMA into the BPCA. This legislation had important provisions for infants and children. The BPCA identified the NIH as a major player together with the FDA in supporting drug studies in infants and children. The act made provisions to address new (on-patent) drugs, but also asked the NIH and FDA to identify off-patent drugs that need to be evaluated in the pediatric population. A list of 12 off-patent drugs was identified and developed in 2003 by the NICHD in consultation with the FDA and experts in pediatric research. The list will be updated and expanded each year. Modest funds have been made available to the NICHD to support the requisite studies and clinical trials. Greater funding is necessary to accomplish all of the provisions of the BPCA.

A very profound and important component of the BPCA concerns studies in the newborn, especially preterm infants. There is a dearth of pharmacologic clinical trials in this age group. At this point, it is important to remember the very large number of drugs prescribed for sick newborn infants. There are not many studies of drug use and surveillance in neonatal intensive care, but a recent epidemiologic investigation in two large Boston teaching hospitals revealed that among 2,690 infants studied, 91% received at least one drug, and often many more than one, while in the intensive care nursery. Indeed, 99% of infants weighing less than 1,500 g were exposed to drugs. The median number of drugs received was eight. The number of drugs administered was inversely related to birth weight and directly related to both length of hospital stay and the complexity of the infants' clinical condition. This study provides further support for the rationale and justification of undertaking proper efficacy and safety studies in the sick newborn.

To achieve the goal of using drugs in preterm or full-term infants that are both safe and efficacious, a change in attitude is necessary. This will require that academicians as well as practicing neonatologists understand the significance of labeling and the limitations of published studies. Neonatologists will require an expanded knowledge of clinical pharmacology, which goes beyond performing pharmacokinetics studies and their analysis. There are relatively few neonatologists with an in-depth knowledge of clinical pharmacology. Training of individuals in this important subspecialty will be necessary. The challenge is to reverse the trend of the introduction of drugs into the neonatal intensive care unit (NICU) based on minimal and limited clinical studies of knowledge of their safety and efficacy. It is highly objectionable to continue to "experiment" with fragile, sick newborns. Rather than employing retrospective analysis to determine, albeit imperfectly, whether a given drug is effective and/or safe, well-designed prospective studies need to be the rule. Guidelines for the conduct of drug studies in preterm and full-term infants need to be developed and adopted to ensure that the information gathered can be used either singularly or in combination to prove efficacy and safety. It is obvious that multicenter studies will be necessary to recruit the needed number of subjects. Studies of new therapies should be attractive to academicians because they can increase or add to scientific knowledge. The performance of these studies not only should satisfy editors of peer-reviewed journals, but also must meet FDA requirements for establishing efficacy and safety so that information on these drugs can be positively incorporated into the label. It is evident that the most difficult challenge is the study of drugs that are already in use. There is little economic incentive on the part of the pharmaceutical industry to support the studies of off-patent drugs that are needed for label change. Yet, this issue is a major public health problem with ethical overtones. Effectiveness of drugs commonly used in the NICU for life-threatening conditions (e.g., heparin, epinephrine, antiarrhythmic drugs, amino caproic acid, and antithrombotic drugs) has never been established. These drugs must be evaluated properly and, if these are shown to be useless, then their prescription in the NICU should stop.

In Europe, parallel regulatory developments were also occurring. In December 12, 2006, the European Parliament passed the Best Medicines for Children Act which became law in January 2007. The law requires studies of drug in newborns and children and a pediatric investigation plan (PIP) for all drugs being developed. It provides for the creation of a pediatric committee to decide priority drugs to study. The pediatric committee also reviews protocol proposals and study plans for drug development in children. It also provides procedures and funding mechanisms to foster studies of drugs for newborns and children. The EMEA (European Medication Evaluation Agency) reviews data for approval and marketing licensure. Thus, there is an increasing concerted effort in Europe and North America to ensure that requisite data for the safe and effective drug use in children are obtained.

This edition attempted to gather pertinent and recent drug information for clinicians, health care givers, investigators, scientists, regulatory agencies and others to guide them in their work and mission of providing safe and effective therapeutic options. Many subspecialties have references and books focused specifically to these subspecialties. While this current edition provides an overview of neonatal and pediatric therapeutics, it also complements and supplements existing focused subspecialty references.

Finally, we would like to quote from Sir William Osler, who in 1889 said, "The century opened auspiciously and those who were awake, saw signs of the dawn." For those who are visionary, let us project some thoughts regarding future directions and need. With the explosion in molecular biology, we must apply these techniques to developmental pharmacology. Much is to be gained by applying a developmental approach to gene expression, pharmacogenomics, and the development of drug receptors and cellular mechanisms for drug uptake and distribution. It is also important to elucidate the molecular mechanisms underlying changes in drug-metabolizing enzymes as well as changes in drug transporters and receptors.

Clinically, many off-patent drugs require study because industry has no interest in these. The neonate is exposed to a large number of drugs for which there is little scientific information. These needs are highlighted in the BPCA. Pediatric formulations are in need of development as well as studies regarding fetal therapy. To accomplish all of this, training of scientists qualified to pursue these investigations must be supported.

It is evident from the events since the publication of the previous editions of this book that neonatal and pediatric pharmacology has grown and developed. The future appears bright, and therapeutic orphans will finally no longer be applicable to drug use in infants and children.

CHAPTER

2

Edmund V. Capparelli

Clinical Pharmacokinetics in Infants and Children

INTRODUCTION

Considerable growth has occurred in the number of new chemical and biologic treatments during the last 25 years. Appropriate use of these agents in pediatric patients requires determining the safe and effective dosage for infants and children. A rational approach to determining appropriate dosage requires understanding the pharmacokinetic and pharmacodynamic properties of a drug in the population in which it is being used. Optimal therapy utilizes knowledge of a drug's pharmacokinetics to determine the dosage with a given formulation that will achieve desired drug concentrations for a particular infant or child. In this setting, pharmacokinetics represents the mathematical description of drug movement through a pediatric patient. Pharmacodynamics describes the relationship of drug concentrations at the site of action and the magnitude of responses, both therapeutic and toxic. In simplified terms, pharmacokinetics describes what the body does to the drug, and pharmacodynamics describes what the drug does to the body (Fig. 2.1).

Knowing the right dosage for an individual is as important as selection of the correct drug. Determining the dosage for an individual patient that maximizes clinical benefit yet minimizes toxicity requires knowledge of the general pharmacokinetic and pharmacodynamic properties of the drug in the population, the variability of these properties, and important physiologic determinants of this variability. Some of the pharmacokinetic and pharmacodynamic variability may be explained by genetic-, age-, size-, and disease-related effects. Even when the sources of pharmacokinetic and pharmacodynamic variability cannot be identified, understanding the range of concentrations and responses to a dosing regimen is necessary in the development of rational treatment strategies.

The pharmacokinetics of most drugs can be well described by a few key parameters. The two most important are volume of distribution, V_d, and clearance, CL. The elimination half-life, $t_{1/2}$, and associated elimination rate constant, K, are also widely determined and useful to determine dosing frequency. Following nonparenteral administration (such as oral, intramuscular, subcutaneous, or inhaled), bioavailability and absorption rate parameters are also necessary to describe a drug's pharmacokinetic behavior. Through these pharmacokinetic parameters a dosing regimen can be derived to achieve target drug concentrations or range of concentrations where the desirable effect is likely and toxicity is minimal. Clinical pharmacodynamic parameters are often highly variable and can require study of many individuals in multiple studies to understand the exposure–effect relationship. To develop appropriate target concentrations, pharmacodynamic models that describe the maximal effect, E_{max}, and concentration that achieves half of the maximal effect, EC_{50}, as either inhibitory or stimulatory influences on disease processes can be used. Methods for calculating these parameters and clinical (physiologic and pathologic) factors that affect them are presented in this chapter.

VOLUME OF DISTRIBUTION

After a drug is administered, it does not stay confined in the circulating blood pool. The drug diffuses into tissues, organs, and other fluid spaces, where it exerts its actions. However, when measuring drug concentrations, we are usually limited to collecting serum or plasma samples from the circulating blood pool and determining drug concentrations in these matrices. This serves as a surrogate for the drug concentration at the site of action. Therefore, it is useful to relate drug concentration measured in plasma to total amount of drug in the body. The volume of distribution, V_d, is a proportionality constant that relates the drug concentration to the total amount of drug in the body and can be represented as

$$V_d = \frac{A}{C_p}$$

where A is the total amount of drug in the body and C_p is the drug concentration in plasma. The direct clinical

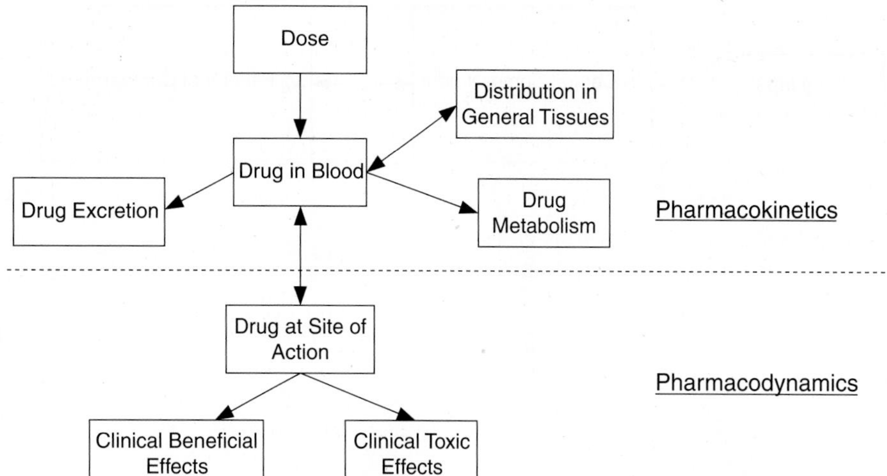

Figure 2.1. Schematic representation of the components that make up the pharmacokinetic–pharmacodynamic interface.

application of this pharmacokinetic parameter is that it can determine a loading dose:

$$\text{Loading dose} = C_{\text{p-desired}} \cdot V_{\text{d}}$$

It can be defined in relation to blood concentrations, plasma or serum concentrations, or unbound concentrations (V_{db}, V_{dp}, V_{du}, respectively). For a given drug, each of these drug concentration measurements may have different values; thus, V_{d} is relative to the matrix from which concentrations were measured. If, after bolus administration, a drug instantaneously equilibrates between plasma and tissues, V_{dp} can easily be estimated as

$$V_{\text{dp}} = \frac{\text{Dose}}{C_{\text{p0}}}$$

where C_{p0} is the drug concentration in plasma at time zero or immediately after drug administration (Fig. 2.2). This represents a *one-compartment* model. Distribution of drug out of blood and into other fluids and tissues takes time; so "true" one-compartment drug behavior is almost never encountered. However, if distribution is very rapid relative to elimination or absorption (following oral administration), a one-compartment model can adequately describe the drug distribution. More commonly, after intravenous administration, a rapid fall in drug concentrations is followed by a slower disappearance of drug. This multiphasic pattern of drug concentrations requires more complicated models and calculation methods. The most common model in this situation is the *two-compartment model* (Fig. 2.3). In this setting, drug concentrations initially fall rapidly because of distribution of the drug out of blood into tissues followed by a slower decline because of elimination. The initial distribution phase is also known as the alpha phase and the elimination period as the beta (β) phase. It is important to recognize that these do not represent true physical tissue or fluid spaces per se but are greatly influenced by body composition, physiologic processes, and the chemical and physical properties of the drug. Therefore, a drug that has a much higher affinity for extravascular tissue than for plasma may have a V_{d} that is in excess of true body size (greater than 1 L per kg). However, it is possible to set a minimum value for V_{d} at the blood or plasma volume. Thus, no drug can have a V_{d} less than total intravascular plasma volume, or about 50 mL per kg. In multiple-compartment models, various methods can be used to calculate V_{d}. A common approach is to estimate V_{d} from the terminal beta phase; it is calculated as follows:

$$V_{\text{d}\beta} = \frac{\text{Dose}}{\text{AUC} \cdot \beta}$$

where AUC is the area under the concentration–time curve after a single dose. An alternative method used to calculate V_{d} is the noncompartmental approach. With this method, V_{d} is defined as V_{d} at steady state, V_{dss}; this is calculated using the following equation:

$$V_{\text{dss}} = \frac{\text{Dose} \cdot \text{AUMC}}{\text{AUC}^2}$$

where AUMC is the area under the first moment curve (concentration × time vs. time). The related fraction

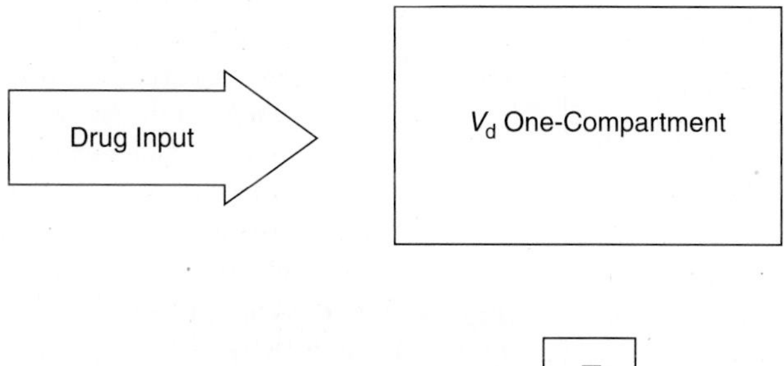

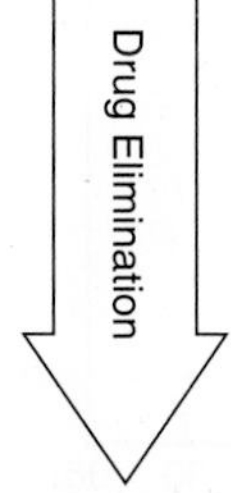

Figure 2.2. Basic one-compartment model.

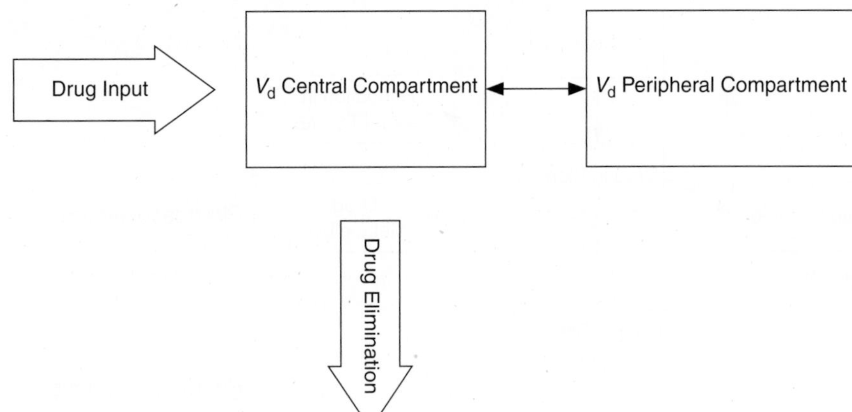

Figure 2.3. Basic two-compartment model. Drug distributes between central and peripheral compartments and is eliminated from central compartment.

AUMC/AUC equals the mean time that drug molecules remain in the body and is referred to as the mean residence time (MRT). From a theoretical basis, $V_{dss} = V_{dc1} + V_{dc2}$, where c1 and c2 are the central and peripheral compartments, respectively. Although this method has the advantage of being relatively independent of terminal-slope determination, it requires a much longer sample collection duration to characterize the AUMC from the first moment curve (because this curve is less "steep" than the concentration vs. time curve, Fig. 2.4). It also requires estimating an absorption input parameter (mean absorption time, MAT) as a correction factor when estimating V_d for drugs that are not administered as an intravenous bolus.

Although the volume of distribution does not represent a true physical space, changes in body composition seen throughout infancy and childhood can have a predictable impact on the volume of distribution based on a drug's chemical and physical properties. Newborn infants have a higher proportion of extracellular and total body water than older populations, and thus drugs that are distributed freely in water have larger volumes of distribution in newborns. Accordingly, aminoglycoside antibiotics, which are highly polar and hydrophilic and are distributed primarily into extracellular fluid, have approximately double the volume of distribution in newborns as in adults. Preterm newborns have a reduced percentage of total body fat. Thus, for lipophilic drugs, the volume of distribution may be reduced compared to that in adults.

Differences in drug binding across age groups can affect its V_d. Whereas drugs can bind to tissue components and plasma proteins, only the free (unbound) drug equilibrates. Thus, in newborns and certain diseases in which albumin and alpha-1 acid glycoprotein levels are low, highly bound drugs will have a greater free-fraction (unbound/total drug concentration) in plasma, and more drug will distribute out of the plasma compartment into tissues. This will have the net effect of a higher V_d for total drug, although the V_{du} may be similar. While free drug concentrations may be more representative of the "effective" concentration seen at the site of action, they are not routinely measured because their measurements require more sensitive, time consuming, expensive assays.

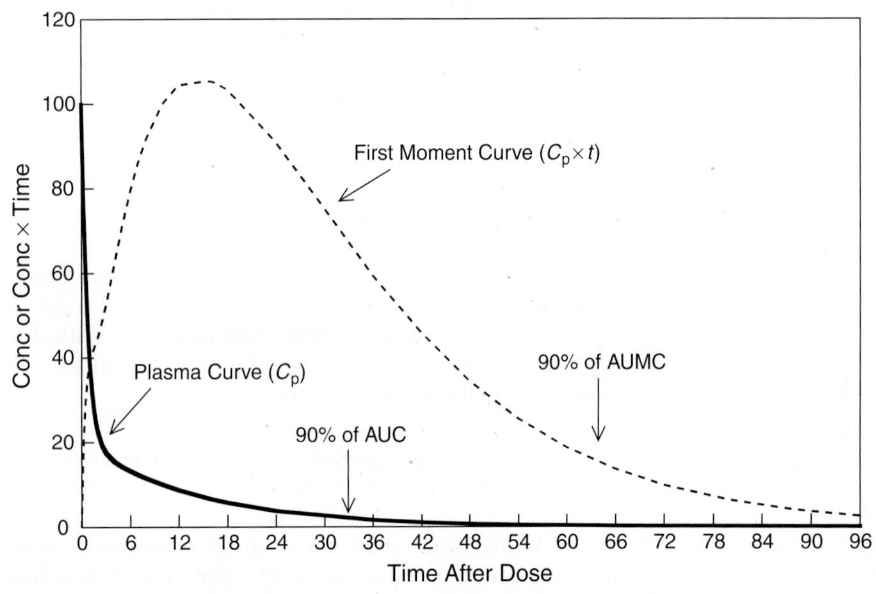

Figure 2.4. Concentration versus time and first moment curve (concentration × time vs. time) for a drug exhibiting pronounced multicompartment pharmacokinetics. Ninety percent of the area under the concentration-versus-time curve (AUC) can be captured with sampling out to 36 hours. To characterize the same portion of the first moment curve (AUMC) requires collecting samples nearly twice as long.

In most clinical situations, alterations in protein binding will not have a significant impact on therapy but can greatly impact the interpretation of measured (total) drug concentrations.

DISTRIBUTION INTO SPECIFIC TISSUES

When acute drug effects are of critical importance, such as in induction of anesthesia or in treatment of shock, the distribution characteristics of a drug are integral to its therapeutic utility. In general, distribution characteristics for drugs used in the treatment of chronic diseases are of lesser clinical importance. One important exception relates to target sites that a drug may not access easily. Whereas most distribution is based on concentration gradients and passive diffusion, in some tissues drug access is limited by tight junctions in the endothelium and active drug transport. For many drugs, free concentrations do not come into true equilibrium within the central nervous system due to these processes. P-glycoprotein and other active transporters pump various drugs out of the central nervous system and greatly reduce the overall effective penetration into this site.

CLEARANCE

Drug clearance (CL) is a measure of drug elimination. It represents the volume of blood or plasma from which drug is completely removed per unit of time. It is analogous to creatinine clearance as an assessment of renal function. It is the ratio of the rate of elimination or extraction divided by the drug concentration and can be mathematically defined as

$$CL = \frac{\text{Rate of elimination}}{C_{\text{p}}}$$

At steady state, where by definition drug input equals drug elimination, this equation can be rearranged to

$$\text{Dose (rate in)} = CL \cdot C_{\text{pave}}$$

Thus, CL dictates the average steady-state concentration, C_{pave}, that will be achieved from a given dosing regimen. It can also be expressed in terms of mass balance for the organ of elimination. The rate of drug clearance from an eliminating organ is the product of the blood flow, Q, and the extraction ratio (ER) from arterial blood of that organ. An organ's ER is determined from arterial concentration, C_{pA}, reaching the organ and venous concentration, C_{pV}, leaving the organ of elimination and can be expressed as

$$ER = \frac{(C_{\text{pA}} - C_{\text{pV}})}{C_{\text{pA}}}$$

It can range from 0 (no extraction) to 1 (complete extraction). An important mathematical property regarding CL is that it can be separated into its individual components. The two most common organs of drug elimination are the liver and the kidney. The liver metabolizes drugs and can also excrete drugs and drug metabolites in bile. The kidney filters and excretes drugs and drug metabolites. Occasionally, other tissues contribute significantly to a drug's clearance. Therefore, overall CL can be expressed as

$$CL_{\text{total}} = CL_{\text{hepatic}} + CL_{\text{renal}} + CL_{\text{other}}$$

For most drugs, CL is constant over the range of concentration encountered clinically. When a drug's CL is independent of concentration, the elimination is referred to as first-order. In this setting, there is a linear relationship between the logarithm of drug concentration and time during drug elimination. With first-order elimination, changes in dosing lead to proportional changes in drug concentrations. Clearance can be estimated by model-based methods through fitting the observed concentration versus time profile to an appropriate model. Following intravenous administration, CL (and V_{d}) can be determined using a *one-compartment* model through iterative fitting of drug concentrations to the following equation:

$$C_{\text{p}(t)} = \frac{\text{Dose}}{V_{\text{d}}} e^{-t \times CL/V_{\text{d}}}$$

Alternatively, CL can be estimated using noncompartmental methods from the area under the concentration versus time curve (AUC). The AUC can be approximated following intensive sampling using the trapezoidal method. This is the summation of the area of trapezoids estimated from sequential, intensively collected plasma concentrations with the area of each individual trapezoid equal to $[(C_{\text{pi}} + C_{\text{pi+1}})/2](t_{\text{i+1}} - t_{\text{i}})$ and the final area after the last trapezoid can be estimated as $C_{\text{p-last}}/\lambda_z$, where λ_z is the terminal slope of the log plasma concentration versus time curve. From the AUC, the CL following a single intravenous dose can be calculated as

$$CL = \frac{\text{Dose}}{\text{AUC}_{0-\infty}}$$

Clearance may also be defined with respect to unbound drug concentrations. For drugs with protein binding, unbound drug concentrations are always less than the total drug concentrations, and thus AUC for unbound drug concentration is always lower than AUC for total drug concentration. Because clearance is inversely related to AUC, the calculated clearance for unbound drug is greater than that for total drug.

RENAL CLEARANCE

Many drugs undergo elimination into the urine by the kidneys. This occurs via filtration through the glomerulus and active secretion of acids and bases, which occurs primarily in the proximal tubule. Typically, only free or unbound drugs are filtered by the glomerulus into the urine. Separate active transport systems exist for acid (anion) and base (cation) secretion by the kidneys. Drug elimination by filtration and active secretion can be mitigated by reabsorption of the drug along the proximal and distal tubules as well as the collecting duct. Reabsorption is primarily a passive process; however, its impact can be pronounced.

Because the great majority of water that is filtered by the glomerulus is reabsorbed, drugs with favorable physical–chemical properties (small, nonpolar) will follow the water and be reabsorbed as well. The reabsorption of drugs with pK_a values in the range of urinary pH can be markedly influenced by acidification or alkalinization of urine. Mathematically, renal clearance equals renal excretion rate divided by average plasma concentration and can be determined from serial blood and urine collections using the equation:

$$CL_{renal} = \frac{A_{e0-t}}{AUC_{0-t}}$$

where A_e is the cumulative drug excreted unchanged in the urine and AUC is derived from the plasma concentration-versus-time profile.

Glomerular filtration rates (GFR) are commonly estimated from serum creatinine in adults and used to individualize dosing of drugs eliminated by renal mechanisms. While GFR can be estimated from serum creatinine in children also, the relationship between measured serum creatinine and GRF is different between pediatric and adult populations. Age-specific equations have been developed for estimating GFR in pediatric populations; however, lower serum creatinine concentrations in children reduce the precision of these equations. In newborn infants, estimating the GFR from serum creatinine is confounded by the transplacental creatinine that infants receive from their mothers in utero. This additional maternally derived creatinine may bias estimates of GFR in newborns during the first few days of life.

HEPATIC CLEARANCE

The liver is the primary site of drug metabolism. Drug biotransformation is influenced by a drug's chemical and structural properties, which determine its affinity to various drug-metabolizing enzymes in the liver. Drug metabolism may also be influenced by hepatic blood flow and protein binding. Drugs with a great affinity for metabolizing enzymes are highly extracted and their metabolism is limited primarily by hepatic perfusion. Their hepatic clearance approaches and parallels hepatic blood flow. Changes in hepatic blood flow have much less impact on the clearance of those drugs with lower affinity for metabolizing enzymes or low hepatic extraction. However, for low-hepatic-extraction drugs, their total hepatic clearance is sensitive to changes in protein binding. Hepatic clearance of unbound drug can be used as a measure of the liver's overall ability to metabolize that drug. Hepatic clearance of unbound drug is also frequently referred to as intrinsic clearance, CL_{hu}. It is mathematically related to total hepatic clearance, CL_h, by multiplying with the fraction unbound:

$$CL_h = CL_{hu} \times f_u$$

Understanding the hepatic extraction of a compound aids in determining the impact that patient-specific factors, including age, liver disease, and cardiac status, may have on hepatic clearance.

SATURABLE ELIMINATION

In some instances, *CL* is not independent of drug concentration, as the metabolizing enzyme or secretory pump gets overwhelmed by excessive drug. This is often referred to as nonlinear or Michaelis–Menten elimination. It is mathematically expressed as

$$\text{Rate of elimination} = \frac{V_{max} \times C_p}{(K_m + C_p)} \quad \text{or} \quad CL = \frac{V_{max}}{K_m + C_p}$$

where V_{max} is the maximum capacity of drug metabolism and K_m is the concentration at which metabolism is half of maximal. This equation is analogous to equations describing enzyme kinetic behavior. An important characteristic of this equation is that as drug input approaches V_{max}, small increases in dose can lead to very large increases in steady-state drug concentrations. Another category of nonlinear pharmacokinetics is zero-order elimination, where metabolism is constant regardless of drug concentration. This represents an extreme version of Michaelis–Menten kinetics where the drug concentration greatly exceeds K_m such that elimination is essentially equal to V_{max} at all experienced concentrations. This pharmacokinetic behavior is seen with ethanol.

DRUG ABSORPTION

Whereas drugs that are administered intravenously are completely available to the systemic circulation, drugs administered by other routes may not enter into the systemic circulation intact. The proportion of a dose that enters into the systemic circulation intact is defined as the drug's bioavailability. By definition, the bioavailability following intravenous administration equals 1. *Absolute bioavailability F* is calculated as the ratio of exposures from an extravenous dose to an intravenous dose, or

$$F = \frac{AUC_{extravenous}}{AUC_{iv}}$$

If extravenous and intravenous doses are of different sizes, then

$$F = \frac{AUC_{extravenous} \times Dose_{iv}}{AUC_{iv} \times Dose_{extravenous}}$$

When pharmacokinetic data following intravenous administration are not available, the *relative bioavailability* between various formulations and routes of administration can be compared. Pharmacokinetic parameters estimated exclusively from oral data are confounded by not knowing the dose of drug absorbed intact. Thus, the relative contribution of bioavailability in estimating *CL* and V_d cannot be determined. Parameters from oral data are typically presented as apparent parameters, specifically *CL*/*F* and V_d/F. Bioavailability less than 100% following oral administration can occur for a number of physiologic and drug formulation–related issues, including problems with drug dissolution or solubility and instability in gastric acid. In addition, gastrointestinal transit time, gastric acid secretion, and biliary and pancreatic exocrine function all can affect drug absorption. These are dynamic processes during the first year of life and can result in age-dependent bioavailability differences. Oral drugs may also undergo metabolism in the gut and liver before reaching the systemic circulation. Blood from the intestinal tract that contains the absorbed drug is carried to the liver by the portal vein, where it can be metabolized before reaching the general systemic circulation. The combined drug metabolism in the gut and in the liver via portal circulation before the drug has reached the systemic circulation is termed first-pass metabolism. Therefore, drugs exhibiting first-pass metabolism, such as morphine, may have excellent absorption but low bioavailability. Whereas most drug absorption from the gut is passive, active transport of drugs in enterocytes back into the lumen of the gut may also limit bioavailability. Other routes of drug administration, including intramuscular, subcutaneous, rectal, and inhaled, may have bioavailability less than 1.

Bioavailability characterizes the extent of absorption but drug entry into the body can also be characterized by the rate of drug absorption. Absorption rate is sometimes confused with bioavailability, as it can be influenced by some of the same formulation and physiologic processes that affect bioavailability. Intuitively, the rate of absorption dictates the onset of effect for rapidly acting drugs, but it can also determine the duration of effect for drugs that are also rapidly eliminated (Fig. 2.5). Absorption rate is most commonly characterized by peak time, t_{max}. Although this is relatively easy to obtain graphically, it reflects both absorption and elimination processes and is different following single-dose and multiple-dose administration. The most common mathematical model used to characterize oral drug absorption is the first-order absorption. This model is characterized by an absorption rate constant K_A, with the amount of drug absorbed per unit of time equal to K_A times the amount of drug remaining in the gut. Because very little drug absorption occurs in the stomach, a delay in the detection of drug in the systemic circulation is often observed during the first few minutes after oral drug administration. In this setting, a lag time can be utilized in conjunction with a first-order absorption model to describe this absorption pattern. Alternative absorption models with constant drug absorption (zero order) and convoluted functions with multiple rate constants affecting various fractions of the dose can also be utilized to describe drug input.

The rate and extent of oral drug absorption is dependent on a drug's chemical properties and formulation as well as physiologic characteristics of the patient and administration circumstances. Oral drug administration to infants and young children requires either liquid or chewable product formulations. These pediatric formulations may have significantly different absorption properties than solid oral dosage forms used in older populations. Extemporaneous compounding liquid pediatric formulations from adult dosage forms may also alter drug stability and thus limit the intended dose administered. The bioavailability of a drug may also be altered by the presence and composition of coadministered food. A true fasting state is difficult to achieve for drug administration in infants and the limited variety in their dietary intake can limit bioavailability of compounds that require high-fat meals for optimal absorption. Based on these factors, large, unanticipated differences between oral absorption in young pediatric and adult populations can be encountered.

HALF-LIFE

The elimination half-life, $T_{1/2}$, is defined as the time necessary for the drug concentration to decrease by 50%. After one half-life, 50% of the initial concentration

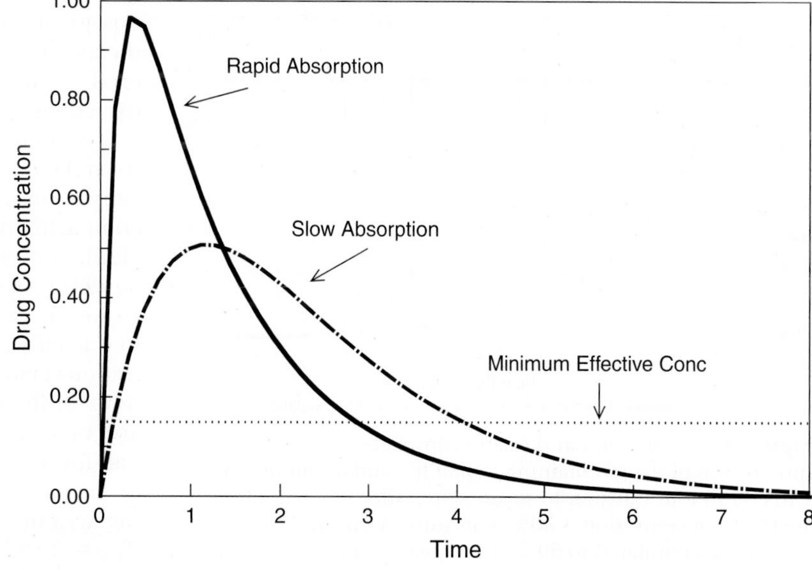

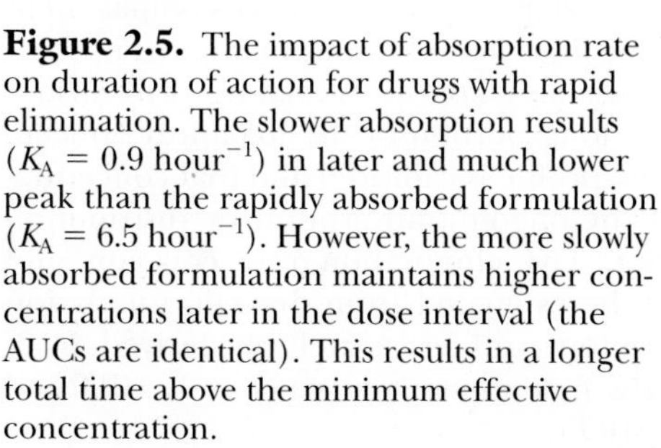

Figure 2.5. The impact of absorption rate on duration of action for drugs with rapid elimination. The slower absorption results (K_A = 0.9 hour^{-1}) in later and much lower peak than the rapidly absorbed formulation (K_A = 6.5 hour^{-1}). However, the more slowly absorbed formulation maintains higher concentrations later in the dose interval (the AUCs are identical). This results in a longer total time above the minimum effective concentration.

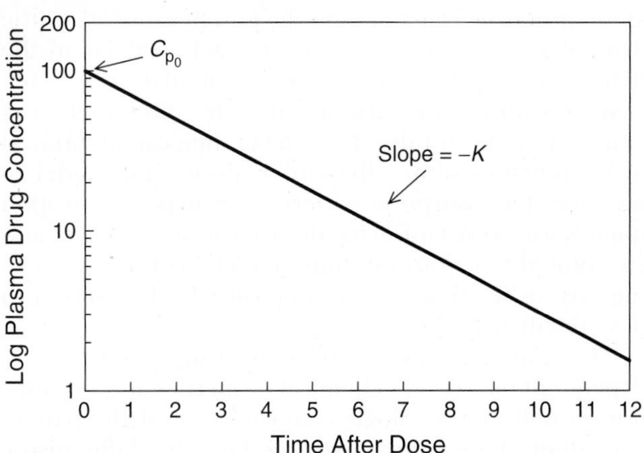

Figure 2.6. Concentration-versus-time profile for one-compartment drug, plotted as log concentration versus time, with the slope representing the elimination rate constant ($-K$).

remains; after two half-lives, 25% of the initial concentration remains; and so on. A related parameter is the elimination rate constant, K, which is related to $T_{1/2}$ by $K = 0.693/T_{1/2}$. During the elimination phase, K can be used to predict concentrations at any time t from the following equation (Fig. 2.6):

$$C_{pi+1} = C_{pi} \times e^{-K \times \Delta t}$$

where Δt is the time between the two concentrations C_{pi} and C_{pi+1} measured during the elimination phase. Half-life can also be used to describe drug accumulation. After one half-life, the drug concentration will be 50% of the ultimate steady-state value; after two half-lives, 75% of the steady-state value; and so on (Fig. 2.7, Table 2.1). Drug accumulation approaches steady state asymptotically; after 3.3 to 5 half-lives on a constant-dosage regimen, drug con-

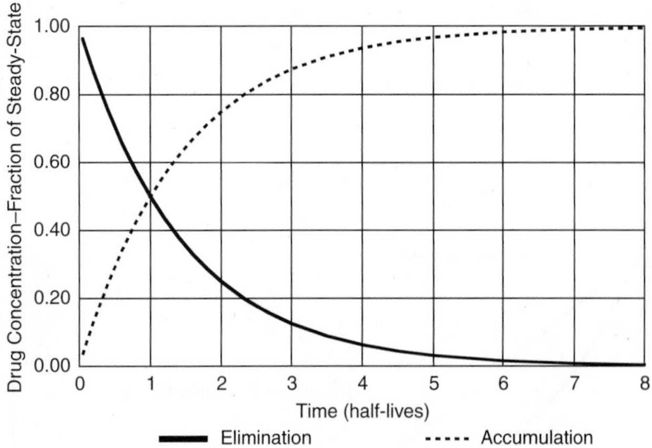

Figure 2.7. Symmetry and relationship between half-life and portion of drug remaining to half-life and accumulation with continuous infusion to steady state. After one half-life, the drug concentration is 50% of its initial value and the drug has accumulated to 50% of the steady-state level.

TABLE 2.1 Relationship Between Half-Life and Portion of Drug Remaining and Accumulation

Half-Lives	*Percentage Remaining*	*Percentage Accumulation*
0.5	71	29
1	50	50
2	25	75
3.3	10	90
4	6	94
5	3	97
6.6	1	99

centrations are 90% to 97% of final steady-state values and can be effectively considered steady state. The exact proportion of steady-state concentration at any time t can be determined from

$$\text{Proportion of steady-state} = 1 - e^{-K \times t}$$

For drugs exhibiting first-order elimination (which includes most drugs), $T_{1/2}$ is independent of dose. It is mechanistically dependent on CL and V_d and can be described as

$$T_{1/2} = \frac{0.693 \cdot V_d}{CL}$$

For drugs with saturable or Michaelis–Menten elimination, $T_{1/2}$ has limited utility as a pharmacokinetic parameter because it is dynamic, increasing at higher drug concentrations. Whereas the general concept of half-life is easily grasped, it is often assumed that any change in half-life reflects a change in drug elimination. This is not necessarily true, as half-life alterations may be entirely due to changes in drug distribution. It is clear from the above equation that clinical situations that reduce a drug's CL or increase its V_d will be associated with an increase in that drug's $T_{1/2}$. Whereas $T_{1/2}$ does not indicate what drug concentrations will result from a given dosage, it is used to determine dosing intervals. Half-life dictates the peak/trough ratio and needs to be considered when constructing an appropriate dosing regimen for a drug.

The elimination $T_{1/2}$ is most commonly determined from the terminal slope or "washout" portion of the concentration–time profile. For drugs that exhibit multicompartment pharmacokinetics, $T_{1/2}$ and the apparent elimination rate constant (λ_z or β for a two-compartment model) can also be determined in this manner (Fig. 2.8). However, care must be taken in estimating β to ensure that a sufficiently long portion of the log-linear concentration-versus-time profile is captured and that concentrations influenced by ongoing absorption or distribution are not included. The elimination rate constant and half-life can also be estimated from drug accumulation or urinary excretion profiles as well as derived from the area under the first moment curve ($K = 1/\text{MRT}$ and $T_{1/2} = 0.693 \times \text{MRT}$).

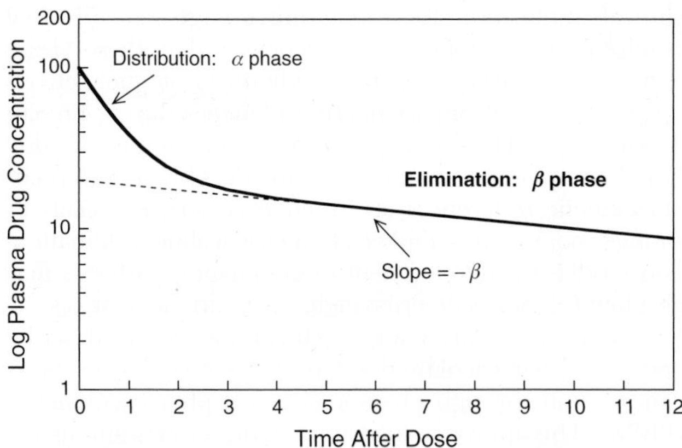

Figure 2.8. Concentration-versus-time profile for a two-compartment drug, plotted as log concentration versus time. The initial slope represents the distribution rate constant, α, and the terminal, linear portion of the curve represents the elimination rate constant β.

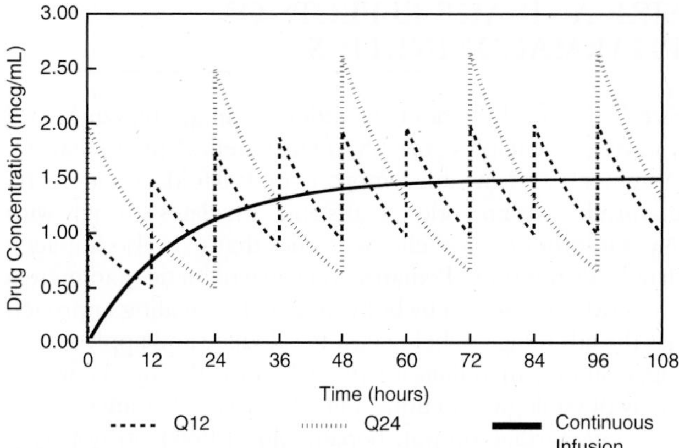

Figure 2.9. Impact of various dosing intervals on concentration-versus-time profile following multiple doses and same total daily dose. Average concentrations for all three regimens are the identical, with peak/trough differences increasing with larger dose intervals.

APPLICATION OF PHARMACOKINETIC PRINCIPLES TO MULTIPLE-DOSE REGIMENS

In most clinical situations, drugs are administered repeatedly at fixed intervals rather than as single doses. The goal is to maintain drug concentrations above a minimum effective target concentration associated with clinical benefit and below concentrations that are likely to result in toxicity, keeping drug concentrations in this "therapeutic range" throughout the dosage interval. For drugs that exhibit linear or dose-independent pharmacokinetics, the pharmacokinetic parameters from a single dose can be used to predict drug concentrations that will result from various multiple-dose regimens. The contribution of each individual dose can be calculated and summed to determine the total concentration following multiple doses. This method of superposition can be used to determine non–steady-state and steady-state concentrations but becomes cumbersome if the number of doses included for steady-state determination is large. However, because the AUC during a dosing interval at steady state equals the sum of AUCs contributed from single doses at dosing intervals of τ ($AUC_{0-\tau}$, + $AUC_{\tau-2\tau}$ + $AUC_{2\tau-3\tau}$ + $\cdots$), the total $AUC_{0-\tau}$ (at steady state) is equal to $AUC_{0-\text{inf}}$ for a single dose. Thus, steady-state clearance can be calculated from the following equation:

$$CL = \frac{\text{Dose}}{AUC_{0-\tau}}$$

Once steady state is achieved, an accumulation factor can determine concentrations at various times in the dosing interval. The rate of accumulation is independent of the dosing interval, but the magnitude of the peak/trough ratio increases with increasing dosing intervals (Fig. 2.9). Peak, trough, and average steady-state concentrations following repeated intravenous boluses can be easily determined using a one-compartment model from the following equations:

$$C_{\text{peak,ss}} = \frac{\text{Dose}}{V_d \cdot (1 - e^{-K \times \tau})}$$

$$C_{\text{trough,ss}} = C_{\text{peak,ss}} \cdot e^{-K \times \tau}$$

$$C_{\text{ave,ss}} = \frac{\text{Dose}}{CL \times \tau}$$

For example, for a drug with V_d = 2.0 L per kg and CL = 0.10 L per hour per kg (K = 0.05 hour^{-1}), a bolus dose of 100 mg per kg every 8 hours yields the following steady-state peak and trough concentrations:

$$C_{\text{peak,ss}} = \frac{100\ \text{mg/kg}}{(2.0\ \text{L/kg}) \times (1 - e^{-0.05 \times 8})} = 152\ \text{mg/L}$$

$$C_{\text{trough,ss}} = 152 \cdot e^{-0.05 \times 8} = 102\ \text{mg/L}$$

$$C_{\text{ave,ss}} = \frac{100\ \text{mg/kg}}{0.10\ \text{L/hr/kg} \times 8\ \text{hr}} = 125\ \text{mg/L}$$

Whereas these equations predict drug concentrations after intravenous bolus administration, they can also approximate drug concentrations following oral administration if bioavailability, F, is added to the numerator and drug absorption is much more rapid than drug elimination (K_A much greater than K). If the absorption rate does not greatly exceed the elimination rate, use of these equations will result in overestimating the true peak and underestimating the true trough concentrations. To characterize drug concentrations following a single-dose oral administration using a one-compartment model with first-order absorption, the following equation can be used:

$$C_p(t) = \frac{F \times K_A \times \text{Dose} \times (e^{-K \times t} - e^{-K_A \times t})}{V_d \times (K_A - K)}$$

SIZE AND AGE EFFECTS ON PHARMACOKINETICS

Size is a critical element in understanding, analyzing, and applying principles of pharmacokinetics in pediatrics. Weight (WT) can range more than 100-fold between premature infants and adolescents and correlates strongly with age and other clinical characteristics that may also impact a drug's disposition. Pediatric pharmacokinetic parameters are most often scaled by body weight. This scaling approach has the advantage of being easy to calculate and apply to dosing resulting in milligram per kilogram dosing. However, many physiologic functions that affect drug clearance (renal function, cardiac output, hepatic blood flow) do not scale directly to weight in a linear manner. Estimated body surface area (BSA) is an alternative scalar for many physiologic processes that affect drug disposition. Using BSA rather than weight to scale for size in children has been found empirically to provide a more linear relationship with clearance for many drugs. However, scaling volume of distribution with BSA may not be as linear as it is with weight. Use of BSA requires height measurements to estimate, is prone to calculation errors, and is primarily reserved for antineoplastics and other agents with very narrow therapeutic indices. A third approach to scaling clearance is the allometric method. Allometric scaling is used extensively in evaluating physiologic and preclinical pharmacokinetic data across animal species. Since the 1940s, it has been applied to adjusting drug doses in humans and is based on relating physiologic functions and morphology to body size. This approach suggests that $WT^{0.75}$ be used to scale clearance, and this scalar correlates closely with percentage of liver weight relative to body weight during the first 18 years of life (Fig. 2.10). It also suggests V_d be scaled by $WT^{1.0}$, which results in shorter half-lives in smaller, younger individuals, which is consistent with what is generally observed. The allometric approach produces similar clearance results to scaling by BSA without requiring a height measurement. However, like BSA, this method is prone to calculation errors and has limited clinical application for estimating dosage in individual children. It is important to recognize that these sizing approaches do not account for additional ontogenic effects on processes that impact pharmacokinetics during human development. Thus, in addition to these size effects, additional components that account for developmental pharmacokinetic differences are often necessary, especially in younger populations. Linked allometric scaling with maturation models for development of elimination pathways may be a helpful tool to describe pediatric pharmacokinetics.

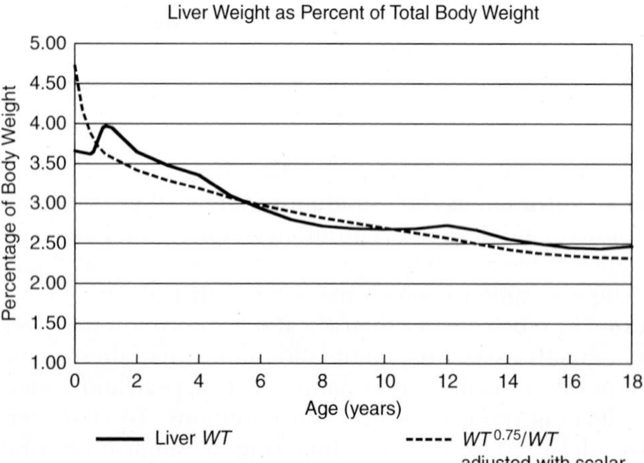

Figure 2.10. Liver size as function of age. The relative liver weight (WT) as percentage of total body weight shows decrease during infancy and childhood. This relationship closely mirrors the shape of the allometric scaling factor $WT^{0.75}/WT$ (adjusted by a scalar to superimpose the two curves).

A more mechanistic approach can be used to describe pediatric pharmacokinetics based on changes in body composition through physiologic-based pharmacokinetics (PBPK). This approach incorporates organ sizes and tissue-specific drug partitioning along with organ blood flows to describe drug disposition in the human body as process of system flows. These models require a large number of differential equations to characterize the drug concentration-versus-time profile and thus cannot be used to estimate PK parameters based on individual patient's PK data. However, the PBPK approach is very useful for predicting the impact of physiologic and maturational changes on drug exposure in plasma and tissues. PBPK modeling is widely used in environmental toxicology to predict the disposition of chemicals in pediatric populations.

PHARMACODYNAMICS

A number of different pharmacodynamic models are used to describe drug action, and most include a monotonic component linking drug exposure and action. The most common are the E_{max} and related sigmoid E_{max} models, which are represented mathematically as

$$\text{Effect} = \frac{E_{max} \cdot C_p^{\gamma}}{EC_{50}^{\gamma} + C_p^{\gamma}}$$

where E_{max} is the maximum effect, EC_{50} is the concentration that produces half-maximal effect, and γ is a shape constant. When γ equals 1, this simplifies to the E_{max} model. This model has its origins in receptor–ligand binding relationships and predicts that effects increase nearly in proportion to drug concentrations at low concentrations (well below EC_{50}), and effects increase in proportion to the logarithm of drug concentrations around the EC_{50}. In situations in which drug concentrations greatly exceed the EC_{50}, drug effects can be maintained despite relatively dramatic changes in drug concentrations (Fig. 2.11).

In some situations, E_{max} and related models can be directly linked to serum concentrations to describe rapidly occurring drug effects. However, a lag or hysteresis between serum drug concentrations and effects often exists. This can be due to two separate phenomena. The first type of lag can be due to distribution. This can be encountered with central nervous system–active drugs, which require distribution into the brain to produce their effects. The second delay occurs when the effects of drugs are mediated through synthesis or metabolism of endogenous moieties. In the latter situation, drug effects can occur through a cascade of processes, and overall homeostasis is altered only after the drug has caused endogenous intermediaries

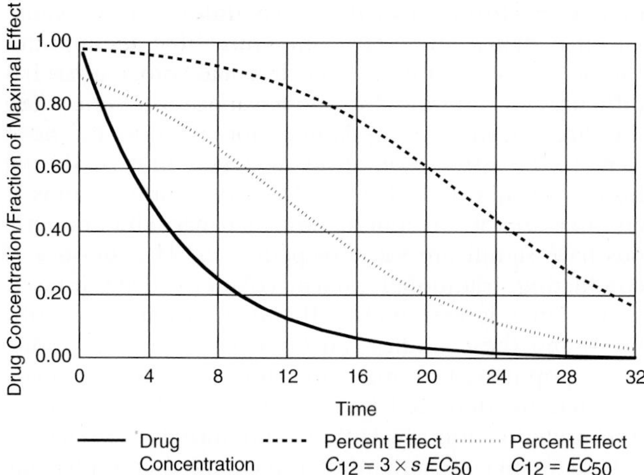

Figure 2.11. The pharmacokinetic–pharmacodynamic relationship of a sigmoid E_{max} model. While the drug concentrations fall rapidly ($T_{1/2}$ = 4 hours), the pharmacodynamic effect persists and drops more slowly when the concentrations are well above the EC_{50}. At 12 hours postdose, the concentration is only 12.5% of the peak value, yet only 50% of the effect has been lost if the 12-hour concentration equals the EC_{50}. If the 12-hour concentration is higher (three times the EC_{50}), less than 15% of the effect is lost in this interval. This persistence of effect allows dosing less frequently than half-life.

of effects to be synthesized or depleted. A group of indirect response pharmacodynamic models with E_{max} equation components can be used to describe these processes. Examples of drugs that have delayed effects through this mechanism include anti-inflammatory effects of glucocorticoids and anticoagulant effects of warfarin. Pharmacodynamic effects may also be related to total drug exposure. In these situations, either very slow accumulation or irreversible changes accrue with continued exposure. This pharmacodynamic relationship commonly describes toxic effects, including those from heavy metals and antineoplastics that irreversibly bind to DNA.

Determining the pharmacodynamic parameters for a drug requires selection of appropriate effect measurements and mechanistically plausible models. Pharmacodynamic parameter estimates are most robust when the effects are relatively direct and reproducible. The range of drug concentrations used to determine the pharmacodynamic parameters is also important. Use of a narrow range of concentrations may limit the ability to fully characterize the concentration–response relationship. A single paired drug concentration and associated response can be described by a variety of E_{max}–EC_{50} value combinations, so broad concentration–response measurements are desired. While this broad dose range approach is used in the early phases of drug development for adults, pharmacodynamic studies in pediatrics typically have limited concentration–effect ranges. In addition, use of indirect markers of drug effects, such as surrogate or biomarkers, can result in different pharmacodynamic parameter values based on the specific biomarker measured. Whereas methods to determine drug concentration are typically consistent across the age continuum studied, biomarkers appropriate in one age group may not be appropriate in another or may change with human development. These potential confounders should be addressed when calculating pediatric pharmacodynamic parameters. Lastly, even with high-quality surrogate markers, disease presentation and progression differences in pediatric subpopulations can lead to pharmacodynamic changes, particularly when the organ system affected undergoes significant development during infancy and childhood.

POPULATION PHARMACOKINETICS/ PHARMACODYNAMICS

Whereas detailed description of pharmacokinetics in individual subjects is determined for regulatory and research purposes, in most clinical circumstances precise determination of an individual's pharmacokinetics to optimize therapy is impractical. Summary data generated from intensive phase 1 pharmacokinetic studies are used to infer individual patient's pharmacokinetic characteristics and drug exposure from a specific dosing regimen. However, most of these studies are performed in relatively healthy and homogeneous populations with limited age ranges and are conducted under tightly controlled environments. Although this approach results in rapid generation of pharmacokinetic data, the patients studied may not reflect subpopulations that will frequently receive the drug clinically. Concomitant drugs, diseases, and patient characteristics encountered clinically with drug use, but avoided in intensive studies, may alter a drug's pharmacokinetics and pharmacodynamics. Thus, the dosing derived from tightly controlled phase 1 and phase 2a clinical trials may provide biased estimates of the larger population of subjects that will ultimately receive therapy. In addition, these studies provide little insight into the extreme pharmacokinetic/pharmacodynamic responses likely to be encountered on a given dose to the larger population. Accordingly, most phase 1 pharmacokinetic studies focus on average or median CL and V_d values with little attention directed to variability and sources of variability.

Recently, emphasis has been placed on the application of sparse pharmacokinetic sampling in larger pediatric populations to better describe pharmacokinetics and pharmacodynamics using population analysis approaches. In this approach, the precision in the pharmacokinetic parameter estimates for individual participants is reduced by taking fewer evaluations per subject. However, less intensive sampling allows inclusion of a wider spectrum of participants likely to receive the drug clinically. Although reduction in frequency and number of samples has obvious appeal in pediatric populations, the ability of population methods to analyze unbalanced data collected at various times is also attractive in these populations. This method allows pooling of data across studies to provide a uniform, robust, single pharmacokinetic analysis rather than attempting to compare results of separate, smaller studies that are complicated by significant analysis methodology differences. The population pharmacokinetic method also regards variability differently than does the traditional intensive approach. Instead of avoiding variability by design, one goal of the population approach is to quantify both within- and

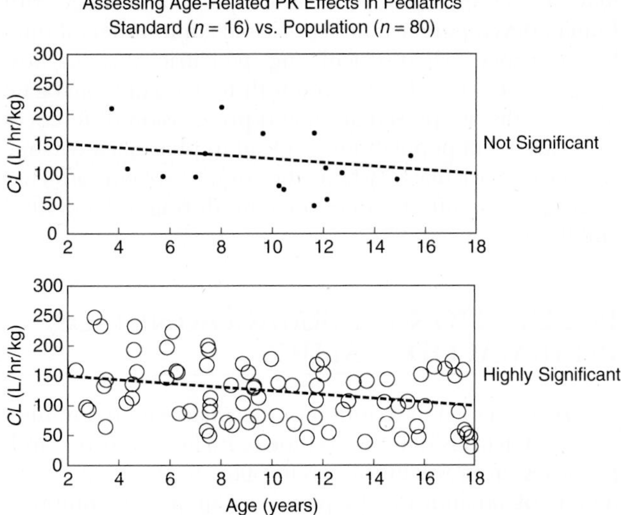

Figure 2.12. A comparison of intensive two-stage and population pharmacokinetic methods for detecting sources of pharmacokinetic variability such as age. This represents a typical simulation using 240 concentrations. In the intensive evaluation, 15 samples were used to precisely calculate the clearance in each of 16 subjects. In the population analysis, three samples collected in 80 subjects were used to describe the population pharmacokinetics. Individual clearance estimates were generated for graphical comparison by a Bayesian method. The size of the symbols is proportional to the relative error of the parameter estimate in each subject. Having fewer samples reduced individual subject parameter precision in the population analysis, but the population analysis was robust in detecting the age effect on clearance.

between-participant variability and examine clinical characteristics that can explain intersubject variability to indicate alternative dosing requirements for specific subpopulations. It is a robust method and can be used to characterize the impact of age and development on drug pharmacokinetics (Fig. 2.12).

The population pharmacokinetic approach in pediatrics has been most widely applied in the newborn population although there has been growing use in older pediatric populations. The ability to accommodate unbalanced designs allows one to incorporate both longitudinal and cross-sectional elements to assess maturation within a study. Whereas traditional pharmacokinetic studies have uniformly been unable to distinguish differences between in utero and postnatal maturation, appropriately designed population studies are able to tease out these different influences. The population method is also particularly useful for drugs with long half-lives or for drugs whose steady-state pharmacokinetics may be difficult to predict from a single-dose pharmacokinetic evaluation (autoinduction or inhibition of metabolism or excretion). In these instances, the logistics and ethical constraints of waiting for the drug to "wash out" to capture $AUC_{0-\text{inf}}$ following a single dose for a traditional pharmacokinetic analysis may preclude its study. Although clearance can be estimated from classically intensive steady-state data collected over a dosage interval, the resulting analyses assume dosing and collection times that are performed exactly on schedule. Even in experienced pediatric study environments, these assumptions can be violated. While the classical intensive analysis has difficultly accounting for these variations, even when they are known, the population approach does not need to make the assumption of steady state if an exact dosing history is collected. The study of drug interactions is another area where population pharmacokinetic methods have significant value in pediatrics. The logistics of conducting traditional pharmacokinetic drug interaction studies is extremely difficult in pediatric populations, and these studies can often be more easily done using population approaches. However, potential drug interactions identified by population methods must be interpreted cautiously. Unless randomized, the relationship between concomitant therapies and altered pharmacokinetics is not causal and may serve only as a marker for other patient characteristics that may be responsible for the pharmacokinetic differences.

Whereas the primary goal of most population pharmacokinetic analyses is to describe the overall pharmacokinetics of the study group, estimates of individual subjects' pharmacokinetic parameters can be obtained through Bayesian post hoc analyses. This allows population pharmacokinetic studies to be nested into traditional phase 3 efficacy studies and provide estimates of individual drug exposure that can be used for exploratory analysis of potential pharmacodynamic relationships. This paradigm is being extensively used for regulatory purposes to look at drug exposure in subjects who experience toxicity or lack clinical benefit. Another outcome from population pharmacokinetic studies is the ability to get more accurate estimates of pharmacokinetic variability. Accurate estimates of the variance and covariance of pharmacokinetic parameters are essential for realistic simulations to evaluate the impact of various dosing strategies on drug exposure and ultimately clinical outcome.

Like other analysis methods, the population pharmacokinetic approach has limitations. It requires a high degree of expertise to perform these analyses, and the analysis process can be time-consuming. The underlying mathematical principles are complex, and if the data are not appropriate for the complexity of the drug, adequate characterization may not be possible. Thus, pharmacokinetic samples that are informative for all of the pharmacokinetic parameters to be estimated must be collected. Random samples or only trough samples may not be sufficient. Frequently, these samples are taken in outpatient settings, so there are additional assumptions of adherence to therapy that are not encountered in single-dose intensive studies. Assessing adherence in younger pediatric populations, where multiple caregivers may be involved, is challenging. Although population analyses allow collection of fewer samples per individual, this reduction of information per subject is compensated by collecting information from a larger number of subjects. As pediatric studies try to maximize the information generated, there is temptation to perform population pharmacokinetic studies from sparse samples in a small number of subjects. The results from these small studies must be viewed critically because they can generate unreliable parameter estimates.

The population method attempts to determine the sources of intersubject variability. Since age, size, and many laboratory measures are highly correlated, it is important that pediatric population–based models have a mechanistic basis. Maturational changes may impact multiple pharmacokinetic parameters simultaneously and be nonlinear. Thus, standard correlation screens of potential covariates and pharmacokinetic parameters may underappreciate important factors that drive the pediatric pharmacokinetic differences. Even after accounting for age, gender, size, renal function, and pharmacogenomic differences, the unexplained pediatric intersubject variability may still be largely due to unidentifiable causes.

SUMMARY

Understanding the pharmacokinetic and pharmacodynamic behavior of a drug in the intended patient population for its use is needed for rational and optimal drug therapy. Application of general pharmacokinetic principles, equations, and models is essential to determining appropriate pediatric dosages. Because the ontogeny of various elimination pathways can differ, detailed knowledge of a drug's pharmacokinetic behavior is important in determining when to expect significant age-specific pharmacokinetics. Significant variability in pharmacokinetic parameters exists and can result in variable drug exposure with similar doses. Defining the determinants of intersubject variability by developmental, genetic, and other clinical characteristics allows optimization of treatment for individual patients. Linking dosing information to the population pharmacokinetic/pharmacodynamic and disease models can facilitate informed and improved therapeutic decision making.

SUGGESTED READINGS

Anderson BJ, Meakin GH. Scaling for size: some implications for paediatric anaesthesia dosing. *Paediatr Anaesth* 2002;12:205–219.

Benet L, Galeazzi R. Noncompartmental determination of the steady-state volume of distribution. *J Pharm Sci* 1979;68:1071–1074.

Benet LZ, Hoener BA. Changes in plasma protein binding have little clinical relevance. *Clin Pharmacol Ther* 2002;71:115–121.

Capparelli EV, Lane JR, Romanowski GL, et al. The influences of renal function and maturation on vancomycin elimination in newborns and infants. *J Clin Pharmacol* 2001;41(9):927–934.

Capparelli EV, Mirochnick M, Dankner WM, et al. Pharmacokinetics and tolerance of zidovudine in preterm infants. *J Pediatr* 2003; 142(1):47–52.

Chiba K, Ishizaki T, Miura H, et al. Michaelis–Menten pharmacokinetics of diphenylhydantoin and application in the pediatric age patient. *J Pediatr* 1980;96:479–484.

Edginton AN, Schmitt W, Voith B, Willmann S. A mechanistic approach for the scaling of clearance in children. *Clin Pharmacokinet* 2006; 45:683–704.

Gibaldi M, Boyes R, Feldman S. Influence of first-pass on the availability of drugs on oral administration. *J Pharm Sci* 1971;60:1338–1340.

Gibaldi M, Perrier D. *Pharmacokinetics*, 2nd ed. New York, NY: Marcel Dekker, 1982.

Haddad S, Restieri C, Krishnan K. Characterization of age-related changes in body weight and organ weights from birth to adolescence in humans. *J Toxicol Environ Health* 2001;64:453–464.

Hoskin PJ, Hanks GW, Aherne GW, et al. The bioavailability and pharmacokinetics of morphine after intravenous, oral and buccal administration in healthy volunteers. *Br J Clin Pharmacol* 1989;27: 499–505.

Johnson TN, Tucker GT, Tanner MS, Rostami-Hodjegan A. Changes in liver volume from birth to adulthood: a meta-analysis. *Liver Transpl* 2005;11(12):1481–1493.

Kearns GL, Reed MD. Clinical pharmacokinetics in infants and children. A reappraisal. *Clin Pharmacokinet* 1989;17(Suppl 1):29–67.

Kim RB. Transporters and xenobiotic disposition. *Toxicology* 2002; 181/182:291–297.

Lundeberg S, Beck O, Olsson GL, et al. Rectal administration of morphine in children. Pharmacokinetic evaluation after a single-dose. *Acta Anaesthesiol Scand* 1996;40:445–451.

Murray DJ, Crom WR, Reddick WE, et al. Liver volume as a determinant of drug clearance in children and adolescents. *Drug Metab Dispos* 1995;23:1110–1116.

Norberg A, Jones WA, Hahn RG, et al. Role of variability in explaining ethanol pharmacokinetics: research and forensic applications. *Clin Pharmacokinet* 2003;42:1–31.

Oie S. Drug distribution and binding. *J Clin Pharmacol* 1986;26: 583–586.

Pelekis M, Gephart L, Lerman S. Physiologic-model-based derivation of the adult and child pharmacokinetic intraspecies uncertainty factors for volatile organic compounds. *Regul Toxicol Pharmacol* 2001;33:12–20.

Schwartz GJ, Brion LP, Spitzer A. The use of plasma creatinine concentration for estimating glomerular filtration rate in infants, children, and adolescents. *Pediatr Clin North Am* 1987;34(3): 571–590.

Sheiner LB, Ludden TM. Population pharmacokinetics/dynamics. *Annu Rev Pharmacol Toxicol* 1992;32:185–209.

Sheiner LB, Rosenberg B, Marathe V. Estimation of population characteristics of pharmacokinetic parameters from routine clinical data. *J Pharmacokinet Biopharm* 1977;5:445–479.

Takasawa K, Terasaki T, Suzuki H, et al. Distributed model analysis of 3′-azido-3′-deoxythymidine and 2′,3′-dideoxyinosine distribution in brain tissue and cerebrospinal fluid. *J Pharmacol Exp Ther* 1997; 282:1509–1517.

Tozer TN, Rowland M. *Introduction to pharmacokinetics and pharmacodynamics. The quantitative basis of drug therapy.* Philadelphia, PA: Lippincott Williams & Wilkins, 2006.

Wu CY, Benet LZ, Hebert MF, et al. Differentiation of absorption and first-pass gut and hepatic metabolism in humans: studies with cyclosporine. *Clin Pharmacol Ther* 1995;58(5):492–497.

CHAPTER

3

Ralph E. Kauffman

Drug Action and Therapy in the Infant and Child

Infancy and childhood extend from 2 months of age to the onset of puberty, which typically occurs at approximately 10 to 12 years in girls and 12 to 14 years in boys. The first 2 to 3 years of life is a period of particularly rapid growth and development. Body weight doubles by 5 months and triples by the first birthday. Body length increases by 50% during the first year. Body surface area doubles by the first birthday. Caloric expenditure increases threefold to fourfold during the first year. The child becomes ambulatory, develops socialization, and learns verbal language.

Substantial changes in body proportions and composition accompany growth and development. Major organ systems differentiate, grow, and mature throughout infancy and childhood. Although growth and development are most rapid during the first several years of life, maturation continues at a slower pace throughout middle and later childhood. This dynamic process of growth, differentiation, and maturation is what sets the infant and child apart from adults, both physiologically and pharmacologically. It should be no surprise, then, that important changes in response to and biodisposition of drugs occur during infancy and childhood. These changes influence the response to, toxicity of, and dosing regimens for drugs.

This chapter focuses on the impact of growth and development on drug actions and biodisposition and the resultant practical implications for pharmacotherapy in children. Comparative pharmacologic data in children and adults are used to illustrate general principles.

DEVELOPMENTAL CHANGES IN BODY COMPOSITION AND PROPORTION

Developmental changes in body composition, body proportions, and relative mass of the liver and the kidneys affect pharmacokinetic characteristics of drugs at different ages. It is therefore important to review the relevant changes that take place between early infancy and pubescence.

The proportions of body weight contributed by fat, protein, and intracellular water, respectively, change significantly during infancy and childhood (Fig. 3.1). Total-body water constitutes approximately 75% to 80% of body weight in the full-term newborn. This decreases to approximately 60% by 5 months of age and remains relatively constant thereafter. Although the percentage of total-body weight constituted by total-body water does not change significantly after late infancy, there is a progressive decrease in extracellular water from infancy to young adulthood. In addition, the percentage of body weight contributed by fat doubles by 4 to 5 months of age, primarily at the expense of total-body water. During the second year of life, protein mass increases, with a compensatory reduction in fat. This corresponds to ambulation and loss of "baby fat" during the transition from infancy to childhood.

Liver and kidney size, relative to body weight, also changes during growth and development (1) (Fig. 3.2). These two organs reach maximum relative weight in the 1- to 2-year-old child, at the period of life when capacity for drug metabolism and elimination also tends to be greatest. Likewise, body surface area is greatest relative to body mass in the infant and the young child compared with the older child and the young adult (1,2) (Fig. 3.3).

DEVELOPMENTAL CHANGES IN ORGAN FUNCTION

GASTROINTESTINAL TRACT

The most common route of drug administration is the gastrointestinal (GI) tract. Therefore, physiologic and structural changes in the GI tract during development may alter both the rate and the extent to which a drug is absorbed. Clinically important developmental changes in the GI tract that may affect drug absorption occur predominantly during the newborn period, infancy, and early childhood. By school age, there is little discernible difference between children and adults.

A number of changes occur in the GI tract during early development that may affect drug absorption (3). Gastric acid production is decreased during infancy (4–7). Gastric

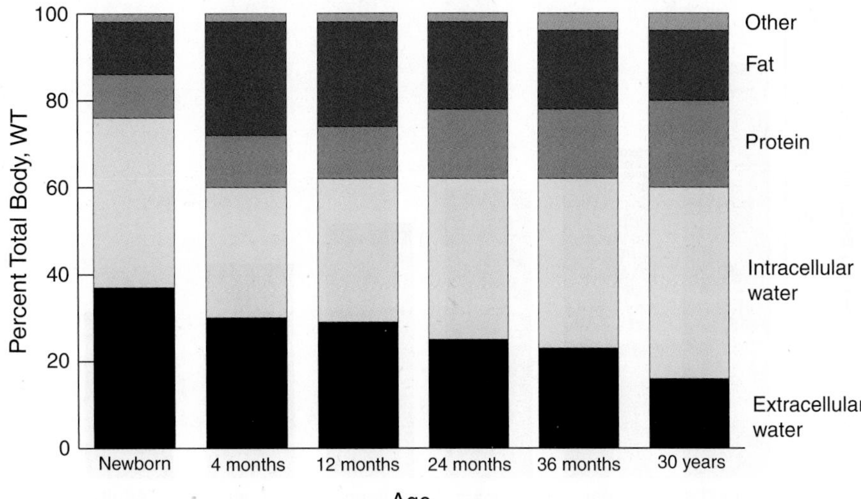

Figure 3.1. Change in proportional body composition during childhood. WT, Weight. (Adapted from Habersang RWO. Dosage. In: Shirkey HC, ed. *Pediatric therapy*, 6th ed. St. Louis, MO: Mosby, 1980:17–20, with permission.)

pH is neutral (6–8) at birth, drops during the first 24 hours, and increases toward neutral in the later newborn period. The capacity for gastric acid production is physiologically decreased during infancy and reaches adult levels sometime during the first 2 years of life. Gastric emptying is irregular and erratic during infancy and approaches adult patterns by 6 to 8 months of age (8). Gut motility in newborns and young infants is irregular with a pattern of peristaltic activity different from that in adults (9,10). This can lead to a longer transit time through the gut. Transit times in premature infants range from 8 to 96 hours, compared to 4 to 12 hours in adults. In the older infant and toddler, coordinated propulsive gut motility is more efficient, resulting in a transit time less than that in adults. Small gut surface area is greater in infants and young children relative to body mass than in adults (11). The gut in the infant is more permeable to large molecules than that of the older child (12). The infant gut has the capability of absorbing intact protein and high–molecular-weight drugs that are not absorbed by the gut of the older child and adult. Pancreatic lipase activity is decreased in newborns and during early infancy. First-pass uptake is presumed to be decreased in infancy, proportional to decreased transport and drug metabolism. Dietary habits of infants are quite different from those of older children and adults. They feed frequently, the diet consists of breast milk or formula for the first 6 months, and gastric contents are easily buffered. The combination of delayed gastric emptying and frequent feeds results in the presence of nutrients in the stomach for the majority of time between feedings.

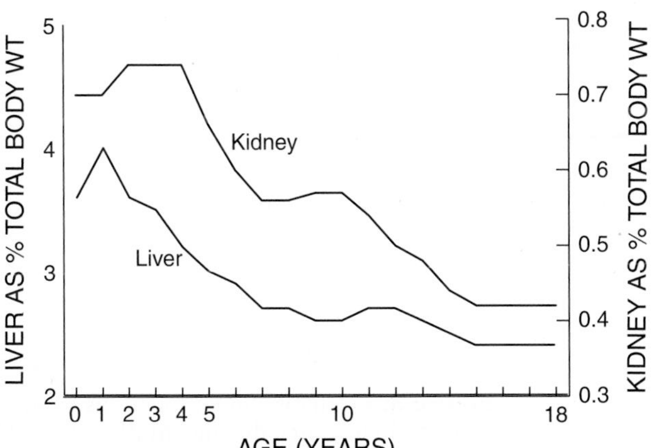

Figure 3.2. Change in relative liver and kidney mass expressed as percentage of body weight (WT) from infancy to young adulthood (1).

ORGANS OF ELIMINATION

The liver and the kidney are the primary organs of drug metabolism and elimination. Although a great deal has been written about the immaturity of hepatic and renal function in the neonate, relatively less emphasis has been placed on maturation of the liver and the kidney during childhood and adolescence and the impact on drug disposition.

Hepatic function is complex, and metabolic pathways for various substrates develop at different rates. Bromsulphalein has been used as a substrate to evaluate maturation of hepatic clearance during infancy and childhood (13,14). Bromsulphalein clearance, normalized for body surface area, increases rapidly during the first 3 months of life, significantly exceeds adult clearance in the preschool child, and declines to adult levels during adolescence (Fig. 3.4). During the last decade a great deal has been learned about the development of drug-metabolizing enzymes, particularly the cytochromes P450, which are responsible for phase I metabolism of most drugs (15,16). The reader is referred to Chapter 4 for a detailed discussion of drug metabolism in the infant and child.

Glomerular filtration rate, as reflected by endogenous creatinine clearance, is physiologically decreased in the newborn but increases rapidly during the first year of life. Creatinine clearance, normalized for body surface area, equals adult clearance by 1 year of life, and there is some evidence that average clearance in prepubescent children exceeds clearance in adults (14,17,18) (Fig. 3.5). Tubular function matures later than glomerular function. However, tubular function is essentially mature by 1 year of age.

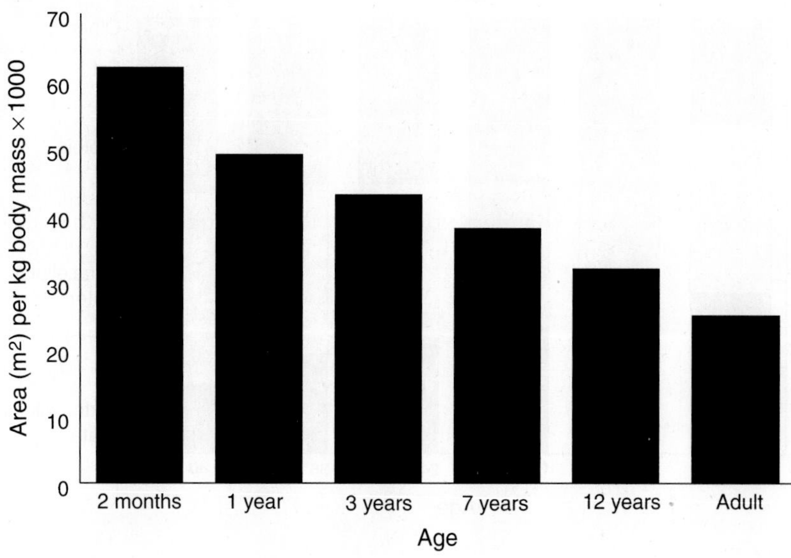

Figure 3.3. Change in the ratio of body surface area to body mass from infancy to young adulthood (1,2).

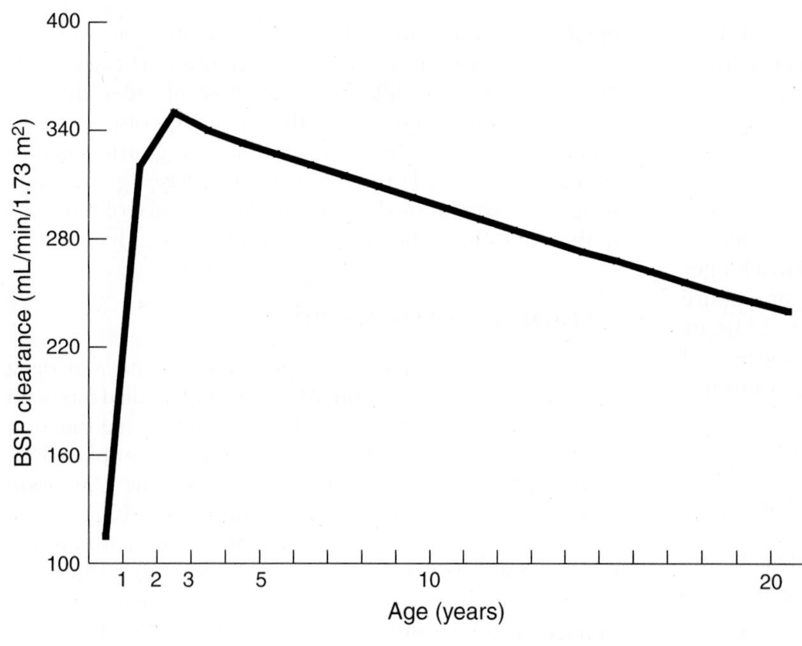

Figure 3.4. Change in hepatic clearance (expressed as mL/min/1.73 m^2) of Bromsulphalein (BSP) during childhood. (Adapted from Habersang RWO. Dosage. In: Shirkey HC, ed. *Pediatric therapy*, 6th ed. St. Louis, MO: Mosby, 1980:17–20, with permission.)

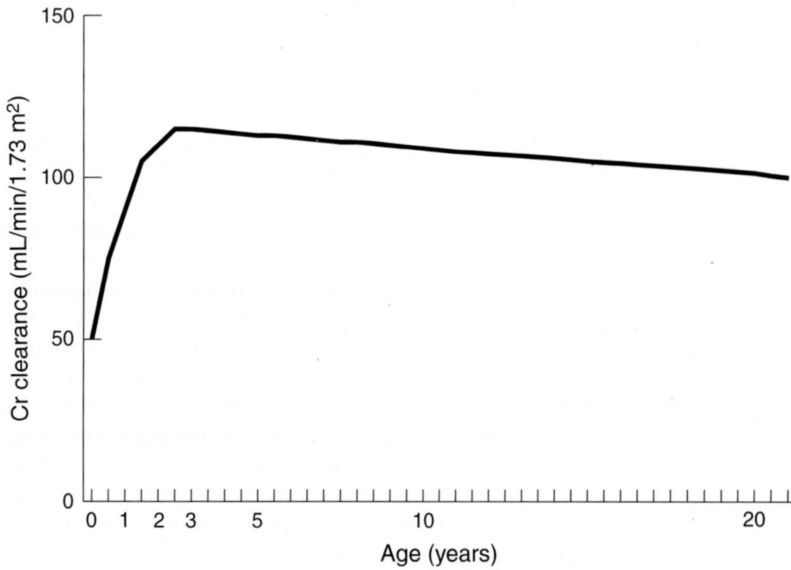

Figure 3.5. Change in endogenous creatinine (Cr) clearance during childhood. (Adapted from Habersang RWO. Dosage. In: Shirkey HC, ed. *Pediatric therapy*, 6th ed. St. Louis, MO: Mosby, 1980:17–20, with permission.)

INFLUENCE OF DEVELOPMENT ON DRUG BIODISPOSITION AND ACTION

DRUG ABSORPTION

Developmental changes in the GI tract are important because medications are commonly administered to children by mouth, and maturational changes may influence drug absorption. It is difficult to generalize, however, because differences in absorption of orally administered drugs associated with growth and maturation are not readily predicted from known drug or developmental characteristics. Nevertheless, it is important to be aware of those aspects of GI tract development that may influence drug absorption.

Most drugs are absorbed from the gut by passive diffusion across a concentration gradient, although active transport mechanisms may be involved for a minority of drugs. The rate and extent of absorption are influenced by physical–chemical properties of the drug and characteristics of the recipient's gut. Important drug properties include molecular weight, lipid solubility, pK_a (dissociation constant of weak acids or bases), formulation in which the drug is administered (e.g., liquid, solid, extended release), and disintegration time and dissolution rate of solid dose forms. Important recipient characteristics include gastric acidity, gastric emptying, gut motility, gut surface area, gut drug-metabolizing enzymes and active transporters, secretion of bile acids and pancreatic lipases, first-pass metabolism, diet at different ages, and diurnal variation.

Reflux of gastric contents retrograde into the esophagus is very common during the first year of life (19). Excessive gastroesophageal reflux may result in regurgitation of medication, resulting in variable and unpredictable loss of an orally administered dose.

Gastric emptying is an important determinant of rate of absorption because most drug absorption takes place in the duodenum. Delayed gastric emptying in infants not only contributes to gastroesophageal reflux but also may result in delayed drug absorption (20–22). On the other hand, gastric emptying in prepubescent children is equal to or exceeds that in adults. This tends to facilitate more rapid drug absorption, other factors being equal (21,23). Administration of medication in liquid as opposed to solid dose forms, as is commonly the case for children, also increases the rate of absorption. In contrast, shorter GI transit time in young children may actually reduce the fraction of dose absorbed when drugs are administered in sustained-release formulations (24,25).

Decreased gastric acid production in the younger infant may result in increased bioavailability of acid-labile drugs such as the penicillins (22,26). For example, increased absorption of penicillin G, ampicillin, and nafcillin in infants compared with older children and adults has been reported (20). However, perturbation of drug absorption due to reduction in gastric acidity is negligible beyond infancy.

Rate and extent of drug absorption are determined to a significant degree by the absorptive surface area of the duodenum. Greater relative small gut surface area in young children tends to enhance drug absorption.

Drugs absorbed from the intestine into the portal circulation are delivered to the liver before entering the systemic circulation. High hepatic extraction of some drugs on the first pass through the liver results in removal of a large fraction of the absorbed drug by the liver, resulting in decreased systemic bioavailability. Intestinal metabolism of drugs also may decrease systemic bioavailability. Little is known about the effect of intestinal and hepatic maturation on first-pass uptake of drugs. However, one would predict, based on increased hepatic clearance in children, that first-pass processes in children beyond infancy would be equal to or exceed uptake in adults. Wilson et al. (27) described wide intersubject variability and low serum concentrations of two high-uptake drugs, propoxyphene and propanolol, when administered orally to children 2 to 13 years of age. This is consistent with extensive first-pass uptake.

Maturation of gut flora during childhood modifies digoxin metabolism. Reduction of digoxin to inactive metabolites by anaerobic GI bacteria accounts for a significant fraction of digoxin clearance in approximately 10% of adult patients (28). Reduction metabolites are not detected in children until after 16 months of age, and the adult metabolite pattern is not found until 9 years of age (29).

The rectum is an alternative route of enteral drug administration in children, which may be used when vomiting or other intervening conditions preclude oral dosing. Drugs administered rectally are absorbed into the hemorrhoidal veins, which are part of the systemic rather than the portal circulation. First-pass uptake, therefore, is not a consideration with rectal administration. However, rectal dosing is less than satisfactory in many cases for other reasons. Absorption of drugs administered in suppository form is typically erratic and incomplete. Furthermore, presence of feces in the rectal vault impedes absorption. In younger children and infants, the dose may be expelled before absorption is complete, thereby reducing bioavailability to a variable extent. Nevertheless, some medications may be successfully administered rectally in solution (30). These include diazepam and valproic acid for seizures and phenobarbital for seizures, sedation, or preanesthesia (31,32). In addition, rectal corticosteroids are routinely used in the treatment of inflammatory bowel disease.

Absorption of drugs from intramuscular or subcutaneous injection sites is influenced by characteristics of the patient as well as properties of the injected drug. Blood flow to the injection site, muscle mass, quantity of adipose tissue, and muscle activity are patient characteristics that determine the rate and extent of absorption. Solubility of the drug at the pH of extracellular fluid, ease with which the drug diffuses across capillary membranes, and surface area over which the injection volume spreads also determine absorption (21,22,30,31,33). Extravascular injection is not an optimal route of administration in the presence of hypoperfusion syndromes, dehydration, vasomotor instability, starvation, or cachexia because all these conditions impede absorption. Some drugs, such as erythromycin and certain cephalosporin antibiotics, are not usually administered intramuscularly because they cause unacceptable pain and tissue trauma. However, many drugs, including most aminoglycoside and penicillin antibiotics, may be administered intramuscularly with resulting plasma concentrations comparable with those achieved with intravenous administration. Conversely, highly hydrophobic drugs such as diazepam and phenytoin are not absorbed well following intramuscular injection and should not be given by this route. Furthermore, phenytoin forms insoluble crystals in intramuscular injection sites, associated with local hemorrhage, muscle necrosis, and minimal systemic absorption (34). Fosphenytoin, which is water soluble, is preferable to phenytoin for parenteral administration.

DRUG DISTRIBUTION

The distribution of a drug throughout the body is influenced by the binding affinity of the drug for plasma and tissue proteins, the lipid/water solubility partition of the drug, the molecular weight of the drug, and the degree of ionization of the drug at physiologic pH. Age-dependent changes in body composition (see earlier in text) may influence drug distribution in the developing child. Highly lipid-soluble compounds such as inhalation anesthetics and lipophilic sedative/hypnotic agents typically exhibit relatively larger distribution volumes in infants during the first year of life compared with older children because of the relatively larger proportion of body fat in infants. Likewise, the apparent distribution volume of drugs such as penicillin, aminoglycoside, and cephalosporin antibiotics, which are distributed primarily in extracellular water, tends to be greater in infants and decreases during maturation coincident with the progressive relative decrease in extracellular water (21,23,33). In general, the apparent volume of distribution of drugs tends to be greater in infants and decreases toward adult values during childhood. However, there is a great deal of interindividual variation, and important exceptions to this general rule exist. Examples of such exceptions are theophylline (35) and phenobarbital (36), which show little consistent age-related change in distribution volume.

Although the plasma protein binding of many drugs is decreased in the fetus and newborn infant relative to adults, age-related differences in plasma protein binding are not clinically significant beyond the newborn period (37). However, maturational changes in tissue binding can significantly affect drug distribution. For example, the myocardial-to-plasma digoxin concentration in infants and children up to 36 months of age is two to three times that of adults (38–40). Using specific assay methods, increased myocardial digoxin concentrations relative to adults have been demonstrated in children and these do not appear to be due to assay interference by endogenous digoxin-like substances (41). In addition, erythrocytes from infants bind three times the quantity of digoxin as adult erythrocytes (40). The increased myocardial and erythrocyte binding of digoxin is associated with a significantly greater volume of distribution of digoxin in infants and children compared with adults.

METABOLISM AND ELIMINATION

Clearance of many drugs is primarily dependent on hepatic metabolism, followed by excretion of parent drug and metabolites by the liver and kidney. Nonpolar, lipid-soluble drugs typically are metabolized to more polar and water-soluble compounds prior to excretion, whereas water-soluble drugs usually are excreted unchanged by glomerular filtration and/or renal tubular secretion.

Phase I metabolic processes involve oxidative, reductive, or hydrolytic reactions that most often are catalyzed by the mixed-function oxidase enzyme systems located in the microsomes. Less commonly, such reactions may be mediated by mitochondrial or cytosolic enzymes. Phase II, or synthetic, metabolism involves conjugation of the substrate to a polar compound such as glucuronic acid, sulfate, or glycine. This usually results in a polar, water-soluble compound that is readily excreted.

Although the capacity to metabolize a number of drug substrates is decreased during the newborn period, with few exceptions, maturation of the various pathways occurs during the first year of life (15,16). The various pathways mature at different times, and there is considerable interindividual variation in rate of maturation of specific pathways. This should not be surprising because other aspects of development proceed at varying rates in different individuals; for example, the chronologic age at which infants sit, crawl, walk, and talk also is quite variable. The reader is referred to Chapter 4 and to cited recent reviews for detailed discussions of the ontogeny of drug metabolism.

In some cases, the dominant metabolic pathway in infants and children is different from that in adults. For example, N_7-methylation of theophylline to produce caffeine is well developed in the newborn infant, whereas oxidative demethylation is deficient (42). Therefore, in contrast to what occurs in older infants and children, theophylline is metabolized to caffeine, which accumulates to pharmacologically active concentrations as a result of its long half-life, when it is administered to newborn infants for longer than 10 days. This pathway is important until 4 to 6 months of age, when the oxidative pathways mature, caffeine clearance increases, and caffeine accumulation no longer occurs. Interestingly, the clearances of theophylline and caffeine increase dramatically coincident with maturation of oxidative N_3-demethylase activity (43). The metabolic profile of acetaminophen also differs in children compared with adults. The dominant metabolic pathway in infants and children younger than 12 years of age is sulfate conjugation, whereas glucuronidation is the major pathway in adolescents and adults (44). Although the major metabolic pathways differ with age, there is no age-related difference in clearance.

Maturation of renal clearance of drugs and their metabolites occurs coincident with maturation of renal function during the first year. With maturation of hepatic and renal function, the clearance of many drugs in young children, when corrected for body surface area, equals or exceeds that in adults after 1 year of age. Table 3.1 compares reported elimination half-lives for a number of drugs among newborns, infants, children, and adults. Typically, the half-life is prolonged in the newborn, decreases during infancy, is shortest in the prepubescent child, and is somewhat longer in adults than in children. With rare exceptions, a shorter half-life reflects greater clearance.

TABLE 3.1 Change in Elimination Half-Life During Development

Drug	Half-Life (hr)				References
	Newborn	Infant	Child	Adult	
Acetaminophen	4.9		4.5	3.6	44
Amikacin	5.0–6.5		1.6	2.3	59–61
Ampicillin	4.0	1.7		1.0–1.5	62
Amoxicillin	3.7		0.9–1.9	0.6–1.5	22
Carbamazepine			8–25	10–20	64
Cefazolin			1.7	2.0	80
Cefotaxime	4.0	0.8	1.0	1.1	80
Cefoxitin	3.8	1.4	0.8	0.8	80
Ceftazidime	4.5	4.5	2.0	1.8	80
Ceftriaxone	17.0	5.9	4.7	7.8	80
Cefuroxime	5.5	3.5	1.2	1.5	80
Cephalothin			0.3	0.6	80
Clindamycin	3.6	3.0	2.4	4.5	81,82
Clonazepam			22–33	20–60	63
Cyclosporine			4.8	5.5	83
Diazepam	30	10	25	30	84–85
Digoxin		18–33	37	30–50	86–88
Ethosuximide			30	52–56	63
Famotidine	11		3.2	3.5	89–90
Gentamicin	4.0	2.6	1.2	2–3	91–94
Ibuprofen			1.0–2.0	2.0–3.0	95–97
Isoniazid			2.9[a]	2.8[a]	98
Mezlocillin	3.7		0.8	1.0	20
Midazolam	6.3	3.1	2.7	4.8	99–100
Moxalactam	5.4	1.7	1.6	2.2	80
Naproxen			11–13	10–17	101,102
Phenobarbital	67–99		36–72	48–120	20,63
Primidone			5–11	12–15	103,104
Piperacillin	0.8	0.5	0.4	0.9	105
Quinidine			4.0	5–7	106
Rifampin			2.9	3.3–3.9	107
Sulfadiazine	40	10		10–15	108
Sulfamethoxypyridazine	280	50	50	50	108
Sulfisoxazole	18	8	8	8	108
Theophylline	30	6.9	3.4	8.1	35,109
Ticarcillin	5–6		0.9	1.3	110
Tobramycin	4.6		1–2	2–3	91,111
Valproate			7.0	6–12	112,113
Vancomycin	4.1–9.1		2.2–2.4	5–6	91,114
Zidovudine			1.0–1.5	1.6	115,116

[a]Slow acetylators.

ONTOGENY OF DRUG ACTION (PHARMACODYNAMICS)

Although a great deal is known about changes in drug distribution, metabolism, and excretion that result in pharmacokinetic changes during development, information regarding developmental changes in pharmacodynamics (e.g., drug action) is limited. Nevertheless, examples from clinical studies and animal data on receptor ontogeny provide strong evidence for changes in drug response during development independent of pharmacokinetic changes.

Opioid receptors are not fully developed in the newborn rat and mature into adulthood (45). A three- to sevenfold increase in opioid binding sites occurs during maturation. Receptor density varies by brain region, with earlier development of caudal and later development in rostral parts of the central nervous system (CNS). Earlier development of opioid receptors in the medulla and pons, where respiratory and cardiovascular centers are located, is consistent with clinically observed higher incidence of opioid-related respiratory depression and bradycardia in the neonate who receives opioids. For example, morphine induced a 75% depression of respiration in immature rats with no analgesia, whereas adult rats given the same weight-adjusted dose exhibited complete analgesia with only a 33% decrease in respiratory rate. These observations have important implications for response to opioid analgesics in the infant and the young child, independent of drug pharmacokinetics.

A distinct pattern of adenosine A1 receptor ontogeny has been observed in the immature rat. Receptor number is decreased in higher centers in the newborn, with an increase in receptor number from birth to adulthood in the thalamus, cerebellum, and hippocampus and little change in lower brain centers. The increase in receptor number is accelerated by neonatal exposure to caffeine (46).

A switch in expression of receptor subgroup type may occur during early postnatal life. Type 2 angiotensin II receptor (AT_2R), which does not mediate vascular contraction, predominates in vascular and cardiac tissue of fetal sheep. However, expression of AT_2R is downregulated shortly after birth, and type 1 angiotensin receptor (AT_1R), a potent vasoconstrictor, becomes dominant by 3 months of age (47,48). Although the therapeutic implications of this postnatal shift in receptor type have not been investigated in humans, it suggests that pharmacologic response to angiotensin receptor blockers or angiotensin-converting enzyme inhibitors may change during the first months of life.

Serotonin is an important neurotransmitter implicated in a number of behavioral and psychiatric disorders. It also is a critical trophic agent in the developing nervous system. In rats, cortical serotonergic neurons decline markedly at 3 weeks of age (49). Serotonin receptor density in the human brain stem also decreases dramatically between infancy and adulthood (50). However, no data are available for the period between infancy and adulthood. Although serotonergic receptors are the target of a number of psychoactive drugs, the pharmacologic implications of this change in serotonin receptors remain to be determined. The high density of receptors in the fetus may simply reflect the critical trophic role of serotonin during fetal neurodevelopment.

Dopamine is an important catecholamine with wide-ranging effects peripherally as well as in the CNS. It acts through a family of receptors that includes at least five subtypes, D_1, D_2, D_3, D_4, and D_5. Studies in several animal species have demonstrated an important difference in pharmacodynamic response to dopamine between newborn and mature animals (51). Dopamine does not elicit D_1-mediated renal vasodilatation in the newborn as it does in the adult animal. In fact, low doses of dopamine that produce renal vasodilatation in the adult actually may induce vasoconstriction in the newborn from stimulation of α-adrenergic receptors, which are well developed at term. Likewise, the natruretic response to D_1 agonists is blunted in the newborn. It is unclear whether the decreased response to dopamine in immature animals is due to differences in receptor density, affinity for the agonist, coupling to second messengers, or distal intracellular mechanisms. In addition, the ontogenic profile of the different dopamine receptor subgroups in various organs and tissues beyond the newborn period is not known. Nevertheless, differences in response to dopamine between the newborn and the adult have important therapeutic implications because dopamine is commonly used to support blood pressure and perfusion in the very ill neonate.

Studies of D_1 and D_2 ontogeny in the CNS are inconclusive. Most studies have been done in rats, with some studies of D_1 receptors showing an increasing number of receptors during maturation and others showing an increase to 35 to 40 days of age followed by a decline. Studies of D_2 receptors in the CNS are also inconsistent, but more recent studies have shown peak expression in the rat at 28 days with subsequent decline to adult levels (52). There are no human data and the functional significance of these changes in early life remains to be elucidated. However, a number of neurologic, psychiatric, and behavioral disorders are related to dopaminergic pathways in the CNS that are targets for a number of psychoactive drugs. This raises the possibility of pharmacodynamic differences in response to these therapeutic agents during infancy and childhood.

Expression of adrenergic receptors during embryonic and postnatal development varies with receptor subtype and CNS locus. In general, α-1B receptors are present during embryonic life in the rat, with intense expression at birth. Expression declines to adult levels after postnatal day 21. In contrast, α-1A/D receptor is absent during embryonic development but increases markedly postnatally. Both receptor subtypes decrease after postnatal day 21 to adulthood (53). $\beta 1$ and $\beta 2$ receptors appear by embryonic day 16 in the rat, with 10% to 20% of adult levels at birth. Postnatally, there is a fivefold increase to adult levels by postnatal day 21 (52). Corollary human data are not available. Although the adrenergic system appears to be important for embryonic development and essential for neonatal survival, the functional significance of changes during later postnatal development is not known.

The $GABA_A$ receptor complex is the site of action of numerous drugs, including benzodiazepines, barbiturates, anesthetics, and several antiepileptic drugs. Studies in nonhuman primates and more recently in children with seizure disorders have shown that major changes in $GABA_A$ receptor binding and subunit expression occur during postnatal development. In positron emission tomography studies of GABA receptor ontogeny in children 2 to 17 years of age, flumazenil brain tissue volume of distribution due to specific receptor binding was highest in children 2 years of age and declined exponentially through childhood to 50% of peak values by 17 years of age (54). The greatest differences between children and adults occur in the temporal lobe, visual cortex, and thalamus. These developmental changes have important implications for understanding differences among children of different ages in the pharmacodynamics of drugs acting through the $GABA_A$ receptor complex.

The anticoagulant response to warfarin is greater in prepubertal children than in adults independent of plasma S-warfarin levels and vitamin K concentrations. Greater inhibition of thrombin generation and lower plasma concentrations of protein C associated with a significantly greater international normalized ratio (INR) was observed in prepubertal patients compared with adults even though mean vitamin K and S-warfarin concentrations were not different between the two age groups. This suggests a greater sensitivity to warfarin in children, although the mechanism remains to be determined (55).

Infants have a greater immunosuppression response to cyclosporine than do older children and adults. The IC_{50} (concentration at which 50% inhibition occurs) for peripheral blood monocyte proliferation was less than half that in older children and adults. In addition, inhibition of interleukin-2 expression by peripheral blood monocytes was significantly greater in infants than in adults. This likely is related to immaturity of the T-lymphocyte response in the infant and has important therapeutic implications for dosing cyclosporine in infants independent of pharmacokinetic differences (56).

The antipyretic response to ibuprofen is greater in children younger than 1 year of age compared with children older than 6 years of age. The onset of antipyresis was earlier and decreases in temperature greater in the younger age group even though the baseline temperature and plasma ibuprofen concentrations were not different. This may be due to greater body surface area relative to body mass in the younger child, which provides more efficient heat dissipation following administration of the antipyretic (57).

THERAPEUTIC IMPLICATIONS OF DEVELOPMENTAL CHANGES

The onset and intensity of effect of most drugs are related to the drug concentration at the site of action, which, in turn, for many drugs (but not all) is reflected by the plasma concentration. The drug concentration at any point in time after a dose is determined by the dose and the pharmacokinetic characteristics of the drug in a particular patient. As described earlier, developmental changes in drug disposition result in significant changes in the pharmacokinetics of many drugs, which must be considered when calculating doses for children of different ages. Dose requirements vary with age as volume of distribution, half-life, and clearance change during development. The dose of many drugs must be adjusted not only for increased body mass but also to compensate for increased clearance and shorter half-life. This is particularly important for drugs that are administered chronically, such as anticonvulsants, cardiovascular agents, and drugs for behavioral disorders. The loading dose of a drug is primarily determined by its volume of distribution, whereas the maintenance dose is determined by the clearance. In addition, the dosing interval relative to the half-life determines the degree of fluctuation of drug concentration between doses. The following examples illustrate these concepts.

Recommended loading and maintenance doses for digoxin reflect changes in volume of distribution and clearance with age. The digitalizing dose for premature infants is 20 μg per kg; for full-term newborns, 30 μg per kg; for infants younger than 2 years of age, 40 to 50 μg per kg; and for children older than 2 years of age, 30 to 40 μg per kg. The maintenance dose for premature infants is 5 μg per kg; for full-term newborns, 8 to 10 μg per kg; for infants younger than 2 years of age, 10 to 12 μg per kg; and for children older than 2 years of age, 8 to 10 μg per kg (58).

The dose of aminoglycoside antibiotics in children required to achieve equivalent plasma concentrations typically is 50% to 100% greater than that in adults because of greater renal clearance in children (59–62). The dosing interval in children also may need to be shorter, for example, every 6 hours versus every 8 hours. Likewise, dose requirements of the anticonvulsants carbamazepine, ethosuximide, phenobarbital, and phenytoin are also significantly greater on a milligram per kilogram basis in prepubescent children compared with adults (63,64) because of the greater metabolic capacity in children (Tables 3.1 and 3.2). In contrast to newborn patients, there is a greater risk of underdosing than overdosing older infants and children unless age-related changes in clearance are considered.

TABLE 3.2 Change in Phenytoin Metabolism with Development

Age (yr)	*K_m (mg/L)*	*V_{max} (mg/kg/d)*
≤1	4.54	17.9
1–4	5.23	12.0
4–8	3.85	10.4
8–12	5.69	11.1
12–16	5.14	7.9
16–22	7.15	9.6

Note: Data from Dodson (117).

Use of sustained-release oral dosage formulations presents unique problems in young children. Absorption may be unpredictable and incomplete, leading to therapeutic failures. In addition, even though the formulation is designed for slow absorption, concentrations may exhibit greater fluctuations between doses than in adults because of the greater clearance in children (35).

GROWTH, DEVELOPMENT, AND DRUG TOXICITY

EXAMPLES OF INCREASED TOXICITY

The complex processes involved in growth and development frequently make the child uniquely vulnerable to mechanisms of toxicity that are not present in mature individuals. Chronic treatment with adrenocorticosteroids (65), amphetamine, and methylphenidate impedes linear growth, an adverse effect that obviously occurs only in the growing individual (66). Tetracycline antibiotics are not recommended for children younger than 9 years of age because they cause enamel dysplasia in developing teeth (67). Use of the fluoroquinolone antibiotics in children is limited because of potential toxicity to growing cartilage (68).

Since cisapride became unavailable because of safety concerns, metoclopramide has been commonly used as a prokinetic agent to treat gastroesophageal reflux in infants. Metoclopramide and prochlorperazine also are occasionally used as antiemetic agents. Both these drugs are dopamine-2 antagonists and in excessive dose can produce acute dystonic reactions or seizures. Haloperidol also has this adverse side effect. Younger children seem to be more susceptible to dystonic reactions associated with dopamine antagonists than do adults. This may be related to greater concentration of dopamine-2 receptors in the brain of young patients (69). Infants and young children are more prone than adults to acute CNS and hyperpyrexic reactions to anticholinergic drugs such as atropine and scopolamine (70). Toxicity associated with topical ocular administration has been described.

Children younger than 1 year of age are more susceptible to respiratory depression from weight-adjusted doses of opioid drugs, which are generally safe in older children and adults. For this reason, opioid antitussive agents such as codeine and dextromethorphan are not recommended for use in this age group (71).

Verapamil is used for the treatment of supraventricular arrhythmias in older children and adult patients. However, infants with supraventricular tachyarrhythmias appear to be at increased risk of sudden cardiac arrest. The mechanism for this increased risk is poorly understood. Verapamil is not recommended for treatment of acute arrhythmias in infants younger than 1 year of age (72).

Valproic acid is one of the anticonvulsants most commonly used in children. In rare cases, it can cause acute hyperammonemia associated with hepatoencephalopathy. Children younger than 5 years of age are at greatest risk for developing this life-threatening adverse reaction, particularly if they are receiving concurrent therapy with other anticonvulsant drugs (73).

EXAMPLES OF DECREASED TOXICITY

Immaturity does not invariably predispose to increased risk of toxicity. Although infants and children may be more susceptible than adults to certain types of drug toxicity, there are important examples in which differences in drug disposition appear to result in decreased risk of toxicity in immature individuals.

Infants and young children appear to be less susceptible to ototoxicity and renal toxicity from aminoglycoside antibiotics compared with older patients (74). This may be due, in part, to reduced intracellular accumulation of the aminoglycoside in renal tubular epithelial cells (75).

Children tend to experience relatively mild liver toxicity from acute acetaminophen overdose. Weight-adjusted doses and serum concentrations that invariably are associated with severe hepatotoxicity in young adults produce much less hepatocellular damage in preschool children (76). There is evidence that this is due to a greater capacity of children to metabolize acetaminophen by nontoxic pathways (77).

Hepatotoxicity from halothane is relatively rare in children, even following multiple exposures, whereas it is not uncommon in adults. The mechanism of reduced hepatotoxicity in children is not known (78).

The risk of isoniazid-induced hepatitis is age related. An incidence of 0 per 1,000 patients younger than 20 years of age was reported by the Food and Drug Administration, whereas the incidence was 23 per 1,000 in patients 50 to 65 years of age (79). It is usually unnecessary to routinely check liver function tests in children receiving isoniazid.

SUMMARY

The prepubescent child is clearly different from the newborn infant and the adolescent. From a pharmacotherapy perspective, the dynamic processes of growth and development create a moving target for the physician. In contrast to newborn infants, young children typically have a greater capacity to metabolize and excrete drugs than at any other time during their life. This, in turn, requires that appropriate dosage regimens be designed to compensate for developmental changes. It is also important to keep in mind that developing human beings may be uniquely susceptible to some types of drug toxicity while being protected from other toxic mechanisms by their immaturity. A knowledge of the developmental changes in drug disposition and action that influence therapeutic response and toxicity is essential to optimize therapy at different stages of childhood.

ACKNOWLEDGMENTS

Supported in part by grant no. 1 U01 HD31313-09, Pediatric Pharmacology Research Unit Network, National Institute of Child Health and Human Development, Bethesda, Maryland.

REFERENCES

1. Maxwell GM. *Principles of paediatric pharmacology.* New York, NY: Oxford University Press, 1984:96.
2. Spino M. Pediatric dosing rules and nomograms. In: MacLeod SM, Raddle IC, eds. *Textbook of pediatric clinical pharmacology.* Littleton, MA: PSG, 1985:118–128.
3. Hamilton JR. The pediatric patient: early development and the digestive system. In: Walker WA, Durie PR, Hamilton JR, Walker-Smith JA, Watkins JB, eds. *Pediatric gastrointestinal disease,* 3rd ed. Hamilton, Canada: BC Decker, 2000:5–8.
4. Agunod M, Yamaguchi N, Lopez R, et al. Correlative study of hydrochloric acid, pepsin, and intrinsic factor secretion in newborns and infants. *Am J Dig Dis* 1969;14:400–414.
5. Harada T, Hyman PE, Everett S, et al. Meal-stimulated gastric acid secretion in infants. *J Pediatr* 1984;104:534–538.
6. Hyman PE, Clarke DD, Everett SL, et al. Gastric acid secretory function in preterm infants. *J Pediatr* 1985;106:467–471.
7. Rodbro P, Kraslinikoff PA, Christiansen PM. Parietal cell secretory function in early childhood. *Scand J Gastroenterol* 1967;2:209–213.
8. Cavell B. Gastric emptying in infants fed human milk or infant formula. *Acta Paediatr Scand* 1981;70:639–641.
9. Ittman PI, Amarnath RA, Berseth CL. Maturation of antroduodenal motor activity in preterm and term infants. *Dig Dis Sci* 1992;37:14–19.
10. Berseth CL. Gestational evolution of small intestine motility in preterm and term infants. *J Pediatr* 1989;115:646–651.
11. Weaver LT, Austin S, Cole TJ. Small intestinal length: a factor essential for gut adaptation. *Gut* 1991;32:1321–1323.
12. Heimann G. Enteral absorption and bioavailability in children in relation to age. *Eur J Clin Pharmacol* 1980;18:43–50.
13. Wichmann HM, Rind H, Gladtke E. Die elimination von Bromsulphalein beim kind. *Z Kinderheilk* 1968;103:262–276.
14. Habersang R, Kauffman RE. Drug doses for children: a rational approach to an old problem. *J Kans Med Soc* 1974;75:98–103.
15. Hines RN, McCarver DG. The ontogeny of human drug-metabolizing enzymes: phase I oxidative enzymes. *J Pharmacol Exp Ther* 2002;300:355–360.
16. McCarver DG, Hines RN. The ontogeny of human drug metabolizing enzymes: phase II conjugation enzymes and regulatory mechanisms. *J Pharmacol Exp Ther* 2002;300:361–366.
17. Arant BS Jr. Developmental patterns of renal functional maturation in the human neonate. *J Pediatr* 1978;92:705–712.
18. Gladtke E, Heimann G. The rate of development of elimination functions in kidney and liver of young infants. In: Morselli PL, Garattini S, Sereni F, eds. *Basic and therapeutic aspects of perinatal pharmacology.* New York, NY: Raven Press, 1975:393–403.

19. Sondheimer JM. Gastroesophageal reflux: update on pathogenesis and diagnosis. *Pediatr Clin North Am* 1988;35:103–116.
20. Milsap RL, Szefler SJ. Special pharmacokinetic considerations in children. In: Evans WE, Schentag JJ, Jusko WJ, eds. *Applied pharmacokinetics: principles of therapeutic drug monitoring.* Spokane, WA: Applied Therapeutics, 1986:294–328.
21. Green TP, Mirkin BL. Clinical pharmacokinetics: pediatric considerations. In: Benet LZ, Massoud N, Gambertoglio JG, eds. *Pharmacokinetic basis for drug treatment.* New York, NY: Raven Press, 1984:269–282.
22. Morselli PL, Franco-Morselli R, Bossi L. Clinical pharmacokinetics in newborns and infants: age-related differences and therapeutic implications. *Clin Pharmacokinet* 1980;5:484–527.
23. Kearns GL, Abdel-Rahman SM, Alander SW, et al. Developmental pharmacology: drug disposition, action, and therapy in infants and children. *N Engl J Med* 2003;349:1157–1167.
24. Pederson S, Moller-Petersen J. Erratic absorption of a slow-release theophylline spinkle product. *Pediatrics* 1984;74:534–538.
25. Rogers RJ, Kalisker A, Wiener MB, et al. Inconsistent absorption from a sustained-release theophylline preparation during continuous therapy in asthmatic children. *J Pediatr* 1985;106:496–501.
26. Huang NN, High RH. Comparison of serum levels following the administration of oral and parenteral preparations of penicillin to infants and children of various age groups. *J Pediatr* 1953;42: 657–668.
27. Wilson JT, Atwood HGF, Shand DG. Disposition of propoxyphene and propranolol in children. *Clin Pharmacol Ther* 1976;19: 264–270.
28. Lindenbaum J, Rund DG, Butler VP Jr, et al. Inactivation of digoxin by the gut flora: reversal by antibiotic therapy. *N Engl J Med* 1981;305:789–827.
29. Linday L, Dobkin JF, Wang TC, et al. Digoxin inactivation by the gut flora in infancy and childhood. *Pediatrics* 1987;79:544–548.
30. Notterman DA. Pediatric pharmacotherapy. In: Chernow B, ed. *The pharmacologic approach to the critically ill patient,* 2nd ed. Baltimore, MD: Williams & Wilkins, 1988:131–155.
31. Raddle IC. Mechanisms of drug absorption and their development. In: MacLeod SM, Raddle IC, eds. *Textbook of pediatric clinical pharmacology.* Littleton, MA: PSG, 1985:25–26.
32. Steward DJ. Anaesthesia in childhood. In: MacLeod SM, Raddle IC, eds. *Textbook of pediatric clinical pharmacology.* Littleton, MA: PSG, 1985:365–378.
33. Koren G. Clinical pharmacology of antimicrobial drugs during development. How are infants and children different? In: Koren G, Prober CG, Gold R, eds. *Antimicrobial therapy in infants and children.* New York, NY: Marcel Dekker, 1988:47–52.
34. Dill WA, Kazenko A, Wolf LM, et al. Studies on 5,5-diphenylhydantoin (Dilantin) in animals and man. *J Pharmacol Exp Ther* 1956;118:270–276.
35. Hendeles L, Weinberger M. Theophylline: a state of the art review. *Pharmacotherapy* 1983;3:2–44.
36. Heimann G, Gladtke E. Pharmacokinetics of phenobarbital in childhood. *Eur J Clin Pharmacol* 1977;12:305–310.
37. Pacifici GM, Viani A, Teddencci-Brunelli G, et al. Effects of development, aging, and renal and hepatic insufficiency as well as hemodialysis on the plasma concentrations of albumin and $alpha_1$ acid glycoprotein: implications for binding of drugs. *Ther Drug Monit* 1986;8:259–263.
38. Andersson KE, Bertler A, Wettrell G. Post-mortem distribution and tissue concentrations of digoxin in infants and adults. *Acta Paediatr Scand* 1975;64:497–504.
39. Park MK, Ludden T, Arom KV, et al. Myocardial vs serum digoxin concentrations in infants and adults. *Am J Dis Child* 1982;136:418–420.
40. Gorodischer R, Jusko WJ, Yaffe SJ. Tissue and erythrocyte distribution of digoxin in infants. *Clin Pharmacol Ther* 1976;19:256–263.
41. Wagner JD, Dick M, Behrendt DM, et al. Determination of myocardial and serum digoxin concentrations in children by specific and nonspecific assay methods. *Clin Pharmacol Ther* 1983;33:577–583.
42. Brazier JL, Salle B, Ribon B, et al. *In vivo* N_7-methylation of theophylline to caffeine in premature infants. *Dev Pharmacol Ther* 1981;2:137–144.
43. Aranda JV, Scalais E, Papageorgiou A, et al. Ontogeny of human caffeine and theophylline metabolism. *Dev Pharmacol Ther* 1984; 7(Suppl 1):18–25.
44. Miller RP, Roberts RJ, Fischer LJ. Acetaminophen elimination kinetics in neonates, children, and adults. *Clin Pharmacol Ther* 1976;19:284–294.
45. Freye E. Development of sensory information processing. *Acta Anaesthesiol Scand* 1996;109(Suppl):98–101.
46. Etzel BA, Guillet R. Effects of neonatal exposure to caffeine on adenosine A1 receptor ontogeny using autoradiography. *Dev Brain Res* 1994;82:223–230.
47. Cox BE, Rosenfeld CR. Ontogeny of vascular angiotensin 2 receptor subtype expression in ovine development. *Pediatr Res* 1999;45(3):414–424.
48. Samyn ME, Petershack JA, Kurt AB, et al. Ontogeny and regulation of cardiac angiotensin types 1 and 2 receptors during fetal life in sheep. *Pediatr Res* 1998;44(3):323–329.
49. Herlenius E, Lagercrantz H. Neurotransmitters and neuromodulators during early human development. *Early Hum Dev* 2001; 65:21–37.
50. Zec N, Filiano JJ, Panigrahy A, et al. Developmental changes in [3H]lysergic acid diethylamide binding to serotonin receptors in the human brainstem. *J Neuropathol Exp Neurol* 1996;55(1):114–126.
51. Cheung PY, Barrington KJ. Renal dopamine receptors: mechanisms of action and developmental aspects. *Cardiovasc Res* 1996; 31:2–6.
52. Rho JM, Storey TW. Molecular ontogeny of major neurotransmitter receptor systems in the mammalian central nervous system: norepinephrine, dopamine, serotonin, acetylcholine, and glycine. *J Child Neurol* 2001;16(4):271–279.
53. McCune SK, Hill JM. Ontogenic expression of two α-1 adrenergic receptor subtypes in the rat brain. *J Mol Neurosci* 1995;6:51–62.
54. Chugani DC, Muzik O, Juhasz C, et al. Postnatal maturation of human GABA receptors measured with positron emission tomography. *Ann Neurol* 2001;49(5):618–626.
55. Takahashi H, Ishikawa S, Nomoto S, et al. Developmental changes in pharmacokinetics and pharmacodynamics of warfarin enantiomers in Japanese children. *Clin Pharm Ther* 2000; 68:541–555.
56. Marshall JD, Kearns GL. Developmental pharmacodynamics of cyclosporine. *Clin Pharm Ther* 1999;66:66–75.
57. Kauffman RE, Nelson MV. Effect of age on ibuprofen pharmacokinetics and antipyretic response. *J Pediatr* 1992;121:969–973.
58. Park MK. Use of digoxin in infants and children with specific emphasis on dosage. *J Pediatr* 1986;108:871–877.
59. Clarke JT, Libke RD, Regamey C, et al. Comparative pharmacokinetics of amikacin and kanamycin. *Clin Pharmacol Ther* 1974;15:610–616.
60. Howard JB, McCracken GH Jr. Pharmacological evaluation of amikacin in neonates. *Antimicrob Agents Chemother* 1975;8:86–90.
61. Vogelstein B, Kowarski A, Lietman PS. The pharmacokinetics of amikacin in children. *J Pediatr* 1977;91:333–339.
62. Brown RD, Campoli-Richards DM. Antimicrobial therapy in neonates, infants, and children. *Clin Pharmacokinet* 1989;17 (Suppl 1):105–115.
63. Morrow JI, Richens A. Disposition of anticonvulsants in childhood. *Clin Pharmacokinet* 1989;17(Suppl 1):89–104.
64. Riva R, Contin M, Albani F, et al. Free concentration of carbamazepine and carbamazepine-10,11-epoxide in children and adults: influence of age and phenobarbitone cometabolism. *Clin Pharmacokinet* 1985;10:524–531.
65. Elders MJ, Wingfield BS, McNatt ML, et al. Glucocorticoid therapy in children. *Am J Dis Child* 1975;129:1393–1396.
66. Mattes J, Gittleman R. Growth of hyperactive children on maintenance regimen of methylphenidate. *Arch Gen Psychiatry* 1983;4: 317–322.
67. Stewart DJ. Prevalence of tetracyclines in children's teeth. II. Resurvey after five years. *Br Med J* 1973;3:320–322.
68. Adam D. Use of quinolones in pediatric patients. *Rev Infect Dis* 1989;11(Suppl 5):S1113–S1116.
69. Wong DF, Wagner HN, Dannals RF, et al. Effects of age on dopamine and serotonin receptors measured by positron tomography of the living human brain. *Science* 1984;226:1393.
70. Morton HG. Atropine intoxication. Its manifestations in infants and children. *J Pediatr* 1939;14:755–760.
71. American Academy of Pediatrics. Use of codeine and dextromethorphan-containing cough syrups in pediatrics. *Pediatrics* 1978;62:118–122.

72. Garson A Jr. Medicolegal problems in the management of cardiac arrhythmias in children. *Pediatrics* 1987;79:84–88.
73. American Academy of Pediatrics. Valproic acid: benefits and risks. *Pediatrics* 1982;70:316–319.
74. McCracken GH Jr. Aminoglycoside toxicity in infants and children. *Am J Med* 1986;8:172–175.
75. Hermann G. Renal toxicity of aminoglycosides in the neonatal period. *Pediatr Pharmacol* 1983;3:251–254.
76. Peterson RG, Rumack GH. Age as a variable in acetaminophen overdose. *Arch Intern Med* 1981;141:390–398.
77. Lieh-lai MW, Sarnaik AP, Newton JF, et al. Metabolism and pharmacokinetics of acetaminophen in a severely poisoned young child. *J Pediatr* 1984;105:125–128.
78. Warner LO, Beach TP, Garvin JP. Halothane and children: the first quarter century. *Anesth Analg* 1984;63:838–842.
79. Food and Drug Administration. Hepatitis associated with isoniazid—warning. *FDA Drug Bull* 1978;8:11.
80. Leeder JS, Gold R. Cephalosporins. In: Koren G, Prober CG, Gold R, eds. *Antimicrobial therapy in infants and children.* New York, NY: Marcel Dekker, 1988:173–235.
81. Bell MJ, Shackelford P, Smith R, et al. Pharmacokinetics of clindamycin phosphate in the first year of life. *J Pediatr* 1984;105: 482–486.
82. Kauffman RE, Shoeman DW, Wan SH, et al. Absorption and excretion of clindamycin phosphate in children after intramuscular injection. *Clin Pharmacol Ther* 1973;13:704–709.
83. Fahr A. Cyclosporin clinical pharmacokinetics. *Clin Pharmacokinet* 1993;24:472–495.
84. Greenblatt DJ, Shader RI, Divoll M, et al. Benzodiazepines: a summary of pharmacokinetic properties. *Br J Clin Pharmacol* 1981; 11:11S–16S.
85. Langslet A, Meberg A, Bredesen JE, et al. Plasma concentrations of diazepam and *n*-desmethyldiazepam in newborn infants after intravenous, intramuscular, rectal and oral administration. *Acta Paediatr Scand* 1978;67:699–704.
86. Wettrell G, Andersson KE. Clinical pharmacokinetics of digoxin in infants. *Clin Pharmacokinet* 1977;2:17–31.
87. Aronson JK. Clinical pharmacokinetics of digoxin. *Clin Pharmacokinet* 1980;5:137–149.
88. Linday LA, Engle MA, Reidenberg MM. Maturation and renal digoxin clearance. *Clin Pharmacol Ther* 1981;30:735–738.
89. Marotti JLP, Stowe CD, Farrar HC, et al. Pharmacokinetics and pharmacodynamics of famotidine in infants. *J Clin Pharmacol* 1998;38:10089–10095.
90. Marshall JLP, Heulitt MJ, Wells TG, et al. Pharmacokinetics and pharmacodynamics of famotidine in children. *J Clin Pharmacol* 1996;36:48–54.
91. Benet LZ, Massoud N, Gambertoglio JG, eds. *Pharmacokinetic basis for drug treatment.* New York, NY: Raven Press, 1984:435–438.
92. Evans WE, Feldman S, Ossi M, et al. Gentamicin dosage in children: a randomized prospective comparison of body weight and body surface area as dose determinants. *J Pediatr* 1979;94:139–143.
93. McCracken GH. Clinical pharmacology of gentamicin in infants 2 to 24 months of age. *Am J Dis Child* 1972;124:884–887.
94. Paisley JW, Smith AL, Smith DH. Gentamicin in newborn infants. *Am J Dis Child* 1973;126:473–477.
95. Kauffman RE, Sawyer LA, Scheinbaum ML. Antipyretic efficacy of ibuprofen vs acetaminophen. *Am J Dis Child* 1992;146:622–625.
96. Walson PD, Galletta G, Braden NJ, et al. Ibuprofen, acetaminophen, and placebo treatment of febrile children. *Clin Pharmacol Ther* 1989;46:9–17.
97. Benvenuti C, Cancellieri V, Gambaro V, et al. Pharmacokinetics of two new oral formulations of ibuprofen. *Int J Clin Pharmacol Ther Toxicol* 1986;24:308–312.
98. Kergueris MF, Bourin M, Larousse C. Pharmacokinetics of isoniazid: influence of age. *Eur J Clin Pharmacol* 1986;30:335–340.
99. De Wildt SN, Kearns GL, Hop WC, et al. Pharmacokinetics and metabolism of intravenous midazolam in preterm infants. *Clin Pharmacol Ther* 2001;70(6):525–531.
100. Reed MD, Rodarte A, Blumer JL, et al. The single-dose pharmacokinetics of midazolam and its primary metabolite in pediatric patients after oral and intravenous administration. *J Clin Pharmacol* 2001;41:1359–1369.
101. Brogden RN, Pinder RM, Sower PR, et al. Naproxen: a review of its pharmacological properties and therapeutic efficacy and use. *Drugs* 1975;9:326–363.
102. Kauffman RE, Bolinger RO, Wan SH, et al. Pharmacokinetics and metabolism of naproxen in children. *Dev Pharmacol Ther* 1982;5:143–150.
103. Cloyd JC, Loeppik IE. Primidone absorption, distribution, and excretion. In: Levy RH, Mattson R, Meldrum B, et al., eds. *Antiepileptic drugs*, 3rd ed. New York, NY: Raven Press, 1989:391–400.
104. Kauffman RE, Habersant R, Lansky L. Kinetics of primidone metabolism and excretion in children. *Clin Pharmacol Ther* 1977;22:200–205.
105. Thirumoorthi MC, Asmar BI, Buckley JA, et al. Pharmacokinetics of intravenously administered piperacillin in preadolescent children. *J Pediatr* 1983;102:941–946.
106. Szefler SJ, Pieroni DR, Gingell RL, et al. Rapid elimination of quinidine in pediatric patients. *Pediatrics* 1982;70:370–375.
107. Shalit I. Rifampin. In: Koren G, Prober CG, Gold R, eds. *Antimicrobial therapy in infants and children.* New York, NY: Marcel Dekker, 1988:373–403.
108. Vree TB, Hekster YA, Lippens RJJ. Clinical pharmacokinetics of sulfonamides in children: relationship between maturing kidney function and renal clearance of sulfonamides. *Ther Drug Monit* 1985;7:130–147.
109. Aranda JV, Grondin D, Sasyniuk BI. Pharmacologic considerations in the therapy of neonatal apnea. *Pediatr Clin North Am* 1981;28:113–133.
110. Lisby SM, Nahata M. Penicillins. In: Koren G, Prober CG, Gold R, eds. *Antimicrobial therapy in infants and children.* New York, NY: Marcel Dekker, 1988:117–152.
111. Kaplan JM, McCrackin GH, Thomas ML, et al. Clinical pharmacology of tobramycin in newborns. *Am J Dis Child* 1973;125:656–660.
112. Bruni J, Wilder BJ, Willmore LJ, et al. Steady-state kinetics of valproic acid in epileptic patients. *Clin Pharmacol Ther* 1978; 2324–2332.
113. Hall K, Otten N, Irvine-Meek J, et al. First-dose and steady-state pharmacokinetics of valproic acid in children with seizures. *Clin Pharmacokinet* 1983;8:447–455.
114. Milliken JF. Vancomycin. In: Koren G, Prober CG, Gold R, eds. *Antimocrobial therapy in infants and children.* New York, NY: Marcel Dekker, 1988:265–285.
115. Balis FM, Pizzo PA, Eddy J, et al. Pharmacokinetics of zidovudine administered intravenously and orally in children with human immunodeficiency virus infection. *J Pediatr* 1989;114:880–884.
116. Langtry HD, Campoli-Richards DM. Zidovudine. A review of its pharmacodynamic and pharmacokinetic properties and therapeutic efficacy. *Drugs* 1989;37:408–450.
117. Dodson WE. Nonlinear kinetics of phenytoin in children. *Neurology* 1982;32:42–48.

CHAPTER

4

Anders Rane

Drug Metabolism and Disposition in Infants and Children

The new regulatory framework for development of drugs for children has promoted the interest in pediatric pharmacology and left behind the traditional pediatric pharmacotherapeutics based on cautious and conservative empiricism. Not only economical incentives but also new guidelines on ethics for pediatric age groups have contributed to this positive development. Several investigations in recent years have evidenced the great dearth of documentation on drugs for children and the extensive off-label use of drugs for pediatric age groups. This situation is metabolised by enzymes with genetic polymorphisms.

The aim of all treatment with drugs is to obtain a specific pharmacologic response with a minimum risk of adverse effects. This is best achieved by selection of well-documented drugs based on comprehensive knowledge about drug behavior and sensitivity in the target group of patients. Due consideration of the large interindividual variability in drug response (pharmacodynamics) and disposition (pharmacokinetics) as well as of disease state and other patient features is required. For most drugs, interindividual variability in drug response is less pronounced than the variability in drug disposition. It is also evident that the age-dependent variation in drug kinetics is larger than the genetic variation for most drugs, except for drugs.

Therapeutic disasters with sulfonamides (1) and chloramphenicol (2) involving toxic effects in the newborn after administration of the same body-weight–related doses as to adult patients are examples of the clinical consequences of altered drug disposition in the young. These events have contributed to the dogma that the infant has an augmented response to drugs throughout development. We know that this is not always the case.

Age-related changes in drug disposition are related to maturational increases in liver and kidney function and variations in plasma protein binding, tissue distribution, and gastrointestinal absorption. Other physiologic parameters also contribute to the rapid changes. Development of drug analytical techniques has been a perequisite for detailed pharmacokinetic studies. However, there is a dearth of understanding and knowledge about the concentration–effect relationships in infants and children. These aspects of developmental pharmacology are important areas for future research because it is not possible to extrapolate these relationships from adult patients to children.

This chapter discusses how the development of certain constitutional features may affect drug disposition in infants and children. To illustrate this, several examples from important pharmacotherapeutic areas are presented.

DRUG METABOLISM AS REFLECTED BY CLINICAL PHARMACOKINETIC DATA

CONCEPTS

Elimination of drugs and other xenobiotics terminates their effects. Elimination involves various excretory pathways with or without a preceding chemical alteration of the drug molecule, enzymatically or nonenzymatically. The elimination processes may be seen as part of the body's defense mechanism. Without these processes, drug accumulation and toxicity would ensue. The sum of all elimination processes is equal to the total-body intravenous (IV) clearance (Cl_{IV}) of the drug. This, by definition, is the volume of blood or plasma that is irreversibly cleared of drug per unit time. If an IV dose D of the drug is administered to the patient and the area under the plasma concentration-versus-time curve (AUC_{IV}) is assessed, the Cl_{IV} can be calculated from

$$Cl_{IV} = \frac{D}{AUC_{IV}} \quad (1)$$

The Cl_{IV} reflects the sum of the different elimination routes. Thus, Cl_{IV} may be the sum of hepatic (Cl_H) and renal (Cl_R) clearance as well as other clearance mechanisms. If the drug is administered orally, the apparent oral clearance

(Cl_O) (consider the fraction F of the oral dose that reaches the systemic circulation) is:

$$Cl_O = \frac{F \times D}{\text{AUC}_O} \quad (2)$$

It follows that $1 - F$ is the fraction of the oral dose that is metabolized or otherwise eliminated in the liver and/or gut wall during passage from the gut to the systemic circulation. This phenomenon is called first-pass elimination. If all the drug in the gut reaches the portal vein, then

$$1 - F = E \quad (3)$$

where E is the hepatic extraction ratio. This is the proportion of the dose that is eliminated during one passage through the liver. The endothelial cells lining the villi harbor drug-metabolizing enzymes that may contribute to the first-pass elimination. In addition, many drugs are acted on by ATP-binding cassette (ABC) transporter proteins or organic anion-transporting polypeptides (OATP) in the endothelial cells and pumped out of the cells back into the gut lumen. If only part of the oral dose reaches the portal vein, the deficient absorption or uptake must be corrected for in the calculations of E and F.

The relationship between Cl_H, the liver blood flow Q, and the total intrinsic hepatic clearance Cl_i is defined by the perfusion-limited clearance model (3), (4) for drug clearance in the liver. This relation is defined as

$$Cl_H = Q \times E = Q\left(\frac{Cl_i}{Q + Cl_i}\right) \quad (4)$$

The intrinsic clearance is defined as the maximum capacity of the liver (or any other organ) to remove drug from the blood in the absence of flow limitations. From Equation (4) it is obvious that changes in liver blood flow will preferentially affect the clearance of drugs with high values of Cl_i, which may be observed as changes in plasma half-life $t_{1/2}$. In contrast, changes in enzyme activity will affect the $t_{1/2}$ only of drugs with low values of Cl_i. In addition, such changes will affect the AUC both after oral and IV administration such that the AUC is decreased when the enzyme activity is enhanced.

The drug clearance from an organ is also dependent on drug binding in the blood by modification of Equation (4):

$$Cl_H = Q\left(\frac{f_B \times Cl'_i}{Q + f_B \times Cl'_i}\right) \quad (5)$$

where f_B denotes the unbound fraction in blood and Cl'_i is the intrinsic hepatic clearance of unbound drug. If Cl'_i is high, drug binding in blood has little importance for the Cl_H. In contrast, drug binding has a limiting (restrictive) influence on Cl_H if the value of Cl'_i is low (5). As a corollary, hepatic drug extraction from the blood is denoted as nonrestrictive or restrictive, respectively. The derivation of the hepatic clearance is important since the determinants are subject to age-dependent development.

CLINICAL DATA

Estimation of metabolic clearance is of interest in pediatric pharmacology since many enzymatic fractions develop slowly in neonatal life. As the hepatic blood flow varies, *in vitro* estimates such as intrinsic clearance ($Cl_i = V_{max}/K_m$) are not very useful. Therefore, *in vivo* methods for estimating Cl_i are preferred. By definition, Cl_O is equivalent to the intrinsic hepatic clearance Cl_i of the drug, provided the drug is eliminated only by liver metabolism and is completely bioavailable to the portal vein. However, very few drugs fulfill these criteria, and in children, no data on the apparent oral clearance of such drugs seem to exist.

The plasma half-life $t_{1/2}$ may serve as an estimate of the hepatic drug-metabolizing activity only under certain criteria. The $t_{1/2}$ gives no information about the efficiency of drug elimination processes even though it provides a rough estimation of duration of effect. If the drug is solely eliminated by hepatic metabolism, that is, if systemic clearance Cl_s is equal to Cl_H, then

$$t_{1/2} = \frac{0.693 \times V_d}{Cl_H} \quad (6)$$

This relationship demonstrates that $t_{1/2}$ depends on Cl_H as well as on the apparent volume of distribution V_d of the drug.

As is evident from Equation (5), hepatic clearance Cl_H is a function not only of enzyme activity (Cl_i) and drug binding in blood (f_B) but also of blood flow (Q). Therefore, to interpret kinetics data from systemic administration of drugs at different stages of development, it is important to differentiate between low-extraction and high-extraction drugs. A number of drugs have been classified according to this system on the basis of adult human pharmacokinetic data (Table 4.1).

Drug distribution is affected by a variety of physiologic factors, including vascular tissue perfusion, body composition, plasma protein binding, and tissue binding. Because the V_d may be subject to developmental changes, caution must be exercised in the interpretation of data on $t_{1/2}$ in infants and children. However, if we make a reasonable assumption that V_d is constant, then $t_{1/2}$ after an IV administration of the drug is virtually proportional to the hepatic enzyme activity (for low-extraction drugs), the hepatic blood flow (for high-extraction drugs), or both (for drugs with intermediate values of Cl_i).

The steady-state concentration C_{ss} of a drug administered orally and metabolized only by the liver is given by the following equation:

$$C_{ss} = \frac{F \times D}{Cl_H \times \Delta} \quad (7)$$

where Δ denotes the dosing interval and F is the drug bioavailability. Rearranging this equation gives

$$C_{ss} = \frac{D}{f_B \times Cl'_i \times \Delta} \quad (8)$$

This relationship shows that the only biologic determinants of C_{ss} of a drug that is given orally and solely metabolized

TABLE 4.1 Comparison of Half-Lives in Newborns and Adults of Drugs with Low or High Hepatic Extraction

Drug	$t_{1/2}$ (hr) Newborns	Adults	References
Drugs with low hepatic clearance			
Aminophylline	24–36	3–9	18
Amylobarbitone	17–60	12–27	105
Caffeine	103	6	17, 19
Carbamazepine	8–28	21–36	10
Diazepam	25–100	15–25	11
Mepivacaine	8.7	3.2	106
Phenobarbitone	21–100	52–120	107–113
Phenytoin	21	11–29	114
Tolbutamide	10–40	4.4–9	115
Drugs with intermediate or high hepatic clearance			
Bromosulfophthalein	0.16		44
Meperidine	22	3–4	116, 117
Nortriptyline	56	18–22	118
Morphine	2.7	0.9–4.3	119
Lidocaine	2.9–3.3	1.0–2.2	120
Propoxyphene	1.7–7.7	1.9–4.3	121

by the liver are the Cl_i' and the binding, irrespective of the extraction ratio (3), (6). In this context, any discussion about blood flow is superfluous.

Most pharmacokinetic data in children were obtained through classical studies requiring "rich" data from the individual patient. Modern therapeutic drug monitoring, improvements in drug assay methodology, and large-scale therapeutic drug monitoring in children have promoted the introduction of population pharmacokinetic modeling methods to achieve optimization and safety of pediatric drug treatment. Population pharmacokinetics is particularly useful in pediatric therapy since it is possible to use and analyze sparse data from a large number of subjects. The mixed-effects model includes fixed effects as well as random effects on variability between subjects. Data capture from a large number of subjects and application of statistical programs such as nonlinear mixed-effects model have yielded a lot of clinically useful pharmacokinetic information in children (7) and been applied in studies of, for example, pantoprazol (8), levetiracetam (9), and other drugs in children. Population modeling can also be used to explore different components of the developmental variation in pharmacokinetics such as maturation of clearance pathways, receptor functions, and so forth. This approach will be increasingly used in investigations of drugs for children.

LOW-CLEARANCE DRUGS

Among the drugs that belong to this group are antiepileptics and certain benzodiazepines. They are frequently used in infants, and their $t_{1/2}$ values are predominantly dependent on the drug-metabolizing enzyme activity. The C_{ss} of these agents is determined by the hepatic enzyme activity and by drug binding in blood according to Equation (8). Inasmuch as the values of f_B and V_d are not age dependent, the $t_{1/2}$ and C_{ss} may serve as rough estimates of the capacity to metabolize the drug. Some of the drugs of this group that have been studied in newborns and adults are listed in Table 4.1.

The $t_{1/2}$ of carbamazepine and phenytoin in newborn infants of epileptic mothers treated with these agents during pregnancy is similar to the $t_{1/2}$ in adults (10), (11). This is probably due to intrauterine induction of the drug metabolism. As judged from the $t_{1/2}$ values, the capacity to metabolize phenytoin in the newborn seems to be well developed at birth, as the V_d of phenytoin does not change from the neonatal to the adult stage (12).

The V_{max} for oxidation of phenytoin is higher in children than in adults (13), and the capacity to oxidize phenytoin decreases with age (14). The recommendation of higher weight-related doses of these antiepileptics in children compared with adults is therefore logical (see later discussion).

Theophylline and caffeine have comparatively long plasma half-lives in the neonatal period (Table 4.1), whereas in adults the corresponding values are only 3.8 to 8 (15–16) and 4 hours (17), respectively. This difference (17–19) is consistent with the extremely low and undeveloped fetal hepatic *in vitro* activity of cytochrome P4501A (20), which is the major catalyst of the oxidation of theophylline and caffeine (21), (22).

HIGH-CLEARANCE DRUGS

The $t_{1/2}$ of drugs belonging to this group is dependent to a large extent on hepatic blood flow, whereas variation in enzyme activity has less influence on the elimination of an IV dose. However, enzyme activity does determine the AUC and C_{ss} values after single and multiple oral administration, respectively. Although the use of these drugs is limited in children, some kinetic data for these agents have been published (Table 4.1).

Table 4.2 lists the half-lives of some drugs unclassified with respect to their clearance values. The general impression is

TABLE 4.2 Comparison of Plasma Half-Lives in Newborns and Adults of Some Drugs that are Unclassified with Respect to Hepatic Clearance

Drug	*$t_{1/2}$ (hr)*		*References*
	Newborns	*Adults*	
Aminopyrine	30–40	2–4	122
Bupivacaine	25	1.3	123
Diazepam	25–100	15–25	11
Furosemide	7.7–19.9	0.5	124–126
Gabapentin	14	7–9	127, 128
Indomethacin	14–20	2–11	129
Levetirazepam	5.3	6–8	130
Oxazepam	21.9	6.5	131
Primidone	7–28.6	3.3–12.5	132, 133
Phenylbutazone	21–34	12–30	134
Valproic acid	23–35	10–16	135, 136

that the half-life of most drugs in the neonate is longer than in the adult patient. This strongly suggests that most investigated drugs have a lower metabolic clearance in neonates and infants than in the adult (as judged from the values of the $t_{1/2}$). The rate of maturation of this capacity varies from drug to drug. As a corollary, attempts to predict the drug-metabolizing activity in children from adult data are bound to fail.

DRUG BINDING TO PLASMA PROTEINS

Because a drug's pharmacologic effects and side effects are related to the unbound fraction of drug in blood f_B, it is relevant to know how f_B varies in different age groups. Routine analyses of drugs in plasma generally account only for the total concentration. As long as the drug binding does not vary substantially between individuals in the same age group, specific analysis of the unbound fraction is generally not warranted. However, such analysis may have a clinical value in special patients, for example, if the plasma protein level is perturbed by compromised kidney function or liver disease.

Most investigated drugs are less bound in cord/infant plasma than in adult plasma (Table 4.3). This may have several explanations. The plasma protein may be qualitatively or quantitatively different at this age. The albumin concentration in neonates appears to be equivalent to the adult concentration (23), but α_1-acid glycoprotein concentrations are lower (24). In addition, hypoproteinemia is frequently observed in premature infants (23). The possible influence of competing ligands on drug binding has been discussed for bilirubin (25) and free fatty acids (26). Such factors may be the reason for the lower serum protein binding of many drugs, such as clonazepam (27). For clonazepam, adults have a lower binding capacity but a higher affinity to serum proteins than children.

As pointed out earlier, the clearance term, Equation (5), is affected by drug binding in blood and plasma. For low-clearance drugs, the hepatic elimination is usually restrictive and the systemic clearance of total drug will depend on binding. The $t_{1/2}$ is prolonged when binding increases. The concentration of unbound drug is essentially unchanged. On the other hand, for drugs with a high clearance, a decreased binding leads to a higher unbound concentration and more pronounced pharmacologic effects (4).

TABLE 4.3 Protein Binding of Some Drugs in Cord Plasma in Relation to Adult Plasma

Lower Binding	*Higher Binding*
Acid drugs	
Ampicillin (154)	Valproic acid[a,b] (136,137)
Benzylpenicillin (154)	Salicylic acid[a] (138)
Nafcillin (155)	Sulfisoxazole[a] (139)
Salicylates (42)	Cloxacillin[a] (140)
Phenytoin[c] (136)	Flucloxacillin[a] (140)
Phenylbutazone (134)	
Phenobarbitone (156)	
Pentobarbitone (157)	
Cloxacillin (140)	
Flucloxacillin (140)	
Sulfamethoxypyrazine (158)	
Sulfaphenazole (159)	
Sulfadimethoxine (159)	
Sulfamethoxydiazine (159)	
Neutral drugs	
Digoxin (56,57)	
Dexamethasone (139)	
Basic drugs	
Diazepam (24,160)	Diazepam[a] (23), (139)
Imipramine (161)	
Desmethylimipramine (162)	
Bupivacaine (123)	
Lidocaine (120)	
Propranolol (121)	
Metocurine[a] (121)	
D-Tubocurarine[a] (121)	

[a]Compared with maternal plasma.
[b]Indirect evidence.
[c]Same or lower binding.

The differential effect of altered drug binding on the total plasma concentration of high-clearance and low-clearance drugs needs consideration in studies of drug concentration–effect relationships.

The steady-state concentration C_{ss} of phenytoin that is attained for a given dose per kilogram body weight is considerably lower in infants than in adults, even though the infant dose is twice as high on a body-weight basis (25), (28). This may be due, in part, to binding alterations, because a lower binding yields a lower total plasma concentration. However, it is believed that a higher metabolic rate at this age contributes substantially to the low C_{ss} in these infants. The issue of the appropriate therapeutic concentration of the drug in infants is one of great interest. It is conceivable that the higher f_B compensates partially for the lower total C_{ss} values that are attained (25).

BIOAVAILABILITY: DRUG ABSORPTION AND TRANSPORTER PROTEINS

The drug absorption process at various ages is not well understood. The gastric pH is alkaline at birth but falls to pH 1 to 3 within 1 or 2 days (29). Adult levels of gastric acid secretion are reached at ages 5 to 12 years (for a review, see reference 27). Although the nonionic diffusion principle would favor absorption of acidic drugs in the stomach, a substantial part of the important absorption takes place in the duodenum. The absorption of penicillin G and semisynthetic penicillins is higher in newborn infants than in adults (29). This may be explained, in part, by the higher pH in newborn infants.

The motility of the gut and the gastric emptying time have been reported to be delayed in newborn infants (30). Although this may affect the absorption–time profile rather than the degree of absorption, it has been proposed as an explanation for the erratic absorption of certain sustained-release theophylline formulations in children (31). There are data to support this assumption. Heimann (32) studied the bioavailability of sulfonamides, digoxin, and some other drugs in infants and children. Although the rate of absorption was significantly lower in neonates, the amount of drug absorbed was not correlated with age.

The fetal gastrointestinal tract is rapidly colonized by bacteria after birth. The level of the gastrointestinal microorganism flora is related to bile acid deconjugation and β-glucuronidase activity, both of which are significantly higher in neonates than in adults (33). Other intestinal enzymes that may affect the drug absorption and are subject to age-dependent alterations include lipase and α-amylase (34), both of which are low in the neonatal period.

Many drugs are substrates of the ABC-transporter system, of which *p*-glycoprotein is the best known and most investigated member. These protein pumps transport drugs across membranes, for example, in the blood–brain barrier and placenta, where they can be protective against foreign compounds in the (maternal) circulation, or in the endothelial cells of the gastrointestinal tract, where they can pump drugs back into the gut lumen. The function of these pumps affects the oral bioavailability, F, as do the drug-metabolizing enzymes that are co-located with the *p*-glycoprotein in the endothelium. Another large family of influx transporters is the organic anion transporting proteins (OATP) which have a role in the transport of several drugs, e.g. statins, across many membranes in the body. Little is known about the development of these transporter systems during maturation.

DEVELOPMENTAL CHANGES IN METABOLISM PATTERN

As is evident from the preceding discussion, the metabolic disposition of most drugs is reduced in the neonatal period, as judged from the plasma half-lives. However, some drugs do not conform to this trend. *In utero* exposure to drugs may induce the fetal metabolizing enzymes. Alternatively, other metabolic pathways that are minor in adults may play a quantitatively more significant role in early life and compensate for the deficient "normal adult" metabolic pathway.

The latter phenomenon is illustrated in Figure 4.1 for two drugs, morphine (35), (36) and acetaminophen (paracetamol). In adulthood, the major metabolic pathway for the latter drug includes glucuronidation. In the early newborn period, glucuronidation is deficient, whereas sulfate conjugation is pronounced (37–39). This leads to an apparently "normal" half-life in newborns. Interestingly, this pattern is consistent with *in vitro* findings in human fetal liver preparations (40). By using liver microsomal preparations or isolated hepatocytes, it was found that acetaminophen was conjugated with sulfate but not with glucuronic acid. It is of clinical importance to note that acetaminophen seems to be less toxic in children than in adults. This may be explained, in part, by the compensatory routes of metabolism, although other mechanisms may also be operating.

Morphine is increasingly used in pediatric pain treatment, for example procedural or surgical pain in premature infants. In adult patients, glucuronidation catalyzed by uridine diphospho-glucuronosyl transferase (UGT) 2B7 is the major route of metabolism. In newborns and small infants, however, morphine is partly sulfated (35), (36). This pathway from the fetal period disappears and is virtually nonexisting in adult patients. It is to be noted that morphine 3-sulfate has a substantial binding affinity in preparations of rat-brain Mu receptor preparations (41).

Developmental changes in metabolic pattern have also been demonstrated for salicylic acid (42), *p*-aminobenzoic acid (43), bromosulfophthalein (44), diazepam (45), and theophylline (46), (47). As shown in Figure 4.1, the hydroxylation reactions of diazepam are relatively deficient in both premature and full-term neonates (45). Theophylline is also subject to extensive age-dependent changes in its metabolism (Fig. 4.1). In premature infants, theophylline is eliminated virtually only through renal excretion, which is marginal in the adult (46), (47). A small part is methylated to caffeine, consistent with findings in fetal liver preparations (17). The formation of 1,3-dimethyluric acid gains increasing importance with age.

The oxidative pathways of caffeine mature at various rates (48). The N_3-demethylation is more important in young infants than in adults, whereas the N_1-demethylation is low and develops later than 19 months of age (Fig. 4.2).

Age	Theophylline	Diazepam	Acetaminophen	Morphine
Premature 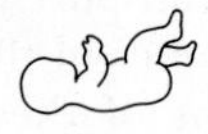		0.62 → *N*-Demethyldiazepam - - → Methyl-oxazepam - - → Oxazepam		
Full-term 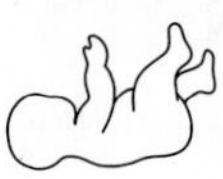	98(~50) → Renal excretion 2 → Caffeine ~10 → 1-Methyluric acid - - → Methylxanthine ~30 → 1,3-Dimethyluric acid	0.84 → *N*-Demethyldiazepam 0.12 → Methyl-oxazepam 0.02 - - → Oxazepam	→ Sulphate conjugation → Glucuronic acid conjugation	→ Sulphate conjugation → Glucuronic acid conjugation
Child 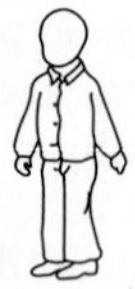	7 → Renal excretion - - → Caffeine 24 → 1-Methyluric acid 16 → 3-Methylxanthine 53 → 1,3-Dimethyluric acid	1.46 → *N*-Demethyldiazepam 1.26 → Methyl-oxazepam 1.77 → Oxazepam		
Adult 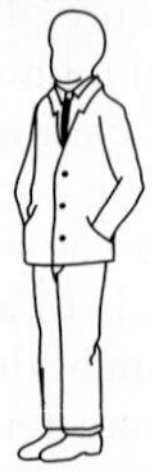	10 → Renal excretion - - → Caffeine 20 → 1-Methyluric acid 13 → Methylxanthine 55 → 1,3-Dimethyluric acid		- - → Sulphate conjugation → Glucuronic acid conjugation	→ Glucuronic acid conjugation

Figure 4.1. Age-dependent changes in the metabolism pattern of some drugs at different developmental stages. From top to bottom, a premature neonate, a full-term neonate, a prepubertal child, and an adult. The numbers indicate the percentage of metabolites retrieved in urine. The thickness of the arrows indicates the relative importance of the respective pathway. Data from references (37–39), (42), and (45–47).

Developmental changes in metabolic patterns are not only of academic interest. Because many drugs are bioactivated to toxic metabolites, the differential maturation of various pathways may put the infant at risk during a limited developmental stage. Further studies to identify such therapeutic situations are required.

MATURATIONAL CHANGES OF RENAL DRUG ELIMINATION

The dosing of drugs that are predominantly eliminated by the kidneys must be adjusted to the immaturity of renal function in early life. To some extent, the problem is similar to the treatment of elderly with decreased renal elimination. Both these risk groups of patients at the extremes of age require that the dose and/or dose frequency be decreased to avoid drug accumulation and toxicity. Several nomograms and dosing tables have been developed to facilitate the dosing of these types of drugs in infants.

The glomerular filtration rate (as measured with inulin) is low at birth and reaches adult levels at 5 months of age (49). The glomerular filtration rate is also a function of the postconceptional age, so there may be a two- to fourfold difference between premature and full-term

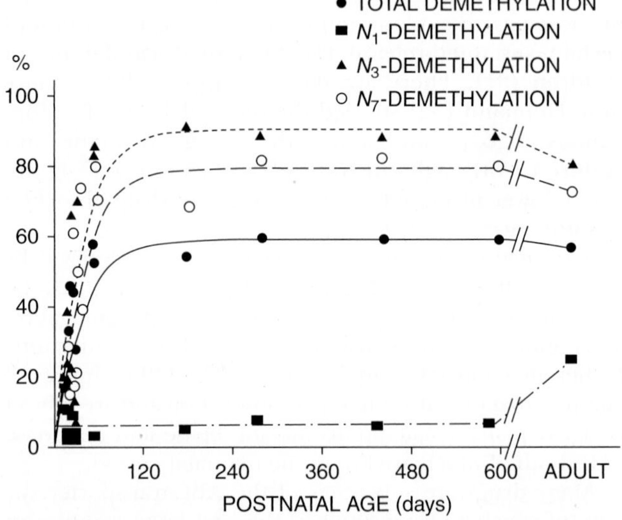

Figure 4.2. Developmental changes in the metabolism of caffeine during the first 600 days of life. Demethylation at different positions is given as the ratio of the number of methyl groups absent in the metabolites recovered in the urine to the number of methyl groups contained in the moles of caffeine from which they originated. (Adapted from Carrier et al. Maturation of caffeine metabolic pathways in infancy. *Clin Pharmacol Ther* 1988;44(2):145–151, with permission from the authors and publishers.)

newborns (50), (51). The difference in inulin clearance persists throughout the neonatal period.

The tubular secretion rate reaches adult levels somewhat later than the glomerular filtration rate (49). With *p*-aminohippuric acid as test agent, adult rates were attained by 7 months. With other drugs, the maturity may be achieved at other ages. This physiologic situation requires special clinical consideration in dosing drugs that are dependent on the kidneys for their elimination. This is the case for penicillins (52) and several aminoglycosides (53), the half-lives of which are extensively prolonged in neonates. The elimination of some cephalosporins, such as ceftriaxone, is also significantly longer in newborns (54), (55).

Digoxin provides an interesting example of bidirectional changes in clearance during the first 5 years of life. It is only 1.8 mL per minute per kg of body weight during the first week. It then increases to 10.7 mL per minute per kg of body weight during the first year and decreases again to 3.8 mL per minute per kg of body weight at 2 to 5 years of age (56). The half-lives vary consistently with the renal clearance. Variation in apparent volume of distribution V_d is less than the clearance changes, and therefore changes in half-lives may be essentially ascribed to maturation of kidney function (57).

Dosing of drugs exerting their desired clinical effect in the kidney has been extensively discussed. A drug's effect may be insufficient because of deficient kidney function. Furosemide is actively secreted in the tubules and exerts its diuretic effect in the intraluminal space (58). It has been suggested (59) that elevated plasma levels may be required to ensure adequate intraluminal delivery of furosemide. This has also been suggested for thiazides and organic mercuric compounds (60), (61).

DOSING PRINCIPLES IN CHILDREN

Optimal tailoring of the dose to the newborn infant and child is a delicate obligation of the treating physician. All suggestions and dosing rules that have been proposed reveal the complexity of the problem. No universal dosage rule can be recommended. If age is used as the basis for dosing, errors may be introduced because of the variability in weight among children in the same age group. Administration of a drug based on an infant's weight is seldom appropriate. With this rule, infants will generally be underdosed. Clinical experience with most drugs has shown that dosing according to the "surface rule" is more appropriate than dosing according to the weight rule. For many drugs sold today this is evident from the manufacturers' dose recommendations. The "surface rule" calculates the dose based on the surface area rather than the weight of the patient. Because surface area is greater relative to volume and weight in small individuals, the dose will be greater than when it is based on body weight. As the child grows, the weight increases and so does the surface area, albeit at a slower rate. The surface area may be estimated from nomograms using body weight and height. Alternatively, an approximation of the dose according to the surface rule is obtained if the

TABLE 4.4 Examples of Drugs Given in Higher Weight-Related Doses to Children than to Adults

Drug	*References*
Phenytoin	141
Phenobarbitone	141
Carbamazepine	133
Ethosuximide	142
Clonazepam	143
Diazepam	133
Lorazepam	144
Theophylline	145
Enprofylline	146
Digoxin	56
Some anticancer drugs	147
Topiramate	148
Imipramine	149
Clomipramine	149
Haloperidol	149
Chlorpromazine	150

dose is calculated to follow the weight ratio (child/adult) to the 0.7 power (62), (63):

$$\mathrm{Dose}_{\mathrm{pediatr}} = \mathrm{dose}_{\mathrm{adult}}\left(\frac{\mathrm{weight}_{\mathrm{pediatr}}}{\mathrm{weight}_{\mathrm{adult}}}\right)^{0.7} \qquad (9)$$

The rationale for using the surface rule is not well understood. However, many physiologic parameters, such as cardiac output, respiratory metabolism, blood volume, extracellular water volume, glomerular filtration rate, and renal blood flow, correlate closely with the body surface area. Many of these functions are of direct importance for drug elimination. The clinical impression and experience that infants and small children often need higher doses than adults have now been verified in several pharmacokinetic investigations showing increased rate of metabolism and renal elimination at lower ages. A list of drugs that are usually administered at higher doses (on a weight basis) to children than to adults is given in Table 4.4. The reader is referred to the reference literature for the pharmacokinetic explanations. Table 4.5 shows the relative doses according to the surface rule, Equation (9), at various ages and body weights.

PEDIATRIC PHARMACOGENETICS

The variability of drug disposition in children is even more complex than in adults since the expression of genetic factors and environment is modified by the impact of physiological development and maturation. The definition of pharmacogenetics has been expressed as "... a monogenic trait caused by the presence in the same population of more than one allele at the same gene locus, and more than one phenotype regarding drug interaction with the organism with the frequency of the less common allele being greater than 1%" (64).

Variability in treatment outcome and adverse drug reactions are often associated with different genotypes. There is

TABLE 4.5 Calculation of Drug Dose to Children According to the Surface Rule [Equation (9)]

		Pediatric Dose (in Arbitrary Units) for a Given Dose to an Adult (70 kg) Patient (in Column Head)										
Body Weight (kg)	*Age (yr)*	*40*	*60*	*80*	*100*	*125*	*150*	*175*	*200*	*250*	*300*	*400*
3		4	7	9	11	14	17	19	22	28	33	44
4		5	8	11	13	17	20	24	27	34	40	54
5	1/4	6	9	13	16	20	24	28	32	39	47	63
6	1/4	7	11	14	18	22	27	31	36	45	54	72
7	1/2	8	12	16	20	25	30	35	40	50	60	80
8	1/2	9	13	18	22	27	33	38	44	55	66	88
9	3/4	10	14	19	24	30	36	42	48	59	71	95
10	1	10	15	20	26	32	38	45	51	64	77	102
15	3	14	20	27	34	43	51	60	68	85	102	136
20	6	17	25	33	42	52	62	73	83	104	125	166
25	8	19	29	39	49	61	73	85	97	122	146	195
30	9–10	22	33	44	55	69	83	97	111	138	166	221
35	11	25	37	49	62	77	92	108	123	154	185	246
40	12	27	41	54	68	84	101	118	135	169	203	270
45	13–15	29	44	59	73	92	110	128	147	183	220	294
50	13–15	32	47	63	79	99	119	138	158	198	237	316
55	13–15	34	51	68	85	106	127	148	169	211	253	338

a dearth of information about the maturation of polymorphic traits during ontogenesis. Increased knowledge in this field is of great value in pediatric drug therapy because several drug substrates of polymorphic enzymes are also used in infants and children. For many such drugs, the treatment results may not be monitored by objective parameters.

Many enzymes as well as drug receptor targets are subject to genetic polymorphisms. The cytochrome P450 (CYP) family is the major enzyme system for oxidation of drugs. Important polymorphisms in this family include the CYP2D6, CYP2C9, and CYP2C19 enzymes. These were among the first to be described (Table 4.6) and are based on enzyme gene mutations that may compromise or delete the enzyme activity. Many pharmacogenetic polymorphisms have also been described in phase II enzyme genes, for example, *N*-acetyltransferase 2 and members of the UGT and glutathione *S*-transferase enzyme families. The clinical importance of the phase II enzyme polymorphisms for drug therapy is not as well explored as for phase I enzymes.

THE CYP2D6 POLYMORPHISM

This polymorphism is inherited as an autosomal recessive trait (65). A large number of mutations have been described in about 70 different alleles conveying poor metabolism to the individual. There are large ethnic differences in frequency (66). Whereas 7% to 10% of Caucasians are poor metabolizers, only 1% to 2% of Asians belong to this group. The third group includes the "ultrarapid metabolizers" which constitute 2% to 3% of the population due to gene duplications or gene multiplications (67).

Homozygous mutated individuals are denoted as poor metabolizers and are deficient in the metabolism of a variety of drugs (Table 4.7). The CYP2D6 polymorphic metabolism pattern is seen for many important groups of drugs, for example, several β-adrenoceptor-blocking agents (68–70), antidepressants (71), neuroleptic drugs (72), and opiates (73–75). The CYP2D6 gene may also be present in two or more copies, leading to the "ultrarapid metabolism" phenotype (67).

In children the number of clinically used drugs that are substrates of CYP2D6 is limited. Even so, clinical implications need to be considered. Thus, codeine and tramadol which are metabolized to active compounds do not have full analgesic effects in poor metabolizer children, whether the poor metabolism is due to immaturity of the enzyme or pharmacogenetic phenotype.

Little is known about the development of the extensive metabolizer phenotype during ontogenesis. *In vitro* studies in human fetal liver have demonstrated that the *N*-demethylation of codeine and dextromethorphan precedes the development of the O-demethylation reaction (76). Whereas the *N*-demethylation is catalyzed by the nonpolymorphic CYP3A, the O-demethylation of these drugs is catalyzed by CYP2D6. Other studies indicate that the

TABLE 4.6 Some Polymorphisms of Drug-Metabolizing Enzymes

Enzyme	*Function*	*Discovered Through Geno/Phenotyping*	*References*
Pseudocholinesterase	Hydrolysis	Pronounced clinical effect (apnea) of succinylcholine/suxamethonium	151
N-acetyltransferase 2	Acetylation	High concentration of isoniazid	152
Cytochrome P450 2D6	Oxidation	Orthostatic hypotension of debrisoquine	65
Cytochrome P450 2C19	Oxidation	Pronounced sensitivity to mephenytoin	79
Cytochrome P450 2C9	Oxidation	—	
Cytochrome P450 2B6	Oxidation	Variable kinetics and bio-activation of certain drug substrates	153

TABLE 4.7 Drug Substrates of the Polymorphic Cytochrome P450 2D6 Enzyme

Cardiovascular agents	**β-Adrenoreceptor blockers**
Debrisoquine	Metoprolol
Sparteine	Propranolol
Propafenone	Timolol
Flecainide	**Antiemetics**
Mexiletine	Tropisetron
Neuroleptics	**Tricyclic antidepressants**
Haloperidol	Amitriptyline
Perphenazine	Nortriptyline
Thioridazine	Clomipramine/desmethylclomipramine
Chlorpromazine	Imipramine/desipramine
Remoxipride	**Other antidepressants**
Zuclopentixol	Paroxetine
Opiates	Fluoxetine
Codeine	Desmethylcitalopram
Dextromethorphan	Mianserin
Ethylmorphine	

TABLE 4.8 Drug Substrates of the Polymorphic Cytochrome P450 2C19 Enzyme

Antiepileptics
Mephenytoin
Benzodiazepines
Diazepam/desmethyldiazepam
β-Adrenoreceptor blockers
Propranolol
Antiulcer agents
Omeprazole
Antidepressants
Citalopram
Imipramine
Clomipramine
Moclobemide
Antimalarials
Proguanil[a]

[a]Bioactivated by cytochrome P450 2C19 to cycloguanil.

CYP2D6 enzyme is expressed in a minority of liver specimens from late gestational period and from newborn infants, and that the catalytic *in vitro* activity of CYP2D6 develops postnatally over a period of several months (77). However, studies of dextromethorphan metabolic ratios in infants as a measure of CYP2D6 activity indicate that there is no change in activity after 2 weeks of age (Blake et al., 2007). The gene expression of CYP2D6 seems to precede the formation of the enzyme protein. Only in adulthood is there a positive correlation between mRNA and enzyme protein, suggesting a transcriptional regulation in adults.

It is evident that the immature development of the polymorphic enzyme will change the phenotype distribution in young infants in relation to the adult distribution pattern. It is unclear when the enzyme maturation takes place. In an early study of dextromethorphan in children aged 3 to 21 years and in adolescents, about 9% of the subjects were classified as poor metabolizers (78), which is similar to the proportion in adult individuals.

Given this background, it is evident that infants and small children may have an increased risk of adverse effects of these important groups of drugs when given at therapeutic doses. In contrast, for drugs that are bioactivated by CYP2D6, such as codeine, there is a potential for lack of efficacy.

THE CYTOCHROME P450 2C19 POLYMORPHISM

This polymorphism was discovered in studies of the kinetics of the antiepileptic drug mephenytoin (79). The enzyme deficiency is inherited as an autosomal recessive trait. The CYP2C19 enzyme catalyzes the oxidation of a limited number of drugs (Table 4.8), of which phenytoin, omeprazole, and certain antidepressants have some relevance in pediatric drug therapy. It is deficient in 2% to 5% of whites (80). Studies in different populations have revealed ethnic differences in the prevalence of the poor metabolizer phenotype. Approximately 20% of Chinese and Japanese individuals are poor metabolizers (80), (81). More than five dysfunctional alleles with different ethnic distribution have been identified. No systematic studies on the ontogeny of this polymorphism are available.

THE CYTOCHROME P450 2C9 POLYMORPHISM

This enzyme is the major catalyst of the oxidation of phenytoin, many nonsteroidal anti-inflammatory drugs, tolbutamide, warfarin, and losartan (Table 4.9). Investigations of phenytoin kinetics at different pediatric ages have revealed a higher biotransformation rate in infants and small children than in adults (13). This gene harbors two major dysfunctional alleles, CYP2C9*2 and CYP2C9*3, of which the first is linked to the CYP2C8*3 allele (82). There is a dearth of information about the enzyme development and the pharmacogenetic ontogeny in the immediate postnatal period; however, adult activity is attained at about half a year of age. At 3 years of age the activity exceeds that of adult individuals.

THE CYTOCHROME P4503A SUBFAMILY

The members of this subfamily account for 30% of all cytochromes in the liver and more than 50% of cytochromes

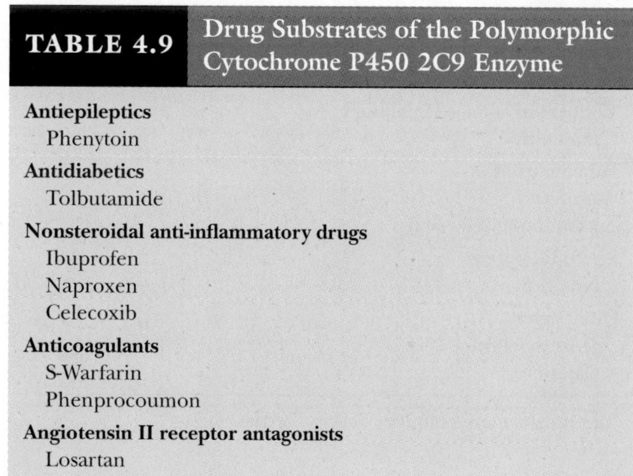

TABLE 4.9 Drug Substrates of the Polymorphic Cytochrome P450 2C9 Enzyme

Antiepileptics
Phenytoin
Antidiabetics
Tolbutamide
Nonsteroidal anti-inflammatory drugs
Ibuprofen
Naproxen
Celecoxib
Anticoagulants
S-Warfarin
Phenprocoumon
Angiotensin II receptor antagonists
Losartan

in the small intestine (83). The CYP3A enzymes are rather promiscuous and are involved in the metabolism of at least two thirds of commonly used drugs.

In adults the predominant form is CYP3A4 which is variably expressed (84–86), however, without any known relation to identified genetic polymorphisms. A large number of drug interactions take place at the level of CYP3A4.

CYP3A5 is under genetic control such that the CYP3A5*1 allele is highly expressed and observed in 10% to 30% of livers in Caucasian individuals (87).

CYP3A7 is the isoform that is predominantly expressed in embryonic tissue and fetal and newborn liver and is soon replaced by CYP3A4 after birth (88).

THE *N*-ACETYLTRANSFERASE POLYMORPHISM

Adult subjects are grouped into slow or rapid acetylators according to their capacity to acetylate isoniazid, sulfonamides, dapsone, and other drug substrates of this enzyme (Table 4.10). The frequency of slow acetylators varies widely among different ethnic groups, from 50% to 70% in whites to only 5% in Eskimos, and less than 25% in the Japanese population (89).

Divergent data on the maturation of the rapid acetylation trait have been published. The rapid acetylation phenotype is expressed when none or only one allele of the *N*-acetyltransferase 2 (NAT2) gene carries a mutation (90). This trait is also seen *in vitro* in adult liver enzyme preparations classified as slow and rapid acetylators, whereas no such dichotomy seems to be developed in the fetal NAT2 assay system with 7-aminoclonazepam as substrate (91).

These results are consistent with attempts to phenotype infants and children with caffeine as probe drug of the NAT2 enzyme (48). In this study of premature newborn infants and older infants it appeared that all individuals but one (the oldest) were slow acetylators, using an antimode of 0.4. The authors concluded that the *N*-acetyltransferase is immature and that caffeine acetylation phenotype cannot be determined with certainty in infants younger than 1 year of age.

The cumulative percentage of rapid acetylators with caffeine as substrate increases with age (92). The plateau was still not achieved at 15 months, as assessed by the 5-acetylamino-6-formylamino-3-methyluracil (AFMU)/1X and AFMU/(AFMU + 1U + 1X + 1,7U + 1,7X) ratios (1X, 1-methylxanthine; 1U, 1-methyluric acid; 1,7U, 1,7-dimethyluric acid; 1,7X, 1,7-dimethylxanthine). It was concluded that acetylation status cannot be determined with certainty before the age of 15 months.

Sulfadimidine has also been used as probe drug in phenotyping of the acetylation capacity (93). With this drug, a significantly higher proportion (83%) of newborn infants was classified as slow acetylators compared with adults (50%). This difference was partly ascribed to deficient dietary intake of pantotenic acid, which is required for coenzyme A in the reaction.

One may conclude that the slow phenotype predominates in newborn infants and infants during the first year. Slow postnatal maturation of the rapid acetylation phenotype may result in higher sensitivity in infants to pharmacologic and toxic effects of drugs that are substrates of the *N*-acetyltransferase 2 (Table 4.10). Uncritical dosing of these drugs may be a potential risk.

TABLE 4.10 Drug Substrates of the Polymorphic *N*-Acetyltransferase (NAT2) Enzyme

Cardiovascular agents
Procainamide
Hydralazine
Sulfonamides
Dapsone
Sulfasalazine
Sulfamethoxazole
Sulfadiazine
Sulfacetamide
Antihormones
Aminoglutethimide
Monoamine oxidase inhibitors
Phenelzine
Tuberculostatics
Isoniazid
p-Aminosalicylic acid
Benzodiazepines
Nitrazepam[a]
Other agents
p-Aminobenzoic acid
Caffeine[a]

[a]Biotransformed to amines before acetylation.

THIOPURINE METHYLTRANSFERASE

This enzyme metabolizing thiopurine drugs is clinically important in treatment of children with acute lymphoblastic leukemia (94), (95) and certain inflammatory disorders (96) as the genetic polymorphism may lead to negligible or severely compromised enzyme activity in one individual in 300. Eighty-nine percent of individuals have a normal enzyme activity which is important for the detoxication of the thiopurine prodrug 6-mercaptopurine (6-MPT). Eleven percent have an intermediate enzyme activity. If the thiopurine methyltransferase (TPMT) activity is compromised, patients treated with standard doses of 6-mercaptopurine are running a high risk of developing myelosuppression. Genotyping for TPMT is considered to be very cost-effective in the care of these patients. The TPMT phenotype may be measured in red blood cells.

5-URIDINE-DIPHOSPHO-GLUCURONOSYL TRANSFERASES

This large superfamily of conjugating enzymes comprises at least 10 different enzymes that catalyze the conjugation of drugs with glucuronic acid. UGTs catalyze the conjugation of bilirubin, sex hormones, and also many drugs including morphine, paracetamol, and so forth.

Decreased activity of UGT1 compromises the glucuronidation of bilirubin which is observed in patients with Crigler-Naijar or Gilbert syndrome (97). The famous chloramphenicol disaster was ascribed to serious adverse reactions caused by immature glucuronidation capacity in newborns.

POLYMORPHISM OF ATP-BINDING CASSETTE TRANSPORTERS

The ABC transporter proteins are significant determinants of absorption, distribution, and elimination of many drugs (98). The most well-known of these proteins is the P-glycoprotein (P-gp) which is encoded by the *ABCB1* (*MDR1*) gene. In the gastrointestinal tract it contributes to the chemical defense of the organism since many drugs are transported back into the gastrointestinal lumen by this transporter. A large number of drugs are substrates pf P-gp. They include several anticancer drugs, immunosuppressants, HIV1-protease inhibitors, glucocorticoids, and so forth.

A multitude of genetic polymorphisms have been described in the *ABCB1* gene, such as the C3435CT mutation in exon 26 (99), which is of relevance for the bioavailability of digoxin.

Other transporter protein genes of potential interest in pharmacogenetics/pharmacokinetics include the *SLCO1B1* gene encoding the hepatic uptake transporter organic anion-transporting polypeptide 1B1 (OATP1B1) (100) and the *ABCC2* gene encoding the efflux transporter multidrug resistance–associated protein 2 (MRP2) (101).

To date, relatively few pharmacological functional implications of these polymorphisms have been described. Clinical data from pediatric pharmacotherapy in respect of the genetic variation in these transporters are virtually absent. However, a recent publication (102) has described the influence of polymorphisms of the *ABCB1* gene on cyclosporine disposition in children. The authors reported an association between oral bioavailability of cyclosporine and two polymorphisms in this gene in children with end-stage renal disease. Carriers of variant alleles had an oral bioavailability almost 2-fold higher compared to patients without these variant alleles. Interestingly, this association was observed only in children older than 8 years of age, suggesting an age-dependent effect of these genetic polymorphisms.

The reasons for this age dependency are unclear. The oral bioavailability and prehepatic and hepatic extraction ratio are also dependent on drug metabolizing enzymes. The ontogenetic development of CYP3A4 and CYP3A5 enzymes acting on cyclosporine and other immunosuppressants may interact in a way to generate this age dependency.

Future research should also focus on the role of ABC transporter proteins in the blood–brain barrier which may relate in a clinically significant way to the CNS toxicity of certain drugs.

PHARMACOGENETICS AND ADVERSE DRUG REACTIONS AND TOXICITY

Pediatric pharmacogenetics aims to study the relation not only between genetic constitution and effects but also between genetics and adverse reactions and toxicity of drugs. The ultimate aim is to incorporate pharmacogenomic forecasting into the clinical routine to minimize the risk of under- or overtreatment.

The bone marrow toxicity of 6-mercaptopurine in children with leukemia with congenital deficiency in TPMT is an ample example of such an application (see above). Other examples include the cytochrome P4502C9 and vitamin K epoxide reductase (*VKORC1*) genes that determine some 50% of the variation in dose requirement of warfarin (103) and the HLA-B 5701 polymorphism which is highly predictive of serious reactions to the antiviral abacavir HIV drug (104).

In future, the above and many other adverse drug reactions with a genetic basis will certainly be possible to predict through pharmacogenetic forecasting.

CONCLUSION AND PERSPECTIVE

The maturation of organ function together with endogenous and environmental factors is the most important cause of variation in drug metabolism in infants and children. Genetic polymorphisms of drug-metabolizing enzymes give an additional dimension to the variation in duration and intensity of drug effects. The limited information about the functional maturation of polymorphic enzymes fuels an increasing interest in this field because this is clinically important in treatment with a variety of widely used drugs. Inasmuch as many of these drugs are used in infants and children, the phenotypic expression is of even greater interest in these groups because effects and side effects of drugs in children are often not possible to monitor by objective means. More information is needed to minimize the risk of therapeutic hazards in this age group. There are several apparent indications for therapeutic drug monitoring, genotyping, or phenotyping (Table 4.11) in clinical drug therapy. If an enzyme pathway is polymorphic and the drug to be used is for long-term treatment, if signs of toxicity are difficult to detect and monitor, or if effect parameters are not measurable by objective methods, phenotyping may help improve the tailoring of the dose according to the patient's need. Low therapeutic index, toxicity problems, and unexpected outcome of therapy are other potential indications for phenotyping. The complexity of the drug-metabolic pattern precludes any attempts to make generalizations from drug to drug. Therefore, we have to accept that safe and rational therapeutics must be founded on solid knowledge in the clinical pharmacology of each drug.

New solid documentation of drugs for children is highly needed. Blind use of agents with unknown behavior and

TABLE 4.11 Indications for Phenotyping

Children and Adults	*Additional Indications in Children*
Polymorphic pathway	Age-dependent kinetics
Long-term treatment	Subjective signs of toxicity
Low therapeutic index	Subjective effect parameters
Toxicity problems	
Unexpected outcome of therapy	
Unexpectedly low or high concentration per dose unit	
Drug–drug interactions	

effects in the pediatric patient does not increase our knowledge about their clinical pharmacology in the pediatric population. Therefore, the performance of controlled clinical studies in children is strongly recommended.

REFERENCES

1. Silverman W, Anderson D, Blanc W, et al. A difference in mortality rate and incidence of kernicterus among premature infants allotted to two prophylactic antibacterial regimens. *Pediatrics* 1956;18:614–621.
2. Weiss C, Glazco A, Weston J. Chloramphenicol in the newborn infant, a physiologic explanation of its toxicity when given in excessive dose. *N Engl J Med* 1960;262:787–794.
3. Rowland M, Benet LZ, Graham GG. Clearance concepts in pharmacokinetics. *J Pharmacokinet Biopharm* 1973;1(2):123–136.
4. Wilkinson GR, Shand DG. Commentary: a physiological approach to hepatic drug clearance. *Clin Pharmacol Ther* 1975; 18(4):377–390.
5. Rane A, Shand DG, Wilkinson GR. Disposition of carbamazepine and its 10,11-epoxide metabolite in the isolated perfused rat liver. *Drug Metab Dispos* 1977;5(2):179–184.
6. Wilkinson GR, Schenker S. Effects of liver disease on drug disposition in man. *Biochem Pharmacol* 1976;25(24):2675–2681.
7. Anderson BJ, Allegaert K, Holford NH. Population clinical pharmacology of children: general principles. *Eur J Pediatr* 2006; 165(11):741–746.
8. Pettersen G, Mouksassi MS, Theoret Y, et al. Population pharmacokinetics of intravenous pantoprazole in paediatric intensive care patients. *Br J Clin Pharmacol* 2009;67(2):216–227.
9. Toublanc N, Sargentini-Maier ML, Lacroix B, et al. Retrospective population pharmacokinetic analysis of levetiracetam in children and adolescents with epilepsy: dosing recommendations. *Clin Pharmacokinet* 2008;47(5):333–341.
10. Rane A, Bertilsson L, Palmér L. Disposition of placentally transferred carbamazepin (Tegretol). *Eur J Clin Pharmacol* 1975;8: 283–284.
11. Morselli PL, Principi N, Tognoni G, et al. Diazepam elimination in premature and full term infants, and children. *J Perinat Med* 1973;1(2):133–141.
12. Loughnan PM, Watters G, Aranda J, et al. Age-related changes in the pharmacokinetics of diphenylhydantoin (DPH) in the newborn and young infants: implication regarding treatment of neonatal convulsions. *Aust Paediatr J* 1976;12:204–205.
13. Eadie MJ, Tyrer JH, Bochner F, et al. The elimination of phenytoin in man. *Clin Exp Pharmacol Physiol* 1976;3(3):217–224.
14. Chiba K, Ishizaki T, Miura H, et al. Apparent Michaelis-Menten kinetic parameters of phenytoin in pediatric patients. *Pediatr Pharmacol* 1980;1:171–180.
15. Vaucher Y, Lightner ES, Walson PD. Theophylline poisoning. *J Pediatr* 1977;90(5):827–830.
16. Ellis EF, Koysooko R, Levy G. Pharmacokinetics of theophylline in children with asthma. *Pediatrics* 1976;58(4):542–547.
17. Aranda JV, Cook CE, Gorman W, et al. Pharmacokinetic profile of caffeine in the premature newborn infant with apnea. *J Pediatr* 1979;94(4):663–668.
18. Aranda JV, Sitar DS, Parsons WD, et al. Pharmacokinetic aspects of theophylline in premature newborns. *N Engl J Med* 1976; 295(8):413–416.
19. Parsons WD, Neims AH. Effect of cigarette smoking in caffeine elimination. *Clin Res* 1978;25:676A.
20. Pelkonen O, Karki NT. 3,4-Benzpyrene and aniline are hydroxylated by human fetal liver but not by placenta at 6-7 weeks of fetal age. *Biochem Pharmacol* 1973;22(12):1538–1540.
21. Lohmann SM, Miech RP. Theophylline metabolism by the rat liver microsomal system. *J Pharmacol Exp Ther* 1976;196(1):213–225.
22. Aldridge A, Parsons WD, Neims AH. Stimulation of caffeine metabolism in the rat by 3-methylcholanthrene. *Life Sci* 1977; 21(7):967–974.
23. Hyvarinen M, Zeltzer P, Oh W, et al. Influence of gestational age on serum levels of alpha-1 fetoprotein, IgG globulin, and albumin in newborn infants. *J Pediatr* 1973;82(3):430–437.
24. Wood M, Wood AJJ. Changes in plasma drug binding and a_1-acid glycoprotein in mother and newborn infant. *Clin Pharmacol Ther* 1981;29(4):522–526.
25. Rane A, Lunde P, Jalling B, et al. Plasma protein binding of diphenylhydantoin in normal and hyperblirubinemic infants. *J Pediatr* 1971;78(5):877–882.
26. Fredholm B, Rane A, Persson B. Diphenylhydantoin binding to proteins in plasma and its dependence on free fatty acid and bilirubin concentration in dogs and newborn infants. *Pediatr Res* 1975;9:26–30.
27. Pacifici GM, Taddeucci-Brunelli G, Rane A. Clonazepam serum protein binding during development. *Clin Pharmacol Ther* 1984; 35:354–359.
28. Jalling B, Boréus L, Rane A, Sjöqvist F. Plasma concentrations of diphenylhydantoin in young infants. *Pharmacologia Clinica* 1970; 2:200–202.
29. Weber WW, Cohen S. Aging effects and drugs in man. In: Gillette J, Mitchell J, eds. *Concepts in biochemical pharmacology*. New York, NY: Springer Verlag, 1975:213–233.
30. Gupta M, Brans YW. Gastric retention in neonates. *Pediatrics* 1978;62(1):26–29.
31. Hendeles L, Iafrate RP, Weinberger M. A clinical and pharmacokinetic basis for the selection and use of slow release theophylline products. *Clin Pharmacokinet* 1984;9(2):95–135.
32. Heimann G. Enteral absorption and bioavailability in children in relation to age. *Eur J Clin Pharmacol* 1980;18(1):43–50.
33. Yaffe SJ, Juchau M. Perinatal pharmacology. *Annu Rev Pharmacol* 1974;14:219–238.
34. Lebenthal E, Lee PC, Heitlinger LA. Impact of development of the gastrointestinal tract on infant feeding. *J Pediatr* 1983; 102(1):1–9.
35. Choonara IA, McKay P, Hain R, et al. Morphine metabolism in children. *Br J Clin Pharmacol* 1989;28:599–604.
36. Choonara I, Ekbom Y, Lindström B, et al. Morphine sulphation in children. *Br J Clin Pharmacol* 1990;30(6):897–900.
37. Levy G, Khanna NN, Soda DM, et al. Pharmacokinetics of acetaminophen in the human neonate: formation of acetaminophen glucuronide and sulfate in relation to plasma bilirubin concentration and D-glucaric acid excretion. *Pediatrics* 1975;55(6): 818–825.
38. Miller RP, Roberts RJ, Fischer LJ. Acetaminophen elimination kinetics in neonates, children, and adults. *Clin Pharmacol Ther* 1976;19(3):284–294.
39. Howie D, Adriaenssens PI, Prescott LF. Paracetamol metabolism following overdosage: application of high performance liquid chromatography. *J Pharm Pharmacol* 1977;29(4):235–237.
40. Rollins DE, von Bahr C, Glaumann H, et al. Acetaminophen: potentially toxic metabolite formed by human fetal and adult liver microsomes and isolated fetal liver cells. *Science* 1979; 205(4413):1414–1416.
41. Chen ZR, Irvine RJ, Somogyi AA, et al. Mu receptor binding of some commonly used opioids and their metabolites. *Life Sci* 1991;48(22):2165–2171.
42. Garrettson LK, Procknal JA, Levy G. Fetal acquisition and neonatal elimination of a large amount of salicylate. Study of a neonate whose mother regularly took therapeutic doses of aspirin during pregnancy. *Clin Pharmacol Ther* 1975;17(1): 98–103.
43. Vest M, Rossier R. Detoxification in the newborn: the ability of the newborn infant to form conjugates with glucuronic acid, glycine, acetate, and glutathione. *Ann N Y Acad Sci* 1963;111: 183–197.
44. Wichmann HM, Rind H, Gladtke E. The elimination of bromsulphalein in children. *Z Kinderheilkd* 1968;103(4):263–276.
45. Sereni F, Morselli PL, Pardi G. Postnatal development of drug metabolism in human infants. In: Bossart H, Cruz J, Huber A, Prodhom L, Sistek J, eds. *Perinatal medicine*. Bern: Hans Huber Publishers, 1972:63–67.
46. Bonati M, Latini R, Marra G, et al. Theophylline metabolism during the first month of life and development. *Pediatr Res* 1981; 15(4, pt 1):304–308.
47. Grygiel JJ, Birkett DJ. Effect of age on patterns of theophylline metabolism. *Clin Pharmacol Ther* 1980;28(4):456–462.
48. Carrier O, Pons G, Rey E, et al. Maturation of caffeine metabolic pathways in infancy. *Clin Pharmacol Ther* 1988;44(2):145–151.

49. West J, Smith H, Chasis H. Glomerular filtration rate, effective renal blood flow, and maximal tubular excretory capacity in infancy. *J Pediatr* 1948;32:10–18.
50. Morselli PL, Franco-Morselli R, Bossi L. Clinical pharmacokinetics in newborns and infants. Age-related differences and therapeutic implications. *Clin Pharmacokinet* 1980;5(6):485–527.
51. Guignard JP. Drugs and the neonatal kidney. *Dev Pharmacol Ther* 1982;4(Suppl):19–27.
52. Barnett H, McNamara H, Schultz S, et al. Renal clearance of sodium penicillin G, procaine penicillin G. *Pediatrics* 1949;3: 418–422.
53. Axline SG, Yaffe SJ, Simon HJ. Clinical pharmacology of antimicrobials in premature infants. II. Ampicillin, methicillin, oxacillin, neomycin, and colistin. *Pediatrics* 1967;39(1):97–107.
54. Nakazawa S, Satoh H, Narita A, et al. Evaluation on ceftriaxone administered intravenously in neonates. *Jpn J Antibiot* 1988;41(3): 225–235.
55. Iwai N, Nakamura H, Miyazu M, et al. Pharmacokinetic and clinical evaluations on ceftriaxone in neonates. *Jpn J Antibiot* 1988; 41(3):262–275.
56. Morselli PL, Assael BM, Gomeni R, et al. Digoxin pharmacokinetics during human development. In: Morselli PL, Garattini S, Sereni F, eds. *Basic and therapeutic aspects of perinatal pharmacology.* New York, NY: Raven Press, 1975:377–392.
57. Nyberg L, Wettrell G. Digoxin dosage schedules for neonates and infants based on pharmacokinetic considerations. *Clin Pharmacokinet* 1978;3(6):453–461.
58. Burg M, Stoner L, Cardinal J, et al. Furosemide effect on isolated perfused tubules. *Am J Physiol* 1973;225(1):119–124.
59. Mirochnick MH, Miceli JJ, Kramer PA, et al. Furosemide pharmacokinetics in very low birth weight infants. *J Pediatr* 1988; 112(4):653–657.
60. Braunlich H, Kersten L. Influence of diuretics on renal water and ion excretion in rats of different ages. IV. Excretion of sodium potassium, H-ions, ammonium, phosphates, calcium and chloride. *Acta Biol Med Ger* 1971;27(1):149–169.
61. Frenzel J, Braunlich H, Schramm D, et al. Renal effects of cyclopenthiazide in the newborn period. *Acta Paediatr Acad Sci Hung* 1974;15(2):157–164.
62. Dawson W. Relation between age and weight and dosage of drugs. *Ann Intern Med* 1940;13:1594–1615.
63. Gyllenswärd Å, Vahlqvist B. Läkemedelsdosering till barn. *Nord Med* 1948;40:2248–2261.
64. Meyer UA. Genotype or phenotype: the definition of pharmacogenetic polymorphisms. *Ann Rev Pharmacol Toxicol* 1991;1:66.
65. Mahgoub A, Idle J, Dring L, et al. Polymorphic hydroxylation of debrisoquine in man. *Lancet* 1977;2:584–586.
66. http://www.cypalleles.ki.se.
67. Johansson I, Lundqvist E, Bertilsson L, et al. Inherited amplification of an active gene in the cytochrome P450 CYP2D locus as a cause of ultrarapid metabolism of debrisoquine [see comments]. *Proc Natl Acad Sci U S A* 1993;90(24):11825–11829.
68. Alvan G, von Bahr C, Seidemann P, et al. High plasma concentrations of beta-receptor blocking drugs and deficient debrisoquine hydroxylation. *Lancet* 1982;1(8267):333.
69. Dayer P, Kubli A, Kupfer A, et al. Defective hydroxylation of bufuralol associated with side-effects of the drug in poor metabolisers. *Br J Clin Pharmacol* 1982;13(5):750–752.
70. Lennard MS, Jackson PR, Freestone S, et al. The relationship between debrisoquine oxidation phenotype and the pharmacokinetics and pharmacodynamics of propranolol. *Br J Clin Pharmacol* 1984;17(6):679–685.
71. Bertilsson L, Eichelbaum M, Mellstrom B, et al. Nortriptyline and antipyrine clearance in relation to debrisoquine hydroxylation in man. *Life Sci* 1980;27(18):1673–1677.
72. Scordo MG, Spina E. Cytochrome P450 polymorphisms and response to antipsychotic therapy. *Pharmacogenomics* 2002;3(2): 201–218.
73. Mortimer O, Lindstrom B, Laurell H, et al. Dextromethorphan: polymorphic serum pattern of the O-demethylated and didemethylated metabolites in man. *Br J Clin Pharmacol* 1989; 27(2):223–227.
74. Rane A, Modiri AR, Gerdin E. Ethylmorphine O-deethylation cosegregates with the debrisoquin genetic metabolic polymorphism. *Clin Pharmacol Ther* 1992;52(3):257–264.
75. Yue QY, Svensson JO, Alm C, et al. Codeine O-demethylation cosegregates with polymorphic debrisoquine hydroxylation. *Br J Clin Pharmacol* 1989;28(6):639–645.
76. Ladona MG, Lindstrom B, Thyr C, et al. Differential foetal development of the O- and N-demethylation of codeine and dextromethorphan in man. *Br J Clin Pharmacol* 1991;32(3):295–302.
77. Treluyer JM, Jacqz-Aigrain E, Alvarez F, et al. Expression of CYP2D6 in developing human liver. *Eur J Biochem* 1991;202(2): 583–588.
78. Evans WE, Relling MV, Petros WP, et al. Dextromethorphan and caffeine as probes for simultaneous determination of debrisoquin-oxidation and N-acetylation phenotypes in children. *Clin Pharmacol Ther.* 1989;45(5):568–573.
79. Kupfer A, Preisig R. Pharmacogenetics of mephenytoin: a new drug hydroxylation polymorphism in man. *Eur J Clin Pharmacol* 1984;26(6):753–759.
80. Wilkinson GR, Guengerich F, Branch R. Genetic polymorphism of S-mephenytoin hydroxylation. In: Kalow W, ed. *Pharmacogenetics of drug metabolism.* New York, NY: Pergamon Press, 1992:657–685.
81. Bertilsson L. Ethnic differences in drug disposition. In: Breimer DD, Crommelin DJA, Midha KK, eds. *Topics in pharmaceutical sciences.* Amsterdam: Amsterdam Medical Press, 1989:555–561.
82. Yasar U, Lundgren S, Eliasson E, et al. Linkage between the CYP2C8 and CYP2C9 genetic polymorphisms. *Biochem Biophys Res Commun* 2002;299(1):25–28.
83. Paine MF, Khalighi M, Fisher JM, et al. Characterization of interintestinal and intraintestinal variations in human CYP3A-dependent metabolism. *J Pharmacol Exp Ther* 1997;283(3): 1552–1562.
84. Wacher VJ, Silverman JA, Zhang Y, et al. Role of P-glycoprotein and cytochrome P450 3A in limiting oral absorption of peptides and peptidomimetics. *J Pharm Sci* 1998;87(11):1322–1330.
85. Koch I, Weil R, Wolbold R, et al. Interindividual variability and tissue-specificity in the expression of cytochrome P450 3A mRNA. *Drug Metab Dispos* 2002;30(10):1108–1114.
86. Lown KS, Mayo RR, Leichtman AB, et al. Role of intestinal P-glycoprotein (mdr1) in interpatient variation in the oral bioavailability of cyclosporine. *Clin Pharmacol Ther* 1997;62(3): 248–260.
87. Paulussen A, Lavrijsen K, Bohets H, et al. Two linked mutations in transcriptional regulatory elements of the CYP3A5 gene constitute the major genetic determinant of polymorphic activity in humans. *Pharmacogenetics* 2000;10(5):415–424.
88. Lacroix D, Sonnier M, Moncion A, et al. Expression of CYP3A in the human liver—evidence that the shift between CYP3A7 and CYP3A4 occurs immediately after birth. *Eur J Biochem* 1997; 247(2):625–634.
89. Price-Evans D. In: Kalow W, ed. *N-acetyltransferase; pharmacogenetics of drug metabolism.* New York, NY: Pergamon Press, 1992: 95–178.
90. Smith CA, Wadelius M, Gough AC, et al. A simplified assay for the arylamine N-acetyltransferase 2 polymorphism validated by phenotyping with isoniazid. *J Med Genet* 1997;34(9):758–760.
91. Peng DR, Birgersson C, von Bahr C, et al. Polymorphic acetylation of 7-amino-clonazepam in human liver cytosol. *Pediatr Pharmacol (New York)* 1984;4(3):155–159.
92. Pariente-Khayat A, Pons G, Rey E, et al. Caffeine acetylator phenotyping during maturation in infants. *Pediatr Res* 1991;29(5): 492–495.
93. Szorady I, Santa A, Veress I. Drug acetylator phenotypes in newborn infants. *Biol Res Pregnancy Perinatol* 1987;8(1 1ST Half):23–25.
94. Lennard L, Lilleyman JS, Van Loon J, et al. Genetic variation in response to 6-mercaptopurine for childhood acute lymphoblastic leukaemia. *Lancet* 1990;336(8709):225–229.
95. Dervieux T, Medard Y, Verpillat P, et al. Possible implication of thiopurine S-methyltransferase in occurrence of infectious episodes during maintenance therapy for childhood lymphoblastic leukemia with mercaptopurine. *Leukemia* 2001;15(11):1706–1712.
96. Colombel JF, Ferrari N, Debuysere H, et al. Genotypic analysis of thiopurine S-methyltransferase in patients with Crohn's disease and severe myelosuppression during azathioprine therapy. *Gastroenterology* 2000;118(6):1025–1030.
97. Mackenzie PI, Miners JO, McKinnon RA. Polymorphisms in UDP glucuronosyltransferase genes: functional consequences and clinical relevance. *Clin Chem Lab Med* 2000;38(9):889–892.

98. Tanigawara Y. Role of P-glycoprotein in drug disposition. *Therc Drug Monit* 2000;22(1):137–140.
99. Hoffmeyer S, Burk O, von Richter O, et al. Functional polymorphisms of the human multidrug-resistance gene: multiple sequence variations and correlation of one allele with P-glycoprotein expression and activity in vivo. *Proc Natl Acad Sci U S A* 2000;97(7):3473–3478.
100. Niemi M, Schaeffeler E, Lang T, et al. High plasma pravastatin concentrations are associated with single nucleotide polymorphisms and haplotypes of organic anion transporting polypeptide-C (OATP-C, SLCO1B1). *Pharmacogenetics* 2004;14(7):429–440.
101. Niemi M, Arnold KA, Backman JT, et al. Association of genetic polymorphism in ABCC2 with hepatic multidrug resistance-associated protein 2 expression and pravastatin pharmacokinetics. *Pharmacogenet Genomics* 2006;16(11):801–808.
102. Fanta S, Niemi M, Jonsson S, et al. Pharmacogenetics of cyclosporine in children suggests an age-dependent influence of ABCB1 polymorphisms. *Pharmacogenet Genomics* 2008;18(2):77–90.
103. Wadelius M, Chen LY, Lindh JD, et al. The largest prospective warfarin-treated cohort supports genetic forecasting. *Blood* 2009; 113(4):784–792.
104. Mallal S, Phillips E, Carosi G, et al. HLA-B*5701 screening for hypersensitivity to abacavir. *N Engl J Med* 2008;358(6):568–579.
105. Krauer B, Draffan GH, Williams FM, et al. Elimination kinetics of amobarbital in mothers and their newborn infants. *Clin Pharmacol Ther* 1973;14(3):442–447.
106. Moore RG, Thomas J, Triggs EJ, et al. The pharmacokinetics and metabolism of the anilide local anaesthetics in neonates. III. Mepivacaine. *Eur J Clin Pharmacol* 1978;14(3):203–212.
107. Butler T, Mahafee C, Wadell W. Phenobarbital: studies on elimination, accumulation tolerance, and dosage schedules. *J Pharmacol Exp Ther* 1954;111:425–435.
108. Garrettson LK, Dayton PG. Disappearance of phenobarbital and diphenylhydantoin from serum of children. *Clin Pharmacol Ther* 1970;11(5):674–679.
109. Heinze E, Kampffmeyer HG. Biological half-life of phenobarbital in human babies. *Klin Wochenschr* 1971;49(20):1146–1147.
110. Jalling B. Plasma and cerebrospinal fluid concentrations of phenobarbital in infants given single doses. *Dev Med Child Neurol* 1976; 16:781–793.
111. Lous P. Blood serum and cerebrospinal fluid levels and renal clearance of phenemal in treated epileptics. *Acta Pharmacol* 1954;10:261–280.
112. Minagawa K, Miura H, Chiba K, et al. Pharmacokinetics and relative bioavailability of intramuscular phenobarbital sodium or acid in infants. *Pediatr Pharmacol* 1981;1:279–289.
113. Wilson JT, Wilkinson GR. Chronic and severe phenobarbital intoxication in a child treated with primidone and diphenylhydantoin. *J Pediatr* 1973;83(3):484–489.
114. Rane A, Garle M, Borg O, et al. Plasma disappearance of transplacentally transferred diphenylhydantoin in the newborn studied by mass fragmentography. *Clin Pharmacol Ther* 1974; 15(1):39–45.
115. Nitowsky HM, Matz L, Berzofsky JA. Studies on oxidative drug metabolism in the full-term newborn infant. *J Pediatr* 1966; 69(6):1139–1149.
116. Caldwell J, Wakile L, Notarianni L, et al. Maternal and neonatal disposition of pethidine in childbirth—A study using quantitative gas chromatography-mass spectrometry. *Life Sci* 1978;22(7): 589–596.
117. Tomson G, Garle M, Thalme B, et al. Maternal kinetics and placental passage of pethidine during labour. *Br J Clin Pharmacol* 1981;13:653–659.
118. Sjoqvist F, Bergfors PG, Borga O, et al. Plasma disappearance of nortriptyline in a newborn infant following placental transfer from an intoxicated mother: evidence for drug metabolism. *J Pediatr* 1972;80(3):496–500.
119. Dahlstrom B, Bolme P, Feychting H, et al. Morphine kinetics in children. *Clin Pharmacol Ther* 1979;26(3):354–365.
120. Mihaly GW, Moore RG, Thomas J, et al. The pharmacokinetics and metabolism of the anilide local anaesthetics in neonates. I. Lignocaine. *Eur J Clin Pharmacol* 1978;13(2):143–152.
121. Wilson JT, Atwood GF, Shand DG. Disposition of propoxyphene and propranolol in children. *Clin Pharmacol Ther* 1976;19(3): 264–270.
122. Reinicke C, Rogner G, Frenzel J, et al. Die Wirkung von Phenylbutazon und Phenobarbital auf die Amidopyrin-Elimination, die Bilrubin-Gesamt-konzentration im Serum und einige Blutgerinnungsfaktoren bei neugeborenen Kindern. *Pharmacologia Clinica* 1970;2:167–172.
123. Caldwell J, Mofatt J, Smith R. Pharmacokinetics of bupivacaine administered epidurally during childbirth. *Br J Clin Pharmacol* 1976;3:956–957.
124. Aranda JV, Perez J, Sitar DS, et al. Pharmacokinetic disposition and protein binding of furosemide in newborn infants. *J Pediatr* 1978;93(3):507–511.
125. Cutler RE, Forrey AW, Christopher TG, et al. Pharmacokinetics of furosemide in normal subjects and functionally anephric patients. *Clin Pharmacol Ther* 1974;15(6):588–596.
126. Peterson RG, Simmons MA, Rumack BH, et al. Pharmacology of furosemide in the premature newborn infant. *J Pediatr* 1980; 97(1):139–143.
127. Ohman I, Vitols S, Tomson T. Pharmacokinetics of gabapentin during delivery, in the neonatal period, and lactation: Does a fetal accumulation occur during pregnancy? *Epilepsia* 2005;46(10): 1621–1624.
128. Tallian KB, Nahata MC, Lo W, et al. Pharmacokinetics of gabapentin in paediatric patients with uncontrolled seizures. *J Clin Pharm Ther.* 2004;29(6):511–515.
129. Traeger A, Noschel H, Zaumseil J. Pharmacokinetics of indomethacin in pregnant and parturient women and in their newborn infants. *Zentralbl Gynakol* 1973;95(1):635–641.
130. Glauser TA, Mitchell WG, Weinstock A, et al. Pharmacokinetics of levetiracetam in infants and young children with epilepsy. *Epilepsia* 2007;48(6):1117–1122.
131. Tomson G, Lunell NO, Sundwall A, et al. Placental passage of oxazepam and its metabolism in mother and newborn. *Clin Pharmacol Ther* 1979;25(1):74–81.
132. Otani K, Kaneko S, Shimada S, et al. The pharmacokinetics of primidone during pregnancy. In: Sato T, Shinagawa S, eds. *Antiepileptic drugs and pregnancy.* Tokyo: Excerpta Medica, 1984: 33–37.
133. Morselli PL. *Drug disposition during development.* New York, NY: Spectrum, 1977.
134. Gladtke E. Pharmacokinetic studies on phenylbutazone in children. *Farmaco Sci* 1968;23(10):897–906.
135. Gugler R, von Unruh GE. Clinical pharmacokinetics of valproic acid. *Clin Pharmacokinet* 1980;5(1):67–83.
136. Ishizaki T, Yokochi K, Chiba K, et al. Placental transfer of anticonvulsants (phenobarbital, phenytoin, valproic acid) and the elimination from neonates. *Pediatr Pharmacol* 1981; 1:291–303.
137. Nau H, Helge H, Luck W. Valproic acid in the perinatal period: decreased maternal serum protein binding results in fetal accumulation and neonatal displacement of the drug and some metabolites. *J Pediatr* 1984;104(4):627–634.
138. Hamar C, Levy G. Factors affecting the serum protein binding of salicylic acid in newborn infants and their mothers. *Pediatr Pharmacol (New York)* 1980;1(1):31–43.
139. Hamar C, Levy G. Serum protein binding of drugs and bilirubin in newborn infants and their mothers. *Clin Pharmacol Ther* 1980;28(1):58–63.
140. Herngren L, Ehrnebo M, Boreus LO. Drug distribution in whole blood of mothers and their newborn infants: studies of cloxacillin and flucloxacillin. *Eur J Clin Pharmacol* 1982;22(4): 351–358.
141. Svensmark O, Buchtal F. Diphenylhydantoin and phenobarbital: serum levels in children. *Am J Dis Child* 1964;108:82–87.
142. Sherwin A, Robb P. Ethosuximide: relation of plasma levels to clinical control. In: Woodbury D, Penry J, Schmidt R, eds. *Antiepileptic drugs.* New York, NY: Raven Press, 1972: 443–448.
143. Rane A. The role of drug metabolism in therapeutic drug monitoring (TDM). Pediatric aspects. In: Tanaka K, Mimaki T, Walson PD, et al., eds. *Advances in therapeutic drug monitoring.* Tokyo: Enterprise, 1990:359.
144. Muchohi SN, Obiero K, Newton CR, et al. Pharmacokinetics and clinical efficacy of lorazepam in children with severe malaria and convulsions. *Br J Clin Pharmacol* 2008;65(1): 12–21.

145. Ahrens R, Hendeles L, Weinburger M. The clinical pharmacology of drugs used in treatment of asthma. In: Yaffe SJ, ed. *Pediatric pharmacology*. New York, NY: Grund & Stratton, 1980:233–280.
146. Watson WT, Simons KJ, Simons FE. Pharmacokinetics of enprofylline administered intravenously and as a sustained-release tablet at steady state in children with asthma. *J Pediatr* 1988; 112(4):658–662.
147. Evans WE, Crom WR, Sinkule JA, et al. Pharmacokinetics of anticancer drugs in children. *Drug Metab Rev* 1983;14(5):847–886.
148. Battino D, Croci D, Rossini A, et al. Topiramate pharmacokinetics in children and adults with epilepsy: a case-matched comparison based on therapeutic drug monitoring data. *Clin Pharmacokinet* 2005;44(4):407–416.
149. Morselli PL, Bianchetti G, Dugas M. Therapeutic drug monitoring of psychotropic drugs in children. *Pediatr Pharmacol (New York)* 1983;3(3–4):149–156.
150. Rivera-Calimlim L, Griesbach PH, Perlmutter R. Plasma chlorpromazine concentrations in children with behavioral disorders and mental illness. *Clin Pharmacol Ther* 1979;26(1):114–121.
151. Kalow W, Genest K. A method for the detection ofatypical forms of human serum cholinesterase. Determination of dibucaine numbers. *Can J Biochem Physiol* 1957;35:339–346.
152. Price-Evans D, Manley K, McKusick V. Genetic control of isoniazid metabolism in man. *Br Med J* 1960;2:485–491.
153. Ariyoshi N, Miyazaki M, Toide K, et al. A single nucleotide polymorphism of CYP2b6 found in Japanese enhances catalytic activity by autoactivation. *Biochem Biophys Res Commun* 2001;281(5): 1256–1260.
154. Ehrnebo M, Agurell S, Jalling B, et al. Age differences in drug binding by plasma proteins: studies on human foetuses, neonates and adults. *Eur J Clin Pharmacol* 1971;3(4):189–193.
155. Krasner J, Giacoia GP, Yaffe SJ. Drug-protein binding in the newborn infant. *Ann N Y Acad Sci* 1973;226:101–114.
156. Boréus L, Jalling B, Kållberg N. Clinical pharmacology of phenobarbital in the neonatal period. In: Morselli PL, Garattini S, Sereni F, eds. *Basic and Therapeutic Aspects of the Perinatal Pharmacology*. New York, NY: Raven Press, 1975:331–340.
157. Short CR, Sexton RL, McFarland K. Binding of 14-C-salicylic acid and 14-C-pentobarbital to plasma proteins of several species during the perinatal period. *Biol Neonate* 1975;26(1–2): 58–66.
158. Sereni F, Perletti L, Marubini E, et al. Pharmacokinetic studies with a long-acting sulfonamide in subjects of different ages. A modern approach to drug dosage problems in developmental pharmacology. *Pediatr Res* 1968;2(1):29–37.
159. Ganshorn A, Kurz H. [Differences between the protein binding of newborns and adults and their importance for pharmacological action]. *Naunyn Schmiedebergs Arch Exp Pathol Pharmakol.* 1968; 260(2):117–118.
160. Kanto J, Erkkola R, Sellman R. Letter: Perinatal metabolism of diazepam. *Br Med J* 1974;1(908):641–642.
161. Pruitt AW, Dayton PG. A comparison of the binding of drugs to adult and cord plasma. *Eur J Clin Pharmacol* 1971;4(1):59–62.
162. Rane A, Lunde PKM, Jalling B, et al. Plasma protein binding of diphenylhydantoin in normal and hyperbilirubinemic infants. *J Pediatr* 1971;78:877–882.

CHAPTER

5

J. Steven Leeder

Pharmacogenetics, Pharmacogenomics, and Pharmacoproteomics

INTRODUCTION

It is readily accepted that genetic factors play an important role in influencing a child's potential physical characteristics such as height, weight, or hair color. Genetic factors are also important (although not sole) determinants of inter- and intraindividual variability in susceptibility to pediatric diseases as well as in the disposition of and response to medications used to treat those diseases. Pharmacotherapy in adults has benefited from knowledge of pharmacogenetic principles acquired over the past 50 to 60 years, but application to pediatric therapeutics is still in its infancy. On April 14, 2003, the International Human Genome Sequencing Consortium announced successful completion of the Human Genome Project initiated in 1990, 2 years after being presented in draft form (1). There is considerable hope that morbidity and mortality will be decreased through the development of more effective strategies to diagnose, treat, and prevent human disease, and society has every right to expect that children and adults will benefit equally from this investment of public funds. However, children present unique challenges in this context since developmental changes in drug disposition and response are superimposed upon a basal level of pharmacogenetic variability. The purpose of this chapter is to introduce the concepts of pharmacogenetics, pharmacogenomics, and pharmacoproteomics (and other "-omic" fields of endeavor spawned in the genome era) in the context of the changes in growth and development characteristic of the pediatric population.

HISTORICAL CONSIDERATIONS

In 1841, Alexander Ure reported that hippuric acid was formed from benzoic acid in the body leading physiological chemists to discover that many foreign substances excreted by humans were chemically altered relative to the forms that had been administered—the process we now refer to as drug biotransformation (or less properly, drug metabolism). At the beginning of the 20th century, Archibald Garrod proposed that enzymes were implicated in the detoxification of foreign substances. A key element of his later work was the concept that disproportionate responses to foreign substances could result from deficiency of the required detoxifying enzyme. A variation in the theme of altered responses to foreign substances (*xenobiotics*) became apparent with the synthesis of phenylthiocarbamide in 1931 when, in the process searching out artificial sweeteners, A. L. Fox discovered that some people found the chemical intensely bitter whereas others found it tasteless (2). It was not until the 1950s, however, that certain adverse drug reactions, such as unusually prolonged respiratory muscle paralysis due to succinylcholine, hemolysis associated with antimalarial therapy, and isoniazid-induced neurotoxicity, were recognized to be a consequence of inherited variation in enzyme activities as reviewed by Arno Motulsky in 1957 (3).

In 1959, Fridriech Vogel coined the term *pharmacogenetics* to describe the study of genetically determined variations in drug response and the first book on the subject was published in 1962 by Werner Kalow (4). Through a series of twin studies conducted during the late 1960s and early 1970s, Elliott Vesell illustrated the importance of genetic variation in drug disposition by observing that the half-lives of several drugs were more similar in monozygotic twins than in dizygotic twins (5). With the discovery of the debrisoquine/sparteine hydroxylase polymorphism (6,7), due to inherited defects in the cytochrome P450 2D6 gene (*CYP2D6*), and mephenytoin hydroxylase deficiency (*CYP2C19*) (8) in the late 1970s and early 1980s, the importance of genetic polymorphisms in drug-metabolizing enzymes has become increasingly apparent. This is particularly true in recent years due to an enhanced awareness of the number of clinically useful drugs that are metabolized by polymorphically expressed enzymes and the proportion of treated patients who are affected.

In the 1970s, an increasing appreciation of genetic influences on variability in drug disposition and response was accompanied by heightened awareness that environmental factors (e.g., diet, smoking status, and concomitant drug or toxicant exposure), physiologic variables (e.g., age, gender, disease, and pregnancy), and patient compliance also played important roles. Advances in analytic tools to accurately measure drugs and drug metabolites in biological fluids and the development of mathematical models to characterize and predict changes in drug concentration over time (*pharmacokinetics*) led to the application of pharmacokinetic principles to optimize drug therapy in individual patients. Introduction of *therapeutic drug monitoring* programs was the first application of personalized medicine—recognition that all patients were unique and that utilizing serum concentration–time data for an individual patient theoretically could be used to optimize pharmacotherapy was a significant advance over the concept of "one dose fits all." However, routine therapeutic drug monitoring does not necessarily translate to improved patient outcome in all situations (9).

At a molecular level, the pharmacokinetic properties of a drug are determined by the genes that control its disposition in the body (e.g., absorption, distribution, metabolism, and excretion) with drug-metabolizing enzymes and drug transporters assuming particularly important roles. Over the past 25 years, the functional consequences of genetic variation in several drug-metabolizing enzymes have been described in subjects representative of different ethnic groups (10). Whereas the most common clinical

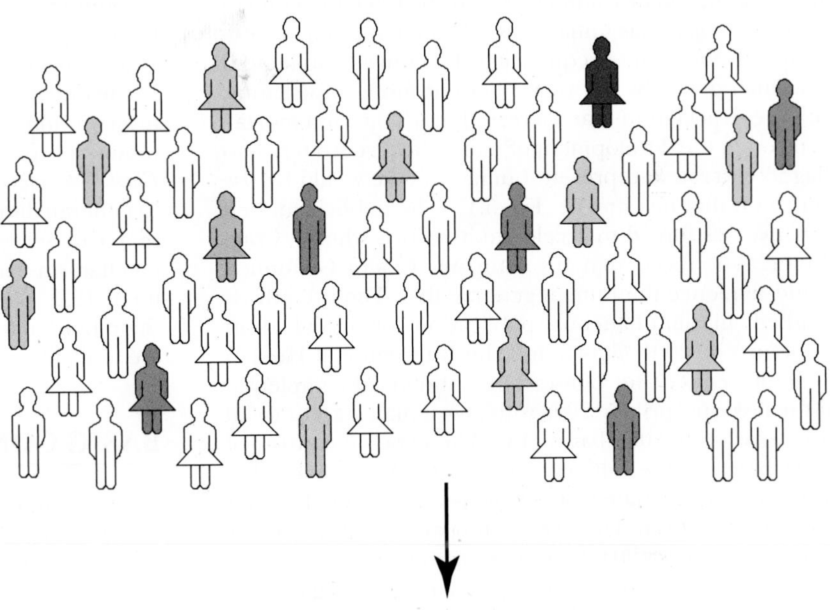

Figure 5.1. The promise of genomic medicine to human health and disease. The goal of personalized medicine will be achieved by identifying subgroups of patients who will respond favorably to a given drug with a minimum of side effects, as well as those who will not respond or who will show excessive toxicity with standard doses. A further benefit of pharmacogenomics will be the ability to select the most appropriate alternative drug for those patients who fail treatment with conventional drugs and doses.

manifestation of pharmacogenetic variability in drug biotransformation is an increased risk of concentration-dependent toxicity due to reduced clearance and drug accumulation, it has become more apparent in recent years that the concentration–effect relationship (*pharmacodynamics*) is more relevant for optimizing drug efficacy. Therefore, the pharmacogenetics of drug receptors and other target proteins involved in signal transduction or disease pathogenesis can also be expected to contribute significantly to interindividual variability in drug response (11,12). However, the most important concept is that the pharmacogenetic determinants of drug response involve multiple genes and therefore, for a particular individual, polymorphisms in a single gene are unlikely to be predictive of response.

In 1987, the term "*genomics*" was introduced to describe the study of the structure and function of the entire complement of genetic material—the genome—including chromosomes, genes, and DNA (13). In 1990, the Human Genome Project was initiated as a $3 billion public investment with the goal of sequencing the entire complement of human genes by the year 2005 but more importantly, with the expectation that decreased morbidity and mortality through the development of more effective strategies to diagnose, treat, and prevent human disease would be the return on that investment (Fig. 5.1). The publicly funded initiative was forced to accelerate its efforts when J. Craig Venter announced that his company, Celera Genomics, would sequence the human genome first. The two efforts resulted in simultaneous publication of initial draft sequences in 2001 (1,14), and the International Human Genome Sequencing Consortium announced completion of the task on April 15, 2003 with an estimated accuracy of one error in 100,000 bases (15). The genome consists of 3 gigabases (three billion bases) of DNA sequence that code for approximately 30,000 genes, far fewer than was originally expected. However, it appears that this number of genes encodes 100,000 proteins through the process of *alternative splicing* whereby a gene's *exons* or coding regions are spliced together in different ways to produce variant mRNA molecules that are translated into different proteins or isoforms of the same protein. Thus, the vast amounts of genomic data generated by the Human Genome Project have laid the foundation for an "-omic" revolution that includes, but is not limited to, the *transcriptome*, the set of expressed genes from a genome (16,17), the *proteome*, the set of proteins encoded by the genome (18), and the *physiome*, in which biochemical, biophysical, and anatomic information from cells, tissues, and organs will be integrated using computational methods to provide a model of the human body (19). Metabolomics and metabonomics are related terms that are sometimes used interchangeably in the literature. *Metabolomics* refers to the complete set of low–molecular-weight molecules (metabolites) present in a living system (cell, tissue, organ, or organism) at a particular developmental or pathological state. *Metabonomics* has been defined as the study of how the metabolic profile of biological systems changes in response to perturbations due to pathophysiologic stimuli, toxic exposures, dietary changes, among others (20,21). *Pharmacometabonomics* has been defined as "the prediction of the outcome, efficacy or toxicity, of a drug or xenobiotic intervention in an individual based on a mathematical model of preintervention metabolite signatures" (22), *Chemogenomics* is the application of combinatorial chemistry to generate libraries of small molecular weight compounds that can serve both as probes to investigate biological mechanisms and as lead compounds for drug development (23). Several resources that define these fields and their potential application to human health and disease are available on the Internet (Table 5.1).

BASIC CONCEPTS AND DEFINITIONS

Genetic variability results from gene mutation and the exchange of genetic information between chromosomes that occurs during meiosis. With the exception of sex-linked genes (genes occurring on the X or Y chromosomes), every individual carries two copies of each gene he or she

TABLE 5.1 Internet Resources for Pharmacogenetics and Pharmacogenomics

Introduction to pharmacogenomics	
http://www.ornl.gov/TechResources/Human_Genome/medicine/pharma.html	
http://www.ncbi.nlm.nih.gov/About/primer/pharm.html	
http://learn.genetics.utah.edu/content/health/pharma/	
http://www.pharmgkb.org/	
Pharmacogenetics: allelic variants of drug-metabolizing enzymes	
CYP2C9	http://www.imm.ki.se/CYPalleles/cyp2c9.htm
CYP2C19	http://www.imm.ki.se/CYPalleles/cyp2c19.htm
CYP2D6	http://www.imm.ki.se/CYPalleles/cyp2d6.htm
CYP3A4	http://www.imm.ki.se/CYPalleles/cyp3a4.htm
CYP3A5	http://www.imm.ki.se/CYPalleles/cyp3a5.htm
UGTs	http://som.flinders.edu.au/FUSA/ClinPharm/UGT/allele_table.html
NAT1 and NAT2	http://www.louisville.edu/medschool/pharmacology/NAT.html
Pharmacogenetics: substrates of drug-metabolizing enzymes	
http://medicine.iupui.edu/flockhart/	

Note: All sites were accessible on August 26, 2009. CYP, Cytochrome P450; UGTs, glucuronosyl transferases; NATs, *N*-acetyltransferases.

possesses. All copies of a specific gene present within a population may not have identical nucleotide sequences and these genetic *polymorphisms* contribute to the variability observed in that population. The presence of different nucleotides at a given position within a gene is called a *single nucleotide polymorphism* or "SNP" and SNPs are rapidly becoming an important component of the genomics lexicon. More recently, focus has shifted to characterizing *haplotypes*, collections of SNPs, and other allelic variations that are located close to each other and inherited together; creating a catalogue of haplotypes or "HapMap" is also a goal of the Human Genome Project (24). In genes where polymorphisms have been detected, alternative forms of the gene are called *alleles*. When the alleles at a particular gene locus are identical, a *homozygous* state exists whereas the term "*heterozygous*" refers to the situation in which different alleles are present at the same gene locus. The term *genotype* refers to an individual's genetic constitution while the observable characteristics or physical manifestations constitute the *phenotype*, which is the net consequence of genetic and environmental effects.

Human genetic variation can take many forms but is broadly divided into two general classes of variation: single nucleotide variations and *structural variations*. SNPs are the most prevalent class of genetic variation, and it has been estimated that there are approximately 11 million SNPs in the human genome. Structural variations encompass all differences in DNA sequence that involve more than one nucleotide. Insertions–deletions variants (*indels*) occur when a contiguous set of one or more nucleotides is absent in some individuals and present in others. *Block substitutions* involve variation of a string of contiguous nucleotides (or "block") that differs between two genomes. Sequence *inversions* occur when the order of an entire block of nucleotides is reversed in a specific region of the genome. Finally, *copy number variations* (CNVs) refer to the deletion or duplication of identical or near-identical DNA sequences that may be thousands to millions of bases in size. Although they occur less frequently than SNPs, structural variations may constitute 0.5% to 1% of an individual's genome and thus are the subject of intensive investigation for their contribution to phenotypic variation (25,26).

Pharmacogenetics, the study of the role of genetic factors in drug disposition, response, and toxicity, essentially relates allelic variation in human genes to variability in drug responses at the level of the individual patient. In other words, the promise of pharmacogenetics is to identify the right drug for the right patient. The field of pharmacogenetics classically has focused on the phenotypic consequences of allelic variation in single genes but often in the past, there was confusion between genotypic and phenotypic definitions of "polymorphism," and thus a need to clarify the relationship between genetic concepts and the clinical relevance of a given phenotype. In 1991, Meyer proposed that *pharmacogenetic polymorphism* be defined as a monogenic trait caused by the presence in the same population of more than one allele at the same locus and more than one phenotype in regard to drug interaction with the organism. The frequency of the least common allele should be at least 1% (27). According to this definition, the key elements of pharmacogenetic polymorphisms are heritability, the involvement of a single gene locus, and the fact that distinct phenotypes are observed within the population *only after drug challenge*.

The vast majority of our current understanding of pharmacogenetic polymorphisms involves enzymes responsible for drug biotransformation. Clinically, individuals are classified as being "fast," "rapid" or "extensive" metabolizers at one end of the spectrum, and "slow" or "poor" metabolizers at the other end of a continuum that may, depending on the particular enzyme, also include an intermediate metabolizer group. *Pediatric pharmacogenetics* involves an added measure of complexity since fetuses and newborns may be phenotypically "slow" or "poor" metabolizers for certain drug-metabolizing pathways, acquiring a phenotype consistent with their genotype at some point later in the developmental process as those pathways mature [e.g., glucuronidation, some cytochrome P450 activities (28–30)].

Although some authors use the terms "pharmacogenetics" and "pharmacogenomics" interchangeably, the latter term represents the marriage of pharmacology with genomics and is therefore considerably broader in scope. *Pharmacogenomics* can be defined as the study of the genome-wide response to small molecular weight compounds administered with therapeutic intent—finding the right drug for the right disease. *Proteomics* represents the systematic investigation of qualitative and quantitative changes in protein expression in a cell or tissue in response to disease or disease treatment. In this context, *pharmacoproteomics* involves characterizing the response of the proteome to therapeutic agents. Similarly, *toxicogenomics* and *toxicoproteomics* investigate the analogous response to environmental contaminants and other toxicants (31,32). In contrast to the focus of "pharmacogenetics" on single gene events, "pharmacogenomics" involves understanding how interacting systems or networks of genes influence drug responses (33). This definition is particularly appealing to pediatric health and disease since the concept of many genes acting in concert captures the essence of the developmental processes that characterize maturation from the time of birth through adulthood while retaining a focus on the individual.

It is safe to say that application of pharmacogenomic principles to pediatric medicine has received far less attention than its application to diseases affecting adults, and the scope of the field remains to be completely defined. However, *developmental* and *pediatric pharmacogenomics* necessarily must take into consideration the dynamic changes in gene expression that accompany maturation from embryonic life through fetal development, the neonatal period, infancy, childhood, and adolescence, for example, during organogenesis, as receptor systems and neural networks become established, and functional drug biotransformation capacity is acquired, among others. In other words, patterns of gene expression and the nature of the gene interactions that contribute to the pathogenesis of pediatric diseases (and thereby serve as potential targets for pharmacologic intervention) may only be discernable or relevant at specific critical points in the developmental continuum. Furthermore, variability in drug disposition (i.e., pharmacokinetics) and action (i.e., pharmacodynamics) that ultimately impact drug response in pediatric patients can also be expected to change as children grow and develop. Finally, developmental and pediatric pharmacogenomic investigations can be distinguished from similar studies conducted in adults by the fact that drug or toxicant exposure at critical points in development may disrupt or alter the normal patterns of development—a genome-wide response to drug/toxicant exposure. This may have immediate, observable consequences, for example, fetal demise or major structural abnormalities such as those associated with retinoids (34) or other human teratogens. Of equal concern, however, is the possibility that drug exposure, or lack of effective drug treatment (35), may have unintended consequences on cognitive or behavioral development that do not manifest until much later in maturation. The remainder of this chapter will highlight examples of how pharmacogenomic approaches are currently improving pediatric pharmacotherapy and present several opportunities for future application.

PHARMACOGENETIC, PHARMACOGENOMIC, PHARMACOPROTEOMIC, AND METABOLOMIC TOOLS

Completion of the Human Genome Project was facilitated by several technological advances; the demands of genomic, proteomic, pharmacogenetic, and pharmacogenomic analyses have driven the development of an industry dedicated to the discovery and refinement of technologies capable of generating large datasets of information derived from DNA, RNA, proteins, and small endogenous molecules. These tools are used widely to investigate disease pathogenesis but are equally applicable to investigations of variability in drug disposition and response.

PHARMACOGENETIC TOOLS

Historically, pharmacogenetic analyses have been dependent upon phenotyping studies to estimate enzyme activity *in vivo* at a specific time point as well as genotyping strategies to identify and characterize SNPs and other forms of genetic variation. Phenotyping studies are best conducted with a probe compound carefully selected to ensure that its biotransformation is primarily dependent upon a single target enzyme and varies quantitatively with the level of protein expression (i.e., phenotyping data correlate with the level of enzyme activity *in vitro*, the fractional clearance of the probe and other substrates of the target enzyme *in vivo*, and biotransformation of the probe is increased or decreased in the presence of inducers and inhibitors, respectively) (36). An ideal probe should involve noninvasive sampling strategies, such as collection or urine or expired air rather than blood samples, especially when phenotyping studies are to be conducted in children. Finally, candidate phenotyping probes should be widely available (nonprescription status, preferably) and have a wide margin of safety. For pediatric studies, the phenotyping probe should be selected from compounds that are likely to be administered to children and perceived as safe by parents, caregivers, and ethics committees (e.g., dextromethorphan as opposed to debrisoquine or sparteine for CYP2D6). The advantages and disadvantages of phenotyping probes commonly utilized in adult studies have been comprehensively and critically evaluated by Streetman et al. (37). Dextromethorphan and caffeine are commonly used in pediatric phenotyping studies with nontherapeutic intent (38–41). However, other accepted phenotyping probes, such as midazolam for CYP3A4 and omeprazole for CYP2C19, may be utilized in selected patient populations where their use is required for therapeutic purposes.

The genotyping component of pharmacogenetic studies has undergone tremendous change over the past 30 years. Historically, studies were conducted at the level of individual genes using rather insensitive DNA hybridization techniques (42) to detect differences in the patterns of DNA fragments generated following digestion of genomic DNA with restriction endonucleases (enzymes that cleave DNA molecules at specific nucleotide sequences). The restriction fragment length polymorphism (RFLP) technique was later coupled with the polymerase chain reaction (PCR–RFLP) to allow a specific region surrounding the SNP of interest to be amplified from small amounts of genomic DNA followed by endonuclease digestion to identify the allelic variant(s) present (43). PCR–RFLP techniques have been widely used to study cytochrome P450 polymorphisms (44–46), among others, but they are too labor-intensive for routine use in genomic applications, such as fine-mapping of disease loci or candidate gene association studies, which involve the analysis of multiple SNPs in thousands of genes. Many innovative genotyping technologies continue to be developed, and some have received approval by the Food and Drug Administration for use in clinical settings. The Roche Amplichip CYP450 Test was the first such device to receive FDA approval (December 17, 2004 and January 10, 2005), followed by products from Third Wave Technologies, Inc. (August 18, 2005), Verigene (September 17, 2007), Autogenomics, Inc. (January 23, 2008), ParagonDx, LLC (April 28, 2008), Osmetech Molecular Diagnostics (July 17, 2008), and Trimgen Corporation (February 6, 2009). In general, applications are limited to one or two genes, such as *CYP2C9* and *VKORC1* genotyping to guide warfarin therapy or genotyping of *UGT1A1* to reduce the risk of irinotecan toxicity.

PHARMACOGENOMIC TOOLS

In contrast to pharmacogenetic studies that typically target single genes, pharmacogenomic analyses are considerably broader in scope since they focus on complex and highly variable drug-related phenotypes (e.g., valproic acid hepatotoxicity or weight gain, tumor response to cancer chemotherapy, drug response in asthma, epilepsy, attention deficit and hyperactivity disorders). Comparison of gene expression profiles in cells from treatment-responsive and nonresponsive patients is a readily accessible pharmacogenomic phenotype. These types of studies utilize *microarray* or "*gene-chip*" *technology* to monitor global changes in expression of thousands of genes simultaneously—"global gene profiling." In essence, a microarray consists of a matrix of DNA fragments (probes) precisely positioned (i.e., coordinates are known) at high density on a solid support, such as a glass slide or a filter. The probes serve as molecular detectors for mRNA in the sample. Common experimental designs involve labeling mRNA (or cDNA) from a control sample with one fluorescent dye and mRNA (or cDNA) from the disease/treatment sample with a second fluorescent dye, using an experimental strategy that allows expression to be compared between the sample pair. Alternatively, samples from many patients can be run, each on a single chip, and the results from all the chips subjected to normalization procedures that allow the gene expression patterns from treated patients and controls, or responders and non-responders, to be compared. Thus, the expression pattern of thousands of genes can be analyzed in a single sample with the underlying hypothesis that the measured intensity for each arrayed gene represents its relative expression level. Because of the massive amounts of data generated in these experiments, sophisticated computational methods and data-mining tools are necessary to reveal patterns of expression that distinguish between the populations under investigation. Potential applications of gene expression profiling include improved disease classification and risk stratification in oncology; pathogen detection, subtyping, and characterization of antibiotic resistance; neonatal screening for genetic disorders and prediction of drug response and adverse drug reactions (47). As an example, this approach has been widely used to address treatment resistance in acute lymphoblastic leukemia and has provided new insights into the mechanistic basis of drug resistance and the genomic basis of interindividual variability in drug response (48,49).

Whole genome genotyping technologies now make it possible to interrogate genetic variation more than a million sites throughout an individual genome for SNP and CNV analyses using a single "chip." The majority of genome-wide association (GWA) studies are conducted with "SNP chips" utilizing one of two commercial platforms, and the approach recently has been applied to several pediatric diseases. A study of Kawasaki disease identified a set of functionally related genes potentially related to inflammation, apoptosis, and cardiovascular pathology (50). The results of the study provide novel insights into the pathogenesis of the disorder and lead to the possibility of identifying new targets for therapeutic intervention. Similarly, GWA studies in patients with early onset asthma (51) and pediatric inflammatory bowel disease (52) have been implemented as a new strategy to identify novel genes in disease pathogenesis. Genome-wide association studies (GWAS) are also being applied to identify genetic associations with drug dosing, response and efficacy, as reported for warfarin (53) and clopidogrel (54), and risk for drug-induced toxicity, as has been described for statin-induced myopathy (55). One of the features of GWAS that is becoming more prevalent is the use of Manhattan plots. An example is presented in Figure 5.2.

The most recent addition to the genomic toolbox is next-generation sequencing technology (56). The major difference between next-generation sequencing methods and the older, more established Sanger capillary sequencing method is the vast amount of sequencing data that can be generated by the next-generation technologies, which utilize massively parallel and short read strategies to sequence DNA and RNA templates. Whereas it has been estimated that 500 days of runtime were required to generate one gigabase (one billion nucleotides) of data, the newer next-generation sequencers can produce this same amount of data in half a day at 1/100th of the cost. However, the short 50 to 75 bp-read lengths provide computational challenges related to assembly of the short sequence reads to produce an accurate contiguous genomic

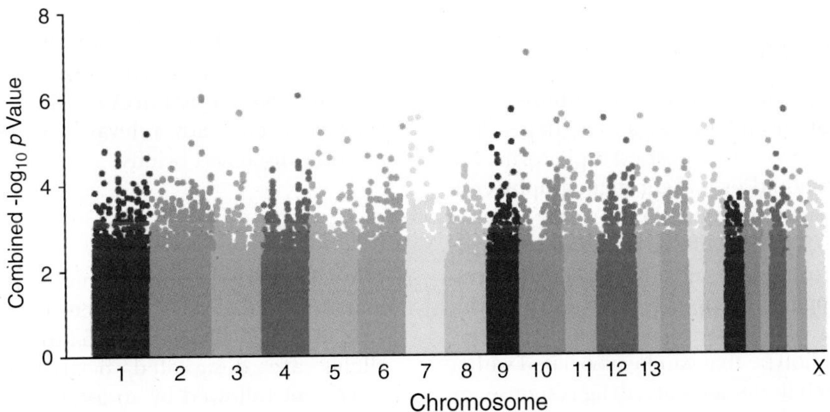

Figure 5.2. Example of a Manhattan plot from a genome-wide association study. This type of plot gains its name from the similarity of such a plot to the Manhattan skyline and presents the genome-wide significance of several hundred thousand SNPs distributed throughout the genome with the trait or phenotype of interest. Along the abscissa, each SNP is plotted according to its chromosomal coordinate, with each color representing an individual chromosome from chromosome 1 to the X chromosome. The ordinate axis represents the inverse $\log_{10}$ of the p value for the association. SNPs exceeding a particular threshold are subject to further verification and validation. (Originally published as Figure 2 in Yang JJ et al., Genome-wide interrogation of germline genetic variation associated with treatment response in childhood acute lymphoblastic leukemia. *JAMA* 2009;301: 393–403 (164). Reprinted with permission.)

sequence. Application of next-generation sequencing to RNA templates referred to as RNA-Seq allows deeper coverage and higher resolution of RNA sequence compared to microarray technology and has revolutionized *transcriptomics.* RNA-Seq has provided new insights into gene regulation, alternative splicing, and allelic variation of transcripts increasing dramatically our understanding of the diversity of protein products encoded by the genome (57,58).

PHARMACOPROTEOMIC TOOLS

Proteomic studies face limitations that are not experienced in genomic or transcriptomic applications. For example, no amplification method analogous to PCR exists to increase the quantity of protein from small amounts of starting material, and the final protein product in a sample may be the result of alternative splicing events and several posttranslational modifications. Therefore, many different techniques are required to detect, quantify and identify proteins in a sample (*expression proteomics*) and to characterize protein function in terms of activity and protein–protein or protein–nucleic acid interactions (*functional proteomics*) (59). At present, two-dimensional electrophoresis (2DE) coupled with mass spectral detection (2DE-MS) represents the mainstay of expression proteomics. Matrix-assisted laser desorption ionization time-of-flight (MALDI-TOF) mass spectrometry is a commonly used approach, and data generated are compared with theoretically derived peptide mass databases for protein identification. Proteomic analyses of drug-induced toxicities of potential relevance to pediatric pharmacotherapy have identified candidate protein targets of acetaminophen hepatotoxicity (60) and gentamicin nephrotoxicity (61). More recently, application of surface-enhanced laser desorption/ionization (SELDI) based approaches has revealed the potential of proteomic technology to identify biomarkers of response to drug treatment in pediatric diseases, such as juvenile idiopathic arthritis (62) and the response of pediatric nephritic syndrome to steroids (63).

METABOLOMIC TOOLS

Several analytical approaches can be utilized for metabolomic and metabonomic investigations, depending on the analytes of interest, but the most used platforms are NMR spectroscopy and liquid or gas chromatography coupled with tandem mass spectral detection (64). One strategy for metabolomic studies is to use a global profiling approach to measure the concentrations of all small molecules present in a sample or changing in response to a perturbation. Subsequent application of pattern recognition algorithms defines a metabolic phenotype that can be associated with a particular end point, such as disease state, drug response, or drug toxicity. Metabolomics can be integrated with other genomic technologies. Combining metabolomic and genome-wide genotyping data has revealed common genetic variations that are associated with variability in metabolic phenotypes involving the corresponding biochemical pathways (65). Metabolomics in conjunction with simultaneous gene expression analysis of the transcriptome provides additional mechanistic insights leading to a more "systems-based" understanding of cellular processes, especially in the context of dug-related perturbations (66). Relatively few metabolomic studies have been conducted in children, but NMR has been used to investigate age-related changes in the metabolome between newborns and children 12 years of age (67).

APPLICATIONS OF PEDIATRIC PHARMACOGENETICS AND PHARMACOGENOMICS

DRUG BIOTRANSFORMATION AND CONCENTRATION-DEPENDENT TOXICITY

Clinical observation of patients with high drug concentrations/excessive or prolonged drug responses, together with the realization that the biochemical traits (subsequently identified as proteins involved in drug biotransformation) were inherited, provided the origins of the concept of pharmacogenetics. Indeed, with few exceptions, the major consequence of pharmacogenetic polymorphisms in drug-metabolizing enzymes is concentration-dependent toxicity due to impaired drug clearance and, to a lesser extent, reduced conversion of prodrugs to therapeutically active compounds. For most cytochromes P450, genotype–phenotype relationships are influenced by development in that fetal expression is limited (with the exception of CYP3A7) and functional activity is acquired postnatally in isoform-specific patterns. Furthermore, clearance of some compounds appears to be greater in children relative to adults, obscuring the correlation between genotype and phenotype in neonatal life through adolescence (28). The ontogeny of several phase I and phase II drug biotransformation pathways has been exhaustively reviewed (68), and comprehensive reviews of cytochromes P450 pharmacogenetics in general (69) and for individual drug biotransformation enzymes, such as CYP2B6 (70), CYP2C9 (71), CYP2C19 (72), CYP2D6 (73,74), the CYP3A subfamily (75), uridine diphosphoglucuronosyl transferases or UGTs (76,77), sulfotransferases or SULTs (78), *N*-acetyltransferases or NATs (79), and thiopurine *S*-methyltransferase or TPMT (80) are also available. Salient features of the more common polymorphisms of clinically relevant drug-metabolizing enzymes are now discussed briefly.

CYP2D6

The *CYP2D6* gene locus is highly polymorphic with more than 75 allelic variants identified to date (http://www.imm.ki.se/CYPalleles/cyp2d6.htm; see Table 5.1). Individual alleles are designated by the italicized gene name (*CYP2D6*) followed by an asterisk and an Arabic number; *CYP2D6*1* designates, by convention, the fully functional wild-type allele. Allelic variants are the consequence of point mutations, single-base pair deletions or additions, gene rearrangements, or deletion of the entire gene that result in a reduction or complete loss of activity. Inheritance of two recessive loss-of-function alleles results in the "poor-metabolizer phenotype," which is found in about 5% to 10% of Caucasians and about 1% to 2% of Asian subjects. In Caucasians, the *3, *4, *5, and *6 alleles are the most common loss of functional alleles and account for approximately 98% of poor metabolizer phenotypes (81). CYP2D6 activity is lower, on a population basis, in Asian and African-American populations due to a lower frequency of nonfunctional alleles (*3, *4, *5, and *6) and a relatively high frequency of alleles that are associated with decreased activity relative to the wild-type *CYP2D6*1* allele. In Asians, *CYP2D6*10* has an allele frequency of approximately 50%, whereas *CYP2D6*17* and *CYP2D6*29* occur at relatively high frequencies in subjects of black African origin. At the other end of the spectrum, the presence of *CYP2D6* gene duplication/multiplication events, which occur at a frequency of 1% to 2% in Caucasians (73,74), most often is associated with enhanced clearance of CYP2D6 substrates although cases of increased toxicity due to increased formation of pharmacologically active metabolites have also been reported (82).

CYP2D6 is involved in the biotransformation of more than 40 therapeutic entities including several β-receptor antagonists, antiarrhythmics, antidepressants, and antipsychotics and morphine derivatives (for updated list, see http://medicine.iupui.edu/flockhart/, Table 5.1). Of these, serotonin selective reuptake inhibitors (SSRIs), codeine, and dextromethorphan are commonly encountered in pediatrics. *In vitro* studies indicate that fetal liver microsomes have very limited CYP2D6 activity (approximately 1% of adult values) but CYP2D6 protein is detectable in all samples from newborns. Thereafter, both CYP2D6 protein and catalytic activity progressively increase over the first 28 days of life to 20% of activity observed in adult samples (83). One consequence of CYP2D6 developmental pharmacogenetics may be the syndrome of irritability, tachypnea, tremors, jitteriness, increased muscle tone, and temperature instability in neonates born to mothers receiving SSRIs during pregnancy. Controversy currently exists as to whether these symptoms reflect a neonatal withdrawal (hyposerotonergic) state (84) or whether they represent manifestations of serotonin toxicity (85,86) analogous to the hyperserotonergic state associated with the SSRI-induced serotonin syndrome in adults (87). Delayed expression of CYP2D6 (and CYP3A4) in the first week of life is consistent with a hyperserotonergic state due to delayed clearance of paroxetine and fluoxetine (CYP2D6) or sertraline (CYP3A4) in neonates exposed to these compounds during pregnancy. Furthermore, decreases in plasma SSRI concentrations and resolution of symptoms would be expected with increasing postnatal age and maturation of these pathways. Given that treatment of a "withdrawal" reaction may include administration of an SSRI, there is considerable potential for increased toxicity in affected neonates. As a result, resolution of the hyperserotonergic–hyposerotonergic pathogenesis is essential for appropriate management of SSRI-induced neonatal adaptation syndromes, but further research should also consider genetic and developmental factors beyond drug disposition given the recent report of a role for genetic variation in the serotonin transporter SLC6A4 in the clinical manifestations of the syndrome (88).

Drug accumulation and resultant concentration-dependent toxicities in genotypic poor metabolizers should be anticipated in children just as they are in adults due to the risk for significant morbidity and mortality (89). A recent analysis of CYP2D6 ontogeny *in vitro* utilizing a relatively large number of samples revealed that CYP2D6 protein and activity were similar between fetal liver samples obtained during the third trimester of pregnancy and liver samples obtained from infants in the first week of life, and both protein and activity remained relatively constant after 1 week of age up to 18 years. The data further imply that genetic variability, rather than ontogeny, is primarily responsible for the observed variability in catalytic activity (90). Similar results have been observed in an *in vivo* longitudinal phenotyping study involving more than 100 infants over the first year of life. This study utilized dextromethorphan as a probe compound and the urinary ratio of dextromethorphan to dextrorphan as a measure of CYP2D6 activity. Although considerable interindividual variability in CYP2D6 activity was observed, no relationship between CYP2D6 activity and postnatal age was apparent between 2 weeks and 12 months of age (91). Similarly, a cross-sectional study involving 586 children (480 Caucasians and 106 African Americans) indicated that the distribution of CYP2D6 phenotypes in children was comparable to that observed in adults by at least 10 years of age, and probably much earlier (38). Cumulatively, these *in vitro* and *in vivo* indicate that developmental factors are less important than genetic variation as determinants of CYP2D6 variability in children.

Drug accumulation with an increased risk of concentration-dependent toxicity is of particular concern in CYP2D6 poor metabolizers. Indeed, a fluoxetine-related death has been reported in a 9-year-old child with multiple neuropsychiatric disorders who was subsequently determined to be a CYP2D6 poor metabolizer by genotype analysis. Measurements of blood and liver concentrations of fluoxetine at autopsy were several-fold higher than expected, consistent with *CYP2D6* genotype (89). On the other hand, poor metabolizers may experience decreased efficacy or therapeutic failure when prescribed drugs that are dependent upon functional CYP2D6 activity for conversion to the pharmacologically active species, such as codeine and tramadol (92,93). Infants and children appear capable of converting codeine to morphine (94) achieving morphine:codeine ratios comparable to those of adults (95). However, in one study, morphine and its metabolites were not detected in 36% of children receiving codeine, and codeine analgesia was found to be unreliable in the studied pediatric population and not related to CYP2D6 phenotype (96).

CYP2C9

Although several clinically useful compounds are substrates for CYP2C9 (for updated list, see http://medicine.iupui.edu/flockhart/, see Table 5.1), the effects of allelic variation are most profound for drugs with narrow therapeutic indices such as phenytoin (97,98), warfarin (99), and tolbutamide (100,101). Several allelic variants of CYP2C9 have been observed in population studies. The *CYP2C9*2* allele results in an amino acid substitution at position 144 of the CYP2C9 protein and is associated with approximately 5.5-fold decreased intrinsic clearance for (*S*)-warfarin relative to the wild-type enzyme (102). The conservative isoleucine to leucine change at position 359 characteristic of the CYP2C9*3 allele occurs within a region of the protein that affects substrate orientation in the active site and, as a result, produces a considerable (27-fold) decrease in intrinsic (*S*)-warfarin clearance (103). A similar decrease in activity has been observed for *CYP2C9*5* due to an aspartate to glutamate change at position 360, also within the active site of the enzyme (104). Approximately one-third of the Caucasian population carries a variant *CYP2C9* allele (*2 and *3 alleles, most commonly) whereas the *2 and *3 alleles are less common in African-Americans, Chinese, Japanese, or Korean populations. In contrast, the *5 allele has been detected in African-Americans but not in Caucasians (45). The risk of bleeding complications in patients treated with warfarin and concentration-dependent phenytoin toxicity is most pronounced for individuals with a *CYP2C9*3/*3* genotype (45). Although the relationship between *CYP2C9* genotype and warfarin dosing/pharmacokinetics has not been as extensively studied in children, consequences of allelic variation can be expected to be similar to those observed in adults (105).

CYP2C19

Also known as "mephenytoin hydroxylase deficiency", the CYP2C19 poor-metabolizer phenotype is present in 3% to 5% of the Caucasian population and 20% to 25% of Asians. Although several defective alleles have been identified, the two most common variant alleles, *CYP2C19*2* and *3, result from single-base substitutions that introduce premature stop codons and consequently, truncated polypeptide chains that possess no functional activity (44,106). In Japanese adults treated with lansoprazole, amoxicillin, and clarithromycin for *Helicobacter pylori* infection, the eradication rate for CYP2C19 poor metabolizers (97.8%) and heterozygous extensive metabolizers (one functional *CYP2C19* allele; 92.1%) was significantly greater than that observed in homozygous extensive metabolizers (72.7%; $p < .001$). Of the 35 patients in whom initial treatment failed to eradicate *H. pylori*, 34 had at least one functional *CYP2C19* allele and eradication could be achieved with higher lansoprazole doses in almost all cases (107). Given that the frequency of the functional *CYP2C19*1* allele is considerably greater in Caucasians (~0.84) compared with Japanese (~0.55) (44,106), eradication failure can be expected to occur more frequently in Caucasians.

More recently, a novel allele characterized by two variants in the 5′-upstream region of the *CYP2C19* gene has been described. This allele, designated *CYP2C19*17*, occurs at a frequency of 18% in Swedish and Ethiopian populations and approximately 4% in a Chinese population (108). *CYP2C19*17* is associated with "ultrarapid" activity as measured by omeprazole metabolite ratio (108) and decreased serum concentrations of substrates, such as escitalopram (109). As proton pump inhibitors and antidepressants are used clinically in pediatric patient populations, pharmacogenetic considerations should guide dosing strategies in children as well as in adults.

CYP3A4, CYP3A5, and CYP3A7

The CYP3A subfamily consists of four members in humans (CYPs3A4, 3A5, 3A7, and 3A43) and is quantitatively the most important group of CYPs in terms of human hepatic drug biotransformation. These isoforms catalyze the oxidation of many different therapeutic entities, several of which are of potential importance to pediatric practice (for updated list, see http://medicine.iupui.edu/flockhart/, see Table 5.1). CYP3A7 is the predominant CYP isoform in fetal liver and can be detected in embryonic liver as early as 50 to 60 days gestation (110,111). CYP3A7 activity is maximal in the early neonatal period with a progressive decline thereafter. In contrast, CYP3A4 activity, the major CYP3A isoform in adults, is essentially absent in fetal liver but increases during the first week of postnatal life (112). CYP3A4 is also abundantly expressed in intestine where it contributes significantly to the first-pass metabolism of orally administered substrates such as midazolam (113,114). CYP3A5 is polymorphically expressed, being present in approximately 25% of adult liver samples studied *in vitro* (115,116).

Several methods have been proposed for CYP3A phenotyping, and the advantages and limitations of each have been reviewed in detail (36,37). Using these various phenotyping probes, CYP3A4 activity has been reported to vary widely (up to 50-fold) among individuals but the population distributions of activity are essentially unimodal and evidence for polymorphic activity has been elusive. Several allelic variants have been identified (http://www.imm.ki.se/CYPalleles/cyp3a4.htm; see Table 5.1), but they occur relatively infrequently and appear to be of minimal clinical consequence. Of interest to pediatrics is the *CYP3A4*1B* allele present in the CYP3A4 promoter region, (117,118). The clinical significance of this allelic variant appears limited with respect to drug biotransformation activity (119–121) despite being associated with two-fold increased activity over the wild-type *CYP3A4*1* allele in reporter gene assays *in vitro* (122). Although there does not appear to be an association between the *CYP3A4*1B* allele and age of menarche as recalled in adulthood in one study (123), a significant relationship does exist between the number of *1B alleles and onset of puberty as defined by Tanner breast score (odds ratio = 3.21; 95% confidence interval 1.62 to 6.89) (124). In this study, 90% of 9-year-old girls with a *CYP3A4*1B/*1B* genotype had a Tanner breast score ≥2 compared with 56% of *CYP3A4*1A/*1B* heterozygotes and 40% of girls homozygous for the *CYP3A4*1A* allele. Since CYP3A4 plays an important role in testosterone catabolism, the authors of the latter study proposed that the estradiol:testosterone ratio may be shifted toward higher values in the presence of the *CYP3A4*1B* allele and trigger the hormonal cascade that accompanies puberty.

Polymorphic CYP3A5 expression is largely due to an SNP in intron 3 that creates a cryptic splice site and gives rise to splice variants that carry premature stop codons thereby accounting for the lack of expression in most Caucasian livers (116). While the role of CYP3A5 in hepatic drug biotransformation is thought to be underestimated by one group (116), this issue currently is controversial (125).

CYP3A7 is expressed at high levels in human fetal liver (126) and plays a critical role during pregnancy through the formation of 16α-hydroxy dehydroepiandrosterone sufate (DHEA-S), the process by which a third hydroxyl group is added to DHEA-S prior to final formation of estriol by placental syncytiotrophoblasts. Other substrates of CYP3A7 include retinoic acid and foreign compounds that gain access to the fetal compartment from the maternal circulation. The *CYP3A7*2* allele occurs at a relatively low frequency in Caucasians (8%) and Asians (28%) compared with Africans (68%). Although the CYP3A7.2 protein product has been associated with 20% to 25% higher activity than the CYP3A7.1 enzyme *in vitro* (127), no significant differences in DHEA 16α-hydroxylation activity was observed in livers genotyped for *CYP3A7*1* and *CYP3A7*2* (128). Given the recent observation of sex-dependent effects of genetic variants in *CYP3A4* and *CYP3A7* (129), the functional consequences of genetic variation in fetal liver *CYP3A7* warrant further investigation. Persistence of fetal CYP3A7 mRNA in adult liver has been partially attributed to the *CYP3A7*1C* allele in which a set of seven tightly linked variants essentially replace 60 bp of the *CYP3A7* promoter with the identical sequence from *CYP3A4* (116).

Glucuronosyl Transferases

The uridine diphospho-glucuronosyl transferase (UGT) gene superfamily catalyzes the conjugation of substrates with glucuronic acid. UGT1A1 is the major *UGT* gene product responsible for bilirubin glucuronidation and more than 60 genetic alterations have been reported, most of which are rare and are more properly considered mutations rather than gene polymorphisms. Inheritance of two defective alleles is associated with reduced bilirubin conjugating activity and gives rise to clinical conditions such as Crigler-Najjar syndrome and Gilbert syndrome. More frequently occurring polymorphisms involve a dinucleotide (TA) repeat in the atypical TATA box of the *UGT1A1* promoter. The wild-type *UGT1A1*1* allele has six repeats (TA_6), and the TA_5 (*UGT1A1*33*), TA_7 (*UGT1A1*28*), and TA_8 (*UGT1A1*34*) variants are all associated with reduced activity. *UGT1A1*28* is the most frequent variant and is a contributory factor to prolonged neonatal jaundice (130,131) and is associated with impaired glucuronidation and thus toxicity of the irinotecan active metabolite, SN-38 (132,133). Two members of the UGT2B subfamily involved in the glucuronidation of androgens and other steroid molecules, *UGT2B17* and *UGT2B28*, are subject to CNVs in which gene deletion events occur frequently (134). Several allelic variants of important UGTs involved in drug biotransformation (UGT1A6 and UGT2B7) have been reported, but the lack of isoform-specific probe compounds analogous to dextromethorphan for CYP2D6 has precluded a clear understanding of the clinical impact of polymorphisms in these genes (76,135).

Arylamine N-Acetyltransferases

One the earliest discovered and most widely recognized genetic polymorphisms is the arylamine *N*-acetyltransferase-2 (NAT2) polymorphism. Approximately 50% of Caucasians and African-Americans residing on the North American continent are phenotypically slow metabolizers placing a substantial number of individuals at increased risk for the development of adverse drug effects such as sulfasalazine-induced hemolysis, hydrazine or arylamine-induced peripheral neuropathy, procainamide- or isoniazid-induced lupus erythematosus, and Stevens-Johnson syndrome or toxic epidermal necrolysis associated with sulfonamide administration (136). NAT2 function is inherited in an autosomal dominant fashion with the inheritance of two "slow" alleles required for expression of the slow metabolizer phenotype. The relative proportion of rapid and slow metabolizers varies considerably with ethnic or geographic origin. For example, the percentage of slow acetylators among Canadian Eskimos is 5% but approaches 90% in some Mediterranean populations (137). According to the standardized NAT2 nomenclature, the wild-type and three additional "fast" alleles give rise to the rapid acetylator phenotype, whereas nine "slow" alleles have been described (138).

In vivo, using caffeine as a phenoptyping probe, all infants between 0 and 55 days of age appear to be phenotypically slow acetylators, whereas 50% and 62% of infants between 122 to 224 and 225 to 342 days of age, respectively, can be characterized as fast acetylators (39). Several independent studies indicate that maturation of the NAT2 phenotype occurs during the first 4 years of life (38,139,140). Thus, phenotype–genotype discordance is likely to be most apparent in the first 2 to 4 months of life, and drugs highly dependent upon NAT2 function for their elimination should be used with caution.

Thiopurine S-Methyltransferase

TPMT is a cytosolic enzyme that catalyses the S-methylation of aromatic and heterocyclic sulfur-containing compounds such as 6-mercaptopurine, azathioprine, and 6-thioguanine that are used in the treatment of several pediatric diseases and disorders including acute lymphoblastic anemia (ALL), inflammatory bowel disease, and juvenile arthritis, and to prevent renal allograft rejection. To exert its cytotoxic effects, 6-mercaptopurine requires metabolism to thioguanine nucleotides (TGNs) by a multistep process that is initiated by hypoxanthine guanine phosphoribosyl transferase. TPMT prevents TGN production by methylating 6-mercaptopurine (Fig. 5.3A). TPMT activity is usually measured in blood with activity in erythrocytes reflecting that found in other tissues including liver and leukemic blasts. While approximately 89% of Caucasians and African-Americans have high TPMT activity and 11% have intermediate activity, 1 in 300 individuals inherits TPMT deficiency as an autosomal recessive trait (Fig. 5.3B) (141). In patients with intermediate or low activity, more drug is shunted toward production of cytotoxic TGNs. TPMT can also methylate 6-thioinosine 5′-monophosphate to generate a methylated metabolite that is capable of inhibiting *de novo* purine synthesis. (Fig. 5.3C). In the small population (i.e., 0.3%) of treated patients with relative TPMT deficiency, severe and potentially life-threatening myelosuppression can develop in

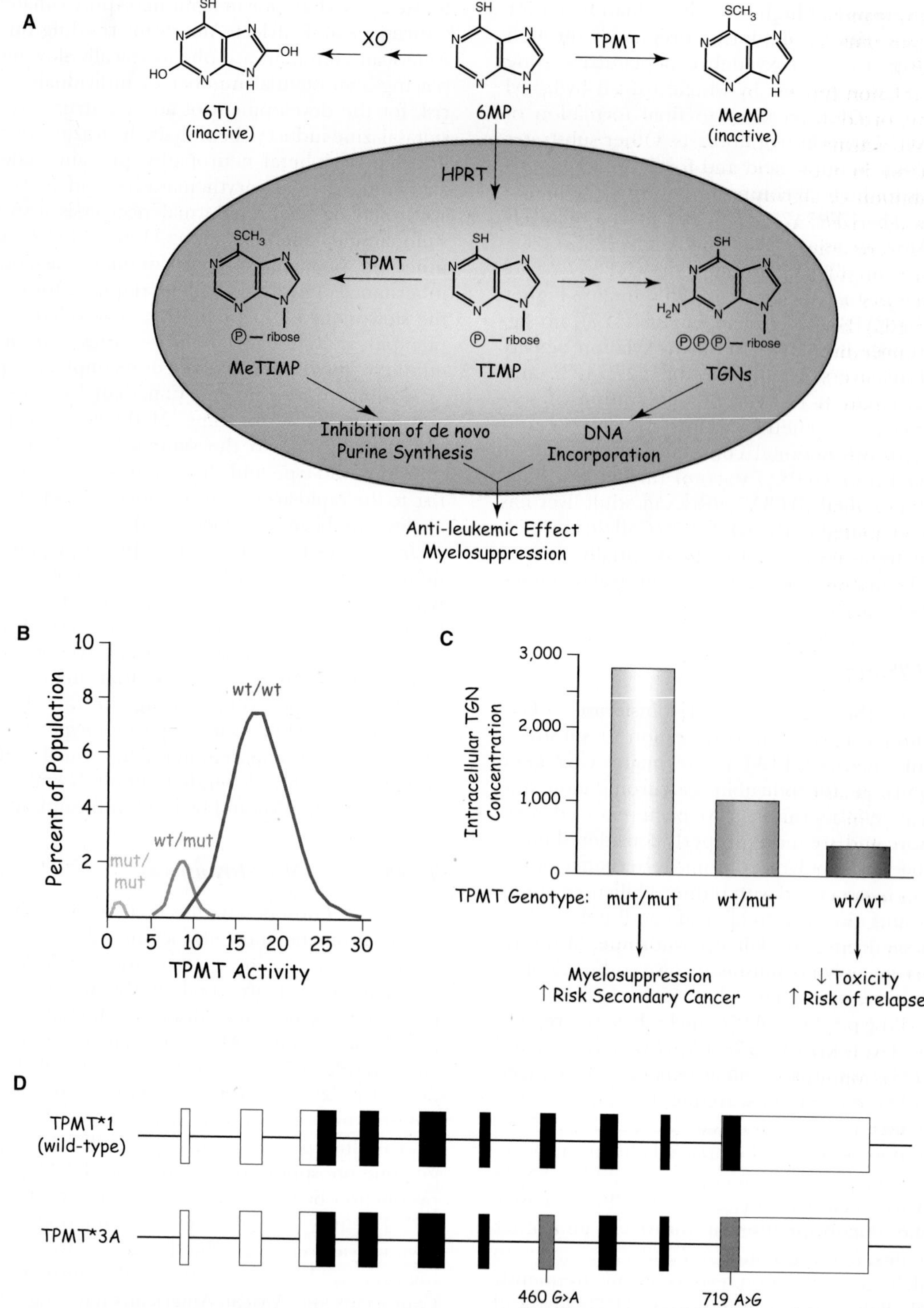

Figure 5.3. The thiopurine *S*-methyltransferase (TPMT) polymorphism. **A:** 6-Mercaptopurine (6MP) undergoes metabolism to thioguanine nucleotides (TGNs) to exert its cytotoxic effects. TPMT and xanthine oxidase (XO) reduce the amount of 6MP available for the bioactivation pathway to TGNs. TPMT can also methylate 6-thioinosine 5′-monophosphate (TIMP) to generate a methylated compound capable of inhibiting *de novo* purine synthesis. 6TU: 6-thiouric acid; MeMP: methylmercaptopurine; HPRT: hypoxanthine guanine phosphoribosyl transferase. **B:** Distribution of TPMT activity in humans. Eighty-nine percent of the population has high activity and 11% has intermediate activity. Approximately 1 in 300 individuals is homozygous for two loss-of-function alleles and has very low activity. wt, wild type; mut, mutant. **C:** Correlation between TPMT genotype and intracellular TGN concentrations. In TPMT poor metabolizers, more 6MP is available to go down the bioactivation pathway to form TGNs and is associated with an increased risk of myelosuppression. **D:** The most common variant TPMT allele is the result of two mutations that give rise to an unstable protein product, which undergoes proteolytic degradation. (Modified from Relling MV, Dervieux T. Pharmacogenetics and cancer therapy. *Nat Rev Cancer* 2001;1:99–108, with permission. Copyright 2001, Macmillan Magazines Ltd.)

patients receiving standard doses of thiopurine (142,143), and starting doses must be reduced to 6% to 10% of the normal dose (59).

Conflicting relationships between age and TPMT activity have been reported in children. In one study, peripheral blood TPMT activity in newborns was reported to be 50% greater than in race-matched adults and demonstrated a distribution of activity consistent with the polymorphism characterized in adults (144). In contrast, TPMT activities were comparable to previously reported adult values in a population of Korean school children ($n = 309$) aged 7 to 9 years (145) and in French Caucasian children ($n = 165$) hospitalized for day surgery (146). Considerable interindividual variability in TPMT activity exists in both pediatric and adult populations consistent with genetic variation being the primary driver of the observed variability.

*TPMT*3A* is the most common variant *TPMT* allele and is characterized by two nucleotide transition mutations, G460A and A719G, that lead to two amino acid substitutions Ala154Thr and Tyr240Cys (Fig. 5.3D). Although the **3A* allele has only a frequency of 0.03% in the general population, it represents 55% of all mutant alleles. Either mutation alone results in loss of functional activity through the production of unstable proteins that are subject to accelerated proteolytic degradation (147,148). Less frequent allele variants involve SNPs that produce amino acid substitutions in the coding region and defective intron–exon splicing (141). A polymorphic locus has been identified in the promoter region of the *TPMT* gene involving four to eight repeats of a specific nucleotide sequence in tandem (149). While these repeats appear to modulate TPMT activity when expressed *in vitro*, their role in regulating activity *in vivo* has not been clearly established (150).

The small percentage of patients with low to absent TPMT activity is at increased risk for developing severe myelosuppression if treated with routine doses of thiopurines and thus requires a 10- to 15-fold reduction in dose to minimize this risk. Furthermore, these patients may be at increased risk of relapse consequent to inadequate or absent treatment with the thiopurines. Given the expanding use of 6-mercaptopurine and azathioprine in pediatrics to treat inflammatory bowel disease and juvenile arthritis and to prevent renal allograft rejection, TPMT deficiency is not a trivial matter. However, the exact role for *a priori* TPMT genotype and phenotype determinations remains to be determined, especially for conditions like inflammatory bowel disease, as risk–benefit considerations differ compared to ALL. In children with inflammatory bowel disease, pretreatment assessment of *TPMT* genotype did not predict azathioprine toxicity in one study (151), whereas azathioprine dose adjustments based on 6-mercaptopurine metabolite concentrations were associated with improved disease control in another. This situation illustrates the limitations of genotype data (genotype does not change with age or changes due to environment, disease, etc.) and the value of continuously monitoring changes in a phenotype or biomarker that accurately reflects the end point of interest. Nevertheless, anecdotal experience suggests that patients classified as having intermediate TPMT activity frequently require more thiopurine dosage reductions in response to drug-induced myelosuppression.

CURRENT AND FUTURE APPLICATIONS FOR PHARMACOGENOMICS IN PEDIATRICS

There are many opportunities to apply pharmacogenomic and pharmacoproteomic strategies to investigate any of several disease processes that affect newborn infants (e.g., patent ductus arteriosus) or that have no close correlates in adults, such as Kawasaki disease. In fact, a genome-wide association study of Kawasaki disease identified a set of functionally related genes potentially related to inflammation, apoptosis, and cardiovascular pathology (50). It is anticipated that the insights gained from this type of study will lead to a better understanding of disease pathogenesis and, ultimately, new targets for therapeutic intervention. Similar strategies may be applied to diseases like ALL, Wilms' tumor, and neuroblastoma that are encountered during childhood and rarely, if at all, in adults. Other opportunities for application of genomic approaches include diseases with complex etiologies such as asthma, autism, attention deficit and hyperactivity disorder, juvenile rheumatoid arthritis, and type I diabetes mellitus that have their origins during childhood, and idiosyncratic toxicities such as Reye syndrome associated with aspirin use (152), valproate hepatotoxicity (153), and lamotrigine-induced cutaneous events (154) that occur predominantly or at a considerably higher frequency in children. Finally, it is important that advances in the development of pharmacogenomic algorithms to aid in the dosing of drugs with narrow therapeutic indices, such as warfarin (155), also be applied to the use of those medications in children of different ages and developmental stages.

As patterns of gene expression and the nature of the gene interactions that contribute to the pathogenesis of pediatric diseases (and thereby serve as potential targets for pharmacologic intervention) may be discernable only at specific critical points in the developmental continuum, a major challenge for pediatric pharmacogenomics will be to identify the critical period during development when deviations from normal patterns of gene expression will be most apparent. To illustrate this point further, it is not unreasonable to expect that the neurobiological differences between the developing brain of young children and the mature brain of adults may lead to differential responses to SSRIs and other neuropsychiatric medications (156).

ACUTE LYMPHOBLASTIC LEUKEMIA

ALL is perhaps the best example of how pharmacogenetics and pharmacogenomics have been applied to a pediatric disease. Of the 3,000 to 4,000 cases of ALL diagnosed each year in the United States, two thirds are children (157), and long-term disease-free survival of childhood ALL has reached 80% because of improvements in the efficacy of combination chemotherapy. Despite improved understanding of the genetic determinants of drug response, many complexities remain to be resolved. For example, ALL patients with one wild-type allele and intermediate TPMT activity tend to have a better response to mercaptopurine therapy than do patients with two wild-type alleles and full activity (158). However, reduced

TPMT activity also places patients at risk of developing irradiation-induced secondary brain tumors (159) and etoposide-induced acute myeloid leukemias (160). Pharmacogenetic polymorphisms of several additional genes also have the potential to influence successful treatment of ALL (161). Thus, multiple genetic and treatment-related factors interact to create patient subgroups with varying degrees of risk and represent an opportunity for pharmacogenomic approaches to identify those subgroups that will tolerate specific treatment regimens and those who will be at risk for short- and long-term toxicities (162).

The 20% of ALL patients who do not respond to chemotherapy represent an additional challenge for pharmacogenomic research. Gene expression (microarray) studies in ALL blasts are able to discriminate among phenotypic subtypes and identify some individuals at risk for treatment failure (163). A recent analysis of acute treatment-induced changes in the gene response of ALL blasts obtained 1 day after initiation of 6-mercaptopurine and methotrexate as single agents, or in combinations of high-dose or low-dose methotrexate and 6-mercaptopurine, revealed several new, important insights into the cellular response to these treatments (48). For example, changes in gene expression were treatment-specific and could accurately discriminate among the four treatments. Subsequent expression profiling analysis has identified a set of genes that is differentially expressed in primary ALL cells from patients' good and poor initial responses to methotrexate. Low activity of three genes in the folate pathway (*DHFR, TYMS,* and *CTPS*) was associated with poor *in vivo* response (49). Using minimal residual disease as a treatment response phenotype, genome-wide analysis of germ line DNA from two cohorts of ALL patients identified SNPs associated with the phenotype (Fig. 5.2), including five in the interleukin 15 gene. The analysis also revealed several SNPs associated with hematologic relapse and drug disposition and implied that greater drug exposure contributed to disease eradication (164). Based on this recent progress, it may, indeed, be possible to personalize treatment strategies in ALL.

SUMMARY AND CONCLUSIONS

The postgenomic era represents an unprecedented opportunity to translate the increasing volume of untapped genomic, transcriptomic, proteomic, and metabonomic data into discoveries that favorably impact the care and treatment of children. Many diseases have their onset during childhood, and effective early intervention may have unforeseen benefits later in life. On the other hand, pharmacologic management of disease or unintended exposure to environmental toxins at critical stages of development may have consequences that are not immediately apparent due to the profound changes that occur as a fetus develops and as newborn infants mature through childhood to adolescence and ultimately adulthood. Given the complexity of human development, a focus on the influence of a single gene or gene product is likely to be of limited value in terms of understanding the consequences of small molecule interactions with a dynamic developmental environment. Rather, the developmental process should be perceived, at a minimum, as networks of interacting genes and different networks being operative at different developmental stages. Furthermore, the repertoire of genes operative within a given network may vary at different developmental stages, and the phenotypic manifestations of gene variants may not manifest until much later in the process of maturation. In the context of identifying new target genes or gene networks for therapeutic intervention, the most compelling challenge to pediatric pharmacogenomic research will be to identify the essential network or pathway (knowing where to look) at the appropriate developmental stage (knowing when to look). There is reason to be optimistic that new strategies and technologies will help unravel the complexities of pediatric disorders since this new knowledge is essential for children to benefit as much as adults from new treatment modalities.

REFERENCES

1. Lander ES, Linton LM, Birren B, et al. Initial sequencing and analysis of the human genome. *Nature* 2001;409:860–921.
2. Guo SW, Reed DR. The genetics of phenylthiocarbamide perception. *Ann Hum Biol* 2001;28:111–142.
3. Motulsky AG. Drug reactions, enzymes, and biochemical genetics. *J Am Med Assoc* 1957;165:835–837.
4. Kalow W. *Pharmacogenetics: heredity and the response to drugs.* Philadelphia, PA: W.B. Saunders, 1962.
5. Vesell ES. Twin studies in pharmacogenetics. *Hum Genet* 1978; 1:19–30.
6. Mahgoub A, Idle JR, Dring LG, et al. Polymorphic hydroxylation of debrisoquine in man. *Lancet* 1977;1:584–586.
7. Eichelbaum M, Spannbrucker N, Steincke B, et al. Defective N-oxidation of sparteine in man: A new pharmacogenetic defect. *Eur J Clin Pharmacol* 1979;16:183–187.
8. Küpfer A, Preisig R. Pharmacogenetics of mephenytoin: a new drug hydroxylation polymorphism in man. *Eur J Clin Pharmacol* 1984;26:753–759.
9. Ensom MHH, Davis GA, Cropp CD, Ensom RJ. Clinical pharmacokinetics in the 21st century. Does the evidence support definitive outcomes? *Clin Pharmacokin.* 1998;34:265–279.
10. Weinshilboum R. Inheritance and drug response. *New Engl J Med* 2003;348:529–537.
11. Johnson JA. Drug target pharmacogenomics: an overview. *Am J Pharmacogenomics* 2001;1:271–281.
12. Evans WE, McLeod HL. Pharmacogenomics–drug disposition, drug targets, and side effects. *New Engl J Med* 2003;348:538–549.
13. McKusick VA, Ruddle FH. A new discipline, a new name, a new journal. *Genomics* 1987;1:1–2.
14. Venter JC, Adams MD, Myers EW, et al. The sequence of the human genome. *Science* 2001;291:1304–1351.
15. Pennisi E. Reaching their goal early, sequencing labs celebrate. *Science* 2003;300:409.
16. Velculescu VE, Zhang L, Zhou W, et al. Characterization of the yeast transcriptome. *Cell* 1997;88(2):243–251.
17. Velculescu VE, Madden SL, Zhang L, et al. Analysis of human transcriptomes. *Nat Genet* 1999;23(4):387–388.
18. Kahn P. From genome to proteome: looking at a cell's proteins. *Science* 1995;270(5235):369–370.
19. Hunter PJ, Borg TK. Integration from proteins to organs: the physiome project. *Nat Rev Mol Cell Biol* 2003;4:237–243.
20. Tweedale H, Notley-McRobb L, Ferenci T. Effect of slow growth on metabolism of *Escherichia coli,* as revealed by global metabolite pool ("metabolome") analysis. *J Bacteriol* 1988;180:5109–5116.
21. Nicholson JK, Lindon JC, Holmes E. "Metabonomics": understanding the metabolic responses of living systems to pathophysiologic stimuli via multivariate analysis of biological NMR data. *Xenobiotica* 1999;29:1181–1189.
22. Clayton TA, Lindon JC, Clorec O, et al. Pharmaco-metabonomic phenotyping and personalized drug treatment. *Nature* 2006;440: 1073–1077.

23. Agrafiotis DK, Lobanov VS, Salemme FR. Combinatorial informatics in the post-genomics era. *Nat Rev Drug Discov* 2002; 1(5):337–346.
24. Daly MJ, Rioux JD, Schaffner SF, et al. High-resolution haplotype structure in the human genome. *Nat Genet* 2001;2:229–232.
25. Beckmann JS, Estivill X, Antonarakis SE. Copy number variants and genetic traits: closer to the resolution of phenotypic to genotypic variability. *Nat Rev Genet* 2007;8:639–646.
26. Frazer KA, Murray SS, Schork NJ, Topol EJ. Human genetic variation and its contribution to complex traits. *Nat Rev Genet* 2009; 10:241–251.
27. Meyer UA. Genotype or phenotype: the definition of a pharmacogenetic polymorphism. *Pharmacogenetics* 1991;1:66–67.
28. Leeder JS. Pharmacogenetics and pharmacogenomics. *Pediatr Clin North Am* 2001;48:756–781.
29. Hines RN, McCarver DG. The ontogeny of human drug-metabolizing enzymes: phase I oxidative enzymes. *J Pharmacol Exp Ther* 2002;300:355–360.
30. McCarver DG, Hines RN. The ontogeny of human drug-metabolizing enzymes: phase II conjugation enzymes and regulatory mechanisms. *J Pharmacol Exp Ther* 2002;300:361–366.
31. Nuwaysir EF, Bittner M, Trent J, et al. Microarrays and toxicology: the advent of toxicogenomics. *Mol Carcinog* 1999;24(3): 153–159.
32. Kennedy S. The role of proteomics in toxicology: identification of biomarkers of toxicity by protein expression analysis. *Biomarkers* 2002;7:269–290.
33. Klein TE, Chang JT, Cho MK, et al. Integrating genotype and phenotype information: an overview of the PharmGKB project. *Pharmacogenomics J* 2001;1:167–170.
34. Collins MD, Mao GE. Teratology of retinoids. *Annu Rev Pharmacol Toxicol* 1999;39:399–430.
35. Nulman I, Rovet J, Stewart DE, et al. Child development following exposure to tricyclic depressants or fluoxetine throughout fetal life: a prospective, controlled study. *Am J Psychiatry* 2002; 159:1889–1895.
36. Watkins PB. Role of cytochromes P450 in drug metabolism and hepatotoxicity. *Semin Liver Dis* 1990;10:235–250.
37. Streetman DS, Bertino JS, Nafziger AN. Phenotyping of drug-metabolizing enzymes in adults: a review of in-vivo cytochrome P450 phenotyping probes. *Pharmacogenetics* 2000;10:187–216.
38. Evans WE, Relling MV, Petros WP, et al. Dextromethorphan and caffeine as probes for simultaneous determination of debrisoquin-oxidation and N-acetylation phenotypes in children. *Clin Pharmacol Ther* 1989;45(5):568–573.
39. Pariente-Khayat A, Pons G, Rey E, et al. Caffeine acetylator phenotyping during maturation in infants. *Pediatr Res* 1991;29(5): 492–495.
40. Relling MV, Cherrie J, Schell MJ, et al. Lower prevalence of the debrisoquin oxidative poor metabolizer phenotype in American black versus white subjects. *Clin Pharmacol Ther* 1991; 50:308–313.
41. Bosso JA, Liu Q, Evans WE, et al. CYP2D6, *N*-acetylation, and xanthine oxidase activity in cystic fibrosis. *Pharmacotherapy* 1996;16:749–753.
42. Skoda RC, Gonzalez FJ, Demierre A, et al. Two mutant alleles of the human cytochrome P450dbl gene associated with genetically deficient metabolism of debrisoquine and other drugs. *Proc Natl Acad Sci USA* 1988;85:5240–5243.
43. Heim MH, Meyer UA. Genetic polymorphism of debrisoquine oxidation: restriction fragment analysis and allele-specific amplification of mutant alleles of CYP2D6. *Methods Enzymol* 1991;206: 173–183.
44. Xie HG, Stein CM, Kim RB, et al. Allelic, genotypic and phenotypic distributions of *S*-mephenytoin 4′-hydroxylase (CYP2C19) in healthy Caucasian populations of European descent throughout the world. *Pharmacogenetics* 1999;9:539–549.
45. Lee CR, Goldstein JA, Pieper JA. Cytochrome P450 2C9 polymorphisms: a comprehensive review of the in-vitro and human data. *Pharmacogenetics* 2002;12:251–263.
46. Gaedigk A, Bradford LD, Marcucci KA, et al. Unique CYP2D6 activity distribution and genotype-phenotype discordance in black Americans. *Clin Pharmacol Ther* 2002;72:76–89.
47. Bates MD. The potential of DNA microarrays for the care of children. *J Pediatr* 2003;142:235–239.
48. Cheok MH, Yang W, Pui C-H, et al. Treatment-specific changes in gene expression discriminate *in vivo* drug response in human leukemia cells. *Nat Genet* 2003;34:85–90.
49. Sorich MJ, Pottier N, Pei D, et al. In vivo response to methotrexate forecasts outcome of acute lymphoblastic leukemia and has a distinct gene expression profile. *PLoS Med* 2008;5(4):e83. doi:10.1371/journal.pmed.0050083.
50. Burgner D, Davila S, Breunis WB, et al. A genome-wide association study identifies novel and functionally related susceptibility loci for Kawasaki disease. *PLoS Genet* 2009;5(1):e1000319.
51. Moffatt MF, Kabesch M, Liang L, et al. Genetic variants regulating ORMDL3 expression contribute to the risk of childhood asthma. *Nature* 2007;448:470–473.
52. Kugathasan S, Baldassano RN, Bradfield JP, et al. Loci on 20q13 and 21q22 are associated with pediatric-onset inflammatory bowel disease. *Nat Genet* 2008;40:1211–1215.
53. Takeuchi F, McGinnis R, Bourgeois S, et al. A genome-wide association study confirms *VKORC1*, *CYP2C9*, and *CYP4F2* as principal genetic determinants of warfarin dose. *PLoS Genet* 2009; 5(3):e1000433.
54. Shuldiner AR, O'Connell JR, Bliden KP, et al. Association of cytochrome P450 2C19 genotype with the antiplatelet effect and clinical efficacy of clopidogrel therapy. *JAMA* 2009;302(8):849–857.
55. Search Collaborative Group. SLCO1B1 variants and statin-induced myopathy—a genomewide study. *N Engl J Med* 2008; 359(8):789–799.
56. Marguerat S, Wilhelm BT, Bähler J. Next-generation sequencing: applications beyond genomes. *Biochem Soc Trans* 2008;36: 1091–1096.
57. Wang Z, Gerstein M, Snyder M. RNA-Seq: a revolutionary tool for transcriptomics. *Nat Rev Genet* 2009;10:57–63.
58. Zhang K, Li JB, Gao Y, et al. Digital RNA allelotyping reveals tissue-specific and allele-specific gene expression in human. *Nat Methods* 2009;6:613–618.
59. Witzman FA, Grant RA. Pharmacoproteomics in drug development. *Pharmacogenomics J* 2003;3:69–76.
60. Ruepp SU, Tonge RP, Shaw J, et al. Genomics and proteomics of acetaminophen toxicity in mouse liver. *Toxicol Sci* 2002;65:135–150.
61. Charlwood J, Skehel JM, King N, et al. Proteomic analysis of rat kidney cortex following treatment with gentamicin. *J Proteome Res* 2002;1(1):73–82.
62. Miyamae T, Malehorn D, Lemster B, et al. Serum protein profile in systemic-onset juvenile idiopathic arthritis differentiates response versus nonresponse to therapy. *Arthritis Res Ther* 2005; 7(4):R746–R55.
63. Woroniecki RP, Orlova TN, Mendelev N, et al. Urinary proteome of steroid-sensitive and steroid-resistant idiopathic nephrotic syndrome of childhood. *Am J Nephrol* 2006;26:258–267.
64. Kaddurah-Douk R, Kristal BS, Weinshilboum RM. Metabolomics: a global biochemical approach to drug response and disease. *Annu Rev Pharmacol Toxicol* 2008;48:653–683.
65. Geiger C, Geistlinger L, Altmaier E, et al. Genetics meets metabolomics: a genome-wide association study of metabolite profiles in human serum. *PLoS Genet* 2008;4(11):E1000282.
66. Xu EY, Perlina A, Vu H, et al. Integrated pathway analysis of rat urine metabolic profiles and kidney transcriptomic profiles to elucidate the systems toxicology of model nephrotoxicants. *Chem Res Toxicol* 2008;21:1548–1561.
67. Gu H, Pan Z, Xi B, et al. ^{1}NMR metabolomics study of age profiling in children. *NMR Biomed* 2009. Online ahead of print; doi: 10.1002/nbm.395.
68. Hines RN. The ontogeny of drug metabolism enzymes and implications for adverse drug events. *Pharmacol Ther* 2008;118: 250–267.
69. Zanger UM, Turpeinen M, Klein K, et al. Functional pharmacogenetics/genomics of human cytochromes P450 involved in drug biotransformation. *Anal Bioanal Chem* 2008;392: 1093–1108.
70. Zanger UM, Klein K, Saussele T, et al. Polymorphic *CYP2B6*: molecular mechanisms and emerging clinical significance. *Pharmacogenomics* 2007;8:743–759.
71. Kirchheiner J, Brockmöller J. Clinical consequences of cytochrome P450 2C9 polymorphisms. *Clin Pharmacol Ther* 2005;77:1–16.
72. Furuta T, Sugimoto M, Shirai N, et al. CYP2C19 pharmacogenomics associated with therapy of Helicobacter pylori infection

and gastro-esophageal reflux diseases with a proton pump inhibitor. *Pharmacogenomics* 2007;8:1199–1210.
73. Zanger UM, Raimundo S, Eichelbaum M. Cytochrome P450 2D6: overview and update on pharmacology, genetics, and biochemistry. *Naunyn Schmiedebergs Arch Pharmacol* 2004;369:23–37.
74. Sistonen J, Sajantila A, Lao O, et al. *CYP2D6* worldwide genetic variation shows high frequency of altered activity variants and no continental structure. *Pharmacogenet Genomics* 2007;17:93–101.
75. Lee SJ, Goldstein JA. Functionally defective or altered *CYP3A4* and *CYP3A5* single nucleotide polymorphisms and their detection with genotyping tests. *Pharmacogenomics* 2005;6:357–371.
76. Guillemette C. Pharmacogenomics of human UDP-glucuronosyltransferase enzymes. *Pharmacogenomics J* 2003;3:136–158.
77. Nagar S, Blanchard RL. Pharmacogenetics of uridine diphosphoglucuronsyltransferase (UGT) 1A family members and its role in patient response to irinotecan. *Drug Metab Rev* 2006;38: 393–409.
78. Hildebrandt MA, Carrington DP, Thomae BA, et al. Genetic diversity and function in the human cytosolic sulfotransferases. *Pharmacogenomics J* 2007;7:133–143.
79. Sim E, Lack N, Wang CJ, et al. Arylamine N-acetyltransferases: structural and functional implications of polymorphisms. *Toxicology* 2008;254:170–183.
80. Wang L, Weinshilboum R. Thiopurine S-methyltransferase pharmacogenetics: insights, challenges and future directions. *Oncogene* 2006;25:1629–1638.
81. Gaedigk A, Gotschall RR, Forbes NS, et al. Optimization of cytochrome P450 2D6 (CYP2D6) phenotype assignment using a genotyping algorithm based on allele frequency data. *Pharmacogenetics* 1999;9:669–682.
82. Koren G, Cairns J, Chitayat D, et al. Pharmacogenetics of morphine poisoning in a breastfed neonate of a codeine-prescribed mother. *Lancet* 2007;368:704–705.
83. Treluyer JM, Jacqz-Aigrain E, Alvarez F, et al. Expression of *CYP2D6* in developing human liver. *Eur J Biochem* 1991;202: 583–588.
84. Stiskal JA, Kulin N, Koren G, et al. Neonatal paroxetine withdrawal syndrome. *Arch Dis Child Fetal Neonatal Ed* 2001;84: F134–F135.
85. Spencer MJ. Fluoxetine hydrochloride (Prozac) toxicity in a neonate. *Pediatrics* 1993;92:721–722.
86. Mhanna MJ, Bennet JB, Izatt SD. Potential fluoxetine chloride (Prozac) toxicity in a newborn. *Pediatrics* 1997;100:158–159.
87. Lane R, Baldwin D. Selective serotonin reuptake inhibitor-induced serotonin syndrome: review. *Clin Psychopharmacol* 1997;17: 208–221.
88. Oberlander TF, Bonaguro RJ, Misri S, et al. Infant serotonin transporter (SLC6A4) promoter genotype is associated with adverse neonatal outcomes after prenatal exposure to serotonin reuptake inhibitor medications. *Mol Psychiatry* 2008;13:65–73.
89. Sallee FR, DeVane CL, Ferrell RE. Fluoxetine-related death in a child with cytochrome P-450 2D6 genetic deficiency. *J Child Adolesc Psychopharmacol* 2000;10:27–34.
90. Stevens JC, Marsh SA, Zaya MJ, et al. Developmental changes in human liver CYP2D6 expression. *Drug Metab Dispos* 2008;36: 1587–1593.
91. Blake MJ, Gaedigk A, Pearce RE, et al. Ontogeny of dextromethorphan O- and N-demethylation in the first year of life. *Clin Pharmacol Ther* 2007;81:510–516.
92. Sindrup SH, Brøsen K. The pharmacogenetics of codeine hypoalgesia. *Pharmacogenetics* 1995;5:335–346.
93. Poulsen L, Arendt-Nielsen L, Brøsen K, et al. The hypoalagesic effect of tramadol in relation to CYP2D6. *Clin Pharmacol Ther* 1996;60:636–644.
94. Quiding H, Olsson GL, Boreus LO, et al. Infants and young children metabolise codeine to morphine. A study after single and repeated rectal administration. *Br J Clin Pharmacol* 1992;33: 45–49.
95. Quiding H, Anderson P, Bondesson U, et al. Plasma concentrations of codeine and its metabolite, morphine, after single and repeated oral administration. *Eur J Clin Pharmacol* 1986;30: 673–677.
96. Williams DG, Patel A, Howard RF. Pharmacogenetics of codeine metabolism in an urban population of children and its implications for analgesic reliability. *Br J Anaesth* 2002;89:839–845.
97. Kutt H, Wolk M, Scherman R, et al. Insufficient parahydroxylation as a cause of diphenylhydantoin toxicity. *Neurology (NY)* 1964;14:542–548.
98. Kidd RS, Curry TB, Gallagher S, et al. Identification of a null allele of *CYP2C9* in an African-American exhibiting toxicity to phenytoin. *Pharmacogenetics* 2001;11:803–808.
99. Steward DJ, Haining RL, Henne KR, et al. Genetic association between sensitivity to warfarin and expression of *CYP2C9*3*. *Pharmacogenetics* 1997;7:361–367.
100. Sullivan-Klose TH, Ghanayem BI, Bell DA, et al. The role of the *CYP2C9*-Leu^{359} allelic variant in the tolbutamide polymorphism. *Pharmacogenetics* 1996;6:341–349.
101. Bhasker CR, Miners JO, Coulter S, et al. Allelic and functional variability of cytochrome P4502C9. *Pharmacogenetics* 1997;7:51–58.
102. Rettie AE, Wienkers LC, Gonzalez FJ, et al. Impaired (S)-warfarin metabolism catalysed by the R144C allelic variant of CYP2C9. *Pharmacogenetics* 1994;4:39–42.
103. Haining RL, Hunter AP, Veronese ME, et al. Allelic variants of human cytochrome P4502C9: baculovirus-mediated expression, purification, structural characterization, substrate stereospecificity and prochiral selectivity of the wild-type and I359L mutant forms. *Arch Biochem Biophys* 1996;333:447–458.
104. Dickman LJ, Rettie AE, Kneller MB, et al. Identification and functional characterization of a new CYP2C9 variant (CYP2C9*5) expressed among African Americans. *Mol Pharmacol* 2001; 60:382–387.
105. Takahashi H, Ishikawa S, Nomoto S, et al. Developmental changes in pharmacokinetics and pharmacodynamics of warfarin enantiomers in Japanese children. *Clin Pharmacol Ther* 2000;68:541–555.
106. Goldstein JA. Clinical relevance of genetic polymorphisms in the human CYP2C subfamily. *Br J Clin Pharmacol* 2001;52(4): 349–355.
107. Furuta T, Shirai N, Takashima M, et al. Effect of genotypic differences in CYP2C19 on cure rates for *Helicobacter pylori* infection by triple therapy with a proton pump inhibitor, amoxicillin, and clarithromycin. *Clin Pharmacol Ther* 2001;69:158–168.
108. Sim SC, Risinger C, Dahl ML, et al. A common novel CYP2C19 gene variant causes ultrarapid drug metabolism relevant for the drug response to proton pump inhibitors and antidepressants. *Clin Pharmacol Ther* 2006;79:103–113.
109. Rudberg I, Mohebi B, Hermann M, et al. Impact of the ultrarapid *CYP2C19*17* allele on serum concentration of escitalopram in psychiatric patients. *Clin Pharmacol Ther* 2008;83(2): 322–327.
110. Wrighton SA, VandenBranden M. Isolation and characterization of human fetal liver cytochrome P450HLp2: a third member of the P450III gene family. *Arch Biochem Biophys* 1989;268: 144–151.
111. Yang HY, Lee QP, Rettie AR, et al. Functional cytochrome P4503A isoforms in human embryonic tissues: expression during organogenesis. *Mol Pharmacol* 1994;46:922–928.
112. Lacroix D, Sonnier M, Moncion A, et al. Expression of CYP3A in the human liver. Evidence that the shift between CYP3A7 and CYP3A4 occurs immediately after birth. *Eur J Biochem* 1997;247: 625–634.
113. Thummel KE, O'Shea D, Paine MF, et al. Oral first-pass elimination of midazolam involves both gastrointestinal and hepatic CYP3A-mediated metabolism. *Clin Pharmacol Ther* 1996;59: 491–502.
114. Paine MF, Shen DD, Kunze KL, et al. First-pass metabolism of midazolam by the human intestine. *Clin Pharmacol Ther* 1996; 60:14–24.
115. Wrighton SA, Ring BJ, Watkins PB, et al. Identification of a polymorphically expressed member of the human cytochrome P-450III family. *Mol Pharmacol* 1989;36:97–105.
116. Kuehl P, Zhang J, Lin Y, et al. Sequence diversity in *CYP3A* promoters and characterization of the genetic basis of polymorphic CYP3A5 expression. *Nat Genet* 2001;27:383–391.
117. Rebbeck TR, Jaffe JM, Walker AH, et al. Modification of clinical presentation of prostate tumors by a novel genetic variant in CYP3A4. *J Natl Cancer Inst* 1998;90:1225–1229.
118. Felix CA, Walker AH, Lange BJ, et al. Association of *CYP3A4* genotype with treatment-related leukemia. *Proc Natl Acad Sci USA* 1998;95:13176–13181.

119. Ball SE, Scatina J, Kao J, et al. Population distribution and effects on drug metabolism of a genetic variant in the 5′ promoter region of *CYP3A4*. *Clin Pharmacol Ther* 1999;66:288–294.
120. Westlind A, Löfberg L, Tindberg N, et al. Interindividual differences in hepatic expression of CYP3A4: relationship to genetic polymorphism in the 5′-upstream regulatory region. *Biochem Biophys Res Commun* 1999;259:201–225.
121. Wandel C, Witte JS, Hall JM, et al. CYP3A activity in African American and European American men: population differences and functional effect of the *CYP3A4*1B* 5′-promoter region polymorphism. *Clin Pharmacol Ther* 2000;68:82–91.
122. Amirimani B, Weber BL, Rebbeck TR. Regulation of reporter gene expression by a CYP3A4 promoter variant in primary human hepatocytes. *Proc Am Assoc Cancer Res* 2000;60:114.
123. Lai J, Vesprini D, Chu W, et al. *CYP* gene polymorphisms and early menarche. *Mol Genet Metab* 2001;74:449–457.
124. Kadlubar FF, Berkowitz GS, Delongchamp RR, et al. The *CYP3A4*1B* variant is related to the onset of puberty, a known risk factor for the development of breast cancer. *Cancer Epidemiol Biomarkers Prev* 2003;12:327–331.
125. Westlind-Johnsson A, Malmebo S, Johansson A, et al. Comparative analysis of CYP3A expression in human liver suggests only a minor role for CYP3A5 in drug metabolism. *Drug Metab Dispos* 2003;31:755–761.
126. Stevens JC, Hines RN, Gu C, et al. Developmental expression of the major human hepatic CYP3A enzymes. *J Pharmacol Exp Ther* 2003;307:573–582.
127. Rodríguez-Antona C, Jande M, Rane A, et al. Identification and phenotype characterization of two *CYP3A* haplotypes causing different enzymatic capacity in fetal livers. *Clin Pharmacol Ther* 2005;77:259–270.
128. Leeder JS, Gaedigk R, Marcucci KA, et al. Variability of CYP3A7 in human fetal liver. *J Pharmacol Exp Ther* 2005;314:626–635.
129. Schirmer M, Rosenberger A, Klein K, et al. Sex-dependent genetic markers of CYP3A4 expression and activity in human liver microsomes. *Pharmacogenomics* 2007;8:443–453.
130. Monaghan G, McLellan A, McGeehan A, et al. Gilbert's syndrome is a contributory factor in prolonged unconjugated hyperbilirubinemia of the newborn. *J Pediatr* 1999;134:441–446.
131. Kadakol A, Sappal BS, Ghosh SS, et al. Interaction of coding region mutations and the Gilbert-type promoter abnormality of the UGT1A1 gene causes moderate degrees of unconjugated hyperbilirubinaemia and may lead to neonatal kernicterus. *J Med Genet* 2001;38(4):244–249.
132. Gagne JF, Montminy V, Belanger P, et al. Common human UGT1A polymorphisms and the altered metabolism of irinotecan active metabolite 7-ethyl-10-hydroxycamptothecin (SN-38). *Mol Pharmacol* 2002;62:608–617.
133. Iyer L, Das S, Janisch L, et al. UGT1A1*28 polymorphism as a determinant of irinotecan disposition and toxicity. *Pharmacogenomics J* 2002;2:43–47.
134. Ménard V, Eap O, Harvey M, et al. Copy-number variations (CNVs) of the human sex steroid metabolizing genes *UGT2B17* and *UGT2B28* and their associations with a *UGT2B15* functional polymorphism. *Hum Mutat* 2009;30:1310–1319.
135. Burchell B. Genetic variation of human UDP-glucuronosyltransferase. Implications in disease and drug glucuronidation. *Am J Pharmacogenomics* 2003;3:37–52.
136. May G. Genetic differences in drug disposition. *J Clin Pharmacol* 1994;34:881–897.
137. Meyer UA. Genetic polymorphisms of drug metabolism. *Fund Clin Pharmacol* 1990;4:595–615.
138. Pompeo F, Brooke E, Kawamura A, et al. The pharmacogenetics of NAT: structural aspects. *Pharmacogenomics* 2002;3:19–30.
139. Hadasova E, Brysova V, Kadlcakova E. *N*-Acetylation in healthy and diseased children. *Eur J Clin Pharmacol* 1990;39:43–47.
140. Pariente-Khayat A, Rey E, Gendrel D, et al. Isoniazid acetylation metabolic ratio during maturation in children. *Clin Pharmacol Ther* 1997;62:377–383.
141. McLeod HL, Siva C. The thiopurine S-methyltransferase gene locus—implications for clinical pharmacogenomics. *Pharmacogenomics* 2002;3:89–98.
142. Lennard L, Gibson BES, Nicole T, et al. Congenital thiopurine methyltransferase deficiency and 6-mercaptopurine toxicity during treatment for acute lymphoblastic leukaemia. *Arch Dis Child* 1993;69:577–579.
143. Lennard L, Lewis IJ, Michelagnoli M, et al. Thiopurine methyltransferase deficiency in childhood lymphoblastic leukaemia: 6-mercaptopurine dosage strategies. *Med Pediatr Oncol* 1997;29: 252–255.
144. McLeod HL, Krynetski EY, Wilimas JA, et al. Higher activity of polymorphic thiopurine S-methyltransferase in erythrocytes from neonates compared to adults. *Pharmacogenetics* 1995;5:281–286.
145. Park-Hah JO, Klemetsdal B, Lysaa R, et al. Thiopurine methyltransferase activity in a Korean population sample of children. *Clin Pharmacol Ther* 1996;60:68–74.
146. Ganiere-Monteil C, Medard Y, Lejus C, et al. Phenotype and genotype for thiopurine methyltransferase activity in the French Caucasian population: impact of age. *Eur J Clin Pharmacol* 2004; 60:89–96.
147. Tai HL, Krynetski EY, Schuetz EG, et al. Enhanced proteolysis of thiopurine *S*-methyltransferase (TPMT) encoded by mutant alleles in humans (TPMT*3A, TPMT*2): mechanisms for the genetic polymorphism of TPMT activity. *Proc Natl Acad Sci USA* 1997;94:6444–6449.
148. Tai HL, Fessing MY, Bonten EJ, et al. Enhanced proteasomal degradation of mutant human thiopurine S-methyltransferase (TPMT) in mammalian cells: mechanism for TPMT protein deficiency inherited by TPMT*2, TPMT*3A, TPMT*3B or TPMT*3C. *Pharmacogenetics* 1999;9:641–650.
149. Spire-Vayron de la Moureyre C, Debuysère H, Sabbagh N, et al. Detection of known and new mutations in the thiopurine *S*-methyltransferase gene by single-strand conformation polymorphism analysis. *Hum Mutat* 1998;12:177–185.
150. Spire-Vayron de la Moureyre C, Debuysère H, Fazio F, et al. Characterization of a variable number tandem repeat region in the thiopurine *S*-methyltransferase gene promoter. *Pharmacogenetics* 1999;9:189–198.
151. De Ridder L, van Dieren JM, van Deventer HJH, et al. Pharmacogenetics of thiopurine therapy in pediatric IBD patients. *Aliment Pharmacol Ther* 2006;23:1137–1141.
152. Belay ED, Bresee JS, Holman RC, et al. Reye's syndrome in the United States from 1981 through 1997. *N Engl J Med* 1999; 340:1377–1382.
153. Bryant AE, Dreifuss FE. Valproic acid hepatic fatalities. III. U.S. experience since 1986. *Neurology* 1996;46:465–469.
154. Messenheimer JA. Rash in adult and pediatric patients treated with lamotrigine. *Can J Neurol Sci* 1998;25:S14–S18.
155. The International Warfarin Pharmacogenetics Consortium. Estimation of the warfarin dose with clinical and pharmacogenetic data. *N Engl J Med* 2009;360:753–764.
156. Kronenberg S, Frisch A, Rotberg B, et al. Pharmacogenetics of selective serotonin reuptake inhibitors in pediatric depression and anxiety. *Pharmacogenomics* 2008;9:1725–1736.
157. Pui CH, Evans WE. Acute lymphoblastic anemia. *N Engl J Med* 1998;339:605–615.
158. Relling MV, Hancock ML, Boyett JM, et al. Prognostic importance of 6-mercaptopurine dose intensity in acute lymphoblastic leukemia. *Blood* 1999;93:2817–2823.
159. Relling MV, Rubnitz JE, Rivera GK, et al. High incidence of secondary brain tumours after radiotherapy and antimetabolites. *Lancet* 1999;354:34–39.
160. Relling MV, Yanishevski Y, Nemec J, et al. Etoposide and antimetabolite pharmacology in patients who develop secondary acute myeloid leukemia. *Leukemia* 1998;12:346–352.
161. Wall AM, Rubnitz JE. Pharmacogenomic effects on therapy for acute lymphoblastic leukemia in children. *Pharmacogenomics J* 2003;3:128–135.
162. Relling MV, Dervieux T. Pharmacogenetics and cancer therapy. *Nat Rev Cancer* 2001;1:99–108.
163. Yeoh EJ, Ross ME, Shurtleff SA, et al. Classification, subtype discovery, and prediction of outcome in pediatric acute lymphoblastic leukemia by gene expression profiling. *Cancer Cell* 2002;1(2):133–143.
164. Yang JJ, Cheng C, Yang W, et al. Genome-wide interrogation of germline genetic variation associated with treatment response in childhood acute lymphoblastic leukemia. *JAMA* 2009;301: 393–403.

CHAPTER

6

Hakan Ergün
Daniel A.C. Frattarelli
Doreen Matsui

Adherence with Pediatric Medication Regimens

INTRODUCTION

In pharmacotherapy, the terms "compliance" and "adherence" are often used interchangeably, although the latter term is preferred by some as it acknowledges the patient's role in the decision-making process. Adherence has been defined as "the extent to which a person's behavior—taking medication, following a diet, and/or executing lifestyle changes—corresponds with agreed recommendations from a healthcare provider" (1).

Deviations from medical advice on the part of the patient (such as using the wrong route of administration, taking too low or too high a dose, or taking the medication at the wrong times or for an inappropriate length of time) is defined as noncompliance. Besides these types of noncompliance, other factors, such as comedication or the intake of certain foods or nutritional supplements, can affect the pharmacokinetics (absorption, distribution, metabolism, or elimination) or pharmacodynamics (drug effect on the body) of the prescribed drug and can result in either a suboptimal effect or unforeseen side effects, both of which can be serious. Once it is known that a particular drug should not be taken with another drug or food (e.g., grapefruit juice*), avoidance of this other drug or food becomes a part of the therapy, and lack of adherence to this recommendation can be considered a form of noncompliance as well. Compliance issues have been well studied in adults, but comparatively little data exist about pediatric compliance.

Despite the best efforts on the part of the physician to diagnose and appropriately treat a condition, treatment failure can still occur if the patient fails to follow medical advice. Adherence is therefore an extremely vulnerable step in the therapeutic process, and one that often receives little consideration. However, attention to matters of adherence can have a very real and beneficial effect on the overall outcome. In this chapter, we describe the impact of compliance on patient care, how to measure it, the types of noncompliance, the factors that contribute to noncompliance in pharmacotherapy, and means of reducing this behavior.

IMPACT OF NONCOMPLIANCE

Noncompliance is a significant problem in all areas of medicine. Studies show that noncompliance for medications ranges from 13% to 93% in adults and from 25% to 82% in children (3). Noncompliance should therefore be viewed more as the rule than the exception. As a result of noncompliance, misjudgment of the efficacy of therapy on the part of the physician who assumes compliance with the medication regimen may result in additional consultations and investigations, alterations of dose or drug, hospitalization, loss of productivity (lost work or school days), and increased risk of adverse effects related to prolonged therapy.

When assessing the prevalence of noncompliance, it is also important to take into account the way in which compliance is determined. Patient self-report, pill count, biological assays, and electronic monitoring devices may vary significantly from each other in terms of the data obtained. Difficulties also arise from the lack of truly objective definitions for compliance, as the dividing line between adherence and nonadherence is not uniformly agreed upon.

The question of whether a patient will comply with the prescribed medication regimen introduces an element of uncertainty into the decision-making process of the physician. When a patient's condition improves, compliance is usually assumed on the part of the physician. However, when things do not go as planned, questions arise and the physician must decide whether the poor response represents a failure at the stages of diagnosis or treatment or in adherence to medical advice. Exploration of issues of compliance can make physicians and patients uncomfortable and is therefore often deferred or avoided. As a result,

*Grapefruit juice is an inhibitor of intestinal cytochrome P450 (CYP) 3A4 enzyme, which is responsible for the first-pass metabolism of many drugs (2).

extra and potentially unnecessary therapies may be used on the noncompliant patient, when an honest discussion may have proved sufficient.

Because there is an overall noncompliance rate of about 50% for the millions of prescriptions written annually, this issue becomes a general public health problem. Noncompliance translates into additional expenditures in terms of wasted medication, repeated or changed courses of medications due to a perceived treatment failure, and extra physician visits. The cost of noncompliance to society is not solely a financial one. The spread of infections such as tuberculosis is an important public health problem and must be treated appropriately (4,5). Untreated or inadequate therapy may result in epidemics or resistance to drugs leading to potentially serious consequences.

HOW TO MEASURE COMPLIANCE

Our knowledge of any phenomenon is dependent on the reliability of the data provided and thus on the means of assessing it. The accuracy and reliability of measurements of compliance vary with the method used. This determination is further complicated by the lack of a clear consensus as to what defines compliance and noncompliance. The simplest way to get information about adherence to therapy is to ask the patient, but the nature of compliance is complex and does not always allow easy accurate assessment. A significant amount of noncompliance happens without the awareness of the patient; as a result, other techniques must be employed to get an accurate assessment of patient compliance.

PATIENT SELF-REPORT

Several studies have been done to compare the differences among methods of measuring compliance (6). One of the most commonly used methods is patient self-report. The validity of the patient interview depends on various factors. The patient's ability to recall events and/or willingness to report these accurately are potentially confounding issues. The use of a medication diary can, to a certain extent, overcome these factors and is a feasible and more reliable way to evaluate compliance. In most studies, the diary method has been found to underestimate noncompliance when compared with other methods (7).

The skill of the interviewer may affect the report as well, because the way in which the question is posed to the patient can have a marked influence on the response. It is also important to ask the questions in a nonjudgmental and nonthreatening manner.

Parent reporting of adherence has been shown to be overrated. Both children and parents overreported adherence with inhaled corticosteroids by computerized-assisted self-interviewing, face-to-face interview, and self-administered questionnaire (8). Parent and caregiver reports of adherence were not predictive of any of the outcome measures in a study of pediatric and adolescent liver transplant recipients (9). Similarly, in children with HIV, caregiver self-report of adherence with antiretroviral therapy was higher than that measured by electronic monitoring (Medication Event Monitoring System, MEMS) (10).

PHYSICIAN ESTIMATES OF PATIENT COMPLIANCE

Many physicians assume noncompliance when a treatment appears to have failed or when an expected side effect does not occur. From a scientific perspective, estimation of compliance by the physician is not an objective measurement technique. Several studies have investigated the reliability of physician estimates of compliance, and they have shown similarly disappointing results (9,11). Charney et al. reported that predictions of compliance by pediatricians in private practice were no better than chance alone (12). Blackwell's review lent credence to this observation and added that physicians tended to overestimate compliance (13).

OUTCOME

Outcome is occasionally used to measure compliance but can be unreliable. Because of the many factors that determine response to therapy, a patient may be noncompliant and improve anyway, or may be quite compliant and not respond at all. Compliance may also change as a function of response. When a patient's condition is improving, compliance tends to increase, whereas when there is a poor response, compliance tends to decrease (14).

PILL COUNT

This method is one of the most frequently used to measure compliance, especially in clinical trials of new drugs, where the remaining drug has to be accounted for and returned. The calculation is simply done by taking the percentage of pills taken versus the total prescribed for a specified period of time. This method tends to overestimate compliance and is limited by factors such as the patient forgetting to return the bottle, the patient losing some or all of the pills, or the possibility of deception on the part of the patient (pill dumping).

ANALYSIS OF BODY FLUIDS

Analysis of body fluids for a particular drug and/or its metabolite has been viewed as an objective method for assessment of compliance. Such assays can be qualitative or quantitative. Measurement of drug levels in body fluids can be employed, for example, in the clinical trial of a new medication to ensure that it is correctly taken, but there are several limitations to this approach. One of the most important of these involves the timing of the measurement. The physician does not know whether this monitoring at a single point in time or at periodic intervals represents uniform and consistent compliance, or whether the patient has taken medications only in the period before the sample was drawn (whitecoat compliance or toothbrush effect). Morrow and Rabin found that compliance was lower when measured by collections from random home visits as compared with scheduled measurements in a clinic (15). Other studies of this issue have been more equivocal (16,17). Individual differences in bioavailability, metabolism, and excretion can also introduce uncertainty into these tests.

Other limitations of this method include that it may involve an invasive and painful means of collecting the sample, which may be particularly concerning in the pediatric population. Assaying for the presence of a medication in a body fluid requires the existence of a method for its detection (which is not always readily available) and the equipment and personnel to perform the assay. These resources are frequently centered at certain institutions, requiring these specimens to be sent out, introducing a time delay in knowing the result, and incurring extra expense.

ELECTRONIC MONITORS

Electronic monitors, such as the MEMS, were introduced for measuring compliance with therapy in the 1980s (18). Microprocessors in the medication container record and store information of the date and time of medication removal as a presumptive dose. Data can be downloaded to computers for analysis. These devices allow for evaluation of temporal dosing patterns and correlation with clinical events.

Electronic compliance monitors have been used to study compliance in several pediatric conditions including epilepsy (19), asthma (8), HIV infection, renal transplantation (20), and acute lymphoblastic leukemia (21). Despite their potential advantages, limitations to their use include expense, the potential for mechanical failure (22), and lack of patient acceptability (23).

TYPES OF NONCOMPLIANCE

There are several types of noncompliance, which can be subclassified and ranked in terms of the disease, the status of the patient, and the characteristics of the therapeutic regimen. It should be understood that compliance is a dynamic process, and that the degree of compliance will change over time. Compliance is also not a binary process. Some children or families will be quite compliant with some aspects of therapy and completely noncompliant with others.

The reasons for a patient not following his or her treatment regimen can be divided into two groups: conscious and unconscious noncompliance. In general, most noncompliance is not a conscious deliberate act. Willingness to be treated is accepted as normal behavior, and patients believe they are following the description of the treatment. However, many factors (to be discussed) related to the disease or the age of the patient may affect the compliance rate. For example, others must care for a small child who is unable to take his or her medicine. In this case, the compliance is not primarily related to the patient but more to other people, often the parents who are caring for the child. Noncompliance in such a case is considered a form of unconscious noncompliance. Unfortunately, there does not appear to be a difference between the parent's behavior in terms of their compliance and compliance with their children's therapy. Kleinteich reported the results of an anonymous questionnaire given to mothers (24). He showed that only half of the prescribed drug had been administered to the children according to the instructions. In a subanalysis, compliance was found to vary with the type of drug as well (24).

Psychological factors affecting compliance with therapy may fall under unconscious noncompliance as well. These complicated factors have been investigated in many studies, especially in adolescents (25). Other factors, such as poor explanation of the therapy on the part of the physician or pharmacist, may result in decreased compliance with therapy and should not be classified as conscious noncompliance.

Unconscious noncompliance may relate to environmental and economic issues. Despite the development of therapeutic alternatives, in many parts of the world, appropriate therapies are not available. A patient may not be able to afford the therapy or may not have access to it in his or her neighborhood. Physicians should take time to ask questions to screen for the availability of the therapy and to check whether there are financial barriers to obtaining the medication.

FACTORS AFFECTING COMPLIANCE

Because of the many multifactorial interactions that affect and determine compliance, it is almost impossible to broadly identify which factors are the more involved. Among those factors that have been found to have some association with compliance, none has been found to be either necessary or sufficient to produce noncompliance. At their best, these factors are useful clues to the astute clinician but are not reliable measures or predictors of compliance. A summary of factors affecting compliance is given in Table 6.1. It has been shown that initial compliance is the best predictor of subsequent compliance with therapy, but compliance is a dynamic process and may change over time within the same patient (17,24–26).

Forgetfulness is often the most commonly cited reason for not taking one's medication or for parent's not administering their children's medication (9,27–29).

DRUG-RELATED FACTORS

Route of Administration

As a general rule, the simpler the administration, the better is the compliance. Spector reported that in asthma

TABLE 6.1 Factors Affecting Compliance

Drug-related factors	Patient-related factors
Taste	Age
Administration route	Health history
Cost	Environment
Dosing frequency	Education
Duration	Family
Side or adverse effect	Insurance
Physician-related factors	Religion
Illness-related factors	Motivation
In- or outpatient therapy	Pharmacist-related factors
Acute or chronic illness	
Comorbidities	

patients, where drugs may be given orally or via inhalation, oral therapy had better compliance, with patients preferring tablets to inhalers (30). Development of oral iron chelators may be advantageous in some patients with thalassemia and other transfusion-dependent anemias, as compliance with deferoxamine is hindered by the requirement for nightly subcutaneous infusions (31).

Dosing Frequency

Greenberg reviewed studies to observe the effects of different dosing regimens. The results demonstrated that there is a negative correlation between dosing frequency and compliance. The once-daily, twice-daily, three-times-daily, and four-times-daily doses showed compliance rates of 73%, 70%, 52%, and 42%, respectively (32). The effect of dosing frequency was subsequently confirmed by a systematic review of studies in which compliance was measured by an electronic monitoring device. Compliance with once-daily dosing was found to be significantly higher than that with drugs dosed three or four times a day, and twice-daily dosing had a superior rate to four-times-daily daily dosing as well. No difference has been found between once-daily and twice-daily dosing (33).

In a study comparing twice-daily and three-times-daily amoxicillin/clavulanate therapy regimens in acute otitis media patients aged 2 months to 12 years (34), the results showed that both regimens had equal efficacy but the twice-daily regimen had a higher level of compliance and lower incidence of drug-related adverse events than did the three-times-daily regimen (34). Block et al. compared two drugs in three daily frequencies in nonrefractory acute otitis media patients aged between 6 months and 12 years (35). They reported that all three groups had equivalent efficacy and that once-daily dosing of same drug seemed to be more favorable (35). Parents prefer less frequent dosing, in particular avoiding the middle of the day (36).

Duration

Duration of therapy is primarily based on the characteristics of the illness. In many chronic diseases, treatment may be lifelong or at least last for a long period of time and it is not possible to reduce the duration of therapy. However, for some conditions (e.g., in infectious diseases), therapy may be required only for a short period of time. Any decrease in the duration of therapy may improve patient satisfaction and compliance, leading to a more favorable clinical outcome while decreasing cost and the incidence of side effects (37). In ambulatory pediatric patients prescribed oral antibiotics for various bacterial infections, compliance was better when treatment lasted for 7 days or less, whereas longer regimens lead to decreased compliance (38). A shorter antibacterial course may result in better adherence with the treatment of pneumonia in children (39). Adherence was higher in children with respiratory tract illness treated with short-course (5 days), high-dose amoxicillin therapy than in children treated with a standard 10-day regimen (40).

Compliance with treatment for acute infection as well as with long-term therapy tends to decrease over time (36). In a questionnaire study of antibiotic use, 31% of patients or parents claimed that they did not complete the antibiotic course with the most common reason for stopping prematurely being that the patients felt better (87%) (41).

Taste

Although few studies have documented the effect of palatability on compliance, parents commonly report difficulty in administering medications due to resistance from the child. It is not unreasonable to assume that if the child refuses to take the medication the adherence may suffer. In a study of adherence issues in children and adolescents receiving antiretroviral therapy for HIV infection, the majority of parents (78%) reported difficulty associated with administering highly active antiretroviral therapy (HAART) medications with taste being one of the most common reasons (42). In pediatric renal transplant patients, a negative association was found between patients' level of agreement that their medicine tastes bad and medication adherence (43).

PATIENT-RELATED FACTORS

The relation between patient and physician generally begins with a willingness to be treated on the part of the patient. The expectation of the patient is that the best and most appropriate therapy will be prescribed in accordance with the practice of evidence-based medicine and the experience and judgment of the physician. Independent of the therapy itself, other factors, such as the explanation of the therapy given by the physician, can affect the success of treatment.

Religion

Aslam and Healy investigated Asian Muslim's behavior during their religious month of Ramadan. Thirty-seven out of 81 patients (46%) changed their drug dosage patterns during the daytime fasting period (44). Although, there are no controlled studies in the literature about the pediatric population yet, adolescents, who have reached the age of puberty and are also fasting during Ramadan, may present a behavior similar to that of adults (45). Physicians should be aware of Ramadan and determine fasting practices and their potential complications among their Muslim adolescent patients to prevent these complications that may arise.

Family

Tebbi et al. reported on 46 cancer patients aged 2.5 to 23 years who were interviewed to determine the causes of their noncompliance. In this study (in contrast to many others), they did not find any correlation between compliance and drug-related factors (type or number of days) or illness-related factors (stage of the disease). Instead, a significant negative correlation was found between compliance and the number of children in the family. As has been seen in other studies, age was found to be an important variable, and adolescent patients were less compliant than were other age groups (46).

Level of maternal education was shown not to affect administration of medication but rather to be associated with other variables, such as knowing the name of the drug, the schedule for its administration, and when the follow-up appointment was scheduled (47). In another study, the amount of formal education (more vs. less than 8 years) was found to be predictive of adherence to therapy in asthmatics (48). These associations, as well as the problem of illiteracy and the presence of caretakers who may not understand the language, should prompt the clinician to evaluate the family situation and make arrangements as necessary. Socioeconomic status has not been shown to correlate with noncompliance in the majority of studies.

Another factor is the degree of family conflict and disorganization (49). In a study of 88 children with diabetes, Miller-Johnson et al. noted no association between discipline, warmth, or emotional support and compliance but did notice a correlation between parent–child conflict and noncompliance (50). Parental involvement has been associated with better adherence with blood glucose monitoring (51,52) and the medical regimen (53,54) in children and adolescents with diabetes mellitus.

Family factors have also been shown to be important in pediatric transplant patients. Adolescents with renal transplants reported fewer missed doses when their parents were in charge than when they were solely responsible for their medications (27). Similarly, Feinstein et al. found that noncompliance was higher in adolescents who were responsible for their own medications and that insufficient family support was more common in the noncompliant group (55). Poorer family cohesion has been reported in nonadherent pediatric liver transplant patients (56,57).

Age

Age has been investigated in many studies to determine whether it is a predictor of compliance (58). Several other factors, such as the characteristics of the illness and social factors, can confound the assessment of age as a variable.

Adolescence seems to be a particularly difficult time to maintain compliance. This was summed up best by Litt and Cuskey, who noted that "teens are abusers of nonprescribed drugs and nonusers of prescribed ones" (59). Noncompliance in this population has been associated with low self-esteem, poor socialization, and psychological problems (17,60). Conflict may occur between the adolescent's growing independence and parental involvement in his or her medication regimen (61). There is also considerable noncompliance with any therapy that results in the adolescent appearing different from or unattractive to his or her peers, even if the lack of therapy will result in significant morbidity or mortality (e.g., cancer). Morse et al. analyzed reasons for noncompliance and found that pill taking in public is an important barrier to many, who feel that they are being stigmatized as ill or different (62). Half of adolescents and young adults with HIV infection acknowledged on a questionnaire that they skipped doses of medications because they feared that family or friends would discover their status (63).

Tamaroff et al. investigated psychologic variables in 34 adolescent and young adult patients (64). Their results indicate that a poor complier has significantly less developed concepts of his or her illness, less perceived vulnerability, higher levels of denial, and less cohesive future orientation. The authors suggested that adolescents and young adults construct their own subjective view of the illness and its treatment, which then has implications for compliance with medication regimens (64).

Jonasson et al. studied 161 children between 7 and 16 years old with mild asthma (65). According to their medication diaries, compliance was found to be 93%, whereas counting the remaining doses revealed a much lower rate of 77%. Age played a significant role in compliance, as children 9 years old and younger were found to have better adherence than were older children (65). Older age was a major predictor for poor adherence to immediate-release methylphenidate in children with attention-deficit hyperactivity disorder (66). More adolescent patients with acute lymphoblastic leukemia were found to be poorly compliant with oral 6-mercaptopurine maintenance therapy than were younger children (67).

PHYSICIAN-RELATED FACTORS

The perception of the behavior of the physician by the patient may play an important role in therapy. A study by Hoppe et al. reported a comparison of different antibiotic regimens and the factors affecting medication compliance (38). The results indicated that age, living in city, the choice of drug and dosing regimen, and the perceived sympathy of the pediatrician were highly scored by the parents of the patient as factors that affect the compliance rate (38). Adherence depends on trust in the health professional–patient relationship and effective communication is a central element (68).

Factors other than those typically thought of as being a direct part of the time spent with the patient may play a significant role as well. DiMatteo et al. showed that physician job satisfaction, the number of patients seen per week, the scheduling of follow-up appointments, and the physician's specialty were all correlated with compliance (26). Compliance was found to be higher when the physician was a specialist rather than a generalist (69). It was also high among parents who had faith in the physician's ability to make a correct diagnosis and who felt that the physician understood their concerns for the child (70,71).

Compliance is greater in private practices than in clinics (72). This may reflect the importance of continuity of care and the establishment of a good doctor–patient relationship, or may represent those patients who have confidence in a particular physician and therefore stay with him or her. However, some aspects of practices are associated with poorer compliance. Specifically, waiting time (either due to block scheduling or physician lateness) is correlated with decreased compliance (73).

Assumption of comprehension and recall on the part of the patient or his or her family must never be assumed. Roughly two-thirds of patients interviewed immediately after an office visit had forgotten the diagnosis and treatment explanations, and half had forgotten the instructional statements (74). This same study also showed that the amount of information retained was inversely proportional to the amount given. At the same time, it has been shown that parents want discussion of the illness (and to a lesser extent the treatment), and that giving this information increases compliance (75). Clinicians should therefore be careful to give detailed written instructions for key parts of therapy including diagnosis, therapeutic recommendations, reasons to come back, and when to follow up.

Factors such as the level of patient anxiety should also be taken into consideration. Hazzard et al. analyzed 35 pediatric seizure patients and found that parents' worry was correlated with behavioral restrictions placed on the child, and turned out to be a negative factor in compliance with therapy (76). They also hypothesized that anxiety-based denial and perceived threats to patient autonomy may interfere with adherence to therapy (76).

ILLNESS-RELATED FACTORS

Chronic illnesses have overall lower compliance rates than do time-limited conditions, and if the disease is asymptomatic, the compliance rates are lower still. In children in an area with a high incidence of tuberculosis, adherence to antituberculosis treatment for disease was significantly better than was adherence to chemoprophylaxis (82.6% vs. 44.2%) (77). In children diagnosed with vesicoureteral reflux prescribed prophylactic antibiotics to prevent urinary tract infections, only 17% of patients were more than 80% compliant with an overall rate of compliance of 41.4% (78).

Taken together, it is not possible to judge the relative importance of these various factors in determining compliance. Clinical research results do not perfectly reflect the realities of daily clinical practice. Because these studies are specially designed to investigate certain variables and are comparatively well monitored, the outcome may very well be different than what is seen in the real world.

HOW TO IMPROVE COMPLIANCE

The most practical and sought-after scenario in pharmacotherapy is that of treatment effectively given by a single dose of an inexpensive drug, free of any side effects, and which can easily be administered by the patient or parent (preferably by the oral route). Unfortunately, this option is not available for the majority of diseases. The reality in most cases is that the drug has to be taken more than once, has a fairly strict time schedule, and sometimes cannot be given orally. Still, there are steps physicians can take to foster compliance. The International Expert Forum on Patient Adherence assigned the highest priority to the development of simple interventions that can be easily implemented in everyday practice (79).

It is important to have a high index of suspicion for noncompliance when the anticipated clinical response does not occur. Improved communication between the physician and patient and/or parents may enhance adherence by identifying potential barriers to medication taking. Family concerns and questions should be elicited. Negotiation and mutual agreement on a medication regimen tailored to the child and family's lifestyle and daily routine may be helpful. Linking medication administration times to routine daily events such as teeth brushing or bedtime may also assist patients in remembering to take their medication. Education of the patient and/or family regarding the disease and its management should be undertaken with provision of a clearly written explanation of the treatment plan. Continuous feedback and reinforcement at subsequent visits of the information provided may also be useful. A multidisciplinary approach is often best acknowledging the significant role of other health care providers.

Physicians should make every attempt to streamline the medication regimen whenever possible, in particular when there are multiple caregivers involved or the child is at daycare or school. Decreasing the number of doses the patient must take per day may result in significantly higher compliance without sacrificing efficacy (80). In a meta-analysis that involved pediatric and adult patients, it was reported that a 10-day twice-daily regimen of penicillin for streptococcal pharyngitis was as effective as more frequent dosing (81). If feasible, once- or twice-daily medication schedules are preferable (82). Consideration should be given to the taste and formulations of medications prescribed for young children. It has been stated that "treatments that are easier to take invite better adherence" (83).

SUMMARY

Compliance with the prescribed medication regimen is as important as selecting the appropriate therapy in effecting a cure for a patient. This issue is not solely the responsibility of the physician. Other parties in the health care system (nurses, pharmacists, regulatory agencies, reimbursement authorities, and insurance companies) have a responsibility to create effective and applicable programs such as public education programs. Implementation of this and the other practices described in this chapter will help ensure that prescribed medication regimens are followed and that optimal patient outcome is achieved.

REFERENCES

1. World Health Organization. Adherence to long-term therapies: evidence for action, 2003. http://www.who.int/chp/knowledge/publications/adherence_full_report.pdf. Accessed January 4, 2009.
2. Drug interactions. Cytochrome P450 system. http://medicine.iupui.edu/flockhart/table.htm. Accessed January 16, 2009.
3. Sclar DA, Tartaglione TA, Fine MJ. Overview of issues related to medical compliance with implications for the outpatient management of infectious diseases. *Infect Agents Dis* 1994;3:266–273.
4. Siafakas NM, Bouros D. Consequences of poor compliance in chronic respiratory diseases. *Eur Respir J* 1992;5:134–136.
5. Smirnoff M, Goldberg R, Indyk L, et al. Directly observed therapy in an inner city hospital. *Int J Tuberc Lung Dis* 1998;2:134–139.
6. Roth HP. Historical review: comparison with other methods. *Control Clin Trials* 1984;5(Suppl 4):476–480.
7. Berg J, Dunbar-Jacob J, Rohay JM. Compliance with inhaled medications: the relationship between diary and electronic monitor. *Ann Behav Med* 1998;20:36–38.
8. Bender BG, Bartlett SJ, Rand CS, et al. Impact of interview mode on accuracy of child and parent report of adherence with asthma-controller medication. *Paediatrics* 2007;120:e471–e477.
9. Shemesh E, Shneider E, Savitzky JK, et al. Medication adherence in pediatric and adolescent liver transplant recipients. *Pediatrics* 2004;113:825–832.

10. Muller AD, Bode S, Myer L, et al. Electronic measurement of adherence to pediatric antiretroviral therapy in South Africa. *Pediatr Infect Dis J* 2008;27;257–262.
11. Murri R, Antinori A, Ammassari A, et al. Physician estimates of adherence and the patient–physician relationship as a setting to improve adherence to antiretroviral therapy. *J Acquir Immune Defic Syndr* 2002;31(Suppl 3):S158–S162.
12. Charney E, Bynum R, Eldredge D, et al. How well do patients take oral penicillin? A collaborative study in private practice. *Pediatrics* 1967;40:188–195.
13. Blackwell B. Drug therapy: patient compliance. *N Engl J Med* 1973;289:249–252.
14. Rickels K, Briscoe E. Assessment of dosage deviation in outpatient drug research. *J Clin Pharmacol J New Drugs* 1970;10:153–160.
15. Morrow R, Rabin DL. Reliability in self medication with isoniazid I & II. *Clin Res* 1965;14:362A.
16. Gordis L, Markowitz M, Lilienfeld AM. Why patients don't follow medical advice: a study of children on long-term antistreptococcal prophylaxis. *J Pediatr* 1969;75:957–968.
17. Friedman IM, Litt IF, King DR, et al. Compliance with anticonvulsant therapy by epileptic youth. Relationships to psychosocial aspects of adolescent development. *J Adolesc Health Care* 1986;7:12–17.
18. Dusing R, Lottermoser K, Mengden T. Compliance with drug therapy—new answers to an old question. *Nephrol Dial Transplant* 2001;16:1317–1321.
19. Modi AC, Morita DA, Glauser TA. One-month adherence in children with new-onset epilepsy: white-coat compliance does not occur. *Pediatrics* 2008;121:e961–e966.
20. Blowey DL, Hebert D, Arbus GS, et al. Compliance with cyclosporine in adolescent renal transplant recipients. *Pediatr Nephrol* 1997;11:547–551.
21. Lau RC, Matsui D, Greenberg M, et al. Electronic measurement of compliance with mercaptopurine in pediatric patients with acute lymphoblastic leukemia. *Med Pediatr Oncol* 1998;30:85–90.
22. Berkovitch M, Papadouris D, Shaw D, et al. Trying to improve compliance with prophylactic penicillin therapy in children with sickle cell disease. *Br J Clin Pharmacol* 1998;45:605–607.
23. Shellmer DA, Zelikovsky N. The challenges of using medication event monitoring technology with pediatric transplant patients. *Pediatr Transplant* 2007;11:422–428.
24. Kleinteich B. Reliability of ambulatory drug therapy in childhood. *Padiatr Grenzgeb* 1993;31:171–174.
25. Staples B, Bravender T. Drug compliance in adolescents: assessing and managing modifiable risk factors. *Paediatr Drugs* 2002;4:503–513.
26. DiMatteo MR, Sherbourne CD, Hays RD, et al. Physicians' characteristics influence patients' adherence to medical treatment: results from the Medical Outcomes Study. *Health Psychol* 1993; 12:93–102.
27. Zelikovsky N, Schast AP, Palmer J, et al. Perceived barriers to adherence among adolescent renal transplant candidates. *Pediatr Transplant* 2008;12:300–308.
28. Burgess SW, Sly PD, Morawska A, et al. Assessing adherence and factors associated with adherence in young children with asthma. *Respirology* 2008;13:559–63.
29. Murphy DA, Sarr M, Durako SJ, et al. Barriers to HAART adherence among human immunodeficiency virus-infected adolescents. *Arch Pediatr Adolesc Med* 2003;157:249–255.
30. Spector S. Noncompliance with asthma therapy—are there solutions? *J Asthma* 2000;37:381–388.
31. Neufeld EJ. Oral chelators deferasirox and deferiprone for transfusional iron overload in thalassemia major: new data, new questions. *Blood* 2006;107:3436–3441.
32. Greenberg RN. Overview of patient compliance with medication dosing: a literature review. *Clin Ther* 1984;6:592–599.
33. Claxton AJ, Cramer J, Pierce C. A systematic review of the associations between dose regimens and medication compliance. *Clin Ther* 2001;23:1296–1310.
34. Damrikarnlert L, Jauregui AC, Kzadri M. Efficacy and safety of amoxycillin/clavulanate (Augmentin) twice daily versus three times daily in the treatment of acute otitis media in children. The Augmentin 454 Study Group. *J Chemother* 2000;12:79–87.
35. Block SL, McCarty JM, Hedrick JA, et al. Comparative safety and efficacy of cefdinir vs amoxicillin/clavulanate for treatment of suppurative acute otitis media in children. *Pediatr Infect Dis J* 2000;19(Suppl 12):S159–S165.
36. Winnick S, Lucas DO, Hartman AL, et al. How do you improve compliance? *Pediatrics* 2005;115:e718–e724.
37. Pichicero M. Short courses of antibiotic in acute otitis media and sinusitis infections. *J Int Med Res* 2000;28(Suppl 1):25A–36A.
38. Hoppe JE, Blumenstock G, Grotz W, et al. Compliance of German pediatric patients with oral antibiotic therapy: results of a nationwide survey. *Ped Infect Dis J* 1999;18:1085–1091.
39. Qazi S. Short-course therapy for community-acquired pneumonia in paediatric patients. *Drugs* 2005;65:1179–1192.
40. Schrag SJ, Pena C, Fernandez J. Effect of short-course, high-dose amoxicillin therapy on resistant pneumococcal carriage: a randomized trial. *JAMA* 2001;286:49–56.
41. Pechere JC. Patients' interviews and misuse of antibiotics. *Clin Infect Dis* 2001;33(Suppl 3):S170–S173.
42. Goode M, McMaugh A, Crisp J, et al. Adherence issues in children and adolescents receiving highly active antiretroviral therapy. *AIDS Care* 2003;15:403–408.
43. Tucker CM, Fennell RS, Pederson T, et al. Association with medication adherence among ethnically different pediatric patients with renal transplants. *Pediatr Nephrol* 2002;17:251–256.
44. Aslam M, Healy MA. Compliance and drug therapy in fasting Moslem patients. *J Clin Hosp Pharm* 1986;11:321–325.
45. Tazi I. Ramadan and cancer. *J Clin Oncol* 2008;26:5485.
46. Tebbi CK, Cummings KM, Zevon MA, et al. Compliance of pediatric and adolescent cancer patients. *Cancer* 1986;58:1179–1184.
47. Becker M, Drachman R, Kirscht J. A new approach to explaining the sick role behavior in low-income populations. *Am J Public Health* 1974;64:205–216.
48. Radius SM, Becker MH, Rosenstock IM, et al. Factors affecting mothers' compliance with a medication regimen for asthmatic children. *J Asthma Res* 1978;15:133–149.
49. Haynes RB. A critical review of the "determinants" of patient compliance with therapeutic regimens. In: Sackett DL, Haynes RB, eds. *Compliance with therapeutic regimens.* Baltimore, MD: Johns Hopkins University Press, 1976:26–50.
50. Miller-Johnson S, Emery RE, Marvin RS, et al. Parent–child relationships and the management of insulin-dependent diabetes mellitus. *J Consult Clin Psychol* 1994;62:603–610.
51. Anderson B, Ho J, Brackett J, et al. Parental involvement in diabetes management tasks: relationships to blood glucose monitoring adherence and metabolic control in young adolescents with insulin-dependent diabetes mellitus. *J Pediatr* 1997;130: 257–265.
52. Anderson BJ, Vangsness L, Connell A, et al. Family conflict, adherence, and glycaemic control in youth with short duration Type 1 diabetes. *Diabet Med* 2002;19;635–642.
53. Ellis DA, Podolski CL, Frey M, et al. The role of parental monitoring in adolescent health outcomes: impact on regimen adherence in youth with type 1 diabetes. *J Pediatr Psychol* 2007; 32:907–917.
54. Pereira MG, Berg-Cross L, Almeida P, et al. Impact of family environment and support on adherence, metabolic control, and quality of life in adolescents with diabetes. *Int J Behav Med* 2008; 15:187–193.
55. Feinstein S, Keich R, Becker-Cohen R, et al. Is noncompliance among adolescent renal transplant recipients inevitable? *Pediatrics* 2005:115:969–973.
56. Fredericks EM, Lopez MJ, Magee JC, et al. Psychological functioning, nonadherence and health outcomes after pediatric liver transplantation. *Am J Transplant* 2007;7:1974–1983.
57. Fredericks EM, Magee JC, Opipari-Arrigan L, et al. Adherence and health-related quality of life in adolescent liver transplant recipients. *Pediatr Transplant* 2008;12:289–299.
58. Imanaka Y, Araki S, Nobutomo K. Effects of patient health beliefs and satisfaction on compliance with medication regimens in ambulatory care at general hospitals. *Nippon Eiseigaku Zasshi* 1993;48: 601–611.
59. Litt IF, Cuskey WR. Compliance with medical regimens during adolescence. *Pediatr Clin North Am* 1980;27:3–15.
60. Korsch BM, Fine RN, Negrete VF. Noncompliance in children with renal transplants. *Pediatrics* 1978;61:872–876.
61. Matsui D. Current issues in pediatric medication adherence. *Pediatr Drugs* 2007;9(5):283–288.

62. Morse EV, Simon PM, Balson PM. Using experiential training to enhance health professionals' awareness of patient compliance issues. *Acad Med* 1993;68:693–697.
63. Rao D, Kekwaletswe TC, Hosek S, et al. Stigma and social barriers to medication adherence with urban youth living with HIV. *AIDS Care* 2007;19:28–33.
64. Tamaroff MH, Festa RS, Adesman AR, et al. Therapeutic adherence to oral medication regimens by adolescents with cancer. II. Clinical and psychologic correlates. *J Pediatr* 1992;120:812–817.
65. Jonasson G, Carlsen KH, Sodal A, et al. Patient compliance in a clinical trial with inhaled budesonide in children with mild asthma. *Eur Respir J* 1999;14:150–154.
66. Gau SSF, Shen HY, Chou MC, et al. Determinants of adherence to methylphenidate and the impact of poor adherence on maternal and family measures. *J Child Adolesc Psychopharmacol* 2006;16: 286–297.
67. Lancaster D, Lennard L, Lilleyman JS. Profile of non-compliance in lymphoblastic leukaemia. *Arch Dis Child* 1997;76:365–366.
68. DiMatteo MR. The role of effective communication with children and their families in fostering adherence to pediatric regimens. *Patient Educ Couns* 2004;55:339–344.
69. Heinzelmann F. Factors in prophylaxis behavior in treating rheumatic fever: an exploratory study. *J Health Hum Behav* 1962;3:73–81.
70. Francis V, Korsch BM, Morris MJ. Gaps in doctor–patient communication. Patients' response to medical advice. *N Engl J Med* 1969;280:535–540.
71. Korsch BM, Gozzi EK, Francis V. Gaps in doctor–patient communication. 1. Doctor–patient interaction and patient satisfaction. *Pediatrics* 1968;42:855–871.
72. Emans SJ, Grace E, Woods ER, et al. Adolescents' compliance with the use of oral contraceptives. *JAMA* 1987;257:3377–3381.
73. Feinstein AR, Wood AF, Epstein JA, et al. A controlled study of three methods of prophylaxis against streptococcal infection in a population of rheumatic children. II. Results of the first three years of the study, including methods for evaluating the maintenance of oral prophylaxis. *N Engl J Med* 1959;260: 697–702.
74. Joyce CRB, Capla G, Mason M, et al. Quantitative study of doctor–patient communication. *Q J Med* 1969;38:183–194.
75. Freeman M, Negrete V, Davis M, et al. Gaps in doctor–patient communication: doctor–patient interaction analysis. *Pediatr Res* 1971;5:298–311.
76. Hazzard A, Hutchinson SJ, Krawiecki N. Factors related to adherence to medication regimens in pediatric seizure patients. *J Pediatr Psychol* 1990;15:543–555.
77. Van Zyl S, Marais BJ, Hesseling AC, et al. Adherence to anti-tuberculosis chemoprophylaxis and treatment in children. *Int J Tuberc Lung Dis* 2006;10:13–18.
78. Hensle TW, Hyun G, Grogg, Eaddy M. Part 2: Examining pediatric vesicoureteral reflux: a real-world evaluation of treatment patterns and outcomes. *Curr Med Res Opin* 2007;23(Suppl 4): S7–S13.
79. van Dulmen S, Sluijs E, van Dijk L, et al. Furthering patient adherence: a position paper of the international expert forum on patient adherence based on an internet forum discussion. *BMC Health Serv Res* 2008;8:47.
80. Dajani AS. Adherence to physicians' instructions as a factor in managing streptococcal pharyngitis. *Pediatrics* 1996;97:976–980.
81. Lan AJ, Colford JM, Colford JM Jr. The impact of dosing frequency on the efficacy of 10-day penicillin or amoxicillin therapy for streptococcal tonsillopharyngitis: a meta-analysis. *Pediatrics* 2000;105:e19.
82. Gardiner P, Dvorkin L. Promoting medication adherence in children. *Am Fam Physician* 2006;74:793–798.
83. Bender BG. Overcoming barriers to nonadherence in asthma treatment. *J Allergy Clin Immunol* 2002;109:S554–S559.

CHAPTER

7

Steven Hirschfeld

Clinical Trials Involving Children: *History, Rationale, Regulatory Framework, and Technical Considerations*

BRIEF HISTORY OF RESEARCH INVOLVING CHILDREN

Children have been utilized to test new therapies for thousands of years, but prospective clinical investigations to test hypotheses were a development of the 18th century. While living in Constantinople in 1718, Lady Mary Montague, daughter of the Duke of Kinston, observed the Turkish procedure of inoculation against smallpox and had her 6-year-old son inoculated. Upon her return to London, she requested a surgeon to inoculate her 5-year-old daughter. The surgeon used a thread soaked in pustular secretions bound to the skin. This technique was replaced by scarring with a lance tip dipped in pus. The resulting plaque was then covered until it healed, and experimental research in pediatric preventive medicine began in Europe (1).

The American clergymen Cotton Mather also became interested in the procedure after hearing from the slave Onesimus about a practice of using fluid from a patient with mild smallpox to inoculate uninfected people in Africa. Subsequently, he read about the European experience in his correspondence with members of the Royal Society of London. An outbreak of smallpox in Boston in 1721, despite efforts at quarantining the index case, provided an opportunity to experiment. Mather persuaded Boston physician Zabdiel Boylston to proceed with what may have been the first clinical trial in North America. Boylston inoculated his 6-year-old son by lancing the skin and applying to it 9- to 14-day-old pustular material from a smallpox patient, then wrapped the skin in a cabbage leaf. Subsequently, he inoculated 280 people, including 65 children. Unfortunately, six of the adults, although none of the children, subsequently died, with a case fatality rate of approximately 2%. Despite the fact that the smallpox fatality rate for the general population in Boston was 14%, a great controversy about the value of inoculation followed, including the hurling of a bomb into Rev. Mather's home. Fortunately, the explosive did not detonate, but the practice of inoculation did not become public policy (2).

Experimental immunotherapy evolved further with the work of Edward Jenner in England. In 1796, Jenner injected James Phipps, an 8-year-old boy, with extract from pustules from the hand of Sarah Nelmes, a milkmaid. Jenner had been told by milkmaids that cowpox protected them against smallpox. The word vaccination is derived from the Latin word for cow-vaccine. Jenner examined his patient every day, and then 2 weeks after the cowpox injection; Jenner applied a challenge of smallpox extract and found that the boy was protected. He expanded his study from the initial child to "a number" of others ranging in age from 11 months to 8 years. None of the children became ill. Over the course of the next 50 years, vaccination became compulsory in some areas of England (3).

During the 19th century, children's hospitals were established in Europe and the United States in cities including Paris, Vienna, London, Philadelphia, Boston, and New York. Concurrently, pediatrics became an academic specialty, and textbooks were published. Ludwig Friedrich Meissner of Leipzig, Germany, published a survey of texts and monographs pertaining to pediatric medicine, in 1826 noting that prior to 1,775 there were 200 publications and subsequently there were at least almost 7,000 (1).

In 1828, Charles-Michel Billard of the Hospice des Infants Trouvts in Paris published a revolutionary treatise classifying pediatric diseases on the basis of pathology rather than symptoms. In addition, he included a catalogue of height, weight, and vital signs (4). This was followed by surveys by Quetelet in Belgium and Chadwick in England on growth rates of children showing that lower socioeconomic class was associated with less growth, most probably due to nutritional deficiencies (5,6). Comparative pharmacology began about the middle of the 19th century.

In 1834, the first periodical devoted entirely to the care of children, Aizalekteiz iiber Kinderkrankheiten (Annals of Diseases of Children), was published in Stuttgart; it ceased publication in 1837 after publishing 12 volumes. Over the course of the following decades, many journals appeared in several countries as academic societies and publishing houses developed interest in the field of pediatric research (7).

In 1847, John Snow began to administer anesthesia with ether to children aged 4 through 16 years. He also experimented with chloroform and by 1857 had successfully anesthetized hundreds of children, including 186 infants under the age of 1 year. He first described differences in metabolism between adults and children, noting that the effects of chloroform were more quickly produced and also subsided more quickly in children, explaining the observation in terms of the quicker breathing and circulation in pediatric patients (1).

Frederik Theodor Berg was appointed the first European professor of pediatrics at the Karolinska Institute in Stockholm, Sweden, in 1845. In 1858, he resigned from the post to become Director of the Central Bureau of Statistics. In that capacity, he expanded the bureau's data banks to include not only population, but also welfare, agricultural, and industrial data. He founded a statistical journal in 1869, and in the same year, utilizing parish records, he published a paper analyzing infant mortality rates in Sweden (8).

The first course in the United States at an academic institution devoted to pediatrics was offered at the Yale College of Medicine in 1813 by Eli Ives (9). In 1860, Abraham Jacobi, an émigré from Germany, was appointed as professor of infantile pathology and therapeutics at the New York Medical College, which may have been the first full academic pediatric appointment in America. A pediatric clinic with the first use of bedside teaching was founded in 1862 (10).

The first institution for sick children in the United States was founded in 1855 in Philadelphia. Boston and New York followed in 1869, and the District of Columbia in 1871. By 1880, Jacobi had been instrumental in the establishment of several hospitals for children in the United States—Chicago, San Francisco, St Louis, and Cincinnati—so that by 1895 there were 26 children's hospitals in this country. In 1868, Jacobi wrote an article on croup in the first issue of the American Journal of Obstetrics and Diseases of Women and Children, published by the American Medical Association. The first American journal dedicated totally to pediatric research. Archives of Pediatrics began publication in 1884.

In 1880, Jacobi organized the pediatric section of the American Medical Association (AMA) and in 1885, he became President of the New York Academy of Medicine. In 1888, he became a founding member of the American Pediatric Society, which limited membership to 110. The society published its Transactions, which, for the first third of the 20th century, was the major American journal devoted to pediatric research. Jacobi was among the first to recognize the potential of using government resources to advance clinical science. He is credited with persuading the US Congress to appropriate the funds for the first printing of Index Medicus, compiled by his friend John Shaw Billings (11).

TRANSITION INTO THE TWENTIETH CENTURY AND THE BEGINNING OF ETHICAL CONCERNS AND REGULATION

Claude Bernard wrote in 1865, "It is our duty and our right to perform experiments on man whenever it can save his life, cure him, or give him some personal benefit" (12). This statement has been interpreted that ethically only studies that provide direct benefit to the participants should be undertaken, but the principle had no legal authority. The question of prior permission to participate was not addressed.

The last decades of the 19th century saw further experimentation in immunotherapy for the treatment of infectious diseases, with many of the major advances resulting from studies on children. In 1885, Pasteur injected 9-year-old Joseph Meister of Alsace, who had been bitten by a rabid dog, with extract of rabbit spinal cord from a rabbit that had died of rabies 2 weeks before. Thirteen inoculations were given daily with the last an extract from a rabid dog. The boy recovered and a second shepherd boy was similarly cured (13).

In 1892, an immunologic approach to reduce transmission of venereal disease was attempted in a study by Albert Neisser, professor of dermatology and syphilis in Breslau and discoverer of the organism responsible for gonorrhea. He subcutaneously and intravenously injected eight women and girls, the youngest being 10 years old, with cell-free extract of syphilis in an attempt to stimulate an immune response.

Subsequently, four of the women became infected, leading to the speculation that the cause of their illness could have been Neisser and his experiment, and a subsequent public scandal followed (14). The debate continued primarily in the press for several years until December 19, 1900, when the Prussian Ministry of Education and Medicine issued a policy statement about human experimentation. The proclamation stated that research may not be performed without the permission of the patient and that research on children was forbidden. It further stated that research should have as its goal the diagnosis, treatment, or prevention of disease.

This was probably the first government edict about human research, and although a potent statement had been made, enforcement powers did not follow (15). The rise of the chemical industry, particularly in Germany, fed the hope of targeting diseases through the administration of manufactured compounds. As an example, the recognition of genital infections as a source of infant morbidity led Karl Sigmund Franz Crede in 1884 to use silver nitrate solution to prevent gonorrhea infections of the eyes of the newborn (16,17).

There was a rush to examine the medical (and potential commercial) activity of many newly synthesized products, spurred by Paul Ehrlich's vision of a "magic bullet" and a permissive social climate. In 1902, the psychiatrist Albert Moll published a monograph, Aertzliche Ethik (Medical

Ethics), in which he catalogued some 600 publications of medical experiments where, he argued, there was no possible benefit to the subject. Moll criticized not only the dangers of the experiments, but the lack of advantage to the patient (18,19). Despite the Prussian edict and Moll's book, however, there would be no translation of patient protection into public policy for another third of a century.

EVOLUTION OF ETHICAL PRINCIPLES AND THEIR APPLICATION TO RESEARCH

Health crises involving children have played a major role in the evolution of food and drug law in the United States. The first major domestic controls occurred early in the 20th century, following more than 100 attempts in the 19th century to pass federal legislation, regulating the manufacture and sale of foods and drugs. In the autumn of 1901 in St Louis, more than a dozen children died of tetanus after receiving diphtheria antitoxin that had been recovered from a tetanus-infected horse. Subsequently, another 100 cases of tetanus were reported, including the deaths of nine more children. This led to the passage of the Biologics Control Act of 1902, which called for the licensing, labeling, and supervision of biological products intended for humans (20).

In the autumn of 1905, Collier's Weekly published an exposé of fraud in the manufacture and sale of patent medicines, citing cases of infants who died following administration of syrup that contained morphine that was intended to treat colic. Although concern was widespread, public documentation of specific cases of death or morbidity due to commercial drugs was lacking due to contract clauses on publications by drug manufacturers threatening to cancel advertisements if legislation regulating drug marketing was passed. Nevertheless, through the efforts of a coalition of chemists, women's clubs, state officials, civic organizations, and writers, in June 1906, President Theodore Roosevelt signed the first Pure Food and Drug Act into law. The Act established the need for product labels, prohibited interstate commerce in adulterated or misbranded drugs, and established the need to maintain standards (20). There was, however, a provision in the Act that permitted deviation from the standards if they were stated on the label. Enforcement was to be by the courts.

This led to the case of US versus Johnson in 1911, in which a majority of the Supreme Court ruled in favor of the defendant, the manufacturer of Dr. Johnson's Mild Combination Treatment for Cancer, this claimed as its ingredients a mixture of substances with the names like Cancerine tablets, Antiseptic tablets, Blood purifier, Special No. 4, Cancerine No. 17, and Cancerine No. 1. The Court stated that prosecution was to be limited to false and misleading statements about the ingredients or the identity of a product and was not intended to extend to false therapeutic claims (21). In an effort to address the gap, the 1912 Sherley Amendment to the Pure Food and Drug Act stated that false therapeutic claims could be prosecuted, but only if intent to defraud could be proven in court (22). The rising political prominence of pediatrics led to the first White House Conference on the Care of Dependent Children in 1909. Based on a recommendation from the Conference, the United States Children's Bureau was established by Congress in 1912 to coordinate health care policy (23).

World War I had multiple aftereffects, including recognition of the poor physical condition of many of the young men recruited to serve in the armed forces. A political response was the Sheppard-Towner bill in 1921 to provide funding for the health care of poor mothers and infants and extend health supervision from infancy to preschool children (24). The question of the role of government and how much support it should provide for health care and children's issues was debated for much of the 20th century, primarily on philosophical and political grounds.

The next major change in regulations occurred in 1927 when the Federal Caustic Poisons Act was passed in an effort to protect children from lye and other dangerous chemicals by requiring labeling with warnings and antidotes.

The American Medical Association was not sheltered from this discussion and at the 1928 meeting there was planning for a society that would be open to any physician trained in pediatrics. Two years later a schism occurred within the AMA on the issue of government support for clinics to treat infants and children with the goal of reducing mortality. A group of pediatricians withdrew and formed a new organization, the American Academy of Pediatrics (25).

In 1930, the US Congress established the National Institutes of Health by renaming the US Hygiene Laboratory in Washington, DC (26). In addition the Food, Drug and Insecticide Administration was established as an enforcement agency. The name was shortened in 1930 to the Food and Drug Administration. Legislation to revise the 1906 Food and Drug Act was proposed in 1933, but became mired in Congress (20).

In 1931, the German Ministry of the Interior issued the first guidelines published for the conduct of research on children. These were part of general guidelines for the conduct of clinical research that were issued in response to allegations by the press and members of the national legislature of questionable and even unethical conduct by physicians. The guidelines were the initial governmental statement of requirements for the ethical conduct of clinical research, which are found in subsequent statements such as the Helsinki Declaration.

The general principles were the primary obligation and duty of the experimenter to protect the subject, the need for informed consent in all circumstances, the principle of preclinical testing in animals prior to human use, and the principle of accurate publication of findings. An experimental compound was defined as any intervention that did not contribute directly to the treatment of an individual patient. No mention is made of peer review in either the experimental or publication process, although the Berlin medical board, which earlier in the century had issued its own recommendations on protection of research subjects, had proposed a regulatory oversight body. This proposal was not incorporated into the final guidelines.

The German guidelines contained two sentences specifically about children: "Application of the new treatment must be considered particularly carefully if it involves infants or adolescents of less than 18 years" and "Experimentation on infants or persons of less than 18 years is forbidden even if it will only expose them to a very slight danger" (27).

In September 1937, the Samuel E. Massengill Pharmaceutical Company in St Louis marketed the newly discovered antibiotic sulfanilamide as a 10% solution, substituting 72% diethylene glycol for the usual solute of ethanol and sweetening it with sugar and raspberry syrup. The resulting elixir killed more than 100 people, including many children, due to glycol-induced renal failure and resulted in the suicide of the chemist who made it. The product was only labeled as an elixir, which implied ethyl alcohol and did not state the full list of ingredients, and thus the company was charged with misbranding. The absence of an applicable law meant that there was no culpability for the deaths.

This tragedy led to the passage of the Food, Drug and Cosmetic Act, which was signed into law by President Franklin Roosevelt in June 1938. The Act gave authority to the Food and Drug Administration (FDA) to require that safety is established before marketing, required disclosure of all active ingredients, required directions for use and warnings about misuse unless the product was sold by prescription, allowed federal inspections of manufacturing facilities, established procedures for the formal review of applications for marketing, explicitly prohibited false claims, and extended the scope of the regulation to cosmetics and devices. There were no provisions for premarketing review, and only those products that were to be sold for interstate commerce were covered. All applications were automatically approved if the FDA did not act within 60 days. The regulation of advertising of therapeutics was assigned to the Federal Trade Commission (28).

International recognition of the need to protect participants in clinical experiments surfaced during the Nuremberg military tribunals in 1946. Evidence was given that up to 200 German doctors had performed experiments with prisoners of war and civilians, which had no protections for the participants and caused harm without any prospect of benefit. The subsequent court proceedings led to the development of the Nuremberg Code, which established international standards for the treatment of one human by another. The guiding principle was that, "The voluntary consent of the human subject is absolutely essential." This statement has been widely interpreted as precluding research on children, although the Nuremberg Code is silent on the specific subject of pediatric research (29).

In 1962, the tragedy of the births of malformed children, primarily in Europe and Canada due to the effects of thalidomide taken as a sedative by their mothers while pregnant resulted in part in Congress passing the Kefauver-Harris amendment to the Food, Drug and Cosmetic Act.

This amendment added an important new facet—the requirement that a product demonstrates efficacy prior to approval of a marketing claim. Additional provisions in the amendment were the need to establish good manufacturing practice (GMP) and maintain production records, the requirement to file an application with the FDA prior to clinical testing (Investigational New Drug application, or IND), an increase in the time for FDA marketing authorization review from 60 to 180 days, the transferral of regulatory authority for drug advertising to the FDA, and withdrawal of approval if new evidence indicated lack of safety or effectiveness (30). The addition of an efficacy requirement prompted a retrospective study by the National Academy of Sciences of FDA approvals between 1938 and 1962, which showed that 40% of the drugs were not effective (31). The new aspect in analysis of product use by adding an efficacy requirement was that benefit and risk could be assessed and acceptable ratios of risk to benefit determined for the intended use at the prescribed dose.

To summarize, the three principles of regulation—labeling, safety, and efficacy—were formalized during the first two-thirds of the 20th century. Formal guidelines for the protection of participants in research and children, in particular, are a product of the last third of the 20th century.

As a point of reference, protection for animals goes back to the 19th century. For example, in the United Kingdom, the Cruelty to Animals Act became law in 1876 (32). In 1960, Louis G. Welt, of the Department of Medicine at Yale University, sent a questionnaire regarding practices for clinical research to university departments of medicine. Sixty-six replied, of which 24 (36%) either already had or were in favor of establishing a committee to review studies involving human experimentation (33). In 1962 the Medical Research Council of the United Kingdom made a statement in its annual report that drew a distinction between research interventions intended to be of direct benefit to the subject of the research and those that are not so intended. These two categories of research were referred to as "therapeutic" and "nontherapeutic," respectively. The report went on to state that, "In the strict view of the law, parents and guardians of minors cannot give consent on their behalf to any procedures which are of no particular benefit to them and which may carry some risk of harm." This statement has regularly been interpreted as placing a complete embargo on nontherapeutic research on children. A follow-up report in 1963 addressed some of the perceived legal and ethical problems in clinical research.

The World Medical Association adopted in 1964 the Declaration of Helsinki: Recommendations Guiding Medical Doctors in Biomedical Research Involving Human Subjects. The document made a distinction between therapeutic and nontherapeutic research, and stated that protocols, independent review of the proposed research, and informed consent should be part of the protection of participants in research. Third-party consent for a participant unable to consent was described, thus offering an approach to pediatric research (34).

Henry Beecher, professor of anesthesia at Harvard Medical School, published an article titled "Ethics and clinical research" in the New England Journal of Medicine in 1966 (35). He drew attention to 22 reports that contained clinical research with a variety of ethical problems, most of which put patients at considerable risk. One of these was the Willowbrook study in New York, which exposed institutionalized children to serum infected with hepatitis. The study was performed with institutional approval, and parents gave permission. The rationale was that hepatitis was so prevalent that the children were likely to become infected and that it was scientifically important to study the early phases of the infectious process.

The Willowbrook approach of using institutionalized children as experimental subjects was not unprecedented. Other studies with institutionalized children in Massachusetts during the 1950s exposed children to radioactive compounds, in one case to study mineral absorption and in another case to study the protective effect of nonradioactive iodine in blocking radioactive iodine in the event of a nuclear explosion. Both studies had federal funding, and the former study had additional funding from the Quaker Oats Company because one of the study questions was to examine the effect of cereal composition on mineral absorption (36).

In 1966, the Surgeon General of the United States, Dr. William H. Stewart, issued a memo based on recommendations by his predecessor, Dr. Luther Terry, and the National Institutes of Health (NIH) director, Dr. James Shannon, requiring institutions accepting federal funds to certify to establish independent review of research projects before they were started. In addition, institutions had to provide the relevant federal funding agency assurance that procedures were in place for consent and review.

In December 1966, the policy was expanded to include behavioral as well as medical research (37). In 1967, the Public Health Service required that intramural research, including that conducted at NIH, abides by similar requirements. Even institutions with existing review committees had to improve their procedures to comply with the new regulations (38).

Also in 1967, the UK Royal College of Physicians Committee on the Supervision of the Ethics of Clinical Investigation in Institutions published a first report recommending that every hospital or institution in which clinical research was undertaken has a research committee that should satisfy itself of the ethics of all proposed investigations. The proposed research committees, with at least one lay member, should be established in every region to review the ethics of proposed investigation, and by law they should be responsible to the General Medical Council (39). In the same year, M. H. Pappworth published Human Guinea Pigs, which detailed several hundred reports of questionable ethics in human experimentation (40).

In 1973 in Great Britain, the chief medical officer of the Department of Health and Social Security requested the Royal College of Physicians Committee to again make a recommendation. The subsequent committee report reflected a shift in attitude. It stated,

> If advances in medical treatment are to continue, so must clinical research investigation. It is in this light, therefore that it is recommended that clinical research investigations of children or mentally handicapped adults which is not of direct benefit to the patients should be conducted, only when the procedures entail negligible risk or discomfort and subject to the provisions of any common and statute law prevailing at the time. The parent or guardian should be consulted and his agreement recorded.

This revision appears to suggest that it is permissible to conduct nontherapeutic research on children, provided this is perceived to be of negligible risk (41). In 1974, the US Department of Health, Education, and Welfare issued regulations requiring institutions that receive federal funds for research to establish institutional review boards and described procedures and criteria for informed consent (42).

Also in 1974, Congress passed the National Research Act. All federally funded clinical research proposals as well as the adequacy of informed consent had to be reviewed by an institutional review board with oversight and enforcement dependent on the particular federal funding agency, meaning there was no global oversight of federally funded research (43).

The National Research Act established a National Commission for the Protection of Human Subjects of Medical and Behavioral Research. The National Commission had a mandate to develop ethical guidelines for the conduct of research on human subjects, in particular children, and to make recommendations to the Secretary of Health, Education, and Welfare. To prepare the report, the National Commission, over the next several years, held public hearings, commissioned papers and other reports, commissioned a survey of the practice of more than 400 investigators engaged in pediatric research, and convened a national conference to ensure that the views of various constituencies were heard (44).

When the UK Department of Health and Social Security issued a circular titled Supervision of the Ethics of Clinical Research Investigations and Fetal Research in 1975, it drew attention to this point, stating, "(one) ought not to infer from this recommendation that the fact that consent has been given by the parent or guardian and that the risk involved is considered negligible will be sufficient to bring such clinical research investigation within the law as it stands" (45). The British chief medical officer wrote in another publication that it was not legitimate to perform an experiment on a child that was not in the child's interests.

The 1975, revision of the Declaration of Helsinki addresses this point by stating, "the potential benefits, hazards and discomfort of a new method should be weighed against the advantage of the best current diagnostic and therapeutic methods." It provides no clear guidance on the subject of nontherapeutic research on children or any other potential subject deemed legally incompetent. The final statement of the Declaration concerning nontherapeutic research states, "In research on man, the interest of science and society should never take precedence over considerations related to the well-being of the subject" (46).

The US National Commission for the Protection of Human Subjects of Biomedical and Behavioral Research was established in 1974 and began publishing reports beginning in 1976 on research involving prisoners and in 1977 on research involving children (44). The latter report contains an analysis of law as it applies to research of children and considerable discussion of the ethical bases of various viewpoints.

The conclusions were that research involving children was important for the health of all children and that such research could be conducted ethically within the general conditions outlined in documents such as the Helsinki Declaration. The rationale for pediatric research was based on two factors: (a) children are different than adults

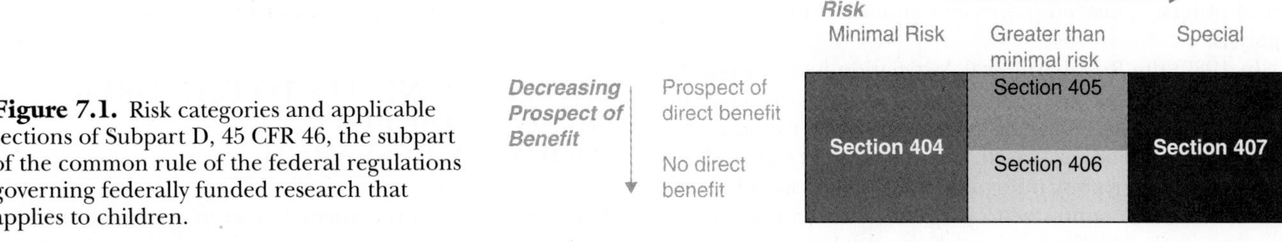

Figure 7.1. Risk categories and applicable sections of Subpart D, 45 CFR 46, the subpart of the common rule of the federal regulations governing federally funded research that applies to children.

and animals in general, and some diseases only occur in children, and (b) the risk of harm from treatments and practices is increased without research. Part of the mission was to develop guidelines. These included a determination by an institutional ethical review board that the proposed study is scientifically sound and significant; that appropriate studies must be conducted first on animals, subsequently in adult humans, and then on older children before involving infants; and that the risks must be minimized by using the safest method consistent with sound research design and by using procedures performed for diagnostic or treatment purposes whenever feasible.

Parents must provide permission for children to participate in research and the child, when feasible, should provide assent. Assent was considered feasible for a normal child at 7 years of age. The Commission report, in an innovative approach, categorized risk and made the following recommendations:

1. Research not involving greater than minimal risk might be conducted on children subject to permission obtained from parents.
2. Research greater than minimal risk might be conducted if it held out the prospect of direct benefit to the subject.
3. Research not holding the prospect of benefit to the subject might be conducted so long as the risk involved was no more than a minor increase over minimal.
4. An additional category for research that was not included in the previous categories is research that carries no prospect of direct benefit to the subject, but carries a risk greater than a small increase over minimal. Such research could be carried out provided it was approved by a national ethics advisory board and was open to public review and comment.

The Commission also recommended that adolescents could have the requirement for parental permission waived in particular circumstances. The Commission published a report in 1978 on institutional review boards, and in 1979 the Belmont Report (named after the donor of the conference room where the Commission met) reviewed the Commission's findings and outlined the ethical basis for clinical research (47,48). These can be summarized in the following three principles:

1. Respect for the personal dignity and autonomy of individuals, with special protections for those with diminished autonomy.
2. Beneficence to maximize benefit and minimize harm.
3. Justice to distribute fairly and equitably the benefits and burdens of research.

The recommendations of the Commission were adopted in June 1983 as federal regulations that apply to all federally funded research (45 CFR 46), with only some minimal changes, for example, excluding the waivers for parental permission for adolescents. Subpart A applies to all research participants, Subpart B applies to research enrolling fetuses and pregnant women, Subpart C applies to research with prisoners, and Subpart D applies to research with children. Sections within Subpart D describe the risk categories and are shown in Figure 7.1 (49).

In 1978, the British Paediatric Association set up a working party on the ethics of research on children. Their report was published in 1980 as guidelines to aid ethical committees considering research involving children. The guidelines were based on the following four premises:

1. Research involving children is important for the benefit of all children and should be supported and encouraged and conducted in an ethical manner.
2. Research should never be done on children if the same investigation could be done on adults.
3. Research that involves a child and is of no benefit to that child (nontherapeutic research) is not necessarily unethical or illegal. This statement had no evidence presented to support the premise. Reference was made without discussion to a single paper that argued that courts were likely to take a more lenient view of the practice of nontherapeutic research on children than had been supposed.
4. The degree of benefit resulting from research should be assessed in relation to the risk of disturbance, discomfort, or pain—in other words, the risk-to-benefit ratio.

The rest of the report is a broader discussion of the concept of risk-to-benefit ratio. It states, for example, that more than negligible risk of nontherapeutic research in children may be justified provided that the anticipated benefits are sufficiently great. In examples, the report gives circumstances where, for instance, a renal biopsy might be taken during abdominal surgery or nontherapeutic blood sampling including repeated glucose tolerance tests in diabetic children may be done to answer important research questions.

The key concept is the definition of negligible risk, which is "risk of less than that run in everyday life." The key components to be considered in assessing risk are the degree and the probability. The report stated that both degree and probability are part of the definition (50). Another aspect of the British Paediatric Association guideline is any absence of any specific mention of the supremacy of the research subject's interest over the interest of others. It instead places an emphasis on risk-benefit analysis.

In 1980, the British Medical Association issued a handbook of medical ethics. It has a brief discussion of research in children. There is no distinction between therapeutic and nontherapeutic research. It does state, however, that adequate background information must be provided to the local ethics committee to judge the scientific merit of the proposal. Although it may be argued that research projects must have scientific merit to be considered ethical, it is unclear that research ethics committees are the most competent forums to evaluate the issue.

The handbook also states that "The investigator should indicate the method he will use to obtain consent, i.e., for the parents or the general practitioner or consultant in charge of the case." This implies that there are occasions when an investigator may obtain consent from another doctor for a research procedure to be carried out on a child without any attempt to obtain either the child's assent or the parent's' consent. There is no legal basis to this in British law. Consent given by another physician would not carry any weight in a court of law. It is more likely to result in a charge of assault (51).

Tyson et al. (52) published a study in 1983 that evaluated the quality of perinatal research. The object of the investigation was to determine the quality of the studies because the treatment methods recommended were widely and rapidly incorporated into clinical practice after publication in a respected obstetric and pediatrics journal. They found that many of the studies failed to meet the criteria for quality perinatal therapeutic research, as shown in Table 7.1.

The report of the working group on Ethics of Clinical Research Investigations on Children by the Institute of Medical Ethics in Great Britain 1986 made a number of detailed recommendations including comments on the effects on the emotions and behavior of children who participate in research and encouragement to not separate children from their parents during procedures (32).

LACK OF BENEFITS TO CHILDREN OF PHARMACEUTICAL INDUSTRY RESEARCH

The US Federal government has been systematically supporting clinical trials with children since the 1950s. Early studies on childhood leukemia were sponsored by the National Cancer Institute, on rheumatic heart disease by the National Heart, Blood and Lung Institute, on retrolental fibroplasias by the National Institute of Neurological Diseases and Blindness, on diabetic retinopathy by the National Eye Institute, on diabetes by the National Institute of Arthritis and Metabolic Diseases, on extra cranial to intracranial arterial anastomosis (a clinical trial) by the National Institute of Neurological and Communicative Disorders and Stroke, and on hereditary angioedema (a clinical trial) by the National Institute of Allergy and Infectious Diseases (53). An NIH institute dedicated to pediatric investigation was founded in 1960, the National Institute of Child Health and Human Development (NICHD). The first director was Dr. Robert Aldrich (54).

As noted previously, in 1962, the Food, Drug and Cosmetic Act was amended to include efficacy data in the FDA approval process and in the approved product package insert. Despite the growing interest in pediatric research, the majority of medications used in children were not studied in children. In 1968, Dr. Harry Shirkey coined the term "therapeutic orphan" to refer to the situation in which sick children were deprived of access to medications because the drugs had not been adequately tested in children (55).

In 1972 at the annual meeting of the American Academy of Pediatrics, Dr. Charles Edwards, former commissioner of the Food and Drug Administration, stated

TABLE 7.1 Summary of Review of 88 Therapeutic Trials

% of Studies Fulfilling Criteria	*Yes*	*Unclear*	*No*
Statement of purpose	94	6	0
Clearly defined outcome variables	74	1	25
Planned prospective data collection	48	30	22
Predetermined sample size (or a sequential trial)	3	16	71
Sample size specified	93	6	1
Disease/health status of subjects specified ($n = 85$)	51	20	29
Exclusion criteria specified ($n = 81$)	46	9	45
Randomization (if feasible) appropriately performed and documented ($n = 69$)	9	12	79
Blinding used, or lack or blinding unlikely to have biased results ($n = 83$)	49	47	4
Adequate sample size	15	44	41
Statistical methods identified, appropriately used, and interpreted	26	0	74
Recommendations/conclusions justified	10	71	19

From Tyson JE, Furzan JA, Reisch JS, et al. An evaluation of the quality of therapeutic studies in perinatal medicine. *J Pediatr* 1983;102(1):10–13.

that a large percentage of the drugs used in sick infants and children are prescribed on empirical grounds (56). In 1973, a report from the National Academy of Sciences emphasized the different nature of the response of an immature organ to pharmacologic agents and suggested that innovative investigative programs were needed to supply information on the use of pharmacologic agents in the pediatric population. Among the reasons cited was that children are different from adults in the process of drug disposition and receptor sensitivity. As an example, the plasma concentrations of the drug theophylline change with the age of the patient.

In 1974, the American Academy of Pediatrics (AAP) issued a report commissioned by the FDA: General Guidelines for the Evaluation of Drugs to Be Approved for Use During Pregnancy and, for the Treatment of Infants and Children (57). In the following year, Dr. John Wilson found that 78% of prescription drugs had a statement in the package insert that the use in infants and children had not been adequately studied or there was no statement and the label was silent on the issue (58).

The FDA adapted the AAP report and in 1977 published it as a guidance document titled General Considerations for the Clinical Evaluation of Drugs in Infants and Children. The major points were an emphasis on anticipating and describing unexpected toxicities in the pediatric population, an expectation that reasonable evidence for efficacy should exist prior to study in infants and children, that only sick children should be enrolled in studies, a preference for active or historical controls over placebo controls, and a recommendation for studying patients in decreasing age order so that experience is gained with older children first (59). Concurrently, the AAP issued Guidelines for the Ethical Conduct of Studies to Evaluate Drugs in Pediatric Populations (60).

In 1979, the FDA issued a regulation adding a Pediatric Use Subsection to the Product Package Insert Precautions Section (61). The intent was to highlight differences in adverse event profiles and to note whether any pediatric use information existed.

Although not directed exclusively at pediatric patients, an important regulatory change occurred in 1983 with passage of the Orphan Drug Act (62). The Act outlined criteria whereby rare diseases, many of them pediatric, and defined as having a prevalence of less than 200,000 in the United States, could benefit from incentives to develop new therapeutics. The program is administered by the FDA and provides both a longer period of marketing exclusivity (7 years for an "orphan" indication compared to 5 years for the first approved indication of a new molecular entity) and subsidies in the way of grants and technical advice for clinical development. An orphan designation is given to the combination of a rare disease and a product. This allows the same disease to have multiple products qualify for orphan designation and does not restrict a product to only treat an orphan disease. The Orphan Drug Act established the principle of government incentives to promote product development in areas of public health need.

Despite the initiative to encourage pediatric data, in 1988 Dr. Franz Rosa, an FDA epidemiologist, surveyed product labels for drugs that are used in infants and found that only 50% had been formally evaluated. Of these, half had been considered safe and effective and the other half had a caution or risk statement in the product label. Of the 50% that had not been evaluated, 60% had a disclaimer about not being indicated for use in children and 40% had no information (63). An independent survey in 1991 found that, just as in 1975, about 80% of product labels had either limited pediatric dosing information or had a disclaimer for use in children (64).

FEDERAL PEDIATRIC INITIATIVES

To further encourage pediatric therapeutic development and the inclusion of pediatric information in product package inserts (product labels), in 1994 the FDA revised the Pediatric Use Section of the regulations, adding a subsection (iv) permitting extrapolation of efficacy data if the disease course in adult and pediatric patients was similar (65).

An FDA guidance document issued in 1996 on the Content and Format of Pediatric Use Section noted that extrapolation should be considered, that the effects of the drugs, both beneficial and adverse, in adult and pediatric patients should be described, and that critical literature references should be included. Compliance was voluntary and did not result in an increase in the proportion of products with pediatric labeling (66).

Also in 1995, the American Academy of Pediatrics Committee on Drugs issued a revision of its Guidelines for the Ethical Conduct of Studies to Evaluate Drugs in Pediatric Populations with detailed discussion of institutional review boards, informed consent, risk and benefit determination, investigator competence. scientific validity and special cases of the dying patient, the newly dead patient, and patients with chronic progressive and potentially fatal diseases (67).

The NICHD established the Pediatric Pharmacology Research Network in 1994 as the first national network for pediatric research, with seven institutions. The network was expanded to 13 institutions in 2001 (68).

As part of the 1997 Food and Drug Administration Modernization Act (FDAMA), an incentive, similar in spirit to the Orphan Drug Act, was added as an option for certain types of products for which pediatric data were submitted to the FDA in response to a written request from the agency.

The incentive was a 6-month extension to existing marketing or patent exclusivity for any product that had the active moiety that was studied in the written request. To qualify for the incentive, a study report must be submitted to the FDA that fairly responds to the terms of the written request.

The results of the submitted studies must be interpretable and informative, but do not need to demonstrate a positive outcome. A negative study can be part of the submission and still contribute to the granting of pediatric exclusivity because the intent is to provide appropriate pediatric information. Existing and newly approved products could qualify with the exception of biologicals, certain antibiotics, and devices (69).

In 1998, a pediatric rule was issued that mandated pediatric studies under particular circumstances. Unlike the pediatric incentive program in the FDAMA, this could apply to any pediatric disease independent of what adult indication a product was approved for; the pediatric rule only applied to the approved adult indication if it occurred in children. If the adult disease or condition did not apply to children, a waiver from compliance could be granted. If the adult indication did not apply to a pediatric subpopulation, for example children younger than 5 years, a partial waiver could be granted.

One of two additional conditions had to be met before the pediatric rule would apply. Either the product had to be a therapeutic advance or it had to be likely to have widespread use defined as 50,000 or more children. The pediatric rule did apply to biologicals, but products with orphan drug designation were exempted (63).

In October 2002, the rule was invalidated in a court decision that ruled that the FDA did not have authority to mandate studies in a population to which a drug sponsor did not intend to market (70). In November 2003, the FDA gained the statutory authority to mandate pediatric studies with the signing of the Pediatric Research Equity Act into law (71). The death of a patient with an inherited metabolic deficiency, Jesse Gelsinger, in a gene therapy experiment in Philadelphia in September 1999 (72) was a catalyst for the formation of a new agency within the Department of Health and Human Services, the Office for Human Research Protection, in June 2000 (73).

The responsibilities for supervising federally funded research were previously in the Office of Protection from Research Risks in the National Institutes of Health. The Office of Human Research Protection has both enforcement and educational roles. The FDA published an adaptation of Subpart D of 45 CFR 46 in the Federal Register in 2001 that would extend the principles and risk categories of the original regulations with some modification to all FDA-regulated research and not just federally funded research (74).

The Best Pharmaceuticals for Children Act (BPCA), signed into law in January 2002, renewed the incentive program contained in the FDAMA and extended the time for the FDA to issue written requests until October 2007. Study reports will be due whenever the written request states and are independent of the last date for issuing written requests. In addition, the BPCA in 2002 endorsed the principle of public disclosure of information regarding the effects of medications in children and provides mechanisms such as Federal Register notices, posting of FDA review summaries on the Internet, product labeling, and advisory committee discussion to promote this goal. A further provision in the BPCA provides mechanisms for the study of off-patent drugs in pediatric populations and a plan for adverse event tracking and reporting (75).

The federal pediatric initiatives were renewed, revised, and extended in September 2007 with the enactment of Public Law 110-85, The Food and Drug and Administration Amendment Act of 2007 (FDAAA). Within FDAAA, Title IV, The Pediatric Medical Device Safety and Improvement Act; Title V, The Pediatric Research Equity Act; and Title VI, The Best Pharmaceuticals for Children Act are all directed at pediatric populations, while Title VIII, Clinical Trial Databases, has implications for pediatric research through the mandatory listing and posting of summary results of clinical studies using FDA-regulated products.

The Pediatric Medical Device Safety and Improvement Act extends the pediatric initiatives to medical devices. The definition of child for research purposes is up to and including 21 years of age. The interpretation of the definition is that if other pediatric populations are enrolled, the upper limit should include patients through 21 years. The interpretation is not to consider a study that enrolls patients between 18 and 21 years in a pediatric study or one that enrolls children. The law recognizes that some studies of childhood diseases and conditions that enroll patients through 21 years acknowledge the late changes in adolescence and that inclusion of these patients can be informative. The primary features of the Pediatric Medical Device Safety and Improvement Act are as follows:

1. Requirement to perform pediatric studies in relevant populations.
2. Applicability of the law to "patients" who "suffer from" a disease or condition.
3. Specific monitoring requirements.
4. Funding of demonstration projects.
5. Development of a federal pediatric medical device plan.
6. Designation of a pediatric medical device point of contact at the National Institutes of Health.

As of early 2009, about 370 drugs had been issued written requests, about 160 drugs had been granted an incentive based on pediatric data, and about 160 product package inserts had been changed as a result of the pediatric incentive programs over the last decade. The pediatric mandate in the 2003 and 2007 laws has produced about 80 product package insert changes.

The package insert or label changes have specified pediatric doses, noted safety information, and, in some cases, extended or established indications for pediatric use (76).

SCIENTIFIC AND ETHICAL RATIONALE FOR CLINICAL STUDIES

For thousands of years, medicine relied on tradition and eminence-based practices. Interventions that were highly active were readily adopted, but other treatments were promulgated without formal establishment of their effectiveness. As a result, the history of medicine is populated with practices that harmed patients and diverted resources. General recognition that a demonstration of effectiveness based on scientific principles is necessary came in the mid-20th century.

The current status of knowledge of biology and pharmacology is insufficient to allow deduction of therapeutic effects, risk, and clinical outcome. Observations are necessary to predict the risks and benefits, and observations are limited for technical and psychological reasons including false expectations, inability to observe events, and bias. The goals of clinical research are to maximize the validity of the observations so that they can be generalized to other patients and minimize the major confounding influences of bias and uncertainty.

Bias is the tendency, intentionally or unintentionally, to influence the outcome by the study design or implementation. Uncertainty is a measure of the confidence in a result. It is defined as the amount that the apparent result differs from what would be a "true" result. The larger the uncertainty, the less confidence there is in the apparent result. Even if the "true" result is not known, there are various analytic methods to determine the level or degree of uncertainty.

Among the ethical reasons for conducting unbiased research are minimizing exposure of patients to unjustified risk and avoiding the consequences of publishing misleading results, which include not only unjustified risk, but the potential delay of superior alternative interventions.

Clinical trials should be undertaken with the concept of equipoise—no prior knowledge of what the results will be. The concept of equipoise has multiple interpretations and may vary with perspective, but is generally taken to reflect that the information needed to make a determination is not available and the planned study is intended to provide that information (77).

Randomized controlled clinical trials were developed in the United States and the United Kingdom during the 1920s and 1930s, but Dr. Austin Bradford Hill initiated the practice of using random numbers to assign patients to treatment arms to study infectious disease therapy, which grew out of a need to treat malaria during World War 2 (78).

In 1948, the Medical Research Council of Britain reported on the use of streptomycin to treat pulmonary tuberculosis in a randomized controlled trial (79). Following the war, randomized controlled studies began in the United States in academia with a study at Johns Hopkins University comparing tetracycline to penicillin for the treatment of pneumococcal pneumonia and in government with the Veterans Administration study of tuberculosis (80,81).

The first pediatric study, as noted previously, was organized by the US National Institutes of Health as a multicenter controlled trial for rheumatic heart disease in 1951 (82).

In 1954, Congress established the Cancer Chemotherapy National Service Center (CCNSC). Subsequently, a clinical trial network was initiated with one section devoted to pediatrics. In the establishment of the clinical program, the CCNSC agreed upon the importance of the following principles:

1. Combination of data from all institutions to rapidly accumulate the necessary number of patients.
2. Standard criteria of diagnosis, treatment, and measurement of effect.
3. Statistical design of the study with randomly assigned patients to different treatment groups.
4. Statistical analysis and collaborative reporting of results.

The rationale for these principles was that randomized studies generally provide more persuasive evidence of benefit than alternative study designs such as single-arm studies. Improvements in outcome ascribed to treatment may be due to other factors such as patient selection (selection bias), other medications or therapies, diet, genetics, and other environmental factors. In addition, historical control populations may differ from current study populations with regard to demographics, precision of diagnosis, and changes in the general practice of medicine (83,84).

The design and analysis of clinical trials continue to evolve, but the value of careful observation and recording of results is timeless. Independent of trial design, clinical studies must address ethical requirements. The varied published international documents have overlapping characteristics and elements, and these have been analyzed by Emanuel et al. of the NIH, leading to a recommendation of seven requirements for ethically conducting a clinical study. These are value, scientific validity, fair subject selection, favorable risk-benefit ratio, independent review, informed consent, and respect (85). With regard to children, the issue of informed consent, as previously discussed, is redirected to parental permission and assent.

SPECIFIC RATIONALE FOR CLINICAL STUDIES IN CHILDREN

It is considered a truism in medicine that children are not small adults. Indeed, results of studies in one adult population may not be translatable to another adult population. The differences between children and adults are many, and vary according to age and developmental stage. These include physical and psychological vulnerability, continuing changes in physiologic development, evolving surface-to-volume ratio, changes in integrity of the skin and other anatomic barriers, maturation of metabolic function, changes in skeletal structure and composition, alterations in penetrability of the central nervous system, maturation of the neurohumoral-immune axis, alterations in protein binding and displacement, and risks that vary with age and development.

The continuing metabolic changes and alterations in surface-to-volume ratio limit the use of fixed doses in children and are the basis for the need to study dosing at different ages, sizes, and developmental stages. Among the reasons to study drugs in children of various ages and sizes are the increased risk of adverse reactions or decreased effectiveness due to inappropriate dose and the potential reluctance of practitioners to prescribe potentially useful products without adequate information. Without adequate information, it is not possible to ensure that the use of a product in children is appropriate.

Additional general factors to address in pediatric studies are the sampling challenges of obtaining meaningful clinical material such as blood, serum, tissue, and images in patients of various sizes, degrees of maturation, and developmental stages (86).

The American Academy of Pediatrics issued updated Guidelines for the Ethical Conduct of Studies to Evaluate Drugs in the Pediatric Population in 1995, which can be summarized as follows (67).

> The premise of studying drugs in children is that it is morally imperative so that children can have equal access to therapeutic agents. In most cases, adults should be

studied prior to children except for agents that are specific for pediatric diseases. Proposed pediatric research must by design protect children and encompass the following six conditions:

- The proposed research must be of value to children in general and, in most instances, to the individual child subject. The value may be a potential benefit in the treatment of the subject's disease, or may be improved understanding of basic biology of the disease state or of children in general.
- The research design must be appropriate for the stated purposes. Poorly designed research may not provide scientifically valid or useful data and may place the subjects at risk with no potential benefits.
- The research design must take into consideration the unique physiology, psychology, and pharmacology of children and their special needs and requirements as research subjects. The design should minimize risk while maximizing potential benefit.
- The study design must take into account the racial, ethnic gender, and socioeconomic characteristics of the children and their parents and, when appropriate, should include input from the community or appropriate advocacy representatives.
- The study must be designed to conform to the local, state, and federal laws of the jurisdiction of the study's location and the investigators' home jurisdiction, and to their local and national ethical guidelines.

The document further states that research studies may be considered ethically permissible when they can be shown to have a potential benefit to the individual child or provide generalizable knowledge, and when potential benefits outweigh potential risks. Benefits should be construed broadly. The investigator's competence and ethical conduct are the most important safeguards for the protection of the child. The primary responsibility of the institutional review board (IRB) is to protect the rights of the research participant.

Additional subsections address specific populations that may be at increased risk for abuse and exploitation, including the child with handicaps, institutionalized children, patients requiring emergency care, the dying patient, patients with chronically progressive or potentially fatal disease, and the brain-dead patient. The following paragraphs have brief comments for each population.

The child with handicaps (mentally, physically or emotionally) must be stringently protected from disproportionate representation in research studies either through exclusion or through inclusion. Institutionalized children should rarely be considered for participation in research studies because of the possibility of not having sufficient safeguards.

The International Conference on Harmonization document on pediatric studies, discussed later, is consistent with the AAP guidelines, noting that information that can be obtained in a less vulnerable, consenting population should not be obtained in a more vulnerable population or one in which the patients are unable to provide individual consent. Studies in populations with handicaps or institutionalized pediatric populations should be limited to diseases or conditions found principally or exclusively in these populations, or to situations in which the disease or condition in these pediatric patients would be expected to alter the disposition or pharmacodynamic effects of a medicinal product.

Patients requiring emergency care may participate in research and have the usual procedures for informed consent or permission or assent altered or waived if the clinical condition is potentially life-threatening or permanently disabling and the only available therapy is investigational or not validated, if no accepted therapy is known to be superior to the experimental therapy, and if permission cannot be obtained in a timely manner. In addition, the relevant IRB should receive assurance that the risk is not more than a minimal added risk, equipoise exists among therapeutic alternatives, and the waiver will not affect the rights and welfare of participants.

The dying patient may be enrolled on a study if the question being addressed is extremely important, the therapy being proposed is well founded in animal and clinical research, or there is good expectation that the therapy may be beneficial and the potential benefits exceed the potential risks. In addition, physicians not involved in the research must document that death appears inevitable and that standard therapy has not improved the patient's prognosis.

Patients with chronically progressive or potentially fatal disease and their parents or guardians are potentially prone to feel an obligation to participate in research proposed by physicians that care for these patients due to the dependent relationship that can develop. Investigators who are not involved in the care of the patient should obtain approval for participation. The brain-dead patient is legally dead in most jurisdictions.

The circumstance of considering research would involve some measurements on remaining body functions. The AAP document stipulates that research may proceed if the death certificate has been signed by a physician independent of the planned research, the medical question addressed by the research is of utmost importance, permission is received from the parents, the research procedure is brief, the drugs are intended for human use, and the research will not compromise either organ donation or an autopsy, if either is planned.

DESIGNING CLINICAL TRIALS: GENERAL CONSIDERATIONS

To be ethical, a clinical trial must be informative. To be informative, a specific question must be asked. To answer a question, the trial must measure an outcome in an unbiased, valid, and interpretable manner. The sequence of steps can vary, but an effective approach to designing a clinical trial is to first decide what the question is, then determine whether there is an end point or small collection of end points that can provide an answer; assess the reproducibility and applicability to the disease condition of measuring the end point; decide what type of study design would be most resource effective, minimize bias, and maximize certainty; and then select the appropriate elements to write a study protocol.

There are multiple statistical approaches to clinical trial analysis, with the distinctions dependent on whether a normal, or parametric, distribution of results is expected and whether prior information is incorporated.

All measurements have associated confidence intervals, which are calculated from statistical tables. The smaller or narrower the confidence intervals, the greater is the certainty of the result. This can be achieved through either a large study population size or a large therapeutic effect. The most difficult results to interpret are from a small population size with a small effect. It is unlikely that the most thorough design will be the least resource intensive. A truism in clinical research, as it is for software development, is "good, fast, cheap-pick any two" (87).

OUTCOME MEASURES

Outcome measures, sometimes referred to as end points, are the informative assessments analyzed to answer the study question or questions for a clinical trial. A trial may have more than one outcome measure, but as the number of outcome measures increase, the complexity of the study and the analysis increases. Clinical outcomes that directly demonstrate patient benefit such as improvement in survival, improvement of functioning, improvement of symptoms, or delay of disease progression are generally preferable because interpretation is simplest.

The National Institutes of Health Definition Working Group defined the terms "clinical end point," "biomarker," and "surrogate end point" in 2001 as follows:

1. A clinical end point is a characteristic or variable that reflects how a patient feels, functions, or survives.
2. A biomarker is a characteristic that is objectively measured and evaluated as an indicator of normal biological processes, pathogenic processes, or pharmacological responses to a therapeutic intervention.
3. A surrogate end point is a biomarker intended to substitute for a clinical end point that should predict clinical benefit or harm or lack of both. (88)

The Biomarkers Consortium, a public private partnership dedicated to developing biomarkers for general use, defines biomarkers as "characteristics that are objectively measured and evaluated as indicators of normal biological processes, pathogenic processes, or pharmacologic responses to therapeutic intervention" (89).

A biomarker needs to be qualified, meaning that the assessment results are reproducible and consistent and independent of who is performing the assessment or where the assessment is done. Qualification usually involves the establishment of standard operating procedures, calibration of the outcome measures, a training procedure and, if applicable, specifications for reagents and equipment.

Once a biomarker is qualified, it can be a candidate for a surrogate marker. The process of establishing a surrogate marker is termed validation. Validation requires clinical studies where the direct measure of the clinical outcome is statistically compared to values of the candidate biomarker. Changes in both a positive and a negative direction are correlated between the candidate biomarker and the clinical outcome measure and interpreted in the context of plausible biological mechanisms and what is known about the causal pathway of the intended clinical outcome. The validation process may not apply to all populations; therefore, it should be accepted only for the population in which the surrogate was studied and validated. This caveat is particularly relevant for pediatric populations.

Operationally, a surrogate end point substitutes for another outcome variable. The ideal surrogate end point is a disease marker that directly reflects what is happening, both positively and negatively, with the underlying disease. A surrogate end point, to be credible, must predict the benefit based on scientific evidence. Usually, a surrogate end point is a laboratory measurement or an observation or event that serves as a substitute for direct measure of a clinically meaningful end point. Some examples of surrogates are blood glucose or hemoglobin A, C for diabetes, intraocular pressure for glaucoma, and blood pressure for hypertension.

Surrogates are often employed as substitutes for efficacy variables, but may also serve as substitutes for safety variables. Among the reasons to use surrogate end points in a particular study are that a clinical event may be difficult to measure, a clinical event may have a low event rate, and it may be faster or cheaper to measure a surrogate. The use of surrogates in an overall development plan can accelerate the determination of benefit and provide patients earlier access to therapy than waiting for a direct demonstration of clinical benefit.

Presumptive surrogate markers can be misleading. Patients who have a positive outcome based on the surrogate may not have true clinical benefit. This can arise in several circumstances when the association of a surrogate end point with clinical outcome may not be causal, but is based on a statistical correlation. Possibilities include alternate mechanisms or multiple pathways for the pathophysiology and alternate or multiple pathways for the action of a drug. A misleading surrogate assumes patient benefit, yet exposes patients to risk.

In addition, the safety of long-term exposure may not be adequately assessed (88). Unexpected results relying on surrogates can occur in almost any clinical setting, such as cardiology [flosequinan for treatment of heart failure (PROFILE study); encainide, flecainide, and moricizine for treatment of arrhythmias in patients after a myocardial infarction (CAST study); and milrinone for treatment of heart failure (PROMISE study)], infectious diseases (interferon gamma for chronic granulomatous disease), and metabolism (sodium fluoride for osteoporosis) (88).

In the heart failure study, the surrogate end points were cardiac output and ejection fraction, whereas the clinical end point was survival. The lack of correlation between changes in the surrogates and survival could be due to actions of the drug that are independent of the disease process, such as postulated for flosequinan on survival in chronic heart failure (89).

A similar scenario may exist for arrhythmia studies, where the surrogate end points were electrocardiographic readings, whereas the clinical end point was survival (90–92). For chronic granulomatous disease, the end point was superoxide production and in vitro bacterial killing, whereas the clinical end point was incidence of serious infection. The lack of correlation may be due to the disease process having an effect on clinical outcome that is independent of the pathway that the drug acts on and which contains the surrogate (93). The metabolism study with sodium fluoride for osteoporosis used bone mineral density as a surrogate for the clinical outcome of fractures. The lack of correlation could be due to the surrogate not being in the causal pathway of the disease process (88,94,95).

PATIENT-REPORTED OUTCOMES

Patient-reported outcomes are descriptions of what happens to the patient based on his or her own assessment, usually through answering a list of standard questions or indicating a perception on some type of a scale. Patient-reported outcomes address the goals of improvement in function or improvement in symptoms.

From a scientific perspective, desirable properties of patient-reported outcomes are that they be disease-related, specifically validated for the disease and population including improvement and worsening of clinically meaningful changes, have real-time assessments (not based on recall) can have confirmation by other assessments and can be measured in controlled studies.

Some examples are changes in pain or changes in symptoms that are disease-related and limit activity or function. Valid reproducible measurements are still required to interpret the results. General advice about the systematic collection of patient-reported outcomes is available from the Food and Drug Administration in the form of a guidance document (www.fda.gov/downloads/Drugs/GuidanceComplianceRegulatoryInformation/Guidances/UCM071975.pdf).

The general principles are that a series of questions are structured during an interview or administration of a questionnaire and organized according to topic. Pediatric-specific aspects of patient-reported outcomes are discussed later.

The accompanying tables list end points on the basis of their relationship to time. If time is variable, then the outcome that is being measured is usually expressed in units of time and is duration. In general, the longer the therapeutic effect or benefit, the more favorable is the outcome. Another way to express the concept is time to event, where the event is either the duration of benefit or the appearance of an unfavorable outcome.

Examples include overall survival, time to disease progression, and duration of favorable response. If time is fixed, then the outcome that is being measured is a rate of events, where, in general, the more events that occur in a population during the study period or some other predefined time interval, the more favorable is the outcome. Examples include percentage of responders, survival at 5 years, and percentage of patients not progressing at 2 years (Tables 7.2 and 7.3, Figs. 7.2 through 7.5).

STUDY GOALS

Study goals will depend upon the question being asked, the expectations for the size of the effect, the available resources, and the feasibility of implementation of the study design. Studies are often categorized by type based on the goals.

TABLE 7.2 Types of Time-Dependent End Points

Time Dependent or Variable Time Expressed as Units of Time Usually the Median Time to an Event for a Population	*Population*	*Comment*
Pharmacokinetics	All patients	A series of parameters that describe the absorption, distribution, metabolism and elimination of a drug as a function of time and exposure.
Overall survival	All patients	Typically, time between study entry and death. Measurement is usually unambiguous. Cause of death may be difficult to determine. Effective therapies can result in long follow-up times for completing studies.
Progression-free survival/ time to progression	All patients that progress	Typically, time between study entry and time to progression first date of disease progression with death being considered as progression. The parameters for progression must be reliably defined and the assay validated—may be symptom-based, imaging study, biomarker, or patient-reported outcome.
Disease-free survival	Only complete responders	Parameter for progression must be reliably defined and assay validated—may be symptom-based, imaging study, biomarker, or patient-reported outcome.
Time to treatment failure	All patients that change treatment	Treatment failure must be reliably defined and may include disease progression or unacceptable toxicity. Unacceptable toxicity can be a highly individual assessment and treatment failure can be due to multiple factors, not all of which are objective. Time to treatment failure is particularly difficult to interpret.
Duration of response	Only responders	Typically, time between first date of response and first date of disease progression. Response is usually defined as having a minimum duration (typically 4 wk) to be considered a response.
Time to response	Only responders	Typically, time between date of study entry and first date of response. Response is usually defined as having a minimum duration (typically 4 wk) to be considered a response.

TABLE 7.3 Types of Time Independent End Points

Time Independent or Time is Fixed[a]	*Population*	*Comment*
Pharmacokinetic/ pharmacodynamic relationships	All patients where measurements are taken	Description of relationship between drug exposure and a clinical or biochemical effect.
Response	Percentage of all patients or a continuous variable such as drug level	Criteria are extremely variable—may be drug levels, symptom-based, imaging a study, biomarker, or patient reported outcome. Response is often subdivided into categories that may be ordered (for example, complete response, partial response, stable disease, progression). Ordered categories require additional analyses and in some cases are combined.
Adverse events	Usually percentage of all patients	Standard reporting criteria are available from several sources.
Landmark	Percentage of all patients	Highly variable—paradigm—an example would be percentage of patients alive at 2 yr for a life-threatening illness, but must be meaningful with regard to disease and patient population.

[a]Expressed as a rate of events per unit time (usually length of the study) such as percentage of the population with an event during the fixed time period.

Pharmacokinetic studies have a series of predefined parameters that describe the fate of a drug and its metabolites at different doses in different patient populations. Exposure response studies examine the relationship between exposures to a product and physiologic or clinical events (both beneficial and adverse) associated with its use. If pharmacodynamics are also measured, then the study may be considered a pharmacokinetic/pharmacodynamic study. Pharmacokinetic studies and exposure response studies are generally considered exploratory. A case where they may not be considered exploratory is when extrapolation of efficacy is feasible between two populations, and pharmacokinetic and exposure response studies are used to extend the use of the product to the new population.

Efficacy studies are by design adequate with regard to power and planned analysis to demonstrate patient benefit and to assess risks. The results of efficacy studies are usually expressed as a calculated number, often called the point estimate, with associated confidence intervals. Confidence intervals are by convention based on the 95% probability that the true result is within a range between an upper and a lower limit.

Efficacy studies may be designed to demonstrate superiority to available therapies or no inferiority. To demonstrate

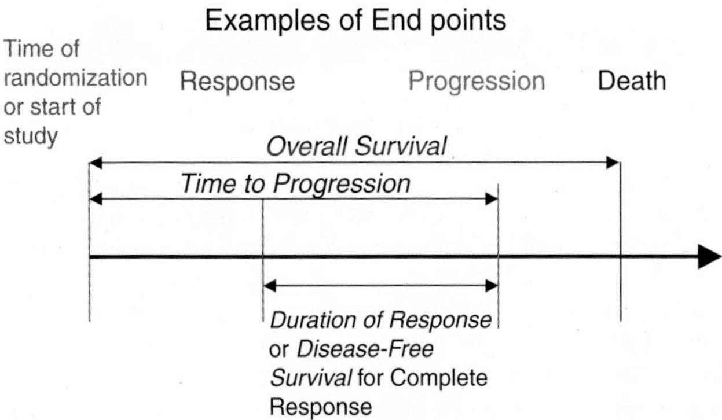

Figure 7.2. Illustration of typical definitions of some time-dependent end points.

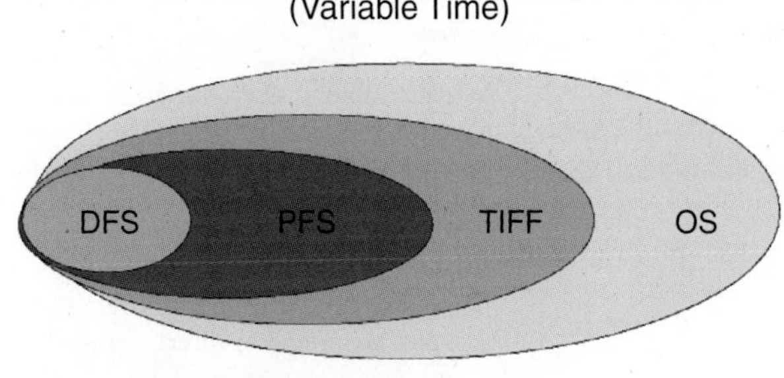

Figure 7.3. Illustration of relative proportions of population size of some time-dependent end points.

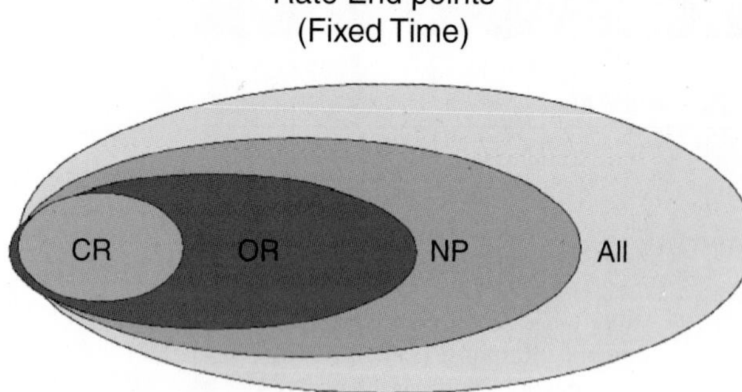

CR = Complete Responders
OR = Overall Response
NP = Nonprogressors
All = All Patients Intended to Treat

Figure 7.4. Illustrations of relative proportions of population size of some time-independent end points.

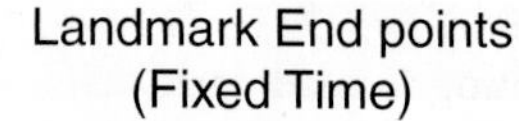

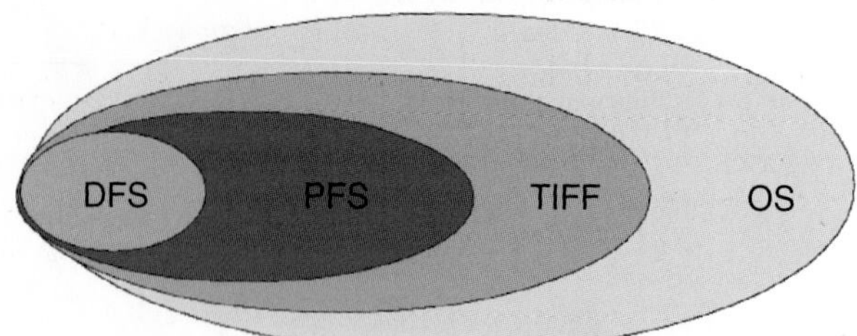

DFS = Disease-Free Survival = Complete Responders
PFS = Progression-Free Survival = Nonprogressors
TTF = Time to Treatment Failure = Nonprogressors Plus Not Tolerated Toxicity
OS = Overall Survival = All Survivors

Figure 7.5. Illustrations of relative proportions of population size of some time-independent end points.

superiority, the 95% confidence intervals of a therapy should not overlap with a comparator, that is, the lower limit of one result must be greater than the upper limit of the comparator. All studies have by implication a historical comparator, although historical comparators can be difficult to determine and not appropriate for direct comparison due to differences in study populations and standards of medical care. The most persuasive and credible comparator is one that is measured concurrently with the study regimen. Several design strategies exist to minimize bias in assigning patients to comparative treatments.

To demonstrate equivalence would usually require large numbers of patients and precise measurements. To conserve resources and maintain a level of confidence in being able to substitute one product for another, a noninferiority approach is employed. Noninferiority implies that the difference in benefit and outcome between a standard therapy and the new therapy is within a predefined and acceptable margin of effect. It requires that the standard has an effect that is measurable, clinically meaningful, and reproducible.

There are several approaches to setting the margin of acceptable difference and analyzing the results of a study. As an example, it may be considered acceptable to preserve at least 80% of the effect of the standard therapy or have a margin of 20%. A caution is that if serial studies use different standards, the efficacy effect could drift down. To be specific, if a new product preserves 80% of the effect of a standard and the next new product preserves 80% of the effect of the first new product, the result is a reservation of about 60% of the original standard. Safety studies are intended to demonstrate the relationship between exposure to a product and adverse events associated with its use. All clinical studies are in one form or another safety studies.

Since the 1950s, clinical studies have been classified into phases on the basis of this study. Initial drug dose finding and safety studies have been termed Phase 1. Exploratory studies to determine biological or clinical activity of a drug have been termed Phase 2. Confirmatory studies to compare an investigational regimen with an established regimen that are powered to establish efficacy have been termed Phase 3. Studies that have been

TABLE 7.4 Types of Clinical Trial Goals

Type	*Comment*
Superiority	The test treatment is better than a comparator. The confidence intervals around the measurement for the test treatment and for the comparator should not overlap. For example, if the standard treatment shows that median survival for a population is 22 mo and the confidence intervals are ± 3 mo, then the test treatment must have a lower confidence interval that is greater than 25 mo (22 + 3) to be considered superior. Results of 29 mo ± 3 mo or 28 mo ± 2 mo would qualify.
Noninferiority	The test treatment is not worse than a comparator. Exact equivalence is difficult to prove requiring large study populations and precise measures. The usual approach is to consider that a treatment is not worse than an accepted treatment by direct comparison with the understanding that: 1. The effect of the accepted treatment is measurable, reproducible, and meaningful. 2. An acceptable difference between the accepted treatment and the new treatment is defined before beginning the study and is smaller than the total effect of the accepted treatment. For example, if the accepted treatment increases median survival by 6 mo and the acceptable difference is 1 mo, then the new treatment in direct comparison to the accepted treatment must not differ by more than 1 mo and the accepted treatment must have a median survival that is consistent with previous results.
Exploratory	A study to examine biological or clinical activity but not designed to establish efficacy.

requested by the Food and Drug Administration to comply with postmarketing commitments following approval of a claim for marketing exclusivity have been termed Phase 4.

Alternative nomenclature such as learning phase and confirming study (96) or initial exposure phase, development phase, and validation phase may also be acceptable (Table 7.4).

PROTOCOL CONSTRUCTION

The mechanics of implementing a study begins with writing a study protocol consistent with International Conference of Harmonization guidelines and relevant regulations. A summary of applicable FDA regulations may be found at http://www.fda.gov/oc/gcp/regulations.html (97).

The general features of a study protocol are that it poses a question, identifies a study population for which the question is relevant, proposes an intervention, has safety monitoring and escape rules for individual patients, assesses outcome based on meaningful and validated end points, utilizes systematic and validated measurement techniques to assess the end points, and contains an analytic plan that minimizes bias and uncertainty. Some elements to address in trial design and protocol writing are listed in Table 7.5.

A protocol must be approved by an institutional review board and, if an investigational agent is used or if an FDA-approved product is used under some conditions, then an Investigational New Drug (IND) application must be filed and the protocol reviewed by the FDA. Detailed information can be found at: http://www.fda.gov/BiologicsBloodVaccines/DevelopmentApprovalProcess/InvestigationalNewDrugINDorDeviceExemptionIDEProcess/default.htm (98).

There are many possible and plausible design variations that include having multiple stages where continuation of

TABLE 7.5 Trial Design Elements

Trial Design Elements	*Comment*
Time frame	
Prospective	A protocol is written and the study is performed following the approval of the protocol. Opportunity to collect all data that is required to test the hypothesis.
Retrospective	A protocol is written to systematically analyze historical data. Often unable to locate all the data required to test the hypothesis.
Controls	
Historical	Comparison is made with either a specific study that is considered to be an appropriate match for the current therapy or with a valid meta-analysis of a series of previous studies. Major problems are as follows: 1. Changes in medical practice (secular effect) that affect results over time 2. Differences in eligibility criteria in different protocols 3. Differences in assessment in different studies 4. Differences in analysis in different studies
Placebo	
Supportive care	If no active antitumor therapy exists for the patient population, then it may be ethical to provide supportive care plus a placebo versus supportive care plus the test therapy. Examples may include testing a symptom benefit therapy.
Add on	All arms receive the same standard therapy with the control arm receiving in addition a placebo and the experimental arm receiving in addition the test therapy.
Active	
Standard therapy	Direct comparison between a standard therapy and the test therapy.
Add on	All arms receive the same standard therapy with the experimental arm eceiving in addition the test therapy.
Withdrawal	All arms receive the same therapy until a predetermined time when one arm has the test therapy withdrawn. The end point of interest is usually the appearance of an event that would be prevented if the test therapy were still present. This type of design is often used in measuring the effect of lowering blood pressure.
Dose comparison	Different doses of the same drug are compared. Generally a trend in benefit or response that follows the exposure to the drug is considered evidence of activity—the greater the exposure the greater the response.
Arms	
Single	A single series of patients.
Multiple	Treatment arms are compared concurrently to one another.
Crossover	Patients can change from one treatment arm to another based on predetermined criteria. If the critical evaluation occurs after the crossover, it may be difficult to interpret due to factors such as the sequence of therapy having an effect or one therapy having a delayed effect.
Analyses	
Single	Study analysis occurs when either a particular time or predefined landmark is reached.
Multiple	Study analysis will incorporate one or more interim analyses triggered by events, landmarks, or time schedule.
Adaptive	The study design may alter in a prospectively defined manner based on the outcome of an interim analysis; for example, a study arm may be closed to accrual, the overall sample size may be increased, or a new study arm may open. All adaptive designs are based on rules described in detail in the original protocol and are not based on protocol amendments developed subsequent to any data analysis.

the trial from an early to a later stage is dependent on interim results.

Such an approach is termed an adaptive design. Among the more common is a two-stage design for clinical activity where an initial cohort of patients is assessed with prespecified rules for a minimum level of activity to justify an expansion of the study to enroll more patients. Another variation on an adaptive design would assign subsequent interventions or observations to patients depending on the results of the initial intervention or other events.

Some study designs are not intended to assess a specific intervention, but are intended to systematically collect data in a prospective manner to describe natural history or make long-term observations. Such a study design may be applicable as a follow-up study to a study that assessed an intervention.

CLINICAL TRIAL MONITORING

The risks of investigational therapy can be unknown. Extrapolation from preclinical models for safety are about 65% predictive (99). The predictive value of preclinical models for children is a field under development. Although preclinical models for teratogenicity exist, several acceptable preclinical models for pediatric specific toxicities such as the impact on growth and organ maturation are still being developed.

In addition, children, particularly the youngest, may not be able to communicate adverse effects. As a consequence, the monitoring of clinical studies in children merits greater vigilance than monitoring in adult populations.

The Eunice Kennedy Shriver National Institute of Child Health and Human Development has analyzed and developed policies and recommendations for monitoring studies that enroll children, which are summarized here (100).

The rationale for monitoring is based on two general research principles:

- Ensuring and enhancing the safety of the study, that is, to protect the study participant from unacceptable risk; and
- Assuring the scientific validity of the study, that is, to protect the data and preserve its integrity.

The most critical component is investigator integrity, which can be actualized by a proactive, comprehensive, and integrated monitoring plan.

To uphold and implement these principles, a monitoring plan must:

- be proactive and anticipate a range of outcomes and responses; and
- include a communication plan to support dynamic interaction between relevant parties, including monitors, investigators, sponsors, regulatory authorities, and others.

Monitoring is assuming responsibility for reviewing events and outcomes during the implementation of a study in two domains: (a) safety of participants and (b) integrity and quality of data including study accrual. Study monitoring encompasses comparing events and outcomes to predefined criteria. If the study events and outcomes indicate deviance from those criteria, study monitoring would mandate making a recommendation to alter the study implementation.

Routine monitoring is when the study team has primary responsibility for monitoring the study typically based on a monitoring plan incorporated in the study protocol or study plan, IRB oversight, institutional oversight in compliance with applicable institutional, state and federal guidelines, policies, regulations, and laws.

Each study should develop a monitoring plan that is included in the overall study plan or protocol that defines the following:

- How the study will comply with regulatory requirements?
- The specific events and activities that will be monitored.
- The roles and responsibilities for everyone on the team who is involved in monitoring.
- Who has responsibility for reporting (and who they report to)?
- A schedule for monitoring.
- Any escape and stopping rules.

Escape rules are criteria for an individual patient to leave the study based on disease progression, toxicity, or lack of efficacy. Escape rules may define alternative regimens. Stopping rules are criteria for either halting accrual or closing a study for toxicity, lack of efficacy, or sufficient efficacy that further enrollment is not required to determine a conclusion. If applicable, the type and number of events that would halt accrual and would generate a review of eligibility, monitoring, assessments, intervention, and how the resumption of accrual would occur in each study plan or protocol will include a list of expected adverse events regardless of whether these adverse events are referenced or explained in other types of study documentation.

A list or description of *expected events* should be in the following forms:

- A description of the scope of expected adverse events of the underlying condition based on either a recent literature review or textbook. If none are expected during the study time frame, simply state that no adverse events are expected;
- If interventional products are administered, a description of the safety profile for *each* product administered in the study (investigational and marketed) including, if known, the frequency, severity, and duration of adverse events;
- If assessments (for example, a blood test, imaging study, and survey instrument) that are not part of the routine care of the disease or underlying condition are scheduled in the study, then the known risks and complications from those assessments should be listed in the study protocol.

The best quality information to include in the study protocol regarding research-specific assessments would be individual institutional experience using the assessment at the study site, which includes the total number of people that received the assessment plus the complication rates. If institutional experience is not available, published data from similar studies and published data on the general use of the assessment tool or technique may be substituted.

An integrated listing of adverse events containing those anticipated from the natural history plus those anticipated from any and all interventions and assessments that may occur on study should conclude the anticipated risks' section of the study plan or protocol. The potential advantages of an integrated list of expected events are that IRBs could readily assess the overall risks from a study, the informed consent process and documents could be prepared to better inform prospective study participants of potential risks, and adverse event reporting could be simplified by comparison of an event with a single source document.

Supplemental monitoring can be implemented in addition to routine monitoring, and depending on the nature of the research, monitoring can be effectively augmented through mechanisms and independent external entities such as a single-person medical monitor, a small study monitoring committee, a multidisciplinary committee, or a chartered multidisciplinary team such as an Independent Data Monitoring Committee (IDMC). Alternative terms include Data and Safety Monitoring Board, Data Monitoring Board, or Data Monitoring Committee.

The NICHD recommends any of the following criteria to establish a supplemental monitoring program:

- Late phase clinical trials statistically powered to establish efficacy. Late phase clinical trials are generally large studies, but not necessarily so, and are designed to affect current medical practice, product labeling if applicable, or public health policy.
- Multisite/multicenter clinical trials. Multisite/multicenter clinical trials involve separate institutions using the same study protocol. Several sites that are within the same legally established institution are not generally considered to be a multisite study.
- Clinical trials involving randomized treatments. Multiarm clinical trials that use randomization are designed to minimize potential bias in the interpretation of the results. Randomization implies scrupulous attention to the details of study implementation to avoid any compromise in data integrity.
- Clinical trials involving vulnerable populations, such as those who are children, pregnant women, elderly and ill, terminally ill, or of diminished mental capacity, or any population otherwise unable or unlikely to provide informed consent that are at greater than minimal risk. If the clinical trial involves only minimal risk to participants, as defined by 45 CFR Subpart A, Sec. 46.102 and minimal risk to data integrity and quality (for example, small number of sites, small sample size, few data elements, short duration), monitoring can be accomplished through alternative mechanisms, such as the use of a detailed monitoring plan in the protocol.
- Clinical trials in which the treatment is particularly invasive or has other serious safety concerns (e.g., may result in serious toxicity).
- Clinical research studies in which an assessment that is used solely for research purposes is considered greater than minimal risk.
- Clinical research studies, including observational studies in which participants are already at elevated risk of (a) death, (b) life-threatening conditions (that is immediate risk of death), (c) in-patient hospitalization or prolongation of existing hospitalization, (d) persistent or significant disability/incapacity, or (e) congenital anomaly or birth defect. These events are considered serious adverse events by regulatory authorities.
- A clinical research project that is of sufficiently long duration that protocol changes may need to be considered based on changing medical practice or interim analyses.
- Any clinical trial in which members of the study team have a stated or perceived conflict of interest.

An Independent Data Monitoring Committee is a structured multidisciplinary mechanism for supplemental monitoring that may be dedicated to a single study or may serve multiple studies. The role of the board or committee is established before a clinical trial begins. Its functions typically include review of the protocol before it is implemented, review of study implementation and progress, and ongoing review of the accumulating data to detect evidence of early, significant benefit or harm for participants while the trial is in progress. This latter review serves as an additional protection for participants, beyond that provided by the IRB, but does not take the place of regulatory requirements for investigators to report serious and unanticipated adverse events to the FDA.

Examples of IDMC responsibilities are as follows:

- Review the research protocol, review model informed consent documents, and plans for data and safety monitoring, including all proposed revisions.
- Review methodology used to help maintain the confidentiality of the study data and the results of monitoring by reviewing procedures put in place by investigators to ensure confidentiality.
- Monitor study design, procedures, and events that will maximize the safety of the study participants and minimize the risks.
- Evaluate the progress of the study, including periodic assessments of data quality and timeliness, participant recruitment, accrual and retention, participant risk versus benefit, performance of the study site(s), and other factors that may affect study outcome.
- Consider factors external to the study when relevant information becomes available, such as scientific or therapeutic developments that may have an impact on the safety of the participants or the ethics of the studies.
- Review serious adverse event documentation and safety reports and make recommendations regarding protection of the safety of the study participants.
- Report on the safety and progress of the study.
- Evaluate and report on any perceived problems with study conduct, enrollment, sample size, and/or data collection.
- Provide a recommendation regarding continuation, termination, or other modifications of the study based on the cumulative experience including the observed beneficial or adverse effects.

An Independent Data Monitoring Committee operates under a charter outlining the roles, responsibilities, and standard operating procedures for the group. The charter:

- will define the roles, responsibilities, and relationships for each of the members, such as who are voting members or

advisory members, who may attend open and closed sessions, the line of authority for reviews and decision making, who is granted access to certain data (e.g., blinded and unblinded), the compensation for IDMC members, and any potential conflicts of interest;
- will outline the responsibilities of the group including familiarizing group members with the study protocol and monitoring of adverse events, data quality, participant recruitment and enrollment, the risks and benefits, reporting, etc.;
- may also include an organizational chart depicting the relationships between all of the major stakeholders of the study team, the study sponsor, the funding organization, and the IDMC;
- will identify the standard procedures for each items such as meeting frequency and format, including logistics and required attendees/quorum, procedures for unscheduled evaluations, including types of events that would trigger an unscheduled evaluation, expected information, involvement of the study chair, required number of members, and communication of recommendations;
- will have statistical procedures that may be utilized by the IDMC, including any stopping rules based on benefit or harm, futility analysis, or decision points in adaptive designs;
- will monitor recruitment goals; and
- will have methods for making recommendations to the study sponsor and investigators, funding organization, and other relevant parties.

ADDITIONAL PEDIATRIC-SPECIFIC CONSIDERATIONS FOR RESEARCH STUDIES

Studies in pediatric populations require additional considerations on ethical, technical, and scientific grounds. For these reasons, pediatric research should be led by investigators trained and experienced in studying children and performed at facilities that have the staffing and infrastructure to support and comfort children. In such a facility, children can feel positive about participation in clinical research (101).

The ideal circumstance in clinical research is that consent, risk, and benefit are vested in the same individual. This is the case with adult volunteers. In pediatric research, formal consent does not apply, but permission is provided by a third party, usually parents or legal guardians, the risk is always borne by the child, and the benefit may or may not accrue to the child. The consequence of permission process is always imperfect, especially in multiarm studies, because if neither the subject nor the researcher knows which therapy is being consented to or what the possible risks may be, the process of being "informed" cannot be considered complete. A need to educate parents and patients about clinical trials should be a component of the process (86,102).

The institutional approval of pediatric studies is also a challenge and would require pediatric expertise on IRBs and ethics committees. The question of whether children who are not affected by a disease or condition under study should be enrolled was formally addressed by an FDA Advisory Subcommittee on November 15, 1999.

The Pediatric Subcommittee of the Anti-Infectives Advisory Committee, supplemented by a number of ethicists, was charged with providing guidance on the ethical consideration for the conduct of pediatric clinical trials, namely the role of pediatric volunteers who do not have the disease under study (100). The consensus areas of the discussion were as follows:

1. In general, pediatric studies should be conducted in subjects who may benefit from participation in the trial. Usually, this implies that the participant has or is susceptible to the disease under study. The advisory subcommittee utilized a broad definition of potential benefit. For example, almost any child has the potential to benefit from a treatment for otitis media.
2. In general, children who can give assent should be enrolled in a study in preference to, or prior to, children who cannot give assent. Careful consideration must be given to the importance of the potential benefit of the study. In certain circumstances, the potential benefit that may be derived from studying children who cannot give assent may override the preference for first enrolling assenting children (103).

As a result of the subcommittee discussions, it is considered appropriate and preferable to refer to children enrolled in clinical research as patients rather than subjects or participants to emphasize the expectation of potential benefit. The subcommittee also recommended that the federal regulations that apply to protecting children enrolled in research studies that receive federal funding, 45 CFR 46, be adapted and extended to studies that receive other sources of funding.

In April 2001, the FDA published in the Federal Register an adaptation of 45 CFR 46 Subpart D that applies to all children enrolled in studies that are FDA-regulated (104).

Placebo-controlled studies have been formally addressed by the American Academy of Pediatrics 1995 guidelines and subsequently by an FDA Advisory Subcommittee.

The American Academy of Pediatrics guidelines from 1995 state that placebo or untreated observational control groups can be used in pediatric studies if their use does not place children at increased risk. Acceptable conditions include when there is no commonly accepted therapy for the condition, or when the commonly used therapy is of questionable efficacy, or when the commonly used therapy has a high frequency of undesirable side effects and the risk may be greater than the benefits. A placebo is also considered acceptable in a comparative add-on study design where a new treatment or placebo is added to an established regimen (67).

The FDA Pediatric Subcommittee of the Anti-Infectives Advisory Committee, supplemented by ethicists and international experts, discussed placebo-controlled studies in children in 2000. The major points of discussion are summarized as follows. Comparison with a placebo may be acceptable if there are no approved or adequately studied therapies for children with the condition under study. For serious or life-threatening illness, a data monitoring committee with planned interim analysis and study-topping rules should be used.

In all studies, each patient should have escape criteria to minimize exposure to ineffective treatment. If an adult and pediatric condition are similar in history, response to therapy, and outcome, placebo should be considered primarily for symptomatic or pharmacodynamic end points.

Add-on trials do not deny any elements of the standard of care if individual patient discontinuation rules are defined. For serious and life-threatening illness, a data monitoring committee may be advisable. For minor illness or discomfort symptoms, a randomized withdrawal study may minimize exposure to placebo. Individual patient escape rules should be defined. A data monitoring committee would generally not be needed unless there was a specific safety concern (105).

Criteria for enrolling children in phase 1 or initial exposure studies was commented upon by the Pediatric Subcommittee of the FDA Oncologic Drugs Advisory Committee in 2002 as it pertains to children with cancer who have relapsed or who are refractory to available anticancer therapy and would be candidates for investigational drugs. The consensus was that the evidence burden for initiating clinical studies in children with cancer should include biological plausibility of the product having activity against a pediatric tumor (which could be obtained from preclinical data), some expectation of potential benefit, and a reasonable expectation of safety, and sufficient information to choose an appropriate starting dose.

If a scientific rationale and a population of pediatric cancer patients with no available anticancer therapy exist, then pediatric oncology clinical studies should be initiated, in most cases, immediately following adult phase 1 studies (106). Although the committee only commented on children with cancer, the same principles may be applicable to children with other diseases.

The International Conference on Harmonization (ICH) began work on a guideline for pediatric research in 1998. These guidelines were adopted as a recommendation by all participating regions in the year 2000 (107). The document is identified as E11, which is the 11th document in a series of recommendations related to the conduct of clinical studies. The letter "E" stands for efficacy. Major provisions of the document, due to its global importance are summarized in the following paragraphs.

The general principles are that pediatric patients should be given medicines that have been properly evaluated for their use in the intended population; that product development programs should include pediatric studies when pediatric use is anticipated; that pediatric development should not delay adult studies or adult availability; and that pediatric therapeutic development is a shared responsibility among companies, regulatory authorities, health professionals, and society as a whole.

The default state is that data on the appropriate use of medicinal products in the pediatric population should be generated unless the use of a specific medicinal product in pediatric patients is clearly inappropriate. Factors to consider when deciding to begin a pediatric development program are the prevalence and seriousness of the condition to be treated in the pediatric population, whether there are unique pediatric indications, age ranges of probable patients, availability and suitability of alternatives (including adverse events and pediatric-specific safety concerns), pediatric knowledge about the class of compounds, potential need for a pediatric formulation, and the need to develop pediatric-specific end points for study.

The timing of initiation of pediatric studies will be dependent on the prevalence, seriousness, and availability and suitability of alternatives. E11 states that the most important factor is the presence of a serious or life-threatening disease for which the medicinal product represents a potentially important advance in therapy and should initiate an urgent and early introduction of pediatric studies in the development program. For products that are predominantly or exclusively intended for pediatric use, all phases of development may occur in children.

Products intended for serious or life-threatening conditions occurring in adults and children for which there are no or limited therapies should begin pediatric studies following initial adult safety and preliminary evidence of potential benefit (early phase 2). This recommendation differs from the FDA Advisory Committee recommendation of October 2002 that pediatric studies begin immediately after adult phase 1.

For all other conditions, pediatric studies should begin when safety and efficacy have sufficient data to justify exposing children to a product. Exposure of children to a product that will be of no benefit should be avoided. In all studies, accurate dosing and patient compliance must be assured; thus, a pediatric formulation may be required. In developing a formulation, the variability of susceptibility of patients of different ages and developmental stages to the toxicity of recipients must be addressed.

Four types of studies are discussed: pharmacokinetics, pharmacokinetics/pharmacodynamics, efficacy, and safety. A pharmacokinetic study in pediatric patients with additional safety data may be adequate to establish pediatric use when the disease process is similar in adults and children and the outcome of therapy is likely to be comparable. In such a case, extrapolation from adult efficacy data may be appropriate. An approach based only on pharmacokinetics is likely to be insufficient when product blood levels are known or expected not to correspond with efficacy or when there is concern that those concentration-response relationships vary with age.

If the comparability of the disease and outcome of therapy are similar, a combined pharmacokinetic/pharmacodynamic approach may be possible. Although relative bioavailability comparisons of formulations should be done in adults, definitive pharmacolunetic studies for dose selection for pediatric patients should be done in the intended population.

In general, dosing should be based on a per-kilogram basis (body weight) because errors in measuring height or length are common and lead to errors in the calculation of body surface area. However, some medications with a narrow therapeutic index may require dosing based on body surface area. In all studies, principles of good clinical practice and other design and statistical considerations in other ICH including other relevant documents as well as general considerations for safety monitoring and adverse event reporting apply.

Clinical end points must be age and developmentally appropriate and validated. End points that rely on patient self-assessment are generally unreliable. Age-appropriate laboratory and clinical values should be used. Some efficacy studies may be simplified by extrapolation of efficacy findings from older to younger patients. The pediatric adverse event profile of a product may differ from the adult profile in types of events and magnitude of severity or duration due to different surface-to-volume ratio in children of varying ages and different levels of maturation of organ function and metabolism.

Unintended exposure such as accidental ingestion may provide additional opportunity for dose and safety information. Long-term or surveillance studies should be considered, particularly for chronic therapies, to observe effects on growth and development. Dimensions to consider are skeletal growth, cognitive function, maturation, postmarketing surveillance, and/or long-term follow-up studies, which may provide safety and/or efficacy information for subgroups within the pediatric population or additional information for the entire pediatric population.

E11 discusses age classification with particular attention to the neonate. Any age classification is arbitrary, and therefore decisions on how to stratify studies and data by age should take into consideration developmental biology and pharmacology. A flexible approach and reassessment is necessary to ensure that studies reflect current knowledge. Common categories are preterm infants (term: neonates) (0 to 27 days), infants and toddlers (28 days to 23 months), children (2 to 11 years), adolescents (older than 12 years). The category of preterm newborn infants is not a homogeneous group of patients, and protocol development should incorporate expert input from neonatologists and neonatal pharmacologists. A child of 25 weeks' gestational age and weighing 500 g is very different in terms of metabolism and response to therapy than a newborn of 30 weeks' gestational age weighing 1,500 g.

A distinction should also be made for low-birth-weight babies as to whether they are immature or growth retarded. Extrapolation of study findings from other populations is generally not feasible. This is due to the immaturity of renal and hepatic clearance mechanisms, protein binding and displacement issues (particularly bilirubin), the integrity of the blood-brain barrier, and subsequent penetration of medicinal products into the central nervous system, transdermal absorption, and rapid and variable maturation of all physiologic and pharmacologic processes leading to different dosing regimens with chronic exposure. Neonatal disease states and susceptibilities such as respiratory distress syndrome of the newborn, patent ductus arteriosus, primary pulmonary hypertension, necrotizing enterocolitis, intraventricular hemorrhage, and retinopathy of prematurity add further complexity. Adolescence has a variable upper age limit that depends on the context. The International Conference on Harmonization Guidance E11 notes that the age is 16 to 18 years depending upon the region. The World Health Organization notes that the age may be up to 20 years (http://www.who.int/bulletin/volumes/87/5/08–059808/en/index.html).

The Food and Drug Administration Amendments Act of 2007 includes people through 21 years as a target population for pediatric product development. The intent is not to recast the 16- or 18-year-old to 21-year-old population as a child but to allow extension of the upper age limit in pediatric studies, particularly for chronic diseases or those with growth delay, to gain additional follow-up information.

For all age groups, risk, discomfort, and distress can be minimized if studies are designed and conducted by investigators trained and experienced in the treatment of pediatric patients. Specific suggestions on minimizing distress include the use of trained personnel, the use of topical anesthetics, minimization of sample collection volume and frequency, comforting physical settings, and the availability and cooperation of parents.

PEDIATRIC STUDY OUTCOMES

Pediatric clinical trials are easiest to implement and interpret when the outcome measures are objective and do not require active patient participation. Outcome measures that are physical signs may be sufficiently precise and reproducible to substitute for symptom evaluation in some cases (e.g., respiratory rate and presence and extent of retractions for shortness of breath). However, when objective outcomes are not available, trials with subjective outcome measures or outcome measures that require active patient participation may be the most feasible option.

Patient-reported outcomes can be direct or indirect, particularly in younger children. Indirect or proxy reporting can be complex to design, analyze, and interpret. Rigorous statistical analyses apply, although the methods to analyze pediatric patient-reported outcomes may differ from the analyses for other types of clinical trial end points.

Several variables can affect patient-reported outcome. Using pain as a paradigm can be instructive. Pain is a combination of perception plus sensation. Therapy can usually be effective, and there are multiple scales available for assessment by the patient or an observer. A literature review shows that age (108–114), gender (115–119), and type of instrument (109,110) are variables that affect outcome in published studies (120,121). These reports collectively demonstrate that particular variables can affect patient-reported outcome and must be accounted for in the design and analysis of studies. Validation is context- and treatment-specific.

EXTRAPOLATION OF EFFICACY

The goal in pediatric clinical studies is to follow Einstein's dictum of making things as simple as possible, but not simpler. In 1994, the FDA published a pediatric rule that allowed extrapolation of adult efficacy to a pediatric population if the course of the disease and the beneficial and adverse effects of the drug are "sufficiently similar" in the pediatric and adult populations (65). The goal was to reduce the barrier to pediatric labeling of products by encouraging the use of borrowed data under appropriate circumstances to eliminate the need for separate adequate and well-controlled studies in children.

A 1996, FDA guidance document on the subject notes that the determination of "sufficiently similar" will depend on numerous factors including pathophysiology, natural history, drug action, and metabolism and would be easier to conclude for brief or acute disorders than for chronic disorders or those with a lengthy and variable history (66,122). Recent explorations into factors that may provide a basis for extrapolation have identified four domains that could provide supporting evidence—nonclinical evidence, pathophysiology, natural history, and response to therapy. Establishing a consistent framework for extrapolation is an area of development, and, if done effectively, could contribute to the sharing of data among study populations that would diminish the resource burden for conducting clinical trials.

INTERNATIONAL STUDIES

Performing a study in several countries could have multiple advantages including faster accrual, potentially greater confidence in the results due to replicability and sharing of resources. Engagement in international studies could also provide opportunities for professional development and cooperation as well as support better acceptance of study findings. In addition, best practices could be disseminated based on the clinical trial experience, which would quickly and directly benefit pediatric patients. The implementation of international studies, to be informative for all participants, should meet several criteria. The study question should be of value to all communities that participate. All assessment techniques should be available and validated at all sites. Eligibility criteria should be standardized. The data repository and analysis should be centralized.

Among the considerations in the design and implementation of an international study are the types of diseases relevant to each region, priority of any new proposed agents, types of studies, and incorporation of study end points that are demonstrative or predictive of clinical benefit. There are also several barriers that include, but are not limited to, regional differences in health care systems and practice, lack of common informatics standards, different languages and different medical terms, logistics and speed of protocol development, regulatory requirements and inconsistencies, compliance with good clinical practice and assurances, logistical challenges to sample processing, access to new agents, data sharing and credit, and funding.

Cooperative and collaborative studies in the 21st century will be feasible on the basis of development and acceptance of international standards for data acquisition, data transmission, and adherence to infrastructure and systems that are interoperable as a result of standards.

COMMON WEAKNESSES OR ERRORS IN TRIAL DESIGN OR ANALYSIS

It is a rare pediatric study outside vaccine trials that enrolls large numbers of patients, so designs and analytic plans must anticipate a limited patient population size. Techniques are available to address the problems associated with limited population size (123).

Hayden noted a trend over the prior 30 years of pediatric research to increasingly use a variety of statistical techniques and offered a critique of published studies (124). Pocock et al. later published a survey of statistical problems in clinical trials that noted that studies tended to have excessive hypothesis testing, which increased the number of false-positive findings (125).

An FDA survey in 1999 noted a number of weaknesses in submissions of clinical trial data for review. These included invalid assumptions, analytic methods, incomplete data, no dictionary for data fields, absence of a protocol with the submission, no statistical plan stated in the protocol, incomplete submissions of data, inconsistent field names across studies, multiple terms for the same type of adverse event, unexplained dropouts, lack of follow-up, treating categorical data as continuous data, mixing dose exposure and dose response, inventing new response variables, unspecified subgroup analysis, analyzing only "evaluable" patients displaying only adjusted analyses, stating results as percentage change or percentage change in hazard ratio, site bias, expressing efficacy per patient and adverse events per dose, and pooling analyses of distinct patient populations (126). Given the preciousness of the resource of pediatric patients, it is imperative that studies be informative and include an analytic plan that minimizes assumptions, is consistent with the end points, adheres to accepted statistical principles, and is prospective.

CONCLUSION

Scientific and ethical rationales support the use of clinical investigations to minimize risk and maximize benefit for the use of therapeutic products or interventions. Children of various ages have sufficient differences in metabolism, organ maturation and function, emotional and psychological function, that studies are necessary to extend the benefits of therapeutics while minimizing the potential for harm.

Clinical studies in pediatric patients should be designed to minimize risk, distress, and discomfort. This is best done by trained and experienced pediatric investigators at facilities that can support the special needs of pediatric patients and by adherence to accepted principles of patient protection and respect. Enrolling children in studies is a combination of educating and gaining the permission of parents or legal guardians and educating the child while obtaining assent if appropriate.

There are conditions when the permission/assent process can be postponed or waived due to emergent circumstances. Approaches to minimize nontherapeutic interventions such as sparse population sampling for pharmacokinetics and special imaging studies in lieu of tissue sampling are preferred. Study design should incorporate escape rules for individual patients, stopping rules for the entire population, and an independent data monitoring committee, if appropriate, particularly for life-threatening diseases. Assessments, both clinical and laboratory, need to be age and developmental stage appropriate. Multiple factors may affect study results. Patient-reported outcomes are generally not sufficiently reliable to serve as the only end point and should be confirmed by other objective findings. Strategies to minimize exposure and risk include studying older populations before younger ones and using extrapolation of efficacy when scientific evidence warrants.

Diseases or conditions that are specific to a particular age group require studies in that population. Study designs and analytic approaches need to address the limitations of small numbers of patients and variability among patient populations. International cooperation can share resources but has many challenges to address before multinational pediatric studies become routine.

Clinical studies in pediatric patients are a necessary component of therapeutic development unless the product is unsafe or addresses only a condition that does not exist in children. The responsibility for clinical studies in pediatrics is shared with pharmaceutical firms, regulatory authorities, health professionals, and society as a whole. The most vulnerable populations merit the most protection and deserve the benefits available to others, which is achieved through careful and persistent pursuit of further knowledge.

REFERENCES

1. Colon AR, Colon PA, eds. *Nurturing children: a history of pediatrics.* Westport, CT: Greenwood, 1999:189, 201, 210.
2. Aronson SM, Newman L. Smallpox in the Americas 1492 to 1815: contagion and controversy. Published December 2002. http://www.brown.edu/Administration/News_Bureau/2002-03/02-017t.html. Accessed June 5, 2009.
3. The Jenner Museum. Edward Jenner and smallpox. http://www.jennermuseum.comlsvlsmallpox2.shtm1. Accessed May 2009.
4. Beckwith J. Charles-Michel Billard (1800–1832): pioneer of infant pathology. *Pediatr Dev Pathol* 2003;5(3):248.
5. Ouetelet A. *Sur l'hornrne et le develoomenr de ses facultés. 011 essai de physique sociale.* Paris, France: Bachelier, 1835.
6. Bogin B. *Patterns of human growth,* 2nd ed. Cambridge, MA: Cambridge University Press, 1999:30–32.
7. Ganison FH, ed. *History of pediatrics.* Philadelphia, PA: WB Saunders, 1965:125.
8. Karolinska Institute. The history of Swedish child and adolescent psychiatry and of the department of child and adolescent psychiatry at the Karolinska Institute. http://www.ki.se/kbh~psyluatri/history~en.htm. Accessed May 2009.
9. Pearson HA. Lectures on diseases of children by Eli Ives, MD, of Yale and New Haven: America's first academic pediatrician. *Pediatrics* 1986;77(5):680–686.
10. Burke EC, Abraham Jacobi MD. The man and his legacy. *Pediatrics* 1998;101(2):309–312.
11. Haggerty RJ, Abraham Jacobi MD. Respectable rebel. *Pediatrics* 1997;99(3):462–466.
12. Bernard C, ed. *An introduction to the shady of medicine.* New York, NY: Macmillan, 1927.
13. Seppa N. With new vaccine, scientist prevents rabies in boys. (Louis Pasteur tests a rabies vaccine in 1885). *Sci News* 1999;156.
14. Silver JR. The decline of German medicine 1933–1945. *J R Coll Physicians Edinb* 2003;33:5466.
15. Vollman J, Winan R. The Prussian regulation of 1900: early ethical standards for human experimentation in Germany. *IRB* 1996; 18(4):9–11.
16. Schaller UC, Klauss V. Is Crede's prophylaxis for ophthalmia neonatorum still valid? *Bull World Health Organ* 2001;79(3): 262–263.
17. Crede CSF. Die Verhiitung der Augenentziindung der Neugeborenen. *Arch Gynaekol* 1881;17:50–53.
18. Vollmann J, Winau R. Informed consent in human experimentation before the Nuremberg code. *Br Med J* 1996;313(7070): 1445.
19. Moll A. Ar:tliche Erhik. Stuttgart: Enke. 1902. 20. 100 years of biologics regulation. FDA Corurrmer Mag 2002 (July). http://www.fda.govlfdaclfeatures/2002/4022bio.html. Accessed June 5, 2009.
20. Janssen WF. The story of the laws behind the labels. *FDA Consumer* June 1981;15(5):32–45.
21. *United States v Johnson,* 433.191 SCt 248, 221 (1911). http://www.druglibrary.org/schaeregaWl191Osvjohnson.htm.
22. Center for Drug Evaluation and Research. FDA History Office. http://www.fda.gov/AboutFDA/WhatWeDo/History/Overviews/ucm056044.htm. Accessed June 5, 2009.
23. The story of the White House conferences on children and youth: the US Department of Health, Education, and Welfare, 1967. In: *Highlights from conferences on children and youth.* Washington, DC: White House, 1981.
24. Duxbury M, Adams LR. *Nursing research contributions to improve VICU care in neonate intensive cure: a history of excellence.* Washington, DC: US Dept of Health and Human Services, National Institutes of Health, 1992. No. 92-2786.
25. American Academy of Pediatrics history. http://www.aap.org/new/aaphistory.pdf. Accessed May 2009.
26. Swain DC. The rise of a research empire: NIH. 1930–1950. *Science* 1962;138:1233–1237.
27. Sass HM. Reichsrundschreiben 1931: pre-Nuremberg German regulations concerning new therapy and human experimentation. *J Med Philos* 1983;8:99–111.
28. Ballentine C. Taste of raspberries, taste of death. The 1937 elixir sulfanilamide incident. *FDA Consumer* June 1981:18–21.
29. Kopelman LM. Children as research subjects: a dilemma. *J Med Philos* 2000;25(6):745–764.
30. US Food and Drug Administration. History of Drug Efficacy Study Implementation. http://www.fda.gov/cdedabout/history/page37.htm. Accessed May 2009.
31. Nicholson RH. *Medical research with children: ethics, law, and practice.* Oxford, England: Oxford University Press, 1986:13.
32. Welt LG. Reflections on the problems of human experimentation. *Conn Med* 1961;25:75–91.
33. Medical Research Council. *Responsibility in investigations on human subjects: report of the 35 Medical Research Council for the year 1962–1963.* London, England: Her Majesty's Stationery Office, 1964:21–26.
34. World Medical Association. Declaration of Helsinki (1964). Recommendations guiding physicians in biomedical research involving human subjects. http://www.wma.nete/policy/b3.htm.1 Accessed May 2009.
35. Beecher HK. Ethics and clinical research. *N Engl J Med* 1966; 274(24):1354–1360.
36. Advisory Committee on Human Radiation Experiments. Nontherapeutic research on children. In: *Advisory Committee on Human Radiation Experiments report.* Washington, DC: Advisory Committee on Human Radiation Experiment, 1995; chap 7. http://www.gwu.edu/~nsarchiv/radiation/.
37. Surgeon General. *Public Health Service to the heads of the institutions contracting research with Public Health Service grants, 8 February 1966: Bureau of Medical Services Curriculum.* Washington, DC: US Dept of Health and Human Services, 1996. ACHRE No. HHS-090794-A. Also available as: No. 38, 1966:23.
38. PHS policy for intramural programs and for contracts when investigations involving human subjects are included (HHS-072894-B). Washington, DC: DHHS, 1966.
39. Royal College of Physicians. Supervision of clinical investigations. *Lancet* 1967;2(7511):357–358.
40. Pappworth MH, ed. *Human guinea pigs.* Boston, MA: Beacon Press, 1967.
41. Royal College of Physicians. *Supervision of the ethics of clinical research investigation in institutions.* London, England: Royal College of Physicians, 1973.
42. US Department of Health, Education, and Welfare. Protection of human subjects. *Fed Regist* 1974;39(105):18914–18920.
43. National Research Act. Pub L No. 93-348 (1974).
44. National Commission for the Protection of Human Subjects of Biomedical and Behavioral Research. *Research involving children: report and recommendations.* Washington, DC: Dept of Health, Education, and Welfare, 1977. No. 77-0004, Appendix 77-0005.
45. National Health Service (United Kingdom) Department of Health and Social Security. *Supervision of the ethics of clinical research investigations and fetal research.* London, England: National Health Service (United Kingdom) Department of Health and Social Security, 1975. HSC(IS)153.
46. World Medical Association. Declaration of Helsinki. Recommendations guiding physicians in biomedical research involving human subjects. 1975 to be revised. http://www.wnia.net/e/policy/b3.htm. Accessed May 2009.

47. National Commission for the Protection of Human Subjects of Biomedical and Behavioral Research. *Institutional national boards: reports and recommendations.* Bethesda, MD: National Commission for the Protection of Human Subjects of Biomedical and Behavioral Research, 1978.
48. National Commission for the Protection of Human Subjects of Biomedical and Behavioral Research. *The Belmont report: ethical principals and guidelines for the protection of human subjects of research.* Washington, DC: National Commission for the Protection of Human Subjects of Biomedical and Behavioral Research, 1979.
49. Department of Health and Human Services. 45 CFR part 46. Additional protections for children involved as subjects in research. *Fed Regist* 1983;48:9814–9820.
50. British Paediatric Association. Guidelines to aid ethical committees considering research involving children. *Arch Dis Child* 1980; 55:75–77.
51. British Medical Association. *The handbook of medical ethics.* London, England: British Medical Association, 1980:25–26.
52. Tyson JE, Furzan JA. Reisch JS, et al. An evaluation of the quality of therapeutic studies in perinatal medicine. *J Pediatr* 1983; 102(1):10–13.
53. Greenhouse SW. Some historical and methodological developments in early clinical trials at the National Institutes of Health. *Stat Med* 1990;9(8):893–901.
54. Obituaries. Aldrich, first NICHD director, dies [Obituary of Dr. Robert Aldrich]. *NIH Record* 1998;L(22). http://wwul.nih.gov/news/NIH-record/11.03~98/obits.htm. Accessed May 2009.
55. Shirkey H. Therapeutic orphans. *Pediatrics* 1968;72(1):119–120.
56. Marks I. Drugs (e.g., hexachlorophene), the FDA, and the AAP. *Pediatrics* 1972;50(2):338.
57. American Academy of Pediatrics Committee on Drugs. *General guidelines for the evaluation of drugs to be approved for use during pregnancy and for the treatment of infants and children.* Chicago, IL: American Academy of Pediatrics, 1974.
58. Wilson JT. Pragmatic assessment of medicines available for young children and pregnant or breast-feeding women. In: Morselli PL, Garattini S, Sereni F, eds. *Basic and therapeutic aspects of perinatal pharmacology.* New York, NY: Raven, 1975:411–421.
59. Department of Health, Education, and Welfare. *General considerations for the clinical evaluation of drugs in infants and children.* Washington, DC: Dept of Health, Education, and Welfare, 1977. DHEW 77-3041.
60. American Academy of Pediatrics, Committee on Drugs. Guidelines for the ethical conduct of studies to evaluate drugs in pediatric populations. *Pediatrics* 1977;60:91–101.
61. Labeling and prescription drug advertising: content and format for labeling for human prescription drugs. *Fed Regist* 1979;44: 37434–37462.
62. Orphan Drug Act. Pub L No. 97-414, 21 USC §360aa–360ee.
63. Regulations requiring manufacturers to assess the safety and effectiveness of new drugs and biological products in pediatric patients—FDA. Final rule. *Fed Regist* 1998;63:66631.
64. Gilman JT, Gal P. Pharmacokinetic and pharmacodynamic data collection in children and neonates. A quiet frontier. *Clin Pharmacokinet.* 1992;23:1–9.
65. Department of Health and Human Services, Food and Drug Administration. Specific requirements on content and format of labeling for human prescription drugs; revision of "pediatric use" subsection in the labeling. *Fed Regist* 1994;59:64240–64250.
66. Center for Drug Evaluation and Research. Center for Biologics Evaluation and Research. Guidance for industry: the content and format for pediatric use supplements. Published May 1996. http://www.fda.gov/cder/guid&ce/clin1.pdf. Accessed May 2009.
67. American Academy of Pediatrics. Guidelines for the ethical conduct of studies to evaluate drugs in the pediatric population. *Pediatrics* 1995;95(2):286–294.
68. Pediatric Pharmacology Research Unit Network. A child is not just a miniature adult. http://www.nichd.nih.gov/rm/eng/ped/ped2.htm. Accessed May 2009.
69. Food and Drug Administration Modernization Act of 1997. Pub L No. 105–115.
70. US District Count for the District of Columbia Civil Action 130-02898 October 17, 2002. http://www.dcd.uscourts.g0/00–02898.pdf. Accessed May 2009.
71. Pediatric Research Equity Act. http://www.fda.gov/opacom-laws/prea.html. Accessed May 2009.
72. Stolberg SG. The biotech death of Jesse Gelsinger. *N Y Times Mag* 1999:136–140, 149–150.
73. Office of Public Health and Science, and the National Institutes of Health, Office of the Director. Statement of organization, functions, and delegations of authority. *Fed Regist* 2000;65(114): 37136–37137.
74. Department of Health and Human Services. Food and Drug Administration. Additional safeguards for children in clinical investigations of FDA regulated products. *Fed Regist* 2001;66(79): 20589.
75. Best Pharmaceuticals for Children Act. Pub L No. 107–109.
76. Food and Drug Administration Pediatric Exclusivity Statistics. http://www.fda.gov/Drugs/DevelopmentApprovalProcess/DevelopmentResources/ucm049867.htm. Accessed May 2009.
77. Ashcroft R. Equipoise, knowledge, and ethics in clinical research and practice. *Bioethics* 1999;13(34):314–326.
78. Hill AB, ed. *Controlled clinical trials.* Oxford, England: Blackwell, 1960.
79. Medical Research Council. Streptomycin treatment of pulmonary tuberculosis. *Br Med J* 1948;2:769–783.
80. Austrian R, MirickG, Rogers D, et al. The efficacy of modified oral penicillin therapy of pneumococcal lobar pneumonia. *Bull Johns Hopkins Hosp* 1951;88:264–269.
81. Tucker WB. Experiences with controls and the study of the chemotherapy of tuberculosis. In: *Transactions of the 13th Veterans Administration Conference on chemotherapy of tuberculosis.* Washington, DC: Veteran's Administration, 1954:50.
82. Rheumatic Fever Working Party. The evolution of rheumatic heart disease in children: five-year report of a cooperative clinical trial of ACTH, cortisone, and aspirin. *Circulation* 1960:22: 505–515.
83. National Program of Cancer Chemotherapy. *Cancer Chemotherapy Rep* 1960;1:5–34.
84. Gehan EA, Schneiderman MA. Historical and methodological developments in clinical trials at the National Cancer Institute. *Stat Med* 1990;9(8):871–880.
85. Emanuel EJ, Wendler D, Grady C. What makes clinical research ethical? *JAMA* 2000;283(20):2701–2711.
86. Sutcliffe A. Testing new pharmaceutical products in children. *Br Med J* 2003;325:64–65.
87. Chiappa JN. http://sailfish.exis.net/-jnc/.
88. NIH Definition Working Group. Biomarkers and surrogate endpoints: preferred definitions and conceptual framework. *Clin Pharmacol Ther* 2001;69:89–95.
89. http://www.biomarkersconsortium.org/index.phpoption=com_content&task=view&id=132&Itemid=184.
90. Fleming TR, DeMets DL. Surrogate end points in clinical trials: are we being misled? *Ann Intern Med* 1996;125(7): 605–613.
91. Packer M, Rouleau J, Swedberg K, et al. Effect of flosequinan on survival of chronic heart failure: preliminary results of the PROFILE study. *Circulation* 1993;88(suppl 1):1301.
92. The Cardiac Arrhythmia Suppression Trial (CAST) Investigators. Preliminary report: effect of encainide and flecainide on mortality in a randomized trial of arrhythmia suppression after myocardial infarction. *N Engl J Med* 1989;321:406–412.
93. Echt DS, Liebson PR, Mitchell LB, et al. Mortality and morbidity in patients receiving encainide, flecainide, or placebo. The Cardiac Arrhythmia Suppression Trial. *N Engl J Med* 1991;324: 781–788.
94. The Cardiac Arrhythmia Suppression Trial II Investigators. Effect of the anti-arrhythmic agent moricizine on survival after myocardial infarction. *N Engl J Med* 1992;327:227–233.
95. The International Chronic Granulomatous Disease Cooperative Study Group. A controlled trial of interferon gamma to prevent infection in chronic granulomatous disease. *N Engl J Med* 1991; 321:509–516.
96. Riggs BL, Hodgson SF, O'Fallon WM. Effect of fluoride treatment on the fracture rate in postmenopausal women with osteoporosis. *N Engl J Med* 1990;321:802–809.
97. Riggs BL, Seeman E, Hodgson SF, et al. Effect of the fluoride/calcium regimen on vertebral fracture occurrence in postmenopausal osteoporosis. Comparison with conventional therapy. *N Engl J Med* 1982;306:446–450.
98. Sheiner LB, Steimer JL. Pharmacokinetic/pharmacodynamic modeling in drug development. *Annu Rev Pharmacol Toxicol* 2000; 40:67–95.

99. US Food and Drug Administration. FDA regulations relating to good clinical practice and clinical trials. Updated August 13, 2009. http://www.fda.gov/oc/gcp/regulations.html. Accessed June 5, 2009.
100. NICHD Clinical Research Monitoring Policy http://www.nichd.nih.gov/funding/policies/datasafety.cfm. Accessed May 2009.
101. Food and Drug Administration. Investigational New Drug Application Process. http://www.fda.gov/cder/regulatoq/applications/indpagel.html. Accessed May 2009.
102. Johnson DE, Wolfgang GH. Predicting human safety: screening and computational approaches. *Drug Discov Today* 2000;5(10): 445–154.
103. Kauffman RE. Clinical Research involving children. *Bioethics Forum* 2000:16(4):45–46.
104. Hirschfeld S. Comment—disclosing a diagnosis of HIV in pediatrics: providing the best possible care. *J Clin Ethics* 2001;12(2): 150–157.
105. Pediatric Subcommittee of Anti-infective Advisory Committee. Discussion of ethical issues. http://www.fda.gov/ohrms/docketslac/99/transcpt/3563tI.pdf. Published November 15, 1999. Accessed May 2009.
106. Food and Drug Administration Ethics Working Group. Consensus statement on the Pediatric Advisory Subcommittee's November 15, 1999 meeting. http://www.fda.govlcder/pediatriclethics-statement.htm. Accessed May 2009.
107. 45 CFR 46 Title 45-Public welfare. Subtitle DHHS Part 46-Protection of human subjects. http://www.access.gpo.gov/nara/cfr/waisidx99/45cfr46–99.html. Accessed May 2009.
108. Food and Drug Administration Pediatric Ethics Working Group. Consensus statement on Pediatric Advisory Subcommittee's September 11, 2000 meeting. http://www.fda.govlcderlpediatriclethics-statement-2000.htm. Accessed May 2009.
109. Pediatric Oncology Subcommittee. Consensus statement on initiating studies with investigational drugs in children with cancer. http://www.fda.gov/cder/cancer/Presentations/phaseone.htm. Accessed May 2009.
110. Guidance for industry El I. Clinical investigation of medicinal products in the pediatric population. Published December 2000. http://www.fda.gov/cder/guidance/4099FNL.pdf. Accessed May 2009.
111. Arts SE, Abu-Saad HH. Champion GD, et al. Age-related response to lidocaine-prilocaine (EMLA) emulsion and effect of music distraction on the pain of intravenous cannulation. *Pediatrics* 1994;93(5):797–801.
112. Chambers CT, Craig KD. An intrusive impact of anchors in children's Faces Pain Scales. *Pain* 1998;78(1):27–37.
113. Johnston CC, Stevens B, Arbess G. The effect of the sight of blood and use of decorative adhesive bandages on pain intensity ratings by preschool children. *J Pediatr Nurs* 1993;8(3): 147–151.
114. Kotiniemi LH, Ryhanen PT, Moilanen IK. Behavioral changes in children following day-case surgery: a 4-week follow-up of 551 children. *Anesthesia* 1997;52(10):970–976.
115. Lander J, Fowler-Kerry S. TENS for children's procedural pain. *Pain* 1993;52(2):209–216.
116. Ljunzman G, Kreuger A, Andreasson S, et al. Midazolam nasal spray reduces procedural anxiety in children. *Pediatrics* 2000;105 (1, pt 1):73–78.
117. Santavina N, Bjorvell H, Solovieva S, et al. Coping strategies, pain, and disability in patients with hemophilia and related disorders. *Arthritis Rheum* 2001;15(1):18–55.
118. Aho AC, Erickson MT. Effects of grade, gender, and hospitalization on children's medical fears. *J Dev Behav Pediatr* 1985;6(3): 146–153.
119. Bruusgaard D, Smedbraten BK, Natvig B. Bodily pain, sleep problems and mental distress in school children. *Ann Pediatr* 2000;89(5):597–600.
120. Goodenough B, Thomas W, Champion GD, et al. Unraveling age effects and sex differences in needle pain: rating of sensory intensity and unpleasantness of venipuncture pain by children and their parents. *Pain* 1999;80(1–2):179–190.
121. Guite JW, Walker LS, Smith CA, et al. Children's perceptions of peers with somatic symptoms: the impact of gender, stress, and illness. *J Pediatr Psychol* 2000;25(3):125–135.
122. Chambers CT, Craig KD, Bennett SM. The impact of maternal behavior on children's pain experiences: an experimental analysis. *J Pediatr Psychol* 2002;27(3):293–301.
123. Pett M. *Nonparametric statistics in health care research: clinical statistics for small samples and unusual distribution.* Thousand Oaks, CA: Sage, 1997.
124. Hayden GF. Biostatistical trends in pediatrics: implications for the future. *Pediatrics* 1983;72(1):84–87.
125. Pocock SJ, Hughes MD, Lee RJ. Statistical problems in the reporting of clinical trials. A survey of three medical journals. *N Engl J Med* 1987;317:426–432.
126. Hirschfeld S. *Drug Information Association workshop on electronic submissions.* Washington, DC: Drug Information Association, Horsham PA, 1999.

Bruce A. Russell
Sanford N. Cohen
Virginia Delaney-Black

CHAPTER

8

Ethics of Drug Research in Pediatric Populations

WHY RESEARCH ON CHILDREN IS NEEDED

The majority of pharmacologic agents and pharmaceutical preparations currently marketed in the United States cannot be advertised as safe and effective for infants and children. Many of the agents and preparations that are commonly prescribed for pediatric patients contain disclaimers in their labeling regarding the lack of information concerning appropriate dosage recommendations, side effects, and so on. This inequity in the protection afforded children when compared with that available to adults has been termed unethical. Indeed, the US Food and Drug Administration (FDA), the regulatory agency charged with the responsibility for certifying that drugs are safe and effective for use as claimed, has established a policy of requiring that new drugs that are likely to be used widely in infants and children be evaluated properly so that they can be labeled accordingly prior to approval for marketing, and the Congress has acted to ensure that this will occur.

The American Academy of Pediatrics (AAP) first published guidelines for the ethical conduct of drug research studies in infants and children in 1977 in an attempt to ease the transition between the situation that existed then and the ideal one, in which labeling of all drugs necessary for the treatment of pediatric patients contains enough information for their safe and effective use (1). The US Department of Health and Human Services (DHHS) issued regulations to control such experimentation in 1991 (2). The AAP guidelines were revised, updated, and reissued in 1995 (3). As we shall see, the US Office of Human Research Protection (OHRP) issued new regulations that reinterpret and clarify how Title 45 Code of Federal Regulations Part 46 (45 CFR 46) must be implemented in 2005.

Nonetheless, there continues to be concern and debate regarding the moral, ethical, and legal issues that surround drug research and evaluation in infants and children. All investigators who engage in experiments involving human participants frequently find themselves in a conflict between their scientific and professional quest for new knowledge and future understanding and their moral (indeed legal) obligation to be mindful and protective of the inviolability of the individual. Thus, there is a potential value conflict inherent in investigations in humans. Few areas exemplify this conflict between the pursuit of knowledge and ethics so strikingly as research in infants and children. Furthermore, research in pediatric populations frequently introduces questions concerning both the legality of investigators' actions and the responsibility of institutions and society at large to protect the interests of those who lack competence under the law to protect themselves.

THE GUIDELINES FOR RESEARCH ON CHILDREN

GENERAL GUIDELINES

One of the basic standards that must be adhered to in drug research in pediatric populations is that all studies must be carried out according to an appropriate scientific design. A poorly designed experiment or one in which there is no potential for a direct benefit to the participant or to society (indirect benefit) is unethical because there is no chance of obtaining valuable scientific knowledge from it, while at the same time the investigator exposes experimental participants to needless risk or, at the very least, inconvenience.

A second basic standard is that the investigator must be both competent and ethical. The competence and ethical nature of the investigator are the most important safeguards for the protection of the interest and well-being of the child participant. The investigator who wishes to conduct studies utilizing human participants who are in the pediatric age groups must not only be knowledgeable and well trained, but also must understand the feelings and attitudes of the parties involved in the research and be especially sensitive to the special needs and fears of young children.

A third standard requires that the investigator must be fully aware of the need for any research plan to include a consideration of the concept of distributive justice and that this be adhered to in its execution. Thus, infants and children should not be exposed to unwarranted risks, no matter how minimal, for the convenience of the investigator, and no subgroup of children (e.g., racial, ethnic, and socioeconomic) should bear a greater share of the research burden than others, except as dictated by the clinical and scientific requirements of the investigation itself or of the disease process under study.

A study conducted to evaluate appropriate dosages and/or effects for pediatric patients who require a specific form of therapy should therefore include patients from as wide a segment of society as is practical, whereas a study to evaluate dosages and/or effects of agents used to treat specific diseases should involve individual subjects in reasonable proportion to the risk or incidence of that disease in their subgroup of society.

Legal restraints imposed by the centuries-old common-law standard, based on the Magna Carta, that permission to act on a minor, or his or her property, can only be given when the action can be construed as being to the minor's own benefit complicated the development of guidelines and standards for many years. However, since the rule was designed in the 13th century to solve a specific political problem of the times, thinking on the issue has undergone significant changes in modern times. Indeed, societal attitudes toward research on children have moved to the current discussion concerning how to define "harm" in a research situation as distinct from "discomfort" or "mere inconvenience" in such a setting. Since social forces lead to changes in public policy, a clearer set of guidelines has been developed to guide investigators, as the legal standards of professional behavior in this area have changed.

We believe that these guidelines, when properly interpreted and modified, can be utilized to carry out necessary studies so that advances can be made for pediatric patients in an ethical manner. Society must continue to afford maximal protection to all individuals (especially to those individuals who are not capable of protecting themselves) while maintaining systems that are seen as equitable by all groups in the society.

SPECIFIC GUIDELINES

The National Commission for the Protection of Human Subjects was mandated by the Congress in 1974. That body debated whether to use the terms "therapeutic" and "nontherapeutic" to describe forms of research in human participants. In the end, the Commission chose not to use these terms but rather to refer to the two classes of research as "research that holds out the prospect of direct benefit for the individual subjects" and its opposite (4). The Canadian Medical Research Council's Working Group on the matter also decided against the older terminology because "therapeutic" research can be confounded with treatment or care (5). They were rightly concerned that potential participants in experimentation or their parents or guardians might be misled into thinking that there would be a greater probability of benefit in "therapeutic" experiments than would actually be the case.

The AAP guidelines and the DHHS regulations for research on children distinguish between experiments where there is some prospect of direct benefits to the participants themselves (sometimes called therapeutic experiments) and those in which there is not (sometimes called nontherapeutic experiments). They also distinguish between research that does not involve greater than minimal risk to individuals and research that does. We could distinguish, further, research that involves subjects competent to give free and informed consent and research involving subjects not competent to give such consent. Using these three different pairs of distinctions, we can construct the following matrix:

	Prospect of Direct Benefit		*No Such Prospect*	
	≤Minimal Risk	*>Minimal Risk*	*≤Minimal Risk*	*>Minimal Risk*
Competent	1a	1b	1c	1d
Incompetent	2a	2b	2c	2d

Minimal risk is risk where "the probability and magnitude of harm or discomfort anticipated in the research is not greater in and of themselves than those ordinarily encountered in daily life or during the performance of routine physical or psychological examinations" (6). The AAP understands minimal risk to be "a level of risk similar to the risk encountered in the child's usual daily activity" (3). OHRP defines these risks in 45 CFR 46 in the same way (CFRs 46.102). However, if harm or discomfort is relativized to the individual child as suggested in this definition, it could lead some to conclude that it is permissible to subject children to research which will involve very painful procedures when those children are already undergoing a painful treatment regimen. However, there is a moral basis for rejecting this conclusion and interpreting "minimal risk" in a general way. It is not morally acceptable to put afflicted children at an even greater disadvantage than healthy children in order to benefit other children. That is, it is never morally acceptable to enroll a child in a study that involves significant pain *when there is no prospect of direct benefit to that child*, even when that child is already subjected to painful treatments/procedures as a part of a therapeutic regimen.

Sometimes it is permissible to expose afflicted children to substantially more harm than most children are exposed to, but this will either be because there is a good prospect that they will directly benefit from being so exposed or there is the potential for obtaining information that cannot be acquired in any other manner and the information is likely to lead to useful information concerning the disorder or condition being investigated. For example, we believe that it can be permissible to take an extra bone marrow aspirate from an adolescent with cancer if the adolescent is capable of assenting, or consenting, to being exposed to more than minimal risk (3). If it were a younger child, one without this capability, we believe that it would not be permissible in an experiment *with no prospect of directly benefiting that child*, for it would violate the basic moral obligation to protect the defenseless. However, such a procedure could be permissible in a younger child if the research has the prospect of benefiting that child. [We are aware that some institutional review boards (IRBs) now also permit collection of blood samples from young children for the sole purpose of developing a database.]

Many different grounds have been offered for and against the limit of minimal risk in experiments *with no prospect of direct benefit.* Ramsey argued that allowing children to be placed at minimal risk where that will not likely benefit them . . . violates a requirement of respect for persons (7). The Belmont Report says that "respect for persons divides into two separate moral requirements: the requirement to acknowledge autonomy and the requirement to protect those with diminished autonomy." The Report goes on to say that respect for autonomy requires giving "weight to autonomous persons' considered opinions," and this is what founds the requirement of obtaining free and informed consent. According to the Belmont Report, questions about protecting those with diminished autonomy concern "the risks of harm and the likelihood of benefits." Because very young children are not autonomous individuals, some have reasonably thought that respect for autonomy is not relevant to actions involving them. However, others have thought that what is relevant is *hypothetical,* or *counterfactual,* consent, that is, what the young child *would want* with respect to treatment or becoming a subject of some experiment, *if he or she were autonomous* (8). For instance, McCormick wrote ". . . that it is permissible for children to be subjected to minimal risk because they *would want* to help others, if they could consent, because they *ought* to aid others when providing that aid requires little of them" (9). In other words, if children could rationally consent, they would want to do what they morally should do. For him, and for others, hypothetical consent (i.e., what the person would want if capable of rationally consenting) is enough; actual consent is not required.

Ackerman argued against both the requirements of actual and hypothetical consent (10). He approached the question about permissible imposition of risk in nontherapeutic experiments (see categories 1c, 1d, 2c, and 2d in the matrix given earlier) by focusing on what sorts of risk or harm parents are permitted to impose on their children to enhance their personal, physical, social, and moral development and also to enhance the interests of other people (10). He argued that the risk of harm that a child encounters in everyday life may be greater than the risk that we can *intentionally* impose on a child. Children normally engage in certain dangerous recreational activities, for example, skateboarding, swimming in polluted or unsafe lakes, and hopping on and off railroad cars, but it would not be permissible to impose such risks on them if they are not needed to benefit them. He suggested that "minimal risk" be taken to mean "no more than that to which it is appropriate to expose a child for educational purposes in the family situation" (10).

The DHHS regulations (cited in the AAP guidelines of 1995) take the position that all cases of at least *no greater than minimal risk* involving children who are *unable to give their free and informed consent,* that is, 2a and 2c, should be treated alike. According to the regulations, appropriate permission and assent is nonetheless required in all such cases. Permission is always required of parents or guardians for all children except for those who are considered to be emancipated or mature minors, as noted later. These regulations also require appropriate assent from children 7 years of age or older, where assent is defined as "active agreement." The child's assent must be free and informed, just as consent must be when it is required. The difference between assent and consent in this context is that a lower level of understanding of the risks and benefits involved may suffice for assent than for informed consent.

Ackerman questioned whether assent is required for those between 7 and around 12 to 14 years of age. Starting with the idea that the primary obligation of parents is to the moral, social, personal, and physical development of their child, Ackerman argued that we are not required to go along with a child's wishes, especially if they are founded on interests that are still developing. However, he did think we should *not go against* the wishes of children in that age bracket, that is, it is not permissible to include them in *nontherapeutic experiments* (categories 2c and 2d) *against* their wishes. This might be called the requirement of no dissent. Ackerman was rightly concerned that involving a child between 7 and 14 years of age in an experiment in one of these categories against the child's wishes may create so much fear and anxiety (and we would add mistrust) that it could not be justified.

We agree with Ackerman that assent should not be required for those aged between 7 and 14 years, but, instead, that it be required that there is *no* informed *dissent* by the child. This clearly deviates from the DHHS regulations, which require assent, where assent is explicitly distinguished from "failure to object" (11). We also agree with his views on subjecting children to more than minimal risk in "nontherapeutic" experiments. He argued that children between 7 and 14 years of age cannot be exposed to more than minimal risk in a research situation, for if they were, given his understanding of minimal risk, they would be exposed to more risk in this situation than it is permissible for parents to expose their children to in nonexperimental situations.

Furthermore, Ackerman argued that assent *is* required from preadolescent youths aged 12 to 14 years. Their judgment is sufficiently developed that parents and others must pay attention to their wishes. He indicated that they are so developed that they can even assent to a risk that is slightly more than minimal to benefit others by participating in a nontherapeutic experiment. We agree with Ackerman's views on nontherapeutic experiments, namely that (a) assent is *not* required for children aged between 7 and 12 years (though lack of dissent is) and no more than minimal risk may be imposed on them and (b) assent *is* required for preadolescents aged 12 to 14 years and we can permissibly involve them in nontherapeutic experiments involving slightly more than minimal risk.

It cannot be permissible to involve a child in an experiment without her or his free and informed consent if that child is capable of giving such consent. However, such consent is not by itself sufficient to make the inclusion of that child permissible. In some states, emancipated and mature minors are sometimes considered to be capable of giving their free and informed consent to participate in an experiment. But, because there is a high risk that they will be exploited, we think the best *policy* regarding emancipated or mature minors is that they should *not* be permitted to be participants in nontherapeutic experiments, that is, experiments where there is no prospect of direct benefit to them and where they are subject to more than minimal risk, that is, category 1d. Thus, our recommendation is more stringent than the AAP guidelines, which permit emancipated and mature minors to participate in nontherapeutic experiments if the knowledge sought cannot be obtained by using another group of children where parental consent is obtainable (3).

When it comes to research with the prospect of direct benefit to the research participants (categories 1a, 1b, 2a, and 2b), the DHHS requires that "the risk is justified by the anticipated benefits to the subjects" and that there is no other available alternative with a more favorable risk–benefit ratio (3,12). Of course, the problem is that in situations where experiments are in order, the relevant risks and benefits will largely be unknown because one cannot extrapolate directly from results of animal or adult human studies.

There must be equipoise to ethically assign participants to alternative therapies in any research trial. Equipoise is defined as the condition where none of the possible research options or "arms" is known to outweigh the alternative(s). Perhaps, under these conditions of uncertainty, the requirement should be that the risk–benefit ratio is *not known to be unfavorable* and *not known to be worse* than that of available alternatives. This is different from requiring that *it be known to be favorable* in itself and in comparison to other available alternatives.

The DHHS regulations also address research that involves no prospect of direct benefit to individual participants but which is likely "to yield generalizable knowledge about *the subject's disorder or condition*." Here, the DHHS requires that the risks "represent only a minor increase over minimal risk," that the pain or discomfort that an experiment imposes on participants be similar to what they would experience if they were not participants in the experiment, and that the experiment is likely to "yield generalizable knowledge about the subject's disorder or condition which is of vital importance for the understanding or amelioration of the subject's disorder or condition." Of course, appropriate permission, assent, or consent must also be obtained (3,13).

The question here is why must experiments with no prospect of direct benefit to individual participants in the experiment be restricted to those that focus on the *participant's disorder or condition*. Why distinguish nontherapeutic experiments that are about the participant's disorder or condition from those that are not? Suppose someone wanted to analyze the breath of children with leukemia and, as a control, the breath of children known to be free of any sort of malignancy, including some who are in a hospital for some other reason. Then it seems permissible to have the children without cancer breathe into a device that analyzes their breath even though that experiment would not yield knowledge about those (control) subjects' disorder or condition. Knowledge might be acquired that is vital for understanding how to ameliorate some condition, without that knowledge being *about* the *participant's* disorder or condition, and that might be vital in learning how to ameliorate or treat other conditions.

The AAP guidelines do include another category of experiments with no prospect of direct benefit to the participants in the experiment, that are not likely to yield important knowledge *about the participant's disorder*, but do promise to yield important knowledge about *a serious problem* affecting children. These experiments "present an opportunity to understand, prevent, or alleviate a serious problem affecting the health or welfare of children." They require that these sorts of experiment present "a reasonable opportunity to further the understanding, prevention, or alleviation of a serious problem affecting the health or welfare of children"; that appropriate permission, assent, and consent be given; and that they be "conducted in accordance with sound ethical principles." Of course, the reference to sound ethical principles does not offer much guidance. We propose that the principles are the same as those that apply to any sort of experimentation that is not of direct benefit to the participants (3,14).

Although we have discussed the general guidelines that apply to any experiment, and the specific ones that apply to the types of experiments indicated by the cells of the foregoing matrix, there are special populations of children who are at "increased risk of abuse and exploitation and therefore require special consideration." The AAP includes children with handicaps and institutionalized children under this category and suggests that institutionalized children "only be involved in studies of specific conditions unique to them or the type of institution in which they reside." Further, the AAP recommends that the interests of children with handicaps in experiments be "stringently protected" (3). Because of the dangers of exploitation, we agree with these recommendations.

The AAP recognizes that in cases of emergency care, the requirement of informed permission/assent/consent may not apply. If the child is incapable of giving assent or consent and the parents are not available, then research might still be conducted provided that the child does not face a life-threatening or permanently disabling condition, there is no more than a minimal difference in risk between the proposed treatment and other available ones, and there is at most a minimal added risk from participation in the research (3). Each IRB should have regulations that address emergency use of study protocols. Typically, as soon as a parent or guardian is available, the researcher must explain the study and obtain signed, informed consent. When the youth has recovered adequately to comprehend the assent materials, his or her formal or verbal assent can then be elicited. Termination of the child's research participation may be required for children for whom appropriate consent documents are not obtained once the emergency period has passed.

There is a special class of experiments that attempt to find a better treatment when there is already a proven and effective treatment on hand. An ethical issue arises when the best-known treatment is too expensive to be available to most people in poor, underdeveloped countries. For instance, it is now accepted that a treatment regimen involving AZT called ACTG 076 is the best treatment to give pregnant women who are HIV positive in order to prevent them from passing the disease on to their fetuses. But that treatment regimen is too expensive for most people in poor countries to afford. The issue is whether it is permissible to run a placebo study in such countries where the control group gets no treatment and the test group the proposed alternative treatment to ACTG 076 or whether, instead, we are required to give the control group the ACTG 076. The argument for the permissibility of the placebo trial is that it does not make members of the control group worse off than they would have been had they not participated in the experiment. Assuming that the subjects in the placebo trial give their free and informed consent, how can it be wrong to run such an experiment?

We think the proper reply is that insofar as you are going to do something that affects someone else, you should not perform an action that does not benefit them if you could perform another action that costs you about the same and promises to produce substantial benefits for that other person. Suppose, for instance, that you have been incapacitated and as a result your lawn is considerably overgrown. Although I have no obligation to mow your lawn, I offer to mow it for you, and you accept. If I set the mower deck high at about 5 in., I will spare the valuable crop of morel mushrooms that are coming up in your lawn. If I set it lower at about 3 in., I will chop off the heads of those mushrooms, and you will never be able to harvest and sell the valuable crop. Insofar as I mow your lawn, I should do it with the mower deck set high, since putting it there costs me little and benefits you a lot. This is true even if we assume that if I had set the deck lower I would not have made you worse off than you would have been had I not mowed your lawn at all, for assume that in that case the mushrooms would have dried up by the time you were well enough to harvest them. Mowing it high provides just the amount of mulch the mushrooms need to stay alive until you are able to pick them. Not mowing them provides no mulch and mowing them low kills them.

This analogy implies that if an investigator is going to conduct an experiment in a poor, third-world country involving an alternative to some effective but expensive treatment, or preventative, he or she should not conduct a placebo trial, where the control group gets nothing. Instead, he must conduct what has been called an equivalency trial, where the control group gets the expensive, but most effective known treatment, available. If they do not get that treatment, some in the control group will die, but no more will die than would have died had they not been part of any experiment. However, several will be saved from death and disease if the control group gets the expensive treatment, and that is why running the equivalency experiment is morally required and running the placebo trial morally prohibited. Much more harm can be prevented if the control group gets the ACTG 076, it will cost the investigators little, and as much scientific knowledge will be produced as would be produced if the placebo trial had been run.

FETAL RESEARCH

Fetal research poses special ethical problems because, arguably, at least at some point in pregnancy, there are two and perhaps three people involved. Decisions concerning what experiments may be carried out on either a fetus or a pregnant woman depend crucially on how one views the moral status of the fetus. If we view the relationship between the mother and the fetus as being like that between conjoined twins, one of whom is competent to make free and informed choices while the other is not (say, because that twin is mentally retarded), it would seem that any experiment on the fetus, with prospects of direct benefit to it (i.e., any therapeutic experiment on the fetus) but with no benefit to the mother and with more than a minimal risk to her, could not be carried out without her free and informed consent. However, unlike in most experiments that may be therapeutic to the second party, it would be permissible for a woman to consent to an experiment on her fetus that posed more than "a minor increase over minimal risk" to herself. If the mother wants to incur a substantial risk in order to benefit her fetus, it is not permissible to prohibit her from exercising her altruistic choice. Of course, we need to make certain that her choice is free and fully informed.

The other side of this coin concerns whether a mother can permissibly *refuse* experiments on her fetus that might prevent great harm, or even death, from befalling it. Although we think that in certain circumstances a mother cannot permissibly refuse life-saving, or even harm-preventing, treatment for her child (say, involving a blood transfusion or the administration of a life-saving drug), the same is not true of the woman's refusal of therapeutic experimentation on her fetus. The two crucial differences are (a) that this situation involves *experimentation,* not treatment (so the chances of benefiting are lower and the risks may be higher) and (b) the fetus is attached to the mother's body, whereas the child is not. You could permissibly refuse treatment on your retarded, conjoined twin that you could not refuse if you were your twin's guardian and your twin was not physically joined to you.

Of course, if the moral status of the fetus is less than that of a retarded and conjoined twin, then there is an even stronger case for saying that the mother may even refuse therapeutic experimentation on her fetus. On the other hand, it still is permissible for her to consent to therapeutic experimentation on her fetus even when it may pose great risk to herself. If we denied this, we would have to deny that it is permissible for someone in wartime to undertake a dangerous mission behind enemy lines designed to save the lives of civilians or his or her fellow soldiers.

OHRP revised its guidance with respect to research on pregnant women, human fetuses, and neonates in 2005. Research offering only potential benefit, but some risk, to the fetus must now, with a few specific exceptions, also have the approval of the father of the fetus. However, if there is no benefit to either participant and the risk to the fetus is no more than minimal, then the pregnant woman alone may consent for herself and the fetus (15).

So far, we have discussed mainly experiments on the fetus where there are prospects of direct benefit to that fetus. But what about cases where there are not such prospects, but prospects of benefiting other fetuses or even children or adults? That is, what about nontherapeutic experimentation on fetuses? Are any of those sorts of experiments morally permissible?

Here, we have to distinguish two pairs of cases. First, there is the case where the fetus is going to be aborted anyway and the case where it is not. Second, we can either assume that the fetus has the same moral status as a born child or assume that it does not. From these two pairs of distinctions, we can construct the following two-by-two matrix:

	Fetus Will Not Be Aborted	*Fetus Will Be Aborted*
Does not have the status of a child	I	III
Does have the status of a child	II	IV

The abortion debate includes lengthy and sophisticated discussions of what the moral status of the fetus is and the relevance of this status to the morality of abortion. We do not intend to address the question of the moral status of the fetus here, but we will offer our views on the relevance of that status to questions concerning the moral permissibility of nontherapeutic experimentation on the fetus.

In category I, the fetus does not have the moral status of a child, but because it will not be aborted, at some point in the future it will have that status (e.g., after it is born). So we should make sure that it is not exposed to risks that can result in permanent harm to it later. Here, the standards for nontherapeutic experimentation on children that were discussed earlier (categories 2c and 2d) should apply. That means that fetuses in category I should not be exposed to more than minimal risk *even if doing so is needed to benefit, or prevent harm, to the mother.* We cannot expose others to risks to benefit, or even to prevent harm to, ourselves. If this is true of category I, then it also holds of II. If the *future* moral status of the child can found restrictions on nontherapeutic experimentation on fetuses, then so can the fact that it presently has that status. In category III, we might think of the fetus as having the moral status that most people attribute to mice, cats, or dogs. *If* it did have that status, then, since it will be aborted, it will never have a greater moral status. So in category III, we could expose the fetus to greater than minimal risk in nontherapeutic research, and such research would be permissible with the relevant consent of the mother. In category IV, the fetus seems comparable to an innocent man on death row who is going to be executed even though he has lost his capacity to consent. In this case, it would seem impermissible to experiment on the innocent man without his consent to benefit others, or even to benefit him. Respect for him would seem to require leaving him alone. Therefore, we conclude that no research that is not therapeutic for the fetus should be conducted in the situation described in category IV.

In summary, we have argued that nontherapeutic experiments on fetuses should be prohibited if the fetus has the moral status of a child but is going to be aborted, and that the normal requirements for nontherapeutic experimentation be applied if the fetus either does or will have the moral status of a child and will not be aborted. The only case where those requirements can be lowered is if the fetus does not have the moral status of a child and is to be aborted, that is, in case III. Of course, in all these cases, we assume that the free and informed consent of the pregnant woman must be obtained.

THE VIRTUES OF A GOOD RESEARCHER AND THE ROLE OF THE INSTITUTIONAL REVIEW BOARD

An investigator's competence and moral compass are among the most important building blocks in the assurances that child-research participants will be protected from unethical behaviors. The AAP's statement comments on a number of characteristics that might be used to define a clinical investigator of the highest ethical standards in the following manner.

The investigator should make every attempt to appreciate the feelings of all parties concerned and attempt to understand the fears and concerns of the children. The investigator should be an effective communicator to the subjects and their parents in order to decrease fears about the clinical protocol and its procedures. These considerations are important because children and their parents may be unable or unwilling to voluntarily communicate their feelings and fears. The investigator should endeavor to understand the attitudes and motivations of the parent and other individuals qualified to act on the child's behalf.

The investigator must be aware of possible conflicts between their own academic, professional, and financial interests—the "need to know"—and the interests of the child subject. The investigator cannot be free from bias or self-interest, but he or she must strive to prevent bias from affecting the study design, the execution of the study, or the presentation of the study results and conclusions. The investigator must present a balanced view of the risks and benefits when seeking participation in the study.

The investigator must vigilantly guard against scientific misconduct. When an investigator knowingly allows personal bias to alter the study, to deviate from the protocol, or to bias the interpretation of the data, this not only places the study patient at unnecessary risk but also places other children at risk whose care may be altered by a fraudulent report (3).

Although the vast majority of investigators are ethical, a researcher's enthusiasm for new and innovative ways to improve patient outcomes may not provide the clearest analysis of their own research protocols. The AAP's position is that the primary responsibility of the IRB is to protect the rights of the research subject. One of the first questions in this process of protecting subjects is what IRB has jurisdiction.

Local, regional, or national IRBs are required to develop and implement policies that regulate research at their participating site(s). For human research that is conducted or supported by any Federal Department or Agency, the US DHHS published and has since revised regulations known as the Common Rule. Although these regulations were originally approved by 18 federal agencies and published initially in the Federal Register in 1991 (2), subparts B, C, and D have been adopted by some, but not all, of these federal agencies. Although the regulations in subpart A of 45 CFR 46 were specifically designed to regulate research conducted or funded by the US government, in fact, IRBs operating under a Federal-Wide Assurance now use these same policies for all of their human research studies, irrespective of funding source. Although these standard policies have helped to reduce differences in review between institutions, they have not eliminated them, since each institution and, in fact, each IRB must individually interpret the meanings of these regulations.

Institutions that perform research on human subjects, either conducted or supported by any agency of DHHS, must have an OHRP-approved assurance of compliance with 45 CFR 46. Institutions without their own IRB or its equivalent Independent Ethics Committee may designate an alternative IRB that will provide both initial and continuing review of their human research process under their own Federal-Wide Assurance. However, whenever changes are made with respect to the review process, the institutions must notify OHRP. Allowing another institution to be the "IRB of record" is also possible and sometimes advisable, even when both institutions have their own IRB. Those charged with administering the same protocol in multicenter studies that involve many different institutions may find it more convenient to allow one of the facilities take the lead in obtaining IRB review and continued oversight. Particularly when children may obtain part of their care at more than one facility, the use of a single "IRB of record" allows the child and family to move between sites seamlessly to obtain treatment under the research protocol.

One example of the utility of identifying an IRB of record is currently being discussed with regard to the National Children's Study (NCS) (16). The NCS will address environmental influences on the health and development of US children through an innovative strategy based on door-to-door canvassing—a strategy that does not rely upon institution-specific participant recruitment. The NCS will recruit more than 100,000 children from 105 counties and will follow these children from before their birth to 21 years of age. It is anticipated that 25% or more of the participants will be identified before their mother becomes pregnant. Although the NCS is an observational study presenting no more than minimal risk, imagine the complexity if each of the institutions involved—obstetrician's office, delivery hospital, pediatric office practice(s), and subspecialists over 21 years—all required their own separate IRB review and consent. Instead, contracting sites are working together to develop an IRB of record that will review the research locally (including across county lines) for this important and unique study.

Substantial differences in IRB reviews between institutions may also exist when children are recruited for multicenter studies. While a child's care is likely to be limited to only one site throughout the course of their study participation, because of differences in institutional review at the local IRB level, families at some sites may be asked to sign consent documents that differ substantially from the proposed study consent developed nationally. Some multicenter studies have sought to reduce this variability by utilizing either a commercial IRB or by developing a central IRB process such as the Central Institutional Review Board Initiative for the National Cancer Institute. One of the caveats for utilization of a central or commercial review board is that both OHRP and the FDA require assurances that adequate review with respect to the specific study site are considered in the review process. This requirement may place a substantial burden on the investigator who may be asked to provide documentation not only of his/her capability to conduct the research but also the local research environment and potential study participants. Mechanisms to provide this insight include having a local consultant sit on the central IRB for the review or through subsequent review by appropriate designated institutional officials from the local IRB.

Whether a local or central IRB review is obtained, DHHS regulations address the membership of the IRB. All IRBs must consist of a minimum of five members whose backgrounds are adequate to review the proposed studies and who provide diversity of review. Specifically, diversity in "race, gender, cultural backgrounds, and sensitivity to such issues as community attitudes . . ." is required (17). These revised regulations further require that the IRB can address the acceptability of the proposed research with regard to "institutional commitments and regulations, applicable law, and standards or professional conduct and practice." IRBs that regularly review research enrolling vulnerable subjects including children, pregnant women, prisoners, or mentally disabled persons should provide additional representation to address the special protections these individuals require. At least one member of the IRB must have no institutional affiliation nor can an immediate member of his/her family be affiliated with the institution; one member must be a nonscientist and one member must be a scientist. To adequately review a protocol, the IRB may request that a nonmember consultant review and address the committee; however, consultants may not take part in the committee's vote.

IRBs can approve children's participation in research in three categories. Category 1 (those that present no more than minimal risk) and category 2 (present more than minimal risk but offer the potential for direct benefit) are the most common criteria for IRB approval. For studies presenting no direct benefit and having the potential for more than minimal risk, additional requirements must be in place (18). The risks for the child's study participation must represent only a minor increase over category 1 studies, and the results of the study must be likely to produce generalizable knowledge about the subject's disorder or condition. All of the studies approved under these three categories must make provisions for appropriate consent and assent. A fourth category of research risk (19) established a process of review by a panel of experts. OHRP conducts the review and reports to DHHS (20). As of 2008, only nine protocols had been reviewed by this process. Rosenfield's discussion of his experience with 45 CFR 46.407 reports that the review of his protocol took 3 years. Others have argued that IRBs should allow more self-judgment for participants and avoid paternalistic thinking (21). While the authors are persuasive, the important vulnerability of children who cannot act independently must also be considered. Importantly, while the recent technical report from the AAP's Committee on Bioethics addresses key components of the role of pediatric professionalism, review of pediatric research is not addressed (22).

Although it is the responsibility of an IRB to assess the risks and benefits of participation in human research, even under the best of circumstances, IRBs cannot foresee all risks of study participation. The death of an 18-year-old man during a gene therapy clinical trial in 1999 brought the issue of conflict of interest to the forefront of discussion for institutional programs designed to protect participants. Both the university and the investigator in that case had an equity interest in one of the companies that supplied materials for the trial. While some institutions are now publishing a list of relations between their staff members and industry, not all such relationships have been clearly disclosed. Recently, National Institutes of Health suspended a 9.3 million dollar grant because an investigator allegedly failed to report private income (24). Nor are these problems limited to only a few institutions. OHRP provides guidance for the scientific community stating that the "ethical principles described in the Belmont Report (e.g. respect for persons, beneficence, and justice) ... should not be compromised by financial relationships. Openness and honesty are indicators of respect for persons, characteristics that promote ethical research and can only strengthen the research process." To that end, institutions, IRB members, and investigators are all being called upon to disclose financial relationships with study sponsors. As a result of these strategies to "manage risk," participants may find new language in the consent documents they are asked to sign identifying not only that such relationships exist but also in some cases the magnitude of the financial stake of the investigator. In some cases, the institution's Conflict of Interest Committee may require that the principal investigators have no contact with participants in order to reduce the potential for coercion or that the patients' long-term physician not be the individual obtaining consent (25).

Financial benefits are not the only potential reward for academic investigators who also seek publications and professional recognition. Another important question to be addressed is does the IRB's review of pediatric proposals have a significant impact on the medical literature? In a European study of 98 articles addressing neonatal pain research, 94% of the studies noted parental informed consent and 87% review by an ethics board. However, the authors suggest that 25% of the journals did not adequately address the ethical guidelines for study participation and many of the newborns received little or no treatment for pain (26). Others have pointed out that journals still have room for improvement, but there has been a substantial change with respect to adherence to ethical guidelines during the decade from 1995 to 2005 (27). This study of 103 English language journals revealed that the notation of IRB approval increased from 42% to 76% and an additional 9% referred to adherence to one or more international ethical guidelines as a requirement for publication. Required statements for conflict of interest also rose from 72% in the earlier time period to 94%. Interestingly, journals with the highest impact factors were more likely to have stringent rules.

Even with the best IRB review, it is the responsibility of each family to ultimately make the decision with regard to their child's participation in clinical trials. In one study of asthma and cancer trials, more than 90% of the children aged 7 to 14 years believed that they should be involved in the decision with respect to their own participation (28). Even when there was no potential for direct benefit but no more than minor risk, children who were participating in research trials and their parents expressed willingness to participate (82% and 79%, respectively). For category III studies, 47% of the children and 24% of their parents remained willing to have the child participate (29). But do children and their parents understand the consent documents? Several investigative teams have suggested that we can do more to improve the process. While the purpose, risks, and benefits of a study were understood by more than half of the child participants, procedures and alternatives to participation were understood by less than a third in one study (30). In other studies, modification of both the children's assent documents (31) and parents' permission (32) using pictures, bullet points, and larger font improved understanding for all. Parents overwhelmingly preferred the modified version of the consent document and among children the youngest study participants reported the greatest benefit.

SUMMARY

We have briefly reviewed some of the issues associated with carrying out drug research in pediatric participants in an ethical manner. We have included a review of salient literature and our interpretation of the current state of thinking in some difficult areas of human conduct. For the most part, we have agreed with the guidelines published as policy statements by the AAP and the regulations published by DHHS, but we have differed in four areas. (a) We do not think minimal risk should be relativized to either the particular subject of the experiment or even to what is normally encountered in daily life. (b) We do not think that minimal risk, when properly understood in Ackerman's terms as "no more than that to which it is appropriate to expose a child for educational purposes in the family situation," should be exceeded in nontherapeutic experiments involving children before 12 years of age. (c) We think that "no dissent," and not "assent," should be required of children between 7 and 14 years of age for any sort of experiment. (d) We think it is permissible to expose a child to slightly more than minimal risk in a nontherapeutic experiment if the child is capable of assenting, or consenting, and gives his or her free and informed assent, or consent, to that exposure.

Although we made no attempt to determine what the moral status of a fetus is, we have stated our view of the issues surrounding research on fetuses, both for the fetus' benefit and for the benefit of others. Our view here is that the parents may refuse therapeutic experimentation on their fetus and at the same time may consent to experimental procedures that put the mother at great risk but are intended to benefit her fetus. Although a mother may refuse to do what might benefit her fetus, she must not put her fetus at more than minimal risk of present or future harm if her fetus has or will have the moral status of, say, a 3-year-old child. Hence, she cannot agree to experiments that pose more than a minimal risk to such a fetus. The only time that she can permissibly put her fetus at more than minimal risk is if it does not have the moral status of a child and never will.

ACKNOWLEDGMENT

The authors thank Ronald L. Poland, M.D., for his major contributions as a coauthor of an earlier version of this chapter.

REFERENCES

1. American Academy of Pediatrics. Guidelines for the ethical conduct of studies to evaluate drugs in pediatric populations. *Pediatrics* 1977;60(1):91–101.
2. Public Welfare. Protection of human subjects (45 CFR 46.101–46.409). *Fed Reg* 1991.
3. American Academy of Pediatrics. Guidelines for the ethical conduct of studies to evaluate drugs in pediatric populations. *Pediatrics* 1995;95:286–294.
4. McCartney JJ. Research on children: national commission says 'Yes, if . . .'. *Hastings Cent Rep* 1978;8:26–31.
5. Miller JR. Recommendations on experimentation with children: some differences in Canadian and American approaches. *Bioethics Q* 1980;2:141–147.
6. Public Welfare. Protection of human subjects (45 CFR 46.102(i)) *Fed Reg* 1991.
7. Ramsey P. Children as research subjects: a reply. *Hastings Cent Rep* 1977;7:40–41.
8. Van deVeer D. Experimentation on children and proxy consent. *J Med Philos* 1981;6:281–293.
9. McCormick RA. Experimentation in children: starting in sociality. *Hastings Cent Rep* 1976;6:41–46.
10. Ackerman TF. Moral duties of parents and nontherapeutic clinical research procedures involving children. *Bioethics Q* 1980;2:94–111.
11. Public Welfare. Protection of human subjects (45 CFR 46.402(b)). *Fed Reg* 1991.
12. Public Welfare. Protection of human subjects (45 CFR 46.405(a)). *Fed Reg* 1991.
13. Public Welfare. Protection of human subjects (45 CFR 46.406(c)). *Fed Reg* 1991.
14. Public Welfare. Protection of human subjects (45 CFR 46.407 (b)(ii)). *Fed Reg* 1991.
15. Public Welfare. Protection of human subjects (45 CFR 46(b)). *Fed Reg* 2005.
16. http://www.nationalchildrensstudy.gov.
17. Public Welfare. Protection of human subjects (21 CFR 56.107) *Fed Reg* 2008.
18. Public Welfare. Protection of human subjects (45 CFR 46.406). *Fed Reg* 2001.
19. Public Welfare. Protection of human subjects (45 CFR 46.407). *Fed Reg* 2001.
20. Rosenfield RL. Improving balance in regulatory oversight of research in children and adolescents. A clinical investigator's perspective. *Ann N Y Acad Sci* 2008;1135:287–295.
21. Edwards SJL, Kirchin S, Huxtable R. Research ethics committees and paternalism. *J Med Ethics* 2004;30:88–91.
22. Fallat ME, Glover J; American Academy of Pediatrics, Committee on Bioethics. Professionalism in pediatrics. *Pediatrics* 2007;120:e1123-e1133.
23. NY Times October 3, 2008.
24. Morin K, Rakatansky H, Riddick FA, et al. Managing conflicts of interest in the conduct of clinical trials. *JAMA* 2002;287:78–84.
25. Axelin A, Salantera S. Ethics in neonatal pain research. *Nurs Ethics* 2008;15:492–499.
26. Rowan-Legg A, Weijer C, Gao J, et al. A comparison of journal instructions regarding institutional review board approval and conflict-of-interest disclosure between 1995 and 2005. *J Med Ethics* 2009;35:74–78.
27. Varma S, Jenkins T, Wendler D. How do children and parents make decisions about pediatric clinical research? *J Pediatr Hematol Oncol* 2008;30:823–828.
28. Wendler D, Jenkins T. Children's and their parents' views on facing research risks for the benefit of others. *Arch Pediatr Adolesc Med* 2008;162:9–14.
29. Chappy H, Doz F, Blanche S, et al. Children's views on their involvement in clinical research. *Pediatr Blood Cancer* 2008;50:1043–1046.
30. Tait AR, Voepel-Lewis T, Malviya S. Presenting research information to children: a tale of two methods. *Anesth Analg* 2007;105:358–364.
31. Tait AR, Voepel-Lewis T, Malviya S, et al. Improving the readability and processability of a pediatric informed consent document. Effects of parents' understanding. *Arch Pediatr Adolesc Med* 2005;159:347–352.
32. Bartholome WG. Parents, children, and the moral benefits of research. *Hastings Cent Rep* 1976;6:44–45.

SUGGESTED READINGS

Levine RJ. *Ethics and regulation of clinical research,* 2nd ed. Baltimore, MD: Urban & Schwarzenberg, 1986.

Peart N. Health Research with children. *N Z Bioeth J* 2000;1:3–9.

Robinson WM. Ethical issues in pediatric research. *J Clin Ethics* 2000;11:145–150.

CHAPTER

9

Alexander A. Vinks
Philip D. Walson

Therapeutic Drug Monitoring

INTRODUCTION

The simplest way to identify interindividual variability in drug response is to objectively measure the degree of effect and then adjust the dosing regimen accordingly. However, such a straightforward approach is seldom feasible, as simple and reliable therapeutic effect measures are not always available in routine clinical situations. In addition, many serious conditions require rapid attainment of adequate clinical effect without excessive dosing, and effects are especially difficult to document in some patients, especially newborns and other nonverbal or uncooperative patients. Rational pharmacotherapy is dependent on a basic understanding of the way patients handle drugs (pharmacokinetics, PK) and their response (effect) to specific drug concentrations (pharmacodynamics, PD) (1). PK may be simply defined as what the body does to the drug, as opposed to PD, which may be defined as what the drug does to the body (2). Advances in the fields of PK and PD, including the development of sensitive and specific methods for concentration measurements in biological fluids, have expanded our understanding of the time course of drug concentrations in plasma and the processes (absorption, distribution, metabolism, and excretion) that influence the amount of drug that reaches target organs and tissues. The ultimate goal of understanding dose–exposure–effect relationships is to derive optimum individualized dosing regimens with maximal therapeutic and minimal side effects with the simplest dosage regimen possible. This can best be achieved by linking PK and PD information to better understand or predict the exposure–effect–time relationship. The proper measurement and interpretation of drug concentrations [therapeutic drug monitoring (TDM) or better "management"] in a specific patient can help us better understand how a particular drug is behaving and will also allow for further individualization of the dosing regimen in that patient as well as how to best select an initial dosing regimen in future patients (3).

THE TARGET CONCENTRATION STRATEGY

Drug actions (effects) are directly related to the drug concentration at the site(s) of action. Although imperfect, there is almost always a better relationship between the effect of a given drug and its concentration in the blood than between the dose of the drug given and the effect. PK is the science that can explain and predict the relationship between a dosing regimen and the concentration of a drug in various body compartments over time. A basic understanding of PK principles and how these principles are altered in the developing child are required to better understand and predict drug actions. In Figure 9.1, the interrelationship among drug input (dose), PK, PD, and clinical effects is schematically conceptualized.

There are many practical, physiologic, and pathophysiologic factors that determine how much drug effect will be associated with a drug prescription. Clinicians make a diagnosis and then prescribe a dosing regimen: drug, dose, formulation, route, frequency, and duration. Once a drug is prescribed, there are many factors that determine how much effect, either therapeutic or toxic, is seen in the individual patient. Prescriptions must be filled correctly, the prescription filled must contain the correct drug and amount, the dosage regimen must be taken/given (adherence), and the drug must get into the patient and reach the site(s) of action. There are many reasons why concentrations and drug exposure (and therefore the effects) that result from prescriptions differ among patients. Even if taken or given exactly as desired, effects produced will depend on many factors including the patient's physiology, prior history, and other drugs present. Patients/parents may never fill the prescription. Up to 25% of patients do not fill prescriptions, and even more do not take medication as indicated. Children and adolescents with chronic illness have great difficulty completing prescribed treatment regimens, which can be complex and burdensome. High rates of nonadherence to treatment (up to 50% or more) have been reported for various pediatric chronic conditions, such as asthma, epilepsy, transplantation, juvenile rheumatoid arthritis (JRA), and diabetes (4–6). Different formulations of the same drug may have different absorption characteristics. Manufacturing problems can and do occur. Pharmacy or pharmaceutical errors can alter the amount of drug delivered or in fact which drug is given, and parents or patients may or may not comply with instructions. All of these factors can alter the amount of drug that reaches the site of action. Several studies have

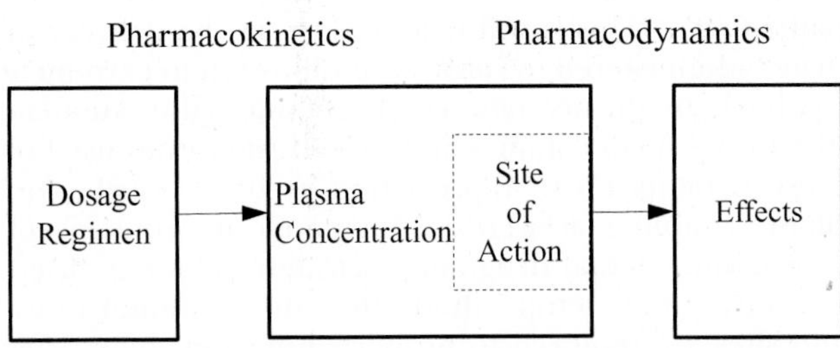

Figure 9.1. Schematic representation of the interrelationship among drug input (dose), pharmacokinetics (concentration), pharmacodynamics, and clinical effects.

TABLE 9.1 Indications for Therapeutic Drug Monitoring

Inadequate response
Higher than standard dose required
Serious or persistent side effects
Suspected toxicity
Suspected nonadherence
Suspected drug–drug interactions
New preparation, changing brands
Other illnesses, for example, hepatic/renal problems, inflammatory diseases

documented the unpredictable drug delivery in neonates. This is especially relevant for antibiotics such as aminoglycosides that are used frequently to treat bacterial infections in this population. A lack of appreciation of drug delivery issues such as the small volumes and low infusion rates used in these patients can result in a much lower than expected blood concentrations and much lower than what is required for optimal antimicrobial therapy (7). Drug concentration measurements can provide an objective way to identify, explain, or eliminate uncertainty caused by a number of these factors, especially in patients who have unusual or unexpected drug responses. However, even patients who actually take or are given the same amount of a drug may also have very different amounts of drug in their body or blood at different times after dosing. The ability to predict and explain the inter- and intraindividual differences in drug concentrations over time requires knowledge of basic PK principles.

Much of our current knowledge of pediatric PK comes from the ability to measure serum concentrations for drugs, especially those with narrow therapeutic ranges or low safety margins (8–10).

THE CONCEPT OF THERAPEUTIC DRUG MONITORING

TDM is defined as the measurement made in the laboratory of a parameter that, with appropriate interpretation, will directly influence dosing. Commonly, the measurement is of a prescribed drug in a biological matrix, but it may also be of a drug taken as a result of a medication error or poisoning or of an endogenous compound prescribed as replacement therapy in an individual who is physiologically or pathologically deficient in that compound (11). It is perhaps more appropriate to consider TDM as therapeutic drug management (C. Pippenger, personal communication, May 2003). The rationale for TDM of a given drug is based on three important requirements: (a) there is a better association between the concentration and the therapeutic effect than between the dose and the effect, (b) TDM and dose individualization will reduce variability and will better predict the patient's concentration–time profile, and (c) maintenance of drug concentrations within desired target ranges (see later discussion) improves clinical outcome by either increasing efficacy, reducing toxicity, or both (12). Proper TDM requires that dosing regimens are then further individualized based on individual measured concentrations and responses. The criteria for monitoring (managing) drugs in children are similar to those in adults. Generally accepted indications for concentration measurements are summarized in Table 9.1.

In pediatrics, use of TDM has been common in (a) the treatment of epilepsy (13,14), (b) transplantation (15), and (c) drug therapy in neonates (16) as opposed to adult medicine, where TDM is used in the management of many more diseases including psychiatric and cardiac diseases. Evolving areas where pediatric TDM has important uses include the anticancer drugs, psychiatric conditions, and infectious diseases including antifungal (17) and anti-HIV therapy with drugs such as protease inhibitors (18,19).

THE THERAPEUTIC RANGE CONCEPT

Despite decades of TDM, recommended concentrations (therapeutic ranges) are largely empirical, population rather than individually based, independent of assay method used, seldom consider time after dosing, and seldom are the result of evidence-based studies. The therapeutic range is also commonly misunderstood even for commonly monitored drugs such as digoxin, aminoglycosides, phenobarbital, phenytoin, and theophylline. Interpretation of TDM results is still almost exclusively focused on altering dosing to get measured concentrations within a published "therapeutic range" (20). The "therapeutic range" is defined as the range of drug concentrations associated with a *high* degree of efficacy and a *low* risk of dose-related toxicity in the *majority* of patients. This is not the same as the optimal concentration for each individual patient. Furthermore, the emphasis in measuring drug concentrations has been mostly toxicity oriented and for drugs with narrow therapeutic indexes. The "therapeutic range" concept is hampered by some important problems (21). First, defining a single, time-independent concentration range leaves the physician with the uncertainty of how to choose the optimal dose when in fact a range of dosing regimens would produce a "therapeutic concentration" at some time in the regimen. Second, the definition of a therapeutic range does not differentiate among concentrations but assumes that all concentrations within the range may be equally desirable. Third, the ranges depend on a number of other things, including time after a dose, time on a particular regimen, the condition being treated, the assay used, and the possibility of active metabolites. Problems created by assays with different specificity for active and inactive metabolites or interfering substances are more commonly a problem in pediatric than in adult patients. Poor understanding of the therapeutic range has led to a rather naive and even potentially dangerous "numbers-only," three-step, all-or-nothing interpretation of the concentration–effect relationship. This simplistic approach assumes that any concentration below the lower end of the range will be of no benefit to the patient, that anywhere within the range the patient will be okay, and that above the upper end of the range the patient will experience unacceptable adverse reactions. None of these may be true in any given patient.

DISTRIBUTION PHASE

Immediately after administration, drugs must distribute into the blood and then to tissues in the body. This results in initial concentrations that are much higher than, and which do not show a log linear correlation with, postdistributional concentrations. This is true for most, if not all, drugs given intravenously, and for several drugs (e.g., digoxin and clonazepam), this phenomenon also occurs after oral administration. There are large differences between trough and distribution concentrations even for very long half-life drugs. Digoxin, for example, can have postdose peak concentrations of 3 to 5 ng per mL in patients with trough concentrations of less than 1 ng per mL. There are also greatly different concentration effect relationships between distribution and postdistributional concentrations at the site of action (22). If not appreciated, this can lead to inappropriate decreases in digoxin doses or even use of digibind (personal experience). Unfortunately, many physicians believe, and teach, that sampling time is not important for drugs with long half-lives because concentrations are not expected to change much when dosing intervals are much less than the drug's half-life. Although true well after completion of the distribution phase, this is not true when comparing trough values with concentrations obtained during distribution. Randomly collected clonazepam concentrations have been used to claim that there is a poor relationship between concentrations and effect. However, it is highly likely that this conclusion is based on the fact that clonazepam, despite having relatively slow clearance, also has very high distribution concentrations relative to predose (trough) concentrations even after oral administration (23). Concentrations drawn during the distribution phase (4 to 6 hours after dosing) will not correlate with effects because they do not reflect the effect site concentration. PK modeling of digoxin or clonazepam with respect to concentrations at their sites of action (heart muscle and brain, respectively) is needed to attempt to correlate concentrations and effect. Bayesian modeling, but not linear correlation methods, can deal with sampling during the distribution phase, but sampling and accurate information on administration time becomes even more critical (22,24). Unfortunately, in pediatrics the time of drug administration is not as easy to determine as it is in adults. Decades ago, Leff and Roberts showed that it can take hours for drugs put into an intravenous setup to actually reach the patient (25). This is still true to date, as the delivery of drugs administered by intravenous infusion in extremely low-birth-weight neonates can be substantially extended due to the small volumes and low infusion rates used in these patients (26). Appreciation of both distribution phase sampling as well as the practical problems of ascertaining actual drug administration time for different intravenous setups, fluids and administration rates, and sites are required to properly interpret some drug concentrations.

REACTIONARY THERAPEUTIC DRUG MONITORING

Many clinical laboratories offer some form of TDM menu. However, test results are commonly reported as "numbers only," in a similar fashion as general chemistry test results (e.g., serum sodium). This type of reporting is misleading and does not optimally use what we know about drug concentrations. As opposed to most endogenous compounds, drug concentrations are not stable over time and are governed by known and predictable PK principles. In addition, more in-depth interpretations (i.e., PK consultation), with the possible exception of aminoglycosides and vancomycin, are seldom offered. As a result, dose adjustments frequently are made on an ad hoc basis relying on one or more "numbers" (i.e., concentration measurements) within or outside a "therapeutic range." This can best be described as "reactionary TDM," where a standard dose is administrated and a concentration is checked to verify whether it is "therapeutic." The process is often toxicity driven; if the level is "toxic" (i.e., above the "therapeutic range"), the dose will be lowered and the level will be checked again. If the level is "subtherapeutic," the dose may be increased, with measurements being repeated until "therapeutic." If the first measurement is within the therapeutic range, things are considered "okay" and no further action is taken. It is obvious that this reactionary TDM does not take into consideration the full concentration–time profile, individual differences, time to attain steady-state, or patient-specific PD targets. It does not lead to efficient use of resources, and has not been shown to produce optimal outcomes. However, many studies have documented that proper pharmacokinetic/pharmacodynamic (PK/PD) guidance, but not "reactionary TDM," is effective. Such guidance can improve overall use of resources and produce better and more cost-efficient outcomes, fewer inappropriately drawn samples, more levels within the desired range, fewer dose adjustments, and reduction in the incidence of adverse events (27–29).

DEVELOPMENTAL PHARMACOKINETIC ASPECTS*

Proper PK/PD guidance is especially important in patients with rapidly changing handling of drugs (PK) and responses (PD). Although this applies to most seriously ill, hospitalized patients, it applies especially to neonates and children because of large, often rapid developmental

*See Chapters 2, 3 and 4.

TABLE 9.2 Age-Related Differences in Pharmacokinetic Parameters for Aminoglycosides and Vancomycin

	CL	V_d	$t_{1/2}$	*Targets*
Aminoglycosides				
Neonates	↓	↑↑	↑	↓
Children	↑	↑	↓/~	↓/~
Cystic fibrosis patients	↑↑	↑	↓/~	↑↑
Vancomycin				
Neonates	↓	↑	↑	↓/~
Children	↑	↑/~	↓	~

CL, clearance; V_d, volume of distribution; $t_{1/2}$, half-life.

changes in both PK and PD (30,31). The developmental changes in PK of medications that occur between birth and adolescence/adulthood create challenges for physicians who desire to prescribe medications on a rational, age-appropriate, individual basis. Routine TDM of prescribed drugs and their active metabolites can be of great help to individualize dose requirements during long-term treatment (12). In addition, the ratio of metabolite(s) to parent drug can also give important information on (non)adherence and can reveal unusual metabolic patterns.

Increasingly, proper interpretation of measured drug concentrations is being used to provide important insights into the different PK behavior in neonates, children, and adolescents (32). Of all routinely monitored drugs, the aminoglycosides have been studied most extensively. PK data for gentamicin, tobramycin, netilmicin, and amikacin are available across (arbitrary) pediatric age categories: preterm newborns, term newborn infants (0 to 27 days), infants and toddlers (28 days to 23 months), children (2 to 11 years), and adolescents (12 to 16 or 18 years) (33). These studies have demonstrated that in the premature neonate, drug clearance is reduced and volume of distribution increased as compared with older children and adults, and glomerular filtration (the predominant route of elimination) by the immature kidney is reduced (10,34). Volumes of distribution are larger than those in older pediatric patients because of larger body water fat content and higher body surface-to-weight ratios. An overview of age-related PK changes and PK parameter estimates for gentamicin and vancomycin as index drugs is summarized in Table 9.2. Drug clearance rapidly increases with age as the kidney develops and the total body water decreases. For renally cleared drugs, after the first postnatal day, the creatinine concentration in plasma or calculated creatinine clearance can be a good a priori indicator of individual drug elimination (35). Individual differences in renal drug clearance can therefore be predicted before or during dosing and used to individualize dosing (both dose and dosing frequency). In addition, however, clearance of renally cleared drugs such as gentamicin can be used to predict renal function more accurately than creatinine clearance calculations used in adults (36). This is especially useful in the newborn, where maternal creatinine influences neonatal creatinine measurements (see case presentation in later discussion). As opposed to renally cleared drugs, we do not have good indicators for drugs that are predominantly metabolized. Drugs that are metabolized often show large, unpredictable interindividual and sometimes intraindividual differences in PK behavior. This interpatient as well as intrapatient variability may be further increased if the drug is taken orally, because of differences in absorption, transport, as well as intestinal metabolism. TDM can detect such interindividual as well as intraindividual variations. However, a single measurement will only describe the net results of all the different underlying processes (e.g., bioavailability, absorption, distribution, metabolism, and excretion) involved. For instance, a concentration that is lower than expected based on data for that patient population can be the result of poor adherence absorption problems, increased metabolism and excretion, or any combination of these.

DOSAGE ADJUSTMENTS BASED ON THERAPEUTIC DRUG MONITORING VALUES

The decision to alter a generally accepted dosing regimen either before or during ongoing therapy is frequently based on an empirical trial-and-error decision-making process where different pieces of clinical information are considered. Patients in whom a rapid onset of effect is required or patients who exhibit lower or higher effects than expected after initiation or alteration of therapy can clearly benefit from proper TDM. In the nonresponding patient, concentration measurements will help the clinician decide whether nonadherence is present, whether a medication error is possible, whether a drug–drug or drug–diet interaction has occurred, or whether individual differences in PK or PD require a different dose or frequency of dosing or whether alternate therapy is indicated. This is true even for drugs for which a well-described "therapeutic range" is unknown.

Appropriate timing of sample collection is crucial for the appropriate interpretation of drug concentrations. Within a dosing interval, the predose or trough concentration is usually the sampling time after steady state is achieved, but efficacy is questioned. In the case of adverse events or (suspected) toxicity, sampling is preferably done at the time maximal side effects are experienced. Other sampling strategies may be required for drugs (such as anticancer and antirejection drugs) where a more accurate measure of drug exposure such as an estimate of the area under the concentration–time curve (AUC) during a dosing interval is needed. Lack of all necessary information, such as the actual time of drug intake, how long after dosing was started, whether a loading dose was used, timing of concomitant medications, and time of sampling, makes it more difficult, or sometimes impossible, to interpret results. TDM laboratories and services can play an important role in improving patient outcomes and the efficient use of TDM by providing up-to-date guidelines and teaching physicians and other health care providers about what information is necessary to properly interpret any result. This information must either be accurately provided with laboratory requests or obtained by TDM service personnel. Unless the ordering professional is thoroughly familiar with PK and analytical principles, all drug concentrations should include an individualized PK interpretation (37–41). For several drug classes, the use of population models and the application of Bayesian optimization algorithms have been shown to be a clinically useful and cost-effective way to provide such interpretations (22,29). These algorithms are quite different from dosing nomograms, which are used to predict "average" or initial doses in various populations.

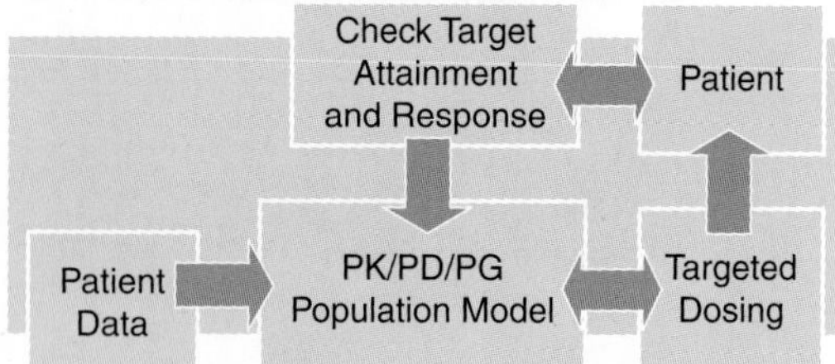

Figure 9.2. Flow diagram of the goal-oriented model-based strategy. A computer program is used with a patient-specific population model describing absorption, distribution, and elimination of the drug in relation to patient-specific parameters. Patient data and desired target concentrations are entered into the system. Next, a model-based loading dose and maintenance regimen required to optimally achieve the target concentrations is determined. This regimen is administered to the patient, and subsequent concentration measurement(s) are used as feedback to update the initial model and design a new dosing regimen if necessary. PD, pharmacodynamic; PG, pharmacogenetic; PK, pharmacokinetic.

BAYESIAN FORECASTING

Bayesian analysis is a particularly useful tool for information-sparse environments such as the neonatal intensive care unit. The method of Bayesian forecasting is derived from Bayes theorem, and is based on the concept that prior PK knowledge of a drug, in the form of a population model, can be combined with individual patient data, such as drug concentrations (24,42,43) (Table 9.3). The idea is to make an individualized model of the behavior of the drug in a particular patient to see how the drug will be or has been handled and to obtain the necessary information to make rational dose adjustments so as to best achieve the selected target goal(s).

Figure 9.2 shows a diagram of the goal-oriented, model-based optimization process. Drug dosage optimization requires (a) population PK parameters (PK model), defined as mean values, standard deviations, covariates, and information on the statistical distribution necessary to select the initial dosing regimen for that particular patient based on chosen goals; (b) measurement of a performance index related to the therapeutic goal, generally one or more plasma concentrations or effects as feedback information to update the system; and (c) availability of reliable software for an adaptive control strategy (maximum a posteriori probability [MAP] Bayesian fitting) and calculation of the subsequent optimal dosage regimen. An example of the use of a population model with Bayesian feedback is described by the following case report:

> *Vignette:* Model-based individualization of gentamicin therapy in a newborn. A term baby girl (2.9 kg) with pulmonary atresia, a serum creatinine of 1.0 mg per dL 1 day after birth, and a suspected gram-negative infection was started on gentamicin (load 4 mg per kg and a maintenance dose of 2.5 mg per kg twice daily). The initial gentamicin concentration was reported as 2.7 mg per L. Based on the initial measurement, patient demographics, and the clinical information, a population PK model predicted that the initial and subsequent dosing changes were inappropriate. A regimen of 9 mg every 36 hours would have been appropriate.

This patient was transferred to another major university hospital, where the levels were repeated (4.3 mg per L, 24 hours after the last dose, and 2.3 mg per L, 11.5 hours later). An off-the-cuff interpretation by a pharmacist without the use of any PK tools resulted in a dosing regimen recommendation of 9 mg every 24 hours. This dosing regimen resulted in a sustained high concentration over several days (Fig. 9.3) despite or because follow-up concentration measurements were done without appropriate PK interpretation. The child eventually developed bilateral hearing loss, which resulted in a malpractice suit against the physicians, the pharmacist, and the hospital (authors' personal, court protected confidential information).

In this example, simulation of the initial gentamicin serum concentration based on published population PK

TABLE 9.3 Flow Scheme for Bayesian Goal-Oriented Model-Based Dosing (24)

Prior probability	→ New information	→ Consider prior and new	→ Posterior probability	→ Therapy goals	→ Therapy control
Population model	→ Drug levels	→ Objective function	→ Individual model	→ Look at patient, think	→ Calculate new dose

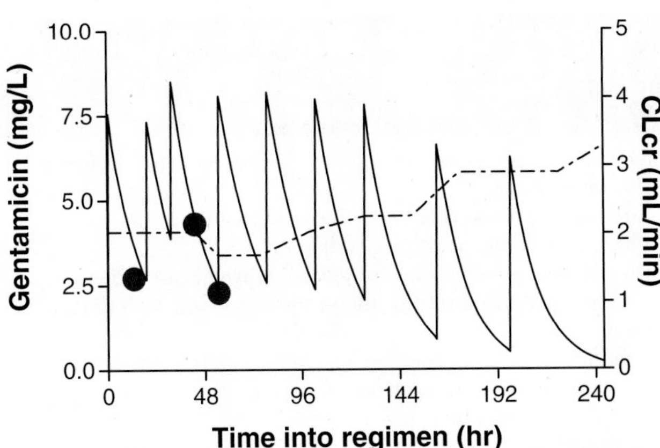

Figure 9.3. Population model-based mean concentration–time profile of gentamicin in a term newborn with renal complication (serum creatinine 1.0 mg/dL and initial creatinine clearance of approximately 2.0 mL/min) given a dose of 2.5 mg/kg twice daily. The large dots indicate measured gentamicin concentrations. The solid line represents the concentration–time profile predicted by the pharmacokinetic model and the dotted line represents the predicted creatinine clearance (CLcr) (see text for further details).

data would have revealed that this patient had a much lower than normal clearance. This possibility was suggested by the elevated creatinine level for age (1.0 mg per dL). However, on the first day of life, neonatal creatinine levels, unlike gentamicin clearance, are influenced largely by maternal creatinine. The initial gentamicin level, if appropriately modeled, would have provided clear evidence of decreased renal function regardless of the reliability of the creatinine. Furthermore, the first level was at a random time after dosing and not a trough level. Nontrough concentrations can be misinterpreted without appropriate calculation, as occurred in this child. A model-based profile and subsequent Bayesian individualization process would have prevented this newborn from being exposed to prolonged, higher than necessary, and potentially toxic concentrations (44).

Population model-based dosing recommendations in a group of less complicated patients were generated in the study of van Lent-Evers et al. (29). In this study, the model-based regimen was administered and a set of two drug levels was drawn at $t = 1$ hour and 8 to 12 hours after the first dose. The concentration measurements were used as feedback, and if necessary the dosing regimen was adjusted according to the patients' clinical condition and selected target concentrations. This approach proved less costly and more effective than traditional, often nomogram-based dosing. It reduced mortality and hospital stay in patients who were admitted with a suspected or proven gram-negative infection. This method is greatly superior to the common "start gentamicin and get a level after 3 to 5 doses" approach used in many neonatal units. This inappropriate monitoring is based on a misunderstanding of the difference between the number of half-lives and the number of "doses" necessary to reach steady state. This approach misses inappropriate doses (such as 10-fold errors) or inadequate clearance for days after they could have been detected with proper TDM done at appropriate time after the initial dose. The authors have also been involved in litigation involving patient harm that was caused by this inappropriate but surprisingly commonly used aminoglycoside monitoring method. Another example of common poorly done TDM involves the misinterpretation of aminoglycoside therapeutic ranges in children given once or less frequent doses. Trough (predose) concentrations in such children should be undetectable using most assays and not "less than 2 mg per L." This "trough" concentration is what is expected with every 8-hour dosing. A child who has 1 to 2 mg per L 24 or more hours after a single dose has been supratherapeutic for many hours and has either received a massive overdose or has decreased renal function.

Bayesian methods can be more cost-effective than other techniques because they require fewer drug measurements for individual PK parameter estimation. They can also handle sparse and random samples (45). TDM, when applied appropriately, can also be used to detect and quantify clinically relevant drug–drug interactions (46,47) as well as medication errors.

However, regardless of what PK dose individualization techniques are used, all are superior to a simple reactionary comparison of a reported result to a "therapeutic range." Simply reporting results as "numbers" that are below, within, or above a published range is usually uninformative, not cost saving, and can lead to inappropriate or even dangerous actions.

OVERCOMING PRACTICAL PROBLEMS IN NEONATAL AND PEDIATRIC THERAPEUTIC DRUG MONITORING

INCOMPLETE INFORMATION FOR INTERPRETATION OF THE DOSE–CONCENTRATION–EFFECT RELATIONSHIP

Unfortunately, incorrect sample collection, handling, or analysis as well as improper interpretation of results can diminish the clinical value of TDM results and have negative economic implications. This can, and has, lead to incorrect opinions about the use of TDM. There are ample studies showing that, when properly ordered, assayed, and interpreted, TDM can often be useful in all patients, and even always useful in selected clinical situations (13). Although there are few studies of the cost-effectiveness of TDM, those that have been done have shown very positive results (27,29,48–52). When poorly done, TDM can be useless or even harmful.

Despite the fact that TDM concepts are relatively simple, most laboratories are not set up to perform the necessary data collection that would allow unambiguous clinical interpretation of drug concentration measurements (53). For instance, simple information such as the time of sampling in relation to the time of last dose needs to be reported with the result. In addition, demographic data (date of birth, weight, height), route of administration, and dosing regimen (time and dates of recent intake) should also be available. Additional factors that may influence proper TDM interpretation are summarized in Table 9.4. Over the years, institutions have struggled with ways of collecting and reporting this type of information. In the outpatient setting, a useful way of data collection can be a questionnaire administered by staff or filled out by the patients, parents, or guardians while waiting for phlebotomy. Figure 9.4 shows an example of a questionnaire that has been successfully used in an antiepileptic TDM service at the author's institutions (54). The TDM system should be set up in such a way that information from the questionnaire is processed with the test request and ultimately reported in a user-friendly format. An important item on this questionnaire is space for patient, parent, or guardian feedback on any issues related to the medication. This is a valuable tool for adverse event monitoring as well as documenting therapeutic response.

ADHERENCE AND VARIATIONS IN PHARMACOKINETICS ARE DIFFICULT TO CONTROL REFERENCES!

In an outpatient setting, nonadherence can represent a major problem in patient management. TDM will contribute to detecting nonadherence, although this will be dependent

TABLE 9.4 Practical Problems in Neonatal and Pediatric Therapeutic Drug Monitoring

Sample collection—access, volume, skin contamination, line or catheter draws
Interference—maternal (Cr, DLIS, maternal Rx)
Altered metabolic patterns as well as rates
Dietary differences, fasting, stomach emptying, gastrointestinal transit-prolonged release, inappropriate dosage alteration
Position changes
Administration uncertainty—cooperation, spillage, measurement, extemporaneous formulation, inappropriate concentrations, measurement errors
Analytical differences (e.g., phenobarbital glucuronide interference missed in adult samples)
Day-to-day variation—weight, pharmacokinetics
Intravenous administration problems, no dose or sample before dose

Cr, serum creatinine; DLIS, digoxin-like immunoreactive substances; maternal Rx, maternal drug therapy.

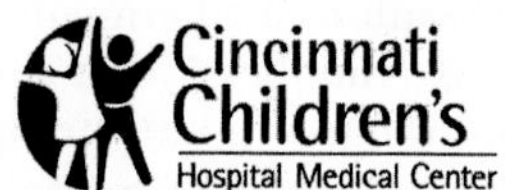

DEPARTMENT OF CLINICAL PHARMACOLOGY
THERAPEUTIC DRUG MANAGEMENT (TDM)

Outpatient Information (to be completed by parent, guardian, or caretaker)

Patient Name: ____________________

Patient Date of Birth: ____________________

Please answer the following questions to the best of your knowledge. Feel free to add comments you feel may be helpful in the interpretation of your child's drug level.

1. Please list all medications your child takes regularly:

2. Your child's weight (please note pounds or kilograms):____________________

3. **FOR THE DRUG BEING MEASURED:**

   Name of Drug: ____________________

   Dose: ____________________
   (in mg's and/or cc'c/mL's, or tsp, Tbl if liquid)

   Frequency: ____________________
   (at what times of the day do you give this medication)

   Formulation: ____________________
   (tablet, capsule, liquid)

   Date This Dose was Started: ____________________
   (Important if recently started or changed)

   Date and Time of Last Dose: ____________________
   (Very important for most drugs)

4. If we have questions about your child may we call you?

   Parent Name: ____________________

   Phone Number: ____________________

5. Any Comments (Does the drug seem to be working? Are there any side effects?):

Figure 9.4. Questionnaire that has been successfully used in an antiepileptic therapeutic drug management service at Cincinnati Children's Hospital Medical Center.

on the clearance of the drug. For instance, skipping doses and only taking medication shortly before a visit may not show for highly cleared drugs but will result in much lower than expected concentrations for more slowly eliminated drugs. Metabolite profiles, when measured, will almost always change and be indicative for poor or nonadherence. In inpatients, adherence should not be an issue, but can occur, and inaccurate recording of the timing of the dose in relation to the blood draw may result in confusion and mistakes. For instance, samples drawn supposedly as "peaks' but actually taken before the actual dose was given will give lower than expected results and may sometimes have people question adherence, whereas a PK consult would clearly predict the measured concentration when assuming a "missed" dose. Over adherence, such as in drug overdose, can also be identified.

The interindividual variability (variability *between* patients) in PK has been documented for many drugs. This variability is, for example, summarized in the population PK models developed. Intraindividual variability (the variability in the same patient), on the other hand, is equally important when interpreting TDM data in lifelong treatments such as in epilepsy, transplantation, and HIV. Causes for intraindividual variability in PK have not been systematically studied but can be attributed to temporary changes in physiology, drug absorption variability, enterohepatic recycling, or, sometimes, part of the clinical noise in the system. Population model-based methods, with the additional use of a graphic presentation of the concentration–time profile, will be of great help in the clinical management of patients and identify outliers, that is, patients with unusual PK as well as potential candidates who would benefit from more intensive monitoring.

SUGGESTIONS FOR MODEL THERAPEUTIC DRUG MANAGEMENT: A TEAM APPROACH

Proper TDM requires cooperation among informed, skilled patients or parents/caregivers and nursing, pharmacy, medical, and laboratory staff. It is best done by a team approach with everyone involved in helping provide accurate information, proper sample collection, analysis, interpretation, response, and follow-up. The best computer PK/PD modeling cannot overcome inaccurate information or incorrect laboratory analysis. The most accurate laboratory analysis is not useful without all the necessary information, proper interpretation, and appropriate clinical response and follow-up. The most cost-efficient, effective TDM will come when all members of the health care team (and this should include patients and their parents/guardians as well) are familiar with, and provide, what is necessary to properly collect, analyze, interpret, and follow-up drug concentration measurements.

This section presents the components for a pediatric therapeutic drug management service. Table 9.5 shows the drugs that should be routinely monitored. Most of these drugs have reasonably well established concentration–effect and adverse events relationships. The suggested target concentration ranges are not to be viewed as "fixed" but rather as a useful starting point. Several drugs and important drug classes have not been included because their assay is not readily available or because there is no consensus on the clinical utility of routine TDM. For instance, we have not included HIV drugs such as the protease inhibitors, as additional data are needed to establish child-specific reference values and to assess the optimal method of TDM (55). Yet TDM is considered a useful tool in the treatment of HIV-1-infected children. TDM has clearly been useful in individual patients (56). Also not included are antifungal (57) or psychoactive drugs [antidepressants and neuroleptics (58–61)] and drugs routinely used in pediatric oncology (62). However, these drugs are rapidly becoming part of TDM menus and should become common in the near future.

GENTAMICIN AND OTHER ANTIBIOTICS

For decades, TDM of the aminoglycosides (gentamicin, tobramycin, amikacin, and netilmicin) has been primarily focused on avoiding potential nephro- and ototoxicity (3). With intermittent dosing (e.g., every 8 hours or every 12 hours), a trough concentration of 2 mg per L is broadly used as the cutoff point above which toxicity is likely to occur, although good clinical evidence-based studies are lacking (63). In addition, it must be realized that aminoglycoside-related toxicity typically develops slowly, and that reducing the duration of exposure to a maximum of 7 to 10 days will reduce incidence of this adverse event (64,65). Few early studies documented clinically effective concentrations, which resulted in the 5 to 10 mg per L postdose target concentrations (66,67). However, recent better understanding of the PD of aminoglycosides, has shifted focus to optimizing efficacy as well (68,69). The new paradigm for this class of "concentration-dependent" drugs is to achieve rapid bacterial killing with as high as possible initial concentrations. The new target concentrations include high peak concentrations [i.e., 10 times the minimum inhibitory concentration (MIC)] and virtually nondetectable trough concentrations. These targets can be achieved with once-daily and extended interval dosing regimens, where the traditional total daily dose is given in one dose instead of as multiple doses. The transition to higher doses given less frequently is ongoing and has generated ongoing discussion about whether to keep using the well-established peak-and-trough monitoring concept, which is still being used in many institutions, or to go back to less informative midpoint nomogram methods or trough-only strategies for the sake of simplicity (70). The traditional dosing interval in newborns and children is every 8 to 12 hours, but once-daily dosing is also now being used in the pediatric population (71,72). Much of the increased efficacy of once-daily dosing arises because seriously ill patients are not underdosed because of a lack of appreciation of the higher volume of distribution (V_d) in septic adults as well as younger children. Giving a single 5 mg per kg dose is the only way to achieve 10 mg per L concentrations in someone with a $V_d = 0.5$ L per kg. Often renal patients, for example, are underdosed because of a misunderstanding of the difference between low clearance and high V_d in renal patients—one determines the interval needed and the other determines how much should be given to achieve a given concentration. We have seen renal

TABLE 9.5 Menu for Pediatric Therapeutic Drug Management[a]

Drug	*Target Range*	*Comments*
Antiepileptic drugs (3,14)		
Carbamazepine	4–9 mg/L	More favorable adverse events profile; has active CBZ-10,11-epoxide metabolite; autoinduction and in combination with other AEDs
Ethosuximide	40–100 mg/L	Treatment of absence (petit mal) seizures; poorly established concentration–effect relationship
Phenobarbital	20–40 mg/L	Negative effects on cognitive and psychomotor function; relatively slow clearance; half-life 4–5 days in neonate and ~2 days in children; inactive glucuronide metabolite may accumulate in newborn. Ranges differ for seizure prophylaxis, for treatment of hyperbilirubinemia (undetectable), and sedation. Long-term treatment leads to tolerance causing the concentration–effect relationship to change over time.
Phenytoin	5–20 mg/L	Concentration-dependent elimination; slower elimination at high concentrations; highly protein bound; free level monitoring useful in specific cases
Primidone	5–12 mg/L	Metabolized to phenobarbital
Valproic acid	50–100 mg/L	Complex concentration–effect relation; several drug–drug interactions with other AEDs
Antibiotics (3,70)		
Gentamicin	MDD: >5–10 mg/L peak <1–2 mg/L trough >20 mg/L peak ODD: <0.1–0.5 mg/L	Use short courses; preferably maximal duration of therapy 5–7 days; toxicity may occur despite therapeutic drug management
Tobramycin	MMD: >5–10 mg/L peak <1–2 mg/L trough ODD: >20 mg/L peak <0.1–0.5 mg/L	Better intrinsic activity against *Pseudomonas aeruginosa* use short courses; preferably maximal duration of therapy 5–7 days; toxicity may occur despite therapeutic drug management
Vancomycin	<10–15 mg/L trough 20–40 mg/L peak	Rapid infusion may give "red man" syndrome; increased toxicity when combined with aminoglycoside
Immunosuppressants		Ranges depend on time posttransplant as well as transplant organ (kidney, liver, heart, or bone marrow)
Cyclosporine	100–200 μg/L (trough)	Target AUC (118): <D30: 6.0 ± 2.2; D30–M3: 5.5 ± 1.7; M3–1 year: 4.7 ± 1.2; >1 year: 3.8 ± 1.0 mg/hr/L In pediatric patients, ranges have been reported as: <M30: 7.4 ± 2.4; D30–1 year: 5.2 ± 1.4; >1 year: 3.9 ± 1.2 mg/hr/L
Sirolimus	4–12 μg/L (with CsA) 10–20 μg/L (without CsA)	No AUC target consensus range has been established yet (107,119).
Tacrolimus	5–20 μg/L	Target AUC: (120) First week posttransplantation: 0.15–0.21 mg/hr/L Long term: 0.12–0.15 mg/hr/L
Mycophenolic acid	1–3.5 mg/L	Target AUC (121): 30–60 mg/hr/L
Mycophenolic acid glucuronide	35–100 mg/L	
Miscellaneous (3)		
Caffeine	5–15 mg/L	Prevention of apneas in premature neonates
Digoxin	0.8–2.0 μg/L	Concentration–effect relationship with peripheral compartment; detection of accumulation in renal compromised patient; endogenous digoxin-like immunoreactive substances are present in neonates and may interfere with assay
Methotrexate	Depends on therapeutic regimen	Light sensitive; protect sample from daylight
Theophylline	5–20 mg/L	Saturation kinetics; *Note 1*: methylation to caffeine in neonate will lead to two active drugs—theophyllin and caffeine. Depending on the assay method, only one will be detected and reported (122) *Note 2*: Target range depends on condition (asthma requires much lower amounts than apnea) (123,124)

CBZ, carbamazepine; AED, antiepileptic drug; MDD, multiple-daily dosing (dosing interval, 8 or 12 hr); ODD, once-daily dosing; CsA, cyclosporin A (cyclosporine); AUC, area under the curve; D30, first 30 days posttransplantation; D30–M3, 30 days to 3 months posttransplant.

[a]This table is included as an example of what a basic TDM service could provide in terms of routing assays. For more comprehensive service overview, the reader is referred to websites: http://www.clinchem.med.uni-goettingen.de/downloads/Referenzwerte-2008_06_25.pdf http://www.umcg.nl/Professionals/dienstverlening/85932/157322/Pages/Default.aspx

patients given only 1 mg per kg gentamicin "because they have slow clearance"—not a problem if the patient is not septic, but a fatal mistake if the patient is really infected. This is what Moore et al. showed many years ago (67). Although many studies in adults have reported equivalent efficacy and equal or less toxicity with once-daily dosing, this approach has not become standard of practice in pediatric hospitals. Limited clinical and efficacy data in children and the difference in PK (e.g., higher clearance) are among the reasons for lack of acceptance (73). As a result of several studies, the extended interval-dosing concept has received much broader acceptance in specific populations such as neonates and patients with cystic fibrosis (74–79). In our view, aminoglycosides are particularly suited for PK model-based monitoring using aminoglycoside level-predicted clearance, serum creatinine, or creatinine clearance PK methods (80). This will also require as mentioned previously that "therapeutic ranges" be specific for the dosing regimen used. If the goal is to truly individualize, then a TDM strategy should be adopted that will enable this to be done. This is not the case when nomograms are implemented. Similar strategies would also work for vancomycin and other antibiotics.

ANTIEPILEPTIC DRUGS

Although TDM of antiepileptic drugs has been performed since the 1950s, no studies have prospectively evaluated the best way for TDM to be delivered as part of a patient's drug management (27,81). The few studies that have been performed to evaluate the use of TDM of epileptic drugs are hampered by design issues. For example, instead of individualized dosing based on well-defined targets and PK interpretation, protocols have used dose titration until the "therapeutic range," and did not include a consult to the participating neurologists as to how to interpret the measured concentrations such as to decide what concentration or combination of concentrations was efficacious or toxic in which individual patient (82). Recent initiatives have evaluated approaches designed to deliver better TDM support as part of epilepsy management (53,83). This renewed interest has resulted in the publication of practice guidelines (14). TDM is useful in several clinical situations: establishing baseline effective concentrations, evaluating potential causes for lack of efficacy, evaluating potential causes for toxicity, evaluating potential causes for loss of efficacy, judging "room to move" or when to change antiepileptic drugs, and minimizing predictable problems. TDM remains a valuable tool in the modern treatment of epilepsy. It can be selectively and appropriately utilized to help maximize seizure control and minimize side effects if levels are obtained in response to a patient-specific PK or PD issue or problem (84). For phenytoin, anticonvulsant activity and neurotoxic effects correlate well with the serum concentration. Target concentrations have been fairly well established. Concentrations above 20 mg per L are associated with increased incidence of nystagmus, ataxia, and drowsiness. The lower limit of concentration response is less well defined, but is generally set at 8 to 10 mg per L. Some children may be well controlled at lower concentrations. Long-term side effects such as gingival overgrowth, coarsening of facial features, and peripheral neuropathy are not well correlated with serum concentrations and may have a genetic basis (85). PK optimization is particularly helpful for a drug such as phenytoin that is subject to nonlinear or saturation kinetics (86). This phenomenon is the result of enzyme saturation at higher concentrations and is also present in children (87). As a consequence, it is difficult to dose phenytoin because small dose changes may result in disproportionally large changes in concentration. Several useful nomograms, graphic as well as derived from Bayesian methods, have been published to deal with this nonlinear behavior (40,88). Again all methods are better than simply comparing a measured level to a therapeutic range (89). Computerized methods such as Bayesian methods hold substantial potential, particularly as more institutions develop better information systems, but other approaches may also be effective and complementary (53,90). Phenytoin is also highly protein bound (90%) and can easily be displaced by drugs with high affinity for albumin-binding sites. Interestingly, when phenytoin is displaced from its binding, the free and pharmacologic active concentration increases, whereas the total concentration may go down as a result of increased metabolism. In such cases, measurement of the free and total concentration is indicated. Published therapeutic ranges cannot necessarily be used for patients with a protein binding different from that of the population used to generate these ranges.

For the newer antiepileptics (felbamate, gabapentin, lamotrigine, levetiracetam, oxcarbazepine, tiagabine, topiramate, vigabatrin, and zonisamide), routine monitoring is generally not recommended mainly because of incomplete data on the concentration–effect relationship. However, measurement of these newer drugs is undoubtedly of help with individualization of treatment in selected cases in a particular clinical setting (91–94).

IMMUNOSUPPRESSANTS

One of the most rapidly advancing areas in TDM in recent years has been the immunosuppressive drugs used to avert rejection of transplanted organs (95–98). Cyclosporine has been available and routinely measured for some 20 years. Despite the fact that the concentration–effect relationship is not well established, clear associations have been made between predose or trough level (C0) monitoring and clinical endpoints. In recent years, there have been major changes in cyclosporine TDM with the advent of area under the curve (AUC) and abbreviated AUC and especially C2 monitoring strategies (99–101). Recent Bayesian methods show great potential and also allow more flexible sampling (50,102,103). Trough (C0) monitoring of tacrolimus has been well established; however, there appears to be an emerging consensus that tacrolimus, too, may benefit from alternatives to C0 monitoring. Mycophenolic acid was originally marketed as "not requiring monitoring." However, the evidence supports the benefits for its TDM as well (15,104). A recent consensus meeting organized by the Transplant Society has clearly identified the need for monitoring guidelines for dose individualization of mycophenolic acid and will be published soon (105). Sirolimus monitoring has fewer sampling-time issues because there is a reasonable relationship between C0 and AUC.

Yet the most optimal way to establish the dose–exposure relationship is by using a limited sampling strategy (106). The limitations for routine introduction of immunosuppressant TDM are the current lack of a reliable immunoassays and metabolite activity and interferences (107). This is especially relevant in children, as developmental changes may result in different metabolite patterns depending on age. For instance, the metabolism of sirolimus in children is very distinct for that reported in adults. This should be considered when monitoring sirolimus exposure using immunoassays as cross-reactivity issues may interfere with the assay and subsequent interpretation of results (108).

DRUG DETERMINATION IN ALTERNATIVE FLUIDS

Blood, either serum or plasma, has been the preferred biological matrix for TDM (109). However, a number of other fluids can and have been used, including tears, saliva, and urine (110). In addition, transcutaneous and continuous microdialysis sampling techniques hold promise for the future, especially for small children, where sampling can be problematic.

DETERMINATION OF UNBOUND CONCENTRATIONS OF DRUGS

Typically, in routine TDM, total drug concentration (protein bound and free) is measured. Because only the free concentration can diffuse to the extracellular and intracellular space to exert its pharmacologic action, measurement of free concentrations may be of value for highly protein bound drugs, for example, phenytoin (~90%), valproic acid (~90%), and possibly carbamazepine (~75%). Changes in free concentration may be the result of hypoalbuminemia, displacement due to endogenous compounds (such as bilirubin), or a drug–drug interaction (e.g., phenytoin–valproic acid). Several methods are available to measure unbound concentrations even in microsamples. Some of the reasons to measure unbound concentrations as well as some problems with interpretation are given in the foregoing discussion on phenytoin. A TDM service should be helpful in deciding which patients would benefit from unbound measurements, but clinicians should consider such monitoring for drugs with high binding, especially if there is clinical suspicion of abnormal binding proteins, including albumin and alpha acid glycoprotein.

FUTURE DEVELOPMENTS

A number of developments have promise for improving the use and usefulness of TDM. These include the development of therapeutic drug management teams, web-based support tools, cost-effectiveness studies, and emerging data on new drug classes such as antifungal, antiviral, and anticancer drugs and pharmacogenetics. TDM is likely to become more effective and popular with the development of modern analytical techniques such as liquid chromatography/tandem mass spectrometry, which can rapidly and reliably quantify a number of drugs and metabolites simultaneously in single, small (less than 1 mL) samples. This will be especially true as the cost and complexity of this instrumentation decreases and its reliability increases. The sensitivity of such instruments promises to allow noninvasive (e.g., transcutaneous or respiratory) monitoring of all drug and metabolite concentrations simultaneously. When combined with stable isotope techniques, they could also simultaneously measure absorption from multiple sites or bioavailability. Linkage of powerful analytical techniques with powerful computer modeling and patient management software promises to revolutionize drug therapy. Eventual linkage with pharmacogenetic and pharmacogenomic information could revolutionize how patients are dosed, both initially and repetitively, prophylactically or therapeutically (111).

HIV therapy has much to gain from properly applied TDM (18,112,113). Protease inhibitor monitoring can be a valuable tool as demonstrated by several groups. Even brief exposure of HIV to inadequate protease concentrations is associated with rapid development of tolerance and poor therapeutic response. Exposure to excessive protease concentrations is associated with increased incidence of toxicity. Measuring multiple protease concentrations in small samples can help clinicians identify causes of low (including "none detected") or excessive concentrations, leading to more effective and less toxic individualized dosing regimens, less resistance, better outcomes, fewer adverse effects, and some cost savings. Although it has been generally thought that TDM of other HIV drugs is less useful because of their mechanisms of action, recent data (114) have again confirmed that TDM of nonprotease anti-HIV drugs can also do much to improve individual therapy.

Methotrexate (MTX) monitoring after high-dose MTX has been done routinely for years. More recently, other drugs are being measured routinely, including mycophenolic acid, sirolimus, everolimus, 6-mercaptopurine, and thioguanine nucleotide. Other anticancer drugs such as the tyrosine kinase inhibitors (e.g. imatinib) may soon be measured routinely to the benefit of patients. In addition, some anticancer drug targets are also being measured (e.g., TPMT).

TDM teams and model TDM services have been in existence for decades in only a few institutions. However, as modern quality control methods are applied (belatedly) to medicine and more data become available on cost-effectiveness of TDM in terms of outcomes rather than laboratory revenue, there is hope that they will become more common. An interesting recent development in terms of data management, reporting of TDM results, and interpretation has been the use of information technology and the design of web-based tools that allow health care providers access real-time data for their patients 24/7 from any place in the world. An example of such web-based approach is the ImmunoSuppressants Bayesian dose Adjustment (ISBA) support tool offered through the Department of Pharmacology and Toxicology at the University Hospital of Limoges, France (115). Through this resource, population model-based data interpretation is being provided using a Bayesian algorithm including a numerical report and graphical representation of the predicted exposure–time relationship (Fig. 9.5). This program provides support for several different immunosuppressive drugs and transplant indications and uses validated sparse sampling strategies to estimate dose–exposure relationships. The developed Bayesian estimators are each prospectively validated in ongoing studies as exemplified for mycophenolic acid therapeutic drug management (50). Another recent web-based support initiative focused on pediatric therapeutics is the Pediatric Knowledgebase program developed by investigators at the Children's Hospital of Philadelphia. One of the features of this program is its "dashboards," a drug-oriented webpage that provides real-time evaluation of patient status using all available TDM and relevant laboratory data with a population model-based Bayesian estimator running in the background (116).

Population model-based individualized therapy can be important extensions of TDM. Application of PK/PD models that relate drug exposure to biomarkers, whether microbiologic, antiviral, or immunosuppressive, and ultimately to clinical outcomes will provide a better rationale for the proper dose selection and therapeutic intervention in different patient populations.

For example, bacterial MICs have been used for years to individualize drug concentration targets such as peaks, troughs, and AUCs. These same methods are being used for other infectious agents such as viruses and fungi. Pharmacogenetics offers the promise of individualizing patient-specific targets as well. For example, genetic predisposition to aminoglycoside ototoxicity has been well described (117). Studies are beginning to demonstrate that determination of individual susceptibility can be used to predict and eventually prevent drug- and patient-specific toxicity. For aminoglycoside ototoxicity, susceptibility is transmitted by maternal mitochondrial DNA. It should therefore be possible to predict or prevent such toxicity by maternal testing and altering maternal or newborn dosing or exposure. This is only one example of what will be possible in the posthuman genome era.

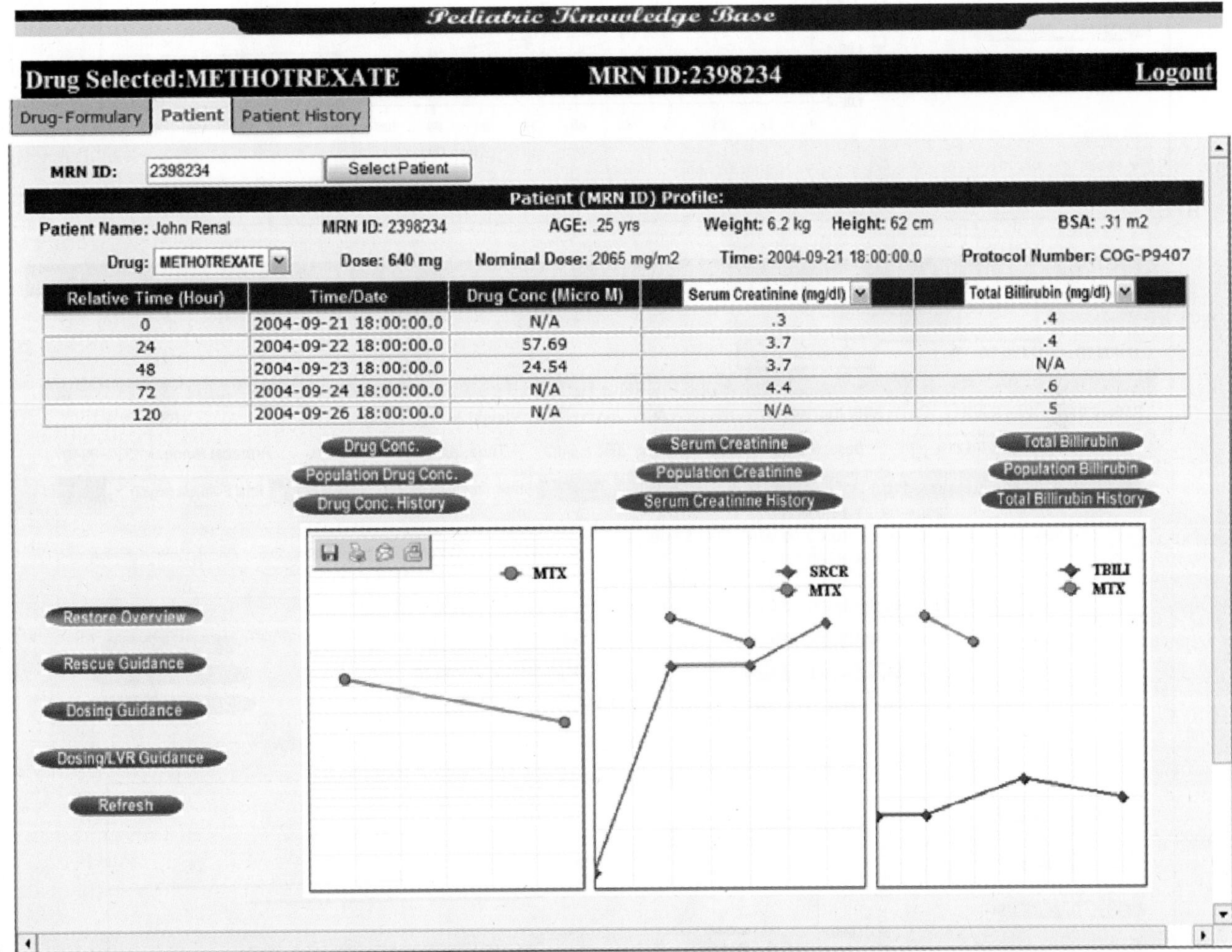

Figure 9.5. Screen captures from the current methotrexate (MTX) dashboard design showing **(A)** the most recent MTX dose event with the complementary monitored MTX plasma concentrations and safety markers serum creatinine and bilirubin, **(B)** current MTX exposure projected versus previous dosing regimens, **(C)** model-based projection of the concentration–time profile overlaid against a nomogram used to assess the potential for MTX toxicity with consideration for drug rescue with leucovorin, and **(D)** the update of the model fit when the additional blood collection time points were added to the final patient data set. (*continued*)

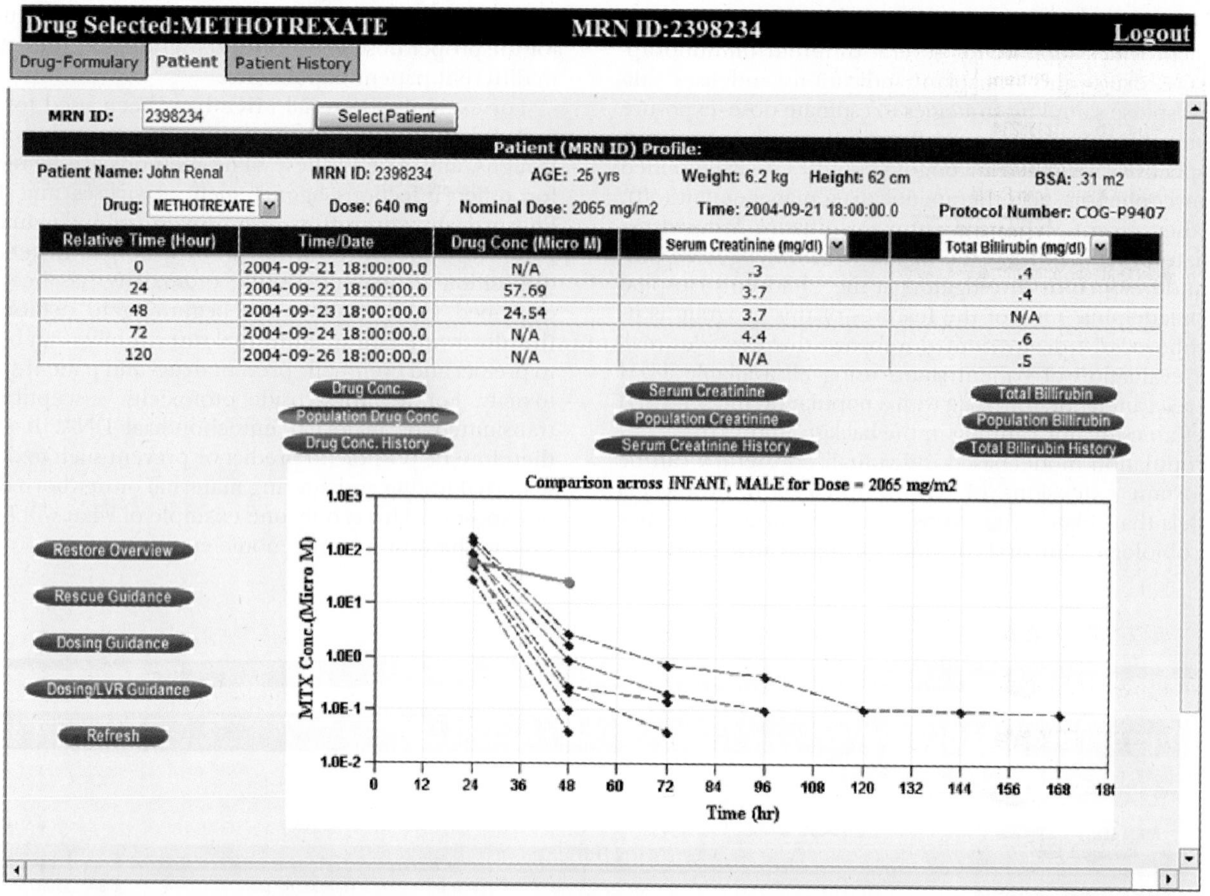

Drug Selected:METHOTREXATE MRN ID:2398234 Logout

Drug-Formulary | Patient | Patient History

MRN ID: 2398234 Select Patient

Patient (MRN ID) Profile:

Patient Name: John Renal **MRN ID:** 2398234 **AGE:** .25 yrs **Weight:** 6.2 kg **Height:** 62 cm **BSA:** .31 m2

Drug: METHOTREXATE **Dose:** 640 mg **Nominal Dose:** 2065 mg/m2 **Time:** 2004-09-21 18:00:00.0 **Protocol Number:** COG-P9407

Relative Time (Hour)	Time/Date	Drug Conc (Micro M)	Serum Creatinine (mg/dl)	Total Billirubin (mg/dl)
0	2004-09-21 18:00:00.0	N/A	.3	.4
24	2004-09-22 18:00:00.0	57.69	3.7	.4
48	2004-09-23 18:00:00.0	24.54	3.7	N/A
72	2004-09-24 18:00:00.0	N/A	4.4	.6
120	2004-09-26 18:00:00.0	N/A	N/A	.5

Drug Conc. | Population Drug Conc | Drug Conc. History | Serum Creatinine | Population Creatinine | Serum Creatinine History | Total Billirubin | Population Billirubin | Total Billirubin History

Restore Overview | Rescue Guidance | Dosing Guidance | Dosing/LVR Guidance | Refresh

Comparison across INFANT, MALE for Dose = 2065 mg/m2

MTX Conc.(Micro M): 1.0E3, 1.0E2, 1.0E1, 1.0E0, 1.0E-1, 1.0E-2

Time (hr): 0, 12, 24, 36, 48, 60, 72, 84, 96, 108, 120, 132, 144, 156, 168, 180

B

Drug Selected:METHOTREXATE MRN ID:2398234 Logout

Drug-Formulary | Patient | Patient History

MRN ID: 2398234 Select Patient

Patient (MRN ID) Profile:

Patient Name: John Renal **MRN ID:** 2398234 **AGE:** .25 yrs **Weight:** 6.2 kg **Height:** 62 cm **BSA:** .31 m2

Drug: METHOTREXATE **Dose:** 640 mg **Nominal Dose:** 2065 mg/m2 **Time:** 2004-09-21 18:00:00.0 **Protocol Number:** COG-P9407

Relative Time (Hour)	Time/Date	Drug Conc (Micro M)	Serum Creatinine (mg/dl)	Total Billirubin (mg/dl)
0	2004-09-21 18:00:00.0	N/A	.3	.4
24	2004-09-22 18:00:00.0	57.69	3.7	.4
48	2004-09-23 18:00:00.0	24.54	3.7	N/A
72	2004-09-24 18:00:00.0	N/A	4.4	.6
120	2004-09-26 18:00:00.0	N/A	N/A	.5

Drug Conc. | Population Drug Conc. | Drug Conc. History | Serum Creatinine | Population Creatinine | Serum Creatinine History | Total Billirubin | Population Billirubin | Total Billirubin History

Restore Overview | Rescue Guidance | Dosing Guidance | Dosing/LVR Guidance | Refresh

Patient at increased risk of METHOTREXATE toxicity.
Consider therapeutic monitoring.

MTX Conc (Micro M): 1.0E3, 1.0E2, 1.0E1, 1.0E0, 1.0E-1, 1.0E-2

Predicted
Observed
LVR (1000 mg/m2 - q6)
LVR (100 mg/m2 - q3)
LVR (10 mg/m2 - q3)
LVR (10 mg/m2 - q6)

Time (hr): 0, 12, 24, 36, 48, 60, 72, 84, 96, 108, 120, 132, 144

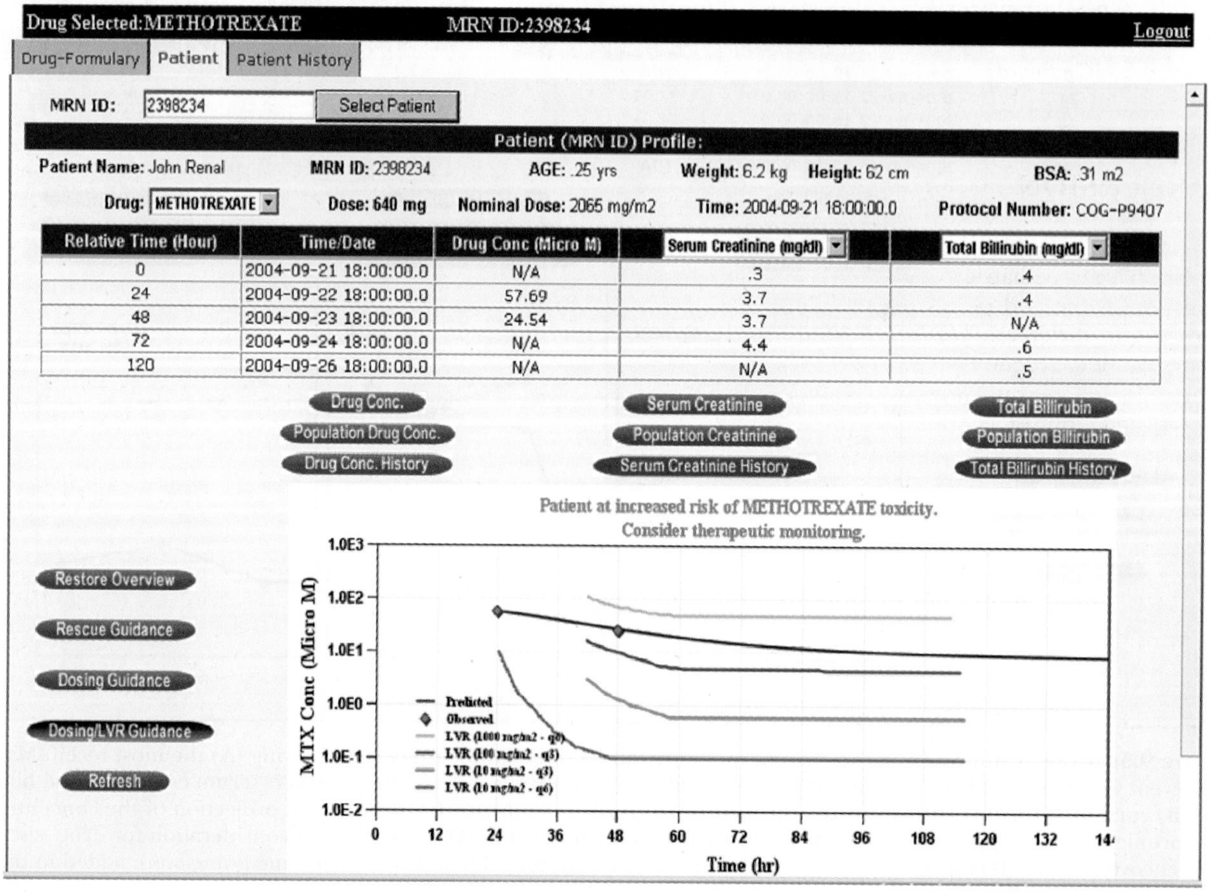

C

Figure 9.5. *(Continued)*

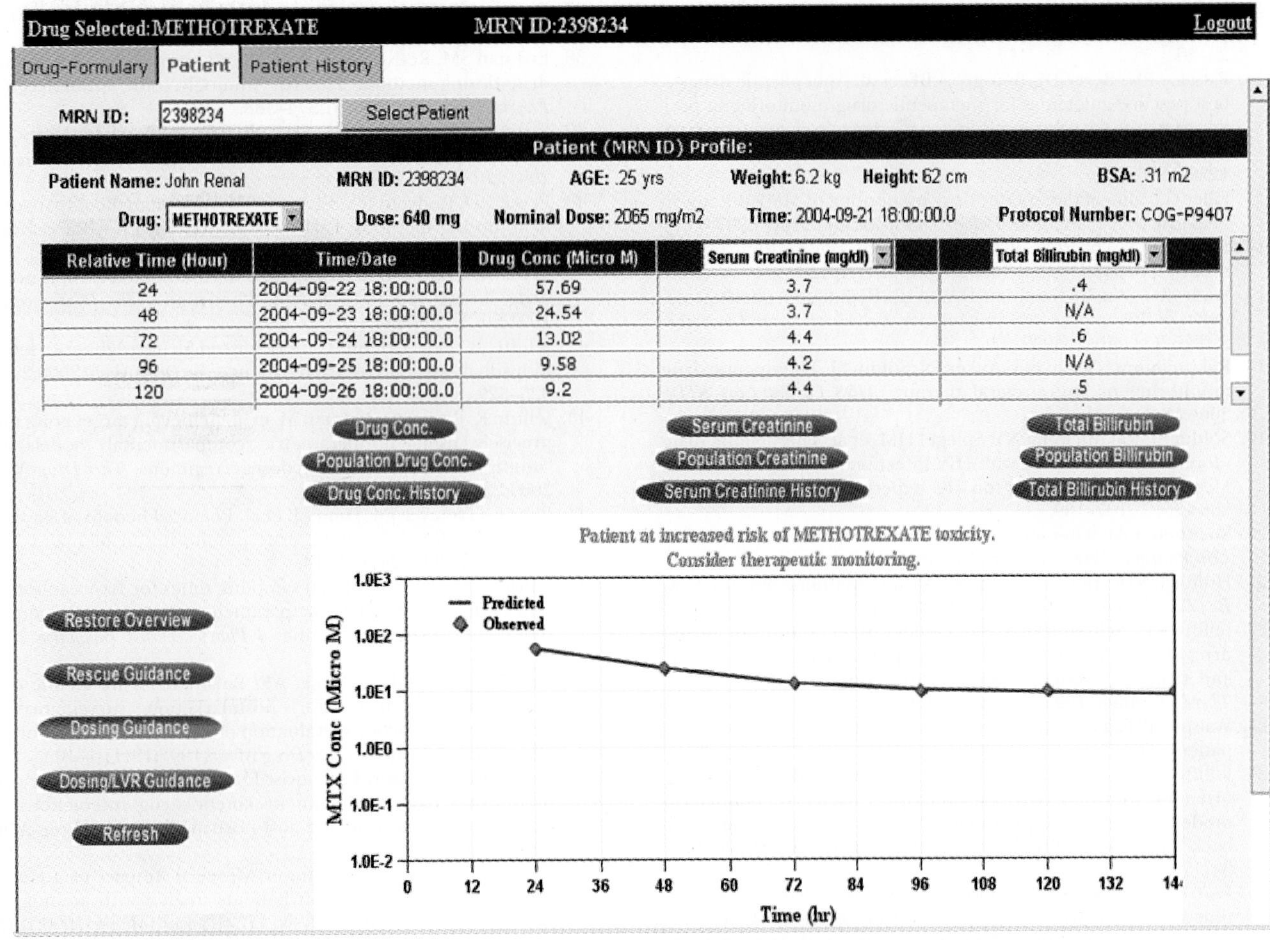

Figure 9.5. (*Continued*)

CONCLUSION

Properly done, TDM has been and will continue to be useful, especially in pediatric populations. However, there are many knowledge and performance deficits that must be corrected in order for TDM to reach its full potential. Simple-minded, reactionary TDM may not be useful and can even be dangerous. However, modern modeling, prediction, and control combined with modern analytical techniques can clearly provide better, more cost-effective pediatric care. In addition, in the future, the combination of analytical, PK/PD modeling, pharmacogenetics, and information technology techniques offers tremendous promise for true optimization of individual therapy beginning with the initial dose of medication and continuing thereafter.

REFERENCES

1. Ritschel WA, Kearns GL. *Handbook of basic pharmacokinetics—including clinical applications*, 5th ed. Washington, DC: American Pharmaceutical Association (APHA), 1998.
2. Benet LZ. Pharmacokinetics: basic principles and its use as a tool in drug metabolism. In: Mitchell JR, Horning MG, eds. *Drug metabolism and drug toxicity*. New York, NY: Raven Press, 1984:199.
3. Burton ME, Shaw LM, Schentag JJ, et al. *Applied pharmacokinetics & pharmacodynamics. Principles of therapeutic drug monitoring*, 4th ed. Philadelphia, PA: Lippincott Williams & Wilkins, 2006.
4. Kahana S, Drotar D, Frazier T. Meta-analysis of psychological interventions to promote adherence to treatment in pediatric chronic health conditions. *J Pediatr Psychol* 2008;33(6):590–611.
5. Modi AC, Morita DA, Glauser TA. One-month adherence in children with new-onset epilepsy: white-coat compliance does not occur. *Pediatrics* 2008;121(4):e961–e966.
6. Quittner AL, Modi AC, Lemanek KL, et al. Evidence-based assessment of adherence to medical treatments in pediatric psychology. *J Pediatr Psychol* 2008;33(9):916–936; discussion 937–938.
7. Sherwin CM, McCaffrey F, Broadbent RS, et al. Discrepancies between predicted and observed rates of intravenous gentamicin delivery for neonates. *J Pharm Pharmacol* 2009;61(4): 465–471.
8. Besunder JB, Reed MD, Blumer JL. Principles of drug biodisposition in the neonate. A critical evaluation of the pharmacokinetic-pharmacodynamic interface (Part II). *Clin Pharmacokinet* 1988;14 (5):261–286.
9. Besunder JB, Reed MD, Blumer JL. Principles of drug biodisposition in the neonate. A critical evaluation of the pharmacokinetic-pharmacodynamic interface (Part I). *Clin Pharmacokinet* 1988;14 (4):189–216.
10. Paap CM, Nahata MC. Clinical pharmacokinetics of antibacterial drugs in neonates. *Clin Pharmacokinet* 1990;19(4):280–318.
11. Watson I, Potter J, Yatscoff R, et al. Editorial therapeutic drug monitoring. *Ther Drug Monit* 1997;19:125.
12. Soldin OP, Soldin SJ. Review: therapeutic drug monitoring in pediatrics. *Ther Drug Monit* 2002;24(1):1–8.

13. Walson PD. Role of therapeutic drug monitoring (TDM) in pediatric anti-convulsant drug dosing. *Brain Dev* 1994;16(1):23–26.
14. Patsalos PN, Berry DJ, Bourgeois BF, et al. Antiepileptic drugs—best practice guidelines for therapeutic drug monitoring: a position paper by the subcommission on therapeutic drug monitoring, ILAE Commission on Therapeutic Strategies. *Epilepsia* 2008;49(7):1239–1276.
15. Filler G. Value of therapeutic drug monitoring of MMF therapy in pediatric transplantation. *Pediatr Transplant* 2006;10(6):707–711.
16. Boreus LO. The role of therapeutic drug monitoring in children. *Clin Pharmacokinet* 1989;17(Suppl 1):4–12.
17. Wade KC, Wu D, Kaufman DA, et al. Population pharmacokinetics of fluconazole in young infants. *Antimicrob Agents Chemother* 2008;52(11):4043–4049.
18. Rakhmanina NY, van den Anker JN, Soldin SJ. Therapeutic drug monitoring of antiretroviral therapy. *AIDS Patient Care STDS* 2004;18(1):7–14.
19. Soldin SJ, Rakhmanina NY, Spiegel HM, et al. Therapeutic drug monitoring for patients with HIV infection: Children's National Medical Center, Washington DC experience. *Ther Drug Monit* 2004;26(2):107–109.
20. Shenfield GM. Therapeutic drug monitoring beyond 2000. *Br J Clin Pharmacol* 2001;52(Suppl 1):3S–4S.
21. Holford NH. Target concentration intervention: beyond Y2K. *Br J Clin Pharmacol* 1999;48(1):9–13.
22. Jelliffe RW, Schumitzky A, Van Guilder M, et al. Individualizing drug dosage regimens: roles of population pharmacokinetic and dynamic models, Bayesian fitting, and adaptive control. *Ther Drug Monit* 1993;15(5):380–393.
23. Walson PD, Edge JH. Clonazepam disposition in pediatric patients. *Ther Drug Monit* 1996;18(1):1–5.
24. Jelliffe RW, Schumitzky A, Bayard D, et al. Model-based, goal-oriented, individualised drug therapy. Linkage of population modelling, new 'multiple model' dosage design, Bayesian feedback and individualised target goals. *Clin Pharmacokinet* 1998;34(1):57–77.
25. Leff RD, Roberts RJ. Methods of intravenous drug administration in the pediatric patient. *J Pediatr* 1981;98(4):631–635.
26. Sherwin CM, McCaffrey F, Broadbent RS, et al. Discrepancies between predicted and observed rates of intravenous gentamicin delivery for neonates. *J Pharm Pharmacol* 2009;61(4):465–471.
27. Ensom MH, Davis GA, Cropp CD, et al. Clinical pharmacokinetics in the 21st century. Does the evidence support definitive outcomes? *Clin Pharmacokinet* 1998;34(4):265–279.
28. Sjoqvist F, Eliasson E. The convergence of conventional therapeutic drug monitoring and pharmacogenetic testing in personalized medicine: focus on antidepressants. *Clin Pharmacol Ther* 2007;81(6):899–902.
29. van Lent-Evers NA, Mathot RA, Geus WP, et al. Impact of goal-oriented and model-based clinical pharmacokinetic dosing of aminoglycosides on clinical outcome: a cost-effectiveness analysis. *Ther Drug Monit* 1999;21(1):63–73.
30. Kearns GL, Abdel-Rahman SM, Alander SW, et al. Developmental pharmacology—drug disposition, action, and therapy in infants and children. *N Engl J Med* 2003;349(12):1157–1167.
31. Kearns GL, Reed MD. Clinical pharmacokinetics in infants and children. A reappraisal. *Clin Pharmacokinet* 1989;17(Suppl 1):29–67.
32. Loebstein R, Koren G. Clinical pharmacology and therapeutic drug monitoring in neonates and children. *Pediatr Rev* 1998;19(12):423–428.
33. Guidelines for industry. E11 Clinical Investigation of medicinal products in the pediatric population. Rockville, MD: US Department of Health and Human Services, Food and Drug Administration, Center for Drug Evaluation and Research (CDER), Center for Biologics Evaluation and Research (CBER), 2000.
34. Butler DR, Kuhn RJ, Chandler MH. Pharmacokinetics of anti-infective agents in paediatric patients. *Clin Pharmacokinet* 1994;26(5):374–395.
35. Rhodin MM, Anderson BJ, Peters AM, et al. Human renal function maturation: a quantitative description using weight and postmenstrual age. *Pediatr Nephrol* 2009;24(1):67–76.
36. Koren G, James A, Perlman M. A simple method for the estimation of glomerular filtration rate by gentamicin pharmacokinetics during routine drug monitoring in the newborn. *Clin Pharmacol Ther* 1985;38(6):680–685.
37. Burton ME, Vasko MR, Brater DC. Comparison of drug dosing methods. *Clin Pharmacokinet* 1985;10(1):1–37.
38. Erdman SM, Rodvold KA, Pryka RD. An updated comparison of drug dosing methods. Part III: Aminoglycoside antibiotics. *Clin Pharmacokinet* 1991;20(5):374–388.
39. Erdman SM, Rodvold KA, Pryka RD. An updated comparison of drug dosing methods. Part II: Theophylline. *Clin Pharmacokinet* 1991;20(4):280–292.
40. Pryka RD, Rodvold KA, Erdman SM. An updated comparison of drug dosing methods. Part IV: Vancomycin. *Clin Pharmacokinet* 1991;20(6):463–476.
41. Pryka RD, Rodvold KA, Erdman SM. An updated comparison of drug dosing methods. Part I: Phenytoin. *Clin Pharmacokinet* 1991;20(3):209–217.
42. Jelliffe R. Goal-oriented, model-based drug regimens: setting individualized goals for each patient. *Ther Drug Monit* 2000;22(3):325–329.
43. Jelliffe R, Bayard D, Milman M, et al. Achieving target goals most precisely using nonparametric compartmental models and "multiple model" design of dosage regimens. *Ther Drug Monit* 2000;22(3):346–353.
44. Pons G, Treluyer JM, Dimet J, et al. Potential benefit of Bayesian forecasting for therapeutic drug monitoring in neonates. *Ther Drug Monit* 2002;24(1):9–14.
45. Merle Y, Mentre F. Optimal sampling times for Bayesian estimation of the pharmacokinetic parameters of nortriptyline during therapeutic drug monitoring. *J Pharmacokinet Biopharm* 1999;27(1):85–101.
46. Gex-Fabry M, Balant-Gorgia AE, Balant LP. Therapeutic drug monitoring databases for postmarketing surveillance of drug–drug interactions: evaluation of a paired approach for psychotropic medication. *Ther Drug Monit* 1997;19(1):1–10.
47. Jerling M, Bertilsson L, Sjoqvist F. The use of therapeutic drug monitoring data to document kinetic drug interactions: an example with amitriptyline and nortriptyline. *Ther Drug Monit* 1994;16(1):1–12.
48. Destache CJ, Meyer SK, Bittner MJ, et al. Impact of a clinical pharmacokinetic service on patients treated with aminoglycosides: a cost-benefit analysis. *Ther Drug Monit* 1990;12(5):419–426.
49. Destache CJ, Meyer SK, Rowley KM. Does accepting pharmacokinetic recommendations impact hospitalization? A cost-benefit analysis. *Ther Drug Monit* 1990;12(5):427–433.
50. Le Meur Y, Buchler M, Thierry A, et al. Individualized mycophenolate mofetil dosing based on drug exposure significantly improves patient outcomes after renal transplantation. *Am J Transplant* 2007;7(11):2496–2503.
51. Destache CJ. Economic aspects of pharmacokinetic services. *Pharmacoeconomics* 1993;3(6):433–436.
52. Bertino JS Jr., Rodvold KA, Destache CJ. Cost considerations in therapeutic drug monitoring of aminoglycosides. *Clin Pharmacokinet* 1994;26(1):71–81.
53. Bates DW, Soldin SJ, Rainey PM, et al. Strategies for physician education in therapeutic drug monitoring. *Clin Chem* 1998;44(2):401–407.
54. Cox S, Team T. Gathering outpatient data for therapeutic drug monitoring. In: 3rd International Congress of Therapeutic Drug Monitoring and Clinical Toxicology. Philadelphia, PA, 1993.
55. Fraaij PL, Rakhmanina N, Burger DM, et al. Therapeutic drug monitoring in children with HIV/AIDS. *Ther Drug Monit* 2004;26(2):122–126.
56. Walson PD, Cox C, Utkin I, et al. Clinical use of a simultaneous HPLC assay for indinavir, saquinavir, ritonavir, and nelfinavir in children and adults. *Ther Drug Monit* 2003;25(6):650–656.
57. Smith J, Andes D. Therapeutic drug monitoring of antifungals: pharmacokinetic and pharmacodynamic considerations. *Ther Drug Monit* 2008;30(2):167–172.
58. Mann K, Hiemke C, Schmidt LG, et al. Appropriateness of therapeutic drug monitoring for antidepressants in routine psychiatric inpatient care. *Ther Drug Monit* 2006;28(1):83–88.
59. Hiemke C. Clinical utility of drug measurement and pharmacokinetics: therapeutic drug monitoring in psychiatry. *Eur J Clin Pharmacol* 2008;64(2):159–166.
60. Hiemke C. Therapeutic drug monitoring in neuropsychopharmacology: does it hold its promises? *Eur Arch Psychiatry Clin Neurosci* 2008;258(Suppl 1):21–27.

61. Baumann P, Ulrich S, Eckermann G, et al. The AGNP-TDM Expert Group Consensus Guidelines: focus on therapeutic monitoring of antidepressants. *Dialogues Clin Neurosci* 2005;7(3): 231–247.
62. Rousseau A, Marquet P, Debord J, et al. Adaptive control methods for the dose individualisation of anticancer agents. *Clin Pharmacokinet* 2000;38(4):315–353.
63. McCormack JP, Jewesson PJ. A critical reevaluation of the "therapeutic range" of aminoglycosides. *Clin Infect Dis* 1992;14(1):320–339.
64. De Broe ME, Giuliano RA, Verpooten GA. Choice of drug and dosage regimen. Two important risk factors for aminoglycoside nephrotoxicity. *Am J Med* 1986;80(6B):115–118.
65. Rougier F, Claude D, Maurin M, et al. Aminoglycoside nephrotoxicity: modeling, simulation, and control. *Antimicrob Agents Chemother* 2003;47(3):1010–1016.
66. Moore RD, Smith CR, Lietman PS. Association of aminoglycoside plasma levels with therapeutic outcome in gram-negative pneumonia. *Am J Med* 1984;77(4):657–662.
67. Moore RD, Smith CR, Lietman PS. The association of aminoglycoside plasma levels with mortality in patients with gram-negative bacteremia. *J Infect Dis* 1984;149(3):443–448.
68. Nicolau DP, Freeman CD, Belliveau PP, et al. Experience with a once-daily aminoglycoside program administered to 2,184 adult patients. *Antimicrob Agents Chemother* 1995;39(3):650–655.
69. Craig W. Pharmacodynamics of antimicrobial agents as a basis for determining dosage regimens. *Eur J Clin Microbiol Infect Dis* 1993;12(Suppl 1):S6–S8.
70. Maglio D, Nightingale CH, Nicolau DP. Extended interval aminoglycoside dosing: from concept to clinic. *Int J Antimicrob Agents* 2002;19(4):341–348.
71. Hansen A, Forbes P, Arnold A, et al. Once-daily gentamicin dosing for the preterm and term newborn: proposal for a simple regimen that achieves target levels. *J Perinatol* 2003;23(8): 635–639.
72. Contopoulos-Ioannidis DG, Giotis ND, Baliatsa DV, et al. Extended-interval aminoglycoside administration for children: a meta-analysis. *Pediatrics* 2004;114(1):e111–e118.
73. Knoderer CA, Everett JA, Buss WF. Clinical issues surrounding once-daily aminoglycoside dosing in children. *Pharmacotherapy* 2003;23(1):44–56.
74. de Hoog M, Mouton JW, Schoemaker RC, et al. Extended-interval dosing of tobramycin in neonates: implications for therapeutic drug monitoring. *Clin Pharmacol Ther* 2002;71(5):349–358.
75. Touw DJ, Vinks AA, Mouton JW, et al. Pharmacokinetic optimisation of antibacterial treatment in patients with cystic fibrosis. Current practice and suggestions for future directions. *Clin Pharmacokinet* 1998;35(6):437–459.
76. Hennig S, Norris R, Kirkpatrick CM. Target concentration intervention is needed for tobramycin dosing in paediatric patients with cystic fibrosis—a population pharmacokinetic study. *Br J Clin Pharmacol* 2008;65(4):502–510.
77. Lam W, Tjon J, Seto W, et al. Pharmacokinetic modelling of a once-daily dosing regimen for intravenous tobramycin in paediatric cystic fibrosis patients. *J Antimicrob Chemother* 2007;59(6): 1135–1140.
78. Touw DJ, Knox AJ, Smyth A. Population pharmacokinetics of tobramycin administered thrice daily and once daily in children and adults with cystic fibrosis. *J Cyst Fibros* 2007;6(5):327–333.
79. Burkhardt O, Lehmann C, Madabushi R, et al. Once-daily tobramycin in cystic fibrosis: better for clinical outcome than thrice-daily tobramycin but more resistance development? *J Antimicrob Chemother* 2006;58(4):822–829.
80. Vinks AA. The application of population pharmacokinetic modeling to individualized antibiotic therapy. *Int J Antimicrob Agents* 2002;19(4):313–322.
81. Warner A, Privitera M, Bates D. Standards of laboratory practice: antiepileptic drug monitoring. National Academy of Clinical Biochemistry. *Clin Chem* 1998;44(5):1085–1095.
82. Jannuzzi G, Cian P, Fattore C, et al. A multicenter randomized controlled trial on the clinical impact of therapeutic drug monitoring in patients with newly diagnosed epilepsy. The Italian TDM Study Group in Epilepsy. *Epilepsia* 2000;41(2):222–230.
83. Schoenenberger RA, Tanasijevic MJ, Jha A, et al. Appropriateness of antiepileptic drug level monitoring. *JAMA* 1995;274(20): 1622–1626.
84. Glauser TA, Pippenger CE. Controversies in blood-level monitoring: reexamining its role in the treatment of epilepsy. *Epilepsia* 2000;41(Suppl 8):S6–S15.
85. Brunet L, Miranda J, Roset P, et al. Prevalence and risk of gingival enlargement in patients treated with anticonvulsant drugs. *Eur J Clin Invest* 2001;31(9):781–788.
86. Ludden TM. Nonlinear pharmacokinetics: clinical Implications. *Clin Pharmacokinet* 1991;20(6):429–446.
87. Battino D, Estienne M, Avanzini G. Clinical pharmacokinetics of antiepileptic drugs in paediatric patients. Part II. Phenytoin, carbamazepine, sulthiame, lamotrigine, vigabatrin, oxcarbazepine and felbamate. *Clin Pharmacokinet* 1995;29(5):341–369.
88. Ludden TM, Hawkins DW, Allen JP, et al. Letter: optimum phenytoin-dosage regimens. *Lancet* 1976;1(7954):307–308.
89. Johannessen SI, Landmark CJ. Value of therapeutic drug monitoring in epilepsy. *Expert Rev Neurother* 2008;8(6):929–939.
90. Chen P, Tanasijevic MJ, Schoenenberger RA, et al. A computer-based intervention for improving the appropriateness of antiepileptic drug level monitoring. *Am J Clin Pathol* 2003;119(3): 432–438.
91. Johannessen SI, Battino D, Berry DJ, et al. Therapeutic drug monitoring of the newer antiepileptic drugs. *Ther Drug Monit* 2003;25(3):347–363.
92. Johannessen SI, Tomson T. Pharmacokinetic variability of newer antiepileptic drugs: when is monitoring needed? *Clin Pharmacokinet* 2006;45(11):1061–1075.
93. Perucca E. Is there a role for therapeutic drug monitoring of new anticonvulsants? *Clin Pharmacokinet* 2000;38(3):191–204.
94. Anderson GD. Pharmacokinetic, pharmacodynamic, and pharmacogenetic targeted therapy of antiepileptic drugs. *Ther Drug Monit* 2008;30(2):173–180.
95. Filler G. Optimization of immunosuppressive drug monitoring in children. *Transplant Proc* 2007;39(4):1241–1243.
96. Kahan BD, Keown P, Levy GA, et al. Therapeutic drug monitoring of immunosuppressant drugs in clinical practice. *Clin Ther* 2002;24(3):330–350; discussion 329.
97. Oellerich M, Armstrong VW, Schutz E, et al. Therapeutic drug monitoring of cyclosporine and tacrolimus. Update on Lake Louise Consensus Conference on cyclosporin and tacrolimus. *Clin Biochem* 1998;31(5):309–316.
98. del Mar Fernandez De Gatta M, Santos-Buelga D, Dominguez-Gil A, et al. Immunosuppressive therapy for paediatric transplant patients: pharmacokinetic considerations. *Clin Pharmacokinet* 2002; 41(2):115–135.
99. David O, Johnston A. Limited sampling strategies. *Clin Pharmacokinet* 2000;39(4):311–313.
100. Johnston A, Chusney G, Schutz E, et al. Monitoring cyclosporin in blood: between-assay differences at trough and 2 hours post-dose (C2). *Ther Drug Monit* 2003;25(2):167–173.
101. Morris RG, Ilett KF, Tett SE, et al. Cyclosporin monitoring in Australasia: 2002 update of consensus guidelines. *Ther Drug Monit* 2002;24(6):677–688.
102. Monchaud C, Rousseau A, Leger F, et al. Limited sampling strategies using Bayesian estimation or multilinear regression for cyclosporin AUC(0–12) monitoring in cardiac transplant recipients over the first year post-transplantation. *Eur J Clin Pharmacol* 2003;58(12):813–820.
103. Rousseau A, Monchaud C, Debord J, et al. Bayesian forecasting of oral cyclosporin pharmacokinetics in stable lung transplant recipients with and without cystic fibrosis. *Ther Drug Monit* 2003;25(1):28–35.
104. Oellerich M, Shipkova M, Schutz E, et al. Pharmacokinetic and metabolic investigations of mycophenolic acid in pediatric patients after renal transplantation: implications for therapeutic drug monitoring. German Study Group on Mycophenolate Mofetil Therapy in Pediatric Renal Transplant Recipients. *Ther Drug Monit* 2000;22(1):20–26.
105. Kuiypers DRJ, Le Meur Y, Cantarovich M, et al., for The Transplant Society (TTS) Consensus Group on TDM of MPA (2010). Consensus report on therapeutic drug monitoring of mycophenolic acid in solid organ transplantation. *Clin J Am Soc Nephrol* in press.
106. Forbes N, Schachter AD, Yasin A, et al. Limited sampling strategies for sirolimus after pediatric renal transplantation. *Pediatr Transplant* 2008;13:1020–1026.
107. Shaw LM, Kaplan B, Brayman KL. Advances in therapeutic drug monitoring for immunosuppressants: a review of sirolimus. Introduction and overview. *Clin Ther* 2000;22(Suppl B): B1–B13.

108. Filler G, Bendrick-Peart J, Strom T, et al. Characterization of sirolimus metabolites in pediatric solid organ transplant recipients. *Pediatr Transplant* 2009;13(1):44–53.
109. Gorodischer R, Koren G. Salivary excretion of drugs in children: theoretical and practical issues in therapeutic drug monitoring. *Dev Pharmacol Ther* 1992;19(4):161–177.
110. Langman LJ. The use of oral fluid for therapeutic drug management: clinical and forensic toxicology. *Ann N Y Acad Sci* 2007; 1098: 145–166.
111. Ensom MH, Chang TK, Patel P. Pharmacogenetics: the therapeutic drug monitoring of the future? *Clin Pharmacokinet* 2001;40(11):783–802.
112. Aarnoutse R, Schapiro J, Boucher C, et al. Therapeutic drug monitoring: an aid to optimising response to antiretroviral drugs? *Drugs* 2003;63(8):741–753.
113. van Rossum AM, Bergshoeff AS, Fraaij PL, et al. Therapeutic drug monitoring of indinavir and nelfinavir to assess adherence to therapy in human immunodeficiency virus-infected children. *Pediatr Infect Dis J* 2002;21(8):743–747.
114. Soldin SJ, Steele BW. Mini-review: the rapeutic drug monitoring in pediatrics. *Clin Biochem* 2000;33(5):333–335.
115. ISBA IBDA. Department of Pharmacology and Toxicology at the University Hospital of Limoges, France 2009 [updated 2009]; Available at: https://pharmaco.chu-limoges.fr/abis.htm. Accessed June 26, 2009.
116. Barrett JS, Mondick JT, Narayan M, et al. Integration of modeling and simulation into hospital-based decision support systems guiding pediatric pharmacotherapy. *BMC Med Inform Decis Mak* 2008;8:6.
117. Guan MX, Fischel-Ghodsian N, Attardi G. A biochemical basis for the inherited susceptibility to aminoglycoside ototoxicity. *Hum Mol Genet* 2000;9(12):1787–1793.
118. Oellerich M, Armstrong VW, Kahan B, et al. Lake Louise Consensus Conference on cyclosporin monitoring in organ transplantation: report of the consensus panel. *Ther Drug Monit* 1995;17(6):642–654.
119. Schubert M, Venkataramanan R, Holt DW, et al. Pharmacokinetics of sirolimus and tacrolimus in pediatric transplant patients. *Am J Transplant* 2004;4(5):767–773.
120. Wallemacq P, Armstrong VW, Brunet M, et al. Opportunities to optimize tacrolimus therapy in solid organ transplantation: report of the European consensus conference. *Ther Drug Monit* 2009;31(2):139–152.
121. van Gelder T, Le Meur Y, Shaw LM, et al. Therapeutic drug monitoring of mycophenolate mofetil in transplantation. *Ther Drug Monit* 2006;28(2):145–154.
122. Boutroy MJ, Vert P, Monin P, et al. Methylation of theophylline to caffeine in premature infants. *Lancet* 1979;1(8120):830.
123. Holford N, Black P, Couch R, et al. Theophylline target concentration in severe airways obstruction—10 or 20 mg/L? A randomised concentration-controlled trial. *Clin Pharmacokinet* 1993; 25(6):495–505.
124. Holford N, Hashimoto Y, Sheiner LB. Time and theophylline concentration help explain the recovery of peak flow following acute airways obstruction. Population analysis of a randomised concentration controlled trial. *Clin Pharmacokinet* 1993;25(6): 506–515.

CHAPTER

10

Milap C. Nahata

Drug Formulations

A continuing decline in the morbidity and mortality in the pediatric population can be attributed, in part, to the availability of effective drugs for preventing and treating various diseases. Over the last 50 years, many drugs have been developed and marketed to manage conditions including fever; pain; infections; diabetes; gastrointestinal, heart, lung, and kidney diseases; and seizure disorders. For proper administration of drugs, however, the medications must be available in age-appropriate formulations to achieve the desired therapeutic outcomes and avoid adverse effects.

Infants and young children often require liquid formulations for oral administration because they are unable to swallow solid (tablet and capsule) dose forms and need doses based on body weight. Infants also need intravenous formulations at suitable concentrations so that small doses can be accurately and precisely measured prior to administration (1,2).

NEED FOR DRUG FORMULATIONS

Nearly three-fourths of the commercially available drugs in the United States have not been labeled for use in infants and children. When a drug has not been approved by the US Food and Drug Administration (FDA) for the pediatric population, it is most likely not commercially available in an appropriate formulation. Many of these unapproved drugs, however, are useful for the treatment of pediatric patients. Thus, these drugs must be reformulated or compounded in an appropriate dosage form extemporaneously by pharmacists, often for one patient at a time.

When gabapentin, lamotrigine, tiagabine, and topiramate were approved by the FDA for adults with seizure disorders, many pediatricians found one or more of these important for use in pediatric patients whose seizures could not be adequately controlled by the previously available anticonvulsants. None of these four drugs were available in liquid dose forms for several years, and three of the four are still not available in a liquid formulation. These are compounded for individual patients by the pharmacists. Table 10.1 provides a partial list of drugs that are not available commercially in a liquid formulation and must be compounded by the pharmacists.

Infants younger than the age of 6 months are not capable of ingesting solid or pureed food from a spoon. Thus, the contents of a capsule or triturated tablet mixed in applesauce or ice cream cannot be successfully given to young infants. Similarly, children below the age of 6 to 8 years have difficulty swallowing a tablet or a capsule. Liquid formulations of all oral drugs are needed for such infants and children. Furthermore, the doses of drugs in infants and young children are not fixed, but are given in milligrams per kilogram of body weight. For example, captopril is commercially available only as 12.5-, 25-, 50-, and 100-mg tablets. These meet the need of adult patients requiring fixed doses. The dose in infants, however, may be 0.1 to 0.3 mg per kg, and thus the required dose in a patient weighing 3 kg would be different from that for a patient weighing 5 kg. Furthermore, it will be impossible to use a 12.5-mg tablet to provide 0.3 mg or 1.5 mg of captopril to these patients. This emphasizes the need to develop liquid formulations, as was done for captopril at a concentration of 1 mg per mL. Table 10.2 provides examples of drugs, commercially available dose forms, normal pediatric doses, and the liquid formulations developed at appropriate concentrations for use in infants and children (3–18).

Intravenous drugs marketed for adult patients (but not labeled for pediatric patients) are often too concentrated for accurate measurement of small doses for newborn infants. For example, injectable morphine is available at 2 to 50 mg per mL and phenobarbital at 30 to 130 mg per mL. Measurement of small volumes to provide the needed doses in premature infants can be associated with inaccurate administration of these drugs. In fact, intoxication has been reported in infants with the use of concentrated digoxin and morphine (19,20). Thus, the intravenous drugs marketed for adults should be diluted prior to the measurement of the needed dose. Table 10.2 provides examples of some intravenous dose formulations for use in infants and young children. Morphine injection was diluted from 10 to 1 mg per mL in bacteriostatic 0.9% sodium chloride injection and found to be stable for 60 days (14). Phenobarbital sodium injection was diluted from 65 to 10 mg per mL in bacteriostatic water for injection and found to be stable for 90 days (15).

TABLE 10.1 Examples of Medications Not Available in a Liquid Formulation

Albendazole	Hydroxyurea	Phenobarbital
Amitriptyline	Irbesartan	Phenoxybenzamine
Arginine	Lansoprazole	Prazosin
Aspartate	Leucovorin	Primidone
Biotin	Lisinopril	Probenecid
Bupropion	Lomustine	Procarbazine
Busulfan	Mefloquine	Propafenone
Carbenicillin	Methimazole	Pyridoxine
Cholestyramine/aquaphor	Methotrexate	Riboflavin
	Methylphenidate	Saquinavir
Clindamycin	Minoxidil	Scopolamine
Clobazam	Neomycin	Sildenafil
Clonidine	Nicardipine	Sodium benzoate
Coenzyme Q	Nimodipine	Squaric acid
Dantrolene	Ofloxacin	Testosterone
Ethambutol	Olanzapine	Vigabatrin
Ethionamide	Pancrelipase	Warfarin
Famciclovir	Paromomycin	Zinc sulfate
Glutamine		

It is important to realize that when a commercially available formulation is altered or modified in any form, the modified formulation must be tested for potency of the active ingredient (drug). Stability studies must be done under the normal conditions of storage and use for all modified formulations. For intravenous drugs, the modified formulations must also be tested for sterility and pyrogens. Finally, the efficacy and safety of the modified formulations must be assured by close monitoring of patients' response to therapy.

REASONS FOR LACK OF DRUG FORMULATIONS

The cost of drug development (more than $800 million) is enormous. The overall size of the pediatric market is much smaller than for adults for many common diseases such as hypertension. It may take 7 to 8 years to develop and market a drug for only the adult population. Thus, unless a condition occurs frequently in the pediatric population (e.g., fever or acute otitis media), the industry may not seek labeling for infants and children. A manufacturer cannot market a formulation unless it has been adequately studied for efficacy and safety in pediatric patients. Therefore, additional costs, limited financial returns, potential delay in marketing for adults, and perceived greater legal liability and regulatory requirements are impediments to developing and marketing a pediatric drug formulation.

OPTIONS IN THE ABSENCE OF DRUG FORMULATIONS

When an appropriate formulation is not available, the options include the following:

1. Refusing or delaying therapy with a potentially efficacious new drug when the available drugs are not fully effective.
2. Calling the manufacturer for data on any extemporaneous formulation.
3. Using an adult formulation somehow.
4. Preparing an extemporaneous formulation based on limited data in the literature or in consultation with peers.

An acceptable option in most cases is to prepare an extemporaneous oral formulation with documented stability and palatability. Ideally, the formulation should have been studied for bioavailability, efficacy, and safety. Such data, however, are often missing.

CLINICAL IMPLICATIONS

Many generic and brand medicines frequently used in infants and children are not available in suitable formulations (Table 10.1). This poses important clinical dilemmas. Captopril is used for the treatment of hypertension

TABLE 10.2 Examples of Extemporaneously Prepared Oral Formulations

Drug	*Available Dose Form*[a]	*Strength (mg)*	*Dose Range (mg/kg)*	*References*
Amiodarone	TAB	200, 400	2.5–15	3
Amlodipine	TAB	2.5, 5, 10	NK[b]	4
Captopril	TAB	12.5, 25, 50, 100	0.01–6	5–7
Clindamycin	INJ	150, 600	5–15	8
Enalapril	TAB	2.5, 5, 10, 20	0.05–5	9
Fumagillin	OPH		NK[b]	10
Gabapentin	CAP	100, 300, 400	5–12	11
Mercaptopurine	TAB	50	1.5–5	12
Mexiletine	CAP	150, 250	1.4–5	13
Morphine	INJ	2, 3, 4, 8, 10, 50	0.05–0.5	14
Phenobarbital	INJ	130	2.5–8	15
Spironolactone	TAB	25, 50, 100	0.04–3.0	16,17
Terbinafine	TAB	250	NK[b]	18

[a]CAP, capsule; INJ, injection; OPH, ophthalmic; TAB, tablet.
[b]Dose not clearly known.

or congestive heart failure in infants. It is available, however, only as a tablet. When we received a prescription for an infant, we got in touch with the manufacturer. The manufacturer had no data on its stability in any liquid vehicles except that "it underwent oxidation in aqueous medium." Two actions were taken:

1. Tablets were triturated and mixed with lactose to prepare powder packets of individual doses to be administered just prior to each dose.
2. A stability study was initiated in water and ascorbic acid (as antioxidant).

Powder packets are extremely time-consuming to prepare and the caretaker must take responsibility to accurately administer the entire dose. A liquid formulation in water and ascorbic acid provided consistency and stability for at least 6 weeks at 4°C and 25°C, and thus has become a standard formulation for the treatment of pediatric patients (7).

The excipients used to prepare drug formulations are generally considered as inert substances; however, some of these may be associated with adverse effects. Propylene glycol is used as a vehicle in many formulations, and excessive use of this agent has led to hyperosmolality in patients. Benzyl alcohol has been used as a preservative and has been associated with severe toxicity in infants. Finally, increased use of sorbitol as an excipient can lead to diarrhea and pneumatosis intestinalis (21).

Because of limited resources, the bioavailability, efficacy, and safety of extemporaneous formulations are rarely studied. Sustained- or extended-release formulations should not be used to prepare extemporaneous formulations because they may lose the delayed-release characteristics of the drugs. Patients receiving an extemporaneous formulation should be closely monitored to assure expected therapeutic outcomes.

DOCUMENTED NEEDS FOR DRUG FORMULATIONS IN PEDIATRIC PATIENTS

A survey of 57 hospitals, with 36 to 350 licensed pediatric beds (mean ± SD = 146 ± 83), conducted during 1998 to 1999 identified the needs for drug formulations for pediatric patients. Table 10.3 provides a list of drugs for which greater than 5% of hospitals indicated that no compounding and/or stability data were available or more data were needed. Table 10.4 identifies additional drugs for which a liquid formulation was needed (2).

PREPARATION AND TESTING OF DRUG FORMULATION

The physicochemical properties of the drug and the characteristics of the available dose form (e.g., tablet or capsule) should be considered in preparing the extemporaneous dose form. Most drugs are not completely water soluble. Thus, a suspension is generally prepared to yield a uniformly dispersed oral formulation. Carboxymethylcellulose and methylcellulose are commonly used suspending agents. We have used commercially available carboxymethylcellulose in a ready-to-use suspension (Ora-Plus, Paddock Laboratories, Minneapolis, MN) and extemporaneously prepared 1% methylcellulose suspension (6) at our hospital. The pH of Ora-Plus is about 4.4, whereas that of methylcellulose is nearly 6.8. We routinely mix the suspending agent with an equal volume of commercially available simple syrup or Ora Sweet (sugared or sugar free). Sweetners containing sucrose and fructose can increase blood sugar and those containing sorbitol and xylitol may cause osmotic diarrhea. Lactrose should be avoided in patients with lactrose intolerance. Flavors and preservatives may be added, as necessary. The commercially available parenteral drugs are normally diluted in sterile or bacteriostatic water for injection or 0.9% sodium chloride injection.

PHYSICAL AND CHEMICAL STABILITY

The physical and chemical stability of the extemporaneous formulations is determined at clinically simulated conditions. For example, about 1 oz of the prepared formulation is stored in each of 10 plastic prescription bottles. Five bottles are stored at 4°C in a refrigerator and five at 25°C to simulate a room temperature condition. Small aliquots are collected and normally studied on day 0 (soon after preparation) and on days 3, 7, 14, 28, 42, 56, 70, and 91 during storage. Physical stability is determined by visual appearance against a white and black background to rule out any changes in color and appearance; odor is also assessed. The chemical stability is determined by measuring the concentration of the drug using an accurate, specific, reproducible, and stability-indicating analytical method (e.g., high-performance liquid chromatography). The stability-indicating nature of the method is confirmed by subjecting samples of the extemporaneous formulation to extremes of temperature by heating and to different pH by mixing with an acid and a base. The degradation products should not interfere with the measurement of the drug for a method to be stability-indicating (22). The pH is also measured on each study day. The drug is considered stable if its physical characteristics have not changed and its concentration has remained above 90% of the initial concentration.

PALATABILITY

The child's acceptance of a liquid dose form is primarily dependent on its palatability. A better-tasting drug is easier to administer to infants and young children, and thus loss of drug from spillage during dose administration is minimized. In general, ease of administration and adherence may be enhanced with improved taste.

The taste of drug formulations should be evaluated in children by using a 5-point hedonic (facial expression) scale (23). The overall taste perception should reflect initial taste, aftertaste, flavor, and texture of the formulations. Interestingly, taste is rarely studied in children, even for commercially available formulations. These studies

TABLE 10.3 Drug Formulations Chosen by 5% or More of the Respondents for Which No Information Was Available or More Information Was Needed for Compounding and/or Stability

Drug Formulation	*Drug Status*	*Number of Respondents (%)*	*Usual Route of Administration*
Acetazolamide	M	4 (8.5)	p.o., p.t.
Allopurinol	M	12 (25.5)	p.o., p.t.
Amiodarone[a]	N	6 (11.5)	p.o., p.t.
Amlodipine[b]	N	6 (11.5)	p.o., p.t.
Aspirin	N	3 (5.8)	p.o., p.t.
Azathioprine	M	4 (8.5)	p.o.
Baclofen	M	5 (10.6)	p.o.
Caffeine (base)	M	6 (12.8)	p.o., p.t.
Caffeine citrate[c]	M	7 (14.9)	p.o., i.v.
Calcitriol[c]	N	3 (5.8)	p.o.
Captopril	M	24 (51.0)	p.o., p.t.
Ciprofloxacin[c]	N	6 (11.5)	p.o., p.t.
Ciprofloxacin[c]	M	4 (8.5)	p.o.
Clonazepam	M	8 (17.0)	p.o., p.t.
Dantrolene[f]	N	8 (16)	p.o., p.t.
Dexamethasone[d]	M	3 (6.4)	p.o.
Enalapril[b]	N	14 (26.9)	p.o.
Ethambutol	N	3 (5.8)	p.o., p.t.
Flecainide	M	4 (8.5)	p.o.
Flucytosine	M	4 (8.5)	p.o.
Gabapentin[a]	N	4 (7.7)	p.o.
Ganciclovir[a]	N	4 (7.7)	p.o., p.t.
Glycopyrrolate[e]	N	3 (5.8)	p.o.
Hydralazine[b]	N	3 (5.8)	p.o., p.t.
Labetalol	M	3 (6.4)	p.o.
Labetalol[b]	N	5 (9.6)	p.o., p.t.
Lansoprazole	N	5 (9.6)	p.o.
Leucovorin	N	3 (5.8)	p.o., p.t.
Levothyroxine[b]	N	10 (19.2)	p.o.
Lorazepam[d]	N	3 (5.8)	p.o., i.v.
Metolazone	M	6 (12.8)	p.o., p.t.
Metoprolol	M	3 (6.4)	p.o.
Metronidazole	M	18 (38.3)	p.o.
Midazolam	M	3 (6.4)	p.o., i.v.
Mycophenolate mofetil[c]	N	5 (9.6)	p.o.
Mycophenolate mofetil[c]	M	5 (10.6)	p.o.
Nifedipine	N	11 (21.2)	p.o.
Omeprazole[a]	N	11 (21.2)	p.o., p.t.
Omeprazole[a]	M	7 (14.9)	p.o.
Paroxetine[c]	N	3 (5.8)	p.o., p.t.
Prazosin	N	3 (5.8)	p.o., p.t.
Procainamide	M	4 (8.5)	p.o.
Rifabutin[c]	N	3 (5.8)	p.o., p.t.
Rifampin	M	11 (23.4)	p.o.
Sotalol	N	5 (9.6)	p.o., p.t.
Spironolactone	M	33 (70.2)	p.o., p.t.
Spironolactone/hydrochlorothiazide	M	5 (10.6)	p.o., p.t.
Tacrolimus	M	6 (12.8)	p.o.
Topiramate	N	3 (5.8)	p.o.
Ursodiol	M	20 (42.6)	p.o.
Ursodiol[b]	N	3 (5.8)	p.o., p.t.
Verapamil	M	3 (6.4)	p.o.
Warfarin	N	6 (11.5)	p.o., p.t.

i.v., intravenous; M, more information needed; N, no information available, p.o., oral; p.t., per tube (gastric or nasogastric).
[a]Stability data published during the survey.
[b]Stability data (by analytical methods) available.
[c]Manufacturer marketed product during the survey.
[d]Currently marketed.
[e]No stability data.
[f]Stability data as "experience" only, not confirmed by analytical means.

TABLE 10.4 Drug Formulations and Routes of Administration Chosen by 5% or Less of the Respondents When a Liquid Dose Form Was Needed

Drug Formulations for Which Adequate Information is Available	*Route of Administration*	*Drug Formulations for Which Longer and Better Information is Needed*	*Route of Administration*	*Drug Formulations for Which Compounding and Stability Information is Needed*	*Route of Administration*
Acetic acid[a] (3%)	t.p.	Acyclovir[b]	p.o.	Acetaminophen (≤40 mg)	p.r.
Aminophylline[b] (10 mg/ml)	p.o., i.v.	Alum (aluminum potassium sulfate)[a]	Bladder irrigation	Albendazole	p.o.
Amiodarone[c]	p.o.	Amitriptyline[b]	p.o., i.v.	Amiloride[d]	p.o.
Amlodipine	p.o.	Amlodipine	p.o.	Amitriptyline[b]	p.t.
Atovaquone[e]	p.o.	Amphotericin B[e]	p.o.	Aspartate (6.25%)	i.v.
Bethanechol	p.o.	Arginine[b]	i.v.	Atropine	p.o.
Biotin[a]	p.o.	Atenolol	p.o.	Biotin	p.o.
Busulfan[a]	p.o.	Busulfan[a]	p.o.	Bupropion	p.o.
Butt paste (1:1:1 corn starch, zinc oxide, petrolatum)[a]	t.p.	Butt paste (1:1:1 corn starch, zinc oxide, petrolatum)[a]	t.p.	Busulfan	p.o.
Clark's solution[a]	p.o.	Caffeine (base)	p.o.	Caffeine citrate	p.o.
Clonidine[a]	p.o., p.t.	Caffeine citrate[f]	p.o.	Calcium carbonate	p.o.
Codeine (3 mg/mL)[e]	p.o.	Carbenicillin[a]	p.o.	Carbamazepine	p.r.
Dakins's solution[a]	t.p.	Cefepime[b]	i.v.	Carbenicillin	p.o.
Dantrolene[g]	p.o.	Cholestyramine/Aquaphor[a]	t.p.	Chlorothiazide[e]	p.o.
Dexamethasone[e]	p.o.	Ciprofloxacin[f]	p.o.	Chloroquine[d]	p.o.
Diltiazem[a]	p.o.	Cisapride[e]	p.o.	Cholestyramine[e]	p.o.
Dinoprostone gel	p.v.	Clonidine[a]	p.o.	Clindamycin mouthwash (300 mg/L)	p.o. (t.p.)
Enalapril					
Coenzyme Q[a]	p.o.	Clobazam	p.o.		
Ferinsol drops[e]	p.o.	Cyclophosphamide	p.o.	Clonazepam[d]	p.o.
Folic acid	p.o.	Desmopressin[b]	i.v.	Clonidine	p.o., p.t.
Glutamine[a]	p.o.	Dexamethasone (1 mg/mL)[e]	p.o.	Cyclophosphamide[d]	p.o.
Glycopyrrolate[a]	p.o.	Dextroamphetamine[a]	p.o.	Cycloserine	p.o.
Hydralazine	p.o.	Digoxin[b]	i.v.	Dantrolene[g]	p.o.
Hydrochlorothiazide[e]	p.o.	Doxapram[b]	i.v.	Desmopressin[b]	p.o.
Hydrocortisone cypionate[e]	p.o.	Enalapril	p.o.	Dexamethasone (≥0.5 mg/mL)[e]	p.o.
Insulin (NPH) (10 or 50 units/mL)[b]	s.c.	Enalaprilat[b]	i.v.	Diazepam[e]	p.r.
Insulin (regular) (10 or 50 units/mL)[b]	s.c.	Ephedrine[e]	p.o.	Diltiazem	p.o.
Isradipine	p.o.	Ethambutol[a]	p.o.	Enoxaparin[b,e]	s.c.
Leucovorin[a]	p.o.	Famotidine[e]	p.o.	Erythromycin (base, 100 mg/mL)	p.o.
Lidocaine/adrenaline/tetracaine[a]	t.p.	Filgrastim[b,e]	i.v.	Ethionamide	p.o.
Lorazepam[e]	p.o.	Flecainide	p.o.	Famciclovir	p.o.
Magic mouthwash[a]	t.p.	Flucytosine	p.o.	Flucytosine[d]	p.o.
Methylcellulose 1%[a,g]	p.o.	Folic acid	p.o.	Fludrocortisone	p.o.
Mineral oil/glycerin[a]	p.r.	Furosemide[e]	i.v.	Folic acid[d]	p.o.
Morphine (1 mg/mL)[b]	i.v.	Gentamicin[a]	p.o.	Glutamate (7.32%)	i.v.
Neomycin (1 g/10 mL)[b]	p.o.	Glutamine[a]	p.o.	Granisetron[c]	p.o.
Phenazopyridine	p.o.	Hydrochlorothiazide[e]	p.o.	Happy Hiney (Maalox, nystatin, cholestyramine)	t.p.
Phenobarbital (10 mg/mL)[b]	p.o.	Hydrocortisone suspension[e]	p.o.	Hydroxyurea	p.o.
Prednisone (10 mg/mL)[b]	p.o.	Indomethacin[b]	i.v.	Ibuprofen	p.r.
Propranolol[e]	p.o.	Itraconazole (40 mg/mL)[b]	p.o.	Ketoconazole[d]	p.o.
Sodium benzoate[a]	p.o.	Labetalol	p.o.	Lamotrigine[c]	p.o.
Sodium bicarbonate (1 mEq/L)	p.o.	Lamotrigine[c]	p.o.	Lisinopril	p.o.

(*continued*)

TABLE 10.4 Drug Formulations and Routes of Administration Chosen by 5% or Less of the Respondents When a Liquid Dose Form Was Needed (*Continued*)

Drug Formulations for Which Adequate Information is Available	*Route of Administration*	*Drug Formulations for Which Longer and Better Information is Needed*	*Route of Administration*	*Drug Formulations for Which Compounding and Stability Information is Needed*	*Route of Administration*
Sodium chloride (2.5 mEq/L)[a]	p.o.	Lidocaine/epinephrine/tetracaine gel	t.p.	Lomustine	p.o.
Sotalol[a]	p.o.	Lidocaine buffered[a]	t.p.	Maalox (30 mL)/hyoscyamine sulfate (10 mL)/lidocaine (20%, 5 mL)	p.o. (t.p.)
Squaric acid[a]	t.p.	Lomustine[a]	p.o.	Magnesium oxide	p.r.
Testosterone (2%)[a]	t.p.	Magnesium oxide[a]	p.o.	Mefloquine	p.o.
Thioguanine	p.o.	Magnesium sulfate[e]	p.o.	Mesalamine	p.o.
Vancomycin (5 mg/mL)[b]	i.v.	Meropenem[b]	i.v.	Methimazole	p.o.
Vitamin infant drops[e]	p.t.	Methadone[b]	i.v.	Methotrexate	p.o.
Zinc sulfate[a]	p.o.	Methylprednisolone (1, 4, 10 mg/mL)[b]	i.v.	Methyldopa[e]	p.o.
		Metoprolol	p.o.	Methylphenidate	p.o.
		Mexiletine	p.o.	Metronidazole[d]	t.p.
		Minoxidil[a]	p.o.	Mexiletine[d]	p.o.
		Mycophenolate mofetil	p.o.	Morphine (0.1 mg/mL)[b]	p.o.
		Myle's Magic Mix (nystatin, erythromycin, hydrocortisone, lidocaine, sterile water)[a]	p.o. (t.p.)	Neomycin (250 mg/5 mL)[b]	p.o., p.t.
		Nifedipine[a]	p.o.	Nevirapine[f]	p.o.
		Nitrofurantoin[e]	p.o.	Niacin[e]	p.o.
		Phenobarbital (10 mg/mL)[b]	i.v.	Nicardipine	p.o.
		Phytonadione[g]	p.o.	Nimodipine	p.o.
		Pink Magic (diphenhydramine, Maalox, lidocaine)[a]	p.o. (t.p.)	Ofloxacin	p.o.
		Prazosin[a]	p.o.	Olanzapine	p.o., p.t.
		Probenecid[a]	p.o.	Parcrease	p.o., p.t.
		Propafenone[a]	p.o.	Paromomycin	p.o., p.t.
		Propranolol[e]	p.o.	Pentobarbital[e]	p.o., p.t.
		Prostaglandin E2 gel	p.v.	Phenazopyridine[d]	p.o., p.t.
		Pyrazinamide	p.o.	Phenobarbital (nonalcoholic)	p.o.
		Riboflavin[a]	p.o.	Phenytoin	p.r.
		Rifabutin[f]	p.o.	Phenoxybenzamine	p.o.
		Sodium bicarbonate (1 mEq/mL)[e]	p.o.	Phytonadione	p.o., p.t.
		Sotalol[a]	p.o.	Prednisone (≥1 mg/mL)[e]	p.o.
		Sulfadiazine[g]	p.o.	Prednisolone (10 mg/mL)	p.o.
		Sulfasalazine[a]	p.o.	Primidone	p.r.
		Tacrolimus	p.o.	Procarbazine[g]	p.o.
		Terbutaline[e]	i.v.	Propafenone	p.o.
		Thioguanine	p.o.	Propranolol[e]	p.o., p.t.
		Tissue plasminogen activator[e]	i.v.	Propylthiouracil[c]	p.o.
		Tobramycin[a]	o.a.	Pyridoxine[g]	p.o.
		Triflupromazine[b]	i.v.	Rifampin[d]	p.o.
		Tropicamide 1%/cyclopentolate 1%/phenylephrine 10%[a]	o.u.	Saquinavir	p.o.
		Vancomycin[a]	o.a.	Scopolamine	p.o., t.p. (gel)
		Vancomycin paste (0.5% methylcellulose)[a]	t.p.	Sertraline	p.o.

(*continued*)

TABLE 10.4 Drug Formulations and Routes of Administration Chosen by 5% or Less of the Respondents When a Liquid Dose Form Was Needed (*Continued*)

Drug Formulations for Which Adequate Information is Available	*Route of Administration*	*Drug Formulations for Which Longer and Better Information is Needed*	*Route of Administration*	*Drug Formulations for Which Compounding and Stability Information is Needed*	*Route of Administration*
		Verapamil	p.o.	Silver nitrate in water for irrigation	t.p.
		Vitamin A (aquasol A 10,000 units/mL)[b]	p.o.	Sodium bicarbonate (1 mEq/mL)[d]	p.o.
		Zinc sulfate[a]	p.o.	Sodium chloride (2.5 mEq/mL)[a]	p.o.
				Sodium polystyrene sulfonate[e]	p.o.
				Spironolactone[d]	p.o.
				Tacrolimus[d]	p.o.
				Valproate	p.r.
				Vigabatrin	p.o.
				Zinc sulfate	p.o.

i.v., intravenous; o.a., in the ears (otic); o.u., in the eyes (ophthalmic); p.o., oral; p.r., per rectal; p.t., per tube (gastric or nasogastric); p.v., per vaginal; t.p., topical; s.c., subcutaneous; NPH, neutral protamine hagedron.
[a]No stability data.
[b]Marketed, but some strengths with no stability data.
[c]Stability data published during the survey.
[d]Stability data (by analytical methods) available.
[e]Currently marketed.
[f]Manufacturer marketed product during the survey.
[g]Stability data as "experience" only, not confirmed by analytical methods.

generally are performed in adult volunteers. It is difficult to predict whether the Human Subjects Research Committee would approve such comparative studies in children.

STERILITY AND PYROGEN TESTING

Intravenous drug formulations must be tested for sterility and pyrogens. When a commercially available concentrated drug is diluted to 1/10 of the original concentration, the preservative is also diluted to 1/10. Such a modified formulation may not contain a sufficient amount of preservative to retard the growth of microorganisms during storage or clinical use. Furthermore, the modified formulation may be contaminated during its preparation from the commercially available product. US Pharmacopeia (USP) procedures should be used for the testing of sterility and pyrogens.

FUNDING OF RESEARCH

When a new drug is marketed for adults, the manufacturer may have little interest in supporting research on developing a liquid formulation for infants and children. Unfortunately, this lack of interest continues for years and decades unless the drug is labeled for pediatric patients. There are many reasons for this lack of enthusiasm, including limited resources and small size of the pediatric market. In some cases, the manufacturer may not share the stability data of a drug in a liquid dose form because it has not evaluated its efficacy and safety in pediatric patients. In addition, some manufacturers may believe that supporting an independent researcher to develop a drug formulation may violate FDA regulations because this would lead to its use in children without adequate efficacy and safety studies in the pediatric population.

The FDA's Orphan Drug Program is designed to support clinical studies, not to develop stable liquid dose forms. In addition, the funding from this program is not targeted toward the labeling of drugs for pediatric patients. This type of research may also be considered to be applied for the typical National Institutes of Health applications for funding.

Professional associations have made a plea to manufacturers to make the appropriate formulations available to children. However, they do not have sufficient financial resources to support research in this area. The Council on Professional Affairs of the American Society of Health-System Pharmacists (ASHP) urged the organization to "directly fund such research" because "errors can occur in dilutions and formulations, leading to patient harm." However, the Board of Directors felt that the "direct funding of such research" was not the primary responsibility of ASHP and that "ASHP should encourage others to develop pediatric dosage forms of drug products" (24). Universities have supported pilot projects for their faculty, but such support generally is not sustained.

The National Institute of Child Health and Human Development, through its Pediatric Pharmacology Research

Units grant, should commit a small portion of its budget to developing stable liquid dose forms of drugs for infants and children. Once the studies are conducted and results disseminated through peer-reviewed journals, any pharmacist can prepare the dose form for their patients (6,25,26).

REGULATIONS FOR PEDIATRIC DRUG FORMULATIONS

The FDA has issued new regulations requiring manufacturers to conduct pediatric studies and seek labeling for new drugs in pediatric patients. However, the requirement can be waived for a number of reasons, including difficulty in developing a pediatric formulation, as long as "reasonable efforts" are made (27). It is unclear what would be sufficient as "reasonable efforts."

The small size of the pediatric market for most drugs is perhaps the leading reason for the lack of investment in drug development for this population. The FDA provides incentives to the industry (6-month extension of exclusivity and waiver of fees for the supplemental new drug application) for pediatric drug development. This may lead to increased availability of pediatric formulations of new drugs; however, extemporaneous formulations will still be needed for generic drugs and for new drugs with limited market size.

The FDA Modernization Act of 1997 also has provisions for bulk drug substances. Effective November 21, 1998, the FDA must develop and publish regulations to address various aspects of pharmacy compounding. The compounding law stipulates that the bulk substances used in compounding should be (a) components of an FDA-approved drug product, (b) in a USP or National Formulary (NF) monograph, or (c) included in a list developed by the FDA, with the input from its Pharmacy Compounding Advisory Committee (28). A request for inclusion of substances on this list was published by the FDA in April 1998. The efforts of the FDA and USP compounding advisory committees are ongoing.

SHARING OF DATA INFORMATION RESOURCES

The results should continue to be disseminated through presentations at national meetings, in publications in peer-reviewed journals, in books, and on the Internet (1,29,30). In addition, the data from stability, palatability, and microbial studies should be included in the drug monographs. For example, compatibility data on most intravenous drugs and stability data on oral rifampin in a liquid are included in the manufacturers' package information (31). It is critical, however, to indicate the details of all the excipients and methods for preparation and storage in the monograph to ensure reproducibility. Finally, lack of bioavailability data and clinical experience should be clearly indicated. The clinical experience with extemporaneous formulations should continue to be shared through publications, as is done for off-label use of drugs in pediatric patients.

A study involving 10 highly cited journals reported that less than 40% of the articles published in these journals provided adequate information about the formulations of oral medications used in drug trials among patients younger than 2 years of age (32). This would limit the use of data from these studies in patient care.

CONTINUED NEED FOR EXTEMPORANEOUS FORMULATIONS

The need for extemporaneous formulations will continue unless all medicines have been approved for newborn infants, infants, children, and adults. This is unlikely to happen for both new and generic drugs. Thus, stability studies would be required to assure the potency of extemporaneously prepared medicines during storage and use in patients. The studies should provide specific details about ingredients and methods so that variability in the preparation of formulations can be prevented. Studies on the bioavailability, efficacy, and safety would be desirable, although the funding for such studies would be difficult to generate. It is important, however, to monitor efficacy and safety of all extemporaneous drug formulations in patients.

The adverse event reporting systems (the USP's MEDMARX system or the FDA's MedWatch program) in the United States are voluntary and were designed to record adverse events from commercially available drug products, not from extemporaneous formulations. Thus, a mechanism to capture adverse events associated with the use of extemporaneous drug formulations in pediatric patients is needed so that such events can be minimized in the future.

SUMMARY

Availability of an appropriate formulation is a rate-limiting step for the clinical use of medicines in infants and children. Funding of research on extemporaneous formulations should be increased. The studies on these formulations should simulate clinical conditions for their use and utilize reproducible and rigorous methodologies. The results and clinical experience with pediatric drug formulations should be shared through presentations, publications, and the Internet.

REFERENCES

1. Nahata MC, Pai V, Hipple TF. *Pediatric drug formulations*, 5th ed. Cincinnati, OH: Harvey Whitney, 2003.
2. Pai V, Nahata MC. Need for extemporaneous formulations in pediatric patients. *J Pediatr Pharmacol Ther* 2001;6:107–119.
3. Nahata MC, Morosco RS, Hipple TF. Stability of amiodarone in extemporaneously oral suspension prepared from commonly available vehicles. *J Pediatr Pharm Pract* 1999;4:186–189.
4. Nahata MC, Morosco RS, Hipple TF. Stability of amlodipine besylate in two liquid dosage forms. *J Am Pharm Assoc* 1999;39: 375–377.
5. Pereira CM, Tam YK. Stability of captopril in tap water. *Am J Hosp Pharm* 1992;49:612–615.
6. Nahata MC, Hipple TF, Morosco RS. Stability of captopril in three liquid dosage forms. *Am J Hosp Pharm* 1994;51:95–96.

7. Nahata MC, Morosco RS, Hipple TF. Stability of captopril in liquid containing ascorbic acid or sodium ascorbate. *Am J Hosp Pharm* 1994;51:1707–1708.
8. Nahata MC, Morosco RS, Hipple TF. Stability of cimetidine hydrochloride and of clindamycin phosphate in water for injection stored in glass vials at two temperatures. *Am J Hosp Pharm* 1993;50:2559–2561.
9. Nahata MC, Morosco RS, Hipple TF. Stability of enalapril maleate in three extemporaneously prepared oral liquids. *Am J Health Syst Pharm* 1998;55:1155–1157.
10. Abdel-Rahman SM, Nahata MC. Stability of fumagillin in an extemporaneously prepared ophthalmic solution. *Am J Health Syst Pharm* 1999;56:547–550.
11. Nahata MC. Stability of gabapentin in extemporaneously prepared suspensions at two temperatures. *Pediatr Neurol* 1999;20: 195–197.
12. Dressman JB, Poust RI. Stability of allopurinol and 5 antineoplastics in suspension. *Am J Hosp Pharm* 1983;40:616–618.
13. Nahata MC, Morosco RS, Hipple TF. Physical and chemical stability of mexiletine in two extemporaneous liquid formulations stored under refrigeration and at room temperature. *J Am Pharm Assoc* 2000;40:257–259.
14. Nahata MC, Hipple TF, Morosco RS. Stability of morphine sulfate diluted in 0.9% NaCl for injection. *Am J Hosp Pharm* 1992;49: 2785–2787.
15. Nahata MC, Hipple TF, Strausbaugh S. Stability of phenobarbital sodium diluted in 0.9% NaCl for injection. *Am J Hosp Pharm* 1986;43:384–385.
16. Nahata MC, Morosco RS, Hipple TF. Stability of spironolactone in an extemporaneously prepared suspension at two temperatures. *Ann Pharmacother* 1993;27:1198–1199.
17. Allen LV Jr, Erickson MA. Stability of ketoconazole, metolazone, metronidazole, procainamide hydrochloride, spironolactone in extemporaneously compounded oral liquids. *Am J Health Syst Pharm* 1996;53:2073–2078.
18. Abdel-Rahman SM, Nahata MC. Stability of terbinafine hydrochloride in an extemporaneously prepared oral suspension at 25 and 4 degrees C. *Am J Health Syst Pharm* 1999;56:243–245.
19. Berman W, Whitman V, Marks KH, et al. Inadvertent over administration of digoxin to low birth weight infants. *J Pediatr* 1978; 92:1024–1025.
20. Zenk KE, Anderson S. Improving the accuracy of mini-volume injections. *Infusion* 1982;6:7–11.
21. Duncan B, Barton LL, Eicher ML, et al. Medication-induced pneumatosis intestinalis. *Pediatrics* 1997;99:633–636.
22. Trissel LA. Assay reliability [letter]. *Am J Health Syst Pharm* 1998;55:491.
23. Mastsui D, Baron A, Rieder MJ. Assessment of the palatability of antistaphyloccal antibiotics in pediatric volunteers. *Ann Pharmacother* 1996;30:586–588.
24. The American Society of Health-System Pharmacists Reports. Council on professional affairs. *Am J Health Syst Pharm* 1997;54: 819–826.
25. Wintermeyer S, Nahata MC. Stability of flucytosine in an extemporaneously compounded oral liquid. *Am J Health Syst Pharm* 1996;53:407–412.
26. Nahata MC, Morosco RS, Hipple TF. Stability of cisapride in a liquid dosage form at two temperatures. *Ann Pharmacother* 1995;29: 125–127.
27. US Department of Health and Human Services, Food and Drug Administration. 21 CFR Parts 201, 312, 314, and 601 (Docket No. 97N-0165; RIN 0910-AB20). Regulations requiring manufacturers to assess the safety and effectiveness of new drugs and biological products in pediatric patients; final rule. *Fed Regist* 1998; 63(231):66631–66672.
28. English T. Compounding symposium covers all the bases. *Pharmacy Today* 1998;4:13.
29. Trissel L. *Trissel's stability of compounded formulations.* Washington, DC: American Pharmaceutical Association, 1996.
30. Allen LV. *The art, science, and technology of pharmaceutical compounding.* Washington, DC: American Pharmaceutical Association, 1998.
31. *Physicians' desk reference,* 52nd ed. Montvale, NJ: Medical Economics Co, 1998.
32. Standing JF, Khaki ZF, Wong IC. Poor formulation information in published pediatric drug trials. *Pediatrics* 2005;116:e559–e562.

CHAPTER

11

Donald R. Mattison

Developmental Toxicology

INTRODUCTION

The United States has made progress in maternal and infant health (1–4); infant mortality has fallen (Fig. 11.1) as a consequence of pediatric nutrition, enhanced sanitation and food safety, and improvements in care for premature infants (5–12). Despite these advances, the United States has the worst rate of infant mortality among industrialized nations and ranks 30th internationally (Table 11.1) (12–14). In addition, substantial disparities in infant mortality have persisted despite attempts to alleviate these differences (Fig. 11.2) (15–20).

As a consequence of the decrease in overall infant mortality, the leading cause of infant death in the United States and in many developed countries today is birth defects (21–23), which account for ~25% of all infant deaths (Fig. 11.3). Prematurity and its consequences, including low birth weight and respiratory distress syndrome, is the second leading cause of infant mortality overall. Among African Americans, prematurity is the primary cause of infant mortality, accounting in part for the substantially higher infant mortality rates in that community.

The increasing relative impact of birth defects on infant mortality is drawing more attention to this public health problem. For example, there is mounting concern about environmental pollutants and their impact on pregnancy outcome and infant health (24,25). Similarly, there is growing interest in the effect of disasters (Katrina, Ike, and World Trade Center) on pregnancy outcome and infant health (26). The Trust for America's Health has mounted a campaign to critically evaluate the ability of state health departments to monitor birth defects and use the data in public health decision making (27). The Birth Defects Prevention Act of 1998 (Public Law 105-168) authorized the Centers for Disease Control and Prevention (CDC) to collect, analyze, and make available data on birth defects. The Children's Health Act of 2000 established a National Center on Birth Defects and Developmental Disabilities (NCBDDD) at the CDC (28). The CDC provides funding to address problems that hinder birth defect surveillance programs (29) which are critical to identification of causes and interventions. Unfortunately, the causes of many birth defects are poorly understood (30–33). When the cause of a particular birth defect is unknown, health scientists suspect the possibility that environmental or occupational exposures may play a substantial role (31–36).

This chapter summarizes knowledge about (a) causes of birth defects and other adverse developmental outcomes (including death and abnormalities of function or growth); (b) levels of exposure to potential developmental hazards; (c) ways to determine whether an exposure to a chemical, physical, or a biological agent may be capable of producing embryo or fetal death, structural malformations, functional abnormalities, or alterations in growth; and (d) the level of certainty (or uncertainty) with regard to various data and risk assessments (37).

BACKGROUND ON DEVELOPMENTAL DISEASE

Developmental diseases may be described in terms of origins or outcomes. Table 11.2 provides definitions of terms associated with developmental diseases.

ORIGINS OF DEVELOPMENTAL DISEASE

Some birth defects occur because an embryo or fetus is destined to develop abnormally from the time of fertilization (36–38). These are called *malformations.* The risk of developing a malformation sometimes can be reduced. For example, folic acid supplements (400 μg) taken prior to fertilization (conception) may reduce the risk of neural tube defects, a serious and common malformation (39–45), by as much as 70% (35,42–45). Of interest are recent data suggesting that increasing the dose (up to 4 mg) may further reduce the risk of developmental disease (42–45). Note, however, that not all neural tube defects result from deficiencies in folic acid (46–49).

Other developmental diseases occur because fetal growth is physically restricted (*deformation*) (50). An infant with a deformation would have been normal if the physical restriction of growth had not occurred during intrauterine development (51,52). One example of a deformation is Potter syndrome (53), a deformation produced by inadequate formation of amniotic fluid, which results in abnormal skeletal and lung development (54–57).

An infant who might have been normal at birth but instead is born with a developmental disease because of

TABLE 11.1	Comparison of Infant Mortality Rates (Deaths/1,000 Live Births) and International Rankings for Selected Countries	
Country	*Infant Mortality Rate*	*International Ranking*
Australia	5.0	21
Belgium	3.7	10
Canada	5.4	25
Denmark	4.4	17
England and Wales	5.0	21
France	3.6	9
Germany	3.9	12
Japan	2.8	4
Sweden	2.4	2
United States	6.9	30

Data from Health, United States 2008, with Special Feature on the Health of Young Adults. http://www.cdc.gov/nchs/data/hus/hus08.pdf. Accessed March 13, 2009.

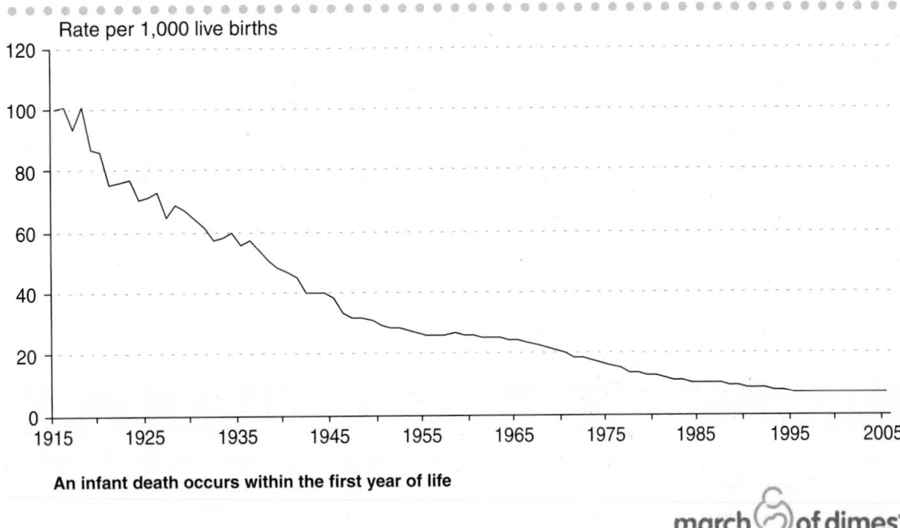

Figure 11.1. Infant mortality in the United States during the period 1915 through 2000. (Data from the National Center for Health Statistics, Centers for Disease Control and Prevention, Department of Health and Human Services, prepared by the Perinatal Data Center of the March of Dimes.)

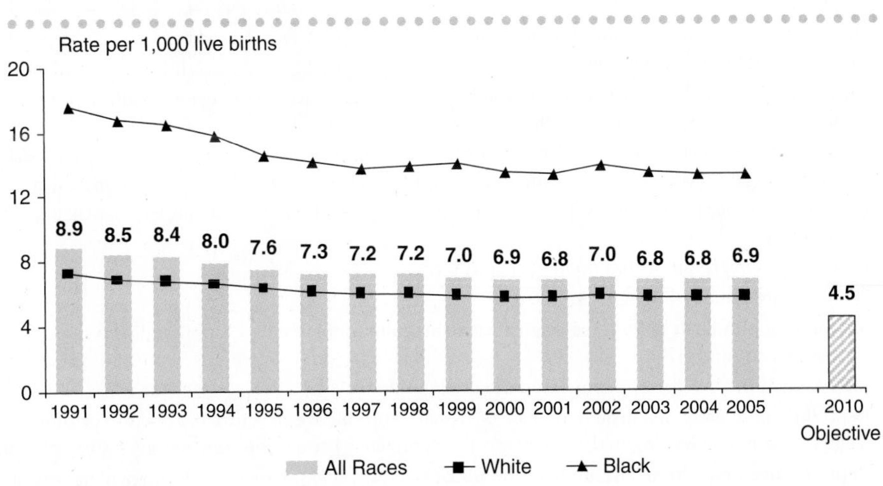

Figure 11.2. Infant mortality by maternal race during the period 1989 through 2000. (Data from the National Center for Health Statistics, Centers for Disease Control and Prevention, Department of Health and Human Services, prepared by the Perinatal Data Center, March of Dimes.)

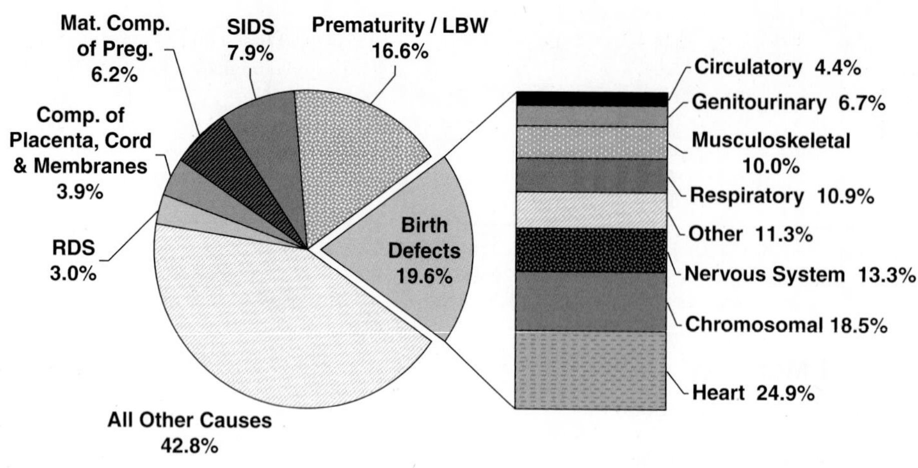

Figure 11.3. Leading cause of infant deaths in the United States during 1999. LBW, low birth weight; RDS, respiratory distress syndrome. SIDS, sudden infant death syndrome. (Data from the National Center for Health Statistics, Centers for Disease Control and Prevention, Department of Health and Human Services, prepared by the Perinatal Data Center, March of Dimes.)

exposure to a chemical, physical, or a biological agent has a preventable developmental disease called a *disruption.* Examples of disruptions include congenital rubella syndrome, neurodevelopmental abnormalities produced by exposure to lead, and those produced by exposures to ionizing radiation (31,32,36,58–60).

Estimates of the percentage of birth defects that might be related to environmental risks have evolved over time as scientists' understanding of developmental processes and causes of disease have progressed (Table 11.3). However, all estimates are problematic when one considers that many birth defects may have more than one cause. Earliest estimates

TABLE 11.2 Working Definitions of Terms Used in this Chapter

Birth defect: A physical/structural, functional, or metabolic abnormality in an embryo or fetus that results in physical or mental disability or is fatal; it may be manifested at any time, from just before or after birth through sexual maturation

Deformation: A structural or functional developmental abnormality (birth defect) resulting from physical forces acting on the fetus

Development: The process of growth and maturation from an immature to a more mature stage

Developmental disease: Any alteration in the growth, life span, structure, or function of an embryo or fetus either before or after birth up to the time of sexual maturation

Developmental hazard: A chemical, biological, or physical agent that produces developmental disease when exposure occurs to a parent prior to conception, a mother following conception, or the infant or child

Disruption: A birth defect caused by an exposure to a developmental hazard

Environment: Most broadly includes the social, chemical, physical, economic, infectious, and cultural exposures experienced by an individual

Functional abnormality: An alteration in the function (e.g., behavior, intelligence, kidney, or lung function) of an individual that occurs as a consequence of exposure to a developmental hazard

Gene: A specific portion of an inherited pattern of chemicals repeated in every cell of an animal or plant, which is transmitted from parent to offspring, and which may determine development, structure, or function of the organism

Gene–environment interactions: Interactions among chemical, physical, social, biological, and other influences within an organism so as to modify gene expression

Infant mortality: Death within the first year of life

Low birth weight: Birth weight ≤2,500 g

Malformation: A birth defect resulting from intrinsically abnormal developmental processes, for example, due to a genetic abnormality (e.g., Down syndrome)

Prematurity: Birth before 37 completed weeks of gestation.

Reproductive disease: Impairment of male or female reproductive structure or function produced by exposure to a chemical, physical, or a biological agent and leading to decreased fertility, completely preventing conception or survival of the fertilized egg, or preventing implantation

Reproductive toxicology: The study of the impact of chemical, physical, or biological agents on the reproductive processes, including formation, release, and interactions of the gametes, the sperm, and the egg; reproductive processes are generally considered to end when fertilization takes place

Teratogen: A chemical, physical, or biological agent capable of producing a disruption in an embryo or fetus (see also developmental hazard)

TABLE 11.3 Estimates of the Environmental Impact on Birth Defects

Reference	*Genetic or Chromosomal (%)*	*Teratogen (%)*	*Gene–Environment (%)*	*Unknown (%)*	*Comment*
30, 58, 61	25	10	Not estimated	65	These estimates were based on hospital data and inadequate population data
62	17	3	37	43	Hospital-based survey
(Shaw, oral communication, 2000	Not estimated	Not estimated	75	25	Estimate based on research birth defects program

(30,58,61) suggested that about 10% of birth defects were due to teratogens, 25% were due to genetic/chromosomal abnormalities, and 65% were of unknown origin. These estimates were widely cited in most publications about the origin of developmental abnormalities until a 1989 study by Nelson and Holmes (62) estimated that about 3% of birth defects are due to teratogens, 17% are genetic/chromosomal, 37% are due to gene–environment interactions, and 43% are of unknown origin. Each of these estimates was consistent with the scientific understanding at the time, which suggested that single factors were important causal agents (e.g., infectious agents, physical factors, chemicals, or maternal conditions responsible for most birth defects.

Our current scientific understanding has evolved. Thus, while earlier estimates of etiology or causation of developmental abnormalities emphasized the small number of birth defects caused by known teratogens (less than 10%), more recent estimates have included an increasing percentage of birth defects produced by gene–environment interactions (62,63). Gene–environment interactions refer to the fact that the individual carries genetic factors that modify the susceptibility of the fetus to the disruptive effect of an environmental agent that produces the birth defect or developmental abnormality observed (24,64–66). This leads to a model for developmental disease like that illustrated in Figure 11.4, in which the risk for a developmental disease is a consequence of an interaction among environmental, social, and biological factors (67–69). G. Shaw (oral communication, 2000), using data from the California Birth Defects Monitoring system, estimated that many birth defects (up to 75%) are due to gene–environment interactions. In contrast, estimates of structural malformations of unknown origin have decreased from 65% to 43% to 25%, suggesting an increase in knowledge. However, there remains much uncertainty about the diseases thought to be caused through gene–environment interaction.

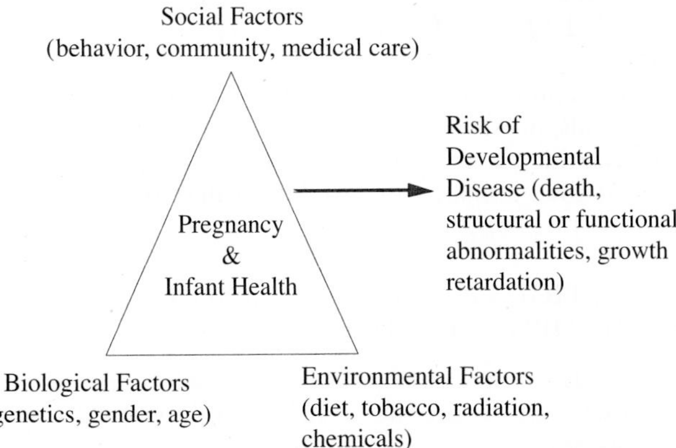

Figure 11.4. Factors associated with adverse pregnancy outcome. Single factors, while prominent in earlier thinking about birth defects and developmental disabilities, are being displaced by growing understanding of the multiple interacting factors now known to be responsible.

Why do scientists think environmental factors play any role in birth defects? Studies have demonstrated that animals treated with chemicals found in the environment and for which there is human exposure produce birth defects in the animals; human epidemiologic studies have also demonstrated an association between such exposures and developmental disease (31,32,36,60,70). In addition, epidemiologists have explored the relationship between the environment and birth defects, with results that suggest that the environment appears to play a significant but poorly defined role, in part due to inadequate investment in biomarker-based epidemiologic research.

OUTCOMES

At least four health outcomes result from birth defects: death, structural abnormalities, functional abnormalities, and alteration of growth. A fifth outcome, premature birth, is also discussed briefly, although it is not usually categorized as a birth defect. Each type of outcome is illustrated in the following discussion.

Death

One class of drugs used to treat hypertension acts by inhibiting the angiotensin-converting enzyme (ACE). When experimental animals are treated with ACE inhibitors, fetal death rates increase (31,32,36,38,71,72). Similar observations have been made in women treated with ACE inhibitors during pregnancy (73,74). It is thought that fetal death results from a substantial reduction in renal blood flow and inhibition of renal development produced by these drugs. Because of the impact on fetal renal blood flow, despite the potential benefit for management of hypertension in some pregnant women, it is recommended that ACE inhibitors not be used during pregnancy.

Structural Malformation

It has been estimated that there are approximately 75 chemicals and drugs that are known to produce human structural malformations (31,32,36,38,63,71,72). One well-known chemical that is associated with structural malformations of both male and female reproductive systems is diethylstilbestrol (DES). DES was used to treat women early in pregnancy because it was thought that it would prevent miscarriage and other pregnancy complications. Unfortunately, not only was DES unable to prevent pregnancy complications, it produced malformations of the male and female reproductive systems and increased the risk for vaginal cancer. Some investigators believe that the structural malformations were unlikely to have been identified if a randomized clinical trial had not been conducted to determine the therapeutic effectiveness of DES.

Functional Abnormality

Over the last three decades, there has been increased recognition that in addition to structural malformations produced by agents that are developmental hazards, functional abnormalities may also be produced. Areas of concern include intelligence, behavior, and performance of various tissues, organs, and systems. Prevention of functional abnormalities will require understanding of exposures known to modify the functional parameter being studied. One clear example is lead, which has been demonstrated cause lowered intelligence and produce behavioral abnormalities (31,32,36,38,63,71,72).

Growth

Growth, including birth weight and rate of weight gain after birth, appears to be a sensitive indicator of various insults during pregnancy and early postnatal development. While measures of growth are thought to be sensitive, they are not specific to chemical exposures because many different factors can influence growth both before and after birth. Prenatal exposure to tobacco smoke and alcohol are known to decrease fetal growth and increase the incidence of low birth weight (31,32,36,38,63,71,72).

Prematurity

Although premature birth is not traditionally included in the spectrum of adverse outcomes considered as developmental toxicology, there is growing evidence that it should be included (75). Premature birth is the second leading cause of death during the first year of life, and there is mounting evidence that environmental and social exposures may play a role in premature delivery (24,76,77). For example, it is known that smoking is associated with premature birth, some agricultural chemicals have been suggested to decrease the length of gestation, and it has been suggested that there are potential interactions between minor variations in the structure of genes (polymorphisms) and length of gestation (78–82). Data from Wang and her coworkers suggest that the length of gestation is decreased because of interactions between polymorphisms in genes involved in metabolism (cytochrome P450 and glutathione S-transferase) and benzene exposures that are below the permissible exposure limit set by the Occupational Safety and Health Administration. In addition, there is mounting evidence that air pollution may also play a role in prematurity (83).

It is not necessary that all of these endpoints of developmental toxicity be present or produced by an agent that causes developmental disease; the presence of one endpoint in humans (identified in an epidemiologic study) or observed in an animal experiment is sufficient to identify the agent as a developmental hazard.

EXPOSURE

To what agents (drugs, chemicals, biologicals, and physical agents) are people exposed at home or at work, outside, or while pursuing hobbies? What are the levels and duration of exposures? What do we know about developmental toxicity produced from agents that may be released into the environment or to which humans may be exposed? Unfortunately, until recently, we had little or no data on the amounts of any industrial chemicals in our bodies. However, an innovative and important program to track the concentrations of chemicals in the US population has been initiated by the National Center for Environmental Health at the CDC (84). This effort may begin to help us understand the impact of environmental chemicals on birth defects and premature delivery (85).

Because birth defect surveillance systems are incomplete in most communities, it is difficult to get well-defined estimates of the actual number of pregnancies affected. Inadequacies in birth defects tracking systems also impair our ability to define human developmental hazards. For example, if there are differences in exposure to an industrial, agricultural, or household chemical in various regions of the United States, comparing differences in birth defect rates with differences in body exposure levels may help describe the causal relationship (if any). This task has been complicated by the recognition that many birth defects may be a consequence of complex interactions (e.g., gene–environment interactions) rather than a single agent (63). However, over the last six decades, it has been possible to identify some single-agent exposures that produce birth defects and developmental disease in humans. Examples are described in the next section.

SELECTED AGENTS AND THEIR HUMAN DEVELOPMENTAL CONSEQUENCES

Clinical and epidemiologic studies of humans exposed to chemicals, physical agents, drugs, or infectious agents that found evidence of developmental toxicity provide some insight into human vulnerability to developmental toxicants (31,32,36,72).

INFECTIOUS AGENTS THAT PRODUCE DEVELOPMENTAL DEFECTS

Table 11.4 summarizes data on four selected infectious agents known to produce human developmental disease (71,86–88).

Cytomegalovirus

Up to 2% of newborns are infected in utero with cytomegalovirus (CMV). Of those infected, as many as 10%

TABLE 11.4 Infectious Agents Known to Produce Human Developmental Disease

Infectious Developmental Hazard	*Developmental Defect(s) Observed Following Maternal and Fetal Infection*	*Estimated Risk*
Cytomegalovirus	Deafness Brain damage Eye disorder	Up to 10% of fetuses develop the indicated developmental defects from an infected pregnancy
Rubella	Eye and heart defects Deafness Brain damage	Up to 90% of fetuses develop a developmental abnormality after confirmed infection of mother in first 10 wks of pregnancy
Toxoplasmosis	Brain damage Eye disorder Deafness	From 30% to 40% of fetuses will be infected and develop developmental disease or abnormalities after maternal seroconversion in pregnancy without treatment
Varicella zoster	Brain damage Eye disorder Cutaneous scara	Up to 2% of fetuses become infected and develop defects after varicella infection of the mother

Modified from Murray CJL, Lopez AD, eds. *Health dimensions of sex and reproduction: the global burden of sexually transmitted diseases, HIV, maternal conditions, perinatal disorders and congenital anomalies (Global Burden of Disease and Injury, No 3).* Harvard University Press, 1998, with permission.

are symptomatic at birth. Characteristic effects include growth retardation and central nervous system and cardiovascular system damage. Additional long-term consequences include hearing and neurodevelopmental impairment. Because there is no treatment for an infected fetus, prevention focuses on minimizing maternal CMV exposure when possible.

Rubella

Prior to the development of the rubella vaccine in the mid-1960s, rubella epidemics occurred every 6 to 9 years and resulted in fetal death and congenital rubella syndrome in thousands of pregnancies. Infection in the first trimester is associated with spontaneous abortion. Fetal infections later in pregnancy are associated with organ damage resulting in hearing loss, cardiovascular impairment, mental retardation, and eye abnormalities. Vaccination of all children and of women of childbearing age prevents infection and consequently congenital rubella syndrome.

Toxoplasmosis

Toxoplasma gondii, a protozoan parasite, can infect the fetus, with the risk of congenital toxoplasmosis increasing as pregnancy progresses. Exposure occurs most frequently via cat feces and infected undercooked meat. Fetal infection is associated with spontaneous abortion, premature delivery, growth retardation, and central nervous system damage. Current treatments are not completely effective; prevention of exposure with hygienic measures appears to be the best approach.

Varicella Zoster

Varicella, or chickenpox, is highly contagious. Most infections and consequent immunity are acquired during childhood. Women who have not acquired immunity during childhood are susceptible and at risk of pneumonia, especially if pregnant. Maternal varicella pneumonia during pregnancy is serious and life threatening. Fetal infection is associated with spontaneous abortion, growth retardation, central nervous system damage, and scarring of skin. A vaccine is available.

MEDICATIONS THAT PRODUCE DEVELOPMENTAL ABNORMALITIES

There are medications that are known to produce developmental abnormalities (31,32,71,72,87,89), some of which are summarized in Table 11.5. Medications used during pregnancy are typically used to treat a specific disease, either in the mother, or the fetus, or, in rare cases, the placenta. In all cases, it is essential to critically consider the benefit of the medication for the disease being treated, whether the disease is maternal, fetal, or placental. In these instances, it is necessary to define the interaction of pregnancy and the disease and subsequently how the complex physiologic alterations of pregnancy influence the use of the medication chosen to treat the disease of interest. A full discussion of obstetric risk–benefit analysis is beyond the scope of this review, and the interested reader is referred to standard obstetric texts. One advance in clinical care relevant to this topic is preconception counseling (31,32,71,72, 87,90). Given that there may be several different therapeutic strategies to treat a chronic maternal disease (e.g., hypertension, seizure disorder, and diabetes), it is important to adjust medications prior to pregnancy to assure the best possible outcome (91). Because most treatment in pregnancy is for maternal disease that exists prior to conception, it is important for the physician caring for reproductive-age women to carefully counsel on treatment benefits as well as risks prior to pregnancy.

Anticonvulsants

The use of anticonvulsants by women of childbearing age clearly illustrates the utility of preconception counseling

TABLE 11.5 Selected Drugs Associated with Developmental Disease

Chemical Developmental Hazard	*Developmental Defect(s) Observed Following Maternal Treatment*	*Estimated Risk of Developmental Abnormality*
Anticonvulsants	Spina bifida after valproate Oral clefts Cardiovascular defects	The risk of developmental defect is about 4% overall, but varies with number and nature of anticonvulsant(s) used; as the number of anticonvulsant drugs used to control the seizure disorder increases, the risk of developmental defect in the fetus also increases; some teratologists believe that the risk of developmental abnormalities is increased in women with seizure disorders irrespective of treatment
Warfarin derivatives	Nasal hypoplasia Epiphyseal stippling Brain damage	Nasal hypoplasia and epiphyseal stippling occur in 8% of fetuses after use in the first trimester, and brain damage in 5% of fetuses after use in the second trimester
Diethylstilbestrol	Genital anomalies in women includes small intrauterine volume, abnormal cervix, substantially increased risk for premature delivery, and increased risk of vaginal adenocarcinoma	Up to 20% of male fetuses and 40% of female fetuses after increasing doses between 7 and 34 wks, with greatest effect in the first trimester of pregnancy

as well as the risk–benefit analysis needed to determine which medications should be used (92–100). Seizure disorders occur in about 800,000 to 1.1 million US women of childbearing age. Most of these women need to use an anticonvulsant to control their seizures, which can be life threatening. Exposure to various anticonvulsants during pregnancy results in the risk of developmental disease approximately doubling.

However, among the medications available for the treatment of the various types of seizure disorders, the risk for malformations appears to vary substantially. There is also disagreement among investigators about the impact of the seizure disorders on development. It has also been suggested that gene–environment interactions may play a significant role.

Warfarin Derivatives

The warfarin derivatives (coumarin, warfarin sodium, Marevan, Panwarfin, Coumadin, and Sofarin) include a group of anticoagulant compounds that act by interrupting the vitamin K-dependent clotting factors, and as a consequence are used to treat disorders of coagulation (31,72,87). These disorders are present among women of reproductive age, and so women are treated with these medications. Treatment is necessary because untreated coagulation disorders can be life threatening. Use of these drugs has a demonstrated increased risk for selected developmental abnormalities including underdevelopment of the nose, growth retardation, and vertebrae abnormalities. As a result, women who are attempting pregnancy typically switch to another anticoagulant, heparin, which appears to have no adverse effect on the developing fetus (101–102).

Diethylstilbestrol

During the 1940s and 1950s, it was thought that spontaneous abortion or miscarriage occurred among some women because of insufficient estrogen production by the placenta (31,32,72,77). As a consequence, some clinicians began to treat women who had previously had a pregnancy that ended in a miscarriage with a synthetic estrogen, DES. It was suggested by these clinicians that the use of this synthetic estrogen would decrease the risk that a subsequent pregnancy would end with a miscarriage. To test the hypothesis that DES decreased the risk of miscarriage, a group of clinical investigators at the Chicago Lying-In Hospital designed a randomized control trial. The outcome of this study demonstrated clearly that DES had no effect on the risk of spontaneous miscarriage, but subsequent studies of this population demonstrated that the use of DES increased the risk of abnormal development of the genitalia in both women and men (103–106). In addition, among the women, there was an increased risk of developing an unusual vaginal carcinoma as a consequence of the abnormal development of the vagina.

These examples of drugs that produce developmental abnormalities have taught us several important lessons concerning the identification of developmental toxicants. A key lesson is that in every case of known human developmental abnormality, the drug has been observed to also produce developmental toxicity in an animal model. A second lesson is that a history of exposure to a chemical or of human use does not necessarily demonstrate safety with respect to fetal development. As an example, consider the effects of alcohol on fetal development (31,32,72,87). Although humans have used alcohol for thousands of years, it was only in 1973 that data demonstrating fetal developmental toxicity was published (107–116). (See next section for more discussion of this topic.)

ENVIRONMENTAL EXPOSURE LEVELS

We have very little data on the potential of most chemicals to produce developmental toxicity, even in experimental

TABLE 11.6 Environmental Exposures Associated with Developmental Disorders in Humans

Teratogen	*Developmental Defect(s) Observed in Infants Exposed in Utero*	*Estimated Risk*
Methyl mercury	Brain damage	6% of infants in fishing village where seafood was contaminated
Hypoxia	Persistent ductus arteriosus	1%–5% of schoolchildren born and living ≥4 km above sea level
Ethyl alcohol	Brain damage; cardiac and joint defects	30% of infants of women with manifest chronic alcoholism

animals (31,32,72,87). As a consequence, we know little about their ability to interfere with human development. It is even more difficult to identify the impact of environmental levels of exposure to chemicals on developmental processes. Data on selected chemicals are summarized in Table 11.6.

METHYL MERCURY

When mercury is dumped into seawater, aquatic organisms metabolize it to methyl mercury. Methyl mercury is fat soluble and concentrates in the fatty tissues of sea animals. When consumed by humans, it is concentrated in fat-rich tissues including the brain. Two acute accidental human exposures to methyl mercury provided information about its developmental effects (31,32,72,87,117–119). Iranians were exposed when they accidentally consumed seed grain that had been treated with methyl mercury to repel rodents. Japanese villagers were exposed to methyl mercury when they consumed fish and other aquatic species living in Minimata Bay. The bay was polluted with industrial releases of mercury that aquatic animals converted to methyl mercury. The mercury concentrated in the fatty tissue of fish. Children exposed to in utero displayed the neurodevelopmental effects predominant when there is damage to the central nervous system.

HYPOXIA

There are several different types of hypoxia (oxygen deprivation) that may occur during pregnancy (120–122). In communities at high altitude, the amount of oxygen in the air is less than that found in the atmosphere of communities at sea level. In the communities at high altitude, it has been observed that there are particular pregnancy complications related to the oxygen deprivation. Lack of oxygen also results from carbon monoxide exposure, frequently a consequence of a faulty combustion device—an unventilated space heater, for example. Carbon monoxide displaces oxygen from hemoglobin in the bloodstream and decreases the amount of oxygen available to the mother as well as the fetus. Carbon monoxide exposure, depending on level and duration, may produce headache, nausea, and ultimately unconsciousness. At the level producing unconsciousness, carbon monoxide can clearly produce damage to the fetus with impact on the developing nervous system (123–129).

ETHYL ALCOHOL

Although alcohol has been used socially for thousands of years, and its adverse effect on embryonic and fetal development had been suggested, it was not until the early 1970s that the impact on fetal development was defined. Exposure to ethyl alcohol occurs as a consequence of ingestion in social settings, but is considered to be environmental exposure in the broadest sense. In some settings, occupational exposure can occur during the production of alcohol or products containing alcohol. It is thought that alcohol produces abnormal development of the face and central nervous system in a dose-dependent fashion across multiple species including humans. It is not known what is the safe dose of alcohol during pregnancy or what is the largest safe dose during development. However, it is known that alcohol is the most significant preventable cause of mental retardation during pregnancy.

For most other chemicals and health outcomes, information on developmental toxicity at environmentally relevant levels of exposure is not available. Some situations and chemicals that have been associated with, or suspected to produce, developmental defects are shown in Table 11.7.

CLASSES OF EVIDENCE FOR DEVELOPMENTAL TOXICITY

This section reviews the four general classes of data available for predicting that an agent might be a developmental hazard and as a consequence be capable of producing human developmental disease. The classes of evidence include human data, animal data, in vitro data, and theoretical data (identified in Table 11.8 as structure–activity relationships, SAR). Within each class of data, the evidence supporting the assertion of developmental safety or risk is variable. In some instances, high-quality, well-designed, and well-conducted animal studies may have considerably more certainty in predicting human risk than anecdotal human observations.

HUMAN DATA

Human data on the developmental impact of an agent, whether chemical, biological, or physical, generally are thought to provide the strongest evidence demonstrating either safety or harm in well-designed and well-conducted studies (31,32,72,87). This is because the data are gathered in the relevant species. There frequently are difficulties in obtaining adequate human data, however. For example, it is generally considered unethical to experimentally expose women prior to or during pregnancy to uncharacterized agents to determine developmental hazard, although pharmacological studies to define dosing safety and efficacy are considered ethical (130,131). The cost of human studies can be quite high, and the time and

TABLE 11.7 Summary of Situations and Substances that Have Been Associated with or Suspected to Produce Developmental Defects

Substance/Situation	*Birth Weight*	*Gestation Length*	*Birth Defect*
Toxic substances			
Electronics assembly	X		
Hair dye			Cardiac defects
Lead	X	X	Total anomalous pulmonary venous return
Polychlorinated biphenyls	X		"Yusho" syndrome
Soldering			Cardiac defects
Styrene monomer	X		
Solvents	X		Anencephaly, gastroschisis
Paint/paint stripping			Total anomalous pulmonary venous return, anencephaly
Benzene	X		Neural tube defects and major cardiac defects
Carbon tetrachloride	X		Central nervous system defects, neural tube defects, and oral cleft defects
Toluene	X		Microcephaly, central nervous system defects
Tetrachloroethylene			Oral cleft defects
Trichloroethylene			Central nervous system defects, neural tube defects, and oral cleft defects
Pesticides			
Agricultural work	X		Total anomalous pulmonary venous return, anencephaly
Triazine herbicides	X		Orofacial clefts
Pollutants			
Carbon monoxide	X		
Chloroform and other trihalomethanes	X		Central nervous system defects, oral cleft defects, and major cardiac defects
Hazardous waste	X	X	Cardiac and circulatory defects, neural tube defects, hypospadias, gastroschisis
Methyl mercury			Central nervous system defects, cerebral palsy, and cleft lip and palate
Particulate matter	X		

effort required to complete those studies can be very long. Confounding factors, such as other exposures (e.g., women who smoke are also frequent coffee drinkers, and women who consume drugs typically consume more than one drug, such as narcotics and alcohol), may also weaken the evidentiary nature of the epidemiologic study. However, it is possible to get relevant information from studies in which women are treated with a drug for its therapeutic effect during pregnancy. In addition, it may be possible to observe the outcome of pregnancy among women accidentally exposed to the agent of concern.

Although the predictive value of data gathered from epidemiologic studies is high, it is important to note that even if an agent has been demonstrated to produce developmental disease in humans, not all those either exposed or treated will get the disease. For example, among women treated with ACE inhibitors during pregnancy, agents that increase the risk of fetal death, there will be infants born who are unaffected. That is also the case for infectious agents such as rubella and environmental exposures such as methyl mercury. In addition, there are clear dose effects, with smaller doses producing lower risk for adverse developmental consequences, as seen with fetal alcohol syndrome and fetal alcohol effects.

Even when data are gathered in humans, there are critical questions that must be asked about the nature of the evidence gathered. For example, because human research usually involves relatively small numbers of human subjects who have been exposed or who have health effects of interest, one critical question is the statistical power of the study, that is, how large an effect would have had to be done before the study could have detected it. This is especially important when reviewing a study that suggests that exposure to the agent of concern produces no adverse developmental

TABLE 11.8 General Qualities of Various Types of Evidence for Evaluating Developmental Risks to Human Health

Data	*Cost*	*Predictive Value*	*Certainty*	*Health Protective*
Human	High	High	High	No
Animal	Moderate	Moderate	Moderate	Yes
In vitro	Low	Low	Low	Yes
SAR	Very low	Low	Low	Yes
Animal + in vitro + SAR	Moderate	High	Moderate to high	Yes

SAR, structure–activity relationships.

effect. Some investigators believe that it is important to indicate that there are actually no truly negative studies of adverse developmental consequence among humans. Instead, negative studies are unable to demonstrate an effect within the designed statistical power of the study. For example, small studies may only be able to identify agents that substantially increase the risk for abnormal development by as much as 10- or 100-fold, but we know that many agents increase the risk for developmental disease by several fold at most. Thus, although the result of such a small study might be characterized by some as "negative," it is clearly only negative for agents whose potency for producing developmental disease is greater than the power of the study, and the study cannot inform decision makers about the safety of an agent with lower or smaller impacts on abnormal development.

Another item of concern with respect to interpreting data from human studies is exposure characterization, especially time, duration, amount, and timing with respect to pregnancy and the developmental stages of the fetus. Relationship of exposure to fetal development may also affect the biological plausibility of exposure being a cause of an adverse health effect.

Finally, a significant critique of the utility of relying on human studies to evaluate safety is the moral concern that data demonstrating human developmental abnormalities only become available when enough people have been sufficiently harmed to be measured at a scientifically acceptable level of certainty, usually 95%. Contrary to public health principles and to the ethics of medical practice, reliance on scientific proof of harm to human health means relying on the failures of preventive medicine.

ANIMAL DATA

If they are of similar quality and quantity, animal data on developmental hazards are clearly inferior to human data as a basis for judging the potential effects on humans of chemical exposure. However, the quantity and quality of animal data frequently are far superior, and therefore animal data have many advantages over human epidemiologic data (31,32,72,87). For example, it is possible to design animal experiments with exposure only to the agent of concern, removing the issue of confounding found in human studies, and to treat groups of animals with measured and increasing doses of the agent. Control groups are more easily formed and better matched to tested animals. Various doses and duration and timing of exposures can be manipulated to delineate the sensitive windows that are frequently difficult to identify using human data. Moreover, animal data can generally be collected relatively quickly and at substantially lower cost than human data using epidemiologic studies. Animals are integrated biological systems that generally respond developmentally in ways relevant to human toxicity.

The quality of data from animal experiments varies. To test for developmental effects of animal exposure, generally it is necessary to expose sexually mature animals throughout at least one egg and sperm production cycle prior to mating. At least three doses and one control group are used. The highest dose should be selected to produce evidence of maternal toxicity, generally a 10% reduction in weight during the course of gestation. Choice of lower doses will depend on knowledge of toxicity of the agent. Exposure continues during mating and throughout gestation for the female animal. Just prior to birth, the mother is sacrificed and the pups delivered. Some of the pups are sacrificed to examine the skeleton and internal organs; others are allowed to grow and develop. Examination of the skeleton and internal organs should carefully evaluate weight, size, and macroscopic, microscopic, and ultrastructural anatomy. In some instances, it may be necessary to evaluate the functional characteristics of individual organs or tissues in the intact animal. Pups raised by foster parents should be evaluated for functional characteristics at various stages of life. In some instances or for some agents, it may be necessary to conduct multigeneration treatments to characterize the full impact of a chemical agent on genetic and developmental processes.

Key criteria for evaluating the quality of animal data include the number of animals in each treatment group, number of treatment groups, number of variables evaluated, number of control groups, species used, appropriateness of the species used for the chemical agent considered, appropriateness of the route of exposure considered or used in the animal model, the route of exposure relative to likely route of human exposure, and the number of generations exposed.

Research conducted by Fabro and colleagues (132–137) and Hashemi et al. (138) described the utility of animal data in estimating human risk for developmental toxicity. In general, these studies demonstrated that all known human developmental toxicants are developmental toxicants in at least one experimental animal, but they are not positive in all animal test species. Animal tests are also quite accurate in identifying chemicals that are not developmental toxicants. A detailed analysis by Schardein (31) found that approximately 4,153 chemicals have been tested for developmental toxicity in experimental animals. Among that group, 66% (2,760) were not developmental toxicants, and the remaining 1,393 (34%), which were considered to be teratogenic, were either clearly teratogenic (291, or 7%), or probably teratogenic (730, or 18%), or possibly teratogenic (372, or 9%).

IN VITRO DATA

Over the last 50 years, developmental biology has benefited from the emergence of a broad array of in vitro models for exploring the effects of chemical, biological, and physical agents on cells and cellular constituents (70,139–142). In vitro models subject isolated organs, tissues, cells, or subcellular fragments to possibly harmful agents in a laboratory (e.g., in a glass plate or test tube).

These in vitro model systems have been useful in exploring mechanisms of normal development using either animal or human cells and the impact of an agent on that developmental process. Depending on the nature of the in vitro experiment, researchers can consider a single chemical interaction, such as chemical binding to a particular type of receptor, with a high degree of control of concentration. Based on in vitro data, chemical agents can be classified into various classes depending on their structure, which determines their physical properties. Some examples of chemical classes include water soluble versus fat soluble, acidic versus basic, and volatile versus nonvolatile. Other examples of chemical classes that are especially relevant to developmental toxicity include estrogenic versus nonestrogenic (depending on whether a chemical interacts with estrogen receptors on cells) and similar to vitamin A versus not similar to vitamin A (depending on whether the chemical agent interacts with retinol receptors). In this manner, in vitro tests are useful screening tools for excluding clearly innocuous chemicals from further scrutiny, at least with regard to specific classes of health impact. There might remain concern about nonspecific toxicity, however. Another benefit of collecting in vitro data is that such data can provide support for the relevance of animal testing for human developmental risk. Two important advantages of these laboratory approaches to toxicity testing are low cost and speed with which they can be established and provide data.

There are also disadvantages to use of in vitro data. For example, it is more difficult to extrapolate to human populations from in vitro data, and any risk estimate made on that basis will be highly uncertain, in part because cultures do not behave like whole animals. Although the data can be used to determine that a chemical agent is, or is not, likely to have a particular effect in humans and to infer whether there is a need to understand how the agent acts in an intact biological system, in vitro data are not sufficient to conduct a full risk assessment unless a chemical agent clearly will not interact with human tissues, regardless of exposure.

THEORETICAL DATA

There are various types of biochemical and theoretical data that may be of value in predicting whether a chemical agent is likely to be a developmental toxicant [see the EPA efforts in computational toxicology as an example (143)]. Perhaps, the best known and most useful is the study of chemical SAR (144–149). It has been known for many years that the biological impact of a chemical is dependent on its structure. Knowledge of chemical structure and of how structure relates to cellular activity, therefore, provides information about chemical class and mechanism of action. Researchers use SAR to evaluate the potential toxicity of chemicals for which other data are lacking. Structure may be used to predict the impact of a previously unsynthesized or untested chemical agent on the biological process of interest. Like many in vitro tests, SAR data probably are most useful for predicting chemical structures of interest for further analysis.

The main drawback to using SAR data with respect to characterizing human developmental toxicity is the uncertainty of any risk estimate. Certainty may be high if analysis identifies chemical agents as belonging to a known class of developmental toxicants, but most often classification is tentative and risk estimates are highly uncertain.

Several chemical classes have been characterized through SAR. Kavlock and colleagues explored the structure and activity of phenols (150–155). Their data were reanalyzed by Hansch et al. (156), who also evaluated aniline mustards, another chemical group. Enslein and colleagues analyzed the impact of heteroaromatic, carboaromatic, alicyclic, and acyclic organic compounds on development (157).

A group of investigators at the University of Pittsburgh and Case-Western Reserve University developed a unique approach to SAR, which they used to analyze a broad range of effects, beneficial as well as toxicologic, in evaluating chemical agents associated with developmental disease (101,102,158–171). They created a database of chemicals associated with developmental toxicity in humans as well as in specific animals, then developed an extensive database of human developmental impacts of chemical agents and drugs.

CONCLUSIONS: HOW DO WE IDENTIFY DEVELOPMENTAL TOXICANTS?

There are testing systems available for identification of agents that are likely to cause human developmental disease. Clearly, the highest degree of certainty (or the smallest degree of uncertainty) in the likelihood that a chemical, physical, or a biological agent is a human teratogen comes from studies in which it is shown that a substance produces birth defects in human populations. However, human data are only available when exposure already has occurred and birth defects discovered. Medical ethics does not allow public health practitioners to wait to evaluate potential chemical toxicity until human data are available.

In all but a few cases, human epidemiologic research data are too sparse to support chemical risk assessments for developmental toxicity. However, experimental animal research data, in vitro experimental data, and theoretical data based on SAR can be effectively utilized to identify potential developmental toxicants. Thus, preliminary conclusions can be drawn about the likelihood that birth defects are due to environmental hazards. However, given the number of known developmental toxicants relative to the number of chemical agents that have been tested for developmental toxicity and the number of chemical agents in commerce for which there is no toxicity data, it is likely that additional developmental toxicants remain to be identified.

ACKNOWLEDGMENTS

I thank my colleague at the Perinatal Data Center of the March of Dimes, Dr. Joanne Petrini, for assistance in preparing figures presented in this chapter.

REFERENCES

1. US Department of Health and Human Services. *Healthy people 2010: understanding and improving health.* Washington, DC, 2000. http://www.healthypeople.gov/. Accessed March 13, 2009.
2. US Department of Health and Human Services. *Tracking healthy people 2010.* Washington, DC, 2000. http://www.healthypeople.gov/Document/tableofcontents.htm#tracking. Accessed March 13, 2009.
3. Black RE, Michaelsen KF. *Public health issues in infant and child nutrition.* Philadelphia, PA: Lippincott Williams & Wilkins, 2002.
4. Alexander GR, Kotelchuck M. Assessing the role and effectiveness of prenatal care: history, challenges, and directions for future research. *Public Health Rep* 2001;116(4):306–316.
5. Wallace RB, Doebbeling BN, eds. *Maxcy–Rosenau–Last. Public health and preventive medicine,* 14th ed. Stamford, CT: Appleton & Lange, 1998.

6. McCormick MC, Siegel JE, eds. *Prenatal care: effectiveness and implementation.* Cambridge: Cambridge University Press, 1999.
7. Taylor HG, Klein N, Hack M. School-age consequences of birth weight less than 750g: a review and update. *Dev Neuropsychol* 2000;17(3):289–321.
8. Mattison DR, Damus K, Fiore E, et al. Preterm delivery: a public health perspective. *Paediatr Perinat Epidemiol* 2001;15(Suppl 2): 7–16.
9. Detels R. *Oxford textbook of public health.* New York, NY: Oxford University Press, 2002.
10. Hack M, Flannery DM, Schluchter M, et al. Outcomes in young adulthood for very-low-birth-weight infants. *N Engl J Med* 2002; 346(3):149–157.
11. Wilson-Costello D, Friedman H, Minich N, et al. Improved neurodevelopmental outcomes for extremely low birth weight infants in 2000–2002. *Pediatrics* 2007;119(1):37–45.
12. Meckel RA. *Save the babies: American public health reform and the prevention of infant mortality, 1850–1929.* Ann Arbor, MI: University of Michigan Press, 1998.
13. Canadian Perinatal Surveillance System, Arbuckle TE. Canadian perinatal health report, 2000. Ottawa, ON: Reproductive Health Division, Bureau of Reproductive and Child Health, Centre for Healthy Development, Population and Public Health Branch, Health Canada, 2000.
14. Bale JR, Stoll BJ. *Improving birth outcomes: meeting the challenges in the developing world.* Washington, DC: National Academy Press, 2003.
15. US Congress Senate Committee on Labor and Human Resources. Oversight of the Healthy Start demonstration project: Hearing before the Committee on Labor and Human Resources, United States Senate, One Hundred Fourth Congress, second session, on the implementation of the Healthy Start demonstration project of the Department of Health and Human Services, created to reduce infant mortality, and its proposed authorization for fiscal year 1997, May 16, 1996. Washington, DC: US Government Printing Office, 1996.
16. US Congress House Committee on Government Reform and Oversight, Subcommittee on Human Resources. The Healthy Start Program: implementation lessons and impact on infant mortality: hearing before the subcommittee on Human Resources of the Committee on Government Reform and Oversight, House of Representatives, One Hundred Fifth Congress, first session, March 13, 1997. Washington, DC: US Government Printing Office, 1997.
17. Anachebe NF, Sutton MY. Racial disparities in reproductive health outcomes. *Am J Obstet Gynecol* 2003;188(4):S37–S42.
18. Fuller KE. Health disparities: reframing the problem. *Med Sci Monit* 2003;9(3):SR9–SR15.
19. Lu MC, Halfon N. Racial and ethnic disparities in birth outcomes: a life-course perspective. *Matern Child Health J* 2003;7(1): 13–30.
20. Wise PH. The anatomy of a disparity in infant mortality. *Annu Rev Public Health* 2003;24:341–362.
21. Petrini J, Damus K, Russell R, et al. Contribution of birth defects to infant mortality in the United States. *Teratology* 2002;66(Suppl 1): S3–S6.
22. Yang Q, Chen H, Correa A, et al. Racial differences in infant mortality attributable to birth defects in the United States, 1989–2002. *Birth Defects Res A Clin Mol Teratol* 2006;76(10):706–713.
23. Copeland GE, Kirby RS. Using birth defects registry data to evaluate infant and childhood mortality associated with birth defects: an alternative to traditional mortality assessment using underlying cause of death statistics. *Birth Defects Res A Clin Mol Teratol* 2007; 79(11):792–797.
24. Stillerman K P Mattison DR, Giudice LC, et al. Environmental exposures and adverse pregnancy outcomes: a review of the science. *Reprod Sci* 2008;15(7):631–650.
25. Woodruff TJ, Parker JD, Darrow LA, et al. Methodological issues in studies of air pollution and reproductive health. *Environ Res* 2009;109(3):311–320.
26. Xiong X, Harville EW, Mattison DR, et al. Exposure to Hurricane Katrina, post-traumatic stress disorder and birth outcomes. *Am J Med Sci* 2008;336(2):111–115.
27. Birth Defects and Developmental Disabilities. The Search for Causes and Cures. July 2005. Trust for Americas' Health. http://healthyamericans.org/reports/birthdefects05/. Accessed January 4, 2010.
28. National Center on Birth Defects and Developmental Disabilities. Centers for Disease Control and Prevention. http://www.cdc.gov/ncbddd/index.html. Accessed January 4, 2010.
29. Tracking Birth Defects. National Center on Birth Defects and Developmental Disabilities. Centers for Disease Control and Prevention. http://www.cdc.gov/ncbddd/bd/monitoring.htm. Accessed January 4, 2010.
30. Brent RL, Beckman DA, eds. *Teratology.* Philadelphia, PA: WB Saunders, 1986.
31. Schardein JL. *Chemically induced birth defects,* 3rd ed., Revised and Expanded. New York, NY: Marcel Dekker, 2000.
32. Shepard TH, Lemire RJ. *Catalog of teratogenic agents,* 12th ed. Baltimore, MD: The Johns Hopkins University Press, 2007.
33. Shepard TH, Brent RL, Friedman JM, et al. Update on new developments in the study of human teratogens. *Teratology* 2002; 65(4):153–161.
34. Brent RL. Addressing environmentally caused human birth defects. *Pediatr Rev* 2001;22(5):153–165.
35. Czeizel E. Prevention of developmental abnormalities with particular emphasis of primary prevention. *Tsitol Genet* 2002;36(5):58–72.
36. Kalter H. *Teratology in the twentieth century: congenital malformations in humans and how their environmental causes are established.* Amsterdam: Elsevier, 2003.
37. National Research Council, Committee on Risk Assessment of Hazardous Pollutants. *Science and judgment in risk assessment.* Washington, DC: National Academy Press, 1994.
38. O'Rahilly R, Meuller F. *Human embryology and teratology.* New York, NY: Wiley-Liss, 2001.
39. Botto LD, Moore CA, Khoury MJ, et al. Neural-tube defects. *N Engl J Med* 1999;341(20):1509–1519.
40. Koren G, Klinger G, Ohlsson A, et al. Fetal pharmacotherapy. *Drugs* 2002;62(5):757–773.
41. McDonald SD, Ferguson S, Tam L, et al. The prevention of congenital anomalies with periconceptional folic acid supplementation. *J Obstet Gynecol Can* 2003;25(2):115–121.
42. Berry RJ, Li Z, Erickson JD, et al. Prevention of neural-tube defects with folic acid in China. China–US Collaborative Project for Neural Tube Defect Prevention. *N Engl J Med* 1999;341(20):1485–1490.
43. Mattison DR. Folic acid requirements for women of childbearing age. *Am Fam Physician* 1999;60(9):2510–2515.
44. Lumley J, Watson L, Watson M, et al. Periconceptional supplementation with folate and/or multivitamins for preventing neural tube defects. *Cochrane Database Syst Rev* 2001;3:CD001056.
45. Wald NJ, Law MR, Morris JK, et al. Quantifying the effect of folic acid. *Lancet* 2001;358(9298):2069–2073.
46. Heseker HB, Mason JB, Selhub J, et al. Not all cases of neural-tube defect can be prevented by increasing the intake of folic acid. *Br J Nutr* 2008:1–8.
47. Sayed AR, Bourne D, Pattinson R, et al. Decline in the prevalence of neural tube defects following folic acid fortification and its cost-benefit in South Africa. *Birth Defects Res A Clin Mol Teratol* 2008;82(4):211–216.
48. Mosley BS, Cleves MA, et al. Neural tube defects and maternal folate intake among pregnancies conceived after folic acid fortification in the United States. *Am J Epidemiol* 2009;169(1):9–17.
49. Toepoel M, Steegers-Theunissen RP, Ouborg NJ, et al. Interaction of PDGFRA promoter haplotypes and maternal environmental exposures in the risk of spina bifida. *Birth Defects Res A Clin Mol Teratol* 2009;85(7):629–636.
50. Smith DW. Recognizable patterns of human deformation. Identification and management of mechanical effects on morphogenesis. *Major Probl Clin Pediatr* 1981;21:1–151.
51. Peitsch WK, Keefer CH, LaBrie RA, et al. Incidence of cranial asymmetry in healthy newborns. *Pediatrics* 2002;110(6):e72.
52. Panchal J, Uttchin V. Management of craniosynostosis. *Plast Reconstr Surg* 2003;111(6):2032–2048; quiz, 2049.
53. Arthur FH. Edith L. Potter, M.D.—Pathologist. *J Am Med Womens Assoc* 1974;29(11):508–510.
54. Greenwood RD, Rosenthal A, Nodas AS. Cardiovascular malformations associated with congenital anomalies of the urinary system. Observations in a series of 453 infants and children with urinary system malformations. *Clin Pediatr (Phila)* 1976;15(12): 1101–1104.
55. Witters I, Moerman P, Natens R, et al. Multiple congenital anomalies syndrome with multicystic renal dysplasia, postaxial polydactyly and lumbosacral meningocele. Difficulties in nosological classification and genetic counseling. *Genet Couns* 2002;13(2): 147–149.

56. Huang CW, Yang AH, Lai CR, et al. Renal tubular dysgenesis in siblings. *J Chin Med Assoc* 2003;66(5):299–302.
57. Potter EL. Bilateral absence of ureters and kidneys: a report of 50 cases. *Obstet Gynecol* 1965;25:3–12.
58. Wilson JG, Fraser FC. *Handbook of teratology: general principles and etiology.* New York, NY: Plenum Press, 1977.
59. Persaud TVN, Chudley AE, et al. *Basic concepts in teratology.* New York, NY: Liss, 1985.
60. Akhurst RJ, Kavlock RJ, Daston G, et al. Drug toxicity in embryonic development: advances in understanding mechanisms of birth defects. Berlin: Springer, 1997.
61. Wilson JG. Embryologic considerations in teratology. *Ann N Y Acad Sci* 1965;123:219–227.
62. Nelson K, Holmes LB. Malformations due to presumed spontaneous mutations in newborn infants. *N Engl J Med* 1989;320(1): 19–23.
63. Thorogood P. *Embryos, genes, and birth defects.* Chichester, New York: J. Wiley, 1997.
64. Shi M, Wehby GL, et al. Review on genetic variants and maternal smoking in the etiology of oral clefts and other birth defects. *Birth Defects Res C Embryo Today* 2008;84(1):16–29.
65. Tan KB, Tan KH, et al. Gastroschisis and omphalocele in Singapore: a ten-year series from 1993 to 2002. *Singapore Med J* 2008;49(1):31–36.
66. Root ED, Meyer RE, Emch ME, et al. Evidence of localized clustering of gastroschisis births in North Carolina, 1999–2004. *Soc Sci Med* 2009; 68(8):1361–1367.
67. Carmichael SL, Shaw GM, et al. Maternal reproductive and demographic characteristics as risk factors for hypospadias. *Paediatr Perinat Epidemiol* 2007;21(3):210–218.
68. Carmichael SL, Shaw GM, et al. Maternal stressful life events and risks of birth defects. *Epidemiology* 2007;18(3):356–361.
69. Carmichael SL, Yang W, et al. Maternal food insecurity is associated with increased risk of certain birth defects. *J Nutr* 2007; 137(9):2087–2092.
70. Daston GP. *Molecular and cellular methods in developmental toxicology.* Boca Raton, FL: CRC Press, 1997.
71. Whittle MJ, Rodeck CH. *Fetal medicine: basic science and clinical practice.* London: Churchill Livingstone, 1999.
72. Yankowitz J, Niebyl JR. *Drug therapy in pregnancy.* Philadelphia, PA: Lippincott Williams & Wilkins, 2001.
73. Bowen ME, Ray WA, et al. Increasing exposure to angiotensin-converting enzyme inhibitors in pregnancy. *Am J Obstet Gynecol* 2008;198(3):291 e1–e5.
74. Martin U, Foreman MA, et al. Use of ACE inhibitors and ARBs in hypertensive women of childbearing age. *J Clin Pharm Ther* 2008;33(5):507–511.
75. Treolar SA, Macones GA, Mitchell LE, et al. Genetic influences on premature parturition in an Australian twin sample. *Twin Res* 2000;3(2):80–82.
76. Buekens P, Klebanoff M. Preterm birth research: from disillusion to the search for new mechanisms. *Paediatr Perinat Epidemiol* 2001;15(Suppl 2):159–161.
77. Rowley DL. Closing the gap, opening the process: why study social contributors to preterm delivery among black women? *Matern Child Health J* 2001;5(2):71–74.
78. Yang CY, Cheng BH, Hsu T, et al. Association between petrochemical air pollution and adverse pregnancy outcomes in Taiwan. *Arch Environ Health* 2002;57(5):461–465.
79. Yang CY, Chiu HF, Tsai SS, et al. Increased risk of preterm delivery in areas with cancer mortality problems from petrochemical complexes. *Environ Res* 2002;89(3):195–200.
80. Moutquin JM. Socio-economic and psychosocial factors in the management and prevention of preterm labour. *Br J Obstet Gynaecol* 2003;110(Suppl 20):56–60.
81. Wilhelm M, Ritz B. Residential proximity to traffic and adverse birth outcomes in Los Angeles county, California, 1994–1996. *Environ Health Perspect* 2003;111(2):207–216.
82. Yang CY, Chang CC, Tsai SS, et al. Preterm delivery among people living around Portland cement plants. *Environ Res* 2003;92(1): 64–68.
83. Lin MC, Chiu HF, Yu HS, et al. Increased risk of preterm delivery in areas with air pollution from a petroleum refinery plant in Taiwan. *J Toxicol Environ Health A* 2001;64(8):637–644.
84. National Center for Environmental Health. Centers for Disease Control and Prevention. http://www.cdc.gov/nceh/. Accessed January 4, 2010.
85. National Report on Human Exposure to Environmental Chemicals. National Center for Environmental Health. Centers for Disease Control and Prevention. http://www.cdc.gov/exposurereport/. Accessed January 4, 2010.
86. Taeusch HW, Ballard RA. *Avery's diseases of the newborn.* Philadelphia, PA: WB Saunders, 1998.
87. Gabbe SG, Niebyl JR, et al. *Obstetrics: normal and problem pregnancies.* New York, NY: Churchill Livingstone, 2002.
88. Pickering LK, ed. *Report of the Committee on Infectious Diseases.* Evanston, IL: American Academy of Pediatrics, 2003.
89. Scialli AR, Lione A, et al. *Reproductive effects of chemical, physical, and biologic agents: Reprotox.* Baltimore: The Johns Hopkins University Press, 1995.
90. Winterbottom J, Smyth R, et al. The effectiveness of preconception counseling to reduce adverse pregnancy outcome in women with epilepsy: what's the evidence? *Epilepsy Behav* 2009;14(2):273–279.
91. Griffiths F, Lowe P, et al. Becoming pregnant: exploring the perspectives of women living with diabetes. *Br J Gen Pract* 2008; 58(548):184–190.
92. Penovich PE. The effects of epilepsy and its treatment on sexual and reproductive function. *Epilepsia* 2000;41(Suppl 2):S53–S61.
93. Sabers A, Gram L. Newer anticonvulsants: comparative review of drug interactions and adverse effects. *Drugs* 2000;60(1):23–33.
94. Pschirrer ER, Monga M. Seizure disorders in pregnancy. *Obstet Gynecol Clin North Am* 2001;28(3):601–611.
95. Crawford P. Epilepsy and pregnancy. *Seizure* 2002;11(Suppl A): 212–219.
96. McAuley JW, Anderson GD. Treatment of epilepsy in women of reproductive age: pharmacokinetic considerations. *Clin Pharmacokinet* 2002;41(8):559–579.
97. Pack AM, Morrell MJ. Treatment of women with epilepsy. *Semin Neurol* 2002;22(3):289–298.
98. Pennell PB. Pregnancy in the woman with epilepsy: maternal and fetal outcomes. *Semin Neurol* 2002;22(3):299–308.
99. Morrow JI, Craig JJ. Anti-epileptic drugs in pregnancy: current safety and other issues. *Expert Opin Pharmacother* 2003;4(4): 445–456.
100. Yerby MS. Clinical care of pregnant women with epilepsy: neural tube defects and folic acid supplementation. *Epilepsia* 2003; 44(Suppl 3):33–40.
101. Ghanooni M, Mattison DR, Zhang YP, et al. Structural determinants associated with risk of human developmental toxicity. *Am J Obstet Gynecol* 1997;176(4):799–805.
102. Gomez J, Macina OT, Mattison DR, et al. Structural determinants of developmental toxicity in hamsters. *Teratology* 1999; 60(4):190–205.
103. Herbst AL. The current status of the DES-exposed population. *Obstet Gynecol Ann* 1981;10:267–278.
104. Herbst AL. Diethylstilbestrol and other sex hormones during pregnancy. *Obstet Gynecol* 1981;58(Suppl 5):35S–40S.
105. Propst AM, Hill JA III. Anatomic factors associated with recurrent pregnancy loss. *Semin Reprod Med* 2000;18(4):341–350.
106. Swan SH. Intrauterine exposure to diethylstilbestrol: long-term effects in humans. *APMIS* 2000;108(12):793–804.
107. Kaufman MH. The teratogenic effects of alcohol following exposure during pregnancy, and its influence on the chromosome constitution of the pre-ovulatory egg. *Alcohol Alcohol* 1997; 32(2):113–128.
108. Abel EL. Prevention of alcohol abuse-related birth effects. I. Targeting and pricing. *Alcohol Alcohol* 1998;33(4):411–416.
109. Abel EL. Prevention of alcohol abuse-related birth effects. II. Targeting and pricing. *Alcohol Alcohol* 1998;33(4):417–420.
110. Chan DQ. Fetal alcohol syndrome. *Optom Vis Sci* 1999;76(10): 678–685.
111. Cramer C, Davidhizar R. FAS/FAE: impact on children. *J Child Health Care* 1999;3(3):31–34.
112. Murphy-Brennan MG, Oei TP. Is there evidence to show that fetal alcohol syndrome can be prevented? *J Drug Educ* 1999;29(1): 5–24.
113. NIAAA Report to Congress. Prenatal exposure to alcohol. *Alcohol Res Health* 2000;24(1): 32–41.
114. Hagberg H, Mallard C. Antenatal brain injury: etiology and possibilities of prevention. *Semin Neonatol* 2000;5(1):41–51.
115. Streissguth AP, O'Malley K. Neuropsychiatric implications and long-term consequences of fetal alcohol spectrum disorders. *Semin Clin Neuropsychiatry* 2000;5(3):177–190.

116. May PA, Gossage JP. Estimating the prevalence of fetal alcohol syndrome. A summary. *Alcohol Res Health* 2001;25(3):159–167.
117. Stern L. In vivo assessment of the teratogenic potential of drugs in humans. *Obstet Gynecol* 1981;58(Suppl 5):3S–8S.
118. Auroux M. Behavioral teratogenesis: an extension to the teratogenesis of functions. *Biol Neonate* 1997;71(3):137–147.
119. Eley BM. The future of dental amalgam: a review of the literature. Part 6: Possible harmful effects of mercury from dental amalgam. *Br Dent J* 1997;182(12):455–459.
120. Longo LD, Pearce WJ. High altitude, hypoxic-induced modulation of noradrenergic-mediated responses in fetal and adult cerebral arteries. *Comp Biochem Physiol A Mol Integr Physiol* 1998; 119(3):683–694.
121. Rees S, Mallard C, Breen S, et al. Fetal brain injury following prolonged hypoxemia and placental insufficiency: a review. *Comp Biochem Physiol A Mol Integr Physiol* 1998;119(3):653–660.
122. Moore LG, Armaza F, Niermeyer S, et al. Comparative aspects of high-altitude adaptation in human populations. *Adv Exp Med Biol* 2000;475:45–62.
123. Robkin MA. Carbon monoxide and the embryo. *Int J Dev Biol* 1997;41(2):283–289.
124. Aubard Y, Magne I. Carbon monoxide poisoning in pregnancy. *Br J Obstet Gynaecol* 2000;107(7):833–838.
125. Raub JA, Mathieu-Nolf M, Hampson NB, et al. Carbon monoxide poisoning—a public health perspective. *Toxicology* 2000; 145(1):1–14.
126. Greingor JL, Tosi JM, Ruhlmann S, et al. Acute carbon monoxide intoxication during pregnancy. One case report and review of the literature. *Emerg Med J* 2001;18(5):399–401.
127. Ravindra A, Mittal K, Van Grieben R. Health risk assessment of urban suspended particulate matter with special reference to polycyclic aromatic hydrocarbons: a review. *Rev Environ Health* 2001;16(3):169–189.
128. Morse D, Sethi J. Carbon monoxide and human disease. *Antioxid Redox Signal* 2002;4(2):331–338.
129. Townsend CL, Maynard RL. Effects on health of prolonged exposure to low concentrations of carbon monoxide. *Occup Environ Med* 2002;59(10):708–711.
130. McCullough LB, Coverdale JH, et al. A comprehensive ethical framework for responsibly designing and conducting pharmacologic research that involves pregnant women. *Am J Obstet Gynecol* 2005;193(3 Pt 2):901–907.
131. Coverdale JH, McCullough LB, et al. The ethics of randomized placebo-controlled trials of antidepressants with pregnant women: a systematic review. *Obstet Gynecol* 2008;112(6):1361–1368.
132. Brown NA, Shull G, Kao J, et al. Teratogenicity and lethality of hydantoin derivatives in the mouse: structure–toxicity relationships. *Toxicol Appl Pharmacol* 1982;64(2):271–288.
133. Fabro S, Shull G, Brown NA. The relative teratogenic index and teratogenic potency: proposed components of developmental toxicity risk assessment. *Teratog Carcinog Mutagen* 1982;2(1):61–76.
134. Brown NA, Fabro S. The value of animal teratogenicity testing for predicting human risk. *Clin Obstet Gynecol* 1983;26(2):467–477.
135. Fabro S. Reproductive toxicology: state of the art, 1982. *Am J Ind Med* 1983;4(1–2):391–393.
136. Fabro S, McLachlan JA, Dames NM. Chemical exposure of embryos during the preimplementation stages of pregnancy: mortality rate and intrauterine development. *Am J Obstet Gynecol* 1984;148(7):929–938.
137. Fabro S. On predicting environmentally-induced human reproductive hazards: an overview and historical perspective. *Fundam Appl Toxicol* 1985;5(4):609–614.
138. Hashemi RR, Jelovsek FR, et al. Developmental toxicity risk assessment: a rough sets approach. *Methods Inf Med* 1993;32(1):47–54.
139. Zbinden G, Gross FH. *Pharmacological methods in toxicology*. Oxford: New Pergamon Press, 1979.
140. Goldberg AM, Principe ML. *In vitro toxicology: mechanisms and new technology*. New York, NY: Mary Ann Liebert, 1991.
141. Jolles G, Cordier A. *In vitro methods in toxicology*. San Diego, CA: Academic Press, 1992.
142. Benigni R. *Quantitative structure–activity relationship (QSAR) models of mutagens and carcinogens*. Boca Raton, FL: CRC Press, 2003.
143. National Center for Computational Toxicology, US Environmental Protection Agency. http://www.epa.gov/comptox/. Accessed January 4, 2010.
144. Devillers J. *Comparative QSAR*. Washington, DC: Taylor & Francis, 1998.
145. Nendza M. *Structure–activity relationships in environmental sciences*. New York: Chapman & Hall, 1998.
146. Salem H, Katz SA. *Toxicity assessment alternatives: methods, issues, opportunities*. Totowa, NJ: Humana Press, 1999.
147. Zupan J, Gasteiger J. *Neural networks in chemistry and drug design*. Weinheim, Germany: Wiley-VCH, 1999.
148. Hayes AW. *Principles and methods of toxicology*, 5th ed. Boca Raton: CRC Press/Taylor & Francis Group, 2008.
149. Devillers, J. Endocrine disruption modeling. Boca Raton, CRC Press, 2009.
150. Kavlock RJ. Structure–activity relationships in the developmental toxicity of substituted phenols: in vivo effects. *Teratology* 1990;41(1):43–59.
151. Kavlock RJ, Greene JA, Kimmel GL, et al. Activity profiles of developmental toxicity: design considerations and pilot implementation. *Teratology* 1991;43(2):159–185.
152. Kavlock RJ, Oglesby LA, Hall LL, et al. In vivo and in vitro structure–dosimetry–activity relationships of substituted phenols in developmental toxicity assays. *Reprod Toxicol* 1991;5(3): 255–258.
153. Fisher HL, Sumler MR, Shrivastava SP, et al. Toxicokinetics and structure–activity relationships of nine para-substituted phenols in rat embryos in vitro. *Teratology* 1993;48(4):285–297.
154. Kavlock RJ. Structure–activity approaches in the screening of environmental agents for developmental toxicity. *Reprod Toxicol* 1993;7(Suppl 1):113–116.
155. Narotsky MG, Francis EZ, Kavloch RJ. Developmental toxicity and structure–activity relationships of aliphatic acids, including dose–response assessment of valproic acid in mice and rats. *Fundam Appl Toxicol* 1994;22(2):251–265.
156. Hansch C, Telzer BR, Zhang L. Comparative QSAR in toxicology: examples from teratology and cancer chemotherapy of aniline mustards. *Crit Rev Toxicol* 1995;25(1):67–89.
157. Gombar VK, Enslein K, Blake BW. Assessment of developmental toxicity potential of chemicals by quantitative structure-toxicity relationship models. *Chemosphere* 1995;31(1) 2499–2510.
158. Rosenkranz HS, Klopman G. Evaluating the ability of CASE, an artificial intelligence structure–activity relational system, to predict structural alerts for genotoxicity. *Mutagenesis* 1990;5(6): 525–527.
159. Rosenkranz HS, Klopman G. Predictions based upon the CASE structure–activity relational method are independent of the nature of the chemicals in the data base. *Qual Assur* 1993;2(3): 251–254.
160. Takihi N, Zhang YP, Klopman G, et al. An approach for evaluating and increasing the informational content of mutagenicity and clastogenicity data bases. *Mutagenesis* 1993;8(3):257–264.
161. Takihi N, Rosenkranz HS, Klopman G, et al. Structural determinants of developmental toxicity. *Risk Anal* 1994;14(4):649–657.
162. Cunningham A, Klopman G, Rosenkranz HS, et al. The carcinogenicity of diethylstilbestrol: structural evidence for a non-genotoxic mechanism. *Arch Toxicol* 1996;70(6):356–361.
163. Cunningham A, Klopman G, Rosenkranz HS. A study of the structural basis of the carcinogenicity of tamoxifen, toremifene and their metabolites. *Mutat Res* 1996;349(1):85–94.
164. Rosenkranz HS, Zhang YP, Macina OT, et al. Human developmental toxicity and mutagenesis. *Mutat Res* 1998;422(2):347–350.
165. Zhu X, Zhang YP, Klopman G, et al. Thalidomide and metabolites: indications of the absence of 'genotoxic' carcinogenic potentials. *Mutat Res* 1999;425(1):153–167.
166. Rosenkranz HS, Cunningham AR. A new approach to evaluate mechanistic relationships among genotoxic phenomena: validation. *Mutagenesis* 2000;15(4):325–328.
167. Rosenkranz HS. Computational toxicology and the generation of mechanistic hypotheses: gamma-butyrolactone. *SAR QSAR Environ Res* 2001;12(5):435–444.
168. Rosenkranz HS, Cunnignham AR. Chemical categories for health hazard identification: a feasibility study. *Regul Toxicol Pharmacol* 2001;33(3):313–318.
169. Rosenkranz HS. A paradigm for determining the relevance of short-term assays: application to oxidative mutagenesis. *Mutat Res* 2002;508(1–2):21–27.
170. Thampatty BP, Rosenkranz HS. SAR modeling: effect of experimental ambiguity. *Comb Chem High Throughput Screen* 2003;6(2): 161–166.
171. Rosenkranz HS, Thampatty BP. SAR: flavonoids and COX-2 inhibition. *Oncol Res* 2003;13(12):529–535.

CHAPTER

12

Olga Zharikova
Tatiana Nanovskaya
Mahmoud S. Ahmed

Biotransformation of Medications by Human Placenta

INTRODUCTION

Human placenta is a tissue of fetal origin located at the interface between the maternal and fetal circulations. The structure and diverse functions of human placenta undergo changes with gestation to accommodate and ensure normal fetal growth and development. Through gestation, the placenta assumes the functions of several organs that include the exchange of gasses (lungs), uptake of nutrients (gut), elimination of waste products (kidneys), and others. Other functions, such as the biosynthesis of human chorionic gonadotropin (hCG) and human placental lactogen (hPL), are specific to trophoblast tissue.

Historically, the placenta has been viewed as a protective barrier that decreases fetal exposure to endogenous metabolic waste products, xenobiotics, environmental pollutants and toxins (1). However, this view, following instances of birth defects related to the administration of medications/drugs to pregnant patients, was revised and the placenta was considered as a passive organ which allows molecules to indiscriminately pass across to the fetal circulation (2). For that reason, one of the major concerns of health care providers and researchers is the extent to which the placenta could protect the fetus from exposure to the medications that are administered to a patient during pregnancy. Current information indicates that human placenta "regulates" fetal exposure to xenobiotics by the existence of trophoblast/basal membrane layers and the activity of its metabolic enzymes responsible for the biotransformation of endogenous and exogenous compounds as well as the activity of its efflux transporters that extrude these compounds from the tissue and fetal circulation back to the maternal circulation.

This chapter will focus on the placental enzymes that are responsible for the biotransformation of medications administered to the pregnant woman. Several of these enzymes also catalyze reactions in metabolic pathways for the biosynthesis of important compounds. In this chapter, the term "biotransformation" will be used to describe the conversion of a medication/drug to its metabolite(s) and the term "metabolism" for conversion of one endogenous compound to another.

OVERVIEW OF XENOBIOTICS BIOTRANSFORMATION

Human liver is the primary organ responsible for the metabolism of endogenous compounds and the biotransformation of xenobiotics including drugs/medications. Other organs which are involved in the biotransfomation of medications are the intestine, pancreas, lungs, brain, skin, mammary glands, kidneys, testes, prostate, uterus, ovary, and the placenta (3–11).

The hepatic and extrahepatic enzymes responsible for the biotransformation of medications are classified according to the type of reaction they catalyze as well as their involvement in either phase I or II metabolism. The largest class of enzymes responsible for the biotransformation of medications and other compounds is the cytochrome P450 (CYP450) family of isozymes. The biotransformation of medications by CYP isozymes results in the formation of a metabolite that is either pharmacologically active, inactive (12), or toxic (13,14). The metabolites formed during phase I can be eliminated from the body unchanged or could be conjugated with the endogenously derived glucuronic acid, sulfate, glutathione, amino acids, or acetate (phase II) to form water-soluble conjugates (15). Most of these conjugated compounds are pharmacologically inactive and are rapidly excreted.

In human placenta, the expression and activity of enzymes involved in phase I (15–21) and phase II metabolic reactions were determined (17,20,22–24). However, their role in the biotransformation of medications administered during pregnancy is less investigated.

DETERMINING THE ACTIVITY OF ENZYMES RESPONSIBLE FOR THE BIOTRANSFORMATION OF MEDICATIONS

Information on the activity of hepatic and extrahepatic tissue enzymes responsible for the biotransformation of a medication is essential for the better understanding of its pharmacokinetics (PK) and pharmacodynamics (PD).

The placental enzymes are mainly localized in the endoplasmic reticulum of trophoblast tissue (microsomes), in the mitochondrial membranes, and to a lesser extent in the brush border membranes and cytoplasm. The expression of these enzymes in the tissue can be determined in vitro at the protein, mRNA (messenger RNA), or DNA levels. However, the presence of an enzyme as determined by its expression does not reflect its activity.

The activity of an enzyme can be determined in vivo and or in vitro. In vivo, the activity is determined by the administration of a probe compound that is a specific substrate of the enzyme. A change in enzyme activity will result in altering the PK of the probe substrate and will be revealed by the change in the area under the time-concentration curve (AUC) (25). However, this approach cannot differentiate between the activities of hepatic versus extrahepatic (including placental) enzymes.

The metabolic activity of a placental enzyme can be determined only by in vitro reactions utilizing subcelleular fractions (mitochondrial, microsomal or cytosolic) prepared from postpartum trophoblast tissue homogenates. The data obtained provides information on the kinetic parameters of the reaction, that is, its maximum rate/velocity (V_{max}) and the affinity of the substrate/medication to the enzyme (apparent K_m). Another valuable parameter, for characterization of the enzyme activity, is its intrinsic clearance (Cl_{in}), which is calculated from K_m/V_{max}. The intrinsic clearance of an enzyme can be used for comparing its activities between tissues or the activity of two different enzymes in the biotransformation of the same substrate.

In addition, in vitro experiments allow the identification of the enzymes involved in the biotransformation of xenobiotics. The identification of enzyme(s) in a subcellular fraction (e.g., microsomal or mitochondrial) can be achieved by utilizing inhibitors of its activity. These inhibitors are chemicals that are selective/specific for the enzyme catalyzing the reaction and antibodies raised against these enzymes. The chemical or antibody causing the greatest inhibition suggests the identity of the enzyme involved. Confirmation of enzyme identification is achieved by comparing of the values of the kinetics parameters of the reaction catalyzed by the microsomes with those catalyzed by the cDNA (complementary DNA) expressed/recombinant or the purified enzyme. The above is true for the identification of the enzyme in question whether in placental or any other tissue preparation.

REGULATION OF ENZYME ACTIVITY

The activity of metabolic enzymes is regulated at the DNA, mRNA, and/or protein level and varies between different cells and tissues. In human placenta, the expression and activities of its enzymes varies with gestational age to accommodate the diverse requirements of the fetus during organogenesis and development (26–31). Consequently, it was assumed that several CYP isozymes expressed during embryogenesis could be "switched off" during the period of fetal development (32,33).

The placenta contains both constitutive and inducible CYP isozymes. The constitutive enzymes are expressed and their activity could be detected during most of the gestational period. On the other hand, the expression and activity of inducible enzymes are subject to an individual's exposure to environmental and/or endogenous stimuli. An induced enzyme exhibits a transient increase in its activity for variable periods of time but usually returns to its basal level when the stimulus ceases to exist. The increase or decrease in the activity of an enzyme is referred to as enzyme up- or down-regulation and occurs at two levels namely, transcriptional (DNA to mRNA) or translational (mRNA to protein).

ENZYME ACTIVATION

The in vivo induction of a hepatic enzyme increases its activity and results in enhancing the biotransformation of a medication and consequently decreasing its efficacy (12,34,35). A similar in vivo induction of a placental enzyme that catalyzes the biotransformation of a medication is usually unnoticed because it is usually overshadowed by the activity of hepatic enzymes. However, the increase in the expression and/or activity of a placental enzyme following its induction can be determined in vitro utilizing postpartum tissue obtained from term or preterm placentas.

Alternatively, the increase in the activity of an allosteric enzyme does not require its induction. An allosteric enzyme has a substrate and an effector binding sites. The first is the active site to which the substrate binds and is biotransformed to a metabolite. The other site (allosteric) is located at a separate part of the quaternary structure of the enzyme where a ligand (the effector molecule) binds. The binding of the effector molecule causes either an increase in the activity of the enzyme in its biotransformation of the substrate (positive cooperativity) or a decrease (negative cooperativity). To the best of our knowledge, the allosteric type of enzymes has not been documented for CYP enzymes though data on the kinetics of several of their reactions revealed atypical steady state kinetics and suggested their existence (36). Several authors hypothesized the presence of two substrates binding sites, and a separate allosteric binding site (25,37,38).

In general, an increase in the activity of an enzyme that biotransforms a medication will result in enhanced first pass-metabolism, reduced bioavailability, decreased plasma concentration, and ultimately efficacy. On the other hand, for medications that are biotransformed to more active or reactive metabolites, increase in the enzyme activity could cause adverse effects and will be further discussed in this chapter.

ENZYME INHIBITION

The simultaneous administration of two medications that are substrates of the same enzyme will result in their biotransformation at lower rates. The medication with higher affinity (lower K_m) will be initially/preferentially biotransformed by the enzyme but the second medication will eventually compete with the first for the same substrate-binding site of the enzyme (competitive inhibition). The result is a higher plasma concentration of the two drugs than that predicted by their PK parameters, the prolongation of the pharmacological effects, and an increase in the likelihood of side effects.

The biotransformation of medication may be also inhibited by a component present in the diet. For example, grapefruit juice inhibits activity of hepatic CYP3A4 enzyme responsible for the biotransformation of numerous medications.

On the other hand, the administered medication could be pharmacologically inactive but is biotransformed to an active metabolite by a metabolic enzyme. In this example, inhibition of the responsible enzyme decreases the efficacy of the medication (12,35).

Activation or inhibition of an enzyme that occurs due to the concomitant administration of two or more medications is often referred to as drug-drug interactions (DDI).

FACTORS AFFECTING PLACENTAL BIOTRANSFORMATION OF MEDICATIONS

The activity of placental enzymes, determined in vitro, varies widely between individuals. This variability in enzyme activity could be explained by one or more factors that include—but not limited to—fetal race, frequency of single nucleotide polymorphisms (SNPs) in the gene coding for the enzyme, maternal exposure to environmental factors, dietary components and contaminants, as well as the administration of a medication that acts as an activator or inhibitor. For example, a wide range of activity was reveled for placental microsomal CYP19 responsible for the biotransformation of methadone and buprenorphine, the opiates used for treatment of the pregnant heroin/opiate addict. The observed variability in enzyme activity was due to differences in the rates of formation of the metabolites (V_{max}) rather than changes in the affinity of the substrates to the enzyme (apparent K_m) (5–7).

Single nucleotide polymorphisms (SNP) in a gene encoding a placental enzyme may also affect the expression of its mRNA, protein, or activity. For example, in nonpregnant women, the coding sequence variants in CYP19—which is also the major placental CYP enzyme—resulted in a decrease in its activity in catalyzing the aromatization of androgens, thus decreasing estrogen levels (39). This phenotype variant of CYP19 was associated with conditions related to low estrogen levels such as the risk of osteoporosis in postmenopausal women (40) and higher breast cancer survival (41). On the other hand, other variants in CYP19 coding sequences were associated with an increase in the activity of CYP19 and higher risk of premenopausal breast cancer (39).

Gestational age is another factor that could also affect the activity of placental enzymes. For example, the activity of placental CYP19 in the biotransformation of methadone increased with gestational age (11). However, this reported increase in CYP19 activity was not based on its determination in the same placenta at sequential periods of gestation. Rather, the activity of CYP19 at a gestational age represented the mean of several individual placentas delivered within a period of 3 to 4 weeks. The interpretation of the data obtained could be misleading since the etiology of preterm birth, as well as the reasons for each preterm delivery, is often unknown. In other words, it is unclear whether the determined expression/activity of the placental enzymes at early gestational ages is a factor of age or a result of the medical condition leading to the preterm delivery.

The activity of placenta enzymes could be also affected by drug interactions. There are numerous examples of DDI involving hepatic enzymes but much less is known for those in extrahepatic tissues including the placenta. Our knowledge of DDI involving placental enzymes is limited because of their smaller contribution to the total amount of the metabolites formed in vivo by hepatic enzymes. Another type of drug interaction observed in trophoblast tissue was for an enzyme catalyzing a reaction in a placental metabolic pathway being also responsible for the biotransformation of a medication. For example, placental CYP19 is a key enzyme in the conversion of androgens to estrogens and provides approximately 50% of their concentration in the maternal circulation. In addition, CYP19 is the major placental microsomal enzyme responsible for the in vitro biotransformation of methadone and buprenorphine, the opiates used for maintenance of the pregnant opiate addict (5,7). Evidence for this type of interaction in vivo was also provided in the report indicating lower levels of estriol in plasma of pregnant women maintained on methadone (42). The in vitro inhibition of placental conversion of androgens to estrogens by methadone and buprenorphine supported the dual role of CYP19 in the biosynthesis of estrogens and the biotransformation of opiates (43). Other medications that inhibit placental CYP19 activity are aminoglutethimide, an inhibitor of adrenocortical steroid synthesis; azoles, which are used as antifungal (e.g., econazol and miconazol) or cytostatic agent (fadrozole) (44–66); natural substances such as components of grapefruit juice, plant flavones, α-naphthoflavone (45); and others.

The above information indicates that human placenta could be a site for drug interactions and underscores the importance of identifying the enzymes responsible for the biotransformation of medications administered during pregnancy.

SIGNIFICANCE OF PLACENTAL BIOTRANSFORMATION OF MEDICATIONS

The placenta is exposed to all compounds present in the maternal blood including medications administered during pregnancy. The extent of fetal exposure to these compounds depends on their transfer across the placenta. The major determinants for xenobiotics transfer across human placenta have been extensively reviewed by several investigators (15,47) and can be divided into three major groups: properties of the drug, functions of placental enzymes and transporters, and maternal and fetal factors/medical conditions. It should be noted here that our knowledge of the concentration of a medication in the fetal circulation is limited to that in cord blood at delivery or the newborn.

Of direct relevance to this chapter is the relation between the activity of placental enzymes in the biotransformation of a medication and the extent of fetal exposure to the drug and its metabolites. The rates and amounts of metabolite formed, for each medication, vary widely between placentas (3–9). Moreover, the activity of placental enzymes constitutes a fraction of that of hepatic enzymes and is often considered as insignificant. However, this smaller amounts of the metabolites formed should not negate their importance because they are in close proximity to the fetal capillaries and consequently are more accessible to the fetal circulation than those formed by maternal hepatic enzymes (9,48). Consequently, if one or more metabolites formed in the placenta is pharmacologically active or toxic (13,14), then their effects on the fetus, whether favorable or unfavorable, might be more pronounced than those formed by hepatic enzymes. In general, the placenta contributes 10% or less of the total metabolites formed for a given medication (49,50). In that respect, the placenta should be viewed as a second line of defense that protects fetus from exposure to xenobiotics, the first being maternal liver. The rationale behind this view is as follows: the weight of a newborn averages between 4% and 8% of the mother's at delivery and the volume of the newborn circulation at term (500 mL or less) is approximately 7% to 8% of that of the pregnant woman (6 to 7 L). Therefore, the "lower" activity of the placental enzymes in the biotransformation of medications should be adequate for protecting the fetus from exposure to xenobiotics/medications in the maternal circulation.

Placental and hepatic enzymes could biotransform the same medication to structurally different metabolites as reported for 17-α-hydroxyprogesterone caproate (17-HPC), used for treatment of recurrent preterm deliveries. Human hepatic enzymes biotransform 17-HPC to several mono-, di-, and trihydroxylated metabolites. On the other hand, placental microsomal enzymes biotransforformed 17-HPC to monohydroxylated derivatives only and two of these metabolites were unique to the tissue, that is, were not formed by hepatic enzymes (10).

Another example for the differences between hepatic and placental enzymes is the biotransformation of the hypoglycemic drug glyburide. The metabolites formed by hepatic microsomes were identical in their structure to those formed by placental microsomes (Table 12.1) (51–112), but the rate of formation of each metabolite and its ratio to the total formed was different between two tissues (8,50). These differences were attributed to the CYP isoforms involved in the formation of each metabolite. Placental CYP19 was the major enzyme responsible for the biotransformation of

TABLE 12.1 Metabolites Formed In Vivo and In Vitro

Drug	*In Vivo*	*Hepatic Microsomes*	*Media of Perfused Placenta*	*Placental Microsomes*
17-hydroxyprogesterone caproate (17-HPC)	Urine and feces: free and conjugated metabolites (51)	21 metabolite: 5 mono-, 6 di-, 10 tri-OH-derivatives of 17-HPC (10); 3 metabolites (in microsomes) and 5 (in fresh human hepatocytes) (52)	2 metabolites (9)	5 metabolites (10)
Betamethasone (BM)	11-DeH-, 11-DeH-20-DH-, 6β-OH-17-oxo-, 20-DH-, □ 6 β-OH-, 6β-OH-20βξ-DH-BM (53)	11-K-BM (54)	11-K-BM (55)	11-K-BM (54,56,57)
Buprenorphine (BUP)	NorBUP (plasma [58]; urine, feces [59]); norBUP; BUP-G; OH-BUP-G; OH-norBUP-G (urine) (60) (*R,R*)-, (*S,S*)-OHB (62); THB; ETB (63,64)	NorBUP; OH-BUP; OH-nor-BUP (60)	NorBUP (61)	NorBUP (5)
Bupropion (B)	THB-G; ETB-G; G of OH-, H-, and DH- metabolites; -S of OH- and H- metabolites (65)	(*S,S*)-, (*R,R*)-OHB (66); ETB (64,67)	THB in media and tissue (68)	No reports
Carbamazepine (CBZ)	10,11-D; CBZ-E; 9-OH-Me-10-carbamoyl acridan (plasma) (3)	CBZ-E; 3-OH-CBZ; 2-OH-CBZ (69); 9-OH-Me-10-carbamoyl acridan; 10-OH-CBZ (70)	ND (3)	ND (70)
Cortisol (COR)	CT/11-K-, 6β-OH-, 1β-OH-TH-COR (71–73) (urine); free metabolites: CT; TOH-COR/3α,11β,17α,21-TOH-5βpregnan-20-one; 6β-OH-COR/6β,11β,17α,21-TOH-pregn-4-ene-3,20-dione; their oxidation products; COR-S; COR-G; -S and -G of metabolites (blood) (74)	CT (75); 3α,5β-TH-, 6β-OH-, 20β-DOH-CT; 6α-OH-, 6β-OH-, 20β-DOH-, 3α,5β-TH-COR (76)	CT (55,77,78)	CT (55–57, 77–79)

(*continued*)

TABLE 12.1 Metabolites Formed In Vivo and In Vitro (*Continued*)

Drug	*In Vivo*	*Hepatic Microsomes*	*Media of Perfused Placenta*	*Placental Microsomes*
Dexamethasone (DEX)	6β-OH-, 20-DH-, 11-DeH-DEX (plasma) (80, 81); 9α-fluoro-11β-OH-16α -Me-1,4-androstadiene-3, 17-dione (eye) (82); mostly unconjugated (83); 6β-OH-DEX; 6α-OH-DEX (urine) (84)	6β-OH-, 6α-OH-DEX; 6-OH-9α-fluoro-androsta-1,4-diene-11β -OH-16α -Me-3,17-dione; 9α-fluoro-androsta-1,4-diene-11β-OH-16α-Me-3,17-dione (85,86); DeH-DEX (71)	11-K-metabolite (55,87)	11-K-metabolite (55–57)
Glyburide (glibenclamide) (GLY)	4-*t*-, 3-*c*-OH-cyclohexyl-GLY (plasma, urine) (88–90), (urine, feces) (91)	4-*t*-, 3-*c*-(89), 4-*c*-, 3-*t*-, 2-*t*-OH-cyclohexyl-GLY and ethylene-OH-GLY (8,50)	ND (94)	ethylene-OH-GLY (major metabolite) and 4-*t*-, 3-*c*-, 4-*c*, 3-*t*-, 2-*t*-OH-cyclohexyl-GLY (8,50)
L-α-Acetylmethadol (LAAM)	NorLAAM and dinorLAAM (plasma) (92)	NorLAAM → dinorLAAM (93)	ND (95)	NorLAAM (6)
Methadone	EDDP (plasma, urine) (96,97) EDDP and EMDP(urine) (98,99)	EDDP (100,101) EDDP → EMDP (97) (*R*)- and (*S*)-EDDP	ND (102)	EDDP (7)
Olanzapine (OLZ)	10-*N*-OLZ-G; *N*-DM-, *N*-oxide-, 2-OH-Me-OLZ (plasma); 9 metabolites: 10-*N*-OLZ-G, *N*-DM-2-CO-, 2-CO-, *N*-oxide-OLZ (urine); 10-*N*-OLZ-G (major in feces) (103)	*N*-oxide-, *N*-DM-, 2-OH-Me-, 7-OH-OLZ (104)	10-*N*-OLZ-G (4)	No reports
Oxcarbazepine (OCBZ)	10-OH-CBZ; 10,11-D; (plasma) (3,105) 10-OH-CBZ; 10-OH-CBZ-G and -S; OCBZ-G (urine) (106)	10-OH-CBZ (70)	10-OH-CBZ (3)	10-OH-CBZ and unknown metabolite (70)
Prednisolone (PDN)	PD/11-K-PDN; 11β,17α,20α,21-, 11β,17α,20b,21-TOH-pregna-1, 4-dien-3-one; 3α,11β,17α,21-TOH-5β-pregnan-20-one; 17α, 20β,21-TrOH-pregna-1,4-dien-3, 11-dione; 3α,17α,21-TrOH-5β-pregnane-11,20-dione; 11b,17α, 21-TrOH-pregna-1,4-dien-3,20-dione; 17α,21-DOH-5β-pregn-1-ene-3,11,20-trione; 3α,11β-DOH-etiocholan-17-one; 3α,-OH-etiocholane-11,17-dione; 6β-OH-PDN; PDN-S; PDN-G (107)	PD; 11b,17α,21-TrOH-allopregnane-3,20-dione; 11β,17α,20b,11-TOH-4-pregnene-3-one (108)	PD (2,63) → 20α-DOH-PD; 20β-DOH-PD → 20β-DOH-PDN (109)	PD (55–57)
Propoxyphen	Norpropoxyphene (110,111)	Norpropoxyphene (111)	ND in media, (Norpropoxyphene determined in placental tissue) (112)	No reports

10,11-D, 10,11-trans-dihydroxy-10,11-dihydro-carbamazepine; *c*, cis; CO, carboxy-; CT, cortisone; DeH, dehydro-; DH, dihydro-; DM, desmethyl; DOH, dihydroxy-; E, expoxide; EDDP, 2-ethylidine-1,5-dimethyl-3,3-diphenyl-pyrrolidine; EMDP, 2-ethyl-5-methyl-3,3-diphenylpyrroline; ETB, erythrohydrobupropion; -G, glucuronide conjugate; H, hydrogenated; K, keto-; Me, methyl-; ND, not determined; OH, hydroxy-; OHB, hydroxybupropion; PD, prednisone; -S, sulphate conjugate; *t*, trans; TH, tetrahydro-; THB, threohydrobupropion; TOH, tetrahydroxy-; TrOH, trihydroxy-.

glyburide whereas the major hepatic enzymes were identified as CYP3A4, 2C9, and 2C8 (O. Zharikova, oral communication, 2009). Moreover, the predominant metabolite of glyburide formed by placental enzymes (ethylene-hydroxylated derivative) should have greater access to the fetal circulation because of its proximity. However, its pharmacologic activity remains unknown. In addition, hepatic enzymes biotransform glyburide to several metabolites and the amount of two of them, 4-trans and 3-cis hydroxylcyclohexyl glyburide, constituted 50% of the total and are pharmacologically active (i.e., cause hypoglycemia). On the other hand, the amounts of these two metabolites formed by placental enzyme were extremely small.

It is apparent that the major metabolite formed by the placenta, namely, the ethylene-hydroxylated derivative of glyburide, is different from that formed by hepatic enzymes. Also, its pharmacological activity needs to be determined to better understand the factors affecting fetal euglycemia in women treated with glyburide for gestational diabetes.

In conclusion, there are differences between the hepatic and the placental enzymes responsible for the biotransformation of a medication, which could lead to the formation of metabolite(s) structurally unique to each tissue. These differences underscore the importance of the identification of the placental enzymes involved, and the metabolites formed, for each medication used for treatment of the pregnant patient.

METHODS AND MODEL SYSTEMS UTILIZED IN INVESTIGATIONS OF PLACENTAL BIOTRANSFORMATION OF MEDICATIONS

In vivo investigations of the biotransformation of medications by human placental enzymes are limited because of ethical and safety considerations that exclude pregnant patients from clinical trials. Moreover, it is impossible to determine the tissue responsible for the formation of the metabolites (liver, placenta, or other extrahepatic tissues) identified in the blood or urine samples obtained from patients or volunteers. It is not then surprising that most of the data on human placental biotransformation of medications, the identification of the metabolites formed and the enzymes catalyzing each reaction are obtained from in vitro investigations.

The following is a summary of the methods and techniques utilized to obtain this data, their advantages, limitations, and difficulties encountered in providing information.

Placentas obtained from the most common laboratory animals (rats, mice, and other rodents) provide information that cannot be extrapolated to humans because of differences in the anatomy of their placentas. Only primates, among mammals, have placentas that are structurally similar to those of humans (113). Indeed, the biotransformation of medications by human placentas revealed similarities to those of rhesus macaques (114) and baboons (50). Therefore, subcellular fractions obtained from term or preterm placentas should be utilized. Placentas obtained from nonhuman primates could be also utilized but the data obtained should be validated for each medication.

The ex vivo technique of dual perfusion of human placental lobule (DPPL) provides valuable information on the transfer of drugs and is considered the best simulation of in vivo conditions. The method can also provide information on the biotransformation of a medication by placental enzymes in absence of maternal and fetal hepatic enzymes. However, its use to obtain the latter type of information has several limitations. First, the small size of the perfused placental cotolydon (4% to 5% of the placental total surface area) limits the access of a medication to the tissue's metabolic enzymes. Second, the selection of concentration of the perfused medication is based on its levels achieved in the maternal circulation and does not consider its affinity to placental enzymes. Third, the minimum amount of metabolite formed or medication transferred across the placenta that can be detected by the analytical method utilized e.g. spectrophotometric (HPLC-U.V./vis.), mass (LC-MS) or radioactive isotope.

The detection limit of the method used to determine the concentration of a medication and/or its metabolites is of paramount importance. The first step is usually extracting the medication and metabolites from the biological fluid obtained from the patient or from the medium of the perfusion system. In most cases, the detection, identification, and quantitative determination of a compound (medication or metabolite) are achieved by utilizing a high-performance liquid chromatography (HPLC) instrument equipped with a detector (spectrophotometer). The retention time of the drug or its metabolite on the HPLC stationary column is determined by utilizing that for the synthesized standard under identical conditions and serves as a guide for identification of the medication and its metabolites. The detection of the drug and its metabolites relies on their absorption of light at an appropriate wavelength (UV or visible), which is an intrinsic property of the compound (drug or metabolites). The detection limits of the spectrophotometer are usually in the microgram range and can be enhanced by 100 to 1000 times by the use of a mass spectrometer (LC-MS [liquid chromatography-mass spectrometry]), that is on line with the HPLC detector. This will also provide data on the mass of the compound, thus confirming its structure and identification (8,50). The detection of the quantity of the metabolite formed could be further increased by another 100 to 1000 times by using a radioisotope (tritium or 14C) of the medication, but it is crucial that the metabolite formed retains the radiolabeled atom present in the parent compound (9,61,115). The ability to detect this minute amount of the metabolite (pico- or femtograms), though crucial, should be carefully considered together with the biological significance of such a concentration before arriving to a conclusion on the extent to which the medication has crossed the placenta or has been biotransformed by its enzymes.

Most of the available information on the biotransformation of medications by term and preterm placentas has been obtained from in vitro methods that utilized microsomal and mitochondrial subcellular fractions prepared from trophoblast tissue homogenates. Several xenobiotics that are biotransformed by placental and hepatic enzymes are shown in Table 12.2 (5–7,50,52,55,57,60,65–67,69,71, 75–78,85,93,100,101,104,111,116–123).

TABLE 12.2 Enzymes, K_m, V_{max}

Drug	Human Placental Microsomes: Enzymes	K_m (μM)	V_{max} ($pmol. mg^{-1}. min^{-1}$)	References	Human Hepatic Microsomes: Enzymes	K_m (μM)	V_{max} ($pmol. mg^{-1}. min^{-1}$)	References
17-HPC	No reports				CYP3A	78		52
Betamethasone	11β-HSD type 2			57,77	11β-HSD type 1			75
Buprenorphine (BUP)	CYP19	12	3	5	CYP3A4	89	3,460	117
					CYP3A4,5	39	710	118
					CYP3A4 (65%), CYP2C8 (30%), (CYP3A5, 7)	15	1,224	60

Bupropion	No reports				CYP2B6	For (*R,R*)-OHB: □40–68
						For (*S,S*)-OHB: □63–90
						For total OHB: □109–162
							30–216
							56–448
							85–662
								66,119

Carbamazepine (CBZ)	Does not inhibit human expressed CYP19			119	CYP2B6 (CYP3A4 minor)	For 2-OH-CBZ: 349	30	67
	Inhibits CYP19 (in microsomes)			120	CYP3A4 (CYP2C8 minor)	For 3-OH-CBZ: 338	75	69
Cortisol	11β-HSD type 2	0.046		77,78	CYP3A (6β-hydroxylase)	15	6.43	76
					4-ene-reductase (cytosolic)	27	108	
					11β-HSD type 1	Oxydation: 0.98 Reduction: 1.4	95,000 187,000	71
Dexamethasone (DEX)	11β-HSD type 2			57	CYP3A4	For 6β-OH-DEX: 23 For 6α-OH-DEX: 25	14 4	85
					11β-HSD type 1	1.6	741,000	71,75
Glyburide (glibenclamide) (GLY)	CYP19	12	11	50	CYP2C9, 2C8, and 3A4 (OH-cyclohexyl-GLY)	4	213	50
				121				122
					CYP3A4 (ethylene-OH-GLY)			122,123
L-α-Acetylmethadol (LAAM)	CYP19	105	86	6	CYP3A4	Biphasic kinetics: 1. 19 2. 600	700–1,800 1,600–3,300	93
Methadone	CYP19	424	420	7	CYP3A4	545	745	101
					CYP3A4 (CYP2C9 and 2C19 possibly)	125–252	333–1,283	100
					CYP3A4, CYP2C8, CYP2D6			65
					CYP2B6, CYP3A4, CYP2C19	(*R*)-methadone: □48–62 (*S*)-methadone: 45–50	501–948 412–1,407	124
Olanzapine (OLZ)	No reports				Flavin mono-oxygenase 3			
					CYP1A2	For *N*-DM-OLZ: 42	41	04
					CYP2D6	For 2-OH-Me-OLZ: 49	8	
Oxcarbazepine	Inhibits human expressed CYP19			119	Inhibits CYP2C19, CYP3A4/5			120
Prednisolone	11β-HSD type 2			55	11β-HSD type 1			75
Propoxyphen	No reports				CYP34A	179–225	700–1,033	111

11β-HSD, 11β-hydroxysteroid dehydrogenase; CYP, cytochrome P; DM, desmethyl; Me, methyl-; OH, hydroxy-; OHB, hydroxybupropion.

PLACENTAL CYTOCHROME P450 ENZYMES

Placental CYP isozymes are localized in the endoplasmic reticulum (microsomal) and mitochondrial membranes of the syncytiotrophoblast layer. In term human placenta, the content of microsomal CYP enzymes is between 10% and 30% of that in adult human liver (16,49). It had been assumed that human placenta expresses a limited number of CYP isoforms but recent investigations, utilizing more sensitive methods for determining the expression of their mRNA (reverse transcriptase-PCR-based), allowed the identification of more than 30 CYP isoforms (18,19). A correlation between CYP mRNA expression and protein levels has been reported for hepatic and other tissues (19). Therefore, it is reasonable to assume that a similar correlation exists for human placenta. The major CYP isozymes identified in human placenta are those responsible for the biosynthesis of female steroid hormones. Based on analysis of the data (18), CYP19 mRNA comprises the majority (approximately 70%) of the total placental CYP isoforms, followed by mitochondrial CYP11A1/CYP450$_{scc}$ (approximately 25%), and the remaining isoforms (3% to 5%) with CYP2J2 being the highest. Interestingly, the expression of mRNA of the major hepatic drug-metabolizing CYP enzymes is low in term human placenta. For example, the expression of mRNA for CYP3A4 and 2C in placenta was close to, or below, the detection limit of the assay used while CYP1A2 was not detected (18,19,32,33). Other members of the CYP1 family of isozymes namely, CYP1A1 and 1B1, are expressed in extrahepatic tissue, including the placenta, and will be further discussed below.

The expression of placental enzymes appears to be dependent on gestational age. For example, mRNA of CYP1A2, 2F1, 4F2, and 4F8 are expressed in first trimester placentas but not at term suggesting their role, together with other enzymes, in cell proliferation and tissue differentiation during fetal organogenesis (18,19,32,33). It should be empathized that the expression of a CYP isozyme at the mRNA or protein level does not provide information on the extent of its activity. Indeed, the activities of only a limited number of CYP isozymes have been determined in preterm and term placentas.

The two major placental enzymes, mitochondrial CYP11A1/P450$_{scc}$ and microsomal CYP19, catalyze key reactions in the biosynthesis of female steroid hormones. CYP11A1 is responsible for the conversion of cholesterol to pregnenolone and CYP19 for androgens to estrogens. Over the last 2 decades, it became apparent that placental CYP isozymes and in particular CYP1A1 are also responsible for the biotransformation of several medications and xenobiotics (5–7,11,14,124,125). Recently, the ability of placental CYP2E1 to metabolize ethanol to acetaldehyde was demonstrated (22). Accordingly, the activity of many other CYPs identified in human placenta is yet to be determined.

CYP19/AROMATASE

The constitutive expression of CYP19 in human placenta is at a level greater than any other CYP isozyme (16,126). CYP19 was initially named aromatase because of its function in the aromatization of ring A in the cyclopentanophenanthrene nucleus of the cholesterol molecule. It is a key enzyme in the conversion of C-19 androgens to C-18 estrogens that are essential for maintenance of pregnancy (127–129). The conversion of androgens to estrogens is a three-step process; the first two steps are hydroxylation reactions typical of other cytochrome P450 isozymes. The third step is postulated to be a ferric peroxide removal of the intermediary aldehyde group, which results in the aromatization of the steroid A-ring (130). Data obtained using immunohistochemistry methods revealed that placental CYP19 is located in the endoplasmic reticulum of the syncytiotrophoblast (126). CYP19 is also highly expressed in the ovary (131), testis (132), adipose (28), and other tissues (29,126, 131,132). The distribution of CYP19 in mammalian tissues appears to be species-specific, as it has been identified in placentas of primates but not those of other mammals including rodents (133,134).

Recent and current investigations established the role of placental CYP19 in the biotransformation of several medications including those used for treatment of the pregnant opiate-dependent or -abusing patient (Tables 12.1 and 12.2). Buprenorphine is a partial opiate agonist that was introduced to the market as an alternative to methadone for treatment of this patient population. CYP19 was identified as the major term placental enzyme responsible for the biotransformation of buprenorphine to norbuprenorphine (5), while the hepatic enzymes responsible for the same reaction are CYP3A4 (59,101,117) and to a lesser extent CYP2C8 (60). Interestingly, the activity of CYP3A4 in human placental microsomes has not been reported.

Another opiate, methadone, has been the preferred medication for pharmacotherapy of heroin/opiate-dependent patients over the last 4 to 5 decades. Methadone maintenance programs for the pregnant opiate addict improve maternal and neonatal outcome and are recognized as the "gold standard" for treatment of this patient population. Nevertheless, an unexplained clinical observation is associated with methadone maintenance programs namely, the lack of a correlation between the dose of methadone administered to a patient during pregnancy, its concentration in the maternal blood, and the incidence and/or intensity of neonatal abstinence syndrome (NAS). An explanation for this observation is offered, namely, the concentration of methadone in the fetal circulation and not the maternal should correlate with NAS. This explanation is based on the following: Placental transfer of methadone from the maternal to fetal circulation depends on the thickness of the trophoblast/basal membrane layer, which is related to gestational age, the activity of placental microsomal enzymes in the biotransformation of methadone, and the activity of the efflux transporters located in the apical membranes in extruding the opiate from the tissue back to the maternal circulation.

An investigation of the biotransformation of methadone by microsomes prepared from placentas obtained from term healthy pregnancies revealed that CYP19 was the major enzyme responsible for its biotransformation to the metabolite 2-ethylidine-1, 5-dimethyl-3, 3-diphenylpyrrolidine (EDDP) (7). Placental biotransformation of methadone is different from that by human hepatic microsomes where the responsible enzymes were identified as

CYP2B6 and 2C19 (97,123,135,136), CYP3A4 (100,116, 137,138), and CYP2C8 and 2D6 (138). Moreover, several of these hepatic enzymes catalyzed the biotrasformation of EDDP to 2-ethyl-5-methyl-3, 3-diphenylpyrroline (EMDP).

L-α-Acetylmethadol (LAAM) is a congener of methadone that was used for treatment of opiate dependence but was withdrawn from the market because of its association with cardiac complications. LAAM is biotransformed by placental CYP19 to norLAAM (6), whereas human hepatic microsomal CYP3A4 sequentially biotransform LAAM to norLAAM and dinorLAAM (93,137,139). The above-mentioned reports demonstrate the differences between placental and hepatic enzymes responsible for the biotransformation of these three opiates. Similar differences between placental and hepatic biotransformation of other medications are sited in Tables 12.1 and 12.2. It should be noted that in human placenta, CYP19 assumes the functions of several hepatic enzymes in the biotransformation of medications, in addition to its role in the biosynthesis of estrogens.

There are several opiates that are used as analgesics, or for other indications, during pregnancy but for shorter periods of time by comparison to methadone maintenance programs. However, the rapid increase in the abuse of these prescription opiates in the United States by the public, including pregnant women, has raised concern over their effects on maternal and neonatal outcome (140) and prompted investigations of their effects on the activity of placental CYP19. The opiates methadone, buprenorphine, sufentanil, L-α-Acetylmethadol, fentanyl, oxycodone, codeine, and (+)-pentazocine inhibited the in vitro conversion of androgens to estradiol (E_2) and estriol (E_3) by placental CYP19 (43,121). However, the affinity of most of these opiates to CYP19 was lower than its endogenous substrates (high K_i, inhibition constant). Therefore, the administration of these opiates as prescription medications for a short period of time renders their effects on the in vivo biosynthesis of estrogens to be unlikely. On the other hand, the illicit use of fentanyl and sufentanil, both have higher affinity to CYP19 than the above-mentioned opiates, for longer durations could decrease placental biosynthesis of estrogens. Moreover, the opiates morphine, hydromorphone, oxymorphone, hydrocodone, propoxyphene, meperidine, levorphanol, dextorphan, (−)-pentazocine, and heroin increased the in vitro activity of CYP19 in the conversion of 16α-hydroxy-testosterone to estriol (E_3) but had no effect on the conversion of testosterone to estradiol (E_2) (121). Accordingly, it is unlikely that these opiates will have an adverse effect on the in vivo biosynthesis of estrogens by the placenta.

Medications, other than opiates, could also affect the expression and/or activity of CYP19. For example, glucocorticoids caused a significant decrease in the levels of its mRNA and activity (141). Alternatively, cigarette smoking (49) and drinking of alcohol during pregnancy (124) did not affect CYP19 gene expression but the in vitro activities of microsomes obtained from placentas of women who smoked during pregnancy and at the same time abused drugs (including opiates) were increased (142). Interestingly, these activities did not correlate with the activation of either CYP19 or CYP1A1.

Therefore, it appears that the activity of placental CYP enzymes in general—and those responsible for steroid-metabolism in particular—could be affected by medications administered during pregnancy.

CYP1 ISOZYMES

The CYP1 isozymes identified in most extrahepatic tissues including the placenta are CYP1A1 and CYP1B1 and they constitute a small fraction of hepatic CYP isozymes (18,19). CYP1A2 is mainly hepatic and constitutes between 10% and 12% of the total CYP450 isozymes (143) and is responsible for the biotransformation of approximately the same percentage of known medications (25,34,144).

CYP1 isozymes are involved in the biosynthesis of steroids and all three metabolize β-estradiol by its hydroxylation in different positions, thus giving rise to several metabolites (145). CYP1B1 is responsible for the metabolism of testosterone and progesterone (146–148). It is also responsible for the metabolism of retinoic acid (an essential compound for eye development), and a mutation in the gene coding for CYP1B1 could result in the development of primary congenital glaucoma (149).

A property shared between CYP1 isozymes is that their induction is mediated via the aryl hydrocarbon receptors (AhR) (31,150–153). Numerous and ubiquitous environmental xenobiotics were identified as ligands of these receptors (AhR). The environmental sources of these compounds include cigarette smoke (16,154,155), car exhaust containing polycyclic aromatic hydrocarbons (PAHs), smoked food products (156–158); food contaminated with dioxins (159,160), and charcoal-cooked food that contains aryl amines (161,162). The above-mentioned xenobiotics, as ligands of the aryl hydrocarbon receptors, induce CYP1 isozymes and most interestingly also become their substrates that are biotransformed to metabolites. The biotransformation of these xenobiotics does not always lead to their detoxification. On the contrary, CYP1 isozymes biotransform procarcinogens to metabolites that bind covalently to DNA and form mutagenic adducts that could be the first step in the chemically induced carcinogenesis (35).

Alternatively, the induction of CYP1 mono-oxydase activity could result in the detoxification of a compound by forming metabolites that are nontoxic or less toxic than the parent compound (34,152). This effect was demonstrated in laboratory animals where an intraperitoneal injection of compounds that induce CYP1A resulted in decreased tumorigenesis caused by the highly carcinogenic compound 7,12-dimethylbenz[α]anthracene (DMBA) (35,163).

Most CYP1 substrates, including several medications, are biotransformed by more than one isozyme. For example, dacarbazine, phenacetin, and propranalol are biotransformed by both recombinant CYP1A2 and CYP1A1 (164,165). Similarly, theophylline and caffeine are biotransformed by recombinant CYP1A2 and CYP1B1 (166,167). It is interesting to note that caffeine and phenacetin are biotransformed by CYP1A1 and 1B1, respectively but are used as probe substrates for determining the in vivo activity of CYP1A2 (16). It is therefore apparent that the determination of the metabolites of CYP1 substrates, formed in vivo, in biological fluids of individuals usually indicates the induction/activity of hepatic CYP1A2 only. This is due to the relative abundance of hepatic CYP1A2 over the other members of CYP1 isozymes and the lack of a probe substrate that is selective or specific for each one of these isozymes.

The exposure of individuals to polycyclic aromatic hydrocarbons or tobacco smoke induces the expression of CYP1 isozymes. The increase in the activity of CYP1 isozymes is determined in vitro by utilizing the following reactions: O-deethylation of 7-ethoxy-coumarin (ECOD), O-deethylation of 7-ethoxyresorufin (EROD), O-deethylation of phenacetin (POD), and/or hydroxylation of the aryl hydrocarbon benzo[α]pyrene (168–170). In general, these deethylation and hydroxylation reactions are catalyzed by all recombinant CYP1 isozymes. However, the kinetic constants of the reaction (apparent K_m and V_{max}) for each CYP1 isozyme are different from those catalyzed by the others (165,166,171). The unique kinetic constants for the biotransformation of a substrate by a particular CYP1 isozyme together with the determination of its expression allow its identification and localization in a tissue. For example, the hydroxylation of aryl hydrocarbons (AHH) is attributed to the activity of CYP1A1 and CYP1B1. Accordingly, a tissue sample obtained from human placenta or other extrahepatic organ that demonstrates an increase in the rate of any of the three reactions, EROD, POD or ECOD, and correlates with an increase in the rate of AHH indicates that either CYP1A1 or CYP1B1 has been induced (34,170,172). Alternatively, if the sample is from hepatic tissue, then the lack of such a correlation suggests that CYP1A2 has been induced (34,168,172).

The expression of CYP1 isozymes has been determined in term and preterm placentas of different gestational ages (18,19). However, CYP1A2 mRNA was only identified in placentas obtained from first trimester deliveries (20,33) but not in those obtained at term (18,19,32). On the other hand, there are no reports on the activity of CYP1A2 in placentas obtained from preterm or term placentas. The expression of CYP1B1 mRNA was detected in first trimester (33) and term placentas (18–20), but its expression was not induced by maternal cigarette smoking (154,173).

The expression of CYP1A1 in human placenta is constitutive during gestation but is also induced by environmental factors that include maternal smoking (17,20,23,32,33, 49,170,174,175). The induction of CYP1A1 by tobacco smoking results in a 10-fold or more increase in its activity as determined in vitro by AHH and EROD (170,172,173, 176,177). CYP1A1 is also induced by maternal exposure to the following environmental pollutants: polychlorinated biphenyls present in contaminated rice oils as well as their thermal degradation products including dibenzofurans (172,178); organochlorines accumulating in fish (179); and polycyclic aromatic hydrocarbons (PAHs) in the air (141,142,180).

Maternal smoking is considered a factor associated with the high levels of DNA adducts in their placentas (181–183). Interestingly, DNA adducts of compounds related to polyaromatic hydrocarbons were also identified in placentas obtained from women who did not report cigarette smoking during pregnancy, suggesting that other sources of PAH can cause similar effects (184). Indeed, the ingestion of seafood containing organochlorines that were identified in the placental tissue and cord blood also resulted in the formation of DNA adducts (179). Accordingly, the presence of carcinogens in the maternal circulation or in the placenta could lead to their biotransformation to metabolites that form adducts with DNA and could be an indication of damage to fetal DNA and possible predisposing an individual to the development of serious diseases later in life (183).

There are several reports that associate the activity of placental CYP1A1 with intrauterine toxicity in human. Lower birth weight of neonates of mothers who smoked cigarettes during pregnancy was associated with an increase in the activity of placental aryl hydrocarbon hydroxylation (AHH) (185) and higher levels of DNA adducts (181). On the other hand, AHH activity was significantly lower in placentas obtained from mothers delivering infants with abnormalities such as anencephaly (186). In addition, the metabolic activity of CYP1A1 is lower in placentas obtained from older mothers. The authors suggested that the decrease in the activity of placental CYP1A1 could be one of the reasons for the higher risk of fetal complications in "older" mothers (23).

It is apparent that CYP1A1 and CYP1B1 as well as other CYP isozymes in the feto-placental unit should have a role in the metabolic pathways that provide essential intermediates for normal fetal organogenesis, growth, and development. Placental CYP isozymes are also responsible for the biotransformation of xenobiotics, including medications, present in the maternal circulation, and their activities are a major contributor to the role of human placenta as a functional barrier that decreases fetal exposure to medications.

In conclusion, the activity of placental enzymes in the biotransformation of a medication is a fraction of that of hepatic enzymes. In addition, the biotransformation of a medication by placental enzymes could lead to the formation of a metabolite that is structurally different from that formed by a hepatic enzyme. The metabolites formed by the placenta are also more accessible to the fetal circulation and their potential effect on the fetus could be more pronounced. Moreover, the placenta can be a site for drug interactions when one of its enzymes that catalyzes a reaction in a metabolic pathway is also responsible for the biotransformation of an administered medication.

The aforementioned information underscores the importance of identifying the placental enzymes responsible for the biotransformation of medications administered to a pregnant woman as well as their metabolites and their effects on fetal growth and development.

ACKNOWLEDGMENTS

This chapter was supported, in part, by the following grants: the Obstetric-Fetal Pharmacology Research Units Network (OPRU, U10-HD0478, NICHD), the National Institute on Drug Abuse (Grants DA13431 and DA024094). The authors express their gratitude to Sarah Hemauer, M.D., Ph.D., combined degree student and Mrs. Svetlana Patrikeeva, B. S., for their assistance in preparation of the text, tables, and references.

REFERENCES

1. Yaffe SJ. Introduction. In: Briggs G, Freeman RK, Yaffe SJ, eds. *Drugs in pregnancy and lactation.* Baltimore, MD: Williams & Wilkins, 1998.

2. Young AM, Allen CE, Audus KL. Efflux transporters of the human placenta [review]. *Adv Drug Deliv Rev* 2003;55(1):125–132.
3. Pienimäki P, Lampela E, Hakkola J, et al. Pharmacokinetics of oxcarbazepine and carbamazepine in human placenta. *Epilepsia* 1997;38(3):309–316.
4. Schenker S, Yang Y, Mattiuz E, et al. Olanzapine transfer by human placenta. *Clin Exp Pharmacol Physiol* 1999;26:691–697.
5. Deshmukh SV, Nanovskaya TN, Ahmed MS. Aromatase is the major enzyme metabolizing buprenorphine in human placenta. *J Pharmacol Exp Ther* 2003;306:1099–1105.
6. Deshmukh SV, Nanovskaya TN, Hankins GDV, et al. N-demethylation of levo-α-acetylmethadol by human placental aromatase. *Biochem Pharmacol* 2004;67:885–892.
7. Nanovskaya TN, Deshmukh SV, Nekhaeva IA, et al. Methadone metabolism by human placenta. *Biochem Pharmacol* 2004;68: 583–591.
8. Ravindran S, Zharikova OL, Hill RA, et al. Identification of glyburide metabolites formed by hepatic and placental microsomes of humans and baboons. *Biochem Pharmacol* 2006;72:1730–1737.
9. Hemauer SJ, Yan R, Patrikeeva SL, et al. Transplacental transfer and metabolism of 17-alpha-hydroxyprogesterone caproate. *Am J Obstet Gynecol* 2008;199(2):169.e1–169.e5.
10. Yan R, Nanovskaya TN, Zharikova OL, et al. Metabolism of 17-alpha-hydroxyprogesterone caproate by hepatic and placental microsomes of human and baboons. *Biochem Pharmacol* 2008; 75(9):1848–1857.
11. Hieronymus TL, Nanovskaya TN, Deshmukh SV, et al. Methadone metabolism by early gestational age placentas. *Am J Perinatol* 2006;23(5):287–294.
12. Leucuta SE, Vlase L. Pharmacokinetics and metabolic drug interactions. *Curr Clin Pharmacol* 2006;1(1):5–20.
13. Manchester DK, Wilson VL, Hsu IC. Synchronous fluorescence spectroscopic, immunoaffinity chromatographic and 32P-postlabeling analysis of human placenta DNA know to contain benzo[a]pyrene diol epoxide adducts. *Carcinogenesis* 1990;11: 553–559.
14. Sawada M, Kitamura R, Norose T, et al. Metabolic activation of aflatoxin B1 by human placental microsomes. *J Toxicol Sci* 1993; 18(2):129–132.
15. Syme MR, Paxton JW, Keelan JA. Drug transfer and metabolism by human placenta. *Clin Pharmacokinet* 2004;43:487–514.
16. Hakkola J, Pelkonen O, Pasanen M, et al. Xenobiotic-metabolizing cytochrome P450 enzymes in the human feto-placental unit: role in intrauterine toxicity [review]. *Crit Rev Toxicol* 1998;28(1): 35–72.
17. Pasanen M. The expression and regulation of drug metabolism in human placenta. *Adv Drug Deliv Rev* 1999;38:81–97.
18. Nishimura M, Yaguti H, Yoshitsugu H, et al. Tissue distribution of mRNA expression of human cytochrome P450 isoforms assessed by high-sensitivity real-time reverse transcription PCR. *Yakugaku Zasshi* 2003;123(5):369–375.
19. Bièche I, Narjoz C, Asselah T, et al. Reverse transcriptase-PCR quantification of mRNA levels from cytochrome (CYP)1, CYP2 and CYP3 families in 22 different human tissues. *Pharmacogenet Genomics* 2007;17(9):731–742.
20. Myllynen P, Pasanen M, Vähäkangas K. The fate and effects of xenobiotics in human placenta [review]. *Expert Opin Drug Metab Toxicol* 2007;3(3):331–346.
21. Huuskonen P, Storvik M, Reinisalo M, et al. Microarray analysis of the global alterations in the gene expression in the placentas from cigarette-smoking mothers. *Clin Pharmacol Ther* 2008;83(4): 542–550.
22. Collier AC, Ganley NA, Tingle MD, et al. UDP-glucuronosyltransferase activity, expression and cellular localization in human placenta at term. *Biochem Pharmacol* 2002;63(3):409–419.
23. Collier AC, Tingle MD, Paxton JW, et al. Metabolizing enzyme localization and activities in the first trimester human placenta: the effect of maternal and gestational age, smoking and alcohol consumption. *Hum Reprod* 2002;17(10):2564–2572.
24. Zusterzeel PL, Nelen WL, Roelofs HM, et al. Polymorphisms in biotransformation enzymes and the risk for recurrent early pregnancy loss. *Mol Hum Reprod* 2000;6(5):474–478.
25. Wienkers LC, Heath TG. Predicting in vivo drug interactions from in vitro drug discovery data. *Nat Rev Drug Discov* 2005;4(10): 825–833.
26. Kilgore MW, Means GD, Mendelson CR, et al. Alternative promotion of aromatase P-450 expression in the human placenta. *Mol Cell Endocrinol* 1992;83(1):R9–R16.
27. Simpson ER, Mahendroo MS, Means GD, et al. Tissue-specific promoters regulate aromatase cytochrome P450 expression [review]. *J Steroid Biochem Mol Biol* 1993;44(4–6):321–330.
28. Simpson ER, Zhao Y, Agarwal VR, et al. Aromatase expression in health and disease. *Recent Prog Horm Res* 1997;52:185–213.
29. Simpson ER, Michael MD, Agarwal VR, et al. Cytochromes P450 11: expression of the CYP19 (aromatase) gene: an unusual case of alternative promoter usage [review]. *FASEB J* 1997;11(1):29–36.
30. Mendelson CR, Jiang B, Shelton JM, et al. Transcriptional regulation of aromatase in placenta and ovary. *J Steroid Biochem Mol Biol* 2005;95(1–5):25–33.
31. Pavek P, Dvorak Z. Xenobiotic-induced transcriptional regulation of xenobiotic metabolizing enzymes of the cytochrome P450 superfamily in human extrahepatic tissues [review]. *Curr Drug Metab* 2008;9(2):129–143.
32. Hakkola J, Pasanen M, Hukkanen J, et al. Expression of xenobiotic-metabolizing cytochrome P450 forms in human full-term placenta. *Biochem Pharmacol* 1996;51(4):403–411.
33. Hakkola J, Raunio H, Purkunen R, et al. Detection of cytochrome P450 gene expression in human placenta in first trimester of pregnancy. *Biochem Pharmacol* 1996;52(2):379–383.
34. Pelkonen O, Mäenpää J, Taavitsainen P, et al. Inhibition and induction of human cytochrome P450 (CYP) enzymes [review]. *Xenobiotica* 1998;28(12):1203–1253.
35. Lin JH, Lu AY. Inhibition and induction of cytochrome P450 and the clinical implications [review]. *Clin Pharmacokinet* 1998; 35(5):361–390.
36. Atkins WM. Non-Michaelis-Menten kinetics in cytochrome P450-catalyzed reactions [review]. *Annu Rev Pharmacol Toxicol* 2005;45: 291–310.
37. Szklarz GD, Halpert JR. Molecular basis of P450 inhibition and activation. Implications for drug development and drug therapy. *Drug Metab Dispos* 1998;26:1179–1184.
38. Lee CA, Manyike PT, Thummel KE, et al. Mechanism of cytochrome P450 activation by caffeine and 7,8-benzoflavone in rat liver microsomes. *Drug Metab Dispos* 1997;25(10):1150–1156.
39. Talbott KE, Gammon MD, Kibriya MG, et al. A CYP19 (aromatase) polymorphism is associated with increased premenopausal breast cancer risk. *Breast Cancer Res Treat* 2008;111(3):481–487.
40. Gennari L, Masi L, Merlotti D, et al. A polymorphic CYP19 TTTA repeat influences aromatase activity and estrogen levels in elderly men: effects on bone metabolism. *J Clin Endocrinol Metab* 2004;89(6):2803–2810.
41. Huang CS, Kuo SH, Lien HC, et al. The CYP19 TTTA repeat polymorphism is related to the prognosis of premenopausal stage I–II and operable stage III breast cancers. *Oncologist* 2008;13(7): 751–760.
42. Facchinetti FG, Comitini F, Petraglia A, et al. Reduced estriol and dehydroepianrosterone sulphate plasma levels in methadone-addicted pregnant women. *Eur J Obstet Gynecol Reprod Biol* 1986; 23:67–73.
43. Zharikova OL, Deshmukh SV, Nanovskaya TN, et al. The effect of methadone and buprenorphine on human placental aromatase. *Biochem Pharmacol* 2006;71(8):1255–1264.
44. Bossche HV, Moereels H, Koymans Luc MH. Aromatase inhibitors—mechanisms for non-steroidal inhibitors. *Breast Cancer Res Treat* 1994;30:43–55.
45. Stresser DM, Turner SD, McNamara J, et al. A high-throughput screen to identify inhibitors of aromatase (CYP19). *Anal Biochem* 2000;284:427–430.
46. Trösken ER, Fischer K, Völkel W, et al. Inhibition of human CYP19 by azoles used as antifungal agents and aromatase inhibitors, using a new LC–MS/MS method for the analysis of estradiol product formation. *Toxicology* 2006;219:33–40.
47. Audus KL. Controlling drug delivery across the placenta. *Eur J Pharm Sci* 1999;8(3):161–165.
48. Karl P, Gordon B, Lieber C, et al. Acetaldehyde production and transfer in perfused human placental cotyledon. *Science* 1988; 242:273–275.
49. Pasanen M, Pelkonen O. Xenobiotic and steroid-metabolizing monooxygenases catalyzed by cytochrome P450 and glutathione S-transferase conjugations in the human placenta and theft relationships to maternal cigarette smoking. *Placenta* 1990; 11:75–85.
50. Zharikova OL, Ravindran S, Nanovskaya TN, et al. Kinetics of glyburide metabolites by hepatic and placental microsomes of humans and baboons. *Biochem Pharmacol* 2007;73:2012–2019.

51. Davis EM, Plotz JE, Lupu CI. The metabolism of progesterone and its related compounds in human pregnancy. *Fertil Steril* 1960; 11:18–48.
52. Sharma S, Ou J, Strom S, et al. Identification of enzymes involved in the metabolism of 17-alpha-hydroxyprogesterone caproate: an effective agent for prevention of preterm birth. *Drug Metab Dispos* 2008;36(9):1896–1902.
53. Butler J, Grey CH. The metabolism of betamethasone. *J Endocrinol* 1970;46(3):379–390.
54. Anderson AB, Gennser G, Jeremy JY, et al. Placental transfer and metabolism of betamethasone in human pregnancy. *Obstet Gynecol* 1977;49(4):471–474.
55. Levitz M, Jansen V, Dancis J. The transfer and metabolism of corticosteroids in the perfused human placenta. *Am J Obstet Gynecol* 1978;132(4):363–366.
56. Blanford TA, Murphy BE. In vitro metabolism of prednisolone, dexamethasone, betamethasone, and cortisol by the human placenta. *Am J Obstet Gynecol* 1977;127:264–267.
57. Murphy VE, Fittock RJ, Zaezycki PK, et al. Metabolism of synthetic steroids by the human placenta. *Placenta* 2007;28:39–46.
58. Moody DE, Slawson MH, Strain EC, et al. A liquid chromatographic-electrospray ionization-tandem mass spectrometric method for determination of buprenorphine, its metabolite, norbuprenorphine, and a coformulant, naloxone, that is suitable for in vivo and in vitro metabolism studies. *Anal Biochem* 2002;306(1):31–39.
59. Cone EJ, Gorodetzky CW, Yousefnejad D, et al. The metabolism and excretion of buprenorphine in humans. *Drug Metab Dispos* 1984;12(5):577–581.
60. Picard N, Cresteil T, Djebli N, et al. In vitro metabolism study of buprenorphine: evidence for new metabolic pathways. *Drug Metab Dispos* 2005;33(5):689–695.
61. Nanovskaya TN, Deshmukh SV, Brooks M, et al. Transplacental transfer and metabolism of buprenorphine. *Pharmacology* 2002; 300(1):26–33.
62. Coles R, Kharasch ED. Stereoselective analysis of bupropion and hydrocybupropion in human plasma and urine by LC/MS/MS. *J Chromatogr B Analyt Technol Biomed Life Sci* 2007;857:67–75.
63. Loboz KK, Gross AS, Ray J, et al. HPLC assay for bupropion and its major metabolites in human plasma. *J Chromatogr B Analyt Technol Biomed Life Sci* 2005;823:115–121.
64. Schroeder DH. Metabolism and kinetics of bupropion. *J Clin Psychiatry* 1983;45:79–81.
65. Petsalo A, Turpeinen M, Tolonen A. Identification of bupropion urinary metabolites by liquid chromatography/mass spectrometry. *Rapid Commun Mass Spectrom* 2007;21:2547–2554.
66. Coles R, Kharasch ED. Stereoselective metabolism of bupropion by cytochrome P4502B6 (CYP2B6) and human liver microsomes. *Pharm Res* 2008;25(6):1405–1411.
67. Faucette SR, Hawke RL, Shord SS, et al. Evaluation of the contribution of cytochrome P450 3A4 to human liver microsomal bupropion hydroxylation. *Drug Metab Dispos* 2001;29: 1123–1129.
68. Earhart AD, Patrikeeva S, Wang X, et al. Transplacental transfer and metabolism of bupropion. *J Matern Fetal Neonatal Med* 2009;31:1–10.
69. Kerr BM, Thummel KE, Wurden CJ, et al. Human liver carbamazepine metabolism. Role of CYP3A4 and CYP2C8 in 10,11-epoxide formation. *Biochem Pharmacol* 1994;47(11):1969–1979.
70. Myllynen P, Pienimaki P, Raunio H, et al. Microsomal metabolism of carbamazepine and oxcarbazepine in liver and placenta. *Hum Exp Toxicol* 1998;17:668–676.
71. Deiderich S, Hanke B, Burkhardt P, et al. Metabolism of synthetic corticosteroids by 11β-hydroxysteroid-dehydrogenases in man. *Steroids* 1998;63:271–277.
72. Dixon R, Jones S, Pennington GW. The in vivo transformation of cortisol to 1b-hydroxytetrahydrococtisone. *Steroids* 1968;11(5): 693–697.
73. Pal SB. 6-hydroxylation of cortisol and urinary 6β-hydroxycortisol. *Metabolism* 1978;27(8):1003–1011.
74. Kornel L, Moore J, Noyes I. Corticosteroids in human blood: IV. Distribution of Cortisol and its metabolites between plasma and erythrocytes in vivo. *J Clin Endocrinol Metab* 1970;30(1):40–50.
75. Diederich S, Eigendorff E, Burkhardt P, et al. 11β-hydroxysteroid dehydrogenase types 1 and 2: an important pharmacokinetic determinant for the activity of synthetic mineralo- and glucocorticoids. *J Clin Endocrinol Metab* 2002;87(12):5695–5701.
76. Abel SM, Back DJ. Cortisol metabolism in vitro-III. Inhibition of microsomal 6β-hydroxylase and cystolic 4-ene-reductase. *J Steroid Biochem Mol Biol* 1993;46(6):827–832.
77. Benediktsson R, Calder AA, Edwards CRW, et al. Placental 11β-hydroxysteroid dehydrogenase: a key regulator of fetal glucocorticoid exposure. *Clin Endocrinol* 1997;46:161–166.
78. Stewart PM, Rogerson FM, Mason JI. Type 2 11β-hydroxysteroid dehydrogenase messenger ribonucleic acid and activity in human placenta and fetal membranes: its relationship to birth weight and putative role in fetal adrenal steroidogenesis. *J Clin Endocrinol Metab* 1995;80:885–890.
79. Osincki PA. Steroid 11beta-ol dehydrogenase in human placenta. *Nature* 1960;187:777.
80. Best R, Nelson SM, Walker BR. Dexamethasone and 11-dehydrodexamethasone as tools to investigate the isozymes of 11β-hydroxysteroid dehydrogenase in vitro and in vivo. *J Endocrinol* 1997;153:41–48.
81. Lowy MT, Meltzer HY. Dexamethasone bioavailability: implications for DST research. *Biol Psychiatry* 1987;22:373–385.
82. Ichigashira N, Yamaga N. Intraocular fate of dexamethasone disodium phosphate topically applied to the eyes of rabbits. *Steroids* 1978;32:615–628.
83. Haque N, Thrasher K, Werk E, et al. Studies on dexamethasone metabolism in man: effect of diphenylhydantoin. *J Clin Endocrinol Metab* 1972;34(1):44–50.
84. Zurbonsen K, Bressolle F, Solassol I, et al. Simultaneous determination of dexamethasone and 6beta-hydroxydexamethasone in urine using solid-phase extraction and liquid chromatography: applications to in vivo measurement of cytochrome P450 3A4 activity. *J Chromatogr B Analyt Technol Biomed Life Sci* 2004; 804(2):421–429.
85. Gentile DM, Tomlinson ES, Maggs JL, et al. Dexamethasone metabolism by human liver in Vitro. Metabolite identification and inhibition of 6-hydroxylation. *J Pharmacol Exp Ther* 1996;277: 105–112.
86. Tomlinson ES, Lewis DFV, Maggs JL, et al. In vitro metabolism of dexamethasone (DEX) in human liver and kidney: the involvement of CYP3A4 and CYP17 (17,20 LYASE) and molecular modeling studies. *Biochem Pharmacol* 1997;54:605–611.
87. Smith MA, Thomford PJ, Mattison DR, et al. Transport and metabolism of dexamethasone in the dually perfused human placenta. *Reprod Toxicol* 1988;2(1):37–43.
88. Rupp W, Christ O, Heptner W. Resorption, excretion and metabolism after intravenous and oral administration of HB 419–14C in man [in German]. *Arzneimittelforschung* 1969;19:1428–1434.
89. Fuccella LM, Tamassia V, Valzelli G. Metabolism and kinetics of the hypoglycemic agent glipizide in man—comparison with glibenclamide. *J Clin Pharmacol* 1973;13:68–75.
90. Rydberg T, Wåhlin-Boll E, Melander A. Determination of glibenclamide and its two major metabolites in human serum and urine by column liquid chromatography. *J Chromatogr* 1991; 564:223–233.
91. Balant L, Fabre J, Zahnd GR. Comparison of the pharmacokinetics of glipizide and glibenclamide in man. *Eur J Clin Phamacol* 1975;8:63–69.
92. Kharasch ED, Whittington D, Hoffer C, et al. Paradoxical role of cytochrome P450 3A in the bioactivation and clinical effects of levo-alpha-acetylmethadol: importance of clinical investigations to validate in vitro drug metabolism studies. *Clin Pharmacokinet* 2005;44(7):731–751.
93. Oda Y, Kharasch ED. Metabolism of levo-alpha-acetylmethadol (LAAM) by human liver cytochrome P450: involvement of CYP3A4 characterized by atypical kinetics with two binding sites. *J Pharmacol Exp Ther* 2001;297(1):410–422.
94. Nanovskaya TN, Nekhayeva I, Hankins GD, et al. Effect of human serum albumin on transplacental transfer of glyburide. *Biochem Pharmacol* 2006;72(5):632–639.
95. Nanovskaya TN, Deshmukh SV, Miles R, et al. Transfer of L-alpha-acetylmethadol (LAAM) and L-alpha-acetyl-N-normethadol (norLAAM) by the perfused human placental lobule. *J Pharmacol Exp Ther* 2003;306(1):205–212.
96. Moody DE, Lin S, Chang Y, et al. An enantiomer-selective liquid chromatography-tandem mass spectrometry method for methadone and EDDP validated for use in human plasma, urine, and liver microsomes. *J Anal Toxicol* 2008;32(3):208–219.
97. Kharasch ED, Hoffer C, Whittington D, et al. Role of hepatic and intestinal cytochrome P450 3A and 2B6 in the metabolism,

disposition, and miotic effects of methadone. *Clin Pharmacol Ther* 2004;76:250–269.

98. Beckett AH, Taylor JF, Casy AF, et al. The biotransformation of methadone in man: synthesis and identification of a major metabolite. *J Pharm Pharmacol* 1968;20(10):754–762.
99. Pohland A, Boaz HE, Sullivan HR. Synthesis and identification of metabolites resulting from the biotransformation of DL-methadone in man and in the rat. *J Med Chem* 1971;14(3):194–197.
100. Foster DJ, Somogyi AA, Bochner F. Methadone N-demethylation in human liver microsomes: lack of stereoselectivity and involvement of CYP3A4. *Br J Clin Pharmacol* 1999;47:403–412.
101. Iribarne C, Picard D, Dréano Y, et al. Involvement of cytochrome P450 3A4 enzyme in the N-demethylation of buprenorphine in human liver microsomes. *Life Sci* 1997;60(22):1953–1964.
102. Nekhayeva IA, Nanovskaya TN, Deshmukh SV, et al. Bidirectional transfer of methadone across human placenta. *Biochem Pharmacol* 2005;69(1):187–197.
103. Kassahun K, Mattiuz E, Nyhart E, et al. Disposition and biotransformation of the antipsychotic agent olanzapie in humans. *Drug Metab Dispos* 1996;25(1):81–93.
104. Ring BJ, Catlow J, Lindsay TJ, et al. Identification of the human cytochromes P450 responsible for the in vitro formation of the major oxidative metabolites of the antipsychotic agent olanzapine. *J Pharmacol Exp Ther* 1996;276(2):658–666.
105. Myllynen P, Pienimaki P, Jouppila P, et al. Transplacental passage of oxcarbazepine and its metabolites in vivo. *Epilepsia* 2001;42(11):1482–1485.
106. Schutz H, Feldmann KF, Faigle JW. The metabolism of C14-oxcabazepine in man. *Xenobiotica* 1986;16(8):769–778.
107. Frey FJ. Kinetics and dynamics of prednisolone. *Endocr rev* 1987;8(4):453–473.
108. Vermeulen A, Caspi E. The metabolism of prednisolone by homogenates of rat liver. *J Biol Chem* 1958;233(1):54–56.
109. Addison RS, Maguire DJ, Mortimer RH, et al. Pathway and kinetics of prednisolone metabolism in the human placenta. *J Steroid Biochem Mol Biol* 1993;44(3):315–320.
110. Barkin RL, Barkin SJ, Barkin DS. Propoxyphene (dextropropoxyphene): a critical review of a weak opioid analgesic that should remain in antiquity. *Am J Ther* 2006;13(6):534–542.
111. Somogyi A, Menelaou A, Fullston SV. CYP3A4 mediates dextropropoxyphene N-demethylation to nordextropropoxyphene: human in vitro and in vivo studies and lack of CYP2D6 involvement. *Xenobiotica* 2004;34(10):875–887.
112. Weigand UW, Chou RC, Maulik D, et al. Assessment of biotransformation during transfer of propoxyphene and acetaminophen across the isolated perfused human placenta. *Pediatr Pharmacol (New York)* 1984;4(3):145–153.
113. Benirschke K, Kaufmann P. *Pathology of the human placenta,* 4th ed. New York, NY: Springer-Verlag Inc, 2000.
114. Caldwell BV, Behrman HR. Prostaglandins in reproductive processes [review]. *Med Clin North Am* 1981;65(4):927–936.
115. Nanovskaya TN, Patrikeeva S, Hemauer S, et al. Effect of albumin on transplacental transfer and distribution of rosiglitazone and glyburide. *J Matern Fetal Neonatal Med* 2008;21(3):197–207.
116. Iribarne CF, Berthou S, Baird S, et al. Involvement of cytochrome P450 3A4 enzyme in the N-demethylation of methadone in human liver microsomes. *Chem Res Toxicol* 1996;9:365–373.
117. Kobayashi K, Yamamoto T, Chiba K, et al. Human buprenorphine N-dealkylation is catalyzed by cytochrome P450 3A4. *Drug Metab Dispos.* 1998;26(8):818–821.
118. Hesse LM, Venkatakrishnan K, Court MH, et al. CYP2B6 mediates the in vitro hydroxylation of bupropion: potential drug interactions with other antidepressants. *Drug Metab Dispos* 2000;28:1176–1183.
119. Jacobsen NW, Halling-Sorensen B, Birkved FK. Inhibition of human aromatase complex (CYP19) by antiepileptic drugs. *Toxicol In Vitro* 2008;22(1):146–153.
120. Ohnishi T, Ichikawa Y. Direct inhibitions of the activities of steroidogenic cytochrome P-450 mono-oxygenase systems by anticonvulsants. *J Steroid Biochem Mol Biol* 1997;60(1–2):77–85.
121. Zharikova OL, Deshmukh SV, Kumar M. The effect of opiates on activity of human placental aromatase/CYP19. *Biochem Pharmacol* 2007;73:279–286.
122. Fischer V, Rodríguez-Gascón A, Heitz F, et al. The multidrug resistance modulator valspodar (PSC 833) is metabolized by human cytochrome P450 3A: implications for drug-drug interactions and pharmacological activity of the main metabolite. *Drug Metab Dispos.* 1998;26(8):802–811.
123. Totah RA, Sheffels P, Roberts T, et al. Role of CYP2B6 in stereoselective human methadone metabolism. *Anesthesiology* 2008;108(3):363–374.
124. Roe DA, Little BB, Bawdon RE, et al. Metabolism of cocaine by human placentas: implications for fetal exposure. *Am J Obstet Gynecol* 1990;163(3):715–718.
125. Osawa Y, Higashiyama T, Yarborough C. Diverse evictions of aromatase CYT P450: catecholestrogen synthesis, cocaine N-demethylation, and other selective drug metabolism. In: *The 8th International Conference on Cytochrome P450.* 1992:251.
126. Fournet-Dulguerov N, MacLusky NJ, Leranth CZ, et al. Immunohistochemical localization of aromatase cytochrome P-450 and estradiol dehydrogenase in the syncytiotrophoblast of the human placenta. *J Clin Endocrinol Metab* 1987;65:757–764.
127. Ryan KJ. Biological aromatization of steroids. *J Biol Chem* 1959;234(2):268–272.
128. Ryan KJ. Metabolism of C-16-oxygenated steroids by human placenta: the formation of estriol. *J Biol Chem* 1959;234(8):2006–2008.
129. Thompson Jr EA, Siiteri PK. The involvement of human placental microsomal cytochrome P450 in aromatization. *J Biol Chem* 1974;249:5373–5378.
130. Kragie L. Aromatase in primate pregnancy: a review. *Endocr Res* 2002;28(3):121–128.
131. Steinkampf MP, Mendelson CR, Simpson ER. Regulation by follicle-stimulating hormone of the synthesis of aromatase cytochrome P-450 in human granulosa cells. *Mol Endocrinol* 1987;1:465–471.
132. Krasnow JS, Hickey GJ, Richards JS. Regulation of aromatase mRNA and estradiol biosynthesis in rat ovarian granulosa and luteal cells by prolactin. *Mol Endocrinol* 1990;4:2–13.
133. Simpson ER, Mahendroo MS, Means GD, et al. Aromatase cytochrome P450, the enzyme responsible for estrogen biosynthesis. *Endocr Rev* 1994;15(3):342–355.
134. Nelson LR, Bulun SE. Estrogen production and action. *J Am Acad Dermatol* 2001;45(suppl 3):s116–s124.
135. Gerber JG, Rhodes RJ, Gal J. Stereoselective metabolism of methadone N-demethylation by cytochrome P450 2B6 and 2C19. *Chirality* 2004;16:36–44.
136. Totah RA, Allen KE, Sheffels P, et al. Enantiomeric metabolic interactions and stereoselective human methadone metabolism. *J Pharmacol Exp Ther* 2007;321(1):389–399.
137. Moody DE, Alburges ME, Parker RJ, et al. The involvement of cytochrome P450 3A4 in the N-demethylation of L-alpha-acetylmethadol (LAAM), norLAAM, and methadone. *Drug Metab Dispos* 1997;25(12):1347–1353.
138. Wang JS, DeVane CL. Involvement of CYP3A4, CYP2C8, and CYP2D6 in the metabolism of (R)- and (S)-methadone in vitro. *Drug Metab Dispos* 2003;31:742–747.
139. Oda Y, Kharasch ED. Metabolism of methadone and levo-alpha-acetylmethadol (LAAM) by human intestinal cytochrome P450 3A4 (CYP3A4): potential contribution of intestinal metabolism to presystemic clearance and bioactivation. *J Pharmacol Exp Ther* 2001;298(3):1021–1032.
140. Dormitzer CM, Tonning JM, Szarfman A, et al. Data mining FDA's post-marketing adverse event reports data to examine drug-dependence reporting. In: Proceedings of the 68th Annual Scientific Meeting of College on Problems of Drug Dependence; June 17–22, 2006; Scottsdale, AZ.
141. Paakki P, Kirkinen P, Helin H. Antepartum glucocorticoid therapy suppresses human placental xenobiotic and steroid metabolizing enzymes. *Placenta* 2000;21:241–246.
142. Paakki P, Stockmann H, Kantola M. Maternal drug abuse and human term placental xenobiotic and steroid metabolizing enzymes in vitro. *Environ Health Perspect* 2000;108:141–145.
143. Shimada T, Yamazaki H, Mimura M, et al. Interindividual variations in human liver cytochrome P-450 enzymes involved in the oxidation of drugs, carcinogens and toxic chemicals: studies with liver microsomes of 30 Japanese and 30 Caucasians. *J Pharmacol Exp Ther* 1994;270:414–423.
144. Parkinson A. Biotransformation of xenobiotics. In: Klaassen CD, ed. *Casarett and Doull's toxicology. The basic science of poisons,* 6th ed. New York, NY: McGraw-Hill, 2001:133–224, chap 6.

145. Spink DC, Eugster HP, Lincoln DW II, et al. 7 beta-estradiol hydroxylation catalyzed by human cytochrome P450 1A1: a comparison of the activities induced by 2,3,7,8-tetrachlorodibenzo-p-dioxin in MCF-7 cells with those from heterologous expression of the cDNA. *Arch Biochem Biophys* 1992;293(2):342–348.
146. Spink DC, Spink BC, Cao JQ, et al. Differential expression of CYP1A1 and CYP1B1 in human breast epithelial cells and breast tumor cells. *Carcinogenesis* 1998;19(2):291–298.
147. Spink BC, Fasco MJ, Gierthy JF, et al. 12-O-tetradecanoylphorbol-13-acetate upregulates the Ah receptor and differentially alters CYP1B1 and CYP1A1 expression in MCF-7 breast cancer cells. *J Cell Biochem* 1998;70(3):289–296.
148. Jönsson A, Hallengren B, Rydberg T, et al. Effects and serum levels of glibenclamide and its active metabolites in patients with type 2 diabetes. *Diabetes Obes Metab* 2001;3:403–409.
149. Choudhary D, Jansson I, Sarfarazi M, et al. Characterization of the biochemical and structural phenotypes of four CYP1B1 mutations observed in individuals with primary congenital glaucoma. *Pharmacogenet Genomics* 2008;18(8):665–676.
150. Okey AB, Riddick DS, Harper PA. Molecular biology of the aromatic hydrocarbon (dioxin) receptor. *Trends Pharmacol Sci* 1994; 15(7):226–232.
151. Hayashi S, Watanabe J, Nakachi K, et al. Interindividual difference in expression of human Ah receptor and related P450 genes. *Carcinogenesis* 1994;15(5):801–806.
152. Schmidt JV, Bradfield CA. Ah receptor signaling pathways [review]. *Annu Rev Cell Dev Biol* 1996;12:55–89.
153. Hasler JA, Estabrook R, Murray M, et al. Human cytochromes P450. *Mol Aspects Med* 1999;20:1–137.
154. Hakkola J, Pasanen M, Pelkonen O, et al. Expression of CYP1B1 in human adult and fetal tissues and differential inducibility of CYP1B1 and CYP1A1 by Ah receptor ligands in human placenta and cultured cells. *Carcinogenesis* 1997;18(2):391–397.
155. Whyatt RM, Bell DA, Jedrychowski W, et al. Polycyclic aromatic hydrocarbon-DNA adducts in human placenta and modulation by CYP1A1 induction and genotype. *Carcinogenesis* 1998;19(8): 1389–1392.
156. Pelkonen O, Nebert D. Metabolism of polycyclic aromatic hydrocarbons: etiologic role in carcinogenesis. *Pharmacol Rev* 1982;34: 189–208.
157. Shimada T, Hayes CL, Yamazaki H, et al. Activation of chemically diverse procarcinogens by human cytochrome P450 1B1. *Cancer Res* 1996;56(13):2979–2984.
158. Kim JH, Stansbury KH, Walker NJ, et al. Metabolism of benzo[a]pyrene and benzo[a]pyrene-7,8-diol by human cytochrome P450 1B1. *Carcinogenesis* 1998;19(10):1847–1853.
159. Iwanari M, Nakajima M, Kizu R, et al. Induction of CYP1A1, CYP1A2, and CYP1B1 mRNAs by nitropolycyclic aromatic hydrocarbons in various human tissue-derived cells: chemical-, cytochrome P450 isoform-, and cell-specific differences. *Arch Toxicol* 2002;76:287–298.
160. Toide K, Yamazaki H, Nagashima R, et al. Aryl hydrocarbon hydroxylase represents CYP1B1, and not CYP1A1, in human freshly isolated white cells: trimodal distribution of Japanese population according to induction of CYP1B1 mRNA by environmental dioxins. *Cancer Epidemiol Biomarkers Prev* 2003;12:219–222, v.
161. Yamazoe Y, Abu-Zeid M, Toyama S, et al. Metabolic activation of a protein pyrolysate promutagen 2-amino-3,8-dimethylimidazo[4,5-f]quinoxaline by rat liver microsomes and purified cytochrome P450. *Carcinogenesis* 1988;9:105–109.
162. Liska DJ. The detoxification enzyme systems [review]. *Altern Med Rev* 1998;3(3):187–198.
163. Wattenberg LW, Leong JL. Inhibition of the carcinogenic action of benzo(a)pyrene by flavones. *Cancer Res* 1970;30(7): 1922–1925.
164. Reid JM, Kuffel MJ, Miller JK, et al. Metabolic activation of dacarbazine by human cytochromes P450: the role of CYP1A1, CYP1A2, and CYP2E1. *Clin Cancer Res* 1999;5(8):2192–2197.
165. Ching MS, Blake CL, Malek NA, et al. Differential inhibition of human CYP1A1 and CYP1A2 by quinidine and quinine. *Xenobiotica* 2001;31(11):757–767.
166. Shimada T, Gillam EM, Sutter TR, et al. Oxidation of xenobiotics by recombinant human cytochrome P450 1B1. *Drug Metab Dispos* 1997;25(5):617–622.
167. Crespi CL, Penman BW. Use of cDNA-expressed human cytochrome P450 enzymes to study potential drug-drug interactions. *Adv Pharmacol* 1997;43:171–188.
168. Pelkonen O, Pasanen M, Kuha H, et al. The effect of cigarette smoking on 7-ethoxyresorufin O-deethylase and other monooxygenase activities in human liver: analyses with monoclonal antibodies. *Br J Clin Pharmacol* 1986;22:125–134.
169. Boobis AR, Brodie MJ, Kahn GC, et al. Monooxygenase activity of human liver in microsomal fractions of needle biopsy specimens. *Br J Clin Pharmacol* 1980;9:11–19.
170. Sesardic D, Pasanen M, Pelkonen O, et al. Differential expression and regulation of members of the cytochrome P450IA gene subfamily in human tissues. *Carcinogenesis* 1990;11(7):1183–1188.
171. Lewis DF, Lake BG. Molecular modelling of CYP1A subfamily members based on an alignment with CYP102: rationalization of CYP1A substrate specificity in terms of active site amino acid residues. *Xenobiotica* 1996;26(7):723–753.
172. Wong TK, Domin BA, Bent PE, et al. Correlation of placental microsomal activities with protein detected by antibodies to rabbit cytochrome P450 isozyme 6 in preparations from humans exposed to polychlorinated biphenyls, quarterphenyls, and dibenzofurans. *Cancer Res* 1986;46:999–1004.
173. Zhu BT, Cai MX, Spink DC, et al. Stimulatory effect of cigarette smoking on the 15 alpha-hydroxylation of estradiol by human term placenta. *Clin Pharmacol Ther* 2002;71(5):311–324.
174. Pasanen M, Pelkonen O. The expression and environmental regulation of P450 enzymes in human placenta [review]. *Crit Rev Toxicol* 1994;24(3):211–229.
175. Pasanen M, Haaparanta T, Sundin M, et al. Immunochemical and molecular biological studies on human placental cigarette smoke-inducible cytochrome P450-dependent mono-oxygenase activities. *Toxicology* 1990;62(2):175–187.
176. Welch RM, Harrison YE, Gommi BW, et al. Stimulatory effect of cigarette smoking on the hydroxylation of 3,4-benzo[a]pyrene and the N-demethylation of 3-methyl-4-monomethylaminoazobenzene by enzymes in human placenta. *Clin Pharmacol Ther* 1968;10:100–109.
177. Manchester DK, Jacoby EH. Sensitivity of human placental monooxygenase activity to maternal smoking. *Clin Pharmacol Ther* 1981;30(5):687–692.
178. Wong TK, Everson RB, Hsu ST. Potent induction of human placental mono-oxygenase activity by previous dietary exposure to polychlorinated biphenyls and their thermal degradation products. *Lancet* 1985;1(8431):721–724.
179. Lagueux J, Pereg D, Ayotte P, et al. Cytochrome P450 CYP1A1 enzyme activity and DNA adducts in placenta of women environmentally exposed to organochlorines. *Environ Res* 1999; 80(4):369–382.
180. Hincal F. Effects of exposure to air pollution and smoking on the placental aryl hydrocarbon hydroxylase (AHH) activity. *Arch Environ Health* 1986;41(6):377–383.
181. Everson RB, Randerath E, Santella RM, et al. Quantitative associations between DNA damage in human placenta and maternal smoking and birth weight. *J Natl Cancer Inst* 1988;80(8):567–576.
182. Manchester DK, Bowman ED, Parker NB, et al. Determinants of polycyclic aromatic hydrocarbon-DNA adducts in human placenta. *Cancer Res* 1992;52:1499–1503.
183. Hansen C, Asmussen I, Autrup H. Detection of carcinogen-DNA adducts in human fetal tissues by the 32-postlabeling procedure. *Environ Health Perspect* 1993;99:229–231.
184. Hatch MC, Warburton D, Santella RM. Polycyclic aromatic hydrocarbon-DNA adducts in spontaneously aborted fetal tissue. *Carcinogenesis* 1990;11:1673–1675.
185. Pelkonen O, Kärki NT, Koivisto M, et al. Maternal cigarette smoking, placental aryl hydrocarbon hydroxylase and neonatal size. *Toxicol Lett* 1979;3:331–335.
186. Manchester DK, Jacoby EH. Decreased placental mono-oxygenase activities associated with birth defects. *Teratology* 1984;30:31–38.

CHAPTER

13

Nada Djokanovic
Rada Boskovic
Gideon Koren

Maternal Drug Intake and the Newborn

INTRODUCTION

The use of prescription drugs during pregnancy has become a concern since the thalidomide tragedy. However, medication use by pregnant women and females of reproductive age is common, and often necessary and unavoidable in chronic conditions. Recent studies have suggested that between 64% and 83% of women use at least one medication during pregnancy (1–3). The most commonly prescribed drugs in pregnancy include anti-infectives, analgesics, and drugs for the respiratory system. Recent Canadian study found that one in every five pregnant women was exposed to prescription drugs with potential fetal risk (4). Because, approximately 50% of pregnancies are unplanned, women whose pregnancies are unintended and unexpected are more likely to be exposed to a wide range of potential teratogens (5,6).

It has been assumed for decades that the human placenta serves as a barrier between mother and fetus, protecting the fetus from exposure to xenobiotics circulating in the mother; however, the thalidomide-induced embryopathies, recognized in 1960, reversed this concept. With the development of appropriate analytical methods, it has become apparent that the placenta not only allows most xenobiotics and their metabolites to cross from the maternal to the fetal circulation, but that it also has an extensive metabolizing capacity and can itself serve also as a site storage for chemicals (7).

The devastating lifelong impact an adverse pregnancy outcome may have on the infant reinforces the critical need for more knowledge about the pharmacokinetics of the maternal–placental–fetal unit. This chapter reviews mechanisms and factors that are involved in the transfer of pharmacologically active substances from the mother to the fetus, undesirable effects of known teratogens, and methods available to study placental drug transfer.

PHARMACOKINETICS OF THE MATERNAL–FETAL UNIT

One cannot discuss the pharmacokinetics of the maternal–fetal unit without considering the placental anatomy and pregnancy-induced physiologic changes.

PLACENTAL ANATOMY

The placenta is a multifaceted organ that plays critical roles in optimal growth and development of the embryo and fetus during pregnancy. It is virtually the sole contact that the fetus has with the mother. The placenta not only "supplies" the embryo and fetus with oxygen, water, electrolytes, and nutrients, but also "excretes" the waste products from the fetus (8). It is also an endocrine organ that produces various steroid hormones (e.g., estrogens and progesterone) and polypeptide hormones (e.g., chorionic gonadotropin and placental lactogen) that are vital for successful pregnancy.

Shortly after fertilization, the zygote (fertilized ovum) undergoes rapid mitotic cell division to form the morula. The outer cells of the morula, called the *trophoblast*, contribute to the formation of the placenta, and a group of centrally located cells, known as the inner cell mass (*embryoblast*), differentiate to form the fetus. There are two layers of trophoblastic cells: the *syncytiotrophoblast* does not undergo mitosis and the *cytotrophoblast* continuously replenishes the growing mass of the syncytiotrophoblast (9). Placental functions are generally related to the syncytiotrophoblast (10). The syncytiotrophoblast consists of two distinct transport regions: a brush border membrane that is facing the maternal side and a basal membrane that is facing the fetal side (11). The transfer of any compound from the maternal blood into fetal blood across the syncytiotrophoblast has to involve transport across the brush border membrane followed by transport across the basal membrane, and vice versa in the case of transfer from the fetal to maternal blood. As the syncytiotrophoblast is the interface of exchange between the maternal and fetal circulations, it may act as a barrier through a large number of ATP (adenosine triphosphate)-binding cassette (ABC) drug transporters such as P-glycoprotein, multidrug resistance-associated proteins (MRPs) and breast cancer resistance protein (BCRP) (12,13).

Although the conceptus is implanted in the endometrium of the uterus by the end of the first week after conception, there is still no interface established for fetal–maternal exchange. The uteroplacental circulation begins to be established by the second week after fertilization, but it is not until the fourth week that the essential arrangements necessary for the physiologic exchange between mother and the embryo are well established (14). From the fourth week of gestation, the syncytiotrophoblast layers become thinner. The surface area for exchange increases dramatically to meet the demands of the growing fetus. At term, the human placenta has only a single cell layer separating the fetal capillary endothelium and the maternal blood; hence it does not pose a hermetic barrier to transport.

There are anatomic and functional differences between animal and human placentae; therefore, it is critically important to consider those differences when considering the applicability of animal data as an approximation of human placental transfer (9,15).

PHARMACOKINETIC CHANGES DURING PREGNANCY

Pregnancy is a dynamic state with complex physiologic alterations that may affect the uptake, distribution, metabolism, and clearance of drug in the mother. During pregnancy the mother's intestinal motility is decreased, the gastric emptying time is increased, and the extent of drug absorption may be reduced (16). As a result of increased maternal blood volume, body mass, and decreased plasma protein binding, the volume of distribution of most drugs increases during pregnancy. Albumin levels are reduced due to plasma dilution, but α-acid glycoprotein remains constant during pregnancy.

Drugs can be distributed into the amniotic fluid and may achieve there even higher values than those in the maternal and fetal plasma (17). In addition, the clearance rate of lipophobic and polar drugs is accelerated due to either an enhanced rate of hepatic metabolism or of renal elimination (increased glomerular filtration rate or increased renal blood flow). In contrast, elimination of lipophilic drugs may be decreased during pregnancy (18). All these changes in pharmacokinetics during pregnancy will affect the rate and extent of fetal drug exposure, and drug dosing during pregnancy should take into account all these alterations. Typically both peak and steady-state serum concentrations of drugs tend to be lower during pregnancy than in the nonpregnant state. For a small number of drugs (e.g., theophylline), there is evidence of a slower metabolic rate in the pregnant mother (19). Major pharmacokinetic changes during pregnancy and their potential clinical effects are summarized in Table 13.1. Compared to the nonpregnant state, there are relatively few specific pharmacokinetic data during pregnancy due to perceived ethical issues in research during pregnancy (20).

MECHANISMS OF PLACENTAL DRUG TRANSFER

It is generally accepted that most chemical substances administered to the mother are able to permeate, to some degree, across the placenta (21). For some compounds, the placenta offers a protective barrier for the developing fetus by reducing the entry from the mother to the fetus, while for others it facilitates their passage both to and from the fetal compartment (22). Hence, the placenta may act in a similar manner to the kidney and liver in the elimination of different substances.

Transplacental exchanges may involve passive transfer, facilitated diffusion, active transport, phagocytosis, and pinocytosis. Passive transfer is the main form of exchange through the placenta. However, passive diffusion alone is not adequate to fulfill the fetal requirements for nutrients, and these are achieved through specific transport proteins for several nutrients, including the transport of amino acids, fatty acids, and glucose. Facilitated diffusion is only a minor role in the transfer of some drugs. It is likely that phagocytosis and pinocytosis are too slow to be important in the transfer of drugs, and therefore they have received little attention in the scientific literature.

Under some circumstances, the comparison of drug concentration in maternal and fetal plasma may give some idea of the exposure of the fetus to drugs that have been administered to the mother. Some drugs rapidly cross the placenta, and their concentrations in fetal and maternal plasma are similar to maternal levels, whereas other drugs cross incompletely and their fetal concentrations are lower than those in the maternal circulation. Many of the drugs fit into these two models. A limited number of drugs reach greater concentrations in fetal than in maternal plasma

TABLE 13.1 Major Pharmacokinetic Changes During Pregnancy (17,40)

Change in Pregnancy	*Pharmacokinetic Effect*	*Potential Clinical Effect*
Greater body weight	Lower serum concentrations	Smaller effects if dose not increased
Lower serum albumin levels	Higher free (unbound) fraction leads to greater transport, clearance	No change in steady-state concentration of free drug (e.g., phenytoin)
Increased hepatic metabolic rate	Faster clearance rate of some drugs metabolized by the liver	Smaller effects if dose is not increased; for example, dexamethasone is not metabolized in the liver and hence is more likely to cross placenta at higher concentrations
Decreased hepatic metabolic rate	Slower clearance rate	For example, theophylline metabolized more slowly
Higher liver blood flow	Faster clearance rate of high-extraction-ratio drugs	Smaller effects if dose is not increased
Higher glomerular filtration rate	Faster clearance rate of renally excreted drugs or their active metabolites	Smaller effects if dose is not increased (e.g., lithium, digoxin)
Lower compliance (because of fears of teratogenicity)	Lower drug concentrations	More therapeutic failures

(23). Ceftizoxime may serve as an example as the only antibiotic known so far with concentrations that are higher in the cord than in maternal plasma (24). This type of transfer is called "exceeding" transfer.

Simple Diffusion

Many of the pharmacologically active compounds cross the human placenta by simple diffusion, which means that the crossing of molecules is a passive process occurring without the use of energy, and is described by Fick's equation:

$$\text{Rate of diffusion} = \frac{KA(C_m - C_f)}{X}$$

where K is the diffusion constant of the investigational drug, A is the surface area available for transfer, C_m is the maternal concentration of the drug, C_f is the fetal concentration of the drug, and X is the thickness of the membrane. Transfer in this case is proportional to the concentration gradient between maternal and fetal plasma. The rate of transfer is also affected by the surface area, the thickness of the membrane, the physicochemical characteristics of the drugs, and placental factors (25). Generally, compounds that have low molecular weight, are lipid soluble, unionized, and unbound to proteins, are able to readily cross the placenta (22). Physiologic substances such as water, urea, carbon dioxide, and hormones are mainly cleared from the fetus by passive diffusion (26). In addition to many pharmacologically active compounds that cross the placenta by simple diffusion, larger molecules such as antibodies may also be transported by this way (27).

Facilitated Diffusion

Facilitated diffusion is a mechanism of transplacental transfer that is carrier-mediated, but not dependent on energy. Transfer occurs down a concentration gradient. Compounds that are structurally related to endogenous substances are assumed to be transported by this mechanism, glucose being the most important example (28). Some drugs that do not necessarily mimic endogenous compounds use this mechanism of transport with the assistance of carriers; examples are cephalexin (28) and ganciclovir (29). Theoretically, facilitated diffusion would enable the drug to reach a higher peak of concentration in the fetus than would be expected from simple diffusion, and hence it may be important for fetal therapy.

Active Transport

Active transport is a carrier-mediated process that requires energy to transfer compounds against an electrochemical or concentration gradient (26). Active transporters are located either in the brush border (apical) membrane facing the maternal blood space or the basal membrane facing the fetal capillaries, where they transfer compounds in and out of the syncytiotrophoblast (22).

There have been more than 20 different transporter proteins identified in the human placenta (30,31). The identified physiological role of most of these transporters is to transport nutrients to the fetus and to eliminate metabolic waste products from the fetus; however many of them are able to interact with pharmacological agents (11). Exogenous compounds that interact with placental transporters are often structurally similar to endogenous substrates. Therefore, if such compounds are present in the maternal blood, placental transporters may facilitate their transfer from the mother to the fetus. In other words, these influx transporters may increase the fetal exposure to such drugs. Similarly, there are placental transporters that mediate the efflux of endogenous substrates from the fetus to the mother and these transporters may protect the fetus from drug exposure. Over the last decade, increasing efforts have been devoted to investigation of the ABC (ATP–binding cassette) efflux transporters in the placenta, including P-glycoprotein, multidrug resistance-associated proteins (MRPs), and breast cancer resistance protein (BCRP). The generally accepted function of ABC transporters is that they act as a protective mechanism against a large variety of xenobiotics, as well as protecting tissues from adverse effects of endogenous compounds (32,33).

P-Glycoprotein (MDR1)

P-glycoprotein, the multidrug-resistant gene (MDR1) product, is the first discovered and so far best characterized of drug efflux transporters. P-glycoprotein is able to actively pump drugs and other xenobiotics from trophoblast cells back to the maternal circulation, thus decreasing fetal exposure (32,31). P-glycoprotein has been detected in human placental trophoblasts from the first trimester to term, however its expression decreases as gestation advances (34,35). It is conceivable that higher P-glycoprotein expression in early pregnancy protect the fetus from xenobiotic toxicity at the sensitive period of embryogenesis. Because of this, the fetus will typically be able to tolerate maternal concentrations of drugs that have a high affinity with P-glycoprotein than drugs that have poor affinity (36).

P-glycoprotein is able to transport an extremely wide variety of chemically and structurally diverse compounds. Recent studies suggest that P-glycoprotein at the apical maternal–fetal interface may provide the mechanism to protect the developing fetus from xenobiotics that are substrates for this efflux pump, including digoxin, azytromycin, anticancer drugs, human immunodeficiency virus (HIV) protease inhibitors, opioids, and antiemetics (32). Inhibition of placental P-glycoprotein (e.g., verapamil, cyclosporine) may therefore increase the fetal exposure to these compounds (37). In addition to specific inhibitors, some herbal drugs including St. John's wort are capable of affecting P-glycoprotein function, and thus may affect the placental transfer of other compounds (32,38). Important elements to consider when studying P-glycoprotein are glucocorticosteroids, which are generally regarded as P-glycoprotein substrates. Young et al. (39) reported that steroid hormones directly influence the level of expression of some of these transporters, and therefore the investigation of this link may be key in developing a strategy for drug delivery to the mother with minimal fetal exposure (39). On the other hand, in some cases, use of P-glycoprotein inhibitors may be theoretically effective in enhancing drug availability to the fetus, while minimizing drug exposure to the mother (32). This new knowledge may lead to methods for increasing drug concentration in the fetal compartment, which is necessary for fetal therapy (e.g., digoxin for fetal tachyarrhythmia) (40). As example, one may consider the treatment of fetal tachyarrhythmia with both digoxin and verapamil. Verapamil has the potential to enhance digoxin transfer to the fetus by inhibiting placental drug efflux through P-glycoprotein (22). However, this must be carefully monitored to ensure that digoxin toxicity to the fetus does not occur. In addition, concerns about possible drug-drug and drug-endogenous substances interactions when they compete for the same transporter have been expressed (22). Thus, caution should be taken when a substrate and an inhibitor of P-glycoprotein are concomitantly administered to pregnant women.

Nevertheless, it is conceivable that assessment of P-glycoprotein activity in the placenta may improve drug choice in pregnancy. For instance, drugs that are actively transported by P-glycoprotein may be preferred to limit fetal drug exposure. In contrast, efflux of HIV protease inhibitors by P-glycoprotein may decrease fetal defense against the virus (36). To increase drug concentrations in the fetal compartment, future use of appropriate P-glycoprotein inhibitors may be advantageous since they would increase drug availability to the fetus and improve therapy outcomes.

Multidrug Resistance-Associated Proteins and Breast Cancer Resistance Protein

Other major drug efflux transporters identified in the placenta are the multidrug resistance-associated proteins (MRPs) and breast cancer resistance protein (BCRP).

The family of MRP transporters currently comprises nine members (MRP1–9) (32). These transporters are involved in the transport of numerous clinically important anionic drugs as well as their glucuronide and glutathione metabolites. Drugs transported by MRPs are the anticancer agents methotrexate, etoposide, vincristine, vinblastine and cisplatin, HIV protease inhibitors, acetaminophen glucuronide, and the antibacterials grepafloxacin and ampicillin (22). Physiologically, MRPs mediate the removal of bilirubin glucuronides from the placenta (11).

The BCRP is highly expressed in the placenta and has a similar role and substrates to P-glycoprotein. It is involved in the efflux of drugs away from the fetus, acting as a protective mechanism for the fetus (39). Functional studies in the last decade have documented that BCRP can transport a large number of drugs from various therapeutic categories including anticancer drugs, antibiotics, antihypertensive, and antidiabetics (41). Of particular interest is that various drugs commonly administered to pregnant women, including nitrofurantoin (42) and glyburide (43) are BCRP substrates. It has been demonstrated that BCRP-mediated placental transport of glyburide is at least one of the mechanisms by which fetal exposure of the drug is limited (41,43). Physiologically, the BCRP may function in the homeostasis of porphyrins (11). Recent studies have suggested that BCRP may also regulate placental estrogen synthesis through modulating intracellular concentrations of estrogen precursors, dehydroepiandrosterone sulfate (DHEAS), and estrone-3-sulfate (E3S) (41,44).

A wide variety of other transporters have also been discovered in the placenta, including the organic anion transporter (OAT), serotonin transporter (SERT), norepinephrine transporter (NET), several organic cation transporters (OCTs), and sodium/multivitamin transporter (SMVT) (30,31). Current knowledge about their pharmacological role is limited.

FACTORS AFFECTING PLACENTAL TRANSFER

Several factors affect the rate of transfer of drugs across the placenta.

Lipid Solubility

As with other biological membranes, lipid-soluble drugs cross the placenta more rapidly than water-soluble agents. For this reason, drugs that are generally well absorbed when taken orally cross the placenta readily.

Size of the Molecule

In general, most drugs with a molecular weight of less than 100 Da cross the placenta quite readily. Compounds with a molecular weight of up to 1,000 Da cross the placenta at slower rates (45). Compounds with a molecular weight greater than 1,000 Da do not cross the placenta or have only a limited transfer. Heparin is an example, and hence it can be used safely throughout pregnancy.

Blood Flow

Blood flow through the placenta increases during gestation from 50 mL per minute at 10 weeks of pregnancy to 600 mL per minute at 38 weeks to meet the growing demands of the developing fetus for nutrients and oxygen (46). Placental rate of drug transfer is determined by blood flow for most unionized and lipophilic compounds. Changes in placental blood flow on either side of the placenta may influence the rate of drug transfer. A decrease in blood flow has the possibility of decreasing the transfer of drugs from the mother to the fetus, but also has the potential to reduce the clearance of drugs from the fetus (22). It was shown that the fetal uptake of the anesthetic agent propofol could be profoundly altered by changes in placental blood flow (47). In addition, changes in blood flow may occur as a result of pathophysiologic conditions (maternal hypertension, abruptio placentae) or due to pharmacologic manipulation. Patients who are cocaine users may exhibit partially altered rates of placental blood flow due to cocaine vasoconstrictive effects.

Although the placenta does not have own innervations, there is evidence that placental blood flow may be partially regulated by acetylcholine-like activities in the human placenta (48).

Protein Binding

It is the free (unbound) fraction of drugs that crosses the placenta, and hence drugs that are highly protein bound tend to cross the placenta slowly. During late pregnancy, the albumin concentration in maternal blood is lower than in the nonpregnant state. As a result, unbound drug concentrations are higher during gestation, making more drugs available for transfer across the placenta. Furthermore, endogenous substances that increase during pregnancy (e.g., free fatty acids) compete with drugs for plasma albumin binding and further increase the free fraction of the drug (49). This can be clinically significant for drugs that are highly protein bound such as propranolol, salicylates, and diazepam. In particular conditions, low protein binding also may be clinically important for drugs used in fetal therapy. Differences in the binding capacity between maternal and fetal serum proteins also influence the concentration gradient of free drugs (50).

In general, fetal albumin has lower binding abilities for drugs than the protein in the maternal circulation, resulting in higher fractions of free drug in the fetus.

Effects of pH

The pH of maternal and fetal blood can influence the transfer of drugs across the human placenta. Fetal blood is more acidic (pH = 7.3) than maternal blood (pH = 7.4); hence, weak basic drugs are more ionized in the fetal circulation, and this leads to a net transfer and accumulation in the fetal circulation (ion trapping). For example, the local anesthetic agent mepivacaine leaves the maternal circulation and becomes ionized. The opposite is true for weakly acidic drugs, where fetal concentrations are lower than those measured in the maternal circulation. Strongly ionized drugs have incomplete transfer; however, this is not an absolute rule, as other factors also play a role. Hence, ampicillin and methicillin, which are strongly acidic, exhibit complete placental transfer.

Placental Binding

The placenta acts as a depot for various compounds due to its ability to bind and retain compounds. Drugs with extensive placental binding may exert a greater effect on the placenta. Placental tissue retention has been demonstrated to reduce the transfer of spiramycin, resulting in its efficacy in placental toxoplasmosis infections (51).

Maternal–Fetal Conditions

Various maternal and fetal conditions may produce histopathologic changes in the placenta that may affect drug transfer from the maternal to the fetal circulation. Fetal hydrops or maternal hypertension, for example, may change the vascularity and perfusion of the placenta. Fetal hydrops and placental edema decrease the transfer of digoxin from the mother to the fetus, which explains the relative resistance of fetal arrhythmia to digoxin in cases of hydrops (52,53).

PLACENTAL METABOLISM

The human placenta has the capacity to biotransform many xenobiotics and endogenous substances, and hence the nature of the compounds reaching the fetal circulation depends on placental biotransformation reactions. Although the number of drug-metabolizing enzymes and their substrate specificity is limited compared to those in the adult liver, many substances are reported to be metabolized by the human placenta (54). The placenta contains many forms of cytochrome P450 (CYP) enzymes in the mitochondria and the endoplasmic reticulum (microsomes), and over the years more cytochromes P450 have been isolated from the placenta (55–57). It appears that more CYP isoforms are expressed in the first trimester than at term (22). Therefore, it has been proposed that the expression of CYP genes is maximal during the early development and growth of the fetus, when it is most susceptible to the effects of teratogens, but as pregnancy progresses enzymes that are not critical for fetal well-being may be switched off. Considering that, Paakki et al. (58) postulated that maternal drug abuse, by acting as an enhancing stimulus, might maintain the expression of specific CYP forms that would normally be switched off.

Drug biotransformation reactions are commonly grouped into two phases: phase I and phase II reactions. The phase I reactions include oxidation, reduction, and hydrolysis, which may increase, decrease, or not alter the pharmacologic activities of a drug (59). In general, phase I reactions introduce a functional group (e.g., amine, hydroxyl) that makes a drug more polar. Although the ultimate role of phase I reactions is to enhance the elimination of xenobiotics, there is evidence that some cytochromes P450 may bioactivate compounds to potentially toxic metabolites. Cigarette smoke has been shown to induce the P450 enzyme CYP1A1 at the mRNA (messenger RNA) level, particularly in the second and third trimesters (60). It was reported that such inductions start during the first trimester of pregnancy (61). It has been suggested that smoking and drinking synergistically elevate placental CYP1A1 activity (62). This suggests that the placenta may be able to increase its protective defenses through increasing metabolism of toxic substances to protect fetus (31). There are two placental cytochrome P450 species identified in the synthesis of steroid hormones (CYP11A1 and CYP19). CYP11A1 (P450scc) converts cholesterol to pregnenolone by the cholesterol side-chain cleavage reaction (CSCC), the activity of which is localized in mitochondria. The aromatization of androgens to estrogens is mediated by CYP19 (P450arom), which is found predominantly in placental microsomes. Placental aromatase (CYP19), which is actively expressed throughout pregnancy, has been significantly suppressed by antepartum glucocorticoid therapy (58). Although other CYP gene products (CYP, 1B1, 2E1, 3A) have been detected in the human placenta, their expression does not appear to be regulated as in the liver. Quantitatively, therefore, the contribution of cytochromes P450 to the elimination of drugs administered to the mother is minor and does not significantly affect fetal exposure.

Phase II reactions involve the coupling of a drug or drug metabolites with endogenous substances. This reaction requires the participation of the specific transferase enzymes that are localized in the microsomal or cytosolic fraction and high-energy-activated endogenous substances. Bioinactivation of xenobiotics includes conjugation with glutathione or glycine, glucuronidation, sulfation, acetylation, and methylation. In the placenta, the enzymes that mediate these activities are present in limited quantities (63). Major enzymes of phase II reactions are gluthathione *S*-transferase (GST), epoxide hydrolase, sulfotransferase, *N*-acetyltransferase, and uridine diphosphate glucuronosyltransferase (UGT) (54,58). GST plays an important role in detoxification, protects against oxidative stress, and is highly expressed throughout pregnancy (64).

Epoxide hydroxylase is expressed during the first trimester and may provide a placental barrier to toxic effects of some maternal epoxides. Placental estrogen sulfotransferase exhibits activity in the sulfate conjugation of both steroids and phenolic compounds. Recent data suggest that the human placenta primarily expresses *N*-acetyltransferase I, which is an important pathway for a number of drugs and food-derived heterocyclic amines. UGT conjugates glucuronic acid to xenobiotics, making the drug more polar and thus more prone to excretion. UGTs are present in the placenta throughout the entire gestation and probably play a major role in placental metabolic activity (22,30). UGT activity is induced by maternal smoking and is greatest in mothers who both smoke and drink alcohol (62).

In general, several conjugating enzymes have been identified in the human placenta, but they probably play a minor role in the bioinactivation of compounds present in the maternal circulation. It appears that placental metabolism is not a significant factor in limiting the transfer of drugs in the placenta (30).

KNOWN HUMAN TERATOGENS

The direct effect of a drug in the fetus depends on the concentration of the drug in the fetal circulation and on the drug's action. Fetal drug concentration, which determines the fetal response, is a function of the maternal concentration, fetal drug clearance, placental permeability, biotransformation, differences in protein binding, and degree of ionization of maternal and fetal plasma. Although a limited number of compounds have been proven to cause malformations in humans, the majority of compounds taken by pregnant women do not pose a significant risk when used in recommended doses (8). In the first 12 weeks of conception, the major body structures of the fetus are formed, and interference in these processes may cause teratogenic effect. Later in fetal development, exposure to a teratogen will not produce a major anatomic defect, but may result in functional abnormalities (e.g., in brain development). The incidence of major malformations in the general population is 1% to 3% of all births (65). Compared to known genetic causes of congenital malformation (25%), the part played by drugs is only around 1% (66). Forty years after thalidomide-associated embryopathy, fewer than 30 drugs have been proven to be teratogenic in humans when used in clinically effective doses. Some of them are no longer in clinical use (Table 13.2) (67).

STUDYING DRUG TRANSFER ACROSS THE HUMAN PLACENTA

IN VIVO APPROACHES

In the past, research on placental transfer was conducted mainly on pregnancies that were terminated voluntarily shortly after a drug of interest was administered. A bolus dose was administered to the mother and drug levels were measured in cord blood or fetal tissue. Such studies were quite limited, however, because only a single set of data was collected; this made it difficult to characterize the kinetics of placental drug transfer. In addition, these data do not have applicability to different gestational ages. It has been observed that phenytoin crosses the placenta more readily during the first and third trimesters than in the middle trimester (68).

TABLE 13.2 Drugs With Proven Teratogenic or Other Adverse Effects in Humans (7,67)

Drug	*Teratogenic Effect*
Aminopterin, methotrexate	CNS and limb malformations
Angiotensin-converting-enzyme inhibitors	Prolonged renal failure in neonates, decreased skull ossification, renal tubular dysgenesis
Carbamazepine	Neural tube defects
Cyclophosphamide	CNS malformations, secondary cancer
Danazol and other androgenic drugs	Masculinization of female fetus
Diethylstilbestrol	Vaginal carcinoma and other genitourinary defects in female and male offspring
Hypoglycemic drugs	Neonatal hypoglycemia
Lithium	Ebstein's anomaly
Mycophenolate mofetil	Microtia, cleft lip/palate, hypoplastic fingers and toenails, heart defects, micrognathia
Misoprostol	Moebius sequence
Nonsteroidal anti-inflammatory drugs	Constriction of the ductus arteriosus, necrotizing enterocolitis
Paramethadione	Facial and CNS defects
Phenytoin	Growth retardation, CNS deficits
Psychoactive drugs (e.g., barbiturates, opioids, and benzodiazepines)	Neonatal withdrawal syndrome when drug is taken in late pregnancy
Systemic retinoids (isotretinoin, etretinate)	CNS, craniofacial, cardiovascular, and other defects
Tetracycline	Anomalies of teeth and bone
Thalidomide	Limb-shortening defects, internal organ defects
Trimethadione	Facial and CNS defects
Valproic acid	Neural tube defects
Warfarin	Skeletal and CNS defects, Dandy–Walker syndrome

CNS, Central nervous system.

Current research techniques aim at sampling both, umbilical venous and arterial blood, yielding information on the extent of transfer, the metabolism, and the elimination of a drug to and from the fetus. Drugs with a high ratio of fetal to maternal concentration are theoretically more appropriate for treatment of life-threatening disease to both fetus and mother; treatment of chorioamnionitis with ceftriaxone is an example (69). Drugs with a low fetal to maternal ratio may be preferable for treating the pregnant mother (e.g., cyclosporine) (70). In addition, drugs can be measured in amniotic fluid to yield fetal to amniotic fluid and maternal to amniotic fluid ratios.

A novel approach to studying drug and toxin transfer across the early human placenta is coelocentesis. Jauniaux et al. (71) demonstrated that selective embryonic fluids can be successfully aspirated to measure drugs under ultrasonographic guidance from exocoelomic cavities from the 5th to the 12th weeks of gestation. Although this technique may be important for measuring of drugs during the first trimester of pregnancy, it is ethically possible only in limited situations, such as pregnancy termination.

Most in vivo research on placental drug transfer has been performed at a later gestational age in human pregnancy. These results are complicated by potential cofounders, such as anesthesia, surgery, or changes of uteroplacental blood flow during labor. Furthermore, in vivo studies of placental drug transfer in humans carry unacceptable risks to both mother and fetus, making it ethically unviable. Because of these concerns, most published data on drug transfer across the placenta are based on animal studies. Animal data are difficult to extrapolate to humans because of wide variations in physiology and morphology of the placenta amongst species.

IN VITRO APPROACHES

Because of limitations of human in vivo studies and the inappropriateness of animal models, several in vitro techniques have been developed to study placental drug transfer.

Cell Culture

Although chorionic cells (72) and decidual cells (73,74) have been cultured, the primary focus of in vitro techniques has been on trophoblast cell cultures. The villous trophoblast is washed and maintained in culture for several days. This technique is suitable for studying different aspects of receptor regulation in the placenta. Trophoblast grows in two or three dimensions and can be studied using a monolayer system. The majority of these studies focus on mechanisms of development and characterization of cell phenotypes in terms of morphology and function, such as the profile of gonadotropins and steroid release (75).

Subcellular Tissue Preparation

Isolated cell fractions had been widely used to study nuclear binding, enzyme functions, protein/membrane isolation, and metabolism in the placenta. There are various types of preparations in this category, including placental slices, microvillous membrane vesicles, dissected syncytiotrophoblastic tissue, and subcellular fractions including microsomes (26). Smith and colleagues (76,77) described a technique for isolating placental brush border vesicles. This technique has been widely used to study transport processes including carrier mediation and membrane configuration required for transport. The membrane technique provides an excellent opportunity to study transport across the placenta and can be important in the evaluation of fetal therapy targeted at specific transporters (e.g., P-glycoprotein).

In Vitro Placental Perfusion

Limitations in studying placental drug transfer in vivo are circumvented by the in vitro human placenta perfusion technique, which makes it possible to collect in a noninvasive manner a broad spectrum of information regarding placental transfer of drugs. Because the model approximates the in vivo situation more closely than the use of subcellular preparations or cell culture systems, it is ideal for evaluation of drug transfer across the intact placenta. Even after undergoing the trauma of delivery, the human placenta has been shown to maintain its structural and functional integrity for perfusion for as long as 12 hours (45,78,79). The dually perfused, isolated human placental cotyledon was introduced by Schneider et al. (80). Placenta perfusion models are used for several purposes: to measure placental transfer of nutrients, therapeutic agents, drugs of abuse and toxic chemicals, effects of endogenous and exogenous substances on fetal perfusion pressure, release of endogenous substances into maternal and fetal perfusate, and adverse effects on the placenta itself.

Immediately after delivery, human term placenta is perfused with heparinized Krebs–Ringer bicarbonate buffer to remove fetal blood components. A single cotyledon with intact tissue is chosen for the experiment. Experiments can be performed using either the closed (recirculated) or the open (nonrecirculated) method. Figure 13.1 is a schematic diagram of the placental perfusion setup.

The majority of the drugs cross the placenta. Table 13.3 compares the placental transfer of medications of therapeutic interest using the in vitro placental perfusion model and in vivo results using maternal and cord blood.

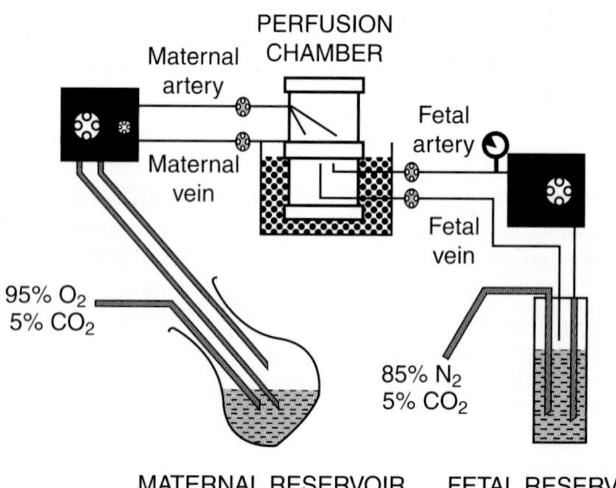

Figure 13.1. Experimental setup for perfusing a human placental lobule in vitro.

TABLE 13.3 Examples of In Vitro and In Vivo Transplacental Transfer of Drugs of Therapeutic Interest

Group	*Drug*	*Transfer*	*Fetal/Maternal Ratio*[a] *In Vitro*	*In Vivo*	*References*
Cardiac glycoside	Digoxin		0.36–1.00	1.00, 0.35	81,82
Antiarrhythmic β-antagonist	Amiodarone		0.30	0.03	83,84
	Verapamil		<0.25	0.35	85
	Flecainide		0.6–0.8		86,87
	Propranolol		0.1–0.3		88,89
	Atenolol	$T = 3.1\%–3.4\%$			89
	Timolol	$T = 17\%–21\%$			89
Analgesic	Aspirin	$T = 15\%$			90,91
	Indometacin	$T = 36\%$			91
	Naproxen			0.002	92
Antibiotic	Penicillins	$CL_A = 0.13–0.22$			93
	Cephalosporins	$CL_A = 0.04–0.03$			94,95
	Sulfonamide	$CL_A = 0.06$			96
	Trimetoprim	$T_f = 0.08\%$			96
β-Agonist	Solbutamol	$T = 2.8\%$			97
	Ritodrine	$T = 2.4\%$		0.69	98,99
	Fenoterol	$T = 2.3\%$			97
Corticosteroid	Dexamethasone	$CL_A = 0.37$			100
	Prednisolone	$CL_A = 0.38$			101
	Cortisol	$CL_A = 0.48$			102
	Betamethasone	$CL_A = 0.41$			102
Respiratory	Theophylline	$T = 22\%$	0.45		103
Gastrointestinal	Cimetidine	$CL_A = 0.23–0.4$	0.46		104
Minor tranquilizer	Diazepam	$T_f = 0.85\%$		1.0	105–107
	Clorazepate	$T_f = 0.84\%$			105
	Midazolam			0.6–0.7	108
Selective serotonin uptake inhibitor	Fluoxetine	$T(SS) = 5.6\%$			109
	Citalopram	$T(SS) = 9.1\%$			109
Anticonvulsant	Phenytoin	$CL_A = 1.08, 1.6$	0.94	0.91	110–112
	Carbamazepine	$CL_A = 0.24$		0.73	112,113
	Valproic acid	$CL_A = 0.95$		1.59	112–115
	Phenobarbital	$CL_A = 0.12–52$	1	~1, 0.86	112
Antiviral	Acyclovir	$CL_A = 0.18$		0.3	116
	Ganciclovir	$CL_A = 0.18$			29,117
	AZT + 3TC + NFV			0–0.3	118
	Nelfinavir			0.0.2	118
	Ritonavir	$CL_G = 0.08$			118,119
	Saquinavir			0.0.1	119
Systemic pain medication	Fentanyl			0.57	120
	Morphine	$CL_A = 0.89$		0.92	121,122
	Propofol			0.65–0.85	123
	Bupivacaine			0.3	124,125
Miscellaneous	Heparin	$CL_A = 0.02$	0.12		126
	Cyclosporine	$T < 5\%$			127

AZT + 3TC + NFV, zidovudine plus lamivudine plus nelfinavir; CL, clearance index; CL_A, CL compound/antipirine; CL_G, CL compound/L-glucose; T, percentage transfer from maternal to fetal direction; T_f, percentage transfer from fetal to maternal direction; $T(SS)$, percentage mean steady-state transfer from maternal to fetal direction.

[a]In vitro study: the fetal/maternal ratio is the mean fetal/maternal ratio of the drug of interest in the fetal and maternal reservoir in the placental perfusion model. In vivo study (cord blood sampling): the fetal/maternal ratio is the mean fetal/maternal ratio of the drug of interest in cord blood and maternal venous sample.

SUMMARY

Because many women use medications during pregnancy either inadvertently or for therapeutic purposes, it is critical to understand the pharmacokinetics of the maternal–fetal unit. Significant progress has been made in the past few years with respect to understanding the role of efflux transporters in placental drug transfer. Medications administered to the mother but designed to work on the fetus are now being used increasingly, demonstrating an important clinical implication in which drug transport across the placenta is desirable. It is apparent that increased knowledge of physiology and pharmacology of placental transporters will be advantageous in implementing therapeutic strategies to control fetal drug exposure and optimize drug therapy during pregnancy. There is still much unknown about drug transport and metabolism in the placenta, and further research is therefore needed to identify substrate drugs of efflux transporters and to determine how high their affinity is to these transporters. The use of in vitro placental perfusion has tremendous potential to enable us to better understand the dual role of the placenta in protecting against and contributing to fetotoxicity.

ACKNOWLEDGMENTS

This work was supported by a grant from the Canadian Institutes for Health Research (CIHR) and the Research Leadership for Better Pharmacotherapy During Pregnancy and Lactation.

REFERENCES

1. Andrade SE, Gurwitz JH, Davis RL, et al. Prescription drug use in pregnancy. *Am J Obstet Gynecol* 2004;191(2):398–407.
2. Hardy JR, Leaderer BP, Holford TR, et al. Safety of medications prescribed before and during early pregnancy in a cohort of 81,975 mothers from the UK General Practice Research Database. *Pharmacoepidemiol Drug Saf* 2006;15(8):555–564.
3. Engeland A, Bramness JG, Daltveit AK, et al. Prescription drug use among fathers and mothers before and during pregnancy. A population-based cohort study of 106,000 pregnancies in Norway 2004–2006. *Br J Clin Pharmacol* 2008;65(5):653–660.
4. Wen SW, Yang T, Krewski D, et al. Patterns of pregnancy exposure to prescription FDA C, D and X drugs in a Canadian population. *J Perinatol* 2008;28(5):324–329.
5. Daniel KL, Honein MA, Moore CA. Sharing prescription medication among teenage girls: potential danger to unplanned/undiagnosed pregnancies. *Pediatrics* 2003;111:1167–1170.
6. Naimi TS, Lipscomb LE, Brewer RD, et al. Binge drinking in the preconception period and the risk of unintended pregnancy: implications for women and their children. *Pediatrics* 2003;111: 1136–1141.
7. Koren G, Pastuszak A, Ito S. Drugs in pregnancy. *N Engl J Med* 1998;338:1128–1137.
8. Koren G, ed. *Maternal–fetal toxicology: a clinician's guide*, 3rd ed. New York, NY: Marcel Dekker, 2001.
9. van der Aa EM, Peereboom-Stegeman JH, Noordhoek J, et al. Mechanism of drug transfer across the human placenta. *Pharm World Sci* 1998;20(4):139–148.
10. Derewlany LO, Koren G. The role of the placenta in perinatal pharmacology and toxicology. In: Radde IC, MacLeod SM, eds. *Pediatric clinical pharmacology*, 2nd ed. St Louis, MO: Mosby-Year Book, 1994:405–422.
11. Ganapathy V, Prasad PD. Role of transporters in placental transfer of drugs. *Toxicol Appl Pharmacol* 2005;207(suppl 2): 381–387.
12. Unadkat JD, Dahlin A, Vijay S. Placental drug transporters. *Curr Drug Metab* 2004;5(1):125–131.
13. Gedeon C, Behravan J, Koren G, et al. Transport of glyburide by placental ABC transporters: implications in fetal drug exposure. *Placenta* 2006;27(11–12):1096–1102.
14. Moore JL, Baker JV, Whitsett. CAMP dependent protein kinase and cAMP, cGMP and calcium stimulated phosphorylation in human placenta. *Trophoblast Res* 1983;1:185.
15. Beck F. Comparative placental morphology and function. In: Kimmel CA, Buelke-Sam J, eds. *Developmental toxicology*. New York, NY: Raven Press, 1981:35.
16. Mattison DR, Malek A, Cistola C. Physiologic adaptations to pregnancy: impact on pharmacokinetics. In: Yaffe SJ, Aranda JV, eds. *Pediatric pharmacology*, 2nd ed. Philadelphia, PA: WB Saunders, 1992:81–96.
17. Loebstein R, Lalkin A, Koren G. Pharmacokinetic changes during pregnancy and their clinical relevance. *Clin Pharmacokinet* 1997;33:328–343.
18. Reynolds F, Knott C. Pharmacokinetics in pregnancy and placental drug transfer. *Oxf Rev Reprod Biol* 1989;11:389–449.
19. Thuy LP, Belmont J, Nyhan WL. Prenatal diagnosis and treatment of holocarboxylase deficiency. *Prenat Diagn* 1999;19: 108–112.
20. Dawes M, Chowienczyk PJ. Drugs in pregnancy. Pharmacokinetics in pregnancy. *Best Pract Res Clin Obstet Gynecol* 2001;15(6): 819–826.
21. Pacifici GM, Nottoli R. Placental transfer of drugs administered to the mother. *Clin Pharmacokinet* 1995;28(3):235–269.
22. Syme MR, Paxton JW, Keelan JA. Drug transfer and metabolism by the human placenta. *Clin Pharmacokinet* 2004;43(8):487–514.
23. Bourget P, Roulot C, Fernandez H. Models for placental transfer studies of drugs. *Clin Pharmacokinet* 1995;28(2):161–180.
24. Pacifici GM. Placental transfer of antibiotics administered to the mother: a review. *Int J Clin Pharmacol Ther* 2006;44(2):57–63.
25. Szeto HH, Mann LA, Ghakthavathsalan A. Meperidine pharmacokinetics in the maternal fetal unit. *J Pharmacol Exp Ther* 1978; 206(2):448–459.
26. Rama Sastry BV. Techniques to study human placental transport. *Adv Drug Deliv Rev* 1999;38:17–39.
27. Malek A, Sager R, Schneider H. Transport of proteins across the human placenta. *Am J Reprod Immunol* 1998;40(5):347–351.
28. Simone C, Derewlany LO, Koren G. Drug transfer across the placenta: considerations in treatment and research. *Perinatol Clin North Am* 1994;21:463–481.
29. Henderson GI, Hu ZQ, Yang Y, et al. Ganciclovir transfer by human placenta and its effects on rat fetal cells. *Am J Med Sci* 1993;306(3):151–156.
30. Myllynen P, Pasanen M, Vähäkangas K. The fate and effects of xenobiotics in human placenta. *Expert Opin Drug Metab Toxicol* 2007;3(3):331–346.
31. Weier N, He SM, Li XT, et al. Placental drug disposition and its clinical implications. *Curr Drug Metab* 2008;9(2):106–121.
32. Ceckova-Novotna M, Pavek P, Staud F. P-glycoprotein in the placenta: expression, localization, regulation and function. *Reprod Toxicol* 2006;22(3):400–410.
33. Behravan J, Piquette-Miller M. Drug transport across the placenta, role of the ABC drug efflux transporters. *Expert Opin Drug Metab Toxicol* 2007;3(6):819–830.
34. Mathias AA, Hitti J, Unadkat JD. P-glycoprotein and breast cancer resistance protein expression in human placentae of various gestational ages. *Am J Physiol Regul Integr Comp Physiol* 2005;289 (4):R963–R969.
35. Sun M, Kingdom J, Baczyk D, et al. Expression of the multidrug resistance P-glycoprotein, (ABCB1 glycoprotein) in the human placenta decreases with advancing gestation. *Placenta* 2006; 27(6–7):602–609.
36. Gedeon C, Koren G. Designing pregnancy centered medications: drugs which do not cross the human placenta. *Placenta.* 2006; 27(8):861–868.
37. St-Pierre MV, Serrano MA, Macias RIR, et al. Expression of members of the multidrug resistance protein family in human term placenta. *Am J Physiol Renal Physiol* 2001;281:F197–F205.

38. Pal D, Mitra AK. MDR- and CYP3A4-mediated drug-herbal interactions. *Life Sci* 2006;78(18):2131–2145.
39. Young AM, Allen CE, Audus KL. Efflux transporters of the human placenta. *Adv Drug Deliv Rev* 2003;55(1):125–132.
40. Koren G, Klinger G, Ohllson A. Fetal pharmacotherapy. *Drugs* 2002;62(5):757–773.
41. Mao Q. BCRP/ABCG2 in the placenta: expression, function and regulation. *Pharm Res* 2008;25(6):1244–1255.
42. Merino G, Jonker JW, Wagenaar E, et al. The breast cancer resistance protein (BCRP/ABCG2) affects pharmacokinetics, hepatobiliary excretion, and milk secretion of the antibiotic nitrofurantoin. *Mol Pharmacol* 2005;67(5):1758–1764.
43. Gedeon C, Anger G, Piquette-Miller M, et al. Breast cancer resistance protein: mediating the trans-placental transfer of glyburide across the human placenta. *Placenta* 2008;29(1):39–43.
44. Grube M, Reuther S, Meyer Zu Schwabedissen H, et al. Organic anion transporting polypeptide 2B1 and breast cancer resistance protein interact in the transepithelial transport of steroid sulfates in human placenta. *Drug Metab Dispos* 2007;35(1):30–35.
45. Miller RK, Wier PJ, Maulik D. Human placenta in vitro: characterization during 12 hours of dual perfusion. *Contrib Gynecol Obstet* 1985;13:77–84.
46. Garland M. Pharmacology of drug transfer across the placenta. *Obstet Gynecol Clin North Am* 1998;25(1):21–42.
47. Yan-Ling H, Hiroshi S, Saburo T, et al. The effects of uterine and umbilical blood flows on the transfer of propofol across the human placenta during in vitro perfusion. *Anesth Analg* 2001; 93:151–156.
48. Sastry BV. Human placental cholinergic system. *Biochem Pharmacol* 1997;53(11):1577–1586.
49. Bardy AH, Hiilesmaa VK, Teramo K, et al. Protein binding of antiepileptic drugs during pregnancy, labor and puerperium. *Ther Drug Monit* 1990;12:40–46.
50. Einarson A, Shuhaiber S, Koren G. Effect of antibacterials on the unborn child. *Pediatr Drugs* 2001;3(11):803–816.
51. Stray-Pedersen B. Treatment of toxoplasmosis in the pregnant mother and newborn child. *Scand J Infect Dis Suppl* 1992;84: 23–31.
52. Gembruch U, Hasmann M, Redel DA, et al. Intrauterine therapy in fetal tachyarrhythmias: intraperitoneal administration of antiarrhythmic drugs to the fetus in fetal tachyarrhythmias with severe hydrops fetalis. *J Perinat Med* 1988;16:39–44.
53. Younis JS, Grant M. Insufficient transplacental digoxin transfer in severe hydrops fetalis. *Am J Obstet Gynecol* 1987;157:1268–1269.
54. Pasanen M. The expression and regulation of drug metabolism in human placenta. *Adv Drug Deliv Rev* 1999;38:81–97.
55. Challier JC, Guerre-Millo M, Nandacumaran M, et al. Clearance of compounds of different molecular size in the human placenta *in vitro*. *Biol Neonate* 1985;48(3):143–148.
56. Chung B, Matteson KJ, Voutilainen R, et al. Human cholesterol-side-chain cleavage enzyme, P450: cDNA cloning, assignment of the gene to chromosome 15, and expression in the placenta. *Proc Natl Acad Sci U S A* 1986;83:8962–8966.
57. Yokotani N, Sogawa K, Matsubara S, et al. cDNA cloning of cytochrome P-450 related to P-450 p-2 from the cDNA library of human placenta: gene structure and expression. *Eur J Biochem* 1990;187:23–29.
58. Paakki P, Stockmann H, Kantola M, et al. Maternal drug abuse and human term placental xenobiotic and steroid metabolizing enzymes in vitro. *Environ Health Perspect* 2000;108(2):141–145.
59. Riddick DS. Drug biotransformation. In: Harold K, Waller HE, eds. *General principles of pharmacology*. New York, NY: Oxford University Press, 1998:38–54.
60. Juchau MR, Rettie AE. The metabolic role of the placenta. In: Fabro S, Scialli AR, eds. *Drug and chemical action in pregnancy*. New York, NY: Marcel Dekker, 1986:153–166.
61. Shiverick KT, Salafia C. Cigarette smoke and pregnancy. I: Ovarian, uterine and placental effects. *Placenta* 1999:20:265–272.
62. Collier AC, Tingle MD, Paxton JW, et al. Metabolizing enzyme localization and activities in the first trimester human placenta: the effect of maternal and gestational age, smoking and alcohol consumption. *Hum Reprod* 2002;17(10):2564–2572.
63. Scialli AR. The fetoplacental unit. In: *A clinical guide to reproductive and developmental toxicology*. Boca Raton, FL: CRC Press, 1992: 45–54.
64. St-Pierre MV, Ugele B, Gambling L, et al. Mechanism of drug transfer across placenta—a workshop report. *Placenta* 2002;23 (suppl A):S159–S164.
65. Ekelund H, Kullander S, Kallen B. Major and minor malformation in newborns and infants up to 1 year of age. *Acta Pediatr Scand* 1970;59:297–302.
66. Backmen DA, Brent RL. Mechanism of teratogenesis. *Annu Rev Pharmacol Toxicol* 1984;24:483–500.
67. Briggs GG, Freeman RK, Yaffe SJ, eds. *Drugs in pregnancy and lactation*, 8th ed. Philadelphia, PA: Lippincott Williams & Wilkins, 2008.
68. Stevens MW, Harbison RD. Placental transfer of diphenylhydantoin: effect of species, gestational age and route of administration. *Teratology* 1974;9:317–326.
69. Bourget P, Quinquis-Desmaris V, Fernadez H, et al. Ceftriaxone distribution and protein binding between maternal blood and milk postpartum. *Ann Pharmacother* 1993;27:294–297.
70. Bourget P, Fernadez H, Bismut E, et al. Transplacental passage of cyclosporin after liver transplantation. *Transplantation* 1990;49: 663–664.
71. Jauniaux E, Gulbis B. *In vivo* investigation of placental transfer early in human pregnancy. *Eur J Obstet Gynecol Reprod Biol* 1990; 92(1):45–49.
72. Poisner AM, Agrawal P, Poisner R. Renin release from human chorionic trophoblasts in vitro: the role of cyclic AMP and protein kinase C. *Trophoblast Res* 1987;2:45–57.
73. Braverman MB, Gurpide E. In vitro effects of human prolactine and oxitocine on sulfatase activity in isolated human decidual cells. *J Clin Endocrinol Metab* 1986;63:725–729.
74. Delvin EE, Arabin A, Glorieux FH, et al. In vitro metabolism of 25-hydroxycholecalciferol by isolated cells from human deciduas. *J Clin Endocrinol Metab* 1985;60:880–885.
75. Wier PJ, Miller RK. In vitro evaluation of human placental function and toxic responses. In: Kimmel GI, Kocchar DM, eds. *In vitro methods in developmental toxicology: use in defining mechanism and risk parameters*. Boca Raton, FL: CRC Press, 1989:1–8.
76. Smith NC, Brush M. Preparation and characterization of human syncytiotrophoblast plasma membrane. *Med Biol* 1978;56:272–276.
77. Smith NC, Brush M, Luckett S. Preparation of human placental villous surface membrane. *Nature* 1974;252:302–303.
78. Schneider H, Panigel M, Dancis J. Transfer across the perfused human placenta of antipyrine sodium and leucine. *Am J Obstet Gynecol* 1972;113:822–828.
79. Cannell GR, Kluck SE, Hamilton SE, et al. Markers of physical integrity and metabolic viability of the perfused human placental lobule. *Clin Exp Pharmacol Physiol* 1988;15:837–844.
80. Schneider H. Techniques: in vitro perfusion of human placenta. In: Sastry BVR, ed. *Placental toxicology*. Boca Raton, FL: CRC Press, 1995:1–26.
81. Derewlany LO, Leeder JS, Kumar R, et al. The transport of digoxin across the perfused human placental lobule. *J Pharmacol Exp Ther* 1991;256:1107–1111.
82. Kanhai HH, van Kamp IL, Moolenaar AJ, et al. Transplacental passage of digoxin in severe rhesus immunization. *J Perinat Med* 1990;18:339–343.
83. Azancot-Benisty A, Jacqz-Aigrain E, Guirgis NM, et al. Clinical and pharmacologic study of fetal supraventricular tachyarrhythmias. *J Pediatr* 1992;121(4):608–613.
84. Schmolling J, Renke K, Richter O, et al. Digoxin, flecainide, and amiodarone transfer across the placenta and the effects of an elevated umbilical venous pressure on the transfer rate. *Ther Drug Monit* 2000;22(5):582–588.
85. Wolff F, Breuker KH, Schlensker KH, et al. Prenatal diagnosis and therapy of fetal heart rate anomalies with a contribution on the placental transfer of verapamil. *J Perinat Med* 1980;8:203–208.
86. Allan LD, Chita SK, Sharland GK, et al. Flecainide in the treatment of fetal tachycardias. *Br Heart J* 1991;65(1):46–48.
87. Wren C, Hunter S. Maternal administration of flecainide to terminate and suppress fetal tachycardia. *Br Med J* 1988;296–249.
88. Erkkola R, Lammintausta R, Liukko P, et al. Transfer of propranolol and sotalol across the human placenta: their effect on maternal and fetal plasma renin activity. *Acta Obstet Gynecol Scand* 1982;61:31–34.
89. Schneider H, Proegler M. Placental transfer of β-adrenergic antagonist studied an *in vitro* perfusion system of human placental tissue. *Am J Obstet Gynecol* 1988;159:42–47.

90. Jacobson RL, Brewer A, Eis A, et al. Transfer of aspirin across the perfused human placental cotyledon. *Am J Obstet Gynecol* 1991; 165:939–944.
91. Akbaraly R, Leng JJ, Brachet-Liermain A, et al. Passage transplacentaire de quatre anti-inflamatoires—son étude per perfusion *in vitro. J Gynecol Obstet Biol Reprod (Paris)* 1981;10:7–11.
92. Siu SS, Yeung JH, Lau TK. In vivo study on placental transfer of naproxen in early human pregnancy. *Hum Reprod* 2002;17(14): 1056–1059.
93. Akbaraly JP, Guilbert S, Leng JJ, et al. Etude du passage transplacentaire de cinq antibiotiques per perfusion in vitro du placenta humain. *Pathol Biol* 1985;33:368–372.
94. Fortunato SJ, Roger MD, Bawdon E, et al. Placental transfer of cefoperazone and sulbactam in the isolated in vitro perfused human placenta. *Am J Obstet Gynecol* 1988;159:1002–1006.
95. Fortunato SJ, Bowdon RE, Maberry MC, et al. Transfer of cefrizoxime surpasses that of cefoperazone by the isolated human placenta perfused in vitro. *Obstet Gynecol* 1990;75:830–833.
96. Bawdon RE, Maberry MC, Fortunato SJ, et al. Trimethoprim and sulfamethoxazole in the in vitro perfused human cotyledon. *Gynecol Obstet Invest* 1991;31:240–242.
97. Sodha EJ, Schneider H. Transplacental transfer of beta-adrenergic drugs studied by an in vitro perfusion method of an isolated human placental lobule. *Am J Obstet Gynecol* 1983;147:303–310.
98. Urbach J, Mor L, Fuchs S, et al. Transplacental transfer of ritodrine and its effect on placental glucose and oxygen consumption in an in vitro human placental cotyledon perfusion. *Gynecol Obstet Invest* 1991;32:10–14.
99. Fujimoto S, Tanaka T, Akahane M. Levels of ritodrine hydrochloride in fetal blood and amniotic fluid following long-term continuous administration in late pregnancy. *Eur J Obstet Gynecol Reprod Biol* 1991;38(1):15–18.
100. Smith MA, Thomford PJ, Mattison DR, et al. Transport and metabolism of dexamethasone in the dually perfused human placenta. *Reprod Toxicol* 1988;2:37–43.
101. Addison RS, Maguire DJ, Mortimer RH, et al. Metabolism of prednisolone by the isolated perfused human placental lobule. *J Steroid Biochem Mol Biol* 1991;39:83–90.
102. Levitz M, Jansen V, Dancis J. The transfer and metabolism of corticosteroids in the perfused human placenta. *Am J Obstet Gynecol* 1978;132:363–366.
103. Omarini D, Barzago MM, Bartolotti A, et al. Placental transfer of theophylline in an in vitro closed perfusion system of human placental isolated lobule. *Eur J Drug Metab Pharmacokinet* 1993; 18:369–374.
104. Schenker S, Dicke J, Johnson RF, et al. Human placental transport of cimetidine. *J Clin Invest* 1987;80:1428–1434.
105. Guerre-Millo M, Challier JC, Rey A, et al. Maternofetal transfer of two benzodiazepines: effect of plasma protein binding and placental uptake. *Dev Pharmacol Ther* 1982;4:158–172.
106. Crawford JC. Premedication for elective caesarean section. *Anaesthesia* 1979;34:892–897.
107. Jauniaux E, Jurkovic D, Lees C, et al. In vivo study of diazepam transfer across the first trimester human placenta. *Hum Reprod* 1996;11(4):889–892.
108. Wilson CM, Duindee J, Moore PJ, et al. A comparison of the early pharmacokinetics of midazolam in pregnant and non-pregnant women. *Anaesthesia* 1987;42:1057–1062.
109. Heikkine T, Ekblad U, Laine K. Transplacental transfer of citalopram, fluoxetine, and their primary demethylated metabolites in isolated perfused human placenta. *Br J Obstet Gynaecol* 2002; 109(9):1003–1008.
110. Kluck RM, Cannell GR, Hooper WD, et al. Disposition of phenytoin and phenobarbital in the isolated perfused human placenta. *Clin Exp Pharmacol Physiol* 1988;15:827–836.
111. Shah YG, Miller RK. Pharmacokinetics of phenytoin in perfused human placenta. *Pediatr Pharmacol (New York)* 1985;5: 165–179.
112. Takeda A, Okada H, Tanaka H, et al. Protein binding of four antiepileptic drugs in maternal and umbilical cord serum. *Epilepsy Res* 1992;13(2):147–151.
113. Pienimaki P, Hartikainen AL, Arvela P, et al. Carbamazepine and its metabolites in human perfused placenta and in maternal and cord blood. *Epilepsia* 1995;36:241–248.
114. Fowler DW, Eadie MJ, Dickinson RG. Transplacental transfer and biotransformation studies of valproic acid and its gluceronides in the perfused human placenta. *J Pharmacol Exp Ther* 1989;249: 318–323.
115. Barzago MM, Bortolotti A, Stellari FF, et al. Placental transfer of valproic acid after liposome encapsulation during in vitro human placenta perfusion. *J Pharmacol Exp Ther* 1996;277(1): 9–86.
116. Henderson GI, Hu ZQ, Yang Y, et al. Acyclovir transport by the human placenta. *J Lab Clin Med* 1992;120:885–892.
117. Gilstrap LC, Bawdon RE, Roberts SW, et al. The transfer of nucleoside analog ganciclovir across the perfused human placenta. *Am J Obstet Gynecol* 1994;170:967–973.
118. Marzolini C, Rudin C, Decostered LA, et al. Transplacental passage of protease inhibitors at delivery. *AIDS* 2002;16(6): 889–893.
119. Casey BM, Bawdon RE. Placental transfer of ritonovir with zidovudine in the ex vivo placental perfusion model. *Am J Obstet Gynecol* 1998;179(3, pt 1):758–761.
120. Bang U, Helbo-Hansen HS, Lindholm P, et al. Placental transfer and neonatal effects of epidural fentanyl-bupivacaine for cesarean section. *Anesthesiology* 1991;75:A847.
121. Gerdin E, Rane A, Lindberg B. Transplacental transfer of morphine in man. *J Perinat Med* 1990;18:305–312.
122. Kopecky EA, Simone C, Knie B, et al. Transfer of morphine across the human placenta and its interaction with naloxane. *Life Sci* 1999;65(22):2359–2371.
123. Gin T, Gregory MA, Chjan K, et al. Maternal and fetal levels of propofol at cesarean section. *Anaesth Intensive Care* 1990;18: 180–184.
124. Datta S, Camann W, Bader A, et al. Clinical effects and maternal and fetal plasma concentration of epidural ropivacaine versus bupivacaine for cesarean section. *Anesthesiology* 1995;82: 1346–1352.
125. Johnson RF, Cahana A, Oleinick M, et al. A comparison of the placental transfer of ropivacaine versus bupivacaine. *Anesth Analg* 1999;89(3):703–708.
126. Bajoria R, Contractor SF. Transfer of heparin across the human perfused placental lobule. *J Pharm Pharmacol* 1999;44: 952–959.
127. Nandakumaran M, Eldeen AS. Transfer of cyclosporine in the perfused human placenta. *Dev Pharmacol Ther* 1990;15:101–105.

CHAPTER

14

Jeffrey L. Blumer
Michael D. Reed

Principles of Neonatal Pharmacology

INTRODUCTION

The history of drug therapy is replete with examples of adverse reactions to drugs in children. Virtually all the drug-related legislation in effect in this country stems directly from these onerous experiences (1), which served as the foundation for the Pediatric Rule (1994), the Food and Drug Act, and, most recently, the Best Pharmaceuticals for Children Act (2).

In 1956, Silverman et al. (3) at Columbia reported an excessive mortality rate and an increased incidence of kernicterus among premature babies receiving a sulfonamide antibiotic compared with those receiving chlortetracycline. In 1959, Sutherland (4) described a syndrome of cardiovascular collapse in three newborns receiving high doses of chloramphenicol for presumed infections. More recently, the therapeutic misadventures experienced by low-birth-weight infants exposed to a parenteral vitamin E formulation (5) and the "gasping syndrome" in infants who received excessive amounts of benzyl alcohol (6,7) serve to underscore the generally held perception that newborn infants are more likely to experience adverse reactions to drugs.

This preconception is espoused even more ardently when the xenobiotic exposure occurs during the embryonic or fetal periods of development. The thalidomide tragedy reported in 1962, in which more than 10,000 babies were born with the rare malformation phocomelia, created an international outcry and changed forever the way in which drug safety is evaluated (8,9). More recently, therapeutic issues surrounding the retinoic acid embryopathy and maternal antidepressant drug use have refocused attention on the effects of drugs on the fetus and newborn (10).

As a result of these experiences, perinatologists, neonatologists, and pediatricians have become extremely conservative in their use of drug therapy. They have recognized that rational drug therapy for pregnant women and newborns is often confounded by a combination of unpredictable and often poorly understood pharmacokinetic and pharmacodynamic interactions (11–14). Although this conservative approach has permitted the fulfillment of the physician's oath to "do no harm," it also has prevented the adoption of newer therapeutic modalities and their adaptation to pediatric patients.

A more specific approach to neonatal therapeutics requires a thorough understanding of human developmental biology as well as insights regarding the dynamic ontogeny of the processes of drug absorption, drug distribution, drug metabolism, and drug excretion. In addition, there must be a rigorous appreciation of the developmental aspects of drug–receptor interactions, including the ontogenetic changes in receptor number, receptor affinity, receptor–effector coupling, and receptor modulation and regulation.

The purpose of this chapter is to develop a therapeutically relevant foundation for neonatal drug therapy based on the physiologic characteristics of extrauterine adaptation. The chapter focuses on the pharmacokinetic determinants of neonatal drug therapy rather than on any developmental variations in pharmacodynamics because only the former are amenable to clinical manipulation. Furthermore, specific discussion of the impact of growth on hepatic and renal function and the resultant important influences these ontogenic changes have on drug disposition and pediatric dosing are specifically addressed in Chapters 4 and 15, respectively, and thus are addressed only briefly here.

DRUG ABSORPTION

Absorption refers to the translocation of a drug from its site of administration into the bloodstream. Drugs administered extravascularly, including the sublingual, buccal, oral, intramuscular, subcutaneous, rectal, and topical routes, must cross multiple membranes to reach the systemic circulation and ultimately be distributed to sites of action. Absorption into the systemic circulation depends on both the physicochemical properties of a drug and a variety of host factors (Table 14.1).

TABLE 14.1 Factors Affecting Drug Absorption

Physicochemical factors
- Formulation characteristics
  - Disintegration of tablets or solid phase
  - Dissolution of drug in gastric or intestinal fluid
  - Release from sustained-release preparations
- Molecular weight
- pK_a and number of ionizable groups
- Degree of lipid solubility

Patient factors
- Gastric content and gastric emptying time
- Gastric and duodenal pH
- Surface area available for absorption
- Size of bile salt pool
- Bacterial colonization of the lower intestines
- Underlying disease states

ONTOGENY OF GASTRIC ACID PRODUCTION

Hess (15) was the first to describe the presence of hydrochloric acid in the newborn stomach several hours after birth. At birth, gastric pH is usually between 6 and 8, but it falls rapidly to between 1.5 and 3.0 within several hours (16). From the available data, this fall in gastric pH is quite variable but appears to be independent of both birth weight and gestational age. Despite beliefs to the contrary, Kelly et al. (17) clearly demonstrated gastric acid secretion in preterm infants at 24 to 29 weeks of gestational age. All of the 22 preterm infants studied on multiple occasions (71 recordings) from 1 to 17 days postnatal life were able to produce and maintain an intragastric median pH below 4, with an inverse relationship between gestational age and initial acid production (17). Grahnquist et al. (18) described the presence of gastric H,K-adenosine triphosphatase in stomach biopsies from infants of 25 to 42 weeks' gestation, with expression increasing with increasing gestational age.

Extrauterine factors (e.g., nutrition) are most likely responsible for initiating acid production, as basal acid output correlates with postnatal but not postconceptual age. The subsequent pattern of gastric acid secretion remains controversial. Initial descriptions suggested that, postnatally, acid secretion displays a biphasic pattern; the highest acid concentrations occur within the first 10 days and the lowest between the 10th and 30th day of extrauterine life. Agunod et al. (19), using betazole stimulation, essentially confirmed these early descriptions and found that the volume of gastric juice and acid concentration were dependent on age, and that gastric acid secretions (corrected for body weight) approached the lower limit of adult values by 3 months of age. Secretion of pepsin and intrinsic factor was also found to parallel that of gastric acid. In contrast, the longitudinal data of Kelly et al. (17) demonstrated a more constant amount of gastric acid (intragastric pH 0.6 to 3.9) over the first 17 days of life in very premature infants. Clearly, more study is necessary to fully elucidate the ontogeny of gastric acid secretion during the first month of life (18). However, these data also demonstrate the large degree of variability in the intragastric pH over the first 30 days of life and its dependence upon extrauterine factors.

Gastric and duodenal pH values affect drug solubility and ionization as well as gastrointestinal motility (20,21). An acid pH favors absorption of acid drugs (low pK_a) because in such an environment, the drug will be largely in an unionized, more lipid-soluble form. In contrast, a relatively high pH (as in state of achlorhydria) will enhance the translocation of basic drugs and retard the absorption of acidic drugs.

GASTRIC EMPTYING

Because most orally administered drugs are absorbed in the small intestine, the rate of gastric emptying is an important determinant of the rate and extent of drug absorption. If it is slowed down, the rate of intestinal drug absorption may be reduced; this will, in turn, reduce the peak serum drug concentration. On the other hand, if gastric emptying is hastened, the extent of intestinal absorption may be reduced as a result of decreased contact time with the absorptive surface. Of course, both these effects presuppose that intestinal motility remains constant.

Gastric emptying rate during the neonatal period is variable and is characterized by irregular and unpredictable peristaltic activity (22–24). It is prolonged relative to that of the adult. The rate of gastric emptying appears to be directly affected by gestational and postnatal age as well as the type of feeding use (16,22–24) (Table 14.2). Gastric emptying time appears to approach adult values within the first 6 to 8 months of life. Similarly, small intestinal motility in the perinatal period is variable and is influenced by the presence or absence of food (23,25).

An inverse relationship between gestational age and the amount of gastric retention 30 minutes after a 5% glucose-in-water feeding has been demonstrated. This relationship was independent of intrauterine growth. With human milk feedings, a characteristic biphasic pattern of gastric emptying in both preterm and term infants, with an initial rapid phase followed by a slower prolonged second phase, is observed. In contrast, a liner pattern of gastric emptying was noted when infant formula was used (22,23).

Gastric emptying is also affected by the composition of the meal. Slower gastric emptying times have been reported with increasing caloric density in premature infants (gestational age 25 to 35 weeks). Significant differences were noted between formulas containing 0 and 6.5, 6.5 and 13, and 13 and 20 calories per 100 g. These differences were significant at all times following the meal (20, 40, 60, 80, and 100 minutes). The difference in gastric emptying between a 20- and a 24-calories/oz (71.5 and 86 calories per 100 g, respectively) formula was significant only at 80 minutes.

TABLE 14.2 Factors Affecting Gastric Emptying Rate

Increase	*Decrease*	*No Effect*
Human milk	Prematurity	Osmolality
Hypocaloric feedings	Gastroesophageal reflux	Posture
	Respiratory distress syndrome	
	Congenital heart disease	
	Long-chain fatty acids	

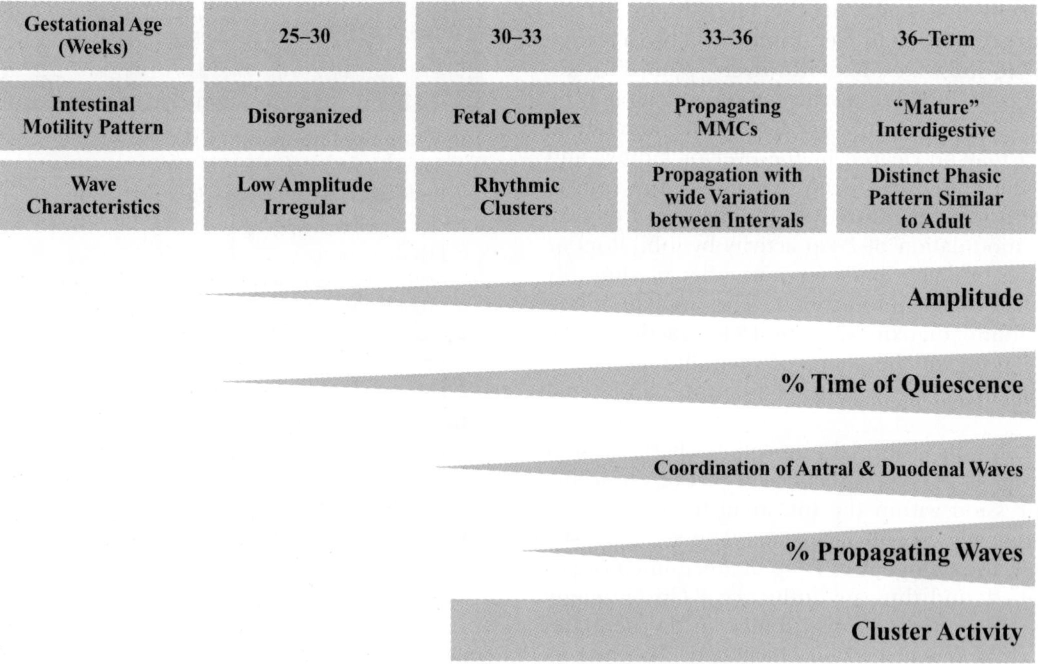

Figure 14.1. Diagrammatic representation of the quantitative changes in small intestinal motility patterns in the human infant as a function of increasing postconceptional age. Amplitude, percentage of time of quiescence, coordination of antral and duodenal waves, and percentage of propagating waves all increase through gestation. MMC, migrating motor complex. (Reproduced from Dumont RC, Rudolph CD. Development of gastrointestinal motility in the infant and child. *Gastroenterol Clin North Am* 1994;23:655–671, with permission.)

Similar findings with slower gastric emptying times have been reported in infants given a 10% glucose solution versus a 5% solution. Interestingly, although reduction in emptying rate is observed with higher caloric density substrates, the quantity of calories delivered to the duodenum from the stomach increased with increasing formula concentration (23).

In contrast to the effect of caloric density on gastric emptying rates, the osmolality of the meal does not appear to be a factor. However, slower emptying is seen in feeding with long-chain fatty acids compared with medium-chain triglycerides, an important variable, considering that infant formulas differ in their fatty acid content (23).

EXOCRINE PANCREATIC FUNCTION

The ontogeny of other physiologic processes may further influence the gastrointestinal absorption of drugs and other compounds. The rate of synthesis, pool size, and intestinal transport of bile acids are less in neonates than in adults (26), as is their character. At birth, pancreatic enzyme activity is low, and enzyme activities are lower in premature than in full-term neonates. Interestingly, at 1 week of postnatal age, fluid output and pancreatic enzyme activity are greater in premature than in full-term neonates. Lipase activity is present by 34 to 36 weeks of gestation, and increases fivefold during the first week and 20-fold during the first 9 months of postnatal life (27). In contrast, amylase activity has been detected as early as 23 weeks of gestation but remains very low even after birth (approximately 10% of adult values). Numerous investigators have shown decreased duodenal amylase activity in both fasting and fed infants during the first year of life. Trypsin secretion in response to pancreozymin and secretin administration is blunted in term infants but develops during the first year of life (16).

Duodenal contractions in term neonates appear to occur at rates similar to those observed in fasting adults, although the number of contractions per burst may be less (28). Fasting or interdigestive motor activity also appears to be shorter in children (29). A diagrammatic representation of the quantitative changes in small intestinal motility patterns in the human infant relative to postconceptional age is shown in Figure 14.1.

PHOSPHORYLATED-GLYCOPROTEIN

One area that has received considerable attention relative to drug absorption (and distribution) is the presence and functional capacity of phosphorylated-glycoprotein (P-Gp). In human, P-Gp is the most prominent member of the adenosine triphosphate–binding cassette family of proteins and is responsible for cellular drug efflux, translocating substances from the intracellular to the extracellular compartment (30,31). Initially considered to be responsible only for primary drug resistance in tumors (cellular resistance to "cancer" chemotherapeutic agents), subsequent studies confirmed that P-Gp is abundant within the human, and is normally found within the cellular membranes of the intestinal tract (duodenum, ileum, jejunum, and colon), apical membrane of heptocytes, renal proximal tubular cells, and on the luminal side of the capillary endothelial cells that make up the blood-brain barrier (30–32). This efflux protein has affinity for a broad range of hydrophobic substrates, and effectively "pumps" xenobiotics out of cells, influencing the amount a drug may be absorbed into systemic circulation, influencing the rate at which a drug may be cleared by the liver or kidney, and influencing the amount of drug that enters the central nervous system (30–33). Moreover, the degree of expression and/or modulation of P-Gp activity by inhibitors or inducers is the probable basis for a number of clinically important drug–drug interactions. The well-described digoxin–quinidine/digoxin–verapamil interactions are most likely a result of the ability of quinidine and verapamil to antagonize the activity of intestinal and renal P-Gp activity.

The variability in intestinal absorption characteristics for many drugs is likely a direct result of the variability of P-Gp expression within the intestinal tract as well as the presence or absence of P-Gp modulators (30,31,34). Unfortunately, the ontogeny of P-Gp in any human organ is not described, and thus any influence P-Gp ontogeny has on drug absorption and distribution in the neonate, infant, and child remains to be elucidated. The importance of this cannot be overemphasized considering the important role that P-Gp plays in the absorption, distribution, and clearance of many clinically important drugs.

ADDITIONAL PHYSIOLOGIC PROCESSES

Colonization of the gastrointestinal tract by bacteria, a process that influences the metabolism of bile salts and drugs as well as intestinal motility, varies with age, type of delivery, type of feeding, and concurrent drug therapy (35–37). All full-term, formula-fed, vaginally delivered infants are colonized with anaerobic bacteria by 4 to 6 days of postnatal life. By 5 to 12 months of age, an adult pattern of microbial reduction products is established. Despite the description of these maturational changes, there are only limited data on the metabolic activity of the gut flora (36,37). For example, children are colonized with intestinal bacteria capable of metabolizing digoxin; the capacity to inactivate the drug appears to develop gradually with age (38).

The diseases that will most likely have the greatest impact on oral drug absorption are those affecting the total surface area available for absorption (39), such as the short-bowel syndrome (Table 14.3). This syndrome often results from massive bowel resection complicating necrotizing enterocolitis, from malrotation with volvulus, or from certain congenital anomalies of the gastrointestinal tract during the neonatal period. In addition, drug absorption may be altered during periods of protein–calorie malnutrition, a condition leading to loss of available surface area due to villous atrophy, delayed gastric emptying, and increased intestinal transit time (40,41).

Multiple systemic diseases may also affect gastrointestinal drug absorption. Congestive heart failure may cause mucosal edema, or it may, by means of various hemodynamic compensations, affect drug absorption by delaying gastric emptying or by shunting blood flow away from visceral organs to accommodate the metabolite needs of the heart and the brain. In addition, hypo- or hyperthyroidism

TABLE 14.3 Selected Disease States Affecting Gastrointestinal Absorption of Drugs

Decreased surface area
Short-bowel syndrome
Protein–calorie malnutrition
Delayed gastric emptying
Pyloric stenosis
Congestive heart failure
Protein–calorie malnutrition
Bile salt excretion
Cholestatic liver disease
Extrahepatic biliary obstruction
Intestinal transit time
Protein–calorie malnutrition
Thyroid disease
Diarrheal disease
Gastric acid secretion
Proximal small-bowel resection

may influence drug absorption by prolonging or reducing intestinal transit time, respectively. Table 14.3 summarizes the effects of specific intestinal and extraintestinal disease states on the processes involved in oral drug absorption.

DRUG ABSORPTION FOLLOWING PARENTERAL ADMINISTRATION

The parenteral route of drug administration is important when oral therapy is physiologically precluded or the bioavailability of an oral formulation is poor. The intravenous route for drug delivery is preferred over intramuscular injection. In the absence of cardiovascular decompensation, intramuscular injection then becomes a viable and effective alternative for the administration of many drugs (Table 14.4). In addition to the ontogenetic factors controlling absorption addressed previously, most extravascular routes share physiochemical and physiologic constraints (Table 14.5) that may affect the rate and/or extent of drug bioavailability. The following subsections highlight pharmacokinetic considerations of several nonoral extravascular routes of administration.

ABSORPTION OF DRUGS GIVEN INTRAMUSCULARLY

Curves of serum concentration versus time following intramuscular drug administration may depend on factors germane to the drug, the site of administration, the presence of concomitant pathophysiology, and/or the developmental status of the patient (Table 14.5). Both physicochemical and physiologic factors affect the rate of drug absorption from the injection site (42). Lipophilicity of a drug favors rapid diffusion into the capillaries; however, the drug must retain a degree of water solubility at physiologic pH to prevent precipitation at the injection site (Table 14.4).

Another important factor influencing absorption of drugs from an intramuscular injection site is the blood flow to and from the injection site. This may be compromised in

TABLE 14.4 Drugs Demonstrating Effective Systemic Absorption Following Intramuscular Drug Administration

Antibacterials
- Amikacin
- Ampicillin
- Benzathine penicillin (penicillin benzathine)
- Benzylpenicillin (penicillin G)
- Carbenicillin
- Cefazolin
- Cefotaxime
- Ceftazidime
- Ceftriaxone
- Clindamycin
- Gentamicin
- Kanamycin
- Latamoxef (moxalactam)
- Methicillin
- Oxacillin
- Nafcillin
- Piperacillin
- Ticarcillin
- Tobramycin

Antituberculous agents
- Isoniazid
- Streptomycin

Anticonvulsants
- Diazepam
- Phenobarbital

Sedatives/tranquilizers
- Chlorpromazine
- Promethazine

Cardiovascular drugs
- Hydralazine
- Procainamide

Diuretics
- Furosemide
- Bumetanide

Endocrine
- Corticotropin (adrenocorticotropic hormone)
- Cortisone
- Desoxycorticosterone
- Glucagon

Pituitary
- Vasopressin (tannate oil)

Narcotics
- Meperidine
- Morphine

Vitamins
- K
- D

Adapted from Blumer JL. Therapeutic agents. In: Fanaroff AA, Martin RJ, eds. *Neonatal–perinatal medicine: diseases of the fetus and infant*, 4th ed. St. Louis, MO: Mosby, 1987:1248, with permission.

newborns with poor peripheral perfusion from low-cardiac-output states or the respiratory distress syndrome (43). The rate and extent of absorption from an intramuscular injection site are also influenced by the total surface area of muscle coming into contact with the injected solution (18), similar to the dependence of oral absorption on the total available absorptive area in the intestines. The ratio of skeletal muscle mass to body mass is less for neonates than for adults (43).

TABLE 14.5 Considerations for Extravascular Routes of Drug Administration that May Affect Drug Absorption

Physicochemical factors
- Molecular weight
- pK_a and degree of ionization
- Lipid–water partition coefficient
- pH and viscosity at the site(s) membrane translocation
- Particle size
- Number and diameter of membrane pores
- Thickness and surface area of membranes at site(s) of translocation
- Relative differences in solute concentration around membranes

Physiologic factors
- Presence or absence of facilitated or active transport mechanisms
- Relative surface area at sites of membrane translocation
- Volume of fluid at administration site
- Presence or absence of metabolic pathways and/or enzymes necessary for biotransformation
- Determination of residence time at absorptive sites (i.e., gastrointestinal motility, bulk flow of cerebrospinal fluid, etc.)
- Blood supply to site(s) of membrane translocation
- Affinity of drug for binding to plasma and/or tissue constituents
- Concomitant pathophysiology

A final consideration relative to intramuscular drug absorption is muscle activity, which may affect the rate of absorption and therefore affect the peak serum concentration. Sick, immobile neonates or those receiving a paralyzing agent to facilitate mechanical ventilation may show reduced absorption rates following intramuscular drug administration.

Intramuscular and intravenous dosing for a given drug may be associated with differences in both the serum concentrations and the pharmacokinetic parameter estimates (i.e., half-life and apparent volume of distribution). Consequently, these potential differences must be considered where serum concentration data following intramuscular administration are used for pharmacokinetic calculations.

PERCUTANEOUS ABSORPTION

The skin represents an often overlooked, but important, organ for systemic drug absorption (44). Chemical agents applied to the skin of a premature infant may result in inadvertent poisoning. There are numerous reports in the literature of neonatal toxicity related to the cutaneous exposure to drugs and chemicals. They include hexachlorophene (45), pentachlorophenol-containing laundry detergents (46), hydrocortisone (47), and aniline-containing disinfectant solution (48). Therefore, extreme caution should be exercised in using topical therapy in newborn infants (44).

The morphologic and functional development of the skin (49) as well as the factors that influence penetration of drugs into and through the skin (50) have been reviewed

(44). Basically, the percutaneous absorption of a compound is directly related to the degree of skin hydration and relative absorptive surface area and inversely related to the thickness of the stratum corneum (51). The integument of the full-term neonate possesses intact barrier function (52) and is similar to that of an older child or adult. However, the ratio of surface area to body weight of the full-term neonate is much higher than that of an adult. Thus, the infant will be exposed to a relatively greater amount of drug topically than do older infants, children, or adults (44). Theoretically, if a newborn receives the same percutaneous dose of a compound as an adult, the systemic availability per kilogram of body weight will be approximately 2.7 times greater in the neonate.

In contrast, studies in premature infants suggest the existence of an immature barrier to percutaneous absorption (44,52). Nachman and Esterly (53) studied the blanching response to topical 10% phenylephrine in preterm and term infants. Newborn infants of 28 to 34 weeks of gestational age had a rapid response lasting from 30 minutes to as long as 6 to 8 hours. No response was apparent under the same study conditions at 21 days of postnatal age. Newborns of gestational age 35 to 37 weeks had a less dramatic response with a longer latency period, and term infants failed to demonstrate a blanching response.

Finally, if the integrity of the integument is compromised (e.g., denuded, burned, or inflamed skin), then percutaneous translocation of compounds into the blood will be enhanced.

RECTAL ABSORPTION

Rectal administration of drugs is of potential therapeutic importance if a patient cannot take an agent orally and intramuscular or intravenous access for drug administration is impractical. The rectal vault may serve as an important alternative site for systemic drug administration when nausea, vomiting, seizure activity, and/or preparation for surgery preclude the use of oral dosage forms (54). General principles regarding the physicochemical factors (55,56), clinical pharmacokinetics (57), and therapeutic use of the rectal route in children (58) have been reviewed. It is important to note that drug absorption via the rectal route can be erratic, and, depending on the specific formulation used (solid suppository, liquid, etc.) and retention time within the rectal vault, drug bioavailability may be unpredictable.

Knowledge of the venous drainage system for the lower gastrointestinal tract is imperative in understanding the potential bioavailability of drugs administered rectally. The inferior and middle rectal veins, which drain the anus and lower rectum, respectively, drain directly into the systemic circulation by means of the inferior vena cava, whereas the superior rectal vein, which drains the upper part of the rectum, empties into the portal vein by means of the inferior mesenteric vein. Therefore, drugs administered into the superior aspect of the rectum will be subjected to the hepatic first-pass effect because portal blood enters the liver, whereas drugs administered lower into the rectum will initially bypass the liver.

The predominant mechanism for drug absorption from the rectum is probably similar to that observed in the upper gastrointestinal tract, that is, passive diffusion. Theoretically, the physicochemical and host factors discussed earlier with respect to oral drug absorption also influence rectal drug absorption (see Table 14.1). In general, absorption from aqueous or alcoholic solutions is more rapid than from suppositories.

Lipophilic drugs with pK_a values between 7 and 8, such as barbiturates and benzodiazepines, seem to be ideally suited for rectal administration because they will be mostly in an unionized form and will readily cross cell membranes. Rectal administration of 0.25 to 0.5 mg per kg of a diazepam solution to children 2 weeks to 11 years old produced serum concentrations comparable with those observed following intravenous administration. In addition, peak serum concentrations occurred within 6 minutes of administration. The rapid attainment of effective systemic drug concentrations with rectal drug administration has been effectively applied to the treatment of status epilepticus (59,60).

DRUG ADMINISTRATION TECHNIQUES

Certainly other routes of drug administration besides the oral, intravenous, intramuscular, percutaneous, and rectal routes may be employed when treating newborns; however, there has been little work systematically evaluating drug absorption from the endotracheal, epidural, intrathecal, and intraperitoneal routes.

An issue of equal importance to the route of administration is the actual method employed to administer the drug. For optimal therapeutics to be realized, a method of drug administration must be used that will enable the drug to reach its site of action at the desired time and in an effective concentration (61,62). The technique or method of drug administration is often the most crucial factor to consider when serum concentrations are used for pharmacokinetic analysis. The lack of awareness of or attention to critical aspects of drug administration techniques can lead to therapeutic misadventures even in the face of the most sophisticated analytical and pharmacokinetic methods (63) (Table 14.6).

Several steps can and should be taken to minimize problems with drug administration. These may include one or more of the following: standardization and documentation of complete administration times, documentation of the volume and content of the solution used to "flush" an intravenous or oral dose, tailoring of the concentrations of drug solutions for desired osmolalities, standardization of specific infusion techniques for drugs with a narrow therapeutic index, standardization of dilution and infusion volumes for drugs given by intermittent intravenous injection, avoidance of attaching lines for drug infusion to a central hub with other solutions being infused at widely disparate rates, maintenance of the recommended solution head height for gravity controllers, and the use of low-volume tubing and the most distal sites for access of drug into an existing intravenous line. In every situation where monitoring of serum drug concentrations is to be employed, the method of drug administration should be noted before these data are used in pharmacokinetic calculations.

TABLE 14.6 Potential Errors in Drug Administration Techniques

Factors involving drug (dose) preparation
Inappropriate dilutions
Similarity in appearance of dose units
Loss of potentially large amounts of drug dose in the dead space of a syringe; infusion Y site, etc.
Unsuitable drug formulations for administration
Unlabeled or undesirable ingredients in dose forms
Undesirable drug concentrations and/or osmolalities
Errors in interpreting drug orders and/or dose calculations
Factors involving intravenous drug administration
Loss of drug consequent to routine changing of intravenous sets
Reduction in serum concentration for drugs with rapid plasma clearance that are infused slowly
Extreme increase in plasma drug concentrations consequent to rapid infusion of drugs with small central compartment volume of distribution
Delayed infusion of total dose when intravenous line is not flushed
Inadvertent admixture of drugs by the manual intravenous retrograde method
Large distance between the site of drug infusion into an intravenous line and the insertion of the line into the patient
Potential loss of large-volume doses in the overflow syringe with the intravenous retrograde technique
Possible loss of drug because of binding to intravenous tubing
Use of large-intraluminal-diameter tubing for small patients
Infiltrations not detected by pump alarms
Infusion of multiple medications/fluids at different rates by means of a common "hub"
Oscillations in fluid/dose rate of potent medication infused with piston-type pumps
Factors involving other routes of drug administration
Loss in delivery (nasogastric tube dead space) or from oral cavity
Leakage of drug from intramuscular or subcutaneous injection site
Expulsion of drug from the rectum
Misapplication to external sites (i.e., ophthalmic ointment in young infants)

DRUG DISTRIBUTION

The movement of drugs and other compounds from the systemic circulation into various body compartments, tissues, and cells is termed *distribution.* The distribution of most drugs in the body is influenced by a variety of age-dependent factors, including protein binding, body compartment sizes, hemodynamic factors such as cardiac output and regional blood flow, and membrane permeability (64,65).

The apparent volume of distribution V_d describes the relationship between the amount of drug in the body and its plasma concentration. V_d is the volume needed to contain the total-body store of drug if the concentration throughout the whole body were the same as in plasma. This is represented by the following mathematical relationship:

$$V_d = \frac{DF}{C_0} \qquad (1)$$

where D is the dose administered, F is the bioavailability, and C_0 is derived by extrapolating the slope of the curve of plasma concentration versus time to time zero. Several factors, including plasma protein concentration and tissue binding, affect V_d. This relationship is expressed by the following equation:

$$V_d = V_b + V_t f_B / f_t \qquad (2)$$

where V_b is the blood volume, V_t is the tissue volume, f_B is the fraction of unbound drug in the blood, and f_t is the fraction of unbound drug in the tissue. Therefore, any factor that increases the blood volume or the fraction of unbound drug in the blood or reduces the fraction of unbound drug in the tissue will increase V_d.

DEVELOPMENTAL ASPECT OF PROTEIN BINDING

The binding of drugs to plasma protein is dependent on the concentration of available binding proteins, the affinity constant of the protein(s) for the drug, the number of available binding sites, and the presence of pathophysiologic conditions or endogenous compounds that may alter the drug–protein binding interaction (66–68) (Table 14.7).

The affinity of albumin for acidic drugs increases, as do total plasma protein levels, from birth into early infancy (51). These values do not reach normal adult levels until 10 to 12 months of age (69). In addition, although plasma albumin may reach adult levels shortly after birth (70), the albumin level in blood is directly proportional to gestational age, reflecting both placental transport and fetal synthesis (71).

Different degrees of drug–protein binding between newborn and adult plasma have been demonstrated (Table 14.8). Four mechanisms have been proposed to explain these differences: (a) displacement of drugs from binding sites by bilirubin in cord plasma, (b) different binding properties of cord and adult albumin, (c) different binding properties of globulins, and (d) decreased binding properties of albumin due to interaction with globulins in newborns.

TABLE 14.7 Physiologic Variables Influencing Drug–Protein Binding in Infancy and Childhood

	Value Relative to Adult Value		
Parameter	*Neonate*	*Infant*	*Child*
Total protein	Decreased	Decreased	Equivalent
Plasma albumin	Decreased	Equivalent	Equivalent
Fetal albumin	Present	Absent	Absent
Plasma globulin	Decreased	Decreased	Equivalent
Unconjugated bilirubin	Increased	Equivalent	Equivalent
Free fatty acids	Increased	Equivalent	Equivalent
Blood pH	Low	Equivalent	Equivalent
α_1-Acid glycoprotein	Decreased	Data not available	Equivalent

Adapted from Radde IC. Drugs and protein binding. In: MacLeod SM, Radde IC, eds. *Textbook of pediatric clinical pharmacology.* Littleton, MA: PSG Publishing, 1985:32–43, with permission.

Albumin is not the only plasma protein that binds drugs. Basic drugs are bound by several plasma proteins, including α_1-acid glycoprotein (67). Piafsky and Mpamugo (72) showed significant reductions in both α_1-acid glycoprotein plasma concentrations and in binding of the basic drugs lidocaine and propranolol to cord blood as compared with adult controls. When the α_1-acid glycoprotein concentration in cord blood was increased to adult values, the protein binding of lidocaine and propranolol approached adult levels, suggesting the reduced plasma concentration of α_1-acid glycoprotein as the primary reason for the decreased protein binding.

INFLUENCE OF ENDOGENOUS SUBSTANCES ON PROTEIN BINDING

There are a number of endogenous molecules that, such as drugs, may bind to plasma proteins (64) and displace drugs from these binding sites. The effect is generally transient and may increase the apparent volume of distribution of the displaced drug. More important, the increase in the fraction of free drug that occurs may result in a transiently intensified pharmacologic response at a given drug dose or serum total drug concentration. Although most clinicians perceive this "interaction" as a primary mechanism of drug toxicity, the clinical significance of protein displacement drug–drug interactions is usually very limited or none (68) due to the increased V_d and concurrent change (increase) in body clearance. However, during the neonatal period, this interaction may be of greater importance due to immaturity in clearance organ function (as discussed later).

Clinically significant protein-binding displacement reactions will occur only when (a) a drug is more than 80% to 90% protein bound, (b) the drug's clearance is capacity limited, (c) the drug's clearance is binding sensitive, and (4) the V_d is small, usually less than 0.15 L per kg, because above this value, only a small percentage of total drug in the body is found in plasma.

Under these conditions, the following sequence of events may occur: The displacement reaction increases the amount of free drug, which may result in a heightened pharmacologic response if the drug's concentration–effect curve is reasonably steep. However, as described previously, this intensified pharmacologic effect is often transient because the displacement reaction increases the amount of free drug available for metabolism and/or excretion. The net result, once steady state is achieved, is a decreased concentration of total drug in plasma accompanied by an unchanged free drug concentration (68).

TABLE 14.8 Comparative Protein Binding of Some Representative Drugs

	Percentage Bound	
Drug	*Newborn*	*Adult*
Ampicillin	10	18
Diazepam	84	99
Lidocaine	20	70
Phenytoin	80	90
Propranolol	60	93
Theophylline	36	56

FREE FATTY ACIDS

Nonesterified fatty acids are reversibly bound to albumin (73) and are present at relatively high concentrations in the plasma of newborn infants. Significant reductions in albumin binding of phenylbutazone, dicoumarol (bishydroxycoumarin), and phenytoin have been demonstrated at high serum levels of free fatty acids (FFAs), approximately 2,000 μEq per L or at an FFA/albumin molar ratio of 3.5. Although these values are rarely attained, they have been observed under certain pathophysiologic conditions such as gram-negative septicemia.

Interestingly, similar elevations in FFA levels have not been reported with gram-positive septicemia, which is common in newborns. Displacing effects of FFAs on the unbound fraction of diazepam have been reported in newborns, and a linear correlation between unbound plasma

TABLE 14.9 Principles Related to Drug-Induced Bilirubin Displacement and the Risk of Kernicterus

Drugs that are administered in low doses such as hormones, cardiac glycosides, and potent loop diuretics are not dangerous because a certain molar amount of the drug is required to occupy a significant fraction of the reserve albumin

Cationic drugs and most electroneutral substances, such as aminoglycosides, antihistamines, general anesthetics, and benzodiazepines, are not bound competitively to the bilirubin-binding site

Sulfonamides show a highly variable effect; sulfadiazine is the weakest competitor and is probably safe at usual doses

Several analgesics and anti-inflammatory drugs are potent displacers

The highest degree of displacement is observed with x-ray contrast media for cholangiography

phenytoin concentrations and the ratio of serum FFA to albumin concentration in neonates has been described.

BILIRUBIN

Bilirubin is noncovalently bound to albumin, and this association is freely reversible (74,75). The bilirubin-binding affinity of albumin at birth is independent of gestational age (76,77) and is less in the newborn than in the adult (78). The binding affinity of albumin for bilirubin increases with age (76,79) and reaches that of adult serum by approximately 5 months of age (79). Ebbesen and Nyboe (76) found that this increased affinity, at least during the first week of life, is related to gestational age. The lower bilirubin-binding affinity of albumin in neonates is believed to be a contributing factor in their susceptibility to kernicterus (79). However, other factors, such as the effect of hypothermia, acidosis, hypoglycemia, hypoxemia, sepsis, birth asphyxia, and hypercapnia, on the permeability of the blood-brain barrier and on bilirubin–albumin binding must be considered (80). Furthermore, the apparent importance of function and concentration of blood-brain barrier P-Gp to bilirubin transport remains to be more fully elucidated (33).

A number of drugs are thought to be able to compete with and displace bilirubin from binding sites on the albumin molecule, thus increasing the risk of the infant's developing kernicterus (80) (Table 14.9).

DEVELOPMENTAL ASPECTS OF FLUID COMPARTMENT SIZES

Total-Body Water

Alterations in body water compartment sizes will affect the volume of distribution of a drug. Age-dependent changes in the various fluid compartments have been reviewed and are summarized in Table 14.10. Total-body water varies inversely with the amount of fat tissue in the body. In the young fetus, total-body water comprises nearly 92% of body weight, with the extracellular fluid volume responsible for 25% of body weight; body fat is less than 1% (81). The results of more recent studies focusing on fat mass relative to age (82,83) are consistent with these earlier findings.

At term, total-body water falls to approximately 75% of body weight, and the amount of fat increases to approximately 15%. By 6 months of age, total-body water and fat comprise 60% and 30% of body weight, respectively. In the second year of life, there is a small increase in total-body water due to sudden increase in the intracellular fluid volume (84). Except for a small increase prior to puberty in males, a gradual reduction in total-body water occurs in both sexes, approaching adult values of 50% to 60% of body weight at puberty.

Extracellular Fluid Volume

The extracellular fluid volume can be estimated from the distribution of chloride or bromide ions because both these elements are distributed primarily in extracellular fluid, entering the intracellular fluid to only a minor extent. By 40 weeks of gestation, measurements of extracellular fluid volume range from 350 to 440 mL per kg of body weight (84) and correlate more closely with body weight than with gestational age. By 1 year of age, the extracellular fluid volume decreases to approximately 26% to 30% of body weight, and after the first year, it decreases slowly and gradually approaches the adult value of 20% of body weight by puberty.

Intracellular Fluid Volume

The intracellular fluid volume cannot be measured directly, and thus it must be estimated by subtracting the extracellular fluid volume from total-body water. The intracellular fluid volume increases from 25% of body weight in the young fetus to 33% at birth to approximately

TABLE 14.10 Fluid Compartment Size as a Function of Age

Age	*Total-Body Water*[a]	*Extracellular Fluid*[a]	*Intracellular Fluid*[a]
<3-mo fetus	92	65	25
Term gestation	75	35–44	33
4–6 mo	60	~23	37
12 mo		26–30	
Puberty	~60	20	40
Adult	50–60	20	40

[a]As a percentage of body weight.

37% of body weight at 4 months of age (81). Except for a sudden increase during early childhood, the intracellular fluid volume remains relatively constant, approximating 40% of body weight.

The clinical relevance of this gradual reduction in the size of body water compartments with age cannot be overemphasized. To achieve comparable plasma and tissue concentrations of drugs distributed into the extracellular fluid, higher doses per kilogram of body weight must be given to infants as compared with adults.

DRUG METABOLISM

The process of drug removal from the body starts the instant a drug molecule is present within the body. The primary organ for drug metabolism is the liver, but the kidneys, intestine, lungs, and skin are also capable of transformation (85). Although the metabolism of most drugs generally results in pharmacologically weaker or inactive compounds, parent compounds may be transformed into active metabolites (e.g., theophylline to caffeine or procainamide to *N*-acetyl procainamide). Furthermore, pharmacologically inactive compounds, or prodrugs, may be converted to their active moiety (e.g., chloramphenicol succinate or palmitate to the active chloramphenicol base) (Table 14.11).

Hepatic xenobiotic metabolism assumes an extremely important role in determining the pharmacokinetic and pharmacodynamic properties of a drug. The pharmacokinetic parameter of estimated clearance describes the overall rate of drug removal. It can be described in terms of plasma clearance, organ clearance, or total-body clearance (86). Plasma clearance is the volume of plasma from which a drug is completely removed per unit of time. Drugs can be cleared by several mechanisms, with hepatic biotransformation, renal excretion, and exhalation by the lungs representing the primary routes. The clearance (CL) of a drug by an individual organ is dependent on the blood flow to the organ (Q) and the organ's extraction ratio (E), and can be described as follows:

$$\mathrm{CL} = QE \qquad (3)$$

where E is the ratio of the arteriovenous concentration difference divided by the arterial concentration, as expressed by the following relationship:

$$E = \frac{C_a - C_v}{C_a} \qquad (4)$$

TABLE 14.11 Active Metabolites of Drugs Used in Neonates

Parent Drug	*Active Metabolite(s)*
Diazepam	Desmethyldiazepam, oxazepam
Lidocaine	Mono- and didesethyl lignocaine
Meperidine	Normeperidine
Procainamide	*N*-Acetyl procainamide
Propranolol	4-Hydroxypropranolol
Theophylline	Caffeine

where C_a and C_v are the arterial and venous concentrations, respectively. Hepatic clearance depends on hepatic blood, plasma free-drug concentration, cellular uptake, hepatic metabolism, and biliary excretion. The hepatic clearance of a drug can be expressed by the following equation:

$$\mathrm{CL_H} = Q\,\frac{f_B \times \mathrm{CL_{int}}}{Q + (f_B \times \mathrm{CL_{int}})} \qquad (5)$$

where $\mathrm{CL_H}$ is the hepatic clearance, Q is the hepatic blood flow, f_B is the fraction of free drug, and $\mathrm{CL_{int}}$ is the intrinsic clearance, which is a measure of hepatocellular metabolism. Drugs that are primarily cleared by the liver can be classified as *flow limited* or *capacity limited.* If a drug displays a high $\mathrm{CL_{int}}$ and E, then doubling the $\mathrm{CL_{int}}$ will have little effect on $\mathrm{CL_H}$, whereas a change in blood flow will produce a proportional change in $\mathrm{CL_H}$. In other words, for drugs that are highly extracted (>80%) and are metabolized by the liver, $\mathrm{CL_H}$ reflects the amount and rate of the drug delivered to the liver.

Drugs with high extraction ratios will be subjected to the *first-pass effect* when administered orally. This term, coined by Harris and Riegelman (87) for aspirin, signifies that a drug is rapidly metabolized or altered when passing through the intestinal mucosa or liver for the first time. Therefore, the parent compound is found in lower concentrations in the systemic circulation than if the drug were administered intravenously, and, conversely, metabolites that are frequently inactive are the predominant form of the parent drug found in the circulation. Examples of drugs that exhibit such high extraction rates include lidocaine, propranolol, acetylsalicylic acid, and isoproterenol.

Capacity-limited drugs display low extraction ratios (<20%) and low intrinsic metabolic clearance. Hepatic clearance is therefore dependent on the degree of hepatic uptake and metabolism of the drug and is independent of hepatic blood flow. Capacity-limited drugs can be further subdivided into binding-sensitive and binding-insensitive drugs. For *binding-sensitive drugs,* such as clindamycin, extraction ratios approach the free drug concentration ($E = f_B$). Therefore, factors that increase f_B, such as decreased protein binding, will increase hepatic clearance. In contrast, other drugs may display extraction ratios that are much less than that of the free drug, and therefore the hepatic clearance is only a function of the intrinsic clearance and is independent of protein binding. These drugs are referred to as *binding insensitive* (e.g., chloramphenicol).

DEVELOPMENTAL ASPECTS OF HEPATIC CLEARANCE

At every level, from the ontogenetic changes in hepatic blood flow and portal oxygen tension to the developmental alterations in protein binding and xenobiotic-metabolizing enzyme activities, there is a real effect of age and various pathophysiologic states on the processes associated with hepatic clearance. Very dramatic developmental changes in the physiologic and biochemical process that

TABLE 14.12 Drug Disposition in Infants Compared with Adults: Potential Influence of Pharmacokinetics

Disposition Parameter	*Newborn versus Adult*	*Possible Pharmacokinetic Result*	*Example Drugs*
Absorption	↓	↓AUC	Penicillins, sulfonamides
Volume of distribution	↑	↓Peak	Gentamicin, digoxin
Percentage protein binding	↓	↑Free fraction	Clindamycin, theophylline
Metabolism	↓	↓Clearance	Chloramphenicol, theophylline
Excretion	↓	↑AUC ↑$t_{1/2}$	Gentamicin, furosemide

↓, Less in newborns than in adults; ↑, greater in newborns than in adults; AUC, area under the concentration-versus-time curve; $t_{1/2}$, elimination half-life.

govern drug disposition occur during the first year of life. These important processes and a description of the ontogeny of hepatic function, including the ontogeny of cytochrome P450 hepatic enzymes (phase I) and conjugation pathways (phase II), are critically addressed in Chapter 4 and have been expertly reviewed by Alcorn and McNamara (86) and Kearns et al. (88).

DEVELOPMENTAL ASPECTS OF RENAL DRUG CLEARANCE

The elimination half-life ($t_{1/2\beta}$) of a drug is commonly used to describe its disappearance from the blood and is measured as the time required for half the amount of drug present in the blood to disappear. The following equation can be used to describe $t_{1/2\beta}$:

$$t_{1/2\beta} = \frac{0.693V}{\mathrm{CL}} \qquad (6)$$

The $t_{1/2\beta}$ of a drug is a parameter that may be employed clinically to devise initial drug dosing guidelines. Recognition of an unusual half-life due to pathophysiologic changes should prompt the clinician to assess the need for dosage and/or dosing interval alterations.

RENAL EXCRETION

Most drugs and/or their metabolites are excreted from the body by the kidneys. Renal excretion is dependent on glomerular filtration, tubular reabsorption, and tubular secretion (Table 14.12). The amount of a drug that is filtered per unit time is influenced by the extent of protein binding and renal plasma flow. If the latter is constant, then the greater the extent of protein binding, the smaller will be the fraction of circulating drug that is filtered. The influence of renal function maturation on drug disposition in the premature and newborn infant is addressed in Chapter 16 and thus will not be addressed here (86,88).

SUMMARY

There exist marked differences in drug biodisposition in the newborn compared with the adult with respect to all pharmacokinetic processes (Table 14.12). Furthermore, the importance of an infant's gestational and postnatal age on drug disposition cannot be overemphasized. These differences and the ontogenetic changes in these processes must be considered carefully when developing therapeutic strategies for newborn and young infants.

ACKNOWLEDGMENT

The authors were supported in part by the National Institutes of Health, National Institute of Child Health and Human Development, Pediatric Pharmacology Research Units grant HD31323-9.

REFERENCES

1. Shirkey H. Editorial comment: therapeutic orphans. *J Pediatr* 1968;72:119–120.
2. Wilson JT. An update on the therapeutic orphan. *Pediatrics* 1999;104(Suppl):585–590.
3. Silverman WA, Anderson DH, Blanc WA, et al. A difference in mortality rate and incidence of kernicterus among premature infants allotted to two prophylactic antibacterial regimens. *Pediatrics* 1956;18:614–624.
4. Sutherland JM. Fatal cardiovascular collapse of infants receiving large amount of chloramphenicol. *Am J Dis Child* 1959;97: 761–767.
5. Lorch V, Murphy D, Hoersten LR, et al. Unusual syndrome among premature infants: association with a new intravenous vitamin E product. *Pediatrics* 1985;75:598–602.
6. Lovejoy FH. Benzyl alcohol poisoning in neonatal intensive care units. A new concern for the pediatrician. *Am J Dis Child* 1982; 136:974–975.
7. Christensen ML, Helms RA, Chesney RW. Is pediatric labeling really necessary? *Pediatrics* 1999;104(Suppl):593–597.
8. Speirs AL. Thalidomide and congenital abnormalities. *Lancet* 1962;10:303–305.
9. Taussig H. A study of the German outbreak of phocomelia. *J Am Med Assoc* 1962;198:1106–1114.
10. Einarson A, Portnoi G, Koren G. Update on Motherisk updates: seven years of questions and answers. *Can Fam Physician* 2002;48: 1301–1304.

11. Lobstein R, Koren G. Clinical relevance of therapeutic drug monitoring during pregnancy. *Ther Drug Monit* 2002;24:15–22.
12. Garland M. Pharmacology of drug transfer across the placenta. *Obstet Gynecol Clin North Am* 1998;25:21–42.
13. Berlin Jr CM. Advances in pediatric pharmacology and toxicology. *Adv Pediatr* 1997;44:545–574.
14. Kearns GL. Impact of developmental pharmacology on pediatric study design: overcoming the challenges. *J Allergy Clin Immunol* 2000;106(3 Suppl):S128–S138.
15. Hess AF. The gastric secretion of infants at birth. *Am J Dis Child* 1913;6:264–284.
16. Grand RJ, Watkins JB, Torti FM. Development of the human gastrointestinal tract: a review. *Gastroenterology* 1976;70:790–810.
17. Kelly EJ, Newell SJ, Brownlee KG, et al. Gastric acid secretion in preterm infants. *Early Hum Dev* 1993;35:215–220.
18. Grahnquist L, Ruuska T, Finkel Y. Early development of human gastric H,K adenosine triphosphatase. *J Pediatr Gastroenterol Nutr* 2000;305:533–537.
19. Agunod M, Yomahuchi N, Lopez R, et al. Correlative study of hydrochloric acid, pepsin and intrinsic factor secretion in newborns and infants. *Am J Dig Dis* 1969;14:400–414.
20. Martinez MN, Amiden GL. A mechanistic approach to understanding the factors affecting drug absorption: a review of fundamentals. *J Clin Pharmacol* 2002;42:620–643.
21. Zhou H. Pharmacokinetic strategies in deciphering atypical drug absorption profiles. *J Clin Pharmacol* 2003;43:211–227.
22. Cavell B. Gastric emptying in infants fed human milk or infant formula. *Acta Paediatr Scand* 1981;70:639–641.
23. Dumont RC, Rudolph CD. Development of gastrointestinal motility in the infant and child. *Pediatr Clin North Am* 1994;23:655–671.
24. Carlos MA, Babyn PS, Macron MA, et al. Changes in gastric emptying in early postnatal life. *J Pediatr* 1997;130:931–937.
25. Tawil YA, Berseth CL. Gestational and postnatal maturation of duodenal motor responses to intragastric feeding. *J Pediatr* 1996;129:374–381.
26. Heubi JE, Babistrern WF, Suchy FJ. Bile salt metabolism in the first year of life. *J Lab Clin Med* 1982;100:127–136.
27. Cavell B. Gastric emptying in preterm infants. *Acta Paediatr Scand* 1979;68:725–730.
28. Morris FH Jr, Moore M, Weisbroadt NW, et al. Ontogenetic development of gastrointestinal mortality. IV. Duodenal contractions in preterm infants. *Pediatrics* 1986;78:1106–1113.
29. Milla PJ, Fenton TR. Small intestinal motility patterns in the perinatal period. *J Pediatr Gastroenterol Nutr* 1983;2(Suppl 1):5141–5144.
30. Kim RB. Drugs as P-glycoprotein substrates, inhibitors, and inducers. *Drug Metab Rev* 2002;34:47–54.
31. Johnson WW. P-glycoprotein-mediated efflux as a major factor in the variance of absorption and distribution of drugs: modulation of chemotherapy resistance. *Methods Find Exp Clin Pharmacol* 2002; 24:501–514.
32. Anthony V, Skach WR. Molecular mechanism of P-glycoprotein assembly into cellular membranes. *Curr Protein Pept Sci* 2002;3: 485–501.
33. Watchko JF, Daood MJ, Mahmood B, et al. P-glycoprotein and bilirubin distribution. *J Perinatol* 2001;21:S43–S47.
34. Schuetz EG, Furuya KN, Schuetz JD. Interindividual variation in expression of P-glycoprotein in normal human liver and secondary hepatic neoplasms. *J Pharmacol Exp Ther* 1995;275:1011–1018.
35. Edwards CA, Parrett AM. Probiotics, prebiotics, and synbiotics: approaches for modulating the microbial ecology of the gut. *Am J Clin Nutr* 1999;69(Suppl):1052S–1057S.
36. Rowland IR. Factors affecting metabolic activity of the intestinal microflora. *Drug Metab Rev* 1988;19:243–261.
37. Ilett KF, Tee LB, Reeves PT, et al. Metabolism of drugs and other xenobiotics in the gut lumen and wall. *Pharmacol Ther* 1990;46: 67–93.
38. Lindenbaum J, Rund D, Butler VP. Inactivation of digoxin by the gut flora: reversal by antibiotic therapy. *N Engl J Med* 1981;305: 789–794.
39. Lebenthal A, Lebenthal E. The ontogeny of the small intestinal epithelium. *JPEN Parenter Enteral Nutr* 1999;23:S3–S6.
40. Krishnaswamy K. Drug metabolism and pharmacokinetics in malnutrition. *Clin Pharmacokinet* 1978;3:216–240.
41. Seth V, Beotra A, Bagga A, et al. Drug therapy in malnutrition. *Indian Pediatr* 1992;29(11):1341–1346.
42. Greenblatt DJ, Koch-Weaser J. Intramuscular injection of drugs. *N Engl J Med* 1976;295:542–546.
43. Radde IC. Mechanisms of drug absorption and their development. In: MacLeod SM, Radde IC, eds. *Textbook of pediatric clinical pharmacology*. Littleton, MA: PSG Publishing, 1985:17–43.
44. Choonara I. Percutaneous drug absorption and administration. *Arch Dis Child* 1994;71:F73–F74.
45. Tyrala EE, Hillman LS, Hillman RE, et al. Clinical pharmacology of kerochlorophene in newborn infants. *J Pediatr* 1977;91: 481–486.
46. Armstrong RW, Eichner ER, Klein DE, et al. Pentachlorophenol poisoning in a nursery for newborn infants. II. Epidemiologic and toxicologic studies. *J Pediatr* 1969;75:317–325.
47. Feinblatt BI, Aceto T, Beckhorn G, et al. Percutaneous absorption of hydrocortisone in children. *Am J Dis Child* 1966;112:218–224.
48. Fisch RO, Berglund EB, Bridge AG, et al. Methemoglobinemia in a hospital nursery. *J Am Med Assoc* 1963;185:760–763.
49. Radde IC, McKercher HG. Transport through membranes and development of membrane transport. In: MacLeod SM, Radde IC, eds. *Textbook of pediatric clinical pharmacology*. Littleton, MA: PSG Publishing, 1985:1–16.
50. Marks J, Rawlins MD. Skin diseases. In: Speight TM, ed. *Avery's drug treatment: principles and practice of clinical pharmacology and therapeutics*, 3rd ed. Aucklan, NZ: ADIS Press, 1987:439–479.
51. Morselli PL, Franco-Morselli R, Bossi L. Clinical pharmacokinetics in newborns and infants: age-related differences and therapeutic implications. *Clin Pharmacokinet* 1980;5:485–527.
52. Lester RS. Topical formulary for the pediatrician. *Pediatr Clin North Am* 1983;30:749–765.
53. Nachman RL, Estlerly NB. Increased skin permeability in preterm infants. *J Pediatr* 1980;96:99–103.
54. van Lingen RA, Deinum HT, Quak CME, et al. Multiple-dose pharmacokinetics of rectally administered acetaminophen in term infants. *Clin Pharmacol Ther* 1999;66:509–515.
55. Senior N. Review of rectal suppositories: formulation and manufacture. *Pharm J* 1969;203:703–706.
56. Williams CN. Role of rectal formulations: suppositories. *Scand J Gastroenterol Suppl* 1990;172:60–62.
57. de Boer AG, Moolenaar F, de Leede LGJ, et al. Rectal drug administration: clinical pharmacokinetic considerations. *Clin Pharmacokinet* 1982;7:285–311.
58. Choonara IA. Giving drugs per rectum for systemic effects. *Arch Dis Child* 1987;62:771–772.
59. Fisher RS, Ho J. Potential new methods for antiepileptic drug delivery. *CNS Drugs* 2002;16:579–593.
60. Wheless JW, Venkataraman V. New formulations of drugs in epilepsy. *Expert Opin Pharmacother* 1999;1:49–60.
61. Roberts RJ. Intravenous administration of medication in pediatric patients: problems and solutions. *Pediatr Clin North Am* 1981;28:23–24.
62. Santerio ML, Stromquist C, Copolla L. Guidelines for continuous infusion medications in the neonatal intensive care unit. *Ann Pharmacother* 1992;26:671–674.
63. Roberts RJ. Pharmacologic principles in therapeutics in infants. In: Roberts RJ, ed. *Drug therapy in infants*. Philadelphia, PA: WB Saunders, 1984:1–12.
64. Radde IC. Drugs and protein binding. In: MacLeod SM, Radde IC, eds. *Textbook of pediatric clinical pharmacology*. Littleton, MA: PSG Publishing, 1985:32–43.
65. Bjorkman S. Prediction of the volume of distribution of a drug: which tissue-plasma partition coefficients are needed? *J Pharm Pharmacol* 2002;54:1237–1245.
66. Muller WE, Wollert V. Human serum albumin as a silent receptor for drugs and endogenous substances. *Pharmacology* 1979;19: 59–67.
67. Piakfsky KM. Disease-induced changes in the plasma binding of basic drugs. *Clin Pharmacokinet* 1980;5:246–262.
68. Benet LZ, Hoener BA. Changes in plasma protein binding have little clinical significance. *Clin Pharmacol Ther* 2002;71:115–121.
69. Windorfer A Jr, Keunzer W, Urbanek R. The influences of age on the activity of acetylsalicylic acid esterase and protein salicylate binding. *Eur J Clin Pharmacol* 1974;7:227–231.
70. Gitlin D, Boseman M. Serum alpha fetoprotein, albumin, and YG-globulin in the human conceptus. *J Clin Invest* 1966;45: 1826–1838.

71. Hyvarinen M, Zeltzer P, Oh W, et al. Influence of gestational age on serum levels of alpha-1-fetoprotein, IgG globulin, and albumin in newborn infants. *J Pediatr* 1973;82:430–437.
72. Piafsky KM, Mpamugo L. Dependence of neonatal drug binding on α-acid glycoprotein concentration. *Clin Pharmacol Ther* 1981;29:272.
73. Thiessen H, Jacobsen J, Brodersen R. Displacement of albumin-bound bilirubin by fatty acids. *Acta Paediatr Scand* 1972;61:285–288.
74. McDonagh AF, Lightner DA. Like a shriveled blood orange—bilirubin, jaundice, and phototherapy. *Pediatrics* 1985;75:443–455.
75. Hansen TW. Mechanisms of bilirubin toxicity: clinical implications. *Clin Perinatol* 2002;29:765–778.
76. Ebbesen F, Nyboe J. Postnatal changes in the ability of plasma albumin to bind bilirubin. *Acta Paediatr Scand* 1983;72:665–670.
77. Rittes DA, Kenny JD. Influence of gestational age on cord serum bilirubin binding studies. *J Pediatr* 1985;106:118–121.
78. Keenan WJ, Arnold JE, Sutherland JM. Serum bilirubin binding determined by Sephadex column chromatography. *J Pediatr* 1969; 74:813.
79. Kapitulnik J, Horner-Mboshan R, Blondheim SH, et al. Increase in bilirubin binding affinity of serum with age of infant. *J Pediatr* 1975;86:442–445.
80. Brodersen R. Bilirubin transport in the newborn infant reviewed with relation to kernicterus. *J Pediatr* 1980;96:349–356.
81. Friis-Hansen B. Water distribution in the fetus and newborn infant. *Acta Paediatr Scan* 1983;305(Suppl):7–11.
82. Butte N, Heinz C, Hopkinson J, et al. Fat mass in infants and toddlers: comparability of total body water, total body potassium, total body electrical conductivity, and dual-energy X-ray absorptiometry. *J Pediatr Gastroenterol Nutr* 1999;29:184–189.
83. Butte NF, Hopkinson JM, Wong WW, et al. Body composition during the first 2 years of life: an updated reference. *Pediatr Res* 2000;47:578–585.
84. Fink CW, Cheeck DB. The corrected bromide space (extracellular volume) in the newborn. *Pediatrics* 1960;26:397–401.
85. Litterst CL, Minnaugh EG, Reagan RL, et al. Comparison of *in vitro* drug metabolism by lung, liver, and kidney of several common laboratory species. *Drug Metab Dispos* 1975;3:259–265.
86. Alcorn J, McNamara PJ. Ontogeny of hepatic and renal systemic clearance pathways in infants. *Clin Pharmacokinet* 2002;41: 959–998, 1077–1094.
87. Harris PA, Riegelman S. Influence of the route of administration on the area under the plasma concentration time curve. *Pharm Sci* 1969;58;71–75.
88. Kearns GL, Abdel-Rahman SM, Alander SW, et al. Developmental pharmacology—drug disposition, action, and therapy in infants and children. *N Engl J Med* 2003;349:1157–1167.

CHAPTER

15

Bernard H. Shapiro

Perinatal Origins of Adult Defects in Drug Metabolism

One of the hot topics in medicine today is the so-called fetal origins of adult diseases. This intriguing topic is not so much new but rather has just begun to raise considerable interest. It has been known for decades that the fetal and early neonatal period is unique in that developmental insults during this time can result in permanent and irreversible structural, behavioral, and biochemical abnormalities. Clearly, then, any disruption in the developmental process could have repercussions throughout the life of the individual. Whereas the consequences of structural abnormalities have always been apparent, we are now starting to appreciate the effects of subtle biochemical disruptions in the developing perinate that could lead to the enhanced occurrence or early onset of certain diseases. Recent high-profile features in both biomedical and lay publications have reported that "endocrine disruptors," that is, environmental compounds with hormonal activities, particularly estrogenic, can be teratogens, producing both permanent abnormalities in the reproductive tracts of males and females and physiologic and behavioral defects in reproductive potential and sexuality (1). Similarly, early exposure to drugs and dietary components that inadvertently disrupt endocrine differentiation could also induce malformations as well as long-lasting hormone-dependent dysfunctions (2). In this chapter, I present evidence demonstrating the plasticity of the developing drug-metabolizing enzyme system, its dependence on growth hormone, and its susceptibility to perinatal insult leading to permanent, often sexually dimorphic dysfunctions.

DELAYED TERATOGENIC EFFECTS

Historically, teratogens have been considered to be prenatal toxic agents that either kill the embryo or produce congenital malformations during the critical period of organogenesis. Using classical definitions, *congenital malformations* have been defined as anatomic abnormalities present at birth. Since its arrival as a bona fide scientific discipline, and even before that, *teratology*, as derived from the Greek *terat-*, meaning "monster," has emphasized the study of gross anatomic anomalies. Understandably, there has been a major concern for those teratogens that produce obvious and devastating structural malformations.

However, there is now a growing awareness that many teratogens may act after the period of organogenesis, through birth and into lactation. Since a preponderance of drugs easily pass through the placental "barrier" as well as the mammary epithelium into the milk, the developing mammal remains susceptible to the teratogenic effects of maternally administered drugs from conception through fetal development and parturition and during nursing. With this awareness has come an understanding that teratogens, often at far lower doses than those needed to produce anatomic anomalies, can induce more subtle biochemical, physiologic, and behavioral defects (2). Furthermore, many of these subtle defects are not apparent at birth and may lie dormant or latent until years later. Like the classic teratogens, those compounds that interfere with normal biochemical, physiologic, or behavioral development are active at only limited critical times during development, and their adverse effects are permanent and irreversible. However, the critical fetal periods for what might be called *subtle teratogens* usually occur sometime after organogenesis, and, depending on the species, this may be as late as the prepubertal period. Furthermore, the effects of the teratogens are latent. That is, at the time of administration, the teratogen appears to produce a "programming" or "imprinting" defect in a developing tissue or organ. This programming defect need not be expressed until adulthood, since the "program" may not be required until that time. Consequently, in the absence of any anatomic anomalies, there is the danger that these later-onset dysfunctions will either go undiagnosed or simply be considered idiopathic.

Several alarming studies of the use of drugs by pregnant women in the 1950s, 1960s, and 1970s suggested that drug taking had become culturally fashionable. During those decades the average number of drugs taken by pregnant women in the United States was 11 (3–5), and their offspring now make up a large fraction of the population. Although epidemiologic surveys in the late 1980s and

1990s revealed that a disappointing 86% of women continued to consume antenatal drugs (6), the average number had declined to 4.7 (7), with the highest rate of ingestion occurring in the final trimester (8), representing the critical developmental period of biochemical differentiation (2,9). Moreover, children during the first year of life take approximately five prescription drugs per annum (10). A study by the American Psychological Association (11) reported that almost 1 million American women of childbearing age are regular, high-frequency users of psychoactive drugs (not to mention nonneuroleptics); 585,000 are regular users of barbiturates; 675,000 use prescription stimulants and appetite depressants; and about 100,000 use prescription antidepressants. The enormity of the problem is further dramatized by the fact that Americans spent $153 billion on prescription drugs during 2002, a number expected to double by the year 2010 (12). There is unlimited self-administration of over-the-counter drugs, minerals, vitamins, herbals, supplements, and metabolites to the tune of more than $2.2 billion in 2002 (13).

As a possible result of its prolonged developmental period extending into early childhood (9,14), both clinical and experimental findings have shown the brain to be highly susceptible to the delayed expression of teratogens. Maternal alcohol consumption can result in retarded development, impaired learning capability (15,16), and a decreased reproductive potential (17) without obvious anatomic anomalies. Prenatal administration of morphine has been reported to alter locomotor activity (18), tolerance to the analgesic effects of morphine in adulthood (19), activity in the open-field test, pubertal onset, and the adrenal stress response (20). Moreover, the prenatal administration of D-amphetamine results in postnatal brain abnormalities in motor behavior and brain biogenic amine levels (21).

This is not to indicate that the brain is unique in its ability to exhibit latent responses to fetal insults. It has been shown from highly publicized studies in humans (22,23) and animals (24) that exposure in utero to diethylstilbestrol (DES) results in subsequent abnormalities in the reproductive structures of both female and male offspring when they become adults. In the case of female offspring, prenatal exposure to maternally administered DES (used in the 1950s through the 1970s to prevent miscarriage and premature birth) is associated with an enhanced risk of clear-cell adenocarcinoma of the vagina and cervix and a dramatic increase in abnormal vaginal cytology (22,25). Furthermore, about half of all DES daughters have less successful pregnancies (26), a greater risk of menstrual irregularities (27), and/or an increase in psychopathologies, especially depression (28), during adult life. DES sons are more likely to have testicular abnormalities, such as undescended or underdeveloped testes, gonadal cysts, and reduced sperm count (29). Some evidence indicates reproductive abnormalities in DES grandchildren (29). Two decades had to pass before the congenital defects produced by the DES teratogen were expressed. Just what DES did in utero to the approximately 2 to 4 million exposed American men and women (30) is still a matter of investigation; only the delayed consequences are now sadly clear.

Equally alarming, and perhaps more insidious, having no recognized etiology, is the dramatic increase in childhood cancers. Depending on the type, during the last 30 years there has been an 18% to 53% increase in cancers in children 4 years and younger and a 29% to 128% increase in 15- to 19-year-olds (31). In this regard, during the last 50 years we have been exposed to 75,000 new synthetic chemicals, fewer than half having been tested for potential toxicity or carcinogenicity in adults, and a fraction of which have been tested in children and pregnant women (32).

In 1979, the National Foundation–March of Dimes reported that more than 250,000 American babies, about 7% of all live births, were born with congenital defects each year (33). In agreement, the National Health Interview Survey (34) reported a 100% increase in the number of birth defects in the 25-year period starting in the late 1950s. Of relevance to this chapter is the finding that the majority of birth defects are no longer obvious malformations apparent in the newborn but represent more subtle biochemical and behavioral anomalies, such as learning disabilities, that are not diagnosed until several years after birth (34,35).

In this chapter, I discuss the latently expressed defects produced by neonatal exposure to phenobarbital and monosodium glutamate (MSG), paradigms for similar-acting compounds (2). Our laboratory is particularly interested in these compounds because of their widespread use; phenobarbital has been a commonly prescribed drug and MSG is a ubiquitous food additive (2). Moreover, neither phenobarbital nor MSG is considered a "hard" teratogen, and thus they are unlikely to produce congenital malformations (35,36). Lastly, we have reported that neonatal administration of normal exposure-like levels of both phenobarbital and MSG can produce delayed but permanent defects in hormone secretion and drug metabolism contributing to long-term, serious health consequences (2). In its broadest sense, we are investigating the unrecognized perinatal origins of adult disease.

THE CASE FOR ANIMAL MODELS

Imagine the difficulty of trying to identify an environmental pollutant or drug ingested for a brief critical period during pregnancy as the cause of some biochemical or behavioral abnormality expressed in adulthood in an individual seemingly free of any anatomic malformations. Who would suspect that the abnormality expressed in adulthood was actually a congenital defect? This inability even to perceive of a link between cause and effect explains why it took decades to identify in utero exposure to DES as the cause of reproductive anomalies in the exposed offspring.

Realizing, then, how profoundly important and long-lasting are the effects of development on the adult, the concept of delayed teratogenic expression seems almost intuitively irrefutable. Nevertheless, numerous drugs identified as teratogens in laboratory species appear to be harmless to the human embryo. The skeptic might recall Albert Szent-Györgyi's comment (37) that "a drug is a substance which, if injected into a rabbit, produces a paper." However, in defense of animal studies, it should be noted that the converse is not true. That is, all human teratogens have been shown to produce congenital defects in experimental animals (35). Although somewhat in hindsight, we have now learned that prenatal exposure to DES produces the same reproductive defects in laboratory animals as previously reported in humans (24). Moreover, it should be noted that drugs considered as nonteratogenic in humans are so classified because they produce no observable structural defects in the newborn.

Our lack of knowledge regarding the causes and effects of latently expressed drug metabolism defects is more a reflection of the paucity of studies in the field than anything else. It was not until 1999 that the Food and Drug Administration (FDA) was given authority to require pharmaceutical companies to conduct target studies on pregnant women and children to learn about side effects and set proper doses. However, the FDA has relied on incentive programs to overcome the unwillingness of companies to include these targeted populations in clinical trials. By 2002, a mere 50 drugs had been reexamined, requiring that 29 be relabeled because of either adverse effects or ineffectual responses (38). Thus, under the present circumstances, assessing the long-term health consequences of perinatal exposure to drugs and environmental chemicals is almost speculative. How do we know that the increasing incidence of infertility in our population is not a delayed result of our increased in utero exposure to drugs and environmental toxins? Perhaps, certain patterns of aging that are expressed near the end of our lives are a legacy of some developmental insult. The heterogeneous influences and the time frame of our lives make it exceedingly difficult to identify latent teratogenic defects in human populations. In contrast, it seems reasonable to conduct these studies on environmentally and genetically controlled laboratory species whose life spans are sufficiently short to allow for the completion of experimental protocols. If perinatal exposure to a drug at therapeutic-like levels for that species produces long-lasting biochemical or behavioral defects in the adult offspring, it seems judicious to consider the drug as a potential threat to the unborn, requiring additional studies in alternate species and already exposed human populations.

DRUG METABOLISM

Two seminal discoveries in the mid to late 1970s altered our concepts of drug metabolism and rejuvenated research in the field. First, it was found that cytochrome P-450 (CYP) was not a single enzyme but a family, or, as we now know, a superfamily of hundreds of forms, having existed for several billion years and distributed across every phylum (39). It is now clear that drug-metabolizing enzymes like hexobarbital hydroxylase, benzphetamine demethylase, aniline hydroxylase, and aminopyrine demethylase are only functional descriptions, and no such enzymes exist. In reality, the activities of these monooxygenases represent the sum of activities of several forms of CYP, each with a different specificity for the substrate, which combine to contribute to the final metabolism of the drug. Thus, when we measure hexobarbital hydroxylase activity, we are actually measuring the total activities of several forms of CYP (40). This important discovery has led to now-routine investigations by pharmaceutical and academic laboratories identifying the individual CYP isoforms contributing to the metabolism of both marketed and investigational drugs.

The realization that individuals express 40 to 50 different isoforms of CYP (39) can explain the occurrence of gender differences in drug metabolism. It is not, as previously thought, that one gender may have "more" hexobarbital hydroxylase enzyme than another. Rather, male and female livers each contain many CYPs, some of which, depending on the species, may be exclusively or predominantly expressed in one sex over the other. In the case of the rat, it just so happens that the isoforms with the greatest hexobarbital hydroxylase activity are predominant in male rats (40). Although most of the studies characterizing gender differences in CYP expression have been conducted in rats, at least a half dozen sex-dependent isoforms, two identified by our laboratory (41,42), have been found in mice (39,43) and smaller numbers in other species (39,44).

In spite of the discovery of sexually dimorphic expression of CYPs in almost every species examined, it is commonly assumed that these gender differences are operative only in the rat, and similar investigations in humans would be unproductive and of little clinical value. However, such assumptions contradict a growing body of literature demonstrating gender differences in human hepatic isoforms CYP1A2, 2C19, 2D6 and the predominant 3A4 (45–49) and their association with gender differences in the incidence of some cancers (50–52), adverse drug effects (53–55), and even longevity (56).

The identification of endogenous regulators of drug metabolism is the second important advance in the field. Compared to other major metabolic pathways, surprisingly little is known about endogenous factors maintaining CYP homeostasis. The generally accepted role of androgens in regulating sex differences in rat hepatic monooxygenases came into question when it was reported that hypophysectomy abolished the gender differences in drug metabolism (i.e., enzymatic activities declined to female levels) and testosterone was completely ineffective in restoring the dimorphism (57,58). After almost 10 more years of investigations, growth hormone was identified as the pituitary factor responsible for maintaining the sexual dimorphisms of hepatic monooxygenases in the rat (59). More specifically, it was determined that the sexually dimorphic ultradian rhythms in circulating growth hormone maintained gender-dependent expression levels of rat CYPs (60,61). Male rats secrete growth hormone in episodic bursts every 3.5 to 4 hours. Between the peaks, growth hormone levels are undetectable. In female rats the hormone pulses are more frequent and irregular and are of lower magnitude than in male rats, whereas the interpeak concentration of growth hormone is always measurable. Exposure to the "continuous" feminine secretory profile of growth hormone produces the characteristic pattern of CYPs expressed in female rats. Conversely, the "episodic" rhythm of growth hormone secretion characterized as masculine is responsible for the expression of CYP isoforms observed in male rats and resulting in a faster rate of drug metabolism. In fact, growth hormone regulation of drug metabolism is far more exquisite. Using laboratory species, we have reported (62–64) that the expression or suppression of each isoform of CYP is regulated by a different "signal," or, perhaps, a differential sensitivity to the "signal" in the sexually dimorphic growth hormone profile. These signals are recognized by the hepatocyte in the frequencies and/or durations of the pulse or interpulse periods. Alternatively, the hepatocyte can monitor the mean plasma concentration of the hormone (62–64). We have observed that expression of some rat CYP isoforms is regulated by the duration of the growth hormone–devoid interpulse period, with the amount of hormone secreted in the pulses of no importance (63,64), while expression levels of other CYPs are proportional to the amplitudes of the growth hormone pulse (63), and other isoforms of CYP are regulated by the mean concentration of growth hormone (62).

Just as many investigators consider gender differences in drug metabolism a "rat phenomenon," sexually dimorphic growth hormone secretion and its regulation of drug metabolism is likewise considered to be limited to the rat. Actually, the contrary is true. Sexually dimorphic growth hormone secretory patterns have been reported in turkeys (65), sheep (66), and horses (67). We have measured and analyzed the plasma growth hormone profiles in mice and chickens (68,69) and reported that, like the female rat, female mice, and hens secrete hormone profiles characterized by more frequent peaks separated by shorter interpulse periods than do males animals of the species. Moreover, like the rat, these sexually dimorphic growth hormone profiles are responsible for the gender differences in drug metabolism and CYP expression observed in mice and chickens (70–73). Not surprisingly then, there are many reports describing sexually dimorphic growth hormone profiles in humans (74–79). In agreement with observations in other species, secretory growth hormone profiles in women compared to men are characterized by more frequent pulses, separated by elevated and briefer interpulse periods.

However, does growth hormone regulate CYP expression in humans as it does in other species? A search of the literature indicates that this question has received little attention. There are a few studies with growth hormone-deficient individuals, before and after hormone replacement therapy, which clearly show that growth hormone alone can restore drug-metabolizing enzymes to normal levels (80–82). Recently, we have reported, using primary human hepatocytes (82), that like other species examined, (1) growth hormone can regulate expression of human isoforms of CYP; (2) the sex-dependent secretory profiles of growth hormone can differentially regulate expression levels of some isoforms; (3) there are intrinsic sexual differences in hepatocytes of men nd women, resulting in both different levels of CYP isoforms (e.g., CYP3A4, 1A2 and 2D6) and their responsiveness to growth hormone; and (4) in agreement with most species but not the rat, growth hormone effects on CYP, although real, can be subtle and easily concealed by the heterogeneous background of human populations. Accordingly, these findings suggest, small developmentally induced defects in the endogenous human growth hormone profiles could permanently alter expression levels of CYP isoforms metabolizing cholesterol, corticosteroids, sex hormones, thyroid hormone, and prostaglandins, not to mention consumed drugs and environmental compounds. Small changes in the metabolism of these endogenous and exogenous bioactive chemicals over a lifetime could seriously affect the long-term health of the affected individual. We have demonstrated this scenario in experimental animals (discussed later) and propose that it is just as likely to occur in humans.

ANTICONVULSANTS

For the physician, there is a particular moral dilemma of treating pregnant and nursing women whose medical conditions require drug therapy. Moreover, we are all concerned about the teratogenic effects of environmental pollutants. However, what can the individual—physician included—do? Surely, this is a societal problem requiring political remedy. The excessive use of over-the-counter medications, alcoholic beverages, cigarettes, recreational drugs, and so on during pregnancy is a serious threat to the unborn, and physicians have unequivocally condemned their excessive use. In contrast, how do you treat women whose medical conditions require drug therapy but who incidentally happen to be pregnant? Who would want to restore the health of the mother at the cost of compromising her child's long-term well-being?

In this regard, there are drugs whose widespread use and teratogenic potential make them likely candidates for long-term birth defects studies. Approximately 1 of every 200 women is epileptic (83), and 95.7% of them are on anticonvulsant therapy (84), which is invariably continued throughout pregnancy and lactation (85,86). Moreover, approximately 1% of children and adolescents, still susceptible to developmental disruptors, are epileptic (87). In other words, about 50 million people globally are epileptic, contributing to an aggregate burden of approximately 0.5% of total world disease (88). In this regard, the evidence indicates that anticonvulsant drugs are responsible for producing a two to three times greater incidence of malformations in the children of epileptic mothers (89,90). With the exception of the fetal alcohol syndrome, anticonvulsant-induced malformations, specifically the fetal hydantoin syndrome, represent the most commonly recognized teratogen-induced malformations (91).

Phenytoin (diphenylhydantoin) is one of the most efficacious and widely used anticonvulsants in North America (92). Considering that phenytoin easily passes through the placenta into the fetal tissues and through the mammary epithelium into the milk (86,93), there has been a justifiable concern that the drug could be teratogenic. In this regard, animal studies have demonstrated clearly that prepartum administration of phenytoin can produce congenital malformations (4,35,89,92). Studies in humans (84,85,90,91) have indicated that in utero exposure to phenytoin may be responsible for inducing such anatomic malformations as cleft lip and palate, microcephaly or trigonocephaly, and various anomalies of the face and fingers, often referred to as the fetal hydantoin syndrome. In addition, there is evidence to suggest that peripartum exposure to phenytoin can produce more subtle long-term biochemical and behavioral defects at doses too low to induce structural malformations (94,95). It has been reported that in the absence of anatomic malformations, adult rats exposed perinatally to maternally administered phenytoin have several behavioral and neurologic deficits resulting in delayed motor development, persistent locomotor dysfunction, and abnormal maze learning (94,96) as well as reduced fertility (97,98). Our findings of normal developmental profiles of serum androstenedione, testosterone, and dihydrotestosterone in phenytoin-exposed male offspring (99) suggest that the delayed reproductive dysfunctions found by others (97,98) are like the behavioral defects (94,96), a result of phenytoin's teratogenic action on the developing brain.

Unrelated to its anticonvulsant properties, phenytoin is also an inducer of hepatic CYP-dependent monooxygenase enzymes that normally metabolize fatty acids, prostaglandins, steroids, and xenobiotics (100,101). In fact, we have reported that maternal treatment with therapeutic-like doses of phenytoin for the rat induces significant elevations in the Michaelis constants and maximal velocities of hepatic aminopyrine-*N*-demethylase in the dam's 8-day-old offspring (102). Similarly, administration of the anticonvulsant to pregnant women has been shown to increase aminopyrine metabolism in their newborn (103). The long-term effects of early exposure to phenytoin on liver function also have been investigated in animal models. Maternal administration of the anticonvulsant at therapeutic-like doses that do not produce morphologic anomalies was found to cause permanent defects in the drug-metabolizing capacity of the exposed adult offspring (95). Perhaps of greater significance is the finding that peripartum exposure to subtherapeutic-like doses of phenytoin for the rat produced, in adulthood, so-called silent defects in the hepatic monooxygenase system. That is, adult rats exposed perinatally to these low doses of phenytoin exhibited very few abnormalities in the basal levels of hepatic drug-metabolizing enzymes. However, when the hepatic monooxygenases of these adults were challenged with various threshold doses of phenobarbital, the silent defect became apparent: Peripartum exposure to phenytoin resulted in a significant block in the response of the hepatic monooxygenases to phenobarbital induction.

In this regard, organisms are constantly exposed to subtle levels of environmental inducing agents (i.e., drugs, carcinogens, food additives, hormones, insecticides, industrial pollutants, etc.) that may be capable of altering the activities of the hepatic drug-metabolizing enzymes. Thus, by disrupting the development of hepatic enzyme induction mechanisms, perinatal exposure to phenytoin may irreversibly alter an important homeostatic mechanism that is normally responsive to daily exposure to low levels of various endogenous and exogenous inducing agents.

Particular concern relates to the use of barbiturates. For at least 30 years, 190 compounds containing barbiturates have been suggested for the treatment of more than 77 different disorders (104). The number of people perinatally exposed to phenobarbital is not trivial. Between 1950 and the late 1970s, it has been estimated that in the United States alone, 23 million children were born to mothers taking prescribed barbiturates during pregnancy (105). Barbiturate-containing drugs are still administered to approximately 2% of all neonates admitted to intensive care units (106) and to pregnant women and newborns for a variety of often commonly occurring maladies, such as convulsive disorders, which complicate 1 of every 200 pregnancies (107,108).

Perinatal exposure of laboratory animals to therapeutic-like, subteratogenic doses (i.e., not producing malformations) of phenobarbital can result in a multitude of long-term reproductive, growth, hepatic, and neural dysfunctions. These defects include reduced sexual behavior (109), decreased serum gonadotropin levels and infertility (110,111), abnormal circulating testosterone secretory profiles (112), subnormal growth rates and associated decreased growth hormone secretion (110,113), elevated aflatoxin B_1 adduct formation increasing carcinogenesis (114), decreased hepatic monoamine oxidase levels (115), altered seizure susceptibility, and elevated brain concentrations of neurotransmitters and locomotor and learning deficits (96,116–118). Of particular relevance to this discussion are reports, including our own, demonstrating that neonatal administration of phenobarbital can induce a delayed but permanent elevation in the activities of several hepatic drug-metabolizing enzymes, for example, total CYP, ethoxycoumarin *O*-deethylase, ethylmorphine *N*-demethylase, and hexobarbital hydroxylase (113,119,120). As expected, neonatal administration of the barbiturate induces an almost immediate increase in the activities of drug-metabolizing enzymes, which declines to noninduction levels when treatment ceases. Contrary to the well-known transient effects of phenobarbital, at approximately the time of sexual maturity when gender-dependent differences in drug metabolism appear, a second round of enzyme induction occurs that persists throughout life.

Since phenobarbital is a potent inducer of CYP2B1 and 2B2 [the prototypic and most responsive isoforms to phenobarbital induction (121)], it seemed reasonable to propose that the barbiturate may have imprinted the developing liver, altering expression levels of CYP2B1 and 2B2. Perhaps the usual nominal constitutive expression levels of CYP2B1 and 2B2 would be sufficiently elevated to explain the overexpressed drug-metabolizing enzymes in affected rats. Indeed, transcript levels for both isoforms remained at concentrations twofold higher in phenobarbital-imprinted male and female rats than controls through adulthood. However, analyses of CYP2B1 and 2B2 protein levels and specific catalytic activity (androstenedione 16β-hydroxylase) demonstrated no such above-normal increases, excluding the isoforms as contributors to the overexpressed drug-metabolizing enzymes induced by neonatal phenobarbital (122).

In a continued attempt to identify the CYP(s) responsible for the permanent elevation in drug-metabolizing enzymes induced by neonatal phenobarbital, we examined expression levels of nine constitutive isoforms. We found that neonatal exposure to the barbiturate produced a permanent overexpression of CYP2C7, 2C6, and 2A2 (123). None of these isoforms is expressed before puberty (123), but postpubertally they are expressed in neonatally phenobarbital-treated rats of both sexes at levels 30% to 50% above normal. The fact that CYP2C7 and 2C6 are female predominant (male to female ratio 1:2–3) and CYP2A2 is a minor male-specific isoform (62–64) could explain why neonatal phenobarbital produces a greater percentage increase in drug-metabolizing capacity in female than in male rats (113,120).

Although we had not identified CYP2B1 and 2B2 as the overexpressed isoforms in the neonatally phenobarbital-treated rats, we did find that early exposure to the barbiturate permanently altered (i.e., imprinted) the inductive responsiveness of the CYP2B isoforms to subsequent barbiturate challenge in adulthood (122). That is, neonatal administration of therapeutic-like levels of phenobarbital caused an overinduction (~30% to 40%) of CYP2B1 and 2B2 mRNAs, proteins, and specific catalytic activity levels when the rats were rechallenged as adults with the barbiturate at doses reflecting either the possible inducing activities of environmental agents (1 mg per kg) or at the minimal anticonvulsant therapeutic dose for the rat (10 mg per kg). Expressions of other isoforms were also significantly elevated by both rechallenge doses of phenobarbital (10 and 1 mg per kg). CYP2C6, 2C7, 3A1, and 3A2 levels were increased an additional 30% to 50% when the animals were neonatally exposed to the barbiturate, demonstrating, for the first time, that inductive mechanisms expressed in adulthood for even constitutive CYP isoforms are developmentally plastic and may be predetermined by neonatal imprinting (124).

The mechanism(s) by which phenobarbital produces these latently expressed defects is unknown. Because the half-life of the barbiturate in adult rats is measured in hours (125) and is no more than 1 day or so in newborns (126), it is unlikely, for example, that the delayed postpubertal elevation in hepatic drug metabolism can be explained by the persistence of the neonatally administered phenobarbital. In this regard, as discussed previously, we have observed that each isoform of CYP appears to be expressed and/or suppressed by different "signaling elements" in the masculine and feminine growth hormone profiles (62–64). Similar to clinical findings (127,128), we reported that neonatal phenobarbital administration results in a permanent reduction of the pulse amplitudes in the masculine circulating growth hormone profile and the mean plasma growth hormone concentration in the feminine profile that are further altered (though not so in control animals neonatally exposed to diluent) by the adult, rechallenge dose of the barbiturate (113,122). Accordingly, these anomalies, often subtle, in the circulating growth hormone profiles could explain, at least in part, both the overexpression and overinduction of individual CYPs contributing to the irreversible above-normal drug-metabolizing capacity of the adult phenobarbital-imprinted rat.

Although there are no reports investigating the long-term effects of perinatal exposure to phenobarbital on drug metabolism in humans, clinical reports have shown that boys perinatally exposed to phenobarbital have a considerably higher incidence of delayed puberty, undescended testes, and genital abnormalities (129,130). Women perinatally exposed to the barbiturate are twice as likely to have irregular menstrual cycles and more problems during subsequent pregnancies (130). Prenatal exposure to phenobarbital causes a significantly greater number of subjects exhibiting cross-gender behaviors and transsexualism, resulting in an unusually high percentage of sex reassignment surgeries (131). As adults, both sexes score significantly lower on intelligence tests (132,133), have persistent learning disabilities, and are more likely to be mentally retarded (134).

We have proposed that perinatal exposure to seemingly innocuous therapeutic levels of drugs could be the origins of subtle, but permanent biochemical defects having long-term health consequences. It is likely that the most dramatic, and possibly ultimate, clinical consequence of any treatment is its effect on health and longevity. Because neonatal treatment with phenobarbital induced a delayed but permanent elevation in baseline expression levels of CYP2C7, 2C6, and 2A2 (123) as well as an overinductive response of CYP2B1, 2B2, 2C6, 2C7, 3A1, and 3A2 (122,124), which could increase the formation of hepatotoxic epoxides and mutagenic and carcinogenic metabolites (124), we examined the long-term consequences of the treatment on longevity (135). Bimonthly determinations of body weight, linear growth, and obesity (i.e., Lee index) for 700 days (equivalent to an octogenarian) in both male and female rats treated with therapeutic-like doses of phenobarbital during the first week of life indicated no effect of the treatment. Moreover, organ weights (liver, kidneys, adrenals, seminal vesicles, or uterine) at 2 years of age were statistically indistinguishable between vehicle control and neonatal phenobarbital-treated rats of the same sex. In contrast, a statistically ($p < .01$) larger number of barbiturate-exposed rats of both sexes died at a younger age than the controls, resulting in a 20% reduced mean life expectancy. At the time of death, necropsy results demonstrated a two- to threefold increase in the incidence of tumors in barbiturate-exposed rats compared with same-sex controls. Whereas no female had blood in her urine at the time of death, it was found in 10% of vehicle-treated males and 37% of phenobarbital-treated males, indicating an enhanced susceptibility to kidney or urinary tract pathologies in old male rats neonatally exposed to phenobarbital.

We observed that the imprinted elevation in drug metabolism (e.g., hexobarbital hydroxylase) is truly permanent, remaining 35% and 60% higher in neonatally phenobarbital-treated male and female rats, respectively, at 2 years of age. As reported in young adults, we found a persistent 25% to 30% overexpression of CYP2C7 in 2-year-old males neonatally exposed to phenobarbital, and a 20% and 30% overexpression of CYP2C7 and 2C6, respectively, in similarly treated 2-year-old female rats. Given that CYP2C7 and 2C6 comprise 14% and 30%, respectively, of the total hepatic CYP content in female rats and CYP2C7 contributes 7% to the total CYP content in male liver (62,136), their overexpression could account, at least in part, for the permanent elevation in drug-metabolizing capacity in the affected rats. To demonstrate that the phenobarbital-imprinted overexpression of multi–CYP-dependent drug-metabolizing enzymes and specific CYP isoforms was not simply a curious test-tube phenomenon, we measured the pharmacologically functional end point of hexobarbital-induced sleeping times. If the permanent overexpression of hexobarbital hydroxylase and contributing CYP isoforms were biologically significant, we should observe a commensurate decline in hexobarbital-induced sleeping times. Indeed, we did observe a permanent, postpubertal 20% to 30% decline ($p < .01$) in sleeping times in both senescent male and female rats neonatally exposed to phenobarbital.

Since a person's hepatic CYP profile could affect her or his longevity (56), it seemed reasonable that a lifetime of overexpressed CYP2C7 and 2C6 resulting in the continuous, above-normal accumulation of reactive intermediary metabolites (40,137) could promote tumorigenesis and a shorter life expectancy in our phenobarbital-exposed rats. In addition, we also considered the contribution of inducible isoforms of CYP known to be implicated in drug and environmentally induced cancers (138–140) and whose response levels to phenobarbital challenge are generally age independent (141). Accordingly, we challenged the senescent animals with a subtherapeutic dose of phenobarbital (1 mg per kg) that equaled approximately 1% of its optimal inductive dose (142) and evoking the insidious dangers to human health of comparable low levels of harmful environmental compounds. Whereas this nominal dose of the barbiturate stimulated a minimal induction of CYP2B1 and 2B2 in the control rats, the inductive response was severalfold greater in the 2-year-olds neonatally treated with the barbiturate. In addition, and in agreement with our findings using young adults (124), the responsiveness of the inducible CYP3A1 and constitutive CYP2C7, 2C6, and 3A2 remained considerably ($p < .01$) greater in the senescent phenobarbital-imprinted rats of both sexes. The results suggest that exposure of newborns to even therapeutic-like doses of phenobarbital can program the liver to continuously overexpress constitutive CYP isoforms, and, when challenged by a lifetime of drug consumption and environmental insults, the liver will overexpress inducible isoforms, all contributing to the long-term, virtual disconnect effect of increasing tumorigenesis and reducing life expectancy. Coincidentally, phenobarbital is a known carcinogen, which can increase the metabolism of innocuous compounds into carcinogenic and toxic metabolites (139,140). In fact, perinatal exposure to the barbiturate has been reported to subsequently increase the risk of cancer in adult rats (114,143) and children (144). Thus, it seems likely that millions of pregnant and nursing women have taken and continue to take drugs that expose their children, those yet to be born and those born within the last five decades, to the risk of long-lasting developmental defects affecting health and longevity (145).

FOOD ADDITIVES

Of equal concern to the growing use of drugs is the enormous consumption of food additives. One need only to go up and down the aisles of modern supermarkets and examine the shopping carts to appreciate our basic reliance on packaged and processed foods, a reliance that is steadily increasing as more homemakers enter the workplace. Like preservatives, some forms of flavor-enhancing chemicals can be found in almost all commercially prepared foods (146). Although its teratogenic potential resulted in its voluntary removal from baby food in 1969, this was a belated action for millions of adults who had already consumed MSG in childhood. Americans continue to consume at least 200 million pounds of it per year (147), which makes it highly likely that human perinates are still being exposed to MSG. The fact that MSG is added to a food is sometimes disclosed on the label and sometimes not, but the amounts used are rarely disclosed. Nevertheless, independent analyses have shown that such commercially available foods as soups contain around 1.1 g of MSG per 6-oz serving (148). Moreover, Chinese and Korean restaurants were found to add 10 g of MSG to a single dish (149).

Aspartame, the ubiquitous artificial sweetener, is a dipeptide which is rapidly hydrolyzed in the gut and quickly absorbed as its constituent amino acids, phenylalanine and aspartic acid (150). [Neonatal exposure to aspartate induces similar latently expressed defects as MSG and has been discussed elsewhere (151)]. The statistics concerning aspartame consumption are nearly as worrisome as those regarding MSG. Studies have reported that children consume almost 100 mg of aspartame per kilogram of body weight per day (152), a level approaching the adverse doses found in our animal studies. Because aspartame's use (cereals, soft drinks, candies, desserts, etc.) includes the major components of a child's diet not currently containing glutamate (frozen dinners, processed lunch meats, canned soups, etc.), there has been a justifiable concern that consumption of both aspartame and glutamate could produce developmental defects in children (146–150). These concerns have been refuted by demonstrating that aspartate and/or glutamate consumption at the highest possible human dietary levels does not induce congenital anomalies in primates (151–154) or produce toxic effects in the large majority of the adult population (155). On the other hand, our studies with rats and mice have shown that either amino acid could produce more subtle developmental defects in growth hormone secretion and drug metabolism (61,72,151,156,157). Accepting the assumption that glutamate and aspartate are not developmentally harmful to most perinates, it is possible, as stated in a Federation of American Societies for Experimental Biology (FASEB) report for the FDA (155), that a subset of the population could be highly sensitive to the effects of the food additives. All smokers do not develop lung cancer, and all children exposed in utero to ethanol do not develop the fetal alcohol syndrome. Thus, we are concerned that early exposure to low levels of food additives like MSG and aspartame, in addition to anticonvulsants and broader-spectrum neuroleptics (e.g., phenobarbital) from before birth until 5 years of age, when hepatic and neuroendocrine differentiation are still incomplete (2–4), could permanently alter the expression of hepatic drug-metabolizing enzymes and/or their response to inducing agents. Such defects could unknowingly affect the efficacy of drug therapy or the susceptibility to chemically induced cancers in adulthood.

Earlier, we reported that neonatal administration of MSG at a rather high exposure dose of 4 mg per g produced obesity as well as latently expressed (postpubertal) defects in multi–CYP-dependent drug-metabolizing enzyme activities (e.g., hexobarbital hydroxylase, aminopyrine demethylase) (156,157) without affecting phase II conjugating enzymes (94), cytochrome b_5, or NADPH–CYP reductase (157). We observed that expression of male-specific CYP2C11, the predominant isoform comprising up to 50% of the total CYP content in male liver (158), as well as male-specific CYP2A2 and 3A2, were completely suppressed in adult male rats by neonatal exposure to high-dose MSG (156,157). The absence of these three major male-specific CYP isoforms explains an 80% to 90% reduction in the drug-metabolizing capacity of the MSG-treated male rats (61,157). Since the complete suppression of CYP2C11, 2A2, and 3A2 was observed at the mRNA, protein, and catalytic levels (156,157), it would appear that the MSG-induced defects in male-specific CYP expression occur transcriptionally. Clearly, a contributing factor, if not the basis for the loss of the CYP isoforms, is the suppression of growth hormone secretion resulting in the absence of a detectable circulating episodic growth hormone profile (61,156,157). [Surprisingly, in spite of a similar MSG-induced depletion of circulating growth hormone in female rats, female-dependent CYPs and associated drug metabolism are unaffected, supporting the contention that birth defects, including latently expressed ones, are gender sensitive (61,159)].

Hypothalamic growth hormone–releasing hormone (GHRH) and somatostatin (growth hormone–inhibiting hormone) regulate the episodic growth hormone secretory profile (160), and we have reported (161) that neonatal MSG produces developmental hypothalamic lesions in nuclei synthesizing and/or secreting GHRH that are responsible for the permanent absence of plasma growth hormone in affected rats. However, restoration of gender-dependent, physiologic GHRH or growth hormone plasma profiles to adults neonatally exposed to MSG is ineffective in restoring normal CYP expression levels (161–163), suggesting that the developing liver and its drug-metabolizing enzymes are irreversibly damaged by early exposure to the food additive. Lastly, we selectively inhibited the neuronal effects of MSG by simultaneously administering the noncompetitive *N*-methyl-D-aspartate (NMDA) receptor blocker dizocilpine maleate (MK-801), which is known to antagonize glutamate disruption of growth hormone secretion (164,165). We found that the long-lasting deleterious effects of neonatal exposure to MSG, including a doubling of hexobarbital-induced sleeping times, repression of hepatic CYP2C11, 3A2, and 2A2 expression, and suppression of plasma growth hormone secretion to undetectable concentrations, were completely prevented by MK-801 (166), suggesting that postnatal growth hormone normally imprints adult expression levels of CYPs.

Paradoxically, when we reduced the dose of MSG by 50% to 80% we observed a considerable elevation in drug metabolism characterized by 40% to 50% increase in CYP2A2 and 3A2 and a far more dramatic overexpression of CYP2C11 (156,157). Concentrating our efforts on CYP2C11, we found that the overexpression was characterized by a 300% increase in mRNA and a much smaller, but highly significant ($p < .01$), 30% to 40% elevation in protein levels and specific CYP2C11-dependent testosterone 2α-hydroxylase (167). Since CYP2C11 expression, as well as those of CYP3A2 and 2A2, is regulated transcriptionally by the masculine episodic growth hormone profile (62–64), we measured the circulating concentrations of the hormone in adult male rats neonatally treated with 1 or 2 mg MSG per g. Male rats treated with these lower MSG doses exhibited typical masculine-like patterns of growth hormone release, except that the amplitudes of the ultradian pulses were reduced to approximately 10% of normal male levels. Otherwise, like those of normal male rats, the peaks occurred about every 3 to 4 hours and the intervening troughs had undetectable levels of growth hormone (167). Moreover, we discovered that the minipulses were responsible for the severalfold overexpression of CYP2C11 mRNA and 30% to 40% increase in CYP2C11 protein levels and dependent catalytic activities observed in the low-dose MSG-treated rats (63,167). Similarly, the circulating minipulses of growth hormone were capable of increasing expression of CYP3A2 and 2A2 mRNA, protein, and catalytic activities by approximately 50% (63,64).

We were surprised by the apparent uncoupling of CYP2C11 translation from transcription and examined the possibility that the minipulses of growth hormone secreted in the MSG rats could result in an aberrant, untranslatable form of the transcript. Using hepatic tissue from low-dose MSG-treated male rats, we cloned a variant species of CYP2C11 mRNA containing all the essential elements of a full-length cDNA, including initiation codon, termination codon, and poly-A tail. In addition, the transcript contained a 742-base pair intervening sequence (we found to be identical to the terminal intron) between the last and penultimate exons. Associated with the overexpression and intron retention of the transcript was a 50% reduction in the nuclear splicing capacity of the liver for CYP2C11 (168). Thus, the difference between the increased expression of mRNA and protein can be explained by the dramatic accumulation of an intron-retained, intermediate precursor mRNA and the smaller, although still above-normal amount of completely processed mRNA responsible for the 30% to 40% increase in CYP2C11 protein. The very presence of the terminal intron may have been sufficient to block the transport and/or translation of the mRNA variant to cytosolic ribosomes, thus accounting for the disproportionately lower levels of CYP2C11 protein observed in low-dose MSG-treated rats. In this regard, using an unregulated in vitro translation system, we found that the variant CYP2C11 mRNA containing an additional termination codon (TAA) as well as a *Hind*III site (AAGCTT) in the retained intron resulted in the translation of a truncated protein, not normally found in the rat hepatocyte, which did not cross-react with anti-CYP2C11 and had no testosterone-metabolizing activity (unpublished material).

CONCLUSIONS

The purpose of this chapter is to introduce the reader to a little-known but potentially very serious health hazard to children. I refer to the ability of perinatally consumed drugs and food additives to produce the subtle biochemical or microstructural defects, undetectable in the newborn, but expressed years or perhaps decades after exposure. Human studies indicate that a higher-than-normal incidence of mental retardation and childhood and adult cancers can be attributed to in utero exposure to alcohol, narcotics, DES, phenobarbital, and various industrial chemicals. Similarly, compelling evidence from animal models shows that peripartum exposure to such drugs as diazepam, phenytoin, sex steroids, and so on can produce latently expressed abnormalities and diseases in the adult offspring.

The question is not whether in utero exposure to drugs can produce latently expressed defects, but how serious is the problem. How do we establish a cause-and-effect relationship between the onset of an isolated disease and exposure to a teratogen that occurred decades earlier? In truth, this clinical problem is complicated by more than a temporal factor. Latently expressed teratogenic defects are not necessarily associated with congenital malformations or recognized syndromes, making it unlikely for the physician to suspect that the adult disease is actually a birth defect. The offending drug may have been considered innocuous when taken and was ingested for only a brief period, albeit a developmentally critical one, so that the consumption is forgotten. Because the actual clinical manifestation expressed in adulthood is merely a consequence of the perinatally induced defect, it becomes more difficult to identify the true developmental lesion(s). Extrapolating from animal models, in utero exposure to phenobarbital would cause a permanent elevation in the activities of drug-metabolizing enzymes. Not only would the affected individual be less responsive to normal drug therapy, but there would also be an enhanced conversion of inactive environmental pollutants (e.g., benzopyrene) to carcinogens, resulting in an increased incidence of cancers. Thus, we cannot ignore the reality of diseases resulting from the delayed expression of birth defects. We shall find that this type of disease is not unique and is similar in consequence to those subtle genetic defects that predispose the carrier to cancer, heart disease, arthritis, and so on. Indeed, these may be the unrecognized health problems of the future. We should continue to develop animal models as sentinels to warn us of the potential teratogenic dangers of drugs and environmental toxins. Moreover, for the present, a little old-fashioned 1960s consciousness raising would be appropriate.

REFERENCES

1. Crews D, Willingham E, Skipper JK. Endocrine disruptors: present issues, future directions. *Q Rev Biol* 2000;75:243–260.
2. Shapiro BH. Delayed teratogenic expression. In: Yaffe SJ, Arand JV, eds. *Pediatric pharmacology. Therapeutic principles in practice*, 2nd ed. Philadelphia, PA: WB Saunders, 1992:111–121.
3. Bleyer WA, An WA, Lange WA, et al. Studies on the detection of adverse drug reactions in the newborn: fetal exposure to maternal medication. *JAMA* 1970;213:2046–2048.
4. Hill RM, Stern L. Drugs in pregnancy: effects on the fetus and newborn. *Drugs* 1979;17:182–197.
5. Doering PL, Stewart RB. The extent and character of drug consumption during pregnancy. *JAMA* 1978;239:843–846.
6. Collaborative Group on Drug Use in Pregnancy. Medication during pregnancy: an intercontinental cooperative study. *Int J Gynecol Obstet* 1992;39:185–186.
7. Bonati M, Bortolus R, Marchetti F, et al. Drug use in pregnancy: an overview of epidemiological (drug utilization) studies. *Eur J Clin Pharmacol* 1990;38:325–328.
8. Rubin PC, Craig GF, Gavin K, et al. Prospective survey of use of therapeutic drugs, alcohol, and cigarettes during pregnancy. *Br Med J* 1986;292:81–83.
9. Shapiro BH, Goldman AS. New thoughts on sexual differentiation of the brain. In: Vallet HL, Porter IH, eds. *Genetic mechanisms of sexual development.* New York: Academic Press, 1979:221–251.
10. Anonymous. Chains still lead, but food stores, mail-order delivery hefty gains. *Drug Store News* 2001;23:33.
11. Russo NF. In: *A women's mental health agenda.* Washington, DC: American Psychological Association, 1985:19–29.
12. Anonymous. Charting health care's future. *Hosp Health Netw* 2002;76:65.
13. Anonymous. New and improved diet supplements tone down cure-all approach. *DSN Retailing Today* 2002;41:816.
14. Moore KL. *The developing human: clinically oriented embryology.* Philadelphia, PA: WB Saunders, 1973.
15. Auroux M, Dehaupas M. Influence de la nutrition de la mère sur le développement tardif du système nerveux central de la progeniture. I. Amelioration chez le rat de la capacité d'apprentissage de la progeniture par alcoolisation de la mère. *CR Soc Biol* 1970;164:1432–1436.
16. Randall L. Teratogenic effects of *in utero* ethanol exposure. In: Blum K, ed. *Alcohol and opiates: neurochemical and behavioral mechanisms.* New York: Academic Press, 1977;91–107.
17. Stockard CR, Papanicolaou GN. Further studies on the modification of the germ cells in mammals: the effect of alcohol on treated guinea pigs and their descendants. *J Exp Zool* 1918;26: 119–226.
18. Davis WM, Lin CH. Prenatal morphine effects on survival and behavior of rat offspring. *Res Commun Chem Pathol Pharmacol* 1972;3:205–214.
19. O'Callaghan JP, Holtzman SG. Prenatal administration of morphine to the rat: tolerance to the analgesic effect of morphine in the offspring. *J Pharmacol Exp Ther* 1976;197:533–544.
20. Zimmerman E, Sonderegger T, Bromley B. Development and adult pituitary–adrenal function in female rats injected with morphine during different postnatal periods. *Life Sci* 1977;20:639–646.
21. Hitzemann RA, Hitzemann RJ, Brase DA, et al. Influence of prenatal D-amphetamine administration on development and behavior of rats. *Life Sci* 1976;8:605–612.
22. Herbst AL, Scully RE, Robboy SJ. Prenatal diethylstilbestrol exposure and human genital tract abnormalities. *Natl Cancer Inst Monogr* 1979;51:25–35.
23. Henderson BE, Benton B, Cosgrove M, et al. Urogenital tract abnormalities in sons of women treated with diethylstilbestrol. *Pediatrics* 1976;58:505–507.
24. Bern HA, Jones LA, Mori T, et al. Exposure of neonatal mice to steroids: long-term effects on the mammary gland and other reproductive structures. *J Steroid Biochem* 1976;6:673–676.
25. O'Brien PC, Noller KL, Robboy SJ, et al. Vaginal epithelial changes in young women enrolled in the National Cooperative Diethylstilbestrol Adenosis (DESAD) Project. *Obstet Gynecol* 1979; 53:300–308.
26. Kaufman RH, Noller KL, Adam E, et al. Upper genital tract abnormalities and pregnancy outcome in diethylstilbestrol-exposed progeny. *Am J Obstet Gynecol* 1984;148:973–984.
27. Peress MR, Tsai CC, Mathur RS, et al. Hirsutism and menstrual patterns in women exposed to diethylstilbestrol *in utero. Am J Obstet Gynecol* 1982;144:135–140.
28. Meyer-Bahlburg HFL, Ehrhardt AA. A prenatal hormone hypothesis for depression in adults with a history of fetal DES exposure. In: Halbreich U, ed. *Hormones and depression.* New York: Raven Press, 1987:325–328.
29. Tunick B. DES legacy may extend to a third generation. *The Philadelphia Inquirer.* April 16, 2001:C1–C4.
30. Department of Health, Education, and Welfare. *DES Task Force summary report.* Washington, DC: Author, 1978:1679–1688.
31. Ries LAG, Kosary CL, et al., eds. SEER cancer statistics review 1973–1996. National Cancer Institute. http://www-seer.ims.nci.nih.gov.
32. U.S. EPA conference on preventable causes of cancer in children. Arlington, VA, September 1997.
33. *Facts.* White Plains, NY: National Foundation-March of Dimes, 1979.
34. Birth defects doubled since '50s, study finds. *The Philadelphia Inquirer* (Suburban North Edition). July 19, 1983:1A.
35. Tuchmann-Duplessis H. Drugs and other xenobiotics as teratogens. *Pharmacol Ther* 1984;26:273–344.
36. Hood RD. *Handbook of developmental toxicology.* Boca Raton, FL: CRC Press, 1996.
37. Szent-Györgyi A. Some reminiscences of my life as a scientist. *Int J Quantum Chem* 1976;3:7–12.
38. Marshall E. Pediatric drug trials. Challenge to FDA's authority may end up giving it more. *Science* 2002;296:820–821.
39. Nelson DR, Koymans L, Kamataki T, et al. P450 superfamily: update on new sequences, gene mapping, accession number and nomenclature. *Pharmacogenetics* 1996;6:1–42.

40. Ryan DE, Levin W. Purification and characterization of hepatic microsomal cytochrome P450. *Pharmacol Ther* 1990;45:153–239.
41. Sharma MC, Shapiro BH. Purification and characterization of constituent testosterone 2α-hydroxylase (cytochrome P450$_{2}\alpha$) from mouse liver. *Arch Biochem Biophys* 1995;316:478–484.
42. Sharma MC, Sharma MR, Jeong SJ, et al. Purification and characterization of constituent androstenedione 15α-hydroxylase (cytochrome P450$_{15}\alpha_{AD}$) from mouse liver: sex- and tissue-dependent expression. *Biochem Pharmacol* 1996;52:901–910.
43. Negishi M, Burkhart B, Aida K. Expression of genes within mouse IIA and IID subfamilies: simultaneous measurement of homologous mRNA. *Methods Enzymol* 1991;206:267–273.
44. Guengerich FP. *Mammalian cytochromes P-450.* Boca Raton, FL: CRC Press, 1987.
45. Gleiter CH, Gundert-Remy U. Gender differences in pharmacokinetics. *Eur J Drug Metab Pharmacokinet* 1996;21:123–128.
46. Wrighton SA, VandenBranden M, Ring BJ. The human drug metabolizing cytochromes P450. *J Pharmacokinet Biopharm* 1996; 24:461–473.
47. Xie HG, Huang SL, Xu ZH, et al. Evidence for the effect of gender on activity of (S)-mephenytoin 4′-hydroxylase (CYP2C19) in a Chinese population. *Pharmacogenetics* 1997;7:115–119.
48. Tamminga WJ, Werner J, Oosterhuis B, et al. CYP2D6 and CYP2C19 activity in a large population of Dutch healthy volunteers: indications for oral contraceptive-related gender differences. *Eur J Clin Pharmacol* 1999;55:177–184.
49. Ou-Yang DS, Huang SJ, Wang W, et al. Phenotypic polymorphism and gender-related differences of CYP1A2 activity in a Chinese population. *Br J Clin Pharmacol* 2000;49:145–151.
50. Bloom HJG. Hormone-induced and spontaneous regression of metastatic renal cancer. *Cancer* 1973;32:1066–1071.
51. Castegnaro M, Bartsch H, Chernozemsky I. Endemic nephropathy and urinary tract tumors in the Balkans. *Cancer Res* 1987;42: 3608–3609.
52. Iba MM, Fung J, Thomas PE, et al. Constitutive and induced expression by pyridine and β-naphthoflavone of rat CYP1 A is sexually dimorphic. *Arch Toxicol* 1999;73:208–216.
53. Elfarra AA, Krause RJ, Last AR, et al. Species- and sex-related differences in metabolism of trichloroethylene to yield chloral and trichloroethanol in mouse, rat, and human liver microsomes. *Drug Metab Dispos* 1998;26:779–785.
54. Kando JC, Yonkers KA, Cole JO. Gender as a risk factor for adverse events to medications. *Drugs* 1995;50:1–6.
55. Luzier AB, Killian A, Wilton JH, et al. Gender-related effects on metoprolol pharmacokinetics and pharmacodynamics in healthy volunteers. *Clin Pharmacol Ther* 1999;66:594–601.
56. Bathum L, Andersen-Ranberg K, Boldsen J, et al. Genotypes for the cytochrome P450 enzymes CYP2D6 and CYP2C19 in human longevity. *Eur J Clin Pharmacol* 1998;54:427–430.
57. Colby HD, Gaskin JH, Kitay JI. Requirement of the pituitary gland for the gonadal hormone effects on hepatic corticosteroid metabolism in rats and hamsters. *Endocrinology* 1973;95:891–896.
58. Gustafsson JA, Stenberg A. Masculinization of rat liver enzyme activities following hypophysectomy. *Endocrinology* 1974;95: 891–896.
59. Gustafsson JA, Edén S, Eneroth P, et al. Regulation of sexually dimorphic hepatic steroid metabolism by the somatostatin–growth hormone axis. *J Steroid Biochem* 1983;19:691–698.
60. Legraverend C, Mode A, Wells T, et al. Hepatic steroid hydroxylating enzymes are controlled by the sexually dimorphic pattern of growth hormone secretions in normal and dwarf rats. *FASEB J* 1992;6:711–718.
61. Shapiro BH, Agrawal AK, Pampori NA. Gender differences in drug metabolism regulated by growth hormone. *Int J Biochem Cell Biol* 1995;27:9–20.
62. Pampori NA, Shapiro BH. Feminization of hepatic cytochrome P-450 by nominal levels of growth hormone in the feminine plasma profile. *Mol Pharmacol* 1996;50:1148–1156.
63. Agrawal AK, Shapiro BH. Differential expression of gender-dependent hepatic isoforms of cytochrome P-450 by pulse signals in the circulating masculine episodic growth hormone profile of the rat. *J Pharmacol Exp Ther* 2000;292:228–237.
64. Agrawal AK, Shapiro BH. Intrinsic signals in the sexually dimorphic circulating growth hormone profiles of the rat. *Mol Cell Endocrinol* 2001;173:167–181.
65. Bacan WL, Vasilatos-Younken R, Nestor KE, et al. Pulsatile patterns of plasma growth hormone in turkeys: effects of growth rate, age, and sex. *Gen Comp Endocrinol* 1989;75:417–426.
66. Gatford KL, Fletcher TP, Rao A, et al. GH-releasing factor and somatostatin in the growing lamb: sex differences and mechanisms for sex differences. *J Endocrinol* 1997;152:19–27.
67. Stewart F, Goode JA, Allen WR. Growth hormone secretion in the horse: unusual pattern at birth and pulsatile secretion through to maturity. *J Endocrinol* 1993;138:81–89.
68. MacLeod JN, Pampori NA, Shapiro BH. Sex differences in the ultradian pattern of plasma growth hormone concentrations in mice. *J Endocrinol* 1991;131:395–399.
69. Pampori NA, Shapiro BH. Testicular regulation of sexual dimorphisms in the ultradian patterns of circulating growth hormone in the chicken. *Eur J Endocrinol* 1994;131:313–318.
70. MacLeod JN, Shapiro BH. Growth hormone regulation of hepatic drug-metabolizing enzymes in the mouse. *Biochem Pharmacol* 1989;38:1673–1677.
71. Pampori NA, Shapiro BH. Sexual dimorphism in avian hepatic monooxygenases. *Biochem Pharmacol* 1993;46:885–890.
72. Pampori NA, Shapiro BH. Effects of neonatally administered monosodium glutamate on the sexually dimorphic profiles of circulating growth hormone regulating murine hepatic monooxygenases. *Biochem Pharmacol* 1994;47:1221–1229.
73. Sharma MC, Agrawal AK, Sharma MR, et al. Interactions of gender, growth hormone, and phenobarbital induction on murine Cyp2b expression. *Biochem Pharmacol* 1998;56:1251–1258.
74. Asplin CM, Faria ACS, Carlsen EC, et al. Alterations in the pulsatile mode of growth hormone release in men and women with insulin-dependent diabetes mellitus. *J Clin Endocrinol Metab* 1989;70:1678–1686.
75. Winer LM, Shaw MA, Baumann G. Basal plasma growth-hormone levels in man: new evidence for rhythmicity of growth hormone secretion. *J Clin Endocrinol Metab* 1990;70:1678–1686.
76. Hartman ML, Iranmanesh A, Thorner MO, et al. Evaluation of pulsatile patterns of growth hormone release in humans: a brief review. *Am J Hum Biol* 1993;5:603–614.
77. Albertsson-Wikland K, Roseberg S, Karlberg J, et al. Analysis of 24-hour growth hormone profiles in healthy boys and girls of normal stature: relation to puberty. *J Clin Endocrinol Metab* 1994;78:1195–1201.
78. Van den Berg G, Veldhuis JD, Frolich M, et al. An amplitude-specific divergence in the pulsatile mode of growth hormone (GH) secretion underlies the gender difference in mean GH concentrations in men and premenopausal women. *J Clin Endocrinol Metab* 1996;81:2460–2467.
79. Engstrom BE, Karlsson FA, Wide L. Marked gender differences in ambulatory morning growth hormone values in young adults. *Clin Chem* 1998;44:1289–1295.
80. Redmond GP, Bell JJ, Nichola PS, et al. Effect of growth hormone on human drug metabolism: time course and substrate specificity. *Pediatr Pharmacol* 1980;1:63–70.
81. Levitsky LL, Schoeller DA, Lambert GH, et al. Effect of growth hormone therapy in growth hormone-deficient children on cytochrome P-450-dependent 3-N-demethylation of caffeine as measured by the caffeine CO_2 breath test. *Dev Pharmacol Ther* 1989;12:90–95.
82. Dhir RN, Dworakowski W, Thangavel C, et al. Sexually dimorphic regulation of hepatic isoforms of human cytochrome P450 by growth hormone. *J Pharmacol Exp* Ther 2006;316:87–94.
83. Kalter H, Warkany J. Congenital malformations: etiologic factors and their role in prevention. *N Engl J Med* 1983;308: 491–497.
84. Kelly TE, Edwards P, Rein M, et al. Teratogenicity of anticonvulsant drugs. II. A prospective study. *Am J Med Genet* 1984;19: 435–443.
85. Janz D. Antiepileptic drugs and pregnancy: altered utilization patterns and teratogenesis. *Epilepsia* 1982;23(Suppl 1):553–563.
86. Nau H, Kuhnz W, Egger HJ, et al. Anticonvulsants during pregnancy and lactation: transplacental, maternal, and neonatal pharmacokinetics. *Clin Pharmacokinet* 1982;7:508–543.
87. Fejerman N. Epilepsy in children and adolescents. *Epilepsia* 2002;43(Suppl 6):44–46.
88. Leonardi M, Ustun TB. The global burden of epilepsy. *Epilepsia* 2002;43(Suppl 6):21–25.

89. Bossi L. Fetal effects of anticonvulsants. In: Morselli PL, Pippenger CE, Penry JK, eds. *Antiepileptic drug therapy in pediatrics.* New York: Raven Press, 1983:37–63.
90. Kelly T. Teratogenicity of anticonvulsant drugs. I. Review of the literature. *Am J Med Genet* 1984;19:413–434.
91. Smith DW. Hydantoin effects on the fetus. In: Hassel TM, ed. *Phenytoin-induced teratology and gingival pathology.* New York: Raven Press, 1980:35–40.
92. Wells PG. Physiological and environmental determinants of phenytoin teratogenicity: relation to glutathione homeostasis, and potentiation by acetaminophen. In: MacLeod SM, Okey AB, Speilberg SP, eds. *Developmental pharmacology.* New York: Raven Press, 1983:367–371.
93. Gabler WL, Falace D. The distribution and metabolism of Dilantin in non-pregnant, pregnant and fetal rats. *Arch Int Pharmacodyn Ther* 1970;184:45–58.
94. Vorhees CV. Developmental effects of anticonvulsants. *Neurotoxicology* 1986;7:235–244.
95. Shapiro BH, Lech GM, Bardales RM. Persistent defects in the hepatic monooxygenase system of adult rats exposed, perinatally, to maternally administered phenytoin. *J Pharmacol Exp Ther* 1986;238:68–75.
96. Vorhees CV. Fetal anticonvulsant syndrome in rats: effects on postnatal behavior and brain amino acid content. *Neurobehav Toxicol Teratol* 1985;7:471–482.
97. Sonawane BR, Yaffe SJ. Delayed effects of drug exposure during pregnancy: reproductive function. *Biol Res Pregnancy Perinatol* 1983;2:48–55.
98. Takagi S, Alleva FR, Seth PK, et al. Delayed development of reproductive functions and alteration of dopamine receptor binding in hypothalamus of rats exposed prenatally to phenytoin and phenobarbital. *Toxicol Lett* 1986;34:107–113.
99. Shapiro BH, Babalola GO. Developmental profile of serum androgens and estrous cyclicity of male and female rats exposed perinatally to maternally administered phenytoin. *Toxicol Lett* 1987;36:165–175.
100. Eling TE, Harbison RD, Becker BA, et al. Diphenylhydantoin effect on neonatal and adult rat hepatic drug metabolism. *J Pharmacol Exp Ther* 1970;171:127–134.
101. Heinicke RJ, Stohs SJ, Al-Turk W, et al. Chronic phenytoin administration and the hepatic mixed function oxidase system in female rats. *Gen Pharmacol* 1984;15:85–89.
102. Shapiro BH, Bardales RM, Lech GM. Perinatal induction of hepatic aminopyrine-*N*-demethylase by maternal exposure to phenytoin. *Pediatr Pharmacol* 1985;5:201–207.
103. Rating D, Jäger-Roman E, Nau H, et al. Enzyme induction in neonates after fetal exposure to antiepileptic drugs. *Pediatr Pharmacol* 1983;3:209–218.
104. Barnhart ER, ed. *Physicians' desk reference.* Oradell, NJ: Medical Economics, 1967.
105. Reinisch JM, Sanders SA. Early barbiturate exposure: the brain, sexually dimorphic behavior and learning. *Neurosci Biobehav Rev* 1982;6:311–319.
106. Painter MJ, Scher MS, Stein AD, et al. Phenobarbital compared with phenytoin for the treatment of neonatal seizures. *N Engl J Med* 1999;341:485–489.
107. Yerby MS. Pregnancy and epilepsy. *Epilepsia* 1991;32(Suppl 6): S51–S59.
108. Lindout D, Omtzigt JGC. Pregnancy and the risk teratogenicity. *Epilepsia* 1992;33(Suppl 4):S41–S48.
109. Clemens LG, Popham TV, Ruppert PH. Neonatal treatment of hamsters with barbiturate alters adult sexual behavior. *Dev Psychobiol* 1979;12:49–59.
110. Gupta C, Sonawane BR, Yaffe SJ, et al. Phenobarbital exposure *in utero*: alternations in female reproductive function in rats. *Science* 1980;208:508–510.
111. Gupta C, Yaffe SJ, Shapiro BH. Prenatal exposure to phenobarbital permanently decreases testosterone and causes reproductive dysfunction. *Science* 1982;216:640–642.
112. Wani JH, Agrawal AK, Shapiro BH. Neonatal phenobarbital-induced persistent alterations in plasma testosterone profiles and testicular function. *Toxicol Appl Pharmacol* 1996;137:295–300.
113. Agrawal AK, Pampori NA, Shapiro BH. Neonatal phenobarbital-induced defects in age- and sex-specific growth hormone profiles regulating monooxygenases. *Am J Physiol* 1995;268:E439–E445.
114. Faris RA, Campbell TC. Long-term effects of neonatal phenobarbital exposure on aflatoxin B_1 disposition in adult rats. *Cancer Res* 1983;43:2576–2583.
115. Soliman KFA, Richardson SD. Effects of prenatal exposure to phenobarbital on the development of monoamine oxidase and glucocorticoids. *Gen Pharmacol* 1983;14:369–371.
116. Sobrian SK, Nandedkar AKN. Prenatal antiepileptic drug exposure alters seizure susceptibility in rats. *Pharmacol Biochem Behav* 1986;24:1381–1391.
117. Middaugh LD, Thomas TN, Simpson LW, et al. Effects of prenatal maternal injections of phenobarbital on brain neurotransmitters and behavior of young C57 mice. *Neurobehav Toxicol Teratol* 1981;3:271–275.
118. Vorhees CV. Fetal anticonvulsant syndrome in rats: dose- and period-response relationships of prenatal diphenylhydantoin, trimethadione and phenobarbital exposure on the structural and functional development of the offspring. *J Pharmacol Exp Ther* 1983;227:274–287.
119. Yanai J. Long-term induction of microsomal drug oxidizing system in mice following prenatal exposure to barbiturate. *Biochem Pharmacol* 1979;28:1429–1430.
120. Bagley DM, Hayes JR. Neonatal phenobarbital administration results in increased cytochrome P450-dependent monooxygenase activity in adult male and female rats. *Biochem Biophys Res Commun* 1983;114:1132–1137.
121. Waxman DJ, Azaroff L. Phenobarbital induction of cytochrome P-450 gene expression. *Biochem J* 1992;281:577–592.
122. Agrawal AK, Shapiro BH. Imprinted overinduction of hepatic CYP2B1 and 2B2 in adult rats neonatally exposed to phenobarbital. *J Pharmacol Exp Ther* 1996;279:991–999.
123. Agrawal AK, Shapiro BH. Latent overexpression of hepatic CYP2C7 in adult male and female rats neonatally exposed to phenobarbital: a developmental profile of gender-dependent P450s. *J Pharmacol Exp Ther* 2000;293:1027–1033.
124. Agrawal AK, Shapiro BH. Phenobarbital-imprinted overinduction of adult constituent CYP isoforms. *Pharmacology* 2003;68: 204–215.
125. Valerino DM, Vesell ES, Aurori KC, et al. Effects of various barbiturates on hepatic miscrosomal enzymes: a comparative study. *Drug Metab Dispos* 1974;2:448–457.
126. Ishizaki T, Yokochi K, Chiba J, et al. Placental transfer of anticonvulsants (phenobarbital, phenytoin, valproic acid) and the elimination from neonates. *Pediatr Pharmacol* 1981;1: 291–303.
127. Franceschi M, Perego L, Cavagnini F, et al. Effects of long-term antiepileptic therapy on the hypothalamic–pituitary axis in men. *Epilepsia* 1984;25:46–52.
128. Kaneko S, Hirane T, Muramatsu E, et al. Fetal and neonatal effects of antiepileptic drugs—the physical and psychomotor developments in the offspring of epileptic parents. In: Fujii T, Adams PM, eds. *Functional teratogenesis.* Tokyo, Japan: Teikyo University Press, 1987:205–215.
129. Yaffe SJ, Dorn LD. Effects of prenatal treatment with phenobarbital. *Dev Pharmacol Ther* 1990;15:215–223.
130. Dessens AB, Cohen-Kettenis PT, Mellenbergh GJ, et al. Association of prenatal phenobarbital and phenytoin exposure with genital anomalies and menstrual disorders. *Teratology* 2001; 64:181–188.
131. Dessens AB, Cohen-Kettenis PT, Mellenbergh GJ, et al. Prenatal exposure to anticonvulsants and psychosexual development. *Arch Sex Behav* 1999;28:31–44.
132. Reinisch JM, Sanders SA, Mortensen EL, et al. In utero exposure to phenobarbital and intelligence deficits in adult men. *JAMA* 1995;274:1518–1525.
133. Koch S, Titze K, Zimmermann RB, et al. Long-term neuropsychological consequences of natural epilepsy and anticonvulsant treatment during pregnancy for school-age children and adolescents. *Epilepsia* 1999;40:1237–1243.
134. Dessens AB, Cohen-Kettenis PT, Mellenbergh GJ, et al. Association of prenatal phenobarbital and phenytoin exposure with small head size at birth and with learning problems. *Acta Paediatr* 2000;89:533–541.
135. Agrawal AK, Shapiro BH. Neonatal phenobarbital imprints overexpression of cytochrome P450 with associated increase in tumorigenesis and reduced life span. *FASEB J* 2005;19:470–472.

136. Bandiers S, Ryan DE, Levin W, et al. Age- and sex-related expression of cytochromes P450f and P450 g in rat liver. *Arch Biochem Biophys* 1986;248:658–676.
137. Henderson CJ, Russell AL, Allan JA, et al. Sexual differentiation and regulation of cytochrome P-450 CYP2C7. *Biochem Biophys Acta* 1992;1118:99–106.
138. Okey AB. Enzyme induction in the cytochrome P-450 system. *Pharm Ther* 1990;45:241–298.
139. Diwan BA, Rice JM, Nims RW, et al. P-450 enzyme induction by 5-ethyl-5-phenylhydantoin and 5,5-diethylhydantoin, analogues of barbiturate tumor promoters phenobarbital and barbital, and promotion of liver and thyroid carcinogenesis initiated by *N*-nitrosodiethylamine in rats. *Cancer Res* 1988;48: 2492–2497.
140. Lubet RA, Nims RW, Ward JM, et al. Induction of cytochrome P450b and its relationship to liver tumor promotion. *J Am Coll Toxicol* 1989;8:259–268.
141. Agrawal AK, Shapiro BH. Constitutive and inducible hepatic cytochrome P450 isoforms in senescent male and female rats and response to low-dose phenobarbital. *Drug Metab Dispos* 2003; 31:612–619.
142. Tavoloni N, Jones MJT, Berk PD. Dose-related effects of phenobarbital on hepatic microsomal enzymes. *Proc Soc Exp Biol Med* 1983;174:20–27.
143. Diwan BA, Anderson LM, Ward JM, et al. Transplacental carcinogenesis by cisplatin in F344/NCR rats—promotion of kidney tumors by postnatal administration of sodium barbital. *Toxicol Appl Pharmacol* 1995;132:115–121.
144. Gold E, Gordis L, Tonascia J, et al. Increased risk of brain cancer in children exposed to barbiturates. *J Natl Cancer Inst* 1978;61: 1031–1034.
145. Dessens AB, Boer K, Koppe JG, et al. Studies on long-lasting consequences of prenatal exposure to anticonvulsant drugs. *Acta Paediatr* 1994;404(Suppl):54–64.
146. Olney JW. Excitatory neurotoxins as food additives: an evaluation of risk. *Neurotoxicology* 1981;2:163–192.
147. The Glutamate Association. Washington, DC. http://www.msgfacts.com/facts/msgfact09.html.
148. Dried soup mixes (this is soup?). *Consum Rep* 1978:615–619.
149. Citizens' Alliance for Consumer Protection of Korea. *A study of the use of MSG in Korea*. UNICEF, 1986.
150. Stegink LD. Interactions of aspartame and glutamate metabolism. In: Stegink LD, Filier LJ Jr, eds. *Aspartame: physiology and biochemistry*. New York: Marcel Dekker, 1984:607–632.
151. Agrawal AK, Shapiro BH. Gender, age and dose effects of neonatally administered aspartate on the sexually dimorphic plasma growth hormone profiles regulating expression of sex-dependent hepatic CYP isoforms. *Drug Metab Dispos* 1997;25: 1249–1256.
152. Pardridge WM. Potential effects of the dipeptide sweetener aspartame on the brain. *Nutr Brain* 1986;7:199–241.
153. Stegink LD. Aspartate and glutamate metabolism. In: Stegink LD, Filier LJ Jr, eds. *Aspartame: physiology and biochemistry*. New York: Marcel Dekker, 1984:47–76.
154. Reynolds WA, Parsons L, Stegink LD. Neuropathology studies following aspartame ingestion by infant nonhuman primates. In: Stegink LD, Filier LJ Jr, eds. *Aspartame: physiology and biochemistry*. New York: Marcel Dekker, 1984:363–378.
155. FDA backgrounder: FDA and monosodium glutamate. http://vm.cfsan.fda.gov/~lrd/msg.html. Published August 31, 1995.
156. Shapiro BH, MacLeod JN, Pampori NA, et al. Signaling elements in the ultradian rhythm of circulating growth hormone regulating expression of sex-dependent forms of hepatic cytochrome P450. *Endocrinology* 1989;125:2935–2944.
157. Pampori NA, Agrawal AK, Waxman DJ, et al. Differential effects of neonatally administered glutamate on the ultradian pattern of circulating growth hormone regulating expression of sex-dependent forms of cytochrome P450. *Biochem Pharmacol* 1991; 41:1299–1309.
158. Morgan ET, MacGeoch C, Gustafsson JÄ. Hormonal and developmental regulation of expression of the hepatic microsomal steroid 16α-hydroxylase cytochrome P-450 apoprotein in the rat. *J Biol Chem* 1985;260:11895–11898.
159. Waxman DJ, Morrissey JJ, MacLeod JN, et al. Depletion of serum growth hormone in adult female rats by neonatal monosodium glutamate treatment without loss of female-specific hepatic enzymes P450 2d (IIC12) and steroid 5α-reductase. *Endocrinology* 1990;126:712–720.
160. Jansson JO, Edén S, Isaksson O. Sexual dimorphism in the control of growth hormone secretion. *Endocrine Rev* 1985;6:128–150.
161. Dhir RN, Dworakowski W, Shapiro BH. Middle-age alterations in the sexually dimorphic plasma growth hormone profiles: involvement of growth hormone-releasing factor and effects on CYP expression. *Drug Metab Dispos* 2002;30:141–147.
162. Shapiro BH, Pampori NA, Ram PA, et al. Irreversible suppression of growth hormone-dependent cytochrome P450 2C11 in adult rats neonatally treated with monosodium glutamate. *J Pharmacol Exp Ther* 1993;267:979–984.
163. Waxman DJ, Ram PA, Pampori NA, et al. Growth hormone regulation of male-specific rat liver P450s 2A2 and 3A2: induction by intermittent growth hormone pulses in male but not female rats rendered growth hormone deficient by monosodium glutamate. *Mol Pharmacol* 1995;48:790–797.
164. Lehmann A, Jonsson T. MK-801 selectively protects mouse arcuate neurons in vivo against glutamate toxicity. *Neuroreport* 1992;3: 421–424.
165. Pinilla L, Gonzales L, Tena-Sempere M, et al. Gonadal and age-related influences on NMDA-induced growth hormone secretion in male rats. *Neuroendocrinology* 1999;69:11–19.
166. Kaufhold A, Nigam PK, Dhir RN, et al. Prevention of latently expressed CYP2C11, CYP3A2, and growth hormone defects in neonatally MSG-treated male rats by *N*-methyl-D-aspartate receptor antagonist MK-801. *J Pharmacol Exp Ther* 2002;302:490–496.
167. Pampori NA, Shapiro BH. Over-expression of CYP2C11, the major male-specific form of hepatic cytochrome P450, in the presence of nominal pulses of circulating growth hormone in adult male rats neonatally exposed to low levels of monosodium glutamate. *J Pharmacol Exp Ther* 1994;271:1067–1073.
168. Pampori NA, Shapiro BH. Nominal growth hormone pulses in otherwise normal masculine plasma profiles induce intron retention of overexpressed hepatic CYP2C11 with associated nuclear splicing deficiency. *Endocrinology* 2000;141:4100–4106.

CHAPTER

16

John N. van den Anker
Karel Allegaert

Renal Function and Excretion of Drugs in the Newborn

A thorough understanding of the developmental changes in neonatal renal function is needed to estimate the renal clearing capacity for the many drugs used in the neonatal period. At birth, anatomic and functional immaturity of the kidney limits glomerular and tubular functional capacity, which results in inefficient drug elimination and a prolonged elimination half-life (1,2). Rapid increases in glomerular and tubular functions occur during the postnatal period, greatly enhancing renal drug elimination. The main factors involved in the development of renal function are gestational age (GA) and the dramatic sequential hemodynamic changes after birth in a situation initially dominated by high vascular resistance and extremely low blood flow. At birth, the glomerular filtration rate (GFR) is 2 to 4 mL per min in term neonates, and it may be as low as 0.6 to 0.8 mL per min in preterm infants. The increase in GFR after birth is important and is usually greater in term than in preterm infants (3–6). This increase is due to the increase in cardiac output associated with specific changes in renal vascular resistances, resulting in an increase in renal blood flow, changes in renal blood flow distribution, and a higher permeability of the glomerular membrane.

In addition to these rapid developmental changes in GFR, a wealth of new information concerning mechanisms of tubular drug transport has recently become available (7). Transporter protein science is a rapidly evolving field of pharmacology, and new transporter proteins are continuously being discovered. However, the clinical implications of many of these new discoveries are not yet established.

RENAL CLEARANCE

Renal clearance contributes to the elimination of a significant number of water-soluble drugs and their metabolites. The rate of renal clearance is expressed as the sum of the rate of glomerular filtration and the rate of tubular secretion minus the rate of tubular reabsorption. This relationship between renal clearance (CL_R) and these processes can be expressed as the following equation:

$$CL_R = f_u \times GFR + CL_S - CL_{RA}$$

where GFR, CL_S, and CL_{RA} are glomerular filtration rate, secretion clearance, and reabsorption clearance, respectively, and f_u is the unbound fraction of the drug in plasma. All these mechanisms exhibit independent rates and patterns of development. Glomerular filtration involves the unidirectional diffusion of unbound drug from the glomerular blood supply into the glomerular filtrate and is dependent on renal blood flow and the extent of plasma protein binding of drugs in the circulation. Tubular reabsorption and secretion are bidirectional processes involving active transport mechanisms and, additionally in the case of tubular reabsorption, passive transport processes. Arterial blood passes through the glomerulus—the part of the nephron that filters plasma water and some of its contents. The pores within the capillary endothelium and the ultrafiltration membrane of the glomerulus allow only small molecules ($<$400 to 600 Å in diameter, or about 5 kDa in molecular weight) to be filtered into the tubular fluid. Therefore, large macromolecules, such as most proteins and hence the drugs bound to them, cannot pass through the filter.

Although the GFR is about 120 mL per min in adults, reabsorption along the proximal, distal, and collecting tubules leads to only 1 to 2 mL per min of the filtered water being eliminated as urine. The tubular epithelium is the site of reabsorption of many substances, with the net effect that these molecules pass through the renal interstitial fluid and back to the plasma. Lipid-soluble or nonionized substances are able to diffuse across cell membranes, whereas charged molecules (including most drugs) are usually not and are subsequently excreted in the urine. The pH of tubular fluid is an important factor influencing the reabsorption of drugs because it may affect the ratio of drug in nonionized form to ionized form. For example, alkalinization of urine may be used to promote drug excretion in cases of acidic drug overdose, such as with salicylate.

Renal secretion is mostly an active process because the transport of drugs is against a concentration gradient (6). Therefore, transporter proteins must be located within the tubules and so must the sources of energy, cotransporters, and countertransport molecules (7). Furthermore, saturation of these transport mechanisms and competition among a variety of drugs using them may affect the rate of renal drug elimination and lead to drug interactions and toxicity (7,8).

GLOMERULAR FILTRATION RATE

The newborn kidney's main physiologic limitation is its very low GFR, maintained by a delicate balance between vasoconstrictor and vasodilatory renal forces. These forces recruit maximal attainable filtration pressure in the face of minimal renal blood supply resulting from a combination of a low mean arterial blood pressure and a high intrarenal vascular resistance. The low GFR of the newborn kidney, although sufficient for growth and development under normal conditions, limits the postnatal renal functional adaptation to endogenous and exogenous stress (9). Such stress may result from renal hypoperfusion caused by anoxia, sepsis, and/or exposure to nephrotoxic medications. Vasoactive forms of nonsteroidal anti-inflammatory drugs (NSAIDs) such as aspirin, indomethacin, and ibuprofen [nonspecific cyclooxygenase (COX) inhibitors] and the new selective COX-2 inhibitors such as rofecoxib can induce renal hypoperfusion resulting in generally reversible, oliguric acute renal failure (ARF). This adverse renal effect of COX inhibition appears to be specific for the term and most prominent in the premature newborn (10,11). The mechanism of action of these drugs abolishes the vasodilatory effect of prostaglandins, which allows maintenance of an effective neonatal GFR. When prostaglandin synthesis is inhibited, the vasoconstrictor state of the newborn kidney is unopposed. These observations are of great clinical importance because NSAIDs are prescribed during pregnancy for the management of preeclampsia, polyhydramnios, and premature birth. These drugs easily pass the placenta, so the fetus is readily exposed to their toxic effects. Postnatally, recurrent boluses of NSAIDs are administered to promote the pharmacologic closure of a hemodynamically significant patent ductus arteriosus (PDA). Indomethacin has traditionally been the drug of choice, but recently ibuprofen has been advocated for its decreased renal toxicity (12). However, Chamaa et al. (10) showed in the newborn rabbit (a well-established model for evaluating developmental changes in neonatal renal function) that ibuprofen is not less nephrotoxic than indomethacin. Because all specific and nonspecific COX inhibitors can cause ARF in the newborn, caution is advised when administering any of these compounds to the very young. Specific and nonspecific COX inhibition in utero may lead to renal morphologic changes and even end-stage renal disease at birth (13,14).

The most important factors that influence the GFR in the neonatal period are GA, prenatal drug exposure (i.e., betamethasone, angiotensin I-converting enzyme inhibitors, angiotensin II-receptor inhibitors, and NSAIDs), postnatal age, the existence of a PDA, and postnatal exposure to indomethacin or ibuprofen, dopamine, furosemide, and more recently genetic polymorphisms of proteins that play a role in neonatal physiology and may contribute to individual susceptibility to ARF and its risk factors (15,16).

THE EFFECTS OF GENETIC POLYMORPHISMS ON THE RISK OF ACUTE RENAL FAILURE IN PRETERM NEONATES

ARF affects approximately 10% of severely ill neonates (17). The majority of ARF cases are prerenal, also called vasomotor nephropathy. Hypovolemia, hypotension, and hypoxemia are some of the main causes of prerenal ARF. In addition to the well-known risk factors (i.e., PDA, intracerebral hemorrhage, respiratory distress syndrome, necrotizing enterocolitis, pharmacotherapy), recent studies have shown that the genetic polymorphisms may contribute to ARF too. The major substances implicated in the pathogenesis of ARF in the neonate are vasoactive agents such as angiotensin II, adenosine or renal prostaglandins, and factors participating in the regulation of inflammatory pathways, called cytokines.

Angiotensin II is a potent pressor agent that increases intraglomerular pressure in the kidneys by constricting mainly postglomerular vessels (18). This effect plays a key role in the maintenance of neonatal glomerular filtration at very low perfusion pressure, as demonstrated by the deleterious effects of angiotensin-converting enzyme (ACE) inhibitors (19) and angiotensin II-receptor antagonists (20). Nobilis et al. looked at genetic variants in the ACE and the angiotensin II-receptor 1 (AT1-receptor) genes but could not detect an impact on the risk of ARF in preterm infants with a birth weight of less than 1,500 g (21). However, Harding et al. showed a relation between genetic variants in the ACE gene and the postnatal adaptation of preterm infants with GAs between 30 and 32 weeks. They found that patients with a certain genotype were at an increased risk for poor postnatal adaptation (22). Cytokines may affect renal function in several different ways (23). The body's ability to produce cytokines varies greatly. Several studies have offered evidence supporting the contribution of genetic polymorphisms of cytokine-encoding genes to this individual variance and have postulated an association with risk for cytokine-mediated disorders in adults. Treszl et al. showed in 92 very low-birth-weight infants with severe systemic infection that high tumor necrosis factor α producer and low interleukin 6 producer genotypes were more prevalent (26%) in neonates with ARF as compared with neonates without ARF (6%) suggesting that preterm infants with systemic infection may be at increased risk for ARF if they possess the aforementioned haplotype (24).

The currently available data on the effect of genetic polymorphisms on the risk of ARF in preterm neonates are still very limited, but the investigation of polymorphisms of genes encoding for other receptors and peptides potentially involved in the complexity of the pathogenesis of ARF might increase our knowledge on the relevance of this variants in neonates who develop ARF.

THE EFFECT OF GESTATIONAL AGE ON THE GLOMERULAR FILTRATION RATE

Developmental changes in the GFR of preterm infants have been the subject of many studies (4,25,26). Despite the fact that most studies included only a limited number of infants with a wide variation of postnatal age, almost all reports showed the presence of a GA-dependent increase in the GFR. Recently, the effects of GA and body weight on the GFR on day 3 of life were studied (27). GFR measurements were performed in 147 preterm infants with a GA between 23.4 and 37.0 weeks by means of a continuous inulin infusion technique. Mean GFR values increased significantly with GA and body weight. Multivariate analysis indicated that GA, but not body weight, was the major determinant for this increase in GFR. The clinical implications of this GA-dependent maturation of the GFR become apparent when one considers drugs that are primarily eliminated by glomerular filtration. Recent studies have investigated the pharmacokinetics of cephalosporins and penicillins in preterm infants (28–30) and showed that the clearance of ceftazidime and amoxicillin increased significantly with increasing GA (28,30). In infants with the lowest GAs, this resulted in drug accumulation, necessitating dosage adjustments base on GA (28). For aminoglycosides and glycopeptides, which are potentially more toxic than cephalosporins and other β-lactam antibiotics, the urge to adapt prescribing practices is even higher (31–36).

THE EFFECT OF PRENATAL EXPOSURE TO BETAMETHASONE ON THE GLOMERULAR FILTRATION RATE

Betamethasone is a synthetic glucocorticoid with a potency equivalent to dexamethasone. The drug is prescribed to pregnant women with an increased risk of preterm delivery before week 34 of gestation. The objective of this treatment is to accelerate maturation of the alveolar epithelium and stimulate synthesis of lipid and protein components of the pulmonary surfactant complex to prevent hyaline membrane disease. Much of the data regarding renal responses to antenatal glucocorticoid treatment are derived from animal studies. For example, prolonged fetal betamethasone infusions have been shown to increase GFR and urine flow in both near-term fetal and newborn lambs (37). Although fetal cortisol infusion may increase fetal renal blood flow, betamethasone-induced increases in GFR result primarily from an increase in filtration fraction (37). Thus, although glucocorticoids increase blood pressure and thus will indirectly alter renal perfusion pressure, glucocorticoid-induced increases in GFR are primarily related to changes in renal vasculature resistance. This phenomenon is of interest because an increase in filtration fraction, rather than total renal blood flow, appears to be the primary mechanism for the marked perinatal increase in GFR observed in term newborn lambs (38). Antenatal betamethasone treatment significantly increases GFR in preterm newborn lambs supported by mechanical ventilation (39). The effects of prenatal exposure to betamethasone on the GFR of preterm infants have been studied by several investigators (27,40–42). The majority of these studies did not show an increase of the GFR during the first week of life after prenatal exposure to glucocorticoids. However, in three of these studies, creatinine clearance was used as a less reliable marker for the GFR in preterm infants, and a small number of children were studied (40–42). This might have prevented the authors from demonstrating an increase in the GFR in the first week of life after prenatal exposure to glucocorticoids. The only study that showed an increase in GFR was hampered by the fact that most pregnant women who were treated with betamethasone were also treated with indomethacin, thereby minimizing the number of women who were treated with betamethasone alone (27). However, betamethasone reversed indomethacin-induced decreases in GFR (27). It was hypothesized that an increase in renal plasma flow due to betamethasone may overcome intrarenal vasoconstriction secondary to the decreased synthesis of intrarenal prostaglandins by indomethacin. More recently, Allegaert and Anderson reported no impact of prenatal exposure to betamethasone on postnatal amikacin clearance in preterm neonates indicating the need for a prospective study investigating the impact of prenatal exposure to betamethasone on GFR (43).

THE EFFECT OF PRENATAL EXPOSURE TO ANGIOTENSIN I-CONVERTING ENZYME INHIBITORS AND ANGIOTENSIN II-RECEPTOR INHIBITORS ON THE GLOMERULAR FILTRATION RATE

All components of the renin–angiotensin system (RAS) exist within the fetal kidney during the early stages of development and participate as promoting factors for the growth of this organ, more specifically its angiogenesis, and have an important role in controlling intrarenal hemodynamics (44–46). In the early fetal stage, renin-containing cells are present in the developing intrarenal branches of the renal artery. Renin is also distributed in other vascular parts including the arcuate, interlobar, and afferent arterioles. Renin mRNA gene expression markedly increases throughout the fetal life to peak in the perinatal period. This gene could be under the influence of adrenergic input, as its expression is abolished with renal denervation (45). In early life, renin is almost exclusively detected in the juxtaglomerular apparatus. Renin acts on plasma angiotensinogen to form angiotensin I.

Angiotensin I-converting enzyme is a dipeptidyl carboxypeptidase that releases the pressor peptide angiotensin II (ANG II) from angiotensin I and inactivates bradykinin as well (47). ACE is present in both vascular and extravascular tissues (brush border) of the kidney. Although the extravascular localization of ACE is not fully known, this enzyme is found on glomerular endothelial cells at the place where the capillary invades the inferior cleft of the S-shaped body. ACE may participate in the tubular handling process of ANG II, as it has been found on the apical and basolateral membranes already in the early nephron stage. This glomerular distribution in the fetal kidney looks different as compared with the more mature kidney, where ACE is essentially found in the peritubular endothelial cells. The switch of ACE from glomerular to peritubular vessel with maturation has been well documented and occurs progressively during infancy. In addition to the renal hemodynamic regulation, the ANG II locally generated in the glomerulus also stimulates angiogenesis through the stimulation of its receptors.

It has been demonstrated that ANG II acts as a growth factor for renal cells and therefore plays a crucial role in the development of the kidney through its two receptors: AT1-R and angiotensin II receptor 2 (AT2-R) (48). Both receptors are indeed independently present in mammalian fetal kidney tissues, and AT2-R seems to predominate (48–52). AT2-R mRNA has been found in almost all fetal tissues, including the metanephros and undifferentiated mesenchymal and connective tissues. AT1-R has been found more specifically in the adrenal glands, liver, and kidney. Within the kidney, both AT1-R and AT2-R mRNAs are expressed in the metanephros at 14 days of gestation, when branching of the ureter bud has already started. AT1-R expression in the immature glomeruli coincides with mesangial cell differentiation from the pericyte, and continues throughout adulthood in the glomeruli and in the tubulointerstitium, whereas AT2-R expression decreases after birth except in large cortical blood vessels. AT1-R mRNA is expressed in mature glomeruli, in maturing S-shaped bodies, and in the proximal and distal tubule as well. Early in the embryologic period, AT2-R mRNA is first expressed in mesenchymal cells adjacent to the stalk of the ureter epithelium. The expression is then extended in the mesenchyme cells of the nephrogenic area and in the collecting ducts. AT2-R is also invariantly expressed in the epithelial cells of the macula densa.

Studies performed to determine the localization of AT1-R and AT2-R will help identify the specific and crucial role of ANG II for kidney development. Via AT1-R, ANG II stimulates proliferation, regulates nitric oxide synthase expression, has growth-promoting effects, and acts on glomerular mesangial and tubular cell differentiation during nephrogenesis (53). It further mediates biological actions such as maintenance of circulatory homeostasis and cell proliferation (54). Furthermore, ANG II participates in the downregulation of AT2-R and renin gene expression. In the growth-retarded fetus, AT2-R expression has been downregulated, and it has been postulated that this downregulation is associated with a higher risk of hypertension in adulthood.

Given the fundamental role of the RAS either in utero for general renal morphogenesis or during the first days of life to promote adequate glomerular filtration, administration of drugs with ACE inhibitory effects or acting as AT1-R or AT2-R inhibitors during pregnancy or during the first days of life is strictly contraindicated.

THE EFFECT OF PRENATAL EXPOSURE TO NONSTEROIDAL ANTI-INFLAMMATORY DRUGS ON THE GLOMERULAR FILTRATION RATE

Two COX isoforms are known: COX-1, which is expressed constitutively in almost all organs, and COX-2, which is usually absent in most organs but can be induced by various stimuli (55). These enzymes have a key role in the biosynthesis of prostanoid derivatives (56). In adults, renal prostaglandin synthesis is thought to counterbalance vasoconstrictive agents (e.g., ANG II), and renal vasodilatory prostanoids are primarily derived from COX-2 (57).

In the fetus, prostaglandins are crucial in the early phase of nephrogenesis, more specifically in the glomerulogenesis and in the differentiation of the nephrons. For example, metabolites of arachidonic acid modulate the activity of Na^+/K^+/ATPase along the nephron, and this action is age dependent (58). Vasodilator prostanoids counteract the high vascular resistance in utero and during the first days of life. Prostaglandin E_2 (PGE_2) and prostaglandin I_2 could also act as potent and rapid stimulators of renin secretion through prostaglandin receptors located on renal juxtamedullar cells, as has been demonstrated in more mature animals (59). Experimental studies show that a constitutive cortical as well as a medullary COX-2 are overexpressed in fetal life and during the first days of life, and this accounts for the high excretion of vasodilator prostaglandins (60,61).

Numerous prostaglandin receptors have been identified, and their role in renal development has become increasingly clear (62). Four PGE_2-receptor subtypes have been identified in the kidney as well: EP1, EP2, EP3, and EP4. They are localized both on glomerular vessels (EP1, EP2, and EP4) and on different parts of the tubule (EP1, EP3, and EP4). Overexpression of some prostaglandin receptors (EP2 and EP4) has been demonstrated in the glomerular afferent vessels of the developmental kidney, allowing for increased activity of vasodilator prostanoids. The vasodilation of the afferent arteriole via these receptors is the way by which prostaglandins counteract the high vascular resistance generated by the ANG II-mediated vasoconstriction of efferent arteriola. It is the main mechanism for maintaining glomerular filtration in fetal and early postnatal life. Overexpression of the tubular EP3 receptor (located in the distal tubule and collecting duct) is needed for amniotic fluid formation and to excrete water during the first days of life (63–65). In addition, it has been postulated that the downregulation of the apical collecting duct water channel AQP2 also results in the excretion of hypotonic urine in utero and during the first days of life (66,67). Embryonic calcium-sensing receptor expression is another mechanism involved in the blockade of arginine vasopressin action, resulting in hypotonic urine, during antenatal life (68).

NONSTEROIDAL ANTI-INFLAMMATORY DRUGS AND RENAL ADVERSE EFFECTS

NSAIDs inhibit the enzymatic activity of both COX-1 and COX-2 and thereby block the formation of prostanoids (56). COX-2-selective NSAIDs as well as the conventional nonselective NSAIDs such as indomethacin may cause a reversible decline in GFR and renal perfusion (69). Experimental data have also shown that endogenous PGE_2 downregulates inducible nitric oxide synthase (iNOS) induction and that the decrease of PGE_2 production by indomethacin COX inhibition results in enhancement of interleukin-1β-induced steady-state iNOS mRNA levels and NO production in mesangial cells (70). Although it has not yet been demonstrated in glomerular vessels, this mechanism highlights a possible feedback mechanism that could exist between prostaglandins and NO, as has been shown for ANG II.

In the perinatal period, NSAIDs are used (a) as a tocolytic agent, (b) for closure of a PDA, and (c) to reduce polyuria in patients with congenital salt-losing tubulopathies.

Numerous case reports have shown transient fetal/neonatal oliguria following exposure to nonselective NSAIDs (13,71–73). In addition, Butler-O'Hara et al. (74) reported a significant prolonged rise in plasma creatinine in infants exposed prenatally to indomethacin. Moreover, Allegaert et al. showed that prophylactic administration of ibuprofen or acetylsalicylic acid had the same impact (20% reduction) on the clearance of aminoglycosides in the preterm neonate (75). NSAIDs may even cause fatal renal failure in the neonate (73). The renal pathology associated with this antenatal NSAIDs exposure is characterized by small and immature glomeruli and cystic dilations in the renal cortex (13,73). Whether these functional and histologic changes can also be attributed to an imbalance of vasodilatory prostanoids and vasoconstrictive agents needs to be demonstrated.

The availability of COX-2-selective inhibitors made some investigators believe that the detrimental effects of the nonselective NSAIDs possibly could be related to inhibition of COX-1, and that administration of COX-2-selective inhibitors would not result in perinatal renal impairment (76). However, following this initial enthusiasm about the fact that COX-2 inhibitors could be renal sparing in the perinatal period, data from recent studies have shown severe fetal oliguria (77) and even fatal renal failure in neonates antenatally exposed to the COX-2-selective inhibitor nimesulide (14,78). This might even indicate that COX-2 is more essential for normal renal development and function than COX-1. In rodents, the essential role of COX-2, but not COX-1, for proper renal development during the perinatal period has been well established, indicating that COX-2 might be more essential for normal renal development and function than COX-1 (79–82).

Based on the current literature, NSAIDs should not be used during renal development. However, indomethacin is still frequently prescribed to inhibit preterm uterine contractions before week 34 of gestation. Short-term exposure to indomethacin leads to a reduction of the GFR, whereas conflicting data exist about the effect on the GFR after long-term exposure (72,83–87). Animal studies have indicated that the inhibition of prostaglandin synthesis by indomethacin increases renal vascular resistance (88). This subsequently results in an impaired renal blood flow and a concomitant reduction in the GFR (88). To investigate the impact of prenatal exposure to betamethasone and indomethacin on the pharmacokinetics of ceftazidime, 136 preterm infants were studied (28). Twenty-five of these infants were treated with indomethacin alone, and 21 infants were treated with both indomethacin and betamethasone. The results of this study clearly demonstrated that prenatal exposure to indomethacin alone significantly decreases ceftazidime clearance and increases serum half-life of ceftazidime. The coadministration of betamethasone prevented these changes. These results indicate that after prenatal exposure to indomethacin alone, additional dosage adjustments are indicated (28).

NSAID-induced reduction of neonatal GFR is an important example that in utero exposure to drugs can have a profound effect on the pharmacokinetics of drugs administered to the newborn infant. Prescribing clinicians should be aware of possible fetal drug exposure and its potential consequences on neonatal renal clearing capacity.

THE EFFECT OF POSTNATAL AGE ON THE GLOMERULAR FILTRATION RATE

It is recommended not to adjust dosage regimens for therapeutic agents during the first 4 weeks of life (89). Despite the fact that these recommendations are derived from studies that did not stratify infants according to postnatal age, this recommendation was made on the assumption that no significant postnatal increment in GFR has been documented in preterm infants. Previous studies on the postnatal development of GFR in preterm infants indeed show conflicting data (4,6,25,90,91). However, several investigators reported the presence of a significant increase in the GFR in the first 10 days after birth (4,6,90). This postnatal age-dependent increase in GFR could be used to predict the pharmacokinetics of drugs that are mainly eliminated by glomerular filtration.

Recent data indicate that there is a significant increase in GFR postnatally (92). GFR values in infants increase with a mean of 0.19 mL per min during the 7-day period between day 3 and day 10 after birth. In utero the weekly increase is 0.035 mL per min (27). This indicates that the postnatal increase of the GFR between days 3 and 10 after birth is 5.4 times higher compared to the intrauterine changes. Therefore, postnatal age seems to be associated with an acceleration of the maturation of the GFR. Our studies showed that this increase in the GFR resulted in a significant increase in the clearance of ceftazidime (92). These findings are consistent with the results of some investigators (93,94), whereas other studies could not find any relation with postnatal age (95,96). Kenyon et al. (96) reported that postnatal renal function maturation exerts a significant influence on the developmental pharmacokinetics of amikacin. These authors speculated, however, that the rapid maturation of the renal function in the first week of life is not present in the extremely preterm population. We showed that the rapid postnatal change in the GFR is also present in very young preterm infants and is primarily responsible for the increase in the clearance of ceftazidime (92). Dosage adjustments seem therefore already indicated during the first weeks of life despite the current recommendation not to adjust dosage regimens for therapeutic agents during the first 4 weeks of life.

THE EFFECT OF A PATENT DUCTUS ARTERIOSUS AND POSTNATAL ADMINISTRATION OF INDOMETHACIN OR IBUPROFEN ON THE GLOMERULAR FILTRATION RATE

PDA is a common clinical problem among preterm infants (97). The ductus arteriosus is a normal fetal vascular connection between the left pulmonary artery and the descending aorta. In utero, the ductus serves to allow the majority of blood flow leaving the right ventricle to circumvent the high-resistance pulmonary circulation and flow directly into the descending aorta. This directs oxygen-deprived blood to flow toward the placenta, the fetal source for reoxygenation. After birth, the elimination of the low-resistance placenta results in an increase in systemic vascular resistance, and the exchange of air for fluid in the lungs creates decreased pulmonary resistance. Constriction of the ductus arteriosus and functional closure generally are spontaneous after birth, redirecting blood flow toward the lungs, which then assumes oxygenation. Factors crucial to the closure of this vessel appear to be oxygen tension, concentrations of circulating prostaglandins, and available muscle mass in the ductus. In preterm infants, higher circulating concentrations of prostaglandins, an immature ductus, and/or an immature respiratory system contribute to continued patency of the ductus (97). After birth, the increased systemic vascular resistance combined with the fall in pulmonary vascular resistance result in a shift of blood flow across the ductus from what previously was a right-to-left shunt (before birth) to a left-to-right shunt (after birth) if the ductus remains patent. This hemodynamic change can lead to a left ventricular overload, increased left-ventricular end-diastolic pressure and volume, increased left atrial pressure, and congestive heart failure (97). The physiologic consequences of PDA relate primarily to hypoxia, hypoperfusion, fluid overload, and acidosis (97,98). Although pharmacokinetic studies directly examining the differences between newborns with and without PDAs are sparse, potential pharmacokinetic changes can be easily predicted. A complicating factor, however, is the varying degree to which these changes occur among neonates with PDA, obviously leading to quite variable drug disposition. Our data showed that a PDA and postnatal exposure to indomethacin altered the aforementioned rapid postnatal increase in GFR (92). This phenomenon will probably delay the need for dosage adjustment during the first 2 postnatal weeks in these preterm infants.

The volume of drug distribution may be altered in neonates with a PDA. Drugs that distribute primarily into body water may demonstrate an increased volume of distribution, as fluid overload is common in newborns with PDA. The presence of acidosis may decrease protein binding of some drugs (e.g., theophylline) and consequently increase volume of distribution (99). Concurrent acidosis may alter the ionization of agents with a pK_a close to 7.4 (e.g., phenobarbital), permitting increased concentrations of unionized molecules that are available to cross biological membranes more freely and potentially distribute more extensively into tissue (100). Comparisons of neonatal pharmacokinetic data reveal that volume of distribution apparently is increased in the presence of a PDA for several drugs (101–103).

In healthy newborns, elimination of most drugs is usually diminished because of immature excretory functions. In the presence of a hemodynamically significant PDA, decreased renal and hepatic blood flow can be anticipated, potentially leading to further reductions in drug elimination capacity (98). The interpretation of drug clearance data in neonates with PDA often is confounded by the effects of mechanical ventilation, indomethacin or ibuprofen therapy, or surgical ligation, which may also influence blood flow to the liver and the kidneys (92,101–104).

The pharmacologic treatment of PDA with indomethacin further confounds pharmacokinetic interpretations because drug disposition changes related to drug interactions may be difficult to separate from those altered by the underlying disease state (92,104). The apparent accumulation of digoxin, gentamicin, amikacin, and vancomycin with concurrent use of indomethacin appears to be the consequence of the dual effect of decreasing renal elimination secondary to indomethacin and decreased volume of distribution once the PDA closes. As either or both interactions may play a role, drug concentrations should be monitored closely when indomethacin therapy is started and after it is discontinued.

Other NSAIDs have also been used to treat PDA in preterm infants but were associated with adverse effects, as in the case of sulindac (105) and mefenamic acid (106), or were less effective than indomethacin at closing the duct, as was shown for acetylsalicylic acid (107).

A relevant number of studies with ibuprofen for the treatment of PDA in preterm infants have been performed in the meanwhile. However, it was concluded from studies in neonates that ibuprofen as compared with indomethacin is effective at closing the duct and is associated with fewer cerebral and renal adverse effects (12,108–110). These conclusions are under debate based on animal studies that did not show any difference in renal side effects between animals treated with ibuprofen and those treated with indomethacin (10). Another large-scale randomized, controlled trial in preterm infants is being conducted aiming at several unresolved issues including very limited information on the pharmacokinetics of ibuprofen in the preterm neonate (104,111,112).

Drug disposition may be altered by the presence of a PDA and/or concomitant use of indomethacin. Close therapeutic drug monitoring is indicated because the changes in drug disposition may be abrupt with PDA closure or initiation of indomethacin therapy (92,104). More recent data have shown that the impact of prophylactic or therapeutic administration of ibuprofen on aminoglycoside or glycopeptides clearance is of a similar magnitude (113).

THE EFFECT OF DOPAMINE ADMINISTRATION ON THE GLOMERULAR FILTRATION RATE

Dopamine has been widely used in neonatal intensive care for the treatment of hypotension or oliguria in sick preterm infants (114–117). Through stimulation of the adrenergic and dopaminergic receptors, dopamine exerts dose-dependent cardiovascular, renal, and endocrine effects that combat the clinical manifestations of shock. This discussion will be focused on the renal effects of dopamine therapy.

As long as renal perfusion pressure is within the autoregulatory range, the direct tubular rather than the renal hemodynamic action of dopamine is mostly responsible for the diuretic and saluretic effects of the drug (116). These effects are brought about by activation of the renal tubular dopamine receptors along the nephron. Data indicate the presence and functional integrity of these receptors and postreceptor mechanisms in the human kidney from as early as week 24 of gestation (114–116). Through selective activation of the renal vascular DA_1 and DA_2 receptors, low doses of dopamine induce an approximately 20% to 40% increase in renal blood flow without significantly influencing systemic blood pressure

(118). Whole-kidney GFR shows a variable, approximately 5% to 20% rise (118). Findings of micropuncture studies indicate that the mechanism of the drug-induced increase in the GFR is the enhancement of glomerular ultrafiltration pressure caused by a more pronounced vasodilation of the afferent than the efferent arteriole (119).

In cases of aminoglycoside toxicity, dopamine, by increasing renal blood flow and GFR, may be useful in facilitating renal excretion of these antibiotics. Dopamine also modifies the renal effects of furosemide and indomethacin (120,121). The recently discovered mechanisms of the renal actions of dopamine enable us to better understand the cellular basis and nature of these interactions. Independent of age and maturation, dopamine enhances the diuretic effect of furosemide in the anuric–oliguric patient (120). This interaction is thought to be the consequence of the dopamine-induced selective augmentation of medullary circulation and thus the enhancement of the delivery of furosemide to its site of action in the kidney (120). Inhibition of prostaglandin synthesis by indomethacin may cause severe, although usually transient, renal side effects in preterm infants and volume-depleted children. Although these findings need to be confirmed, dopamine attenuates the indomethacin-induced decrease in urine output and sodium excretion in sick preterm infants with PDA (121). However, the renal vasoconstrictive actions of indomethacin have not been reported to be influenced by dopamine (121). Dopamine interacts with the renal prostaglandin system mainly at the tubular level (122), and it is not surprising that the renal tubular but not the vascular actions of indomethacin are attenuated by the drug. This is further supported by a recent Cochrane analysis showing that there is no evidence from randomized trials to support the use of dopamine to prevent renal dysfunction (primarily GFR) in indomethacin-treated preterm infants and the lack of effect of dopamine administration on amikacin clearance (123,124).

In conclusion, the administration of dopamine will enhance the renal clearing capacity of the preterm infant and can attenuate the detrimental side effects of high levels of potentially nephrotoxic drugs (i.e., aminoglycosides, indomethacin). Whether it should be administered prophylactically as a protective agent during, for example, indomethacin treatment needs to be prospectively validated. Moreover, the effect of dopamine administration on recommended dosing schemes of, for example, antibacterial agents have not been studied. The clinician should be aware that the use of dopamine might lead to subtherapeutic drug concentrations due to the increase in GFR.

THE EFFECT OF FUROSEMIDE ADMINISTRATION ON THE GLOMERULAR FILTRATION RATE

Furosemide, a loop diuretic, is frequently administered to critically ill newborn infants to augment urine output and relieve pulmonary edema. Furosemide acts on the luminal side of the renal tubule at the thick ascending limb or the loop of Henle (125). It inhibits chloride reabsorption, thereby inhibiting passive reabsorption of sodium, and must be cleared by the kidney into the tubular fluid to exert its diuretic effect (126). Because the diuretic effect of furosemide is directly related to the renal tubular drug concentration, its effectiveness is correlated with the degree of renal function (126). In addition to the distal action, free water clearance is increased by an inhibition of carbonic anhydrase activity in the proximal tubule (127).

A number of hemodynamic responses contribute to the diuretic action of furosemide. Total renal vascular blood flow is increased (128), renal cortical blood flow is redistributed, and renin secretion is stimulated from the juxtaglomerular cells to the kidney (129). The mechanisms controlling each of these responses to furosemide are only partially defined but appear to be mediated, at least in part, through the prostaglandin system, which is activated almost immediately after furosemide administration (130). In a very recent study in critically ill pediatric patients, furosemide was observed to induce a prompt and generalized increase of the arachidonic acid-derived prostaglandins concomitant with increased renin production (131). Furosemide-induced increased prostaglandins may have played an integral role in the causation of the ensuing hemodynamic, diuretic, and neurohormonal changes. There is evidence to support the theory that furosemide increases renin release through an increase in renal prostaglandins (132). Diuresis may occur in response to increased renal blood flow induced by the increase in renal prostaglandin production. Furosemide causes a rapid diuresis in newborns of all GAs after parenteral administration. In premature infants, the onset of action is evident within 1 hour, but peak diuresis does not occur until 1 to 3 hours after dosing, with a duration of diuresis of approximately 6 hours (133). In very low-birth-weight infants, the plasma half-life exceeds 24 hours, and accumulation of furosemide to potentially ototoxic levels can occur when the drug is administered every 12 hours (134). By stimulating prostaglandin synthesis at both vascular and tubular sites in the kidney, furosemide prevents the occurrence of both the renal hemodynamic and the tubular side effects of indomethacin (135). However, the long-term furosemide administration also increases the occurrence of PDA in preterm infants (136), so extensive use of this drug may not be prudent in preterm infants treated with indomethacin to close their duct. In addition, it was recently shown in a study of critically ill pediatric infants that administration of furosemide can induce a decrease in cardiac output and an increase in systemic vascular resistance, potentially increasing the risk for paradoxical pulmonary edema (131). The clinician needs to consider such hemodynamic alterations when administering furosemide in critically ill preterm infants. As an alternative, a continuous infusion with furosemide may perhaps lead to more controlled diuresis with fewer hemodynamic alterations. Very recently this suggestion has been investigated in near-term neonates on extracorporeal membrane oxygenation (137). Clearly, this way of administering furosemide needs clinical investigation in preterm neonates.

ASSESSMENT OF GLOMERULAR FILTRATION RATE

Creatinine clearance remains a widely used clinical tool for evaluating renal glomerular function. Many years ago, creatinine was chosen for clinical clearance determination because serum creatinine can be easily measured in the laboratory and creatinine is totally filtered at the glomerulus, not reabsorbed by the renale tubule, and only slightly secreted by the tubular cells. Creatinine clearance is an excellent endogenous estimate of glomerular filtration in children. However, measures of renal clearance using creatinine clearance do not account for tubular secretion or reabsorption of drugs. Unfortunately, quantitative measures of the relative contributions of tubular and glomerular function are not available for most drugs, and creatinine clearance remains the only guiding factor for drug dosing in renal failure.

To measure GFR for research purposes, the clearance of exogenously infused inulin is used (91,93,138). In the neonate, as in all young children, the creatinine clearance is cumbersome and is unreliable unless a bladder catheterization is used to ensure an accurate, timed urine collection. This invasive procedure is not indicated for routine use in clinical practice. Therefore, it has become standard of care to follow renal function in neonates using repeated serum creatinine concentrations. Reference values for serum creatinine values are provided in Table 16.1 (3,138). Unfortunately, serum creatinine concentrations in the first 3 weeks of life are not reliable. At birth, serum creatinine is high, reflecting maternal concentrations. During the first week of life, the highest concentrations are observed in the most premature infants (3). In term neonates, serum creatinine decreases rapidly to reach stable neonatal levels close to 0.4 mg per dL by 1 to 2 weeks of age. In very premature infants, there is a transient increase in serum creatinine with a peak on day 4 (143) followed by a progressive decline toward normal neonatal values by 3 to 4 weeks of life (Fig. 16.1). This decline is probably caused by the tubular reabsorption of creatinine, as observed in newborn rabbits, before the completion of nephrogenesis (144). This transient increase in serum creatinine might be the consequence of passive back diffusion of creatinine across leaky tubules (145). Finally, it is important to use an appropriate assay for creatinine assessment to prevent interferences with cephalosporins, bilirubin, and ketoacids in the neonate (146). The practical conclusion, therefore, is that repeated determinations of serum creatinine is the only clinically applicable, but a less than ideal, measure of neonatal glomerular function immediately after birth. Serum creatinine concentrations

TABLE 16.1 Reference Values of Plasma Creatinine Concentrations in the Newborn

References	*Gestational Age (wk)*	*Postnatal Age*	*n*	*Creatinine Concentration (μmol/L)*
139	28–32	4–5 d	7	60 (54–85)[a]
		8–10 d	5	73 (65–86)[a]
	33–37	4–5 d	13	63 (60–70)[a]
		8–10 d	6	53 (50–60)[a]
140	25–28	1 wk	10	123 ± 70[b]
		2–8 wk	26	79 ± 44[b]
		>8 wk	9	35 ± 18[b]
	29–34	1 wk	27	79 ± 26[b]
		2–8 wk	27	62 ± 26[b]
		>8 wk	1	31
141	30–40	6–30 d	34	35 (12–62)[a]
142	26–34	1 wk	34	97 (69–141)[c]
		2 wk	34	70 (45–99)[c]
		3–4 wk	34	57 (39–71)[c]
		5–6 wk	34	51 (42–62)[c]
		7–9 wk	34	44 (39–48)[c]
3	28–31	1–2 d	11	95 ± 5[d]
		8–9 d	10	64 ± 5[d]
		15–16 d	8	49 ± 4[d]
		22–23 d	8	35 ± 3[d]
	32–34	1–2 d	15	90 ± 5[d]
		8–9 d	11	58 ± 7[d]
		15–16 d	11	50 ± 8[d]
		22–23 d	9	30 ± 2[d]
138	<28	3 d	26	92 ± 24[b]
	28–32	3 d	76	77 ± 21[b]
	28–32	3 d	42	64 ± 19[b]

[a]Median and range.
[b]Mean and standard deviation.
[c]Mean and 10th–90th percentile.
[d]Mean and the standard error of the mean.

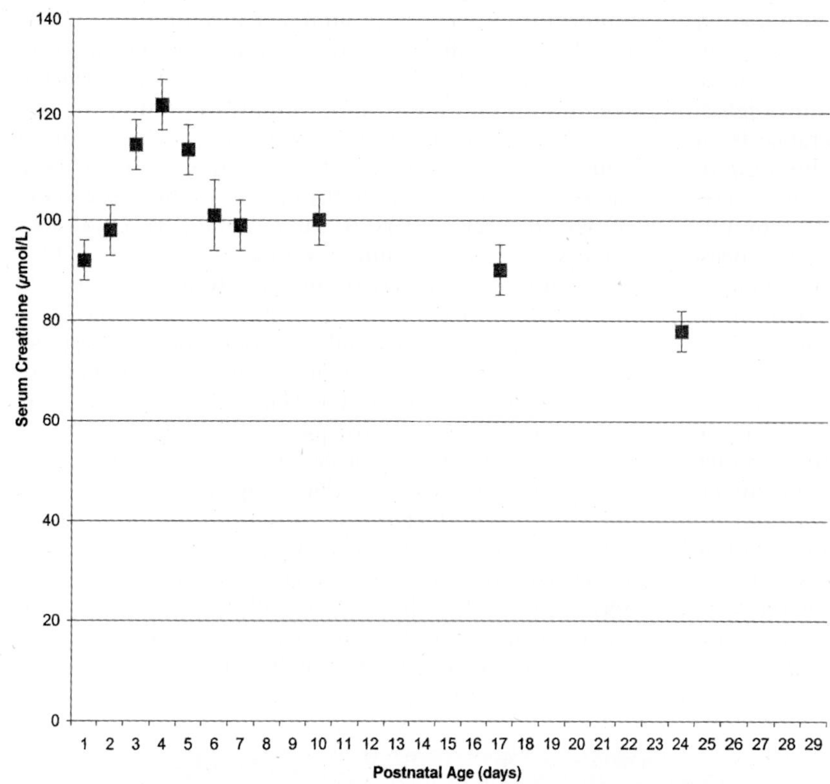

Figure 16.1. Serum creatinine values in 15 preterm infants with gestational ages of less than 26 weeks during the first 28 days of life (van den Anker JN, unpublished data, 2006).

must be interpreted in the context of the clinical renal status of the newborn. Recently, blood levels of cystatin C, a 13-kDa protein produced at a constant rate by all nucleated cells, have been used as a marker for GFR (147–150). However, insufficient data are available to recommend the routine use of cystatin C levels for everyday use in determining neonatal GFR (151).

DRUG TRANSPORTERS AND RENAL TUBULAR SECRETION OF DRUGS

The term drug transporter refers to a protein that affects how drugs get in or out of cells. Secretion or reabsorption of compounds may be against a concentration gradient. Therefore, adenosine triphosphate (ATP) must be consumed by ATPases to produce energy needed for the uphill flow. The movement of molecules that requires ATP consumption is referred to as active transport, whereas passive transport is not energy dependent. Sometimes exchanger proteins are required that replace one ion or atom with another to provide enough substrate to drive cotransport, or to maintain isoelectricity or pH. Cotransporters move two molecules in the same direction across cell membranes. Countertransporters move two molecules in opposite directions. The sodium/hydrogen (Na^+/H^+) antiporter is one such transporter which exchanges sodium for hydrogen ions.

A variety of human transport proteins have been cloned, including proteins for the transport of organic cations [human organic cation transporter (OCT) 1, human OCT2, human OCT3] (152,153); proton–organic cation exchangers [organic cation transporter novel type (OCTN) 1, OCTN2] (152,154); a protein for transport of neutral and cationic hydrophobic compounds, the ATP-dependent drug efflux protein [multidrug resistance (MDR) 1-type P-glycoprotein] (155); proteins for the transport of organic anions, including a sodium-independent organic anion transport protein (OATP) (156); nucleoside transporters (sodium-dependent purine nucleoside transporter); concentrative nucleoside transporter (CNT) 1 and CNT2 (157,158); a prostaglandin transporter (159); and proteins for the transport of anionic conjugates, such as the ATP-dependent drug efflux transporters [MRP1, MRP2, canalicular multispecific organic anion transporter (cMOAT), MRP3/cMOAT3, MRP6] (160,161), often referred to as glutathione S-conjugates (162).

It must be remembered that for renal tubular secretion to occur, a molecule must first pass from the extracellular fluid (ECF) (blood) into the renal tubular cell, and then from the renal tubular cell into the tubular lumen to be excreted in the urine. Thus, two distinct transporters are required, one at the basolateral membrane of the tubular cell to accept molecules from blood and one at the apical (brush border) membrane to mediate the exit of the molecule into the tubular lumen (urine).

TRANSPORTERS AT THE BASOLATERAL MEMBRANE

A proton concentration gradient exists among the three compartments involved in renal drug secretion. The concentration of protons is greater in the urine and lowest in the ECF. Furthermore, an electrical gradient is maintained between the renal tubular lumen (0 mV), renal tubular cell (−70 mV), and blood (−3 mV). The basolateral membrane is in contact with the ECF. Electrogenic pH-independent transport systems located here are able to transport organic cations from ECF into the renal tubular cells (163,164). The transporters are believed to be the proteins coded by the OCT1, OCT2, and OCT3 genes. These OCTs are supposed to mediate the first step in organic cation secretion from the blood into the renal tubule and translocate a variety of organic cations such as endogenous cationic metabolites, monoamine transmitters, cationic drugs, and xenobiotics. Recently, polymorphisms in OCT2 have been linked to adversely affected transporter function, indicating that future studies in humans with OCT2 variants will elucidate the relationship between genetic variation in OCT2 and renal drug elimination and toxicities (165).

At the brush border membrane is a proposed electroneutral pH-dependent hydrogen/organic cation antiporter system energized by the transmembrane hydrogen gradient that is sustained by an Na^+/H^+exchanger and/or hydrogen ATPase. Thus, organic cation transport is mediated by a variety of transmembrane proteins that either sustain or depend on both a pH and an electrical gradient.

Organic anions are able to enter renal tubular cells from the ECF via the dicarboxylate–organic anion exchanger (166). This entry of anions is coupled with a sodium–dicarboxylate (α-ketoglutarate) exchanger, which moves dicarboxylates outward. This exchange process constitutes the first step in the proximal tubular excretion of a large number of organic anions, including widely used drugs such as ACE inhibitors (captoprilate, enalaprilat), angiotensin-receptor blockers (losartan and related compounds), β-lactam antibiotics (penicillins, cephalosporins), antiviral drugs (e.g., acyclovir, amantadine, azidothymidine), diuretics (bumetanide, furosemide, thiazides), sedatives (barbiturates), NSAIDs (e.g., acetylsalicylate, diclofenac, ibuprofen), and a number of test agents such as *p*-aminohippurate, phenol red, and some X-ray contrast agents (156,167,168). These examples underline the physiologic and pharmacologic importance of proximal tubules in the handling of organic anions of diverse chemical structures. The process is driven by an inward sodium gradient established by a sodium–potassium ATPase.

TRANSPORTER AT THE APICAL (BRUSH BORDER) MEMBRANE

The apical membrane is on the luminal side of the tubular cell and thus is in contact with urine. At the luminal membrane, organic cations are exchanged with protons from the urine by transporters such as OCTN1 and OCTN2. Although OCTN2 is coupled with sodium-independent OAT, there also appears to be a sodium-dependent, high-affinity carnitine transport function. Protons for these exchangers are supplied by an Na^+/H^+ antiporter and hydrogen-ATPases. Organic anions that have been exchanged with dicarboxylic acid at the basal membranes are believed to be excreted into urine by two postulated mechanisms. Either a potential-sensitive facilitated diffusion system or a hydroxyl ion exchanger may lead to organic anion elimination. Such a hydroxyl exchange pump is believed to be coded by the OATP gene (156). Although a variety of apical anion transport proteins have been cloned, their functions are not well understood. Peptide transporters (PEPTs) involved in the absorption of oligopeptides are also expressed in the apical membrane. These PEPTs are involved in the electrogenic hydrogen-coupled cotransport of dipeptides and tripeptides. The drive for this comes from an inward hydrogen gradient and a negative transmembrane potential difference. Two homologous PEPTs have been described, PEPT1 and PEPT2, with the latter showing higher affinity for a variety of substrates. PEPTs mediate transport of peptide-like drugs, including β-lactam antibiotics, ACE inhibitors, and the dipeptide chemotherapeutic drug bestatin (152). They are located at the brush border membrane.

Amphipathic anionic conjugates such as glucuronide, sulfate, and glutathione S-conjugates are believed to be moved by ATP-dependent pumps called glutathione S-conjugate export (GS-X) pumps, which belong to the ABC (ATP-binding cassette) family of transporters. The ABC family of transport proteins includes MRP, the cystic fibrosis transmembrane regulator, and P-glycoprotein. GS-X pumps are forms of MRP, and two isoforms have been identified, MRP1 at the basolateral membrane and MRP2 and cMOAT at the apical membrane. These ATP-dependent pumps are able to move conjugated drugs within renal tubular cells either into the urine or back to the ECF. There is also evidence to suggest that cisplatin and daunorubicin may be handled by GS-X transporters (169).

By now, the role of P-glycoprotein and its overexpression in tumor cells that respond poorly to chemotherapy is well known. Recent data suggest that the P-glycoprotein plays an important role in the renal handling of drugs. Also known as MDR, P-glycoprotein is an ATP-dependent, 170-kDa-membrane glycoprotein that belongs to the ABC family of transport proteins. Two human isoforms of P-glycoprotein have been identified: MDR1 can be found on the apical membrane of renal tubular cells and MDR3 is found mostly in liver cells (169). Although the exact mechanism of drug translocation by P-glycoprotein MDR1 is speculative, it is known that drug transport is unidirectional into the urine. In a landmark study by Schinkel et al. (170), genetically altered knockout mice without the MDR1α gene (the murine equivalent to human MDR1) had plasma concentrations of a variety of drugs that were two to three times higher than those measured in the wild-type mice, which expressed *mdr1α* (170).

CLINICAL SIGNIFICANCE OF RENAL TUBULAR SECRETORY MECHANISMS

Drugs can affect the renal excretion of other drugs leading to pharmacokinetic drug interactions. The full spectrum of mechanisms for drug-induced alterations in renal drug clearance is not fully known. However, if two drugs are eliminated through the same tubular secretion protein, then one or both drugs may have reduced excretion,

TABLE 16.2 Renal Tubular Pharmacokinetic Interactions in the Newborn

Transporter	*Sample Drug*	*Precipitant*[a]	*Effect of Interaction*
Organic anion	Benzyl penicillin	Probenecid	Increased penicillin levels
Organic cation	Triamterene	Histamine-2 blockers	Decreased triamterene secretion
P-glycoprotein	Digoxin	Quinidine	Increased digoxin levels

[a]Refers to a drug that causes an alteration of the action or pharmacokinetics of another drug.

TABLE 16.3 Precipitant Drugs in Tubular Secretion-Related Pharmacokinetic Drug Interactions in the Newborn

Amphotericin B
Cephalosporins
Cimetidine
Nonsteroidal anti-inflammatory drugs
Penicillins
Probenecid
Salicylates
Thiazides

TABLE 16.4 Human Organic Anion Transport Proteins Relevant to the Newborn

Transporter	*Substrates*
OAT1	NSAIDs, uric acid, β-lactam antibiotics, and prostaglandin E_2
OAT2	Salicylates and prostaglandin E_2
OAT3	Cimetidine
PEPT1	β-Lactam antibiotics, ACE inhibitors, and valacyclovir
PEPT2	β-Lactam antibiotics and ACE inhibitors
PGT	Prostanoids

ACE, angiotensin-converting enzyme; NSAIDs, nonsteroidal anti-inflammatory drugs; OAT, organic anion transporter; PEPT, peptide transporter; PGT, prostaglandin transporter.

TABLE 16.5 Human Renal Organic Cation Transport Proteins Relevant to the Newborn

Transporter	*Substrates*
OCT1	Dopamine
OCT2	Dopamine, epinephrine, norepinephrine
OCTN1	L-Carnitine, quinidine, verapamil
OCTN2	L-Carnitine

OCT, organic cationic transporter; OCTN, organic cationic transporter novel type.

increased serum levels, and thus a greater chance for causing side effects. Examples of such interactions in the newborn are outlined in Table 16.2. There is also the possibility that a drug may induce or inhibit the expression or function of a particular transport protein. A drug that can cause an altered action or elimination of another drug is often called the precipitant drug in a drug–drug interaction. Table 16.3 lists some examples of common precipitant drugs implicated in drug interactions due to altered active tubular secretion used in the neonatal period.

Tables 16.4 and 16.5 provide a summary of the major cloned human renal tubular transport systems, grouped as having either anionic or cationic substrates, that are relevant to the neonate. Knowing the basic properties of these transport systems may be useful in predicting potential drug interactions. Methotrexate and NSAIDs are organic anions believed to be transported by OAT1. Animal models suggest that OATs are involved in the methotrexate–NSAID interaction (171). Trimethoprim, procainamide, triamterene, and histamine-2 receptor antagonists appear to interact via OCTs. Cimetidine and trimethoprim can inhibit renal secretion of procainamide, whereas ranitidine and famotidine can inhibit renal secretion of triamterene (156).

THE IMPORTANCE OF RENAL P-GLYCOPROTEIN

Immunohistochemical studies reveal that P-glycoprotein is localized at the apical brush border membrane of the proximal renal tubule, which is the major site of renal secretion. The finding of the localization of renal P-glycoprotein has led to recognition of the importance of this transporter in tubular secretion of drugs. MDR1-type P-glycoprotein has been shown to transport a variety of drugs including vinca alkaloids, cyclosporine, colchicine, tacrolimus, anthracyclines, etoposide, verapamil, diltiazem, nifedipine, propafenone, digoxin, chloroquine, and protease inhibitors, including saquinavir, ritonavir, and nelfinavir (172–175).

Inhibition and induction of cytochrome P450 (CYP) enzymes, particularly CYP3A4, are probably the most common causes for documented drug interactions (176). Therefore, CYP-mediated drug interactions have always been a major concern for clinicians and patients. Like CYP-mediated drug interactions, P-glycoprotein-mediated drug interactions may be anticipated when P-glycoprotein substrates and P-glycoprotein inhibitors (or inducers) are coadministered. Inhibition and induction of P-glycoprotein

TABLE 16.6	P-Glycoprotein Substrates in the Newborn
Cimetidine	
Dexamethasone	
Digoxin	
Morphine	
Nifedipine	
Erythromycin	
Hydrocortisone	
Lidocaine	
Propanolol	

have been reported and their pharmacokinetic consequences are similar to those observed for inhibition and induction of CYP enzymes.

Serum digoxin levels may be increased due to reduced renal secretion of digoxin via P-glycoprotein interactions with quinidine (177), verapamil (175,178), clarithromycin (179), propafenone (180), and cyclosporine (181). Cyclosporine may also lead to increased etoposide levels (182).

Tacrolimus concentrations may be raised by diltiazem (183) and reduced by rifampin (184). Early evidence suggests that P-glycoprotein activity and expression can be affected by a variety of drugs including calcium channel blockers and immunomodulators (185). It is an interesting point that many of these unrelated compounds are also substrates for CYP3A4. The inhibition of P-glycoprotein-mediated vinblastine efflux by grapefruit juice components has been reported (186). Grapefruit juice components appear to inhibit P-glycoprotein to the same degree as CYP3A4 (187). Tables 16.6 through 15.8 list drugs used in the neonatal period that are P-glycoprotein substrates, inducers, and inhibitors, respectively.

SUMMARY

Renal clearance of drugs in the newborn is a complex dynamic process involving filtration, secretion, and reabsorption. The clinical importance of renal tubular transport systems is not limited to drug interactions and toxicity. With the advent of new molecular biology techniques, greater knowledge of the molecular transport of drugs within the renal tubular cells has become possible. An understanding of the secretory mechanisms may be useful in predicting drug pharmacokinetics and potential drug interactions in the newborn. The discovery of P-glycoprotein within the renal tubular cell luminal membrane is of particular importance because it offers an explanation for a variety of well-known drug interactions, such as that between digoxin and quinidine, whose mechanisms, until now, had not been understood. Once additional transport mechanisms are identified, specific pharmacologic agents may be selected to predictably alter pharmacokinetics in the hope of increasing drug efficacy, minimizing toxicity, and preventing drug interactions. This ultimately will lead to individualized pharmacotherapy for the neonate and result in optimal treatment and improved short- and long-term clinical outcome.

TABLE 16.7	P-Glycoprotein Inducers in the Newborn
Dexamethasone	
Rifampin	

TABLE 16.8	P-Glycoprotein Inhibitors
Nifedipine	
Erythromycin	
Hydrocortisone	
Lidocaine	
Propranolol	
Clarithromycin	
Ketoconazole	
Local anesthetics	

REFERENCES

1. Besunder JB, Reed MD, Blumer JL. Principles of drug biodisposition in the neonate: a critical evaluation of the pharmacokinetic—pharmacodynamic interface (Part 1). *Clin Pharmacokinet* 1988;4:189–216.
2. Van den Anker JN. Pharmacokinetics and renal function in preterm infants. *Acta Paediatr* 1996;85:1393–1399.
3. Bueva A, Guignard JP. Renal function in preterm neonates. *Pediatr Res* 1994;36:572–577.
4. Coulthard MG. Maturation of glomerular filtration in preterm and mature babies. *Early Hum Dev* 1985;11:281–292.
5. Arant BS Jr. Developmental patterns of renal functional maturation compared in the human neonate. *J Pediatr* 1978;92:705–712.
6. Drukker A, Guignard JP. Renal aspects of the term and preterm infant: a selective update. *Curr Opin Pediatr* 2002;14:175–182.
7. Burckhardt BC, Burckhardt G. Transport of organic anions across the basolateral membrane of proximal tubule cells. *Rev Physiol Biochem Pharmacol* 2003;146:95–158.
8. Perri D, Ito S, Rowsell V, et al. The kidney—the body's playground for drugs: an overview of renal drug handling with selected clinical correlates. *Can J Clin Pharmacol* 2003;10:17–23.
9. Toth-Heyn P, Drukker A, Guignard JP. The stressed neonatal kidney: from pathophysiology to clinical management of neonatal vasomotor nephropathy. *Pediatr Nephrol* 2000;14:227–239.
10. Chamaa NS, Mosig D, Drukker A, et al. The renal hemodynamic effect of ibuprofen in the newborn rabbit. *Pediatr Res* 2000;48:600–605.
11. Drukker A, Mosig D, Guignard JP. The renal hemodynamic effects of aspirin in newborn and young adult rabbits. *Pediatr Nephrol* 2001;16:713–718.
12. Van Overmeire B, Smets K, Lecoutere D, et al. A comparison of ibuprofen and indomethacin for closure of patent ductus arteriosus. *N Engl J Med* 2000;343:674–681.
13. Kaplan BS, Restaino I, Raval DS, et al. Renal failure in the neonate associated with in utero exposure to nonsteroidal anti-inflammatory agents. *Pediatr Nephrol* 1994;8:700–704.
14. Peruzzi L, Gianoglio B, Porcellini MG, et al. Neonatal end-stage renal failure associated with maternal ingestion of cyclooxygenase type 2 selective inhibitor nimesulide as tocolytic. *Lancet* 1999;354:1615.
15. Vasarhelyi B, Toth-Heyn P, Treszl A, et al. Genetic polymorphisms and risks for acute renal failure in preterm neonates. *Pediatr Nephrol* 2005;20:132–135.
16. Treszl A, Kaposi A, Hajdu J, et al. The extent to which genotype information may add to the prediction of disturbed perinatal adaptation: none, minor, or major? *Pediatr Res* 2007;62:610–614.
17. Stapleton FB, Jonse DP, Green RS. Acute renal failure in neonates: incidence, etiology and outcome. *Pediatr Nephrol* 1987;1:314–320.

18. Chevalier RL. Developmental renal physiology of the low birth weight pre-term newborn. *J Urol* 1996;156:714–719.
19. Tack ED, Perlman JM. Renal failure in sick hypertensive premature infants receiving captopril therapy. *J Pediatr* 1988;112: 805–810.
20. Prevot A, Mosig D, Guignard JP. The effects of losartan on renal function in the newborn rabbit. *Pediatr Res* 2002;51:728–732.
21. Nobilis A, Kocsis I, toth-Heyn P, et al. Variance of ACE and AT1 receptor gene does not influence the risk of neonatal acute renal failure. *Pediatr Nephrol* 2001;16:1063–1066.
22. Harding D, Dhamrait S, Marlow N, et al. Angiotensin-converting enzyme DD genotype is associated with worse perinatal cardiorespiratory adaptation in preterm infants. *J Pediatr* 2003;143: 746–749.
23. Thijs A, Thijs LG. Pathogenesis of renal failure in sepsis. *Kidney Int* 1998;66:S34–S37.
24. Treszl A, Toth-Heyn P, Kocsis I, et al. Interleukin genetic variants and the risk of renal failure in infants with infection. *Pediatr Nephrol* 2002;17:713–717.
25. Aperia A, Broberger O, Elinder G, et al. Postnatal development of renal function in pre-term and full-term infants. *Acta Paediatr Scand* 1981;70:183–187.
26. Van der Heijden AJ, Grose WF, Ambagstheer JJ, et al. Glomerular filtration rate in the preterm infant: the relation to gestational and postnatal age. *Eur J Pediatr* 1988;148:24–28.
27. Van den Anker JN, Hop WC, De Groot R, et al. Effects of prenatal exposure to betamethasone and indomethacin on the glomerular filtration rate in the preterm infant. *Pediatr Res* 1994; 36:578–581.
28. Van den Anker JN, Schoemaker RC, Hop WC, et al. Ceftazidine pharmacokinetics in preterm infants: effect of renal function and gestational age. *Clin Pharmacol Ther* 1995;58:650–659.
29. Van den Anker JN, Schoemaker RC, van der Heijden AJ, et al. Once-daily versus twice-daily administration of ceftazidime in the preterm infant. *Antimicrob Agents Chemother* 1995;39:2048–2050.
30. Huisman-de Boer JJ, van den Anker JN, Vogel M, et al. Amoxicillin pharmacokinetics in preterm infants with gestational ages of less than 32 weeks. *Antimicrob Agents Chemother* 1995; 39:431–434.
31. De Hoog M, Mouton JW, Schoemaker RC, et al. Extended-interval dosing of tobramycin in neonates: implications for therapeutic drug monitoring. *Clin Pharmacol Ther* 2002;71:349–358.
32. Treluyer JM, Merle Y, Tonnelier S, et al. Nonparametric population pharmacokinetic analysis of amikacin in neonates, infants, and children. *Antimicrob Agents Chemother* 2002;46:1381–1387.
33. De Hoog M, Schoemaker RC, Mouton JW, et al. Tobramycin population pharmacokinetics in neonates. *Clin Pharmacol Ther* 1997;62:392–399.
34. Rodvold KA, Everett JA, Pryka RD, et al. Pharmacokinetics and administration regimens of vancomycin in neonates, infants and children. *Clin Pharmacokinet* 1997;33:32–51.
35. De Hoog M, Schoemaker RC, Mouton JW, et al. Vancomycin population pharmacokinetics in neonates. *Clin Pharmacol Ther* 2000;67:360–367.
36. Capparelli EV, Lane JR, Romanowski GL, et al. The influences of renal function and maturation on vancomycin elimination in newborns and infants. *J Clin Pharmacol* 2001;41:927–934.
37. Stonestreet BS, Hansen NB, Laptook AR, et al. Glucocorticoid accelerates renal functional maturation in fetal lambs. *Early Hum Dev* 1983;8:331–341.
38. Nakamura KT, Matherne GP, McWeeny OJ, et al. Renal hemodynamics and functional changes during the transition from fetal to newborn life in sheep. *Pediatr Res* 1987;21:29–34.
39. Berry LM, Ikegami M, Woods E, et al. Postnatal renal adaptation in preterm and term lambs. *Reprod Fertil Dev* 1995;7:491–498.
40. MacKintosh D, Baird-Lambert J, Drage D, et al. Effects of prenatal glucocorticoids on renal maturation in newborn infants. *Dev Pharmacol Ther* 1985;8:107–114.
41. Al-Dahhan J, Stimmler L, Chantler C, et al. The effect of antenatal dexamethasone administration on glomerular filtration rate and renal sodium excretion in premature infants. *Pediatr Nephrol* 1987;1:131–135.
42. Zanardo V, Giacobbo F, Zambon P, et al. Antenatal aminophylline and steroid exposure: effects of glomerular filtration rate and renal sodium excretion in preterm newborns. *J Perinat Med* 1990;18:283–288.
43. Allegaert K, Anderson B. Antenatal steroids and neonatal renal function. *Arch Dis Child* 2006;91(5):451.
44. Tufro-McReddie A, Gomez RA. Ontogeny of the renin–angiotensin system. *Semin Nephrol* 1993;13:519–530.
45. Ito H, Wang J, Strandhoy JW, et al. Importance of the renal nerves for basal and stimulated renin mRNA levels in fetal and adult ovine kidneys. *J Soc Gynecol Investig* 2001;8:327–333.
46. Wang J, Rose JC. Developmental changes in renal renin mRNA half-life and responses to stimulation in fetal lambs. *Am J Physiol* 1999;277:R1130–R1135.
47. Berecek KH, Zhang L. Biochemistry and cell biology of angiotensin-converting enzyme and converting enzyme inhibitors. *Adv Exp Med Biol* 1995;377:141–168.
48. Wolf G. Angiotensin as a renal growth promoting factor. *Adv Exp Med Biol* 1995;377:225–236.
49. Kakuchi J, Ichiki T, Kiyama S, et al. Developmental expression of renal angiotensin II receptor genes in the mouse. *Kidney Int* 1995;47:140–147.
50. Shanmugam S, Llorens-Cortes C, Clauser E, et al. Expression of angiotensin II AT2 receptor mRNA during development of rat kidney and adrenal gland. *Am J Physiol* 1995;268:F222–F230.
51. Robillard JE, Page WV, Matthews MS, et al. Differential gene expression and regulation of renal angiotensin II receptor subtypes (AT1 and AT2) during fetal life in sheep. *Pediatr Res* 1995; 38:896–904.
52. Butkus A, Albiston A, Alcorn D, et al. Ontogeny of angiotensin II receptors, types 1 and 2, in ovine mesonephros and metanephros. *Kidney Int* 1997;52:628–636.
53. Fischer E, Schnermann J, Briggs JP, et al. Ontogeny of NO synthase and renin in juxtaglomerular apparatus of rat kidneys. *Am J Physiol* 1995;268:F1164–F1176.
54. Maric C, Aldred GP, Harris PJ, et al. Angiotensin II inhibits growth of cultured embryonic renomedullary interstitial cells through the AT2 receptor. *Kidney Int* 1998;53:92–99.
55. Herschman HR. Prostaglandin synthase 2. *Biochim Biophys Acta* 1996;1299:125–140.
56. Smith W. Prostanoid biosynthesis and mechanism of action. *Am J Physiol* 1992;263:F181–F191.
57. Qi Z, Hao CM, Langenbach RI, et al. Opposite effects of cyclooxygenase-1 and -2 activity on the pressor response to angiotensin II. *J Clin Invest* 2002;110:61–69.
58. Li D, Belusa R, Nowicki S, et al. Arachidonic acid metabolic pathways regulating activity of renal Na(+)-K(+)-ATPase are age dependent. *Am J Physiol* 2000;278:F823–F829.
59. Jensen BL, Schmid C, Kurz A. Prostaglandins stimulate renin secretion and renin mRNA in mouse renal juxtaglomerular cells. *Am J Physiol* 1996;271:F656–F669.
60. Zhang MZ, Wang JL, Cheng HF, et al. Cyclooxygenase-2 in rat nephron development. *Am J Physiol* 1997;273:F994–F1002.
61. Khan KN, Stanfield KM, Dannenberg A, et al. Cyclooxygenase-2 expression in the developing human kidney. *Pediatr Dev Pathol* 2001;4:461–466.
62. Breyer MD, Breyer RM. Prostaglandin E receptors and the kidney. *Am J Physiol* 2000;279:F12–F23.
63. Bonilla-Felix M, Jiang W. Expression and localization of prostaglandin EP3 receptor mRNA in the immature rabbit kidney. *Am J Physiol* 1996;271:F30–F36.
64. Joppich R, Haberle DA, Weber PC. Studies of the immaturity of the ADH-dependent cAMP system in conscious newborn piglets—possible impairing effects of renal prostaglandins. *Pediatr Res* 1981;15:278–281.
65. Bonilla-Felix M, John-Phillip C. Prostaglandins mediate the defect in AVP-stimulated cAMP generation in immature collecting duct. *Am J Physiol* 1994;267:F44–F48.
66. Bonilla-Felix M, Jiang W. Aquaporin-2 in the immature rat: expression, regulation, and trafficking. *J Am Soc Nephrol* 1997;8: 1502–1509.
67. Bonilla-Felix M, Vehaskari VM, Hamm LL. Water transport in the immature rabbit collecting duct. *Pediatr Nephrol* 1999;13: 103–107.
68. Chattopadhyay N, Baum M, Bai M, et al. Ontogeny of the extracellular calcium-sensing receptor in rat kidney. *Am J Physiol* 1996;271:F736–F743.
69. Reinalter S, Jeck N, Brochhausen C, et al. Role of cyclooxygenase-2 in hyperprostaglandin E syndrome/antenatal Bartter syndrome (HPS/aBS). *Kidney Int* 2002;62:253–260.

70. Tetsuka T, Daphna-Iken D, Srivastava SK, et al. Cross-talk between cyclooxygenase and nitric oxide pathways: prostaglandin E_2 negatively modulates induction of nitric oxide synthase by interleukin 1. *Proc Natl Acad Sci USA* 1994;91:12168–12172.
71. Gloor JM, Muchant DG, Norling LL. Prenatal maternal indomethacin use resulting in prolonged neonatal renal insufficiency. *J Perinatol* 1993;13:425–427.
72. Vanhaesebrouck P, Thiery M, Leroy JG, et al. Oligohydramnios, renal insufficiency, and ileal perforation in preterm infants after intrauterine exposure to indomethacin. *J Pediatr* 1988;113:738–743.
73. Van der Heijden BJ, Carlus C, Narcy F, et al. Persistent anuria, neonatal death, and renal microcystic lesions after prenatal exposure to indomethacin. *Am J Obstet Gynecol* 1994;171:617–623.
74. Butler-O'Hara M, D'Angio CT. Risk of persistent renal insufficiency in premature infants following the prenatal use of indomethacin for suppression of preterm labor. *J Perinatol* 2002;22:541–546.
75. Allegaert K, Vanhole C, de Hoon J, et al. Nonselective cyclo-oxygenase inhibitors and glomerular filtration rate in preterm neonates. *Pediatr Nephrol* 2005; 20(11):1557–1561.
76. Sawdy R, Slater D, Fisk N, et al. Use of a cyclo-oxygenase type-2-selective non-steroidal anti-inflammatory agent to prevent preterm delivery. *Lancet* 1997;350:265–266.
77. Holmes RP, Stone PR. Severe oligohydramnios induced by cyclooxygenase-2 inhibitor nimesulide. *Obstet Gynecol* 2000;96: 810–811.
78. Balasubramaniam J. Nimesulide and neonatal renal failure. *Lancet* 2000;355:575.
79. Norwood VF, Morham SG, Smithies O. Postnatal development and progression of renal dysplasia in cyclooxygenase-2 null mice. *Kidney Int* 2000;58:2291–2300.
80. Morham SG, Langenbach R, Loftin CD, et al. Prostaglandin synthase 2 gene disruption causes severe renal pathology in the mouse. *Cell* 1995;83:473–482.
81. Komhoff M, Wang JL, Cheng HF, et al. Cyclooxygenase-2-selective inhibitors impair glomerulogenesis and renal cortical development. *Kidney Int* 2000;57:414–422.
82. Dinchuk JE, Car BD, Focht RJ, et al. Renal abnormalities and an altered inflammatory response in mice lacking cyclooxygenase II. *Nature* 1995;378:406–409.
83. Van der Heijden AJ, Provoost AP, Nauta J, et al. Renal functional impairment in preterm neonates related to intrauterine indomethacin exposure. *Pediatr Res* 1988;24:644–648.
84. Wurtzel D. Prenatal administration of indomethacin as a tocolytic agent: effect on neonatal renal function. *Obstet Gynecol* 1990;76: 689–692.
85. Gerson A, Abbasi S, Johnson A, et al. Safety and efficacy of long-term tocolysis with indomethacin. *Am J Perinatol* 1990;7:71–74.
86. Simeoni U, Messer J, Weisburd P, et al. Neonatal renal dysfunction and intrauterine exposure to prostaglandin synthesis inhibitors. *Eur J Pediatr* 1989;148:371–373.
87. Dudley DK, Hardie MJ. Fetal and neonatal effects of indomethacin used as a tocolytic agent. *Am J Obstet Gynecol* 1985;151:181–184.
88. Duarte-Silva M, Gouyon JB, Guignard JP. Renal effects of indomethacin and dopamine in newborn rabbits. *Kidney Int* 1986; 30:453–454.
89. Prober CG, Stevenson DK, Benitz WE. The use of antibiotics in neonates weighing less than 1200 grams. *Pediatr Infect Dis J* 1990; 9:111–121.
90. Fawer CL, Torrado A, Guignard JP. Maturation of renal function in full-term and premature neonates. *Helv Paediatr Acta* 1979;32: 11–21.
91. Leake RD, Trygstad CW, Oh W. Inulin clearance in the newborn infant: relationship to gestational and postnatal age. *Pediatr Res* 1976;10:759–762.
92. Van den Anker JN, Hop WC, Schoemaker RC, et al. Ceftazidime pharmacokinetics in preterm infants: effect of postnatal age and postnatal exposure to indomethacin. *Br J Clin Pharmacol* 1995;40: 439–443.
93. Mulhall A, De Louvois J. The pharmacokinetics and safety of ceftazidime in the neonate. *J Antimicrob Chemother* 1985;15:97–103.
94. Kacet N, Roussel-Delvallez M, Gremillet C, et al. Pharmacokinetic study of piperacillin in newborns relating to gestational and postnatal age. *Pediatr Infect Dis J* 1992;11:365–369.
95. Aujard Y, Brion F, Jacqz-Aigrain E, et al. Pharmacokinetics of cefotaxime and desacetylocfotaxime in the newborn. *Diagn Microbiol Infect Dis* 1989;12:87–91.
96. Kenyon CE, Knoppert DC, Lee SK, et al. Amikacin pharmacokinetics and suggested dosage modifications for the preterm infant. *Antimicrob Agents Chemother* 1990;34:265–268.
97. Bhatt V, Nahata MC. Pharmacologic management of patent ductus arteriosus. *Clin Pharm* 1989;8:17–33.
98. Huhta JC. Patent ductus arteriosus in the preterm neonate. In: Long WA, ed. *Fetal and neonatal cardiology*. Philadelphia, PA: WB Saunders, 1990:389–400.
99. Vallner JJ, Speir WA, Kolbeck RC, et al. Effects of pH on the binding of theophylline to serum proteins. *Am Rev Respir Dis* 1979;120:83–86.
100. Waddel WJ, Butler TC. The distribution and excretion of phenobarbital. *J Clin Invest* 1957;36:1217–1226.
101. Collins C, Koren G, Crean P, et al. Fentanyl pharmacokinetics and haemodynamic effects in preterm infants during ligation of patent ductus arteriosus. *Anesth Analg* 1985;64:1078–1080.
102. Watterberg KL, Kelly HW, Johnson JD, et al. Effect of patent ductus arteriosus on gentamicin pharmacokinetics in very low birth-weight (<1500 g) babies. *Dev Pharmacol Ther* 1987;10:107–117.
103. Gal P, Ransom JL, Weaver RI, et al. Indomethacin pharmacokinetics in neonates: the value of volume of distribution as a marker of permanent patent ductus arteriosus closure. *Ther Drug Monit* 1991;13:42–45.
104. Van Overmeire B, Touw D, Schepens PJ, et al. Ibuprofen pharmacokinetics in preterm infants with patent ductus arteriosus. *Clin Pharmacol Ther* 2001;70:336–343.
105. Ng PC, So KW, Fok TF, et al. Comparing sulindac with indomethacin for closure of ductus arteriosus in preterm infants. *J Pediatr Child Health* 1997;33:324–328.
106. Sakhalkar VS, Merchant AH. Therapy of symptomatic patent ductus arteriosus in preterms using mefenamic acid and indomethacin. *Indian Pediatr* 1992;29:313–318.
107. Van Overmeire B, Brus F, van Acker KJ, et al. Aspirin versus indomethacin treatment of patent ductus arteriosus in preterm infants with respiratory distress syndrome. *Pediatr Res* 1995;38: 886–891.
108. Mosca L, Bray M, Lattanzio M, et al. Comparative evaluation of the effects of indomethacin and ibuprofen on cerebral perfusion and oxygenation in preterm infants with patent ductus arteriosus. *J Pediatr* 1997;131:549–554.
109. Patel J, Marks KA, Roberts I, et al. Ibuprofen treatment of patent ductus arteriosus. *Lancet* 1995;346:255.
110. Aranda JV, Varvarigou A, Beharry K, et al. The effect of early intravenous ibuprofen on renal function in premature newborns. *Pediatr Res* 1994;37:361A.
111. Aranda JV, Varvarigou A, Beharry K, et al. Pharmacokinetics and protein binding of intravenous ibuprofen in the premature newborn infant. *Acta Paediatr* 1997;86:289–293.
112. Hirt D, van Overmeire B, Treluyer JM, et al. An optimized ibuprofen dosing scheme for preterm neonates with patent ductus arteriosus, based on a population pharmacokinetic and pharmacodynamic study. *Br J Clin Pharmacol* 2008;65(5):629–636.
113. Allegaert K, Rayyan M, Anderson BJ. Impact of ibuprofen administration on renal drug clearance in the first weeks of life. *Methods Find Exp Clin Pharmacol* 2006;28(8):519–522.
114. Cuevas L, Yeh TF, John EG, et al. The effect of low-dose dopamine infusion on cardiopulmonary and renal status in premature newborns with respiratory distress syndrome. *Am J Dis Child* 1991;145:799–803.
115. Emery EF, Greenough A. Efficacy of low-dose dopamine infusion. *Acta Paediatr* 1993;82:430–432.
116. Seri I, Rudas G, Bors Z, et al. Effects of low-dose dopamine infusion on cardiovascular and renal functions, cerebral blood flow, and plasma catecholamine levels in sick preterm neonates. *Pediatr Res* 1993;34:742–749.
117. Seri I. Cardiovascular, renal, and endocrine actions of dopamine in neonates and children. *J Pediatr* 1995;126:333–344.
118. Felder RA, Felder CC, Eisner GM, et al. The dopamine receptor in adult and maturing kidney. *Am J Physiol* 1989;257: F315–F327.
119. Seri I, Aperia A. Contribution of dopamine receptors to the dopamine-induced increase in glomerular filtration rate. *Am J Physiol* 1988;254:F196–F201.
120. Tulassay T, Seri I. Interaction of dopamine and furosemide in acute oliguria of preterm infants with hyaline membrane disease. *Acta Paediatr Scand* 1986;75:420–424.

121. Seri I, Tulassay T, Kiszel J, et al. The use of dopamine for the prevention of the renal side effects of indomethacin in premature infants with patent ductus arteriosus. *Int J Pediatr Nephrol* 1984;5: 209–214.
122. Seri I, Hajdu J, Tulassay T, et al. The effect of low-dose dopamine infusion on urinary PGE_2 excretion in sick preterm infants. *Eur J Pediatr* 1988;147:616–620.
123. Barrington K, Brion LP. Dopamine versus no treatment to prevent renal dysfunction in indomethacin-treated preterm newborn infants. *Cochrane Database Syst Rev* 2002;(3):CD003213.
124. Allegaert K, Debeer A, Cossey V, et al. Dopamine is not an independent risk factor for reduced amikacin clearance in extremely low-birth-weight infants. *Pediatr Crit Care Med* 2006;7(2):143–146.
125. Burg MB, Stoner L, Cardinal J, et al. Furosemide effect in isolated perfused tubules. *Am J Physiol* 1973;225:119–124.
126. Green TP, Mirkin BL. Determinants of the diuretic response to furosemide in infants with congestive heart failure. *Pediatr Cardiol* 1982;3:47–51.
127. Brenner BM, Kaimowitc RI, Wright FS, et al. An inhibitory effect of furosemide on sodium reabsorption by the proximal tubule of the rat nephron. *J Clin Invest* 1969;48:290–300.
128. Gerber JG, Nies AS. Furosemide-induced vasodilatation: importance of the state of hydration and filtration. *Kidney Int* 1980;18: 454–459.
129. Osborne JL, Hook JB, Bailie MD. Control of renin release: effects of *d*-propranolol in renal denervation on furosemide-induced renin release in the dog. *Circ Res* 1977;41:481–486.
130. Weber PC, Scherer B, Larsson C. Increase of free arachidonic acid by furosemide in man as the cause of prostaglandin and renin release. *Eur J Pharmacol* 1977;41:329–332.
131. Yetman AT, Singh NC, Parbtani A, et al. Acute haemodynamic and neurohormonal effects of furosemide in critically ill pediatric patients. *Crit Care Med* 1996;24:398–402.
132. Freeman RH, David JO, Villarreal D. Role of prostaglandins in the control of renin release. *Circ Res* 1984;43:1–9.
133. Ross BS, Pollik A, Oh W. The pharmacologic effects of furosemide therapy in the low-birth-weight infant. *J Pediatr* 1978; 92:149–152.
134. Mirochnick MH, Miceli JJ, Kramer PA, et al. Furosemide pharmacokinetics in very low birth weight infants. *J Pediatr* 1988; 112:653–657.
135. Yeh TF, Wilks A, Singh J, et al. Furosemide prevents the renal side effects of indomethacin therapy in premature infants with patent ductus arteriosus. *J Pediatr* 1982;101:433–437.
136. Green TP, Thompson TR, Johnson D, et al. Furosemide promotes patent ductus arteriosus in premature infants with the respiratory distress syndrome. *N Engl J Med* 1983;308:743–748.
137. Van der Vorst M, den Hartigh J, Wildschut E, et al. An exploratory study with an adaptive continuous intravenous furosemide regimen in neonates treated with extracorporeal membrane oxygenation. *Crit Care* 2007;11(5):R111.
138. Van den Anker JN, de Groot R, Broerse HM, et al. Assessment of glomerular filtration rate in preterm infants by serum creatinine: comparison with inulin clearance. *Pediatrics* 1995;96:1156–1158.
139. Gordjani N, Burghard R, Leititis JU, et al. Serum creatinine and creatinine clearance in healthy neonates and prematures during the first 10 days of life. *Eur J Pediatr* 1988;148:143–145.
140. Brion LP, Fleischman AR, McCarton C, et al. A simple estimate of glomerular filtration rate in low birth weight infants during the first year of life: noninvasive assessment of body composition and growth. *J Pediatr* 1986;109:698–707.
141. Feldman H, Guignard JP. Plasma creatinine in the first month of life. *Arch Dis Child* 1982;57:123–126.
142. Sonntag J, Prankel B, Waltz S. Serum creatinine concentration, urinary creatinine excretion and creatinine clearance during the first 9 weeks in preterm infants with a birth weight below 1500 g. *Eur J Pediatr* 1996;155:815–819.
143. Gallini F, Maggio L, Romagnoli C, et al. Progression of renal function in preterm neonates with gestational age < or = 32 weeks. *Pediatr Nephrol* 2000;15:119–124.
144. Matos P, Duarte-Silva M, Drukker A, et al. Creatinine reabsorption by the newborn rabbit kidney. *Pediatr Res* 1998;44:639–641.
145. Guignard JP, Drukker A. Why do newborn infants have a high plasma creatinine? *Pediatrics* 1999;103:e49.
146. Van den Anker JN. Renal function in preterm infants. *Eur J Pediatr* 1997;156(7):583–584.
147. Stickle D, Cole B, Hock K, et al. Correlation of plasma concentrations of cystatin C and creatinine to inulin clearance in a pediatric population. *Clin Chem* 1998;44:1334–1338.
148. Bokenkamp A, Domanetzki M, Zinck R, et al. Cystatin C—a new marker of glomerular filtration rate in children independent of age and height. *Pediatrics* 1998;101:875–881.
149. Cataldi L, Mussap M, Bertelli L, et al. Cystacin C in healthy women at term pregnancy and in their infant newborns: relationship between maternal and neonatal serum levels and reference values. *Am J Perinatol* 1999;16:287–295.
150. Harmoinen A, Ylinen E, Ala-Houhala M, et al. Reference values for cystatin C in pre- and full-term infants and children. *Pediatr Nephrol* 2000;15:105–108.
151. Randers E, Erlandsen EJ. Serum cystatin C as an endogenous marker of the renal function—a review. *Clin Chem Lab Med* 1999; 37:389–395.
152. Inui K, Masuda S, Saito H. Cellular and molecular aspects of drug transport in the kidney. *Kidney Int* 2000;58:944–958.
153. Gorbouley V, Ulzherimer JC, Akhoundova A, et al. Cloning and characterization of two human polyspecific organic cation transporters. *DNA Cell Biol* 1997;16:871–881.
154. Tamia I, Yabuuchi H, Nezu J, et al. Cloning and characterization of a novel human pH-dependent organic cation transporter, OCTN1. *FEBS Lett* 1997;419:107–111.
155. Gros P, Neriah YP, Croop JM, et al. Isolation and expression of a cDNA that confers multidrug resistance. *Nature* 1986;323: 728–731.
156. Kullak-Ublick GA, Hagenbuch B, Steiger B, et al. Molecular and functional characterization of an organic anion transporting polypeptide cloned from human liver. *Gastroenterology* 1995;109: 1274–1282.
157. Wang J, Su SF, Dresser MJ, et al. Na(+)-dependent purine nucleoside transporter from human kidney: cloning and functional characterization. *Am J Physiol* 1997;273:F1058–F1065.
158. Van Aubel RA, Masereeuw R, Russel FG. Molecular pharmacology of renal organic anion transporters. *Am J Physiol Renal Physiol* 2000;279:F216–F232.
159. Lu R, Kanai N, Bao Y, et al. Cloning, *in vitro* expression, and tissue distribution of a human prostaglandin transporter cDNA (hPGT). *J Clin Invest* 1996;98:1142–1149.
160. Cole SP, Bhardwaj G, Gerlach JH, et al. Overexpression of a novel transporter gene in a multidrug resistant human lung cancer cell line. *Science* 1992;258:1650–1654.
161. Evers R, Kool M, van Deemter L, et al. Drug export activity of the human canalicular multispecific organ anion transporter in polarized kidney MDCK cells expressing cMOAT (MRP2) cDNA. *J Clin Invest* 1998;101:1310–1319.
162. Ishikawa T. The ATP-dependent glutathione S-conjugate export pump. *Trends Biochem Sci* 1992;17:463–468.
163. Schlatter E, Monnich V, Cetinkaya I, et al. The organic cation transporters rOCT1 and hOCT2 are inhibited by cGMP. *J Membr Biol* 2002;189:237–244.
164. Goralski KB, Lou G, Prowse MT, et al. The cation transporters rOCT1 and rOCT2 interact with bicarbonate but play only a minor role for amantadine uptake into rat renal proximal tubules. *J Pharmacol Exp Ther* 2002;303:959–968.
165. Leabman MK, Huang CC, Kawamoto M, et al. Polymorphisms in a human kidney xenobiotic transporter, OCT2, exhibit altered function. *Pharmacogenetics* 2002;12:395–405.
166. Burckhardt BC, Drinkuth B, Menzel C, et al. The renal Na+-dependent dicarboxylate transporter, NADC-3, translocates dimethyl- and disulfhydryl-compounds and contributes to renal heavy metal detoxicifation. *J Am Soc Nephrol* 2002;13:2628–2638.
167. Sekine T, Watanabe N, Hosoyamada, et al. Expression, cloning, and characterization of a novel multispecific organic anion transporter. *J Biol Chem* 1997;272:18526–18529.
168. Dresser MJ, Leabman MK, Giacomini KM. Transporters involved in the elimination of drugs in the kidney: organic anion transporters and organic cation transporters. *J Pharm Sci* 2001;90: 397–421.
169. Ito S. Drug secretion systems in renal tubular cells: functional models and molecular identify. *Pediatr Nephrol* 1999;13:980–988.
170. Schinkel AH, Wagenaar E, van Deemter L, et al. Absence of the mdr1a P-glycoprotein in mice affects tissue distribution and pharmacokinetics of dexamethasone, digoxin, and cyclosporin A. *J Clin Invest* 1995;96:1698–1705.

171. Masuda S, Sait H, Inui K. Interactions of nonsteroidal anti-inflammatory drugs with rat renal organic anion transporter, OAT-K1. *J Pharmacol Exp Ther* 1997;283:1039–1042.
172. Shapiro AB, Ling V. The mechanism of ATP-dependent and multidrug transport by P-glycoprotein. *Acta Physiol Scand* 1998;643: 227–243.
173. Vezmar M, Georges E. Direct binding of chloroquine to the multidrug resistance protein (MRP); possible role for MRP in chloroquine drug transport and resistance in tumor cells. *Biochem Pharmacol* 1998;56:733–742.
174. Washington CB, Duran GE, Man MC, et al. Interaction of anti-HIV protease inhibitors with the multidrug transporter P-glycoprotein (P-gp) in human cultured cells. *J AIDS* 1998;19: 203–209.
175. Rebbeor JF, Senior AE. Effects of cardiovascular drugs on ATPase activity of P-glycoprotein in plasma membranes and purified reconstituted form. *Biochim Biophys Acta* 1998;1369: 85–93.
176. Lin JH, Lu AY. Inhibition and induction of cytochrome P450 and the clinical implications. *Clin Pharmacokinet* 1998;35:361–390.
177. Fromm MF, Kim RB, Stein CM, et al. Inhibition of P-glycoprotein-mediated drug transport: a unifying mechanism to explain the interaction between digoxin and quinidine. *Circulation* 1999;99: 552–557.
178. Ito S, Woodland C, Harpter PA, et al. The mechanism of the verapamil–digoxin interaction in renal tubular cells (LLC-PK1). *Life Sci* 1993;53:PL399–403.
179. Wakasugi H, Yano I, Ito T, et al. Effect of clarithromycin on renal excretion of digoxin: interaction with P-glycoprotein. *Clin Pharmacol Ther* 1998;64:123–128.
180. Woodland C, Verjee Z, Giesbrecht E, et al. The digoxin–propafenone interaction: characterization of a mechanism using renal tubular cell monolayers. *J Pharmacol Exp Ther* 1997;283: 39–45.
181. Okamura N, Hirai M, Tanigawara Y, et al. Digoxin–cyclosporin A interaction: modulation of the multidrug transporter P-glycoprotein in the kidney. *J Pharmacol Exp Ther* 1993;266:1614–1619.
182. Lum BL, Kaubisch S, Yahanda AM, et al. Alteration of etoposide pharmacokinetics and pharmacodynamics by cyclosporine in a phase I trial to modulate multidrug resistance. *J Clin Oncol* 1992;10:1635–1642.
183. Herbert MF, Lam AY. Diltiazem increases tacrolimus concentrations. *Ann Pharmacother* 1999;33:360–362.
184. Herbert MF, Fisher RM, March CL, et al. Effects of rifampin on tacrolimus pharmacokinetics in healthy volunteers. *J Clin Pharmacol* 1999;39:91–96.
185. Tramonti G, Romiti N, Norpoth M, et al. P-glycoprotein in HK-2 proximal tubule cell line. *Ren Fail* 2001;23:331–376.
186. Takanaga H, Ohnishi A, Matsuo H, et al. Inhibition of vinblastin efflux mediated by P-glycoprotein by grapefruit juice components in caco-2 cells. *Biol Pharm Bull* 2001;21:1062–1066.
187. Wang EJ, Casciano CN, Clement RP, et al. Inhibition of P-glycoprotein transport function by grapefruit juice psoralen. *Pharm Res* 2001;18:432–438.

CHAPTER

17

Cheston M. Berlin, Jr.

The Excretion of Drugs and Chemicals in Human Milk

INTRODUCTION

During the 1960s and the early 1970s, the incidence of breastfeeding reached a nadir; in 1972 only 20% of newborns discharged from nurseries were breast-fed, and only 15% were still being breast-fed at 6 months of age (1). Both medical and psychological studies have emphasized the considerable biologic and psychological benefits for breastfeeding infants (2,3). The last 35 years has seen a great increase in the incidence of breastfeeding due to the enthusiastic efforts of both professional (American Academy of Pediatrics) and lay organizations (La Leche League International) with support from the Federal Government (4). The most recent data from the National Health and Nutrition Examination Surveys (NHANES) for 2005 to 2006 show that 77% of infants are discharged from nurseries breastfeeding and at 6 months of age 35% are still being breast-fed (5). Lactating mothers take significantly more medications than pregnant mothers (6). The medications most often used by breastfeeding mothers are multivitamins, nonsteroidal anti-inflammatory drugs, acetaminophen, progestins, antibiotics, and decongestants.

With this increased emphasis and interest in breastfeeding, there has been a parallel increase in concern over the excretion of drugs and chemicals into breast milk. It is very important that this concern, while appropriate, not translate into discouraging nursing when it is necessary for a mother to take medication for a medical condition. In caring for both the mother and her nursing infant, there are two important objectives: (a) protect the nursing infant from adverse effects from maternal medication and (b) permit the mother to receive necessary pharmacotherapy while preserving her ability to breast-feed her infant. A brief review of breast function and milk synthesis will help elucidate the possible mechanisms involved in the excretion of drugs into breast milk.

It must be emphasized that virtually all experimental work on breast function/milk secretion has been done in animal species. The difficulties and limitations of studying human lactation (anatomically and physiologically) using methods of continuous milk collection, serial biopsy of lactation tissue, and the administration of isotopic biochemical precursors are obvious. There are also known biochemical differences among the milk of different species: protein, fat, and carbohydrate content seem related to growth requirements (especially the rate of growth) of the infant of the particular species. Some of these differences will obviously dictate differences in drug transfer from maternal plasma to the milk. The pH of human milk, for example, is usually 7.0 or above; in the cow (where lactation has been most extensively studied), the pH is usually 6.8 or below. As seen later, this will have significant effect on the transport of some drugs depending on their pK_a. However, there is no reason to suppose that the formation of human milk is qualitatively different from that in other animal species.

The lactating breast resembles a bunch of grapes, with each grape being tear-shaped and consisting of a cluster of alveolar cells in which breast milk is synthesized and secreted into a central lumen. The lumens feed into small ducts that meet each other in channels of increasing size until the nipple region is reached. With the possible exception of water transport, little alteration in the composition of milk occurs once it leaves the alveolar lumen. Excretion of drugs and chemicals most likely occurs only within this lumen.

Human milk is a suspension of fat and protein in a carbohydrate (lactose) and mineral solution. A nursing mother can easily produce 600 mL of milk per day (the amount needed for the complete nourishment of a 4-kg infant) containing 6.0 g of protein, 22.2 g of fat, and 42 g of lactose with the correct amount of minerals and most vitamins. Human milk also contains immunoglobulins, macrophages, lymphocytes, transferrin, lactoferrin, interferon, complement, fibronectin, erythropoietin, and many other unusual biologic compounds, all of which are designed to protect the infant and accelerate maturation of many physiologic processes (7). The exact composition of milk varies with duration of lactation, and may even vary within the time of a single feeding. Using a noninvasive computerized breast measurement system, it was demonstrated that infants were self-regulating their milk intake,

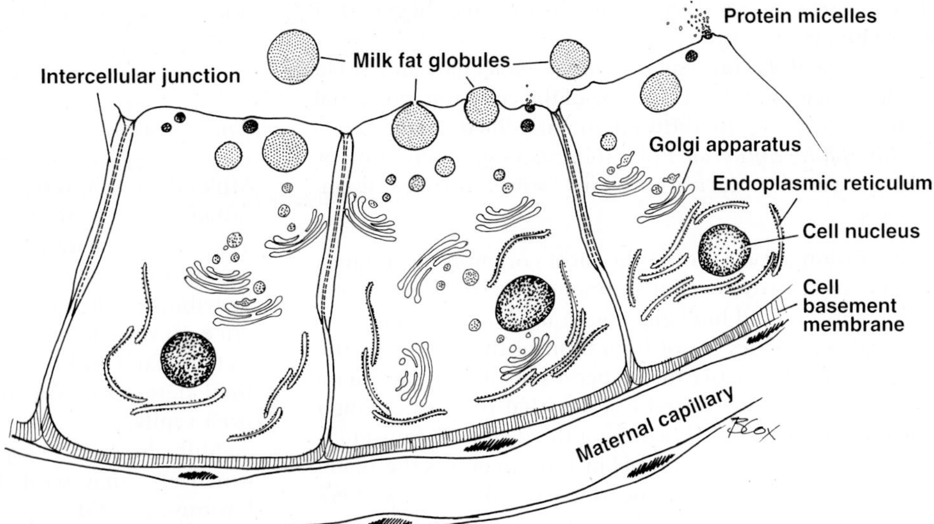

Figure 17.1. Schematic drawing of alveolar breast cells. All cells are actively synthesizing protein, fat, and carbohydrate. The cell on the right has discharged most of the products into the alveolar lumen as milk. Carbohydrate is secreted with protein.

and that the rate of milk synthesis was at a maximum when the breast was empty and a minimum when the breast was full (8–10).

Milk protein is synthesized within the mammary gland. A small amount of maternal plasma protein does enter into breast milk, presumably across the alveolar cell and/or through the extracellular space between these cells. This explains the presence of cow milk protein (β-lactoglobulin from maternal cow milk consumption) in the serum of exclusively breast-fed infants. The major human milk proteins are casein and lactalbumin (the latter is also needed for lactose synthesis). Synthesis is initiated by prolactin and needs insulin and hydrocortisone to continue. The proteins are very digestible and contribute to the low curd tension of human milk. Proteins are transported from the endoplasmic reticulum into the Golgi apparatus, migrate from the base of the cell toward the apex, and are discharged into the alveolar lumen by apocrine secretion. The role of these proteins in binding drugs has yet to be investigated completely. In the two reported studies that specifically measured drug (theobromine and theophylline) binding to human milk protein, it was found to vary between 0% and 24% (11,12).

Short-chain fatty acids are synthesized in the mammary gland from acetate. Long-chain fatty acids are supplied by transfer from plasma. Both classes of fat are esterified in the breast with glycerol (from intracellular glucose). The lipids collect in the endoplasmic reticulum. As they ascend the cell in ever-increasing sizes of droplets, they acquire a three-layered membrane (lipoprotein) and are extruded into milk as milk fat globules (13). It is intriguing to speculate on the possibilities of drug binding to both the protein and fat components of the milk fat globule. It is also possible that some lipid-soluble drugs may be trapped entirely within the milk fat globule.

Lactose is entirely synthesized in the breast alveolar cell. Its synthesis proceeds from UDP-galactose and glucose, with lactose synthetase (galactose transferase plus lactalbumin) as the enzyme. Prolactin is absolutely required. Lactose is excreted from the cell into the alveolar lumen alone and with milk protein. Electrolytes, vitamins, and water are supplied by the cell (from plasma water) to achieve the final concentration.

All the preceding elements achieve a concentration in human milk that provides the ideal nutrient supply to the infant for at least the first 6 months. After 6 months of age, the infant's caloric need usually requires supplemental food.

The transport of drugs into breast milk from maternal tissues and plasma may proceed by a number of routes. Figure 17.1 is a schematic drawing of the alveolar breast cell; it illustrates the cellular structures a substance in maternal plasma must traverse to enter milk contained within the alveolar lumen. After crossing the capillary endothelium, the drug traverses the interstitial space and must cross the basement membrane (consisting mostly of mucopolysaccharides of the alveolar breast cell). The cell plasma membrane is trilaminar with the usual phospholipid–protein membrane structure. After reaching the cell cytoplasm, the compound travels apically and leaves the cell by diffusion, reverse pinocytosis, or apocrine secretion (apical part of cell disintegrates). This entire process is nicely detailed by Vorherr (14). Excellent scanning electron micrographs of this process in the human breast are presented in the paper by Ferguson and Anderson (15).

The following are the most probable mechanisms of drug excretion in milk (16,17):

Transcellular diffusion. Small un-ionized molecules with lipid solubility, such as urea and ethanol, transverse the capillary epithelium, intercellular water, basal cell membrane, alveolar cell, and its apical membrane by diffusion. This mechanism is supported by the observations that milk concentrations of such compounds mirror simultaneous maternal plasma levels (milk/plasma [M/P] ratio = 1) and that the elimination rate constants (as calculated from the elimination phases) are very similar (18).

Intercellular diffusion. This route avoids the breast alveolar cell entirely. Histologic studies in some animal species suggest that such a space may not exist or is very tight. It may be important functionally in the human and may explain how large molecules such as interferon, immunoglobulins, and cow milk protein enter human milk.

The electron microscopic studies in humans suggest that these junctions exist (15).

Passive diffusion. Small ionized molecules and small proteins may enter the basal part of the cell from interstitial water through passive diffusion in water-filled channels.

Ionophore diffusion. Polar substances may penetrate by being bound to carrier proteins within the cell membranes.

Diffusion appears to be the most common mechanism for a drug to cross a cell membrane. The distribution of a drug across a lipid biologic membrane has been shown to depend on the degree of ionization of the drug plus the assumption that a pH difference exists across the membrane; it is the un-ionized fraction that diffuses through the membrane (16–19). Knowing the degree of ionization of the drug (pK_a) plus the pH difference across the mammary alveolar cell membrane, one can calculate the theoretical M/P ratio. [A complete discussion of the distribution of ionized drugs between plasma and milk is given by Rasmussen (20). Acknowledgment must be made of the elegant experiments by Rasmussen in defining this process in the animal models of the lactating cow and goat. Equally, acknowledgment must be made of Wilson et al. (21,22) for pointing out the limitations of using the M/P ratio to predict quantitation excretion of drugs into milk.] Figure 17.2 illustrates the situation for two weakly acidic drugs with markedly different pK_a values: salicylic acid ($pK_a = 3.0$) and phenobarbital ($pK_a = 7.2$). Plasma pH is assumed to be 7.4, and milk pH is assumed to be 7.0 (commonly accepted for human milk). For a weak acid, the Henderson–Hasselbach equation defines the ratio of un-ionized (U) to ionized (I) drug at equilibrium as

$$\log(U/I) = pK_a - pH$$

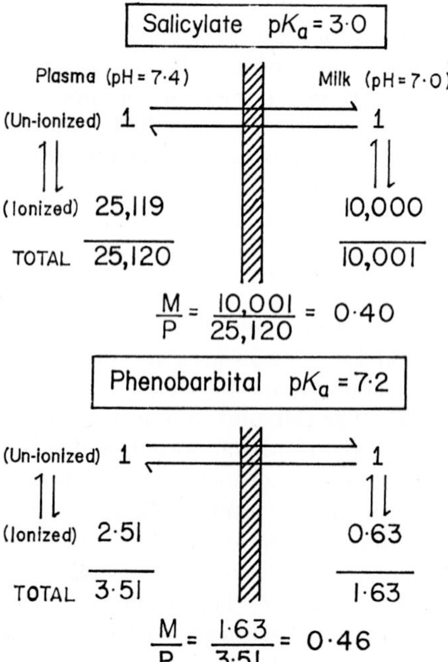

Figure 17.2. Theoretical distribution of weakly acidic drugs across a lipid cell membrane. Units are arbitrary for illustration. M/P, Milk/plasma ratio.

and for a weak base as

$$\log(I/U) = pK_a - pH$$

The theoretical M/P ratio for total salicylate (un-ionized plus ionized) is 0.40; the experimental value obtained by Miller et al. (23) is 0.35. The theoretical ratio for total phenobarbital is 0.46; the experimental value is 0.7 (20,24). This difference for phenobarbital may be explained by the significant lipid solubility of this drug (chloroform/water distribution of un-ionized drug = 4.8). Thus, the presence on one side of a biologic membrane of a substance rich in fat (milk) will introduce another factor in the final determination of the concentration of a drug in breast milk.

Milk also has 1.0 g per 100 mL of proteins, any one of which also may bind drugs. Few data are available, but Rasmussen (25) demonstrated sulfonamide binding in milk to be present from 0% to 40% depending on the sulfonamide. As a general statement, weak acids (e.g., sulfanilamide, phenobarbital, salicylate, and penicillin) have an M/P ratio (both theoretical and experimental) of less than 1.0. Weak bases (e.g., antipyrine, lincomycin, quinine, ephedrine) have an M/P ratio greater than 1.0 (20,21). The precise experimental value will depend on factors such as maternal dosing intervals, milk pH, protein binding in plasma and milk, and lipid solubility of the drug (21,24–27).

The ratio of drug in the ultrafiltrate of milk to that in the ultrafiltrate of plasma was found to be independent of plasma levels (M/P ratio identical at all levels of plasma concentration). The concentration in milk was also found to be constant regardless of the volume of milk in the mammary gland. These observations support the thesis that diffusion is the major mechanism for the appearance of drugs in breast milk (20).

A number of reviews discuss the excretion of drugs in milk, and some provide tables of the concentration of drugs in breast milk (26,28–31). Many of the studies cited in these reviews are single case reports or small series of mother–child pairs. Many of the values consist of a single measurement of the drug concentration in milk; the period of time from maternal ingestion is frequently not defined, nor is maternal dose, frequency of dose, frequency of nursing, or duration of lactation. Measurement of the drug in the nursing infant's blood or urine is frequently not mentioned. Hence, it is usually not possible to determine the risk to the nursling at a single isolated point. Many of the quoted references refer to data from the 1940s and the 1950s, when analytical methods were primitive. The oft-quoted reference to salicylates, for example, dates from 1935 and employed a semiquantitative method ($FeCl_3$) for salicylate analysis; no quantitative values are given (32). The discipline of pharmacokinetics was not developed when many of the drugs in breast milk were initially assayed. Hence, few detailed studies employing drug measurements over a period of time in both maternal and infant body fluids are available. The availability of newer techniques (high-pressure liquid chromatography, mass spectroscopy) coupled with increased interest will result in more comprehensive studies.

TABLE 17.1 Excretion of Drugs in Human Milk

Drug	Maternal Dose[a]	Peak Concentration in Milk	Milk/Plasma Ratio at Peak	Time of Peak Concentration in Milk	$t_{1/2}$ in Milk[b]	Amount Secreted in Milk 24 hr After Single Dose[c]	Maternal Dose (%)[d]
Acetaminophen (88)	650 mg p.o.	10–15 μg/mL	0.8	1–2 hr	2.3 hr	0.88 mg	0.14
Antipyrine (103)	18 mg/kg p.o.	20–30 μg/mL	1.0	10 min	6–22 hr	7–25 mg	0.5–2.4
Caffeine (104)	35–336 mg p.o. as beverage	2–7 μg/mL	0.6–0.8	½–1 hr	6.1 hr	0.57 mg	0.53
Cefazolin (105)	2 g i.v.	1.51 μg/mL	0.023	3 hr		1.5 mg	0.075
	500 mg i.m. t.i. d.	0		Not detected in milk		0	
Chlorothiazide (106)	500 mg p.o.	0		Not detected in milk		<1 mg/d	
Diazepam (107)	Not stated	0.27 μg/mL	0.68	3 d	3 d	0.27 mg (peak) on day 3	
Digoxin (108)	0.25 mg p.o.	0.6–1.0 ng/mL	0.8–0.9	4 hr	12 hr	0.18–0.36 μg/d	0.07–0.14
Ethanol (18)	0.6 g/kg p.o.	777 μg/mL	0.93	90 min	2.9 hr	300 mg	1
Isoniazid (109)	300 mg p.o.	16.6 μg/mL	1.6	3 hr	5.9 hr	7 mg	2.3
Lithium (110)	Chronic: dose not specified, p.o.	0.1–0.6 mmol/L	0.5	Levels fairly constant			
Methadone (111)	70 mg/d p.o.	0.36 μg/mL	0.83			300 μg	0.4
		0.51 μg/mL	1.89				
Metronidazole (112)	2.0 g p.o.	50–57 μg/mL		2–4 hr	9 hr	21.8 mg	1.1
Nicotine (113)	1 pack/d (400 mg)	91 ng/mL (range: 20–512 ng/mL)		No correlation		0.68 mg	0.17
Prednisolone (114)	5 mg p.o.	26 ng/mL		1 hr	8.2 hr	6 μg	0.12
Prednisone (115)	120 mg p.o.	154 ng/mL (prednisone)		2 hr	1.8 hr	47 μg (as both prednisone and prednisolone)	0.04
		473 ng/mL (prednisolone)	2	1.1 hr			
Propranolol (116)	20 mg	10 ng/mL	0.56	3 hr		0.6 μg	0.03
	160 mg	150 ng/mL	0.65	3 hr		90 μg	0.05
Salicylate (117)	20 mg/kg						0.18–0.36
Sulfasalazine (118)	2 g/d p.o.	9–15 mg/mL	0.6	Constant		1.4–2.1 mg	0.16
Sulphone (119)	5 g i.m. sulfetrone or 500 mg p.o. dapsone	14 μg/mL	0.16	4–6 hr		10 mg	2
Theophylline (12)	4.25 mg/kg	4 μg/mL	0.7	2 hr	4.0 hr	8 mg	4
Verapamil (120)	80 mg p.o. t.i.d.		0.6	1–2 hr	4.3	31 μg	0.01

[a]i.m., Intramuscular; i.v., intravenous; p.o., oral; t.i.d., three times a day.
[b]$t_{1/2}$ is calculated from the elimination (β) phase.
[c]Amount excreted in 24 hr is estimated by assuming that the infant ingests 90 mL of milk every 4 hr.
[d]The percentage of maternal dose is calculated by dividing the amount secreted in 24 hr by the maternal dose (single dose or 24-hr total maternal dose).

In spite of the widespread use of drugs by the lactating women, there are only a very small number of reports of adverse reactions in breast-fed infants. Anderson et al. (33) surveyed the literature in Medline from 1966 to 2002. They identified 94 reports involving 100 infants of adverse reactions in nursing infants. Using the Naranjo method (34) they classified 53 of the reports as "possibly" being related to the drugs use by the mother and 47 of the reports as "probable." No report met the criteria for "definite." The age of the infants is of interest: 37% of the case reports occurred in infants younger than 2 weeks of age; 78% of reports were for infants 2 months of age or younger. Only 4% of the reports were for infants older than 6 months of age. Because of the immaturity of the hepatic and renal systems of these very young infant, they would be the most vulnerable to even the small concentrations of drugs excreted in milk. The very young infant, especially neonates, appears to be potentially most vulnerable.

It is important not to become too complacent about the apparent lack of significant adverse effects from maternal drug use. A recent important report describes significant central nervous system depression, including death, as a result of the maternal use of codeine for pain control (35). These authors report 17 infants (24%), 14 younger than the age of 2 weeks, who exhibited central nervous system depression following maternal codeine administration. The mothers of these affected infants took a dose of codeine 59% higher than mothers whose infants were unaffected. Codeine is metabolized to morphine by the cytochrome enzyme *CYP2D6*. Two of the mothers of affected infants were found to be homozygous for the *CYP2D6* ultrarapid metabolizer phenotype. One of these infants died with a postmortem blood level of 70 ng/mL. These cases emphasize a number of important factors in considering possible toxicity of maternal medical medication to the nursing infant. These principles include age of the nursing infant, large interindividual variations in drug response, dose-response relationship (especially the length of time of maternal administration), pharmacogenetics, and interaction of all of these principles (36).

Two critical questions are what dose does the infant absorb (as measured by infant blood and urine concentrations), and does the breast excrete any metabolites of the parent drug. Is mammary tissue, which is so metabolically active, itself capable of drug biotransformation?

Table 17.1 lists some drugs that appear in human milk for which some pharmacokinetic data can be found. The blank spaces in the table cannot be filled using current data. This emphasizes the gaps in knowledge in precisely determining the risk to the nursing infant. The following general points may be made:

1. Most drugs (and environmental chemicals) with molecular weights less than 200 daltons can cross from plasma to milk by the process of simple diffusion (17).
2. Concentrations in milk parallel plasma concentrations in time; milk/plasma ratios usually vary from 0.5 to 1.0. Low–molecular-weight compounds with no electric charge and having lipid solubility are most likely to have a milk/plasma ratio of 1 (18).
3. Following a single maternal dose, $t_{1/2}$ values are similar for plasma and milk. This implies rather rapid transport from plasma to milk (according to M/P ratios).
4. The total amount available for infant absorption is usually less than 1% of maternal dose. This amount may be minimized by planning nursing periods at times of low maternal plasma levels (e.g., just before a maternal dose).
5. There are few data about the situation with repetitive maternal doses over days or weeks (i.e., chronic maternal drug therapy). One infant became salicylate toxic after nursing for 2 weeks from a mother ingesting 650 mg of aspirin four times per day (37). There is a report of an infant with feeding difficulties and having measurable plasma concentrations of fluoxetine and norfluoxetine (38).
6. For most drugs, even those with potent pharmacologic actions, the risk to the infant (with attention to proper nursing scheduling to minimize drug exposure of the infant) is very small (33,39), with possible exceptions of the neonate and the infant younger than 2 months of age (33,35).

Table 17.2 lists those drugs for which adverse effects on the nursing infant have been described. The number

TABLE 17.2 Drugs Associated with Adverse Effects in Nursing Infants

Drug	*Effect*
Acebutolol (121)	Hypotension, bradycardia, tachypnea
Atenolol (122)	Cyanosis, bradycardia
Bromocriptine (123)	Suppresses lactation
Cocaine (124,125)	Cocaine poisoning in infant
Codeine (36)	Central nervous depression, death
Ergotamine (126) (as used in migraine medication)	Vomiting, diarrhea, convulsions
Lithium (110)	Significant blood concentrations in the infant (one-third to one-half maternal levels)
Phencyclidine (127)	Potent hallucinogen
Phenindione (128)	Anticoagulant; bleeding in one case report with increased prothrombin time and increased partial thromboplastin time; not used in United States
Salicylate (aspirin) (37)	Salicylism in infant

is small; note that two are considered drugs of abuse. This list may be expanded as more data are collected and with the introduction of new drugs. There are several drug categories for which much most questions are raised.

RADIOACTIVE ISOTOPES AND CONTRAST MEDIUM

The use of radioactive isotopes and contrast medium for diagnostic purposes is very common All women of child-bearing age should be asked whether they are breast-feeding before a radioactive isotope is given. It may be possible to delay the test, employ an alternate test, or give specific instructions about how long to avoid nursing to ensure the disappearance from the milk of all significant radioactivity (40). Table 17.3 summarizes the excretion of the more commonly used radiopharmaceuticals in human milk. For technetium-99, it is safe to resume nursing 48 hours after maternal injection. For gallium-67 or iodine-131, nursing may have to be terminated because it may be difficult for the mother to continue to hand express (or by breast pump) milk for the 7 to 14 days necessary to achieve background radiation in her breast milk. Women who received therapeutic radiation isotopes (e.g., iodine-131) may have to terminate breastfeeding because the radiation dose to the infant will be too high for too long (e.g., 52 days in the case of the administration of 4,000 MBq of iodine-131 for thyroid carcinoma) (41).

Agents used for contrast studies in radiology are usually iodinated or gadolinium compounds. Less than 1% of the contrast given to the mother is excreted in milk and less than 1% of that ingested by the infant is absorbed from the gastrointestinal tract (42). There have been no reports of adverse effects in the nursing infant that would be traced to the use of these agents for diagnostic studies.

ENVIRONMENTAL CHEMICALS

In 1951, Laug et al. (43) published a report of dichlorodiphenyltrichloroethane (DDT) excretion in human milk samples collected in the United States (Washington, D.C.). This was the first environmental chemical to receive extensive study in human milk. Although this chemical is no longer used in the United States, the research done concerning its excretion into human milk is instructive. Laug et al. found DDT present in 94% of milk samples, with a mean level of 0.13 ppm (mg per kg milk). This was in excess of the level permitted by the World Health Organization (44) and the *US Code of Federal Regulations* (Title 12, 120.147C) of 0.050 ppm. Similar numbers have been reported from other parts of the world, including Norway (45,46), Australia, (47) the Netherlands (48), and Canada (49). Within the United States, similar concentrations of DDT were present in human milk regardless of geographic location or population size (50). In 1951 in the United States, the amount of DDT found by Laug et al. (43) was 0.13 ppm. In 1965, Quinby et al. (50) found levels of 0.12 ppm, and in 1972, Kroger (52) found levels of 0.10 ppm from six areas throughout the United States. Thus, in the United States, there was no change in content over 20 years even though this chemical was no longer being used. In Norway, 7 years after the total ban of DDT (1969/1970), the level in milk in Oslo had fallen from a mean of 0.082 ppm in 1969 to 0.050 ppm in 1976 (46). Other areas of Norway showed similar decreases.

The environmental chemicals are of concern because of their widespread use and their long dwelling time in the environment. The Environmental Protection Agency lists 2,200 chemicals manufactured in or imported into the United States each year in amounts of 1 million pounds or greater (53). Many of these compounds do not have adequate studies concerning their appearance in milk, and data concerning toxicity to living organisms are sparse (54–57).

The studies on DDT were the first to present the following information, which suggests that these highly lipid-soluble chemicals, which are widely available in the environment, are stored in body fat, and that milk may be the only route of elimination from the body (57,58):

1. DDT concentrations are 11-fold higher in body fat samples than in milk.

TABLE 17.3 Secretion of Radioactive Isotopes in Milk

Isotope	*Maternal Dose*[a]	$t_{1/2}$ *(hr)*	*Amount in Milk (μCi/mL)*	*Infant Dose on Day 1*[b] *(μCi/d)*	*Cumulative Dose to Infant*[b] *(μCi)*
Gallium-67 (129)	3 mCi i.v.	78	3 d: 0.15	75	350 (if nursed from day 3 on)
			7 d: 0.045	23	108 (if nursed from day 7 on)
			14 d: 0.010	5	23 (if nursed from day 14 on)
Indium-111 (130)	0.32 mCi i.v.		6 hr: 0.028	0.1	
			20 hr: 0.06		
Iodine-131 (131)	200 μCi i.v.	24	25 hr: 0.028	6	15 (if nursed through day 5)
					7.5% of maternal dose
Sodium-123 iodide (132)	183 mCi i.v.	5.8	6 hr: 0.0128	2.8	2.6% of maternal dose
Technetium-99 (51,133)	15 mCi i.v.	4	8.5 hr: 0.1	95	0.63% of maternal dose
			20 hr: 0.02		
			60 hr: 0.006		

[a] i.v., Intravenous.
[b] Data are calculated by assuming that the infant takes 3 oz of breast milk every 4 hr.

2. DDT concentrations decrease with number of infants nursed by the same mother.
3. DDT concentrations decrease with increasing number of months nursed.
4. DDT concentrations are significantly lower at the end of a single feed.

The group of halogenated aromatic hydrocarbons has received much attention. These include dioxins (contaminants formed during the manufacture of 2,4,5-trichlorophenoxyacetic acid, an ingredient in Agent Orange), furans, and polychlorinated biophenyls (PCBs). The unfortunate contamination of cattle feed with polybrominated biphenyls (PBBs) on Michigan cattle farms in 1973/1974 resulted in detectable levels of PBBs in human milk. For samples from the lower Michigan peninsula (site of heaviest contamination), 96% were positive for PBBs in the range from 0.02 to 1.0 ppm. The upper-peninsula samples were positive for PBB in 43% of samples in a range from 0.02 to 0.5 ppm, with most samples below 0.1 (59). There was a high degree of correlation between values in paired samples of milk and adipose tissue. The degree of risk even at these levels is not known (60). The Jacobson study (61) investigated infants whose mothers had consumed a moderate amount of fish from Lake Michigan compared with mothers who ate fish from another source. The only item noted to be less in the exposed group of children was activity, which was slightly reduced only in those who breast-fed for more than 1 year. IQ was unaffected at ages 4 and 11 years (61). A Dutch PCB/dioxin (1990 to 1992) study also did not show adverse developmental effects of exposure to PCBs. The breast-fed infants experienced no adverse effect on growth or neurologic outcome compared with formula-fed infants (62,63). A large-scale study in the United States was conducted in North Carolina (1978 to 1982). There did not appear to be measurable problems with illnesses, growth, or development. Some of these patients were followed from 10 to 15 years of age (64). A German study (1993 to 1995) did demonstrate subtle differences in Bayley scores from 7 to 30 months (65). The differences may be due to prenatal exposure during pregnancy. The isolation of pregnancy from lactation exposure is a difficult one for these studies, and may not be possible. The foregoing studies, taken collectively, do not show a significant effect on the infant in the areas of growth and development, and, when examined in context of the importance of breastfeeding, support the beneficial effect of breastfeeding in general (66,67).

Other highly lipid-soluble chemicals [e.g., tetrahydrocannabinol (68)] may be expected to act in a similar fashion. For women known to have had high exposure (by occupation or food ingestion), it may be reasonable to assay milk samples to determine exact risk. Because of advances in analytic instrumentation, some of these compounds can be measured in human milk in amounts as small as nanograms and picograms. There must be great care in any biomonitoring projects in how the information is presented to individuals concerned. For breastfeeding mothers (or mothers contemplating breastfeeding) there is great concern that transmitting such information to mothers may result in stopping nursing or not even starting (69). Research needs for a better understanding of the appearance of these chemicals in milk and description of possible biologic effects will require longitudinal studies over the entire woman's lactating period of quantification of the chemicals, disposition and elimination of the chemicals in the infant, identification of biomarkers of the effects of exposure, and a determination of the risk–benefit ratio of breastfeeding versus formula feedings when concern exists of the level of environmental chemical(s) present (54,70).

HERBAL PRODUCTS

Herbal products are widely available and used. The content is not regulated by the United States Food and Drug Administration. Active compounds in these preparations are not entirely defined and purity is widely variable. Concern has been raised over both efficacy and safety. Until the active compounds have been identified and quantified, they should be avoided by nursing mothers (71,72).

ORAL CONTRACEPTIVES

The postpartum use of the oral contraceptive pill by nursing mothers represents a common potential drug exposure to the nursing infant. Vorherr (14) summarized 18 papers published over a 10-year period dealing with this problem. It must be emphasized that these are older publications, in some instances reflecting the use of oral contraceptive pill with amounts of estrogen and progesterone that may no longer be used. Other studies addressed effects on lactation and growth and development (73–76). Neither estrogens nor progesterones seem to interfere with milk composition or with infant growth and development (74,77–82). There are some reports that do indicate that estrogens or the combined estrogen–progesterone pill may decrease milk production (83–85). It is reasonable advice that oral contraceptive treatment be withheld for several weeks until lactation is firmly established. Except for very rare reports (86), nursing infants do not appear to be hormonally affected. Most recently, oral contraceptives have been reformulated with smaller amounts of estrogen. The amount of estrogen excreted is, in most cases, not any greater than that naturally excreted by ovulating women (76). Methods of contraception that do not affect milk composition or production are preferred, especially the lactational amenorrhea method, which provides nearly 98% effective contraception if the mother is both exclusively breastfeeding and amenorrheic (87). The pharmacology of oral contraceptives changes frequently; studies of the effects of these newer agents on milk production and composition are very much needed.

PSYCHOTROPIC DRUGS

The psychotropic drugs include antidepressants, antianxiety agents, and antipsychotic (neuroleptic) drugs. Virtually all drugs in this class have been detected in milk after maternal ingestion (28,88–91). The milk/plasma ratio is usually less than 1. These drugs and, in many cases, their active metabolites usually have long half-lives, which accounts for their measurable appearance in the infant's plasma especially in young infants with maturing hepatic and renal function. These drugs act in the central nervous system by affecting neurotransmitter function, and presumably their presence in the plasma and urine of the nursing infant implies that there may be pharmacodynamic effects in the infant as well. The interesting review by Lauder suggests that neurotransmitters, separate from their neuronal regulatory activity, may act as growth regulatory signals, influencing proliferation, differentiation, and cell motility (92). There appears to be little short-term (15 to 166 days) effect on the infant (see earlier discussion concerning fluoxetine) (91,93). The long-term consequences, if any, to the infant's developing central nervous is unknown. A longer follow-up series by Nulman et al. showing no neurobehavioral effects in children assessed at 18 to 86 months after prenatal exposure to fluoxetine and tricyclic antidepressants is encouraging (94). In future studies it will be important to separate prenatal exposure from lactational exposure.

DRUG METABOLISM IN BREAST TISSUE

Little evidence is available concerning the actual drug-metabolizing activity of human breast tissue. Rasmussen and Linzell (95) described the acetylation of sulfanilamide by the mammary tissue of the lactating goat. Dao (96) was unable to demonstrate metabolism of the carcinogen 3-methylcholanthrene in mammary tissue. Bruder et al. (97) described cytochrome P-420 and cytochrome b_5 in the membranes of the milk fat globule of human milk; the same cytochromes were identified in the rough endoplasmic reticulum of lactating bovine and rat mammary epithelial cells. No cytochrome P-450 was identified in human, bovine, or rat milk or mammary tissue. Liu et al. (98) identified a calcium-stimulated ribonuclease in rat milk and mammary tissue. A reverse transcriptase has been observed in human milk (99). It is intriguing to speculate on its role in light of the observation by Scholm et al. (100) that human milk contains high–molecular-weight RNA particles.

SOURCES OF INFORMATION

The Committee on Drugs of the American Academy of Pediatrics has published a statement on the Transfer of Drugs and Other Chemicals into Human Milk (30). The first statement was published in 1983 with revisions in 1989, 1994, and 2001. It is a comprehensive listing of drugs and chemicals with references to guide the physician in advising nursing mothers. An even more complete compilation of the excretion of drugs in human milk has been published online by the Library of Medicine as their product named LactMed (101). This is a peer reviewed, continually updated database. The text by Briggs et al. is a compendium of information on drug exposure in both pregnancy and lactation (102). Quarterly updates are provided by the publisher (Lippincott Williams & Wilkins).

SUMMARY

Nearly all drugs (or environmental chemicals) may be found in breast milk after maternal ingestion. It is prudent to minimize maternal exposure, although very few are known to be hazardous to the nursing infant (Table 17.2). Chronic maternal drug administration and exposure to environmental chemicals are areas that need further exploration. More sensitive analytical techniques are being used to detect metabolites that may present a greater risk than the parent compound. Nursing mothers should avoid exposure to environmental chemicals. If maternal medication is necessary, drug exposure to the nursing infant may be minimized by the timing of a maternal dose just after nursing and/or at least one half-life of the drug prior to another nursing period. In the older infant who sleeps through the night, medication prescribed on a once-daily frequency would best be taken after the last evening feeding of the baby. Assay for the drug in the infant's plasma may be indicated for some drugs when parent and physician wish to know the extent of transfer from mother to infant. Breast milk, the ideal infant food, must be made as safe as possible. Nursing mothers should not be deprived of needed medication.

REFERENCES

1. Nutrition Committee of the Canadian Paediatric Society and the Committee on Nutrition of the American Academy of Pediatrics. Breast feeding. *Pediatrics* 1978;62:591–601.
2. Gartner LM, Morton J, Lawrence RA et al; American Academy of Pediatrics Section on Breastfeeding. Breastfeeding and the use of human milk. *Pediatrics* 2005;115:496–506.
3. Lawrence RA, Lawrence RB. *Breastfeeding: a guide for the medical profession*, 6th ed. St. Louis, MO: Mosby, 2005.
4. Department of Health and Human Services, Office on Women's Health. *Breastfeeding. HHS blueprint for action on breastfeeding.* Washington, DC: Department of Health and Human Services, Office on Women's Health, 2000.
5. McDowell MA, Wang C-Y, Kennedy-Stephenson J. *Breastfeeding in the United States: findings from the National Health and Nutrition Examination Surveys 1999–2006.* NCHS data briefs, no 5. Hyattsville, MD: National Center for Health Statistics, 2008.
6. Stultz EE, Stokes JL, Shaffer ML, et al. Extent of medication use in breastfeeding women. *Breastfeed Med* 2007;2:145–151.
7. Nestlé Nutrition Services. Bioactive factors in milk. *Ann Nestlé* 1996;54:79–119.
8. Daly SEJ, Owens RA, Hartmann PE. The short-term synthesis and infant-regulated removal of milk in lactating women. *Exp Physiol* 1993;78:209–220.
9. Dewey KG, Lönnerdal B. Infant self-regulation of breast milk intake. *Acta Pediatr Scand* 1986;75:893–898.
10. Daly SEJ, Di Rosso A, Owens RA, et al. Degree of breast emptying explains changes in the fat content, but not fatty acid composition, of human milk. *Exp Physiol* 1993;78:741–755.
11. Resman BH, Blumenthal HP, Jusko WJ. Breast milk distribution of theobromine from chocolate. *J Pediatr* 1977;91:477–480.
12. Yurchak AM, Jusko WJ. Theophylline secretion into breast milk. *Pediatrics* 1976;57:518–520.
13. Patton S, Keenan TW. The milk fat globule membrane. *Biochem Biophys Acta* 1975;415:273–309.
14. Vorherr H. *The breast.* New York, NY: Academic Press, 1974: 107–124.

15. Ferguson DJP, Anderson TJ. An ultrastructural study of lactation in the human breast. *Anat Embryol (Berl)* 1983;168:349–359.
16. Schanker LS. Passage of drugs across membranes. *Pharmacol Rev* 1962;14:501–550.
17. Wilkinson GR. Pharmacokinetics. In: Hardman JG, Limbird LE, Gilman AG, eds. *Goodman & Gilman's the pharmacological basis of therapeutics*, 10th ed. New York, NY: McGraw-Hill, 2001:3–43.
18. Kesaniemi YA. Ethanol and acetaldehyde in the milk and peripheral blood of lactating women after ethanol administration. *J Obstet Gynaecol Br Commonw* 1974;81:84–86.
19. Begg EJ, Atkinson HC. Modeling of the passage of drugs into milk. *Pharmacol Ther* 1993;59:301–310.
20. Rasmussen F. Excretion of drugs by milk. In: Brodie BB, Gilette JR, eds. *Handbook of experimental pharmacology*, Vol. 28. New York, NY: Springer-Verlag, 1971:390–402.
21. Wilson JT, Brown RD, Cherek DR, et al. Drug excretion in human breast milk. *Clin Pharmacokinet* 1980;5:1–66.
22. Wilson JT, Brown RD, Hinson JL, et al. Pharmcokinetic pitfalls in the estimation of the breast milk/plasma ratio for drugs. *Annu Rev Pharmacol Toxicol* 1985;25:667–689.
23. Miller GE, Banejee NC, Stowie CM Jr. Drug movement between bovine milk and plasma as affected by milk pH. *J Dairy Sci* 1967;50:1395–1403.
24. Rasmussen F. *Studies on the mammary excretion and absorption of drugs*. Copenhagen: Martenson, 1966.
25. Rasmussen F. The mechanisms of drug secretion into milk. In: Galli G, Jacini G, Pecile A, eds. *Dietary lipids and postnatal development*. New York, NY: Raven Press, 1973:231–245.
26. Atkinson HC, Begg EJ, Darlow BA. Drugs in human milk; clinical pharmacokinetic considerations. *Clin Pharmacokinet* 1988;14: 217–240.
27. Fleishaker JC, Desai N, McNamara PJ. Factors affecting the milk-to-plasma drug concentration ratio in lactating women: physical interactions with protein and fat. *J Pharm Sci* 1987;76:189–193.
28. Pons G, Rey E, Matheson I. Excretion of psychoactive drugs into breast milk. *Clin Pharmacokinet* 1994;27:270–289.
29. Atkinson HC, Begg EJ. Prediction of drug distribution into human milk from physicochemical characteristics. *Clin Pharmacokinet* 1990;18:151–167.
30. American Academy of Pediatrics Committee on Drugs. Transfer of drugs and other chemicals into human milk. *Pediatrics* 2001;108:776–789.
31. Ito S. Drug therapy for breast-feeding women. *N Engl J Med* 2000;343:118–126.
32. Kwit NT, Harcher RA. Excretion of drugs in milk. *Am J Dis Child* 1935;49:900–904.
33. Anderson PO, Pochop SL, Manoguerra AS. Adverse drug reactions in breastfed infants: less than imagined. *Clin Pediatr* 2003;42(4):325–340.
34. Naranjo CA, Busto U, Sellers EM, et al. A method for estimating the probability of adverse drug reactions. *Clin Pharmacol Ther* 1981;30:239–245.
35. Madadi P, Ross CJD, Hayden MR, et al. Pharmacogenetics of neonatal opiod toxicity following maternal use of codeine during breastfeeding: a case-control study. *Clin Pharmacol Ther* 2008; 85:31–35.
36. Berlin CM Jr, Paul IM, Vesell ES. Safety issues of maternal drug therapy during breastfeeding. *Clin Pharmacol Ther* 2008;85: 20–22.
37. Clark JH, Wilson WG. A 16-day-old breast-fed infant with metabolic acidosis caused by salicylate. *Clin Pediatr (Phila)* 1981;20:53–54.
38. Lester BM, Cucca J, Andreozzi L, et al. Possible association between fluoxetine and colic in an infant. *J Am Acad Child Psychiatry* 1993;32:1253–1255.
39. Ito S, Blajchman A, Stephenson M, et al. Prospective follow-up of adverse reactions in breast-fed infants exposed to maternal medication. *Am J Obstet Gynecol* 1993;168:1393–1399.
40. Stabin MG, Breitz HB. Breast milk excretion of radiophamaceuticals: mechanisms, findings, and radiation dosimetry. *J Nucl Med* 2000;41:863–873.
41. Robinson PS, Barker P, Campbell A, et al. Iodine-131 in breast milk following therapy for thyroid carcinoma. *J Nucl Med* 1994;35:1797–1801.
42. American College of Radiology. *ACR practice guideline. Manual on contrast media. 2008. Version 6.0.* American College of Radiology, 2004:65–66. Available at www.acr.org.
43. Laug EP, Kunze FM, Prickett CS. Occurrence of DDT in human fat and milk. *Arch Ind Hyg Occup Med* 1951;3:245–246.
44. WHO/FAO. Pesticide residues in food (Technical Report Series No. 417). Geneva: WHO/FAO, 1969.
45. Brenik EM, Bjerk JE. Organochlorine compounds in Norwegian human fat and milk. *Acta Pharmacol Toxicol (Copenh)* 1978;43: 59–63.
46. Bakken AF, Seip M. Insecticides in human breast milk. *Acta Paediatr Scand* 1976;65:535–539.
47. Siyali DS. Polychlorinated biphenyls, hexachlorobenzene and other organochlorine pesticides in human milk. *Med J Aust* 1973;2:815–818.
48. Turistra LGMT. Organochlorine insecticide residues in human milk in one Leiden region. *Neth Milk Dairy J* 1971;25:24–32.
49. Holdrinet MVH, Braun HE, Frank R, et al. Organochlorine residues in human adipose tissue and milk from Ontario residents 1969–1974. *Can J Public Health* 1977;68:74–80.
50. Quinby GE, Armstrong JF, Durham WF. DDT in human milk. *Nature* 1965;207:726–728.
51. Rumble WF, Aamodt RL, Jones AE, et al. Accidental ingestion of Tc-99 m in breast milk by a 10-week-old child. *J Nucl Med* 1978;19: 913–915.
52. Kroger M. Insecticide residues in human milk. *J Pediatr* 1972;80: 401–405.
53. U.S. Environmental Protection Agency. High production volume chemicals. OPPT databases. http:/www.epa.gov/chemrtk/index.htm.
54. LaKind JS, Berlin CM. Technical workshop on human milk surveillance and research on environmental chemicals in the United States: an overview. *J Toxicol Environ Health A* 2002;65: 1829–1837.
55. Berlin CM, LaKind JS, Sonawane BR, et al. Conclusions, research needs, and recommendations of the expert panel: technical workshop on human milk surveillance and research for environmental chemicals in the United States. *J Toxicol Environ Health A* 2002;65:1929–1935.
56. Berlin CM, Kacew S. Environmental chemicals in human milk. In: Kacew S, Lambert GH, eds. *Environmental toxicology and pharmacology of human development*. Washington, DC: Taylor & Francis, 1997:67–93.
57. LaKind JS, Berlin CM, Park CN, et al. Methodology for characterizing distributions of incremental body burdens of 2,3,7,8-TCDD and DDE from breast milk in North American nursing infants. *J Toxicol Environ Health A* 2000;59:605–639.
58. LaKind JS, Berlin CM, Naiman DQ. Infant exposure to chemicals in breast milk in the United States: what we need to learn from a breast milk monitoring program. *Environ Health Perspect* 2001;109(1):75–88.
59. Brilliant LB, Amburg GV, Isbister J, et al. Breast-milk monitoring to measure Michigan's contamination with polybrominated biphenyls. *Lancet* 1978;2:643–646.
60. Wolff MS. Occupationally derived chemicals in breast milk. *Am J Ind Med* 1983;4:259–281.
61. Jacobson JL. Behavioral effects of developmental exposure to fish-borne contaminants. *Neurotoxicology* 2000;21:619–620.
62. Patandin S, Lanting CI, Mulder PGH, et al. Effects of environmental exposure to polychlorinated biphenyls and dioxins on cognitive abilities in Dutch children at 42 months of age. *J Pediatr* 1999;134:33–40.
63. Patandin S, Koopman-Esseboom C, de Ridder MA, et al. Effects of environmental exposure to polychlorinated biphenyls and dioxins on birth size and growth in Dutch children. *Pediatr Res* 1998;44:538–545.
64. Gladen BC, Ragan NB, Rogan WJ. Pubertal growth and development and prenatal and lactational exposure to polychlorinated biphenyls and dichlorodiphenyl dichloroethane. *J Pediatr* 2000;136: 490–496.
65. Walkowiak J, Wiener JA, Fastabend A, et al. Environmental exposure to polychlorinated biphenyls and quality of the home environment. *Lancet* 2001;358:1602–1607.
66. Brouwer A, Ahlborg UG, van Leeuwen FXR, et al. Report of the WHO working group on the assessment of health risks for human infant from exposure to PCDDs, PCDFs and PCBs. *Chemosphere* 1998;37:1627–1643.
67. Lakind JS, Berlin CM, Mattison DR. The heart of the matter on breastmilk and environmental chemicals: essential points for

healthcare providers and new parents. *Breastfeed Med* 2008;3: 251–259.

68. Perez-Reyes M, Wall EM. Presence of tetrahydrocannabinol in human milk. *N Engl J Med* 1982;307:819.
69. Geraghty SR, Khoury JC, Morrow AL, et al. Reporting individual test results of environmental chemicals in breastmilk: potential for premature weaning. *Breastfeed Med* 2008;3:207–213.
70. Berlin CM, Kacew S, Lawrence R, et al. Criteria for chemical selection for programs on human milk surveillance and research for environmental chemicals. *J Toxicol Environ Health A* 2002;65:1839–1851.
71. Snodgrass WR. Herbal products: risks and benefits of use in children. *Curr Ther Res Clin Exp* 2001;62:724–737.
72. De Smet PAGM. Herbal remedies. *N Engl J Med* 2002;347: 2046–2056.
73. Zacharias S, Aguillern E, Assenzo JR, et al. Effects of hormonal and nonhormonal contraceptives on lactation and incidence of pregnancy. *Contraception* 1986;33:203–213.
74. Nilsson S, Mellbin T, Hofvander Y, et al. Long-term follow-up of children breast-fed by mothers using oral contraceptives. *Contraception* 1986;34:443–457.
75. Nilsson S, Nygren KG. Transfer of contraceptive steroids to human milk. *Res Reprod* 1979;11:1–2.
76. American Academy of Pediatrics Committee on Drugs. Breastfeeding and contraception. *Pediatrics* 1981;68:138–140.
77. World Health Organization Task Force on Oral Contraceptives, Special Programme of Research, Development and Research Training in Human Reproduction. Effects of hormonal contraceptives on breast milk composition and infant growth. *Stud Fam Plann* 1988;19:361–369.
78. Tankeyoon M, Dusitsin N, Chalapati S, et al. World Health Organization Task Force on Oral Contraceptives, Special Programme of Research, Development and Research Training in Human Reproduction. Effects of hormonal contraceptives on milk volume and infant growth. *Contraception* 1984;30: 505–522.
79. Moggia AV, Harris GS, Dunson TR, et al. A comparative study of a progestin-only oral contraception versus non-hormonal methods in lactating women in Buenos Aires, Argentina. *Contraception* 1991;44:31–43.
80. Pardthaisong T, Yenchit C, Gray R. The long-term growth and development of children exposed to depo-provera during pregnancy or lactation. *Contraception* 1992;45:313–324.
81. Shaaban M. Contraception with progestogens and progesterone during lactation. *J Steroid Biochem Mol Biol* 1991;40:705–710.
82. Shikary ZK, Betrabet SS, Patel ZM, et al. ICMR task force study on hormonal contraception: transfer of levonorgestrel (LNG) administered through different drug delivery systems from the maternal circulation into the newborn infant's circulation via breast milk. *Contraception* 1987;35:477–486.
83. Compodonico I, Guerro B, Landa L. Effect of a low-dose oral contraceptive (150 μg of levonorgestrel and 30 μg ethinylestradiol) on lactation. *Clin Ther* 1978;1:454–459.
84. Koetsawang S, Bhiraleus P, Chiemprajert T. Effects of oral contraceptives in lactation. *Fertil Steril* 1972;23:24–28.
85. Díaz S, Croxatto HB. Contraception in lactating women. *Cur Opin Obstet Gynecol* 1993;5:815–822.
86. Curtis EM. Oral-contraceptive feminization of a normal male infant: report of a case. *Obstet Gynecol* 1964;23:295–296.
87. Perez A, Labbock MH, Queenan JT. Clinical study of the lactational amenorrhea method for family planning. *Lancet* 1992;339: 968–970.
88. Berlin CM, Yaffe SJ, Ragni M. Disposition of acetaminophen in milk, saliva, and plasma of lactating women. *Pediatr Pharmacol (New York)* 1980;1:135–141.
89. Stowe ZN, Owens MJ, Landry J, et al. Sertraline and desmethylsertraline in human breast milk and nursing infants. *Am J Psychiatry* 1997;154:1255–1260.
90. Yoshida K, Smith B, Craggs M, et al. Neuroleptic drugs in breast milk: a study of pharmacokinetics and of possible adverse effects in breast-fed infants. *Psychol Med* 1998;28:81–91.
91. Birnbaum CS, Cohen LS, Bailey J, et al. Serum concentrations of antidepressants and benzodiazepines in nursing infants: a case series. *Pediatrics* 1999;104:e11.
92. Lauder JM. Neurotransmitters as growth regulatory signals: role of receptors and second messengers. *Trends Neurosci* 1993;16:233–240.
93. Taddio A, Ito S, Koren G. Excretion of fluoxetine and its metabolite, norfluoxetine, in human breast milk. *J Clin Pharmacol* 1996;36:42–47.
94. Nulman I, Rovet J, Stewart DE, et al. Neurodevelopment of children exposed in utero to antidepressant drugs. *N Engl J Med* 1997;336:258–262.
95. Rasmussen F, Linzell JL. The acetylation of sulphanilamide by mammary tissue of lactating goats. *Biochem Pharmacol* 1967;16: 918–919.
96. Dao TL. Studies on mechanism of carcinogenesis in mammary gland. *Prog Exp Tumor Res* 1969;11:235–261.
97. Bruder G, Fink A, Jarasch ED. The β-type cytochrome in endoplasmic reticulum of mammary gland epithelium and milk fat globule membranes consists of two components, cytochrome b5 and cytochrome P-420. *Exp Cell Res* 1978;117:207–217.
98. Liu DK, Kulick D, Williams GH. Ca2+ stimulated ribonuclease. *Biochem J* 1979;178:241–244.
99. McCormick JJ, Larson LJ, Rich MA. RNAse inhibition of reverse transcriptase activity in human milk. *Nature* 1974;251:737–740.
100. Scholm J, Spiegelman S, Moore DH. Detection of high-molecular-weight RNA in particles from human milk. *Science* 1972;175: 542–544.
101. United States National Library of Medicine. Toxicology Data Network. Drugs and lactation database (LactMed). http://toxnet.nlm.nih.gov/cgi-bin/sis/htmlgen?LACT.
102. Briggs GG, Freeman RK, Yaffe SJ. *Drugs in pregnancy and lactation*, 8th ed. Philadelphia, PA: Lippincott Williams & Wilkins, 2008.
103. Berlin CM, Vesell ES. Antipyrine disposition in milk or saliva of lactating women. *Clin Pharmacol Ther* 1982;31:38–44.
104. Berlin CM, Denson HM, Daniel CH, et al. Disposition of dietary caffeine in milk, saliva, and plasma of lactating women. *Pediatrics* 1984;73:59–63.
105. Yoshioka H, Cho K, Takimoto M, et al. Transfer of cefazolin into human milk. *J Pediatr* 1979;94:151–152.
106. Werthmann MW, Drees SV. Excretion of chlorothiazide in human breast milk. *J Pediatr* 1972;81:781–783.
107. Cole AP, Hailey DM. Diazepam and active metabolite in breast milk and their transfer to the neonate. *Arch Dis Child* 1975;50: 741–742.
108. Loughnan PM. Digoxin excretion in human breast milk. *J Pediatr* 1978;92:1019–1020.
109. Berlin CM, Lee C. Isoniazid and acetylisoniazid disposition in human milk, saliva and plasma. *Fed Proc* 1979;38:426.
110. Schou M, Amdisen A. Lithium and pregnancy—III. Lithium ingestion by children breast fed by women on lithium treatment. *Br Med J* 1973;2:138.
111. Blinick G, Inturrisi CE, Jerez E, et al. Methadone assays in pregnant women and progeny. *Am J Obstet Gynecol* 1975;121: 617–621.
112. Erickson Sh, Oppenheim GL, Smith FH. Metronidazole in breast milk. *Obstet Gynecol* 1981;57:48–50.
113. Ferguson BB, Wilson DJ, Schaffner W. Determination of nicotine concentrations in human milk. *Am J Dis Child* 1976;130: 837–839.
114. McKenzie SA, Selley JA, Agnew JE. Secretion of prednisolone into breast milk. *Arch Dis Child* 1975;50:894–896.
115. Berlin CM, Demers L, Kaiser D. Prednisone and prednisolone in human milk after large oral dose of prednisone. *Pharmacologist* 1979;13:396.
116. Karlberg B, Lindberg D, Aberg H. Excretion of propranolol in human breast milk. *Acta Pharmacol Toxicol* 1974;34:222–224.
117. Levy G. Salicylate pharmacokinetics in the human neonate. In: Morselli PL, Garactini G, Sereni F, eds. *Basic and therapeutic aspects of perinatal pharmacology*. New York, NY: Raven Press, 1975:319–330.
118. Berlin CM, Yaffe SJ. Disposition of sulfasalazine (Azulfidine) in human breast milk, plasma, and saliva. *Dev Pharmacol Ther* 1980;1:31–39.
119. Dreisbach JA. Sulphone levels in breast milk of mothers on sulphone therapy. *Lepr Rev* 1952;23:101–106.
120. Anderson P, Bondesson U, Mattiasson I, et al. Verapamil and norverapamil in plasma and breast milk during breast-feeding. *Eur J Clin Pharmacol* 1987;3:625–627.
121. Boutry MJ, Bianchetti G, Dubruc C, et al. To nurse when receiving acebutolol: Is it dangerous for the neonate? *Eur J Clin Pharmacol* 1986;30:737–739.

122. Schimmel MS, Erdelman AI, Wilschanski MA, et al. Toxic effects of atenolol consumed during breast feeding. *J Pediatr* 1989;114:476–478.
123. Kulski JK, Hartmann PE, Martin JD, et al. Effects of bromocriptine mesylate on the composition of the mammary secretion in non-breast-feeding women. *Obstet Gynecol* 1978;52:38–42.
124. Chasnoff IJ, Lewis DE, Squires L. Cocaine intoxication in a breast-fed infant. *Pediatrics* 1978;80:836–838.
125. Chaney NE, Franke J, Wadlington WB. Cocaine convulsions in a breast-feeding baby. *J Pediatr* 1988;112:134–135.
126. Fomina POL. Untersuchungen uber den Ubergang des aktiven agens des Mutterkorns in die milch stillender Mutter. *Arch Gynecol Obstet* 1934;157:275–285.
127. Kaufman KR, Petrucha RA, Pitts FN Jr, et al. PCP in amniotic fluid and breast milk: case report. *J Clin Psychiatry* 1983;44:269–270.
128. Eckstein HB, Jack B. Breast-feeding and anticoagulant therapy. *Lancet* 1970;1:672.
129. Tobin RE, Schneider PB. Uptake of 67 Ga in the lactating breast and its persistence in milk: case report. *J Nucl Med* 1976;17:1055–1056.
130. Butt D, Szaz KF. Indium-111 radioactivity in breast milk. *Br J Radiol* 1986;59:80–82.
131. Wyburn JR. Human breast milk excretion of radionuclides following administration of radiopharmaceuticals. *J Nucl Med* 1973;14:115–117.
132. Hedrick WR, DiSimone RN, Keen RL. Radiation dosimetry from breast milk excretion of radioiodine and pertechnetate. *J Nucl Med* 1986;27:1569–1571.
133. Maisels MJ, Gilcher RO. Excretion of technetium in human milk. *Pediatrics* 1983;71:841–842.

David K. Stevenson
Ronald J. Wong
Susan R. Hintz
Hendrik J. Vreman

CHAPTER 18

Drugs for Hyperbilirubinemia

INTRODUCTION

Hyperbilirubinemia is a natural and essentially ubiquitous transitional phenomenon among human newborns. Approximately 60% to 70% of all term infants, and nearly all premature infants, become visibly jaundiced during the first week of life after birth. For term infants, the serum or plasma total bilirubin (PTB) concentration typically peaks 3 to 4 days after birth in the range of 5 to 6 mg per dL (86 to 103 μmol per L). For premature infants, PTB levels peak later and higher after the first several days of life. Although much uncertainty and debate remains concerning the range of PTB considered as benign physiologic jaundice, the consensus places the maximal "safe" peak PTB threshold at approximately 17 mg per dL (291 μmol per L) for otherwise healthy term and late preterm babies. Because hyperbilirubinemia above this threshold is considered to be pathologic, the etiology of the hyperbilirubinemia should be investigated and appropriate therapy considered or initiated depending on the clinical circumstances (1). In immature infants, treatment to decrease PTB levels is often initiated at lower PTB levels because of lower albumin levels and diminished affinity of albumin for bilirubin in these infants. Moreover, binding to albumin is least avid in the early transitional period after birth and is influenced adversely by any confounding conditions, such as infection or acidosis, that increase free bilirubin in circulation and the likelihood of movement into tissues.

Historically, the main therapies for neonatal hyperbilirubinemia have been phototherapy and exchange transfusion. Light could be considered a drug for hyperbilirubinemia, but most physicians pay little attention to the radiometric qualities (effective spectral width and peak emission) and quantities [irradiance (μW per cm^2 per nm)] involved, or the factors that affect the dose of phototherapy (duration, body surface area exposure) (2,3). Finally, issues that are involved in producing phototherapy-related side effects (riboflavin destruction, erythema, and photosensitizing drugs) also deserve attention. A discussion of these topics should include reference to the qualities of light-emitting diodes because of their high intensity and narrowband light in the spectrum of choice with minimal heat generation (3–6), but these issues are beyond the scope of this chapter. In spite of the proven benefits of phototherapy and maximal spatial limitations, the understanding of the biology of newborn jaundice and the existence and further development of alternative pharmacologic therapies for neonatal hyperbilirubinemia are an integral part of the management of neonatal jaundice and its consequences.

NEONATAL JAUNDICE

Neonatal jaundice is the result of an imbalance between the production of bilirubin and its elimination (7–9). Bilirubin production on a body weight basis is increased in the newborn by approximately two to three times that of an adult (10,11). This relative increase in bilirubin production in the newborn is the result of an increased circulating red cell mass and a shortened red cell life span. Consequently, all newborn infants have increased bilirubin production as a contributing cause of their transitional or pathologic jaundice. The pattern of hyperbilirubinemia (its peak and duration) is influenced further by the efficiency with which the pigment is eliminated. The major factor contributing to impaired elimination in the transitional period after birth is decreased hepatic conjugation of bilirubin. The gradual induction of uridine diphosphoglucuronate glucuronosyltransferase (UGT) contributes most importantly to the pattern of hyperbilirubinemia after birth because changes in bilirubin production are slower and more gradual within the time frame of the rapid elevation in PTB levels after birth and the decline in the latter part of the first week and into the second week of life. Thus, because all newborn babies have temporarily impaired conjugation, any pathologic state associated with increased bilirubin production, such as hemolysis, represents a serious risk to the newborn infant, especially in the first several days of life. Even without pathologic elevations in bilirubin production, greater impairments in conjugation associated with conditions such as Gilbert syndrome (12–14) and the Asian G71R mutation in the UGT1A1 gene (14–16) can place infants at risk for kernicterus because of unexpected alterations in the pattern of hyperbilirubinemia, including its peak and duration. In particular, the coexpression of gene polymorphisms involved in bilirubin production, such as $(GT)_n$, repeats in the HO-1 promoter and glucose-6-phosphate dehydrogenase

(G6PD) mutations, and metabolisms, such as OATP1A1 and UGT1A1 and the TATAA box variants, may provide genetic markers for clinical risk assessments, as well as potential therapeutic targets (17,18).

The imbalances in the production of the pigment and its elimination have been well studied, and various methods have been proposed to identify infants at risk for severe hyperbilirubinemia. Because the predominant source of carbon monoxide (CO) in the body is the degradation of heme, which ultimately leads to the production of equimolar amounts of bilirubin, increased bilirubin production can be estimated by measuring the end-tidal CO in breath, or carboxyhemoglobin (COHb) in circulation, after these measurements are corrected for ambient CO (ETCOc or COHbc, respectively) (19,20). The normalization of COHbc to hemoglobin concentration (COHbc/Hb) can serve as an even more sensitive index of excessive red cell destruction (21). For example, the infant with hemolytic anemia would have a higher COHbc/Hb ratio than the infant with anemia caused by blood loss. By measuring the conjugated fraction of bilirubin, another index can be applied, which assesses the relative balance between bilirubin production and conjugation [COHbc/TCB (%)], where TCB is the total conjugated bilirubin (9). Finally, a nomogram plotting hour-specific bilirubin levels is also informed by the balance of bilirubin production and elimination over time (22). Because all infants have impaired conjugation during the transitional period, deviations from the percentile tracks in the first several days of life are most often related to a relative increase in bilirubin production, whereas deviations after the first week of life are more likely the result of persistent impairment in bilirubin conjugation and therefore elimination.

The logic of removing bilirubin from circulation after it has been produced is clear, but it is also only reactionary and may not avoid potential neurologic injury in every circumstance. Another, more rational, treatment strategy would be to inhibit bilirubin production, thus ameliorating the primary contributing factor in neonatal hyperbilirubinemia and the risk for kernicterus. If a safe drug for inhibiting bilirubin production could be identified, its use could be universalized. However, another alternative preventive strategy could involve the early rapid and accurate identification of infants at risk for increased bilirubin production or at least with an imbalance between the production and the elimination of bilirubin. One direct approach would be to measure ETCOc or COHbc as an index of bilirubin formation and, thus, identify high producers of the pigment for targeted therapy. Yet another approach would be to plot hour-specific bilirubin levels and be cognizant of early deviations from the nomogram suggestive of increased bilirubin production or the combination of relatively insufficient conjugation for a given bilirubin load (23). Whether the approach is targeted would depend, at least in part, on the safety, efficacy, and cost of the chemotherapeutic agent.

HEME DEGRADATION PATHWAY

Heme is degraded in a two-step enzymatic pathway, which requires molecular oxygen and NADPH (see Fig. 18.1). The first step is rate limiting and catalyzed by heme oxygenase (HO), a membrane-bound enzyme (24). In this first step, the porphyrin macrocycle is broken at the 9-α-meso carbon bridge after a series of oxidations and reductions, and liberates CO, iron, and biliverdin in equimolar amounts. In the second enzymatic step, biliverdin is immediately reduced in the cytosol by biliverdin reductase in an NADPH-dependent reaction to generate bilirubin. Because HO is the rate-limiting enzyme in the pathway, its inhibition results in decreased production of CO, iron, and biliverdin, thus leading to decreased bilirubin production (25,26).

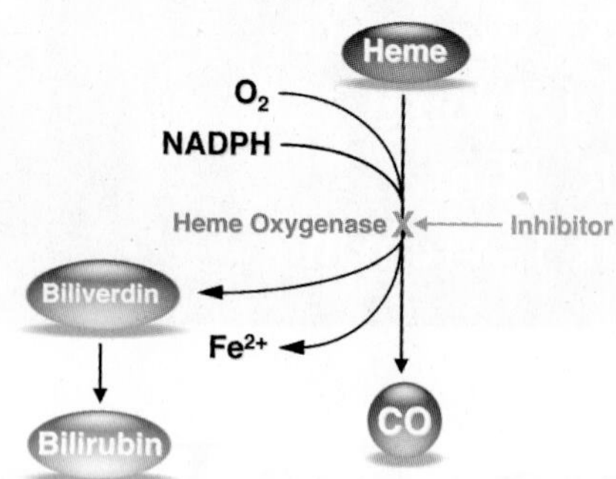

Figure 18.1. Heme catabolic pathway.

HEME OXYGENASE INHIBITORS

METALLOPORPHYRINS

Many synthetic structural analogues or metalloporphyrins (Mps) of heme (ferro-protoporphyrin) are effective in vitro and in vivo competitive inhibitors of HO (Fig. 18.2, Table 18.1). The original idea for using heme analogues (i.e., zinc protoporphyrin, ZnPP) as drugs for modulating bilirubin production was pioneered in 1981 by Maines (27) and has driven nearly three decades of intensive investigation of a variety of related potential chemopreventive agents. These compounds proved to have variable efficacies with respect to the two primary and well-described isoforms of HO, the inducible form (HO-1) and the constitutive form (HO-2), which occur in different relative proportions in tissues (28,29). Moreover, some of

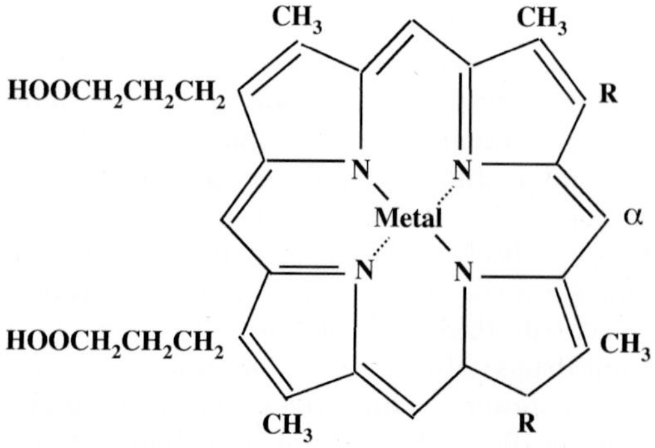

Figure 18.2. Metalloporphyrin structure. (From Vreman HJ, Wong RJ, Stevenson DK. Alternative metalloporphyrins for the treatment of neonatal jaundice. *J Perinatol* 2001; 21(Suppl 1):S108–S113, with permission.)

TABLE 18.1 Porphyrin Type Based on Chelated Metal and Ring Substituent

Metal	*Deuteroporphyrin (DP) (R = –H)*	*Mesoporphyrin (MP) (R = –CH_2–CH_3)*	*Protoporphyrin (PP) (R = –CH = CH_2)*	*Bis Glycol Porphyrin (BG) (R = –CHOH–CH_2OH)*
Metal free	MfDP	MfMP	MfPP	MfBG
Iron (Fe^{2+})	FeDP	FeMP	FePP (hemin)	FeBG
Zinc (Zn^{2+})	ZnDP	ZnMP	ZnPP	ZnBG
Tin (Sn^{4+})	SnDP	SnMP	SnPP	SnBG
Chromium (Cr^{2+})	CrDP	CrMP	CrPP	CrBG
Manganese (Mn^{2+})	MnDP	MnMP	MnPP	MnBG
Copper (Cu^{2+})	CuDP	CuMP	CuPP	CuBG
Nickel (Ni^{2+})	NiDP	NiMP	NiPP	NiBG

these compounds have been found to also inhibit other enzymes, such as nitric oxide synthase (NOS) and soluble guanylyl cyclase (sGC), as well as processes such as lipid peroxidation (30,31). In fact, the products of heme degradation, CO, iron, biliverdin, and bilirubin all have been shown to have important biological roles as antioxidant and anti-inflammatory agents (20,32–34). Thus, the deliberate attenuation of heme degradation for the purpose of controlling the production of bilirubin must be considered in the context of the potential side effects on other important biologic processes in the transitional period and their effects beyond (35).

Tin protoporphyrin (SnPP) was the first synthetic heme analogue used for the purpose of inhibiting HO in human neonates, after intensive investigation in rodents and nonhuman primates (36–38). Although highly efficacious, the photoreactivity of this Mp made it a less desirable drug (39–41). Tin mesoporphyrin (SnMP), which is also photoreactive and more potent, however, has been used in several randomized controlled trials in human neonates at considerably lower doses than was possible with SnPP (42,43). In fact, a single intramuscular dose of 6 and 4.5 μM SnMP per kg body weight has been shown to eliminate the need for phototherapy (42) or for exchange transfusion (44), respectively, during the postnatal period. The efficacy of the compound has been well established, but it still may not represent the ideal therapeutic agent because it is photoreactive and contains a foreign (nonessential) metal, induces the HO-1 gene, and can inhibit other enzyme systems such as NOS and sGC. ZnPP has been proposed as an alternative drug, but its inhibitory potency is much lower and its formulation for administration has been more difficult (26). Nonetheless, it is a naturally occurring Mp and has both in vitro and in vivo inhibitory properties for both HO-1 and HO-2, and has been shown to suppress hyperbilirubinemia in neonatal rodents and nonhuman primates (40). Moreover, this naturally occurring heme analogue has no apparent photoreactivity in vivo. With respect to photoreactivity, many of the heme analogues have already been characterized along with their inhibitory potency (26,40,41,45).

In addition to screening for potential phototoxicity, the impact of these heme analogues on the induction of HO-1 is also important to consider (26,46–48). In fact, the various Mps also differ in their ability to upregulate the HO-1 gene. For example, ZnPP and zinc bis glycol porphyrin (ZnBG) appear to cause minimal induction. The latter compound is a very potent inhibitor, which is orally absorbable (46,47,49,50). Although ZnBG is photoreactive, its substantial potency would allow for its use with minimal clinical risk similar to what has been observed for SnMP. The characteristics of the unique metabolite ZnPP have been reviewed in detail elsewhere (51). Besides its therapeutic potential, it also has clinical applications for assessing nutritional iron status in pediatric patients, pregnant women, and blood donors and for diagnosing other disorders in iron metabolism including lead toxicity (51). With respect to the potential for inducing HO-1, preliminary data on cadmium-induced HO-1 transcription suggest a possible programming effect, with a second exposure to the drug resulting in less of an induction. Whether such an effect is observable and consequential with the other structural analogues of heme, some of which are also strong inducers of HO-1, would be important to understand in the context of selecting a safe drug with a short duration of action, no lingering side effects on other biologic processes, and no long-term alterations in HO-1 gene expression secondary to drug exposure in a critical period.

Besides a wide spectrum of HO inhibitory potential among the different Mps, for the two isozymes, the route of administration can also influence the bioavailability and efficacy of the drugs. For example, oral administration may be possible with ZnBG and with chromium mesoporphyrin (CrMP) (52–54), but with the current formulations, is unlikely to be possible for SnMP or ZnPP. The packaging of Mps for targeting particular tissues, such as the spleen, is also possible. Liposomes have been reported as useful for this purpose (55), and there are probably other targeting approaches that could alter distribution by the various routes of administration.

Another factor to consider when choosing a drug for hyperbilirubinemia is the fact that inhibition of HO in the liver and spleen leads to the proportional excretion of undegraded heme in bile (56). Thus, it is important to inhibit HO activity in the intestine so that heme reaching the intestine is not catabolized to bilirubin, which can be recirculated. Little is known about the effect that most of these drugs have on intestinal HO; however, it is likely that inhibition occurs sufficiently to ensure the overall attenuation of bilirubin production in the clinical setting.

The ideal chemotherapeutic agent should have a relatively short duration of action and have a limited residence time. Unfortunately, little is known about the distribution and duration of action and metabolism of most of the Mps (57,58). Of the synthetic analogues, only cobalt protoporphyrin, besides heme, appears to be a substrate for HO and is therefore metabolized like heme. It is also likely that developmental changes may affect the pharmacokinetics of the various heme analogues, and more information is needed, in particular about the retention of SnMP after administration.

In summary, the ideal compound should have a low I_{50} (dose for 50% inhibition of HO activity); should not be a photosensitizer; should be orally absorbable; should not cross the blood–brain barrier; should be short acting and easily excretable; should not be degraded with subsequent release of the sequestered metal iron; should not substantially upregulate HO-1, mRNA, protein, or activity; and should not affect other enzyme systems (26,41). To date, no compound seems to meet all the ideal characteristics, and compounds vary in their fulfillment of these criteria. Nonetheless, SnMP is the only compound approved as an investigational drug. It has a low I_{50}, does not appear to cross the blood–brain barrier, but it possesses photoreactive properties, and upregulates HO-1 (26,47). ZnPP is naturally occurring but has only moderate inhibitory potency. Nevertheless, it is the least likely to be toxic and is not a photosensitizer in vivo. However, it is also unstable under acid (gastric) conditions, cannot be absorbed orally, and upregulates HO-1, but only very briefly. Its formulation is difficult and may limit its usefulness as a drug. ZnBG has very high potency, is orally absorbable, but it is a photosensitizer (50) and increases HO-1 transcription minimally (48). Thus, this compound has a promising potential, as it also contains a biocompatible, essential metal. CrMP is also an interesting compound, which may have promise. It has high inhibitory potency, is orally absorbable, does not cross the blood–brain barrier, and is photochemically inactive. It also does not upregulate HO-1 (53,54). At low doses, it affects only HO-1 and does not affect the activity of NOS or sGC, like the zinc and tin analogues and their derivatives.

D-PENICILLAMINE

D-Penicillamine is a chelating agent in use since the 1950s in the treatment of Wilson disease and heavy metal intoxication. It has also been used to treat cystinuria and rheumatoid arthritis. In the early 1970s, D-penicillamine was described as a therapy for neonatal hyperbilirubinemia in Europe (59). Further studies provided a likely mechanism of action for its use in the treatment of hyperbilirubinemia, indicating that a 3-day course of the drug significantly reduced HO activity levels in neonatal, but not adult, rats (60). A study of D-penicillamine to reduce severe hyperbilirubinemia was conducted in 120 full-term infants with ABO hemolytic disease over a 5-year period, using 60 untreated infants from the first part of the study period as historical controls (59). If initiated within the first 24 hours of life, treatment with D-penicillamine was associated with significantly reduced PTB levels and a decreased need for exchange transfusion in this population. Although the proposed mechanism in its action in decreasing PTB levels may be through inhibition of HO activity, this finding has not been confirmed through direct measurement. Its administration (300 to 400 mg per kg per day) has been associated with amelioration of neonatal hyperbilirubinemia; however, its efficacy has not been well proven, especially in light of the considerable risks associated with its use in neonates.

Numerous cutaneous lesions, including urticaria, macular or papular reactions, pemphigoid lesions, and dermatomyositis, have been reported with long-term use of D-penicillamine (61). Furthermore, significant renal, hepatic, and hematologic complications, including nephrotic syndrome, Goodpasture syndrome, elevation of liver enzymes, aplastic anemia, and thrombocytopenia, have been associated with prolonged therapy for rheumatoid arthritis. The effect of short-term therapy on liver function has been reported in 20 term or near-term infants and on renal function in 30 term or near-term infants (62). Liver function tests were found to be unchanged after 4.3 ± 1.7 days of treatment with D-penicillamine at a dose of 300 mg per kg per day. Cholesterol, blood urea nitrogen, and creatinine levels were also unaffected after 2.8 ± 1.1 days of D-penicillamine treatment at the same dose. The in vitro effect of the drug on human peripheral granulocytes was also investigated. Superoxide anion generation and β-glucuronidase release were both found to be significantly increased at all concentrations of D-penicillamine; however, phagocytic or killing activity of the granulocytes appeared to be unaffected by the drug.

A decreased incidence of retinopathy of prematurity (ROP) was unexpectedly noted among very low-birth-weight infants treated with D-penicillamine in later studies (63,64). Recently, a meta-analysis of the effect of prophylactic D-penicillamine on the incidence of ROP in infants of less than 2,000 g birth weight was undertaken (65). This review concluded that treatment was unlikely to affect survival and may reduce the incidence of ROP among survivors. It is important to note, however, that these conclusions were based on the findings of only two randomized trials, and that no conclusion could be reached regarding the effect of D-penicillamine on severity of ROP. Further studies are required to fully evaluate the possible efficacy and potential side effects of D-penicillamine in the neonatal population before including this drug in the therapeutic armamentarium.

OTHER NONMETALLOPORPHYRIN INHIBITORS

Peptide inhibitors, originally developed for use in transplantation survival studies from the immunomodulatory peptide 2702.75–84, have been shown to be immunosuppressive in vitro and in vivo (66). Some of these compounds, such as D2702.75–84, can bind heat shock protein 70 and have also been found to inhibit HO activity in vitro in a dose-dependent manner. However, similar to what has been found with some Mps, administration of peptides in mice resulted in an upregulation of HO-1 mRNA and protein, as well as HO activity in liver, spleen, and kidney. Consequently, human studies using these peptides for the treatment of hyperbilirubinemia have not been performed.

Originally designed to inhibit cholesterol production (67–69), imidazole dioxolanes, which are structurally different from Mps, have also been found to inhibit in vitro

(70–73) and in vivo (74) HO activity. These compounds have been observed to have a high selectivity for inhibiting the inducible HO-1. Some of these compounds have been found to affect other important enzymes, such as NOS and sGC, in rat tissues (73), whereas others, such as Azalanstat, inhibit in vivo HO activity, but only at a high dose, and also can induce HO-1 gene transcription (74).

Biliverdin reductase inhibitors have not been studied for the purpose of treating hyperbilirubinemia.

DRUGS INCREASING CONJUGATION OF BILIRUBIN

Several pharmacologic compounds have been found to induce UGT activity in hepatocytes and thereby increase the conjugation and excretion of bilirubin. Phenobarbital and nicotinamide were the first of such agents used for the prevention and treatment of hyperbilirubinemia. Phenobarbital continues to be used in the treatment of Gilbert disease and Crigler–Najjar syndrome type II (Arias) disease. Crigler–Najjar syndrome type I disease does not respond well to this therapy (75).

PHENOBARBITAL

A state of limited bilirubin clearance exists in the immediate neonatal period. The associated causes for this phenomenon include a relatively immature neonatal hepatic enzyme system in general, including UGT, as demonstrated by studies in both humans and animal models (76–80). In addition, it has been suggested that the lack of bilirubin in the in utero environment, owing to mature maternal bilirubin conjugation and elimination systems in the normal state, results in the absence of a potent natural inducer of UGT (81,82).

Phenobarbital has been shown to induce a number of hepatic enzymes, including UGT (83–85). The phenobarbital response enhancer sequence of the UGT1A1 gene has been recently been delineated (86). Further research demonstrated a successful reduction of PTB levels with phenobarbital therapy in patients with mild or moderate Crigler–Najjar syndrome (87–90). These studies, and a retrospective analysis demonstrating a decreased incidence of neonatal jaundice in infants of mothers treated with phenobarbital for seizure disorders (91), led to additional clinical investigations of the efficacy of antenatal and postnatal phenobarbital for neonatal hyperbilirubinemia.

Antenatal Phenobarbital

The available studies of antenatal phenobarbital for the prevention of neonatal hyperbilirubinemia differ broadly in terms of dose, length of treatment, target patient population, and sample size (92–97). Comparison of studies is therefore less than optimal. In general, the studies indicate that antenatal phenobarbital treatment was associated with a lower incidence of neonatal jaundice. A daily dose of 30 mg (92,97) was less effective than a daily dose of 60 to 100 mg in both reducing neonatal PTB levels at 48 hours to 4 days of age and decreasing incidence of significant hyperbilirubinemia or need for phototherapy. In the randomized trial by Rayburn et al. (95), which focused on very low-birth-weight infants, a daily dose of 90 mg of phenobarbital was given to women with arrested premature labor at 26 to 33 weeks of gestation. Conjugated bilirubin levels were found to be significantly higher among infants of the phenobarbital-treated group, and need for phototherapy was significantly decreased. Initiation of phototherapy was also delayed among infants of treated mothers. In the very large randomized controlled trial of antenatal phenobarbital therapy in Greece by Valaes et al. (98), a highly significant decrease in neonatal PTB levels was demonstrated among infants of treated mothers; however, this effect was dependent on the mothers' receipt of at least 10 daily doses of 100 mg of phenobarbital prior to delivery. Among infants exposed to this phenobarbital regimen in utero, the need for exchange transfusion was all but eliminated (1.4% vs. 0.23%, $p < .001$). The three infants who required exchange transfusion in the treatment group were all noted to have hemolytic diseases.

The true need for and actual applicability of such a prophylactic therapy for neonatal hyperbilirubinemia is questionable. For populations at very high risk for severe neonatal hyperbilirubinemia, this approach appears attractive, although alternative therapies have been more recently proposed. Mp treatment for infants would have the advantage of a much shorter course of therapy and would eliminate the need for early prenatal identification of high-risk mothers. It is unclear whether the cost of a single postnatal Mp injection would outweigh that of a full course of antenatal phenobarbital. Similarly, the safety of each therapy remains to be established definitively; however, data regarding the neurodevelopmental outcome of infants exposed to antenatal phenobarbital suggest that risks in this regard are limited. In the Greek antenatal phenobarbital study by Valaes et al. (98), no difference in neurodevelopmental outcome was seen between treated and untreated infants among a small subgroup of infants who were examined at 61 to 82 months of age. Long-term follow-up studies have also been published of premature infants enrolled in a National Institute of Child Health and Human Development Neonatal Research Network-sponsored randomized controlled trial of antenatal phenobarbital for reducing incidence of intraventricular hemorrhage (IVH) (99–101). There were no significant differences in Bayley Scales of Infant Development scores or incidence of cerebral palsy between treatment and control groups at 18 to 22 months corrected age (102). Furthermore, there were no significant differences in McCarthy Scales of Children's Abilities scores or incidence of neurologic deficits noted on exam at 36 months (101). It is crucial to note, however, that although 93% of women enrolled received the entire first infusion dose of 10 mg per kg body weight, only 33% received one or more oral maintenance doses of 100 mg per day (99). Therefore, the cumulative phenobarbital exposure in this study is unlikely to approach what would be required for significant reduction in neonatal PTB levels.

Other potential risks of treatment are of more concern. Antenatal phenobarbital is known to significantly decrease vitamin K-dependent clotting factors in the newborn, as demonstrated by reports of hemorrhagic complications of infants born to epileptic women (102–104) and in the

Greek antenatal phenobarbital trial (105). Vitamin K injection at birth was shown to correct these clotting abnormalities at 48 to 72 hours, but there were significant hemorrhagic findings in two of the phenobarbital-exposed infants, including one with subgaleal hemorrhage. None of the control infants had hemorrhagic complications. Increased somnolence was reported among phenobarbital-treated mothers compared with controls in the trial of antenatal phenobarbital for IVH reduction (101); however, no significant sedation effects have been observed among infants born to mothers treated with phenobarbital to prevent neonatal jaundice.

Postnatal Phenobarbital

The mechanistic basis for postnatal phenobarbital is the same as that for antenatal treatment: UGT activity is induced, enhancing bilirubin conjugation and subsequent elimination. In addition, an increase in bile flow with phenobarbital treatment has been reported, putatively mediated by the induction of multidrug resistance protein-2 (MRP-2) (106). Unfortunately, it is clear that there is a delay from initiation of phenobarbital treatment to clinical effectiveness. From a practical standpoint, the usefulness of phenobarbital for treatment of neonatal hyperbilirubinemia is therefore limited in the era of phototherapy.

Comparison of studies of postnatal phenobarbital therapy are limited by many of the same shortcomings that were described in relation to antenatal treatment studies: sample size in most studies is very small, patient population and treatment regimen differs from study to study, and timing of study endpoint neonatal serum bilirubin levels is not consistent among reports. Studies from the late 1960s and early 1970s (94,96,107–113) reported decreased PTB levels at 3 to 7 days of age, although statistically significant differences between treatment and control groups were not observed in all studies. In general, a decrease in the need for exchange transfusion was also observed in phenobarbital-treated infants compared with control, especially among the low-birth-weight population. Phenobarbital doses used in these studies ranged from 2 to 10 mg per kg per day, and drug was administered intramuscularly or orally. Because of the numerous differences in study designs, it is difficult to ascertain which would be the most efficacious phenobarbital dosage regimen. A randomized controlled study of the effect of different single phenobarbital doses (0 to 12 mg per kg) in preventing neonatal hyperbilirubinemia (114) indicated that patients only in the 12 mg per kg group had a significantly improved total serum bilirubin disappearance rate, which was not evident until day of life 7. However, sample size was extremely small (approximately 10 patients in each of the four groups), and dosing regimen was arguably limited in terms of consistency with clinical practice.

Although postnatal phenobarbital alone is inappropriate for treatment of neonatal hyperbilirubinemia in the current era, the therapeutic combination of phototherapy and phenobarbital has been suggested. Blackburn et al. (115) reported no advantage to phenobarbital with phototherapy compared with phototherapy alone in the premature population. However, in scenarios of ongoing hemolysis, such as clinically significant ABO incompatibility or Rh sensitization, the addition of phenobarbital to the treatment regimen may be of potential benefit.

MINOCYCLINE

Minocycline, a semisynthetic second-generation tetracycline, has been shown to exert beneficial anti-inflammatory effects that are independent of its antimicrobial actions (116). It has also been shown to inhibit matrix metalloproteinases, superoxide production, and iNOS expression (117). In a recent study by Lin et al. (118), minocycline was shown to afford neuroprotection against cerebellar damage due to hyperbilirubinemia in the Gunn rat. In 2007, also using the Gunn rat model, Shapiro and colleagues (119) reported that minocycline protects the central auditory system from acute bilirubin neurotoxicity. However, the exact mechanism by which minocycline might be protective is largely speculative (118,120).

CLOFIBRATE

Clofibrate, the ethyl ester of 2-chlorophenoxy-2-methylpropionic acid, has been primarily used as an antilipemic agent in adult patients with hyperlipoproteinemia (121,122). The drug is an activator of peroxisome proliferator-activated receptors (123) and has also been shown to enhance UGT activity in rats (124), significantly increasing hepatic clearance of bilirubin within hours. Subsequently, clofibrate was shown to decrease unconjugated PTB levels in adult patients with Gilbert syndrome (121). Two randomized controlled trials of clofibrate for treatment or prophylaxis of neonatal jaundice have been performed in Europe. In the first of these studies (125), 93 term infants with hyperbilirubinemia before day 5 of life were randomized to receive either a single 50 mg per kg oral dose of clofibrate or an equal volume of placebo. The treatment group had significantly lower PTB levels than controls from 16 hours after drug or placebo administration. In a later study (126), 89 infants of 31 to 36 weeks estimated gestational age were randomized to receive either a single 100 mg per kg dose of clofibrate or placebo during day of life 2. Significantly reduced PTB levels were reported in the treatment group compared with controls from 48 hours after drug or placebo dosing.

Concerns regarding the safety of clofibrate in the neonatal population have been raised (127). Studies in rats have demonstrated carcinogenic properties primarily affecting the liver and pancreas by an unknown mechanism. However, these properties are likely to be observed only after prolonged therapy and furthermore, two multicenter studies of clofibrate in adults demonstrated no significant increase in cancer-related mortality in treated compared with untreated patients after analyses of long-term follow-up data (128,129). No long-term follow-up studies were undertaken in the two neonatal studies noted previously (125,126). An acute muscular syndrome has also been described but reportedly only in the presence of high serum levels of clofibric acid. Finally, concerns regarding displacement of bilirubin from albumin by clofibric acid have been raised, which have been refuted by Gabilan et al. (130). Many more neonatal-specific pharmacokinetic, safety, and efficacy studies would likely be required before clofibrate treatment for neonatal jaundice could be routinely considered. Given the relatively ready accessibility to phototherapy in the United States, this would seem to be a highly unlikely prospect.

CHINESE HERBAL REMEDIES

A number of traditional Chinese herbal medicines have properties of inducing UGT activity similar to that of phenobarbital (131). It has been common practice among Chinese women to take herbal remedies during pregnancy. These herbs have been shown to accelerate plasma clearance and conjugation of bilirubin but have different effects on other liver enzymes, most likely due to different mechanisms of action. Exposure to herbs either before or after birth has been suspected to be a cause of hemolysis and jaundice in newborns, such that a number of herbs have been implicated in causing hemolysis in infants with G6PD deficiency. It can be concluded that although herbal treatment has been practiced for a long time in China, its effectiveness remains doubtful with no convincing evidence without properly controlled randomized clinical studies.

Herbs and Chinese herbal combinations have for centuries been used for treatment of neonatal jaundice. Only relatively recently, however, have these traditional remedies been critically studied by Western medical researchers. In a review of the Chinese literature (132), *Artemisia* (*Yin-chin*, or Oriental wormwood) was the most commonly used herb for neonatal jaundice. Other commonly used herbs included *Glycyrrhiza* (*Gan-coa*, or licorice), *Scutellaria baicalensis* (*Huang-qin*, or skullcap root), *Rheum officinale* (*Da-huang*, or rhubarb), and *Coptis chinesis* (*Huang-lian*, or goldthread rhizome). In the 1980s, treatment with the herbal combination known as *Yin zhi huang* (YZH), consisting of *Artemisia*, *Gardenia*, *Rheum*, and *Scutellaria*, as well as another traditional herbal combination, was shown to decrease neonatal PTB levels after 3 to 4 days (133,134). Subsequent studies revealed increased conjugation and clearance of bilirubin in animal models after YZH similar to that seen after phenobarbital (135,136), although the pattern of hepatic enzyme induction was different (131). Further delineation of the individual components of YZH revealed that *Artemisia* and *Rheum*, but not *Gardenia* or *Scutellaria*, were potent inducers of UGT (137). Cytochrome P450 levels of animals treated with individual component herbs of YZH were shown to be similar to control and lower among those animals treated with *Gardenia*. This is in sharp contrast to the significant elevation of cytochrome P450 levels seen among animals treated with phenobarbital.

The safety of these traditional remedies has not been adequately studied. However, some of these herbs have been shown to possess potentially extremely dangerous properties in the setting of neonatal hyperbilirubinemia. *Artemisia*, for example, can displace bilirubin from albumin, which could lead to enhanced neurotoxicity (138,139). The alkaloid berberine, which is contained in *Huang-lian*, can cause severe acute hemolysis in patients with G6PD deficiency (132). Contamination of herbal medicines with heavy metals has also been reported (140). In light of the unregulated atmosphere in which these herbal remedies are currently produced, inconsistencies in preparation, and inability to reliably assess concentrations of individual herbal components or presence of contaminants, the use of these therapies cannot be recommended.

ACTIGALL

Actigall, or ursodeoxycholic acid (UDCA), is primarily used for the treatment of cholestatic liver diseases but has been suggested to be useful for the treatment of hyperbilirubinemia in patients with Crigler–Najjar syndrome (141). Experimental evidence suggests that its mechanisms of action may be mediated through the stimulation of hepatobiliary secretion, via Ca^{2+}- and protein kinase C-alpha-dependent mechanisms and/or activation of p38 (mitogen-activated protein kinase) and extracellular signal-regulated kinases, resulting in insertion of transporter molecules [e.g., bile salt export pump and conjugate export pump (MRP-2)]. Future studies need to be performed to investigate dosage regimens as well as to elucidate the mechanisms of action of UDCA at the molecular level (142) and potential toxicities in the newborn.

George et al. (143) conducted a retrospective study reviewing the efficacy of Actigall in the treatment of hyperbilirubinemia in a pediatric intensive care unit population. Actigall administered at a dose of 20 mg per kg per day to five pediatric intensive care unit patients resulted in a decrease in PTB levels with no adverse effects in four patients. These preliminary findings suggest that Actigall is effective in the treatment of hyperbilirubinemia. However, a prospective, randomized trial is warranted to further assess the efficacy of this therapy before use in the neonatal population.

REDUCTION OF ENTEROHEPATIC RECIRCULATION OF BILIRUBIN

Neonatal hyperbilirubinemia is exacerbated and may be caused by enhanced reabsorption of bilirubin in the enterohepatic circulation. The absence of intestinal flora in neonates prevents the degradation of bilirubin in meconium and stool to products such as urobilinogen, which can be excreted. Bilirubin glucuronides entering the intestines are readily deconjugated to bilirubin and subsequently reabsorbed. To circumvent this process, various strategies have been developed to bind the bilirubin in the intestinal lumen to substances that resist absorption.

BILIRUBIN OXIDASE

Bilirubin oxidase (BOX), derived from the fungus *Myrothecium verrucarea*, has been found to interrupt bilirubin reabsorption by oxidizing bilirubin to biliverdin and other less toxic and more water-soluble products in order to be excreted (144,145). A study by Soltys et al. (145) showed that the in vivo administration of 0.1 to 2.0 mg per day of BOX to chronically jaundiced Gunn rats over a 4-day period effectively decreased PTB levels from 11.3 to 6.3 mg per dL (-40%, $n = 5$; $p < .05$). However, the decrease was observed only when the molar ratio of STB to rat serum albumin was greater than 0.35. When BOX was administered to rats with a ratio less than 0.35 (n = 10), there was no statistically significant change in PTB levels. Because large-scale human studies are lacking, the potential for use of BOX for the treatment of neonatal hyperbilirubinemia is still under investigation (146).

ORAL FEEDING

Initiation of oral feedings can ameliorate the accumulation of bilirubin in the intestines and its enterohepatic recirculation. Formula feeding is most influential in this regard, but successful breastfeeding has a similar effect.

CHARCOAL

Activated charcoal administered by gavage feeding can reduce PTB levels by binding bilirubin in the intestinal lumen and reducing the enterohepatic circulation of unconjugated bilirubin. The effectiveness of activated charcoal as an adjunct to phototherapy in reducing PTB levels has been studied in the jaundiced rat (147,148). The administration of charcoal by feeding or gavage was shown to be effective in reducing PTB levels in both the adult and the suckling jaundiced rat. Charcoal feeding and phototherapy administered jointly in the adult rat was shown to be additive in significantly lowering PTB levels when compared with reductions in PTB levels of those given charcoal alone. In the suckling rat, PTB levels were also significantly reduced after the administration of either charcoal alone or charcoal in combination with phototherapy; however, the combination of treatments did not appear to be additive. These findings suggest that charcoal can be used as an adjunct to phototherapy and that charcoal used in combination with phototherapy may also reduce the intensity of phototherapy needed to effectively lower PTB levels.

Amitai et al. (149) prospectively studied the efficacy of multiple-dose oral activated charcoal (OAC) therapy for neonatal hyperbilirubinemia in 30 jaundiced newborns receiving phototherapy. For newborns under phototherapy who received OAC before meals with a total amount of 8.5 ± 0.85 g (mean ± SE, n = 14) and for infants receiving phototherapy only (controls, n = 16), STB levels on initiation of phototherapy were 265 ± 8 and 253 ± 4 μmol per L, respectively. After 24 hours, there was no significant decrease in PTB levels in the control group (240 ± 8 μmol per L), but PTB levels of the study group decreased (235 ± 7 μmol per L; $p < .02$). For both groups, PTB levels were significantly lower than baseline values 48 hours after initiation of phototherapy. However, the decline in PTB levels in the study group (56 ± 10 μmol per L) was greater than that of the controls (21 ± 10 μmol per L; $p < .02$). It was concluded that OAC seems to be an effective adjunct to phototherapy in the treatment of neonatal hyperbilirubinemia.

AGAR

Plain dried agar, an extract of seaweed, has been shown to effectively decrease PTB levels by binding to bilirubin in the gut and increasing stool frequency. Consequently, the enterohepatic circulation of bilirubin is decreased, which in turn leads to an enhanced clearance of intraluminal bilirubin and decreased PTB levels.

An early study (150) investigating the efficacy of oral agar supplementation (600 mg per kg) in low-birth-weight infants (1,500 to 2,500 g) at 12 hours of age for 7 days found that PTB levels were not significantly lower in the agar-fed infants. It was concluded that agar-supplemented oral feeding is not indicated in the management of hyperbilirubinemia in low-birth-weight infants. In 1977, Ebbesen and Moller (151) evaluated the ingestion of agar used as an adjunct to phototherapy and found that PTB levels were decreased regardless of agar ingestion and concluded that oral agar does not supplement the effect of phototherapy alone.

In another study that investigated the effect of oral agar in term and preterm newborns (152), it was observed that agar ingestion decreased PTB levels and increased fecal elimination of the pigment ($p < .001$) only in term newborns and not in preterm newborns.

Odell et al. (153) tested the hypothesis that sequestration of luminal unconjugated bilirubin by enteral agar administration would enhance the efficacy of phototherapy in jaundiced infants. They found that the rate of decline of PTB concentrations after 24 hours of phototherapy was greater and significantly more uniform in the agar-supplemented infants (−1.59 ± 2.3 vs. −2.51 ± 1.44 mg per dL). Stool frequencies were greater in control infants (5.5 vs. 4.3 mg per kg per 24 hours), whereas fecal bilirubin excretions were greater in agar-supplemented infants during the second day of phototherapy (1.32 vs. 3.29 mg per kg per 24 hours). In addition, agar supplementation reduced the duration of phototherapy by 23% (37.6 ± 3.2 vs. 48.1 ± 5.0 hours).

The value of oral agar in the treatment of neonatal hyperbilirubinemia was determined and compared to phototherapy alone and phototherapy plus oral agar (154). Oral agar was found to be as effective as phototherapy, with the most significant decrease in PTB levels in infants treated with both phototherapy and oral agar. It was concluded that the efficacy of phototherapy in decreasing the PTB levels could be enhanced with the use of oral agar. In addition, oral agar can also be used alone for the treatment of neonatal hyperbilirubinemia because it is as effective as phototherapy.

A meta-analysis of nine prospective clinical trials evaluating agar therapy found these studies at risk for biased treatment allocation (155). Although the pooled data analysis suggests that prophylactic agar treatment is associated with reduced peak PTB levels, this observation must be interpreted cautiously in light of heterogeneous patient populations and the methodologic problems. Based on this meta-analysis, agar therapy for neonatal jaundice can neither be recommended nor rejected.

BILIRUBIN BINDING

Bilirubin in circulation is predominantly bound to albumin. Although the binding ratio is potentially 1:1 and avid, albumin levels are lower in premature and sick infants, and binding affinity is often diminished (156). Furthermore, some drugs (e.g., sulfisoxazole, benzoate) can compete with bilirubin for binding to albumin, causing displacement of bilirubin (157,158). Therefore, prior to exchange transfusion, albumin can be administered (1 g per kg) to improve the efficacy of the exchange.

A method has been described by Ahlfors (159–161) for measuring the unconjugated fraction of the unbound bilirubin concentration in plasma by combining the peroxidase method for determining unbound bilirubin with a diazo method for measuring conjugated and unconjugated bilirubin. The accuracy of the unbound bilirubin determination is improved by decreasing sample dilution, eliminating interference by conjugated bilirubin, monitoring changes in bilirubin concentration, and correcting for rate-limiting dissociation of bilirubin from albumin. It was found that the unbound unconjugated bilirubin concentration by this method in plasma from 20 jaundiced newborns was significantly greater than and poorly correlated ($r = 0.7$) with the unbound bilirubin determined by the existing peroxidase method (162). This may be possibly due to differences in sample dilution between the two methods. The unbound unconjugated bilirubin was an unpredictable fraction of the unbound bilirubin in plasma samples from patients with similar total bilirubin concentrations but varying levels of conjugated bilirubin. A bilirubin-binding competitor was readily detected at a sample dilution typically used for the combined test but not at the dilution used for the existing peroxidase method. The combined method is ideally suited to measuring unbound unconjugated bilirubin in jaundiced human newborns or animal models of kernicterus (163).

SUMMARY

Besides phototherapy, the HO inhibitors are the most promising therapeutic agents for prevention and treatment of neonatal jaundice. Whether any of these compounds would be suitable for universal prophylaxis for the essentially ubiquitous phenomenon of transitional hyperbilirubinemia of the neonate would depend upon the relative frequency of pathologic jaundice [>17 mg per dL (291 μmol per L)] in the population and the relative safety and efficacy of the compounds. A targeted approach for infants at higher risk for pathologic jaundice is a more likely scenario. Nonetheless, chemotherapeutic approaches for the management of hyperbilirubinemia may become more important if phototherapy applied to small, very immature, and relatively translucent neonates (<1,500 g) were found to pose previously unrecognized risks (164). Most likely, phototherapy will remain the mainstay of therapy for most jaundiced neonates, but understanding the biology of newborn jaundice and further development of alternative pharmacologic therapies for neonatal hyperbilirubinemia will broaden the options for management of neonatal jaundice and its consequences.

ACKNOWLEDGMENTS

This work was supported by the National Institutes of Health, grants HL68703 and HD/HL58013, the Hess Research Fund, the L. H. M. Lui Research Fund, and the Mary L. Johnson Research Fund.

REFERENCES

1. American Academy of Pediatrics. Management of hyperbilirubinemia in the newborn infant 35 or more weeks of gestation. *Pediatrics* 2004;114:297–316.
2. Maisels MJ. Phototherapy—traditional and nontraditional. *J Perinatol* 2001;21(Suppl 1):S93–S97.
3. Vreman HJ, Wong RJ, Stevenson DK. Phototherapy: current methods and future directions. *Semin Perinatol* 2004;28:326–333.
4. Seidman DS, Moise J, Ergaz Z, et al. A new blue light-emitting phototherapy device: a prospective randomized controlled study. *J Pediatr* 2000;136:771–774.
5. Vreman HJ, Wong RJ, Stevenson DK, et al. Light-emitting diodes: a novel light source for phototherapy. *Pediatr Res* 1998;44: 804–809.
6. Wong RJ, Stevenson DK, Ahlfors CE, et al. Neonatal jaundice: bilirubin physiology and clinical chemistry. *NeoReviews* 2007;8: e58–e67.
7. Yao TC, Stevenson DK. Advances in the diagnosis and treatment of neonatal hyperbilirubinemia. *Clin Perinatol* 1995;22:741–758.
8. Dennery PA, Seidman DS, Stevenson DK. Neonatal hyperbilirubinemia. *N Engl J Med* 2001;344:581–590.
9. Kaplan M, Muraca M, Hammerman C, et al. Imbalance between production and conjugation of bilirubin: a fundamental concept in the mechanism of neonatal jaundice. *Pediatrics* 2002;110:e47.
10. Stevenson DK, Vreman HJ, Oh W, et al. Bilirubin production in healthy term infants as measured by carbon monoxide in breath. *Clin Chem* 1994;40:1934–1939.
11. Vreman HJ, Rodgers PA, Gale R, et al. Carbon monoxide excretion as an index of bilirubin production in rhesus monkeys. *J Med Primatol* 1989;18:449–460.
12. Kaplan M, Renbaum P, Levy-Lahad E, et al. Gilbert syndrome and glucose-6-phosphate dehydrogenase deficiency: a dose-dependent genetic interaction crucial to neonatal hyperbilirubinemia. *Proc Natl Acad Sci U S A* 1997;94:12128–12132.
13. Koiwai O, Nishizawa M, Hasada K, et al. Gilbert's syndrome is caused by a heterozygous missense mutation in the gene for bilirubin UDP-glucuronosyltransferase. *Hum Mol Genet* 1995;4: 1183–1186.
14. Kaplan M, Hammerman C, Maisels MJ. Bilirubin genetics for the nongeneticist: hereditary defects of neonatal bilirubin conjugation. *Pediatrics* 2003;111:886–893.
15. Akaba K, Kimura T, Sasaki A, et al. Neonatal hyperbilirubinemia and mutation of the bilirubin uridine diphosphate-glucuronosyltransferase gene: a common missense mutation among Japanese, Koreans and Chinese. *Biochem Mol Biol Int* 1998;46: 21–26.
16. Beutler E, Gelbart T, Demina A. Racial variability in the UDP-glucuronosyltransferase 1 (UGT1A1) promoter: a balanced polymorphism for regulation of bilirubin metabolism? *Proc Natl Acad Sci U S A* 1998;95:8170–8174.
17. Lin Z, Fontaine J, Watchko JF. Coexpression of gene polymorphisms involved in bilirubin production and metabolism. *Pediatrics* 2008;122:e156–e162.
18. Huang CS, Chang PF, Huang MJ, et al. Glucose-6-phosphate dehydrogenase deficiency, the UDP-glucuronosyl transferase 1A1 gene, and neonatal hyperbilirubinemia. *Gastroenterology* 2002; 123:127–133.
19. Vreman HJ, Mahoney JJ, Stevenson DK. Carbon monoxide and carboxyhemoglobin. *Adv Pediatr* 1995;42:303–325.
20. Vreman HJ, Wong RJ, Stevenson DK. Carbon monoxide in breath, blood, and other tissues. In: Penney DG, ed. *Carbon monoxide toxicity*. Boca Raton, FL: CRC Press. 2000:19–60.
21. Widness JA, Lowe LS, Stevenson DK, et al. Direct relationship of fetal carboxyhemoglobin with hemolysis in alloimmunized pregnancies. *Pediatr Res* 1994;35:713–719.
22. Bhutani VK, Johnson L, Sivieri EM. Predictive ability of a predischarge hour-specific serum bilirubin for subsequent significant hyperbilirubinemia in healthy term and near-term newborns. *Pediatrics* 1999;103:6–14.

23. Stevenson DK, Fanaroff AA, Maisels MJ, et al. Prediction of hyperbilirubinemia in near-term and term infants. *Pediatrics* 2001; 108:31–39.
24. Tenhunen R, Marver HS, Schmid R. The enzymatic conversion of heme to bilirubin by microsomal heme oxygenase. *Proc Natl Acad Sci U S A* 1968;61:748–755.
25. Stevenson DK, Rodgers PA, Vreman HJ. The use of metalloporphyrins for the chemoprevention of neonatal jaundice. *Am J Dis Child* 1989;143:353–356.
26. Wong RJ, Bhutani VK, Vreman HJ, et al. Tin mesoporphyrin for the prevention of severe neonatal hyperbilirubinemia. *NeoReviews* 2007;8:e77–e84.
27. Maines MD. Zinc protoporphyrin is a selective inhibitor of heme oxygenase activity in the neonatal rat. *Biochim Biophys Acta* 1981; 673:339–350.
28. Pierce NW, Wong RJ, Morioka I, et al. Inhibition of *in vitro* heme oxygenase isozyme activity by metalloporphyrins. *EPAS* 2006; 59:5575.483.
29. Vreman HJ, Wong RJ, Williams SA, et al. *In vitro* heme oxygenase isozyme activity inhibition by metalloporphyrins. *Pediatr Res* 1998; 43:202A.
30. Appleton SD, Chretien ML, McLaughlin BE, et al. Selective inhibition of heme oxygenase, without inhibition of nitric oxide synthase or soluble guanylyl cyclase, by metalloporphyrins at low concentrations. *Drug Metab Dispos* 1999;27:1214–1219.
31. Wong RJ, Vreman HJ, Stevenson DK. (Metallo)porphyrin inhibitors of heme oxygenase also inhibit lipid peroxidation (LP). *Pediatr Res* 2000;47:465.
32. Dore S, Snyder SH. Neuroprotective action of bilirubin against oxidative stress in primary hippocampal cultures. *Ann N Y Acad Sci* 1999;890:167–172.
33. Stocker R, McDonagh AF, Glazer AN, et al. Antioxidant activities of bile pigments: biliverdin and bilirubin. *Methods Enzymol* 1990; 186:301–309.
34. Stocker R, Yamamoto Y, McDonagh AF, et al. Bilirubin is an antioxidant of possible physiological importance. *Science* 1987; 235:1043–1046.
35. Stevenson DK, Vreman HJ, Wong RJ, et al. Carbon monoxide detection and biological investigations. *Trans Am Clin Climatol Assoc* 2000;111:61–75.
36. Drummond GS, Galbraith RA, Sardana MK, et al. Reduction of the C2 and C4 vinyl groups of Sn-protoporphyrin to form Sn-mesoporphyrin markedly enhances the ability of the metalloporphyrin to inhibit *in vivo* heme catabolism. *Arch Biochem Biophys* 1987;255:64–74.
37. Drummond GS, Kappas A. Prevention of neonatal hyperbilirubinemia by tin protoporphyrin IX, a potent competitive inhibitor of heme oxidation. *Proc Natl Acad Sci U S A* 1981;78: 6466–6470.
38. Drummond GS, Kappas A. Sn-protoporphyrin inhibition of fetal and neonatal brain heme oxygenase. Transplacental passage of the metalloporphyrin and prenatal suppression of hyperbilirubinemia in the newborn animal. *J Clin Invest* 1986;77: 971–976.
39. Vreman HJ, Cipkala DA, Stevenson DK. Characterization of porphyrin heme oxygenase inhibitors. *Can J Physiol Pharmacol* 1996; 74:278–285.
40. Vreman HJ, Ekstrand BC, Stevenson DK. Selection of metalloporphyrin heme oxygenase inhibitors based on potency and photoreactivity. *Pediatr Res* 1993;33:195–200.
41. Vreman HJ, Wong RJ, Stevenson DK. Alternative metalloporphyrins for the treatment of neonatal jaundice. *J Perinatol* 2001; 21(Suppl 1):S108–S113.
42. Martinez JC, Garcia HO, Otheguy LE, et al. Control of severe hyperbilirubinemia in full-term newborns with the inhibitor of bilirubin production Sn-mesoporphyrin. *Pediatrics* 1999;103:1–5.
43. Valaes T, Petmezaki S, Henschke C, et al. Control of jaundice in preterm newborns by an inhibitor of bilirubin production: Studies with tin-mesoporphyrin. *Pediatrics* 1994;93:1–11.
44. Reddy P, Najundaswamy S, Mehta R, et al. Tin-mesoporphyrin in the treatment of severe hyperbilirubinemia in a very-low-birth-weight infant. *J Perinatol* 2003;23:507–508.
45. Vreman HJ, Gillman MJ, Stevenson DK. *In vitro* inhibition of adult rat intestinal heme oxygenase by metalloporphyrins. *Pediatr Res* 1989;26:362–365.
46. Morioka I, Wong RJ, Abate A, et al. Systemic effects of orally-administered zinc and tin (IV) metalloporphyrins on heme oxygenase expression in mice. *Pediatr Res* 2006;59:667–672.
47. Wong RJ, Abate A, Dennery PA, et al. Direct intestinal administration of metalloporphyrins and heme oxygenase expression. *J Invest Med* 2003;51:S140.
48. Zhang W, Contag PR, Hardy J, et al. Selection of potential therapeutics based on *in vivo* spatiotemporal transcription patterns of heme oxygenase-1. *J Mol Med* 2002;80:655–664.
49. Vallier HA, Rodgers PA, Stevenson DK. Oral administration of zinc deuteroporphyrin IX 2,4 bis glycol inhibits heme oxygenase in neonatal rats. *Dev Pharmacol Ther* 1991;17:220–222.
50. Vreman HJ, Lee OK, Stevenson DK. *In vitro* and *in vivo* characteristics of a heme oxygenase inhibitor: ZnBG. *Am J Med Sci* 1991; 302:335–341.
51. Labbé RF, Vreman HJ, Stevenson DK. Zinc Protoporphyrin: a metabolite with a mission. *Clin Chem* 1999;45:2060–2072.
52. Vallier HA, Rodgers PA, Stevenson DK. Inhibition of heme oxygenase after oral vs intraperitoneal administration of chromium porphyrins. *Life Sci* 1993;52:L79–L84.
53. Morisawa T, Wong RJ, Xiao H, et al. Inhibition of heme oxygenase activity by chromium mesoporphyrin in the heme-loaded newborn mouse. *EPAS* 2008:6130.9.
54. Xiao H, Morisawa T, Wong RJ, et al. Short- and long-term effects of heme oxygenase activity by chromium mesoporphyrin in newborn mice. *EPAS* 2008:6130.8.
55. Hamori CJ, Lasic DD, Vreman HJ, et al. Targeting zinc protoporphyrin liposomes to the spleen using reticuloendothelial blockade with blank liposomes. *Pediatr Res* 1993;34:1–5.
56. Hintz SR, Kwong LK, Vreman HJ, et al. Recovery of exogenous heme as carbon monoxide and biliary heme in adult rats after tin protoporphyrin treatment. *J Pediatr Gastroenterol Nutr* 1987;6: 302–306.
57. Anderson KE, Simionatto CS, Drummond GS, et al. Tissue distribution and disposition of tin-protoporphyrin, a potent competitive inhibitor of heme oxygenase. *J Pharmacol Exp Ther* 1984; 228:327–333.
58. Anderson KE, Simionatto CS, Drummond GS, et al. Disposition of tin-protoporphyrin and suppression of hyperbilirubinemia in humans. *Clin Pharmacol Ther* 1986;39:510–520.
59. Lakatos L, Kover B, Oroszlan G, et al. D-penicillamine therapy in ABO hemolytic disease of the newborn infant. *Eur J Pediatr* 1976; 123:133–137.
60. Oroszlan G, Lakatos L, Szabo L, et al. Heme oxygenase activity is decreased by D-penicillamine in neonates. *Experientia* 1983;39: 888–889.
61. Levy RS, Fisher M, Alter JN. Penicillamine: review and cutaneous manifestations. *J Am Acad Dermatol* 1983;8:548–558.
62. Lakatos L, Szabo I, Csathy L. The effects of D-penicillamine on the renal and liver functions in neonates and the *in vitro* influence on granulocytes. *Acta Paediatr Scand Suppl* 1989;360:135–139.
63. Lakatos L. D-penicillamine and retinopathy of prematurity. *Pediatrics* 1988;82:951–953.
64. Lakatos L, Hatvani I, Oroszlan G, et al. D-penicillamine in the prevention of retrolental fibroplasia. *Acta Paediatr Acad Sci Hung* 1982;23:327–335.
65. Phelps DL, Lakatos L, Watts JL. D-Penicillamine for preventing retinopathy of prematurity in preterm infants. *Cochrane Database Syst Rev* 2001:CD001073.
66. Iyer S, Woo J, Cornejo MC, et al. Characterization and biological significance of immunosuppressive peptide D2702.75–84(E $\rightarrow$ V) binding protein. Isolation of heme oxygenase-1. *J Biol Chem* 1998;273:2692–2697.
67. Burton PM, Swinney DC, Heller R, et al. Azalanstat (RS-21607), a lanosterol 14 alpha-demethylase inhibitor with cholesterol-lowering activity. *Biochem Pharmacol* 1995;50:529–544.
68. Swinney DC, So OY, Watson DM, et al. Selective inhibition of mammalian lanosterol 14 alpha-demethylase by RS-21607 *in vitro* and *in vivo*. *Biochemistry* 1994;33:4702–4713.
69. Walker KA, Kertesz DJ, Rotstein DM, et al. Selective inhibition of mammalian lanosterol 14 alpha-demethylase: a possible strategy for cholesterol lowering. *J Med Chem* 1993;36:2235–2237.
70. DeNagel DC, Verity AN, Madden FE, et al. Identification of non-porphyrin inhibitors of heme oxygenase-1. *Neuroscience* 1998;24: 2058.

71. Vreman HJ, Wong RJ, Stevenson DK, et al. Azalanstat (RS-1607): evidence for a novel class of potential heme oxygenase inhibitors. *Pediatr Res* 2002;51:341A.
72. Vlahakis JZ, Kinobe RT, Bowers RJ, et al. Imidazole-dioxolane compounds as isozyme-selective heme oxygenase inhibitors. *J Med Chem* 2006;49:4437–4441.
73. Kinobe RT, Vlahakis JZ, Vreman HJ, et al. Selectivity of imidazole-dioxolane compounds for *in vitro* inhibition of microsomal haem oxygenase isoforms. *Br J Pharmacol* 2006;147:307–315.
74. Morisawa T, Wong RJ, Bhutani VK, et al. Inhibition of heme oxygenase activity in newborn mice by Azalanstat. *Can J Physiol Pharmacol* 2008;86:651–659.
75. Rubaltelli FF, Griffith PF. Management of neonatal hyperbilirubinaemia and prevention of kernicterus. *Drugs* 1992;43:864–872.
76. Gartner LM, Lee KS, Vaisman S, et al. Development of bilirubin transport and metabolism in the newborn rhesus monkey. *J Pediatr* 1977;90:513–531.
77. Gow PJ, Ghabrial H, Smallwood RA, et al. Neonatal hepatic drug elimination. *Pharmacol Toxicol* 2001;88:3–15.
78. Pacifici GM, Rane A. Intestinal and hepatic morphine glucuronidation in immature and pregnant rats. *Dev Pharmacol Ther* 1981;3:160–167.
79. Pasleau F, Kolodzici C, Kremers P, et al. Ontogenic development of steroid 16 alpha-hydroxylase as a tool for the study of the multiplicity of cytochrome P-450. *Eur J Biochem* 1981;120: 213–220.
80. Yaffe SJ. Antimicrobial therapy and the neonate. *Obstet Gynecol* 1981;58:85S–94S.
81. Thaler MM. Substrate-induced conjugation of bilirubin in genetically deficient newborn rats. *Science* 1970;170:555–556.
82. Valaes T. Bilirubin metabolism. Review and discussion of inborn errors. *Clin Perinatol* 1976;3:177–209.
83. Conney AH, Davison C, Gastell R, et al. Adaptive increases in drug-metabolizing enzymes induced by phenobarbital and other drugs. *J Pharmacol Exp Ther* 1960;130:1–8.
84. Hollman S, Touster O. Alterations in tissue levels of uridine diphosphate glucose dehydrogenase, uridine diphosphate glucuronic acid pyrophosphatase and glucuronyl transferase induced by substances influencing the production of ascorbic acid. *Biochim Biophys Acta* 1962;26:338.
85. Inscoe JK, Axelrod J. Some factors affecting glucuronide formation *in vitro*. *J Pharmacol Exp Ther* 1960;129:128–131.
86. Sugatani J, Kojima H, Ueda A, et al. The phenobarbital response enhancer module in the human bilirubin UDP-glucuronosyltransferase UGT1A1 gene and regulation by the nuclear receptor CAR. *Hepatology* 2001;33:1232–1238.
87. Berthelot P, Erlinger S, Dhumeaux D, et al. Mechanism of phenobarbital-induced hypercholeresis in the rat. *Am J Physiol* 1970; 219:809–813.
88. Crigler JF Jr, Gold NI. Effect of sodium phenobarbital on bilirubin metabolism in an infant with congenital, nonhemolytic, unconjugated hyperbilirubinemia, and kernicterus. *J Clin Invest* 1969;48:42–55.
89. Kreek MJ, Sleiseng MH. Reduction of serum-unconjugated-bilirubin with phenobarbitone in adult congenital nonhaemolytic unconjugated hyperbilirubinaemia. *Lancet* 1968;2:73.
90. Yaffe SJ, Levy G, Matsuzawa T, et al. Enhancement of glucuronide-conjugating capacity in a hyperbilirubinemic infant due to apparent enzyme induction by phenobarbital. *N Engl J Med* 1966;275:1461–1466.
91. Trolle D. Phenobarbitone and neonatal icterus. *Lancet* 1968;1:251.
92. Halpin TF, Jones AR, Bishop HL, et al. Prophylaxis of neonatal hyperbilirubinemia with phenobarbital. *Obstet Gynecol* 1972;40: 85–90.
93. Maurer HM, Wolff JA, Finster M, et al. Reduction in concentration of total serum-bilirubin in offspring of women treated with phenobarbitone during pregnancy. *Lancet* 1968;2:122–124.
94. Ramboer C, Thompson RP, Williams R. Controlled trials of phenobarbitone therapy of neonatal jaundice. *Lancet* 1969;1: 966–968.
95. Rayburn W, Donn S, Piehl E, et al. Antenatal phenobarbital and bilirubin metabolism in the very low birth weight infant. *Am J Obstet Gynecol* 1988;159:1491–1493.
96. Valaes T, Petmezaki S, Doxiadis SA. Effect on neonatal hyperbilirubinemia of phenobarbital during pregnancy or after birth: practical value of the treatment in a population with high risk of unexplained severe neonatal jaundice. *Birth Defects Orig Artic Ser* 1970;6:46–54.
97. Yeung CY, Tam LS, Chan A, et al. Phenobarbitone prophylaxis for neonatal hyperbilirubinemia. *Pediatrics* 1971;48:372–376.
98. Valaes T, Karaklis A, Stravrakakis D, et al. Incidence and mechanism of neonatal jaundice related to glucose-6-phosphate dehydrogenase deficiency. *Pediatr Res* 1969;3:448–458.
99. Shankaran S, Papile LA, Wright LL, et al. The effect of antenatal phenobarbital therapy on neonatal intracranial hemorrhage in preterm infants. *N Engl J Med* 1997;337:466–471.
100. Shankaran S, Papile LA, Wright LL, et al. Neurodevelopmental outcome of premature infants after antenatal phenobarbital exposure. *Am J Obstet Gynecol* 2002;187:171–177.
101. Shankaran S, Woldt E, Nelson J, et al. Antenatal phenobarbital therapy and neonatal outcome. II: Neurodevelopmental outcome at 36 months. *Pediatrics* 1996;97:649–652.
102. Mountain KR, Hirsh J, Gallus AS. Neonatal coagulation defect due to anticonvulsant drug treatment in pregnancy. *Lancet* 1970; 1:265–268.
103. Bleyer WA, Skinner AL. Fatal hemorrhage after maternal anticonvulsant therapy. *JAMA* 1976;235:626.
104. Srinivasan G, Seeler RA, Tiruvury A, et al. Maternal anticonvulsant therapy and hemorrhagic disease of the newborn. *Obstet Gynecol* 1982;59:250–252.
105. Valaes T, Kipouros K, Petmezaki S, et al. Effectiveness and safety of prenatal phenobarbital for the prevention of neonatal jaundice. *Pediatr Res* 1980;14:947–952.
106. Johnson DR, Habeebu SS, Klaassen CD. Increase in bile flow and biliary excretion of glutathione-derived sulfhydryls in rats by drug-metabolizing enzyme inducers is mediated by multidrug resistance protein 2. *Toxicol Sci* 2002;66:16–26.
107. Cao A, Falorni A, Fracassini F, et al. Phenobarbital effect on serum bilirubin levels in underweight infants. *Helv Paediatr Acta* 1973;28:231–238.
108. Carswell F, Kerr MM, Dunsmore IR. Sequential trial of effect of phenobarbitone on serum bilirubin of preterm infants. *Arch Dis Child* 1972;47:621–625.
109. Dortmann A, Haupt H, Kuster F. Barbiturate treatment of neonatal icterus. *Z Kinderheilkd* 1972;112:163–170.
110. Stern L, Khanna NN, Levy G, et al. Effect of phenobarbital on hyperbilirubinemia and glucuronide formation in newborns. *Am J Dis Child* 1970;120:26–31.
111. Valdes OS, Maurer HM, Shumway CN. Controlled clinical trial of phenobarbital and/or light in reducing neonatal hyperbilirubinemia in a predominantly Negro population. *J Pediatr* 1971;79: 1015.
112. Vest M, Signer E, Weisser K, et al. A double blind study of the effect of phenobarbitone on neonatal hyperbilirubinaemia and frequency of exchange transfusion. *Acta Paediatr Scand* 1970;59: 681–684.
113. Zwacka G, Frenzel J. The influence of short time phenobarbital treatment on neonatal jaundice. *Padiatr Padol* 1971;6: 102–107.
114. Wallin A, Boreus LO. Phenobarbital prophylaxis for hyperbilirubinemia in preterm infants. A controlled study of bilirubin disappearance and infant behavior. *Acta Paediatr Scand* 1984;73: 488–497.
115. Blackburn MG, Orzalesi MM, Pigram P. The combined effect of phototherapy and phenobarbital on serum bilirubin levels of premature infants. *Pediatrics* 1972;49:110–112.
116. Ryan ME, Ashley RA. How do tetracyclines work? *Adv Dent Res* 1998;12:149–151.
117. Gabler WL, Smith J, Tsukuda N. Comparison of doxycycline and a chemically modified tetracycline inhibition of leukocyte functions. *Res Commun Chem Pathol Pharmacol* 1992;78:151–160.
118. Lin S, Wei X, Bales KR, et al. Minocycline blocks bilirubin neurotoxicity and prevents hyperbilirubinemia-induced cerebellar hypoplasia in the Gunn rat. *Eur J Neurosci* 2005;22:21–27.
119. Geiger AS, Rice AC, Shapiro SM. Minocycline blocks acute bilirubin-induced neurological dysfunction in jaundiced Gunn rats. *Neonatology* 2007;92:219–226.
120. Arvin KL, Han BH, Du Y, et al. Minocycline markedly protects the neonatal brain against hypoxic-ischemic injury. *Ann Neurol* 2002;52:54–61.

121. Kutz K, Kandler H, Gugler R, et al. Effect of clofibrate on the metabolism of bilirubin, bromosulphophthalein and indocyanine green and on the biliary lipid composition in Gilbert's syndrome. *Clin Sci (Lond)* 1984;66:389–397.
122. Thorp JM, Waring WS. Modifcation of metabolism and distribution of lipids by ethyl chlorophenoxyisobutyrate. *Nature (Lond)* 1962;194:948–949.
123. Brun S, Carmona MC, Mampel T, et al. Activators of peroxisome proliferator-activated receptor-alpha induce the expression of the uncoupling protein-3 gene in skeletal muscle: a potential mechanism for the lipid intake-dependent activation of uncoupling protein-3 gene expression at birth. *Diabetes* 1999;48: 1217–1222.
124. Foliot A, Drocourt JL, Etienne JP, et al. Increase in the hepatic glucuronidation and clearance of bilirubin in clofibrate-treated rats. *Biochem Pharmacol* 1977;26:547–549.
125. Lindenbaum A, Hernandorena X, Vial M, et al. Clofibrate for the treatment of hyperbilirubinemia in neonates born at term: a double blind controlled study (author's transl). *Arch Fr Pediatr* 1981;38(Suppl 1):867–873.
126. Lindenbaum A, Delaporte B, Benattar C, et al. Preventive treatment of jaundice in premature newborn infants with clofibrate. Double-blind controlled therapeutic trial. *Arch Fr Pediatr* 1985; 42:759–763.
127. Erkul I, Yavuz H, Ozel A. Clofibrate treatment of neonatal jaundice. *Pediatrics* 1991;88:1292–1294.
128. Group CDPR. Clofibrate and niacin in coronary heart disease. *JAMA* 1975;231:360–381.
129. Organization WH. WHO cooperative trial on primary prevention of ischaemic heart disease with clofibrate to lower serum cholesterol: final mortality follow-up. Report of the Committee of Principal Investigators. *Lancet* 1984;2:600–604.
130. Gabilan JC, Benattar C, Lindenbaum A. Clofibrate treatment of neonatal jaundice. *Pediatrics* 1990;86:647–648.
131. Yin J, Miller M, Wennberg RP. Induction of hepatic bilirubin-metabolizing enzymes by the traditional Chinese medicine *yin zhi huang*. *Dev Pharmacol Ther* 1991;16:176–184.
132. Ho NK. Traditional Chinese medicine and treatment of neonatal jaundice. *Singapore Med J* 1996;37:645–651.
133. Chen ZL, Guan WH. Approach to the effect and indication of *Yin Zhi Huang* to treat neonatal jaundice (Chinese). *J Clin Pediatr* 1985;3:302–303.
134. Yang SH, Lu CF. Effects of *Artemisia, Rheum, Gardenia, Coptidis*, and *Rhizoma* on neonatal jaundice in Chinese newborn infants. *J Chin Child Med* 1984;25:144–148.
135. Roberts RJ, Plaa GL. Effect of phenobarbital on the excretion of an exogenous bilirubin load. *Biochem Pharmacol* 1967;16:827–835.
136. Yin J, Wennberg RP, Xia YC, et al. Effect of a traditional Chinese medicine, *yin zhi huang*, on bilirubin clearance and conjugation. *Dev Pharmacol Ther* 1991;16:59–64.
137. Yin J, Wennberg RP, Miller M. Induction of hepatic bilirubin and drug metabolizing enzymes by individual herbs present in the traditional Chinese medicine, *yin zhi huang*. *Dev Pharmacol Ther* 1993;20:186–194.
138. Dennery PA. Pharmacological interventions for the treatment of neonatal jaundice. *Semin Neonatol* 2002;7:111–119.
139. Yeung CY, Leung CS, Chen YZ. An old traditional herbal remedy for neonatal jaundice with a newly identified risk. *J Paediatr Child Health* 1993;29:292–294.
140. Chan TY. The prevalence use and harmful potential of some Chinese herbal medicines in babies and children. *Vet Hum Toxicol* 1994;36:238–240.
141. Strauss KA, Robinson DL, Vreman HJ, et al. Management of hyperbilirubinemia and prevention of kernicterus in 20 patients with Crigler–Najjar disease. *Eur J Pediatr* 2006;165:306–319.
142. Paumgartner G, Beuers U. Ursodeoxycholic acid in cholestatic liver disease: mechanisms of action and therapeutic use revisited. *Hepatology* 2002;36:525–531.
143. George R, Stevens A, Berkenbosch JW, et al. Ursodeoxycholic acid in the treatment of cholestasis and hyperbilirubinemia in pediatric intensive care unit patients. *South Med J* 2002;95:1276–1279.
144. Murao S, Tanaka N. A new enzyme "bilirubin oxidase" produced by *Myrothecium verrucarea* MT-1. *Agricult Biolog Chem* 1981;45: 2383–2385.
145. Soltys PJ, Mullon C, Langer R. Oral treatment for jaundice using immobilized bilirubin oxidase. *Artif Organs* 1992;16:331–335.
146. Johnson LH, Dworanczyk R, Abbasi M, et al. Bilirubin oxidase (BOX) feedings significantly decrease serum bilirubin (B) in jaundiced infant Gunn rats. *Pediatr Res* 1988;22:412A.
147. Davis DR, Yeary RA. Activated charcoal as an adjunct to phototherapy for neonatal jaundice. *Dev Pharmacol Ther* 1987;10: 12–20.
148. Davis DR, Yeary RA, Lee K. Activated charcoal decreases plasma bilirubin levels in the hyperbilirubinemic rat. *Pediatr Res* 1983; 17:208–209.
149. Amitai Y, Regev M, Arad I, et al. Treatment of neonatal hyperbilirubinemia with repetitive oral activated charcoal as an adjunct to phototherapy. *J Perinat Med* 1993;21:189–194.
150. Romagnoli C, Polidori G, Foschini M, et al. Agar in the management of hyperbilirubinaemia in the premature baby. *Arch Dis Child* 1975;50:202–204.
151. Ebbesen F, Moller J. Agar ingestion combined with phototherapy in jaundiced newborn infants. *Biol Neonate* 1977;31:7–9.
152. Bueno A, Perez-Gonzalez J, Bueno M. Effect on agar on neonatal bilirubin seric levels (author's transl). *An Esp Pediatr* 1977;10: 721–730.
153. Odell GB, Gutcher GR, Whitington PF, et al. Enteral administration of agar as an effective adjunct to phototherapy of neonatal hyperbilirubinemia. *Pediatr Res* 1983;17:810–814.
154. Caglayan S, Candemir H, Aksit S, et al. Superiority of oral agar and phototherapy combination in the treatment of neonatal hyperbilirubinemia. *Pediatrics* 1993;92:86–89.
155. Kemper K, Horwitz RI, McCarthy P. Decreased neonatal serum bilirubin with plain agar: a meta-analysis. *Pediatrics* 1988;82: 631–638.
156. Brodersen R, Stern L. Deposition of bilirubin acid in the central nervous system—a hypothesis for the development of kernicterus. *Acta Paediatr Scand* 1990;79:12–19.
157. Ahlfors CE. Benzyl alcohol, kernicterus, and unbound bilirubin. *J Pediatr* 2001;139:317–319.
158. Ahlfors CE. Bilirubin–albumin binding and free bilirubin. *J Perinatol* 2001;21(Suppl 1):S40–S42.
159. Ahlfors CE. Measurement of plasma unbound unconjugated bilirubin. *Anal Biochem* 2000;279:130–135.
160. Ahlfors CE, Marshall GD, Wolcott DK, et al. Measurement of unbound bilirubin by the peroxidase test using Zone Fluidics. *Clin Chim Acta* 2006;365:78–85.
161. Ahlfors CE, Vreman HJ, Wong RJ, et al. Effects of sample dilution, peroxidase concentration, and chloride ion on the measurement of unbound bilirubin in premature newborns. *Clin Biochem* 2007;40:261–267.
162. Nakamura H, Yonetani M, Uetani Y, et al. Determination of serum unbound bilirubin for prediction of kernicterus in low birthweight infants. *Acta Paediatr Jpn* 1992;34:642–647.
163. McDonagh AF, Vreman HJ, Wong RJ, et al. Photoisomers—obfuscating factors in clinical peroxidase measurements of unbound bilirubin? *Pediatrics* 2009;123:67–76.
164. Morris BH, Oh W, Tyson JE, et al. A Multi-center randomized trial of aggressive versus conservative phototherapy for extremely low birth weight infants. *N Engl J Med* 2008;359:1885–1896.

CHAPTER

19

Alan H. Jobe
John P. Newnham

Drugs and Lung Development

Lung development is a target for drug therapy only within the context of prematurity. Corticosteroids are standard of care for women at high risk of preterm delivery to decrease the risk of respiratory distress syndrome (RDS) and increase infant survival. Corticosteroids have pleiotropic effects, which can be both beneficial and potentially harmful for the developing lung and other fetal organ systems. Although lung development and maturation are modulated by multiple hormones, growth factors, and disease states, no drug class other than corticosteroids has proven effective as a maturational agent in clinical practice. This chapter reviews the clinical literature on the use of antenatal corticosteroids to induce early lung maturation and emphasizes the areas of uncertainty. Other agents that have not proven to be effective are briefly discussed.

THE DEVELOPMENT OF ANTENATAL CORTICOSTEROID THERAPY

In 1969, Liggins observed that fetal sheep infused with cortisol had lungs that were better aerated than control lungs after preterm delivery (1). Liggins and Howie (2) then reported in 1972 the first randomized control trial of antenatal corticosteroids, which demonstrated decreased RDS and decreased death in preterms, with no increase in complications. The trial was controversial because the obstetric community was concerned about adverse effects of "steroids" on human development after the experience with diethylstilbestrol. Over the next 18 years multiple trials were reported, which generally supported the benefits of antenatal corticosteroid treatments. In 1990, Crowley and colleagues published a meta-analysis of the trials demonstrating compelling benefit with minimal risk (3). However, in that era in the United States and elsewhere, fewer than 20% of women at risk of preterm delivery were treated with antenatal corticosteroids. In 1994, a National Institutes of Health (US) Consensus Conference strongly endorsed the use of antenatal corticosteroids (Table 19.1) (4), and utilization rates increased to current treatment rates of 80% to 90% of women at risk. However, many clinicians began using repetitive courses of antenatal corticosteroids, which resulted in a second Consensus Conference in 2000, which recommended against repetitive courses of corticosteroids until further studies were available (5). Some of those trials of repetitive dosing with maternal corticosteroids are now available and will be reviewed (6,7). Although antenatal corticosteroid treatment is considered the standard of care by obstetric societies worldwide and the NIH, the indication is not approved by the US Food and Drug Administration because no request for approval has been submitted by pharmaceutical companies.

SINGLE-COURSE TREATMENTS WITH ANTENATAL CORTICOSTEROIDS

The clinical indicators for a single course of antenatal corticosteroids were developed by the NIH Consensus Conference in 1994, based primarily on the Crowley meta-analysis (3). The most recent update of that meta-analysis in 2006 by Roberts and Dalziel further strengthens the recommendations for treatment (8). This is now the definitive analysis as further placebo-controlled trials are not ethical. The analysis includes 21 randomized controlled trials of 3,885 women and 4,269 infants. No risks for the mother were identified, even for women with preeclampsia or diabetes, although attention to glycemic control is required after corticosteroids are administered to women with diabetes. The benefits for the newborn are substantial with large decreases in death, RDS, intraventricular hemorrhage, and necrotizing enterocolitis (Fig. 19.1). The risk of developing bronchopulmonary dysplasia is not decreased.

The primary indication for antenatal corticosteroid treatment in most studies was the prevention of RDS. The effect of antenatal corticosteroids on RDS is robust with comparable decreases in RDS independent of gestational age more than 28 weeks of gestation. However, because the risk of RDS decreases as gestational age increases, the number needed to treat to prevent one case of RDS was 4 for deliveries prior to 31 weeks, 15 at 31 to 34 weeks, and 145 at greater than 34 weeks (9). The treatment to delivery interval for the maximal decrease in RDS was 1 to 7 days after initiating treatment, and with loss of benefit after 7 days (Fig. 19.1). The RDS benefit was demonstrated in trials conducted in the 70s, 80s, and 90s, demonstrating persistent benefits across time.

TABLE 19.1 Recommendations of the 1994 and 2000 Consensus Conferences for the Use of Antenatal Corticosteroids

The 1994 conference: antenatal corticosteroids
- All fetuses between 24 and 34 wk of gestation at risk of preterm delivery are candidates for treatment
- The benefits vastly outweigh the risks; the benefits include decreased risks of respiratory distress syndrome, intraventricular hemorrhage, and death
- Patients eligible for tocolytics should receive corticosteroids
- Corticosteroids are indicated unless delivery is imminent because of possible benefit for treatment-to-delivery intervals of <24 hr
- Corticosteroids are indicated for preterm prolonged rupture of membranes to decrease the risk of intraventricular hemorrhage

The 2000 conference: repetitive courses of antenatal corticosteroids
- Reaffirmed that women between 24 and 34 wk of gestation at risk of preterm delivery should receive a single course of corticosteroids
- Insufficient data to support repetitive courses
- Repetitive courses should be used within the context of clinical trials

The clinical literature supports other benefits, which were also demonstrated in experimental animal models (10). Preterm fetal exposure to corticosteroids increased blood pressure and myocardial performance after preterm delivery. The blood pressure was higher despite lower levels of circulating catecholamines in the sheep. Kidney tubular function as measured by an improved ability to handle salt and water loads was also improved by fetal exposure to corticosteroids. A fetal exposure to corticosteroids resulted in an integrated response that made the preterm lamb more tolerant to postnatal asphyxia (11). The pleiotropic organ maturational effects of corticosteroids result in global adaptive responses that benefited the preterm. Within the context of normal development, these effects can be viewed as replicating the normal fetal adaptations to term birth.

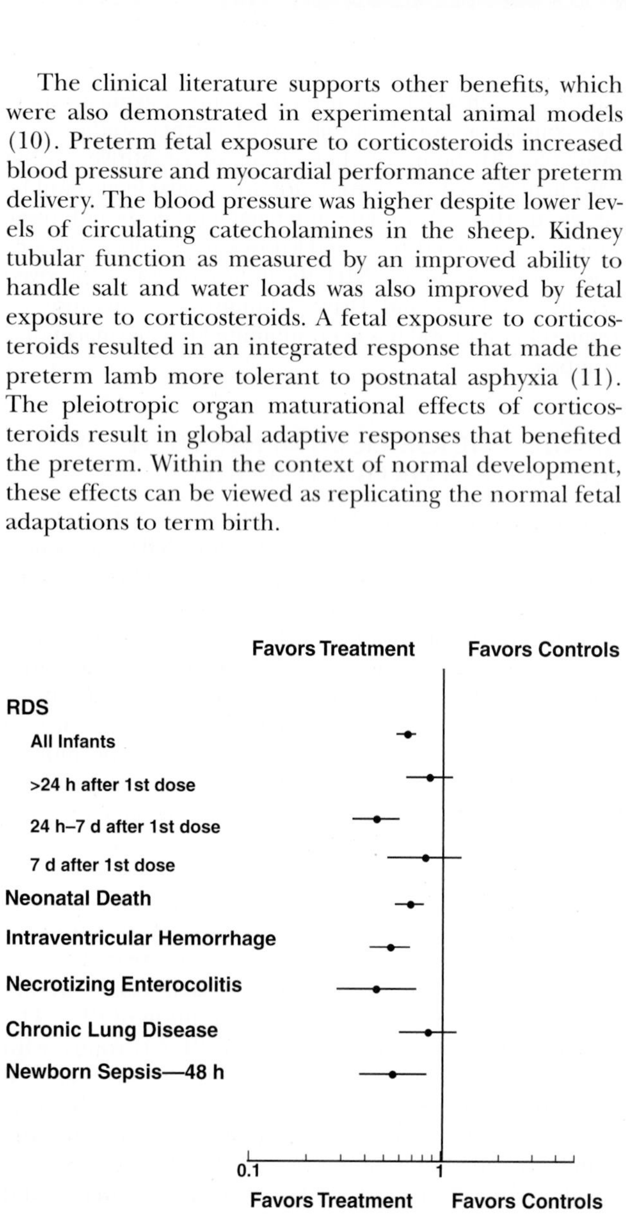

Figure 19.1. Meta-analysis of randomized controlled trials of antenatal corticosteroids. The point estimates for the risk ratios and 95% confidence intervals are the summary values for the composite analysis. Antenatal glucocorticoids improve outcomes for preterm infants. RDS, Respiratory distress syndrome. Based on data from Roberts and Dalziel (8).

A continuing concern has been the potential for harm from hormones that can clearly alter development, cause dysmorphic changes in rodents, and decrease brain and body growth in multiple animal models (12). A single course of corticosteroids did not decrease birth weight in the preterm human in 11 studies of 3,586 infants (weight difference −17.5 g; 95% CI, −62 to 27 g). When used as a single treatment course at gestations more than 28 weeks, antenatal corticosteroids have been remarkably safe. No acute adverse effects after preterm birth have been reported despite widespread use. The risks of infection in the newborn and postpartum infection in the mother were not increased (8). The lingering concern has been potential long-term adverse effects of antenatal corticosteroid exposure of preterm fetuses. Long-term outcomes are available and are reassuring. Children exposed to a single course of antenatal corticosteroids were taller and had better cognitive function than controls at a 14-year follow-up (13). However, they also had higher blood pressures, although few were in the hypertensive range (14). In contrast, in 6-year and 23-year follow-up reports, the steroid exposed young adults had lower systolic blood pressures (15,16). A 30-year follow-up of the newborns from the original Liggins and Howie trial found some evidence of insulin resistance in the steroid-exposed adults, but no other cardiovascular abnormalities relative to controls (17). The remaining concern is corticosteroid effects of very early gestational exposures, which is not addressed by follow-up of children from the early trials.

PHARMACOLOGY AND DOSE OF ANTENATAL CORTICOSTEROIDS

The Consensus Conference recommended maternal treatment with betamethasone or dexamethasone rather than cortisol or methylprednisolone because the fluorinated corticosteroids cross the placenta from the mother to the fetus, have no mineralocorticoid activity, and have a relatively long duration of action (4). Betamethasone and dexamethasone are equivalent structurally except for the isomeric position of the 16-methyl group. Betamethasone was given as the suspension of relatively insoluble acetate and soluble phosphate by Liggins and Howie in the original trial (2), and that formulation,

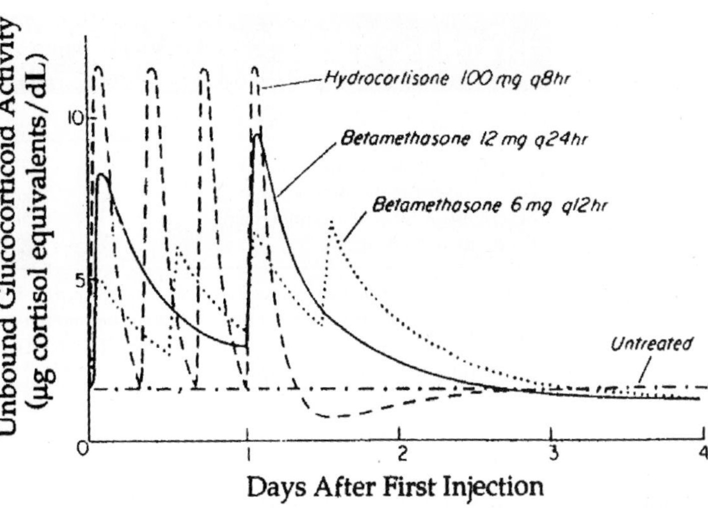

Figure 19.2. Fetal plasma unbound glucocorticoid activity estimated for maternal treatments with corticosteroids. The curves are estimates based on maternal dosing with 12 mg of betamethasone acetate + phosphate given every 24 hours, 6 mg of betamethasone alcohol given every 6 hours, and 100 mg of hydrocortisone given every 8 hours. The curve for betamethasone alcohol should be similar to what would occur with 6 mg of dexamethasone sodium phosphate. (From Ballard PL, Ballard RA. Scientific basis and therapeutic regimens for use of antenatal glucocorticoids. *Am J Obstet Gynecol* 1995;173:254–262, with permission.)

marketed in the United States as Celestone Soluspan® (Schering Plough) is the only betamethasone preparation available for injection. Betamethasone phosphate preparations are available elsewhere. Dexamethasone is given as the soluble sodium phosphate. The soluble phosphates of betamethasone and dexamethasone are prodrugs that are rapidly dephosphorylated to the active forms and have a rapid onset of action when given by intramuscular injection. Two dosing schedules were empirically evaluated in the clinical trials and are currently the recommended dosing schedules. A total dose of 24 mg betamethasone (acetate plus phosphate) is given as a divided dose of 12 mg at the recognition of risk of preterm delivery and 24 hours later. The same total dose of 24 mg of betamethasone sodium phosphate is given as a four-dose treatment, with 6 mg given at the recognition of the risk of preterm delivery and three subsequent doses of 6 mg given at 12-hour intervals. The resulting corticosteroid exposures for the fetus were modeled by Ballard and Ballard (18) (Fig. 19.2). Both agents readily cross the placenta and achieve fetal plasma levels of 30% to 40% of the maternal levels. There are isolated reports of higher corticosteroid doses or shorter treatment intervals to "accelerate" the maturation if delivery cannot be delayed for 48 hours, but no clinical data support these other dosing strategies.

The pharmacology of corticosteroids for the indication of maternal corticosteroids for fetal lung maturation has not been well studied. The dosing schedules were selected quite empirically on the basis of what seemed to work in the initial trial (2). In fetal sheep models, single doses of dexamethasone phosphate or betamethasone phosphate given to the fetus or ewe do not induce lung maturation (19), nor do single fetal doses of cortisol (20). Repetitive dosing with the soluble phosphates or cortisol does induce lung maturation, suggesting that prolonged exposure is important to the response. In sheep, fetal treatments with betamethasone acetate plus phosphate induce some lung maturation, whereas maternal treatments induce more lung maturation and also fetal growth restriction (21). The maternal dosing results in much lower fetal blood levels of betamethasone but causes larger fetal effects. The slow release betamethasone acetate increases blood levels in the ewe minimally but will induce fetal lung maturation in sheep. Low and repeated maternal doses of dexamethasone also cause fetal growth restriction in sheep (22). These observations have not been exploited to develop the minimally effective dose and formulation of corticosteroid for clinical use.

BETAMETHASONE VERSUS DEXAMETHASONE

Antenatal treatments with either agent decrease RDS and intraventricular hemorrhage (8), which means that comparisons of efficacy are evaluating differences in responses against a background of benefit. There are a number of reports comparing the efficacy of maternal treatments with betamethasone or dexamethasone and a recent meta-analysis of the randomized controlled trials (23). The relative efficacy of the treatments can also be compared indirectly by evaluating the responses of each treatment relative to controls using the larger data set from the Roberts and Dalziel meta-analysis (8) (Table 19.2). Either comparison of dexamethasone and betamethasone treatments demonstrates more intraventricular hemorrhage in the betamethasone-treated infants, similar fetal/neonatal deaths, and a better efficacy for betamethasone to decrease RDS than dexamethasone. The increased intraventricular hemorrhage results primarily from the large Elimian trial (24), which contributed about 80% to this outcome in the direct meta-analysis. There are no randomized and controlled data on longer-term outcomes. A recent observational study suggests better neurological outcomes at 2 years for betamethasone-exposed children than for dexamethasone-exposed children (25). Thus, the clinical benefits of one treatment choice versus the other are not compelling. The large trials of repeated courses of antenatal corticosteroids selected betamethasone as the treatment drug.

If these drugs are so similar, should there be any differences in clinical responses? The drug formulations and timing of dosing are different, so any differential clinical

TABLE 19.2 Comparison of Direct and Indirect Estimates of Dexamethasone to Betamethasone

	Direct[a]	*Indirect*[b]
Respiratory distress syndrome	1.06 (0.88–1.28)	1.43 (1.14–1.78)
Any Intraventricular hemorrhage	0.44 (0.21–0.92)	0.31 (0.14–0.73)
Severe intraventricular hemorrhage	0.40 (0.13–1.24)	0.47 (0.09–2.33)
Fetal/neonatal death	1.28 (0.46–3.52)	0.96 (0.71–1.30)

[a]Risk ratios and 95% confidence intervals from Brownfoot, Crowther, Middleton (23) based on randomized controlled trials of dexamethasone versus betamethasone.
[b]Risk ratios and 95% confidence intervals from Roberts, Dalziel (8) based on comparing effects of the agents relative to control groups.

responses may not result from the drugs themselves. However, there is physiologic information indicating that maternal/fetal responses to the treatments differ. (Table 19.2) In sheep, fetal treatment with betamethasone more predictably induced preterm labor than did dexamethasone (26). In mice, betamethasone was a more potent inducer of lung maturation and had less effect on subsequent neurodevelopment than did dexamethasone (27). Both betamethasone and dexamethasone altered fetal heart rates in humans, but betamethasone had less effect on fetal heart rate variability (28). Although the genomic potencies of betamethasone and dexamethasone are similar, these corticosteroids also have rapid effects on cell membrane functions such as ion transport that can alter intracellular signal transduction pathways (29). Corticosteroids can also modulate metabolic pathways that regulate endothelial nitric oxide synthase by nonnuclear effects (30). For some nongenomic effects, dexamethasone is much more potent than betamethasone (31). These drugs are not equivalent and the preferred drug for antenatal treatments remains unclear because of unknown differences in these drugs for this indication as well as formulation and dosing differences.

REPETITIVE COURSES OF ANTENATAL CORTICOSTEROIDS

The Rationale for Repetitive Courses

The maximal benefit from antenatal corticosteroids is when delivery occurs between 1 and 7 days after initiation of therapy (17) (Fig. 19.1). The decrease in risk of RDS following a single treatment course was about 50%, leaving half of the fetuses with a potential for benefit from another course of treatment. As obstetric practice has changed to try to delay deliveries at early gestational ages for as long as possible, about 50% of women assessed to be in preterm labor and at risk of preterm delivery do not deliver for more than 1 week after identification (32). Therefore, a large population of women at risk might benefit from repetitive courses of corticosteroids. Furthermore, in one report a time interval of more than 14 days between the corticosteroid treatment and delivery was associated with increased lung disease in newborns delivered at more than 28 weeks of gestation (33).

Animal models have been used to evaluate the potential for repetitive corticosteroid treatment. Animals with short gestations are of limited value because the duration of action of the synthetic corticosteroid is long relative to the short gestation. The sheep, with a term gestation of 150 days, has been used most effectively to evaluate retreatment strategies (12). The potential for benefit is based on the biology of induced maturation and the goals of treatment (34) (Fig. 19.3). If the maturational effects of a single treatment course are lost in 7 days, then repeated treatments make sense. If the treatment shifts the curve for maturation, there may be benefit of repetitive courses to induce more maturation. If a single course triggers progressive maturation, then there is no reason to retreat. Although some markers of induced maturation such as the mRNAs for the surfactant proteins are reversibly induced (35), net lung maturation in sheep is best approximated by a shift in the maturation curve (34). Repetitive treatments at weekly intervals incrementally improve lung function after preterm delivery, although the amount of growth restriction increases (36). Therefore, there are

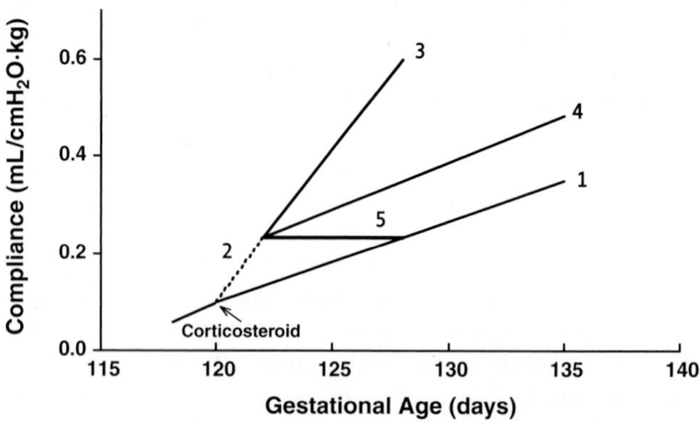

Figure 19.3. Relationship between gestational age and lung compliance in sheep. Curve 1 represents the increase in compliance with gestational age. Curve 2 illustrates the maturational effect of corticosteroid over several days. Curve 3 illustrates the outcome if corticosteroids triggered progressive maturation. Curve 4 demonstrates a shift in the position but not the slope of the maturation curve. Curve 5 represents a loss of compliance over 7 days back to the normal curve. The experimental information from the fetal sheep is best approximated by curve 4.

experimental data to support both added benefit and risk of repetitive corticosteroid treatments.

Clinical Experience with Repetitive Treatments

After the consensus conference of 1994, 7- or 14-day repeated courses of antenatal corticosteroids became virtually standard practice despite no supportive clinical information. Multiple retrospective databases were used to evaluate the risks and benefits. For example, Abbasi et al. (37) reported lower incidences of RDS and patent ductus arteriosis without decreased birth weights with repetitive doses. Thorp et al. (38) found no adverse effects of repetitive courses and increased birth weights. In contrast, French et al. (39) noted reduced birth weights and head circumferences with increasing numbers of corticosteroid courses without any added benefit from decreased incidences of RDS or neonatal death. Disabilities assessed at 3 years were unchanged by repetitive courses of corticosteroids. Banks et al. (40) found a worrisome increase in early severe lung disease. These varied outcomes from retrospective analyses suggest risk and emphasize the need for randomized controlled trials. In 2000, a second consensus conference, held to assess the appropriateness of the shift in clinical practice to repetitive courses of antenatal corticosteroids, concluded that information was insufficient to support repetitive treatment courses (5). Clinical trials were recommended.

A number of those trials are now complete and are combined in a recent meta-analysis (6). All trials used betamethasone, but the retreatment was with either a single dose or with the 2-dose course of betamethasone. The meta-analysis of five trials including more than 2,000 women demonstrated significant decreases in lung disease in the newborns (relative risk 0.82; 95% CI, 0.72 to 0.93) and in composite serous infant morbidity (RR 0.79; 95% CI, 0.67 to 0.93). Mean birth weight was not decreased (−62 g; 95% CI, −129 to +5 g). There were no differences in any other adverse outcomes for the mother or the newborn, suggesting some benefit of repeated treatments. However, the largest trial of 1,858 randomized women was recently published (7). This trial repeated the 2-dose betamethasone treatment at 14 days rather than 7 days intervals, with most of the infants receiving one or two repeated treatments after the initial treatment. Only 4% of infants were delivered before 28 weeks of gestational age. The composite primary outcome for adverse events (odds ratio, 1.04; 95% CI, 0.77 to 1.39) or effects on RDS, bronchopulmonary dysplasia, or intraventricular hemorrhage was not different. This trial demonstrated that the infants exposed to repeated courses of corticosteroids weighed less by an average of 140 g, were shorter by 1 cm, and had a head circumference that was 0.6 cm smaller (all p values <.002). These growth effects are biologically plausible based on the known growth effects of corticosteroids. The 2-year follow-up of children from the Crowther trial of weekly retreatments demonstrated no adverse neurodevelopmental effects (41), whereas the Wapner trial found a concerning trend for increased cerebral palsy for infants exposed to 4 or more weekly courses of betamethasone (2.9% vs. 0.5%) (42). These are very good and large trials that demonstrate conflicting outcomes with respect to neonatal morbidities and fetal growth. The only benefit may be decreased respiratory problems for the infants, and the risks of adverse growth effects and longer-term developmental outcomes remain unclear.

A second strategy has been to give a "rescue" treatment of corticosteroid prior to preterm delivery if the first course was given more than 7 days earlier. This strategy has the advantage of exposing the fetus only twice and targeting only fetuses delivering prematurely. Unfortunately, in a randomized controlled trial of 249 women, there was no indication of benefit, perhaps because the rescue treatment to delivery interval averaged only 8 hours (43). A second trial of 437 randomized women tested whether a rescue course of corticosteroids given 14 or more days after an initial treatment would improve outcomes (44). The rescue course decreased composite neonatal morbidity (RR 0.73; CI, 0.58 to 0.91) and respiratory outcomes without adverse effects on fetal growth or other outcomes.

More trials are ongoing, but to date the benefits of repeated courses of corticosteroids are not compelling. These trials are trying to demonstrate a marginal benefit of repeated or rescue courses of corticosteroids against the background of clear benefit of the initial treatment course. Any marginal benefit may be in select subpopulations of women at risk of preterm delivery. No trials have accessed the need for a repeated treatment by measuring indicators of lung maturation in individual cases, for example. A more targeted approach might demonstrate selective benefit, but the experimental literature demonstrates potential risks.

CORTICOSTEROIDS AT EARLY GESTATIONAL AGES

The meta-analysis gives little guidance about the use of corticosteroids for pregnancies at less than 28 weeks of gestation because most of the trials include few very low-gestation infants (8). The effectiveness of treatment of early-gestation pregnancies is inferential. Corticosteroids accelerate lung maturation in explants of human lungs collected between about 12 and 20 weeks of gestation, indicating that the human lung is responsive at very early gestational ages (45). The primate lung is also matured at early gestations by maternal corticosteroid treatments (46). Information from a number of databases indicated that antenatal corticosteroid treatments increased survival of infants with birth weights less than 1 kg. Survival and outcome information for all infants born at less than 26 weeks of gestation for the United Kingdom and Ireland demonstrated that antenatal corticosteroid treatments decreased death (odds ratio, 0.57; 95% CI, 0.37 to 0.85) and decreased severe head ultrasound abnormalities (odds ratio, 0.39; 95% CI, 0.22 to 0.77) (47). A recent multivariant analysis demonstrated decreased death for infants at 23 weeks of gestational ages who were exposed to antenatal corticosteroid (48). Although not proven by randomized trials, which at this time would probably be considered unethical, antenatal corticosteroids are standard care if an attempt is made to achieve survival of a very low gestation infant. However, the risks of adverse effects of corticosteroids on brain and other organ system development may be increased. These early gestation fetuses will also be exposed to more repetitive treatments if that treatment course is selected, possibly increasing exposure to the highest risk group.

CHORIOAMNIONITIS AND PRETERM PROLONGED RUPTURE OF MEMBRANES

Corticosteroids generally are contraindicated in infected patients or when the risk of infection is high. Nevertheless, low-grade indolent infection of the chorioamnion and amniotic fluid is frequent in women delivering prior to 30 weeks of gestation (49). Preterm prolonged rupture of membranes (PPROM) is also associated with an increase in chorioamnionitis. The clinical conundrum is that the majority of fetuses that may benefit from antenatal corticosteroids may be exposed to an infectious environment. Harding et al. (50) reported the meta-analysis of trial data for antenatal corticosteroids with PPROM (Fig. 19.4). Antenatal corticosteroids were as effective and risk free in women with PPROM as for the overall population of women at risk for preterm delivery. For a population of 457 consecutive deliveries at 23 to 32 weeks of gestation, 45% had chorioamnionitis and 83% received antenatal corticosteroids (51). The antenatal corticosteroid treatment decreased RDS from 72% to 60%, intraventricular hemorrhage from 15% to 10%, and the neonatal systemic inflammatory response syndrome from 66% to 40%. These beneficial effects of corticosteroids may result from the combined effects of induced maturation and suppression of inflammation.

Recent studies in animal models support the complex interactions between pregnancies complicated by infection and inflammation and antenatal corticosteroid treatments. Fetal exposures to proinflammatory mediators such as *Escherichia coli* lipopolysaccharide, interleukin-1, or live Ureaplasma cause lung maturation (52). Simultaneous exposure to maternal corticosteroids initially suppresses the fetal inflammation, but augments the lung maturational response. However, 5 to 15 days after the corticosteroid treatment, fetal inflammation has increased probably because of maturation of fetal inflammatory cells by the inflammatory mediators and corticosteroids (53). These exposures also strikingly modulate the fetal innate immune responses to secondary exposures (54). This complex biology probably contributes to clinical outcomes in presently unknown ways, particularly with repeated courses of antenatal corticosteroids.

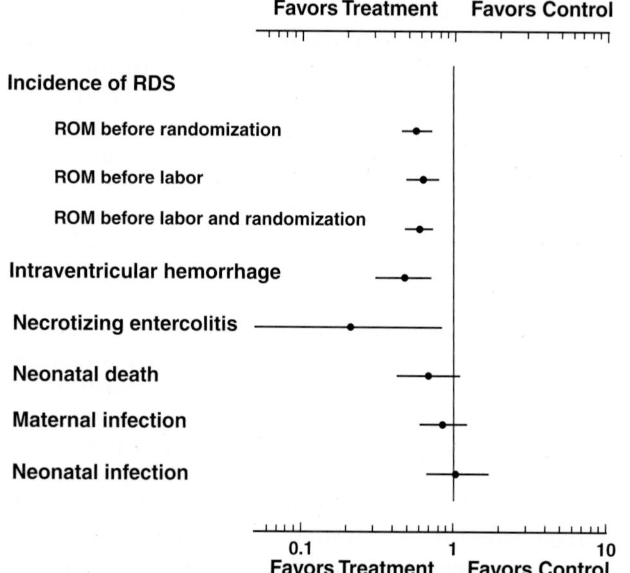

Figure 19.4. Summary meta-analyses of randomized controlled trial data for use of antenatal corticosteroids in women with preterm rupture of membranes. The point estimates for the odds ratios and 95% confidence limits favor treatment. RDS, Respiratory disease syndrome; ROM, rupture of membranes. Data from Harding et al. (50).

MULTIPLE GESTATION

Multiple pregnancies make up a large percentage of the infants at risk of delivery at very early gestations, in part because of assisted reproduction technologies. The meta-analysis of a single treatment course of corticosteroids demonstrated no decrease in RDS, but only 310 multiple pregnancies were included (8). Two other reports indicated either no benefit or considerable benefit for multiple gestations (55,56). An analysis of a population of deliveries that included 4,754 singletons, 2,460 twins, and 906 triplets demonstrated that antenatal corticosteroids decreased respiratory distress in singletons by 15%, by 16% in twins, and by 5% in triplets (57). In this same population, antenatal corticosteroids also decreased intraventricular hemorrhage in multiple births (58). The argument has been made that twins may require higher maternal doses because of increased fetal mass. However, a higher dose should not be required because the major reservoir for the drug is the mother, and that volume far exceeds the incremental volume of distribution of twins, especially at gestational ages of less than 30 weeks. In fact, the same dose of antenatal corticosteroids is given independent of maternal weight. A more likely possibility is that the causes of preterm labor in multiples differ from the causes in singletons. Infection/inflammation may be less likely, for example.

INDICATIONS FOR CORTICOSTEROIDS AT GESTATIONS BEYOND 34 WEEKS

The analysis by Sinclair in 1995 (9) demonstrated that the magnitude of response to decreased respiratory distress was independent of gestation age, but that the number needed to treat increased to more than 100 beyond 34 weeks of gestation. However, the number of infants born by cesarean section prior to labor and at gestations less than 39 weeks has increased strikingly worldwide. Although the incidence of RDS, transient tachypnea of the newborn, and other problems of neonatal adaptation is low, the number of affected infants is large. Stutchfield et al. (59) randomized 998 women to antenatal betamethasone or placebo prior to elective cesarean section. Admissions for special care and for respiratory distress were significantly decreased by antenatal corticosteroids. This strategy is being further evaluated in ongoing trials. Other trials are evaluating antenatal corticosteroids for late preterm deliveries associated with maternal diabetes.

OTHER MEDIATORS OF LUNG MATURATION

THYROID HORMONES

The fetus needs small amounts of thyroid hormones to mature the fetal lung and for normal brain development. Tissue levels of T_3 and reverse T_3 are regulated in part locally by deiodinases. The fetal thyroid is responsive to thyrotropin-releasing hormone (TRH), a tripeptide that can cross the placenta. In contrast, very little T_3 or T_4 crosses the placenta, although that residual small amount is sufficient to sustain fetal brain and lung development (60). Thyroid hormones alone can induce fetal lung maturation, and they act additively or synergistically with corticosteroids in a number of animal and lung explant models (61,62). T_3 or T_4 cannot be given in high dose to women at risk of preterm delivery because of the adverse metabolic effects on the mother. Therefore, TRH has been evaluated primarily as an adjunct to antenatal corticosteroid treatments. The initial small trials were very encouraging, but subsequent large trials showed no benefit (32,63). The meta-analysis of the antenatal use of TRH, which included 13 trials and more than 4,600 randomized women, demonstrated no benefit for the outcomes of RDS, bronchopulmonary dysplasia, or death (64). The TRH–exposed-infants had lower Apgar scores at 5 minutes, and more infants required mechanical ventilation. The TRH exposure was also associated with adverse effects on neurodevelopment in two trials (65,66). There is no indication to use TRH to induce lung maturation and no further trials are justified.

BETA AGONISTS

Beta agonists such as terbutaline and ritodrine are used as tocolytics to delay preterm delivery. These agents increase intracellular cyclic AMP levels and are secretogogues for surfactant. They may also induce lung maturation and can act additively with corticosteroids to promote lung maturation (62). Theoretically, they could also have adverse effects on the fetal lung if induced secretion depleted the surfactant pool available at the time of preterm birth. The beta agonists have not been used with the sole intent of inducing lung maturation in the human. There is no information demonstrating effects of antenatal beta agonists on postnatal lung function.

OTHER HORMONES AND GROWTH FACTORS

Multiple hormones and growth factors have been explored *in vitro* and in experimental animal models. From the clinical perspective, the ideal agent would target specifically the maturational effect that is desired. Pleiotropic agents such as the retinoids are likely to have adverse effects. Large proteins will not cross the placenta and would need to be given by fetal injection. The lung can be targeted by agents injected into the amniotic cavity if the agent is not absorbed from the swallowed amniotic fluid by the gastrointestinal tract. However, the mixing of fetal lung fluid with amniotic fluid is inefficient, and large amounts of an agent might be required. The development of new agents to induce fetal lung maturation is a challenge because the fetus is not readily accessible for treatment, the potential for damage of a developing fetus is high, and pharmaceutical industry is concerned about risk.

REFERENCES

1. Liggins GC. Premature delivery of fetal lambs infused with glucocorticoids. *J Endocrinol* 1969;45:515–523.
2. Liggins GC, Howie RN. A controlled trial of antepartum glucocorticoid treatment for prevention of RDS in premature infants. *Pediatrics* 1972;50:515–525.
3. Crowley P, Chalmers I, Keirse MJ. The effects of corticosteroid administration before preterm delivery: an overview of the evidence from controlled trials. *Br J Obstet Gynaecol* 1990;97:11–25.
4. National Institutes of Health. Consensus development panel on the effect of corticosteroids for fetal maturation on perinatal outcomes. Effect of corticosteroids for fetal maturation on perinatal outcomes. *J Am Med Assoc* 1995;273:413–418.
5. Antenatal Corticosteroids Revisited: Repeat Courses. *NIH Consens Statement Online* 2000;17:1–10.
6. Crowther CA, Harding JE. Repeat doses of prenatal corticosteroids for women at risk of preterm birth for preventing neonatal respiratory disease. *Cochrane Database Syst Rev* 2007:CD003935.
7. Murphy KE, Hannah ME, Willan AR, et al. Multiple courses of antenatal corticosteroids for preterm birth (MACS): a randomised controlled trial. *Lancet* 2009;372:2143–2151.
8. Roberts D, Dalziel S. Antenatal corticosteroids for accelerating fetal lung maturation for women at risk of preterm birth. *Cochrane Database Syst Rev* 2006;3:CD004454.
9. Sinclair JC. Meta-analysis of randomized controlled trials of antenatal corticosteroid for the prevention of respiratory distress syndrome: discussion. *Am J Obstet Gynecol* 1995;173:335–344.
10. Padbury JF, Ervin MG, Polk DH. Extrapulmonary effects of antenatally administered steroids. *J. Pediatr* 1996;128:167–172.
11. Ervin MG, Padbury JF, Polk DH, et al. Antenatal glucocorticoids alter premature newborn lamb neuroendocrine and endocrine responses to hypoxia. *Am J Physiol* 2000;279:R830–R838.
12. Jobe AH, Ikegami M. Fetal responses to glucocorticoids. In: Mendelson CR, ed. *Endocrinology of the lung.* Totowa, NJ: Humana Press, 2000:45–57.
13. Doyle LW, Ford GW, Rickards AL, et al. Antenatal corticosteroids and outcome at 14 years of age in children with birth weight less than 1501 grams. *Pediatrics* 2000;106:E2.
14. Doyle LW, Ford GW, Davis NM, et al. Antenatal corticosteroid therapy and blood pressure at 14 years of age in preterm children. *Clin Sci (Lond)* 2000;98:137–142.
15. Dessens AB, Haas HS, Koppe JG. Twenty-year follow-up of antenatal corticosteroid treatment. *Pediatrics* 2000;105:E77.
16. Dalziel SR, Liang A, Parag V, et al. Blood pressure at 6 years of age after prenatal exposure to betamethasone: follow-up results of a randomized, controlled trial. *Pediatrics* 2004;114:e373–e377.
17. Dalziel SR, Walker NK, Parag V, et al. Cardiovascular risk factors after antenatal exposure to betamethasone: 30-year follow-up of a randomised controlled trial. *Lancet* 2005;365:1856–1862.
18. Ballard PL, Ballard RA. Scientific basis and therapeutic regimens for use of antenatal glucocorticoids. *Am J Obstet Gynecol* 1995;173:254–262.
19. Jobe A, Moss TJM, Nitsos I, et al. Betamethasone for lung maturation: testing dose and formulation in fetal sheep. *Am J Obstet Gynecol* 2007;97:523–526.
20. Jobe AH, Newnham J, Moss TJ, et al. Differential effects of maternal betamethasone and cortisol on lung maturation and growth in fetal sheep. *Am J Obstet Gynecol* 2003;188:22–28.
21. Jobe AH, Newnham J, Willet K, et al. Fetal versus maternal and gestational age effects of repetitive antenatal glucocorticoids. *Pediatrics* 1998;102:1116–1125.
22. Kutzler MA, Ruane EK, Coksaygan T, et al. Effects of three courses of maternally administered dexamethasone at 0.7, 0.75, and 0.8 of gestation on prenatal and postnatal growth in sheep. *Pediatrics* 2004;113:313–319.
23. Brownfoot FC, Crowther CA, Middleton P. Different corticosteroids and regimens for accelerating fetal lung maturation for

women at risk of preterm birth. *Cochrane Database Syst Rev* 2008: CD006764.
24. Elimian A, Garry D, Figueroa R, et al. Antenatal betamethasone compared with dexamethasone (betacode trial): a randomized controlled trial. *Obstet Gynecol* 2007;110:26–30.
25. Lee BH, Stoll BJ, McDonald SA, et al. Adverse neonatal outcomes associated with antenatal dexamethasone versus antenatal betamethasone. *Pediatrics* 2006;117:1503–1510.
26. Derks JB, Giussani DA, Van Dam LM, et al. Differential effects of betamethasone and dexamethasone fetal administration of parturition in sheep. *J Soc Gynecol Investig* 1996;3:336–3341.
27. Rayburn WF, Christensen HD, Gonzalez CL. A placebo-controlled comparison between betamethasone and dexamethasone for fetal maturation: differences in neurobehavioral development of mice offspring. *Am J Obstet Gynecol* 1997;176: 842–851.
28. Senat MV, Minoui S, Multon O, et al. Effect of dexamethasone and betamethasone on fetal heart rate variability in preterm labour: a randomised study. *Br J Obstet Gynaecol* 1998;105: 749–755.
29. Chen YZ, Qiu J. Possible genomic consequence of nongenomic action of glucocorticoids in neural cells. *News Physiol Sci* 2001;16: 292–296.
30. Hafezi-Moghadam A, Simoncini T, Yang E, et al. Acute cardiovascular protective effects of corticosteroids are mediated by non-transcriptional activation of endothelial nitric oxide synthase. *Nat Med* 2002;8:473–479.
31. Buttgereit F, Brand MD, Burmester GR. Equivalent doses and relative drug potencies for non-genomic glucocorticoid effects: a novel glucocorticoid hierarchy. *Biochem Pharmacol* 1999;58:363–368.
32. ACTOBAT. Australian collaborative trial of antenatal thyrotropin-releasing hormone (ACTOBAT) for prevention of neonatal respiratory disease. *Lancet* 1995;345:877–882.
33. Ring AM, Garland JS, Stafeil BR, et al. The effect of a prolonged time interval between antenatal corticosteroid administration and delivery on outcomes in preterm neonates: a cohort study. *Am J Obstet Gynecol* 2007;196:457, e1–e6.
34. Ikegami M, Polk DH, Jobe AH, et al. Effect of interval from fetal corticosteroid treatment to delivery on postnatal lung function of preterm lambs. *J Appl Physiol* 1996;80:591–597.
35. Tan RC, Ikegami M, Jobe AH, et al. Developmental and glucocorticoid regulation of surfactant protein mRNAs in preterm lambs. *Am. J. Physiol* 1999;277:L1142–L1148.
36. Ikegami M, Jobe AH, Newnham J, et al. Repetitive prenatal glucocorticoids improve lung function and decrease growth in preterm lambs. *Am J Respir Crit Care Med* 1997;156:178–184.
37. Abbasi S, Hirsch D, Davis J, et al. Effect of single versus multiple courses of antenatal corticosteroids on maternal and neonatal outcome. *Am J Obstet Gynecol* 2000;182:1243–1249.
38. Thorp JA, Jones AM, Hunt C, et al. The effect of multidose antenatal betamethasone on maternal and infant outcomes. *Am J Obstet Gynecol* 2001;184:196–202.
39. French NP, Hagan R, Evans SF, et al. Repeated antenatal corticosteroids: size at birth and subsequent development. *Am J Obstet Gynecol* 1999;180:114–121.
40. Banks BA, Macones G, Cnaan A, et al. Multiple courses of antenatal corticosteroids are associated with early severe lung disease in preterm neonates. *J Perinatol* 2002;22:101–107.
41. Crowther CA, Doyle LW, Haslam RR, et al. Outcomes at 2 years of age after repeat doses of antenatal corticosteroids. *N Engl J Med* 2007;357:1179–1189.
42. Wapner RJ, Sorokin Y, Mele L, et al. Long-term outcomes after repeat doses of antenatal corticosteroids. *N Engl J Med* 2007;357: 1190–1198.
43. Peltoniemi OM, Kari MA, Tammela O, et al. Randomized trial of a single repeat dose of prenatal betamethasone treatment in imminent preterm birth. *Pediatrics* 2007;119:290–298.
44. Garite TJ, Kurtzman J, Maurel K, Clark R. Impact of a 'rescue course' of antenatal corticosteroids: a multicenter randomized placebo-controlled trial. *Am J Obstet Gynecol* 2009;200:248, e1–e9.
45. Mendelson CR, Johnston JM, MacDonald PC, et al. Multihormonal regulation of surfactant synthesis by human fetal lung in vitro. *J Clin Endocrinol Metab* 1981;53:307–317.
46. Bunton TE, Plopper CG. Triamcinolone-induced structural alterations in the development of the lung of the fetal rhesus macaque. *Am J Obstet Gynecol* 1984;148:203–215.
47. Costeloe K, Hennessy E, Gibson AT, et al. The EPICure study: outcomes to discharge from hospital for infants born at the threshold of viability. *Pediatrics* 2000;106:659–671.
48. Hayes EJ, Paul DA, Stahl GE, et al. Effect of antenatal corticosteroids on survival for neonates born at 23 weeks of gestation. *Obstet Gynecol* 2008;111:921–926.
49. Goldenberg RL, Hauth JC, Andrews WW. Intrauterine infection and preterm delivery. *N Engl J Med* 2000;342:1500–1507.
50. Harding JE, Pang J, Knight DB, et al. Do antenatal corticosteroids help in the setting of preterm rupture of membranes? *Am J Obstet Gynecol* 2001;184:131–139.
51. Goldenberg RL, Andrews WW, Faye-Petersen OM, et al. The Alabama preterm birth study: corticosteroids and neonatal outcomes in 23- to 32-week newborns with various markers of intrauterine infection. *Am J Obstet Gynecol* 2006;195:1020–1024.
52. Kramer BW, Kallapur S, Newnham J, et al. Prenatal inflammation and lung development. *Semin Fetal Neonatal Med* 2009;14:2–7.
53. Kallapur SG, Kramer BW, Moss TJ, et al. Maternal glucocorticoids increase endotoxin-induced lung inflammation in preterm lambs. *Am J Physiol Lung Cell Mol Physiol* 2003;284:L633–L642.
54. Kallapur SG, Jobe AH, Ball MK, et al. Pulmonary and systemic endotoxin tolerance in preterm fetal sheep exposed to chorioamnionitis. *J Immunol* 2007;179:8491–8499.
55. Hashimoto LN, Hornung RW, Lindsell CJ, et al. Effects of antenatal glucocorticoids on outcomes of very low birth weight multifetal gestations. *Am J Obstet Gynecol* 2002;187:804–810.
56. Murphy DJ, Caukwell S, Joels LA, et al. Cohort study of the neonatal outcome of twin pregnancies that were treated with prophylactic or rescue antenatal corticosteroids. *Am J Obstet Gynecol* 2002;187:483–488.
57. Blickstein I, Shinwell ES, Lusky A, et al. Plurality-dependent risk of respiratory distress syndrome among very-low-birth-weight infants and antepartum corticosteroid treatment. *Am J Obstet Gynecol* 2005;192:360–364.
58. Blickstein I, Reichman B, Lusky A, et al. Plurality-dependent risk of severe intraventricular hemorrhage among very low birth weight infants and antepartum corticosteroid treatment. *Am J Obstet Gynecol* 2006;194:1329–1333.
59. Stutchfield P, Whitaker R, Russell I. Antenatal betamethasone and incidence of neonatal respiratory distress after elective caesarean section: pragmatic randomised trial. *BMJ* 2005;331:662.
60. Muglia L, Jacobson L, Dikkes P, et al. Corticotropin-releasing hormone deficiency reveals major fetal but not adult glucocorticoid need. *Nature* 1995;373:427–432.
61. Gross I, Wilson CM. Fetal rat lung maturation: initiation and modulation. *J Appl Physiol* 1983;55:1725–1732.
62. Warburton D, Parton L, Buckley S, et al. Combined effects of corticosteroid, thyroid hormones, and ß-receptor binding in fetal lamb lung. *Pediatr Res* 1988;24:166–170.
63. Ballard RA, Ballard PL, Cnaan A, et al. Antenatal thyrotropin-releasing hormone to prevent lung disease in preterm infants. North American Thyrotropin-Releasing Hormone Study Group. *N Engl J Med* 1998;338:493–498.
64. Crowther CA, Alfirevic Z, Haslam RR. Thyrotropin-releasing hormone added to corticosteroids for women at risk of preterm birth for preventing neonatal respiratory disease. *Cochrane Database Syst Rev* 2004:CD000019.
65. Briet JM, van Sonderen L, Buimer M, et al. Neurodevelopmental outcome of children treated with antenatal thyrotropin-releasing hormone. *Pediatrics* 2002;110:249–253.
66. Crowther CA, Hiller JE, Haslam RR, et al. Australian Collaborative Trial of Antenatal Thyrotropin-Releasing Hormone: adverse effects at 12-month follow-up. ACTOBAT Study Group. *Pediatrics* 1997;99:311–317.

CHAPTER

20

Girija Natarajan
Jose Maria Lopes
J.V. Aranda

Pharmacologic Treatment of Neonatal Apnea

METHYLXANTHINES

Since the initial report in 1973 of a decrease in the frequency of apneic episodes in neonates given theophylline rectally, numerous studies have demonstrated the usefulness of the methylated xanthines in the treatment of neonatal apnea (1). Therefore, caffeine and theophylline have gained universal acceptance in the last few decades as first-line therapy of neonatal apnea.

MECHANISM OF ACTION

Several mechanisms appear to be involved in the decrease in apnea frequency seen after methylxanthine administration. These include the following:

1. Respiratory center stimulation.
2. Improvement in respiratory muscle contraction.
3. Others: altered sleep states, metabolic rate, cardiac output, metabolic homeostasis, and potentiation of catecholamine effect.

Respiratory Center Stimulation

Both caffeine and theophylline produce an increase in minute ventilation, a decrease in partial pressure of arterial CO_2 (P_aCO_2), and an increase in most indices of neural respiratory drive. Davi et al. investigated the effect of theophylline on the control of breathing in newborn infants and found a decreased CO_2 threshold and increased CO_2 sensitivity (2). Gerhardt et al. observed a parallel shift in the slope of the CO_2 response curve after aminophylline administration (3). In both newborn infants and in cats, caffeine has a potent effect on central neural drive (4,5). Caffeine increases mean inspiratory flow (tidal volume/inspiratory time) (V_t/T_i), the pressure generated after airway occlusion ($p < .01$), and minute ventilation. In the cat, when isocapnic conditions were maintained, ventilation was threefold greater, suggesting an interaction between caffeine and CO_2. In the newborn baby, doses as low as 2.5 mg per kg of caffeine increase tidal volume. However, the optimal ventilatory response is observed only with doses of 10 mg per kg (6). The central respirogenic effect of the xanthines is further supported by the observation that they antagonize the depressant effects of narcotics such as codeine, morphine, and meperidine (7–9).

Improved Respiratory Muscle Function

The effect of caffeine and theophylline on muscle contraction has been known for many years (10). However, it was only in the last decade that the effects of these drugs were investigated in relation to respiratory muscle function. Several reports in the literature have described the effects of caffeine and theophylline on diaphragmatic contraction both in vivo and in vitro (11–13). Theophylline improves diaphragmatic efficiency and increases force production with electrical stimulation. The drug not only affected muscle contraction but also decreased the recovery time of fatigued muscles (14). In the newborn, fatigue of the respiratory muscles has been associated with apnea, which is effectively treated by xanthine administration (15–17). Therefore, it is possible that part of the anti-apneic effect of these drugs is due to improvement in respiratory muscle function (15–17).

Other Mechanisms

In addition to the increase in respiratory drive, increased CO_2 sensitivity, and improvement in respiratory muscle contraction, other factors that may facilitate the action of the xanthines include increased neuromuscular transmission, catecholamine release, improved metabolic homeostasis, and changes in sleep states (18–22). The increase in metabolic rate and catecholamine levels after xanthine administration may lead to improved oxygenation and increased cardiac output. Improvement in metabolic homeostasis, such as increased blood glucose, may also lessen the frequency of apneic spells. A decrease in apnea frequency has been described at low doses of theophylline that do not alter ventilation or the CO_2 response curve but may impact the sleep–wake pattern. Increased neuromuscular transmission may lead to improved muscle tone, a well-known in vitro effect of the xanthines. Improved respiratory muscle tone has been related to increased functional residual capacity and better oxygenation in the newborn (23).

Adenosine Receptor Blockade

The methylxanthines appear to exert their effects by (a) blocking adenosine receptors A1 and A2a, (b) inhibition of phosphodiesterase with increased cyclic 3,5 adenosine monophosphate, and (c) translocation of intracellular calcium. Prostaglandin antagonism and upregulation of γ-aminobutyric acid receptor A subunit expression (opposing the effect of hypoxia) have also been described (24,25). Both caffeine and theophylline are able to bind to adenosine receptors; adenosine is now recognized as a neurotransmitter or neuromodulator (21,22,26). Therefore, attention has been directed to the role of this particular neurotransmitter in the control of breathing. Adenosine and its analogues have potent inhibitory effects on respiration. Administration of L-phenylisopropyl adenosine, a stable adenosine analogue, causes respiratory depression in laboratory animals in a dose-dependent manner (27). This effect has been described in several species, including rat, rabbit, cat, and newborn piglet and in both the anesthetized (cat, rabbit, and piglet models) and the awake state (rat model) (28–30). The inhibition of respiration can be partially or completely reversed by the administration of theophylline and caffeine, both of which antagonize adenosine at the receptor level.

The role of intracerebral adenosine levels in the control of ventilatory response to hypoxia was explored in 15 spontaneously breathing piglets, 1 to 5 days old, sedated with chloral hydrate. Animals exposed to 12% oxygen showed a typical biphasic ventilatory response with an initial increase in ventilation followed by a late decrease. Both intravenous caffeine citrate (20 mg per kg) and inhaled CO_2 separately and independently abolished or attenuated the late respiratory depression associated with hypoxia. In the same experiment, administration of dipyridamole, a competitive inhibitor of adenosine receptors, potentiated the ventilatory depression (30). These observations suggest that part of the efficacy of the xanthines in reducing apnea frequency in the neonate may be due to adenosine blockade with consequent central nervous system (CNS) stimulation.

PHARMACOKINETICS AND THERAPEUTIC DRUG MONITORING

Several studies have shown that the plasma clearance and elimination of theophylline and caffeine are both prolonged in newborn babies compared with adults (31–33). The representative kinetic profiles of these two drugs are shown in Table 20.1. The obvious difference between the two drugs is the remarkably slow elimination of caffeine relative to theophylline. The plasma half-life is about 100 hours for caffeine and about 30 hours for theophylline. This difference in drug elimination indicates that caffeine can be given more sparingly (i.e., once daily), and that drug monitoring is probably not as crucial with caffeine as with theophylline. Caffeine half-life may be further prolonged in infants with cholestatic jaundice and breastfed infants (34). The recommended therapeutic plasma concentrations for theophylline and caffeine are about 5 to 15 and 5 to 20 mg per L, respectively. To achieve and maintain these

TABLE 20.1 Pharmacokinetics of Theophylline and Caffeine Used in the Neonatal Period

	Theophylline	*Caffeine*
Plasma half-life (hr)	30	100
Range	12–64	40–230
Mean adult value	6.7	6
Apparent volume of distribution (L/kg)	0.69	0.9
Range	0.2–2.8	0.4–1.3
Mean adult value	0.5	0.6
Clearance (mL/kg/hr)	22	8.9
Range	4.3–68	2.5–17
Adult value	66	94
Dose (mg/kg)		
Loading	5–6 2.5[b]	10[a]
Maintenance	1 q8 hr 0.66 q8 hr+	2.5 q24 hr
Route of administration	i.v., p.o.	i.v., p.o.
Desired plasma level (mg/L)	5–15 3–4[c]	5–20

Note: q8 hr, every 8 hr; q24 hr, every 24 hr; i.v., intravenous; p.o., oral.
[a]Active base.
[b]Low-dose regimen.
[c]Adjusted according to plasma level.

TABLE 20.2 Suggested Guidelines for Respiratory Stimulants in Neonatal Apnea

	Theophylline	*Caffeine*	*Doxapram*
Plasma half-life (hr)	30	100	7
Loading dose (mg/kg)	5–6	10	2.5[a]
Maintenance dose (mg/kg/d)[b]	2–4	2.5	1.0[c]
Therapeutic blood level (mg/L)	5–15	5–20	1.5–3
TD	EMIT/HPLC	EMIT/HPLC	HPLC

EMIT, enzyme-multiplied immunoassay technique; HPLC, high-performance liquid chromatography; TD, technique used.
[a]Intravenous infusion only for 15 min.
[b]Adjusted according to blood level. All doses are in active base.
[c]As intravenous infusion per hour.

plasma concentrations, a loading dose of 4 to 8 mg per kg of theophylline (active base) followed by a maintenance dose of 2 to 4 mg per kg per day in two to four divided doses may be required. There exists substantial interindividual variability in the pharmacokinetic properties of theophylline; thus, it is necessary to monitor plasma concentrations and adjust the dose accordingly (saliva has been proposed as an alternative site for therapeutic drug monitoring in the preterm, with good correlation with blood levels) (35,36). Similarly, caffeine is recommended as a loading dose of 10 to 20 mg per kg of active base or 20 to 40 mg per kg of caffeine citrate salt, intravenously or orally. A maintenance dose of 2.5 to 4 mg per kg per day (or 5 to 8 mg per kg per day of caffeine citrate) is usually needed to maintain plasma concentrations of 5 to 20 mg per L of caffeine (Table 20.2). About 25% of theophylline is methylated to caffeine (37,38), with plasma theophylline-to-caffeine ratios sometimes reaching 0.30 to 0.40 at steady state. A small (3% to 8%) proportion of caffeine is converted to theophylline via CYP1A2. Thus, the overall methylxanthine effect has to account for the sum of the two drugs because both agents are pharmacologically active.

The methylxanthines are powerful CNS stimulants and may interact with anticonvulsants such as phenobarbital at a kinetic or a pharmacodynamic level. Babies given theophylline and phenobarbital have been shown to require higher doses of theophylline to control apnea and higher doses of phenobarbital to control seizures (39). The methylxanthines also have the potential to interact with drugs that are substrates for CYP1A2 such as cimetidine and ketoconazole.

CHOICE OF METHYLXANTHINES

Caffeine and theophylline exert similar pharmacodynamic effects but may vary in their potency concerning a specific organ receptor. Moreover, the differences in their kinetic properties alter the dosing schedules and the need for therapeutic drug monitoring. Table 20.3 lists some of the differences between the two drugs. Controlled comparative trials between theophylline and caffeine indicate that although both drugs are effective in the management of apnea, more adverse effects such as tachycardia are observed with theophylline (40–42). Because caffeine has a more prolonged plasma half-life, the dosing schedule is less frequent and the need for therapeutic monitoring less crucial. Although frequent monitoring is advisable for theophylline, plasma caffeine measurement only if there is lack of clinical response or suspected toxicity is generally acceptable during the neonatal period (43,44). In cases of overdosing with caffeine, the prolonged drug elimination may result in sustained high plasma concentrations of caffeine for a prolonged period. However, observations suggest that caffeine plasma concentrations of up to 50 mg per L may occur with no adverse effects, whereas plasma concentrations of theophylline greater than 15 mg per L may be associated with tachycardia. Some investigators even suggest much higher doses of caffeine to achieve a therapeutic effect. This suggests that caffeine might have a wider therapeutic index relative to theophylline. In practice, caffeine has emerged as the preferred alternative in infants with apnea of prematurity.

In 1998, Steer and Henderson-Smart reviewed three trials comparing theophylline and caffeine in reducing

TABLE 20.3 Theophylline and Caffeine in Neonatal Apnea

Variable	*Theophylline*	*Caffeine*
Efficacy	+++	+++
Peripheral side effects	+++	+/−
Drug clearance	Slow ($t_{1/2}$ = 30 hr)	Very slow ($t_{1/2}$ = 30 hr)
Plasma level at steady state	Fluctuating	Stable
Need for drug monitoring	+++	−
Dosing interval	1–3×/d	Once/day
Drug monitoring	HPLC/EMIT	HPLC/EMIT
Commercial preparation	+++	+

EMIT, enzyme-multiplied immunoassay technique; HPLC, high-performance liquid chromatography.

recurrent apnea and the need for mechanical ventilation (45). There was no difference in the failure rate (<50% reduction in apnea/bradycardia) of treatment with caffeine or theophylline at 1 to 3 days (two studies) or 5 to 7 days (three studies). There was a higher rate of apnea in the standard caffeine group at 1 to 3 days [three studies, mean difference 0.398 (0.334 to 0.72)/100 minutes] but not at 5 to 7 days (two studies). Side effects, as indicated by tachycardia or feed intolerance leading to changed dosing, were lower with caffeine, relative risk (RR) = 0.17 (0.04 to 0.43). One additional study, which has been reported only in abstract form, found that mean rates of apnea (15 seconds or more) and episodes of oxygen desaturation (<85%) were no different in the 13 infants treated with theophylline than in the 11 infants treated with caffeine. However, mean rates of bradycardia were lower with theophylline at 1, 3, and 7 days after the initiation of therapy (46–48). In aggregate, the data favor the use of caffeine for neonatal apnea.

CLINICAL EFFECTS

EFFICACY OF METHYLXANTHINES IN NEONATAL APNEA AND WEANING FROM MECHANICAL VENTILATION

The capability of caffeine to stimulate respiration has been known for a century, and the ability of aminophylline to regulate breathing in adult patients with Cheyne–Stokes respiration was noted by Vogl in 1927. Kuzemko and Paala first described the use of aminophylline in neonates (49). Since then, several clinical trials have confirmed the efficacy of the xanthines in decreasing the number of apneas, cyanotic spells, and episodes of bradycardia (4,50–59) (Table 20.4). Shannon et al. described a reduced incidence of severe apnea, lasting more than 30 seconds, and bradycardia associated with theophylline serum concentrations between 6 and 11 μg per mL (50). Peabody et al. observed less apnea and bradycardia associated with regulating the breathing pattern and less fluctuation in transcutaneous partial pressure of oxygen (PO_2) in infants treated with aminophylline (53). Roberts et al. described a significant reduction in all types of apnea, suggesting that theophylline may act to improve the coordination between upper airway and respiratory muscles (56). This also has been observed in premature infants where diaphragmatic electromyelography (EMG) and laryngeal muscle EMG were recorded simultaneously (60). Similarly, caffeine, which has potent CNS stimulant properties with fewer peripheral effects than theophylline, has also been shown to be effective in neonatal apnea. Caffeine stimulates respiration and decreases episodes of apnea, produces regular breathing patterns, and increases alveolar ventilation (see Table 20.1). Henderson-Smart and Steer reviewed recent randomized controlled trials to evaluate the efficacy of methylxanthines for the treatment of apnea (61).

TABLE 20.4 Clinical Studies and Drug Regimens of Methylxanthines in Neonatal Apnea

			Frequency of Apnea		
Reference (year)	*Drug Preparation*	*Dose and Route*	*Before*	*After*	*Success Rate*
49 (1973)	Aminophylline suppositories	5 mg q6 hr × 3 doses, then q6 hr p.r.n.	63	6	24/24
50 (1975)	Theophylline alcohol elixir (10%)	4 mg/kg q6 hr orally	5.9/13 hr	0/13 hr	17/17
52 (1975)	Theophylline alcohol solution (20%)	4 mg/kg q6 hr orally	10.6/d	0.9/d	15/15
105 (1976)	Aminophylline suppositories	5 mg q6 hr (1.7–4 mg/kg/d) rectally	1.7/hr	0.39/hr	10/13
4 (1977)	Caffeine citrate	I.D.: 20 mg/kg i.v. or orally M.D.: 5–140 mg/kg every day or twice daily	13.6/d	2.1/d	17/18
53 (1978)	Aminophylline	I.D.: 8 mg/kg q12 hr; M.D.: 4 mg/kg q12 hr rectally	115/12 hr	26/12 hr	4/4
2 (1978)	Theophylline	3 mg/kg q6 hr i.v. or orally	55/hr+	11/hr+	8/10
16 (1980)	Theophylline	2 mg/kg/d by nasogastric tube	16.1/hr	5.2/hr	6/7
55 (1981)	Caffeine citrate	20 mg/kg loading i.m., then 5 mg/kg q24 hr p.o.	1.17/hr day 1	0.11/hr day 5	9/9
56 (1982)	Theophylline	6 mg/kg/d orally	80	46	5/20
57 (1985)	Theophylline	6.8 mg/kg i.v. loading, then 1.4 mg/kg q8 hr	11/24 hr	1/24 hr day 5	19/22
58 (1990)	Theophylline	8.0 mg/kg i.v. continuous infusion of 0.5 mg/kg/hr	0.72/hr	0.34/hr	8/10
59 (2000)	Caffeine citrate	10 mg/kg loading, 2.5 mg/kg q24 hr			

I.D., initial dose; i.m., intramuscular; i.v., intravenous; M.D., maintenance dose; p.o., oral; p.r.n., as the situation demands; q6 hr, every 6 hr; q8 hr, every 8 hr; q12 hr, every 12 hr; q24 hr, every 24 hr.

In five studies (three with theophylline and two with caffeine) including a total of 192 infants, they found that compared with control (placebo or no drug), methylxanthine administration to infants with recurrent apnea of prematurity was followed by less treatment failure, RR = 0.43 (0.31 to 0.60), and less use of mechanical ventilation, RR = 0.34 (0.12 to 0.97), in the 2 to 7 days after starting treatment. Both caffeine and theophylline had similar effects in decreasing the number of apneic spells and reducing the need for mechanical ventilation.

Despite optimal plasma concentrations of theophylline, however, significant apnea reduction has been reported in only about 75% of neonates (62). When used as prophylaxis to prevent apnea in preterm infants, two placebo-controlled studies involving 104 infants found no differences between the groups in the proportion of infants with apnea, bradycardia, hypoxemic episodes, or the use of positive pressure ventilation (63,64). The sample sizes in the studies were small, however, and caffeine was used for a total duration of 96 hours in one.

Caffeine and theophylline are also effective respiratory stimulants during weaning from mechanical ventilation. Several clinical trials have suggested that the success rate of extubation is improved if theophylline/caffeine is administered prior to extubation (65–68). The effect is presumed to be related to improvement in respiratory muscle function and decreased pulmonary resistance. Reviews updating information on the prophylactic administration of methylxanthines for extubation of preterm infants reported data from six trials with a total of 187 infants (four trials with theophylline and two with caffeine) (69). The primary outcome was failure of extubation within 1 week of commencing treatment—unable to wean from intermittent positive pressure ventilation (IPPV) and extubate, or reintubation for IPPV, or use of continuous positive airway pressure. Other measured outcomes were side effects and chronic lung disease. Three trials found significant reductions in failure of extubation within 1 week of treatment. One study found that treatment was effective in reducing failed extubation in those infants born with weight less than 1,000 g and who were younger than 1 week. Overall analysis of the six trials showed that methylxanthines treatment resulted in a reduction of failed extubation, RR = 0.47 (0.32 to 0.70). There was an absolute reduction of 27% in the incidence of failed extubation, risk reduction = 0.27 (−0.39, −0.15). The reviews pointed out that the number of infants in each study was small, and only a large difference in outcomes could reliably be detected. More recently, a randomized, double-blind clinical trial of three dosing regimens of caffeine citrate (3, 15, and 30 mg per kg) for periextubation management of 127 ventilated preterm infants younger than 32 weeks of gestation showed no statistically significant difference in the incidence of extubation failure between the dosing groups (70). The infants in the two higher dosing groups did have statistically significant less documented apnea in the immediate peri-extubation period. A larger trial involving 234 neonates younger than 30 weeks of gestation reported a significant reduction in failure to extubate in infants receiving 20 mg per kg per day caffeine citrate compared with 5 mg per kg per day (15% vs. 29.8%, RR = 0.51; 95% CI: 0.31 to 0.85) (71). A significant difference in the duration of mechanical ventilation was observed in infants younger than 28 weeks of gestation who received the higher dose. No differences were noted in short-term adverse effects or at 12-month follow-up.

EFFECT ON LUNG FUNCTION

In an immature baboon model treated with surfactant, early caffeine treatment was associated with better lung function, higher compliance, and significant decreases in ventilator support (72). In a rat pup model that received neonatal caffeine, there was a 22% higher minute ventilation response to hypercapnia in males in the juvenile stage, which persisted until adulthood (73). This reported long-term effect on respiratory control was speculated to be due to a persistent change in adenosinergic neurotransmission. Small studies in infants with bronchopulmonary dysplasia (BPD) have shown a decrease in airway resistance and improved lung mechanics within 1 hour of caffeine therapy (74). An improvement in respiratory system compliance after caffeine has also been reported in preterm infants with resolving respiratory distress syndrome (75). In the multicenter, randomized, controlled Caffeine for Apnea of Prematurity (CAP) trial, the rates of BPD defined as an oxygen need at 36 weeks postconceptional age were 36.3% in the caffeine group compared with 46.9% in the placebo group, a statistically significant difference (76).

EFFECT ON PATENT DUCTUS ARTERIOSUS

There were initial concerns regarding the relaxant effect of the methylxanthines on the ductus arteriosus, presumably because of increased 3′,5′-cyclic AMP caused by phosphodiesterase blockade. The concentration of xanthine required to produce relaxation in vitro (540 to 1,620 mg per L) is far higher than the plasma concentrations achieved in the newborn infant (about 10 mg per L). Caffeine has been shown to be a prostaglandin antagonist at concentrations achieved in plasma (24). In a preterm sheep model of ductus arteriosus, caffeine (0.003 to 0.3 mM) showed no direct effect on ductus arteriosus tension nor the contractile response to increasing oxygen concentrations (77). The CAP trial involving infants weighing less than 1,250 g at birth showed a statistically significant decrease in the incidence of patent ductus arteriosus (30% vs. 40%) and in the rates of surgical ligation (4.5% vs. 12.6%) in the group treated with caffeine citrate (76).

EFFECT ON CARDIAC FUNCTION

Augmentations of cardiac inotropy and chronotropy are reported effects of methylxanthines, although data from systematic human observations are scarce. In an observational study involving 31 premature infants, cardiac index increased by a mean of 14.6% ± 16.3% (SD), stroke volume increased in 24 of 31 trials by 7.8% ± 12.2%, heart rate increased in 28 of 31 trials by 7.7 ± 7.2 beats per minute, and blood pressure increased in 25 of 31 trials by 4.1 ± 5.8 mmHg (all $p < .001$) following an intravenous dose of caffeine

(78). Previously, Hoecker et al. reported no change in left ventricular cardiac output (LVCO), heart rate, or blood pressure following caffeine loading (79,80). Walther et al. demonstrated an increase in LVCO and heart rate in 11 infants treated with aminophylline and an increase in stroke volume by 15% in the first 3 days of treatment, which returned to baseline by the seventh day of treatment (81). An increase in LVCO, stroke volume, and heart rate was also shown in a study of theophylline effect on 15 infants by Fesslova et al. (82).

OTHER PHARMACOLOGIC EFFECTS

Besides effects on respirogenesis, lung and cardiac function, caffeine and theophylline exhibit a variety of pharmacologic actions, including CNS stimulation, smooth muscle relaxation, systemic blood vessel dilation, cerebral vessel vasoconstriction, diuresis, and augmentation of metabolic rate, among others (18,19,83,84) (see Table 20.5). Bronchodilatation has been demonstrated in premature infants with BPD after the administration of both caffeine and theophylline (74). Diuresis caused by increased renal blood flow and increased glomerular filtration rate has not been shown to be significant in premature neonates treated with theophylline (83). Neonates given theophylline and control infants not given theophylline were similar with respect to urine volume, serum osmolality and electrolytes, and urinary electrolyte excretion. Caffeine is a much weaker diuretic and appears to have no effect on serum sodium, potassium, calcium, and phosphorus levels, while urinary calcium excretion increases and serum creatinine decreases significantly in premature neonates (85).

Caffeine can shorten the blood coagulation time resulting from increased clotting factors such as factor V, prothrombin, and fibrinogen. A relatively important effect of the methylxanthines pertains to metabolic homeostasis. In experimental animals, adult volunteers and patients, and pancreatic islet cell cultures, caffeine can stimulate insulin and glucagon release and increase catecholamine release, blood glucose, cortisol secretion, and plasma free fatty acid levels. The increased plasma free fatty acid could potentially compete with bilirubin at albumin-binding sites. Studies suggest that there is a transient hyperglycemia following intravenous infusion of caffeine in the premature infant, with a delayed increase or no change in plasma insulin levels.

Caffeine and theophylline constrict cerebral vessels, increase cerebrovascular resistance, and decrease cerebral blood flow in adults (86,87). Systematic studies in newborn humans and experimental animals (i.e., newborn piglets) to determine the effect of caffeine and theophylline on cerebral blood flow suggest that cerebral blood flow alteration is not a prime concern (18,88,89). In contrast, a significant decrease in blood flow velocities in the internal carotid and anterior cerebral arteries has been reported in 16 preterm infants following a 25 mg per kg dose of oral caffeine (80). No increase in the incidence of cicatricial retrolental fibroplasia was observed in babies treated with caffeine compared with controls.

Caffeine causes a slight increase in basal metabolic rate, which can be observed in the adult habitual coffee drinker. The ingestion of 0.5 g of caffeine may increase the basal metabolic rate to an average of 10% and occasionally to 25%. In the neonate, a mean increase in oxygen consumption of 25% has been observed following the administration of theophylline. Similarly, an increase in oxygen consumption and energy expenditure has been reported after 48 hours of caffeine therapy, which persisted through 4 weeks (84). The CAP trial found that the caffeine-treated group of infants had a reduced weight gain, with the greatest difference noted after 2 weeks (mean difference: −23 g) (76). This effect could be of potential significance, especially in the tiny premature infant with limited calorie intake.

A reduction in mesenteric blood flow velocities in response to a loading dose of caffeine has been reported (80,90). A small trial involving 85 infants had suggested an association between the use of methylxanthines and necrotizing enterocolitis (NEC) (59). In the larger CAP trial, there was no significant difference in the incidence of NEC in the caffeine-treated and placebo groups. Besides, apnea with hypoxemic episodes can, by itself, be a risk factor for the development of NEC (2,91).

TABLE 20.5 Major Pharmacologic Effects of Methylxanthines

Central nervous system: stimulation of all levels
Heart: augmentation of inotropy and chronotropy
Vascular system: pulmonary, dilation, systemic, dilation; cerebral, constriction (in adults)
Smooth muscles: relaxation
Skeletal muscles: stimulation
Kidney: increased renal blood flow and diuresis
Gastrointestinal system: stimulation of gastric acid and fluid secretion
Endocrine system: multiple effects
Hematologic: mild increased clotting and shortened coagulation time
Basal metabolic rate: augmentation

LONG-TERM EFFECTS OF METHYLXANTHINES

The methylated xanthines are some of the most psychoactive agents in the human diet and exert significant CNS excitation and other neuronal effects at a very critical time in human development. Caffeine has been demonstrated to induce neuronal death in neonatal rat brain and cortical cell cultures and theophylline to decrease the rate of anoxic survival in vivo (92,93). In rat pups treated with daily caffeine, transient impairment in motor skills and changes in locomotor activity were observed, depending on the developmental stage (94). In a newborn mouse model, caffeine did not worsen excitotoxic periventricular white matter lesions (95). In human infants, data suggest that there is no independent adverse effect of caffeine on long-term outcome. Gunn et al. followed a group of 21 very low-birth-weight premature neonates treated with caffeine and compared them to a similar group ($n = 21$) not treated with caffeine (96). No differences in growth and development were noted at 12-month follow-up.

Similarly, Ment et al. showed no differences in neurodevelopmental outcome and in Bayley scores at 18 months in 73 infants weighing less than 1,250 g at birth with respect to presence or absence of intraventricular hemorrhage and with or without treatment with methylxanthines (51). In fact, infants who received methylxanthine therapy scored better at 18 months, regardless of hemorrhage status. In the CAP trial, which is the largest follow-up study so far, of the 937 infants in the caffeine group, 377 (40.2%) died or survived with a neurodevelopmental disability, as compared with 431 of the 932 infants (46.2%) in the placebo group [odds ratio adjusted for center, 0.77; 95% confidence interval (CI), 0.64 to 0.93; p = .008]. Treatment with caffeine as compared with placebo reduced the incidence of cerebral palsy (4.4% vs. 7.3%; adjusted odds ratio, 0.58; 95% CI, 0.39 to 0.87; p = .009) and of cognitive delay (33.8% vs. 38.3%; adjusted odds ratio, 0.81; 95% CI, 0.66 to 0.99; p = .04). The rates of death, deafness, and blindness and the mean percentiles for height, weight, and head circumference at follow-up did not differ significantly between the two groups (97). In further analyses, the investigators reported that the size and direction of the caffeine effect on death or disability differed depending on positive pressure ventilation (PPV) at randomization (p = .03) (98). Odds ratios (95% CI) were as follows: no support, 1.32 (0.81 to 2.14); noninvasive support, 0.73 (0.52 to 1.03); and endotracheal intubation (ETT), 0.73 (0.57 to 0.94). Adjustment for baseline factors strengthened this effect (p = .02). There is a substantial placental transfer of caffeine, and significant numbers of neonates are born with therapeutic concentrations of caffeine in their cord blood. Any follow-up studies must account for antenatal and postnatal exposure to the methylated xanthines because these are pervasive components of dietary, including beverage, intake.

DOXAPRAM

Doxapram, an analeptic and respiratory stimulant in adults used clinically since 1962, has been given to neonates with apnea and those resistant to methylated xanthines. Gupta and Moore used doxapram to produce respiratory stimulation in 83 full-term infants born to mothers who received narcotic analgesics or general anesthesia causing respiratory depression (99). The doses varied from 0.5 to 3 mg per kg (as a single dose) immediately after birth. A randomized trial by Peliowski and Finer in 1990 including 11 infants given intravenous doxapram and 10 infants given placebo showed less treatment failures with doxapram compared with placebo (4/11 vs. 8/10) (58). These studies were reviewed by Henderson-Smart and Steer (2004) who suggested that intravenous doxapram might reduce apnea within the first 48 hours of treatment, but there are insufficient data to evaluate the precision of this result or to assess potential adverse effects (100). Moreover, no long-term outcomes have been measured. The same reviewers (Henderson-Smart and Steer, 2000) also analyzed data comparing doxapram and methylxanthine and concluded that intravenous doxapram and intravenous methylxanthine appear to be similar in their short-term effects for treating apnea in preterm infants (101). However, these trials performed are too small to exclude an important difference between the two treatments or to exclude the possibility of less common adverse effects. Longer-term outcome of infants treated in these trials has not been reported. In addition to apnea of prematurity, doxapram has also been used in central hypoventilation, weaning from mechanical ventilation, and in obstructive apnea.

Because of the known safety and efficacy of the methylated xanthines and because of the uncertainty related to the side effects of doxapram, this drug is used only in cases where methylxanthines are not effective and only before considering a more aggressive form of treatment such as mechanical ventilation.

DOSAGE

The dosage regimen of 2.5 mg per kg per hour was basically derived from adult data. A dose–response relationship has been suggested. Barrington et al. showed that incremental doses of continuous intravenous infusion were associated with increased response (102). In 18 premature infants given doxapram, 47% responded at 0.5 mg per kg per hour and up to 89% responded at 2.5 mg per kg per hour. Hayakawa et al. (1986), in a study of 12 premature infants, reported a good correlation between dose and serum concentration and a success rate of 75% with infusion of 1.0 to 1.5 mg per kg per hour (103). The ideal dosage and route of administration remain to be defined, a regimen of a loading dose of 2.5 to 3 mg per kg administered over 15 to 30 minutes followed by a continuous infusion of 1 mg per kg per hour with careful surveillance of blood pressure changes has been used. This maintenance dosage may be increased if necessary by 0.5 mg per kg per hour up to a maximum of 2.5 mg per kg per hour. Some pharmaceutical preparations may contain benzyl alcohol or chlorobutanol, and appropriate caution should be exercised to monitor possible adverse effects of these preservatives.

MODE OF ADMINISTRATION

Doxapram is poorly absorbed enterally and has a short duration of action, despite a relatively apparent long half-life. An intermittent intravenous bolus regimen has been proposed, although continuous intravenous infusion is often used.

THERAPEUTIC PLASMA LEVEL

The ideal plasma therapeutic concentrations need to be defined, but data suggest a possible therapeutic window. Those babies who responded to doxapram all had a serum level of at least 1.5 mg per L; the mean serum concentration related to this response was 2.9 mg per L, with the therapeutic threshold proposed being greater than 2 mg per L. Adverse drug effects become more frequent at plasma levels above 5 mg per L.

METABOLITES

Doxapram is metabolized by the human liver to give at least three metabolites. The oxidation pathway that yields metabolites AHR-5955 (ketodoxapram) and AHR-5904 seems more active than the deethylation pathway producing AHR-0914. Ketodoxapram is also a strong respiratory stimulant, without the side effects reported with doxapram (i.e., increase in blood pressure and excitability). Pharmacokinetic studies in newborn infants indicate prolonged elimination in infants compared with adults (104). The plasma half-life ranges from 6.6 to 8.2 hours, plasma clearance = 0.44 to 0.7 L per kg per hour, and apparent value of distribution = 4.0 to 7.3 L per kg. The pharmacokinetic profile suggests a first-order kinetics in premature infants, with substantial interpatient variability and a decreasing plasma half-life with advancing age. Little doxapram is excreted in the urine, and ketodoxapram is usually detected in every patient receiving doxapram.

SIDE EFFECTS

Adverse reactions to doxapram that have been reported include the following:

- Adverse drug reaction (ADR) definitely related to doxapram: increase in blood pressure, mainly at infusion greater than 1.5 mg per kg per hour, or at a level greater than 5 mg per L.
- ADR probably or possibly related to doxapram: regurgitation, excessive salivation increased agitation, excessive crying, disturbed sleep, jitteriness, increase in gastric residuals, vomiting, and irritability and cardiac conduction blocks; blood in stool, abdominal distension, hyperglycemia, glycosuria, premature teeth buds (lower central incisors).

MECHANISMS OF ACTION

The exact mechanism of action of doxapram is probably via stimulation of the peripheral chemoreceptors, mainly at low doses (<0.5 mg per kg), and the central respiratory and nonrespiratory neurons, mainly at a higher dose. Doxapram also increases respiratory center output. In human infants, doxapram causes a significant fall in PCO_2 and an increase in minute ventilation, tidal volume, and occlusion pressure but no change in respiratory rate, inspiratory, or expiratory time.

CONCLUSION

Available data suggest that doxapram is an effective drug to treat apnea in the premature infant and can be used as a second-line drug in cases of failure with methylxanthine and prior to a much more aggressive form of therapy such as endotracheal intubation and mechanical ventilation. Complications from the latter therapy are significant, particularly in the very small premature infant. Doxapram is used off label and caution should be exercised when using in newborn infants.

GENERAL CONSIDERATIONS FOR APNEA MANAGEMENT

Although drug therapy is a major component of neonatal apnea management, the multicausal (including metabolic, infectious, neurologic, and other pathophysiologic states) nature of neonatal and infantile apnea should be recognized. Treatment should be directed at those physiologic and biochemical perturbations illustrated in Figure 20.1. In this figure, apnea appears as a common pathway by which various noxious or other stimuli exert their effect on an immature respiratory control system not yet ready for the complex integration of various neural inputs. Whatever the mechanism involved in the pathogenesis of neonatal and infantile apnea, correctable factors associated

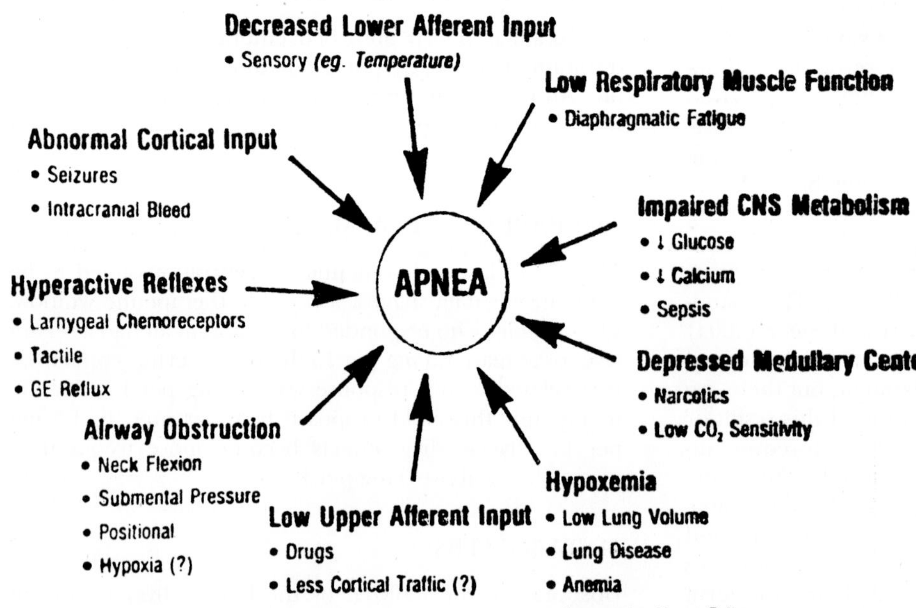

Figure 20.1. Factors associated with the genesis of neonatal apnea. Therapy should be directed toward correction of etiologic factors. GE, gastroenteric.

with the occurrence of apnea should be treated. As the survival of the very low-birth-weight infants at greatest risk for apnea increases with medical advances, the challenge for safe and effective treatment of apnea remains a primary investigative and clinical concern.

REFERENCES

1. Kuzemko JA, Broadhead R, Shaw R. Management of apnoeic attacks in the preterm baby. Presented to the European Perinatal Society; Prague, Czech Republic, August 1974.
2. Davi MJ, Sankaran K, Simons KJ, et al. Physiologic changes induced by theophylline in the treatment of apnea in preterm infants. *J Pediatr* 1978;92:91–95.
3. Gerhardt T, McCarthy J, Bancalari E. Effect of aminophylline on respiratory center activity and metabolic rate in premature infants with idiopathic apnea. *Pediatrics* 1979;63:537–542.
4. Aranda JV, Gorman W, Bergsteinsson H, et al. Efficacy of caffeine in treatment of apnea in the low-birth-weight infant. *J Pediatr* 1977;90:467–472.
5. Mazzarelli M, Jaspan N, Zin WA, et al. Dose effect of caffeine on control of breathing and respiratory response to CO_2 in cats. *J Appl Physiol* 1986;60:52–59.
6. Aranda JV, Forman W, Cook C, et al. Pharmacokinetic profile of caffeine in the premature newborn infant with apnea. *J Pediatr* 1977;50:467–472.
7. Bellville JW, Escarrage LA, Wallenstein SL, et al. Antagonism by caffeine of the respiratory effects of codeine and morphine. *J Pharmacol Exp Ther* 1962;136:8727.
8. Lambertson CJ. Drugs and respiration. *Annu Rev Pharmacol* 1966;6:327–345.
9. Stroud MW III, Lambertson CJ, Ewing JH, et al. The effects of aminophylline and meperidine alone and in combination on the respiratory response to CO_2 inhalation. *J Pharmacol Exp Ther* 1955;114:461–465.
10. Huidobro F, Amenbar L. Effectiveness of caffeine (1,3,7 trimethylxanthines) against fatigue. *J Pharmacol Exp Ther* 1945; 84:82–87.
11. Aubier M, Detroyer A, MacKelem PT, et al. Aminophylline improves diaphragmatic contractility. *N Engl J Med* 1981;305: 249–252.
12. Aubier M, Murciano D, Lecocgnic Y, et al. Diaphragmatic contractility enhanced by aminophylline: role of extracellular calcium. *J Appl Physiol* 1983;54:460–464.
13. Lopes JM, LeSoeuf PN, Heather MH, et al. The effects of theophylline on diaphragmatic fatigue in the newborn [Abstract]. *Pediatr Res* 1982;16:355A.
14. Nassan-Gentina, Parsonneau V, Rappaport S. Fatigue and metabolism of frog muscle fibers during stimulation and in response to caffeine. *Am J Physiol* 1981;241:C160–C166.
15. Heyman E, Ohlsson A, Heyman Z, et al. The effect of aminophylline on the excursions of the diaphragm in preterm neonates. A randomized double-blind controlled study. *Acta Paediatr Scand* 1991;80:308–315.
16. Meyers RF, Milnap RL, Krauss AN, et al. Low dose theophylline therapy in idiopathic apnea of prematurity. *J Pediatr* 1980;5: 99–104.
17. Davis GM, Bureau MA. Pulmonary and chest wall mechanics in the control of respiration in the newborn. *Clin Perinatol* 1987;14:552–579.
18. Dani C, Bertini G, Reali MF, et al. Brain hemodynamic changes in preterm infants after maintenance dose caffeine and aminophylline treatment. *Biol Neonate* 2000;78:27–32.
19. Ritchie JM. Central nervous stimulants. 11. The xanthines. In: Goodman LS, Gilman A, eds. *The pharmacological basis of therapeutics*, 5th ed. London, England: Cassell & Collier Macmillan, 1975:367–378.
20. Curzi-Dascalova L, Aujard Y, Gaultier C, et al. Sleep organization is unaffected by caffeine in premature infants. *J Pediatr* 2002; 140:766–771.
21. Fredholm BB. On the mechanism of action of theophylline and caffeine. *Acta Med Scand* 1985;217:149–153.
22. Aldridge FL, Millhorm DE, Waltrop TG, et al. Mechanisms of respiratory effects of methylxanthines. *Respir Physiol* 1979;53: 239–261.
23. Lopes J, Muller N, Bryan AC, et al. Importance of inspiratory muscle tone in maintenance of FRC in the newborn. *J Appl Physiol* 1981;51:830–834.
24. Manku MS, Horrobin DF. Chloroquine, quinine, procaine, quinidine, tricyclic antidepressants and methylxanthines as prostaglandin agonists and antagonists. *Lancet* 1976;2:1115–1117.
25. Clifford E, Miller M, Chakravarti S, et al. Caffeine and hypoxia have opposing effects on GABA A receptor subunit expression in the neonatal rat brainstem. *Pediatr Res* 2005;403:5466A.
26. Phillis JW, Wu PH. The role of adenosine and its nucleotides in central synaptic transmission. *Prog Neurol* 1981;16:287–289.
27. Runold M, Lagercrantz H, Fredholm BB. Ventilatory effect of an adenosine analogue in unanesthetized rabbits during development. *J Appl Physiol* 1986;61:255–259.
28. Winn HR, Rubio R, Berne RM. Brain adenosine concentration during hypoxia in rats. *Am J Physiol* 1981;241:H235–H242.
29. Darnall RA. Aminophylline reduces hypoxic ventilatory depression: possible role of adenosine. *Pediatr Res* 1985;19:206–210.
30. Lopes JM, Davis GM, Mullahoo K, et al. Role of adenosine in the hypoxic ventilatory depression of the newborn piglet. *Pediatr Pulmonol* 1994;17:50–55.
31. Aranda JV, Grondin D, Sasyniuk B. Pharmacologic considerations in the therapy of neonatal apnea. *Pediatr Clin North Am* 1981;28:113–133.
32. Aranda JV. Maturational changes in theophylline and caffeine metabolism and disposition: clinical implications. In: *Proceedings of 2nd World Congress, Clinical Pharmacology and Therapeutics.* Rockville, MD: American Society for Pharmacology and Experimental Therapeutics, 1984:868–877.
33. De Carolis MP, Romagnoli C, Muzii U, et al. Pharmacokinetic aspects of caffeine in premature infants. *Dev Pharmacol Ther* 1991;16:117–122.
34. Le Guennec JC, Billon B, Pare C. Maturational changes of caffeine concentrations and disposition in infancy during maintenance therapy for apnea of prematurity: influence of gestational age, hepatic disease and breast feeding. *Pediatrics* 1985;76: 834–840.
35. Lee TC, Charles BG, Steer PA, et al. Saliva as a valid alternative to serum in monitoring intravenous caffeine treatment for apnea of prematurity. *Ther Drug Monit* 1996;18:288–293.
36. de Wildt SN, Kerkvliet KT, Wezenberg MG, et al. Use of saliva in therapeutic drug monitoring of caffeine in preterm infants. *Ther Drug Monit* 2001;23:250–254.
37. Bory C, Baltassat P, Porthault M, et al. Metabolism of theophylline to caffeine in premature infants. *J Pediatr* 1979;94: 988–993.
38. Aranda JV, Louridas AT, Vitullo B, et al. Metabolism of theophylline to caffeine in human fetal liver. *Science* 1979;206: 1319–1321.
39. Yazdani M, Kissling GE, Tran TH, et al. Phenobarbital increases theophylline requirement of premature infants being treated for apnea. *Am J Dis Child* 1987;141:97–99.
40. Brouard C, Moriette G, Murat I, et al. Comparative efficacy of theophylline and caffeine in the treatment of idiopathic apnea in premature infants. *Am J Dis Child* 1985;139:698–700.
41. Bairam A, Boutroy MJ, Badonnel Y, et al. Theophylline versus caffeine: comparative effects in treatment of idiopathic apnea in the preterm infants. *J Pediatr* 1987;110:636–639.
42. Scanlon JE, Chin KC, Morgan ME, et al. Caffeine or theophylline for neonatal apnoea? *Arch Dis Child* 1992;67(4 spec no.): 425–428.
43. Natarajan G, Botica ML, Thomas R, et al. Therapeutic drug monitoring of caffeine in preterm neonates: an unnecessary exercise? *Pediatrics* 2007;119(5):936–940.
44. Pesce AJ, Rakhkin M, Kotagal U. Standards of laboratory practice: theophylline and caffeine monitoring. *Clin Chem* 1998;44: 1124–1128.
45. Steer PA, Henderson-Smart DJ. Caffeine versus theophylline for apnea in preterm infants. *Cochrane Database Syst Rev* 2000;(2): CD000273.
46. Kumar SP, Metha PN, Bradley BS, et al. Documented monitoring show theophylline to be more effective than caffeine in prematurity apnea. *Pediatr Res* 1992;31:208A.
47. Bairam A, Boutroy MJ, Badonnel Y, et al. The choice between theophylline and caffeine in the treatment of apnea in premature infants [in French]. *Arch Fr Pediatr* 1990;47:461–465.

48. Larsen PB, Brendstrup L, Skov L, et al. Aminophylline versus caffeine citrate for apnea and bradycardia prophylaxis in premature neonates. *Acta Paediatr* 1995;84:360–364.
49. Kuzemko JA, Paala J. Apnoeic attacks in the newborn treated with aminophylline. *Arch Dis Child* 1973;48(5):404–406.
50. Shannon DC, Gotay F, Stein M, et al. Prevention of apnea and bradycardia in low-birth-weight infants. *Pediatrics* 1975;55:589.
51. Ment LR, Scott DT, Ehrenkranz RA, et al. Early childhood developmental follow-up of infants with GMH/IVH: effect of methylxanthine therapy. *Am J Perinatol* 1985;2:223–227.
52. Uauy R, Shapiro DL, Smith B, et al. Treatment of severe apnea in prematures with orally administered theophylline. *Pediatrics* 1975;55:595–598.
53. Peabody J, Neese AL, Phillip AG, et al. Transcutaneous oxygen monitoring in aminophylline-treated apnoeic infants. *Pediatrics* 1978;62:698.
54. Fang S, Sherwood RA, Gamsu HR, et al. Comparison of the effects of theophylline and caffeine on serum erythropoietin concentration in premature infants. *Eur J Pediatr* 1998;157:406–409.
55. Murat I, Moriwette G, Blin MC, et al. The efficacy of caffeine in the treatment of recurrent apnea in premature infants. *J Pediatr* 1981;99:984–999.
56. Roberts JL, Mathew OP, Thach BT. The efficacy of theophylline in premature infants with mixed and obstructive apnea associated with pulmonary and neurologic disease. *J Pediatr* 1982;100:968–970.
57. Sims ME, Yau G, Rambhatla S, et al. Limitations of theophylline in the treatment of apnea of prematurity. *Am J Dis Child* 1985;139:567–570.
58. Peliowski A, Finer NN. A blinded, randomized, placebo controlled trial to compare theophylline and doxapram for the treatment of apnea of prematurity. *J Pediatr* 1990;116(4):648–653.
59. Erenberg A, Leff RD, Haack DG, et al. Caffeine citrate for the treatment of apnea of prematurity: a double-blind, placebo-controlled study. *Pharmacotherapy* 2000;20(6):644–652.
60. Eichenwald EC, Howell GR, Leszczynski LE, et al. Theophylline improves coordination of laryngeal abduction and inspiratory effort in premature infants [Abstract]. *Pediatr Res* 1989;25:308A.
61. Henderson-Smart DJ, Steer P. Methylxanthine treatment for apnea in preterm infants. *Cochrane Database Syst Rev* 2001;(3):CD000140.
62. Muttitt SC, Tierney AJ, Finer NN. The dose response of theophylline in the treatment of apnea of prematurity. *J Pediatr* 1988;112:115–121.
63. Henderson-Smart DJ, Steer PA. Prophylactic methylxanthine for prevention of apnea in preterm infants. *Cochrane Database Syst Rev* 2000;(2):CD000432.
64. Bucher HU, Duc G. Does caffeine prevent hypoxaemic episodes in premature infants? A randomized controlled trial. *Eur J Pediatr* 1988;147(3):288–291.
65. Harris MC, Baumgart S, Rocklin AR, et al. Successful extubation of infants with respiratory distress syndrome using aminophylline. *J Pediatr* 1983;103:303–305.
66. Viscardi RM, Faix RG, Nicks JJ, et al. Efficacy of theophylline for prevention of post-extubation respiratory failure in very low birth weight infants. *J Pediatr* 1985;107:469–472.
67. Barrington KJ, Finer NN. A randomized, controlled trial of aminophylline in ventilatory weaning of premature infants. *Crit Care Med* 1993;21:846–850.
68. Sims ME, Rangasamy R, Lee S, et al. Comparative evaluation of caffeine and theophylline for weaning premature infants from the ventilator. *Am J Perinatol* 1989;6:72–75.
69. Henderson-Smart DJ, Davis PG. Prophylactic methylxanthines for extubation in preterm infants. *Cochrane Database Syst Rev* 2003;(1):CD000139.
70. Steer PA, et al. Periextubation caffeine in preterm neonates: a randomized dose response trial. *J Paediatr Child Health* 2003;39(7):511–514.
71. Steer P, Flenady V, Shearman A, et al. High dose caffeine citrate for extubation of preterm infants: a randomized controlled trial. *Arch Dis Child Fetal Neonatal Ed* 2004;89:499–503.
72. Yoder B, Thomson M, Coalson J. Lung function in immature baboons with respiratory distress syndrome receiving early caffeine therapy: a pilot study. *Acta Paediatr* 2005;94:92–98.
73. Montandon G, Bairam A, Kinkead R. Long term consequences of neonatal caffeine on ventilation, occurrence of apneas and hypercapnic chemoreflex in male and female rats. *Pediatr Res* 2006;59:519–524.
74. Davis JM, Bhutani VK, Stefano JL, et al. Changes in pulmonary mechanics following caffeine administration in infants with bronchopulmonary dysplasia. *Pediatr Pulmonol* 1989;6:49–52.
75. Laubscher B, Greenough A, Dimitriou G. Comparative effects of theophylline and caffeine on respiratory function of prematurely born infants. *Early Hum Dev* 1998;50:185–192.
76. Schmidt B, Roberts RS, Davis P, et al. Caffeine therapy for apnea of prematurity. *N Engl J Med* 2006;354:2112–2121.
77. Clyman RI, Roman C. The effects of caffeine on the preterm sheep ductus arteriosus. *Pediatr Res* 2007;62(62):167–169.
78. Soloveychik V, Bin Nun A, Ionchev A, et al. Acute hemodynamic effects of caffeine administration in premature infants. *J Perinatol* 2009;29(3):205–208.
79. Hoecker C, Nelle M, Beedgen B, et al. Effects of a divided high loading dose of caffeine on circulatory variables in preterm infants. *Arch Dis Child Fetal Neonatal Ed* 2006;91(1):F61–F64.
80. Hoecker C, Nelle M, Poeschl J, et al. Caffeine impairs cerebral and intestinal blood flow velocity in preterm infants. *Pediatrics* 2002;109(5):784–787.
81. Walther FJ, Sims ME, Siassi B, et al. Cardiac output changes secondary to theophylline therapy in preterm infants. *J Pediatr* 1986;109(5):874–876.
82. Fesslova V, Caccamo ML, Salice P, et al. Assessment of cardiovascular effects to theophylline in premature newborns by means of serial echocardiography. *Acta Paediatr Scand* 1984;73(3):404–405.
83. Shannon DC, Gotay F. Effects of theophylline on serum and urine electrolytes in preterm infants with apnea. *J Pediatr* 1979;94:963–965.
84. Bauer J, Maier K, Linderkamp O, et al. Effect of caffeine on oxygen consumption and metabolic rate in very low birth weight infants with idiopathic apnea. *Pediatrics* 2001;107:660–663.
85. Zanardo V, Dani C, Trevisanuto D, et al. Methylxanthines increase renal calcium excretion in preterm infants. *Biol Neonate* 1995;68:169–174.
86. Lundstrom KE, Larsen PB, Brendstrup L, et al. Cerebral blood flow and left ventricular output in spontaneously breathing, newborn preterm infants treated with caffeine or aminophylline. *Acta Paediatr* 1995;84:6–9.
87. Wechsler RL, Kleiss LM, Kety SS. Effect of intravenously administered aminophylline on cerebral circulation and metabolism in man. *J Clin Invest* 1954;29:28–33.
88. Saliba E, Autret E, Gold F, et al. Effect of caffeine on cerebral blood flow velocity in preterm infants. *Biol Neonate* 1989;56:198–203.
89. Van Bel F, Van de Bor M, Stijnen T, et al. Does caffeine affect cerebral blood flow in the preterm infant? *Acta Paediatr Scand* 1989;78:205–209.
90. Lane AJ, Coombs RC, Evans DH, et al. Effect of caffeine on neonatal splanchnic blood flow. *Arch Dis Child Fetal Neonatal Ed* 1999;80:F128–F129.
91. Davis JM, Abbasi S, Spitzer AR, et al. Role of theophylline in pathogenesis of necrotizing enterocolitis. *J Pediatr* 1986;109:344–347.
92. Kang SH, Lee YA, Won SJ, et al. Caffeine-induced neuronal death in neonatal rat brain and cortical cell cultures. *Neuroreport* 2002;13:1945–1950.
93. Thurston JH, Hauhart RE, Dirgo JA. Aminophylline increases cerebral metabolic rate and decreases anoxic survival in young mice. *Science* 1978;201:649–651.
94. Tchekalarova J, Kubova H, Mares P. Postnatal caffeine exposure: effects on motor skills and locomotor activity during ontogenesis. *Behav Brain Res* 2005;160:99–106.
95. Bahi N, Nehlig A, Evrard P, et al. Caffeine does not affect excitotoxic brain lesions in newborn mice. *Eur J Paediatr Neurol* 2001;5:161–165.
96. Gunn TR, Metrakos K, Riley PS, et al. Sequelae of caffeine treatment in preterm infants with apnea. *J Pediatr* 1979;94:106–110.
97. Schmidt B, Roberts RS, Davis P, et al. Caffeine for Apnea of Prematurity Trial Group. Long-term effects of caffeine therapy for apnea of prematurity. *N Engl J Med* 2007;357(19):1893–1902.

98. Davis PG, Schmidt B, Roberst RS, et al. Caffeine for Apnea of Prematurity Trial Group. Caffeine for Apnea of Prematurity Trial: benefits may vary in subgroups. *J Pediatr* 2010;156(3): 382–387.
99. Gupta PK, Moore J. The use of doxapram in the newborn. *J Obstet Gynaecol Br Commonw* 1973;80(11):1002–1006.
100. Henderson-Smart DJ, Steer PA. Doxapram treatment for apnea in preterm infants *Cochrane Database Syst Rev* 2001;(4): CD000074. Review. Update in: *Cochrane Database Syst Rev* 2004;(4):CD000074.
101. Henderson-Smart DJ, Steer P. Doxapram versus methylxanthine for apnea in preterm infants. *Cochrane Database Syst Rev* 2000;(4): CD000075.
102. Barrington KJ, Finer NN, Torok-Both G, et al. Dose–response relationship of doxapram in the therapy for refractory idiopathic apnea of prematurity. *Pediatrics* 1987;80(1):22–27.
103. Hayakawa F, Hakamada S, Kuno K, et al. Doxapram in the treatment of idiopathic apnea of prematurity: desirable dosage and serum concentrations. *J Pediatr* 1986;109(1):138–140.
104. Jamali F, Barrington KJ, Finer NN, et al. Doxapram dosage regimen in apnea of prematurity based on pharmacokinetic data. *Dev Pharmacol Ther* 1988;11(5):253–257.
105. Bednarek FJ, Roloff DW. Treatment of apnea of prematurity with aminophylline. *Pediatrics* 1976;58:335–339.

CHAPTER

21

Maria Delivoria-Papadopoulos
Agustín Legido
Ignacio Valencia
Om Prakash Mishra

Drugs and Perinatal Brain Injury

Severe fetal asphyxia may have a broad range of effects on the brain from no evident alteration in brain function to profound cerebral palsy. A large amount of information has been collected on the fetal cardiovascular and respiratory response to oxygen limitations, giving rise to a better understanding and management of neonatal deterioration induced by asphyxia. Besides these physiologic studies, cellular and biochemical mechanisms that result in brain cell death are being increasingly explored, particularly in the adult with respect to focal (stroke) and global (cardiac arrest) hypoxia–ischemia (1). These studies have shown that complex and interrelated biochemical alterations are triggered during hypoxia–ischemia in mature subjects that ultimately result in neuronal death. Studies are in progress to investigate mechanisms of hypoxic brain injury in the fetus and newborn brain (2–6). A thorough knowledge of these biochemical events may lead to recognition of certain steps that may be amenable to pharmacologic intervention to limit or even prevent neuronal cell damage during fetal asphyxia.

Hypoxic injury in the fetal and newborn brain results in neonatal morbidity and mortality as well as long-term sequelae such as mental retardation, seizure disorders, and cerebral palsy (2,7). Although the consequences of antepartum or perinatal hypoxia can be observed in babies, the specific mechanisms of pathologic processes preceding the onset of cerebral dysfunction are not well understood. To focus on the cellular and molecular mechanisms of hypoxic injury in the developing brain, it is important to recognize the factors that may determine the susceptibility of the developing brain to prenatal and perinatal hypoxia.

The determinants of the susceptibility of the developing brain to hypoxia include the lipid composition of the brain cell membrane, the rate of lipid peroxidation, the presence of antioxidant defenses, the development and modulation of the excitatory neurotransmitter receptors such as the *N*-methyl-D-aspartate (NMDA) receptor, and the intracellular Ca^{2+} and intranuclear Ca^{2+} influx mechanisms. In addition to the developmental status of these cellular components, the response of these potential mechanisms to hypoxia determines the fate of the hypoxic brain cell in the developing brain in the fetus and the newborn. Elucidating basic cellular mechanisms in response to hypoxia of the developing brain will enable the development of novel strategies for preventing or attenuating the deleterious effects of hypoxia in the human newborn. Several excellent reviews on different aspects of hypoxic/ischemic cell injury in the developing brain have been published recently (4,8–11).

Perinatal hypoxic ischemia is the most common cause of neurologic disease during the neonatal period [hypoxic–ischemic encephalopathy (HIE)], and is associated with a high mortality and morbidity rate, including cerebral palsy, mental retardation, and seizures. The incidence of perinatal asphyxia is about 1.0% to 1.5% in most centers and is usually related to gestational age and birth weight. It occurs in 9.0% of infants less than 36 weeks' gestation and in 0.5% of infants more than 36 weeks' gestation (12–14). The etiology of perinatal HIE includes those circumstances that can affect the cerebral blood flow in the fetus and newborn compromising the supply of oxygen to the brain. They may develop antepartum (20%), intrapartum (30%), intrapartum and antepartum (35%), or postpartum (10%) (1).

HIE develops in the setting of perinatal asphyxia, which is a multiorgan system disease (12–16). Assessment and management of these complications is an integral part of the treatment of perinatal asphyxia/HIE (12–15).

This chapter primarily focuses on the neuroprotective agents that have suggested to be effective in human clinical studies, and highlights alternative approaches for the treatment of HIE in the future.

NEUROPROTECTIVE TREATMENTS WITH SUGGESTED EFFICACY IN HUMANS

MAGNESIUM SULFATE

Magnesium is a naturally occurring NMDA receptor antagonist that blocks the neuronal influx of Ca^{2+} within the receptor ion channel (3,4,17,18). Experimental studies in newborn animals have shown a neuroprotective effect of magnesium sulfate ($MgSO_4$). $MgSO_4$ reduced brain injury in 7-day-old rats when administered 15 minutes after cerebral injection of NMDA (19). $MgSO_4$ administration in newborn piglets prevented hypoxia-induced modification of the NMDA receptor as well as alteration of neuronal membrane structure and function (20). In addition, $MgSO_4$ administration in pregnant guinea pigs prior to hypoxia prevented the hypoxia-induced generation of oxygen free radicals, cell membrane peroxidation, and nuclear DNA fragmentation (21,22). $MgSO_4$ also decreased excitotoxic brain damage in 50-day-old mice when given before or 10 minutes after an injection of ibotenate, a glutamatergic agonist (23). However, in fetal lambs and piglets subjected to hypoxia and/or ischemia, $MgSO_4$ failed to prevent cerebral injury (24,25).

In the clinical setting, $MgSO_4$ has been widely used in obstetrics practice for more than 60 years. Its indications include suppression of preterm labor and management of pregnancy-induced hypertension (26). A retrospective epidemiologic study by Nelson and Grether (27) suggested that premature fetuses whose mothers received $MgSO_4$ for the treatment of preeclampsia or as a tocolytic agent are less likely to develop cerebral palsy compared with a gestational age-matched group of fetuses not exposed to the drug. The Collaborative Eclampsia Trial (28) reported that babies of women who had been given $MgSO_4$ before delivery were significantly less likely to be intubated at the place of delivery or to be admitted to a special care nursery than the babies of mothers who had been given phenytoin. These studies suggested that $MgSO_4$ might provide a protective effect against brain damage in immature fetuses and newborn infants. Randomized, controlled, double-blind trials were established to examine this hypothesis. One was discontinued after interim analysis showed that administration of $MgSO_4$ to mothers in preterm labor before 34 weeks of gestation was associated with significant increase in infants' mortality (29). However, other trials have not shown any difference in the mortality between the placebo and treatment groups (30).

Recent studies have been statistically more powerful. A multicenter randomized controlled trial of $MgSO_4$ versus placebo, for the prevention of cerebral palsy, in 2,241 women at risk of imminent premature delivery at 24 to 31 weeks of gestation carried out in the United States was published in 2008 (31). The primary outcome was the composite of stillbirth or infant death by 1 year of corrected age or moderate or severe cerebral palsy at or beyond 2 years of corrected age. The primary outcome was not significantly different in the $MgSO_4$ group and the placebo group. However, in a prespecified secondary analysis, moderate or severe cerebral palsy occurred significantly less frequently in the $MgSO_4$ group (1.9% vs. 3.5%). A similar study in France followed up 606 infants less than 33 weeks of gestation, whose mothers were treated with $MgSO_4$. Compared to placebo, treated infants showed a decrease of all primary end points (total mortality, severe white matter injury, and their combined outcome) and of all secondary end points (motor dysfunction, cerebral palsy, cognitive dysfunction, and their combined outcomes at 2 years of age). The decrease was nearly significant or significant for gross motor dysfunction and combined criteria: death and cerebral palsy, death and gross motor dysfunction, death, cerebral palsy, and cognitive dysfunction (32). A recent paper by Doyle et al. (33) reviewed the evidence of the neuroprotective effects of $MgSO_4$ given to women considered at risk of preterm birth. The authors concluded that the neuroprotective role for antenatal $MgSO_4$ therapy given to mothers at such risk is now established. The number of women needed to treat to benefit one baby by avoiding cerebral palsy is 63 (95% confidence interval 43 to 87). Given the beneficial effects of $MgSO_4$ on substantial gross motor function in early childhood, outcomes later in childhood should be evaluated to determine the presence or absence of later potentially important neurologic effects, particularly on motor or cognitive function.

ALLOPURINOL

Allopurinol, an inhibitor of the enzyme xanthine oxidase, blocks the synthesis of xanthine from hypoxanthine and therefore prevents the formation of the free radical superoxide. Ischemia–reperfusion results in injury to organs containing the highest amounts of xanthine oxidase, such as the liver and the intestine. The injury results in the release of xanthine oxidase into the circulation. Circulating xanthine oxidase in adults causes damage to remote nonischemic organs that possess low amounts of endogenous xanthine oxidase, such as the heart and the brain. It is not known whether allopurinol inhibits circulating xanthine oxidase or endogenous xanthine oxidase in the brain, or both (3,4,6,8,12).

In experimental animal models, administration of allopurinol to immature rats 30 minutes before inducing focal hypoxia–ischemia reduced the severity of the secondary edema and the extent of the neuropathologic lesion in the treated group compared with a control group (34). Similarly, pretreatment with allopurinol preserved cerebral energy metabolism of the 7-day postnatal rat during hypoxia–ischemia (35). The same group of researchers also found that oxypurinol, the active metabolite of allopurinol, administered at the same dose and at the same time as allopurinol after hypoxia–ischemia reduced brain injury in the immature rat (36). Administration of allopurinol in newborn piglets prevented the hypoxia-induced modification of NMDA receptor as well as cell membrane peroxidation and neuronal dysfunction (37,38).

In the clinical setting, a 7-day course of enteral allopurinol (20 mg per kg) given after birth to 400 infants between 24 and 32 weeks' gestation did not change the incidence of periventricular leukomalacia (39). In a study of 22 asphyxiated newborn infants, intravenous allopurinol in a dose of 40 mg per kg given 4 hours after birth resulted in a decrease in mortality (2/11 vs. 6/11 in the control group), and in a beneficial effect on free radical formation, cerebral blood flow, and electrical brain activity, without toxic side effects (40). Clancy et al. (41) conducted a clinical trial to test the hypothesis that allopurinol could reduce death, seizures, coma, and cardiac events in infants who underwent heart surgery using deep hypothermic circulatory arrest. They studied a total of 318 infants, 131 hypoplastic left heart syndrome (HLHS) and 187 non-HLHS. In HLHS surgical survivors, 40 of 47 (85%) allopurinol-treated infants did not experience any end point event, compared with 27 of 49 (55%) controls ($p = .002$). There were fewer "seizure-only" ($p = .05$) and "cardiac-only" (p = .03) events in the allopurinol versus placebo groups. Allopurinol did not reduce efficacy end point events in non-HLHS infants. Treated and control infants did not differ in adverse events. Recently, Benders et al. (42) investigated whether postnatal allopurinol would reduce free radical induced reperfusion/reoxygenation injury of the brain in severely asphyxiated neonates. In an interim analysis of a randomized, double-blind, placebo controlled study, 32 severely asphyxiated infants were given allopurinol or a vehicle within 4 hours of birth. The analysis showed an unaltered (high) mortality and morbidity in the infants treated with allopurinol. The authors concluded that allopurinol treatment started postnatally was too late to reduce the early reperfusion-induced free radical surge. Allopurinol administration to the fetus with (imminent) hypoxia via the mother during labor may be more effective in reducing free radical–induced postasphyxial brain damage.

Chaudhari and McGuire (43) performed a meta-analysis to evaluate the evidence of the effect of allopurinol on mortality and morbidity in newborn infants with suspected hypoxic–ischaemic encephalopathy. The authors concluded that the available data are not sufficient to determine whether allopurinol has clinically important benefits for newborn infants with hypoxic–ischaemic encephalopathy and, therefore, larger trials are needed. Such trials could assess allopurinol as an adjunct to therapeutic hypothermia in infants with moderate and severe encephalopathy and should be designed to exclude clinically important effects on mortality and adverse long-term neurodevelopmental outcomes.

OPIOIDS

The antinociceptive effects of opioids are mediated through a combination of pre- and postsynaptic hyperpolarization, which produces a decrease in the release of and the sensitivity to endogenous mediators like glutamate (44,45). This suggests that they may have a neuroprotective effect. Indeed, studies in cell cultures have demonstrated that endogenous and exogenous opioids may protect cortical neurons from hypoxia-induced cell death (46,47). Similarly, opioids may induce ischemic tolerance in cerebellar Purkinje cells subject to ischemia-reperfusion (48). Antagonists of opioid receptors increase the survival time during severe hypoxia in intact animals (49,50) and enhance tissue preservation and survival time of organs used for transplants (51).

In 2005, Angeles et al. (52), published the results of a retrospective study of 52 term newborns with perinatal asphyxia, in which they analyzed the relationship between treatment with opioid analgesics (morphine or fentanyl) and neurological damage. A total of 33% of them received opioids; in spite of having a more severe degree of asphyxia (higher levels of lactate, lower 5-minute Apgar score), this group of patients had less severe signs of brain damage on the MRI performed after 7 days of life. Moreover, their neurologic outcome at a mean follow-up of 13 months was better than that of the group of newborns who did not receive opioids. The same group of researchers also performed a follow-up study with MR spectroscopy of 28 term newborns treated with opioids and 20 controls (53). The results showed that occipital gray matter NAA/Cr was significantly decreased and lactate was present in a significantly higher amount in non–opioid-treated neonates compared with opioid-treated neonates. Also, compared with controls, untreated neonates showed larger changes in more metabolites in basal ganglia, thalami, and occipital gray matter with greater significance than treated neonates. The authors concluded that the use of opioids during the first week following perinatal asphyxia has no long-term adverse effects and may increase brain resistance to hypoxic ischemia. The authors speculated that the neuroprotective effect of opioids may be mediated by increasing the levels of adenosine, an endogenous nucleoside with neuroprotective activity, or by inducing neuronal hyperpolarization, which results in diminishing intracellular penetration of calcium.

Despite the potential benefit of opioids on asphyxiated term neonates as indicated in these studies, caution must be exercised in the use of this class of medications. Available literature suggests that the routine use of opioid analgesics can be complicated by problems such as tolerance, withdrawal, and ventilator dependence. Very few studies have examined the long-term effects of exposure to opioids in the neonatal period. In addition, previous reports indicate that endogenous opioids can suppress DNA synthesis in vivo in immature cerebellar and glial cells (opioid receptors are widely distributed in the CNS with functions that include pain modulation, cardiorespiratory regulation), whereas exogenous opioids can exacerbate neurotoxicity in animal models of cerebral ischemia. Future prospective randomized trials are warranted to determine whether there is truly an immediate neuroprotective effect on hypoxic–ischemic brain injury and whether these agents can play a role in improving long-term outcome.

HYPOTHERMIA

Hypothermia has developed during the past few years as an alternative for treating perinatal asphyxia/HIE (54,55). Hypothermia during experimental cerebral ischemia is associated with potent dose-related, long-lasting neuroprotection. Conversely, hyperthermia of only 1°C to 2°C extends and markedly worsens damage, and in particular tends to promote pannecrosis (54). Although the majority of such studies involved global ischemia in adult rodents (56), similar results were reported from studies and hypoxia–ischemia in 7-day-old rats (57) and newborn piglets (58), kittens, rabbits, and puppies (59).

The study of the mechanisms of action of hypothermic neuroprotection suggests that cooling affects many or all of the pathways leading to delayed cell death (54). Hypothermia reduces the rate of oxygen-requiring enzymatic reactions and cerebral oxygen consumption, slows the fall of phosphocreatine/inorganic phosphate (PCr/Pi), and confers a protective effect of the brain after adenosine triphosphate (ATP) exhaustion. In addition, hypothermia decreases oxygen consumption of the brain by 6% to 7% and cerebral energy utilization rate by 5.3% per degree. Additional experimental evidence suggests that hypothermia suppresses cytotoxic excitatory amino acid accumulation, inhibits nitric oxide synthase activity, decreases interleukin-1 levels, decreases the release of other cytotoxic cytokines by microglial cells, and suppresses free radical activity and delayed cell death by apoptosis. Hypothermia also decreases blood–brain barrier permeability and intracranial pressure and facilitates recovery of electrophysiologic function after cerebral ischemia.

The efficacy of hypothermia is dependent on a number of factors, such as the timing of initiation of cooling, its duration, and the depth of cooling attained (54). Mild hypothermia is defined as a reduction in core temperature of 1°C to 3°C, moderate as 4°C to 6°C, severe as 8°C to 10°C, and profound as 15°C to 20°C. Brief (0.5 to 3 hours), mild-to-moderate hypothermia immediately after hypoxia–ischemic injury may be most effective after relatively mild insults. Protection appears to be lost if brief hypothermia is delayed by as little as 15 to 45 minutes after the primary insult. A more recent approach has been to try to suppress the secondary encephalopathic processes by maintaining hypothermia throughout the course of the secondary phase. An extended period of cooling (between 5 and 72 hours) appears to be more consistently effective and remains effective after significant delays (possibly up to 6 hours) between the primary insult and the start of cooling; however, the degree of neuroprotection progressively declines if cooling is initiated more than a few hours postinsult (54). In addition, cerebral hypothermia is not neuroprotective when started after postischemic seizures occur (60).

Potential adverse effects of induced hypothermia (the risk increasing with depth of hypothermia) include increased blood viscosity, mild metabolic acidosis, cardiac arrhythmias, decreased oxygen availability, dysfunction of cellular immunity, coagulation abnormalities and platelet dysfunction, intracellular shift of potassium, and choreic syndrome (55).

The first study on neuroprotection of perinatal HIE with selective head cooling was published in 1998 by Gunn et al. (61), who basically proved the safety of this procedure. Later on, the same group of researchers published the results of other studies in a small number of patients, which confirmed the lack of side effects and a tendency to a better neurologic prognosis in those newborns with moderate or severe HIE treated with this hypothermia technique (62,63).

In 2005, Gluckman et al. (64) published the results of the most important study that has produced reliable and significant data about the neuroprotective effect of selective head cooling hypothermia. It was a multicenter investigation that included 234 newborns with HIE and estimated gestational age (EGA) above 36 weeks. HIE was defined according to the following criteria: pH less than 7.0, base excess equal to or higher than 16 mmol per L, Apgar store at 10 minutes equal to or less than 5, need for cardiorespiratory resuscitation for more than 10 minutes, abnormal neurological examination according to the Sarnat's criteria of moderate or severe encephalopathy, and abnormal amplitude integrated electroencephalogram (EEG) (aEEG). Patients were randomized before 5.5 hours of life into two groups: body normothermia or hypothermia of 34.5°C, induced through selective head cooling during 72 hours. Patients treated with hypothermia had a significantly higher incidence of arrhythmia (mostly sinus bradycardia). A total of 218 infants were followed up until 18 months of age. The presence of death or neurological disability was found in 66% of patients in the control group and 55% in the hypothermia group ($p < .1$). However, when newborns with severe neurological depression or those who had seizures on the aEEG were excluded, 66% of infants in the control group and 48% in the hypothermia group died or had neurological disability ($p < .02$). Moreover, the presence of severe neurological disability was 28% and 12% in each group, respectively. The authors concluded that except in newborns with the most severe forms of HIE, selective head cooling applied immediately following delivery may be a feasible therapeutic technique to decrease neurological sequelae of perinatal HIE.

The first study with generalized body hypothermia in perinatal HIE was published in 2000 by Azzopardi et al. (65), who found that prolonged hypothermia of 33°C to 34°C was associated with minimal physiological changes (e.g., decreased heart rate, increased blood pressure) but was well tolerated. During the next 3 years, other research protocols in a limited number of patients corroborated that generalized body hypothermia was a feasible and clinically safe technique (66–68).

In 2005, Eicher et al. (69,70) published the results of a pilot multicenter study about the safety and efficacy of generalized body hypothermia in the treatment of 32 newborns with perinatal HIE. Adverse effects included bradycardia, hypotension, decreased platelets, increased prothrombin time, and higher incidence of seizures, but none of them was severe, and they all responded to treatment (69). The efficacy results showed a higher incidence of death or severe neurological motor involvement in the control group (82%) compared with the group of hypothermia-treated newborns (52%) ($p = .019$). A severe psychomotor developmental delay (<70%) was seen in 64% of infants in the control group and in 24% of those subjected to hypothermia ($p = .053$).

Also in 2005, Shankaran et al. (71) published a larger multicenter study on the use of body hypothermia to treat perinatal HIE. A total of 208 newborns with HIE, EGA more than 36 weeks, were included. HIE was defined according to the following criteria: need for neonatal resuscitation, abnormal neurologic examination compatible with moderate or severe encephalopathy, pH less than 7.0, and a base excess equal to or above 16 mmol per L. EEG criteria were not included in the diagnostic requirements. Patients were randomized before 6 hours of life into two groups: body normothermia or hypothermia of 33.5°C, induced by body cooling, during 72 hours. Patients were followed up until 18 to 22 months. The incidence of mild complications was similar in both groups. The incidence of death or moderate or severe neurological disability was 62% in the control group and 44% in the hypotermia-treated group ($p = .01$). The incidence of cerebral palsy was 30% in the control newborns and 19% in those treated with hypothermia ($p = .20$). The authors concluded that generalized body hypothermia reduces the risk of death and neurological disability in newborns with moderate or severe HIE. An MRI follow-up study of infants enrolled in the above-mentioned trial (71) aimed to measure relative volumes of subcortical white matter. They were significantly larger in hypothermia-treated than in control infants.

Furthermore, relative total brain volumes correlated significantly with death or neurosensory impairments. Relative volumes of the cortical gray and subcortical white matter also correlated significantly with Bayley scales psychomotor development index (72).

Hypothermia is currently in the process of translating from the clinical research experience to direct clinical application (73,74). However, the clinical trials with hypothermia have also addressed many questions, which need to be answered before it becomes the standard of care to treat newborns with perinatal asphyxia: Which should be the patients' selection criteria? When should hypothermia be initiated? How long should hypothermia last? Which is the most effective technique? Is hypothermia a safe technique? Which is the long-term outcome? Should sedation be administered concomitantly with hypothermia? How should rewarming be done? and Could hypothermia efficacy be enhanced with simultaneously administering other neuroprotective agents? (6,8,75–80).

Some of those questions are tried to be answered with additional research in experimental animals (81–85) and through clinical studies (73,86–89). In the meantime the practical recommendations have been recently established by the National Institute of Child Health and Human Development (NICHD), which published an Executive Summary with the following conclusions:

> Based on the available data and large knowledge gaps, the expert panel suggested that although hypothermia appears to be a potentially promising therapy for HIE, long-term efficacy and safety are yet to be established. Clinicians choosing to offer this treatment should therefore understand all of the limitations of the available evidence, be prepared to keep up-to-date on evidence on this topic as it evolves, and counsel parents and family about the limitations of the current evidence. (90)

FUTURE TREATMENTS

In the future, several of the neuroprotective agents that have been under investigation for a long time (Table 21.1) [i.e., NMDA antagonists; nitric oxide (NO) synthesis inhibitors] may overcome the problems they face today (cognitive and memory side effects of the NMDA antagonists; unavailability of NO synthesis inhibitors) and achieve clinical application in humans. At the same time, clinical and experimental research is providing additional information about the potential to use new compounds or methods of neuroprotection. It seems encouraging that the therapeutic options for protecting neuronal damage in perinatal asphyxia/HIE will improve significantly in the future.

NEW ANTIEPILEPTIC DRUGS

Seizures are the main clinical manifestation of perinatal HIE. On the other hand, the new antiepileptic drugs (AEDs), in particular, have multiple mechanisms of action that block different steps in the biochemical and molecular cascade that causes neuronal damage both in hypoxia–ischemia and in epilepsy. Therefore, there is a

TABLE 21.1 Some Proposed Neuroprotective Agents

Agent Class	*Example*
Adenosine	Adenosine
Adrenergic blockers	Propranolol
Antioxidant/free radical scavengers	Vitamins C, E, superoxide dismutase
Barbiturates	Phenobarbital
Calcium channel blockers	Nimodipine, flunarizine
Cyclooxygenase inhibitors	Indomethacin
Excitatory amino acid blockers	MK-801
Growth factors	Nerve growth factor, insulin growth factor-1
Hypothermia	Systemic or brain only
Lazaroids	U74006F
Magnesium	$MgSO_4$
Monogangliosides	GM1
Nitric oxide inhibitors	*N*-Nitro-L-arginine methyl ester
Opiate antagonists	Naltrexone
Osmotic agents	Mannitol
Phenotiazines	Chlorpromazine
Phosphodiesterase inhibitors	Aminophylline
Platelet-activating factors	Gingko extract
Polyamines	Spermine
Procoagulants	Vitamin K
Serotonin agonists	Ipsapirone
Steroids	Dexamethasone
Xanthine oxidase inhibitors	Allopurinol

Modified from Miller VS. Pharmacologic management of neonatal cerebral ischemia and hemorrhage: old and new directions. *J Clin Neurol* 1993;8:7–18, with permission.

great interest in investigating the possible neuroprotective role of these drugs (91–97).

LAMOTRIGINE

Lamotrigine blocks neuronal sodium channels, inhibits voltage-dependent Ca^{2+} currents, possibly through inhibition of type N Ca^{2+} presynaptic channels, and inhibits the release of the excitatory neurotransmitters glutamate and aspartate (94,98).

Although some animal models of ischemia did not demonstrate a neuroprotective effect for lamotrigine (99), this AED seems to have a neuroprotective efficacy similar to MK-801 (glutamate, NMDA receptor antagonist) in the prevention of neuronal damage mediated by excitatory amino acids (100). In a model of focal hypoxia–ischemia in adult rats, the intraperitoneal administration of 100 mg per kg of lamotrigine between 0.5 and 24.5 hours after the occlusion of the middle cerebral artery reduced the cortical infarct size measured 3 days after by 28% (100). In a similar model in rats, the immediate treatment with 20 mg per kg of intraventricular lamotrigine reduced the volume of the cerebral infarct (101). In a model of global hypoxia–ischemia with bilateral carotid artery ligation in the guinea pig, lamotrigine prevented neuronal loss in the CA1 sector of the hippocampus when administered right after the ligation. This AED also reduced the mortality and improved their cognitive function (102). In the same animal model, lamotrigine administration 30 minutes before and after the carotid ligation produced a histological neuroprotective effect at 7 and 28 days. The behavior on the treated animals was also better. The microdialysis measurement of cerebral glutamate demonstrated a significant reduction of this excitatory amino acid (103). Lamotrigine also had a neuroprotective effect in a rat model of heart arrest when immediately administered within 5 hours of the arrest (104). In a model of focal ischemia followed by global ischemia in the rat, lamotrigine decreased the levels of glutamate and aspartate in the hippocampus and prevented neuronal damage (105). The neuroprotective effect of lamotrigine can be potentiated with the simultaneous administration of calcium antagonist flunarizine (106) or hypothermia (107).

TOPIRAMATE

Topiramate has the following mechanisms of action: It blocks sodium channels, increases γ-amino-butyric acid (GABA) levels and chloride channel-dependent transmission, inhibits the activity of the glutamate α-amino-3-hydroxyl-5-methyl-4-isooxazole-propionic acid (AMPA) receptor, and decreases the voltage-gated calcium currents, which can decrease the release of excitatory neurotransmitters. Topiramate also inhibits the carbonic anhydrase enzyme and opens potassium channels (94,98).

The administration of 20 to 40 mg per kg of topiramate to animals, 2 hours after an embolus of the middle cerebral artery, decreases the volume of the infarct by 55% to 80% when examined 24 hours later (108,109). In a model of focal hypoxia–ischemia induced by middle cerebral artery occlusion in the guinea pig, topiramate treatment with 100 to 200 mg per kg decreased neuronal damage (110). Topiramate also reduced the hippocampal lesion in an experimental model of status epilepticus (111). In neonatal rat models of hypoxia–ischemia, topiramate demonstrated a neuroprotective effect on hypoxia and seizure-induced apoptosis in the hippocampus (112). It also decreased the neuronal damage after hypoxia–ischemia in pigs (113), oligodendrocyte damage in a periventricular leukomalacia glutamatergic rat model (114), and excitotoxic neuronal damage induced by glutamate agonists in mice (115). The therapeutic dose of topiramate has not been toxic to the developing brain (116).

ZONISAMIDE

Zonisamide exerts its anticonvulsant effect by inhibiting sodium and T-type calcium channels, decreasing glutamate-mediated excitotoxicity, and increasing the GABAergic activity of chloride channels. It also inhibits the carbonic anhydrase enzyme and has an antioxidant effect (94,98).

In an adult rat animal model of middle cerebral artery occlusion, treatment with 10 to 100 mg per kg of oral zonisamide, 15 or 30 minutes before and 4 hours after occlusion, significantly reduced the cerebral ischemic damage (117). In a global hypoxic–ischemic model in guinea pigs, administration of zonisamide 150 mg per kg before hypoxia decreased neuronal damage in the CA1 sector of the hippocampus when evaluated at 7 and 28 days of life. Microdialysis measurement of cerebral glutamate showed lower levels in treated animals (118). In a model of focal hypoxia–ischemia in neonatal rats, treatment with 75 mg per kg of intraperitoneal zonisamide 1 hour before hypoxia decreased the volume of the infarct in the cortex and striatum by 90%, independently of its anticonvulsant action (119).

LEVETIRACETAM

The exact mechanism of action of levetiracetam is unknown, although several possibilities have been suggested. They have included its indirect effects in the GABAergic system through binding to a specific receptor, decreasing the electrical discharge in the *pars reticulata* of the *substantia nigra,* activation of Ca^{2+} depended processes, and binding to the synaptic vesicle 2A (SV2A) (94,98).

In a model of focal hypoxia–ischemia in adult rats, intraperitoneal administration of 5.5 to 44 mg per kg of levetiracetam before the occlusion of the middle cerebral artery and 1.25 to 10.2 mg per kg per hour during the following 24 hours decreased the cerebral infarct volume by 33% with the higher dose (120). However, levetiracetam did not show a neuroprotective effect in a pilocarpine-induced status epilepticus model (121).

ROLE OF NITRIC OXIDE IN HYPOXIC BRAIN INJURY

The observation that activation of the NMDA receptor generates NO in a Ca^{2+}-dependent manner led to the hypothesis that NO, a well-known cytotoxin, participates in neuronal excitotoxicity. This hypothesis was further strengthened by the demonstration that inhibition of NO synthesis attenuates NMDA-dependent neurotoxicity in neuronal culture and reduces brain damage produced by middle cerebral artery occlusion in mice (122). We showed that cerebral hypoxia results in generation of nitric oxide free radicals (123) as demonstrated by electron spin resonance spectroscopy of NO. In addition, administration of NO synthase (NOS) inhibitor prevented the hypoxia-induced generation of free radicals, nitration of the NMDA receptor subunits, and calmodulin kinase IV activation, and increased phosphorylation of cAMP response element-binding (CREB) protein at Ser^{133}, expression of proapoptotic protein Bax, and fragmentation of nuclear DNA (124–128).

In view of these observations, NO can play a central role in hypoxia-induced neuronal death by both the necrotic and apoptotic or programmed cell death mechanisms. First, the NO-induced increase in NMDA receptor–mediated intracellular Ca^{2+} potentially initiates a number of reactions leading to increased free radical generation via a number of enzymatic pathways such as Ca^{2+} activation of phospholipase A_2, causing release of arachidonic acid, which then can be metabolized by cyclooxygenase and lipoxygenase, the conversion of xanthine dehydrogenase to xanthine oxidase by Ca^{2+}-dependent activation of proteases, and activation of nitric oxide synthase by Ca^{2+} to further generate NO, leading to formation of peroxynitrite and oxygen free radical species. The increased free radicals generated result in increased peroxidation of cellular and subcellular membranes, leading to necrotic cell death. Second, the increased intracellular Ca^{2+} may lead to increased intranuclear Ca^{2+} by mechanisms of Ca^{2+} influx such as the inositol triphosphate (IP_3) and inositol tetraphosphate (IP_4) receptors and the nuclear-membrane high-affinity Ca^{2+} ATPase. Furthermore, we have demonstrated that NO increases nuclear Ca^{2+} influx (129). In light of these observations, NO is capable of increasing intranuclear Ca^{2+} by more than one mechanism in vivo. Increased intranuclear Ca^{2+} may activate Ca^{2+}-dependent endonucleases, leading to DNA fragmentation. In addition, increased intranuclear Ca^{2+} can activate calmodulin kinase IV in the nucleus, leading to increased phosphorylation of CREB resulting in increased transcription of apoptotic genes such as Bax and initiating the early events of DNA fragmentation and programmed cell death. Thus, a central role for NO is proposed in regulating neuronal function and specifically in hypoxia-induced neuronal death, by altering the nuclear membrane mechanisms of Ca^{2+} influx, resulting in increased nuclear Ca^{2+}.

NEURONAL NITRIC OXIDE SYNTHASE–NMDA RECEPTOR LINK

In mammalian systems, three isoforms of NOS have been identified. NOS I (nNOS) is present in neurons and is a constitutively expressed enzyme whose activity is regulated by Ca^{2+} and calmodulin (130). NOS II (iNOS) is an inducible enzyme whose activity is independent of Ca^{2+}. NOS III (eNOS) is constitutively expressed in endothelial cells and is also regulated by Ca^{2+} and calmodulin. Increasing evidence indicates that NOS expression can be regulated by various physiologic and pathologic conditions. nNOS and mRNA upregulation represents a general response of neuronal cells to stress conditions, including hypoxia (131) and ischemia (132).

In neurons of the central venous system, nNOS is colocalized with NMDA receptors (133). In addition, neuronal NOS is activated by Ca^{2+} influx through the NMDA receptor ion channel; however, nNOS is not efficiently stimulated by activation of non-NMDA receptors that also induce Ca^{2+} influx (134). In synaptic plasma membranes, the nNOS immunoreactivity is associated with the NMDA receptor (135). The synaptic localization of nNOS in brain may be mediated by the postsynaptic density protein PSD-95. Recently, it was demonstrated that nNOS, PSD-95, and NMDA receptor subunit NR2B from the brain coimmunoprecipitate, and that PSD-95 is sufficient to assemble a tight ternary complex with nNOS and the NR2B subunit of the NMDA receptor (136). In summary, results of these studies indicate that NO production in the brain is preferentially activated by Ca^{2+} influx through the NMDA receptor ion channel, and that there is a specific structural and functional link between the NMDA receptor and the neuronal NOS.

ROLE OF INTRANUCLEAR Ca^{2+} IN HYPOXIC BRAIN INJURY

In a recent study, we demonstrated that cerebral hypoxia results in increased Ca^{2+} influx in neuronal nuclei of newborn piglets (129,137). Nuclear Ca^{2+} influx was 2.04 ± 1.10 pmol per mg of protein per 120 s in the normoxic group, compared with 8.57 ± 3.21 pmol per mg of protein per 120 s in the hypoxic group ($p < .005$). Nuclear calcium influx ranged from 4.36 to 14.9 pmol per mg of protein per 120 s in the hypoxic group and correlated inversely as an exponential function with cerebral tissue ATP ($r = .92$) and phosphocreatine ($r = .88$) concentrations.

Nuclear calcium controls a variety of functions in the nucleus, including regulation of gene transcription, DNA synthesis and repair, nuclear envelope breakdown, and cell cycle regulation. Nuclear Ca^{2+} signals can regulate events that lead to hypoxia-induced neuronal death. The increased intranuclear Ca^{2+} may activate Ca^{2+}-dependent endonucleases, leading to nuclear DNA fragmentation. In addition, the increased intranuclear Ca^{2+} can activate Ca^{2+}/calmodulin-dependent protein kinase IV (CaM kinase IV), leading to increased phosphorylation of CREB protein, which triggers transcription of apoptotic proteins such as Bax and Bad and initiates early events of caspase-mediated programmed neuronal death.

Intranuclear Ca^{2+} is differentially regulated from the cytoplasmic calcium. For example, nuclear calcium is higher in some cell systems than the cytosolic ones and lower in smooth muscle cell and neuronal cells. There is some evidence that increased cytosolic Ca^{2+} may lead to increased intranuclear calcium influx. Studies have shown that modification of the NMDA receptor can lead to an increased cytosolic calcium concentration, which may lead to increased production of oxygen free radicals and modification of nuclear membrane and hence increased intranuclear calcium. The results of our study just cited showed that there is an increase in the Ca^{2+} influx in the hypoxic nuclei and there is a curvilinear relationship between the tissue levels of high-energy phosphates and the nuclear Ca^{2+} influx.

There are potential mechanisms that could explain the increase in nuclear Ca^{2+} influx such as modification of nuclear membrane by oxygen free radicals or modification of high-affinity Ca^{2+}-ATPase and the IP_3 and IP_4 receptors. We observed that the activity of neuronal nuclear membrane high-affinity Ca^{2+}-ATPase is increased during hypoxia (138). The increase in enzyme activity is linearly correlated with the increase in the degree of cerebral tissue hypoxia as measured by cerebral tissue high-energy phosphates. In this study, the ATP-dependent nuclear Ca^{2+} influx was measured. However, the curvilinear relationship of the nuclear Ca^{2+} influx with the ATP as well as phosphocreatine relates to the degree of tissue hypoxia and reflects the hypoxia-induced modification of ATP-dependent mechanisms of nuclear Ca^{2+} influx such as high-affinity nuclear membrane Ca^{2+}-ATPase. We also observed that the receptor-mediated mechanisms of Ca^{2+} influx such as IP_4 receptor-dependent and IP_3 receptor-dependent mechanisms are modified (139).

Hypoxia-induced calcium influx in the nucleus may activate several calcium-dependent mechanisms. Increased nuclear Ca^{2+} may activate CaM kinase IV in the nucleus, which phosphorylates CREB, leading to increased expression of apoptotic proteins. In our previous studies we observed that cerebral hypoxia results in increased activity of neuronal nuclear CaM kinase IV as well as increased phosphorylation of CREB. Nuclear calcium, through activation of CREB protein, may alter transcription of apoptotic genes. This may result in altered expression of proapoptotic protein, Bax, and antiapoptotic protein Bcl-2, leading to an altered Bax and Bcl-2 ratio, a determinant of apoptosis or programmed cell death. The role of CREB phosphorylation appears complex and has also been shown to favor cell survival in cell culture models. In our studies we showed that hypoxia results in increased expression of Bax as compared to Bcl-2, thus altering the ratio of these proteins in neuronal nuclei of newborn piglets (140). The Bax expression during hypoxia increased as a function of the increase of the cerebral tissue hypoxia as measured by cerebral tissue high-energy phosphates. The increased ratio of Bax to Bcl-2 may initiate the cascade of activation of initiator caspase-9 through the activation of apoptotic protease activating factor-1 and subsequently activate the executioner caspase-3. Furthermore, the caspase-3-dependent cleavage of caspase-activated DNase (CAD) and inhibitor of CAD (ICAD) may lead to CAD-mediated fragmentation of nuclear DNA. In addition, increased intranuclear Ca^{2+} may activate calcium magnesium-dependent endonucleases, which may lead to DNA fragmentation at internucleosomal sites. Studies from our laboratory have shown that hypoxia results in increased fragmentation of neuronal nuclear DNA, and the degree of DNA fragmentation increases with the degree of cerebral tissue hypoxia (141).

During hypoxia, the hypoxia-induced modification of the NMDA leads to increased intracellular Ca^{2+}, initiating a number of Ca^{2+}-dependent pathways of free radical generation including nitric oxide (5,123,124). Subsequently, modification of nuclear membrane Ca^{2+}-influx mechanisms such as high-affinity Ca^{2+}-ATPase and IP_3 and IP_4 receptors leads to increased intranuclear Ca^{2+}. The increased intranuclear Ca^{2+} leads to activation of CaM kinase IV in the nucleus, leading to phosphorylation of CREB, which triggers transcription of apoptotic proteins as well as fragmentation of nuclear DNA via endonuclease-dependent and CAD-mediated mechanisms. At this point, it is important to mention that these events could be triggered by free radicals during hypoxia. In fact, our studies demonstrate that all of the mentioned events can be prevented or attenuated by the administration of NOS inhibitors, indicating that the events in hypoxic neuronal injury are nitric oxide mediated (124–128,137,138,140).

ANTI-NMDA RECEPTOR IMMUNIZATION

As an alternative to antagonizing NMDA receptors involved in the pathogenesis of hypoxia–ischemia, During et al. (142) investigated the hypothesis that a humoral autoimmune response targeting the NR1 subunit of NMDA receptor might have neuroprotective activity. They also hypothesized that such autoantibodies would have minimal penetration into the central nervous system under basal conditions and thereby avoid the toxicity associated with traditional approaches, but following a cerebral insult, would pass into the brain more efficiently, antagonize the receptor, and thereby attenuate NMDA receptor-mediated injury. The authors used an oral genetic vaccine approach for immunization. For the experimental stroke they used the endothelin-1 model of middle cerebral artery occlusion. The size of the infarct was reduced by approximately 70% in the vaccinated rats in comparison to the control group. The animals had no neurologic impairment. These results suggest the possibility of vaccination for individuals at risk of stroke and other cerebral insults without impairment of neurologic function.

GENETIC TREATMENT

Brain hypoxia–ischemia is one of the most potent stimuli for gene induction. Many of them are related to neuronal damage functions such as excitotoxicity, inflammatory response, and neuronal apoptosis. On the other hand, hypoxia–ischemia is also an important stimulus for neuroprotective genes. The experimental alteration of such genes appears as a promising treatment of hypoxia–ischemia, which is still being studied in the laboratory (143). For example, the genetic expression of the calcium binding protein calbindin D_{28k} (144), oncogen Bcl-2 protein (145–147), or growth factor (148) through viral vectors (143,145,146,148) or transgenic animals (147) in animal models of hypoxia–ischemia has demonstrated a neuroprotective effect.

STEM CELLS TREATMENT

Stem cell transplant holds a great promise as a therapeutic alternative to replace tissue or damaged neurons in patients with hypoxic ischemic injury, trauma, or other neurological diseases. It is not clear whether stem cells work by replacing neurons and glial cells, by having a trophic effect on them, or by modifying the local environment to stimulate a process of neuroprotection and regeneration (149,150).

The stem cell studies in models of hypoxia–ischemia are still in their early stages. In HIE rat models, astrocytic or bone marrow pluripotential stem cells demonstrated that they can survive, migrate to the damage area, and differentiate into neurons and astrocytes (151,152). In China, a group of authors injected fetal brain stem cells into the ventricular system of rats subject to hypoxia–ischemia. They also showed that these cells survived, migrated, and differentiated into neurons and astrocytes (153).

Umbilical cord pluripotential cells have recently been used for hypoxia–ischemia (154–156). Meier et al. (156) induced a cerebral infarct in a neonatal rat model by occluding the carotid artery with resulting contralateral hemiparesis. Human mononuclear cells derived from the umbilical cord were injected at 8 days of life in the peritoneum. These cells migrated to the brain, especially to the damaged area improving the hemiparesis. Borlongan et al. (155) stated that it might not be necessary to directly administer the cells into the brain parenchyma, as long as their secreted molecules cross the brain–blood barrier.

Recently, Comi et al. (157) developed an immature mouse model of stroke with acute seizures and ischemic brain injury. Postnatal day 12 CD1 mice received right-sided carotid ligation. Two or 7 days after ligation, mice received an intrastriatal injection of B5 embryonic stem cell–derived neural stem cells. Four weeks after ligation, hemispheric brain atrophy was measured. Pups receiving stem cells 2 days after ligation had less severe hemispheric brain atrophy compared with either noninjected or vehicle-injected ligated controls. Transplanted cells survived, but 3 out of 10 pups injected with stem cells developed local tumors. No difference in hemispheric brain atrophy was seen in mice injected with stem cells 7 days after ligation. Neural stem cells have the potential to ameliorate ischemic injury in the immature brain, although tumor development is a serious concern.

SUMMARY

HIE develops following perinatal asphyxia, which is a multiorgan system disease. The mechanisms of neuronal damage in HIE are multifactorial and include the participation of circulatory factors (dysregulation of the cerebral blood flow), metabolic factors (increased anaerobic metabolism, decreased ATP, hypoglycemia, hyperlactacidemia), biochemical factors (increased excitatory amino acids, intracellular accumulation of calcium, dysfunction of calcium-binding proteins, activation of nitric oxide synthesis, production of free radicals), and apoptotic factors (pro- and anti-apoptotic proteins, apoptotic factor-1, caspases and caspase-activated DNase). These mechanisms of HIE are the basis for the development of new neuroprotective therapies aimed at preventing neuronal damage. Agents that have suggested in clinical studies efficacy in human newborns include magnesium sulfate, allopurinol, and hypothermia. Strategies for preventing or treating perinatal asphyxia/HIE should explore the efficacy of combination therapies. Future treatments that hold promise or offer a novel approach for treating hypoxia–ischemia are selective nNOS inhibitors, immunization against the NMDA receptor, gene therapy with antiapoptotic agents (Bcl-2), calcium-binding proteins (calbindin-D_{28K}) or growth factors, and stem cells transplant. The treatment of HIE needs concerted effort to develop neuroprotective strategies against perinatal brain damage.

ACKNOWLEDGMENTS

The work was supported by grants from the National Institutes of Health, grant numbers NIH-HD R01-20337 and NIH-HD R01-38079.

REFERENCES

1. Raichle ME. The pathophysiology of brain ischemia. *Ann Neurol* 1983;13:2–10.
2. Vannucci RC. Experimental biology of cerebral hypoxia–ischemia: relation to perinatal brain damage. *Pediatr Res* 1990;27:317–326.
3. Mishra OP, Delivoria-Papadopoulos M. Cellular mechanisms of hypoxic injury in the developing brain. *Brain Res Bull* 1999;48: 233–328.
4. Delivoria-Papadopoulos M, Mishra OP. Mechanisms of cerebral injury in perinatal asphyxia and strategies for prevention. *J Pediatr* 1998;132:S30–S34.
5. Mishra OP, Fritz KI, Delivoria-Papadopoulos M. NMDA receptor and neonatal hypoxic brain injury. *Ment Retard Dev Disabil Res Rev* 2001;7:249–253.
6. Legido A, Katsetos CD, Mishra OP, et al. Perinatal hypoxic ischemic encephalopathy: current and future treatments. *Int Pediatr* 2001;15:143–151.
7. Miller SP, Ramaswamy V, Michelson D, et al. Patterns of brain injury in term neonatal encephalopathy. *J Pediatr* 2005;146: 453–460.
8. Tan S, Parks DA. Preserving brain function during neonatal asphyxia. *Clin Perinatol* 1999;26:733–747.
9. du Plessis AJ, Volpe JJ. Perinatal brain injury in the preterm and term newborn. *Curr Opin Neurol* 2002;15:151–157.
10. McLean C, Ferriero D. Mechanisms of hypoxic-ischemic injury in the term infant. *Semin Perinatol* 2004;28:425–432.
11. Johnston MV. Excitotoxicity in perinatal brain injury. *Brain Pathol* 2005;15:234–240.
12. Legido A, Valencia I, Katsetos CD, et al. Neuroprotection in perinatal hypoxic-ischemic encephalopathy. Effective treatments and future perspectives. *Medicina (B Aires)* 2007;67:543–555.
13. Volpe J. Hypoxic-ischemic encephalopathy. In: Volpe J, ed. *Neurology of the newborn*, 5th ed. Philadelphia, PA: Saunders Elsevier, 2008:247–480.
14. Hill A. Hypoxic–ischemic cerebral injury in the newborn. In: Swaiman KF, Ashwal S, Ferriero DM, eds. *Pediatric neurology. Principles and practice*, 4th ed. Philadelphia, PA: Mosby Elsevier, 2006:279–295.
15. Piazza AJ. Postasphyxial management of the newborn. *Clin Perinatol* 1999;26:749–765.
16. Martin-Ancel A, Garcia-Alix A, Gaya F, et al. Multiple organ involvement in perinatal asphyxia. *J Pediatr* 1995;127:786–793.
17. Vanucci RC, Perlman JM. Interventions for perinatal hypoxic–ischemic encephalopathy. *Pediatrics* 1997;100:1004–1014.
18. Levene MI. Management of the asphyxiated full term infant. *Arch Dis Child* 1993;68:612–616.
19. McDonald JW, Silverstein FS, Johnston MV. Magnesium reduces *N*-methyl-D-aspartate (NMDA)-mediated brain injury in perinatal rats. *Neurosci Lett* 1990;109:234–238.
20. Hoffmann DJ, Marro PJ, McGowan JE, et al. Protective effect of $MgSO_4$ infusion on NMDA receptor binding characteristics during cerebral cortical hypoxia in the newborn piglet. *Brain Res* 1994;644:144–149.
21. Maulik D, Zanelli S, Numagami Y, et al. Oxygen free radical generation during *in-utero* hypoxia in the fetal guinea pig brain: the effects of maturity and of magnesium sulfate administration. *Brain Res* 1999;817:117–122.
22. Maulik D, Qayyum I, Powell SR, et al. Post-hypoxic magnesium decreases nuclear oxidative damage in the fetal guinea pig brain. *Brain Res* 2001;890:130–136.

23. Marrett S, Gressens P, Gadisseux JF, et al. Prevention by magnesium of excitotoxic neuronal death in the developing brain: an animal model of clinical intervention studies. *Dev Med Child Neurol* 1995;37:473–484.
24. de Hann HH, Gunn AJ, Williams CE, et al. Magnesium sulphate therapy during asphyxia in near term lambs does not compromise the fetus but does not reduce cerebral injury. *Am J Obstet Gynecol* 1997;176:18–27.
25. Penrice J, Amess P, Punwani S, et al. Magnesium sulphate after transient hypoxia–ischemia fails to prevent delayed cerebral energy failure in the newborn piglet. *Pediatr Res* 1997;41:443–449.
26. Levene MI, Evans DJ, Mason S, et al. An international network for evaluating neuroprotective therapy after severe birth asphyxia. *Semin Perinatol* 1999;23:226–233.
27. Nelson KB, Grether JK. Can magnesium sulphate reduce the risk of cerebral palsy in very low birthweight infants? *Pediatrics* 1995;95:263–269.
28. The Eclampsia Trial Collaborative Group. Which anticonvulsant for women with eclampsia? Evidence from the Collaborative Eclampsia Trial. *Lancet* 1995;345:1455–1463.
29. Mittendorf R, Covert R, Boman J, et al. Is tocolytic magnesium sulphate associated with increased total pediatric mortality? *Lancet* 1997;350:1517–1519.
30. Benichou J, Zupan V, Fernandez H, et al. Tocolytic magnesium sulphate and paediatric mortality. *Lancet* 1997;351:290–291.
31. Rouse D, Hirtz DG, Thom E, et al. A randomized, controlled trial of magnesium sulfate for the prevention of cerebral palsy. *N Engl J Med* 2008;359:895–905.
32. Moriette G, Barrat J, Truffert P, et al. Effect of magnesium sulphate on mortality and neurologic morbidity of the very preterm newborn (of less than 33 weeks) with two-year neurological outcome: results of the prospective PREMAG trial. *Gynecol Obstet Fertil* 2008;36:278–288.
33. Doyle LW, Crowther CA, Middleton P, et al. Magnesium sulphate for women at risk of preterm birth for neuroprotection of the fetus. *Cochrane Database Syst Rev* 2009;(1):CD004661.
34. Palmer C, Vanucci RC, Towfighi J. Reduction of perinatal hypoxic–ischemic brain damage with allopurinol. *Pediatr Res* 1990;27:332–336.
35. Williams GD, Palmer C, Heitjan DF, et al. Allopurinol preserves cerebral energy metabolism during perinatal hypoxic–ischemia: a 31P NMR study in anaesthetized immature rats. *Neurosci Lett* 1992;144:103–106.
36. Palmer C, Roberts RL. Reduction of perinatal brain damage with oxypurinol treatment after hypoxic–ischemic injury. *Pediatr Res* 1991;29:362A.
37. Marro PJ, McGowan JE, Razdan B, et al. Effect of allopurinol on uric acid levels and brain cell membrane Na^+, K^+-ATPase activity during hypoxia in newborn piglets. *Brain Res* 1994;650:9–15.
38. Marro PJ, Hoffman D, Schneiderman R, et al. Effect of allopurinol on NMDA receptor modification following recurrent asphyxia in newborn piglets. *Brain Res* 1998;787:71–77.
39. Russell GA, Cooke RW. Randomized controlled trial of allopurinol prophylaxis in very preterm infants. *Arch Dis Child Fetal Neonatal Ed* 1995;73:F27–F31.
40. Van Bel F, Shadid M, Moison RM, et al. Effect of allopurinol on postasphyxial free radical formation, cerebral hemodynamics, and electrical brain activity. *Pediatrics* 1998;101:185–193.
41. Clancy RR, McGaurn SA, Goin JE, et al. Allopurinol neurocardiac protection trial in infants undergoing heart surgery using deep hypothermic circulatory arrest. *Pediatrics* 2001;108:61–70.
42. Benders MJ, Bos AF, Rademaker CM, et al. Early postnatal allopurinol does not improve short term outcome after severe birth asphyxia. *Arch Dis Child Fetal Neonatal Ed* 2006;91:F163–F165.
43. Chaudhari T, McGuire W. Allopurinol for preventing mortality and morbidity in newborn infants with suspected hypoxic-ischaemic encephalopathy. *Cochrane Database Syst Rev* 2008;(2): CD006817.
44. Lee J, Kim MS, Park C, et al. Morphine prevents glutamate-induced death of primary rat neonatal astrocytes through modulation of intracellular redox. *Immunopharmacol Immunotoxicol* 2004;26:17–28.
45. Yamakura T, Sakimura K, Shimoji K. Direct inhibition of the N-methyl-D-aspartate receptor channel by high concentration of opioids. *Anesthesiology* 1999;91:1053–1063.
46. Zhang J, Gibney GT, Zhao P, et al. Neuroprotective role of delta-opioid receptors in cortical neurons. *Am J Physiol* 2002;282: C1225–C1234.
47. Zhang J, Haddad GG, Xia Y. Delta-, but not mu- and kappa-, opioid receptor activation protects neocortical neurons from glutamate-induced excitotoxic injury. *Brain Res* 2000;8856:143–153.
48. Lim YJ, Zheng S, Zuo Z. Morphine preconditions Purkinje cells against cell death under in vitro simulated ischemia-reperfusion conditions. *Anesthesiology* 2004;100:562–568.
49. Mayfield KP, D'Alecy LG. Role of endogenous opioid peptides in the acute adaptation to hypoxia. *Brain Res* 1992;582:226–231.
50. Mayfield KP, D'Alecy LG. Delta-1 opioid agonist acutely increases hypoxic tolerance. *J Pharmacol Exp Ther* 1994;268: 683–688.
51. Chien S, Oeltgen PR, Diana JN, et al. Extension of tissue survival time in multiorgan block preparation with a delta DADLE ([D-Ala2, D-leu5]-enkephalin). *J Thorac Cardiovasc Surg* 1994; 107:964–967.
52. Angeles DM, Wycliffe N, Michelson D, et al. Use of opioids in asphyxiated term neonates: effects of neuroimaging and clinical outcome. *Pediatr Res* 2005;57:873–878.
53. Angeles DM, Ashwal S, Wycliffe ND, et al. Relationship between opioid therapy, tissue-damaging procedures, and brain metabolites as measured by proton MRS in asphyxiated term neonates. *Pediatr Res* 2007;61:614–621.
54. Gunn AJ, Gunn TR. The "pharmacology" of neuronal rescue with cerebral hypothermia. *Early Hum Dev* 1998;53:19–35.
55. Wagner CL, Eicher DJ, Katikaneni LD, et al. The use of hypothermia: a role in the treatment of neonatal asphyxia? *Pediatr Neurol* 1999;21:429–443.
56. Coimbra C, Wieloch T. Moderate hypothermia mitigates neuronal damage in the rat brain when initiated several hours following transient cerebral ischemia. *Acta Neuropathol (Berlin)* 1994;87:325–331.
57. Trescher WH, Ishiwa S, Johnston MV. Brief post-HI hypothermia markedly delays neonatal brain injury. *Brain Dev* 1997;19:326–328.
58. Thorensen M, Penrice J, Lorek A. Mild hypothermia after severe transient hypoxia–ischemia ameliorates delayed cerebral energy failure in the newborn piglet. *Pediatr Res* 1995;37:667–670.
59. Miller JA. New approaches to preventing brain damage during asphyxia. *Am J Obstet Gynecol* 1971;110:125–132.
60. Gunn AJ, Bennet L, Gunning MI, et al. Cerebral hypothermia is not neuroprotective when started after postischemic seizures in fetal sheep. *Pediatr Res* 1999;46:274–280.
61. Gunn AJ, Gluckman PD, Gunn TR. Selective head cooling in newborn infants after perinatal asphyxia: a safety study. *Pediatrics* 1998;102:885–892.
62. Battin MR, Dezoete JA, Gunn TR, et al. Neurodevelopmental outcome of infants treated with head cooling and mild hypothermia after perinatal asphyxia. *Pediatrics* 2001;107:480–484.
63. Battin MR, Penrice J, Gunn TR, et al. Treatment of term infants with head cooling and systemic hypothermia (35.0 degrees C and 34.5 degrees C) after perinatal asphyxia. *Pediatrics* 2003;111: 244–251.
64. Gluckman PD, Wyatt JS, Azzopardi D, et al. Selective head cooling with mild systemic hypothermia after neonatal encephalopathy: multicenter randomized trial. *Lancet* 2005;365:663–670.
65. Azzopardi D, Robertson NJ, Cowan FM, et al. Pilot study of treatment with whole body hypothermia for neonatal encephalopathy. *Pediatrics* 2000;106:684–694.
66. Shankaran S, Laptook A, Wright LL, et al. Whole-body hypothermia for neonatal encephalopathy: animal observations as a basis for randomized, controlled pilot study in term infants. *Pediatrics* 2002;110:377–385.
67. Compagnoni G, Pogliani L, Lista G, et al. Hypothermia reduces neurological damage in asphyxiated newborn infants. *Biol Neonate* 2002;82:222–227.
68. Debillon T, Daoud P, Durand P, et al. Whole-body cooling after perinatal asphyxia: a study in term neonates. *Dev Med Child Neurol* 2003;45:17–23.
69. Eicher DJ, Wagner CL, Katikaneni LP, et al. Moderate hypothermia in neonatal encephalopathy: safety outcomes. *Pediatr Neurol* 2005;32:18–24.
70. Eicher DJ, Wagner CL, Katikaneni LP, et al. Moderate hypothermia in neonatal encephalopathy: efficacy outcomes. *Pediatr Neurol* 2005;32:11–17.

71. Shankaran S, Laptook AR, Ehrenkranz RA, et al. Whole-body hypothermia for neonates with hypoxic-ischemic encephalopathy. *N Engl J Med* 2005;353:1574–1584.
72. Parikh NA, Lasky RE, Garza CN, et al. Volumetric and anatomical MRI hypoxic-ischemic encephalopathy: relationship to hypothermia therapy and neurosensory impairments. *J Perinatol* 2009;29:143–149.
73. Zanelli SA, Naylor M, Dobbins N, et al. Implementation of a "hypothermia for HIE" program: 2-year experience in a single NICU. *J Perinatol* 2008;28:171–175.
74. Kapetanakis A, Azzopardi D, Wyatt J, et al. Therapeutic hypothermia for neonatal encephalopathy: a UK survey of opinion, practice and neuron-investigation at the end of 2007 [online publication ahead of print]. *Acta Paediatr* 2009;98:631–635.
75. Gunn AJ, Battin M, Gluckman PD, et al. Therapeutic hypothermia: from lab to NICU. *J Perinat Med* 2005;33:340–346.
76. Gunn AJ, Thoresen M. Hypothermic neuroprotection. *NeuroRx* 2006;3:154–169.
77. Shankaran S, Laptook A. Challenge of conducting trials of neuroprotection in the asphyxiated term infant. *Semin Perinatol* 2003;27:320–332.
78. Wyatt JS, Robertson NJ. Time for a cool head-neuroprotection becomes a reality. *Early Hum Dev* 2005;81:5–11.
79. Edwards AD, Azzopardi DV. Therapeutic hypothermia following asphyxia. *Arch Dis Fetal Neonatal Ed* 2006;91:F127–F131.
80. Sahni R, Sanocka UM. Hypothermia for hypoxic-ischemic encephalopathy. *Clin Perinatol* 2008;35:717–734.
81. Wagner BP, Nedelcu J, Martin E. Delayed postischemic hypothermia improves long-term behavioral outcome after cerebral hypoxia-ischemia in neonatal rats. *Pediatr Res* 2002;51:354–360.
82. Ma D, Hossain M, Chow A, et al. Xenon and hypothermia combine to provide neuroprotection from neonatal asphyxia. *Ann Neurol* 2005;58:182–193.
83. Iwata O, Thornton JS, Sellwood MW, et al. Depth of delayed cooling alters neuroprotection pattern after hypoxia-ischemia. *Ann Neurol* 2005;58:75–87.
84. Kanagawa T, Fukuda H, Tsbouchi H, et al. A decrease of cell proliferation by hypothermia in the hippocampus of the neonatal rat. *Brain Res* 2006;1111:36–40.
85. Hoeger H, Engidawork E, Stolzlechner D, et al. Long-term effect of moderate and profound hypothermia on morphology, neurological, cognitive and behavioural functions in a rat model of perinatal asphyxia. *Amino Acids* 2006;31:385–396.
86. Talati AJ, Yang W, Yolton K, et al. Combination of early perinatal factors to identify near-term and term neonates for neuroprotection. *J Perinatol* 2005;25:245–250.
87. Ambalavanan N, Carlo WA, Shankaran S, et al. Predicting outcomes of neonates diagnosed with hypoxemic-ischemic encephalopathy. *Pediatrics* 2006;118:2084–2093.
88. Schifrin BS, Ater S. Fetal hypoxic and ischemic injuries. *Curr Opin Obstet Gynecol* 2006;18:112–122.
89. van Bel F, Groenendaal F. Long-term pharmacologic neuroprotection after birth asphyxia: where do we stand? *Neonatology* 2008;94:203–210.
90. Higgins RD, Rahu TN, Perlman J, et al. Hypothermia and perinatal asphyxia: executive summary of the National Institute of Child Health and Human Development workshop. *J Pediatr* 2006; 148:170–175.
91. Moshé SL. Neuroprotection and epilepsy. *Medscape.* January 19, 2000:1–12. http://www.medscape.com.
92. Pitkänen A. Efficacy of current antiepileptics to prevent neurodegeneration in epilepsy models. *Epilepsy Res* 2002;50:141–160.
93. Calabresi P, Cupini LM, Centonze D, et al. Antiepileptic drugs as a possible neuroprotective strategy in ischemia. *Ann Neurol* 2003;53:693–702.
94. Leker RR, Neufeld MY. Anti-epileptic drugs as possible neuroprotectants in cerebral ischemia. *Brain Res Brain Res Rev* 2003;42: 187–203.
95. Sankar R. Neuroprotection in epilepsy: the Holy Grail of antiepileptic therapy. *Epilepsy Behav* 2005;7(Suppl 3):S1–S2.
96. Wilmore LJ. Antiepileptic drugs and neuroprotection: current status and future roles. *Epilepsy Behav* 2005;7(Suppl 3):S25–S28.
97. Valencia I, Legido A. Prevention of epilepsy. In: Benjamin SM, ed. *Focus on epilepsy research.* Hauppauge, NY: Nova Biomedical Books, 2004:1–21.
98. Wyllie E, Gupta A, Lachhwani DK, eds. *The treatment of epilepsy. Principles and practice.* Philadelphia, PA: Lippincott Williams & Wilkins, 2006.
99. Traystman RJ, Klaus JA, DeVries AC, et al. Anticonvulsant lamotrigine administered on reperfusion fails to improve experimental stroke outcomes. *Stroke* 2001;32:783–787.
100. Lee WT, Shen YZ, Chang C. Neuroprotective effect of lamotrigine and MK-801 on rat brain lesions induced by 3-nitropropionic acid: evaluation by magnetic resonance imaging and in vivo proton magnetic spectroscopy. *Neuroscience* 2000;95:89–95.
101. Smith SE, Meldrum BS. Cerebroprotective effect of lamotrigine after focal ischemia in rats. *Stroke* 1995;26:117–121.
102. Wiard RP, Dickerson MC, Beek O, et al. Neuroprotective properties of the novel antiepileptic lamotrigine in a gerbil model of global cerebral ischemia. *Stroke* 1995;26:466–472.
103. Shuaib A, Mahmood RH, Wishart T, et al. Neuroprotective effects of lamotrigine in global ischemia in gerbils. A histological, in vivo microdialysis and behavioural study. *Brain Res* 1995;702:199–206.
104. Crumrine RC, Bergstrand K, Cooper AT, et al. Lamotrigine protects hippocampal CA1 neurons from ischemic damage after cardiac arrest. *Stroke* 1997;28:2230–2237.
105. Papazisis G, Kallaras K, Kaiki-Astara A, et al. Neuroprotection by lamotrigine in a rat model of neonatal hypoxic-ischaemic encephalopathy. *Int J Neuropscyhopharmacol* 2008;11:321–329.
106. Lee YS, Yoon BW, Roth JK. Neuroprotective effect of lamotrigine enhanced by flunarizine in gerbil global ischemia. *Neurosci Lett* 1999;265:215–217.
107. Koinig H, Morimoto Y, Zornow MH. The combination of lamotrigine and mild hypothermia prevents ischemia-induced increase in hippocampal glutamate. *J Neurosurg Anethesiol* 2001; 13:106–112.
108. Yang Y, Shuaib B, Li Q, et al. Neuroprotection by delayed administration of topiramate in a rat model of middle cerebral artery embolization. *Brain Res* 1998;804:169–176.
109. Yang Y, Li Q, Miyashita H, et al. Usefulness of postischemic thrombolysis with or without neuroprotection in a focal embolic model of cerebral ischemia. *J Neurosurg* 2000;92:841–847.
110. Lee SR, Kim SOP, Kim JE. Protective effect of topiramate against hippocampal neuronal damage after global ischemia in the gerbils. *Neurosci Lett* 2000;281:183–186.
111. Niebauer M, Gruenthal M. Topiramate reduces neuronal injury after experimental status epilepticus. *Brain Res* 1999;837:263–269.
112. Koh S, Jensen FE. Topiramate blocks perinatal hypoxia-induced seizures in rat pups. *Ann Neurol* 2001;50:366–372.
113. Schubert S, Brandl U, Brodhun M, et al. Neuroprotective effects of topiramate after hypoxia-ischemia in newborn piglets. *Brain Res* 2005;1958:129–136.
114. Follett PL, Deng W, Dai W, et al. Glutamate receptor-mediated oligodendrocyte toxicity in periventricular leukomalacia: a protective role for topiramate. *J Neurosci* 2004;24:4412–4420.
115. Sfaello I, Baud O, Arzimanoglou A, et al. Topiramate prevents excitotoxic damage in the newborn rodent brain. *Neurobiol Dis* 2005;20:837–848.
116. Glier C, Dzietto M, Bittigau P, et al. Therapeutic doses of topiramate are not toxic to the developing brain. *Exp Neurol* 2004;187: 403–409.
117. Minato H, Kikuta C, Fujitani B, et al. Protective effect of zonisamide, an antiepileptic drug, against transient focal cerebral ischemia with middle cerebral artery occlusion-reperfusion in rats. *Epilepsia* 1997;38:975–980.
118. Owen AJ, Ijaz S, Miyashita H, et al. Zonisamide as a neuroprotective agent in an adult gerbil model of global forebrain ischemia: a histological, in vivo microdialysis and behavioral study. *Brain Res* 1997;770:115–122.
119. Hayakawa T, Higuchi Y, Nigami H, et al. Zonisamide reduces hypoxic-ischemic brain damage in neonatal rats irrespective of its anticonvulsant effect. *Eur J Pharmacol* 1994;257:131–136.
120. Hanon E, Klitgaard H. Neuroprotective properties of the novel antiepileptic drug levetiracetam in the rat middle cerebral artery occlusion model of focal cerebral ischemia. *Seizure* 2001; 10:287–293.
121. Klitgaard HV, Matagne AC, Vanneste-Goemare J, et al. Effects of prolonged administration of levetiracetam on pilocarpine-induced epileptogenesis. *Epilepsia* 2001;42(Suppl 7):114–115.

122. Dawson TM, Zhang J, Dawson VL, et al. Nitric oxide: cellular regulation and neuronal injury. *Prog Brain Res* 1994;103:365–369.
123. Mishra OP, Zanelli SA, Ohnishi ST, et al. Hypoxia-induced generation of nitric oxide free radicals in cerebral cortex of newborn guinea pigs. *Neurochem Res* 2000;25:1559–1565.
124. Numagami Y, Zubrow AB, Mishra OP, et al. Lipid free radical generation and brain cell membrane alteration following nitric oxide synthase inhibition during cerebral hypoxia in the newborn piglet. *J Neurochem* 1997;69:1542–1547.
125. Zanelli SA, Ashraf QM, Mishra OP. Nitration is a mechanism of regulation of the NMDA receptor function during hypoxia. *Neuroscience* 2002;112:869–877.
126. Zubrow AB, Delivoria-Papadopoulos M, Ashraf QM, et al. Nitric oxide-mediated Ca^{++}/calmodulin-dependent protein kinase IV activity during hypoxia in neuronal nuclei from newborn piglets. *Neurosci Lett* 2002;335:5–8.
127. Zubrow AB, Delivoria-Papadopoulos M, Ashraf QM, et al. Nitric oxide-mediated expression of Bax protein and DNA fragmentation during hypoxia in neuronal nuclei from newborn piglets. *Brain Res* 2002;954:60–67.
128. Mishra OP, Ashraf QM, Delivoria-Papadopoulos M. Phosphorylation of cAMP response element binding (CREB) protein during hypoxia in cerebral cortex of newborn piglets and the effect of nitric oxide synthase inhibition. *Neuroscience* 2002;115: 985–991.
129. Mishra OP, Delivoria-Papadopoulos M. Nitric oxide-mediated Ca^{++}-influx in neuronal nuclei and cortical synaptosomes of normoxic and hypoxic newborn piglets. *Neurosci Lett* 2002;318:93–97.
130. Forstermann U, Boissel JP, Kleinert H. Expressional control of the “constitutive” isoforms of nitric oxide synthase (NOS I and NOS III). *FASEB J* 1998;12:773–790.
131. Shaul PW, North AJ, Brannon TS, et al. Prolonged *in vivo* hypoxia enhances nitric oxide synthase type I and type III gene expression in adult rat lung. *Am J Respir Cell Mol Biol* 1995;13: 167–174.
132. Zhang ZG, Chopp M, Gautam S, et al. Upregulation of neuronal nitric oxide synthase and mRNA, and selective sparing of nitric oxide synthase-containing neurons after focal cerebral ischemia in rat. *Brain Res* 1994;654:85–95.
133. Bhat GK, Mahesh VB, Lamar CA, et al. Histochemical localization of nitric oxide neurons in the hypothalamus: association with gonadotropin-releasing hormone neurons and co-localization with *N*-methyl-D-aspartate receptors. *Neuroendocrinol Lett* 1997; 62:187–197.
134. Kiedrowski L, Costa E, Wroblewski JT. Glutamate receptor agonists stimulate nitric oxide synthase in primary cultures of cerebellar granule cells. *J Neurochem* 1992;58:335–341.
135. Aoki C, Fenstemaker K, Lubin M, et al. Nitric oxide synthase in the visual cortex of monocular monkey as revealed by light and electron microscopic immunocytochemistry. *Brain Res* 1993;620: 97–113.
136. Christopherson KS, Hillier BJ, Lim WA, et al. PDS-95 assembles a ternary complex with the *N*-methyl-D-aspartic acid receptor and a bivalent neuronal NO synthase PDX domain. *J Biol Chem* 1999;274:27467–27473.
137. Delivoria-Papadopoulos M, Akhter W, Mishra OP. Hypoxia induced Ca^{++}-influx in cerebral cortical neuronal nuclei of newborn piglets. *Neurosci Lett* 2003;342:119–123.
138. Gavini G, Zanelli SA, Ashraf QM, et al. Effect of nitric oxide synthase inhibition on high affinity Ca^{++}-ATPase during hypoxia in cerebral cortical neuronal nuclei of newborn piglets. *Brain Res* 2000;887:385–390.
139. Mishra OP, Qayyum I, Delivoria-Papadopoulos M. Hypoxia-induced modification of the inositol triphosphate (IP_3) receptor in neuronal nuclei of newborn piglets: the role of nitric oxide. *J Neurosci Res* 2003;74:333–338.
140. Ravishankar S, Ashraf QM, Fritz K, et al. Expression of Bax and Bcl-2 proteins during hypoxia in cerebral cortical neuronal nuclei of newborn piglets: effect of administration of magnesium sulfate. *Brain Res* 2001;901:23–29.
141. Akhter W, Zanelli SA, Gavini G, et al. Effect of graded hypoxia on cerebral cortical genomic DNA fragmentation in newborn piglets. *Biol Neonate* 2001;79:187–193.
142. During MJ, Symes CW, Lawlor PA, et al. An oral vaccine against NMDARI with efficacy in experimental stroke and epilepsy. *Science* 2000;287:1453–1460.
143. Millan M, Arenillas J. Gene expression in cerebral ischemia: a new approach for neuroprotection. *Cerebrovasc Dis* 2006;21(Supl 2): 30–37.
144. Yenari MA, Minami M, Huan Sun G, et al. Calbindin D28 K overexpression protects striatal neurons from transient focal cerebral ischemia. *Stroke* 2001;32:1028–1035.
145. Linnik MD, Zahos P, Geschwind MD, et al. Expression of bcl2 from a defective herpes simplex virus-1 vector limits neuronal death in focal cerebral ischemia. *Stroke* 1995;26:1670–1674.
146. Jia WW, Wang Y, Qiang D, et al. A bcl-2 expressing viral vector protects cortical neurons from excitotoxicity even when administered several hours after the toxic insult. *Brain Res Mol Brain Res* 1996;42:350–353.
147. Sasaki T, Kitagawa K, Yagita Y, et al. Bcl2 enhances survival of newborn neurons in the normal and ischemic hippocampus. *J Neurosci Res* 2006;84:1187–1196.
148. Shen F, Su H, Fan Y, et al. Adeno-associated viral vector mediated hypoxia-inducible vascular endothelial growth factor gene expression attenuates ischemic brain injury after focal cerebral ischemia in mice. *Stroke* 2006;37:2601–2606.
149. Tai YT, Svendsen CN. Stem cells as a potential treatment of neurological disorders. *Curr Opin Pharmacol* 2004;4:98–104.
150. Longhi L, Zanier ER, Royo N, et al. Stem cell transplantation as a therapeutic strategy for traumatic brain injury. *Transpl Immunol* 2005;15:143–148.
151. Qu SQ, Luan Z, Yin GC, et al. Transplantation of human fetal neural stem cells into cerebral ventricle of the neonatal rat following hypoxic-ischemic injury: survival, migration and differentiation. *Zhonghua Er Ke Za Zhi* 2005;43:576–579.
152. Zheng T, Rossignol C, Leibovici A, et al. Transplantation of multipotent astrocytic stem cells into a rat model of neonatal hypoxic-ischemic encephalopathy. *Brain Res* 2006;1112:99–105.
153. Yasuhara T, Matsukawa N, Yu G, et al. Transplantation of cryopreserved human bone marrow-derived multipotent adult progenitor cells for neonatal hypoxic-ischemic injury: targeting the hippocampus. *Rev Neurosci* 2006;17:215–225.
154. Jensen A, Vaihinger HM, Meier C. Perinatal brain damage-from neuroprotection to neurodegeneration using cord blood stem cells. *Med Klin (Munich)* 2003;98(Suppl 2):22–26.
155. Borlongan CV, Hadman M, Sanberg CD, et al. Central nervous system entry of peripherally injected umbilical cord blood cells is not required for neuroprotection in stroke. *Stroke* 2004;35:2385–2389.
156. Meier C, Middelanis J, Wasielewski B, et al. Spastic paresis after perinatal brain damage in rats is reduced by human cord blood mononuclear cells. *Pediatr Res* 2006;59:244–249.
157. Comi AM, Cho E, Mulholland JD, et al. Neural stem cells reduce brain injury after unilateral carotid ligation. *Pediatr Neurol* 2008; 38:86–92.

CHAPTER

22

Mark Mirochnick
Brookie M. Best

Antiretroviral Pharmacology in Pregnant Women and Newborns

INTRODUCTION

As infection with human immunodeficiency virus (HIV) continues to spread throughout the world, HIV/AIDS has become a major contributor to global morbidity and mortality. At the end of 2007, 33 million people worldwide were estimated to be living with HIV infection, of whom nearly half are women of childbearing age and 2.0 million are children under the age of 15 years, most of whom acquired HIV infection from mother-to-child transmission (1). Worldwide deaths from AIDS in 2007 were estimated at 2.0 million people, including 290,000 children. Although the number of new HIV infections worldwide likely peaked in the late 1990s at an estimated rate of 3.0 million people per year, in 2007 an estimated 2.7 million people were still newly infected, including 370,000 children (1). Those children who escape mother-to-child HIV transmission may still suffer from the AIDS epidemic. The number of children in sub-Saharan Africa who had lost one or both parents because of AIDS was estimated at 11.4 million in 2007 (1).

INDICATIONS FOR THE USE OF ANTIRETROVIRALS IN HIV-INFECTED PREGNANT AND POSTPARTUM WOMEN AND THEIR NEONATES

Much progress has been made in recent years in treating HIV infection. Currently, more than 20 antiretroviral drugs in five classes are available in the United States (Table 22.1) and new drugs are in development. The use of combination regimens of three or more antiretrovirals, often referred to as highly active antiretroviral therapy (HAART), has resulted in dramatic improvements in HIV morbidity and mortality. However, while antiretroviral therapy improves the health and prolongs the lives of HIV-infected patients, it does not eradicate the virus or cure the infection. Once initiated, antiretroviral therapy generally continues for life. Because of the long asymptomatic phase that generally follows HIV infection, the lifelong duration of antiretroviral treatment, the side effects and toxicities of the drugs, and the frequent development of viral resistance resulting in loss of antiretroviral efficacy, clinical criteria have been established to determine when antiretroviral therapy should be initiated. Guidelines have been published outlining these criteria for the initiation of antiretroviral therapy in HIV-infected adults and children living in areas where the availability of medical resources permits wide-scale access to antiretroviral therapy and in resource poor areas with limited access (2–4). Both sets of adult guidelines recommend initiation of antiretroviral therapy in HIV-infected pregnant women according to the same criteria as those used in nonpregnant adults.

Antiretroviral therapy may also be used in pregnant women for prevention of mother-to-child HIV transmission in those women whose HIV disease is not sufficiently advanced to meet the clinical criteria for initiation of antiretroviral therapy. HIV can be passed from mother to child in three ways: across the placenta during pregnancy (transplacental), from exposure during labor and delivery to maternal blood and other bodily fluids (intrapartum), and from breast milk during nursing (5). In the absence of treatment, 15% to 45% of HIV-infected pregnant women will pass the infection on to their infants, with 5% to 10% of infants born to HIV-infected women infected across the placenta, 10% to 20% infected from exposure at or around the time of delivery, and 10% to 20% infected from breast milk (5).

Effective therapeutic strategies to prevent mother-to-child HIV transmission have been developed. In 1994, the PACTG 076 protocol demonstrated that administration of a zidovudine regimen composed of oral dosing initiated at 14 to 34 weeks' gestation, continuous intravenous infusion during labor, and 6 weeks of oral dosing to the newborn reduced mother-to-child transmission by 67% (transmission rate of 7.6% with zidovudine compared with 22.6% with placebo) (6). The relative importance of the three components (prenatal, intrapartum, and postpartum) of the PACTG 076 regimen in reducing mother-to-child transmission has not been fully defined. A retrospective analysis of the use of abbreviated zidovudine regimens in New York State found that zidovudine was most effective if

TABLE 22.1 Pregnancy Dosing Recommendations for anti-HIV Drugs Available for Use in the United States

		FDA Pregnancy Category[a]	*Pregnancy Dosing Recommendations*
Nucleoside/tide reverse transcriptase inhibitors	Abacavir	C	Standard adult dosing
	Didanosine (ddI)	B	Standard adult dosing; avoid use in combination with d4T due to increased risk of lactic acidosis
	Lamivudine (3TC)	C	Standard adult dosing
	Stavudine (d4T)	C	Standard adult dosing; avoid use in combination with ddI due to increased risk of lactic acidosis
	Tenofovir	B	Standard adult dosing
	Zalcitabine (ddC)	C	No pregnancy pharmacokinetic or safety data available
	Zidovudine (ZDV)	C	Standard adult dosing
Nonnucleoside reverse transcriptase inhibitors	Delavirdine	C	Avoid use during pregnancy—no pregnancy pharmacokinetic data available; teratogenic in animal studies
	Efavirenz	D	Avoid use during pregnancy—no pregnancy pharmacokinetic data available; teratogenic in animal studies
	Etravirine	B	No pregnancy pharmacokinetic or safety data available
	Nevirapine	B	Standard adult dosing
Protease inhibitors	Atazanavir	B	Low concentrations with standard dosing during pregnancy. Consider increased dose in second and third trimesters.
	Darunavir	C	No pregnancy pharmacokinetic or safety data available
	Fosamprenavir	C	No pregnancy pharmacokinetic or safety data available
	Indinavir	C	Avoid use as single PI, consider as part of boosted regimen
	Lopinavir	C	Low concentrations with standard dosing during pregnancy. Consider increased dose in second and third trimesters.
	Nelfinavir	B	Low concentrations with standard dosing during pregnancy. Consider increased dose in second and third trimesters.
	Ritonavir	B	Avoid use as single PI, consider as part of boosted regimen
	Saquinavir	B	Avoid use as single PI, consider as part of boosted regimen
Viral entry inhibitors	Enfuvirtide (T-20)	B	No pregnancy pharmacokinetic or safety data available
	Maraviroc	B	No pregnancy pharmacokinetic or safety data available
Integrase inhibitors	Raltegravir	C	No pregnancy pharmacokinetic or safety data available

[a]The Food and Drug Administration (FDA) categories are as follows: A, adequate and well-controlled studies involving pregnant women failed to demonstrate a risk to the fetus during the first trimester of pregnancy (and there is no evidence of risk during the later trimesters); B, reproduction studies in animals failed to demonstrate a risk to the fetus, and adequate and well-controlled studies involving pregnant women have not been conducted; C, safety in human pregnancy has not been determined, studies in animals are either positive for fetal risk or have not been conducted, and the drug should not be used unless the potential benefit outweighs the potential risk to the fetus; D, there is positive evidence of human fetal risk in the form of data regarding adverse reactions from investigational or marketing experiences, but the potential benefits from the use of the drug in pregnant women may be acceptable despite its potential risks; X, studies in animals or reports of adverse reactions have indicated that the risk associated with the use of the drug for pregnant women clearly outweighs any possible benefit.

initiated during pregnancy, reducing transmission from 26.6% to 6.1%, and had decreased efficacy if begun during labor or within 48 hours after birth, reducing transmission to 9% to 10% (7).

Further reductions in mother-to-child HIV transmission have been associated with the use of elective cesarean delivery performed before rupture of membranes and of combination antiretroviral regimens. Elective cesarean reduces the rate of mother-to-child transmission to 2% or less when used in combination with zidovudine (8,9). Administration of combination regimens of multiple antiretrovirals during pregnancy is associated with reductions in the rate of mother-to-child transmission to 1.5% or less in women who do not breast-feed their infants (10–12). Guidelines for the use of antiretroviral drugs to prevent mother-to-child transmission have been developed (13). Although some variation exists among practitioners, the use of combination antiretroviral regimens during pregnancy, elective cesarean section if the HIV RNA level at the time of delivery is not suppressed to below the level of

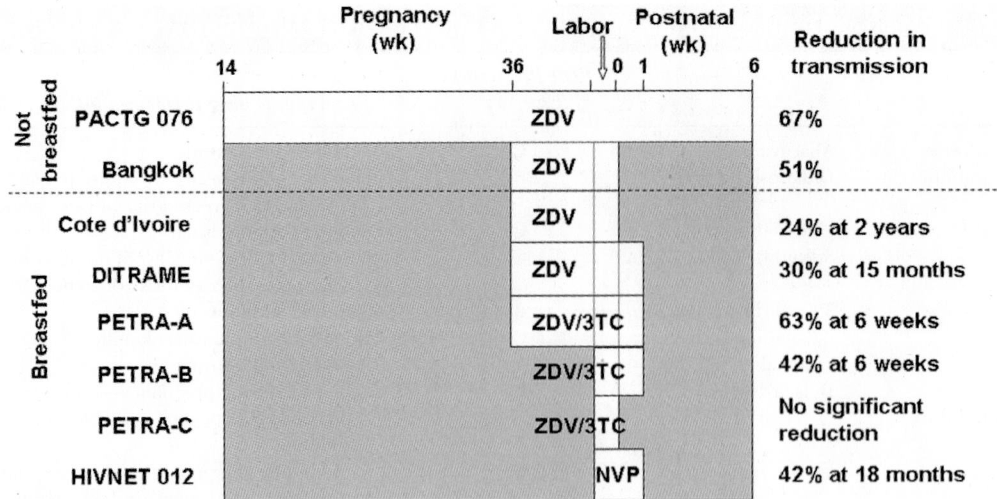

Figure 22.1. Duration of antiretroviral therapy and reduction in mother-to-child HIV transmission. White bar indicates duration of prenatal, intrapartum and/or postnatal dosing. ZDV, zidovudine; 3TC, lamivudine; NVP, nevirapine. From PACTG 076, Wade et al. (7); Bangkok, Shaffer et al. (14); Cote d'Ivoire, Wiktor et al. (15); DITRAME, Dabis et al. (16); PETRA, PETRA Study Team (17); HIVNET 012, Jackson et al. (19).

assay detection, and formula feeding in place of breastfeeding have become standard treatment of HIV-infected pregnant women in areas of the world where medical resources are sufficient to make these interventions readily available.

Unfortunately, those parts of the world most affected by HIV generally lack sufficient health care resources to make these interventions widely available. Less intensive antiretroviral regimens more practical for use in resource poor areas have been developed (3,5) (Fig. 22.1). Shortened zidovudine regimens that start at 36 to 38 weeks of pregnancy, use oral rather than intravenous dosing during labor, and decrease or eliminate postnatal infant dosing have been shown to reduce transmission by 38% to 50%, compared with the 67% reduction seen with the full PACTG 076 regimen (14–16). A short-course regimen combining zidovudine and lamivudine (arm A of the PETRA study—maternal treatment from 36 weeks' gestation through delivery, infant treatment for 1 week after birth) reduced transmission at 6 weeks after birth by 63% compared with placebo (17). Arm B of that study (zidovudine and lamivudine to the mother during labor and to the infant for 1 week after birth) reduced transmission at 6 weeks by 42%, while arm C (intrapartum dosing only) had no impact on transmission (17).

The least intensive, lowest cost antiretroviral regimen shown to be effective in preventing mother-to-child HIV transmission involves two doses of nevirapine—one oral dose to the mother during labor and another oral dose to the infant at 48 to 72 hours after birth. This nevirapine two-dose intrapartum–postnatal regimen reduced mother-to-child HIV transmission by 41% in a breastfeeding population (18,19). In a South African study, mother-to-child transmission at 8 weeks of age was equally low (9% to 12%) with either an abbreviated zidovudine–lamivudine regimen based on arm B of the PETRA study or intrapartum–postnatal nevirapine (20).

In a Thai study, the combination of third trimester zidovudine with intrapartum–postnatal nevirapine and formula feeding resulted in a mother-to-child HIV transmission rate below 2%, nearly equivalent to that seen with the use of HAART during pregnancy (21). The combination of zidovudine starting at 28 weeks' gestation plus intrapartum–postnatal nevirapine is currently recommended by WHO as the first choice antiretroviral regimen for use in resource-constrained settings (22).

In resource-constrained areas where formula feeding is not safe or affordable, prevention of mother-to-child HIV transmission via breast milk remains a major problem. Breastfeeding is the cultural norm in most resource-constrained settings and is critical to infant survival. In a meta-analysis, breastfeeding was associated with a sixfold decrease in mortality due to infectious diseases for infants younger than 2 months (23). If a breastfeeding mother is HIV infected, her infant is at risk of HIV infection from breast milk, with an estimated risk of transmission of 0.6% to 0.9% for every month of breastfeeding (24,25). Breast milk HIV transmission is reduced but not eliminated with exclusive breastfeeding, as opposed to mixed feeding with formula, water, juice, and other liquids or solids in addition to breast milk (26). Preliminary studies of the use of antiretrovirals to prevent breast milk HIV transmission have been reported. Treatment of the lactating mother with combination antiretroviral therapy and the nursing infant with nevirapine both seem to protect against infection of the infant (27–29).

EFFECT OF PREGNANCY ON DRUG DISPOSITION

Maternal physiologic changes associated with pregnancy may have a considerable impact on drug disposition. All four components of drug disposition—absorption, distribution, metabolism, and excretion—may be affected by pregnancy. When antiretrovirals are used during pregnancy, whether for prevention of mother-to-child HIV transmission or treatment of the mother's underlying HIV infection, or both, special consideration must be taken and usual adult dosing may need to be modified.

Pregnancy results in significant changes in gastrointestinal function that may impact drug absorption. Nausea and vomiting, especially pronounced in early pregnancy, may decrease drug absorption. Plasma progesterone increases during pregnancy, associated with a 30% to 50% decrease in intestinal motility and increases in gastric emptying and intestinal transit times (30). The ionization and absorption of weak acids and bases may be affected by increased gastric pH due to a 40% reduction in acid secretion (31). Although these physiologic changes would be expected to result in delayed drug absorption and reduced peak maternal blood concentrations, few studies have evaluated the clinical impact of these changes in a rigorous manner (32).

The profound changes in body composition during pregnancy are well known. During an average pregnancy, total body water increases by 8 L, plasma volume enlarges by 50%, and body fat stores increase, changing volume of distribution of both hydrophilic and lipophilic drugs (33). The dilutional decrease in serum albumin as well as competitive inhibition from steroid hormones results in decreased protein binding (34). As a result of these physiologic changes, volume of distribution generally increases and peak drug concentrations decrease during pregnancy. The decrease in protein binding also results in an increase in the free fraction, or unbound fraction, of drug. Unbound drug is the pharmacologically active drug moiety, available for binding to sites of action and for biotransformation and elimination. The free fraction of many drugs, including theophylline, diazepam, salicylates, and some β-lactam antibiotics, have been shown to increase during pregnancy as a result of changes in protein binding (35–37).

The effect of pregnancy on drug elimination is variable but may be significant. Progesterone may induce hepatic drug metabolic pathways as has been shown for phenytoin (38). Drug metabolism may be reduced due to competition with estrogen and progesterone for metabolic binding sites as has been demonstrated for theophylline and caffeine (39). Renal function increases during pregnancy, with 25% to 50% increases in renal plasma flow and GFR. Clearance of renally excreted drugs, such as ampicillin and gentamicin, and drug metabolites increases during pregnancy (40,41).

Although the disposition of most drugs will be measurably changed by the physiologic changes of pregnancy, the need for dosing adjustment will be determined by the magnitude of these changes and the pharmacokinetic–pharmacodynamic relationship for each drug. Multiple and contradictory effects may coexist (31). Absorption often decreases and volume of distribution and clearance increase, leading to decreased total plasma concentrations, while protein binding decreases, leading to a larger free fraction of drug. Although rigorous pharmacokinetic studies are rare in pregnant women, clinical experience suggests that these effects may be significant. Between one quarter and one-third of pregnant women with epilepsy will have an increase in seizure frequency during pregnancy associated with subtherapeutic drug levels (42). Pregnant women receiving antidepressants often develop increased depressive symptoms and require dose increases to maintain adequate serum drug concentrations during late pregnancy (43). Pharmacokinetic studies are difficult to perform during pregnancy and, until recently, women of reproductive age were excluded from most clinical trials. As a result, published studies of drug disposition in pregnancy are limited, often contradictory and almost always fail to provide clinically relevant guidelines (44). Monitoring of drugs with narrow therapeutic indices, such as phenytoin and theophylline, has been recommended during pregnancy (45). However, routine laboratory drug assays must be interpreted with caution during pregnancy, as they measure total drug concentration, not the free fraction, and therapeutic and toxic effects may occur at lower total concentrations in the face of decreased protein binding.

SAFETY OF ANTIRETROVIRALS DURING PREGNANCY

The current approach to prevention of mother-to-child HIV transmission through the use of antiretrovirals can reduce the rate of mother-to-child HIV transmission below 2% (10,12). The vast majority of fetuses exposed to antiretrovirals during pregnancy will not be infected with HIV, making the safety of these agents for both fetus and mother of paramount importance. The risk or safety of drugs used in pregnancy is difficult to assess. Preclinical drug evaluations include in vitro and animal in vivo studies for carcinogenicity, mutagenicity, and reproductive and teratogenic effects. Direct extrapolation of the results of these preclinical studies to humans is of uncertain value. Of approximately 1,200 known animal teratogens, only about 30 have been shown to be teratogenic in humans (46). However, in at least one case, that of isotretinoin, animal studies demonstrating severe teratogenicity prevented widespread use of this agent in pregnant women and averted a likely epidemic of birth defects (47). Preclinical animal studies are especially concerning for efavirenz, zalcitabine, delavirdine, and tenofovir (see descriptions of the pharmacology of individual antiretroviral agents later) and if possible these agents should be avoided during pregnancy, especially during the first trimester.

Human perinatal phase I, II, and III antiretroviral studies are too small and of too limited duration to adequately assess for adverse effects, especially those effects that are uncommon or first appear outside of infancy. The largest amount of data is available for zidovudine, which has been consistently associated with transient neonatal anemia but otherwise appears to be without harmful effects following in utero and postnatal exposure (48,49). Safety data from perinatal clinical trials specific to individual antiretroviral drugs are included in the descriptions of the pharmacology of individual antiretroviral agents below.

The potentially life-threatening consequences of HIV infection to mother and fetus have compelled the use of many antiretroviral agents, often as part of combination regimens, in pregnant women and their newborns in the absence of definitive safety data. Monitoring of this clinical experience is ongoing in epidemiological cohort studies and in the Antiretroviral Pregnancy Registry, a postmarketing surveillance registry sponsored by the pharmaceutical industry to collect information about major teratogenic effects with exposure to 18 antiretroviral agents (http://www.apregistry.com/). Although these cohorts will include large numbers of exposures and provide useful information, the data include exposure to a large variety of drug combinations, making it difficult to establish safety assessments for individual agents. These monitoring studies are also limited by ethnic, social, and clinical differences in the populations studied, the lack of randomized comparator groups, inadequate information about confounding variables, and uncertain accuracy of outcomes (50).

Published reports of pregnancy outcomes associated with perinatal antiretroviral exposure highlight these difficulties. An initial observational study from Switzerland reported in 1998 on pregnancy outcome in 37 women receiving combination antiretroviral therapy, including 16 women receiving protease inhibitors. Twenty-nine women had adverse events, including preterm delivery in 10 (51). However, a meta-analysis published in 1998 that examined the association of maternal HIV infection and perinatal outcomes in 31 studies found that the risk of premature delivery was increased 1.83-fold among HIV-infected women (52). A collaborative European group reported on 2,414 uninfected children born to HIV-infected mothers between 1985 and 2001, of whom 1,008 were exposed to antiretroviral agents during pregnancy, delivery, and/or the neonatal period (53). No pattern or prevalence of congenital anomalies or low birth weight was associated with antiretroviral exposure, but exposure to any antiretroviral was associated with mild transient anemia in early life. In an updated 2004 report, this group reported that in 4,372 HIV-infected European women delivering between 1986 and 2004, the risk of delivery at less than 37 weeks was 1.9-fold increased with HAART started during pregnancy and 2.1-fold increased with HAART started prepregnancy (54). In contrast, several US studies have shown no association between antiretroviral use and preterm delivery or other adverse pregnancy outcomes (55,56). A recent meta-analysis of 14 studies that examined the association between antiretroviral therapy during pregnancy and premature delivery found no increased risk of premature delivery associated with antiretroviral use (57). Although no clear explanation is available for the inconsistency between the European and US experience, the potential for an increased risk of premature birth in HIV-infected pregnant women receiving combination antiretroviral therapy during pregnancy should be recognized and included in clinical discussions of the risks and benefits of antiretroviral therapy (58).

Nucleoside reverse transcriptase inhibitors (NRTIs) are known to inhibit mitochondrial function (59). Their long-term use may result in toxicity associated with depletion of mitochondrial DNA, although these toxicities generally resolve with cessation of use (60). Investigators in France reported that 8 of 1,754 uninfected infants with in utero and postnatal nucleoside reverse transcriptase exposure had biopsy proven persistent mitochondrial dysfunction (61). All eight infants were exposed to zidovudine, four as zidovudine monotherapy and four in combination with lamivudine. Five, of whom two died, presented with delayed onset of neurological symptoms while three were symptom free but had laboratory abnormalities (61). This report stimulated a worldwide search for other uninfected infants with perinatal antiretroviral exposure and evidence of mitochondrial toxicity. One US infant has been reported who was exposed to antiretrovirals for the last 4 weeks of pregnancy and had severe neurological symptoms present at birth and a muscle biopsy confirming mitochondrial dysfunction (62). Otherwise no cases consistent with mitochondrial dysfunction could be found among the uninfected antiretroviral exposed children in several research cohorts, including 3 US cohorts totaling 19,486 children, 1 African cohort of 1,798 children, 1 Thai cohort of 330 children, and a European cohort of 1,008 children (53,63–66). Although the difficulty in finding cases fitting the description of mitochondrial dysfunction in these other cohorts from around the world is encouraging, the limitations in diagnosing mitochondrial dysfunction without prospective neurologic and laboratory evaluations prevents a definitive conclusion about the relationship between perinatal nucleoside exposure and persistent mitochondrial toxicity from being drawn (67).

The health of the mother must not be forgotten when evaluating the risks and safety of antiretroviral use during pregnancy. The physiologic changes of pregnancy may lead to toxicities unique to pregnancy, such as premature delivery, or may make the mother more susceptible to toxicities described in nonpregnant adults. Abnormalities in carbohydrate metabolism are common side effects in nonpregnant adults receiving combination antiretroviral regimens, especially those including protease inhibitors, raising concerns about an increase in gestational carbohydrate intolerance in pregnant women receiving antiretrovirals (68). However, several studies have shown no significant association between type of antiretroviral treatment and gestational diabetes, including a recent prospective study that performed detailed evaluations for glucose intolerance and insulin resistance in HIV-infected pregnant women receiving protease-inhibitor–containing and nonprotease-inhibitor–containing regimens (69,70). Pregnancy may also predispose to mitochondrial dysfunction associated with nucleoside exposure. Lactic acidosis and hepatic steatosis are rare nucleoside toxicities attributed to mitochondrial dysfunction from nucleoside analogue exposure (71). Three fatal and several less severe cases of lactic acidosis and hepatic steatosis have been reported in pregnant or postpartum women whose antiretroviral regimen during pregnancy included stavudine and didanosine (72,73). Acute fatty liver and HELLP syndrome (hemolysis, elevated liver enzymes, and low platelets), two rare but life-threatening syndromes that occur during pregnancy, have been associated with abnormal mitochondrial fatty acid oxidation in mother and/or fetus (74). Pregnancy may possibly predispose to the mitochondrial dysfunction leading to all three syndromes—acute fatty liver of pregnancy, HELLP syndrome, and nucleoside-associated lactic acidosis/hepatic steatosis. The combination of stavudine and didanosine should be used with caution during pregnancy and only when other drug combinations have failed.

Another risk to the mother from antiretroviral use during pregnancy is the development of viral resistance. Drug-resistant HIV mutants develop when suppression of viral replication is incomplete during antiretroviral therapy, so that ongoing viral replication and genetic mutation leads to the selection of drug-resistant HIV variants (75). Complete viral suppression is achieved in only 40% to 80% of patients beginning HAART regimens and is rare in patients receiving single or dual drug therapy (76,77). Although drug-resistant HIV strains fade after treatment with an individual drug ceases, they generally recur with reexposure to the drug, limiting the efficacy of that antiretroviral agent in the future.

HIV drug resistance develops most easily for the first-generation non-NRTIs, requiring only a single mutation of the HIV genome (78). In individuals with uncontrolled viral replication, instability of the HIV genome results in daily production of single mutation nevirapine-resistant virus even in the absence of nevirapine therapy (79). Nevirapine has a long half-life and can be detected in plasma up to 3 weeks after administration of a single intrapartum dose (80). Under the selective pressure of nevirapine monotherapy, resistant viral strains proliferate and become detectable 1 to 2 weeks after initiation of treatment (79). Among women exposed to a single dose of nevirapine during labor for prevention of mother-to-child transmission, nevirapine-resistant HIV isolates could be detected 6 weeks after delivery in 20% of women receiving no other antiretrovirals and in 15% of women receiving standard perinatal antiretroviral regimens (81,82). The clinical implications of the presence of nevirapine-resistant HIV are unclear. Drug-resistant HIV mutants tend to be less fit than wild-type virus and gradually disappear as wild-type virus reemerges once the selective pressure from continued antiretroviral exposure is removed. Nevirapine-resistant virus could not be detected 1 to 2 years later in any of 11 women who received a single intrapartum nevirapine dose and had detectable nevirapine-resistant HIV shortly after delivery (83). In women who received a second or third course of single-dose intrapartum nevirapine in subsequent pregnancies, resistant virus was detected in 38% within 1 year after delivery but in only 7% at 3 years after exposure (84). Single-dose nevirapine appears to be as effective in preventing HIV transmission in subsequent pregnancies as when it is used for the first time (85,86). Several studies have suggested that efficacy does not decrease when nevirapine-based combination therapy is started at least 6 to 12 months after delivery (87–90). The development of nevirapine resistance can be reduced by administration of a short course of antiretrovirals to the mother after delivery (91,92).

Resistance to zidovudine and protease inhibitors requires multiple mutations and develops more slowly than resistance to the first-generation non-NRTIs (93). In PACTG 076, antenatal zidovudine treatment resulted in low-level genotypic resistance in only 1 of 39 women tested (94). Follow-up of women enrolled in PACTG 076 over 4 years could find no differences in the clinical course or in the incidence of zidovudine-resistance mutations in the women who received zidovudine when compared with those who received placebo (95). In contrast, the development of resistance to the NRTI lamivudine requires only a single mutation, and four of five women receiving dual therapy with lamivudine and zidovudine during pregnancy developed lamivudine resistance by the time of delivery (96). In a larger study, lamivudine resistance was detectable 6 weeks after delivery in 52 of 132 women receiving lamivudine and zidovudine during pregnancy (97).

Drug-resistant HIV may be transmitted from mother to infant. In a group of 91 HIV-infected infants born in New York State in 1998 to 1999, 12.1% were infected with drug-resistant HIV strains (98). However, the presence of resistance mutations does not increase the rate of transmission (58). All pregnant women starting antiretroviral therapy or those on therapy with detectable HIV viral RNA levels should have resistance testing performed to ensure selection of an optimal regimen to suppress HIV viremia and minimize the risk of transmission (2,13).

PHARMACOLOGY OF INDIVIDUAL ANTIRETROVIRAL AGENTS

Nucleoside/tide Reverse Transcriptase Inhibitors

The first antiretroviral agents developed were NRTIs. Structurally similar to endogenous deoxynucleosides, these agents are prodrugs that are inactive until metabolized within the cell to triphosphorylated forms, which then inhibit HIV reverse transcriptase and viral DNA replication (99). Quantification of the intracellular concentrations of these active triphosphorylated forms is difficult, requiring large blood samples and sophisticated assay techniques (100,101). The half-life of these active intracellular metabolites generally exceeds that of the parent drug in plasma (99). Extracellular plasma NRTI concentrations do not correlate well with concentrations of the active intracellular forms, and the plasma pharmacokinetics of NRTIs does not generally correlate with therapeutic effect (102). Tenofovir, the first nucleotide to be approved for use against HIV, is an acyclic analogue of adenosine monophosphate that requires only two phosphorylation steps to reach its active form, tenofovir diphosphate (103).

Prolonged treatment of HIV-infected individuals with either a single agent in this class (monotherapy) or two agents (dual therapy) generally results in only a transient suppression of HIV replication, as resistance mutations develop in the HIV gene that codes for reverse transcriptase. As a result, NRTIs are recommended to be used only as part of a combination regimen of at least three drugs, most commonly two NRTIs with either a protease inhibitor or a non-nucleoside reverse transcriptase inhibitor, when treating HIV infection (2). Less intensive regimens in pregnant women have been shown to protect against mother-to-child HIV transmission, as described earlier.

Zidovudine

Zidovudine, the first antiretroviral to be developed, was also the first drug shown to prevent mother-to-child transmission (6). Zidovudine remains a common component of initial combination regimens to treat HIV infection and of regimens to prevent mother-to-child transmission (4). Absorption of zidovudine is rapid and complete. In nonpregnant adults receiving zidovudine oral doses of

200 mg, the average maximum concentration (C_{max}) is 1.0 μg per mL reached at an average time of maximum concentration (T_{max}) of 0.65 hours (104). Zidovudine is avidly metabolized by the liver by glucuronidation and undergoes extensive first pass metabolism, so that bioavailability averages 63% despite nearly complete absorption (105). Zidovudine is rapidly eliminated from the body, primarily by renal excretion as glucuronide (106). Zidovudine half-life ($t_{1/2}$) averages around 1.1 hours and oral clearance (Cl/F) around 1.3 L per hour per kg in nonpregnant adults (107).

Several studies have evaluated zidovudine pharmacokinetics during pregnancy. In early studies, zidovudine C_{max}, T_{max}, bioavailability, and $t_{1/2}$ appeared no different than in historical values from nonpregnant adults (108,109). In two later studies where pharmacokinetics was compared during pregnancy and at 1 to 4 weeks postpartum in the same women, average Cl/F significantly increased during pregnancy by 47% to 65% while average area under the plasma concentration-time curve (AUC) decreased by 34% to 39% (110,111). The clinical significance of the decrease in zidovudine plasma exposure during pregnancy is not known. Like the other NRTIs, zidovudine is a prodrug that requires intracellular metabolism by cellular enzymes to the active triphosphorylated nucleotide form (102). The rate-limiting step in zidovudine activation is the conversion of zidovudine monophospate to diphosphate, catalyzed by cellular thymidylate kinase (112,113). This enzyme is saturated at relatively low substrate concentrations, so that intracellular concentrations of zidovudine monophosphate greatly exceed those of zidovudine di- and triphosphate, and plasma zidovudine concentrations do not correlate with intracellular concentrations of zidovudine triphosphate (112,113). The half-life of intracellular zidovudine triphosphate exceeds that of zidovudine in plasma, averaging 3 to 4 hours (114,115). As a result, zidovudine dose and plasma zidovudine concentration do not directly correlate with the concentration of intracellular phosphorylated metabolites or clinical effects (102,116). No studies of intracellular zidovudine metabolites have been performed in women receiving chronic oral dosing during pregnancy. The prenatal zidovudine-dosing regimen used in the PACTG 076 study was 100 mg given five times a day, which was the standard adult regimen at that time (6). With awareness of the importance and persistence of intracellular zidovudine triphosphate and the lack of correlation between plasma zidovudine concentrations and clinical effect, less frequent dosing regimens have been developed that appear to be equally effective and encourage adherence (2). The current standard adult zidovudine regimens of either 200 mg every 8 hours or 300 mg every 12 hours are generally used in pregnant women (13).

Zidovudine appears to cross the placenta well, with roughly equivalent concentrations in maternal plasma compared with amniotic fluid during pregnancy and in maternal plasma at the time of delivery compared with cord blood (110,111,117). Primate and human studies suggest that zidovudine moves across the placenta by simple diffusion (118–121). Regimens to prevent mother-to-child HIV transmission generally incorporate antiretroviral dosing during labor to ensure that suppression of HIV viral replication continues throughout labor and that protective plasma antiretroviral concentrations are present in the infant at the time of birth (13). The first intrapartum regimen studied was 140 mg of zidovudine given intravenously every 4 hours (109). This regimen led to average zidovudine concentrations of 1.15 μg per mL at the end of the infusion. However, zidovudine concentrations in umbilical cord and infant plasma at the time of delivery were highly variable and were dependent on the length of time separating birth and the last zidovudine dose (109). As a result, continuous intravenous infusion was investigated as a means of ensuring adequate zidovudine exposure at the time of birth. With continuous intravenous infusion of zidovudine using a 2 mg per kg loading dose followed by 1 mg per kg per hour, the average zidovudine plasma concentration at the time of birth was 0.82 μg per mL in the mother and 0.75 μg per mL in the newborn (109). Continuous intravenous zidovudine infusion during labor was part of the regimen used in the PACTG 076 protocol, the first study to demonstrate the efficacy of antiretrovirals in preventing mother-to-child HIV transmission, and remains part of standard clinical practice for HIV-infected pregnant women (6,13). Zidovudine is the only antiretroviral commercially available in a formulation for intravenous administration.

The human placenta phosphorylates zidovudine to its active metabolite, and the intracellular mechanisms needed to phosphorylate zidovudine are also present in the fetus (99). Intracellular concentrations of phosphorylated metabolites of zidovudine in maternal and cord blood have been studied following administration of continuous infusions during labor. Median levels of zidovudine monophosphate and triphosphate were similar in maternal (1,556 and 67 fmol per 10^6 cells) and cord (1,464 and 70 fmol per 10^6 cells) blood, but considerable variability was observed among study subjects (122). These values are two to three times higher than those reported in HIV-infected adults receiving oral zidovudine and, assuming uniform intracellular distribution of zidovudine triphosphate, around five times the zidovudine triphosphate 50% inhibitory concentration (IC_{50}) for HIV reverse transcriptase (~0.05 μM) (122). Although continuous intravenous infusion of zidovudine during labor provides maternal and cord blood intracellular zidovudine triphosphate levels consistent with high antiviral activity, the relative contributions of maternal, placental, and fetal zidovudine triphosphate in preventing intrapartum and early postpartum mother-to-child transmission are unknown.

Although the full zidovudine regimen used in the PACTG 076 protocol is standard of care in the United States and other developed countries, it is not available in resource poor areas of the world where the majority of HIV-infected women live. Less intensive zidovudine regimens that are more practical for use in these areas have been developed (14,123). These regimens start later in gestation, include oral dosing (rather than intravenous) during labor, and provide short or no postpartum newborn dosing. While these less intensive regimens have been shown to reduce mother-to-child HIV transmission, they are less effective than the full 076 protocol regimen (5). Zidovudine pharmacokinetics following oral dosing during labor has been described. In a study of five US women, trough plasma zidovudine concentrations following oral dosing with 300 mg every 3 hours during labor ranged from 0.11 to 1.34 μg per mL (124). In a study conducted in Bangkok, median cord blood concentrations following zidovudine dosing with 300 mg every 3 hours during labor were 0.25 μg per mL, considerably less than with continuous intravenous infusion (125). Simulations based on the pharmacokinetic parameters observed in the US women suggest that a regimen consisting of an oral loading dose of 600 mg followed by 400 mg every 3 hours during labor would produce plasma concentrations equivalent to those seen with continuous infusion (124). Although this regimen has been used in clinical trials, no data are available describing plasma or intracellular zidovudine concentrations achieved with its use (20).

Zidovudine is rapidly cleared in adults by hepatic glucuronide conjugation, followed by renal excretion of mostly conjugated metabolite and some unchanged drug (104). Both hepatic glucuronidation and renal function are known to be depressed in infants immediately after birth, so not surprisingly, the washout $t_{1/2}$ of transplacentally acquired zidovudine is extremely prolonged, averaging 13 hours (126). Zidovudine elimination increases rapidly during the first days of life, with $t_{1/2}$ averaging 3 hours during days 3 to 10 (126). A population analysis combining zidovudine pharmacokinetic data from six studies demonstrated a further increase in zidovudine clearance over the first 2 months of life, with clearance reaching adult levels by 4 to 8 weeks of life (Fig. 22.2) (127). The developmental pattern of the increase in zidovudine clearance in the infant parallels that of bilirubin, whose primary route of elimination is also via hepatic glucuronidation (128). However, although bilirubin and zidovudine clearance mature in parallel, they are metabolized by different isoenzymes of the uridine diphosphate-glucuronosyltransferase (UGT) family, with zidovudine metabolized primarily by UGT 2B7 and bilirubin by UGT 1A1 (129,130). The current FDA-approved dosing recommendation for zidovudine in infants from birth to 3 months of age is 2 mg per kg PO or 1.5 mg IV every 6 hours. To facilitate adherence, many clinicians and some research protocols have used 4 mg per kg PO every 12 hours (17,131). Zidovudine clearance is further decreased in premature infants (Fig. 22.2) and a dosing reduction is needed to avoid the accumulation of potentially toxic serum zidovudine concentrations (132,133). Infants born before 35 weeks' gestation who require zidovudine should receive initial doses of 2.0 mg per kg PO or 1.5 mg per kg IV every 12 hours. Zidovudine dosing frequency should increase to every 8 hours at 2 weeks of age if gestational age at birth is above 30 weeks or at 4 weeks of age if gestational age at birth is less than 30 weeks (134).

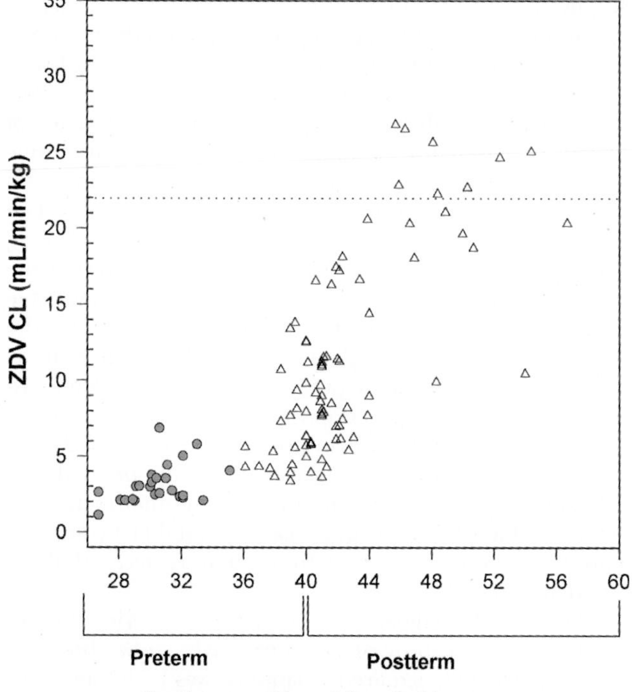

Figure 22.2. Zidovudine clearance plotted against postconceptional age (gestational age at birth plus postnatal age) for infants from birth to age 5 months. *Open triangles,* term infants; *solid circles,* preterm infants; *broken line,* average adult clearance [from Mirochnick et al. (127)].

Zidovudine is the drug with the longest history of use during pregnancy and the most safety information. High dose administration of zidovudine to female adult rodents is associated with the development of vaginal tumors (135). These tumors have not been reported in humans and are thought to result from chronic local exposure of the vaginal epithelium to high urine concentrations of unmetabolized zidovudine due to patterns of zidovudine metabolism and female anatomy unique to rodents. Bone marrow depression is a common toxicity of zidovudine, and mild, transient depression of hematologic parameters has been observed in the newborn after exposure to the full PACTG 076 regimen and to less intensive regimens (6,136). Hemoglobin was decreased by an average of 1 mg per dL at 3 weeks of age in newborns exposed to zidovudine in PACTG 076 compared with those exposed to placebo. By 12 weeks of age, no differences were seen in hemoglobin between the two groups (6). No adverse effects of zidovudine exposure have been detected during follow-up of the PACTG 076 infants followed for up to 5.6 years (48). Eighteen-month follow-up of a group of Thai infants randomized to exposure to a short-course prenatal zidovudine regimen or placebo similarly showed no adverse effects of zidovudine exposure (49). No evidence of cardiac toxicity could be found when comparing zidovudine exposed and unexposed infants born to HIV-infected mothers (137). Sufficient numbers of exposures to zidovudine in humans have been monitored in the Antiretroviral Pregnancy Registry to be able to determine that first trimester zidovudine exposure is not associated with a 1.5-fold or greater increase in the risk of overall birth defects or with a twofold or greater increase in the risk of cardiovascular or genitourinary system defects (138). However, the Women and Infants Transmission Study documented a 10-fold increased risk of hypospadias with first trimester zidovudine use (139). The potential relationship between perinatal zidovudine exposure and persistent infant mitochondrial toxicity has been discussed previously in this chapter.

Lamivudine

Lamivudine is a deoxycytidine analogue commonly used in combination with zidovudine during pregnancy. In nonpregnant adults, lamivudine is rapidly absorbed with bioavailability averaging 85%. Protein binding is low (10% to 50%) and the volume of distribution (V/F) is large (1.3 L per kg) (140,141). Lamivudine is rapidly eliminated via renal excretion as unchanged drug. Overall plasma Cl/F is 0.3 L × hr/mL and $t_{1/2}$ is around 6 hours (141,142). The intracellular $t_{1/2}$ of lamivudine triphosphate is longer than that of zidovudine, with a median of 15 hours (143). In a study of South African women receiving zidovudine and lamivudine, no significant differences were found in lamivudine pharmacokinetic parameters during the 38th week of gestation and the first week after delivery and no pharmacokinetic drug interaction occurred between the two drugs (111). Lamivudine crosses the placenta by simple diffusion, and the ratio of lamivudine concentration in maternal plasma at the time of delivery and cord blood is around 1.0 (144,145). Lamivudine accumulates in amniotic fluid, where the concentration at the time of delivery averages around five times more than the maternal plasma concentration (145). The lamivudine dose used in most pregnancy studies is 150 mg every 12 hours. No data are available with the use of the other approved adult dose of 300 mg once a day during pregnancy.

Infant lamivudine clearance is prolonged immediately after birth, with the elimination $t_{1/2}$ in neonates of transplacentally acquired lamivudine averaging around 14 hours (131). Lamivudine elimination increases as renal function improves after birth, with clearance averaging 0.25 L per hour on day 1 after birth and 0.40 L per kg per hour after 1 week of life, compared with 0.53 L per kg per hour in older children (111,131,146). The recommended lamivudine dose for neonates less than 1 month old is 2 mg per kg every 12 hours, compared with the standard dose in older infants of 4 mg per kg every 12 hours (up to a maximum of 150 mg every 12 hours) (13).

Lamivudine is generally used in combination with zidovudine during pregnancy, making the determination of independent toxicity of this drug difficult. Lamivudine is known to depress bone marrow function, and hematologic toxicity is the most common toxicity reported with perinatal exposure. The only safety data for perinatal lamivudine monotherapy comes from a small phase I study from South Africa where lamivudine monotherapy was given to 10 women starting at 38 weeks' gestation and to their infants for 1 week after birth. The only toxicities noted were mild anemia in one mother and one infant (111). One case of severe anemia in an infant with perinatal exposure to lamivudine and zidovudine has been reported (147). In a larger French observational study, pregnant women received the PACTG 076 zidovudine regimen with lamivudine added at 32 weeks' gestation and their infants were treated for 6 weeks with lamivudine and zidovudine, with a mother-to-child HIV transmission rate of 1.6% (97). The mothers tolerated the regimen well, with only occasional anemia and rare liver function test abnormalities. Hematologic toxicity was common in the infants, with 18% having neutropenia and 15% anemia, and mean hemoglobin level and neutrophil counts were slightly lower than in a historical control group exposed only to zidovudine (97). Three of the infants in this cohort are included in the report of persistent mitochondrial toxicity following perinatal exposure to zidovudine and lamivudine (61). In a Thai study of a shortened regimen of lamivudine and zidovudine (from 34 weeks' gestation until delivery in the mothers and for 4 weeks after birth in the infants), the rate of mother-to-child HIV transmission was 2.8% (148). No serious adverse events were noted in the mothers, while 6% of infants had anemia, 3% had thrombocytopenia, and 1% had elevated transaminase levels (148). Sufficient numbers of exposures to lamivudine in humans have been monitored in the Antiretroviral Pregnancy Registry to be able to determine that first trimester lamivudine exposure is not associated with a 1.5-fold or greater increase in the risk of overall birth defects or with a twofold or greater increase in the risk of cardiovascular or genitourinary system defects (138).

Didanosine

Didanosine is a deoxyadenosine analogue often used as an alternative NRTI in women intolerant or resistant to zidovudine and/or lamivudine (58). Didanosine is degraded by stomach acid and must be administered with antacid. In nonpregnant adults, didanosine bioavailability is poor, averaging around 40% to 45% (149,150). Although the plasma $t_{1/2}$ of didanosine is short (1.5 hours), the $t_{1/2}$ of the intracellular phosphorylated derivative is 12 to 40 hours, longest of all the NRTIs, and once-daily dosing with enteric-coated didanosine capsules has been approved for use in adults (99,151). Didanosine pharmacokinetics has been determined in nine women at 31 weeks' gestation and again at 6 weeks postpartum following both intravenous and oral doses (152). Bioavailability of buffered capsules averaged 50%, but was highly variable, ranging from 15% to 84%. Clearance of intravenous doses was significantly increased during pregnancy compared with postpartum (12.0 ± 2.45 mL per minute per kg vs. 9.4 ± 3.5 mL per minute per kg, $p < .05$). No significant differences were seen in the estimates of clearance of oral doses administered during and after pregnancy, as the large variability in bioavailability obscured the relatively modest difference in clearance (152). The median cord to maternal plasma ratio in 10 women taking didanosine at delivery was 0.38, which is the lowest of the nucleoside agents (118). Although didanosine is available as buffered capsules or an enteric-coated capsule, the improved tolerance and pharmacokinetics of the enteric-coated capsule make it the preferred formulation. Standard adult dosing of 200 mg every 12 hours or 400 mg once daily is recommended during pregnancy (13). The combination of didanosine with stavudine should be used with caution during pregnancy and only when other drug combinations have failed, as three cases of fatal lactic acidosis have been reported in pregnant women treated with these two drugs (72,73).

Data describing didanosine pharmacokinetics in neonates are limited. In a study of 11 infants, average washout $t_{1/2}$ of transplacentally acquired didanosine was 1.7 hours (152). Didanosine pharmacokinetic parameters were determined for four of the infants following single 60 mg per m^2 doses administered on day 1 of life and again at week 6. Didanosine pharmacokinetic parameters in these infants were very variable, and Cl/F averaged 4.5 L per minute per m^2 and $t_{1/2}$ of 1.1 hours on day 1, compared with average

Cl/*F* of 5.0 L per minute per m^2 and $t_{1/2}$ of 0.88 hour at week 6 (152). In a second study, didanosine pharmacokinetics was studied at 2 and 4 weeks of age in eight neonates receiving 100 mg per m^2 didanosine once daily in combination with stavudine and nelfinavir (153). Didanosine pharmacokinetics did not differ at the two ages, with average $t_{1/2}$ of 1.2 hours at 2 weeks and 1.1 hours at 4 weeks. In a study of six neonates taking 25 mg per m^2 twice daily, Cl/*F* was lower in neonates than in eight infants older than 28 days to younger than 120 days (57 vs. 84 L per hour per m^2) (154). However, the lower dose did not achieve the minimum target AUC, so an additional six neonates were studied at a dose of 50 mg per m^2 twice daily, which achieved the target exposure. The recommended dose for didanosine in newborns is 50 mg per m^2 every 12 hours compared with 90 to 150 mg per m^2 every 12 hours in older infants and children (4). An increased frequency of birth defects has been detected for didanosine exposure in the first trimester, with 16 defects in 353 live births (4.5%, 95% CI: 2.6% to 7.3%) as compared with the total population prevalence of birth defects of 2.7% reported by the Centers for Disease Control and Prevention (CDC) (138). No specific pattern of defects with didanosine exposure has been detected; the Antiretroviral Pregnancy Registry continues to monitor didanosine closely.

Stavudine

Stavudine is a deoxythymidine analogue also used as an alternative NRTI (58). In nonpregnant adults, stavudine has good bioavailability (around 86%), a serum $t_{1/2}$ of 1 hour, and an intracellular $t_{1/2}$ of around 3.5 hours (155). In a study of 14 pregnant women, stavudine pharmacokinetic parameters approximated historical values for nonpregnant adults (156). Placental transfer of stavudine was good, with cord blood stavudine concentrations averaging 130% that of the maternal serum concentration at the time of delivery (156). Standard adult dosing of 40 mg twice daily (30 mg if weight is less than 60 kg) should be used during pregnancy (13). The combination of stavudine with didanosine should be used with caution during pregnancy and only when other drug combinations have failed, as three cases of fatal lactic acidosis have been reported in pregnant women treated with these two drugs (72,73).

Stavudine pharmacokinetics in neonates has been described in several studies. In a US study of 11 neonates receiving single 1 mg per kg stavudine doses at 1 and 6 weeks of age, $t_{1/2}$ was longer (2.2 hours vs. 1.5 hours) and Cl/*F* was lower (5.6 mL per minute per kg vs. 6.8 mL per minute per kg) at 1 week compared with 6 weeks (156). In a Thai study of eight neonates receiving 1 mg per kg stavudine twice daily in combination with didanosine and nelfinavir for 4 weeks, stavudine $t_{1/2}$ averaged 1.8 hours at 2 weeks and 1.4 hours at 4 weeks of age (153). Twenty-five neonates younger than 13 days receiving stavudine (0.5 mg per kg per dose every 12 hours) with routine drug monitoring were included in a population pharmacokinetic analysis, which found that current recommended stavudine-dosing regimens in pediatric patients give similar exposure to adult doses (157). Recommended dosing from birth to 13 days old is 0.5 mg per kg per dose twice daily. For infants older than 13 days but with weight less than 30 kg, the recommended dose is 1 mg per kg per dose twice daily. Pediatric patients weighing more than 30 kg should receive the adult dose. Fixed dose combination pediatric formulations including stavudine, lamivudine, and nevirapine have been studied (158). They are dosed by weight bands in 5 kg increments for children 6 to 30 kg, corresponding to stavudine doses of 0.7 to 1.5 mg per kg twice daily that result in expected stavudine concentrations. More data are needed for neonates under 6 kg for weight-band dosing strategies. Sufficient numbers of exposures to stavudine in humans have been monitored in the Antiretroviral Pregnancy Registry to be able to determine that first trimester stavudine exposure is not associated with a twofold or greater increase in the risk of overall birth defects (138).

Abacavir

Abacavir is an oral, synthetic, guanosine analogue NRTI frequently used in pregnancy with potent activity against HIV-1. In nonpregnant adults, it is predictably and extensively absorbed with a mean absolute bioavailability of 83% (159). Protein binding is approximately 50%, and the mean volume of distribution is 0.86 L per kg. Abacavir is metabolized primarily by alcohol dehydrogenase and glucuronyl transferase to inactive metabolites, with no significant metabolism by the cytochrome P450 enzyme system. Plasma Cl/*F* is 0.8 L per hour per kg, and $t_{1/2}$ is 1.5 hours (160,161). Abacavir is metabolized inside cells to its active moiety, carbovir triphosphate, which has a median intracellular half-life of 18 hours (162). A phase I study of 25 women showed decreased maximum concentrations of abacavir in pregnancy with similar overall plasma exposure (AUC) in the third trimester compared with 6 to 12 weeks postpartum and compared with nonpregnant individuals (163). Therefore, standard adult dosing of 300 mg orally twice daily is recommended in pregnancy. Cord blood concentrations are equivalent to maternal concentrations at delivery (163). Abacavir is excreted in the breast milk of lactating rats; breast milk transfer has not been studied in humans. Abacavir pharmacokinetic data for use in neonates are not available. Serious, sometimes fatal, hypersensitivity reactions to abacavir have occurred in nonpregnant adults. Carriage of the HLA-B*5701 allele is associated with a significantly increased risk of a hypersensitivity reaction to abacavir and screening for this allele is recommended prior to initiating treatment with abacavir (159). Sufficient numbers of exposures to abacavir in humans have been monitored in the Antiretroviral Pregnancy Registry to be able to determine that first trimester abacavir exposure is not associated with a twofold or greater increase in the risk of overall birth defects (138).

Tenofovir

Tenofovir, the first nucleotide approved for use against HIV, has been shown to protect newborn macaques against infection following oral exposure to simian immunodeficiency virus (164). In nonpregnant adults, the bioavailability is 25%, with maximum concentrations of 200 to 300 ng per mL reached 1 to 2 hours postdose (165–168). Protein binding is low, and tenofovir is not a substrate for the cytochrome P450 enzyme system. Tenofovir has a plasma half-life of 15 hours and the active moiety, tenofovir diphosphate, has a long intracellular half-life of 60 hours or more (169). Tenofovir and emtricitabine administered as single doses at delivery along with zidovudine and nevirapine reduce the development of viral resistance to non-NRTIs by half (91). A tenofovir dose of 600 mg is needed at delivery to produce the same tenofovir concentrations as 300 mg chronic doses in nonpregnant adults (170,171). Tenofovir pharmacokinetics with chronic dosing in pregnancy (300 mg once daily) was described for 19 women in the third trimester and again 6 to 12 weeks postpartum (172). Tenofovir AUC and C_{max} were lower during the third trimester compared with postpartum, but predose concentrations ($C_{predose}$) and minimum concentrations (C_{min}) were not different. Most women had HIV viral loads of less than 400 copies per mL (88% third trimester, 70% postpartum). Although overall exposure was decreased during pregnancy, minimum threshold concentrations were appropriate and virologic control was maintained, suggesting that the standard adult dose of 300 mg once daily is reasonable to use in pregnancy (172). Transplacental passage of tenofovir is 60% to 70% with a single 600 mg intrapartum dose and is 100% with chronic standard dosing during pregnancy (170–172). No pharmacokinetic data are available describing tenofovir use in neonates.

Unfortunately, primate studies have demonstrated osteomalacia and renal toxicity with prolonged high-dose tenofovir exposure in adult animals and fetal growth retardation and reduction in bone porosity after chronic prenatal exposure (173–175). Renal toxicity has also been described in HIV-infected adults taking tenofovir (176–178). Decreased bone mineral density has been reported in some, but not all, studies of adult and pediatric patients taking tenofovir (179–181). The clinical significance of these findings is unknown. A retrospective case series of 15 heavily treatment-experienced pregnant women taking tenofovir reported that tenofovir was well tolerated in these women and that the infants experienced normal growth and development through the 12 month follow-up period (182). However, another case report described 2 diagnoses of fetal pyelectasis out of 7 pregnant women using tenofovir compared with 0 of 26 pregnant women not using tenofovir (183). Sufficient numbers of exposures to tenofovir in humans have been monitored in the Antiretroviral Pregnancy Registry to be able to determine that first trimester tenofovir exposure is not associated with a twofold or greater increase in the risk of overall birth defects (138).

Emtricitabine

Emtricitabine is an oral, synthetic, cytidine analogue NRTI frequently used in pregnancy with potent activity against HIV-1. In nonpregnant adults, it is well absorbed, has low protein binding, and the standard dose of 200 mg once daily results in an average AUC of 10 μg × hr/mL (184). Less than 15% of emtricitabine is metabolized, primarily by oxidation of the thiol moiety to form the 3′-sulfoxide diastereomers and conjugation with glucuronic acid to form 2′-O-glucuronide, with no significant metabolism by the cytochrome P450 enzyme system. Most is eliminated unchanged in the urine, and its clearance is proportional to renal function. Plasma $t_{1/2}$ is 8 hours and intracellular emtricitabine triphosphate $t_{1/2}$ is 20 to 39 hours (166,169,185). Emtricitabine pharmacokinetics in 35 women receiving a single 400 mg dose at delivery followed by 200 mg once daily for 7 days after delivery showed an AUC, C_{max}, and C_{min} after the 400 mg dose of 14.3 μg × hr/mL, 1,680 and 760 ng per mL, respectively (186). Eighteen women receiving 200 mg once daily during pregnancy and postpartum had slightly lower AUC and C_{min} in the third trimester (8.6 μg × hr/mL and 52 ng per mL) as compared with 6 to 12 weeks postpartum (9.8 μg hour per mL and 86 ng per mL) (187). Emtricitabine crosses into the placenta. In 18 women receiving 200 mg once daily during pregnancy, the mean ratio of cord blood/maternal plasma concentration at delivery was 1.17 (187). In 35 women given a single 400 mg dose at the start of labor, cord blood concentrations were approximately 80% of maternal plasma concentrations (186).

Emtricitabine pharmacokinetics in the first 3 months of life was studied in 20 infants at doses of 3 mg per kg once daily for four days, with two 4-day courses administered at least 2 weeks apart (188). Oral clearance increased with age, with mean values of 13, 22, and 29 mL per minute at postnatal days 0 to 21, 22 to 42, and 43 to 90, respectively. Mean AUCs ranged from 8.55 to 13.44 μg × hr/mL, similar to values seen in older children taking 6 mg per kg once daily and adults taking 200 mg once daily. No serious adverse effects were deemed related to emtricitabine use in these infants. Sufficient numbers of exposures to emtricitabine in humans have been monitored in the Antiretroviral Pregnancy Registry to be able to determine that first trimester emtricitabine exposure is not associated with a twofold or greater increase in the risk of overall birth defects (138).

NONNUCLEOSIDE REVERSE TRANSCRIPTASE INHIBITORS

Non-NRTIs bind directly and noncompetitively to HIV reverse transcriptase without intracellular phosphorylation or activation (189). Four drugs in this class have been approved for clinical use—nevirapine, efavirenz, delavirdine, and etravirine. Use of the first three agents as monotherapy in HIV-infected individuals results in the rapid emergence of resistance, so when used in treatment of HIV infection, they are generally used only as part of combination multiple drug regimens (79). Nevirapine has been shown to be effective in preventing mother-to-child HIV transmission when used as monotherapy in a two-dose intrapartum–postpartum regimen (19,190).

Nevirapine

Nevirapine, a dipyridodiazepinone, is a potent nonnucleoside inhibitor of reverse transcriptase with pharmacokinetic characteristics that make it desirable for use in the perinatal setting (191). Nevirapine absorption is rapid and complete, with bioavailability exceeding 90% following oral administration in tablet or liquid form (192,193). Nevirapine is highly lipophilic at physiologic pH and is rapidly and widely distributed throughout the body (78). Mean apparent volume of distribution exceeds total body water and is significantly higher in adult females than males (1.54 L per kg vs. 1.38 L per kg, $p = .001$) (194). The protein-bound fraction of nevirapine in plasma is approximately 60% (78). The main route of elimination of nevirapine is hepatic metabolism by enzymes of the cytochrome P450 family, primarily CYP3A4 and CYP2B6, followed by renal excretion (78). Elimination following initial doses is slow, with a mean elimination half-life of 40 hours (range: 22 to 84 hours) (192). With chronic therapy, metabolic autoinduction of the elimination pathway occurs, so that after 2 weeks of treatment nevirapine clearance increases 1.5- to 2-fold and mean elimination half-life decreases to 20 to 30 hours (195,196). To avoid elevated nevirapine concentrations and minimize toxicity during this autoinduction phase, the recommended dosing schedule for nevirapine as part of combination antiretroviral regimens in HIV-1-infected adults is 200 mg once daily for the first 2 weeks, followed by an increase to 200 mg twice daily (2).

Nevirapine pharmacokinetics has been evaluated in women taking combination antiretroviral therapy including nevirapine during pregnancy. In a study of 18 pregnant women treated with zidovudine, lamivudine, and nevirapine during the second and third trimesters, steady state concentrations were equivalent to those seen in nonpregnant adults (197). One intensive pharmacokinetic study of nevirapine in 26 pregnant women (7 in second trimester, 19 in third trimester), and in the same women at 4 to 12 weeks postpartum, found that pregnancy did not significantly alter nevirapine pharmacokinetic parameters (198). However, an intensive pharmacokinetic study of 16 pregnant women taking nevirapine found a 20% greater nevirapine clearance, 28% lower area under the curve, and 30% lower C_{max} compared with 13 nonpregnant women (199).

Nevirapine pharmacokinetic parameters following initial doses administered during the third trimester of pregnancy before the onset of labor are equivalent to those seen in nonpregnant adults receiving initial doses (200). When initial doses are administered during labor, the physiologic changes associated with labor and delivery have a significant impact on nevirapine pharmacokinetic parameters, with increases in V/F, Cl/F, and $t_{1/2}$ and decreases in C_{max} and AUC (191). Nevirapine crosses the placenta well. Cord blood concentrations average around 1,000 ng per mL after administration of single doses to the mother during labor, and the ratio of the nevirapine concentrations in cord blood and maternal blood at the time of delivery averages approximately 80% (201,202). Average cord blood concentration doubles to over 2,000 ng per mL with chronic maternal dosing during the last trimester of pregnancy (200).

In newborns, washout elimination (excretion of nevirapine acquired across the placenta following maternal dosing during labor) is prolonged and variable, with a median $t_{1/2}$ of 64.9 hours (range: 35.4 to 330.7 hours) when the data from US and Ugandan studies are combined (191). Elimination accelerates during the first days of life. Following administration of a 2 mg per kg oral dose of nevirapine to infants at 48 to 72 hours after birth, median $t_{1/2}$ was 43.6 hours (range: 23.6 to 81.6 hours) and median Cl/F was 36.1 mL per kg per hour (range: 22.0 to 40.0 mL per kg per hour). Absorption was variable and prolonged in the newborns, with a median T_{max} of 8.2 hours (range: 2.0 to 26.1 hours) (202).

Taking advantage of the rapid maternal absorption and distribution and slow neonatal elimination of nevirapine, a two-dose intrapartum–postnatal regimen was developed to prevent mother-to-child HIV transmission in resource poor areas of the world where more intensive antiretroviral treatment is not available. This regimen, which consists of a single oral 200 mg dose to the mother during labor and a single oral 2 mg per kg dose to the infant after birth, was designed to maintain newborn plasma nevirapine concentrations above 100 ng per mL (5 to 10 times the in vitro IC_{50} against wild-type HIV) from birth through the end of the first week of life (201,202). The two-dose intrapartum–postnatal nevirapine regimen reduced mother-to-child HIV transmission by 41% compared with an equivalently abbreviated zidovudine regimen in a randomized controlled trial in Uganda and by 49% compared with a contemporaneous untreated population in a prospective cohort study in Zambia (19,203).

Despite the rapid absorption and distribution of nevirapine, cord blood nevirapine concentrations may be below 100 ng per mL in many infants if the interval between maternal dosing and delivery is less than 2 hours (204). Infants who are born less than 2 hours after maternal nevirapine dosing should receive an extra dose of nevirapine immediately after birth in addition to the standard infant dose at 48 to 72 hours (204). When pregnant women begin chronic dosing with nevirapine during pregnancy and achieve steady state nevirapine concentrations prior to the onset of labor, nevirapine concentrations in the mother at delivery, in cord blood, and in the infant at 48 to 72 hours after birth are increased two to five times compared with concentrations seen after administration of only single doses during labor (197,200,201). Chronic maternal nevirapine dosing prior to delivery appears to accelerate nevirapine elimination in the infant after birth, presumably due to in utero autoinduction of nevirapine elimination. In a group of 10 infants whose nevirapine exposure began with maternal dosing at 38 weeks' gestation and included a single 2 mg per kg oral dose at 48 to 72 hours, nevirapine concentrations fell below 100 ng per mL before the end of the first week of life in 4 infants (200). If a pregnant woman receives prolonged nevirapine therapy prior to delivery, then an additional nevirapine dose should be given to the newborn at around day 5 of life to maintain infant nevirapine concentrations above 100 ng per mL throughout the first week of life.

A simple, practical regimen to prevent mother-to-child HIV transmission via breast milk in resource poor areas of the world where formula feeding is not possible would be a major therapeutic advance. Nevirapine administration to the infant for the duration of nursing has been proposed as one possible approach. Administration of 2 mg per kg once a day for 2 weeks, followed by 4 mg per kg once a day through age 6 months was shown to be safe and to maintain trough nevirapine concentrations above 100 ng per mL in all infants (205). The efficacy of this daily low-dose nevirapine regimen in preventing breast milk HIV transmission is currently under investigation. An alternative approach to preventing breast milk transmission of HIV is to treat the lactating mother with combination antiretroviral therapy, reducing maternal plasma and breast milk viral load (27). If nevirapine is used as part of the maternal regimen, nevirapine will be excreted into the breast milk, effectively dosing the infant. In 19 lactating women receiving nevirapine, lamivudine, and zidovudine, the median breast milk to maternal plasma concentration ratio was 0.67 (206). Median infant nevirapine plasma concentration at 2 and 5 months of life was 971 ng per mL, which was 40 times the wild-type IC_{50} (24 ng per mL) and may be sufficient to provide protection against infant infection with nevirapine-sensitive strains of HIV (206).

The two-dose intrapartum–postnatal nevirapine regimen is well tolerated in mothers and infants. No adverse effects of this short-course regimen were seen when compared with placebo in Ugandan infants exposed to no other antiretroviral agents and in infants from the United States, Europe, Brazil, and the Bahamas exposed to standard perinatal antiretroviral regimens (11,18). Long-term therapy with nevirapine is associated with rare but significant toxicities. Severe, life-threatening hypersensitivity skin reactions, including Stevens–Johnson syndrome, and severe, life-threatening, and in some cases, fatal hepatotoxicity, including fulminant and cholestatic hepatitis, hepatic necrosis, and hepatic failure, have been reported in HIV-infected patients receiving nevirapine in combination with other drugs for treatment of HIV disease (207). The development of severe nevirapine-associated skin rash is more common in women than in men and has been reported during pregnancy (208–210). Nevirapine-associated hepatic toxicity is also more common in women, is associated with CD4 cell counts above 250 cells per mm^3, and has been reported during pregnancy (211,212). Initiation of nevirapine therapy should be avoided if at all possible in pregnant women with CD4 cell counts above 250 cells per mm^3 (13). Sufficient numbers of exposures to nevirapine in humans have been monitored in the Antiretroviral Pregnancy Registry to be able to determine that first trimester nevirapine exposure is not associated with a twofold or greater increase in the risk of overall birth defects (138).

Delavirdine, Efavirenz, and Etravirine

Studies of efavirenz and delavirdine in pregnant animals have demonstrated significant toxicity, and clinical experience is limited with the use of these drugs during pregnancy. Administration of efavirenz to 20 pregnant cynomolgus monkeys resulted in three with severe malformations, including anencephaly, anophthalmia, microphthalmia, and cleft palate (213). Three cases of myelomeningocele in infants born to women receiving efavirenz early in pregnancy have been reported (214–216). Sufficient numbers of exposures to efavirenz in humans have been monitored in the Antiretroviral Pregnancy Registry to be able to determine that first trimester efavirenz exposure is not associated with a twofold or greater increase in the risk of overall birth defects, but insufficient data are available to make comparisons for specific subgroups of defects (138). The use of efavirenz should be avoided during pregnancy, especially during the first trimester (13). In 13 women in Rwanda given efavirenz during the third trimester and for 6 months postpartum, breast milk concentrations of efavirenz were 54% of mean maternal plasma efavirenz concentrations. Infant plasma concentrations of efavirenz were 13% of maternal plasma levels (217). Additional data for efavirenz use in neonates are not currently available.

Administration of delavirdine to pregnant rats at doses that produced systemic exposures equal to or lower than typical human exposures caused ventricular septal defects and increased infant mortality (218). No human data describing delavirdine pharmacokinetics during pregnancy are available and its use is not recommended. Etravirine is a new non-NRTI with activity against HIV strains resistant to efavirenz and nevirapine (219). Rat and rabbit studies of etravirine have not demonstrated reproductive, teratogenic, or developmental toxicities. No data are available describing etravirine pharmacokinetics during pregnancy, passage into placenta or breast milk, or use in neonates.

PROTEASE INHIBITORS

Protease inhibitors are potent antiretrovirals used as components of combination antiretroviral regimens. Inhibition of HIV protease, the enzyme responsible for cleavage of large polypeptide chains into the smaller proteins needed for production of functional HIV virions, leads to the release of structurally disorganized and noninfectious viral particles (189). Protease inhibitors, when used as part of combination regimens, can produce a sustained suppression of HIV replication and are considered first-line therapies in HIV-infected individuals (2). Protease inhibitors are often used as part of combination antiretroviral regimens used in HIV-infected pregnant women. In the United Kingdom and Ireland in 2006, 95% of HIV-infected pregnant women received combination antiretroviral therapy and 73% of the combination regimens included a protease inhibitor (220).

Protease inhibitors are metabolized by enzymes of the cytochrome P450 enzyme system, especially those of the CYP3A family, with lesser contributions by CYP2C9 and CYP2D6 (221). Some protease inhibitors alter the activity of these enzymes, leading to complex interactions among drugs of this class acting as inducers, competitive inhibitors, and substrates. Ritonavir, a potent cytochrome P450 enzyme inhibitor, increases concentrations of other protease inhibitors when administered together (221). This pharmacokinetic interaction is taken advantage of in "boosted" regimens of low-dose ritonavir in combination with another protease inhibitor (222). Protease inhibitors tend to be difficult to formulate into convenient and palatable dosage forms and generally have poor absorption characteristics. Bioavailability of these agents tends to be very variable. Gastrointestinal side effects (nausea, vomiting, and diarrhea) are common with all agents in this class (2). Protease inhibitors cross the placenta poorly. Most infants born to mothers receiving protease inhibitors have low or undetectable protease inhibitor concentrations in cord blood, suggesting that the primary mechanism of action of protease inhibitors in preventing mother-to-child HIV transmission is by decreasing maternal viral load (223,224). Limited placental transfer of protease inhibitors may protect the fetus against potential toxic or teratogenic effects of these agents. However, if protease inhibitors do not readily cross the placenta to the fetus following maternal dosing, then administration of protease inhibitors to the mother during labor will probably not provide postexposure prophylaxis of the newborn at the time of birth, in contrast to nevirapine or the NRTIs.

Atazanavir

Atazanavir is a potent antiretroviral agent that is among the first-line protease inhibitors recommended for use in adults and adolescents (2). Atazanavir is usually administered to adults as 300 mg once daily in combination with 100 mg ritonavir, although treatment naive adults may receive 400 mg once daily without concomitant ritonavir. The main side effects associated with atazanavir use are gastrointestinal symptoms (e.g., nausea, vomiting, abdominal pain, and diarrhea), jaundice, headache, rash, tingling in hands and feet, and depression (225). Atazanavir inhibits activity of the enzyme UGT 1A1, which is responsible for glucuronidation of bilirubin, and mild reversible unconjugated hyperbilirubinemia is often seen with atazanavir use (225).

The pharmacokinetics of atazanavir 300 mg when administered during pregnancy once daily with ritonavir 100 mg has been investigated in several studies. In a retrospective study of 19 pregnant women, trough atazanavir concentrations were measured at a median of 30 weeks' gestation and all but two women had a mean trough atazanavir concentration above 100 ng per mL (226). Full pharmacokinetic profiles of atazanavir during pregnancy have been evaluated in three studies. In a study of 17 pregnant women, atazanavir AUC and C_{max} were not different during pregnancy compared with 1 to 6 months postpartum (227). In contrast, two studies have shown reductions in plasma atazanavir concentrations of 30% to 40% during pregnancy. Eley et al. determined atazanavir pharmacokinetics in 12 pregnant women and found a mean AUC of 26.6 μg × hr/mL during the third trimester compared with 57.0 μg × hr/mL at 2 weeks postpartum. All subjects had trough atazanavir concentrations above 150 ng per mL (228). In a larger study, atazanavir pharmacokinetics was evaluated in 27 pregnant women, 13 of whom were also receiving tenofovir (229). In nonpregnant adults, administration of concomitant tenofovir has been shown to reduce atazanavir concentrations by around 25% (225). In those women not receiving tenofovir, median AUC was 37.5 μg × hr/mL during pregnancy versus 57.9 μg × hr/mL postpartum. In those women also receiving tenofovir, median AUC was 32.7 μg × hr/mL during pregnancy compared with 41.9 μg × hr/mL postpartum (229). Investigations of atazanavir exposure during pregnancy with the use of an increased dose of 400 mg in combination with 100 mg ritonavir are underway.

The ratio of cord blood atazanavir concentration to maternal serum concentration at the time of delivery averages 13% to 18% (227,229). The prevalence of birth defects reported in the Antiretroviral Pregnancy Registry with first trimester atazanavir exposure was 2.0% (95% CI: 0.7% to 4.7%) compared with total prevalence of birth defects in the US population based on CDC surveillance of 2.7% (138). Several studies have demonstrated that infants born to mothers who received atazanavir during pregnancy do not have pathologic or dangerous bilirubin elevations in the newborn period (226–229). No pharmacokinetic data are available describing atazanavir use in young infants, and atazanavir should not be administered to infants at risk for hyperbilirubinemia.

Indinavir

Published data describing indinavir pharmacokinetic parameters in pregnant women suggest that without ritonavir boosting, indinavir exposure is significantly decreased during pregnancy (230–232). In one report of indinavir pharmacokinetics in two pregnant women receiving standard adults doses of 800 mg thrice daily throughout pregnancy and postpartum, $AUC_{0-8\ hours}$ was reduced by more than 60% during the third trimester compared with 9 to 12 weeks postpartum (230). In a larger study with nine women, pharmacokinetic evaluations following administration of 800 mg thrice daily during pregnancy and again at 6 weeks postpartum demonstrated considerable variability in plasma concentrations during pregnancy and a significant decrease during pregnancy in C_{max} (5,224 ng per mL vs. 9,801 ng per mL) and $AUC_{0-8\ hours}$ (9.1 mg × hr/L vs. 24.7 mg × hr/L) (232). In a third study, an increased ratio of 6β-hydroxycortisol to cortisol in urine during pregnancy, which suggests an increase in cytochrome P450 activity, was associated with a decrease in indinavir AUC (231). These studies suggest that indinavir plasma concentrations may be suboptimal in pregnant women taking standard doses of indinavir without ritonavir boosting during the third trimester of pregnancy.

One study suggests that indinavir boosted with ritonavir may be effective during pregnancy. In a study of pregnant women receiving indinavir 400 mg with 100 mg ritonavir twice daily, the regimen was generally well tolerated and 93% had undetectable viral load at delivery, although 14% had undetectable trough indinavir concentrations (233). The prevalence of birth defects reported in the Antiretroviral Pregnancy Registry with first trimester indinavir exposure was 2.2% (95% CI: 0.8%, 4.7%) compared with total prevalence of birth defects in the US population based on CDC surveillance of 2.7% (138).

Lopinavir

Lopinavir, the most commonly used protease inhibitor in US pregnant women, is available only in fixed dose combination with ritonavir. Lopinavir was originally formulated as capsules containing 133 mg lopinavir and 33 mg ritonavir but is currently available only as heat-stable tablets with improved bioavailability characteristics containing 200 mg lopinavir and 50 mg ritonavir or as an oral solution with 80 mg lopinavir and 20 mg ritonavir per mL (234). Lopinavir may be dosed in adults as two tablets twice daily or, in treatment-naive adults only, as four tablets once daily. The most common side effects associated with lopinavir use are diarrhea, asthenia, and triglyceride and cholesterol elevations (234).

When lopinavir was administered to pregnant women in the third trimester as three capsules twice daily, plasma concentrations were reduced by 40% to 50% during pregnancy compared with postpartum (235). Increasing the dose of lopinavir/ritonavir to four capsules twice daily provided adequate lopinavir exposure during the third trimester but resulted in higher than normal levels at 2 weeks postpartum (236). In a study of pregnant women receiving standard dosing with two of the newer lopinavir/ritonavir tablets twice daily, trough plasma lopinavir levels were adequate in 33 of 36 women (237). In an intensive pharmacokinetic study, lopinavir plasma exposure with an increased dose of three tablets twice daily during the third trimester was equivalent to standard dosing with two tablets twice daily in nonpregnant adults (187).

Lopinavir placental transfer is low, with the ratio of lopinavir concentration in cord blood to maternal plasma at the time of delivery averaging around 20% (235). The prevalence of birth defects reported in the Antiretroviral Pregnancy Registry with first trimester lopinavir with ritonavir exposure was 1.9% (95% CI: 0.8% to 3.7%) compared with total prevalence of birth defects in the US population based on CDC surveillance of 2.7% (138).

Lopinavir clearance is increased in infants 6 weeks to 6 months of age compared with older infants and children; a twice-daily dose of 300 mg per m^2 lopinavir and 75 mg per m^2 ritonavir provides similar exposure to that in older children (238).

Nelfinavir

Nelfinavir pharmacokinetics in nonpregnant adults is characterized by erratic and variable absorption and significant diurnal variation in trough concentrations. The oral bioavailability of nelfinavir ranges from 20% to 80% and increases two to three times when administered with food (239). Nelfinavir is highly protein bound (>98%) and has a volume of distribution of 2 to 7 L per kg (239). Nelfinavir is extensively metabolized by enzymes of the cytochrome P450 system. Its active metabolite M8 is produced by CYP2C19 metabolism, and both nelfinavir and M8 are eliminated via metabolism by CYP3A family enzymes (240,241). The elimination $t_{1/2}$ of nelfinavir in nonpregnant adults is 3 to 5 hours (242). Nelfinavir concentrations exhibit significant diurnal variability. In nonpregnant adults, nelfinavir trough concentrations with 1,250 mg twice daily dosing average 2.2 ± 1.3 μg per mL before morning doses and 0.7 ± 0.4 μg per mL before evening doses (239).

Nelfinavir was originally formulated as 250 mg tablets, which were administered as 750 mg thrice daily or 1,250 mg twice daily. Two studies of nelfinavir pharmacokinetics with use of the 250 mg tablets demonstrated decreased nelfinavir exposure during pregnancy, with reductions in nelfinavir AUC in pregnant women of 25% to 35% compared with the same women postpartum (243,244). Median trough nelfinavir concentrations during pregnancy were around 0.50 μg per mL, below the target trough concentration of 0.80 μg per mL used in therapeutic drug monitoring programs (2). Low nelfinavir exposure with standard tablet dosing in these pharmacokinetic studies has been confirmed by observations from pregnant women participating in a clinical program monitoring nelfinavir concentrations during routine clinical use (245). In nonpregnant populations, lower nelfinavir concentrations are associated with more rapid development of viral resistance and a less durable suppression of viral replication (246–248). Several studies have shown that during pregnancy, there is a greater decrease in circulating concentration of nelfinavir's M8 metabolite relative to nelfinavir, suggesting that pregnancy is associated with an increase in CYP3A activity relative to CYP2C19 activity (243,244,249). Nelfinavir protein binding and pharmacokinetic parameters following intravenous dosing have not been determined in pregnant women, making it impossible to evaluate the contributions of changes in nelfinavir bioavailability, volume of distribution, protein binding, and metabolism to the reduced nelfinavir concentrations observed with standard dosing during pregnancy.

Nelfinavir is currently available as a 625-mg tablet with improved bioavailability compared with the original 250-mg tablet (239). In a study of 27 women who received 1,250 mg of nelfinavir twice daily as 625 mg tablets, nelfinavir exposure was again reduced significantly during pregnancy and trough nelfinavir concentrations exceeded the 0.80 μg per mL target in only 15% of women studied during the third trimester (250). A study using a higher dose of nelfinavir during pregnancy is underway. The prevalence of birth defects reported in the Antiretroviral Pregnancy Registry with first trimester nelfinavir exposure was 3.4% (95% CI: 2.3% to 4.7%) compared with total prevalence of birth defects in the US population based on CDC surveillance of 2.7% (138).

Several studies have investigated nelfinavir pharmacokinetics in infants during the first months of life. In children older than 2 years, dosing with 20 to 30 mg per kg thrice daily or 50 mg per kg twice daily results in plasma nelfinavir exposure equivalent to that seen in adults receiving standard dosing of 750 mg thrice daily or 1,250 mg twice daily (251). Nelfinavir exposure is much lower with similar dosing in children younger than 2 years of age (252). In US infants under 6 weeks of age, dosing with 10 mg thrice daily resulted in extremely low nelfinavir plasma concentrations, with all infants having an $AUC_{0-8\ hours}$ below the 10th percentile for nelfinavir AUC in adults (253). Nelfinavir exposure improved with 40 mg per kg twice daily dosing, although 30% to 40% of infants receiving this dose who were sampled during the first and sixth weeks of life had a nelfinavir $AUC_{0-12\ hours}$ below 15 μg × hr/mL, the 10th percentile for adults (253). Similar results were seen at 2 and 4 weeks of age in Thai infants receiving 45 mg per kg twice daily dosing (254). Both studies demonstrated considerable interpatient variability in nelfinavir pharmacokinetic parameters. Although median nelfinavir clearance did not change between the first and sixth weeks of life in the US study, the ratio of the M8 nelfinavir metabolite to the parent compound in plasma increased significantly, suggesting an increase in CYP2C19 activity over the first weeks of life (253). Dosing with a weight-band–dosing regimen that provided an average dose of nearly 60 mg per kg twice daily has been investigated in a study of Brazilian newborns during the first 2 weeks of life. Although median $AUC_{0-12\ hours}$ was 26 μg × hr/mL, well above the 10th percentile for adults (15 μg × hr/mL), interpatient variability was extreme, with $AUC_{0-12\ hours}$ below 15 $\mu g \times hr/mL$ and trough concentration below the 0.80 μg per mL therapeutic drug monitoring target in 44% of the infants (255).

Saquinavir

Saquinavir is a protease inhibitor with poor bioavailability when administered without ritonavir boosting. Saquinavir was originally introduced as a 200-mg hard gelatin capsule, which, when given without ritonavir, had bioavailability of only around 4% due to incomplete absorption and extensive first-pass metabolism (256). A 200 mg soft gelatin capsule formulation with approximately three times better bioavailability was introduced but was later withdrawn from production. Saquinavir is now available as 200 mg hard gelatin capsules and as 500 mg film-coated tablets, both of which, when administered as 1,000 mg saquinavir with 100 mg ritonavir, have better systemic exposure than does 1,200 mg of the soft gelatin capsules (256). Two reports described inadequate saquinavir concentrations with administration of soft gelatin capsules dosed at 1,200 mg three times daily during pregnancy. In four US women, median saquinavir $AUC_{0-8\ hours}$ was 1,672 ng $\times$ hr/mL (range: 738 to 2,614 ng $\times$ hr/mL), compared with an average of 7,249 ng $\times$ hr/mL in nonpregnant adults, and the protocol was stopped because of the inadequate plasma saquinavir exposure (257). Similar results were found in nine Thai women, with mean AUC of 2,630 ng $\times$ hr/mL and mean C_{min} of less than 10 ng per mL (258). Several subsequent reports have shown adequate saquinavir exposure with doses of current formulations at 800 or 1,000 mg saquinavir with 100 mg ritonavir twice daily and with 1,200 mg saquinavir with 100 mg ritonavir once daily (259–262). Placental transport of saquinavir appears poor. After maternal intrapartum dosing with 800 mg saquinavir and 100 mg ritonavir twice daily, saquinavir was measurable in only four of seven cord blood samples obtained, with a range of 128 to 357 ng per mL (259). The number of first trimester exposures of saquinavir reported to the Antiretroviral Pregnancy Registry is inadequate to be able to detect at least a twofold increase in the risk of overall birth defects (138).

Ritonavir

Ritonavir is perhaps the most difficult protease inhibitor to tolerate because of its frequent and severe gastrointestinal side effects, making it especially unattractive for use at full doses in pregnant women. Ritonavir pharmacokinetics has been studied in a group of 26 pregnant women also receiving lopinavir (236). Median ritonavir AUC and trough concentrations were decreased by 40% to 50% during pregnancy compared to 2 weeks postpartum (236). Ritonavir transport across the placenta is poor, with cord blood ritonavir concentrations averaging 5.3% of maternal plasma concentration at delivery (263). The prevalence of birth defects reported in the Antiretroviral Pregnancy Registry with first trimester ritonavir exposure was 2.7% (95% CI: 1.5% to 4.1%) compared with total prevalence of birth defects in the US population based on CDC surveillance of 2.7% (138).

Other Protease Inhibitors

No pharmacokinetic or safety data during pregnancy are available for the protease inhibitors darunavir, fosamprenavir, and tipranavir.

OTHER CLASSES

For the viral entry inhibitor enfuvirtide (T-20), several reports have described its use during pregnancy to successfully prevent mother-to-child transmission of multidrug-resistant HIV-1 (264–269). However, in one case, perinatal transmission occurred despite maternal viral suppression on an enfuvirtide regimen (270). Placental transfer of enfuvirtide is low, with mean cord blood concentrations of 83 ng per mL in 12 women with mean plasma concentrations of 1,008 ng per mL (264). Cord blood concentrations were undetectable in an ex vivo placental perfusion model and in two other pregnant women (269,271). No pharmacokinetic or safety data during pregnancy are available for the viral entry inhibitor maraviroc or for the integrase inhibitor raltegravir.

SUMMARY

Antiretrovirals are used in pregnant women and their newborns both for treatment of HIV infection and for prevention of mother-to-child HIV transmission. Zidovudine and lamivudine are the antiretrovirals most often used during pregnancy, and addition of a protease inhibitor or nevirapine is common where medical resources permit. When three drug combination antiretroviral regimens are used during pregnancy in combination with cesarean section if the HIV RNA level at the time of delivery is not suppressed to below the level of assay detection and safe formula feeding, the rate of mother-to-child HIV transmission is less than 2%. If these interventions are not available, less intensive regimens with zidovudine (sometimes in combination with lamivudine) and/or nevirapine have been shown to provide a lesser degree of protection against mother-to-child HIV transmission.

Use of antiretrovirals in pregnant women and newborns is complicated by differences in pharmacokinetics and safety profiles compared with nonpregnant adults and older children. Pharmacokinetic and safety data crucial for the safe and effective use of these drugs during pregnancy and the first months of life are incomplete for many currently approved antiretrovirals as well as for new agents now in development. Traditional phase I studies are difficult to perform during pregnancy for ethical and practical reasons. New and innovative methods to assess the pharmacokinetics and safety of antiretrovirals in pregnant women and their newborns are urgently needed.

REFERENCES

1. WHO. 2008 Report on the global AIDS epidemic. http://www.unaids.org/en/KnowledgeCentre/HIVData/GlobalReport/2008/2008_Global_report.asp. Accessed November 11, 2008.
2. Panel on Antiretroviral Guidelines for Adults and Adolescents. Guidelines for the use of antiretroviral agents in HIV-1-infected

adults and adolescents. Department of Health and Human Services. November 3, 2008:1–139. http://www.aidsinfo.nih.gov/ContentFiles/AdultandAdolescentGL.pdf. Accessed November 11, 2008.

3. WHO. Guidance on global scale-up of the prevention of mother-to-child transmission of HIV: towards universal access for women, infants and young children and eliminating HIV and AIDS among children. http://www.who.int/hiv/pub/guidelines/pmtct_scaleup2007/en/index.html. Accessed November 10, 2008.
4. Working Group on Antiretroviral Therapy and Medical Management of HIV-Infected Children. Guidelines for the use of antiretroviral agents in pediatric HIV infection. July 29, 2008: 1–134. http://aidsinfo.nih.gov/contentfiles/PediatricGuidelines.pdf. Accessed November 11, 2008.
5. De Cock KM, Fowler MG, Mercier E, et al. Prevention of mother-to-child HIV transmission in resource-poor countries: translating research into policy and practice. *JAMA* 2000;283(9):1175–1182.
6. Connor EM, Sperling RS, Gelber R, et al. Reduction of maternal–infant transmission of human immunodeficiency virus type 1 with zidovudine treatment. Pediatric AIDS Clinical Trials Group Protocol 076 Study Group. *N Engl J Med* 1994;331(18):1173–1180.
7. Wade NA, Birkhead GS, Warren BL, et al. Abbreviated regimens of zidovudine prophylaxis and perinatal transmission of the human immunodeficiency virus. *N Engl J Med* 1998;339(20):1409–1414.
8. The International Perinatal HIV Group. The mode of delivery and the risk of vertical transmission of human immunodeficiency virus type 1—a meta-analysis of 15 prospective cohort studies. *N Engl J Med* 1999;340(13):977–987.
9. The European Mode of Delivery Collaboration. Elective caesarean-section versus vaginal delivery in prevention of vertical HIV-1 transmission: a randomised clinical trial. *Lancet* 1999;353(9158):1035–1039.
10. Cooper ER, Charurat M, Mofenson L, et al. Combination antiretroviral strategies for the treatment of pregnant HIV-1-infected women and prevention of perinatal HIV-1 transmission. *J Acquir Immune Defic Syndr* 2002;29(5):484–494.
11. Dorenbaum A, Cunningham CK, Gelber RD, et al. Two-dose intrapartum/newborn nevirapine and standard antiretroviral therapy to reduce perinatal HIV transmission: a randomized trial. *JAMA* 2002;288(2):189–198.
12. Townsend CL, Cortina-Borja M, Peckham CS, et al. Low rates of mother-to-child transmission of HIV following effective pregnancy interventions in the United Kingdom and Ireland, 2000–2006. *AIDS* 2008;22(8):973–981.
13. Public Health Service Task Force. Recommendations for use of antiretroviral drugs in pregnant HIV-infected women for maternal health and interventions to reduce perinatal HIV transmission in the United States. July 8, 2008:1–98. http://aidsinfo.nih.gov/contentfiles/PerinatalGL. Accessed November 11, 2008.
14. Shaffer N, Chuachoowong R, Mock PA, et al. Short-course zidovudine for perinatal HIV-1 transmission in Bangkok, Thailand: a randomised controlled trial. Bangkok Collaborative Perinatal HIV Transmission Study Group. *Lancet* 1999;353(9155):773–780.
15. Wiktor SZ, Ekpini E, Karon JM, et al. Short-course oral zidovudine for prevention of mother-to-child transmission of HIV-1 in Abidjan, Cote d'Ivoire: a randomised trial. *Lancet* 1999;353(9155):781–785.
16. Dabis F, Msellati P, Meda N, et al. 6-month efficacy, tolerance, and acceptability of a short regimen of oral zidovudine to reduce vertical transmission of HIV in breastfed children in Cote d'Ivoire and Burkina Faso: a double-blind placebo-controlled multicentre trial. DITRAME Study Group. Diminution de la Transmission Mere-Enfant. *Lancet* 1999;353(9155):786–792.
17. Petra Study Team. Efficacy of three short-course regimens of zidovudine and lamivudine in preventing early and late transmission of HIV-1 from mother to child in Tanzania, South Africa, and Uganda (Petra study): a randomised, double-blind, placebo-controlled trial. *Lancet* 2002;359(9313):1178–1186.
18. Guay LA, Musoke P, Fleming T, et al. Intrapartum and neonatal single-dose nevirapine compared with zidovudine for prevention of mother-to-child transmission of HIV-1 in Kampala, Uganda: HIVNET 012 randomised trial. *Lancet* 1999;354(9181):795–802.
19. Jackson JB, Musoke P, Fleming T, et al. Intrapartum and neonatal single-dose nevirapine compared with zidovudine for prevention of mother-to-child transmission of HIV-1 in Kampala, Uganda: 18-month follow-up of the HIVNET 012 randomised trial. *Lancet* 2003;362(9387):859–868.
20. Moodley D, Moodley J, Coovadia H, et al. A multicenter randomized controlled trial of nevirapine versus a combination of zidovudine and lamivudine to reduce intrapartum and early postpartum mother-to-child transmission of human immunodeficiency virus type 1. *J Infect Dis* 2003;187(5):725–735.
21. Lallemant M, Jourdain G, Le Coeur S, et al. Single-dose perinatal nevirapine plus standard zidovudine to prevent mother-to-child transmission of HIV-1 in Thailand. *N Engl J Med* 2004;351(3):217–228.
22. WHO. Antiretroviral drugs for treating pregnant women and preventing HIV infection in infants in resource-limited settings: towards universal access. Recommendations for a public health approach. 2006 version. http://www.who.int/hiv/pub/guidelines/pmtct/en/index.html. Accessed November 10, 2008.
23. WHO Collaborative Study Team on the Role of Breastfeeding on the Prevention of Infant Mortality. Effect of breastfeeding on infant and child mortality due to infectious diseases in less developed countries: a pooled analysis. *Lancet* 2000;355:451–455.
24. Nduati R, John G, Mbori-Ngacha D, et al. Effect of breastfeeding and formula feeding on transmission of HIV-1: a randomized clinical trial. *JAMA* 2000;283(9):1167–1174.
25. Coutsoudis A, Dabis F, Fawzi W, et al. Late postnatal transmission of HIV-1 in breast-fed children: an individual patient data meta-analysis. *J Infect Dis* 2004;189(12):2154–2166.
26. Coovadia HM, Rollins NC, Bland RM, et al. Mother-to-child transmission of HIV-1 infection during exclusive breastfeeding in the first 6 months of life: an intervention cohort study. *Lancet* 2007;369(9567):1107–1116.
27. Giuliano M, Guidotti G, Andreotti M, et al. Triple antiretroviral prophylaxis administered during pregnancy and after delivery significantly reduces breast milk viral load: a study within the Drug Resource Enhancement Against AIDS and Malnutrition Program. *J Acquir Immune Defic Syndr* 2007;44(3):286–291.
28. Bedri A, Gudetta B, Isehak A, et al. Extended-dose nevirapine to 6 weeks of age for infants to prevent HIV transmission via breastfeeding in Ethiopia, India, and Uganda: an analysis of three randomised controlled trials. *Lancet* 2008;372(9635):300–313.
29. Kumwenda NI, Hoover DR, Mofenson LM, et al. Extended antiretroviral prophylaxis to reduce breast-milk HIV-1 transmission. *N Engl J Med* 2008;359(2):119–129.
30. Morgan DJ. Drug disposition in mother and foetus. *Clin Exp Pharmacol Physiol* 1997;24(11):869–873.
31. Loebstein R, Lalkin A, Koren G. Pharmacokinetic changes during pregnancy and their clinical relevance. *Clin Pharmacokinet* 1997;33(5):328–343.
32. Wright LL, Catz CS. Drug distribution during fetal life. In: Polin RA, Fox WW, eds. *Fetal and neonatal physiology*. Philadelphia, PA: W.B. Saunders Company, 1998:169.
33. Krauer B, Krauer F, Hytten FE. Drug disposition and pharmacokinetics in the maternal-placental-fetal unit. *Pharmacol Ther* 1980;10(2):301–328.
34. Krauer B, Dayer P, Anner R. Changes in serum albumin and alpha 1-acid glycoprotein concentrations during pregnancy: an analysis of fetal-maternal pairs. *Br J Obstet Gynaecol* 1984;91(9):875–881.
35. Connelly TJ, Ruo TI, Frederiksen MC, et al. Characterization of theophylline binding to serum proteins in pregnant and non-pregnant women. *Clin Pharmacol Ther* 1990;47(1):68–72.
36. Dean M, Stock B, Patterson RJ, et al. Serum protein binding of drugs during and after pregnancy in humans. *Clin Pharmacol Ther* 1980;28(2):253–261.
37. Heikkila A, Erkkola R. Review of beta-lactam antibiotics in pregnancy. The need for adjustment of dosage schedules. *Clin Pharmacokinet* 1994;27(1):49–62.
38. Davis M, Simmons CJ, Dordoni B, et al. Induction of hepatic enzymes during normal human pregnancy. *J Obstet Gynaecol Br Commonw* 1973;80(8):690–694.
39. Juchau MR, Mirkin DL, Zachariah PK. Interactions of various 19-nor steroids with human placental microsomal cytochrome P-450 (P-450 hpm). *Chem Biol Interact* 1976;15(4):337–347.
40. Philipson A. Pharmacokinetics of ampicillin during pregnancy. *J Infect Dis* 1977;136(3):370–376.

41. Zaske DE, Cipolle RJ, Strate RG, et al. Rapid gentamicin elimination in obstetric patients. *Obstet Gynecol* 1980;56(5):559–564.
42. Yerby MS. The use of anticonvulsants during pregnancy. *Semin Perinatol* 2001;25(3):153–158.
43. Newport DJ, Wilcox MM, Stowe ZN. Antidepressants during pregnancy and lactation: defining exposure and treatment issues. *Semin Perinatol* 2001;25(3):177–190.
44. Little BB. Pharmacokinetics during pregnancy: evidence-based maternal dose formulation. *Obstet Gynecol* 1999;93(5, pt 2): 858–868.
45. Briggs GG, Freeman RK, Yaffe SJ. *Drugs in pregnancy and lactation.* Baltimore, MD: Williams & Wilkins 1994:695, 814–815.
46. Mills JL. Protecting the embryo from X-rated drugs. *N Engl J Med* 1995;333(2):124–125.
47. Lammer EJ, Chen DT, Hoar RM, et al. Retinoic acid embryopathy. *N Engl J Med* 1985;313(14):837–841.
48. Culnane M, Fowler M, Lee SS, et al. Lack of long-term effects of in utero exposure to zidovudine among uninfected children born to HIV-infected women. Pediatric AIDS Clinical Trials Group Protocol 219/076 Teams. *JAMA* 1999;281(2):151–157.
49. Chotpitayasunondh T, Vanprapar N, Simonds RJ, et al. Safety of late in utero exposure to zidovudine in infants born to human immunodeficiency virus-infected mothers: Bangkok. Bangkok Collaborative Perinatal HIV Transmission Study Group. *Pediatrics* 2001;107(1):E5.
50. Fleming TR. Evaluating the safety of interventions for prevention of perinatal transmission of HIV. *Ann N Y Acad Sci* 2000; 918:201–211.
51. Lorenzi P, Spicher VM, Laubereau B, et al. Antiretroviral therapies in pregnancy: maternal, fetal and neonatal effects. Swiss HIV Cohort Study, the Swiss Collaborative HIV and Pregnancy Study, and the Swiss Neonatal HIV Study. *AIDS* 1998;12(18): F241–F247.
52. Brocklehurst P, French R. The association between maternal HIV infection and perinatal outcome: a systematic review of the literature and meta-analysis. *Br J Obstet Gynaecol* 1998;105(8): 836–848.
53. European Collaborative Study. Exposure to antiretroviral therapy in utero or early life: the health of uninfected children born to HIV-infected women. *J Acquir Immune Defic Syndr* 2003;32(4): 380–387.
54. Thorne C, Patel D, Newell ML. Increased risk of adverse pregnancy outcomes in HIV-infected women treated with highly active antiretroviral therapy in Europe. *AIDS* 2004;18(17):2337–2339.
55. Tuomala RE, Shapiro DE, Mofenson LM, et al. Antiretroviral therapy during pregnancy and the risk of an adverse outcome. *N Engl J Med* 2002;346(24):1863–1870.
56. Tuomala RE, Watts DH, Li D, et al. Improved obstetric outcomes and few maternal toxicities are associated with antiretroviral therapy, including highly active antiretroviral therapy during pregnancy. *J Acquir Immune Defic Syndr* 2005;38(4):449–473.
57. Kourtis AP, Schmid CH, Jamieson DJ, et al. Use of antiretroviral therapy in pregnant HIV-infected women and the risk of premature delivery: a meta-analysis. *AIDS* 2007;21(5):607–615.
58. Watts H. Management of human immunodeficiency virus infection in pregnancy. *N Engl J Med* 2002;346:1879–1891.
59. Martin JL, Brown CE, Matthews-Davis N, et al. Effects of antiviral nucleoside analogs on human DNA polymerases and mitochondrial DNA synthesis. *Antimicrob Agents Chemother* 1994;38(12): 2743–2749.
60. Brinkman K, ter Hofstede HJ, Burger DM, et al. Adverse effects of reverse transcriptase inhibitors: mitochondrial toxicity as common pathway. *AIDS* 1998;12(14):1735–1744.
61. Blanche S, Tardieu M, Rustin P, et al. Persistent mitochondrial dysfunction and perinatal exposure to antiretroviral nucleoside analogues. *Lancet* 1999;354(9184):1084–1089.
62. Cooper ER, DiMauro S, Sullivan M, et al. *Biopsy-confirmed mitochondrial dysfunction in an HIV-exposed infant whose mother received combination antiretrovirals during the last 4 weeks of pregnancy* [Abstract TUPEB4394 2004]. Presented at the 15th International AIDS Conference, Bangkok, Thailand, 2004.
63. Bulterys M, Nesheim S, Abrams EJ, et al. Lack of evidence of mitochondrial dysfunction in the offspring of HIV-infected women. Retrospective review of perinatal exposure to antiretroviral drugs in the Perinatal AIDS Collaborative Transmission Study. *Ann N Y Acad Sci* 2000;918:212–221.
64. Lindegren ML, Rhodes P, Gordon L, et al. Drug safety during pregnancy and in infants. Lack of mortality related to mitochondrial dysfunction among perinatally HIV-exposed children in pediatric HIV surveillance. *Ann N Y Acad Sci* 2000;918: 222–235.
65. Dominguez K, Bertolli J, Fowler M, et al. Lack of definitive severe mitochondrial signs and symptoms among deceased HIV-uninfected and HIV-indeterminate children < or = 5 years of age, Pediatric Spectrum of HIV Disease project (PSD), USA. *Ann N Y Acad Sci* 2000;918:236–246.
66. Lange J, Stellato R, Brinkman K, et al. *Review of neurological adverse events in relation to mitochondrial dysfunction in the prevention of mother to child transmission of HIV: PETRA Study* [abstract]. Presented at the Second Conference on Global Strategies for the Prevention of HIV Transmission from Mothers to Infants, Montreal, September 1–6, 1999.
67. Blanche S, Tardieu M, Benhammou V, et al. Mitochondrial dysfunction following perinatal exposure to nucleoside analogues. *AIDS* 2006;20(13):1685–1690.
68. Dube MP, Sattler FR. Metabolic complications of antiretroviral therapies. *AIDS Clin Care* 1998;10(6):41–44.
69. Watts DH, Balasubramanian R, Maupin RT Jr., et al. Maternal toxicity and pregnancy complications in human immunodeficiency virus-infected women receiving antiretroviral therapy: PACTG 316. *Am J Obstet Gynecol* 2004;190(2):506–516.
70. Hitti J, Andersen J, McComsey G, et al. Protease inhibitor-based antiretroviral therapy and glucose tolerance in pregnancy: AIDS Clinical Trials Group A5084. *Am J Obstet Gynecol* 2007;196(4):331 e1–e7.
71. Powderly WG. Long-term exposure to lifelong therapies. *J Acquir Immune Defic Syndr* 2002;29(Suppl 1):S28–S40.
72. Food and Drug Administration. Important drug warning: retyped text of a letter from Bristol-Myers Squibb, January 5, 2001. http://www.fda.gov/medwatch/safety/2001/zerit&videx_letter.htm. Accessed October 15, 2002.
73. Sarner L, Fakoya A. Acute onset lactic acidosis and pancreatitis in the third trimester of pregnancy in HIV-1 positive women taking antiretroviral medication. *Sex Transm Infect* 2002;78(1):58–59.
74. Ibdah JA, Bennett MJ, Rinaldo P, et al. A fetal fatty-acid oxidation disorder as a cause of liver disease in pregnant women. *N Engl J Med* 1999;340(22):1723–1731.
75. Tobin NH, Frenkel LM. Human immunodeficiency virus drug susceptibility and resistance testing. *Pediatr Infect Dis J* 2002;21(7): 681–683.
76. Ledergerber B, Egger M, Opravil M, et al. Clinical progression and virological failure on highly active antiretroviral therapy in HIV-1 patients: a prospective cohort study. Swiss HIV Cohort Study. *Lancet* 1999;353(9156):863–868.
77. Flexner C. HIV-protease inhibitors. *N Engl J Med* 1998;338(18): 1281–1292.
78. Murphy RL, Montaner J. Nevirapine: a review of its development, pharmacological profile and potential for clinical use. *Expert Opin Investig Drugs* 1996;5(9):1183–1199.
79. Havlir DV, Eastman S, Gamst A, et al. Nevirapine-resistant human immunodeficiency virus: kinetics of replication and estimated prevalence in untreated patients. *J Virol* 1996;70(11): 7894–7899.
80. Cressey TR, Jourdain G, Lallemant MJ, et al. Persistence of nevirapine exposure during the postpartum period after intrapartum single-dose nevirapine in addition to zidovudine prophylaxis for the prevention of mother-to-child transmission of HIV-1. *J Acquir Immune Defic Syndr* 2005;38(3):283–288.
81. Jackson JB, Becker-Pergola G, Guay LA, et al. Identification of the K103N resistance mutation in Ugandan women receiving nevirapine to prevent HIV-1 vertical transmission. *AIDS* 2000;14(11): F111–F115.
82. Cunningham CK, Chaix ML, Rekacewicz C, et al. Development of resistance mutations in women receiving standard antiretroviral therapy who received intrapartum nevirapine to prevent perinatal human immunodeficiency virus type 1 transmission: a substudy of pediatric AIDS clinical trials group protocol 316. *J Infect Dis* 2002;186(2):181–188.
83. Eshleman SH, Mracna M, Guay LA, et al. Selection and fading of resistance mutations in women and infants receiving nevirapine to prevent HIV-1 vertical transmission (HIVNET 012). *AIDS* 2001;15(15):1951–1957.

84. Flys TS, McConnell MS, Matovu F, et al. Nevirapine resistance in women and infants after first versus repeated use of single-dose nevirapine for prevention of HIV-1 vertical transmission. *J Infect Dis* 2008;198(4):465–469.
85. McConnell M, Bakaki P, Eure C, et al. Effectiveness of repeat single-dose nevirapine for prevention of mother-to-child transmission of HIV-1 in repeat pregnancies in Uganda. *J Acquir Immune Defic Syndr* 2007;46(3):291–296.
86. Martinson NA, Ekouevi DK, Dabis F, et al. Transmission rates in consecutive pregnancies exposed to single-dose nevirapine in Soweto, South Africa and Abidjan, Cote d'Ivoire. *J Acquir Immune Defic Syndr* 2007;45(2):206–209.
87. Lockman S, Shapiro RL, Smeaton LM, et al. Response to antiretroviral therapy after a single, peripartum dose of nevirapine. *N Engl J Med* 2007;356(2):135–147.
88. Chi BH, Sinkala M, Stringer EM, et al. Early clinical and immune response to NNRTI-based antiretroviral therapy among women with prior exposure to single-dose nevirapine. *AIDS* 2007;21(8):957–964.
89. Jourdain G, Ngo-Giang-Huong N, Le Coeur S, et al. Intrapartum exposure to nevirapine and subsequent maternal responses to nevirapine-based antiretroviral therapy. *N Engl J Med* 2004;351(3):229–240.
90. Coffie PA, Ekouevi DK, Chaix ML, et al. Maternal 12-month response to antiretroviral therapy following prevention of mother-to-child transmission of HIV type 1, Ivory Coast, 2003–2006. *Clin Infect Dis* 2008;46(4):611–621.
91. Chi BH, Sinkala M, Mbewe F, et al. Single-dose tenofovir and emtricitabine for reduction of viral resistance to non-nucleoside reverse transcriptase inhibitor drugs in women given intrapartum nevirapine for perinatal HIV prevention: an open-label randomised trial. *Lancet* 2007;370(9600):1698–1705.
92. Arrive E, Newell ML, Ekouevi DK, et al. Prevalence of resistance to nevirapine in mothers and children after single-dose exposure to prevent vertical transmission of HIV-1: a meta-analysis. *Int J Epidemiol* 2007;36(5):1009–1021.
93. Hirsch MS, Conway B, D'Aquila RT, et al. Antiretroviral drug resistance testing in adults with HIV infection: implications for clinical management. International AIDS Society—USA Panel. *JAMA* 1998;279(24):1984–1991.
94. Eastman PS, Shapiro DE, Coombs RW, et al. Maternal viral genotypic zidovudine resistance and infrequent failure of zidovudine therapy to prevent perinatal transmission of human immunodeficiency virus type 1 in pediatric AIDS Clinical Trials Group Protocol 076. *J Infect Dis* 1998;177(3):557–564.
95. Bardeguez AD, Shapiro DE, Mofenson LM, et al. Effect of cessation of zidovudine prophylaxis to reduce vertical transmission on maternal HIV disease progression and survival. *J Acquir Immune Defic Syndr* 2003;32(2):170–181.
96. Clarke JR, Braganza R, Mirza A, et al. Rapid development of genotypic resistance to lamivudine when combined with zidovudine in pregnancy. *J Med Virol* 1999;59(3):364–368.
97. Mandelbrot L, Landreau-Mascaro A, Rekacewicz C, et al. Lamivudine–zidovudine combination for prevention of maternal-infant transmission of HIV-1. *JAMA* 2001;285(16):2083–2093.
98. Parker MM, Wade N, Lloyd RM Jr., et al. Prevalence of genotypic drug resistance among a cohort of HIV-infected newborns. *J Acquir Immune Defic Syndr* 2003;32(3):292–297.
99. Sandberg JA, Slikker W Jr. Developmental pharmacology and toxicology of anti-HIV therapeutic agents: dideoxynucleosides. *FASEB J* 1995;9(12):1157–1163.
100. Robbins BL, Waibel BH, Fridland A. Quantitation of intracellular zidovudine phosphates by use of combined cartridge-radioimmunoassay methodology. *Antimicrob Agents Chemother* 1996;40(11):2651–2654.
101. Rodriguez JF, Rodriguez JL, Santana J, et al. Simultaneous quantitation of intracellular zidovudine and lamivudine triphosphates in human immunodeficiency virus-infected individuals. *Antimicrob Agents Chemother* 2000;44(11):3097–3100.
102. Barry MG, Khoo SH, Veal GJ, et al. The effect of zidovudine dose on the formation of intracellular phosphorylated metabolites. *AIDS* 1996;10(12):1361–1367.
103. Grim SA, Romanelli F. Tenofovir disoproxil fumarate. *Ann Pharmacother* 2003;37(6):849–859.
104. Singlas E, Pioger JC, Taburet AM, et al. Comparative pharmacokinetics of zidovudine (AZT) and its metabolite (G.AZT) in healthy subjects and HIV seropositive patients. *Eur J Clin Pharmacol* 1989;36(6):639–640.
105. Klecker RW Jr., Collins JM, Yarchoan R, et al. Plasma and cerebrospinal fluid pharmacokinetics of 3′-azido-3′-deoxythymidine: a novel pyrimidine analog with potential application for the treatment of patients with AIDS and related diseases. *Clin Pharmacol Ther* 1987;41(4):407–412.
106. Yarchoan R, Mitsuya H, Myers CE, et al. Clinical pharmacology of 3′-azido-2′,3′-dideoxythymidine (zidovudine) and related dideoxynucleosides. *N Engl J Med* 1989;321(11):726–738.
107. Collins JM, Unadkat JD. Clinical pharmacokinetics of zidovudine. An overview of current data. *Clin Pharmacokinet* 1989;17(1):1–9.
108. Sperling RS, Roboz J, Dische R, et al. Zidovudine pharmacokinetics during pregnancy. *Am J Perinatol* 1992;9(4):247–249.
109. O'Sullivan MJ, Boyer PJ, Scott GB, et al. The pharmacokinetics and safety of zidovudine in the third trimester of pregnancy for women infected with human immunodeficiency virus and their infants: phase I acquired immunodeficiency syndrome clinical trials group study (protocol 082). Zidovudine Collaborative Working Group. *Am J Obstet Gynecol* 1993;168(5):1510–1516.
110. Watts DH, Brown ZA, Tartaglione T, et al. Pharmacokinetic disposition of zidovudine during pregnancy. *J Infect Dis* 1991; 163(2):226–232.
111. Moodley J, Moodley D, Pillay K, et al. Pharmacokinetics and antiretroviral activity of lamivudine alone or when coadministered with zidovudine in human immunodeficiency virus type 1-infected pregnant women and their offspring. *J Infect Dis* 1998; 178(5):1327–1333.
112. Furman PA, Fyfe JA, St Clair MH, et al. Phosphorylation of 3′-azido-3′-deoxythymidine and selective interaction of the 5′-triphosphate with human immunodeficiency virus reverse transcriptase. *Proc Natl Acad Sci U S A* 1986;83(21):8333–8337.
113. Wattanagoon Y, Na Bangchang K, Hoggard PG, et al. Pharmacokinetics of zidovudine phosphorylation in human immunodeficiency virus-positive Thai patients and healthy volunteers. *Antimicrob Agents Chemother* 2000;44(7):1986–1989.
114. Stretcher BN, Pesce AJ, Frame PT, et al. Pharmacokinetics of zidovudine phosphorylation in peripheral blood mononuclear cells from patients infected with human immunodeficiency virus. *Antimicrob Agents Chemother* 1994;38(7):1541–1547.
115. Ho HT, Hitchcock MJ. Cellular pharmacology of 2′,3′-dideoxy-2′,3′-didehydrothymidine, a nucleoside analog active against human immunodeficiency virus. *Antimicrob Agents Chemother* 1989; 33(6):844–849.
116. Sale M, Sheiner LB, Volberding P, et al. Zidovudine response relationships in early human immunodeficiency virus infection. *Clin Pharmacol Ther* 1993;54(5):556–566.
117. Pons JC, Taburet AM, Singlas E, et al. Placental passage of azathiothymidine (AZT) during the second trimester of pregnancy: study by direct fetal blood sampling under ultrasound. *Eur J Obstet Gynecol Reprod Biol* 1991;40(3):229–231.
118. Chappuy H, Treluyer JM, Jullien V, et al. Maternal-fetal transfer and amniotic fluid accumulation of nucleoside analogue reverse transcriptase inhibitors in human immunodeficiency virus-infected pregnant women. *Antimicrob Agents Chemother* 2004; 48(11): 4332–4336.
119. Schenker S, Johnson RF, King TS, et al. Azidothymidine (zidovudine) transport by the human placenta. *Am J Med Sci* 1990;299(1): 16–20.
120. Patterson TA, Binienda ZK, Lipe GW, et al. Transplacental pharmacokinetics and fetal distribution of azidothymidine, its glucuronide, and phosphorylated metabolites in late-term rhesus macaques after maternal infusion. *Drug Metab Dispos* 1997;25(4): 453–459.
121. Dancis J, Lee J, Mendoza S, et al. Nucleoside transport by perfused human placenta. *Placenta* 1993;14(5):547–554.
122. Rodman JH, Flynn PM, Robbins B, et al. Systemic pharmacokinetics and cellular pharmacology of zidovudine in human immunodeficiency virus type 1-infected women and newborn infants. *J Infect Dis* 1999;180(6):1844–1850.
123. Lallemant M, Jourdain G, Le Coeur S, et al. A trial of shortened zidovudine regimens to prevent mother-to-child transmission of human immunodeficiency virus type 1. Perinatal HIV Prevention Trial (Thailand) Investigators. *N Engl J Med* 2000;343(14): 982–991.

124. Mirochnick M, Rodman JH, Robbins BL, et al. Pharmacokinetics of oral zidovudine administered during labour: a preliminary study. *HIV Med* 2007;8(7):451–456.
125. Bhadrakom C, Simonds RJ, Mei JV, et al. Oral zidovudine during labor to prevent perinatal HIV transmission, Bangkok: tolerance and zidovudine concentration in cord blood. Bangkok Collaborative Perinatal HIV Transmission Study Group. *AIDS* 2000;14(5):509–516.
126. Boucher FD, Modlin JF, Weller S, et al. Phase I evaluation of zidovudine administered to infants exposed at birth to the human immunodeficiency virus. *J Pediatr* 1993;122(1):137–144.
127. Mirochnick M, Capparelli E, Connor J. Pharmacokinetics of zidovudine in infants: a population analysis across studies. *Clin Pharmacol Ther* 1999;66(1):16–24.
128. Kawade N, Onishi S. The prenatal and postnatal development of UDP-glucuronyltransferase activity towards bilirubin and the effect of premature birth on this activity in the human liver. *Biochem J* 1981;196(1):257–260.
129. Rajaonarison JF, Lacarelle B, De Sousa G, et al. In vitro glucuronidation of 3′-azido-3′-deoxythymidine by human liver. Role of UDP-glucuronosyltransferase 2 form. *Drug Metab Dispos* 1991;19(4):809–815.
130. Herber R, Magdalou J, Haumont M, et al. Glucuronidation of 3′-azido-3′-deoxythymidine in human liver microsomes: enzyme inhibition by drugs and steroid hormones. *Biochim Biophys Acta* 1992;1139(1–2):20–24.
131. Moodley D, Pillay K, Naidoo K, et al. Pharmacokinetics of zidovudine and lamivudine in neonates following coadministration of oral doses every 12 hours. *Br J Clin Pharmacol* 2001;41(7):732–741.
132. Mirochnick M, Capparelli E, Dankner W, et al. Zidovudine pharmacokinetics in premature infants exposed to human immunodeficiency virus. *Antimicrob Agents Chemother* 1998;42(4):808–812.
133. Balis FM, Pizzo PA, Murphy RF, et al. The pharmacokinetics of zidovudine administered by continuous infusion in children. *Ann Intern Med* 1989;110(4):279–285.
134. Capparelli EV, Mirochnick M, Dankner WM, et al. Pharmacokinetics and tolerance of zidovudine in preterm infants. *J Pediatr* 2003;142(1):47–52.
135. Ayers KM, Clive D, Tucker WE Jr., et al. Nonclinical toxicology studies with zidovudine: genetic toxicity tests and carcinogenicity bioassays in mice and rats. *Fundam Appl Toxicol* 1996;32(2):148–158.
136. Taha TE, Kumwenda N, Gibbons A, et al. Effect of HIV-1 antiretroviral prophylaxis on hepatic and hematological parameters of African infants. *AIDS* 2002;16(6):851–858.
137. Lipshultz SE, Easley KA, Orav EJ, et al. Absence of cardiac toxicity of zidovudine in infants. Pediatric Pulmonary and Cardiac Complications of Vertically Transmitted HIV Infection Study Group. *N Engl J Med* 2000;343(11):759–766.
138. Antiretroviral Pregnancy Registry Steering Committee. Antiretroviral Pregnancy Registry international interim report for 1 Jan 1989–31 July 2008. Wilmington, NC: Registry Coordinating Center, 2008. http://www.APRegistry.com.
139. Watts DH, Li D, Handelsman E, et al. Assessment of birth defects according to maternal therapy among infants in the Women and Infants Transmission Study. *J Acquir Immune Defic Syndr* 2007; 44(3): 299–305.
140. Perry CM, Faulds D. Lamivudine. A review of its antiviral activity, pharmacokinetic properties and therapeutic efficacy in the management of HIV infection. *Drugs* 1997;53(4):657–680.
141. Barry M, Mulcahy F, Merry C, et al. Pharmacokinetics and potential interactions amongst antiretroviral agents used to treat patients with HIV infection. *Clin Pharmacokinet* 1999;36(4):289–304.
142. Moore KH, Yuen GJ, Raasch RH, et al. Pharmacokinetics of lamivudine administered alone and with trimethoprim–sulfamethoxazole. *Clin Pharmacol Ther* 1996;59(5):550–558.
143. Moore KH, Barrett JE, Shaw S, et al. The pharmacokinetics of lamivudine phosphorylation in peripheral blood mononuclear cells from patients infected with HIV-1. *AIDS* 1999;13(16):2239–2250.
144. Bloom SL, Dias KM, Bawdon RE, et al. The maternal–fetal transfer of lamivudine in the ex vivo human placenta. *Am J Obstet Gynecol* 1997;176(2):291–293.
145. Mandelbrot L, Peytavin G, Firtion G, et al. Maternal–fetal transfer and amniotic fluid accumulation of lamivudine in human immunodeficiency virus-infected pregnant women. *Am J Obstet Gynecol* 2001;184(2):153–158.
146. Mueller BU, Lewis LL, Yuen GJ, et al. Serum and cerebrospinal fluid pharmacokinetics of intravenous and oral lamivudine in human immunodeficiency virus-infected children. *Antimicrob Agents Chemother* 1998;42(12):3187–3192.
147. Watson WJ, Stevens TP, Weinberg GA. Profound anemia in a newborn infant of a mother receiving antiretroviral therapy. *Pediatr Infect Dis J* 1998;17(5):435–436.
148. Chaisilwattana P, Chokephaibulkit K, Chalermchockcharoenkit A, et al. Short-course therapy with zidovudine plus lamivudine for prevention of mother-to-child transmission of human immunodeficiency virus type 1 in Thailand. *Clin Infect Dis* 2002;35(11):1405–1413.
149. Knupp CA, Hak LJ, Coakley DF, et al. Disposition of didanosine in HIV-seropositive patients with normal renal function or chronic renal failure: influence of hemodialysis and continuous ambulatory peritoneal dialysis. *Clin Pharmacol Ther* 1996;60(5):535–542.
150. Knupp CA, Shyu WC, Dolin R, et al. Pharmacokinetics of didanosine in patients with acquired immunodeficiency syndrome or acquired immunodeficiency syndrome-related complex. *Clin Pharmacol Ther* 1991;49(5):523–535.
151. Ahluwalia G, Johnson MA, Fridland A, et al. Cellular pharmacology of the anti-HIV agent 2′,3′-dideoxyinosine [abstract]. *Proc Am Acad Cancer Res* 1988;29:349P.
152. Wang Y, Livingston E, Patil S, et al. Pharmacokinetics of didanosine in antepartum and postpartum human immunodeficiency virus–infected pregnant women and their neonates: an AIDS clinical trials group study. *J Infect Dis* 1999;180(5):1536–1541.
153. Rongkavilit C, Thaithumyanon P, Chuenyam T, et al. Pharmacokinetics of stavudine and didanosine coadministered with nelfinavir in human immunodeficiency virus-exposed neonates. *Antimicrob Agents Chemother* 2001;45(12):3585–3590.
154. Kovacs A, Cowles MK, Britto P, et al. Pharmacokinetics of didanosine and drug resistance mutations in infants exposed to zidovudine during gestation or postnatally and treated with didanosine or zidovudine in the first three months of life. *Pediatr Infect Dis J* 2005;24(6):503–509.
155. Bartlett JG, Gallant JE. *Medical management of HIV infection.* Baltimore, MD: Johns Hopkins University Division of Infectious Diseases, 2001:278.
156. Wade NA, Unadkat JD, Huang S, et al. Pharmacokinetics and safety of stavudine in HIV-infected pregnant women and their infants: Pediatric AIDS Clinical Trials Group protocol 332. *J Infect Dis* 2004;190(12):2167–2174.
157. Jullien V, Rais A, Urien S, et al. Age-related differences in the pharmacokinetics of stavudine in 272 children from birth to 16 years: a population analysis. *Br J Clin Pharmacol* 2007;64(1):105–109.
158. L'Homme RF, Kabamba D, Ewings FM, et al. Nevirapine, stavudine and lamivudine pharmacokinetics in African children on paediatric fixed-dose combination tablets. *AIDS* 2008;22(5):557–565.
159. Ziagen package insert. Research Triangle Park, NC. GlaxoSmithKline, 2008.
160. Kumar PN, Sweet DE, McDowell JA, et al. Safety and pharmacokinetics of abacavir (1592U89) following oral administration of escalating single doses in human immunodeficiency virus type 1-infected adults. *Antimicrob Agents Chemother* 1999;43(3):603–608.
161. McDowell JA, Lou Y, Symonds WS, et al. Multiple-dose pharmacokinetics and pharmacodynamics of abacavir alone and in combination with zidovudine in human immunodeficiency virus-infected adults. *Antimicrob Agents Chemother* 2000;44(8):2061–2067.
162. Hawkins T, Veikley W, St Claire RL III, et al. Intracellular pharmacokinetics of tenofovir diphosphate, carbovir triphosphate, and lamivudine triphosphate in patients receiving triple-nucleoside regimens. *J Acquir Immune Defic Syndr* 2005;39(4):406–411.
163. Best BM, Mirochnick M, Capparelli EV, et al. Impact of pregnancy on abacavir pharmacokinetics. *AIDS* 2006;20(4):553–560.
164. Van Rompay KK, McChesney MB, Aguirre NL, et al. Two low doses of tenofovir protect newborn macaques against oral simian immunodeficiency virus infection. *J Infect Dis* 2001; 184(4):429–438.

165. Viread package insert. Foster City, CA. Gilead Sciences, 2008.
166. Ramanathan S, Shen G, Cheng A, et al. Pharmacokinetics of emtricitabine, tenofovir, and GS-9137 following coadministration of emtricitabine/tenofovir disoproxil fumarate and ritonavir-boosted GS-9137. *J Acquir Immune Defic Syndr* 2007;45(3): 274–279.
167. Blum MR, Chittick GE, Begley JA, et al. Steady-state pharmacokinetics of emtricitabine and tenofovir disoproxil fumarate administered alone and in combination in healthy volunteers. *Br J Clin Pharmacol* 2007;47(6):751–759.
168. Parks DA, Jennings HC, Taylor CW, et al. Pharmacokinetics of once-daily tenofovir, emtricitabine, ritonavir and fosamprenavir in HIV-infected subjects. *AIDS* 2007;21(10):1373–1375.
169. Stevens RC, Blum MR, Rousseau FS, et al. Intracellular pharmacology of emtricitabine and tenofovir. *Clin Infect Dis* 2004;39(6): 877–878; author reply 8–9.
170. Hirt D, Urien S, Ekouevi D, et al. Population pharmacokinetics of tenofovir in HIV-1-infected pregnant women and their neonates (ANRS 12109). *Clin Pharmacol Ther* 2008;85(2):182–189.
171. Rodman J, Flynn P, Shapiro D, et al. for PACTG 394 Study Team. *Pharmacokinetics (PK) and safety of tenofovir disoproxil fumarate (TDF) in HIV-1-infected pregnant women and their infants* [Abstract 708]. Presented at the 13th Conference on Retroviruses and Opportunistic Infections, Denver, CO, February 5–8, 2007. http://www.retroconference.org/2006/PDFs/708.pdf. Accessed December 2, 2008.
172. Burchett SK, Best B, Mirochnick M, et al. for the PACTG P1026s Team. *Tenofovir pharmacokinetics during pregnancy, at delivery and postpartum* [Abstract 738b]. Presented at the 14th Conference on Retroviruses and Opportunistic Infections, Los Angeles, CA, February 25–28, 2007.
173. Antoniou T, Park-Wyllie LY, Tseng AL. Tenofovir: a nucleotide analog for the management of human immunodeficiency virus infection. *Pharmacotherapy* 2003;23(1):29–43.
174. Tarantal AF, Marthas ML, Shaw JP, et al. Administration of 9-[2-(R)-(phosphonomethoxy)propyl]adenine (PMPA) to gravid and infant rhesus macaques (Macaca mulatta): safety and efficacy studies. *J Acquir Immune Defic Syndr Hum Retrovirol* 1999; 20(4):323–333.
175. Tarantal AF, Castillo A, Ekert JE, et al. Fetal and maternal outcome after administration of tenofovir to gravid rhesus monkeys (Macaca mulatta). *J Acquir Immune Defic Syndr* 2002;29(3): 207–220.
176. Lanzafame M, Lattuada E, Rapagna F, et al. Tenofovir-associated kidney diseases and interactions between tenofovir and other antiretrovirals. *Clin Infect Dis* 2006;42(11):1656–1657; author reply 8.
177. Antoniou T, Raboud J, Chirhin S, et al. Incidence of and risk factors for tenofovir-induced nephrotoxicity: a retrospective cohort study. *HIV Med* 2005;6(4):284–290.
178. Izzedine H, Hulot JS, Villard E, et al. Association between ABCC2 gene haplotypes and tenofovir-induced proximal tubulopathy. *J Infect Dis* 2006;194(11):1481–1491.
179. Gafni RI, Hazra R, Reynolds JC, et al. Tenofovir disoproxil fumarate and an optimized background regimen of antiretroviral agents as salvage therapy: impact on bone mineral density in HIV-infected children. *Pediatrics* 2006;118(3):e711–e718.
180. Purdy JB, Gafni RI, Reynolds JC, et al. Decreased bone mineral density with off-label use of tenofovir in children and adolescents infected with human immunodeficiency virus. *J Pediatr* 2008;152(4):582–584.
181. Giacomet V, Mora S, Martelli L, et al. A 12-month treatment with tenofovir does not impair bone mineral accrual in HIV-infected children. *J Acquir Immune Defic Syndr* 2005;40(4):448–450.
182. Nurutdinova D, Onen NF, Hayes E, et al. Adverse effects of tenofovir use in HIV-infected pregnant women and their infants. *Ann Pharmacother* 2008;42(11):1581–1585.
183. Sabbatini F, Prati F, Borghi V, et al. Congenital pyelectasis in children born from mothers on tenofovir containing therapy during pregnancy: report of two cases. *Infection* 2007;35(6): 474–476.
184. Emtriva package insert. Foster City, CA. Gilead Sciences, 2008.
185. Wang LH, Begley J, St Claire RL III, et al. Pharmacokinetic and pharmacodynamic characteristics of emtricitabine support its once daily dosing for the treatment of HIV infection. *AIDS Res Hum Retroviruses* 2004;20(11):1173–1182.
186. Hirt D, Urien S, Rey E, et al. *Population pharmacokinetics of emtricitabine in HIV-infected pregnant women and their neonates: TEmAA ANRS 12109* [Abstract 626]. Presented at the 15th Conference on Retroviruses and Opportunistic Infections, Boston, MA, February 3–6, 2008.
187. Best B, Stek A, Hu C, et al. for the PACTG/IMPAACT P1026S team. *High-dose lopinavir and standard-dose emtricitabine pharmacokinetics during pregnancy and postpartum* [Abstract 629]. Presented at the 15th Conference on Retroviruses and Opportunistic Infections, Boston, MA, February 3–8, 2008.
188. Blum MR, Ndiweni D, Chittick G, et al. *Steady-state pharmacokinetic evaluation of emtricitabine in neonates exposed to HIV in utero* [Abstract 568]. Presented at the 13th Conference on Retroviruses and Opportunistic Infections, Denver, CO, February 5–9, 2006.
189. Temesgen Z, Wright AJ. Antiretrovirals. *Mayo Clin proc* 1999; 74(12):1284–1301.
190. Stringer EM, Sinkala M, Stringer JS, et al. Prevention of mother-to-child transmission of HIV in Africa: successes and challenges in scaling-up a nevirapine-based program in Lusaka, Zambia. *AIDS* 2003;17(9):1377–1382.
191. Mirochnick M, Clarke DF, Dorenbaum A. Nevirapine: pharmacokinetic considerations in children and pregnant women. *Clin Pharmacokinet* 2000;39(4):281–293.
192. Cheeseman SH, Hattox SE, McLaughlin MM, et al. Pharmacokinetics of nevirapine: initial single-rising-dose study in humans. *Antimicrob Agents Chemother* 1993;37(2):178–182.
193. Lamson MJ, Sabo JP, MacGregor TR, et al. Single dose pharmacokinetics and bioavailability of nevirapine in healthy volunteers. *Biopharm Drug Dispos* 1999;20(6):285–291.
194. Lamson MJ, Cort S, Sabo JP, et al. *Effects of food or antacid on the bioavailability of nevirapine 200 mg in 24 healthy volunteers* [abstract]. Presented at the 11th World Conference on AIDS, Vancouver, Canada, July 7–12, 1996.
195. Cheeseman SH, Havlir D, McLaughlin MM, et al. Phase I/II evaluation of nevirapine alone and in combination with zidovudine for infection with human immunodeficiency virus. *J Acquir Immune Defic Syndr Hum Retrovirol* 1995;8(2):141–151.
196. Havlir D, Cheeseman SH, McLaughlin M, et al. High-dose nevirapine: safety, pharmacokinetics, and antiviral effect in patients with human immunodeficiency virus infection. *J Infect Dis* 1995; 171(3):537–545.
197. Taylor GP, Lyall EG, Back D, et al. Pharmacological implications of lengthened in-utero exposure to nevirapine. *Lancet* 2000; 355(9221):2134–2135.
198. Capparelli EV, Aweeka F, Hitti J, et al. Chronic administration of nevirapine during pregnancy: impact of pregnancy on pharmacokinetics. *HIV Med* 2008;9(4):214–220.
199. von Hentig N, Carlebach A, Gute P, et al. A comparison of the steady-state pharmacokinetics of nevirapine in men, nonpregnant women and women in late pregnancy. *Br J Clin Pharmacol* 2006;62(5):552–559.
200. Mirochnick M, Siminski S, Fenton T, et al. Nevirapine pharmacokinetics in pregnant women and in their infants after in utero exposure. *Pediatr Infect Dis J* 2001;20(8):803–805.
201. Mirochnick M, Fenton T, Gagnier P, et al. Pharmacokinetics of nevirapine in human immunodeficiency virus type 1-infected pregnant women and their neonates. Pediatric AIDS Clinical Trials Group Protocol 250 Team. *J Infect Dis* 1998;178(2): 368–374.
202. Musoke P, Guay LA, Bagenda D, et al. A phase I/II study of the safety and pharmacokinetics of nevirapine in HIV-1-infected pregnant Ugandan women and their neonates (HIVNET 006). *AIDS* 1999;13(4):479–486.
203. Stringer JS, Sinkala M, Chapman V, et al. Timing of the maternal drug dose and risk of perinatal HIV transmission in the setting of intrapartum and neonatal single-dose nevirapine. *AIDS* 2003;17(11):1659–1665.
204. Mirochnick M, Dorenbaum A, Blanchard S, et al. Predose infant nevirapine concentration with the two-dose intrapartum neonatal nevirapine regimen: association with timing of maternal intrapartum nevirapine dose. *J Acquir Immune Defic Syndr* 2003;33(2): 153–156.
205. Shetty AK, Coovadia HM, Mirochnick MM, et al. Safety and trough concentrations of nevirapine prophylaxis given daily, twice weekly, or weekly in breast-feeding infants from birth to 6 months. *J Acquir Immune Defic Syndr* 2003;34(5):482–490.

206. Shapiro RL, Holland DT, Capparelli E, et al. Antiretroviral concentrations in breast-feeding infants of women in Botswana receiving antiretroviral treatment. *J Infect Dis* 2005;192(5):720–727.
207. Patel SM, Johnson S, Belknap SM, et al. Serious adverse cutaneous and hepatic toxicities associated with nevirapine use by non-HIV-infected individuals. *J Acquir Immune Defic Syndr* 2004; 35(2):120–125.
208. Mazhude C, Jones S, Murad S, et al. Female sex but not ethnicity is a strong predictor of non-nucleoside reverse transcriptase inhibitor-induced rash. *AIDS* 2002;16(11):1566–1568.
209. Bersoff-Matcha SJ, Miller WC, Aberg JA, et al. Sex differences in nevirapine rash. *Clin Infect Dis* 2001;32(1):124–129.
210. Knudtson E, Para M, Boswell H, et al. Drug rash with eosinophilia and systemic symptoms syndrome and renal toxicity with a nevirapine-containing regimen in a pregnant patient with human immunodeficiency virus. *Obstet Gynecol* 2003;101(5, pt 2): 1094–1097.
211. Hitti J, Frenkel LM, Stek AM, et al. Maternal toxicity with continuous nevirapine in pregnancy: results from PACTG 1022. *J Acquir Immune Defic Syndr* 2004;36(3):772–776.
212. Lyons F, Hopkins S, Kelleher B, et al. Maternal hepatotoxicity with nevirapine as part of combination antiretroviral therapy in pregnancy. *HIV Med* 2006;7(4):255–260.
213. Sustiva package insert. Wilmington, DE: Dupont Pharmaceuticals Company. 2000.
214. Fundaro C, Genovese O, Rendeli C, et al. Myelomeningocele in a child with intrauterine exposure to efavirenz. *AIDS* 2002;16(2): 299–300.
215. De Santis M, Carducci B, De Santis L, et al. Periconceptional exposure to efavirenz and neural tube defects. *Arch Intern Med* 2002;162(3):355.
216. Saitoh A, Hull AD, Franklin P, et al. Myelomeningocele in an infant with intrauterine exposure to efavirenz. *J Perinatol* 2005; 25(8):555–556.
217. Schneider S, Peltier A, Gras A, et al. Efavirenz in human breast milk, mothers', and newborns' plasma. *J Acquir Immune Defic Syndr* 2008;48(4):450–454.
218. Rescriptor package insert. La Jolla, CA: Agouron Pharmaceuticals. 2001.
219. Intelence package insert. Raritan, NJ: Tibotec, Inc., 2008.
220. Townsend CL, Cortina-Borja M, Peckham CS, et al. Trends in management and outcome of pregnancies in HIV-infected women in the UK and Ireland, 1990–2006. *BJOG* 2008;115(9): 1078–1086.
221. Barry M, Gibbons S, Back D, et al. Protease inhibitors in patients with HIV disease. Clinically important pharmacokinetic considerations. *Clin Pharmacokinet* 1997;32(3):194–209.
222. van Heeswijk RP, Veldkamp A, Mulder JW, et al. Combination of protease inhibitors for the treatment of HIV-1-infected patients: a review of pharmacokinetics and clinical experience. *Antivir Ther* 2001;6(4):201–229.
223. Mirochnick M, Dorenbaum A, Holland D, et al. Concentrations of protease inhibitors in cord blood after in utero exposure. *Pediatr Infect Dis J* 2002;21(9):835–838.
224. Marzolini C, Rudin C, Decosterd LA, et al. Transplacental passage of protease inhibitors at delivery. *AIDS* 2002;16(6):889–893.
225. Reyataz package insert. Bristol-Myers Squibb Co., Princeton, NJ. September, 2008. http://packageinserts.bms.com/pi/pi_reyataz.pdf. Accessed November 21, 2008.
226. Natha M, Hay P, Taylor G, et al. *Atazanavir use in pregnancy: a report of 33 cases* [Abstract 750]. Presented at the 14th Conference on Retroviruses and Opportunistic Infections, Los Angeles, CA, February 25–28, 2007.
227. Ripamonti D, Cattaneo D, Maggiolo F, et al. Atazanavir plus low-dose ritonavir in pregnancy: pharmacokinetics and placental transfer. *AIDS* 2007;21(18):2409–2415.
228. Eley T, Vandeloise E, Child M, et al., and The Atazanavir 182 Pregnancy Study Group Steady State Pharmacokinetics and Safety of Atazanavir after Treatment with ATV 300 mg Once Daily/Ritonavir 100 mg Once Daily + ZDV/3TC during the Third Trimester in HIV+ Women [Abstract 624]. Presented at the 15th Conference on Retroviruses and Opportunistic Infections, Boston, MA, February 3–6, 2008.
229. Mirochnick M, Stek A, Capparelli E, et al., and PACTG 1026s Protocol Team. *Atazanavir pharmacokinetics with and without tenofovir during pregnancy.* Presented at the 16th Conference on Retroviruses and Opportunistic Infections, Montreal, Canada, February, 2009.
230. Hayashi S, Beckerman K, Homma M, et al. Pharmacokinetics of indinavir in HIV-positive pregnant women. *AIDS* 2000;14(8): 1061–1062.
231. Kosel BW, Beckerman KP, Hayashi S, et al. Pharmacokinetics of nelfinavir and indinavir in HIV-1-infected pregnant women. *AIDS* 2003;17(8):1195–1199.
232. Unadkat JD, Wara DW, Hughes MD, et al. Pharmacokinetics and safety of indinavir in human immunodeficiency virus-infected pregnant women. *Antimicrob Agents Chemother* 2007;51(2):783–786.
233. Ghosn J, De Montgolfier I, Cornelie C, et al. Antiretroviral therapy with a twice-daily regimen containing 400 milligrams of indinavir and 100 milligrams of ritonavir in human immunodeficiency virus type 1-infected women during pregnancy. *Antimicrob Agents Chemother* 2008;52(4):1542–1544.
234. Lopinavir package insert. Abbott Laboratories, North Chicago, IL. June, 2008. http://www.rxabbott.com/pdf/kaletratabpi.pdf. Accessed November 25, 2008.
235. Stek AM, Mirochnick M, Capparelli E, et al. Reduced lopinavir exposure during pregnancy. *AIDS* 2006;20(15):1931–1939.
236. Mirochnick M, Best BM, Stek AM, et al. Lopinavir exposure with an increased dose during pregnancy. *J Acquir Immune Defic Syndr* 2008;49(5):485–491.
237. Lyons F, Lechelt M, De Ruiter A. Steady-state lopinavir levels in third trimester of pregnancy. *AIDS* 2007;21(8):1053–1054.
238. Chadwick EG, Capparelli EV, Yogev R, et al. Pharmacokinetics, safety and efficacy of lopinavir/ritonavir in infants less than 6 months of age: 24 week results. *AIDS* 2008;22(2):249–255.
239. Nelfinavir Package Insert. La Jolla, CA: Agouron Pharmaceuticals Inc., 2007. http://www.fda.gov/cder/foi/label/2007/020778s027, 020779s048, 021503s0091b1.pdf. Accessed July 23, 2008.
240. Baede-van Dijk PA, Hugen PW, Verweij-van Wissen CP, et al. Analysis of variation in plasma concentrations of nelfinavir and its active metabolite M8 in HIV-positive patients. *AIDS* 2001; 15(8):991–998.
241. Zhang KE, Wu E, Patick AK, et al. Circulating metabolites of the human immunodeficiency virus protease inhibitor nelfinavir in humans: structural identification, levels in plasma, and antiviral activities. *Antimicrob Agents Chemother* 2001;45(4):1086–1093.
242. Pai VB, Nahata MC. Nelfinavir mesylate: a protease inhibitor. *Ann Pharmacother* 1999;33(3):325–339.
243. Bryson YJ, Mirochnick M, Stek A, et al. Pharmacokinetics and safety of nelfinavir when used in combination with zidovudine and lamivudine in HIV-infected pregnant women: Pediatric AIDS Clinical Trials Group (PACTG) Protocol 353. *HIV Clin Trials* 2008;9(2):115–125.
244. van Heeswijk RP, Khaliq Y, Gallicano KD, et al. The pharmacokinetics of nelfinavir and M8 during pregnancy and post partum. *Clin Pharmacol Ther* 2004;76(6):588–597.
245. Nellen JF, Schillevoort I, Wit FW, et al. Nelfinavir plasma concentrations are low during pregnancy. *Clin Infect Dis* 2004;39(5): 736–740.
246. Angel JB, Khaliq Y, Monpetit ML, et al. An argument for routine therapeutic drug monitoring of HIV-1 protease inhibitors during pregnancy. *AIDS* 2001;15(3):417–419.
247. Burger D, Hugen P, Reiss P, et al. Therapeutic drug monitoring of nelfinavir and indinavir in treatment-naive HIV-1-infected individuals. *AIDS* 2003;17(8):1157–1165.
248. Burger DM, Hugen PW, Aarnoutse RE, et al. Treatment failure of nelfinavir-containing triple therapy can largely be explained by low nelfinavir plasma concentrations. *Ther Drug Monit* 2003; 25(1):73–80.
249. Hirt D, Treluyer JM, Jullien V, et al. Pregnancy-related effects on nelfinavir-M8 pharmacokinetics: a population study with 133 women. *Antimicrob Agents Chemother* 2006;50(6):2079–2086.
250. Read JS, Best BM, Stek AM, et al. Pharmacokinetics of new 625 mg nelfinavir formulation during pregnancy and postpartum. *HIV Med* 2008;9(10):875–882.
251. Gatti G, Castelli-Gattinara G, Cruciani M, et al. Pharmacokinetics and pharmacodynamics of nelfinavir administered twice or thrice daily to human immunodeficiency virus type 1-infected children. *Clin Infect Dis* 2003;36(11):1476–1482.
252. Capparelli EV, Sullivan JL, Mofenson L, et al. Pharmacokinetics of nelfinavir in human immunodeficiency virus-infected infants. *Pediatr Infect Dis J* 2001;20(8):746–751.

253. Mirochnick M, Stek A, Acevedo M, et al. Safety and pharmacokinetics of nelfinavir coadministered with zidovudine and lamivudine in infants during the first 6 weeks of life. *J Acquir Immune Defic Syndr* 2005;39(2):189–194.
254. Rongkavilit C, van Heeswijk RP, Limpongsanurak S, et al. Dose-escalating study of the safety and pharmacokinetics of nelfinavir in HIV-exposed neonates. *J Acquir Immune Defic Syndr* 2002;29(5): 455–463.
255. Mirochnick M, Nielsen-Saines K, Pilotto JH, et al., and NICHD/HPTN 040/PACTG 1043 Protocol Team. *Nelfinavir pharmacokinetics with an increased dose during the first two weeks of life.* Presented at the 15th Conference on Retroviruses and Opportunistic Infections, Boston, MA, February, 2008.
256. Saquinavir package insert. Nutley, NJ: Roche Laboratories Inc., July 2007. http://www.rocheusa.com/products/invirase/pi.pdf. Accessed November 26, 2008.
257. Acosta EP, Zorrilla C, Van Dyke R, et al. Pharmacokinetics of saquinavir-SGC in HIV-infected pregnant women. *HIV Clin Trials* 2001;2(6):460–465.
258. Vithayasai V, Moyle GJ, Supajatura V, et al. Safety and efficacy of saquinavir soft-gelatin capsules + zidovudine + optional lamivudine in pregnancy and prevention of vertical HIV transmission. *J Acquir Immune Defic Syndr* 2002;30(4):410–412.
259. Acosta EP, Bardeguez A, Zorrilla CD, et al. Pharmacokinetics of saquinavir plus low-dose ritonavir in human immunodeficiency virus-infected pregnant women. *Antimicrob Agents Chemother* 2004; 48(2):430–436.
260. Burger D, Eggink A, van der Ende ME, et al. *The pharmacokinetics of saquinavir in the new tablet formulation + ritonavir (1000/100 mg twice daily) in HIV-1-infected pregnant women* [Abstract 741]. Presented at the 14th Conference on Retroviruses and Opportunistic Infections, Los Angeles, CA, February 25–28, 2007. http://www.retroconference.org/2007/PDFs/741.pdf. Accessed November 26, 2008.
261. Lopez-Cortes LF, Ruiz-Valderas R, Pascual R, et al. Once-daily saquinavir-hgc plus low-dose ritonavir (1200/100 mg) in HIV-infected pregnant women: pharmacokinetics and efficacy. *HIV Clin Trials* 2003;4(3):227–229.
262. Lopez-Cortes LF, Ruiz-Valderas R, Rivero A, et al. Efficacy of low-dose boosted saquinavir once daily plus nucleoside reverse transcriptase inhibitors in pregnant HIV-1-infected women with a therapeutic drug monitoring strategy. *Ther Drug Monit* 2007;29(2): 171–176.
263. Scott GB, Rodman JH, Scott WA, et al. *Pharmacokinetic and virologic response to ritonavir (RTV) in combination with zidovudine (ZDV) and lamivudine (3TC) in HIV-1-infected pregnant women and their infants* [Abstract 794-W]. Presented at the 9th Conference on Retroviruses and Opportunistic Infections, Seattle, WA, February 24–28, 2002. http://www.retroconference.org/2002/Abstract/13702.htm. Accessed November 26, 2008.
264. Haberl A, Linde R, Reitter A, et al. *Use of enfuvirtide in HIV+ pregnant women* [Abstract 627b]. Presented at the 15th Conference on Retroviruses and Opportunistic Infections, Boston, MA, February 3–6, 2008.
265. Madeddu G, Calia GM, Campus ML, et al. Successful prevention of multidrug resistant HIV mother-to-child transmission with enfuvirtide use in late pregnancy. *Int J STD AIDS* 2008;19(9):644–645.
266. Meyohas MC, Lacombe K, Carbonne B, et al. Enfuvirtide prescription at the end of pregnancy to a multi-treated HIV-infected woman with virological breakthrough. *AIDS* 2004;18(14): 1966–1968.
267. Sued O, Lattner J, Gun A, et al. Use of darunavir and enfuvirtide in a pregnant woman. *Int J STD AIDS* 2008;19(12):866–867.
268. Wensing AM, Boucher CA, van Kasteren M, et al. Prevention of mother-to-child transmission of multi-drug resistant HIV-1 using maternal therapy with both enfuvirtide and tipranavir. *AIDS* 2006;20(10):1465–1467.
269. Brennan-Benson P, Pakianathan M, Rice P, et al. Enfurvitide prevents vertical transmission of multidrug-resistant HIV-1 in pregnancy but does not cross the placenta. *AIDS* 2006;20(2): 297–299.
270. Cohan D, Feakins C, Wara D, et al. Perinatal transmission of multidrug-resistant HIV-1 despite viral suppression on an enfuvirtide-based treatment regimen. *AIDS* 2005;19(9):989–990.
271. Ceccaldi PF, Ferreira C, Gavard L, et al. Placental transfer of enfuvirtide in the ex vivo human placenta perfusion model. *Am J Obstet Gynecol* 2008;198(4):433, e1–e2.

CHAPTER

23

Mary Lieh-Lai
Ashok Sarnaik

Therapeutic Applications in Pediatric Intensive Care

INTRODUCTION

> The worst thing about medicine is that one kind makes another necessary.
>
> Elbert Hubbard

Management of a critically ill child poses a special challenge to the clinician. Most children admitted to an intensive care unit (ICU) have multisystem involvement. The clinician must not only be aware of age-related changes in pharmacokinetics and pharmacodynamics but also be cognizant of various drug–drug and drug–disease interactions. Because of the ongoing pathophysiologic changes, the physician must also deal with changes in volume of distribution and elimination kinetics during the clinical course. A critically ill child is often exposed to 20 or more medications during his or her hospital stay. Practically, every organ system and disease entity is represented in the pathophysiologic derangements of the patients in the ICU. A comprehensive discussion of management of an individual disease entity is beyond the scope of this chapter. Instead, we offer a working outline of management of most commonly encountered disease processes in critically ill children.

I. Central Nervous System
1. Increased intracranial pressure
   Introduction
   Management
   - Osmotherapy
   - Barbiturates
   - Hypertonic saline and glycerol
   - Acetazolamide and furosemide
   - Corticosteroids
2. Status epilepticus
   Introduction
   Management algorithm
   Initial survey
   The role of metabolic abnormalities and toxins in status epilepticus
   Drug therapy of status epilepticus

   - Lorazepam
   - Midazolam
   - Diazepam
   - Phenytoin
   - Fosphenytoin
   - Phenobarbital
   - Levetiracetam
   - Pentobarbital
   - Isoflurane
   - Etomidate
   - Propofol
   - Paraldehyde
3. Myasthenia gravis
   Introduction
   Management

   - Edrophonium
   - Neostigmine
   - Corticosteroids
   - Intravenous immunoglobulin
4. Neuromuscular blocking agents
   Introduction
   Depolarizing neuromuscular blocking agent
   - Succinylcholine

   Nondepolarizing or competitive neuromuscular blocking agents

   - Pancuronium
   - Vecuronium
   - Cisatracurium
   - Mivacurium
   - Rocuronium

   Complications of neuromuscular blocking agents
   Monitoring of neuromuscular blockade: train of four
5. Sedation
   Introduction
   Measures of sedation

   - Ramsay scale
   - COMFORT scale
   - Bispectral index (BIS)
   - Penn State Sedation Algorithm

   Drugs used for sedation

   - Benzodiazepines
   - Propofol
   - Etomidate
   - Ketamine
   - Barbiturates
   - Dexmedetomidine

   Complications of sedation

6. Pain and analgesia
   Introduction
   - Measures of Pain
   - CHEOPS
   - Oucher scale
   - FLACC
   Analgesics
   - Opioids
   - Nonsteroidal anti-inflammatory drugs (NSAIDs)
7. Syndrome of inappropriate antidiuretic hormone (SIADH) secretion
   Definition
   Management
   Conivaptan
8. Central diabetes insipidus
   Introduction
   Management

II. Disorders of the Respiratory System
1. Status asthmaticus
   Introduction
   Management

- β_2-Adrenergic agents
- Ipratropium bromide
- Corticosteroids
- Magnesium sulfate

2. Laryngotracheobronchitis and postextubation stridor
   Introduction
   Management
   - Dexamethasone
   - Budesonide
3. Pulmonary hypertension
   Introduction and definitions
   Management

- Nitric oxide
- Prostacyclin
- Bosentan
- Sildenafil

III. Acute Circulatory Failure
Introduction
1. Augmentation of preload
   - Crystalloids
   - Colloids
2. Reduction of preload
   - Furosemide
   - Bumetanide
   - Nesiritide
3. Enhancement of myocardial contractility
   a. Sympathomimetics
      - Dopamine
      - Dobutamine
      - Epinephrine
      - Isoproterenol
   b. Phosphodiesterase inhibitors
      - Milrinone
   c. Afterload reduction
      - Nitroglycerin
      - Nitroprusside
      - Angiotensin-converting enzyme inhibitors
   d. Miscellaneous agents
      - Prostaglandin E_1
      - Vasopressin
      - β-Blockers: labetalol, esmolol, carvedilol
      - Fenoldopam

IV. Anticoagulation and Thrombolytics
Introduction
Drugs used
1. Unfractionated heparin
2. Low-molecular-weight heparin
3. Oral anticoagulation
4. Recombinant tissue plasminogen activator
Monitoring of anticoagulation

V. Gastrointestinal Hemorrhage
Introduction
Management
1. Vasopressin
2. Octreotide

CENTRAL NERVOUS SYSTEM INJURY AND INCREASED INTRACRANIAL PRESSURE

Management of intracranial hypertension is the cornerstone of modern neurointensive care. Primary brain injury results from a direct insult from the initial event such as trauma, infection, metabolic derangement, and ischemia. Secondary brain damage results from pathophysiologic alterations in response to the primary event. Increased intracranial pressure (ICP) is one of the most important factors which further aggravate the brain damage.

OSMOTHERAPY

Osmotherapy takes advantage of the unique nature of the blood–brain barrier (BBB), which freely allows the transport of water across the capillary endothelium while remaining relatively impermeable in varying degrees to osmotic agents (1). Osmotherapy is most effective in situations where water accumulation is mainly intracellular and the BBB is well preserved. However, disruption of the BBB is neither absolute nor uniform even in conditions such as trauma and infections. Osmotherapy therefore is still effective to varying degrees in decreasing total brain water in such situations.

Mannitol

By far the most commonly used osmotic agent is mannitol (2). Intravenous administration of 0.25 to 0.5 g per kg of 20% mannitol solution reduces ICP within 30 minutes for periods up to 4 to 6 hours. Because the effectiveness of an osmotic agent depends upon the steepness of the osmolal gradient it creates, intermittent administration of a bolus of mannitol over 10 to 15 minutes is preferred to continuous infusion. The dose often needs to be repeated based upon clinical response and/or ICP measurement. In addition to its osmotic effects, mannitol may have other salutary effects on cerebral metabolism by its rheologic and free radical scavenging effects.

The aim of osmotherapy is to decrease brain bulk without causing total body dehydration and hypovolemia. It is important to monitor serum electrolytes, osmolality, and indicators of circulation. Mannitol is also associated with acute tubular necrosis. Inadequate renal function may result in hypervolemia and hyperosmolality that are poorly tolerated by patients requiring osmotherapy. On occasion, mannitol can be combined with intravenous (IV) furosemide (0.5 to 1 mg per kg) to maximize its effects.

Hypertonic Saline and Glycerol

Other osmotic agents such as glycerol and hypertonic saline have been used in brain-injured patients (3,4). Neither of these agents has been shown to be clearly superior to mannitol in randomized controlled trials. Hypertonic saline, however, has been shown to be safe and effective in controlling cerebral edema and seizures associated with severe symptomatic hyponatremia from SIADH and water intoxication. A small (3 to 4 mEq per L) but rapid rise in serum sodium is most effective for this purpose. With an apparent volume of distribution for sodium being 0.6 L per kg, an infusion of 4 to 5 mL per kg of 3% saline given over 10 to 15 minutes will raise serum sodium by approximately 3 to 4 mEq per L. This dose can be repeated two to three times as necessary (5). For hyponatremia associated with syndrome of inappropriate antidiuretic hormone, IV furosemide (1 mg per kg) given before hypertonic saline is effective in eliminating free water in addition to raising serum sodium.

Hypertonic saline has been recommended as an alternative to mannitol for the treatment of intracranial hypertension in brain-injured patients (6). Of the administered drug, mannitol is much more likely to be excreted compared with sodium. If a sustained increase in serum osmolality is desired, hypertonic saline is preferable. If the therapeutic aim is to expose the brain to elevated serum osmolality, mannitol is the preferred agent. There is no convincing evidence that hypertonic saline is superior to mannitol in this setting.

BARBITURATES

High-dose barbiturate therapy is often used in conjunction with osmotherapy for management of intracranial hypertension associated with traumatic brain injury (2). Barbiturates are proposed to exert their beneficial effects by decreasing cerebral metabolic rate and cerebral vasoconstriction, decreasing lactate and excitatory amino acids, and inhibiting free radical mediated lipid peroxidation (7–9). Pentobarbital is by far the most commonly used agent for this purpose. We recommend using pentobarbital in a dose that best controls ICP. This can be accomplished by administering an IV bolus of 3 to 5 mg per kg followed by continuous infusion of 1 to 2 mg per kg per hour. Additional boluses or a higher infusion rate may be necessary. In general, serum levels of 30 to 40 μg per mL are required in most severely brain-injured patients. However, higher levels may be necessary. Barbiturate therapy is associated with significant hypotension and myocardial depression. Most patients require concomitant administration of inotropic agents such as dopamine and dobutamine for hemodynamic stability when high-dose barbiturate therapy is used.

ACETAZOLAMIDE AND FUROSEMIDE

A combination of acetazolamide and furosemide has been proposed to decrease ICP in pseudotumor cerebri (10). Both these drugs reduce cerebrospinal fluid production by inhibiting choroid plexus carbonic anhydrase. Furosemide decreases cerebrospinal fluid production by an additional unknown mechanism. Acetazolamide may be used singly or in combination with furosemide. Acetazolamide is administered orally or intravenously in a dose of 10 to 30 mg per kg given every 6 to 8 hours not to exceed 2 g per day. A randomized controlled trial did not show any benefit of acetazolamide–furosemide combination in posthemorrhagic hydrocephalus in infants (11).

CORTICOSTEROIDS

There is no evidence that corticosteroids favorably impact the outcome in traumatic brain injury. However, high-dose steroid therapy has been shown to confer benefit in terms of improved function in traumatic spinal cord injury (12). For steroids to be effective, they should preferably be given within 8 hours of injury. If given within 3 hours of injury, the recommended dose of methylprednisolone is an IV bolus of 30 mg per kg followed within 1 hour by a continuous infusion of 5.4 mg per kg per hour for 23 hours. If given between 3 and 8 hours from injury, the IV bolus should be followed within 1 hour by a continuous infusion of 5.4 mg per kg per hour for 47 hours.

STATUS EPILEPTICUS

Status epilepticus is defined as continuous or repeated convulsive or nonconvulsive seizures lasting 30 minutes or more. In children, causes include infections, trauma, toxic ingestions, and metabolic disturbances such as hyponatremia and hypocalcemia, brain tumors, epilepsy, and subtherapeutic levels of antiepileptic drugs. Status epilepticus is one of the most common disorders in children requiring ICU admission. Within the first 30 minutes of status epilepticus, sympathetic overactivity results in hypertension, tachycardia, and increased cardiac output. Increased catecholamine activity produces hyperglycemia. A combined respiratory and metabolic acidosis is a result of lactic acidosis and CO_2 retention. Excessive muscle activity can lead to rhabdomyolysis and acute tubular necrosis. The increase in cerebral metabolism often outstrips cerebral blood flow and eventually this discrepancy leads to depletion of brain glucose and oxygen. Status epilepticus should be considered an emergency, and treatment and determination of the etiology should be instituted immediately (Fig. 23.1).

INITIAL SURVEY

Complications of status epilepticus may include vomiting and aspiration, apnea, and increased oxygen requirement. The initial assessment should ascertain that the airway is adequate. Supplemental oxygen should be started, and if there is any concern that airway and breathing are compromised, the patient should be intubated and mechanical ventilation started. Intravenous access is essential. If IV access cannot be established within the first 5 minutes, intraosseous access should be attempted, especially in children younger than 1 year. Blood pressure measurement is

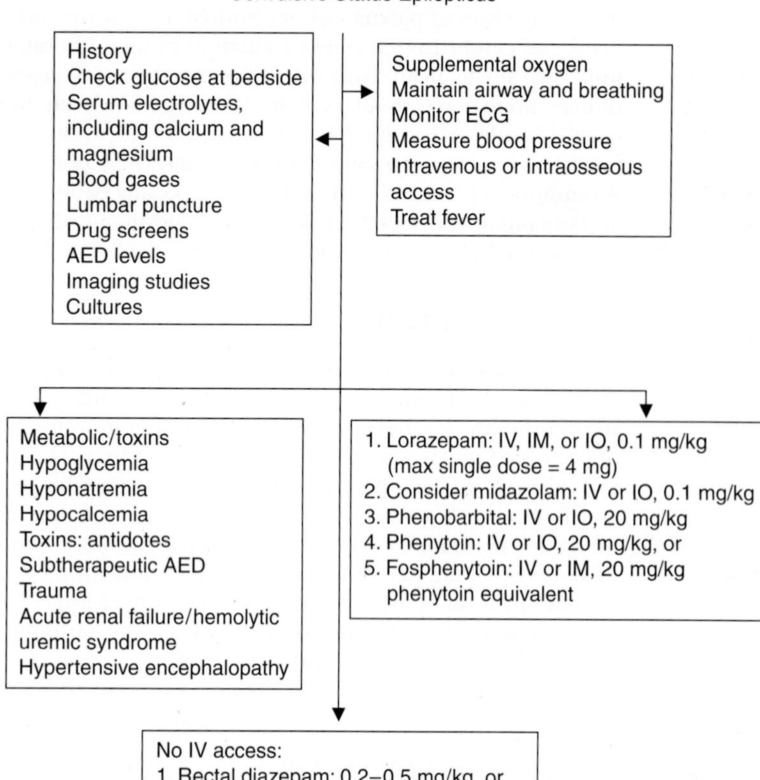

Figure 23.1. Etiology and treatment of status epilepticus. AED, antiepileptic drug; ECG, electrocardiogram; IV, intravenous; IM, intramuscular; IO, intraosseous.

important to determine the presence of hypertension as the cause of seizures. A lumbar puncture can be performed as long as the patient has a stable airway and hemodynamic status, and if there are no other contraindications such as an infection at the puncture site, coagulopathy, and increased ICP with evidence of focal neurologic findings. If imaging studies are needed, patients should first have their airway and hemodynamic status stabilized before studies such as computed tomography scans are obtained. Avoid the use of contrast material if renal failure is suspected.

METABOLIC ABNORMALITIES/TOXINS

Hyponatremia resulting from excessive water supplementation or improper mixing of formula can be a common cause of seizures in infants and should be suspected in an infant presenting with status epilepticus who appears otherwise healthy. A proper history should be elicited immediately and once improper formula mixing or if excessive water administration is confirmed, 3% sodium chloride should be administered pending the results of serum electrolytes determination. Accidental ingestion of toxins should be suspected in toddlers, while intentional overdose should be suspected in older children and adolescents. In addition to removal of the toxin, an appropriate antidote should be administered if available.

BENZODIAZEPINES

A group of drugs that bind to the benzodiazepine receptor on the neuronal γ-aminobutyric acid (GABA) receptors, thereby facilitating the inhibitory action of GABA on neuronal transmission.

Lorazepam (Ativan) is the currently recommended first-line drug of choice for the treatment of status epilepticus because it can be injected rapidly and has a rapid onset of action of 2 to 3 minutes. Respiratory depression is observed in up to 9% of patients. Lorazepam is five times more potent than diazepam, is 90% protein bound, and has dependable absorption, with a serum half-life of up to 20 hours. It is metabolized by hepatic glucuronidation to inactive metabolites, and except in hepatic and renal failure, its metabolism is not significantly altered in critically ill children. Lorazepam is insoluble in water, needing the addition of polyethylene glycol as a solvent. With prolonged and high-dose infusions, lactic acidosis and hyperosmolar coma have been reported (13).

Midazolam (Versed) is an imidazobenzodiazepine that has been successfully used in the treatment of status epilepticus by both intravenous (14) and transmucosal (intranasal or buccal) route at a dose of 0.5 to 1 mg per kg (15–18). Baysun et al. determined that buccal midazolam was as effective as rectal diazepam in stopping seizures; and Harbord et al. found that seizures resolved in 89% of patients given intranasal midazolam. The use of continuous IV infusion of midazolam at 1 to 5 μg per kg per minute has been used for the treatment of prolonged status epilepticus (19). The investigators found that the mean infusion rate required to control seizures was 2 μg per kg per minute. The onset of action is within 1 to 5 minutes, with a serum half-life of 1 to 2 hours. Up to 95% of the drug is protein bound. It is metabolized by hepatic microsomal oxidation, transforming it to active metabolites, α-hydroxymidazolam, and α-hydroxymidazolam-glucuronide. Drugs such as propofol and erythromycin can prolong the clearance of the active metabolites. This and other factors may prolong the effects of midazolam in critically ill children.

Diazepam (Valium) is highly lipophilic and is known to penetrate the BBB quickly. The onset of action is within 1 to 2 minutes, and the serum half-life as long as 60 hours. Although it has been replaced by lorazepam as the first-line drug of choice, 0.2 to 0.5 mg per kg rectal diazepam has its place in the treatment of status epilepticus in patients without IV access or as a drug that caregivers can use at home for children known to have frequent seizures.

Phenytoin: The solution for injection contains propylene glycol, ethanol, and sodium hydroxide resulting in an alkaline pH of about 12. When injected too rapidly, phenytoin has been known to precipitate cardiovascular collapse and arrhythmias. In addition, extravasation of phenytoin into the subcutaneous tissue causes tissue necrosis. Phenytoin follows both first-order and zero-order kinetics and is hydroxylated in the liver. The recommended bolus dose is 20 mg per kg, to be infused not more than 0.5 mg per kg per minute in children younger than 1 month, and not more than 1 mg per kg per minute in children older than 1 month. The onset of action is approximately 10 to 30 minutes, with a half-life of approximately 60 hours. Because of great variability in phenytoin metabolism, subsequent maintenance doses should be titrated to maintain free phenytoin serum levels at 1 to 2 μg per mL.

Fosphenytoin is a prodrug of phenytoin. Fosphenytoin sodium 1.5 mg is equivalent to 1 mg of phenytoin. Therapeutic concentrations can be achieved within 10 minutes following rapid IV injection and within 2 hours after intramuscular (IM) injection. Because fosphenytoin has a pH of 8.6 and is water soluble, it can be injected by IV injection more rapidly, and by IM injection when IV access cannot be obtained. However, in infants, there is extreme variability in therapeutic phenytoin levels (20) and, therefore, careful monitoring of serum levels is indicated.

BARBITURATES

These drugs bind to the barbiturate receptor in the GABA receptor complex, producing sedation, hypnosis, anesthesia, and suppression of epileptiform activity. They are known to decrease cerebral metabolic oxygen demand and intracranial pressure. Adverse effects include suppression of myocardial contractility and peripheral vasodilation that can lead to hypotension. With prolonged infusion and use of high doses, patients often require inotropic drug support. With repeated doses, barbiturates can cause respiratory depression and apnea.

Phenobarbital is less lipophilic and does not enter the brain as rapidly. Onset of action can take as long as 60 minutes, and serum half-life as long as 3 days. A loading dose of 20 mg per kg is recommended, with a maintenance dose of 4 to 5 mg per kg per day. In the management of status epilepticus, serum levels should be monitored and maintained at 20 to 30 μg per mL. Higher therapeutic levels may be necessary for the treatment of prolonged status epilepticus resistant to lower levels and/or other antiepileptic drugs. Like lorazepam and thiopental, phenobarbital is formulated in propylene glycol.

Pentobarbital is formed by desulfurization of thiopental and has a short half-life. For the treatment of status epilepticus, a loading dose of 2 to 4 mg per kg can be administered. Because of a short half-life, a continuous infusion of 1 to 3 mg per kg per hour is often necessary. Some practitioners recommend electroencephalogram (EEG) monitoring, aiming for burst suppression. However, seizures have been known to continue despite burst suppression. All patients who require continuous pentobarbital therapy will need intubation and mechanical ventilation.

Isoflurane is a volatile anesthetic agent that is eliminated through the lungs. The difficulty in using this drug in the ICU is the lack of gas scavenging devices.

Etomidate is an anesthetic agent that has been used successfully in adults with status epilepticus (21). There are no studies evaluating the use of etomidate in children. The advantages of etomidate include its lack of myocardial depressant effects. However, it has been shown to result in significant adrenal suppression with only one dose (22); therefore, its long-term use requires supplementation with corticosteroids.

Propofol: Like etomidate, propofol is a short-acting intravenous anesthetic agent. It is formulated in an egg and soy emulsion and therefore should be avoided in children with egg or soy allergies. It has been found to be effective in stopping status epilepticus in adults but has not been studied in children. Long-term infusion has been reported to cause severe metabolic acidosis and the reports do support a cause and effect basis.

Paraldehyde is a cyclic polymer of acetaldehyde that is rapidly absorbed into the brain. It has been used successfully for over a century in the treatment of seizures. In the United States, however, paraldehyde USP is no longer available for human use. The manufacturers believe it is too expensive to make USP grade paraldehyde and with such limited use in humans, the decision was made to discontinue production. Paraldehyde is available in Canada and Europe.

Valproic acid by intravenous injection has been evaluated in adults with status epilepticus. Seizures were controlled in up to 75% of patients and no adverse cardiorespiratory effects were noted (23,24). However, intravenous valproic acid for the first-line treatment of status epilepticus has not been studied in children and its role is unclear at this time.

Levetiracetam is an anticonvulsant initially approved by the Food and Drug Administration (FDA) in oral form for adjunctive treatment of partial onset seizures in children aged 4 years or more, for myoclonic seizures in those older than 12 years, and for primary generalized tonic–clonic seizures. More recently, an intravenous form of the drug was approved for use as well. Levetiracetam has been shown to be efficacious, with a good safety profile. There are increasing reports that the intravenous administration of the drug may be effective in the treatment of status epilepticus in adults and children, with one report of successful treatment of status epilepticus that was refractory to benzodiazepine (25–27). The mechanism of action of the drug is unclear but may be due to the prevention of hypersynchronization of epileptiform burst firing and propagation of seizure activity. Dosing regimen includes an intravenous loading dose of 15 mg per kg followed by 15 mg per kg per day divided in two doses. Others recommend no loading dose, with IV dose of 10 to 40 mg per kg per dose every 8 hours for infants and every 12 hours for older children. Approximately 66% of the drug is eliminated by the kidneys as unchanged drug. Therefore, dose adjustment is necessary with renal insufficiency.

MYASTHENIA GRAVIS

Myasthenia gravis is an autoimmune disease caused by autoantibodies directed against the nicotinic receptors in the neuromuscular junction. Neonatal myasthenia gravis results from transplacental passage of maternal antibodies to the fetus. Medical therapy of myasthenia gravis consists of inhibition of acetyl cholinesterase inhibitors, immune suppression, and immune modulation. Acetyl cholinesterase inhibitors that are quaternary ammonium compounds (edrophonium, neostigmine, etc.) do not cross the BBB and are therefore appropriate for the management of myasthenia gravis. Tertiary amines such as physostigmine cross the BBB and are not appropriate in this setting.

Edrophonium is used mainly to establish the diagnosis but may also be used to distinguish between myasthenic crisis and cholinergic crisis in children receiving anticholinesterase therapy. An IV dose of 0.04 mg per kg over 1 minute is followed by 0.16 mg per kg (maximum 10 mg) given within 45 seconds if no response is observed. Objective evidence of motor function such as muscle strength and forced vital capacity should be documented. The onset of action is within seconds and duration of action is a few minutes. As with other anticholinesterase agents, severe bradycardia, hypotension, and other cholinergic effects can occur with the use of edrophonium. Atropine (0.01 mg per kg IV, minimum 0.1 mg, maximum 2 mg) should be available at the patient's bedside to counteract serious cholinergic effects if they should occur.

Neostigmine is used both as a diagnostic agent as well as for ongoing therapy. It can be given IM in a dose of 0.025 to 0.04 mg per kg as a diagnostic tool. For ongoing therapy, 0.04 mg per kg can be given IM every 3 to 4 hours. Neostigmine bromide given orally in a dose of 0.4 mg per kg every 4 to 6 hours is preferred for prolonged use. For patients with significant dysphagia, neostigmine should be administered about 30 minutes before meals. *Pyridostigmine* is slightly longer acting than neostigmine. It is administered orally in a dose of 5 mg per kg per day in 4 to 6 divided doses. The doses of both neostigmine and pyridostigmine may have to be adjusted every 48 hours.

Corticosteroids: Long-term therapy may be necessary for immune suppression. A single oral daily dose of prednisone (0.5 to 1 mg per kg per day) is recommended. In resistant cases, combined steroid and azathioprine therapy is utilized to minimize the side effects of steroids. Thymectomy should be considered for patients with high titers of anti-acetylcholine-receptor antibodies.

Intravenous immunoglobulin (IVIG): For immune modulation, plasmapheresis and IVIG are sometimes beneficial. IVIG is administered as 2 g per kg as a single dose over 10 to 12 hours or 400 mg per kg daily for 4 days. Relative benefits of immune modulation are still unconfirmed by randomized controlled studies. Several case series report short-term benefit from plasmapheresis particularly in myasthenic crisis (28).

NEUROMUSCULAR BLOCKING AGENTS

In addition to sedative agents, critically ill children may require neuromuscular blocking agents (NMBAs) to facilitate various mechanical ventilatory modes such as high frequency oscillation, inverse ratio ventilation, and slow rates, all of which can induce significant discomfort and agitation. The addition of neuromuscular blockade may help improve respiratory system compliance and reduce barotrauma by preventing the patient from "fighting" the ventilator. Occasionally, neuromuscular blockade may also be necessary in children following laryngotracheoplasty, or those with extensive facial injuries or following facial reconstructive surgery where movement has to be kept at a minimum to maintain the artificial airway. NMBAs exert either depolarizing or nondepolarizing (competitive) effects on the neuromuscular junction.

Succinylcholine acts similarly to acetylcholine and induces membrane depolarization. Because it is resistant to degradation by acetylcholinesterase, administration of succinylcholine produces initial fasciculations resulting from repetitive excitation, followed by flaccid paralysis. The recommended dose in children is 1 mg per kg per dose. Paralysis occurs in 1 minute after IV injection. Effects dissipate quickly as the drug is metabolized by butyrylcholinesterase in the blood and liver. However, during depolarization induced by succinylcholine, significant amounts of potassium are released, and succinylcholine is therefore contraindicated in conditions that can potentiate hyperkalemia. These include crush injuries, burns, and rhabdomyolysis. It is also contraindicated in patients with ICP, spinal cord injuries, muscular dystrophies, and known or family history of malignant hyperthermia.

Nondepolarizing or competitive NMBAs include pancuronium, vecuronium, atracurium, and mivacurium. These drugs block acetylcholine from binding to receptors on the motor endplate, thereby inhibiting depolarization. Elimination of nondepolarizing NMBAs varies, and this characteristic should be taken into account when using these drugs in critically ill children (Table 23.1).

In using NMBAs, a number of potential complications should be taken into account. It is important to ascertain adequacy of sedation to prevent the frightening consequence of paralyzing a child who has total awareness. The paralysis induced by agents with steroid rings such as pancuronium and vecuronium can result in a myopathy and prolonged paralysis when the patient is on corticosteroids as well (29). There are a number of drugs frequently used in children in the ICU that can potentiate the effects of NMBAs resulting in prolonged paralysis. These include antibiotics such as aminoglycosides; antiarrhythmics such as

TABLE 23.1 Nondepolarizing Blocking Agents

Drug	*Dose*	*Duration of Action (min)*	*Route of Elimination*
Pancuronium	0.1–0.15 mg/kg/dose q 30–60 min p.r.n.	40–60	Kidneys
Vecuronium	0.1 mg/kg/dose q 60 min p.r.n.	30–40	Kidneys
Cisatracurium	0.15–0.2 mg/kg/dose q 40–65 min p.r.n.	35–45	Hoffman elimination
Mivacurium	0.2 mg/kg/dose	9–20	Enzymatic hydrolysis by plasma cholinesterase
Rocuronium	0.6 mg/kg/dose initial dose, then 0.075–0.125 q 20–30 min p.r.n.	26–40	70% by biliary excretion; 30% unchanged via kidneys

p.r.n., as the situation demands.

β-adrenergic blockers; and other drugs such as furosemide, magnesium, and cyclosporine. Abnormalities in renal function and electrolyte disorders such as hypocalcemia and treatment modalities such as hypothermia can all prolong neuromuscular blockade and weakness. Unlike vecuronium or rocuronium, 80% of cisatracurium is metabolized to laudanosine via Hoffman elimination, with less than 20% of unchanged drug excreted in the kidneys, making it the more appropriate NMBA to use in patients with renal insufficiency. In addition, a study comparing vecuronium and cisatracurium in infants after congenital heart surgery showed more rapid spontaneous recovery of neuromuscular function with cisatracurium (30). Occasionally, there may be a need for continuous or frequent neuromuscular blockade. In such patients, the depth of neuromuscular blockade should be monitored. Clinical parameters such as handgrip strength may be used but may not be applicable in infants or those children who are sedated. Stimulating the ulnar nerve and assessing the evoked response of the adductor pollicis can provide a more objective measurement. Monitoring of neuromuscular function with the train-of-four ratio is useful in judging the response to therapy. Train of four is a modality whereby peripheral motor nerve stimulation is applied followed by the observation of muscle movement in response to the stimuli. Nondepolarizing agents such as vecuronium decrease the size of single twitches and both the strength and duration of the response to repetitive stimulation. The train of four consists of four stimuli given at 2 per second and is commonly used to determine the degree of neuromuscular blockade and the number of receptors occupied. If three twitches are observed, approximately 75% to 80% of receptors are occupied; and if one twitch is observed, 90% to 95% of receptors are occupied. One to two twitches indicate approximately 75% to 90% receptor occupancy and are thought to provide the optimum level of neuromuscular relaxation. Monitoring of the train of four in patients who are receiving frequent or continuous dosing of NMBAs helps prevent overdosing and prolonged paralysis.

The injection of aminosteroidal nondepolarizing NMBAs such as rocuronium and vecuronium stimulates the C-nociceptors in the peripheral veins, causing severe pain (31,32). The pain, as indicated by localized withdrawal response, is significant even after loss of consciousness during anesthesia induction. Ahmad et al. assessed the efficacy of fentanyl or lidocaine in the prevention of rocuronium injection–associated pain and found that fentanyl was more effective than lidocaine (33).

Rapid reversal of neuromuscular blockade is sometimes necessary in ICU patients who have received nondepolarizing agents. Neostigmine, 0.05 to 0.07 mg per kg IV (maximum of 5 mg), can be used for this purpose and has a peak action within 5 to 8 minutes. Atropine may have to be administered to counteract excessive muscarinic effects of bradycardia, increased secretions, and bronchospasm.

Sugammadex is a drug-specific modified γ-cyclodextrin that is a selective relaxant binding agent. Unlike neostigmine, which increases cholinergic activity, the selective relaxant binding agent rapidly encapsulates steroidal NMBAs such as rocuronium, thereby directly preventing the pharmacologic actions of NMBAs. Studies have shown that sugammadex is effective and safe (34). The drug has been approved for use in Europe but not in the United States.

SEDATION

Sedation is often necessary in critically ill children because of the need to maintain endotracheal tubes, facilitate mechanical ventilation, and to ensure that chest tubes, central venous, arterial, and bladder catheters are not pulled out by an agitated child. The ICU environment is often a stressful one. Endotracheal tubes prevent children from crying or communicating. Frequent monitor and ventilator alarms and harsh lighting prevent normal sleep. Pain from catheters and procedures may add to the discomfort. However, despite the routine use of sedative agents in ICUs, there are few sedation scales that are designed for, and validated for use in children. A number of scales have been designed to assess sedation, including the Ramsay scale, the Comfort scale, Children's Hospital of Eastern Ontario Pain Scale (CHEOPS), visual analogue scale, and the Riker sedation–agitation scale. More commonly, caregivers use physiologic parameters such as heart rate and blood pressure, or movement to determine a child's need for sedation. Children therefore can be subject to both undersedation and oversedation. The complications of oversedation include hemodynamic instability, severe withdrawal syndromes, and prolongation of mechanical ventilation and ICU stay.

THE RAMSAY SCALE (35)

Awake Levels

Level 1: Patient anxious and agitated, restless, or both.
Level 2: Patient cooperative, oriented, and tranquil.

Asleep Levels

Level 3: Patient awake responds to commands only.
Level 4: Patient asleep, brisk response to a light glabellar tap or loud auditory stimulus.
Level 5: Sluggish response to a light glabellar tap or loud auditory stimulus.
Level 6: No response to a light glabellar tap or loud auditory stimulus.

Shortcomings of the Ramsay scale include overlap between the levels; each level is not described clearly and the scale has not been validated. There are difficulties in using this scale in children at the stage of development where they cannot understand commands or cooperate.

THE COMFORT SCALE (36)

This scale was specifically designed for intubated children in the ICU and scores eight physiologic and behavioral parameters from 1 to 5, with a total range of 8 to 40. The optimal sedation range is 17 to 26. The COMFORT scale (Table 23.2) has advantages over all other scales because of its applicability to children of all ages and developmental status, and it does not require repeatedly awakening a patient to assess the adequacy of sedation.

THE PENN STATE CHILDREN'S HOSPITAL SEDATION ALGORITHM (37)

Popernack et al. instituted the Penn State Children's Hospital Algorithm to provide goal-directed sedation for mechanically ventilated children. Physicians write the order for the goal sedation level along with the appropriate medications that allow the nursing staff autonomy to provide individualized patient sedation regimens. Following implementation of the algorithm, the accidental extubation rates decreased significantly without increasing length of stay (37).

The Penn State Children's Hospital Sedation Algorithm for ventilated children:

Level 1
Goal: Awake and interactive with environment, that is, watches television, communicates (generally for more mature children with neuromuscular cause for assisted ventilation).
Action: PRN anxiolytics/analgesics.

Level 2
Goal: Sleepy, arouses to light stimulation, becomes excited with nursing care/suctioning, moves spontaneously, turns head, consistently breathes above the ventilator.
Action: PRN anxiolytics/analgesics, with or without continuous anxiolytics/analgesics; paralytics only if PRN sedatives fail.

Level 3
Goal: Asleep most of the time, arouses to pain, coughs with suctioning, breathes above ventilator, little spontaneous movement or head turning.

TABLE 23.2 The COMFORT Scale

Scale Component	*Score*	*Scale Component*	*Score*
Alertness		**Calmness/agitation**	
Deeply asleep	1	Calm	1
Lightly asleep	2	Slightly anxious	2
Drowsy	3	Anxious	3
Fully awake and alert	4	Very anxious	4
Hyperalert	5	Panicky	5
Respiratory response		**Physical movement**	
No coughing, no spontaneous respiration	1	No movement	1
Spontaneous effort with little response to ventilator	2	Occasional, slight movement	2
Occasional cough or resistance to ventilator	2	Frequent, slight movement	3
Breathes against ventilator or coughs regularly	4	Vigorous movement limited to extremities	4
Fights ventilator, coughs, or chokes	5	Vigorous movement including head and torso	5
Blood pressure		**Heart rate**	
Blood pressure below baseline	1	Heart rate below baseline	1
Blood pressure consistently at baseline	2	Heart rate consistently at baseline	2
Infrequent elevations ≥15% above baseline	3	Infrequent elevations ≥15% above baseline	3
Frequent elevations ≥15% above baseline	4	Frequent elevations ≥15% above baseline	4
Sustained elevations ≥15% above baseline	5	Sustained elevations ≥15% above baseline	5
Muscle tone		**Facial tension**	
Muscles totally relaxed, no muscle tone	1	Facial muscles totally relaxed	1
Reduced muscle tone	2	Facial muscle tone normal, no tension evident	2
Normal muscle tone	3	Tension evident in some facial muscles	3
Increased muscle tone, flexion of fingers and toes	4	Tension evident throughout facial muscles	4
Extreme muscle rigidity, flexion of fingers and toes	5	Facial muscles contorted and grimacing	5

The COMFORT scale, adapted from Marx CM, Smith PG, Lowrie LH, et al. Optimal sedation of mechanically ventilated pediatric critical care patients. *Crit Care Med* 1994;22(1):163–170.

Action: PRN anxiolytics/analgesics with or without continuous anxiolytics/analgesics; paralytics only if PRN sedation fails.

Level 4

Goal: Asleep, arouses to pain, coughs with suctioning, returns to sleep immediately, does not consistently breathe above ventilator, little spontaneous movement, no head turning.

Action: Continuous anxiolytics/analgesics, PRN anxiolytics/analgesics; paralytics only if PRN sedatives fail.

Level 5

Goal: Asleep, minimal response to pain or suctioning, no respiratory effort, no sustained spontaneous movements.

Action: Continuous anxiolytics/analgesics; liberal use of paralytics if PRN sedatives fail.

Level 6

Goal: Asleep, continuous paralysis, level of paralysis assessed by nerve stimulator or by observing minor movements between supplemental doses.

Action: Continuous anxiolytics/analgesics, continuous paralytics; PRN anxiolytics/analgesics titrated to vital signs. Utilize train-of-four nerve stimulator for serial assessments, or observe motor movements between supplemental doses.

Protocol for using the levels of sedation algorithm:

1. After intubation, the level is established by the team to create an individualized patient behavior goal. The level is written as a physician order.
2. With appropriate medications prescribed, the nurse uses clinical assessment skills to administer pharmacological and age-appropriate psychological support to achieve the established goal.
3. The staff explains the desired level and the plans for implementation to the patient's family. Nonverbal communication is used for levels 1 through 3 based on the patient's cognition and age.
4. Respiratory therapists are responsible to help identify changes in patient status that deviate from the set goal.
5. An evaluation and adjustments are made daily and when dynamic changes occur.
6. Documentation:
   - Physician order on the plan of care.
   - Medications administered.
   - Patient data indicating therapeutic efficacy or required adjustments.
   - Assessment in the progress notes (37).

The BIS Monitor (Aspect Medical Systems, Natick, MA): BIS is a processed EEG variable obtained by computing EEG signals through Fast Fourier transformation, bispectral analysis, and artifact filtering and suppression detection, resulting in a single number—the BIS. BIS allows monitoring of depth of anesthesia or sedation, ranging from 100 (awake) to 0 (isoelectric EEG). Its use has been validated in children (38,39). Crain et al. compared the BIS score to the COMFORT scale and found that BIS may be better than the COMFORT scale in identifying and preventing oversedation of children in the pediatric ICU (PICU) (39). Furthermore, Lamas et al. compared the BIS, middle latency auditory evoked potentials and the modified Ramsay scale, and the Comfort scale to detect the responsiveness of 86 children to painful stimuli and determined that the BIS provided the most sensitive method of assessing responses (40). More importantly, these investigators determined that hemodynamic variables such as heart rate and blood pressure did not change after the application of the stimulus. This confirms the findings of other studies that using such clinical parameters to determine the occurrence of pain is of little use (41,42).

BENZODIAZEPINES

Benzodiazepines offer anxiolysis, hypnosis, and amnesia, characteristics which are desirable in many ICU patients. Midazolam and lorazepam are the most commonly used benzodiazepines. The ideal amount of sedation is that which makes the patient sleepy and quiet but arousable and able to follow commands. More frequently, however, deeper sedation is needed, especially in those children on high-frequency oscillation, those with intracranial hypertension, those who have undergone surgical procedures where minimal movement is required for healing, and those requiring frequent neuromuscular blockade. Benzodiazepines exert their action by binding to GABA receptors. The binding results in increased cellular chloride entry inducing hyperpolarization of neuronal cells, rendering them resistant to excitation.

Lorazepam penetrates the BBB more slowly than other benzodiazepines such as diazepam. This characteristic results in a longer duration of amnestic effect. It is metabolized by hepatic glucuronidation into harmless metabolites and is therefore void of drug interactions, making it an ideal drug to use in the PICU. Lorazepam can be given by continuous infusion (0.06 mg per kg per hour) or intermittent injection (0.1 mg per kg per dose). It is also available in oral form. Lorazepam is the sedative agent most frequently used in both adult and pediatric ICUs.

Midazolam is unique because of its water solubility in an acid pH, becoming lipid soluble in physiologic pH, allowing it to penetrate the BBB rapidly. This accounts for its rapid onset of action. Midazolam is metabolized by hepatic microsomal oxidation, making it prone to interaction with a number of drugs. Drug clearance is decreased in renal failure and may result in accumulation of its active metabolite. Just like lorazepam and other benzodiazepines, midazolam produces respiratory depression, especially when injected rapidly. It can cause hypotension as well. Midazolam is used for procedural sedation as well as for continuous sedation of children in the PICU. The dose for continuous infusion is 0.4 to 6 μg per kg per minute. Abrupt withdrawal after long-term sedation can result in significant adverse effects such as irritability, agitation, tremors, and sleeplessness. We recommend weaning from midazolam by conversion from continuous midazolam infusion to oral lorazepam, as shown in Table 23.3.

OTHER AGENTS USED IN SEDATION

Propofol is an intravenous alkylphenol sedative–hypnotic agent. The advantages of its use for sedation include rapid onset of action and short half-life, allowing patients to wake up rapidly after drug discontinuation. Side effects include pain at the infusion site, hypotension, and apnea.

TABLE 23.3 Conversion of Midazolam to Lorazepam for Weaning off Midazolam

Midazolam Rate	*Lorazepam Equivalent Dosing*
1 μg/kg/min = 1.44 mg/kg/d	0.3 mg/kg/d = 0.1 mg/kg/dose q 8 hr
2 μg/kg/min = 2.88 mg/kg/d	0.6 mg/kg/d = 0.1–0.15 mg/kg/dose q 6 hr
3 μg/kg/min = 4.32 mg/kg/d	0.9 mg/kg/d = 0.1–0.15 mg/kg/dose q 4–6 hr
4 μg/kg/min = 5.76 mg/kg/d	1.2 mg/kg/d = 0.15 mg/kg/dose q 4 hr

From Cyndi Reid, PharmD, Department of Pharmaceutical Services, Children's Hospital of Michigan, Detroit, MI, with permission.

In several studies comparing the use of midazolam, lorazepam, and propofol for prolonged sedation in the ICU, propofol was found to be associated with less hemodynamic instability, was weaned more rapidly, and was not associated with acute withdrawal symptoms. No one developed lactic acidosis. In addition, patients on propofol needed less NMBAs (43,44). Propofol has been found to be safe for use in procedural sedation in children. Vardi et al. compared combinations of propofol/lidocaine with ketamine/midazolam/fentanyl and showed that children who received propofol for procedural sedation scored better on the COMFORT scale, had a much more rapid recovery, smoother emergence, and shorter stay in the procedure area (45). The safety of propofol for long-term sedation in children is unclear. There are reports in literature of propofol infusion syndrome, a rare but fatal condition where metabolic acidosis, bradycardia, rhabdomyolysis, and renal failure develop in children who received propofol for long-term sedation (46). Wolf et al. described a child with propofol infusion syndrome in whom they documented elevated levels of malonyl carnitine, C5-acylcarnitine, creatine phosphokinase, troponin, and myoglobinemia, all of which resolved with hemodialysis. The propofol infusion syndrome was attributed to impaired fatty acid oxidation (47). An open-label, randomized multicenter trial comparing the safety and efficacy of 1% propofol, 2% propofol, and other standard sedative agents showed mortality rates of 11%, 8%, and 4% in each of the groups, respectively. The mortality rates were not statistically significant, and none of the investigators felt that the deaths were related to propofol. More importantly, children who were terminally ill with a "do-not-resuscitate" status were included in the study [(48); also unpublished data available from FDA review of a study conducted by Blumer et al.]. Cornfield et al. reported the use of continuous propofol infusion in 142 children, none of whom developed metabolic acidosis (49). Ghanta et al. conducted a randomized, open-label, controlled trial to compare the use of propofol to a morphine/atropine/suxamethonium (MASux) regimen for neonatal endotracheal intubation. Sixty-three infants were included in the study. The primary study endpoint was time to achieve successful intubation. Successful intubation was more than twice as fast with propofol, taking 120 seconds compared with 260 seconds for the MASux regimen (50). The infants who received propofol had less nasal/oral trauma and a shorter recovery time. In addition, those infants who received the MASux regimen had significantly lower oxygen saturation during the procedure (60% vs. 80%). There was no difference in blood pressure and heart rate between groups, and no significant adverse events were observed.

Etomidate is an imidazole derivative used for induction in anesthesia. It is most often used for patients with hemodynamic instability because of its lack of cardiovascular depressant effects. Sedation is produced through stimulation of the GABA receptor. Etomidate is generally used for rapid sequence intubation, or other procedural sedation. Prolonged infusion has been associated with deaths associated with suppression of adrenal steroid synthesis (51). This may be due to selective adrenocortical 11β-hydroxylase inhibition by etomidate (52). In an editorial, Annane reviewed the adverse effects of etomidate, particularly those that relate to adrenal suppression and suggests that etomidate should be withdrawn from use in preference for other agents, which do not result in adrenal suppression (53).

Ketamine is a phencyclidine derivative that can be given IM or IV for induction for children undergoing anesthesia. The advantages of its use include bronchodilation and cardiovascular stimulation by increasing sympathetic discharges. Ketamine may be the ideal agent to use for sedation of children with status asthmaticus who require intubation. However, because it can increase myocardial oxygen demand, it should be avoided in children with congestive heart failure and arrhythmias. The most unpleasant side effects of using ketamine include psychiatric symptoms such as hallucinations, delirium, and increased salivation. The concurrent administration of a benzodiazepine diminishes the psychiatric symptoms. More recently, concerns have been raised about the neurotoxicity of ketamine (54,55). Exposure to ketamine resulted in apoptotic neurodegeneration and the development of long-term cognitive defects in neonatal animals.

Barbiturates such as thiopental, pentobarbital, and methohexital are seldom used for routine sedation in the ICU. This may be because barbiturates have a long elimination half-life and because of adverse effects such as dose-related myocardial depression, respiratory depression, bronchospasm, and laryngospasm.

Dexmedetomidine is an IV α_2-adrenergic agonist similar to clonidine. It has primarily been used as a sedative agent during the immediate postoperative period. Respiratory depressant effects are minimal. Two double blind randomized controlled studies showed significantly fewer requirements for rescue medications such as midazolam, morphine, and propofol (56,57). Significant untoward effects include bradycardia and the lack of amnesia, and patients have complained of unpleasant memories of their care.

Hypotension seems to occur only in patients with decreased intravascular volume but is long lasting when it does occur (57). Tobias et al. reported the use of dexmedetomidine in four children. The dose of 0.25 to 0.75 μg per kg per hour was found to provide adequate sedation and anxiolysis (58). Koroglu et al. evaluated the sedative, hemodynamic, and respiratory effects of dexmedetomidine compared with midazolam in 80 children undergoing magnetic resonance imaging and found that children who received dexmedetomidine were adequately sedated, required less rescue drug, and the onset of sedation was more rapid (59). There were no adverse hemodynamic or respiratory effects. The other advantages of using dexmedetomidine include lack of effects on the respiratory system and blunting of the sympathetic response, avoiding rebound hypertension after discontinuation of the drug. In addition, unlike other direct acting vasodilators, dexmedetomidine appears to have no effects on intracranial pressure.

Despite the routine use of prolonged sedation for patients in the ICU, there is no consensus as to dosage and degree of sedation. Sedation scales such as the COMFORT scale are available but not routinely used. In addition, there are no parameters regarding the addition of narcotics such as morphine or fentanyl and the use of NMBAs. Frequently, we find that children are oversedated. Prolonged, continuous use of high-dose benzodiazepines can lead to a number of adverse effects. Kollef et al. has shown that the continuous use of IV sedation significantly prolongs the need for mechanical ventilation and ICU stay (60). By assigning a targeted level of sedation, written orders for the appropriate sedatives and analgesics and allowing nursing staff to add or adjust medications to achieve the target, the Penn State Children's Hospital Sedation Algorithm helps in providing adequate sedation for children on mechanical ventilation. More importantly, the study has shown that oversedation and prolongation of mechanical ventilation and ICU stay was avoided (37).

A number of studies have shown withdrawal syndromes in patients who received prolonged sedation with midazolam alone or in combination with fentanyl (61,62). Withdrawal symptoms included movement disorders such as choreoathetosis and dystonic posturing. Irritability and encephalopathy have been reported as well. Risk factors for the occurrence of withdrawal syndromes include use of high doses, prolonged sedation greater than 9 days, and abrupt discontinuation. Creation of standardized sedation protocols may reduce these complications.

The BIS holds promise by its ability to provide objective monitoring of sedation depth. Crain et al. demonstrated the advantage of BIS over the COMFORT scale (39), whereas Simmons et al. showed that BIS correlated to the sedation–agitation scale for evaluation of patients on mechanical ventilation in the ICU (63).

PAIN AND ANALGESIA

Untreated pain can leave the stress response unabated. Anand et al. has clearly shown increased levels of stress hormones and higher mortality and morbidity in neonates who did not receive adequate pain control (64,65). Assessment is central to the treatment of pain. There are a large number of pain scores, but two that are well validated are the CHEOPS or Children's Hospital of Eastern Ontario Pain Scale (66), a behavioral scale suitable for use even in nonverbal infants, and the Oucher scale (67), which is a self-report pain score.

CHEOPS is a behavioral scale designed to measure acute pain in children. A trained observer scores six categories. The categories include assessment of cry (1 to 3), facial expression (0 to 2), verbal (0 to 2), torso (1 to 2), touch (1 to 2), and legs (1 to 2). The child may receive a total score ranging from 4 to 13, depending on specific behaviors, with 4 representing "no pain" and 13 representing "the worst pain."

The Oucher Faces scale is a self-report of pain for children that consists of a laminated poster with photographs consisting of 6 colored pictures of one child's face arranged vertically to show increasing levels of hurt beginning with "no hurt" (scored as 0) and ending with the "biggest hurt you could have" (scored as 5). The photographs are anchored to indicate mild, moderate, or severe pain. The photographs are ethnic specific for Whites, African Americans, and Hispanics. The Oucher analogue scale on the laminated poster contains a 0 to 100 analogue scale, which is recommended for use by older children (Table 23.4).

The **F**ace, **L**egs, **A**ctivity, **C**ry, and **C**onsolability (FLACC) tool was developed for the assessment of pain in children who are unable to verbalize or those with cognitive impairment (68). Behaviors of children in the areas of the face, legs, activity, cry, and consolability are assigned a score of 0 to 2, where 0 indicates "neutral behavior" and 2 indicates "significant distress." FLACC has been shown to provide an objective measure of postoperative pain in children.

Opioids constitute the standard for pain management in the ICU. Opioids produce analgesia by binding to μ-receptors in spinal and paraspinal sites where they inhibit the release of neurotransmitters and output neurons from the spinothalamic tract, preventing pain signals from being transmitted to the brain. Side effects of use include respiratory depression and slowing of gastrointestinal motility. Some opioids are known to cause chest wall rigidity that is mediated through central dopaminergic activity. Other side effects include sedation, peripheral vasodilation, and lower blood pressure. Pruritus is a common symptom and is due to histamine release. Tachyphylaxis and physical dependence occur with prolonged use. Table 23.5 shows commonly used opiates.

TABLE 23.4 Pain Descriptors Associated with Respective Score Ranges

	Oucher (≤7 yr) Faces	*Oucher (>7 yr) Analogue*	*CHEOPS*
None	0	0	4
Little	1	1–29	5–6
Moderate	2	30–59	7
Severe	3–4	60–99	8
Worst	5	100	13

CHEOPS, Children's Hospital of Eastern Ontario Pain Scale.

TABLE 23.5 Commonly Used Opiates

Drug	*Intermittent Dose*	*Continuous Infusion*
Morphine	0.1 mg/kg/dose i.v. q 3–4 hr	Morphine 50 mg/250 mL D5 W to run at 10–40 μg/kg/hr
Fentanyl	1–2 μg/kg/dose i.v. q 1–2 hr	Fentanyl 1 mg in 25 mL of 5% or 10% dextrose in water at 0.5–5 μg/kg/hr
Codeine	0.5 mg/kg/dose p.o.	NA
Methadone	0.1 mg/kg/dose p.o. q 4–8 hr	NA
Hydromorphone	0.03–0.08 mg/kg/dose p.o.	1 μg/kg/hr continuous infusion
	0.01–0.02 mg/kg/dose i.v.	PCA: 2–4 μg/kg with lock out period of 8–15 minutes and basal infusion rate of 1–5 μg/kg/hr

i.v., intravenous; NA, not available; p.o., oral.

NONSTEROIDAL ANTI-INFLAMMATORY DRUGS

NSAIDs provide analgesia by inhibition of cyclooxygenase enzyme, thereby reducing prostaglandin production. Bleeding is a known complication of NSAIDs by inhibition of platelet aggregation. In addition, gastrointestinal bleeding can be induced by inhibition of prostaglandin E_2 (PGE_2) and prostaglandin I_2 (PGI_2) both of which are known protectors of gastric mucosal integrity. NSAIDs have also been implicated in acute renal failure, particularly in patients who are either dehydrated or have decreased cardiac output. It is believed that by inhibition of PGE_2, NSAIDs prevent local release of PGE_2 in the renal vascular bed, decreasing renal blood flow and leading to renal failure. Commonly used NSAIDs include acetaminophen and ibuprofen.

Ketorolac is an NSAID with an IV formulation. We have shown that 0.6 mg per kg per dose of ketorolac is equipotent to 0.1 mg per kg per dose of morphine for analgesia in children following open-heart surgery and other surgeries such as posterior spinal fusion and craniotomies (69).

Other methods of analgesia include patient-controlled analgesia, extradural and intrathecal analgesia, and regional blockade.

SYNDROME OF INAPPROPRIATE ANTIDIURETIC HORMONE SECRETION

The features of the SIADH secretion are well described and consist of inappropriate secretion of ADH in normovolemia or isosmotic states. This results in water retention and concentrated urine, and if left untreated, eventually leads to hyponatremia, hypoosmolality, and cerebral edema. SIADH has been observed with severe pulmonary disease, the use of drugs such as vincristine and morphine, traumatic brain injury, meningitis, and surgical procedures such as spinal fusion and craniotomies. It is therefore a relatively common entity in critically ill children. Asymptomatic SIADH can be treated by fluid restriction and careful monitoring of serum electrolytes. Symptomatic SIADH with a degree of hyponatremia severe enough to cause seizures or encephalopathy requires emergent treatment. Upon documentation of low serum sodium, 5 mL per kg of 3% NaCl should be administered intravenously. This will increase the serum sodium level by 4 mEq per L. In addition, 0.5 to 1 mg per kg of IV furosemide should be given. Three percent NaCl administration may be repeated. We have shown that relatively rapid correction of acute hyponatremia is not likely to lead to central pontine myelinolysis (5). Following the administration of 3% NaCl and furosemide, patients with SIADH require fluid restriction. Some children with SIADH are particularly resistant to management and may require treatment with the demeclocycline, which increases urine output by inhibiting the production and action of cyclic adenosine monophosphate (cAMP). The dose in children is 8 to 12 mg per kg per day PO divided every 6 to 12 hours.

Conivaptan is a nonpeptide dual arginine vasopressin V1A and V2 receptor antagonist that inhibits the effects of arginine vasopressin or antidiuretic hormone on receptors in the kidney, resulting in aquaresis or the excretion of water without solutes, leading to increased serum sodium and osmolality. At a dose of 20 to 40 mg per day, IV conivaptan is approved by the FDA for the treatment of conditions with euvolemic or hypervolemic hyponatremia such as SIADH.

CENTRAL DIABETES INSIPIDUS

Central diabetes insipidus can occur in children in the ICU following surgery for removal of craniopharyngioma or in children following traumatic brain injury. It is also observed in children with significant intracranial hypertension with or without herniation. The decreased level of pitressin leads to uncontrolled excretion of water, producing dilute urine, hypernatremia, dehydration, and hypovolemic shock. During the acute phase, the use of continuous infusion of pitressin provides much better control than intranasal or oral deamino-8-D-arginine-vasopressin (DDAVP). We recommend mixing 10 units of pitressin in 1,000 mL of D5 Water with an infusion rate of 1 to 3 milliunits per kg per hour, increasing as needed. It is important to continue monitoring intravascular volume and serum electrolytes, making adjustments in the dose of pitressin and IV solutions accordingly. Once intravascular volume and serum electrolytes are under better control, the pitressin infusion can be discontinued, and the patient converted to DDAVP intranasally (5 to 30 μg once or divided twice a day), or orally (0.05 mg twice a day).

DISORDERS OF THE RESPIRATORY SYSTEM

SEVERE STATUS ASTHMATICUS

Severe status asthmaticus is one of the commonest causes of admissions to the PICU. Pharmacotherapy in asthma is directed at maintaining adequate oxygenation and prompt reversal of airway obstruction by administration of bronchodilators and amelioration of mucosal inflammation. Supplemental oxygen should be administered to maintain Spo_2 above 90% to 95%.

β_2-agonists are the primary agents used for bronchodilation. In most patients admitted to the ICU for severe asthma exacerbation, continuous aerosol therapy is preferred. Albuterol is the most commonly used drug for this purpose. Continuous nebulization of albuterol in a dose of 0.15 to 0.45 mg per kg per hour (maximum of 15 mg per hour) can be administered via a non rebreather oxygen face mask or through the inspiratory limb of the ventilator tubing.

Ipratropium bromide has local anticholinergic effects and may provide additional bronchodilation when combined with albuterol. Ipratropium aerosol is administered in a dose of 0.25 to 0.5 mg every 30 minutes for three doses and then every 2 to 4 hours as needed. It can be mixed in the same nebulizer with albuterol. Ipratropium is not well absorbed, thus minimizing its systemic anticholinergic effects. It should be considered only as an adjuvant therapy with albuterol in the management of status asthmaticus.

Corticosteroids: The predominant pathophysiologic process in asthma is inflammation. Corticosteroids are therefore indicated in all children with status asthmaticus. Intravenous administration of 1 mg per kg (maximum 60 mg per day) of methylprednisolone every 6 hours for 48 hours followed by 1 to 2 mg per kg per day in two divided doses is a reasonable regimen.

Magnesium sulfate: Some studies have shown benefits of IV administration of magnesium sulfate. A dose of 25 to 50 mg per kg (max 2 g) over 15 to 20 minutes is recommended for this purpose. This dose can be repeated in 2 to 4 hours. For repeated administration, serum magnesium levels should be monitored.

Continuous intravenous terbutaline: Terbutaline is a sympathomimetic amine that has been shown by in vitro and in vivo pharmacologic studies in animals to exert a preferential effect on β_2-adrenergic receptors, such as those located in bronchial smooth muscle. It has been available for clinical use since the 1970s and has been approved by the FDA for use in the treatment of asthma in children. Terbutaline binds to the β_2-adrenergic receptor resulting in G_s-protein stimulation, which in turn activates adenylyl cyclase increasing intracellular levels of 3′-5′ cAMP. cAMP then activates protein kinase A that phosphorylates several proteins that contribute to smooth muscle relaxation and resultant bronchodilation. Carroll and Schramm showed that a protocol-based titration of intravenous terbutaline in children with status asthmaticus decreased ICU and hospital length of stay (70). Recommended dosing includes a loading dose of 5 to 20 μg per kg followed by a continuous IV infusion of 30 μg per kg per hour. A retrospective study of 77 patients who received IV terbutaline showed a significant increase in heart rate and fall in diastolic blood pressure that was not clinically significant. None of the patients in the study developed arrhythmias. However, 10 patients (13%) developed significant hypokalemia that required potassium supplementation. Of those children who were not on mechanical ventilation at the start of terbutaline infusion, none required initiation of ventilatory support (71).

β_2-Adrenergic agents are implicated in development of metabolic acidosis. Worsening respiratory distress in children treated for acute asthma may be due to compensatory hyperventilation response to metabolic acidosis, and it may be mistaken for increasing severity of airway obstruction. Increased rate and depth of breathing along with hypocapnia should alert the physician that a tapering rather than escalating β_2-adrenergic therapy is needed (72).

VIRAL LARYNGOTRACHEOBRONCHITIS AND POSTEXTUBATION STRIDOR

Viral laryngotracheobronchitis and postextubation stridor are managed symptomatically by administration of nebulized aerosol of either L-epinephrine (1:1,000) or racemic epinephrine (2.25%). Racemic epinephrine, although used traditionally, offers no advantage over L-epinephrine. Half milliliter of either of these agents is mixed in 3 mL of normal saline and nebulized depending on the response. Heart rate should be monitored during therapy. A meta-analysis has shown that dexamethasone or nebulized budesonide is effective in ameliorating airway obstruction associated with viral laryngotracheobronchitis (73). A single IM injection of 0.6 mg per kg per day of dexamethasone has been shown to be effective for this purpose. In patients admitted to the ICU, we prefer to administer 0.15 mg per kg dexamethasone IV every 6 hours. Nebulized aerosol of 2 to 4 mg of budesonide solution has also been shown to be as effective as dexamethasone or nebulized epinephrine (74,75). In a randomized controlled study, we have shown that 4 to 6 doses of 0.15 mg per kg dexamethasone administered every 6 hours prior to extubation significantly reduces the incidence of postextubation stridor (76).

PULMONARY HYPERTENSION

There are two types of pulmonary hypertension (PHT) in children: primary and secondary. Secondary PHT is more common than primary pulmonary hypertension (PPHT). Secondary PHT results from congenital heart disease with systemic to pulmonary shunts, increased pulmonary blood flow, and increased pulmonary artery pressure. Noncardiac causes of secondary PHT include HIV infection, drug-induced pulmonary venous abnormalities, and chronic pulmonary disease. PPHT on the other hand is characterized by smooth muscle hypertrophy of the arterial wall, intimal proliferation of the pulmonary arterioles, and in situ thrombosis with small vessel occlusion. The etiology is unknown. Consequences include elevation of pulmonary artery pressure and right ventricular pressure leading to progressive heart failure and death. Prior to 1987, treatment of PHT was mainly palliative, with the use of oxygen, vasodilators such as tolazoline, and other drugs such as digoxin, with anticoagulation, diuresis, and eventually lung transplantation. More recently, inhaled nitric oxide has become available, and drugs such as prostacyclin, sildenafil, sitaxsentan, and bosentan have been shown to provide significant improvement in both adults and children with PHT.

Nitric oxide (NO) gas was approved by the FDA for use in neonates with PPHN in 1999. NO relaxes vascular smooth muscle by activating guanylate cyclase, thereby increasing intracellular levels of cyclic guanosine 3′, 5′-monophosphate, leading to vasodilation. NO has been shown to improve oxygenation and decrease pulmonary vascular resistance. In neonates with meconium aspiration and other causes of PPHN, it has led to a decreased need for more invasive therapy such as extracorporeal membrane oxygenation (ECMO). The recommended dose for NO is 20 ppm. Following inhalation, most of it is absorbed into the pulmonary capillary bed. NO combines with oxyhemoglobin to produce methemoglobin and nitrate. The predominant metabolite of NO metabolism is nitrate, which is excreted via glomerular filtration. NO has been used with some success in older children with PHT due to congenital heart disease and, to a limited degree, in children with acute respiratory distress syndrome (ARDS) (77,78). The disadvantages of its use include methemoglobinemia and the expense.

Prostacyclin (PGI_2) is normally produced by vascular endothelium and is a potent short-acting vasodilator and inhibitor of platelet aggregation. Prostacyclin has been shown to decrease pulmonary pressure and improve cardiac output and oxygenation. Bush et al. (79) first used prostacyclin in 1985 to test pulmonary vasoreactivity in children with secondary PHT from congenital heart disease. Since then, there have been a number of studies (80–82) showing the benefits of long-term continuous PGI_2 infusion for the treatment of PHT or PPHT. PGI_2 has been used as a bridge to lung transplantation. The recommended dose is 2 ng per kg per minute. A number of patients require dose escalation, particularly during the first few months of therapy, some of whom have needed up to 50 to 80 ng per kg per minute. In some patients for whom transplantation may not be an option, the use of PGI_2 has provided significant improvements in hemodynamic parameters, exercise tolerance, and quality of life. The disadvantages of prostacyclin infusion include the need for prolonged IV access and its attendant risks; life-threatening rebound effects if the drug is discontinued abruptly; the need for skilled nursing care, and the expense. Alternative routes of administration have been evaluated and both oral (beraprost) and inhaled (iloprost) forms of prostacyclin show promise (83,84).

Bosentan is a competitive nonpeptide dual endothelin-receptor antagonist approved by the FDA for the treatment of PHT. It acts as a vasodilator and neurohormonal blocker that improves left ventricular function, diminishes cardiac remodeling, and is available in both IV and oral preparations. In studies of adults with PHT, bosentan improved exercise tolerance, increased cardiac index, decreased pulmonary pressures, and improved symptomatology (85). The most common side effect of bosentan is the elevation of serum aminotransferase. Nineteen children who received similar doses of bosentan as that recommended for adults had the same beneficial effects (86). Beghetti et al. reported on the safety experience with bosentan in 146 children aged 2 to 11 years with PHT (87). The data were obtained from the European Postmarketing Surveillance Program. Majority of the children were in New York Heart Association functional class II or III and almost 50% developed PHT related to congenital heart disease. The aminotransferase elevation was much less in children aged 2 to 11 years compared with children older than 12 years (2.7% vs. 7.8%). More importantly, the elevated aminotransferase levels resolved without sequelae. In a study evaluating the effects of long-term (1 year) use of bosentan with or without concomitant prostanoid therapy in 86 children with PHT, Rosenzweig et al. reported an overall decrease in pulmonary arterial pressures and pulmonary vascular resistance (88). Of the 33 children who received bosentan without prostanoids, 76% did not require additional therapy, with 1- and 2-year survival estimates at 98% and 91%, respectively. Twelve percent of these children developed asymptomatic aminotransferase elevation that resolved even with continued use of bosentan.

Sildenafil is a selective inhibitor of type-V phosphodiesterase. Type-V phosphodiesterase inhibits the breakdown of cAMP, thus increasing cyclic guanosine monophosphate (cGMP)-mediated vasodilation by nitric oxide. Sildenafil appears to be well tolerated at the recommended dose of 0.25 to 0.5 mg per kg per dose by mouth every 4 to 6 hours, and is effective in the treatment of acute PHT, and its effects on the pulmonary vasculature are sustained (89). Studies suggest that because of its sustained long-term effects, sildenafil may be most beneficial in preventing rebound PHT, when inhaled nitric oxide or prostacyclin therapy is being weaned (90). Several studies in children show improvement in oxygenation and hemodynamic parameters (91,92).

ACUTE CIRCULATORY FAILURE

Disease states characterized by low cardiac output are often encountered in the ICU. Pharmacologic manipulation of components of cardiac output is necessary in a variety of disorders such as hypovolemia, hypervolemia, myocardial dysfunction, and septic shock. Several agents are commonly employed for these reasons.

AUGMENTATION OF PRELOAD

Despite years of research and clinical experience, the controversy involving the superiority of crystalloids versus colloids for increasing preload has not been resolved. For the most part, crystalloids such as 0.9% saline or Lactated Ringer's solution are satisfactory for rapid intravascular expansion. They are safe, relatively inexpensive, and readily available. An IV bolus of 20 mL per kg crystalloid bolus administered over 20 to 30 minutes is indicated when hypovolemic state accompanied by an overall depletion of extracellular fluid compartment is suspected. Such a bolus can be repeated as required based on the hemodynamic response. While superiority of colloids such as 5% albumin remains to be established, it is often the plasma expander of choice for managing hypovolemia with either normal or expanded interstitial fluid space as in sepsis or after surgical procedures. Because of its colloid oncotic pressure, 5% albumin (10 to 20 mL per kg bolus over 30 to 60 minutes) is expected to preferentially expand the intravascular space. However, it is expensive and occasionally associated with hypotension. Administration of 25% albumin is often utilized in patients with hypoproteinemia, hypovolemia, and edema to draw interstitial fluid into the intravascular space. Adequacy of cardiac and renal function must be ensured to avoid congestive heart failure and pulmonary edema. A continuous infusion of 25% albumin solution (1 to 2 g per kg per day) can be administered along with furosemide for restoring vascular volume and mobilizing the interstitial fluid.

REDUCTION OF PRELOAD

Congestive heart failure and renal insufficiency are major reasons for excessive preload in critically ill children. Decreasing the extracellular fluid space without causing excessive hypovolemia is the goal in such patients. Furosemide is the most commonly employed diuretic to achieve this. The usual dose is 1 mg per kg repeated every 6 to 8 hours as necessary. It has been shown that compared with intermittent doses, continuous infusion of furosemide (0.1 mg per kg per hour) is as effective in increasing the urine output, requires lower total dose, and is associated with less hemodynamic instability (93). Bumetanide (0.015 to 0.1 mg per kg per day IV or PO), chlorothiazide (10 to 20 mg per kg per 12 hour PO, 1 to 4 mg per kg per 12 hour IV), and metolazone (0.1 to 0.2 mg per kg per 12 hour PO) can be given alone or in combination with furosemide for greater effect.

B-type natriuretic peptide (BNP) has been used in the management of acute decompensated heart failure (94). BNP is synthesized in the ventricular myocardium, and its production is increased in patients with congestive heart failure. It causes arterial and venous dilation, natriuresis, and diuresis while maintaining glomerular filtration rate and renal blood flow. Nesiritide is a recombinant form of hBNP. In several clinical trials, nesiritide has been shown to be beneficial in management of acute decompensated heart failure. Use of nesiritide in such patients can decrease pulmonary capillary wedge pressure, systemic vascular resistance, and the amount of additional inotropic agents needed for hemodynamic improvement. Intravenous nesiritide has been used in doses of 0.3 to 2 μg per kg bolus followed by 0.01 to 0.03 μg per kg per minute infusion (95,96).

ENHANCEMENT OF MYOCARDIAL CONTRACTILITY

Sympathomimetics

For decades, natural or synthetic catecholamines have been the mainstay of inotropic support. Dopamine and dobutamine are by far the most commonly used agents. However, other agents are often used in special circumstances.

Dopamine acts directly by stimulation of α- and β-adrenergic as well as dopaminergic receptors and indirectly by releasing norepinephrine from presynaptic sympathetic terminals. Stimulation of the dopamine (DA_1) receptors results in relaxation of renal, cerebral, coronary, mesenteric, and pulmonary vasculature. Stimulation of DA_2 receptors results in renal and mesenteric vasodilation. The effects of dopamine on various receptors are dose dependent. At a low dose (2 to 5 μg per kg per minute), dopamine stimulates mainly the dopaminergic receptors resulting in increased renal, mesenteric, and coronary blood flow without significantly increasing myocardial oxygen consumption. At moderate doses (5 to 10 μg per kg per minute), β-adrenergic receptors are stimulated with an increase in myocardial contractility, heart rate, and norepinephrine release. At a high dose (10 to 20 μg per kg per minute), dopamine causes α-adrenergic stimulation resulting in peripheral vasoconstriction, increases in systemic and pulmonary vascular resistances and blood pressure.

Dobutamine is a synthetic catecholamine that acts predominantly on β_1-receptors increasing myocardial contractility. It also causes β_2-mediated vasodilation. Dobutamine causes greater augmentation of myocardial blood flow for the same increase in myocardial oxygen demand when compared with dopamine (97). The immature cardiovascular system of neonates and infants may not be as responsive to dobutamine as in older children and adults (98). Dobutamine is used as a continuous infusion in doses varying from 2 to 20 μg per kg per minute.

Epinephrine is often used as a continuous infusion in combination with dopamine and dobutamine in patients who require additional inotropic therapy. In low doses (0.02 to 0.03 μg per kg per minute), it acts predominantly on β-adrenergic receptors with an increase in heart rate, contractility, and vasodilation in splanchnic and skeletal muscle vasculature resulting in a decrease in systemic vascular resistance. In increasing doses (up to 1 μg per kg per minute), progressive α-stimulation occurs, increasing the systemic vascular resistance. Myocardial ischemia is a concern in such doses.

Isoproterenol is a synthetic β_1- and β_2-agonist with no alpha effects. Its use is limited by its considerable arrhythmogenic potential and propensity toward causing myocardial ischemia. Treatment with isoproterenol is almost exclusively restricted to the settings of atrioventricular block for which it is useful even in transplanted hearts. It is used as a continuous infusion in a dose of 0.01 to 0.5 μg per kg per minute. Isoproterenol is contraindicated in children with subaortic stenosis because of its inotropic and vasodilatory effects, which can worsen the outflow tract gradient.

Phosphodiesterase (PDE) inhibitors: Inhibition of PDE results in accumulation of 3′5′ cAMP. Drugs in this class, used for increasing cardiac output, inhibit PDE-III, the predominant form of phosphodiesterase in the myocardium. PDE-III is also present in vascular smooth muscle. The action of PDE-III inhibitors is independent of β-receptors that may be downregulated in congestive heart failure. Clinically significant effects of PDE-III inhibitors include positive inotropy, vasodilation, and improved relaxation of myocardium during diastole. PDE-III inhibitors do not increase myocardial oxygen consumption to the same extent as β-agonists. In clinical practice, milrinone is the most commonly used PDE-III inhibitor. Milrinone was shown to decrease the risk of low cardiac output syndrome in infants and young children after repair of congenital heart defects (99). In this study, a dose of 75 μg per kg IV bolus followed by 0.75 μg per kg per minute infusion was found to be superior to placebo. Milrinone is also effective for improving cardiac output in cardiogenic shock from other conditions such as myocarditis and cardiomyopathy. An IV bolus dose of milrinone (50 to 75 μg per kg) is followed by a continuous infusion of 0.375 to 0.75 μg per kg per minute. A significant side effect of milrinone, especially after a bolus dose, is hypotension from vasodilation. Volume augmentation may be required to counteract this effect.

AFTERLOAD REDUCTION

Decreasing the afterload by venous or arterial dilation can augment cardiac output. The main reasons vasodilators are used in critically ill children are for myocardial dysfunction after cardiac surgery, myocarditis, myocardial ischemia, dilated cardiomyopathy, and systemic or PHT. The most common agents used for this purpose are nitroglycerin, sodium nitroprusside, angiotensin-converting enzyme (ACE) inhibitors, and hydralazine.

Nitroglycerin is a potent venous dilator, but it also relaxes the systemic and pulmonary arterial musculature. In the vascular endothelial cell, it is converted to nitric oxide that activates guanylate cyclase thereby increasing the intracellular concentration of cGMP, a potent vascular smooth muscle relaxant. Clinically significant effects of nitroglycerine are decreased afterload and preload, decreased myocardial oxygen consumption, increased cardiac output, and increased myocardial blood flow. Excessive vasodilation may result in hypotension necessitating volume augmentation or decreased dosing. Nitroglycerin is infused intravenously at a rate of 0.5 to 5 μg per kg per minute according to hemodynamic response. The usefulness of nitroglycerin may be limited by the development of tachyphylaxis with prolonged use.

Sodium nitroprusside stimulates guanylate cyclase resulting in the increase in intracellular concentrations of cGMP. Pharmacologically desirable effects result from arterial and venous dilation. Nitroprusside causes greater reduction in systemic and pulmonary arterial pressure than does nitroglycerin. When used to augment cardiac output, both nitroprusside and nitroglycerin are combined with an inotrope. Sodium nitroprusside is especially effective in hypertensive emergencies and after coarctectomy. It is used as a continuous infusion titrated to effect in a dose of 0.5 to 10 μg per kg per minute. With prolonged usage, cyanide and thiocyanate toxicity are a concern especially in those with impaired renal clearance. Significant toxicity is not commonly encountered in children with normal hepatic and renal function. However, to avoid the adverse effects of cyanide toxicity, some institutions routinely add sodium thiosulfate in a ratio of 10:1 nitroprusside to thiosulfate in the solution. Thiosulfate provides the sulfur donor that allows the combination of cyanide with thiosulfate to form less toxic sodium thiocyanate, which is then excreted.

Angiotensin-Converting Enzyme Inhibitors

ACE inhibitors are often utilized for reduction of afterload for prolonged periods of time. They are particularly helpful after heart surgery, dilated cardiomyopathy, and congestive heart failure from left to right shunts and mitral and aortic regurgitation. ACE inhibitors reduce angiotensin II-mediated vasoconstriction and potentiation of sympathetic nervous system activity. In addition, decreased aldosterone release decreases sodium and water retention, myocardial fibrosis, and nitric oxide release. In children, enalapril is currently the most commonly used agent for this purpose. Enalapril can be given either intravenously or orally. When administered orally, infants and children should receive 0.05 mg per kg every 12 hours with dosing increase as required to 0.25 mg per kg every 12 hours. Adolescents and adults should receive a total dose of 1 to 2.5 mg every 12 hours, increased gradually to 5 to 20 mg every 12 hours. The IV dose of enalapril is 5 to 10 μg per kg every 8 to 24 hours in infants and children and a total of 0.625 to 1.25 mg every 6 to 8 hours in adolescents and adults. A study of 63 children with congestive heart failure by Leversha et al. showed improvement in 58% of patients (100). However, eight (12%) patients required discontinuation of the drug because of renal failure that developed within 5 days of institution of enalapril. All eight patients were younger than 4 months and had left-to-right shunts. Because ACE inhibitors abolish vasoconstriction in the renal efferent arterioles necessary for maintaining glomerular filtration pressure, ACE inhibitors should not be used in patients with renal artery stenosis.

MISCELLANEOUS AGENTS

Since its introduction in clinical practice in 1970s, *Prostaglandin E_1* or alprostadil has established itself as a life-saving temporizing pharmacologic measure to keep the ductus arteriosus open in ductal-dependent congenital heart defects. In neonates with left-sided obstructive lesions such as hypoplastic left heart syndrome, coarctation, and interrupted aortic arch, patency of ductus arteriosus is necessary to maintain blood flow through the descending aorta. Similarly, blood flow across the ductus is essential to maintain pulmonary blood flow in neonates with cyanotic heart defects such as pulmonary and tricuspid atresia. Alprostadil is administered as a continuous IV infusion in a dose of 0.05 to 0.2 μg per kg per minute. Side effects include hypotension from vasodilation, apnea, fever, and seizures. Hypotension should be treated initially with volume expansion. Prolonged therapy (>5 days) is associated with gastric antral mucosal hyperplasia, cortical hyperostosis, and soft tissue swelling.

Vasopressin has been recently introduced to improve hemodynamic stability in vasodilatory shock in sepsis and after cardiac surgery (101,102). A continuous infusion of 0.04 units per minute for 16 hours was shown to increase mean arterial pressure, systemic vascular resistance, and urine output in adults with vasodilatory septic shock (101). Continuous infusion of vasopressin (0.0003 to 0.002 units per kg per minute) was used to treat hypotension with adequate myocardial function in 11 infants and children after heart surgery (102). There was an improvement in systolic blood pressure and decreased need for inotropes after vasopressin administration. It appears that myocardial function should be optimized when vasopressin is administered. On the basis of available studies, vasopressin appears to be effective in restoring organ perfusion in the settings of vasoplegia (vasodilatory septic shock) and catecholamine-resistant shock states. In a low dose such as mentioned above, vasopressin retains its predominant systemic vasoconstrictor effects while causing pulmonary, cerebral, and coronary vasodilation (103). Recommended doses in children are extrapolated from adult studies.

Fenoldopam is a benzazepine derivative with selective dopamine-1 receptor (DA-1) agonist activity. As a peripheral dopamine receptor agonist, fenoldopam promotes the relaxation of smooth muscles by increasing intracellular cAMP-dependent protein kinase A activity. It was developed for the treatment of severe hypertension and is approved for such use by the FDA. A number of studies have shown that fenoldopam is safe and effective for the treatment of mild-to-severe hypertension (104–106). In a prospective, randomized multicenter trial that compared fenoldopam to sodium nitroprusside for the treatment of severe hypertension, the investigators found that the efficacy of fenoldopam was similar to sodium nitroprusside (106). In addition, fenoldopam increases cAMP activity in the proximal tubular cells and the medullary part of the thick ascending limb of the loop of Henle with inhibition of the sodium–potassium ATP pump. The vasodilatory effects of fenoldopam on the renal vascular bed results in significant increase in renal blood flow, natriuresis, and hydrostatic pressure with resultant increase in urine output. In a study that compared fenoldopam with sodium nitroprusside for the treatment of hypertension (106), the patients who received fenoldopam more than doubled their urine output. In addition, there were significant increases in sodium excretion and improvement in creatinine clearance. More recent studies on fenoldopam have investigated its role in increasing urine output and renal protection in sepsis. Although information regarding the use of fenoldopam in children is limited, studies in adult patients indicate that fenoldopam increases urine output and possibly has renal protective effects in sepsis and in patients following cardiac surgery (107). In a retrospective review, Costello et al. showed that 25 infants who received fenoldopam following cardiopulmonary bypass had more urine output than those who did not receive the drug (108). Fenoldopam may have a role in the diuretic regimen of children who are unable to achieve an adequate negative fluid balance in spite of maximal conventional diuretic therapy following cardiopulmonary bypass for repair of congenital heart disease. It may also have renal protective effects in sepsis.

β-Blockers are used as continuous infusions for management of hypertensive emergencies and tachyarrhythmias. The advantages of continuous infusion of short-acting β-blockers are the rapid onset of action with a relative brief duration of effects after discontinuation of therapy. Patients should be under close electrocardiographic and blood pressure monitoring. Side effects include hypotension, negative inotropy and potentiation of digitalis effects, hypoglycemia, and bronchospasm.

Labetalol has both α- and β-adrenergic blocking properties. Intravenous infusion of labetalol has been used for hypertensive emergencies. An initial IV bolus of 0.2 to 1 mg per kg (max 20 mg) is followed by a continuous infusion of 0.25 to 1.5 mg per kg per hour with close monitoring of blood pressure. Onset of action is within 5 minutes and the effects last for 2 to 4 hours.

Esmolol has selective β_1-adrenergic blocking properties. It is used as a class II antiarrhythmic agent and to alleviate dynamic left or right outflow tract obstruction such as in hypertrophic cardiomyopathy and cyanotic spells of tetralogy of Fallot. An initial bolus of 0.1 to 0.5 mg per kg over 1 minute is followed by a continuous infusion of 0.025 to 0.1 mg per kg per minute. Infusion may be increased by 0.025 to 0.05 mg per kg per minute every 5 to 10 minutes up to 0.5 mg per kg per minute depending upon the response. Concomitant use of morphine may increase esmolol levels by as much as 50%.

Carvedilol is a nonselective β-adrenoreceptor and α_1-adrenoreceptor antagonist. Traditionally, β-blockers have not been used for the treatment of congestive heart failure because of concerns regarding their negative inotropic effects. However, it is now apparent that heart failure results in widespread neurohumoral activation with increased sympathetic activity that worsens heart failure. The use of β-blockers such as carvedilol can help inhibit sympathetic activity and may reduce progression of congestive heart failure. Carvedilol is the first β-blocker approved by the FDA for the treatment of mild-to-moderate congestive heart failure. The benefits of this drug in adults with congestive heart failure have been shown in several studies (109–112). However, in a study by Shaddy et al., children with congestive heart failure treated with carvedilol showed no significant improvement (113). The recommended dose of carvedilol in children is 0.08 mg per kg twice a day and can be titrated to 0.46 mg per kg twice daily.

ANTICOAGULATION AND THROMBOLYTICS

The benefits of routine use of antithrombotic therapy for prophylaxis of deep vein thrombosis (DVT) and pulmonary embolism (PE) in children are unclear. This is most likely due to the lower incidence of DVT and PE in children (114,115) with estimates ranging from 0.07 events per 10,000 to 5.3 per 10,000 hospital admissions compared with that of 2.5% to 5% in adults (116). More recently, the treatment of thromboembolic disease in children has become better defined, largely in part due to the work of Andrews and colleagues (117). The indications for antithrombotic therapy in children are as follows.

Prophylaxis
- Central venous catheters
- Prosthetic heart valves
- Blalock–Taussig shunt
- Endovascular stents
- Fontan procedure
- Atrial fibrillation
- Continuous arteriovenous hemofiltration
- Hemodialysis
- Extracorporeal membrane oxygenation
- Kawasaki disease

Treatment
- DVT
- PE
- Arterial thromboembolism
- Venous thromboembolism
- Nonhemorrhagic stroke

TABLE 23.6 Protocol for Systemic Heparin Administration and Adjustment for Children

Activated Partial Thromboplastin Time (aPTT)	*Bolus (units/kg)*	*Hold (min)*	*Rate Change (%)*	*Repeat aPTT*
<50	50	0	+10	4 hr
50–59	0	0	+10	4 hr
60–85	0	0	0	Next day
86–95	0	0	−10	4 hr
96–120	0	30	−10	4 hr
>120	0	60	−15	4 hr

Note: Loading dose = heparin 75 units/kg i.v. over 10 min; initial maintenance dose = 28 units/kg/hr for infants ≤ 1 year, 20 units/kg/hr for children older than 1 year. Adjust heparin to maintain aPTT 60–85 s. Adapted from Michelson AD, Bovill E, Andrew M. Antithrombotic therapy in children. *Chest* 1995;108: 506s–522S.

Unfractionated heparin is a naturally occurring mucoitin polysulfuric acid stored in mast cells. The commercially available sources have varying potency and are generally obtained from bovine or porcine lungs or intestinal mucosa. Heparin activity is standardized by a USP reference that is measured as the amount of heparin needed to prevent clotting of citrated sheep plasma with calcium. Heparin is ineffective when given orally and must be administered by IV or IM injection. Heparin inhibits coagulation by acting with antithrombin to inhibit activated coagulation factors (Table 23.6).

The three major complications associated with the use of heparin include bleeding, osteoporosis with long-term use, and heparin-induced thrombocytopenia (HIT). If immediate reversal of heparin effect is needed, protamine sulfate can be given (Table 23.7).

Low-molecular-weight heparin (LMWH) has several advantages over unfractionated heparin, which include predictability of effects, lessening the need for frequent monitoring; subcutaneous route, which obviates the need for IV access; and lower incidence of HIT. The action of LMWH is similar to that of heparin. Therapeutic level of LMWH is indicated by factor Xa level of 0.50 to 1 unit per mL 4 to 6 hours following subcutaneous injection. A study of 900 adults with symptomatic lower extremity DVT showed that once or twice daily enoxaparin was as safe and efficacious as continuously infused unfractionated heparin (118).

TABLE 23.7 Reversal of Heparin Therapy

Time Since Last Heparin Dose (min)	*Protamine Dose (mg/100 units Heparin)*
<30	1
30–60	0.5–0.75
60–120	0.375–0.5
>120	0.25–0.375

Note: Maximum dose = 50 mg. Infusion rate 10 mg/mL, solution should not exceed 5 mg/min.
Adapted from Monagle P, Michelson AD, Bovill E, et al. Antithrombotic therapy in children. *Chest* 2001;119:344–370S.

Heparin-induced thrombocytopenia: Type-I HIT is a condition where mild thrombocytopenia develops soon after exposure to heparin and is due to the pro-aggregating effects of heparin. There is no need to discontinue heparin use. Type-II HIT is more severe and is an immune-mediated condition resulting from the development of antibodies to heparin/platelet factor 4 (HPF4) complexes. The complex then binds and cross-links to the platelet Fcγ-receptor IIA, resulting in platelet activation, leading to thrombosis and thrombocytopenia. In addition, the antibody activates endothelial cells, increasing expression of tissue factor and thrombin generation (119,120). Type-II HIT generally occurs 7 to 10 days after exposure to heparin. Heparin use should be discontinued immediately. Approximately 1% to 5% of adults who receive heparin develop HIT (121–123). The incidence of HIT in children is unclear. Schmugge et al. performed a retrospective cohort study in children admitted to the PICU over a 3-year period and found that HIT-associated thrombosis occurred in 2.3% of children who were exposed to heparin (124).

Oral anticoagulation with warfarin results in anticoagulation by decreasing levels of vitamin K-dependent coagulation factors. Therapeutic effects of warfarin should be monitored using international normalized ratio (INR). Levels of warfarin are affected by many factors including diet and commonly used medications. When first starting coumadin therapy, concomitant heparin infusion is recommended. The anticoagulant effect of coumadin results from inhibition of hepatic production of the vitamin K-dependent factors that include prothrombin and factors VII, IX, and X. Specifically, this process is due to the interference with interconversion of vitamin K and vitamin K 2,3 epoxide, which then leads to depletion of the reduced form of vitamin K. Following dosing, anticoagulant effects precede antithrombotic effects. The anticoagulant effects occur once the decarboxylated vitamin K replaces the normal clotting factors. Specifically, the early anticoagulant effects and increase in INR are due to the loss of the fully carboxylated factor VII, which has a short half-life of 6 hours. The antithrombotic effects of coumadin are dependent on decreased levels of the other vitamin K-dependent coagulation proteins and factors II, VII, and X. However, these factors have a long half-life of 60 hours and therefore, therapeutic effects of coumadin may not be achieved until 2 to 3 days following the start of therapy. The delay in antithrombotic effect is an important consideration when starting coumadin. Since the half-life of protein C is the same as that of factor VII, a prothrombotic state may actually exist at the beginning of coumadin therapy. There are reports that treatment of venous thrombosis with oral coumadin alone results in extension of the thrombus and recurrence of thrombosis. In addition, coumadin-induced skin necrosis may also result from rapid decrease in protein C with relatively normal levels of prothrombin and factor X. The concomitant use of heparin infusion during the initiation phase of oral coumadin helps prevent the early prothrombotic effects of coumadin. Heparin inactivates thrombin and factors Xa, IXa, and XIIa. This not only prevents fibrin formation, thrombin-catalyzed activation of factors V and VIII is inhibited as well.

The major complication of oral anticoagulation is bleeding, for which vitamin K is the antidote.

MONITORING OF ANTICOAGULATION

The laboratory test most commonly used to measure the effects of warfarin is the prothrombin time (PT). However, because of the use of different tissue thromboplastins in various laboratories around the world, there is confusion as what level of PT should be considered therapeutic in patients receiving anticoagulation. For example, rabbit brain thromboplastin, which is widely used in North America, is not as sensitive as human brain thromboplastin, which is used in Europe, accounting for marked differences in PT. To provide standardization, the World Health Organization recommends an INR for expressing the PT ratio based on a reference thromboplastin from human brain tissue. Currently, the INR is the standard for monitoring adequacy of anticoagulation (Table 23.8).

TABLE 23.8 Protocol for Oral Anticoagulation Therapy to Maintain an International Normalized Ratio (INR) between 2 and 3 in Children

I. Day 1: If the baseline INR is 1–1.3, dose = 0.2 mg/kg orally

II. Loading days 2–4: If the INR is

INR	Action
1.1–1.3	Repeat initial loading dose
1.4–1.9	50% of initial loading dose
2–3	50% of initial loading dose
3.1–3.5	25% of initial loading dose
>3.5	Hold until INR < 3.5, then restart at 50% less than previous dose

III. Maintenance oral anticoagulation dose guidelines

INR	Action
1.1–1.4	Increase by 20% of dose
1.5–1.9	Increase by 10% of dose
2–3	No change
3.1–3.5	Decrease by 10% of dose
>3.5	Hold until INR < 3.5, then restart at 20% less than previous dose

Adapted from Michelson AD, Bovill E, Andrew M. Antithrombotic therapy in children. *Chest* 1995;108:506s–522S.

THROMBOLYTIC AGENTS

Thrombolytic agents such as streptokinase, urokinase, and recombinant tissue plasminogen activator (rtPA) exert their therapeutic effects by converting plasminogen to plasmin. Because of the thrombolytic ability of these agents, they are contraindicated in patients with strokes and other neurologic disease such as traumatic brain injury and recent surgery. Streptokinase and urokinase are no longer used, and rtPA is the most commonly used thrombolytic agent.

Recombinant Tissue Plasminogen Activator

Currently, despite its expense, rtPA (Alteplase) is the thrombolytic agent of choice. The benefits of rtPA are a short half-time, minimal antigenicity, lack of inhibition by α_2-antitrypsin, and a local and specific action on plasminogen-bound fibrin. The experience with rtPA for the treatment of myocardial infarction in adults is well described. In the PICU, it is most commonly used for clot lysis in central venous catheters (Table 23.9).

More recently, rtPA has also been used as a continuous intravenous infusion for lysis of intracardiac or large-vessel thrombus. A bolus of 0.7 mg per kg is followed by continuous IV infusion of 0.1 to 0.3 mg per kg per hour with a continuous heparin infusion of 4 to 10 international units per kg per hour. The concomitant use of low-dose heparin serves to prevent reoccurrence of the thrombus. In a study of 14 neonates with catheter-related thrombus, infusion of rtPA resulted in complete clot dissolution in 11 patients

TABLE 23.9 Guidelines for Local Instillation of rtPA

Treatment	*Single Lumen CVC*	*Double Lumen CVC*	*SC Port*
rtPA ≤ 10 kg	0.5 mg diluted in 0.9% NaCl to volume required to fill line	0.5 mg per lumen diluted in 0.9% NaCl to fill volume of line. Treat 1 lumen at a time	0.5 mg diluted with 0.9% NaCl to 3 mL
rtPA ≥ 10 kg	1 mg in 1 mL 0.9% NaCl. Use amount required to fil volume of line to maximum of 2 mL in 2 mg	1 mg/mL. Use amount required to fill volume of line, to a maximum of 2 mL (2 mg/lumen). Treat 1 lumen at a time.	2 mg diluted with 0.9% NaCl to 3 mL

CVC, central venous catheter; rtPA, recombinant tissue plasminogen activator; SC, subcutaneous.
Adapted from Monagle P, Michelson AD, Bovill E, et al. Antithrombotic therapy in children. *Chest* 2001;119:344–370S.

and partial clot lysis in 2 patients (125). Adverse side effects such as intracranial hemorrhage or allergic reactions were not observed.

GASTROINTESTINAL HEMORRHAGE

There are many causes of gastrointestinal hemorrhage in children, including esophageal varices, peptic ulcer disease, intussusception, hemolytic uremic syndrome, necrotizing enterocolitis, and Meckel's diverticulum. Severe gastrointestinal bleeding is accompanied by orthostatic hypotension or shock, or a drop in hematocrit of up to 10%, requiring blood transfusion. Initial management of gastrointestinal hemorrhage includes stabilization of the circulation, followed in most instances by endoscopy or surgical intervention, with the occasional need for angiography. Specific medical management is limited to the treatment of bleeding esophageal varices.

Vasopressin lowers portal pressure by vasoconstriction of the splanchnic arteriolar bed. We recommend a concentration of 10 units of vasopressin in 1,000 mL of IV solution. A bolus of 0.3 units per kg should be followed by a continuous infusion of 70 milliunits per kg per hour. Unfortunately, vasoconstriction mediated by vasopressin is nonspecific, and side effects may include hypertension and arrhythmias.

Octreotide is a long-acting somatostatin that causes venous dilation with decreased splanchnic blood flow resulting in decreased portal venous pressure without altering cardiac output or mean arterial blood pressure. It provides splanchnic vasoconstriction without systemic vasoconstriction, which makes it a safer drug than vasopressin. The recommended dose in adults is 25 to 50 μg per hour. More recently, there have been reports of successful medical treatment of chylothorax using octreotide. The benefits of octreotide in chylothorax are due to the decrease in hydrostatic pressures that drive chylous flow.

REFERENCES

1. Paczynski RP. Osmotherapy: basic concepts and controversies. Update on Neurologic Critical Care. *Crit Care Clin* 1997;13:105–129.
2. Brain Trauma Foundation and the Association of Neurological Surgeons. *Management and prognosis of severe traumatic brain injury: the use of mannitol.* Brain Trauma Foundation, Inc., J Neurotrauma. 2007;24:565–570.
3. Qureshi AI, Suarez JI. Use of hypertonic saline solutions in treatment of cerebral edema and intracranial hypertension. *Crit Care Med* 2000;28:3301–3313.
4. Biestro A, Alberti R, Galli R, et al. Osmotherapy for increased intracranial pressure: comparison between mannitol and glycerol. *Acta Neurochi (Wien)* 1997;139:725–733.
5. Sarnaik AP, Meert KL, Hackbarth R, et al. Management of hyponatremic seizures in children with hypertonic saline: a safe and effective strategy. *Crit Care Med* 1991;19:758–762.
6. White H, Cook D, Venkatesh B. The use of hypertonic saline for treating intracranial hypertension after traumatic brain injury. *Anesth Analg* 2006;102:1836–1846.
7. Kassell NF, Hithon PW, Gerk MK, et al. Alterations in cerebral blood flow, oxygen metabolism, and electrical activity produced by high-dose thiopental. *Neurosurgery* 1980,7:598–603.
8. Goodman JC, Valdka AB, Gopinath SP, et al. Lactate and excitatory amino acids are decreased by pentobarbital coma in head injured patients. *J Neurotrama* 1996;13:549–556.
9. Demopoulous HB, Flamm ES, Pietronigro DD, et al. The free radical pathology and the microcirculation in the major central nervous system. *Acta Physiol Scand Suppl* 1980;492:91–119.
10. Schoeman JF. Childhood pseudotumor cerebri: clinical and intracranial pressure response to acetazolamide and furosemide treatment in a case series. *J Child Neurol* 1994;9:130–134.
11. International PHVD drug Trial group. International randomized controlled trial of acetazolamide and furosemide in posthemorrhagic ventricular dilatation in infancy. *Lancet* 1998;352:433–440.
12. Bracken MB, Holford TR. Effects of timing of methylprednisolone or naloxone administration on recovery of segmental and long-tract neurological function in NASCIS 2. *J Neurosurg* 1993;79:500–507.
13. Laine GA, Hossain SM, Solis RT, et al. Polyethylene glycol nephrotoxicity secondary to prolonged high-dose intravenous lorazepam. *Ann Pharmacother* 1995;29:1110–1114.
14. Pellock JM. Use of midazolam for refractory status epilepticus in pediatric patients. *J Child Neurol* 1998;13:581–587.
15. Kendall JL, Reynolds M, Goldberg R. Intranasal midazolam in patients with status epilepticus. *Ann Emerg Med* 1997;29:415–417.
16. Baysun S, Aydin OF, Atmaca E, et al. A comparison of buccal midazolam and rectal diazepam for the acute treatment of seizures. *Clin Pediatr (Phila)* 2005;44:771–776.
17. McIntyre J, Robertson S, Norris E, et al. Safety and efficacy of buccal midazolam versus rectal diazepam for emergency treatment of seizures in children: a randomized controlled trial. *Lancet* 2005;366:205–210.
18. Harbord MG, Kyrkou NE, Kyrkou MR, et al. Use of intranasal midazolam to treat acute seizures in paediatric community settings. *J Paediatr Child Health* 2004;40:556–558.
19. Koul RL, Aithala GR, Chacko A, et al. Continuous midazolam infusion as treatment of status epilepticus. *Arch Dis Child* 1997; 76:445–448.
20. Takeoka M, Krishnamoorthy KS, Soman TB, et al. Fosphenytoin in infants. *J Child Neurol* 1998;13:537–540.
21. Yeoman P, Hutchinson A, Byrne A, et al. Etomidate infusions for the control of refractory status epilepticus. *Intensive Care Med* 1989;15:255–259.
22. Wagner RL, White PF, Kan PG, et al. Inhibition of adrenal steroidogenesis by the anesthetic etomidate. *N Engl J Med* 1984; 310:1415–1421.
23. Limdi NA, Shimpo AV, Faught E, et al. Efficacy of rapid IV administration of valproic acid for status epilepticus. *Neurology* 2005;64:353–355.
24. Peters CN, Pohlmann-Eden B. Intravenous valproate as an innovative therapy in seizure emergency situations including status epilepticus—experience in 102 adult patients. *Seizure* 2005;14: 164–169.
25. Goraya JS, Khurana DS, Valencia I. Intravenous levetiracetam in children with epilepsy. *Pediatr Neurol* 2008;38:177–180.
26. Michaelides C, Thibert RL, Shapiro MJ, et al. Tolerability and dosing experience of intravenous levetiracetam in children and infants. *Epilepsy Res* 2008;81:143–147.
27. Knake S, Gruener J, Hattemer K, et al. Intravenous levetiracetam in the treatment of benzodiazepine refractory status epilepticus. *J Neurol Neurosurg Psychiatry* 2008;79:588–589.
28. Gajdos P, Chevret S, Toyka K. Plasma exchange for myasthenia gravis. *Cochrane Database Syst Rev* 2002;(4):CD002275.
29. Watling SM, Dasta JF, Seidl EC. Sedatives, analgesics, and paralytics in the ICU. *Ann Pharmacother* 1997;31:148–153.
30. Reisch DL, Hollinger I, Harrington DJ, et al. Comparison of cisatracurium and vecuronium by infusion in neonates and small infants after congenital heart surgery. *Anesthesiology* 2004; 101:1122–1127.
31. Arndt JO, Seifert F, Schmels M, et al. Pain evoked by polymodal stimulation of hand veins in humans. *J Physiol* 1991;440:467–478.
32. Blunk JA, Serifert F, Schmelz M, et al. Injection pain of rocuronium and vecuronium is evoked by direct activation of nociceptive nerve endings. *Eur J Anaesthesiol* 2003;20:245–253.
33. Ahmad N, Choy CY, Aris EA, et al. Preventing the withdrawal response associated with rocuronium injection: a comparison of fentanyl with lidocaine. *Anesth Analg* 2005;100:987–990.
34. Vanacker BF, Vermeyen KM, Struys MMRF, et al. Reversal of rocuronium-induced neuromuscular block with the novel sugammadex is equally effective under maintenance anesthesia with propofol or sevoflurane. *Anesth Analg* 2007;104:563–568.

35. Ramsay MA, Savege TM, Simpson BRJ, et al. Controlled sedation with alphaxalone–alphadolone. *BMJ* 1974;2:656–659.
36. Ambuel B, Hamlett KW, Marx CM, et al. Assessing distress in pediatric intensive care environments: the COMFORT scale. *J Pediatr Psychol* 1992;17:95–109.
37. Popernack ML, Thomas NJ, Lucking SE. Decreasing unplanned extubations: utilization of the Penn State Children's Hospital Sedation Algorithm. *Pediatr Crit Care Med* 2004;5:58–62.
38. Aneja R, Heard AMB, Fletcher JE, et al. Sedation monitoring of children by the bispectral index in the pediatric intensive care unit. *Pediatr Crit Care Med* 2003;4:60–64.
39. Crain N, Slonim A, Pollack MM. Assessing sedation in the pediatric intensive care unit by using BIS and the COMFORT scale. *Pediatr Crit Care Med* 2002;3:11–14.
40. Lamas A, Lopez-Herce J, Sancho L, et al. Responsiveness to stimuli of bispectral index, middle latency auditory evoked potentials and clinical scales in critically ill children. *Anesthesia* 2008;6: 1296–1301.
41. Haberthur C, Lehman F, Ritz R. Assessment of depth of midazolam sedation using objective parameters. *Intensive Care Med* 1996;22:1385–1390.
42. van Dijk M, de Boer JB, Koot HM, et al. The reliability and validity of the COMFORT scale as a postoperative pain instrument in 0–3 year old infants. *Pain* 2000;84:367–377.
43. Chamorro C, de Latorre FJ, Montero A, et al. Comparative study of propofol versus midazolam in the sedation of critically ill patients: results of a prospective, randomized, multicenter trial. *Crit Care Med* 1996;24:932–939.
44. Carrasco G, Molina R, Costa J, et al. Propofol vs midazolam in short-, medium-, and long-term sedation of critically patients. *Chest* 1993;103:557–564.
45. Vardi A, Salem Y, Padeh S, et al. Is propofol safe for procedural sedation in children? A prospective evaluation of propofol versus ketamine in pediatric critical care. *Crit Care Med* 2002;30: 1231–1236.
46. Bray RJ. Propofol infusion syndrome in children. *Paediatr Anaesth* 1998;8:491–499.
47. Wolf A, Weir P, Segar P, et al. Impaired fatty acid oxidation in propofol infusion syndrome. *Lancet* 2001;357:606–607.
48. Reed MD, Blumer JL. Propofol bashing: the time to stop is now! *Crit Care Med* 1996;24:175–176.
49. Cornfield DN, Tegtmeyer K, Nelson MD, et al. Continuous propofol infusion in 142 critically ill children. *Pediatrics* 2002; 110:1177–1181.
50. Ghanta S, Abdel-Latif ME, Lui K, et al. Propofol compared with the morphine, atropine, and suxamethonium regimen as induction agents for neonatal endotracheal intubation: a randomized, controlled trial. *Pediatrics* 2007;119:e1248–e1255.
51. Feldman D. Ketoconazole and other imidazole derivatives as inhibitors of steroidogenesis. *Endocr Rev* 1986;7:409–420.
52. Dorr HG, Kuhnle U, Holthausen H, et al. Etomidate: a selective adrenocortical 11 beta-hydroxylase inhibitor. *Klin Wochenschr* 1984;62:1011–1013.
53. Annane D. ICU physicians should abandon the use of etomidate! *Intensive Care Med* 2005;31:325–326.
54. Young C, Jevtovic-Todorovic V, Qin YQ, et al. Potential of ketamine and midazolam, individually or in combination to induce apoptotic neurodegeneration in the infant mouse brain. *Br J Pharmcol* 2005;146:189–197.
55. Scallet AC, Schmued LC, Slikker W, et al. Developmental neurotoxicity of ketamine: morphometric confirmation, exposure parameters, and multiple fluorescent labeling of apoptotic neurons. *Toxicol Sci* 2004;81:364–370.
56. Bellevile JP, Ward DS, Bloor BC, et al. Effects of intravenous dexmedetomidine in humans. I. Sedation, ventilation and metabolic rate. *Anesthesiology* 1992;77:1125–1133.
57. Bloor BC, Ward DS, Belleville JP, et al. Effects of intravenous dexmedetomidine in humans. II. Hemodynamic changes. *Anesthesiology* 1992;77:1134–1992.
58. Tobias JD, Berkenbosch JW. Initial experience with dexmedetomidine in paediatric-aged patients. *Paediatr Anaesth* 2002;12: 171–175.
59. Koroglu A, Demirbilek S, Teksan H, et al. Sedative, haemodynamic and respiratory effects of dexmedetomidine in children undergoing magnetic resonance imaging examination: preliminary results. *Br J Anaesth* 2005;94:821–824.
60. Kollef MH, Levy NT, Ahrens TS, et al. The use of continuous IV sedation is associated with prolongation of mechanical ventilation. *Chest* 1998;114:541–548.
61. Cammarano EB, Pittet JF, Weitz S, et al. Acute withdrawal syndrome related to the administration of analgesic and sedative medications in adult intensive care unit patients. *Crit Care Med* 1998;26:676–684.
62. Katz R, Kelly HW, His A. Prospective study on occurrence of withdrawal in critically ill children who receive fentanyl by infusion. *Crit Care Med* 1994;22:763–767.
63. Simmons LE, Riker RR, Prato BS, et al. Assessing sedation during intensive care unit mechanical ventilation with the bispectral index and the sedation–agitation scale. *Crit Care Med* 1999; 27:1499–1504.
64. Anand KJS, Hickey PR. Pain and its effects in the human neonate and fetus. *N Engl J Med* 1987;317:1321–1329.
65. Anand KJS, Brown MJ, Causon RC, et al. Can the human neonate mount an endocrine and metabolic response to surgery? *J Pediatr Surg* 1985;20:41–48.
66. McGrath PJ, Johnson G, Goodman JT, et al. CHEOPS: a behavioral scale for rating postoperative pain in children. In: Fiels HL, Dubner R, Ververo F, eds. *Advances in pain research and therapy*, Vol 9. New York, NY: Raven Press, 1985:395–402.
67. Beyer JE. *The Oucher: A user's manual and technical report.* Evanston, IL: Judson Press; 1984.
68. Voepel-Lewis T, Merkel S, Tait AR, et al. The reliability and validity of the face, legs, activity, cry, consolability observational tool as a measure of pain in children with cognitive impairment. *Anesth Analg* 2002;95:1224–1229.
69. Lieh-Lai M, Kauffman R, Uy H, et al. A randomized comparison of ketorolac tromethamine to morphine for postoperative analgesia in critically-ill children. *Crit Care Med* 1999;27:2786–2791.
70. Carroll CL, Schramm CM. Protocol-based titration of intravenous terbutaline decreases length of stay in pediatric status asthmaticus. *Pediatr Pulmonol* 2006;41:350–356.
71. Kambalapalli M, Nichani S, Upadhyayula S. Safety of intravenous terbutaline in acute severe asthma: a retrospective study. *Acta Paediatr* 2005;94:1214–1217.
72. Meert KL, Clark J, Sarnaik AP. Metabolic acidosis as an underlying mechanism of respiratory distress in children with severe acute asthma. *Pediatr Crit Care Med* 2007;8:519–523.
73. Ausejo M, Saenz A, Pham B, et al. The effectiveness of glucocorticoids in treating croup: meta-analysis. *Br Med J* 1999;319: 595–600.
74. Johnson DW, Jacobson S, Edney P, et al. A comparison of nebulized budesonide, intramuscular dexamethasone and placebo for moderately severe croup. *N Engl J Med* 1998;339:498–503.
75. Fitzerald D, Mellis C, Johnson M. Nebulized budesonide is as effective as nebulized adrenaline in moderately severe croup. *Pediatrics* 1996;97:722–725.
76. Anene O, Meert KM, Uy H, et al. Dexamethasone for the prevention of post-extubation airway obstruction. A prospective, randomized, double-blind trial. *Crit Care Med* 1996;24:1666–1669.
77. Atz AM, Adatia I, Lock JE, et al. Combined effects of nitric oxide and oxygen during acute pulmonary vasodilator testing. *J Am Coll Cardiol* 1999;33:813–819.
78. Baldauf M, Silver P, Sagy M. Evaluating the validity of responsiveness to inhaled nitric oxide in pediatric patients with ARDS. *Chest* 2001;119:1166–1172.
79. Bush A, Busst CM. Shinebourne EA: The use of oxygen and prostacyclin as pulmonary vasodilators in congenital heart disease. *Int J Cardiol* 1985;9:267–274.
80. Rozenzweig EB, Kerstein D, Barst RJ. Long-term prostacyclin for pulmonary hypertension with associated congenital heart defects. *Circulation* 1999;99:1858–1865.
81. Wax D, Garofano R, Barst RJ. Effects of long-term infusion of prostacyclin on exercise performance in patients with primary pulmonary hypertension. *Chest* 1999;116:914–920.
82. Barst RJ, Maislin G, Fishman AP. Vasodilator therapy for primary pulmonary hypertension in children. *Circulation* 1999;99: 1197–1208.
83. Ichida F, Uese K, Tsubata S, et al. Additive effect of beraprost on pulmonary vasodilation by inhaled nitric oxide in children with pulmonary hypertension. *Am J Cardiol* 1997;8:662–664.
84. Rimensberger PC, Spahr-Schopfer I, Berner M, et al. Inhaled nitric oxide versus aerosolized iloprost in secondary pulmonary

hypertension in children with congenital heart disease. *Circulation* 2001;103:544.
85. Badesch DB, Bodin F, Channick RN, et al. Complete results of the first randomized placebo-controlled study of bosentan, a dual endothelin receptor antagonist, in pulmonary arterial hypertension. *Curr Ther Res Clin Exp* 2002;63:227–246.
86. Barst RJ, Ivy D, Dingemanse J, et al. Pharmacokinetics, safety and efficacy of bosentan in pediatric patients with pulmonary arterial hypertension. *Clin Pharmacol Ther* 2003;73:372–382.
87. Beghetti M, Hoeper MM, Kiely DG, et al. Safety experience with bosentan in 146 children 2–11 years old with pulmonary arterial hypertension: results from the European Postmarketing Surveillance Program. *Pediatr Res* 2008;64:200–204.
88. Rosenzweig EB, Ivy DD, Widlitz A, et al. Effects of long-term bosentan in children with pulmonary arterial hypertension. *J Am Coll Cardiol* 2005;46:697–704.
89. Michelakis E, Tymchak W, Lien D, et al. Oral sildenafil is an effective and specific pulmonary vasodilator in patients with pulmonary arterial hypertension, comparison with nitric oxide. *Circulation* 2002;105:2398–2403.
90. Stiebellehner L, Petkov V, Vonbank K, et al. Long-term treatment with oral sildenafil in addition to continuous IV epoprostenol in patients with pulmonary arterial hypertension. *Chest* 2003;123:1293–1295.
91. Abrams D, Sculze-Neick I, Magee AG. Sildenafil as a selective pulmonary vasodilator in childhood primary pulmonary hypertension. *Heart* 2000;84:e4.
92. Baquero H, Soliz A, Neira F, et al. Oral sildenafil in infants with persistent pulmonary hypertension of the newborn: a pilot randomized blinded study. *Pediatrics* 2006;117:1077–1083.
93. Luciani GB, Nichani S, Chang AC, et al. Continuous versus intermittent furosemide infusion in critically ill infants after open heart surgery. *Ann Thorac Surg* 1997;64:1133–1139.
94. Adams KF, Mathur VS, Gheorghiade M. B-type natriuretic peptide: from bench to bedside. *Am Heart J* 2003;145(Suppl):34–46.
95. Behera SK, Zuccaro JC, Wetzel GT, et al. Nesiritide improved hemodynamics in chidlren with dilated cardiomyopathy: a pilot study. *Pediatr Cardiol* 2009;30:26–34.
96. Simsic JM, Mahle WT, Cuadrado A, et al. Hemodynamic effects and safety of nesiritide in neonates with heart failure. *J Intensive Care Med* 2008;23:389–394.
97. Fowler MB, Alderman EL, Oesterle SN, et al. Dobutamine and dopamine after cardiac surgery: greater augmentation of myocardial flow with dobutamine. *Circulation* 1984;70(I):103–111.
98. Martinez A, Padbury J, Thio S. Dobutamine pharmacokinetics and cardiovascular responses in critically ill neonates. *Pediatrics* 1992;89:47–51.
99. Hoffman TM, Wernosky G, Atz AM, et al. Efficacy and safety of milrinone in preventing low cardiac output syndrome in infants and children after corrective surgery for congenital heart disease. *Circulation* 2003;107:996.
100. Leversha AM, Wilson MG, Clarkson PM, et al. Efficacy and dosage of enalapril in congenital and acquired heart disease. *Arch Dis Child* 1994;70:35–39.
101. Tsuneyoshi I, Yamada H, Kakihana Y, et al. Hemodynamic and metabolic effects of low-dose vasopressin infusions in vasodilatory septic shock. *Crit Care Med* 2001;29:487–493.
102. Rosenzweig EB, Starc TJ, Chen JM, et al. Intravenous arginine-vasopressin in children with vasodilatory shock after cardiac surgery. *Circulation* 1999;100:II182–II186.
103. Holmes CL, Landry DW, Granton JT. Science review: vasopressin and the cardiovascular system. Part 1—Receptor physiology. *Crit Care* 2003;7:427–434.
104. Taylor AA, Shepherd AM, Polvino W, et al. Prolonged fenoldopam infusions in patients with mild to moderate hypertension: pharmacodynamic and pharmacokinetic effects. *Am J Hypertens* 1999; 12:906–914.
105. Murphy MB, McCoy CE, Weber RR, et al. Augmentation of renal blood flow and sodium excretion in hypertensive patients during blood pressure reduction by intravenous administration of the dopamine 1 agonist fenoldopam. *Circulation* 1987;76: 1312–1318.
106. Panacek EA, Bednarczyk EM, Dunbar LM, et al. Randomized, prospective trial of fenoldopam vs sodium nitroprusside in the treatment of acute severe hypertension. *Acad Emerg Med* 1995;2:959–965.
107. Bove T, Landoni G, Calabro MG, et al. Renoprotective action of fenoldopam in high-risk patients undergoing cardiac surgery: a prospective, double-blind, randomized clinical trial. *Circulation* 2005;111:3230–3235.
108. Costello JM, Thiagarajan RR, Dione RE, et al. Initial experience with fenoldopam after cardiac surgery in neonates with an insufficient response to conventional diuretics. *Pediatr Crit Care Med* 2006;7:28–90.
109. Olsen SL, Gilber TM, Renlund DG, et al. Carvedilol improves left ventricular function and symptoms in chronic heart failure: a double-blind randomized study. *J Am Coll Cardiol* 1995;25: 1225–1231.
110. Metra M, Nardi M, Guibbini R, et al. Effects of short- and long-term carvedilol administration on resta and exercise hemodynamic variables, exercise capacity and clinical condition in patients with idiopathic dilated cardiomyopathy. *J Am Coll Cardiol* 1994;24:1678–1687.
111. Krum H, Sackner-Bernstein JD, Goldsmith RL. Double blind, placebo-controlled study of the long-term efficacy of carvedilol in patients with severe chronic heart failure. *Circulation* 1995;92: 1499–1506.
112. Packer M, Colucci WS, Sackner-Bernstein JC, et al. Double blind placebo-controlled study of the effects of carvedilol in patients with moderate to severe heart failure. *Circulation* 1996;94: 2793–2799.
113. Shaddy RE, Boucek MM, Hsu DT, et al. Carvedilol for children and adolescents with heart failure: a randomized controlled trial. *JAMA* 2007;298:1171–1179.
114. Wise RC, Todd JK. Spontaneous lower-extremity venous thrombosis in children. *Am J Dis Child* 1973;126:766–769.
115. Bernstein D, Coupey S, Schonberg S. Pulmonary embolism in adolescents. *Am J Dis Child* 1989;140:667–671.
116. Coon W, Willis P, Keller J. Venous thromboembolism and other venous disease in the Tecumseh Community Health study. *Circulation* 1973;48:839–846.
117. Monagle P, Michelson AD, Bovill E, et al. Antithrombotic therapy in children. *Chest* 2001;119:344–370S.
118. Merli G, Spiro TE, Olsson CG, et al. Subcutaneous enoxaparin once or twice daily compared with intravenous unfractionated heparin for treatment of venous thromboembolic disease. *Ann Intern Med* 2001;134:191–202.
119. Amiral J, Bridey F, Dreyfus M, et al. Platelet factor 4 complexed to heparin is the target for antibodies generated in heparin-induced thrombocytopenia. *Thromb Haemost* 1992;68:95–96.
120. Visentin GP, Ford SE, Scott JP, et al. Antibodies from patients with heparin-induced thrombocytopenia/thrombosis are specific for platelet factor 4 complexed with heparin or bound to endothelial cells. *J Clin Invest* 1994;93:81–88.
121. Warkentin TE, Levine MN, Hirsh J, et al. Heparin-induced thrombocytopenia in patients treated with low-molecular with heparin or unfractionated heparin. *N Engl J Med* 1995;332:1330–1335.
122. Warkenin TE, Sheppard JA, Horsewood P, et al. Impact of patient population on the risk for HIT. *Blood* 2000;96:1703–1708.
123. Warkenin TE, Kelton JC. A 14-year study of heparin-induced thrombocytopenia. *Am J Med* 1996;101:502–507.
124. Schmugge M, Risch L, Huber AR, et al. Heparin-induced thrombocytopenia-associated thrombosis in pediatric intensive care patients. *Pediatrics* 2002;109. http://www.pediatrics.org/cgi/content/full/109/1/e10.
125. Hartman J, Hussein A, Becker J, et al. Treatment of neonatal thrombus formation with recombinant tissue plasminogen activator: six years experience and review of the literature. *Arch Dis Child Fetal Neonatal Ed* 2001;85:F18–F22.

CHAPTER

24

Shannon F. Manzi
Michael W. Shannon

Drug Therapy in the Pediatric Emergency Department*

INTRODUCTION

Pharmacotherapy is an essential part of pediatric emergency medicine. Although few data are available, an estimated 70% to 85% of emergency department (ED) encounters result in the prescription of a medication. Illnesses range from minor respiratory infections to cardiorespiratory arrest, and the majority have the administration of medications as a critical intervention. In addition, a significant percentage of children who come to pediatric EDs have a chronic or preexisting condition requiring routine medications (e.g., asthma, seizure disorder, cystic fibrosis, or sickle cell anemia). One study describes the use of an urban pediatric ED documented one-quarter of patients presenting for care had a preexisting diagnosis of a chronic condition (1). For example, between 2002 and 2005, one study demonstrated a 100% increase in the number of prescriptions for type 2 antidiabetic agents prescribed to children between the ages of 5 and 19 years (2). Thus, an understanding of the scope of pediatric drug therapy, including the pharmacology of the drugs commonly prescribed in the pediatric ED setting, is crucial.

Weighted data estimate that the percentage of US children requiring a visit to EDs between 2000 and 2002 was 11.4%, and 14.6% for children of low-income families (2). An urban, tertiary care pediatric hospital and trauma center can average more than 60,000 visits annually. According to the Database for Pediatric Studies statistics for 2000, between 9% and 23% of hospital admissions originate from the ED (3).

Although not exhaustive, this chapter will review the more common complaints and associated drug therapies managed in a pediatric ED. Attention to airway, breathing, and circulation (ABCs) is always the first priority in managing all ED patients. The following discussion describes the "D" in the ABCD algorithm, that is, drug therapy.

*This chapter is dedicated in memory of Michael—a great pediatrician and mentor.

ANAPHYLAXIS AND ALLERGIC REACTIONS

Anaphylaxis is a life-threatening emergency in children, requiring urgent intervention. Usually precipitated by an identifiable antigen, anaphylaxis is a systemic allergic response mediated by immunoglobulin E (IgE) and subsequent inflammatory processes (4). Signs and symptoms of anaphylaxis include bronchospasm, urticaria, angiodema, and hypotension. Anaphylactoid reactions present with similar signs and symptoms to anaphylaxis; however, the mechanism is felt to be a direct release of inflammatory components of the cells and not mediated by IgE. For the purposes of this chapter, the term "anaphylaxis" will refer to both true anaphylactic and anaphylactoid reactions.

TREATMENT

The drug of choice for the initial treatment of anaphylaxis is epinephrine. Epinephrine is a potent sympathomimetic agent and stimulates both α- and β-adrenergic receptors. Producing vasoconstriction via α-receptor agonism, epinephrine increases blood pressure and decreases capillary leakage (5). As a bronchodilator (acting via β_2-receptor agonism-induced relaxation of the bronchial muscle), epinephrine improves ventilation in the bronchioles and concomitantly increases tidal volume (5). The β_1-receptor agonism results in greater myocardial contraction.

The ideal route of administration of epinephrine in anaphylaxis is intramuscular (IM). In the United States, many practitioners historically administered epinephrine subcutaneously (SC). Although it is effective via this route, when given subcutaneously, epinephrine induces a local vasoconstriction and resultant slow absorption (6). In Canada, Europe, and the United Kingdom, the majority of practitioners prefer the intramuscular route, citing better blood flow and greater predictability of absorption (6–8). This has now been adopted by leading experts in the United States as well (9). Intravenous (IV) epinephrine is used in advanced anaphylactic shock, when blood flow to the extremities is compromised and SC/IM epinephrine is less effective. Caution should be exercised when calculating and infusing the dose if it is given by the intravenous route. In uncompromised anaphylaxis, administration of epinephrine should not be delayed by placement of an intravenous line.

Practitioners need to be aware of the correct dosing for epinephrine and potential errors associated with the availability of multiple concentrations. Epinephrine exists as 1:10,000 (0.1 mg per mL) and 1:1,000 (1 mg per mL) concentrations. For intramuscular administration in anaphylaxis, 0.01 mg per kg (0.01 mL per kg, max 0.3 mL per dose) of the 1:1,000 concentration is used to minimize the volume injected. If the intravenous route is used, epinephrine 0.005 mg per kg (0.05 mL per kg) of the 1:10,000 concentration is given. Common adverse reactions include tachycardia and arrhythmia, hypertension, tremor, and headache.

All patients who have experienced an anaphylactic reaction should be given a prescription for an epinephrine autoinjector along with proper instruction for use at discharge (4,6). Autoinjectors are available in 0.15-mg strength for children younger than 8 years (weighing <30 kg) and 0.3 mg for those 8 years or older (weighing at least 30 kg).

Other agents used in the mitigation of anaphylaxis include H_1-antagonists. H_1-antagonists block the binding of histamine to the receptors on effector cells in the gastrointestinal (GI) tract, blood vessels, and respiratory tract and inhibit vasodilation and vasoconstriction, increased capillary permeability, and edema formation (10). Diphenhydramine is the most commonly used agent for allergic reactions and is available in both injectable and oral (PO) preparations. Dosing is 1.25 mg per kg per dose (max 50 mg per dose) IV/PO every 6 hours around the clock for 24 to 48 hours. Onset of the intravenous preparation occurs within 1 hour and the duration of action is approximately 6 hours. Side effects include sedation, hypotension, and tachycardia.

Corticosteroids are also useful in the treatment of allergic reactions and anaphylaxis, although it is important to note that the peak of action is delayed, approximately 4 to 6 hours following an intravenous dose (6,11). Corticosteroids mitigate both immediate and delayed phases of hypersensitivity reaction. Chemotaxis of white blood cells (WBCs) and circulating inflammatory mediators such as histamine, kinins, prostaglandins, and leukotrienes are decreased following the administration of a corticosteroid (11). Corticosteroids also decrease both vasodilation and vessel permeability, leading to a reduction in edema. Methylprednisolone sodium succinate injection is usually initiated at 2 mg per kg and then continued at a dose of 0.5 to 1 mg per kg per dose (max 80 mg per dose) IV every 6 hours for 24 hours. Methylprednisolone can be converted to oral prednisone or prednisolone when the patient is able to tolerate oral medications at a dose of 1 mg per kg per dose (max 80 mg per dose) PO every 6 to 12 hours. Given the potentially biphasic nature of anaphylaxis, corticosteroids are generally continued for 24 to 48 hours, although their efficacy in preventing a resurgence of symptoms has been questioned (12). Side effects include mood changes, electrolyte alterations, and hypertension.

H_2-antagonists are adjuvant medications that may also be added to the patient's regimen. These agents competitively antagonize the histamine (predominantly H_2) receptors primarily in the GI tract and include ranitidine, famotidine, and cimetidine. They are available as injectable and oral preparations. Ranitidine injection is dosed at 1 mg per kg per dose (max 50 mg per dose) IV every 8 hours; it can be converted to oral dosing at 2 mg per kg per dose (max 150 mg per dose) PO every 12 hours. Famotidine injection and oral preparations are dosed at 0.5 mg per kg per dose IV/PO every 12 hours (max 40 mg per dose). The dose of intravenous and oral cimetidine is 5 mg per kg per dose IV/PO divided every 6 to 12 hours depending on age. Because cimetidine is a potent inhibitor of several cytochrome (CYP) isozymes, including CYP1A2, 2D6, 2E1, 2C19, and 3A3/4, there is potential for significant drug interactions if it is used (13). Side effects of the H_2-antagonists are similar and include headache, dizziness, GI intolerance, and rare thrombocytopenia.

More often, allergic reactions of a less severe nature are seen in the ED. These may include food, drug, and environmental allergen exposures that result in rash, rhinorrhea, and/or itchy, watery eyes. Often these allergic reactions can be treated with discontinuation or avoidance of the offending agent. In some cases, a traditional antihistamine, such as diphenhydramine, or a nonsedating antihistamine, such as loratadine, fexofenadine, or cetirizine, may be needed. Intranasal steroids and ophthalmic antihistamine preparations may also be helpful.

INFECTION

SEPSIS AND MENINGITIS

Sepsis is defined as the systemic inflammatory response to infection (14). Elevated temperature, tachycardia, hypotension or shock, tachypnea, and elevated WBC count are common findings in a patient with sepsis. Septic infants and children can become seriously ill in a rapid fashion. Infants in particular may present with nonspecific signs and symptoms such as fever and lethargy. Therefore, febrile infants younger than 4 weeks generally require a full "septic workup," consisting of a lumbar puncture and the collection of blood and urine cultures (15).

Sepsis can progress quite rapidly to septic shock. The resultant hypotension leads to decreased organ perfusion, with altered mental status reflecting the lack of oxygen and nutrients reaching the brain (14). Septic shock carries a mortality of 27% to 43%, depending on time of onset and delay in seeking medical attention (16). Treatment should begin with fluid resuscitation and vasopressors (see later discussion of shock), with the early addition of broad-spectrum antibiotics. Acyclovir should be added if the diagnosis of herpes simplex virus (HSV) sepsis is suspected (17). The most recent Surviving Sepsis Campaign update advocates the use of steroids only in children with suspected or proven adrenal insufficiency (18).

Meningitis may have a presentation similar to sepsis in infants and young children. Nonspecific signs and symptoms include irritability, vomiting, decreased oral intake, lethargy, inconsolable crying, and fever. Seizures and a bulging fontanel are late signs of meningitis. Older patients may complain of nuchal rigidity, headache, photophobia, and fever. Meningitis may be bacterial, partially treated bacterial, or aseptic in origin. Aseptic meningitis includes viral, fungal, mycoplasma, and drug-induced causes.

Bacterial colonization of mucosal surfaces with subsequent mucosal invasion leads to bacteremia (19). After crossing the blood—brain barrier (BBB), the bacteria enter the central nervous system (CNS) and induce cytokine production (19). Leukocytes accumulate in the cerebrospinal fluid (CSF), and albumin begins to pass through the intercellular junctions of the meninges. Brain edema ensues, increasing intracranial pressure (ICP) and compromising cerebral blood flow (20). Cranial nerve injury, seizures, ischemic injury, and brain herniation can result if the infection is left untreated. Treatment consists of early administration of intravenous antibiotics and may also include dexamethasone in some cases.

Treatment of Sepsis and Meningitis

Detailed discussion of the anti-infective agents can be found in Chapter 29. A brief overview of the anti-infective agents used for the treatment of sepsis and meningitis follows. Penicillins and cephalosporins, the most commonly prescribed antibiotics, are classified as β-lactam agents based on their essential chemical structure. The β-lactam antibiotics destroy cell wall–containing bacteria by inactivating the enzyme peptidoglycan transpeptidase (21). By binding irreversibly to the penicillin-binding proteins, β-lactam antibiotics interrupt the synthesis of the cell wall and subsequently cause the bacteria to rupture.

A major mechanism of penicillin resistance is bacterial production of a β-lactamase enzyme, usually occurring secondary to gene transfer. The β-lactamase enzyme hydrolyzes the β-lactam ring, destroying the structure of the antibiotic (21). To circumvent β-lactamase production as a means of resistance, a β-lactamase inhibitor such as clavulanic acid or sulbactam is added to the β-lactam antibiotics. Although these inhibitors possess weak or no intrinsic antimicrobial activity, they protect the β-lactam antibiotic from hydrolysis and thus expand the spectrum of activity (22). Examples include amoxicillin–clavulanic acid and ampicillin–sulbactam.

Aminoglycoside antibiotics exert their antimicrobial effect by binding to the 30S ribosome, subsequently inhibiting bacterial protein synthesis (23). The primary target of aminoglycoside antibiotics is gram-negative organisms, although they are often used synergistically with β-lactam antibiotics for certain gram-positive infections. Aminoglycosides are widely distributed in extracellular fluid and have relatively poor tissue penetration. Dosing for obese patients should be based on adjusted body weight. Aminoglycosides are concentration-dependent bactericidal antibiotics and extended-interval dosing (i.e., "once daily") has garnered interest in the pediatric population. Many regimens for extended-interval dosing have been proposed and are still being debated in the literature (24). The elimination of aminoglycosides is dependent on renal function; therefore, patients with reduced creatinine clearance (calculated creatinine clearance of <60 mL per minute per 1.73 m^2) should not receive extended-interval dosed aminoglycosides. Aminoglycosides can be inactivated by penicillin derivatives, possibly from the formation of an inactive amide with the open β-lactam ring (25). Coadministration should be separated by at least 30 minutes.

Vancomycin is a glycopeptide antibiotic primarily effective against gram-positive organisms. Similar to β-lactam antibiotics, vancomycin inhibits synthesis of the cell wall. However, vancomycin binds at the D-alanyl–D-alanine terminus and inhibits the release of building blocks necessary for cell wall synthesis (26). Vancomycin is a large molecule with poor distribution into the CNS, although greater penetration occurs when the meninges are inflamed. The elimination of vancomycin is also dependent on renal function and requires dosage adjustment in patients with calculated creatinine clearances of less than 70 mL per minute per 1.73 m^2.

Age-specific bacterial pathogen patterns for sepsis and meningitis must be appreciated to choose the most appropriate empiric antibiotic therapy. Neonates and infants should receive antimicrobial agents that cover organisms acquired during birth (27). Immunocompromised hosts presenting with fever should be treated with an agent that provides adequate gram-negative antibiotic coverage, including activity against *Pseudomonas aeuriginosa.* Vancomycin should be added if there is evidence of infection around a central line or other indwelling catheter (28) (Table 24.1).

TABLE 24.1 Empiric Treatment of Sepsis

Population	*Empiric Antibiotic(s) of Choice*	*Dosage*	*Comments*
Neonates (<30 d)	Ampicillin + gentamicin	Ampicillin 300 mg/kg/d Gentamicin 4 mg/kg/d	Add acyclovir 60 mg/kg/d if HSV suspected
Infants 1–3 mo	Ampicillin + gentamicin or ampicillin + cefotaxime or ceftriaxone	Ampicillin 200–300 mg/kg/d Gentamicin 6–7.5 mg/kg/d Ceftriaxone 50–100 mg/kg/d	Add aminoglycoside if gram-negative organism suspected Cefotaxime 150 mg/kg/d may be used in place of ceftriaxone
Infants 3 mo to 18 yr	Ceftriaxone	Ceftriaxone 50–100 mg/kg/d	Cefotaxime 150 mg/kg/d may be used in place of ceftriaxone
Febrile immunocompromised	Ceftazidime or piperacillin/tazobactam + gentamicin	Ceftazidime 150 mg/kg/d Piperacillin/tazobactam 300 mg/kg/d (as piperacillin) Gentamicin 6–7.5 mg/kg/d	Add vancomycin if evidence of CVL infection

CVL, central venous line; HSV, herpes simplex virus.

TABLE 24.2 Empiric Treatment of Meningitis (17,27,41,69)

Population	*Empiric Antibiotic(s) of Choice*	*Dosage*	*Comments*
Neonatal (<30 d)	Ampicillin + gentamicin or ampicillin + cefotaxime	Ampicillin 300 mg/kg/d Gentamicin 4 mg/kg/d Cefotaxime 200 mg/kg/d	If gram-negative meningitis suspected: ampicillin and gentamicin as shown + cefotaxime 200 mg/kg/d i.v. divided every 12 hr Ceftriaxone may be used in place of cefotaxime if the infant is not hyperbilirubinemic Acyclovir 60 mg/kg/d should be added if HSV suspected
Infants 1–3 mo	Ampicillin + ceftriaxone + vancomycin	Ampicillin 400 mg/kg/d Ceftriaxone 100 mg/kg/d[a] Vancomycin 60 mg/kg/d	Vancomycin can be omitted if evidence of nonpneumococcal infection exists Cefotaxime 300 mg/kg/d may be used in place of ceftriaxone
Infants 3 mo to 18 yr	Ceftriaxone + vancomycin	Ceftriaxone 100 mg/kg/d[a] (max 4 g/d) Vancomycin 60 mg/kg/d (max 4 g/d, adjust as needed based on serum concentrations)	Vancomycin can be omitted if evidence of nonpneumococcal infection exists Cefotaxime 300 mg/kg/d, max 12 g/d, may be used in place of ceftriaxone
Febrile immunocompromised	Ampicillin + ceftazidime	Ampicillin 400 mg/kg/d (max 12 g/d) Ceftazidime 150 mg/kg/d (max 6 g/d)	
Ventriculoperitoneal shunt, neurosurgery, hardware	Ceftazidime + vancomycin	Ceftazidime 150 mg/kg/d (max 6 g/d) Vancomycin 60 mg/kg/d (max 4 g/d, adjust as needed based on serum concentrations)	

HSV, herpes simplex virus.
[a]Give extra dose of ceftriaxone 100 mg/kg 12 hr after first dose on day 1, then resume every 24-hr schedule.

As with sepsis, age-specific bacterial pathogen patterns for meningitis must be appreciated to choose the most appropriate antibiotic therapy. Neonates and infants younger than 1 month are most likely to develop meningitis secondary to vaginal flora acquired during birth. Group B streptococcus, *Listeria monocytogenes*, and *Escherichia coli* are common causes of neonatal meningitis (27,29). Infants between the ages of 1 and 3 months require coverage for the same pathogens as neonates; however, *Streptococcus pneumoniae* and *Neisseria meningitidis* must also be considered (30). Infants older than 3 months and children are most likely to present with meningitis caused by *S. pneumoniae* and *N. meningitidis* (20). Immunocompromised patients may present with atypical organisms such as *L. monocytogenes* or gram-negative bacilli (30). Cochlear implants have been associated with an increased risk of meningitis, predominantly with *S. pneumoniae* (31,32). Patients with ventriculoperitoneal shunts or other hardware may present with *Staphylococcal* meningitis. All patients with suspected *S. pneumoniae* or staphylococcal meningitis should receive vancomycin until susceptibility results are available.

With meningitis, several factors affect drug penetration into the CNS. Inflammation of the meninges allows larger and more-polar drug molecules to penetrate into the CSF (30). Degree of ionization, lipid solubility, and protein binding are all characteristics that influence the efficacy of antibiotics chosen to treat meningitis. High doses of β-lactam antibiotics and vancomycin are required to achieve necessary CSF concentration to minimum inhibitory concentration ratios for bactericidal activity. A lower pH of the CSF in meningitis decreases the activity of aminoglycoside and macrolide antibiotics (30) (Table 24.2).

Steroid use in childhood meningitis continues to be a controversial topic, reignited in part by recent studies in adults indicating a possible benefit in patients who receive dexamethasone prior to or just at the time of antibiotic administration (33,34). The greatest benefit of dexamethasone in pediatric patients has been demonstrated in *Haemophilus influenzae* meningitis, a disease that is now rarely seen following the widespread immunization of children (34–36). A possible explanation for the positive outcomes in patients receiving dexamethasone is depression of inflammatory response that follows the antibiotic-induced lysis of bacteria. Bacterial cell wall breakdown leads to the release of cytokines such as tumor necrosis factor, interleukin-6 (IL-6), and IL-1 into the subarchnoid space, increasing leukocyte accumulation and inflammation (29,30,33,37). By decreasing inflammation, corticosteroids may mitigate or prevent sequelae such as hearing loss, and therefore should be considered in *S. pneumoniae* and *N. meningitidis* meningitis (29,30). Other experts have cautioned against the use of corticosteroids in children with presumed meningitis who have been vaccinated against *H. influenzae* (38). Concerns around the use of steroids in meningitis include masking of clinical response, GI hemorrhage, and decreases in the CNS penetration of antibiotics with large molecular weights, such as vancomycin (33,37). However, one study in pediatric patients and a recent adult study demonstrated no reduction in cephalosporin or vancomycin CSF penetration with concomitant steroid therapy (39,40).

Acyclovir is an antiviral agent that is incorporated into the viral DNA and competes for DNA polymerase, inhibiting viral replication. Acyclovir should be added in all children in whom the diagnosis of HSV meningoencephalitis is suspected, and particularly in infants younger than 30 days (41,42). Lack of prompt treatment can have devastating consequences, including permanent neurologic damage. Dosing for intravenous acyclovir is doubled to 60 mg per kg per day IV divided every 8 hours when HSV encephalitis/meningitis is suspected. Acyclovir is widely distributed into body tissues, with CSF concentrations reaching 50% of the serum concentrations. Renal excretion accounts for up to 90% of acyclovir elimination, and therefore the dose must be adjusted for renal insufficiency (43). Slow infusions and adequate hydration are necessary to prevent drug crystallization into the renal tubules and subsequent renal damage.

Prophylaxis of day care and household contacts may be necessary when a patient is diagnosed with meningococcal meningitis (44). In addition, persons directly exposed to secretions (e.g., during endotracheal intubation) may also require postexposure prophylaxis (45). In outbreaks caused by a serotype contained in the vaccine (A, C, Y, and W-135), immunization of the exposed groups may be recommended by public health authorities (Table 24.3).

CELLULITIS

Cellulitis is a localized bacterial infection of the skin and soft tissue, most often caused by staphylococcal and streptococcal species (46). The incidence of community-acquired methicillin-resistant staphylococcus aureus (CA-MRSA) has been rising exponentially in the past 5 years. One study demonstrated a rate increase from 9% in 2004 to 21% in 2006, necessitating a shift in empiric treatment (47). Emergent cellulitis infections include orbital and periorbital cellulitis and necrotizing fascitis. Cellulitis secondary to human or animal bites will be covered later in the chapter.

Cellulitis can follow minor trauma, such as a cut or a scratch. Because skin floras are likely to be the causative agents, empiric antibiotic therapy should have adequate staphylococcal and streptococcal coverage. If a mixed anaerobic infection is suspected, ampicillin–sulbactam or clindamycin provide additional coverage. Mild to moderate cellulitis can be successfully treated with oral agents on an outpatient basis (46). First-line antibiotics for cellulitis include oral penicillinase-resistant β-lactams such as dicloxacillin or a first-generation cephalosporin such as cephalexin (46). If CA-MRSA is suspected, first-line agents may include clindamycin or trimethoprim-sulfamethoxazole depending on local resistance patterns. Cellulitis with purulent drainage may require hospitalization and parenteral antibiotics.

Periorbital cellulitis usually occurs secondary to trauma, although it can also be the result of contiguous microbial spread from the sinuses or be hematogenous in origin. The affected eye is red with significant eyelid swelling. Seventy-five percent of patients with periorbital cellulitis have fever (47). If bacteremia is present, the child may have a temperature of more than 39°C and a WBC count of more than 15,000 cells per mm^3 (47). Prior to the introduction of the vaccine, *H. influenzae* was one of the most common pathogens implicated in periorbital and orbital cellulitis. Since 1990, when universal vaccination began, the number of cases of *H. influenzae* periorbital and orbital cellulitis and the overall number of cases have declined (48). Currently, staphylococcal and streptococcal species are responsible for the majority of periorbital cellulitis. Periorbital cellulitis can be treated with intramuscular ceftriaxone or oral antibiotics such as a first-generation cephalosporin, amoxicillin–clavulanate, clindamycin, or bactrim on an outpatient basis if there is no retrobulbar involvement (48).

Orbital cellulitis is typically a complication of sinusitis (47). With these infections, eyelid tissue becomes edematous, and a periorbital purple discoloration may ensue. Proptosis, ophthalmoplegia, pain on movement of the eye, and decreased visual acuity necessitate rapid imaging and ophthalmologic consultation. Orbital cellulitis requires hospitalization and treatment with parenteral antibiotics, primarily ceftriaxone or cefotaxime plus vancomycin (49). Infectious organisms generally include *Staphylococcus aureus*, *Streptococcus pyogenes*, and *S. pneumoniae* (50).

Necrotizing fasciitis is an infection of the skin and subcutaneous soft tissue resulting in necrosis, often caused by invasive group A β-hemolytic streptococcus (GABHS).

TABLE 24.3 *Postexposure Prophylaxis* for Neisseria Meningitidis

Regimen (Choose One)	*Age*	*Medication and Dosage (Choose One)*
1	<1 mo	Rifampin 5 mg/kg p.o. every 12 hr for 2 d
	>1 mo	Rifampin 10 mg/kg (max 600 mg) p.o. every 12 hr for 2 d
2	≤12 yr	Ceftriaxone 125 mg i.m. × 1 dose
	>12 yr	Ceftriaxone 250 mg i.m. × 1 dose
3	>18 yr	Ciprofloxacin 500 mg p.o. × 1 dose

i.m., intramuscular; p.o., oral.

Adapted from American Academy of Pediatrics. Meningococcal infections. In: Pickering LK, ed. *2000 red book: report of the Committee on Infectious Diseases*, 25th ed. Elk Grove Village, IL: Author, 2000:396–401.

Superantigens, in the form of exotoxins, are released by GABHS and induce massive cytokine release (51). Local inflammation produces extensive tissue damage and shock. Despite a high mortality rate for adults of 30% to 80%, childhood mortality from invasive GABHS infections has a rate of 5% to 10% (51). The highest risk factor in children for the development of invasive GABHS is intercurrent varicella infection (51,52).

Treatment of Necrotizing Fasciitis

Treatment of necrotizing fasciitis includes early surgical debridement and administration of parenteral antibiotics. Intravenous penicillin is the drug of choice for GABHS, dosed at 400,000 units per kg per day IV divided every 4 hours. Clindamycin is advocated by many experts as an adjuvant therapy following reports of improved survival in animal trials (53). Theoretically, clindamycin may be more efficacious in overcoming the large inoculum of organisms due to slow replication and decreased number of penicillin-binding proteins, which may inhibit β-lactam antimicrobial efficacy (51). Clindamycin also inhibits exotoxin production via inhibition of protein synthesis by binding to the 50S subunit on bacterial ribosomes (26,53,54). Because of the rising incidence of bacterial resistance and the bacteriostatic properties (dependent on concentration) of clindamycin, it should not be used as the sole agent (51). Clindamycin is dosed at 40 mg per kg per day IV divided every 6 hours (max 4.8 g per day). Although rare, pseudomembranous colitis with severe, persistent diarrhea can occur with clindamycin administration and may be fatal. Prophylaxis of contacts exposed to necrotizing fasciitis is controversial, and data on effectiveness are lacking.

PNEUMONIA

Community-acquired pneumonia is common in children, especially those younger than 5 years (55–58). Signs and symptoms include fever, acute respiratory distress, and infiltrates on chest radiograph. The prevalent bacterial organisms vary based on age, and therefore the most appropriate empiric antibiotics vary (see Table 24.4) (55,59). The resistance patterns of *S. pneumoniae* in pneumonia are similar to that in meningitis, although the serum concentrations of β-lactam antibiotics in the serum generally exceed the minimum inhibitory concentration severalfold (36). Recently, there has been an estimated 35% reduction in the incidence of *S. pneumoniae* pneumonia following the release of the heptavalent pneumococcal vaccine (Prevnar®) (55).

Atypical organisms such as *Chlamydia pneumoniae* and *Mycoplasma pneumoniae* are increasingly common pathogens found in children older than 4 months, particularly those older than 4 years (55,58). Concomitant infection with mixed bacterial organisms or bacterial with viral infection can occur in up to 25% of children with pneumonia, most frequently *S. pneumoniae* with respiratory syncytial virus (RSV) or *M. pneumoniae* (59,60). In cases of severe necrotizing pneumonia, addition of antimicrobial agents with activity against *S. aureus*, such as oxacillin or nafcillin, is warranted (55,56). Vancomycin should be added if the child is at risk for infection with MRSA.

Viral and bacterial pneumonia may have similar appearance on chest radiograph. Clinically, pneumonia accompanied by wheezing is more likely to be viral in origin, whereas chest pain as a result of pleural irritation is likely to be bacterial (55). RSV will be discussed further in the "Respiratory Distress Syndromes" section of this chapter.

TREATMENT

Empiric treatment of community-acquired pneumonia in children includes penicillins, macrolides, and doxycycline (55). Aminoglycosides, cephalosporins, and antistaphylococcal agents are added for severe pneumonia. The pharmacology of penicillins, cephalosporins, vancomycin, and aminoglycosides has been discussed previously.

The most common macrolides used for the treatment of community-acquired pneumonia in children include azithromycin and erythromycin. Azithromycin and erythromycin are bacteriostatic antibiotics that bind to the 50S ribosome in susceptible organisms, inhibiting protein synthesis (26). Azithromycin displays extensive tissue distribution, resulting in a high intracellular concentrations and subsequent long half-life. Erythromycin is widely distributed in body fluids except the CNS, although it has less tissue binding than azithromycin. Both azithromycin and erythromycin are available in intravenous and oral preparations. Erythromycin is acid sensitive and is therefore administered in enteric-coated formulations to improve stability (61). Azithromycin and erythromycin are metabolized in the liver. Erythromycin inhibits isozymes CYP1A2 and 3A3/4, resulting in multiple reported drug interactions (61). Azithromycin is a mild inhibitor of CYP3A3/4 and demonstrates few clinically significant drug–drug interactions (62). Common side effects include nausea, vomiting, and diarrhea, especially with erythromycin. Studies recently published describe pyloric stenosis occurring in neonates who have received erythromycin and suggest that it is not a class effect seen with all macrolides (63,64). Therefore, azithromycin may be a better option for infants requiring a macrolide antibiotic.

Doxycycline is a tetracycline antibiotic, binding to the 30S ribosome in susceptible organisms and inhibiting protein synthesis (26). Doxycycline has a broad spectrum of activity, including gram-positive, gram-negative, and atypical organisms. Distribution is extensive and tissue penetration is excellent, although CNS penetration is poor. Doxycycline is partially chelated in the GI tract and minimally excreted via the kidneys. Side effects include GI distress, photosensitivity, hepatotoxicity, and teeth staining in children younger than 8 years (Table 24.4).

A lower hospital admission rate has been demonstrated in children with pneumococcal pneumonia with associated bacteremia when treated with an initial parenteral dose of antibiotics prior to outpatient oral therapy as compared with those who receive oral antibiotics alone (60). Parenteral antibiotics may achieve higher concentrations in sites of consolidation, resulting in more rapid improvement.

Aspiration pneumonia, especially in children with chronic airway problems or severe reflux, can present in the ED. If antibiotic therapy is necessary, antimicrobial coverage should cover oral anaerobes. Despite concerns over penicillin-resistant *Bacteroides* species, one study has

TABLE 24.4 Empiric Treatment of Community-Acquired Pneumonia (50,54,223)

Age Group	*Likely Infecting Organism*	*Empiric Antibiotic Recommendations*	*Dosage*	*Comments*
Neonatal (<3 wk)	Perinatal: GBS, enteric gram-negative bacteria, *Listeria*	**Inpatient:** ampicillin + gentamicin or ampicillin + gentamicin + cefotaxime	Ampicillin 200–300 mg/kg/d Gentamicin 4 mg/kg/d Cefotaxime 200 mg/kg/d	Ceftriaxone may be used in place of cefotaxime if the infant is not hyperbilirubinemic[a]
Infant 3 wk–3 mo	*Chlamydia trachomatis, Bordetella pertussis, Streptococcus pneumoniae*	**Inpatient:** macrolide + cefotaxime or macrolide + cefuroxime	Azithromycin 10 mg/kg × 1 dose, then 5 mg/kg/d Erythromycin 30–40 mg/kg/d Cefotaxime 200 mg/kg/d Cefuroxime i.v. 75–150 mg/kg/d	Azithromycin should be considered in infants <6 wk in light of reports of pyloric stenosis with erythromycin Ceftriaxone may be used in place of cefotaxime
Child 4 mo–4 yr	*C. trachomatis, Mycoplasma pneumoniae, Chlamydia pneumoniae, S. pneumoniae*	**Outpatient:** amoxicillin **Inpatient:** ampicillin or cefotaxime or cefuroxime	Amoxicillin 80–100 mg/kg/d Ampicillin 200 mg/kg/d Cefotaxime 200 mg/kg/d Cefuroxime i.v. 75–150 mg/kg/d	Viral pneumonia is most common in this age group and requires no antimicrobial therapy May consider adding macrolide to amoxicillin as first-line therapy for children 2–5 yr old Ceftriaxone may be used in place of cefotaxime
Child 5–15 yr	*M. pneumoniae, C. pneumoniae, S. pneumoniae*	**Outpatient:** macrolide ordoxycyline (if patient >8 yr)	Azithromycin 10 mg/kg × 1 dose (max 500 mg/dose), then 5 mg/kg/d (max 250 mg/d) × 4 d	Amoxicillin or ceftriaxone may be added to outpatient treatment if pneumonia is severe
		Inpatient: macrolide + ampicillin or macrolide + cefotaxime or macrolide + cefuroxime	Erythromycin 30–40 mg/kg/d Doxycycline 4 mg/kg/d (max 200 mg/d) Cefotaxime 200 mg/kg/d (max 12 g/d) Cefuroxime i.v. 75–150 mg/kg/d (max 6 g/d)	Doxycycline may be used if patient is >8 yr old Ceftriaxone may be used in place of cefotaxime

GBS, group B streptococcus; i.v., intravenous.
[a]Ceftriaxone directly displaces bilirubin from albumin-binding sites.

shown equivalent efficacy between intravenous penicillin G and intravenous clindamycin (65). Other empiric choices may include ampicillin–sulbactam with or without an aminoglycoside, dependent on severity.

OSTEOMYELITIS AND SEPTIC ARTHRITIS

Bacterial infections of bone (osteomyelitis) and joint (septic arthritis) are a significant cause of morbidity in children (66–68). Presentation may vary from unwillingness to move an extremity, to limp, to pseudoparalysis, to local swelling. Fever, pain, and elevated erythrocyte sedimentation rate and C-reactive protein are common features of both infections, although neonates may present with nonspecific signs such as lethargy and decreased oral intake. Delay in treatment, particularly with septic arthritis, can result in irreversible damage to the articular cartilage (66). As with other infectious processes, *H. influenzae* was the dominant pathogen prior to widespread vaccination against it. Currently, the most common causes of osteomyelitis and septic arthritis are *S. aureus* and *Streptococcus* species (67,68). Neonates and immunocompromised hosts can present with infection by gram-negative organisms; empiric antimicrobial coverage should reflect this possibility. Sickle cell patients demonstrate higher rates of *Salmonella* osteomyelitis than the general population (69).

TREATMENT

Antistaphylococcal β-lactam antibiotics are recommended as first-line agents for the treatment of both osteomyelitis and septic arthritis (67,68). Agents chosen must possess good bone and synovial fluid penetration. Initial intravenous therapy can be transitioned to oral antibiotics. Length of intravenous and subsequent oral therapy is patient specific. Traditionally, 6 to 8 weeks of antibiotic treatment was thought to be necessary, although recent studies have shown similar outcomes with shorter, 3-week courses of antibiotics (70,71).

Patients with sickle cell disease and suspected osteomyelitis should receive coverage for both *Salmonella* and *S. aureus* until culture results are available. Empiric choices include a third-generation cephalosporin or a fluoroquinolone plus an antistaphylococcal β-lactam (67). Puncture wounds with resulting osteomyelitis may require pseudomonal coverage. Four to 6 weeks of therapy is suggested to prevent relapse (72).

OTITIS MEDIA

Otitis media is defined as the inflammation of the middle ear and is classified as either acute otitis media (AOM) or otitis media with effusion (73). AOM is more commonly encountered in the ED and will be discussed here. AOM is characterized by fever, pain in the affected ear(s), otorrhea, or a bulging tympanic membrane. It has been well established that up to 80% of AOM episodes will spontaneously resolve if left untreated, although identifying those cases not requiring therapy may be difficult (36). The most common bacterial causes of AOM include *S. pneumoniae, H. influenzae*, and *Moraxella catarrhalis* (21,74). Given recent resistance patterns of penicillin resistance in *S. pneumoniae* AOM, it is important to achieve adequate antibiotic levels in the middle ear fluid. Pneumococci and other organisms develop resistance through development of penicillin-binding protein mutations. High-dose penicillin (usually amoxicillin) may be efficacious when otitis media secondary to penicillin-resistant organisms.

TREATMENT

In the child older than 2 years, AOM can usually be treated symptomatically with analgesic agents alone. If antibiotic treatment is warranted, the drug of choice for otitis media is high-dose amoxicillin at 80 to 100 mg per kg per day PO divided thrice daily for 5 to 7 days (74–76). The higher dosing range of amoxicillin should provide adequate coverage against penicillin-nonsusceptible *S. pneumoniae* (76). For patients allergic to penicillins, alternative agents include azithromycin 30 mg per kg PO × 1 dose (62). Azithromycin can also be given as a 5-day regimen dosed at 10 mg per kg on the first day, followed by 5 mg per kg per day for 4 days. The primary side effects of azithromycin are GI cramping, vomiting, and diarrhea (62).

Treatment failures following high-dose amoxicillin may be due to resistant *S. pneumoniae* or β-lactamase–producing *H. influenzae*, and may respond to amoxicillin–clavulanic acid, cefuroxime, or intramuscular ceftriaxone (76). Amoxicillin–clavulanic acid distributes well into middle ear effusions, achieving bactericidal concentrations (21). High-dose amoxicillin–clavulanic acid contains 90 mg per kg per day of the amoxicillin component and may be necessary in cases of penicillin-resistant *S. pneumoniae.* Twice-daily administration of the high-dose amoxicillin–clavulanic acid has produced similar response rates as three divided doses per day (21). The recommended length of treatment is generally 5 to 7 days, unless the patient is at risk for treatment failure (36). The patients at risk for treatment failure tend to be younger than 18 to 24 months, have a history of recurrent AOM, or have underlying immunologic or anatomic abnormalities (36). These patients should receive 10 days of treatment. Common side effects of amoxicillin-clavulanic acid include diarrhea, vomiting, and rash.

STREPTOCOCCAL PHARYNGITIS

Symptoms of pharyngitis include sore throat, headache, and fever. Viral pharyngitis can be virtually indistinguishable from bacterial pharyngitis on physical examination. However, the presence of rhinorrhea, conjunctivitis, or cough is more suggestive of a viral etiology. GABHS is the most common causative organism of bacterial pharyngitis and can have serious sequelae, including poststreptococcal glomerulonephritis and acute rheumatic fever/carditis, if left untreated (77,78). Other bacterial causes of pharyngitis do not require treatment, as no benefit from antimicrobial therapy has been demonstrated (77). Therefore, a rapid strep antigen detection test and/or throat culture is necessary to make the diagnosis. A positive result is the criterion for antibiotic therapy (36). The main goal of antibiotic therapy is the prevention of rheumatic fever. This complication can be averted if treatment is instituted within 9 days of onset of symptoms (78).

TREATMENT

First-line treatment with penicillin is recommended due to its efficacy and safety profile, narrow spectrum, and low cost (77,78). Amoxicillin is often substituted due to better tolerability of the oral suspension. Alternatively, benzathine penicillin G can be given intramuscularly to patients who are unlikely to be compliant with therapy. Benzathine penicillin G should never be given via the intravenous route, as fatalities have occurred (79). Peak serum levels are achieved within 12 to 24 hours following intramuscular administration and remain detectable for 1 to 4 weeks. Pain on injection is common and can be ameliorated by warming the injection to room temperature prior to administration.

Macrolides are acceptable alternatives in children with penicillin allergy (78). For patients who are penicillin allergic, but do not exhibit type-I hypersensitivity to penicillin, first-generation cephalosporins may be used. For patients who have failed treatment despite adequate antimicrobial therapy, amoxicillin–clavulanate and clindamycin are excellent choices for eradication of group A streptococcus (77) (Table 24.5).

The course of therapy is traditionally 10 days to eradication of the organism. Shorter courses have been recommended, although concerns regarding equivalence to standard therapy have been raised (77).

TABLE 24.5 Empiric Therapy for Group A β-Hemolytic Streptococcus (GABHS) Pharyngitis (33,71,72)

Patient Characteristics	*Drug and Dosage*
Children <12 yr, no allergy to penicillin	Penicillin VK 250 mg p.o. b.i.d.–t.i.d. for 10 d or Amoxicillin 25 to 50 mg/kg/d divided every 8–12 hr for 10 d
Children >12 yr, no allergy to penicillin	Penicillin VK 500 mg p.o. b.i.d.–t.i.d. for 10 d or Amoxicillin 250–500 mg p.o. t.i.d. for 10 d
Children <27 kg, noncompliance suspected	Benzathine penicillin G 600,000 units i.m. × 1 dose
Children >27 kg, noncompliance suspected	Benzathine penicillin G 1,200,000 units i.m. × 1 dose
Penicillin allergy (non-type-I hypersensitivity)	First-generation cephalosporin for 10 d such as cephalexin 50–100 mg/kg/d p.o. divided q.i.d. (max 4 g/d) for 10 d
Penicillin allergy (true type-I hypersensitivity)	Erythromycin base 40 mg/kg/d p.o. divided b.i.d.–q.i.d. for 10 d (max 2 g/d) or Azithromycin 10 mg/kg p.o. × 1 d (max 500 mg/dose), then 5 mg/kg/d p.o. × 4 d (max 250 mg/dose) or Clarithromycin 15 mg/kg/d p.o. divided b.i.d. (max 1 g/d) for 10 d
Recurrent GABHS pharyngitis	Clindamycin 20–30 mg/kg/d p.o. divided t.i.d.–q.i.d. (max 600 mg/d) for 10 d or Amoxicillin-clavulanic acid 40 mg/kg/d p.o. divided t.i.d. (max 1 g/d) for 10 d

p.o., oral; i.m., intramuscular; b.i.d., twice daily; t.i.d., thrice daily; q.i.d., four times daily.

PAIN

Acute pain is one of the most common adverse experiences among pediatric patients (80). Pain in children presenting to the ED has varied etiologies. Common causes include fractures and sprains, sickle cell disease, and migraine headaches. The goal of pain management is early, effective control with appropriate monitoring (80,81). Pain medication options include opioids, nonsteroidal anti-inflammatory drugs (NSAIDs), acetaminophen, and adjuvant agents such as topical anesthetics. Each drug used for pain has a unique profile and different benefits and risks. Distraction techniques, relaxation, and physical therapy are also important components of effective pain management (80).

Traditionally, practitioners have been reluctant to utilize appropriate doses of pain medications, particularly opioids, for fear of causing respiratory depression and creating addiction from prolonged use (74,81). Although drug-seeking behavior does occasionally occur in those who take opioids regularly, the vast majority of patients who come to the ED reporting pain are truly in distress and require analgesia.

Opioids are classified as centrally acting receptor agonists, partial agonists, or mixed agonist–antagonists (82). The opioid receptors are categorized as mu (μ), kappa (κ), delta (δ), and sigma (σ) (83). μ-Receptor activation results in analgesia, respiratory depression, miosis, decreased GI motility, and euphoria. The κ- and σ-receptors are responsible for analgesia, dysphoria, and psychomimetic reactions, primarily acting in the spinal cord (84). The δ-receptors may be responsible for some analgesic responses to thermal stimuli.

Adverse reactions are similar within the class and include respiratory depression, sedation, nausea and vomiting, and constipation. Histamine release more commonly occurs with morphine, meperidine, and codeine, resulting in urticaria, generalized pruritis, and hypotension (84).

Morphine is the most commonly used opiate (82,84). As a μ-receptor agonist, morphine is a potent pain reliever. Onset occurs within 15 to 30 minutes following IV administration and within 30 to 60 minutes following IM administration (84). Duration is usually 3 to 5 hours after IV, IM, or SC administration. The parenteral dose of morphine is commonly 0.05 to 0.1 mg per kg per dose IV/IM/SC. Hypotension, respiratory depression, miosis, bronchospasm, and decreased GI motility are adverse effects of morphine administration (82,84).

Parenteral hydromorphone is a powerful opioid, approximately 6.5 times as potent as morphine. Onset time is similar to morphine, occurring within 15 to 30 minutes following an intravenous dose. Dosing references have recently revised initial dose recommendations due to reports of adverse effects from clinical experts (85). The initial intravenous dose in an opiate-naive patient should start at 0.015 mg per kg per dose, and the usual maximum first dose range from 0.2 to 0.6 mg. Duration is approximately 4 to 5 hours. Common adverse reactions include hypotension, bradycardia, sedation, and GI disturbances.

Fentanyl is potent lipophilic opioid available in parenteral, transdermal, and oral lozenge forms. As a μ-receptor agonist, fentanyl is 100 times more potent than morphine (86). In the ED, fentanyl injection is commonly used for pain relief and procedural sedation and analgesia (PSA). Fentanyl does not release histamine and thus results in negligible changes in hemodynamic status (86). Therefore, it is the agent of choice for patients with mild hypotension who require pain control. Onset of action is rapid, approximately 30 seconds, following intravenous administration (84). Duration of action is approximately 30 to 60 minutes when given at a dose of 1 to 2 μg per kg intravenously. Hypoxemia and apnea occur more frequently when fentanyl is combined with a sedative, such as midazolam (84,87). Chest wall and tongue rigidity, marked by muscle rigidity, respiratory distress, hypercapnia, hypoxia, and difficult intubation, can occur with rapid administration of fentanyl (88). If it does occur, naloxone at 10 μg per kg per dose can effectively reverse chest wall rigidity (88,89). Neuromuscular blocking agents such as succinylcholine or pancuronium have also been successfully used to reverse chest wall rigidity but will mandate endotracheal intubation (88).

Meperidine is generally not used as a first-line agent in childhood acute pain management. Nausea and vomiting are common side effects and the drug is difficult to titrate (84). Neurotoxicity may occur with meperidine due to formation of its primary metabolite, normeperidine. Accumulation of normeperidine can result in tremors, irritability, and seizures (87). Meperidine is a potent inhibitor of serotonin reuptake into presynaptic neurons and therefore can interact with other medications that also affect serotonin, such as selective serotonin reuptake inhibitors, tricyclic antidepressants (TCAs), and amphetamines (90). Concurrent use of meperidine with monoamine oxidase inhibitors should always be avoided because the combination can lead to severe serotonin syndrome characterized by malignant hypertension and can be fatal (87,90,91).

The oral opioids frequently used in the ED are summarized in Table 24.6.

Acetaminophen is the most commonly used nonopioid analgesic in children. Its mechanism of action involves the inhibition of cyclooxygenase and prostaglandin synthetase in the CNS in a greater proportion than the periphery, therefore accounting for acetaminophen's antipyretic effect and apparent lack of anti-inflammatory effects (82,91). Dosing is 10 to 15 mg per kg per dose PO/PR every 4 to 6 hours as needed. Single-dose protocols for 30 mg per kg oral loading doses have been shown to lower fever more quickly than the traditional 15 mg per kg dose with no increase in adverse effects (92). Maximum daily dose should not exceed 90 mg per kg per day or 4 g per day, whichever is less. Acetaminophen is metabolized in the liver, primarily via the sulfation pathway in children (91). In overdose settings, a greater amount of acetaminophen is metabolized outside the major pathways of sulfation and glucuronidation, via the CYP450 isozyme system (93). The resultant metabolite is toxic to the hepatocytes. Adverse effects are minimal at therapeutic doses, but hepatotoxicity leading to liver failure and death can occur with overdose.

NSAIDs can be used for pain control instead of or in conjunction with opioid analgesics. NSAIDs are cyclooxygenase inhibitors and prevent the formation of prostaglandins. Prostaglandins, particularly PGE_2, are released when cells are damaged or when the level of circulating cytokine increases (82). Therefore, NSAIDs are excellent choices for the treatment of pain associated with inflammation. Ibuprofen is widely used, dosed at 10 mg per kg per dose (max 600 to 800 mg per dose) PO every 6 to 8 hours as needed. Onset occurs in approximately 60 minutes and the duration is usually 6 to 8 hours. Side effects include GI irritation and ulceration, GI hemorrhage, impaired platelet function, and allergy. The propensity to cause GI hemorrhage is greater with ketorolac and naproxen compared with ibuprofen (87).

Ketorolac is the only available injectable nonspecific NSAID in the United States (ibuprofen injection is indicated only for PDA closure in the newborn at this time). Although not approved by the Food and Drug Administration (FDA) for use in children younger than 17 years, ketorolac is commonly used in pediatric patients older than 1 year (84,94). Pain control with 30 mg of intravenous ketorolac has been demonstrated comparable with 4 mg of intravenous

TABLE 24.6 Oral Opioid Agents

Drug	*Equivalent Oral Dose (Immediate Release Only)*	*Onset (min)*	*Duration (hr)*	*Available Forms*	*Available Strength*
Morphine	0.2–0.5 mg/kg/dose (max 30 mg/dose)	60	3–5	Tablet	15 mg, 30 mg
				Solution	10 mg/5 mL, 20 mg/5 mL, 100 mg/5 mL
Codeine	0.5–1 mg/kg/dose (max 60 mg/dose)	30–60	4–6	Tablet	15 mg, 30 mg, 60 mg
				Solution	15 mg/5 mL
Hydromorphone	0.03–0.08 mg/kg/dose (max 6 mg/dose[a])	15–30	4–5	Tablet	2 mg, 4 mg, 8 mg
				Solution	1 mg/mL
Oxycodone	0.2 mg/kg/dose (max 10 mg/dose)	15–30	4–5	Tablet	5 mg, 15 mg
				Solution	5 mg/mL, concentrated solution 20 mg/mL
Oxycodone/ acetaminophen[b]	0.2 mg/kg/dose (max 10 mg/dose) based on oxycodone	10–15	3–6	Tablet	2.5/325, 5/325, 5/500, 7.5/325, 7.5/500, 10/325, 10/650 mg
				Solution	5 mg oxycodone and 325 mg acetaminophen per 5 mL
Hydrocodone/ acetaminophen[b]	0.2 mg/kg/dose (max 10 mg/dose) based on hydrocodone	10–20	3–6	Tablet	Many
				Elixir	2.5 mg hydrocodone and 167 mg acetaminophen per 5 mL

[a]Maximum dose for opiate-naive patients is 6 mg.
[b]Do not exceed 90 mg/kg or 4 g, whichever is less of acetaminophen from all sources per 24-hr period.

morphine (95). Single-dose treatment doses range from 0.4 to 1 mg per kg IV/IM to a maximum of 30 mg in children weighing less than 50 kg and 60 mg in children weighing more than 50 kg. Multiple dosing should be no greater than 0.5 mg per kg per dose (maximum 30 mg per dose) IV/IM every 6 hours not to exceed 20 doses (84). Onset of action occurs 10 minutes after administration, peak effect occurs within 40 to 60 minutes, and the duration of action is approximately 6 hours (84). The risk for GI hemorrhage increases exponentially after day 5 of therapy and is the subject of a "black box" warning for ketorolac (95). Additional adverse effects include hemorrhage outside the GI tract, nausea, diarrhea, headache, and drowsiness.

Local anesthetic agents will be covered later in the chapter during the discussion of laceration management.

PROCEDURAL SEDATION

PSA, also erroneously termed conscious sedation, refers to the process of inducing sedation in a patient for the purpose of obtaining stillness for imaging or for completion of a painful procedure such as laceration repair or fracture reduction. Opioids, benzodiazepines, barbiturates, ketamine, propofol, and chloral hydrate are the most common medications use to facilitate PSA in children. A concern with using procedural sedation is the need for appropriate monitoring of adverse events both during and following the procedure (84,96–98). Death, permanent neurologic injury, and prolonged hospitalization are potential adverse outcomes of procedural sedation (98). Prolonged recovery effects can include ataxia, agitation, GI effects, and restlessness (97). Medication errors and drug interactions can contribute to an increased rate of adverse side effects associated with procedural sedation (98). However, one study demonstrated a low incidence of adverse events (2.3%) associated with procedural sedation in more than 1,000 patients in a pediatric ED (99).

TREATMENT

Fentanyl is the most commonly used opioid for PSA. Fentanyl is frequently used in conjunction with benzodiazepines, primarily midazolam, for procedural sedation. See the "Pain" section for a discussion of fentanyl pharmacology.

Midazolam is a relatively short-acting benzodiazepine, which exerts a sedative effect by binding to the benzodiazepine receptor on the γ-aminobutyric acid (GABA) complex (100). This action enhances GABA binding to the receptor and increases chloride currents into the cell, inhibiting action potential generation (87). Hypnotic effect is usually seen at doses lower than those producing respiratory depression. Midazolam is dosed at 0.05 to 0.1 mg per kg per dose (max 2 mg per dose) IV every 3 to 5 minutes as needed to obtain adequate sedation. It is important to note that adolescents and adults do not require as high a dose of midazolam to achieve sedation as do younger children. Onset of sedation occurs within 1 to 5 minutes after IV administration and within 5 minutes following IM administration. Duration is commonly 20 to 30 minutes after IV administration. Intramuscular administration results in a significantly longer duration of action, ranging from 2 to 6 hours in some cases. Adverse effects include prolonged sedation, hypotension, bradycardia, paradoxical reactions, muscle tremors, and respiratory depression. Because midazolam is a sedative hypnotic and does not possess analgesic effects, fentanyl is often used in conjunction for painful procedures. Fentanyl and midazolam combinations result in greater respiratory depression than midazolam alone (87).

Ketamine is a phencyclidine derivative and produces a dissociative anesthetic state with analgesia; patients often have involuntary movements, spontaneous respirations, and eye opening (101,102). The respiratory drive is not compromised with normal procedural sedative dosing, making ketamine a valuable agent in pediatric sedation (84). Ketamine can be given orally, intravenously, or intramuscularly. The oral dose of ketamine is 6 to 10 mg per kg × 1 dose 30 minutes prior to the procedure. Palatability is improved if ketamine is mixed with cola or other beverage. Intravenous dosing is usually 1 to 1.5 mg per kg with additional 0.5 mg per kg aliquots as needed to maintain sedation. If the intramuscular route is to be used, the dose is 3 to 4 mg per kg. Onset of action occurs within 60 seconds of intravenous administration and within 5 to 10 minutes following intramuscular administration (84). Duration of action lasts for 10 to 15 minutes when given IV and 15 to 30 minutes when given IM. Atropine is recommended by some experts as a premedication for ketamine-induced secretions and may be mixed in the same syringe as intramuscular ketamine (87). Adverse effects from ketamine include laryngospasm, involuntary movements, and emergence reactions. Emergence reactions have been reported to occur in up to 34% of patients older than 16 years but occur in less than 10% of patients younger than 10 years (103). Practice differences exist over the prophylactic use of low-dose midazolam to prevent emergence reactions, as convincing evidence of efficacy is lacking (104).

Pentobarbital is a short-acting barbiturate with no analgesic properties. It is commonly used to facilitate pediatric imaging (84). Barbiturates depress the activity in the CNS by binding to the barbiturate receptor on the GABA complex (105). The customary intravenous dose is 2 to 5 mg per kg in divided aliquots with a cumulative maximum of 6 mg per kg or 100 mg, whichever is less. Onset of action occurs within 3 to 5 minutes of intravenous administration, and duration of action is 15 to 45 minutes (84). Persistent drowsiness, respiratory depression, and rare allergic reactions may occur with pentobarbital administration.

Propofol is a relative newcomer to the procedural sedation armamentarium for children. It is an ultra-short-acting nonopioid, nonbarbituate hypnotic agent with no analgesic property. Structurally unrelated to other general anesthetics, propofol increases the response of $GABA_A$ receptor to GABA, enhancing inhibitory neurotransmission and potentiating glycine-activated currents. Glycine receptors may play a role in mediating response to noxious stimuli. Propofol is insoluble in aqueous solutions, formulated in 10% soybean oil base that also contains glycerol, purified egg phospholipids, and a preservative. Therefore, propofol is contraindicated in patients with egg, soy, lipid, albumin, or metabisulfite allergies. Propofol is attractive in the ED setting due to favorable pharmacokinetic parameters, with an onset of action within 30 seconds, peak within 60 seconds, and a duration of action of 3 to 10 minutes. Because of the short-acting nature of propofol, a continuous infusion is often necessary. As propofol can induce apnea and significant hypotension, a protocol outlining its use is highly recommended (96).

Chloral hydrate is classified as a miscellaneous sedative–hypnotic drug, and likely exerts its effect on the CNS through its primary metabolite, trichloroethanol (97). Trichloroethanol has barbiturate-like effects on the GABA receptors (97). The primary indication for chloral hydrate sedation in children is an imaging procedure, such as head computed tomography in patients younger than 3 years (84). The dose can be given orally or per rectum at 50 to 100 mg per kg, not to exceed 1,000 mg in infants or 2,000 mg in older children. Onset of action occurs over 40 minutes after administration and lasts for 60 to 120 minutes (84). Side-effect rates are high and may include nausea and vomiting, motor imbalance, agitation, and prolonged sedation (84,97). Delayed apneic events are the main complications of chloral hydrate use (97,98).

Reversal agents should be readily available during all procedural sedations involving opioids or benzodiazepines (106,107). Naloxone and nalmefene are opioid-receptor antagonists, reversing the sedative and analgesic effects. Naloxone can be titrated to the degree of reversal desired, depending on the dose used. Doses between 1 and 10 μg per kg can alleviate respiratory depression without fully reversing the analgesic effect of the opioid (108). Doses of 100 μg per kg are used for full reversal in cases of apnea and overdose. Onset of action occurs within 2 minutes, and the effect lasts for 20 to 60 minutes. It is important to realize that the duration of reversal is shorter than the duration of action of most opioids and will likely result in rebound respiratory depression requiring additional doses (108). Side effects of naloxone administration include ventricular arrhythmia and cardiac arrest, primarily in patients with underlying cardiovascular disease or those receiving cardiotoxic drugs (108). This is believed to be secondary to opioid-reversal–induced catecholamine surge, which can result in hypertension, myocardial infarction, and precipitation of withdrawal. Pulmonary edema has been reported with both low-dose (<100 μg) and high-dose (>100 μg) naloxone administration (109).

Nalmefene is a longer-acting μ-receptor antagonist, and has a similar pharmacokinetic profile in children as in adults, with a terminal half-life of 8.7 hours in children and 7.9 to 10.8 hours in adults (110). The longer half-life as compared with naloxone results in less rebound respiratory depression and a decreased need for additional dosing. Nalmefene has been successfully used in the reversal of procedural sedation in children (111). Side effects are similar to those with naloxone.

Flumazenil reverses benzodiazepine effects at the GABA receptor and is useful when reversal of benzodiazepine sedation is desired, for example, after excess sedation. It is dosed at 0.01 mg per kg every minute to a cumulative maximum of 0.05 mg per kg or 1 mg, whichever is less (112). Flumazenil has been shown to safely and effectively reverse benzodiazepine-induced sedation in children following procedural sedation with no significant adverse effects (112). Onset of action generally occurs within 1 to 3 minutes. Resedation can occur because the half-life of flumazenil is shorter than the half-life of most benzodiazepines, and therefore patients should be monitored for the need for additional dosing (112). Adverse effects are rare and may include arrhythmias, hypertension, and seizures, primarily in patients dependent on benzodiazepines or who are receiving TCAs. Caution should be used when considering the use of flumazenil in a patient dependent on benzodiazepines for seizure control due to the risk of precipitating seizures or status epilepticus (SE).

LACERATIONS

Lacerations are a common injury presenting to the pediatric ED. Several pharmacologic tools are available for wound management. These include pain and anxiolysis medications, local anesthetics, topical anesthetics, topical antimicrobials, tissue adhesives, and tetanus immunization.

TREATMENT

Local anesthetics are used to decrease the pain associated with repair of the laceration. Commonly used local anesthetics include lidocaine and bupivacaine, with or without epinephrine. Distractive techniques, warming the solution to body temperature, use of a long, fine-gauge needle, and the rate of infiltration are important factors in the success of a local anesthetic (113). In addition, buffering the lidocaine with sodium bicarbonate 8.4% in a 10:1 dilution decreases the pH of the local anesthetic and may decrease the pain associated with infiltration (114).

Lidocaine and bupivacaine act by blocking nerve impulse generation and conduction by decreasing the cell membrane permeability to sodium (115). Toxicity is related to the amount of free anesthetic released into the circulation, and duration of action is directly related to the contact time with the nerve (115,116). Adverse reactions to local anesthetics are generally related to toxic levels and include seizures, cardiac arrhythmias, and decreased GI motility. Hypersensitivity is rare and occurs more frequently with the ester-type anesthetics such as procaine and tetracaine as compared with the amide-type anesthetics such as lidocaine and bupivacaine (117,118). Hypersensitivity reactions are believed to occur secondary to the metabolite *p*-aminobenzoic acid formed from the ester-type anesthetics (116,119). The preservative methylparaben, which can be found in the amide-type anesthetics, also may be responsible for hypersensitivity reactions (119). If hypersensitivity occurs with the amide-type anesthetics, most patients will tolerate subsequent skin testing, and the reaction may be shown to be due to the preservative (114,120).

Lidocaine has a duration of action of approximately 1 to 2 hours (without epinephrine) and is the most commonly used local anesthetic (114). Lidocaine injection is available in 0.5%, 1%, and 2% solutions. The total amount of lidocaine a patient receives for wound management, including topical and local infiltration, should be kept lower than the toxic range (i.e., no greater than 4.5 mg per kg) (121).

Bupivicaine has a duration of action that is four to six times the duration of lidocaine, but it also has an increased risk of cardiovascular side effects (114). This effect is likely due to the slower dissociation from the sodium channels. Bupivicaine for simple laceration repair is generally not warranted, although it remains a good option for peripheral nerve blocks in prolonged repairs (113).

Most local anesthetics are available with and without low-concentration epinephrine (1:200,000) (116). Epinephrine acts primarily as a local vasoconstrictor, slowing down the rate of absorption of the local anesthetic into the systemic circulation and prolonging the action of the anesthetic (116,122). Concern exists for local tissue damage when using epinephrine as a vasoconstrictor in areas with limited collateral circulation, leading to hypoxic tissue damage, necrosis, and gangrene (115). Therefore, areas such as digits, the pinna of the ear, the nasal alae, the penis, and skin flaps should not be treated with a local anesthetic containing a vasoconstrictor (122). Phentolamine may be used to reverse unintended vasoconstriction if necessary. Vasoconstriction in contaminated wounds may increase the likelihood of infection secondary to hindrance of blood flow (122).

Diphenhydramine injection infiltrated locally can be used as an effective alternative to the ester- and amide-type anesthetics when an allergy truly exists. The structure of the antihistamines is closely related the structure of local anesthetics (123). Diphenhydramine diluted to a 1% solution is painful on injection but provides anesthesia similar to 1% lidocaine (123,124). Skin necrosis is a potential serious side effect of diphenhydramine injection and may be dose related.

Topical anesthetic agents are used either alone or in conjunction with infiltrated local anesthetics. Prior to the introduction of LET (lidocaine, epinephrine, and tetracaine), a solution of tetracaine, epinephrine (adrenaline), and cocaine (TAC) was shown to be efficacious in reducing pain associated with laceration repair (125). However, TAC solutions are associated with significant adverse effects such as seizures and death secondary to cocaine absorption when misapplied, especially when contact with mucous membranes occurred (113,126). TAC solutions are costlier and subject to regulatory control due to the cocaine component.

Comparison of LET solution with placebo has demonstrated significant reduction in pain associated with repair when applied to lacerations prior to lidocaine infiltration (127). A direct comparison of LET with TAC solutions showed equivalent efficacy in pediatric patients (128,129). Subsequent studies demonstrated LET in a gel formulation was at least as effective as the solution and was less likely to drip into the eyes of children with forehead or scalp lacerations (130).

Another topical anesthetic, EMLA (eutectic mixture of local anesthetics) cream, contains prilocaine and lidocaine. EMLA is used for pretreatment on intact skin in an area that will be used for venipuncture, lumbar puncture, or injection. As a liquid at body temperature, EMLA contains a high concentration of local anesthetics and demonstrates good transdermal absorption (131). One study compared EMLA cream with LET gel for simple extremity lacerations and found no difference in pain on injection of lidocaine but found a longer duration needed to achieve anesthesia with EMLA versus LET (60 minutes vs. 15 to 30 minutes) (132). Several important considerations to use exist for EMLA, including the possibility of developing methemoglobinemia secondary to the orthotoluidine metabolite of prilocaine (131). This occurs more frequently in patients with other risk factors for developing methemoglobinemia such as infants receiving medications that induce methemoglobinemia (phenazopyridine, dapsone) or children with glucose-6-phosphate dehydrogenase (G6PD) deficiency (131). Newer lidocaine-only preparations (Elamax, LMX-4) have been shown to be as effective as EMLA, with shorter onset time and fewer drug–drug interactions. A transdermal application of lidocaine and tetracaine (Synera) is indicated for children 3 years and older.

Topical antibiotic ointments are frequently applied to clean and repaired lacerations prior to dressing coverage. Common topical ointments include bacitracin, a combination of bacitracin/neomycin/polymixin B, and silver sulfadiazine. When compared with plain petrolatum, the antibiotic ointments resulted in significantly lower infection rates (133). Several experts recommend bacitracin-only ointments over the triple-antibiotic or silver sulfadiazine ointments due to lower allergic reaction rates with bacitracin alone.

Cyanoacrylates, commonly known as tissue adhesives, are used frequently for wound closure. Primary use in children has been closure of lacerations in the ED (134). The adhesives form a strong bond when exposed to a fluid or basic medium, creating an exothermic reaction resulting in a polymer (134). Dermabond, 2-octyl cyanoacrylate, is approved for use in the United States and has recently become available over the counter. Comparable efficacy to sutures under low tension has been demonstrated with acceptable cosmetic results (134,135). Advantages include ease of application, decreased time of repair, and elimination of needle-induced anxiety and pain of suturing. Dermabond is not recommended for use on nonimmobilized joints.

All patients presenting with puncture wounds should be assessed for tetanus vaccination status.

BITE WOUNDS

Animal bites and/or exposures to saliva of a possibly infected animal are relatively common presentations to the ED. The first concern is the potential rabies status, particularly in wild animals known to be carriers. Bats and carnivores, primarily raccoons, skunks, foxes, and coyotes, are known to carry and transmit rabies to humans (136,137). The rabies virus enters the system via a bite or secretion exposure and travels to the CNS, eventually causing a fatal encephalomyelitis (137).

Preexposure prophylaxis is recommended for persons at high risk secondary to occupation such as veterinarians, animal handlers, and laboratory workers (137). Travelers to highly endemic areas with limited access to medical care and individuals who frequently come in contact with potentially rabid animals should also be considered for preexposure prophylaxis (137). Postexposure prophylaxis is more commonly sought in the ED and will be discussed here.

TABLE 24.7 Rabies Postexposure Prophylaxis

Exposure	*Recommendation*	*Management*	*Drug and Dosage*[a]
Dogs, cats, ferrets	Hold animal for 10-d evaluation	None unless animal determined to be rabid	None
Dogs, cats, ferrets	Animal escaped or suspected rabid	Vaccinate immediately	Rabies vaccine[b] 1 mL i.m. to deltoid[c] on days 0, 3, 7, and 14; and RIG 20 units/kg i.m. × 1 dose; infiltrate one-half of RIG dose into wound, give other one-half i.m.
Skunks, foxes, most carnivores, and bats	Treat as rabid unless laboratory confirmation of negative rabies virus	Vaccinate immediately	Rabies vaccine[b] 1 mL i.m. to deltoid[c] on days 0, 3, 7, and 14; and RIG 20 units/kg i.m. × 1 dose; infiltrate one-half of RIG dose into wound, give other one-half i.m.
Livestock, small rodents, lagomorphs (rabbits and hares), large rodents (woodchucks and beavers), and other mammals	Consult public health officials	Rarely requires vaccination	None unless directed by public health officials

[a]i.m., intramuscular; RIG, rabies immune globulin.
[b]Human diploid cell vaccine (HDCV), rabies vaccine adsorbed (RVA), or purified chick embryo cell-derived vaccine (PCEC).
[c]May be given in midlateral aspect of thigh in infants.
Adapted from Centers for Disease Control and Prevention. Human rabies prevention—United States, 1999 recommendations of the Advisory Commqittee on Immunization Practices (ACIP). *MMWR Morb Mortal Wkly Rep* 1999;48(RR-1):1–21.
Use of a reduced (4-dose) vaccine schedule for postexposure prophylaxis to prevent human rabies: recommendations of the advisory committee on immunization practices.
Rupprecht CE, Briggs D, Brown CM, et al. Centers for Disease Control and Prevention (CDC). *MMWR Recomm Rep* 2010;19;59(RR-2):1–9.

The Advisory Committee for Immunization Practices has set forth guidelines for postexposure prophylaxis (see Table 24.7). Because human rabies is uniformly fatal once symptoms appear, prophylaxis with rabies immune globulin (RIG) and vaccination is imperative if exposure to rabies is suspected. In bat-associated cases of human rabies reported since 1980, at least 17 out of the 21 cases reported no bite, and several of those cases reported no contact (137). Domesticated animals such as dogs and cats may carry rabies, but the incidence varies by region. Therefore, determining the need for postexposure prophylaxis may require assistance from state health department resources, particularly in light of the recent vaccine shortage. Fatalities from human rabies have averaged three cases per year for the last 10 years, with the majority of cases related to bat exposure (136) (Table 24.7).

TREATMENT

Rabies vaccine is available as human diploid cell vaccine (Imovax), rabies vaccine adsorbed (RVA), and purified chick embryo cell-derived vaccine (PCEC). It is important to note that there are dosing and administration route differences for pre- and postexposure prophylaxis. Intradermal injections should **not** be used for postexposure prophylaxis (138). The postexposure treatment schedule consists of 1-mL IM vaccinations on days 0, 3, 7, and 14 (137,138). Injection site should be the deltoid muscle in children and adults; infants may require injection in the midlateral aspect of the thigh (138). Side effects occur in 5% to 40% of recipients and include pain and erythema at the injection site, headache, nausea, muscle ache, and dizziness (138).

RIG provides immediate passive immunity to protect the patient until active immunity is conferred from the vaccine. The immune globulin is dosed at 20 units per kg IM × 1 dose ideally within 72 hours of the bite/wound (139). However, the incubation of human rabies has been reported at more than 1 year, so postexposure presentation should be treated with RIG as well as the vaccine, no matter the length of delay in seeking treatment (137). One-half of the dose should be used to infiltrate the wound (if present), and the remainder is given intramuscularly in the opposite arm from the vaccine. Side effects include local muscle soreness and tenderness at the injection site (139). Individuals who have been previously immunized against rabies should not receive RIG as part of the postexposure treatment because it may interfere with the vaccine efficacy in these individuals (137,139).

Antibiotics are not indicated in every animal bite/wound but are strongly encouraged where there is an increased risk of infection. Cat bites are particularly prone to infection (30% to 40%) due to the deep-puncture wounds inflicted (140). Treatment of choice for cat bites includes a β-lactamase–resistant antibiotics to cover *Pasturella multocida* and *S. aureus*. Commonly, amoxicillin–clavulanic acid is used as first-line therapy because there is a high failure rate for cephalexin against *P. multocida* (140,141). Dog bites have an infection rate of about 15% to 20% and do not generally require prophylactic treatment unless severe crush injury exists or there is bone, joint, tendon, or ligament involvement (140). Immunocompromised patients, patients prone to infectious endocarditis, and highly contaminated wounds are indications for prophylactic antibiotic therapy (113,140).

Human bites in children are usually minor, often inflicted by another child. However, human bites to an area that is not well vascularized such as the hand are highly prone to infection and should be considered for antibiotic prophylaxis (113). Staphylococcal and streptococcal species in addition to oral anaerobes are the focus of antimicrobial coverage for human bites requiring prophylaxis. A β-lactamase–resistant antibiotic such as amoxicillin–clavulanic acid is usually the treatment of choice (141). For penicillin-allergic patients, clindamycin can be used in combination with trimethoprim/sulfamethoxazole.

RESPIRATORY DISTRESS SYNDROMES

STATUS ASTHMATICUS

Status asthmaticus is an acute severe asthma exacerbation requiring emergency treatment. Patients present with significant wheezing, increased work of breathing, and progressive respiratory failure. All attempts to avoid intubation and mechanical ventilation are undertaken, as positive-pressure ventilation will only worsen the underlying hyperinflation of the lungs (142,143). Therefore, many pharmacologic agents are utilized in the treatment of a patient in status asthmaticus in an effort to avoid intubation.

Treatment

Inhaled β_2-adrenergic agonists, generally in the form of inhaled albuterol, are first-line bronchodilating agents in acute asthma exacerbations. Albuterol exhibits significant activity within 15 minutes of inhalation, with no demonstrable difference in efficacy between nebulization or metered dose inhaler with spacer administration (144,145). Initial dosing in status asthmaticus of the undiluted albuterol (0.5%) solution is 0.03 mL per kg (0.15 mg per kg) to a maximum of 1 mL per dose for three doses or 6 to 10 puffs (90 μg spray) with spacer. For patients presenting with acute asthma exacerbations, common regimens consist of three back-to-back treatments together with ipratropium. Continuous nebulized albuterol dosed at 0.5 mg per kg per hour is sometimes required in status asthmaticus and has been shown to result in rapid improvement in select patients (146). The main adverse effect of albuterol treatment is tachycardia from stimulation of β_1-receptors in the heart. Tremors, hypokalemia, and hyperglycemia can also occur (146). Levalbuterol, the R-isomer of albuterol, has not been shown to be more effective in children with status asthmaticus (142,146). Long-acting β-agonists have no role in status asthmaticus and have resulted in fatalities when used for this indication.

Additional bronchodilation is achieved by adding ipratropium, an anticholinergic agent, to albuterol. Ipratropium antagonizes the muscarinic receptors in the airway, decreasing parasympathetic tone by blocking further release of acetylcholine and producing resistance to bronchoconstriction (142,147). By using ipratropium together with albuterol, prolongation of the bronchodilation can be achieved (142). A review of the literature demonstrates a reduction in hospital admissions for children with acute asthma exacerbations receiving multiple-dose ipratropium in addition to standard β_2-agonists and corticosteroids (148). The dose of ipratropium is 0.25 to 0.5 mg inhaled, and it has an onset of 1 to 3 minutes and a duration of action of up to 4 to 6 hours. Clinically significant side effects of ipratropium are rare (148).

Terbutaline, an injectable selective β_2-receptor agonist, has been used successfully in status asthmaticus (142,149). Although not approved by the FDA for status asthmaticus, terbutaline is used by many centers as a continuous intravenous infusion for continued bronchodilation when decreased airflow reduces the amount of nebulized albuterol actually reaching the alveoli. Dosing usually begins with a bolus of 5 to 10 μg per kg given either subcutaneously or intravenously. If response is not adequate, a continuous infusion of 0.05 to 0.1 μg per kg per minute is begun, titrated to a maximum of 10 μg per kg per minute (142,149). Tachycardia is the most common dose-limiting adverse effect. Hypotension generally occurs between 0.4 and 2 μg per kg per minute, disappearing at doses more than 2 μg per kg per minute, perhaps due to downregulation of the β_2-receptors with higher doses (149). Cardiac arrhythmias and seizures are possible although rare. Increased troponin and creatine phosphokinase (CPK) serum levels have been reported, although one study failed to find a relationship between CPK-myocardial band and the dose of terbutaline used (149). Additive β-agonist doses (albuterol and terbutaline) as high as 40 to 45 mg per hour have been used, although most patients will not tolerate more than 20 mg per hour.

Corticosteroids are additional first-line agents in the treatment of asthma exacerbation and exert their effect primarily on the inflammatory response. Several mechanisms, including decreased cytokine and eicosanoid production; reduced accumulation of eosinophils, basophils, and leukocytes in lung tissue; and decreased vascular permeability, contribute to the usefulness of corticosteroids in asthma (147). Systemic administration is preferred for acute asthma exacerbations. Oral prednisone/prednisolone is generally dosed at 2 mg per kg initially, followed by oral prednisone/prednisolone at 2 mg per kg per day divided every 12 hours. For patients who cannot tolerate oral therapy, intravenous methylprednisolone dosed at 2 mg per kg or intravenous dexamethasone dosed at 0.4 mg per kg can be given for the bolus dose. Oral prednisone is available in tablets and solution, although the solution is unpalatable (it can be substituted with oral prednisolone). Recent formulations of oral prednisolone have attempted to improve the palatability of steroid therapy for children, including orally disintegrating tablets (143). Relatively few adverse side effects occur with short-course steroids given for asthma exacerbations; these include GI disturbances, mood changes, and serum electrolyte alterations.

Intramuscular epinephrine is an effective bronchodilator (see discussion of anaphylaxis) but has become less frequently used secondary to cardiac side effects (142). However, it is still used as a first-line agent in children with status asthmaticus who are not moving air.

Magnesium sulfate has bronchodilator effects, presumably secondary to smooth muscle relaxation due to the inhibition of calcium uptake (142). Intravenous magnesium sulfate dosed at 25 to 50 mg per kg (max 2 g) given over 20 minutes has been shown to improve pulmonary function in children with status asthmaticus (144). Toxicity should be monitored by continuous electrocardiograph and assessment of reflexes. Common, less serious side effects include hypotension, flushing, and nausea.

CROUP

Laryngotracheobronchitis, commonly known as croup, is a viral infection frequently seen in the ED. Patients with croup are generally younger than 3 years and present with upper airway stridor, a barking cough, and hypoxia at rest (145). The primary causative agent is the parainfluenza virus (146).

Treatment

First-line therapy for croup has traditionally been inhaled racemic epinephrine, although this agent does not appear to affect outcome (146–148). The goal is to reduce airway obstruction by relaxing the bronchial muscles via β_2-receptor activation. When given by inhalation, racemic epinephrine is largely confined to the airways, although in large doses systemic absorption and resulting cardiac arrhythmias may occur (4). The peak effect occurs approximately 30 minutes after inhalation and the duration is 120 minutes (150). L-Epinephrine can be used in place of racemic epinephrine at an equivalent dose; racemic epinephrine 10 mg = L-epinephrine 5 mg.

Corticosteroid therapy, primarily in the form of dexamethasone, has been shown to lessen the severity and duration of croup (146,150). Oral and parenteral dexamethasone are equally efficacious and are dosed at 0.6 mg per kg IM/PO to a maximum of 10 mg per dose (150). Side effects may include irritability, hypertension, and headache.

Inhaled budesonide has shown to be as effective as oral or IM dexamethasone (143,144). Inhaled budesonide has demonstrated favorable results in decreasing hospital admission rates in children with croup (143). The dose is 1 mg inhaled followed by another 1 mg dose in 30 minutes. Beneficial effects for both dexamethasone and inhaled budesonide were seen as early as 1 hour after treatment (144). Adverse effects including respiratory infections, headache, and otitis media are reported as being similar to placebo (143). Further studies are needed to define the role of inhaled budesonide with or without systemic dexamethasone for the treatment of croup.

BRONCHIOLITIS

Bronchiolitis is inflammation of the lower airways and occurs primarily in children younger than two years (150). Primary manifestations include fever, coryza, wheezing, and respiratory distress (150). Apnea, lethargy, and irritability are common in young infants with this infection (151). Viral etiologies are often causative, especially RSV during the winter and early spring (152). Although diagnostic, laboratory testing for RSV does not add to the management plan and has been discouraged for routine use (153). With the availability of RSV immune globulin such as RSV-IG (Respigam) and a monoclonal antibody preparation, palivizumab (Synagis), high-risk patients can receive preventative treatment for RSV infection.

Treatment

The initial management of bronchiolitis is supportive, with a focus on the ABCs (154). Corticosteroids and antibiotics have shown no benefit in RSV bronchiolitis and are not indicated (150,151,155–157).

Bronchiolitis is characterized by airway edema and generally does not have a bronchospastic component (152). Bronchodilators such as albuterol are of limited benefit in bronchiolitis and are not routinely recommended. They may even cause hypoxia in some infants (152,154,156,158). However, when the distinction between reactive airway disease and bronchiolitis is difficult, a select group of infants may have a salutary response, and albuterol should be given to them (156,159). As in croup, racemic epinephrine appears to offer benefit in bronchiolitis, decreasing respiratory rate and pulmonary resistance (150). Ipratropium, an anticholinergic agent with bronchodilatory effects, has been investigated as a potential treatment option in bronchiolitis. Although ipratropium reduced the work of breathing, there was no effect on outcome (160).

Ribavirin has largely fallen out of favor as a treatment for RSV bronchiolitis. An antiviral agent given as an inhalation treatment, ribavirin carries theoretical risks of teratogenicity to pregnant health care workers (156). Studies have shown a benefit of ribavirin therapy for children with underlying bronchopulmonary disease, congenital heart disease, or immunodeficiency with RSV infection. However, in light of the preventive and potential treatment measures available with RSV-IG and pavilizumab, ribavirin is rarely used.

SEXUAL ASSAULT

There are several pharmacologic interventions to consider for a patient who has been sexually assaulted. Important variables include the age of the victim and whether the assailant was known to the victim, so that the risk for HIV transmission can be assessed.

TREATMENT

Prevention of sexually transmitted disease is the goal of antimicrobial therapy in the postsexual assault victim. Chlamydia, caused by *Chlamydia trachomatis,* can be effectively treated with azithromycin dosed at 1 g PO × 1 dose or alternatively with doxycycline 100 mg PO twice daily for 7 days (161). Resistance to *C. trachomatis* is rare, and resistant strains still respond to treatment with a macrolide (36).

Neisseria gonorrhoeae can be treated with a single dose of cefixime 400 mg PO or alternatively with ceftriaxone 250 mg IM × 1 dose (162). Fluoroquinolone resistance is becoming more prevalent in the United States and in some Asian countries and therefore ciprofloxacin and other fluoroquinolones are no longer recommended for treatment of gonorrhea (161). Although azithromycin has been shown to be effective in treating gonorrhea as well as chlamydia, the required higher dose of 2 g PO × 1 dose is highly emetogenic and also expensive (161). Therefore, current recommendations for treating gonorrhea do not include azithromycin.

Metronidazole is added for coverage of anaerobes, particularly to prevent bacterial vaginosis caused by *Trichomonas vaginalis* (161). Mechanism of action results from the activation of the prodrug form by the anaerobic transfer of electrons. The resultant radical selectively targets the organism DNA and other biomolecules (163). The dose is 2 g PO × 1, and common side effects include metallic taste, GI disturbances, and disulfiram reaction if combined with alcohol.

Pelvic inflammatory disease (PID) may occur in patients who delay seeking treatment for sexual assault. For both chlamydia and gonorrhea associated with PID, longer duration of therapy and higher doses are required for treatment. Recommendations for chlamydia treatment include doxycycline 100 mg PO twice daily for 14 days; gonorrhea should be treated with ceftriaxone 250 mg IM × 1 dose when associated with PID (161).

Hepatitis B prophylaxis should be considered if the patient has not been previously immunized. The initial immunization with hepatitis B vaccine 1 mL (10 μg per mL formulation) IM is given at the acute visit, with follow-up vaccinations at 1 and 6 months (164). Hepatitis B immune globulin is reserved for victims exposed within 14 days with a high-risk exposure (164).

Postexposure prophylaxis for HIV infection is not uniformly applied, and guidelines for exposure in the nonoccupational setting have not been established (153,165, 166). Often, postexposure prophylaxis is offered based on risk assessment of exposure (166,167). The estimated risk of HIV transmission is thought to be low but not zero (166). Recommendations include the antiretrovirals. Preferred regimens include efavirenz and lamivudine or emtricitabine with zidovudine or tenofovir (as a nonnucleoside-based regimen) and lopinavir/ritonavir (Kaletra®) and zidovudine with either lamivudine (Combivir®) or emtricitabine for patients presenting within 72 hours of exposure (164,166). Efavirenz is a nonnucleoside reverse transcriptase inhibitor that blocks RNA and DNA polymerases, inhibiting replication. Zidovudine is a nucleoside reverse transcriptase inhibitor (NRTI) thymidine analogue and becomes incorporated into the viral DNA, thereby inhibiting synthesis (168). Common side effects include headache, dizziness, GI disturbances, leukopenia, anemia, myalgias, and hepatic dysfunction. Lamivudine is an NRTI pyrimidine analogue and competes for incorporation into viral DNA; like zidovudine, it inhibits further synthesis (168). Side effects are less common with lamivudine and include headache, psychomotor disturbances, GI disturbances, myalgias, and pancreatitis. Combivir is a combination product containing both zidovudine and lamivudine. Lopinavir is a combination of emcitrabine and tenofovir (a reverse transcriptase inhibitor). A protease inhibitor such as indinavir, nelfinavir, or a combination such as lopinavir/ritonavir (Kaletra®) should be added for high-risk exposures. Protease inhibitors bind reversibly to the active site of the HIV protease, inhibiting further viral cleavage and maturation (168). Side effects include GI disturbances and electrolyte and lipid abnormalities. Twice-daily regimens should be prescribed to improve compliance; postexposure prophylaxis should be given within 1 hour of exposure if possible (165).

Emergency contraception prophylaxis may also be indicated after sexual assault. The preferred treatment is levonorgestrel (Plan B) 0.75 μg PO every 12 hours × 2 doses (169,170). The WHO recommends administration of both levonorgestrel tablets at one dose, improving compliance without an increase in emesis or decrease in efficacy. Levonorgestrel prevents the implantation or fertilization of the ovum by altering tubule transport (171). Pregnancy prophylaxis is thought to be effective for at least 72 hours after unprotected intercourse (169,172). Although efficacy decreases proportionally with increasing time, studies have suggested that protection from pregnancy remains even when the dose is administered up to 5 days postevent (173). Prior to the introduction of levonorgestrel, high-dose estrogen (Yuzpe method) was commonly used (174). High-dose estrogen was provided with ethinyl estradiol 50 μg (two tablets, Ovral) orally, given immediately and then repeated after 12 hours (173). The Yuzpe regimen was considered effective in reducing the risk of pregnancy by 60% to 90%, although associated with a significant (up to 20%) risk of emesis (164,169,170). Levonorgestrel has been demonstrated to be more effective (crude pregnancy rate 1.1% vs. 3.2% in the Yuzpe regimen group) and cause fewer side effects than high-dose estrogen (nausea 23.1% vs. 50.5%, vomiting 5.6% vs. 18.8%, respectively) (169). Side effects of levonorgestrel therapy include nausea, abdominal pain, alteration in menstrual bleeding, fatigue, and headache (171). No known contraindications exist to hormonal emergency contraception, except allergy to estrogens (173) (Table 24.8).

STATUS EPILEPTICUS

Status epilepticus is defined as any seizure activity lasting for more than 30 minutes without return to baseline mental status, more than 5 minutes of continuous convulsive seizures, or three discrete seizures within 1 hour (175). All seizure types can present "in status," and therefore not all patients will have generalized tonic–clonic movements. Persistent confusion and inability to perform tasks or engage in conversation can represent continual complex partial seizures, also termed "nonconvulsive SE" (176). Absence of SE is characterized by continued staring or blinking (176). *Epilepsia partialis continua* is the term used to describe focal motor SE (175). With this disorder, patients can have continued movement of an extremity for years (176).

There are many potential causes of SE including electrolyte abnormalities such as hypo/hyperphosphatemia and hypo/hypercalcemia, toxin exposures, CNS infection, underlying epilepsy, and trauma (177). Seizures lasting longer than 20 to 30 minutes are associated with cerebral edema and permanent focal damage (175,178). The longer the seizure continues, the more refractory to treatment it becomes, with overall mortality approaching 30% (175). Terminating seizure activity and correcting any underlying disorder is therefore the primary goal of therapy.

TREATMENT

Benzodiazepines are the first-line medications used for the treatment of SE (175,178). Seizure activity is halted when

TABLE 24.8 Postexposure Prophylaxis for Sexual Assault

Chlamydia *Chlamydia trachomatis*	Azithromycin 1 g p.o. × 1 dose or Doxycycline 100 mg p.o. b.i.d. × 7 d
Gonorrhea *Neisseria gonorrhoeae*	Cefixime 400 mg p.o. × 1 dose or Ceftriaxone 125 mg i.m. × 1 dose or Ciprofloxacin 500 mg p.o. × 1 dose
Trichomoniasis *Trichomonas vaginalis*	Metronidazole 2 g p.o. × 1 dose
Hepatitis B	Hepatitis B vaccine 1 mL i.m. × 1 dose In high-risk situations: Hepatitis B immune globulin 0.06 mL (max 5 mL) i.m. × 1 dose
HIV (<13 yr old)	Zidovudine 180 mg/m^2/dose p.o. b.i.d. (max 300 mg/dose) plus Lamivudine 4 mg/kg/dose p.o. b.i.d. (max 150 mg/dose) In high-risk situations add: Indinavir 500 mg/m^2/dose p.o. every 8 hr (max 800 mg/dose) or Nelfinavir 20–30 mg/kg/dose p.o. t.i.d. (max 750 mg/dose)
HIV (>13 yr old)	Zidovudine/lamivudine (Combivir) 1 tablet p.o. b.i.d. In high-risk situations add: Indinavir 800 mg p.o. every 8 hr or Nelfinavir 1,250 mg p.o. b.i.d.
Pregnancy	Levonorgestrel 0.75 μg p.o. × 1 dose immediately, then repeat 0.75 μg p.o. 12 hr later

p.o., oral; i.m., intramuscular; b.i.d., twice daily; t.i.d., three times daily.
Adapted from Weinberg GA. Postexposure prophylaxis against human immunodeficiency virus infection after sexual assault. *Pediatr Infect Dis J* 202;21:959–60; and Petter LM, Whitehall DL. Management of female sexual assault. *Am Fam Physicians* 1998;58(4):920–26.

the drug binds to the benzodiazepine site on the GABA-receptor complex in the brain. Benzodiazepines enhance the activity of GABA, the major inhibitory transmitter in the CNS (179,180). Injectable preparations of lorazepam, diazepam, and midazolam are available. The parenteral benzodiazepine of choice is usually lorazepam due to a rapid onset of 2 to 5 minutes and a duration of 6 to 8 hours (180). The dose of intravenous lorazepam is 0.1 mg per kg to a maximum of 4 mg per dose. Diazepam injection can also be used for SE and has a faster onset (1 to 3 minutes) than lorazepam secondary to increased lipophilicity and the ability to penetrate the BBB rapidly. However, the increased lipophilicity also leads to a shorter duration of action for diazepam (175). Midazolam can be used; however, the short duration of action limits the utility of use during SE, except initial IM dose prior to obtaining IV access or as a continuous infusion. Diazepam injection can also be given successfully per rectum if intravenous access is not possible. The dose of diazepam injection is 0.5 mg per kg when given rectally to a maximum of 20 mg per dose (175). A gel formulation of diazepam (Diastat) is available for home management of seizures but has not been shown to be superior to the rectal administration of diazepam injection. Side effects include excessive sedation and respiratory depression.

Phenytoin has traditionally been the second-line agent used in SE if benzodiazepine therapy is not successful (175,178,180). Fosphenytoin, a prodrug of phenytoin, is now preferred in pediatric patients (181). A more water-soluble drug than phenytoin, fosphenytoin does not contain propylene glycol as a diluent (182). This allows a more rapid intravenous administration of fosphenytoin with less concern for cardiac dysrhythmias and cardiovascular collapse (178,181). Fosphenytoin can also be given via the intramuscular route if intravenous access is not obtainable (178,182). Although dosed the same as phenytoin at 15 to 20 mg per kg, it is important to designate the dose in terms of phenytoin equivalents (PEs) when using fosphenytoin. There have been reports of medication errors when the salt weight of fosphenytoin was used to calculate the dose (183).

The mechanism of action of fosphenytoin is the same as that of phenytoin. Stabilization of the neuronal membranes by blockage of the sodium-dependent voltage channels during depolarization results in cessation of seizure activity (182). Side effects of fosphenytoin include hypotension during infusion, which can be ameliorated by slowing the infusion rate. Fosphenytoin should not be infused faster than 3 mg PE per kg per minute to a max of 150 mg PE per minute (182). Intense pruritus in the perianal region is unique to fosphenytoin and may be secondary to the release and deposition of phosphate during conversion to phenytoin (178). Other side effects are similar to those seen with phenytoin and include nystagmus, ataxia, drowsiness, and hypersensitivity. Because the drug is highly protein bound, unbound concentrations can be higher than expected if hypoalbuminemia is present and may result in toxicity.

Third-line agents for SE include phenobarbital, valproic acid, and levetiracetam. Phenobarbital is a barbiturate used to depress the activity in the CNS by binding to the barbiturate receptor on the GABA complex (105). As with benzodiazepines, modulating GABA activity, the primary inhibitory neurotransmitter in the CNS, halts seizure activity in the majority of patients. The loading dose in SE is generally 20 mg per kg IV given slowly at a rate no faster than 1 mg per kg per minute to a max of 30 mg per minute in children and 60 mg per minute in adults weighing more than 60 kg. Phenobarbital can be repeated to a cumulative maximum of 30 mg per kg. At high doses, respiratory depression is expected, and intubating equipment and supplies must be readily available.

Some experts recommend using valproic acid injection as a third-line alternative in SE, especially in situations in which the patient is allergic or refractory to phenytoin and/or phenobarbital (184,185). Valproic acid acts on both sodium channel recovery time and the GABA receptor, either by increasing the activity of GABA in the brain or by binding directly to the site (105). The loading dose is 20 to 30 mg per kg IV and is given at a rate no faster than 5 mg per kg per minute (186). Although valproic acid is not recommended in patients younger than 2 years due to the increased risk of hepatotoxicity, some case reports document successful cessation of refractory SE in patients younger than 24 months (185,187). Acute side effects include somnolence, ataxia, nausea, and vomiting.

Levetiracetam recently became available as an intravenous preparation, increasing interest in its use for SE (188,189). The exact mechanism of action is unknown, although it has been demonstrated to inhibit burst firing without altering normal neuronal functioning. Levetiracetam is minimally metabolized and primarily eliminated by the kidney, necessitating dose reduction in renal insufficiency. Dosing during SE is still undetermined, but many experts recommend 30 mg per kg as the initial loading dose. Ataxia and mood changes are the most common side effects, with reports of increased suicidality in patients taking levetiracetam as maintenance therapy.

For SE refractory to the foregoing interventions, continuous infusions of short-acting barbiturates, such as pentobarbital, or a benzodiazepine, such as midazolam, may be necessary (175). Pentobarbital continuous infusions commonly result in significant hypotension, often requiring vasopressor support. Propofol infusions have also been used with success (188); however, increased mortality in pediatric patients receiving long-term propofol infusions has been reported (189). Intubation and intensive care monitoring will be necessary for patients requiring continuous infusions.

SHOCK

Shock may follow trauma and can be secondary to blood loss and/or hypovolemia, sepsis, anaphylaxis, cardiogenic etiologies, or traumatic spinal cord injury. The definition of shock includes an inadequate perfusion of tissues and is usually associated with hypotension and, if left untreated, multisystem organ failure (16). Primary therapy of shock begins with fluid resuscitation. Vasopressor infusions are instituted in cases of severe hypotension refractory to fluid resuscitation.

TREATMENT OF SHOCK

Fluid resuscitation is accomplished initially with crystalloid infusions such as normal saline or lactated Ringer's solution. Initial bolus is given at 20 to 30 mL per kg and repeated up to two times (usual total max of 60 mL per kg) if no effect is seen. At this time, colloid infusions should be considered and may include albumin and/or blood.

Vasopressor therapy is instituted if fluid resuscitation alone is not adequate to maintain the patient's blood pressure. Dopamine, dobutamine, epinephrine, norepinephrine, and vasopressin are all used for their action on the cardiovascular system. Each has slightly different properties and side effects. It is important to obtain central access as soon as possible once the decision is made to begin vasopressor therapy. Although central access should not delay the initiation of vasopressors, inadvertent infiltration of soft tissue with dopamine, epinephrine, vasopressin, and norepinephrine can cause significant local tissue damage and necrosis (190,191). Phentolamine, an α-receptor antagonist, should be available for inadvertent infiltrations and injected around the site of extravasation as soon as possible (190).

Dopamine is usually the first vasopressor begun in a patient who has persistent hypotension after adequate fluid resuscitation. A central neurotransmitter, dopamine activates adenylyl cyclase and thus increases cyclic AMP in cells (7). Dopamine acts on the α, β, and dopaminergic receptors in a dose-related response. Dopaminergic D_1-receptors are primarily affected at low doses of 1 to 5 μg per kg per minute (192). At this dose, renal perfusion is increased with minimal effect on the systemic circulation. This may also be secondary to an effect on the β_1-receptors, increasing cardiac output enough to improve circulation to the kidneys, thus improving urine output. At a dose of 5 to 10 μg per kg per minute, β_1-receptors are activated in the myocardium with resultant increase in cardiac output and stroke volume. When the dose is increased to 10 to 20 μg per kg per minute, dopamine activates the α_1-receptors in the peripheral vasculature, producing peripheral vasoconstriction and a rise in systemic blood pressure. For shock states, dopamine should be initiated at a dose that will support the patient's blood pressure. Therefore, a common starting dose is 10 μg per kg per minute and is titrated to effect. Nausea and vomiting, tachycardia, arrhythmias, and hypertension are adverse effects that can occur during dopamine infusions and are secondary to the sympathomimetic effects (7).

Dobutamine is structurally related to dopamine and acts on the α- and β-adrenergic receptors, although the clinical effect is primarily seen on the heart secondary to the increased inotropy (193). Dobutamine exists as a racemic mixture, with the (−) isomer exerting α_1-receptor agonism and the (+) isomer exerting α_1-receptor antagonism and potent β-receptor agonism (7). Peripheral resistance is not greatly affected due to counterbalancing of the α_1-mediated vasoconstriction and β_2-mediated vasodilation (7). Dobutamine is frequently chosen for patients requiring greater inotropic support. In addition, dobutamine may be added to vasoconstrictor therapy such as epinephrine following volume resuscitation (16). The dose must be individually titrated; usual range is 5 to 20 μg per kg per minute (193). Side effects may include severe hypertension, myocardial ischemia, tachycardia, and arrhythmias.

Epinephrine is a potent stimulant of both α- and β-adrenergic receptors (7,16). Dose-related clinical effects include increased blood pressure and increased cardiac output. Blood pressure increases secondary to vasoconstriction by α_1-receptor activation in the systemic vasculature (7). In addition, β_1-receptor activation in the myocardial tissue increases inotropy and chronotropy (7). Small doses may produce vasodilation secondary to the greater sensitivity of the β_2-receptors over the α-receptors (7). Use in pediatric shock is reserved for severe hypotension unresponsive to fluid resuscitation and dopamine. The dose range is generally 0.1 to 1 μg per kg per minute. Adverse effects include tachycardia, arrhythmias, myocardial infarction, and severe hypertension especially in patients receiving β-blocking therapies.

Norepinephrine is structurally related to epinephrine, although the primary action is on the α-receptors, with little effect on β-receptors (7). Peripheral resistance is significantly increased without an increase in cardiac output. Norepinephrine is usually the drug of choice in septic or neurogenic shock with fluid-unresponsive severe hypotension (192). Severe hypertension and ischemia are the principal adverse reactions.

Vasopressin has been used with success as an adjuvant agent in adults with vasodilatory shock (194). It has been demonstrated that patients in prolonged shock have substantially decreased plasma vasopressin levels (194). A potent vasoconstrictor, vasopressin activates the V_1-receptors in the vascular smooth muscle (194,195). When added to patients receiving catecholamine infusions, vasopressin allowed for the reduction in the catecholamine doses and increased systemic vascular resistance and urine output (194). With large doses, vasopressin decreases cardiac output and heart rate as well as decreasing coronary blood flow. Vasopressin may find a place in the treatment of pediatric shock requiring high-dose catecholamines to avoid toxicity, but it is still is controversial and requires more study (16,196,197). Adverse effects include myocardial infarction, arrhythmias, water intoxication, anaphylaxis, and severe hypertension.

MULTIPLE TRAUMA

Trauma is the leading cause of death in children and adolescents (198). Time to treatment has the greatest impact on morbidity and mortality. The overwhelming majority of injuries (approximately 90%) presenting to the pediatric ED are minor (199). Approximately 10% to 15% of children presenting to the ED with significant trauma are at risk of dying from their injuries (200). It is estimated that one out of six hospitalizations in children aged 10 to 14 years are related to traumatic injuries (201). As with all other presentations to the ED, attention to the ABCs is paramount. Establishing a patent airway and obtaining vascular access are primary goals. See discussion on rapid sequence intubation for intubating medications. Vascular access utilizing large-caliber, short catheters are preferred for rapid fluid resuscitation (198). If vascular access cannot be obtained after two to three attempts, an intraosseous (IO) needle should be placed into the bone. All medications and fluids can be administered via this route.

TREATMENT OF MULTIPLE TRAUMATIC INJURIES

Patients with multiple traumatic injuries will likely require pain management and sedation (see "Procedural Sedation" and "Pain" sections). Care must be taken not to compound hypotension in the presence of hemorrhage or shock. Fentanyl is often the drug of choice for pain management due to the relative absence of effects on hemodynamic status (86). Antibiotics are usually given for prophylaxis of open wounds and should include staphylococcal and streptococcal coverage. If the wounds involve the abdomen, gram-negative and anaerobic coverage is necessary (201). Tetanus immunization status should be assessed.

CLOSED HEAD INJURY

Closed head injury with elevated ICP presents a challenge for initial emergency management. As ICP increases, a subsequent decrease in cerebral perfusion occurs. With decreased perfusion, the brain does not receive necessary oxygen and ischemia with cell death occurs, resulting in further edema (200). Without initial intracranial monitoring, the degree of elevation is unknown; suspected intracranial hypertension must be managed in all cases with suggestive clinical manifestation.

Treatment

Initial therapy involves oxygen and fluid resuscitation to ensure adequate cardiac output and perfusion of the brain (200). Treatment of elevated ICP may include mild hyperventilation (PCO_2 30 to 35 torr), lidocaine, mannitol, furosemide, barbiturates (pentobarbital), benzodiazepines, and/or propofol. Mannitol is commonly the first pharmacotherapeutic intervention used to decrease ICP (196). Mannitol is an osmotic diuretic and rapidly decreases ICP by creating a concentration gradient across the BBB (197). Duration of reduction in ICP is dose related and ranges from 2 to 4 hours. Dosing begins with a 1 g per kg load IV and is commonly followed by 0.25 g per kg per dose IV every 4 hours, based on serum osmolality (goal 300 to 330 mOsm per L). Mannitol crystallizes at room temperature and must be filtered prior to administration. Side effects of mannitol include fluid and electrolyte imbalance, acidosis, and hypo/hypertension. Mannitol should not be used in patients with hypotension.

By blunting ICP spikes caused by noxious stimuli such as endotracheal intubation or suctioning, lidocaine is the second medication usually chosen. Lidocaine injection is given at a dose of 1 to 1.5 mg per kg and will reduce ICP without affecting mean arterial pressure.

Pentobarbital is initiated if ICP continues to be elevated despite hyperventilation and mannitol therapy (196). Dosing usually begins with 5 mg per kg IV bolus and subsequent continuous infusion of 1 to 4 mg per kg per hour, titrated to burst suppression of ICP spikes (200).

SPINAL CORD INJURY

Spinal cord injury, resulting in neurologic deficits and sometimes paralysis, is an area of ongoing research. Spinal cord injury without radiologic abnormality may occur in pediatric cervical and thoracic spine injuries (200). These injuries can present with transient neurologic deficits and may be followed by severe deficits several hours after the injury.

Treatment

Protocols may still exist at some institutions outlining the use of high-dose intravenous methylprednisolone for blunt spinal cord injury despite significant debate on the effectiveness of this therapy (200,202–207). The presumed mechanism of action centers around inhibition of membrane lipid breakdown at the site of injury, although it has been suggested that the steroid may act through other mechanisms, including increasing blood flow through the spinal cord and inflammatory modulation (206,207).

Cord injuries can result in neurogenic shock, characterized by profound hypotension, bradycardia, hypothermia, and peripheral vasodilation (195). Treatment consists of fluid resuscitation to restore volume and vasopressor therapy, primarily norepinephrine (see the "Shock" section).

RAPID SEQUENCE INTUBATION

Rapid sequence intubation (RSI) is frequently utilized in emergency care of children who are unable to maintain a patent airway (208). Medications used for RSI include a combination of premedications, sedatives, and neuromuscular blockading agents given concurrently to achieve a loss of consciousness and paralysis, providing ideal intubating conditions. The agents of choice depend on the presentation and age of the patient. This method of intubating pediatric patients in an emergency setting has been shown to be effective with minimal side effects (208,209). Patients presenting in full cardiopulmonary arrest are intubated immediately without medication (210).

Atropine may be considered as a premedication for all patients younger than 7 years who require intubation. Recently, some studies have reported that atropine may not be as useful in preventing bradycardia induced during RSI as previously thought (211,212). The vagolytic properties of atropine may mitigate the effects of vagal stimulation on the heart rate secondary to endotracheal tube placement (212). This is particularly important in young children, who can demonstrate significant bradycardia with vagal stimulation. Dosing of atropine is 0.02 mg per kg to a maximum dose of 0.5 mg. The minimum dose should not be lower than 0.1 mg because doses less than this may cause paradoxical bradycardia.

Lidocaine is another pretreatment consideration, primarily in patients presenting with head trauma who require intubation. Because endotracheal intubation is a noxious stimulus and results in unwanted increases in ICP, lidocaine is a useful premedication (101,213). By providing peripheral anesthesia of cough receptors and stabilizing cerebral cell membranes via blockage of sodium channels, a dose of 1 to 2 mg per kg IV of lidocaine can successfully mitigate rises in ICP during endotracheal intubation (101,213).

Etomidate is an ultra-short-acting, nonbarbiturate hypnotic that anesthetizes the patient within 30 seconds. Duration of action ranges from 4 to 8 minutes (102,214). Etomidate is especially useful in hypotensive patients, as minimal decreases in blood pressure are seen following administration (101,102,215). Pain on injection likely due to the propylene glycol solvent and involuntary muscle movements are common side effects (216). If used in nonhypotensive patients, pretreatment with low-dose fentanyl (1 to 2 μg per kg IV) may be protective against the hypertensive effect produced by sympathetic stimulation during intubation, since etomidate does not have analgesic properties (217). Long-term administration of etomidate in the intensive care unit setting has been associated with decreased adrenal function and increased mortality (218). Clinically significant depressions in serum cortisol have not been demonstrated with single injections of etomidate for pediatric RSI (219). Etomidate dosing for RSI is 0.3 mg per kg IV for children. Although indicated for children older than 10 years, it has been successfully used in younger patients (214,219). Additional adverse effects include small increases in heart rate, nausea, and vomiting.

Sodium thiopental is a barbiturate useful for RSI, particularly in patients with head trauma or SE, who are not hypotensive. Barbiturates bind to the GABA receptor and produce depression of the reticular activating system, resulting in anesthesia (101,102). ICP may be increased secondary to the intracranial process, and therefore an agent such as sodium thiopental that does not increase ICP and may in fact decrease ICP through cerebral vasoconstriction is desirable. Sodium thiopental is a very short acting barbiturate, with high lipid solubility, resulting in an onset of 10 to 30 seconds and a duration of 5 to 8 minutes (101,102). Higher dosing is required in neonates and infants at 5 to 8 mg per kg IV compared with that in older children at 3 to 5 mg per kg IV. Doses should be reduced by 10% to 50% if given concomitantly with benzodiazepines, opioids, or α_2-receptor agonists (102). It is important to note that the barbiturates can cause significant vasodilation and hypotension and therefore should not be used in patients with hypovolemia or hypotension. Other adverse effects include respiratory depression, precipitation of acute porphyria, and rare hypersensitivity reactions.

Another common medication combination used for endotracheal intubation is midazolam and fentanyl. Midazolam provides sedation, and fentanyl can effectively block the increase in blood pressure associated with endotracheal intubation at a dose of 1.5 to 3 μg per kg IV $\times$ 1 dose (101). Fentanyl should not be administered rapidly due to the risk of chest wall rigidity and apnea. See discussion of midazolam and fentanyl in the "Procedural Sedation" section.

Ketamine is the agent of choice for the intubation of a patient in status asthmaticus (103,212,220). Ketamine is a phencyclidine derivative and may block *N*-methyl-D-aspartic acid receptors that mediate airway tone (101,221). It is also a potent bronchodilator and provides adrenergic stimulation due to blockade of norepinephrine reuptake and may inhibit vagal outflow (220). By increasing secretions, ketamine may also improve the pulmonary toilet and decrease mucus plugging in children with asthma. The intubating dose of ketamine is 1 to 2 mg per kg given intravenously. Onset of action occurs within 60 seconds and duration of action is 10 to 15 minutes. Adverse reactions can include emergence reactions, laryngospasm, hypertension, and increased ICP. Ketamine should not be used for RSI of patients with head trauma and/or elevated ICP, secondary to its ability to increase ICP (Table 24.9).

Neuromuscular blockading agents (NMBAs) that are effective for RSI must have a very short onset time. Three NMBAs are recommended for RSI in pediatrics. Succinylcholine, rocuronium, and high-dose vecuronium (0.3 mg per kg) are all useful agents, having onset times of less than 1 minute.

Composed of two acetylcholine molecules, succinylcholine is a depolarizing paralytic agent that opens the receptor channels on the motor end plate of skeletal muscle and remains in place, causing initial fasciculations and then ultimate skeletal muscle paralysis (222,223). Onset occurs within 60 seconds and duration of action is a maximum of 5 to 8 minutes due to hydrolysis by plasma cholinesterases (223). Succinylcholine is commonly dosed at 1 mg per kg IV, although infants younger than 1 year may require 2 mg per kg IV. Intramuscular administration is possible with succinylcholine and should be given at a dose of 3 to 4 mg per kg to a maximum of 150 mg (222).

Significant literature has been published on the risks of using succinylcholine in the pediatric population (224, 225). A black box warning issued by the FDA cautions against the use of succinylcholine in children due to the risk of rhabdomyolysis and hyperkalemia resulting in cardiac arrest (222). Contraindications include use in patients with a history of muscle disease and in patients in the acute phase of injury secondary to burns, multiple trauma, denervation of skeletal muscle, or upper motor neuron injury due to the risk of hyperkalemia (222). Despite the limitations, succinylcholine remains an important paralytic agent particularly in patients with difficult or anticipated difficult airways in the emergency setting (217,226). The ultra-short onset and duration of action enables the patient to regain respiratory control if the intubation attempt is unsuccessful. The short duration of action can be extremely useful in patients in whom a complete neurological examination is important for reassessing extension of injury and clinical status, particularly status posthead trauma.

Adverse events include prolonged paralysis in those with congenital absence of cholinesterases, malignant hyperthermia, masseter muscle spasm, and hyperkalemic cardiac arrest secondary to rapid release of potassium from the cells. Bradycardia can occur in children following repeat succinylcholine doses secondary to an acetylcholine-like effect the drug has on the cardiac postganglionic muscarinic receptors (101). Pretreatment with atropine may prevent bradycardia, although this remains controversial (227). Increased ICP following succinylcholine use in undersedated patients has been reported as a concern (205,225). Histamine release may occur with rapid administration of succinylcholine due to direct mast cell degranulation (222).

A defasciculating dose of a nondepolarizing paralytic such as pancuronium or vecuronium can be used to minimize the depolarization of the skeletal muscle following succinylcholine administration (223). The goal is to decrease muscle injury and therefore reduce the complications associated with succinylcholine, especially in children older than 5 years. The dose is 1/10 of the dose used for induction of paralysis given 1 to 3 minutes prior to succinylcholine. Some paralysis may occur at this dose and may require positive pressure ventilation until the succinylcholine is given.

Rocuronium is a short-acting, nondepolarizing paralytic agent and has been used successfully in pediatric patients for RSI (208). As a nondepolarizing paralytic, rocuronium competitively binds to the nicotinic acetylcholinergic receptor on the motor end plate of the skeletal muscle, inhibiting transmission of impulses (223,224). Rocuronium is an attractive alternative for pediatric RSI due to the relatively short onset of less than 60 seconds with a dose of 1.2 mg per kg and intermediate duration of 30 to 60 minutes (210). In addition, rocuronium can be given intramuscularly if intravenous access cannot be obtained.

TABLE 24.9 Indications and Medications for Rapid Sequence Intubation[a]

Nonhead trauma, normotensive
- Atropine if <7 yr old
- Thiopental
- Rocuronium

Head trauma/elevated ICP, normotensive
- Atropine if <7 yr old
- Lidocaine
- Thiopental
- Rocuronium

Head trauma/elevated ICP, hypotensive
- Atropine if <7 yr old
- Lidocaine
- Etomidate
- Rocuronium

Hypotension/hypovolemia
- Atropine if <7 yr old
- Etomidate (or ketamine)
- Rocuronium

Status asthmaticus
- Atropine if <7 yr old
- Ketamine
- Rocuronium

[a]Succinylcholine can be used in place of rocuronium if no contraindications exist. ICP, intracranial pressure.

Dosing for RSI is 1 to 1.2 mg per kg IV or 1 to 1.8 mg per kg IM × 1 dose. Adverse effects include prolonged paralysis when given with other drugs known to prolong neuromuscular blockade and rare allergic reactions. Rocuronium has been reported to precipitate in IV tubing when thiopental is used concurrently and is not adequately flushed prior to administration.

Vecuronium is structurally related to rocuronium and can be used for RSI but must be given at three times the normal dose (0.25 to 0.3 mg per kg vs. 0.1 mg per kg) to achieve an adequate onset time (208,228). By increasing the dose, the duration of action is also increased to as much as 2 hours in some cases. Vecuronium demonstrates an age-related time to recovery from neuromuscular block that is greater in infants than in children and not seen with rocuronium (223). Histamine release is less likely with vecuronium and rocuronium as compared with succinylcholine.

RESUSCITATION MEDICATIONS

Pediatric advanced life support (PALS) recommendations published by the American Heart Association provide guidelines for the resuscitation of children, with an emphasis on pharmacologic therapies (229). Current treatment algorithms are given as follows (Table 24.10).

ASYSTOLE/PULSELESS ELECTRICAL ACTIVITY

Unfortunately, the outcome in children presenting in asystole from an out-of-hospital arrest is very poor. However, rapid intervention may improve the chances of successful resuscitation. Initial management of asystole includes assessment of the airway and provision of adequate ventilation. Epinephrine is the primary pharmacologic agent used in asystole. Epinephrine may be given via intravenous/intraosseous routes or endotracheally. Dosing of epinephrine for intravenous or intraosseous administration begins at 0.1 mL per kg of a 1:10,000 solution (equivalent to 0.01 mg per kg). If the endotracheal route must be utilized, the higher concentration of epinephrine 1:1,000 is dosed at 0.1 mL per kg (equivalent to 0.1 mg per kg). To ensure adequate dispersal and absorption in the lungs, the epinephrine dose should be diluted in 3 to 5 mL of normal saline prior to administration; installation should be followed by five positive pressure breaths. Epinephrine doses should be repeated every 3 to 5 minutes. Despite years of empiric practice, "high-dose epinephrine" (0.1 mg per kg IV) does not appear to improve outcome unless the underlying cause of the arrest is a condition in which the body becomes relatively resistant to exogenous catecholamines (i.e., β-blocker overdose) (229).

Vasopressin dosed at 40 units IV is advocated for cardiac arrest in adults. There have not been any randomized controlled trials in children using vasopressin for cardiac arrest. A review of two small case series reported survival in three patients following two doses of epinephrine and subsequent vasopressin (230). There are not enough data at this time to recommend routine use of vasopressin in pediatric arrest.

Pulseless electrical activity (PEA) may result from several reversible causes. Most often, these causes are referred to as the 5Hs and 5Ts: hypoxia, hyperthermia, hypovolemia, hydrogen ion (acid/base disorder), and hypo/hyperkalemia and metabolic disorders encompass the 5Hs (229). The 5Ts refer to cardiac tamponade, tension pneumothorax, toxins/poisons/drugs, trauma, and thromboembolism (229). If any of these conditions exist, it is essential to recognize and correct them immediately. The drug of choice for PEA is epinephrine, as discussed in the preceding paragraph.

TABLE 24.10 Pediatric Advanced Life Support Recommendations (224)

Asystole/pulseless electrical activity
Epinephrine
Ventricular fibrillation/pulseless ventricular tachycardia
Defibrillation
Epinephrine + defibrillation
Amiodarone OR lidocaine + defibrillation
Magnesium sulfate if torsades de pointes
Bradycardia
Epinephrine
Atropine
Transcutaneous pacing
Supraventricular tachycardia
Stable
Vagal maneuvers
Adenosine
Amiodarone, lidocaine, or procainamide
Alternative agents
Unstable
Cardioversion

PULSELESS VENTRICULAR TACHYCARDIA AND VENTRICULAR FIBRILLATION

The first and foremost treatment for ventricular fibrillation (VF)/pulseless ventricular tachycardia (VT) is defibrillation followed by immediate cardiopulmonary resuscitation (CPR). This principle is true for both children and adults and is becoming more evident through the increased placement of automatic electrical defibrillators in public venues. A version design for children that delivers lower voltage impulses is becoming commercially available. In the treatment of VF/pulseless VT, a single "shock" is given with immediate resumption of CPR. The amount of electricity delivered is dependent upon the type of defibrillator available, either monophasic or biphasic. Following subsequent shocks, circulation is reassessed. Initial settings for the monophasic defibrillator begin at 2 joules per kg (max 300 joules) with the second defibrillation; the second and all subsequent defibrillations are given at 4 joules per kg (max 360 joules). Adolescent and adult patients should receive the initial and all subsequent shocks at 360 joules. The energy settings on the biphasic defibrillators is reduced and for adults will be set at 150 joules for the initial shock and 200 joules for subsequent shocks.

Secondary treatment of VF/pulseless VT includes epinephrine as dosed for PEA. Each dose of medication given in VF/pulseless VT should be followed by a defibrillating shock. If no response is seen following the initial dose of epinephrine, the PALS algorithm directs the practitioner to use an antiarrhythmic medication, specifically either amiodarone or lidocaine (229,231).

Amiodarone is a class III antiarrhythmic that prolongs the action potential and refractory period in the myocardial tissue primarily via sodium and potassium channel blockade (231). Additional effects include calcium channel blockade and downregulation of β-receptors (232). Conduction through the atrioventricular node is slowed down secondary to the delay in repolarization. Dosing begins at 5 mg per kg (max 300 mg per dose) given as a rapid IV/IO bolus. In stable VT, amiodarone is infused over 20 to 60 minutes. Amiodarone must be diluted in 10 to 15 mL of dextrose 5% in water (D5 W) prior to administration. Onset time is rapid after IV bolus. Amiodarone is very lipophilic and possesses an extended half-life; in cases of chronic oral administration, the elimination half-life may be several months. Adverse side effects are common and can include complete heart block, hypotension, and the development of torsades de pointes if hypomagnesemia or hypokalemia exists. Amiodarone should not be given if the patient is receiving procainamide or other class I antiarrhythmic agents due to its propensity to prolong the QT interval.

Lidocaine is a class Ib antiarrhythmic agent that suppresses the automaticity of ventricles and the His-Purkinje system by directly blocking the conduction of impulses in the myocardial tissues, thereby decreasing sodium ion permeability of the membranes (231). Dosing of lidocaine is recommended at 1 to 1.5 mg per kg via IV/IO as a rapid bolus. Fifty percent of the dose (0.5 to 0.75 mg per kg) can be repeated every 3 to 5 minutes until a maximum of 3 mg per kg is reached. A continuous infusion of lidocaine may be necessary to maintain sinus rhythm.

It is important to note that there is no evidence that amiodarone is superior to lidocaine in pediatric VF/pulseless VT. There is, however, evidence that amiodarone in the out-of-hospital setting is effective and perhaps superior to lidocaine in adults with VF/pulseless VT (233,234).

If torsades de pointes is present, the drug of choice is magnesium sulfate 25 to 50 mg per kg (max 2,000 mg per dose) (229). Magnesium sulfate acts as a calcium channel blocker and influences the Na^{-}K-ATPase activity in the heart, terminating the malignant rhythm. Magnesium sulfate is diluted and run over 10 to 20 minutes in torsades de pointes. Onset of action is nearly immediate.

In cases of acute VF secondary to TCA toxicity, sodium bicarbonate is the drug of choice. Sodium bicarbonate in doses of 1 mEq per kg boluses have been shown to overcome the fast sodium channel blockade produced by the TCAs and other sodium channel blockers such as diphenhydramine. The standard 8.4% solution of sodium bicarbonate is extremely hyperosmolar and should not be used in infants due to the risk of intraventricular hemorrhage (229). The 4.2% solution of sodium bicarbonate (Neut) should be used in infants requiring sodium bicarbonate. A continuous infusion of sodium bicarbonate, 75 to 150 mEq per L, in D5 W may be necessary to control the arrhythmia. For other arrest scenarios, sodium bicarbonate administration is avoided until correctable causes are identified and adequate ventilation can be assured.

BRADYCARDIA

Early correction of possible underlying factors in bradycardia such as hypoxia and hypothermia, among others, is essential.

The first-line pharmacologic agent for bradycardia is epinephrine, as discussed earlier; the second-line medication is atropine. As a vagolytic agent, atropine decreases the depressive vagal influence on the heart, thus increasing cardiac output. Atropine is dosed at 0.02 mg per kg (min dose 0.1 mg, max dose 1 mg) given IV/IO. If the endotracheal route is used, the dose of atropine should be 2 to 10 times the IV/IO dose. As with epinephrine, the dose of atropine should be diluted with 3 to 5 mL of normal saline; administration should be followed by five positive pressure breaths. Atropine may be repeated once, 3 to 5 minutes after the initial dose. The onset of action occurs within 2 to 4 minutes. It is important to note that atropine's dilating effects on the pupils may last several hours, making pupillary examination more difficult to interpret.

Cardiac pacing may be necessary to maintain perfusion for patients in a bradycardic rhythm. Special situations such as calcium channel blocker induced bradycardia may require the administration of calcium or insulin and dextrose. It is also important to note that calcium should not be given to patients also receiving digoxin, as a worsening of the arrhythmia may be seen. Calcium chloride 10% solution is given at a dose of 20 mg per kg (max 1,000 mg per dose) intravenously. It is important to note that calcium chloride must be further diluted before administration and is ideally infused via a central line. Calcium gluconate 10% solution is dosed at 100 mg per kg (max 3,000 mg per dose) and may be infused peripherally, although central administration is preferred wherever possible. Calcium administration may also be required in cases of hyperkalemia, hypocalcemia, and magnesium toxicity.

SUPRAVENTRICULAR TACHYCARDIA

The most common cause of malignant tachycardia in children is supraventricular tachycardia (SVT). If hypotension is also present, the patient is considered to be unstable and should immediately proceed to cardioversion (229). In the stable patient, vagal maneuvers are initially attempted to interrupt the abnormal conduction while an IV line is being placed. Vagal maneuvers may include placing ice on the face directly covering the mouth and nose, blowing through an occluded straw, or bearing down as if having a bowel movement.

The first-line pharmacologic agent for the treatment of SVT is adenosine (229). Because of the ultra-short half-life of adenosine in vivo, all doses must be given as centrally as possible and are immediately followed by a saline flush. Three-way stopcocks are often used to facilitate this process. The dose of adenosine is 0.1 mg per kg to a maximum of 6 mg via rapid IV push for the first dose, followed by 0.2 mg per kg (max 12 mg) via rapid IV push if the initial dose was unsuccessful at converting the patient to normal sinus rhythm. It is important to realize that a few seconds of asystole follow each dose of adenosine. This short period of asystole allows the heart to resume normal sinus rhythm by interrupting the conduction through the atrioventricular node. The onset is nearly immediate, and the duration of action is generally less than 2 minutes.

Amiodarone, lidocaine, and procainamide may also be useful in perfusing SVT. Amiodarone and lidocaine are described earlier, although the infusion times lengthen to avoid severe hypotension when these drugs are given for SVT. As a class Ia antiarrhythmic agent, procainamide has a similar mechanism of action as lidocaine. The dose of procainamide is 15 mg per kg run over 30 to 60 minutes. Adverse effects requiring cessation of infusion include hypotension and prolongation of the QT interval. Continuous infusion of procainamide may also be necessary to control the arrhythmia. Other alternatives for SVT may include β-blockers, verapamil (not for children younger than 1 year), and digoxin (235).

Cardioversion is employed as the next intervention if the drugs are ineffective or if the patient becomes unstable at any time. Different from defibrillation, cardioversion energy settings begin at 0.5 joules per kg (max 50 to 100 joules) and increase incrementally to 2 joules per kg (max 200 joules). As with defibrillation, the energy settings may vary between monophasic and biphasic machines, so it is important to become familiar with the equipment available to you. Sedation and analgesia with agents such as midazolam and fentanyl (see previous section) are preferable when time allows, as cardioversion is extremely unpleasant.

In conclusion, drug therapy in the ED is complex and varied. Conditions can range from a simple otitis media to CPR. Pharmacotherapy plays an important role in the treatment of children in the ED.

REFERENCES

1. Reynolds S, Desquin B, Uyeda A, et al. Children with chronic conditions in a pediatric emergency department. *Pediatr Emerg Care* 1996;12(3):166–169.
2. Cox ER, Halloran DR, Homan SM, et al. Trends in the prevalence of chronic medication use in children: 2002–2005. *Pediatrics* 2008;122:e1053–e1061.
3. Simpson L, Owens PW, Zodet MW, et al. Health care for children and youth in the United States: annual report on patterns of coverage, utilization, quality, and expenditures by income. *Ambul Pediatr* 2005;5(1):6–44.
4. Dibs SD, Baker MD. Anaphylaxis in children: a 5-year experience. *Pediatrics* 1997;99(1):E7.
5. Hoffman BB. Catecholamines, sympathomimetic drugs, and adrengeric receptor antagonists. In: Hardman JG, Limbird LE, eds. *Goodman & Gilman's The pharmacological basis of therapeutics,* 10th ed. New York: McGraw-Hill, 2001:215–268.
6. Simons FE, Roberts JR, Gu X, et al. Epinephrine absorption in children with a history of anaphylaxis. *J Allergy Clin Immunol* 1998; 101:33–37.
7. Project Team of the Resuscitation Council (UK). The emergency medical treatment of anaphylactic reactions. *J Accid Emerg Med* 1999;16:243–247.
8. Muraro A, Roberts G, Clark A, et al. The management of anaphylaxis in childhood; position paper on European Academy of Allergology and Clinical Immunology. *Allergy* 2007;62(8): 857–871.
9. Pongracic JA, Kim JS. Update on epinephrine for the treatment anaphylaxis. *Curr Opin Pediatr* 2007;19(1):94–98.
10. Brown N, Roberts LJ. Histamine, bradykinin and their antagonists. In: Hardman JG, Limbird LE, eds. *Goodman & Gilman's The pharmacological basis of therapeutics,* 10th ed. New York: McGraw-Hill, 2001:651–657.
11. Schimmer BP, Parker KL. Adrenocorticotropic hormone; adrenocortical steroids and their synthetic analogs; inhibitors of the synthesis and actions of adrenocortical hormones. In: Hardman JG, Limbird LE, eds. *Goodman & Gilman's The pharmacological basis of therapeutics,* 10th ed. New York: McGraw-Hill, 2001:1649–1677.
12. Lee JM, Greenes DS. Biphasic anaphylactic reactions in pediatrics. *Pediatrics* 2000;106(4):762–766.
13. Rendiae S. Drug interactions of H2-receptor antagonists involving cytochrome P450 (CYPs) enzymes: from the laboratory to the clinic. *Croat Med J Online* 1999;40(3);357–367.
14. ACCP/SCCM Consensus Conference Committee. American College of Chest Physicians/Society of Critical Care Medicine Consensus Conference: definitions for sepsis and organ failure and guidelines for the use of innovative therapies in sepsis. *Crit Care Med* 1992;20(6):864–874.
15. Kadish HA, et al. Applying outpatient protocols in febrile infants 1–28 days of age: can the threshold be lowered? *Clin Pediatr (Phila)* 2000;39(2):81–88.
16. Butt W. Pediatric critical care: a new millennium. Septic shock. *Pediatr Clin North Am* 2001;48(3):601–625.
17. D'Andrea CC, Ferrera PC. Disseminated herpes simplex virus infection in a neonate. *Am J Emerg Med* 1998;16:376–378.
18. Delinger RP, Levy MM, Carlet JM, et al. Surviving sepsis campaign: international guidelines for the management of severe sepsis and septic shock 2008. *Crit Care Med* 2008;36(1): 1394–1396.
19. Lipton JD, Schafermeyer RW. Evolving concepts in pediatric bacterial meningitis—Part I: Pathophysiology and diagnosis. *Ann Emerg Med* 1993;22(10):1602–1615.
20. Wubbel L, McCracken GH. Management of bacterial meningitis: 1998. *Pediatr Rev* 1998;19(3):78–84.
21. Silverman RB. Enzyme inhibition and inactivation. In: *The organic chemistry of drug design and drug action.* San Diego, CA: Academic Press, 1992:181–185.
22. Easton J, Noble S, Perry CM. Amoxicillin/clavulanic acid: a review of its use in the management of paediatric patients with acute otitis media. *Drugs* 2003;63(3):311–340.
23. Chopra I, Hesse L, O'Neill AJ. Exploiting current understanding of antibiotic action for discovery of new drugs. *J Appl Microbiol Symp* 2002;92(Suppl):4S–15S.
24. Condren M, Luedtke SA. Prescribing patterns for extended interval aminoglycoside dosing in pediatric patients. *J Pediatr Pharmacol Ther* 2001;6:385–391.
25. Konishi H, Goto M, Nakamoto Y, et al. Tobramycin inactivation by carbenicillin, ticarcillin and piperacillin. *Antimicrob Agents Chemother* 1983;23(5):653–657.
26. Chambers HF. Antimicrobial agents: protein synthesis inhibitors and miscellaneous antibacterial agents. In: Hardman JG, Limbird LE, eds. *Goodman & Gilman's The pharmacological basis of therapeutics,* 10th ed. New York: McGraw-Hill, 2001:1239–1271.
27. Bonadio WA, Jeruc W, Anderson Y, et al. Systemic infection due to group B beta-hemolytic streptococcus in children. A review of 75 outpatient-evaluated cases during 13 years. *Clin Pediatr (Phila)* 1992;31(4):230–234.
28. IDSA Practice Guidelines Committee. 1997 guidelines for the use of antimicrobial agents in neutropenic patients with unexplained fever. *Clin Infect Dis* 1997;25:551–573.
29. Lipton JD, Schafermeyer RW. Evolving concepts in pediatric bacterial meningitis—Part II: Current management and therapeutic research. *Ann Emerg Med* 1993;22(10):1616–1629.
30. Quagliarello VJ, Scheld WM. Treatment of bacterial meningitis. *N Engl J Med* 1997;336(10):708–716.
31. Wooltorton E. Cochlear implant recipients at risk for meningitis. *Can Med Assoc J* 2002;167(6):670.
32. Food and Drug Administration. FDA Public Health Web Notification: Cochlear implant recipients may be at greater risk for meningitis. Originally issued July 24, 2002—Updated October 17, 2002. Rockville, MD: Author, 2002.
33. De Gans J, Van De Beek D. Dexamethasone in adults with bacterial meningitis. *N Engl J Med* 2002;347(20):1549–1556.
34. Wald ER, Kaplan SL, Mason EO Jr, et al. Dexamethasone therapy for children with bacterial meningitis. *Pediatrics* 1995;95(1): 21–28.
35. Schaad UB, Lips U, Gnehm HE, et al. Dexamethasone therapy for bacterial meningitis in children. *Lancet* 1993;342:457–461.

36. Bennett J, St. Geme JW. Bacterial resistance and antibiotic use in the emergency department. *Pediatr Clin North Am* 1999;46(6): 1125–1143.
37. American Academy of Pediatrics. Therapy for children with invasive pneumococcal infections (RE9709). *Pediatrics* 1997;99(2): 289–299.
38. Prober CG. The role of steroids in the management of children with bacterial meningitis. *Pediatrics* 1995;95(1):29–31.
39. Klugman K, Friedland IR, Bradley JS. Bactericidal activity against cephalosporin-resistant *Streptococcus pneumoniae* in cerebrospinal fluid of children with acute bacterial meningitis. *Antimicrob Agents Chemother* 1995;39:1988–1992.
40. Ricard JD, Wolff M, Lacherade JC, et al. Levels of vancomycin in cerebrospinal fluid of adult patients receiving adjunctive corticosteroids to treat pneumococcal meningitis: a prospective multicenter observational study. *Clin Infect Dis* 2007;44(2):250–255.
41. Kohl S, James AR. Herpes simplex virus encephalitis during childhood: importance of brain biopsy diagnosis. *J Pediatr* 1985; 107:212–215.
42. Whitley RJ, Lin Cy, Jacobs RF, et al. Herpes simplex virus infection. *Semin Pediatr Infect Dis* 2002;13(1):6–11.
43. Acyclovir sodium package insert. Los Angeles, CA: American Pharmaceutical Partners, Inc., 2002.
44. Kimberlin DW, Lin CY, Jacobs RF, et al. Safety and efficacy of high-dose intravenous acyclovir in the management of neonatal herpes simplex virus infections. *Pediatrics* 2001;108:230–238.
45. American Academy of Pediatrics. Meningococcal infections. In: Pickering LK, ed. *2000 red book: report of the Committee on Infectious Diseases*, 25th ed. Elk Grove Village, IL: American Academy of Pediatrics 2000:396–401.
46. Powers RD. Soft tissue infections in the emergency department: the case for the use of 'simple' antibiotics. *South Med J* 1991; 84(11):1313–1315.
47. Gupta K, MacIntyre A, Vannasse G, et al. Trends in prescribing beta-lactam antibiotics for treatment of community-associated methicillin resistant Staphylococcus aureus infections. *J Clin Microbiol* 2007;45(12):3930–3934.
48. Powell KR. Orbital and periorbital cellulitis. *Pediatr Rev* 1995; 16(5):163–167.
49. Ambati BK, Ambati J, Azar N, et al. Periorbital and orbital cellulitis before and after the advent of *Haemophilus influenzae* type B vaccination. *Ophthalmology* 2000;107(8):1590–1593.
50. Starkey CR, Steele RW. Medical management of orbital cellulitis. *Pediatr Infect Dis J* 2001;20:1002–1005.
51. American Academy of Pediatrics. Severe invasive group a streptococcal infections: a subject review (RE9804). *Pediatrics* 1998; 101(1):136–140.
52. Doctor A, Harper MB, Fleisher GR. Group A beta-hemolytic streptococcal bacteremia: historical overview, changing incidence, and recent association with varicella. *Pediatrics* 1995;96: 428–433.
53. Norrby SR, Norrby-Teglund A. Infections due to group A streptococcus: new concepts and potential treatment strategies. *Ann Acad Med Singapore* 1997;26(5):691–693.
54. American Academy of Pediatrics. Toxic shock syndrome. In: Pickering LK, ed. *2000 red book: report of the Committee on Infectious Diseases*, 25th ed. Elk Grove Village, IL: American Academy of Pediatrics, 2000:580–581.
55. McIntosh K. Community-acquired pneumonia in children. *N Engl J Med* 2002;346(6):429–437.
56. Dellinger RP, Carlet JM, Masur H, et al. Surviving sepsis campaign guidelines for management of severe sepsis and shock. *Crit Care Med* 2004;32(3):853–873.
57. Bradley JS. Management of community-acquired pediatric pneumonia in an era of increasing antibiotic resistance and conjugate vaccines. *Pediatr Infect Dis J* 2002;21(6):592–598.
58. Chumpa A, Bachur RG, Harper MB. Bacteremia-associated pneumococcal pneumonia and the benefit of initial parenteral antimicrobial therapy. *Pediatr Infect Dis J* 1999;18(12):1981–1985.
59. McCracken GH. Etiology and treatment of pneumonia. *Pediatr Infect Dis J* 2000;19(4):373–377.
60. Esposito S, Bosis S, Cavagna R, et al. Characteristics of *Streptococcus pneumoniae* and atypical bacterial infections in children 2–5 years of age with community acquired pneumonia. *Clin Infect Dis* 2002;35:1345–1352.
61. Erythromycin Base Film-tab package insert. Abbott Park, IL: Abbott Laboratories, 2000.
62. Zithromax (azithromycin) package insert. New York: Pfizer, 2002.
63. Hauben M, Amsden GW. The association of erythromycin and infantile hypertrophic pyloric stenosis: causal or coincidental? *Drug Saf* 2002;25(13):929–942.
64. Cooper WO, Griffin MR, Arbogast P, et al. Very early exposure to erythromycin and infantile hypertrophic pyloric stenosis. *Arch Pediatr Adolesc Med* 2002;156(7):647–650.
65. Jacobson SJ, Griffiths K, Diamond S, et al. A randomized controlled trial of penicillin vs clindamycin for the treatment of aspiration pneumonia in children. *Arch Pediatr Adolesc Med* 1997; 158:701–704.
66. Kim MK, Karpas A. Orthopedic emergencies: the limping child. *Clin Pediatr Emerg Med* 2002;3(2):129–137.
67. Perron AD, Brady WJ, Miller MD. Orthopedic pitfalls in the ED: osteomyelitis. *Am J Emerg Med* 2003;21:61–67.
68. Luhmann JD, Luhmann SJ. Etiology of septic arthritis in children: an update for the 1990s. *Pediatr Emerg Care* 1999;15(1):40–42.
69. Chambers JB, Forsythe DA, Bertrand SL, et al. Retrospective review of osteoarticular infections in a pediatric sickle cell age group. *J Pediatr Orthop* 2000;20(5):682–685.
70. Vinod MB. Duration of antibiotics in children with osteomyelitis and septic arthritis. *J Paediatr Child Health* 2002;38(4):363–367.
71. Jaberi FM, Shahcheraghi GH, Ahadzadeh M. Short-term intravenous antibiotic treatment of acute hematogenous bone and joint infection in children: a prospective randomized trial. *J Pediatr Orthop* 2002;22(3):317–320.
72. American Academy of Pediatrics. Salmonella infections. In: Pickering LK, ed. *2000 red book: report of the Committee on Infectious Diseases*, 25th ed. Elk Grove Village, IL: American Academy of Pediatrics, 2000:501–503.
73. American Academy of Pediatrics. Judicious use of antimicrobial agents. In: Pickering LK, ed. *2000 red book: report of the Committee on Infectious Diseases*, 25th ed. Elk Grove Village, IL: American Academy of Pediatrics, 2000:647–648.
74. Hendley JO. Otitis media. *N Engl J Med* 2002;347(10): 1169–1174.
75. American Academy of Pediatrics. Pneumococcal infections. In: Pickering LK, ed. *2000 red book: report of the Committee on Infectious Diseases*, 25th ed. Elk Grove Village, IL: American Academy of Pediatrics, 2000:452–460.
76. Dowell SF, Butler JC, Giebink GS, et al. Acute otitis media: management and surveillance in an era of pneumococcal resistance—a report from the Drug-Resistant *Streptococcus Pneumoniae* Therapeutic Working Group. *Pediatr Infect Dis J* 1999;18(1):1–9.
77. Bisno AL, Gerber MA, Gwaltney JM, et al. Practice guidelines for the diagnosis and management of group A streptococcal pharyngitis. *Clin Infect Dis* 2002;35(2):113–125.
78. American Academy of Pediatrics. Group A streptococcal infections. In: Pickering LK, ed. *2000 red book: report of the Committee on Infectious Diseases*, 25th ed. Elk Grove Village, IL: American Academy of Pediatrics, 2000:526–536.
79. Bicillin LA (penicillin G benzathine) package insert. Bristol, TN: Monarch Pharmaceuticals, 2001.
80. AAP/APS. Policy Statement. The assessment and management of acute pain in infants, children, and adolescents (0793). *Pediatrics* 2001;108(3):793–797.
81. Read JV. Perceptions of nurses and physicians regarding pain management of pediatric emergency room patients. *Pediatr Nurs* 1994;20(3):314–318.
82. Roberts LJ, Morrow JD. Analgesic-antipyretic and antiinflammatory agents. In: Hardman JG, Limbird LE, eds. *Goodman & Gilman's The pharmacological basis of therapeutics*, 10th ed. New York: McGraw-Hill, 2001:687–719.
83. Curtis SM, Curtis RL. Somatosensory function and pain. In: Porth CM, ed. *Pathophysiology: concepts of altered health states*, 3rd ed. Philadelphia, PA: Lippincott Williams & Wilkins, 1990: 839–872.
84. Rodriquez E, Jordan R. Contemporary trends in pediatric sedation and analgesia. *Emerg Med Clin North Am* 2002;20(1):199–222.
85. Institute for Safe Medication Practices. *ISMP Medication Safety Alert!* 2002; October 30, 7(22).
86. Gutstein HB, Akil H. Opioid analgesics. In: Hardman JG, Limbird LE, eds. *Goodman & Gilman's The pharmacological basis of therapeutics*, 10th ed. New York: McGraw-Hill, 2001:595–596.

87. Blackburn P, Vissers R. Pharmacologic advances in emergency medicine: pharmacology of emergency department pain management and conscious sedation. *Emerg Med Clin North Am* 2000;18(4):803–827.
88. Müller P, Vogtmann C. Three cases with different presentation of fentanyl-induced muscle rigidity—a rare problem in intensive care of neonates. *Am J Perinatol* 2000;17(1):23–26.
89. Fahnenstich H, Steffan J, Ku N, et al. Fentanyl-induced chest wall rigidity and laryngospasm in preterm and term infants. *Crit Care Med* 2000;28:836–839.
90. Weiner AL. Meperidine as a potential cause of serotonin syndrome in the emergency department. *Acad Emerg Med* 1999; 6(2):156–158.
91. Boyer E, Shannnon M. The serotonin syndrome. *N Engl J Med* 2005;352(11):1112–1120.
92. Tréluyer JM, Tonnelier S, d'Athis P, et al. Antipyretic efficacy of an initial 30-mg/kg loading dose of acetaminophen versus a 15-mg/kg maintenance dose. *Pediatrics* 2001;108(4):e73.
93. Gladtke E. Use of antipyretic analgesics in the pediatric patient. *Am J Med* 1983;75(5A):121–126.
94. Pierce MC, Fuchs S. Evaluation of ketorolac in children with forearm fractures. *Ann Emerg Med* 1997;4:22–26.
95. Ketorolac tromethamine package insert. Bedford, OH: Bedford Laboratories, 1999.
96. Bassett KE, Anderson JL, Pribble CG, et al. Propofol for procedural sedation in children in emergency departments. *Ann Emerg Med* 2003;42:773–782.
97. Malviya S, Voepel-Lewis T, Prochaska G, et al. Prolonged recovery and delayed side effects of sedation for diagnostic imaging studies in children. *Pediatrics* 2000;105(3):e42.
98. Coté CJ, Karl HW, Notterman DA, et al. Adverse sedation events in pediatrics: analysis of medications used for sedation. *Pediatrics* 2000;106(4):633–644.
99. Peña B, Krauss B. Adverse events of procedural sedation and analgesia in a pediatric emergency department. *Ann Emerg Med* 1999;34:483–491.
100. Charney DS, Mihic SJ, Harris RA. Hypnotics and sedatives. In: Hardman JG, Limbird LE, eds. *Goodman & Gilman's The pharmacological basis of therapeutics*, 10th ed. New York: McGraw-Hill, 2001:399–427.
101. Wadbrook PS. Pharmacologic advances in emergency medicine—advances in airway pharmacology. *Emerg Med Clin North Am* 2000;18(4):767–788.
102. Evers AS, Crowder CM. General anesthetics. In: Hardman JG, Limbird LE, eds. *Goodman & Gilman's The pharmacological basis of therapeutics*, 10th ed. New York: McGraw-Hill, 2001: 337–365.
103. Rock MJ, De La Rocha SR, L'Hommedieu CS, et al. Use of ketamine in asthmatic children to treat respiratory failure refractory to conventional therapy. *Crit Care Med* 1986;14(5):514–516.
104. Wathen JE, Roback MG, Mackenzie T, et al. Does midazolam alter the clinical effects of intravenous ketamine sedation in children? A double-blind, randomized, controlled, emergency department trial. *Ann Emerg Med* 2000;36(6):579–588.
105. McNamara JO. Drugs effective in the therapy of the epilepsies. In: Hardman JG, Limbird LE, eds. *Goodman & Gilman's The pharmacological basis of therapeutics*, 10th ed. New York: McGraw-Hill, 2001:521–548.
106. Task Force on Sedation and Analgesia by Non-Anesthesiologists. Practice guidelines for sedation and analgesia by non-anesthesiologists. *Anesthesiology* 1996;84:459–471.
107. Brent AS. Acute pain in children: the management of pain in the emergency department. *Pediatr Clin North Am* 2000;47(3): 651–679.
108. Naloxone hydrochloride package insert. Abbott Park, IL: Abbott Laboratories, 1999.
109. Johnson C, Mayer P, Grosz D. Pulmonary edema following naloxone administration in a healthy orthopedic patient [Letter]. *J Clin Anesth* 1995;7:356–357.
110. Rosen DA, Morris JL, Rosen KR, et al. Nalmefene to prevent epidural narcotic side effects in pediatric patients: a pharmacokinetic and safety study. *Pharmacotherapy* 2000;20(7):745–749.
111. Chumpa A, Kaplan RL, Burns MM, et al. Nalmefene for elective reversal of procedural sedation in children. *Am J Emerg Med* 2001;19:545–548.
112. Shannon M, Albers G, Burkhart K, et al. Safety and efficacy of flumazenil in the reversal of benzodiazepine-induced conscious sedation. *J Pediatr* 1997;131:582–586.
113. Knapp JF. Updates in wound management for the pediatrician. *Pediatr Clin North Am* 1999;46(6):1201–1213.
114. Hollander JE, Singer AJ. Laceration management. *Ann Emerg Med* 1999;34(3):56–67.
115. Catterall W, Mackie K. Local anesthetics. In: Hardman JG, Limbird LE, eds. *Goodman & Gilman's The pharmacological basis of therapeutics*, 10th ed. New York: McGraw-Hill, 2001:367–384.
116. Covino BG. Pharmacology of local anaesthetic agents. *Br J Anaesth* 1986;58:701–716.
117. Ball IA. Allergic reactions to lignocaine. *Br Dent J* 1999;186(5): 224–226.
118. Gall H, Kaufmann R, Kalveram CM. Adverse reactions to local anesthetics: analysis of 197 cases. *J Allergy Clin Immunol* 1996;97(4): 933–937.
119. Eggleston ST, Lush LW. Understanding allergic reactions to local anesthetics. *Ann Pharmacother* 1996;30(7):851–857.
120. Troise C, et al. Management of patients at risk for adverse reactions to local anesthetics: analysis of 386 cases. *J Invest Allergol Clin Immunol* 1998;8(3):172–175.
121. Xylocaine (lidocaine hydrochloride) package insert. Wilmington, DE: AstraZeneca, 2000.
122. Emslander HC. Local and topical anesthesia for pediatric wound repair: a review of selected aspects. *Pediatr Emerg Care* 1998; 14(2):123–129.
123. Green SM, Rothrock SG, Gorchynski J. Validation of diphenhydramine as a dermal local anesthetic. *Ann Emerg Med* 1994;23 (6):1284–1289.
124. Ernst AA, Anand P, Nick T, et al. Lidocaine versus diphenhydramine for local anesthesia minor laceration repair. *J Trauma* 1993;34:354–357.
125. Smith GA, Strausbaugh SD, Harbeck-Weber C, et al. Comparison of topical anesthetics with lidocaine infiltration during laceration repair in children. *Clin Pediatr (Phila)* 1997; 36(1):17–23.
126. Smith GA, Strausbaugh SD, Harbeck-Weber C, et al. Prilocaine–phenylephrine and bupivicaine–phenylephrine topical anesthetics compared with tetracaine–adrenaline–cocaine during repair of lacerations. *Am J Emerg Med* 1998;16: 121–124.
127. Singer AJ, Stark MJ. Pretreatment of lacerations with lidocaine, epinephrine and tetracaine at triage: a randomized double-blind trial. *Acad Emerg Med* 2000;7:751–756.
128. Schilling CG, Bank DE, Borchert BA, et al. Tetracaine, epinephrine (adrenaline) and cocaine (TAC) versus lidocaine, epinephrine and tetracaine (LET) for anesthesia of lacerations in children. *Ann Emerg Med* 1995;25:203–208.
129. Ernst AA, Marvez-Valls E, Nick TG, et al. LAT (lidocaine–adrenaline–tetracaine) versus TAC (tetracaine–adrenaline–cocaine) for topical anesthesia in face and scalp lacerations. *Am J Emerg Med* 1995;13:158–154.
130. Resch K, Schilling C, Borchert BD, et al. Topical anesthesia for pediatric lacerations: a randomized trial of lidocaine–epinephrine–tetracaine solution versus gel. *Ann Emerg Med* 1998;36(6): 693–697.
131. EMLA Cream (lidocaine 2% and prilocaine 2.5%) package insert. Wilmington, DE: AstraZeneca, 2002.
132. Singer AJ, Stark MJ. LET versus EMLA for pretreating lacerations: a randomized trial. *Acad Emerg Med* 2001;8(3):223–230.
133. Dire DJ, Coppola M, Dwyer DA, et al. Prospective evaluation of topical antibiotics for preventing infections in uncomplicated soft-tissue wound repairs in the ED. *Acad Emerg Med* 1995;2:4–10.
134. Bernard L, Doyle J, Friedlander SF, et al. A prospective comparison of octyl cyanoacrylate tissue adhesive (Dermabond) and suture for the closure of excisional wounds in children and adolescents. *Arch Dermatol* 201;137:1177–1180.
135. Bruns TB, Robinson BS, Smith RJ, et al. A new tissue adhesive for laceration repair in children. *J Pediatr* 1998;132(6): 1067–1070.
136. Centers for Disease Control and Prevention. Human rabies—Tennessee, 2002. *MMWR Morb Mortal Wkly Rep* 2002;51(37): 828–829.
137. Centers for Disease Control and Prevention. Human rabies prevention—United States, 1999 recommendations of the advisory

committee on immunization practices (ACIP). *MMWR Morb Mortal Wkly Rep* 1999;48(RR-1):1–21.
138. Imovax package insert. Swiftwater, PA: Aventis Pasteur, 1991.
139. Rabies Immune Globulin (Human) USP Imogam Rabies–HT package insert. Stillwater, PA: Aventis Pasteur, 1999.
140. Lewis KT, Stiles M. Management of cat and dog bites. *Am Fam Physician* 1995;52(2):479–485.
141. American Academy of Pediatrics. Bite wounds. In: Pickering LK, ed. *2000 red book: report of the Committee on Infectious Diseases*, 25th ed. Elk Grove Village, IL: American Academy of Pediatrics, 2000:155–159.
142. Werner HA. Status asthmaticus in children. *Chest* 2001;119(6): 1913–1929.
143. Hvizdos KM, Jarvis B. Budesonide inhalation suspension: a review of its use in infants, children and adults with inflammatory respiratory disorders. *Drugs* 2000;60(5):1141–1178.
144. Geelhoed GC, Macdonald WBG. Oral and inhaled steroids in croup: a randomized, placebo-controlled trial. *Pediatr Pulmonol* 1995;20:355–361.
145. Hampers LC, Faries SG. Practice variation in the emergency management of croup. *Pediatrics* 2002;109(3):505–508.
146. American Academy of Pediatrics. Parainfluenza viral infections. In: Pickering LK, ed. *2000 red book: report of the Committee on Infectious Diseases*, 25th ed. Elk Grove Village, IL: American Academy of Pediatrics, 2000:419–420.
147. Kunkel N, Baker MD. Use of racemic epinephrine, dexamethasone and mist in the outpatient management of croup. *Pediatr Emerg Care* 1996;12:156–159.
148. Ledwith CA, Shea LM, Mauro RD. Safety and efficacy of nebulized racemic epinephrine in conjunction with oral dexamethasone and mist in the outpatient management of croup. *Ann Emerg Med* 1995;25:331–337.
149. Stephanopoulos DE, Monge R, Schell KH, et al. Continuous intravenous terbutaline for pediatric status asthmaticus. *Crit Care Med* 1998;26(10):1744–1748.
150. Klassen TP. Recent advances in the treatment of bronchiolitis and laryngitis. *Pediatr Clin North Am* 1997;44(1):249–261.
151. American Academy of Pediatrics. Respiratory syncytial virus. In: Pickering LK, ed. *2000 red book: report of the Committee on Infectious Diseases*, 25th ed. Elk Grove Village, IL: American Academy of Pediatrics, 2000:483–487.
152. Perlstein PH, Kotagal UR, Bolling C, et al. Evaluation of an evidence-based guideline for bronchiolitis. *Pediatrics* 1999;104(6): 1334–1341.
153. Babl FE, Cooper ER, Kastner B, et al. Prophylaxis against possible human immunodeficiency virus exposure after nonoccupational needlestick injuries or sexual assaults in children and adolescents. *Arch Pediatr Adolesc Med* 2001;155:680–682.
154. Dawson K, Kennedy D, Asher I, et al. The management of acute bronchiolitis. Thoracic Society of Australia and New Zealand. *J Paediatr Child Health* 1993;29(5):335–337.
155. Le Saux N, Pham B, Bjornson C, et al. Antimicrobial use in febrile children diagnosed with respiratory tract illness in an emergency department. *Pediatr Infect Dis J* 1999;18(12):1078–1080.
156. Rakshi K, Couriel JM. Management of acute bronchiolitis. *Arch Dis Child* 1994;71:463–469.
157. Jartti T, Vanto T, Heikkinen T, et al. Systemic glucocorticoids in childhood expiratory wheezing: relation between age and viral etiology with efficacy. *Pediatr Infect Dis J* 2002;21:873–878.
158. Ho L, Collis G, Landau LI, et al. Effect of salbutamol on oxygen saturation in bronchiolitis. *Arch Dis Child* 1991;66:1061–1064.
159. Hall CB, McBride JT. Bronchiolitis. In: Mandell GL, ed. *Principles and practice of infectious diseases*, 5th ed. Philadelphia, PA: Churchill Livingstone, 2000:710–717.
160. Henry RL, Milner AD, Stokes GM. Ineffectiveness of ipratropium bromide in acute bronchiolitis. *Arch Dis Child* 1983;58: 925–926.
161. Centers for Disease Control and Prevention (CDC). Update to CDC's Sexually transmitted diseases treatment guidelines 2006; Fluoroquinolones No Longer Recommended for Treatment of Gonococcal Infections. *MMWR Morb Mortal Wkly Rep* 2007;56 (14):332–336.
162. Centers for Disease Control and Prevention. Notice to readers: discontinuation of cefixime tablets—United States. *MMWR Morb Mortal Wkly Rep* 2002;51(46):1052.
163. Tracy JW, Webster LT. Drugs used in the chemotherapy of protozoal infections: amebiasis, giardiasis, trichomoniasis, trypanosomiasis, leishmaniasis, and other protozoal infections. In: Hardman JG, Limbird LE, eds. *Goodman & Gilman's The pharmacological basis of therapeutics*, 10th ed. New York: McGraw-Hill, 2001:1097–1120.
164. Centers for Disease Control and Prevention (CDC). Antiretroviral postexposure prophylaxis after sexual, injection drug use, or other non-occupational exposure to HIV in the United States. *MMWR Morb Mortal Wkly Rep* 2005;54(RR02):1–20.
165. Merchant RC, Keshavarz R. Human immunodeficiency virus postexposure prophylaxis for adolescents and children [Abstract]. *Pediatrics* 2001;108(8):e37.
166. Weinberg GA. Postexposure prophylaxis against human immunodeficiency virus infection after sexual assault. *Pediatr Infect Dis J* 2002;21:959–960.
167. American Academy of Pediatrics. Human immunodeficiency virus infection. In: Pickering LK, ed. *2000 red book: report of the Committee on Infectious Diseases*, 25th ed. Elk Grove Village, IL: American Academy of Pediatrics, 2000:347–348.
168. Raffanti S, Haas DW. Antimicrobial agents: antiretroviral agents. In: Hardman JG, Limbird LE, eds. *Goodman & Gilman's The pharmacological basis of therapeutics*, 10th ed. New York: McGraw-Hill, 2001:1349–1380.
169. Task Force on Postovulatory Methods of Fertility Regulation. Randomised controlled trial of levonorgestrel versus the Yuzpe regimen of combined oral contraceptives for emergency contraception. *Lancet* 1998;352:428–433.
170. Wanner MS, Couchenour RL. Hormonal emergency contraception. *Pharmacotherapy* 2002;22(1):43–53.
171. Plan B (levonorgesterol) package insert. Washington, DC: Women's Capital Corporation.
172. Trussell J, Ellertson C, Rodriguez G. The Yuzpe regimen of emergency contraception: how long after the morning after? *Obstet Gynecol* 1996;88:150–154.
173. Grimes DA, Raymond EG. Emergency contraception. *Ann Intern Med* 2002;137:180–189.
174. Yuzpe AA, Lancee WJ. Ethinyl estradiol and dl-norgestrel as a postcoital contraceptive. *Fertil Steril* 1977;28:932–936.
175. Roth HL, Drislane FW. Neurologic emergencies—seizures. *Neurol Clin* 1998;16(2):257–284.
176. Huff JS. The challenge of managing patients with seizures. *Emerg Med* 1996;(Suppl):2–8.
177. LaCroix J, Deal C, Gauthier M, et al. Admissions to a pediatric intensive care unit for status epilepticus: a 10-year experience. *Crit Care Med* 1994;22(5):827–832.
178. Flomembaum NE, ed. Treating acute seizure patients in the emergency department. *Emerg Med* 1996;(Suppl):1–32.
179. Meldrum B. Pharmacology of GABA. *Clin Neuropharmacol* 1982; 5(3):293–316.
180. Treiman DM. The role of benzodiazepines in the management of status epilepticus. *Neurology* 1990;40(Suppl 2):32–42.
181. Meek PD, Davis SN, Collins DM, et al. Guidelines for nonemergency use of parenteral phenytoin products. *Arch Intern Med* 1999; 159:2639–2644.
182. Cerebryx (fosphenytoin) package insert. Morris Plains, NJ: Warner-Lambert Co., 1999.
183. Lilley LL, Guanci R. Equivalence dosing. *Am J Nurs* 1997;97(3): 12.
184. Hovinga CA, Chicella MF, Rose DF, et al. Use of intravenous valproate in three pediatric patients with nonconvulsive or convulsive status epilepticus. *Ann Pharmacother* 1999;33:579–584.
185. Chez MG, Hammer MS, Loeffel M, et al. Clinical experience of three pediatric and one adult case of spike-and-wave status epilepticus treated with injectable valproic acid. *J Child Neurol* 1999;14(4):239–242.
186. Venkataraman V, Wheless JW. Safety of rapid intravenous infusion of valproate loading doses in epilepsy patients. *Epilepsy Res* 1999;35(2):154–153.
187. Depacon (valproic acid) package insert. Abbott Park, IL: Abbott Laboratories, 2002.
188. Hirsch LJ. Levitating levetiracetam's status for status epilepticus. *Epilepsy Curr* 2008;8(5):125–126.
189. Gallentine WB, Hunnicutt AS, Husain AM. Levetiracetam in children with refractory status epilepticus (published online ahead of print October 13, 2008). *Epilepsy Behav* 2008.

190. Stafford PW, Blinman TA, Nance ML. Practical points in evaluation and resuscitation of the injured child. *Surg Clin North Am* 2002;82(2):273–301.
191. Elixhauser A, Machlin SR, Zodet MW, et al. Health care for children and youth in the United States: 2001 anuual report on access, ultilization, quality and expenditures. *Ambulat Pediatr* 2002;2(6):419–437.
192. Fabian TC. Infection in penetrating abdominal trauma: risk factors and preventive antibiotics. *Am Surg* 2002;68:29–35.
193. Dufresne RG. Skin necrosis from intravenously infused materials. *Cutis* 1987;39:197–198.
194. Kahn JM, Kress JP, Hall JB. Skin necrosis after extravasation of low-dose vasopressin administered for septic shock. *Crit Care Med* 2002;30(8):1899–1901.
195. American Heart Association. Fluid therapy and medications for shock and cardiac arrest. In: *PALS provider manual.* Dallas, TX: Author, 2002:127–153.
196. Meyer S, Gortner L, McGuire W, et al. Vasopressin in catecholamine-refractory shock in children. *Anaesthesia* 2008;63(3): 288–234.
197. Baldasso E, Ramos Garcia PC, Piva JP, et al. Hemodynamic and metabolic effects of vasopressin infusion in children with shock. *J Pediatr (Rio J)* 2007;83(Suppl 5):S137–S145.
198. Brown LA, Levin GM. Role of propofol in refractory status epilepticus. *Ann Pharmacother* 1998;32:1053–1059.
199. Parke TJ, Stevens JE, Rice AS, et al. Metabolic acidosis and fatal myocardial failure after propofol infusion in children: five case reports. *Br Med J* 1992;305:613–616.
200. Amick LF. Pediatric trauma: penetrating trauma in the pediatric patient. *Clin Pediatr Emerg Med* 2001;2(1):63–70.
201. Krauss B, Harakal T, Fleisher GR. General trauma in a pediatric emergency department: spectrum and consultation patterns. *Pediatr Emerg Care* 1993;9(3):134–138.
202. Berg RA, Donnerstein RL, Padbury JF. Dobutamine infusions in stable, critically ill children: pharmacokinetics and hemodynamic actions. *Crit Care Med* 1993;21(5):678–685.
203. Dünser MW, Wenzel V, Mayr AJ, et al. Management of vasodilatory shock: defining the role of arginine vasopressin. *Drugs* 2003;63(3):237–256.
204. Jackson EK. Vasopressin and other agents affecting the renal conservation of water. In: Hardman JG, Limbird LE, eds. *Goodman & Gilman's The pharmacological basis of therapeutics,* 10th ed. New York: McGraw-Hill, 2001:789–808.
205. Gedeit R. Head injury. *Pediatr Rev* 2001;22(4):118–123.
206. Boucher BA, Phelps SJ. Acute management of the head injury patient. In: DiPiro JT, Talbert RL, Hayes PE, et al. eds. *Pharmacotherapy: a pathophysiologic approach,* 2nd ed. Norwalk, CT: Appleton & Lange, 1993:904–912.
207. Bracken MB. Methylprednisolone and acute spinal cord injury: an update of the randomized evidence. *Spine* 2001;26(24 Suppl): S47–S54.
208. Sagarin MJ, Chiang V, Sakles JC, et al. Rapid sequence intubation for pediatric emergency airway management. *Pediatr Emerg Care* 2002;18(6):417–423.
209. Marvez-Valls E, Houry D, Ernst AA, et al. Protocol for rapid sequence intubation in pediatric patients—a four year study. *Med Sci Monit* 2002;8(4):CR229–CR234.
210. Nakayama DK, Waggoner T, Venkataraman ST, et al. The use of drugs in emergency airway management in pediatric trauma. *Ann Surg* 1992;216(2):205–211.
211. Bean A, Jones J. Atropine—reevaluating its use during paediatric RSI. *Emerg Med J* 2007;24(5):361–362.
212. Fastle RK, Roback MG. Pediatric rapid sequence intubation: incidence of reflex bradycardia and effects of pretreatment with atropine. *Pediatr Emerg Care* 2004;20(10):651–655.
213. Bracken MB, Shepard MJ, Collins WF, et al. A randomized, controlled trial of methylprednisolone or naloxone in the treatment of acute spinal-cord injury—results of the Second National Acute Spinal Cord Injury Study. *N Engl J Med* 1990;322(20): 1405–1411.
214. Yamamoto LG, Yim GK, Britten AG. Rapid sequence anesthesia induction for emergency intubation. *Pediatr Emerg Care* 1990; 6(3):200–213.
215. Amidate (etomidate) package insert. Abbott Park, IL: Abbott Laboratories, 1998.
216. Doenicke AW, Roizen MF, Hoernecke R, et al. Solvent for etomidate may cause pain and adverse effects. *Br J Anaesth* 1999; 83(3):464–466.
217. McAllister JD, Gnauck KA. Emergency medicine—rapid sequence intubation of the pediatric patient. *Pediatr Clin North Am* 1999;46(6):1249–1284.
218. Fellows IW, Bastow MD, Byrne AJ, et al. Adrenocortical suppression in multiply injured patients: a complication of etomidate treatment. *Br Med J* 1983;287:1835–1837.
219. Sokolove PE, Price DD, Okada P. The safety of etomidate for emergency rapid sequence intubation of pediatric patients. *Pediatr Emerg Care* 2000;16(1):18–21.
220. L'Hommedieu CS. The use of ketamine for the emergency intubation of patients with status asthmaticus. *Ann Emerg Med* 1987; 16(5):568–571.
221. Undem BJ, Lichtenstein LM. Drugs used in the treatment of asthma. In: Hardman JG, Limbird LE, eds. *Goodman & Gilman's The pharmacological basis of therapeutics,* 10th ed. New York: McGraw-Hill, 2001:738–747.
222. Quelicin (succinylcholine) package insert. Abbott Park, IL: Abbott Laboratories, 1999.
223. Taylor P. Agents acting at the neuromuscular junction and autonomic ganglia. In: Hardman JG, Limbird LE, eds. *Goodman & Gilman's The pharmacological basis of therapeutics,* 10th ed. New York: McGraw-Hill, 2001:193–213.
224. Mazurek AJ, Rae B, Hann S, et al. Rocuronium versus succinylcholine: are they equally effective during rapid-sequence induction of anesthesia? *Anesth Analg* 1998;87:1259–1262.
225. Orebaugh SL. Therapeutics—succinylcholine: adverse effects and alternatives in emergency medicine. *Am J Emerg Med* 1999; 17(7):715–721.
226. American Heart Association. Rapid sequence intubation. In: *PALS provider manual.* Dallas, TX: Author, 2002:359–378.
227. McAuliffe G, Bissonnette B, Boutin C. Should the routine use of atropine before succinylcholine in children be reconsidered? *Can J Anaesth* 1995;42:724–729.
228. Brandon BW, Fine GF. Neuromuscular blocking drugs in pediatric anesthesia. *Anesth Clin North Am* 2002;20(1):45–58.
229. American Heart Association & American Academy of Pediatrics. *PALS provider manual.* Dallas, TX: American Heart Association, 2002.
230. de Caen AR, Reis A, Bhutta A. Vascular access and drug therapy in pediatric resuscitation. *Pediatr Clin N Am* 2008;55: 909–927.
231. Dorian P, Cass D, Schwartz B, et al. Amiodarone as compared with lidocaine for shock-resistant ventricular fibrillation. *N Engl J Med* 2002;346(12):884–890.
232. Roden D. Antiarrhythmic drugs. In: Hardman JG, Limbird LE, eds. *Goodman & Gilman's The pharmacological basis of therapeutics,* 10th ed. New York: McGraw-Hill, 2001:651–657.
233. McKee MR. Amiodarone—an "old" drug with new recommendations. *Curr Opin Pediatr* 2003;15:193–199.
234. Kudenchuk PJ, Cobb LA, Copass MK, et al. Amiodarone for resuscitation after out-of-hospital cardiac arrest due to ventricular fibrillation. *N Engl J Med* 1999;341:871–878.
235. Gewitz MH, Vetter VL. Cardiac emergencies. In: Fleisher G, Ludwig S, eds. *Textbook of pediatric emergency medicine,* 4th ed. Philadelphia, PA: Lippincott Williams & Wilkins; 2000:659–700.

SUGGESTED READINGS

Anonymous. Pharmacological therapy after acute cervical spinal cord injury. *Neurosurgery* 2002;50(3 Suppl):S63–S72.

Bracken MB. Steroids for acute spinal cord injury. *Cochrane Database Syst Rev* 2002(3):CD001046.

Bracken MB, Shepard MJ, Holford TR, et al. Administration of methylprednisolone for 24 or 48 hours or tirilazad mesylate for 48 hours in the treatment of acute spinal cord injury—results of the Third National Acute Spinal Cord Injury Randomized Controlled Trial. *J Am Med Assoc* 1997;277(20):1597–1604.

Buck ML. Clinical experience with ketorolac in children. *Ann Pharmacother* 1994;28:1009–1013.

Burstein GR, Berman SM, Blumer JL, et al. Ciprofloxacin for the treatment of uncomplicated gonorrhea infection in adolescents:

does the benefit outweigh the risk? *Clin Infect Dis* 2002;35(Suppl 2): S191–S199.

Ciarallo L, Sauer AH, Shannon MW. Intravenous magnesium therapy for moderate to severe pediatric asthma: results of a randomized, placebo-controlled trial. *J Pediatr* 1996;129:809–814.

Hugenholtz H, et al. High-dose methylprednisolone for acute closed spinal cord injury—only a treatment option. *Can J Neurol Sci* 2002; 29(3):227–235.

Hurlbert RJ, Moulton R. Why do you prescribe methylprednisolone for acute spinal cord injury? A Canadian perspective and a position statement. *Can J Neurol Sci* 2002;29(3):236–239.

Mahabee-Gittens EM. Respiratory emergencies: pediatric pneumonia. *Clin Pediatr Emerg Med* 2002;3(3):200–214.

Mandelberg A, Tsehori S, Houri S, et al. Is nebulized aerosol treatment necessary in the pediatric emergency department? *Chest* 2000; 117(5):1309–1313.

Orapred (prednisolonesodium phosphate) oral solution package insert. Wilmington, MA: Ascent Pediatrics, Inc., 2000.

Petri WA. Antimicrobial agents: sulfonamides, trimethoprim–sulfamethoxazole, quinolones and agents for urinary tract infections. In: Hardman JG, Limbird LE, eds. *Goodman & Gilman's The pharmacological basis of therapeutics,* 10th ed. New York: McGraw-Hill, 2001:1171–1188.

Roberts JS, Bratton SL, Brogan TV. Acute severe asthma: differences in therapies and outcomes among pediatric intensive care units. *Crit Care Med* 2002;30(3):581–585.

Rowe BH, Travers AH, Holroyd BR, et al. Nebulized ipratropium bromide in acute pediatric asthma: does it reduce hospital admissions among children presenting to the emergency department? *Ann Emerg Med* 1999;34:75–85.

Streetman DD, Bhatt-Mehta V, Johnson CE. Management of acute, severe asthma in children. *Ann Pharmacother* 2002;36:1249–1260.

Williams JR, Bothner JP, Swanton RD. Delivery of albuterol in a pediatric emergency department. *Pediatr Emerg Care* 1996;12(4):263–267.

Zemuron (rocuronium) package insert. West Orange, NJ: Organon, Inc., 2002.

CHAPTER

25

Ian M. Paul
Richard L. Levine

Drug Therapy in the Adolescent

Adolescence is a novel period in human development in which marked physical and physiologic changes occur. These are compounded by the psychosocial development and evolution toward social independence that also occur during these years. These changes affect the way medications and therapeutic strategies are initiated, monitored, and maintained as the individual transitions from childhood to adulthood. Because adolescents share many physiologic similarities with adults, they may not quite be the "therapeutic orphans" (1) that younger children continue to be. Still, they are not simply smaller versions of adults. As recently as the early 20th century, it was suggested in medical literature that 15-year-old children should receive three-fourths of adult doses because they were nearly three-fourths as old as the adult age of 21 years (2). Although science has advanced considerably over the last century, the literature focused on therapeutics for adolescents for many decades revealed a paucity of data relating to the pharmacokinetic and pharmacodynamic changes that occur during this distinctive period of life.

Table 25.1 depicts the various factors that the clinician may consider when designing a therapeutic strategy for an adolescent. These physical, physiologic, and environmental factors influence the often delicate balance between desired and undesired drug effects (3). As the understanding of genetics and the human genome improves, pharmacogenetics will increasingly influence the way diseases are diagnosed and therapeutic strategies are designed for all people, including adolescents (4).

PHYSICAL CHANGES DURING ADOLESCENCE

PHYSICAL GROWTH

Adolescents experience marked changes in their physical size and body composition. Pubertal changes during adolescence coincide with significant increases in height, which alone account for nearly 25% of total adult height (5). Male and female adolescents, respectively, average nearly 10 and 8 increases in height per year during the period of maximal growth rate (6). The normal timing and variability of these increases in height, weight, and pubertal development for both genders have been well established (Figs. 25.1 and 25.2) (7–9). The changes in body size often cause difficulty in determining which measure of size should be used for calculating doses of medications. Although most drugs are dosed according to body weight, in other instances the use of body surface area may be more appropriate (10).

Coinciding with the growth acceleration is the significant growth of organs during adolescence (Fig. 25.3), some of which have pharmacologic implications (11,12). For example, urinary clearance of carbamazepine to its metabolites has been shown to be proportional to liver volume relative to body weight (13). Similarly, liver weight was recently shown to be a better parameter for determining warfarin doses than is body weight for growing Japanese children and adolescents (14). In contrast, lorazepam, antipyrine, and indocyanine green did not exhibit age-related changes in clearance based on liver volume when normalized to body surface area (15). Another organ, the small intestine, grows in length and therefore increases its absorptive surface area linearly in relation to body length. Small bowel length has been shown to be the most accurate variable for determining the necessary dose of cyclosporine after liver transplantation for patients younger than 20 years (16,17). Last, the kidneys not only increase in size but also undergo a maturation of their microanatomy that is completed during adolescence (18,19). The growth of the kidney equates with a maximal glomerular volume and absolute number of glomeruli, which both subsequently decline progressively with advancing age (20).

CHANGES IN BODY COMPOSITION

Many of the important changes in body composition that occur during childhood and adolescence have been described by Friis-Hansen (12,21). During the teenage years, differences in composition between males and females may be more pronounced than during any other period of life. Although males increase the percentage of total body water and reduce the percentage of body fat, females experience the opposite trend (Fig. 25.3). Lean body mass and muscle thickness also increase during adolescence, more rapidly in males than in females, reaching their peak before beginning a progressive decline in early adulthood (22,23). Blood flow to the muscle is also greater during this period and then, too, diminishes gradually

TABLE 25.1 Physical, Physiologic, and Environmental Considerations When Prescribing Drug Regimens for the Adolescent

Physical and Physiologic Factors	*Environmental Factors*
Weight	Drug interactions
Height	Tobacco smoking
Body surface area	Alcohol intake
Nutritional status	Drugs of abuse
Lean body mass	Oral contraceptives
Adipose tissue	Occupational exposures
Organ size	Social maturity
Genetics	Compliance
Sex	
Age	
Pubertal stage	
Disease state	
Pregnancy	
Lactation	

with age (24). Similar findings related to tissue perfusion have been reported for the eye (25). The capillary vasculature supplying the musculature also evolves. Adolescents have increased numbers of capillaries per muscle fiber compared with younger children, but less per fiber than in adults (26). Individually and collectively, these changes in body size and composition may influence the pharmacokinetics of drugs and can be part of the source of gender-related differences in drug metabolism, which are seen less in younger children.

CHANGES IN DRUG DISPOSITION AND METABOLISM DURING ADOLESCENCE

During this time of physical growth, numerous physiologic changes occur that affect the way the body processes xenobiotics. This evolution causes differences to varying degrees in each stage of drug metabolism that distinguish this population from those younger and older.

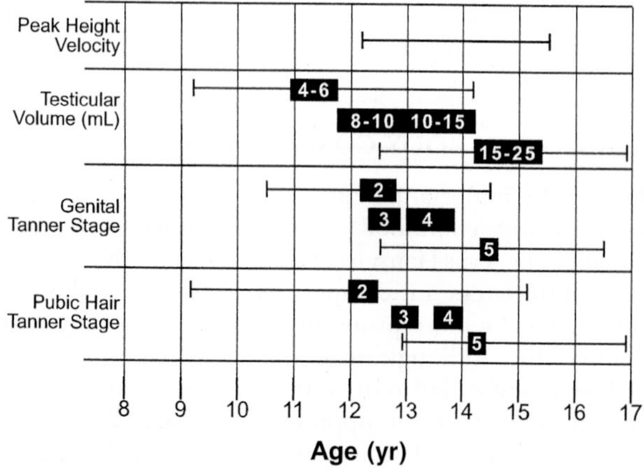

Figure 25.1. The normal timing and variability of the initiation, stages, and completion of pubertal events for males (12). (Adapted from Mansbach JM, Gordon CM. Demystifying delayed puberty. *Contemp Pediatr* 2001;18(4):43–62, with permission.)

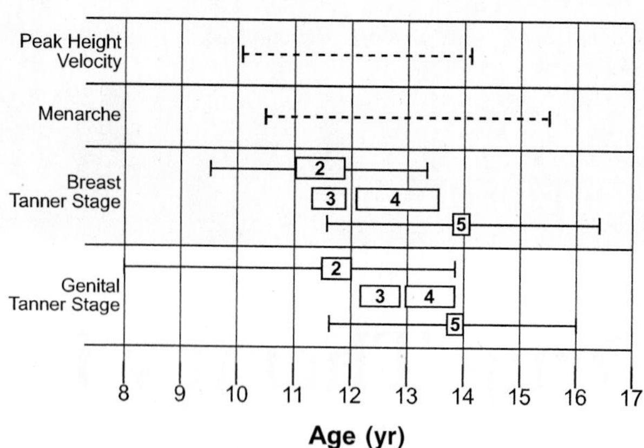

Figure 25.2. The normal timing and variability of the initiation, stages, and completion of pubertal events for females (12). (Adapted from Mansbach JM, Gordon CM. Demystifying delayed puberty. *Contemp Pediatr* 2001;18(4):43–62, with permission.)

ABSORPTION

Oral Administration

Drugs encounter a complex array of digestive enzymes and hostile environments during passage through the gastroin-

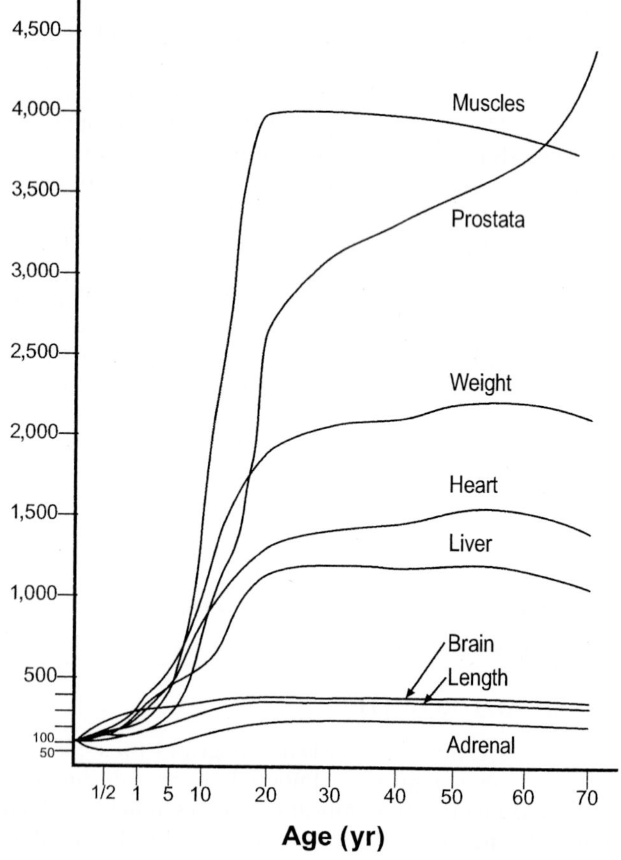

Figure 25.3. The increase in weight of different organs expressed as percentage of their weight in the newborn. (From Friis-Hansen B. Body composition during growth. *In vivo* measurements and biochemical data correlated to differential anatomical growth. *Pediatrics* 1971;47(1, Suppl 2): 264–274, with permission.)

testinal tract. Although similar to adults and younger children in most regards, the adolescent has certain features that differ from other age groups. Digestion and metabolism for drugs taken enterally begins in the mouth from contact with saliva. The rate of parotid gland saliva secretion markedly decreases in childhood, reaching adult levels during adolescence, a rate that is 10% to 15% of that in a 3-year-old child (27). The gastric pH and rate of gastric emptying, in contrast, are relatively constant outside of the neonatal period (28). Distal to the stomach, the small intestinal transit time is also known to be relatively constant, suggesting that the velocity of travel increases as children grow (29,30). In contrast, colonic motility during adolescence is reduced compared with that in younger children (31). Finally, the activity of some enzymes involved in extrahepatic biotransformation located in the intestinal mucosa may differ during this time of life, but the activity of enzymes released by the pancreas does not (32,33).

These physiologic changes may account for some of the variability in bioavailability of drugs after oral administration and for the differing rates of absorption seen during adolescence (34). Just as calcium absorption increases during puberty to account for metabolic needs, the amount of a given drug that is absorbed by the intestine may vary with age (35). For example, lower serum levels of penicillin were found in older children and adolescents compared with infants after oral administration (36). This was partially attributed to a reduced absorption in that population. Next, inconsistent absorption of sustained-released theophylline within and between subjects including adolescents has resulted in variable serum levels (37). In addition to the amount absorbed, significantly slower absorption of midazolam has been demonstrated for children between ages 12 and 16 years when compared with those younger than age 12 (38).

Another factor that may account for differences is the change in gut flora that occurs with age. This evolution can influence the absorption of medications as demonstrated by the increasing ability of these bacteria to metabolize digoxin throughout childhood (39). The adult pattern of metabolism is not reached until adulthood, reflecting the development of enzymes such as β-glucosidase and reductases secreted by these intestinal organisms (40).

Topical Application

As for absorption through the skin, the major change between adolescents and other age groups is the surface area for potential exposure, which proportionally decreases with increasing body size. The physiology and percutaneous absorption of drugs, however, appear to be relatively constant throughout life (41). One potential source of variability may be the known reduction in cutaneous blood perfusion between childhood and adulthood, though limited research has been performed to demonstrate the effect of this variable (42).

DISTRIBUTION

Body Composition

Changes in drug distribution throughout the body that occur during adolescence can largely be attributed to the physical growth and redistribution of body compartments. For example, lipophilic drugs, such as many psychoactive medications, may have shorter half-lives in adolescents than in younger children and adults because of the reduction in body fat that generally occurs during these years (43). Similar results have been seen for lipid-soluble anesthetic agents such as thiopental and propofol, the latter of which was shown to require increased doses for induction of anesthesia for adolescents and those with greater lean body mass than for older, fatter patients (44,45). In contrast, theophylline was shown to have a longer half-life in adolescents related to an increase in lean body mass (46).

Protein Binding

Changes in plasma proteins also influence drug distribution and are known to vary with age. Beginning in adolescence, there is a progressive decline with age of serum levels of albumin but an increase of α_1-acid glycoprotein (47). This causes differences in affinity for medications after adolescence, resulting in increased amounts of some unbound drugs such as desipramine, salicylic acid, phenytoin, and lidocaine but reduced amounts of other unbound drugs, including chlorpromazine (47,48). In contrast, seizure medications such as valproic acid and carbamazepine that have a narrow therapeutic window fortunately do not appear to have changes in protein binding among younger children, adolescents, and adults (49–52).

METABOLISM AND CLEARANCE

During the pubescent years, the liver, where the majority of drugs are metabolized, undergoes significant maturational changes. In addition to an increase in size, there are also changes in the enzymes and metabolic pathways located within the liver that are responsible for the processing of medications. During this time, it is likely that hormones involved with growth and sexual development have an influence on drug metabolism (53). Though mechanisms for hormonal influences on drug metabolizing enzymes are incompletely understood, it is notable that in general, the developmental pattern of enzymatic activity is inversely related to levels of hormones involved in the hypothalamic-pituitary-gonadal axis and corresponding pubertal stage (9). This inverse relationship is most obvious during the two life stages with the greatest levels of hormonal change, early infancy and adolescence.

Phase-1 Reactions

The cytochrome P450 (CYP) enzymes are responsible for the metabolism of many xenobiotics via oxidation and reduction reactions primarily within the liver. Although these enzyme systems have been shown to mature at varying times throughout development, there are contrasting opinions as to whether these changing activities account for the differences in drug clearance seen among different age groups (54–56). Most agree though that age should be considered an important variable for any evaluation of the CYP system (57). A database recently designed to examine the age-related pharmacokinetic variability of 45 drugs found that the CYP enzymes, individually and collectively, did not contribute to overall variability between

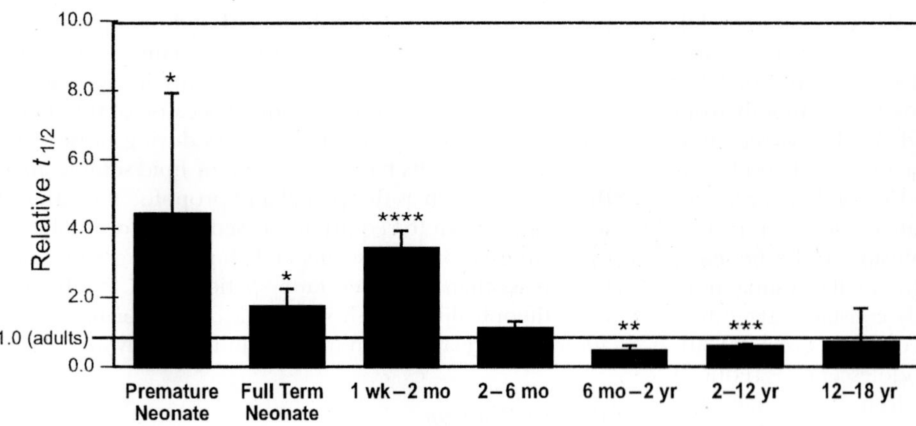

Figure 25.4. Half-life ($t_{1/2}$) results relative to adults for 18 substrates metabolized by cytochrome P450 enzymes. $*p < .05$; $**p < .01$; $***p < .001$; $****p < .0001$. (From Ginsberg G, Hattis D, Sonawane B, et al. Evaluation of child/adult pharmacokinetic differences from a database derived from the therapeutic drug literature. *Toxicol Sci* 2002;66:185–200, with permission.)

adolescents and adults, although significant differences did exist between teenagers and younger age groups (Fig. 25.4) (58). Alternatively, one investigation demonstrated reduced clearance of antipyrine after adolescence (59). Because antipyrine is a widely used marker for overall hepatic drug-metabolizing capacity due to the numerous CYP enzymes involved in its metabolism, this is particularly noteworthy (60). Confounding the issue further, both antipyrine and another drug used as a marker for similar reasons, indocyanine green, demonstrated weight-adjusted clearance values that correlated significantly with age from childhood through adolescence into adulthood (61,62). These correlations disappeared, however, when these values were adjusted for body surface area.

The need for continued investigation in this area is highlighted by several studies that indicate that levels of individual enzyme activity do vary with age including during adolescence. For example, a frequently cited study employed isotopically labeled CO_2 to evaluate cytochrome P450 metabolism of caffeine (63). The (3–^{13}C-methyl) caffeine breath test described in this investigation demonstrated that clearance mediated by CYP1A2 declined to adult levels during adolescence, but that girls achieved this earlier in puberty (Tanner stage 2) than did boys (Tanner stage 5). Similarly, theophylline clearance was found to diminish linearly with increasing age for participants aged 1 to 30 years (64). Proton-pump inhibitors such as omeprazole and lansoprazole, metabolized primarily by CYP2C19, demonstrated a reduction in clearance during adolescence and adulthood when compared with younger children (65,66). Similar results were shown for the metabolism of phenytoin by CYP2C9 and chlorpromazine by CYP2D6 (67,68). Furthermore, two investigations reported that carbamazepine is converted to its epoxide metabolite by CYP3A4 at a faster rate in younger children than in older children and adolescents, with a resultant higher ratio of metabolite to parent compound existing in the younger age groups (69,70). Finally, a progressive decline in cyclosporine clearance by CYP3A4 from childhood through adolescence into adulthood has also been demonstrated, which remained even after adjustment for body surface area (71).

Although hepatocytes are the primary location where these enzymes metabolize drugs, they are also abundant in other tissues (72). Within enterocytes, CYP3A4 levels were recently shown to increase with age throughout childhood into adolescence (73). This potentially could modify drug bioavailability after oral administration.

Phase-2 Reactions

The ontogeny of nonoxidative metabolic reactions, which include acetylation, sulfation, glucuronidation, and glutathione conjugation, has received considerably less attention in adolescent pharmacology despite their significant contribution to the metabolism and clearance of xenobiotics. In contrast to the results described for the CYP enzymes, the pharmacokinetic database described previously was indeed able to detect overall age-related changes in phase-2 reactions, notably glucuronidation, between adolescents and adults (Fig. 25.5) (58). Lorazepam, morphine, valproic acid, and zidovudine were some of the substrates included in this pharmacokinetic analysis.

From individual analyses, when normalized for body surface area, lorazepam was shown to have increased clearance with age through adolescence into adulthood (61). The opposite result was demonstrated for busulfan, where enterocyte glutathione S-transferase activity declined with age through adolescence (74). Conflicting with the collective and individual findings, zidovudine when examined alone was not shown to have age-related variability in conjugation and overall metabolism among young children, adolescents, and adults (61,75).

For acetylation, the presence of a bimodal phenotypic distribution of metabolism has emerged, with individuals classified as either fast or slow acetylators (76). This distribution appears to vary as a function of age, with an increased prevalence of fast acetylators younger than 15 years compared with older individuals (77). During childhood, the distribution also changes, with the frequency of fast acetylators increasing until age 4 and then remaining relatively constant throughout the remainder of childhood and adolescence (78).

Importantly, there are also age-related changes in the predominance of specific metabolic pathways. Overall, the rate of acetaminophen clearance remains constant with age. In contrast to adults and adolescents, however, for young children, sulfation, not glucuronidation, is the principal method of conjugation for both acetaminophen and salicylamide (79,80). It is not until approximately age

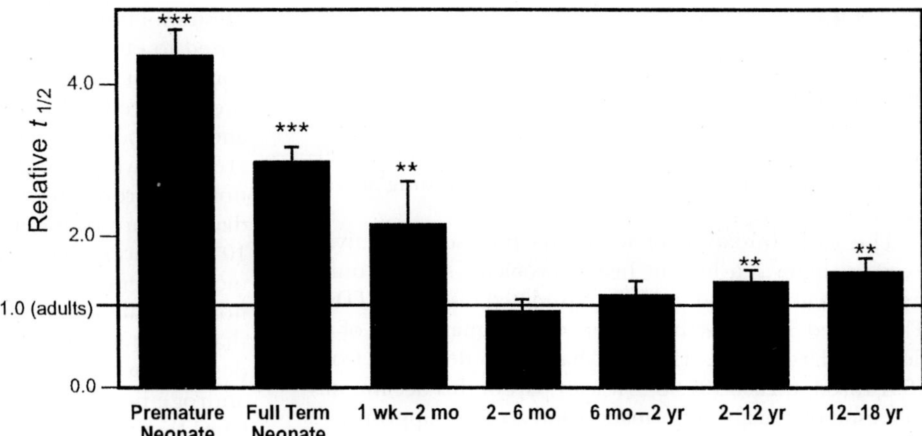

Figure 25.5. Half-life ($t_{1/2}$) results relative to adults for glucuronidation substrates (lorazepam, morphine, oxazepam, trichloroethanol, valproic acid, zidovudine). $^{**}p < .05$; $^{***}p < .01$. (From Ginsberg G, Hattis D, Sonawane B, et al. Evaluation of child/adult pharmacokinetic differences from a database derived from the therapeutic drug literature. *Toxicol Sci* 2002;66:185–200, with permission.)

12 that the adult pattern develops where glucuronidation predominates (79).

ELIMINATION

The kidney is responsible for the elimination of the majority of water-soluble compounds and fat-soluble substrates that are metabolized to hydrophilic agents, though other organs such as the lung, biliary tract, intestines, and skin contribute to the excretion of drugs (81). Kidney function as measured by the glomerular filtration rate is relatively constant outside of infancy. Another important function of the kidney, tubular reabsorption, also varies little throughout childhood into adulthood and is not influenced by pubertal stage (82).

One renal parameter that does appear to develop throughout childhood and adolescence is tubular secretion, which was shown to decline with advancing age for uric acid (83). When this function was tested using digoxin as the substrate, similar results were obtained (84,85). The net tubular secretion of digoxin declined during adolescence to amounts seen in adults, but appeared to better correlate with Tanner staging and therefore sexual maturity than with age alone. Methotrexate, which is excreted by the kidney via glomerular filtration and tubular secretion, also shows reduced clearance as a function of age through adolescence (86). Tubular secretion may also account for the differences in renal ceftriaxone and theophylline clearance that occur during adolescence (87,88).

THERAPEUTIC CONSIDERATIONS

DIFFERENCES BETWEEN SEXES

Because the physical and hormonal disparities between males and females are much greater during adolescence than in other parts of childhood, it is at this age that pharmacokinetic variability between the sexes may first become prominent. Differences may affect nearly all aspects of drug disposition and metabolism. Beginning with absorption, intestinal transit time differs between sexes, which may influence the bioavailability of some drugs when administered orally (89). As for distribution, the significant differences in lipid and lean body compartments between sexes (Fig. 25.6) can affect the pharmacokinetics of many drugs, particularly those that are lipophilic. Numerous sex-related differences in drug metabolism have also been described with distinctive activity levels for some, but not all phase-1 and -2 enzymes (90,91). Because the genes for these enzymes are located on autosomal chromosomes, it is presumed that differences in activity likely result from interactions with endogenous hormones (92). Finally, the influence of the menstrual cycle on pharmacokinetics and pharmacodynamics is controversial, with conflicting data supporting an effect and a lack thereof (93). Although the majority of sex- or menstrual-related differences are minor, there are instances when the disparity can cause significant effects. A frequently cited example is the greater prolongation of the QT interval for women given cardiovascular medications than for men (94,95). The associated increased risk for torsades de pointes may also be influenced by the menstrual cycle (96).

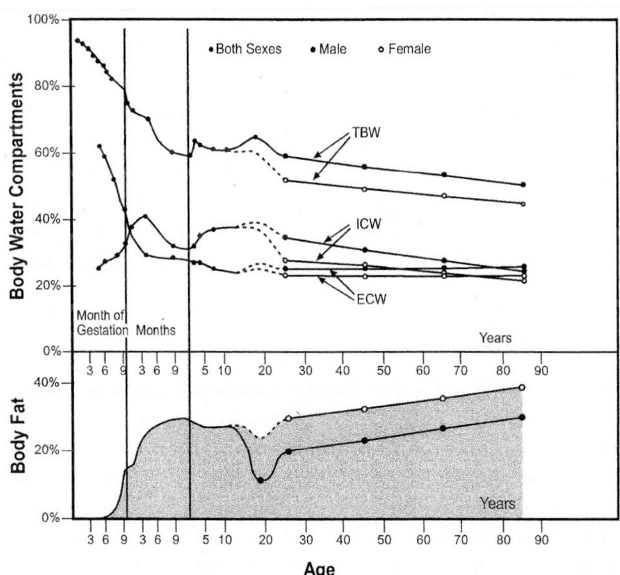

Figure 25.6. Changes in total body water (TBW), intracellular water (ICW), extracellular water (ECW), and fat content of the body from early fetal life to old age. (From Friis-Hansen B. Body composition during growth. In vivo measurements and biochemical data correlated to differential anatomical growth. *Pediatrics* 1971;47(1, Suppl 2):264–274, with permission.)

CONTRACEPTION

The extraordinary changes that occur during adolescence include the development of a sexual identity. In addition, adolescents have feelings of invulnerability as part of their normal development. This combination can lead to significant risk-taking behavior by adolescents including sexual activity.

The early initiation of teenagers into sexual activity exposes them to a host of health problems such as unintended pregnancy and sexually transmitted diseases (STDs). The United States has the highest teen pregnancy rate of all developed countries. This rate had been declining from 1991 through 2005 (97,98). At least part of this decline was the result of available information and access to appropriate contraception. The birth rate for the youngest teens, aged 10 to 14 years, continued this decline in 2006. Unfortunately, the birth rate for teens 15 to 19 years increased 3% in 2006 (99).

There are many effective forms of contraception for adolescents, though none are completely effective at preventing pregnancy or STDs. These include nonhormonal/barrier methods and hormonal methods. A general rule for contraception for adolescents is that the use of two methods simultaneously is better than one alone, and one method should always be a condom to protect against the spread of STDs including the human immunodeficiency virus (HIV).

Contraception efficacy is measured by its success or failure rate (100). This includes its theoretical effectiveness with correct and consistent use and its actual or typical use effectiveness rate (98,100). Because of various developmental and social factors, teens generally have lower actual use efficacy rates (100).

The nonhormonal/barrier methods include the condom, the female condom, the diaphragm, and the cervical cap. Timing ovulation via the rhythm method to avoid pregnancy, withdrawal before male ejaculation, and vaginal douching after intercourse are not effective forms of contraception.

The last several decades have seen an evolution of hormonal methods of contraception, with numerous currently available options. These include oral, injectable, and implantable contraceptives; the intrauterine device (IUD); emergency contraception; and newer forms of contraception including the contraceptive patch and the vaginal ring.

Oral Contraceptives

Oral contraceptives include the combined oral contraceptive (COC) pill and the progestin-only contraceptive pill (Table 25.2). There are two forms of COCs, including fixed dose and multiphasic pills. All of the COCs contain an estrogenic component and a progestational component. Most COCs contain 21 days of combined estrogens and progestin with 7 days of inert pills during which withdrawal bleeding occurs. One formulation (Mircette™) contains only 2 days of placebo pills to limit estrogen withdrawal symptoms, whereas others (Loestrin® Fe, Estrostep® Fe) contain iron during the week without hormones (98,101). The current estrogen component of most COCs is ethinyl estradiol at a dose of 20 to 35 μg per tablet (98,102,103). Mestranol is found in a small number of pills and is metabolized to ethinyl estradiol (98,102,103). The progesterone component includes the older progestins such as norethindrone, norethindrone acetate, norgestrel, levonorgesterol, and ethynodiol diacetate, but the potencies of these agents are somewhat controversial (98,102,103). In general, norethindrone, norethindrone acetate, and ethynodiol diacetate are considered equally potent; norgestrel is 5 to 10 times more potent, and levonorgesterol is 10 to 20 times more potent (103). The newer progestin pills contain norgestimate and desogestrel, and there is some evidence that the new progestins have a greater amount of the desired progestational effect and fewer undesirable androgenic side effects (98,102,103). Two additional COC that are relatively new (Yasmin® and Yaz®) contain drospirenone, which is an antimineralcorticoid derivative of spironolactone developed to limit COC-associated weight gain (103,104). It also has some antiandrogenic effects and might be a good choice for patients with hyperandrogenism such as polycystic ovary syndrome (105). In addition, there are two new extended cycle oral contraceptive on the market called Seasonale® and Seasonique™, which contains ethinyl estradiol and levonorgesterol in a 91-day cycle—84 active pills with 7 placebo pills or very low estrogen pills. These are helpful in patients with menstrual-related medical issues such as menstrual migraines (105). There are no studies in adolescents on the newest extended cycle pill, Lybrel®, which is given continuously, 365 days per year.

Mechanism of Action

The mechanism of action of all of the COCs includes (a) inhibition of ovulation; (b) modification of cervical mucous to make it more viscid, thus limiting spermatic motility; (c) alteration of the endometrium to make it unsuitable for implantation; and (d) reduction of fallopian tubule motility (102,103). The theoretical effectiveness of COCs is 99.9%, but the actual efficacy ranges between 92% and 95% (92% for adolescents) (98,100,102,103). A number of measures are utilized to increase adolescent compliance including comprehensive education about the pills and their health benefits, counseling regarding the logistics of using the pills, and close follow-up (100,102,103).

Health Benefits

It is very important to consider the health benefits of COCs for adolescents. First, there are the menstrual benefits. COCs have an antiproliferative effect on the endometrium and thus reduce menstrual flow, the duration of menstruation, and subsequently the occurrence of menstruation-related anemia (98,102,106). In addition, menstrual periods are more regular, and midcycle pain, or Mittelschmerz, is reduced because ovulation is inhibited (102,106). Young women with anovulation and dysfunctional uterine bleeding have significantly more regular, predictable cycles as well (102,106,107). Dysmenorrhea is also markedly reduced in young women with use of COCs (102,106,108). In fact, many young women primarily use COCs for this purpose. COCs produce this effect through a reduction in the production of prostaglandin $F_{2\alpha}$ by decreasing the proliferation of the endometrium

TABLE 25.2 Oral Contraceptive Formulations Currently Available in the United States

Group	*Brand Name*	*Estrogen*	*Progestin*	*Inactive Tablets Include and Miscellaneous Comments*
Progestin only	Micronor	...	Norethindrone, 0.35 mg	
Estrogen, 20 μg	Loestrin 21 1/20	EE	Norethindrone, 1 mg	
	Loestrin FE 1/20	EE	Norethindrone, 1 mg	75 mg ferrous fumarate
	Mircette	EE	Desogestrel, 0.15 mg	EE 10 μg (last 5 d)
	Alesse	EE	Levonorgestrel, 0.1 mg	
	Lybrel	EE	Levonorgestrel, 0.90 mg	taken continuously 365 d/yr)
	Yaz	EE	Drospirenone, 3 mg	4 inactive pills
	Loestrin 24 Fe	EE	Norethindrone, 1 mg	4 inactive pills, 75 mg ferrous fumarate
Estrogen, 25 μg	Levlen 21	EE	Levonorgestrel, 0.15 mg	
Estrogen, 30 μg	Seasonale	EE	Levonorgestrel, 0.15 mg	84 pills
	Seasonique	EE	Levonorgestrel, 0.15 mg	84 pills, 7 with 10 μg EE
	Loestrin 21 1.5/30	EE	Norethindrone, 1.5 mg	
	Loestrin FE 1.5/30	EE	Norethindrone, 1.5 mg	75 mg ferrous fumarate
	Lo/Ovral-28	EE	Norgestrel, 0.3 mg	
	Low-Ogestrel 21	EE	Norgestrel, 0.3 mg	
	Nordette	EE	Levonorgestrel, 0.15 mg	
	Ortho-Cept	EE	Desogestrel, 0.15 mg	
	Yasmin	EE	Drospirenone, 3 mg	
Estrogen, 35 μg	Demulen 1/35–21	EE	Ethynodiol diacetate, 1 mg	
	Demulen 1/35–28	EE	Ethynodiol diacetate, 1 mg	
	Modicon 28	EE	Norethindrone, 0.5 mg	
	Norinyl 1 + 35, 21 d	EE	Norethindrone, 1 mg	
	Ortho-Cyclen 28	EE	Norgestimate, 0.25 mg	
	Ortho-Novum 1/35–28	EE	Norethindrone, 1 mg	
	Ovcon 35	EE	Norethindrone, 0.4 mg	
	Balziva-21	EE	Norethindrone, 0.4 mg	
Estrogen, 50 μg	Demulen 1/50–21	EE	Ethynodiol diacetate, 1 mg	
	Demulen 1/50–28	EE	Ethynodiol diacetate, 1 mg	
	Ogestrel 0.5/50–21	EE	Norgestrel, 0.5 mg	
	Ogestrel 0.5/50–28	EE	Norgestrel, 0.5 mg	
	Ovcon 50	EE	Norethindrone, 1 mg	
	Norinyl 1+50, 21 d	Mestranol	Norethindrone, 1 mg	
	Ortho-Novum 1/50–28	Mestranol	Norethindrone, 1 mg	
Biphasics	Necon 10/11–21	EE, 35 μg	Norethindrone, 0.5/1 mg	
	Ortho-Novum 10/11–28	EE, 35 μg	Norethindrone, 0.5/1 mg	
Multiphasics	Cyclessa	EE, 25 μg	Desogestrel, 0.1/0.125/0.15 mg	
	Ortho Tri-Cyclen Lo	EE, 25 μg	Norgestimate, 0.18/0.215/0.25 mg	
	Triphasil-28	EE, 30/40/30 μg	Levonorgestrel, 0.050/0.075/0.125 mg	
	Estrostep 21	EE, 20/30/35 μg	Norethindrone, 1 mg	
	Estrostep FE	EE, 20/30/35 μg	Norethindrone, 1 mg	75 mg ferrous fumarate
	Ortho-Novum 7/7/7–28	EE, 35 μg	Norethindrone, 0.5/0.75/1 mg	
	Ortho Tri-Cyclen 28	EE, 35 μg	Norgestimate, 0.18/0.215/0.25 mg	
	Tri-Norinyl-28	EE, 35 μg	Norethindrone, 0.5/1/0.5 mg	

EE, ethinyl estradiol.
Adapted from Nelson AL, Neinstein LS. Combination hormonal contraceptives. In: Neinstein LS, ed. *Adolescent health care: a practical guide*, 5th ed. Philadelphia, PA: Lippincott Williams & Wilkins, 2008:598–600, with permission.

(106,108). Polycystic ovary syndrome is often treated with COCs using continuous dosing for 2, 3, or more months without the placebo weeks (106). This serves to limit androgen excess by decreasing ovarian androgen production via inhibition of luteinizing hormone secretion (106). In addition, COCs increase sex hormone-binding globulin, which decrease free testosterone levels (106).

Other health benefits include (a) a reduction in the risk of benign breast disease including fibroadenomas and fibrocystic disease (109); (b) treatment of mild-to-moderate cystic acne (110,111); and (c) protection against dysfunctional uterine bleeding, ectopic pregnancy, pelvic infections, ovarian cancer, and endometrial cancer (102,106,107,111–114).

Effects on Metabolism and Potential Adverse Effects

Potential adverse effects of COCs include medically significant complications generally related to oncogenic potential, circulatory complications including the risk of thromboembolism, hepatic changes, and lipid abnormalities.

The potential impact of COCs on the development of breast cancer is not clear and has become controversial. Studies have produced conflicting results regarding the incidence of breast cancer in patients who have taken COCs (102,103,115,116). For example, two recent studies indicated a slight increase in the risk of breast cancer in long-term users of COCs (117,118). One of these studies found that the new, lower estrogen pills imparted a lower risk than earlier, higher potency COCs (118). However, another recent investigation found no association between current or former COC use and the risk of breast cancer (119).

There is more certainty regarding the lack of association between COCs and other forms of cancer. As previously mentioned, studies indicate that COCs have a protective effect on the development of endometrial cancer by preventing unopposed stimulation by estrogen (102, 103,115,116). In addition, patients who have taken COCs have a decreased incidence of ovarian cancer, and there seems to be no effect on the development of cervical cancer (102,103,111–113,115,116).

There are also a number of consistent metabolic effects of COCs. One of the most significant is the effect on the extrinsic clotting pathway. Fibrinogen and factors I, V, VII, VIII, and X are increased, and fibrinolytic and anticoagulation factors are increased as well (102,103,115). The balance of these changes can increase the risk of thromboembolism with COC (102,103,115). There is a clear relationship between the dose of estrogen in the COC and the risk of thromboembolism, with higher doses producing an increased risk (101–103,115,116). The overall incidence of venous thromboembolism is 15 to 30 per 10,000 woman-years for the low-dose pill formulations, but is known to be greater for patients with the factor V Leiden gene mutation (101–103,115,117). As for the risk of venous thrombosis with the new progestins desogestrel and gestodene, some epidemiologic studies suggested that they are associated with a higher risk, whereas other researchers claimed that these studies are flawed and that there is no actual increased risk (101,103).

Fortunately, there does not appear to be an increased risk of cerebrovascular accidents or myocardial infarctions in patients on low-dose COCs (102,103,115,116). Smoking does, however, increase the risk of all types of cardiovascular disease with use of COCs (98,102,103,115,116). Clearly, practitioners should discourage smoking for all adolescents, but nevertheless it is not considered a contraindication to the prescription of COCs for teens (98,102,103).

There are several other effects of COCs that can affect their own pharmacology as well as those for other drugs. As previously described, estrogen increases the hepatic synthesis of various binding globulins including sex hormone-binding globulin, thyroid-binding globulin, and corticosteroid-binding globulin (102,103). Estrogen increases the production of renin and results in an increase in angiotensin, but this rarely causes a significant increase in blood pressure for adolescents (102,103). Lipid changes, however, are potentially significant, with increases in total cholesterol, high-density-lipoprotein cholesterol, and triglyceride levels and a decrease in low-density-lipoprotein cholesterol level (102,103,116). This results from the androgen effects of the progestin component of the COC. The new progestins have fewer androgen effects and thus less of an impact on lipids (102,103,116). Both the estrogen and progestin components of COCs can affect glucose metabolism, and the progestins can increase insulin resistance (102,103,116). Clinically, though, the newer COCs have no significant impact on glucose tolerance, and even most patients with diabetes mellitus tolerate COCs without increases in insulin requirements (102,103,116). Finally, COCs can have an impact on laboratory testing. For example, total thyroxine levels can be elevated due to the increase in thyroid-binding globulin, but free thyroxine levels are unaffected and remain normal (102,103).

COCs may produce other minor side effects due to hormonal imbalances related to the estrogenic and progestational components (102,103). Estrogenic-related side effects include nausea and vomiting; headaches including migraines; postmenstrual breakthrough bleeding; and fluid retention, which can result in edema, leg cramps, and bloating (102,103). Progestational-related side effects include fatigue, depression, increased breast size, and pre- or postmenstrual breakthrough bleeding (102,103). There are also side effects from the androgenic effects of the progestins, including acne, increased appetite and weight gain, and hirsutism, which can be limited by selecting one of the new progestins that have fewer androgenic effects (102,103). Changing the formulation of the prescribed COC can usually treat many of these minor complications, and current clinical care deems that the many advantages of COC use during adolescence often outweigh the other, generally small potential risks (102,103,116).

Drug Interactions

Drug–drug interactions are also important to consider with COCs. These may occur because of changes in absorption, alteration of serum protein binding, and changes in hepatic metabolism (102,116). The induction of CYP enzymes can be a significant cause of alterations in drug metabolism (102,116). Drug–drug interactions with COCs can alter both the metabolism and action of the COC as well as the other drug (102,116). Medications that can affect the efficacy of COCs include antibiotics such as rifampin and griseofulvin and the anticonvulsants phenytoin, phenobarbital, carbamazepine, and ethosuximide (102,116,120). Drugs whose activity may be modified by COC use include nonsteroidal anti-inflammatory agents, narcotics, anticoagulants, antidepressants, benzodiazepines, corticosteroids, methylxanthines, and immunomodulating medications (102,116,121).

Contraindications

Absolute contraindications to the use of COCs include (a) a history of a cerebral vascular accident or coronary artery disease, (b) migraines with focal neurologic symptoms, (c) a history of a thromboembolic disorder, (d) impaired liver function including cholestatic jaundice and hepatic tumor, (e) an estrogen-dependent neoplasm including breast cancer or endometrial cancer, (f) undiagnosed genital bleeding, and (g) pregnancy (98,102,103). Relative contraindications include (a) an abnormal breast exam; (b) diabetes mellitus; (c) lipid abnormalities; (d) uncomplicated migraine headaches; (e) depression; and (f) gallbladder, heart, or kidney disease (although in clinical practice, many of these patients tolerate and actually do well on COCs) (98,102,103).

Prescribing Guidelines

Practical guidelines regarding the use of COCs in adolescents include the following (102,103):

1. Use a low-dose-estrogen COC to limit estrogenic side effects.
2. Consider a new progestin to limit the androgenic side effects of the progestational agents.
3. Use a 28-day pack with a Sunday start for ease of compliance.
4. Recommend dosing of the pills at the same time each day; the evening is preferable if nausea is a side effect.
5. Supply missed-pill instructions: Take two pills per day if the previous day's pill was not taken, and take two pills per day for 2 days if the 2 prior days were missed.
6. Provide safe-sex guidelines including the use of spermicidal lubricated condoms with all sexual encounters to protect teens from pregnancy and STDs including HIV.
7. Consideration should be given to the Quick Start Program, which begins the COC at the time of the first visit which may increase compliance (122).

Progestin-Only Pills

The progestin-only pills or minipills contain only norethindrone 0.35 mg or norgestrel 0.075 mg. They have the advantage of containing only the progestational hormonal component and thus avoid the estrogenic side effects (98,102,103). They can be used in patients for whom the COCs are contraindicated such as patients with a history of systemic lupus erythematosus, congenital heart disease, or thromboembolism (98,102,103). In addition, they can be used in adolescent mothers who are breast-feeding. However, they have a significantly higher incidence of breakthrough bleeding and must be taken at the same time each day to be effective because they have a very short half-life (98,102,103,123). These issues preclude their widespread use in adolescents.

Injectable Hormonal Contraceptives

There are two forms of injectable hormonal contraceptives, depot medroxyprogesterone acetate (DMPA) and a new, combined injectable that contains the long-acting estrogen–estradiol cypionate and the progestin medroxyprogesterone in a lipid base. Because of quality control issues, the latter, long-acting agent is not currently available. This is unfortunate because it had a good side effect profile, though the monthly injections limited its potential use in adolescents (102,124).

Mechanism of Action and Prescribing Guidelines

DMPA has been used outside of the United States since the 1970s, and became available in the United States in 1992 (124). It is administered as a 1-mL intramuscular injection with a dose of 150 mg. The medication consists of the progestational agent suspended in a lipid base, which functions as a long-acting delivery system (124,125). The mechanism of action of DMPA is the same as that of the COCs (124,125). It is recommended that patients receive the injection every 12 weeks, although the agent does prevent ovulation for up to 14 weeks. Traditionally, treatment was to be initiated within 5 days of the onset of menstruation to ensure that the patient is not pregnant and to prevent ovulation during the first month of use (124,125). However, there is a new program called Depot Now, which recommends immediate administration of DMPA at the time of the first visit which improves adherence to its continuation and fewer unintentional pregnancies (126). The typical use failure rate is only 0.3%, and there is no long-term effect on fertility (124,125). However, there is a significant delay in the return of ovulation and fertility after use (124,125). Half of patients will establish fertility 10 months after the last injection, but some patients will not ovulate for up to 18 months (124,125). There is a new formulation, Depo-SubQ Provera™ 104, which contains 104 mg of DMPA and is administered subcutaneously (127). This new route makes home administration possible, although there are no studies in adolescents.

Overall, DMPA is a very good contraceptive choice for adolescents for several reasons (98,103,124,125):

1. It is extremely effective.
2. It is not expensive.
3. It is a private method, which does not require personal use in the home.
4. It potentially limits the incidence of pelvic inflammatory disease (PID) due to the thickened cervical mucous.

Contraindications and Potential Adverse Effects

The few contraindications to this method include undiagnosed genital bleeding, pregnancy, active liver disease, known or suspected breast malignancy, and hypersensitivity to the agent (124,125). Thromboembolism is listed as a contraindication, although there is no evidence of an increase in thromboembolism with this agent (124,125). There are very few drug–drug interactions. With regard to effects on metabolism, there is no effect on coagulation factors, a negligible effect on lipid profiles, and a theoretical impact on glucose tolerance that is not usually of clinical significance (124,125).

There may be significant side effects associated with the use of DMPA, however, which must be taken into consideration. The most common is irregular menstrual periods (98,103,124,125). Patients can experience significant irregular and sometimes heavy menstrual bleeding, especially during the first 3 to 6 months of use, but this usually diminishes over time (98,103,124,125). Menstrual irregularity is the most common reason cited for discontinuation of use by patients (98). Prescribing concomitant ethinyl estradiol or low-dose COC for the first 3 weeks of the patient's cycle with the DMPA for several months can reduce the frequency of irregular bleeding (103,124,125). In addition, amenorrhea can frequently occur after regular use of DMPA (103,124,125). Several studies have demonstrated that 50% of patients will experience amenorrhea after 6 months of use, with the rate increasing to more than 70% after 24 months of use (103,124,125). Some adolescents welcome the amenorrhea, but others are disturbed by the absence of menses. It is important to inform patients of this possibility.

Another significant side effect is weight gain (104,108, 128). Studies are somewhat contradictory on this subject. Some reports have documented a 2-kg weight gain after 1 year of use, increasing with continued use, but other investigations have failed to confirm these findings (124,125,129). A retrospective analysis demonstrated significantly more weight gain over a 1-year period in patients taking DMPA than those taking COCs (129). However, 45% of teens receiving DMPA either did not gain weight or even lost weight (129). Obese adolescents may be particularly vulnerable to weight gain with DMPA, as a recent prospective study demonstrated a mean weight gain of 9.4 kg over 18 months with injections compared with 0.2 kg with oral contraceptives and 3.1 kg with no contraceptive therapy (128). Clearly, counseling must be given to adolescents prescribed DMPA to limit the weight gain that may be associated with this agent (103,124,125,129).

One major concern with long-term use of DMPA is its effect on bone density and the risk of osteopenia and osteoporosis. Adolescence is a critical time for the acquisition of peak bone mass, and the majority of bone mineral acquisition occurs during this time. This bone mineral acquisition is influenced by a number of factors including nutrition, exercise, and the hormonal milieu (130). Estrogen production can be suppressed by DMPA because of its effect on the hypothalamus and the pituitary, leading to a hypoestrogenic state, which can hinder bone mineral acquisition (124,125,131). The glucocorticoid effects of DMPA may also result in demineralization of bone (132). There are therefore significant concerns about a lack of sufficient bone mineral acquisition in adolescents receiving DMPA during this critical time. These concerns were realized from investigations that documented reduced bone mineral density in patients receiving DMPA compared with controls (124,125,132–138). A recent overview of the epidemiologic literature on this topic confirmed this finding, though conflicting results have been shown for adolescents (133). It has been found that DMPA may suppress bone mineral acquisition in adolescents when compared with COCs (134). Although two studies have demonstrated no statistical difference in bone mineral density in adolescents prescribed COCs or DMPA, two others did demonstrate a significant decline in bone mineral density of the lumbar spine and/or hip with DMPA (135,139,140). Importantly, the most recent evaluation showed that while there was significant continuous loss of bone mineral density for young women using DMPA, significant gains in bone mass occurred after DMPA was discontinued (140). Clinically, DMPA is still a convenient, effective agent for contraception in adolescents. It remains a very important contraceptive option for teens, and its continued prescription is recommended by the Society for Adolescent Medicine and the American College of Obstetricians and Gynecologists (141–143). Given the concerns about osteopenia, it is prudent to recommend calcium supplementation and moderate weight-bearing exercise to maximize bone mineral acquisition during this critical time in development (125).

Implantable Contraceptives

Another long-acting progestin is implantable etonogestrel, which was approved in 2006 under the brand name Implanon™. This system consists of one 40 mm × 2 mm rod containing 68 mg of the progestin, etonogestrel. It is approved for up to 3 years of use. Insertion and removal are relatively simple (127,144). The capsule steadily release the compound into the surrounding tissue, from which it is absorbed into the circulation. The progestin effects include thickening of cervical mucous, alteration in tubal motility, endometrial atrophy leading to failure of implantation, and suppression of ovulation. It is a very effective contraceptive with an annual failure rate of less than 1%.

Intrauterine Devices

Intrauterine devices (IUDs) have not been typically used in adolescents. They are particularly recommended for multiparous women in a stable, monogamous relationship with a low risk of STDs, and therefore are used infrequently in the usual adolescent population (144,145). Modern IUDs do not contain a polyfilament tail as previously were used in the original Dalkon Shield IUD, and do not facilitate the spread of vaginal flora to the uterus (144,145). However, IUD users at risk for STDs can have an increased incidence of uterine infection and PID (144,145). Contraindications for use include pregnancy, acute PID, unexplained genital bleeding, acute cervicitis, known or suspected uterine or cervical malignancy, or multiple sexual partners (144,145).

There are two types of IUDs available in the United States, the ParaGard T-380A Copper IUD and the Mirena IUD, which contains levonorgesterol (145). The ParaGard IUD is typically inserted during menses and is effective for 10 years with a failure rate of 0.7% in the first year and 2.7% over 10 years (144,145). The mechanism of action is primarily spermicidal from the release of copper, which interferes with sperm transport. It also causes an inflammatory reaction in the endometrium that is spermicidal (144,145). Side effects include menstrual cramping and bleeding, perforation, embedment, and expulsion of the IUD, which occurs more frequently in nulliparous females (144,145).

Mirena is approved for 5 years of use and is also very effective, with failure rates of less than 0.2% (145). The mechanism of action is via progestin and its effect on cervical mucous as well as on tubal motility and the endometrium (145). Side effects are similar to those of ParaGard and include the progestin side effects (145).

Overall, the IUDs are a very effective form of contraception, but their use in teens is limited. Patients desiring this method of contraception must be screened very carefully and cautioned regarding the risks of multiple sexual partners and STDs (144,145).

Emergency Contraception

Emergency contraception is also known as postcoital contraception and the "morning-after pill."

It is a very important method of treatment to prevent pregnancy in sexually active adolescents who have not used contraception, have been sexually assaulted, or experienced a method failure such as a broken condom.

The mechanisms of action of emergency contraception pills (ECPs) involve prevention of ovulation, fertilization, and implantation (146,147). This occurs primarily through disruption of the luteal phase hormone patterns, resulting in an altered endometrium that is unsuitable for egg implantation (146,148). Other actions include changes in cervical mucous and disruption of tubal motility that prevent fertilization (146,148).

ECPs are very effective and reduce the risk of pregnancy with any particular act of intercourse by 75% (146,148). Although the usual expected pregnancy rate for a single act of intercourse is 8%, with ECP this is reduced to 2% (146–149). After intercourse, the more promptly the method is used, the greater is the success rate (146,148). A large trial published in 1999 regarding ECP demonstrated that ECP given within 12 hours produced a 94% reduction in pregnancy; medication administered 60 to 72 hours after intercourse produced a 50% reduction (147). Although earlier use is preferred, the methods might even be somewhat effective after 72 hours (150).

A traditional form of emergency contraception is the Yuzpe method, which is named after the Canadian physician who first described its use (146–149). The Yuzpe method involves taking a number of standard COCs, containing ethinyl estradiol and norgestrel or levonorgesterol, within 72 hours of unprotected intercourse followed by another dose 12 hours later (146–149). The classic regimen was two Ovral with each dose (146–149). Ovral is a high-estrogen pill containing 50 μg of ethinyl estradiol. This pill is not easily available, however, and alternative pill regimens have been developed (146–149). They include taking four Lo-Ovral®, Nordette®, Levlen®, Triphasil®, or Tri-Levlen® pills or five Alesse® tablets followed by the same number of pills 12 hours later (146,148).

The contraindications for the Yuzpe method of emergency contraception are consistent with those for COCs (146,148). Clinicians have questioned those contraindications, however (146,148). Some feel that the risk of thromboembolism with the short term of hormones in ECPs is negligible (146).

The undesired effects of the Yuzpe method are hormonally related. These include nausea in 30% to 66% of patients and vomiting in 12% to 22% of patients (146–149). These side effects can be prevented or modulated by the use of over-the-counter emetics such as dimenhydrinate or prescription emetics such as promethazine hydrochloride and trimethobenzamide hydrochloride (146,148). It is important to note that there is no known effect on an established pregnancy after implantation from ECPs and there is no known teratogenicity (146,148).

More recently, a product has been marketed specifically for emergency contraception, Plan B® (levonorgestrel), which is a progestin-only contraceptive that inhibits ovulation and prevent pregnancy when taken by women within 72 to 120 hours of unprotected intercourse and does not require a pregnancy test. After a long period of discussion and debate, the Food and Drug Administration (FDA) approved the OTC placement of Plan B® (levonorgestrel) for women 18 years and older in August 2006 (151).

Plan B® has been shown to be generally well tolerated by adolescent women with minor side effects such as nausea, fatigue, and vomiting (152). The change in accessibility was supported by the American Academy of Pediatrics (AAP), though the AAP supported improved availability for all teens and young adults in its policy statement (153). Plan B® remains available as a prescription-only product for women aged 17 and younger. No significant contraindications exist for the use of Plan B® except known pregnancy, hypersensitivity, or undiagnosed genital bleeding (146). Plan B® has a decreased incidence of gastrointestinal side effects, which is one of the main advantages to its use (146,148).

Specialists recommend the distribution of prescriptions in advance to teens who are likely to require ECPs (146,148). In addition, the requirement for an examination and pregnancy test before their use has been questioned (146,148). Therefore, ECPs could theoretically be provided when necessary via the telephone after a history is obtained as long as follow-up office visits are assured (140,141). Importantly, one recent study showed that access to emergency contraception from pharmacies did not change women's sexual behavior, frequency of unprotected intercourse, or acquisition of sexually transmitted infections even for those women 16 years or younger (154,155).

Transdermal Patch

The new transdermal contraceptive patch, OrthoEvra®, delivers 20 μg of ethinyl estradiol and 150 μg of norelgestromin (156). The patch is placed weekly for 3 weeks followed by a 7-day free period and may be applied to various areas of the body including the lower abdomen, upper buttocks, upper outer arm, or upper torso (156). The mechanism of action is the same as for COCs, and the efficacy rate is excellent, with 1.24 pregnancies per 100 woman-years (156,157). The side effects are essentially the same as for COCs except for a higher rate of breakthrough bleeding during the first 3 months (156,157). In addition, 2% to 3% of patients can have local application side effects, which can lead to discontinuation of use (156). There is some evidence that the failure rate may be higher in patients weighing more than 90 kg, although this is true for COC as well (156,158). Because of the ease of its use, this form of contraception may be very attractive for many teens, although its relative visibility cannot ensure complete confidentiality (156).

Vaginal Ring

Another new form of contraception is the vaginal ring (NuvaRing®). The ring is composed of an ethylene vinyl acetate copolymer and contains ethinyl estradiol and etonogestrel (156,159,160). It is placed in the vagina for 3 weeks and then removed for 1 week. With each menstrual cycle, a new ring is inserted (156,159,160). Ethinyl estradiol is released at a rate of 15 μg per day, and serum levels reach their peak 2 to 3 days after insertion, with subsequent decline (156,159,160). Etonogestrel is released at a rate of 12 μg per day with levels peaking by 7 days before declining (156,159,160). The mechanism of action is the same as for COCs, primarily via inhibition of ovulation (156,159,160). It is a very effective form of contraception, with a failure rate of 0.65%, and side effects are similar to those of COCs, with the addition of device-related effects (156,159,160). Some patients have discontinued the ring because of vaginitis, foreign body sensation, expulsion of the ring, and problems during coitus (156,159,160). In general, though, the ring has a very high acceptability rate for adult women. One advantage for adolescents is its confidential nature, but some adolescents are uncomfortable with the required placement and removal (156,159,160). A recent study has shown that negative initial reactions can be overcome, however, with proper assessment by providers, discussion of question and concerns, and an adjustment period by the adolescent (161).

OBESITY

The worldwide prevalence of obesity has reached epidemic proportions, and adolescents have not been spared from this worsening trend (162). In the United States, nearly one in every five teenagers is now considered obese, using the definition of above the 95th percentile of body mass index for age (163). More than one in three adolescents are overweight using the 85th percentile for body mass index as the reference point. Minorities are particularly at risk for this problem, which may have significant pharmacokinetic effects (164–166).

As might be expected, lipophilic drugs are most subject to pharmacokinetic differences in obese individuals due to the increase in volume of distribution. A greater effect is thought to occur with increasing obesity, and numerous other physiologic and metabolic disparities have also been demonstrated (164). These changes include differences in the affinity for plasma proteins, specifically α_1-acid glycoprotein (166,167). Increases in organ mass, cardiac output, blood volume, and splanchnic blood flow have been established, as have changes in hepatic phase-I and -II enzyme activities (168–170). Collectively, these differences may affect drug disposition and metabolism and should be considered when prescribing a therapeutic regimen for this population of adolescents.

CIGARETTE SMOKING

During adolescence, the majority of children will experiment with cigarettes, and in the United States, approximately 30% in this age group become regular smokers (171). Because the polycyclic aromatic hydrocarbons in tobacco smoke are thought to induce some phase-I hepatic enzymes, smoking may significantly affect the pharmacokinetics of drugs metabolized by this system (172,173). The enzymes believed to be most affected are CYP1A1, 1A2, and 2E1. The methylxanthines are a class of drugs commonly cited as having an interaction with tobacco smoke. Both theophylline and caffeine are more rapidly eliminated by smokers (174–176). Interactions have also been described with insulin, antipsychotics, and cardiovascular agents.

PERFORMANCE-ENHANCING AGENTS

An important category of drugs taken by adolescents is the performance-enhancing or ergogenic agents (177). These include nutritional supplements, stimulant diet pills, and hormonal supplements. One report describes these agents as "body image drugs" because they are used in an attempt to enhance both appearance and athletic performance (178). A recent large national survey demonstrated that 4.7% of boys and 1.6% of girls have used some kind of product weekly (179,180). Adolescents in our society are under great pressure to achieve and perform, including on the athletic field. This intense pressure can sometimes induce them to take potentially dangerous supplements for ergogenic purposes (178,181). Adolescents are also under societal pressure regarding their appearance, especially influenced by the media's display of athletes and models who are strikingly thin and/or muscular (180,182). The pressure for thinness for women has been well described and can lead to eating disorders such as anorexia nervosa and bulimia nervosa (182). Men are also coming under pressure to achieve a muscular male body ideal (178,182).

A number of studies have correlated ergogenic drug use with other risk-taking behaviors such as substance use and abuse (183,184). Some of the common supplements currently taken by adolescents include creatine, stimulant diet pills, and the hormonal supplements androstenedione and anabolic steroids (oral and injectable).

Creatine

Creatine is a nutritional supplement commonly used by adolescents to improve muscular and athletic performance (181,184–187). As a nutritional supplement, creatine use is neither banned nor tightly regulated by the FDA (181). One study demonstrated that creatine was used by 23% of a study sample of patients aged 17 to 35 years, with a mean age of 21 (184). Another report on high school students demonstrated that creatine was used by 5.6%, with use varying by school from 1.9% to 9.3% (185). Creatine use increased with age, and the use in the 12th-grade student athlete population was 44% (170). Use by boys was more than by girls in both of these studies (184,185).

Creatine, found naturally in muscle tissue, is a tripeptide consisting of arginine, glycine, and methionine (181,185). It exerts its physiologic effect via conversion to phosphocreatine and is utilized in the regeneration of ATP in muscle tissue (181,185). Athletes use creatine to prolong the time until aerobic metabolism is converted to anaerobic metabolism in muscle tissue during exercise, and creatine has been shown to increase myofibril protein synthesis (181,185).

The normal daily requirement is approximately 2 g (181,185). The dose used as a supplement by athletes consists of a loading dose of 20 to 40 g per day in divided doses with a maintenance dose of 20 g per day also in divided doses (181). Peak levels occur approximately 60 to 90 minutes after ingestion, and it is often taken pre- and post-workout (181). A recent meta-analysis demonstrated that creatine did improve maximal resistance exercise performance in previously trained male athletes (188). One study did show that creatine supplementation improved short-term performance on a cycling ergometer (189). In addition, it has been shown that the addition of creatine to a glucose, taurine, and electrolyte supplement promoted greater gains in muscle mass, lifting volume, and sprint performance (190).

The safety of creatine has not been established. Common side effects include muscular and gastrointestinal cramping, and concerns have been raised about renal dysfunction and damage with creatine supplementation (181,185,191). One report has been published detailing interstitial nephritis in a patient taking creatine supplementation, but more information is needed regarding its safety and efficacy (192).

Diet Pills

Stimulant diet pills are another common supplement taken by adolescents for body image purposes (180,186). Many of these compounds contain ephedra and ephedrine used for weight loss and improvement of athletic performance (193). A Chinese herb, *ma huang*, is noted in a number of supplements and also contains ephedra alkaloids (194). Therefore, manufacturers are not required to provide evidence regarding safety and efficacy. As stimulants, these drugs act as sympathomimetic agents with effects on both α- and β-adrenergic receptors (194). They can therefore have profound effects on cardiac function, heart rate, and blood pressure (194). A recent meta-analysis determined that although these compounds did produce short-term weight loss, there was insufficient data to describe their effects beyond 6 months of use (193). With regard to athletic performance, no controlled studies have been reported on ephedra compounds (193). One group of trials did show that although neither caffeine nor ephedrine had any effect on performance, the combination did produce an increase in performance. Other trials have not shown this effect (195–198).

Numerous reports have delineated the side effects of these stimulant compounds. The previously mentioned meta-analysis summarized the side effects and grouped them into categories (193):

1. Psychiatric: euphoria, agitation, irritability, and anxiety.
2. Autonomic hyperactivity: tremor, jitteriness, insomnia, and increased sweating.
3. Gastrointestinal: nausea, vomiting, abdominal pain, and gastroesophageal reflux.
4. Cardiovascular: palpitations, tachycardia, and hypertension.
5. Neurologic: headache.

Other reports have outlined the risk of severe side effects including the risk of severe cardiovascular and cerebrovascular events such as myocardial infarction, arrhythmias, and stroke (199,200). Another sympathomimetic agent, phenylpropanolamine, became unavailable in 2001 in the United States due to the risk of serious side effects (200). Many investigators are recommending, at the very least, the implementation of tighter regulation and standards for these other potentially dangerous compounds (194,195). In response, the FDA has prohibited sales of dietary supplements containing ephedrine alkaloids effective April 12, 2004 (201).

Hormonal Supplements

Adolescents also use hormonal supplements for ergogenic purposes (202–204). This includes the over-the-counter supplement androstenedione, as well as prescription oral and injectable anabolic steroids. The sales of androstenedione increased in 1998 after the revelation that a popular baseball star was taking the supplement (181). Because it is a metabolic precursor, the compound theoretically acts to increase testosterone levels (181,205,206). One study demonstrated no increase in total testosterone levels in a group of 19- to 29-year-old young men, although serum estradiol and estrone levels were elevated (205). Alternatively, a subsequent study suggested that the dose of 300 mg per day of the compound did increase testosterone levels as well as estradiol levels (206). This would indicate that androstenedione could have anabolic effects (206). This easily available over-the-counter supplement could, therefore, have the same side effect profile as the anabolic steroids (206).

Numerous studies have analyzed the incidence of anabolic steroid use by adolescents. The 2001 Youth Risk Behavior Survey by the Centers for Disease Control and Prevention documented the lifetime use as 5%. In this survey, 6% of male students used anabolic steroids compared with 3.9% of female students (207). Another report examined multiple surveys and showed that the use of anabolic steroids by adolescents declined overall between 1989 and 1996 (208). From 1991 to 1996, however, the use for boys remained steady but actually increased for girls (208). Another study of high school football players in Indiana revealed that 6.3% of participants had used or currently were using the compounds (209). Finally, another report describing middle and high school students demonstrated that a 5.4% of boys and 2.9% of girls use anabolic steroids (210). Studies have also documented increased use of other drugs by adolescents using anabolic steroid as well as other risk-taking behavior (183,184). Importantly, these drugs are banned by athletic organizations including the International Olympic Committee, the National Collegiate Athletic Association, and the National Football League, where testing is performed to detect their use (211).

Anabolic steroids can be used orally and/or by injection, and typically adolescents use both methods (212). There are a number of different patterns of use including (a) "cycling," with several weeks on and then off the drugs; (b) "stacking," with simultaneous use of multiple preparations; and (c) "pyramiding," which involves increasing the dose over time up to 10 to 40 times the usual medically therapeutic dose.

Anabolic steroids exert their anabolic effect by binding to androgen receptors and increasing protein synthesis, leading to increased muscle strength and size (212). They have anticatabolic properties as well, accomplished by improving utilization of protein and blocking the catabolic effect of cortisol (181,212). These compounds do increase muscle size and strength in conjunction with adequate nutrition and training, and their potential athletic benefit is greater in strength-dependent sports such as weight lifting and football (212). Although males have traditionally been more likely to use anabolic steroids, a recent report on a nationally representative US sample demonstrated that over 5% of US high school girls have used anabolic steroids (213).

The adverse effects of prescription anabolic steroids have been well documented (212,214,215). They include (a) acne; (b) hirsutism and virilization in women, (c) gynecomastia, testicular failure, and decreased sexual function in men; (d) abnormal liver function test and liver tumors; (e) premature epiphyseal closure, resulting in short stature; (f) lipid abnormalities, thrombosis, and cardiac effects including myocardial infarction; (g) potential infection with injection of steroids; and (h) psychiatric effects including increased aggression, emotional lability, and psychosis (212,214–216). A recent study has investigated the neuroendocrine and behavioral side effects of high-dose anabolic steroids on normal volunteers. This study demonstrated significant decreases in plasma levels of gonadotropins, gonadal steroids, sex hormone-binding globulin, Free T3 and T4, and thyroid-binding globulin. Changes in Free T4 levels correlated with increased aggressiveness in the study participants. In addition, changes in total testosterone correlated with changes in cognitive function. The study concluded that mood and behavioral side effects may be due in part to hormonal changes induced by the anabolic steroids (217). There have also been concerns regarding the potential for physical drug dependence with continued anabolic steroid use (215).

Prevention efforts have focused on education of adolescent and young adult athletes about the serious health consequences of anabolic steroid use (212). In addition, vigorous drug-testing programs at the collegiate, Olympic, and professional levels have been implemented to detect and prevent the use of these dangerous agents (211,212).

COMPLIANCE AND INAPPROPRIATE USE OF MEDICATIONS

Particularly important to consider for adolescent patients is compliance because investigators have demonstrated varied and conflicting adherence to prescribed regimens for teenagers (218–220). Part of the difficulty is that adolescents may be significantly misinformed regarding medications or have incorrect perceptions about their desired purpose or effects (221). Adolescents also appear to frequently share medications inappropriately including those that may be teratogenic (222). These problems may be compounded by the lack of comfort felt by the majority of pharmacists in adolescent-specific issues, thereby limiting a potential source of valuable information for this population (223).

REFERENCES

1. Shirkey H. Therapeutic orphans. *J Pediatr* 1968;72(1):119–120.
2. Dreyer G, Walker EWA. The determination of the minimal lethal dose of various toxic substances and its relationship to the body weight in warm-blooded animals, together with considerations bearing on the dosage of drugs. *Proc R Soc Med Ser B* 1914; 87:319–330.
3. Vesell ES. Sounding board. Why are toxic reactions to drugs so often undetected initially? *N Engl J Med* 1980;302(18):1027–1029.
4. Toriello HV. Effect of the human genome project on the practice of adolescent medicine. *Adolesc Med* 2002;13(2):201–212.
5. Biro F. Physical growth and development. In: Friedman SB, Schonberg SK, Alderman EM, et al., eds. *Comprehensive adolescent health care*, 2nd ed. St. Louis, MO: Mosby, 1998:28–33.
6. Tanner JM, Davies PS. Clinical longitudinal standards for height and height velocity for North American children. *J Pediatr* 1985; 107(3):317–329.
7. Marshall WA, Tanner JM. Variations in pattern of pubertal changes in girls. *Arch Dis Child* 1969;44(235):291–303.
8. Marshall WA, Tanner JM. Variations in the pattern of pubertal changes in boys. *Arch Dis Child* 1970;45(239):13–23.
9. Sizonenko PC. Normal sexual maturation. *Pediatrician* 1987;14 (4):191–201.
10. Rodman JH. Pharmacokinetic variability in the adolescent: implications of body size and organ function for dosage regimen design. *J Adolesc Health* 1994;15(8):654–662.
11. Coppoletta JM, Wolbach SB. Body length and organ weights of infants and children: a study of the body length and normal weights of the more important vital organs of the body between birth and twelve years of age. *Am J Pathol* 1933;9:55–70.
12. Friis-Hansen B. Body composition during growth. *In vivo* measurements and biochemical data correlated to differential anatomical growth. *Pediatrics* 1971;47(1, Suppl 2):264–274.
13. Reith DM, Appleton DB, Hooper W, et al. The effect of body size on the metabolic clearance of carbamazepine. *Biopharm Drug Dispos* 2000;21(3):103–111.
14. Takahashi H, Ishikawa S, Nomoto S, et al. Developmental changes in pharmacokinetics and pharmacodynamics of warfarin enantiomers in Japanese children. *Clin Pharmacol Ther* 2000;68(5):541–555.
15. Murry DJ, Crom WR, Reddick WE, et al. Liver volume as a determinant of drug clearance in children and adolescents. *Drug Metab Dispos* 1995;23(10):1110–1116.
16. Weaver LT, Austin S, Cole TJ. Small intestinal length: a factor essential for gut adaptation. *Gut* 1991;32(11):1321–1323.
17. Whitington PF, Emond JC, Whitington SH, et al. Small-bowel length and the dose of cyclosporine in children after liver transplantation. *N Engl J Med* 1990;322(11):733–738.
18. Macdonald MS, Emery JL. The late intrauterine and postnatal development of human renal glomeruli. *J Anat* 1959;93(3): 331–341.
19. Fetterman GH, Shuplock NA, Philipp FJ, et al. The growth and maturation of human glomeruli and proximal convolutions from term to adulthood: studies by microdissection. *Pediatrics* 1965;35:601–619.
20. Nyengaard JR, Bendtsen TF. Glomerular number and size in relation to age, kidney weight, and body surface in normal man. *Anat Rec* 1992;232(2):194–201.
21. Friis Hansen B. Hydrometry of growth and aging. In: Brozek J, ed. *Human body composition: approaches and applications.* Oxford: Pergamon Press, 1965:191–210.
22. Maresh M. Changes in tissue widths during growth. Roentgenographic measurements of bone, muscle, and fat widths from infancy through adolescence. *Am J Dis Child* 1966;111(2): 142–155.
23. Forbes GB. Growth of the lean body mass in man. *Growth* 1972; 36(4):325–338.
24. Amery A, Bossaert H, Verstraete M. Muscle blood flow in normal and hypertensive subjects. Influence of age, exercise, and body position. *Am Heart J* 1969;78(2):211–216.
25. Ravalico G, Toffoli G, Pastori G, et al. Age-related ocular blood flow changes. *Invest Ophthalmol Vis Sci* 1996;37(13):2645–2650.
26. Carry MR, Ringel SP, Starcevich JM. Distribution of capillaries in normal and diseased human skeletal muscle. *Muscle Nerve* 1986; 9(5):445–454.
27. Lourie RS. Rate of secretion of the parotid glands in normal children: a measurement of function of the autonomic nervous system. *Am J Dis Child* 1943;65:455–479.
28. Stewart CF, Hampton EM. Effect of maturation on drug disposition in pediatric patients. *Clin Pharm* 1987;6(7):548–564.
29. Vreugdenhil G, Sinaasappel M, Bouquet J. A comparative study of the mouth to caecum transit time in children and adults using a weight adapted lactulose dose. *Acta Paediatr Scand* 1986;75(3): 483–488.
30. Murphy MS, Nelson R, Eastham EJ. Measurement of small intestinal transit time in children. *Acta Paediatr Scand* 1988;77(6): 802–806.
31. Di Lorenzo C, Flores AF, Hyman PE. Age-related changes in colon motility. *J Pediatr* 1995;127(4):593–596.
32. van Riet HG, Hoeke JO. Amylase and lipase values in normal subjects. *Clin Chim Acta* 1968;19(3):459–467.
33. Stahlberg MR, Hietanen E, Maki M. Mucosal biotransformation rates in the small intestine of children. *Gut* 1988;29(8):1058–1063.
34. Heimann G. Enteral absorption and bioavailability in children in relation to age. *Eur J Clin Pharmacol* 1980;18(1):43–50.
35. Matkovic V. Calcium metabolism and calcium requirements during skeletal modeling and consolidation of bone mass. *Am J Clin Nutr* 1991;54(1, Suppl):245S–260S.

36. Huang NN, High RH. Comparison of serum levels following the administration of oral and parenteral preparations of penicillin to infants and children of various age groups. *J Pediatr* 1953;42: 657–668.
37. Rogers RJ, Kalisker A, Wiener MB, et al. Inconsistent absorption from a sustained-release theophylline preparation during continuous therapy in asthmatic children. *J Pediatr* 1985;106(3): 496–501.
38. Reed MD, Rodarte A, Blumer JL, et al. The single-dose pharmacokinetics of midazolam and its primary metabolite in pediatric patients after oral and intravenous administration. *J Clin Pharmacol* 2001;41(12):1359–1369.
39. Linday L, Dobkin JF, Wang TC, et al. Digoxin inactivation by the gut flora in infancy and childhood. *Pediatrics* 1987;79(4):544–548.
40. Ilett KF, Tee LB, Reeves PT, et al. Metabolism of drugs and other xenobiotics in the gut lumen and wall. *Pharmacol Ther* 1990;46 (1):67–93.
41. Michel M, L'Heureux N, Auger FA, et al. From newborn to adult: phenotypic and functional properties of skin equivalent and human skin as a function of donor age. *J Cell Physiol* 1997; 171(2):179–189.
42. Fluhr JW, Pfisterer S, Gloor M. Direct comparison of skin physiology in children and adults with bioengineering methods. *Pediatr Dermatol* 2000;17(6):436–439.
43. Tosyali MC, Greenhill LL. Child and adolescent psychopharmacology. Important developmental issues. *Pediatr Clin North Am* 1998;45(5):1021–1035.
44. Benet LZ, Kroetz DL, Sheiner LB. Pharmacokinetics: the dynamics of drug absorption, distribution, and elimination. In: Hardman JG, Limbird LE, eds. *Goodman & Gilman's The pharmacological basis of therapeutics*, 9th ed. New York: McGraw-Hill, 1996:3–27.
45. Kazama T, Ikeda K, Morita K, et al. Relation between initial blood distribution volume and propofol induction dose requirement. *Anesthesiology* 2001;94(2):205–210.
46. Cary J, Hein K, Dell R. Theophylline disposition in adolescents with asthma. *Ther Drug Monit* 1991;13(4):309–313.
47. Verbeeck RK, Cardinal JA, Wallace SM. Effect of age and sex on the plasma binding of acidic and basic drugs. *Eur J Clin Pharmacol* 1984;27(1):91–97.
48. Lerman J, Strong HA, LeDez KM, et al. Effects of age on the serum concentration of alpha 1-acid glycoprotein and the binding of lidocaine in pediatric patients. *Clin Pharmacol Ther* 1989; 46(2):219–225.
49. Kodama Y, Tsutsumi K, Kuranari M, et al. *In vivo* binding characteristics of carbamazepine and carbamazepine-10,11-epoxide to serum proteins in paediatric patients with epilepsy. *Eur J Clin Pharmacol* 1993;44(3):291–293.
50. Cloyd JC, Fischer JH, Kriel RL, et al. Valproic acid pharmacokinetics in children. IV. Effects of age and antiepileptic drugs on protein binding and intrinsic clearance. *Clin Pharmacol Ther* 1993;53(1):22–29.
51. Kodama Y, Kodama H, Kuranari M, et al. No effect of gender or age on binding characteristics of valproic acid to serum proteins in pediatric patients with epilepsy. *J Clin Pharmacol* 1999;39(10): 1070–1076.
52. Kodama Y, Kodama H, Kuranari M, et al. Protein binding of valproic acid in Japanese pediatric and adult patients with epilepsy. *Am J Health Syst Pharm* 2002;59(9):835–840.
53. Kennedy MJ. Hormonal regulation of hepatic drug-metabolizing enzyme activity during adolescence. *Clin Pharmacol Ther* 2008;84:662–673.
54. Tanaka E. *In vivo* age-related changes in hepatic drug-oxidizing capacity in humans. *J Clin Pharmacol Ther* 1998;23(4):247–255.
55. de Wildt SN, Kearns GL, Leeder JS, et al. Cytochrome P450 3A: ontogeny and drug disposition. *Clin Pharmacokinet* 1999;37(6): 485–505.
56. Blanco JG, Harrison PL, Evans WE, et al. Human cytochrome P450 maximal activities in pediatric versus adult liver. *Drug Metab Dispos* 2000;28(4):379–382.
57. Sotaniemi EA, Arranto AJ, Pelkonen O, et al. Age and cytochrome P450-linked drug metabolism in humans: an analysis of 226 subjects with equal histopathologic conditions. *Clin Pharmacol Ther* 1997;61(3):331–339.
58. Ginsberg G, Hattis D, Sonawane B, et al. Evaluation of child/adult pharmacokinetic differences from a database derived from the therapeutic drug literature. *Toxicol Sci* 2002;66(2):185–200.
59. Sotaniemi EA, Pelkonen O, Arranto AJ, et al. Diabetes and elimination of antipyrine in man: an analysis of 298 patients classified by type of diabetes, age, sex, duration of disease and liver involvement. *Pharmacol Toxicol* 2002;90(3):155–160.
60. Vesell ES, Shively CA, Passananti GT. Temporal variations of antipyrine half-life in man. *Clin Pharmacol Ther* 1977;22(6): 843–852.
61. Crom WR, Relling MV, Christensen ML, et al. Age-related differences in hepatic drug clearance in children: studies with lorazepam and antipyrine. *Clin Pharmacol Ther* 1991;50(2): 132–140.
62. Evans WE, Relling MV, de Graaf S, et al. Hepatic drug clearance in children: studies with indocyanine green as a model substrate. *J Pharm Sci* 1989;78(6):452–456.
63. Lambert GH, Schoeller DA, Kotake AN, et al. The effect of age, gender, and sexual maturation on the caffeine breath test. *Dev Pharmacol Ther* 1986;9(6):375–388.
64. Gardner MJ, Jusko WJ. Effect of age and sex on theophylline clearance in young subjects. *Pediatr Pharmacol (New York)* 1982;2: 157–169.
65. Andersson T, Hassall E, Lundborg P, et al. Pharmacokinetics of orally administered omeprazole in children. International Pediatric Omeprazole Pharmacokinetic Group. *Am J Gastroenterol* 2000;95(11):3101–3106.
66. Tran A, Rey E, Pons G, et al. Pharmacokinetic–pharmacodynamic study of oral lansoprazole in children. *Clin Pharmacol Ther* 2002;71(5):359–367.
67. Chiba K, Ishizaki T, Miura H, et al. Michaelis–Menten pharmacokinetics of diphenylhydantoin and application in the pediatric age patient. *J Pediatr* 1980;96(3, pt 1):479–484.
68. Furlanut M, Benetello P, Baraldo M, et al. Chlorpromazine disposition in relation to age in children. *Clin Pharmacokinet* 1990; 18(4):329–331.
69. Riva R, Contin M, Albani F, et al. Free and total serum concentrations of carbamazepine and carbamazepine-10,11-epoxide in infancy and childhood. *Epilepsia* 1985;26(4):320–322.
70. Korinthenberg R, Haug C, Hannak D. The metabolization of carbamazepine to CBZ-10,11-epoxide in children from the newborn age to adolescence. *Neuropediatrics* 1994;25(4):214–216.
71. Yee GC, Lennon TP, Gmur DJ, et al. Age-dependent cyclosporine: pharmacokinetics in marrow transplant recipients. *Clin Pharmacol Ther* 1986;40(4):438–443.
72. Litterst CL, Mimnaugh EG, Reagan RL, et al. Comparison of *in vitro* drug metabolism by lung, liver, and kidney of several common laboratory species. *Drug Metab Dispos* 1975;3(4):259–265.
73. Johnson TN, Tanner MS, Taylor CJ, et al. Enterocytic CYP3A4 in a paediatric population: developmental changes and the effect of coeliac disease and cystic fibrosis. *Br J Clin Pharmacol* 2001; 51(5):451–460.
74. Gibbs JP, Liacouras CA, Baldassano RN, et al. Up-regulation of glutathione S-transferase activity in enterocytes of young children. *Drug Metab Dispos* 1999;27(12):1466–1469.
75. Balis FM, Pizzo PA, Eddy J, et al. Pharmacokinetics of zidovudine administered intravenously and orally in children with human immunodeficiency virus infection. *J Pediatr* 1989;114(5):880–884.
76. Capparelli EV. Pharmacokinetic considerations in the adolescent: non-cytochrome P450 metabolic pathways. *J Adolesc Health* 1994;15(8):641–647.
77. Kergueris MF, Bourin M, Larousse C. Pharmacokinetics of isoniazid: influence of age. *Eur J Clin Pharmacol* 1986;30(3):335–340.
78. Pariente-Khayat A, Rey E, Gendrel D, et al. Isoniazid acetylation metabolic ratio during maturation in children. *Clin Pharmacol Ther* 1997;62(4):377–383.
79. Miller RP, Roberts RJ, Fischer LJ. Acetaminophen elimination kinetics in neonates, children, and adults. *Clin Pharmacol Ther* 1976;19(3):284–294.
80. Alam SN, Roberts RJ, Fischer LJ. Age-related differences in salicylamide and acetaminophen conjugation in man. *J Pediatr* 1977;90(1):130–135.
81. Braunlich H. Excretion of drugs during postnatal development. *Pharmacol Ther* 1981;12(2):299–320.
82. Bangstad HJ, Kierulf P, Kjaersgaard P, et al. Urinary excretion of retinol-binding protein in healthy children and adolescents. *Pediatr Nephrol* 1995;9(3):299–302.
83. Stapleton FB, Linshaw MA, Hassanein K, et al. Uric acid excretion in normal children. *J Pediatr* 1978;92(6):911–914.

84. Linday LA, Engle MA, Reidenberg MM. Maturation and renal digoxin clearance. *Clin Pharmacol Ther* 1981;30(6):735–738.
85. Linday LA, Drayer DE, Khan MA, et al. Pubertal changes in net renal tubular secretion of digoxin. *Clin Pharmacol Ther* 1984; 35(4):438–446.
86. Donelli MG, Zucchetti M, Robatto A, et al. Pharmacokinetics of HD-MTX in infants, children, and adolescents with non-B acute lymphoblastic leukemia. *Med Pediatr Oncol* 1995;24(3):154–159.
87. Hayton WL, Stoeckel K. Age-associated changes in ceftriaxone pharmacokinetics. *Clin Pharmacokinet* 1986;11(1):76–86.
88. Berdel D, Suverkrup R, Heimann G, et al. Total theophylline clearance in childhood: the influence of age-dependent changes in metabolism and elimination. *Eur J Pediatr* 1987;146(1):41–43.
89. Degen LP, Phillips SF. Variability of gastrointestinal transit in healthy women and men. *Gut* 1996;39(2):299–305.
90. Tanaka E. Gender-related differences in pharmacokinetics and their clinical significance. *J Clin Pharmacol Ther* 1999;24(5): 339–346.
91. Meibohm B, Beierle I, Derendorf H. How important are gender differences in pharmacokinetics? *Clin Pharmacokinet* 2002;41(5): 329–342.
92. Smith G, Stubbins MJ, Harries LW, et al. Molecular genetics of the human cytochrome P450 monooxygenase superfamily. *Xenobiotica* 1998;28(12):1129–1165.
93. Kashuba AD, Nafziger AN. Physiological changes during the menstrual cycle and their effects on the pharmacokinetics and pharmacodynamics of drugs. *Clin Pharmacokinet* 1998;34(3):203–218.
94. Makkar RR, Fromm BS, Steinman RT, et al. Female gender as a risk factor for torsades de pointes associated with cardiovascular drugs. *J Am Med Assoc* 1993;270(21):2590–2597.
95. Benton RE, Sale M, Flockhart DA, et al. Greater quinidine-induced QTc interval prolongation in women. *Clin Pharmacol Ther* 2000;67(4):413–418.
96. Rodriguez I, Kilborn MJ, Liu XK, et al. Drug-induced QT prolongation in women during the menstrual cycle. *J Am Med Assoc* 2001;285(10):1322–1326.
97. Neinstein LS, Farmer M. Teenage pregnancy. In: Neinstein LS, ed. *Adolescent health care: a practical guide,* 4th ed. Philadelphia, PA: Lippincott Williams & Wilkins, 2002:810–833.
98. Brooks TL, Shrier LA. An update on contraception for adolescents. *Adolesc Med* 1999;10(2):211–219.
99. Martin JA, Hamilton BE, Sutton PD, et al. Births: Final data for 2006. National Vital Statistics Reports, vol 57, no. 7. Hyattsville, MD: National Center for Health Statistics, 2009.
100. Neinstein LS, Nelson AL. Contraception. In: Neinstein LS, ed. *Adolescent health care: a practical guide,* 4th ed. Philadelphia, PA: Lippincott Williams & Wilkins, 2002:834–856.
101. Hewitt G, Cromer B. Update on adolescent contraception. *Obstet Gynecol Clin North Am* 2000;27(1):143–162.
102. Nelson AL, Neinstein LS. Combination hormonal contraceptives. In: Neinstein LS, ed. *Adolescent health care: a practical guide,* 4th ed. Philadelphia, PA: Lippincott Williams & Wilkins, 2002:857–881.
103. Emans SJ. Contraception. In: Emans SJ, Laufer MR, Goldstein DP, eds. *Pediatric and adolescent gynecology,* 4th ed. Philadelphia, PA: Lippincott Williams & Wilkins, 1998:611–674.
104. Yasmin—an oral contraceptive with a new progestin. *Med Lett Drugs Ther* 2002;44(1133):55–57.
105. Ornstein RM, Fisher MM. Hormonal contraception in adolescents: special considerations. *Pediatr Drugs* 2006;8:25–45.
106. Jensen JT, Speroff L. Health benefits of oral contraceptives. *Obstet Gynecol Clin North Am* 2000;27(4):705–721.
107. Davis A, Godwin A, Lippman J, et al. Triphasic norgestimate–ethinyl estradiol for treating dysfunctional uterine bleeding. *Obstet Gynecol* 2000;96(6):913–920.
108. Davis AR, Westhoff CL. Primary dysmenorrhea in adolescent girls and treatment with oral contraceptives. *J Pediatr Adolesc Gynecol* 2001;14(1):3–8.
109. Charreau I, Plu-Bureau G, Bachelot A, et al. Oral contraceptive use and risk of benign breast disease in a French case–control study of young women. *Eur J Cancer Prev* 1993;2(2):147–154.
110. Thorneycroft IH, Stanczyk FZ, Bradshaw KD, et al. Effect of low-dose oral contraceptives on androgenic markers and acne. *Contraception* 1999;60(5):255–262.
111. The reduction in risk of ovarian cancer associated with oral-contraceptive use. The Cancer and Steroid Hormone Study of the Centers for Disease Control and the National Institute of Child Health and Human Development. *N Engl J Med* 1987;316(11): 650–655.
112. Schlesselman JJ. Net effect of oral contraceptive use on the risk of cancer in women in the United States. *Obstet Gynecol* 1995;85 (5, pt 1):793–801.
113. Narod SA, Risch H, Moslehi R, et al. Oral contraceptives and the risk of hereditary ovarian cancer. Hereditary Ovarian Cancer Clinical Study Group. *N Engl J Med* 1998;339(7):424–428.
114. Wolner-Hanssen P, Eschenbach DA, Paavonen J, et al. Decreased risk of symptomatic chlamydial pelvic inflammatory disease associated with oral contraceptive use. *J Am Med Assoc* 1990;263(1): 54–59.
115. Shulman LP. Oral contraceptives. Risks. *Obstet Gynecol Clin North Am* 2000;27(4):695–704.
116. Grimes DA, Wallach M. *Modern contraception: update from the contraception report.* Totawa, NJ: Emron, 1997.
117. Kumle M, Weiderpass E, Braaten T, et al. Use of oral contraceptives and breast cancer risk: the Norwegian–Swedish Women's Lifestyle and Health Cohort Study. *Cancer Epidemiol Biomarkers Prev* 2002;11(11):1375–1381.
118. Althuis MD, Brogan DR, Coates RJ, et al. Hormonal content and potency of oral contraceptives and breast cancer risk among young women. *Br J Cancer* 2003;88(1):50–57.
119. Marchbanks PA, McDonald JA, Wilson HG, et al. Oral contraceptives and the risk of breast cancer. *N Engl J Med* 2002;346(26): 2025–2032.
120. Dickinson BD, Altman RD, Nielsen NH, et al. Drug interactions between oral contraceptives and antibiotics. *Obstet Gynecol* 2001; 98(5, pt 1):853–860.
121. Carlsson B, Olsson G, Reis M, et al. Enantioselective analysis of citalopram and metabolites in adolescents. *Ther Drug Monit* 2001;23(6):658–664.
122. Westhoff C, Kerns J, Morroni C, et al. Quick start: a novel oral contraceptive initiation method. *Contraception* 2002;66:141–145.
123. McCann MF, Potter LS. Progestin-only oral contraception: a comprehensive review. *Contraception* 1994;50(6, Suppl 1):S1–S195.
124. Kaunitz AM. Injectable contraception. New and existing options. *Obstet Gynecol Clin North Am* 2000;27(4):741–780.
125. Nelson AL, Neinstein LS. Long-acting progestins. In: Neinstein LS, ed. *Adolescent health care: a practical guide,* 4th ed. Philadelphia, PA: Lippincott Williams & Wilkins, 2002:921–934.
126. Rickert VI, Tiezzi L, Lipshutz J, et al. Depo Now: preventing unintended pregnancies among adolescents and young adults. *J Adolesc Health* 2007;40:22–28.
127. Committee on Adolescence. Contraception and adolescents. *Pediatrics* 2007;120:1135–1148.
128. Bonny AE, Ziegler J, Harvey R, et al. Weight gain in obese and nonobese adolescent girls initiating depot medroxyprogesterone, oral contraceptive pills, or no hormonal contraceptive method. *Arch Pediatr Adolesc Med* 2006;160:40–45.
129. Mangan SA, Larsen PG, Hudson S. Overweight teens at increased risk for weight gain while using depot medroxyprogesterone acetate. *J Pediatr Adolesc Gynecol* 2002;15(2):79–82.
130. Levine RL. Endocrine aspects of eating disorders in adolescents. *Adolesc Med* 2002;13(1):129–143.
131. Cundy T, Ames R, Horne A, et al. A randomized controlled trial of estrogen replacement therapy in long-term users of depot medroxyprogesterone acetate. *J Clin Endocrinol Metab* 2003;88 (1):78–81.
132. Ishida Y, Heersche JN. Pharmacologic doses of medroxyprogesterone may cause bone loss through glucocorticoid activity: an hypothesis. *Osteoporos Int* 2002;13(8):601–605.
133. Banks E, Berrington A, Casabonne D. Overview of the relationship between use of progestogen-only contraceptives and bone mineral density. *Br J Obstet Gynaecol* 2001;108(12):1214–1221.
134. Cromer BA, Blair JM, Mahan JD, et al. A prospective comparison of bone density in adolescent girls receiving depot medroxyprogesterone acetate (Depo-Provera), levonorgestrel (Norplant), or oral contraceptives. *J Pediatr* 1996;129(5):671–676.
135. Tharnprisarn W, Taneepanichskul S. Bone mineral density in adolescent and young Thai girls receiving oral contraceptives compared with depot medroxyprogesterone acetate: a cross-sectional study in young Thai women. *Contraception* 2002;66(2):101–103.
136. Scholes D, Lacroix AZ, Ott SM, et al. Bone mineral density in women using depot medroxyprogesterone acetate for contraception. *Obstet Gynecol* 1999;93(2):233–238.

137. Berenson AB, Radecki CM, Grady JJ, et al. A prospective, controlled study of the effects of hormonal contraception on bone mineral density. *Obstet Gynecol* 2001;98(4):576–582.
138. Scholes D, LaCroix AZ, Ichikawa LE, et al. Change in bone mineral density among adolescent women using and discontinuing depot medroxyprogesterone acetate contraception. *Arch Pediatr Adolesc Med* 2005;159:139–144.
139. Scholes D, LaCroix AZ, Ichikawa LE, et al. The association between depot medroxyprogesterone acetate contraception and bone mineral density in adolescent women. *Contraception* 2004;69(2):99–104.
140. Busen NH, Britt RB, Rianon N. Bone mineral density in a cohort of adolescent women using depot medroxyprogesterone acetate for one to two years. *J Adolesc Health* 2003;32(4):257–259.
141. Cromer BA, Scholes D, Berenson A, et al. Depot medroxyprogesterone acetate and bone mineral density in adolescents—the black box warning: a position paper of the Society for Adolescent Medicine. *J Adolesc Health* 2006;39:296–301.
142. American College of Obstetricians and Gynecologists. ACOG Practice Bulletin Number 73: Use of hormonal contraception in women with coexisting medical conditions. *Obstet Gynecol* 2006; 107:453–472.
143. Kaunitz AM. Long-acting hormonal contraceptives—indispensable in preventing teen pregnancy. *J Adolesc Health* 2007;40:1–3.
144. Tolaymat LL, Kaunitz AM. Long-acting contraceptives in adolescents. *Curr Opin Obstet Gynecol* 2007;19:453–460.
145. Nelson AL, Neinstein LS. Intrauterine devices. In: Neinstein LS, ed. *Adolescent health care: a practical guide,* 4th ed. Philadelphia, PA: Lippincott Williams & Wilkins, 2002:882–890.
146. Nelson AL, Neinstein LS. Emergency contraception. In: Neinstein LS, ed. *Adolescent health care: a practical guide,* 4th ed. Philadelphia, PA: Lippincott Williams & Wilkins, 2002:911–920.
147. Piaggio G, von Hertzen H, Grimes DA, et al. Timing of emergency contraception with levonorgestrel or the Yuzpe regimen. Task Force on Postovulatory Methods of Fertility Regulation. *Lancet* 1999;353:721.
148. Gold MA. Emergency contraception. *Adolesc Med* 1997;8(3): 455–462.
149. Schein AB. Pregnancy prevention using emergency contraception: efficacy, attitudes, and limitations to use. *J Pediatr Adolesc Gynecol* 1999;12(1):3–9.
150. Rodrigues I, Grou F, Joly J. Effectiveness of emergency contraceptive pills between 72 and 120 hours after unprotected sexual intercourse. *Am J Obstet Gynecol* 2001;184(4):531–537.
151. http://www.accessdata.fda.gov/drugsatfda docs/nda/2006/021 045s011 Plan B APPROV.pdf. Accessed March 30, 2010.
152. Harper CC, Rocca CH, Darney PD, et al. Tolerability of levonorgestrel emergency contraception in adolescents. *Am J Obstet Gynecol* 2004;191(4):1158–1163.
153. American Academics of Pediatrics Committee on Adolescence. Emergency contraception. *Pediatrics* 2005;116(4):1026–1035.
154. Raine TR, Harper CC, Rocca CH, et al. Direct access to emergency contraception through pharmacies and effect on unintended pregnancy and STIs: a randomized controlled trial. *JAMA* 2005;293(1):54–62.
155. Harper CC, Cheong M, Rocca CH, et al. The effect of increased access to emergency contraception among young adolescents. *Obstet Gynecol* 2005;106(3):483–491.
156. Keder LM. New developments in contraception. *J Pediatr Adolesc Gynecol* 2002;15(3):179–181.
157. Audet MC, Moreau M, Koltun WD, et al. Evaluation of contraceptive efficacy and cycle control of a transdermal contraceptive patch vs an oral contraceptive: a randomized controlled trial. *J Am Med Assoc* 2001;285(18):2347–2354.
158. Holt VL, Cushing-Haugen KL, Daling JR. Body weight and risk of oral contraceptive failure. *Obstet Gynecol* 2002;99(5, pt 1):820–827.
159. Dieben TO, Roumen FJ, Apter D. Efficacy, cycle control, and user acceptability of a novel combined contraceptive vaginal ring. *Obstet Gynecol* 2002;100(3):585–593.
160. Timmer CJ, Mulders TM. Pharmacokinetics of etonogestrel and ethinylestradiol released from a combined contraceptive vaginal ring. *Clin Pharmacokinet* 2000;39(3):233–242.
161. Epstein LB, Sokal-Gutierrez K, Ivey SL. Adolescent experiences with the vaginal ring. *J Adolesc Health* 2008;43:64–70.
162. World Health Organization. *Report of a WHO Consultation on obesity: preventing and managing the global epidemic.* Geneva: World Health Organization, 1997.
163. Ogden CL, Carroll MD, Flegal KM. High body mass index for age among US children and adolescents. *J Am Med Assoc* 2008; 299(20):2401–2405.
164. Blouin RA, Warren GW. Pharmacokinetic considerations in obesity. *J Pharm Sci* 1999;88(1):1–7.
165. Cheymol G. Effects of obesity on pharmacokinetics implications for drug therapy. *Clin Pharmacokinet* 2000;39(3):215–231.
166. Benedek IH, Blouin RA, McNamara PJ. Serum protein binding and the role of increased alpha 1-acid glycoprotein in moderately obese male subjects. *Br J Clin Pharmacol* 1984;18(6):941–946.
167. Benedek IH, Fiske WD III, Griffen WO, et al. Serum alpha 1-acid glycoprotein and the binding of drugs in obesity. *Br J Clin Pharmacol* 1983;16(6):751–754.
168. Abernethy DR, Greenblatt DJ, Divoll M, et al. Enhanced glucuronide conjugation of drugs in obesity: studies of lorazepam, oxazepam, and acetaminophen. *J Lab Clin Med* 1983;101(6): 873–880.
169. Hunt CM, Westerkam WR, Stave GM, et al. Hepatic cytochrome P-4503 A (CYP3 A) activity in the elderly. *Mech Ageing Dev* 1992; 64(1–2):189–199.
170. O'Shea D, Davis SN, Kim RB, et al. Effect of fasting and obesity in humans on the 6-hydroxylation of chlorzoxazone: a putative probe of CYP2E1 activity. *Clin Pharmacol Ther* 1994;56(4): 359–367.
171. Trends in cigarette smoking among high school students—United States, 1991–2001. *MMWR Morb Mortal Wkly Rep* 2002;51 (19):409–412.
172. Schein JR. Cigarette smoking and clinically significant drug interactions. *Ann Pharmacother* 1995;29(11):1139–1148.
173. Zevin S, Benowitz NL. Drug interactions with tobacco smoking. An update. *Clin Pharmacokinet* 1999;36(6):425–438.
174. Hunt SN, Jusko WJ, Yurchak AM. Effect of smoking on theophylline disposition. *Clin Pharmacol Ther* 1976;19(5, pt 1):546–551.
175. Powell JR, Thiercelin JF, Vozeh S, et al. The influence of cigarette smoking and sex on theophylline disposition. *Am Rev Respir Dis* 1977;116(1):17–23.
176. Vistisen K, Loft S, Poulsen HE. Cytochrome P450 IA2 activity in man measured by caffeine metabolism: effect of smoking, broccoli and exercise. *Adv Exp Med Biol* 1991;283:407–411.
177. Calfee R, Fadale P. Popular ergogenic drugs and supplements in young athletes. *Pediatrics* 2006;117:e577–e589.
178. Kanayama G, Pope HG Jr., Hudson JI. "Body image" drugs: a growing psychosomatic problem. *Psychother Psychosom* 2001;70 (2):61–65.
179. Field AE, Austin SB, Camargo CA, et al. Exposure to the mass media, body shape concerns and use of supplements to improve weight and shape among male and female adolescents. *Pediatrics* 2005;116:e214–e220.
180. Holland-Hall C. Performance-enhancing substances: is your adolescent patient using? *Pediatr Clin North Am* 2007;54:651–662.
181. Koch JJ. Performance-enhancing: substances and their use among adolescent athletes. *Pediatr Rev* 2002;23(9):310–317.
182. Labre MP. Adolescent boys and the muscular male body ideal. *J Adolesc Health* 2002;30(4):233–242.
183. DuRant RH, Rickert VI, Ashworth CS, et al. Use of multiple drugs among adolescents who use anabolic steroids. *N Engl J Med* 1993;328(13):922–926.
184. Stephens MB, Olsen C. Ergogenic supplements and health risk behaviors. *J Fam Pract* 2001;50(8):696–699.
185. Metzl JD, Small E, Levine SR, et al. Creatine use among young athletes. *Pediatrics* 2001;108(2):421–425.
186. Lattavo A, Kopperud A, Rogers PD. Creatine and other supplements. *Pediatr Clin North Am* 2007;54:735–760.
187. Gregory AJM, Fitch RW. Sports medicine: performance-enhancing drugs. *Pediatr Clin North Am* 2007;54:797–806.
188. Dempsey RL, Mazzone MF, Meurer LN. Does oral creatine supplementation improve strength? A meta-analysis. *J Fam Pract* 2002;51(11):945–951.
189. Kamber M, Koster M, Kreis R, et al. Creatine supplementation—Part I: Performance, clinical chemistry, and muscle volume. *Med Sci Sports Exerc* 1999;31(12):1763–1769.
190. Kreider RB, Ferreira M, Wilson M, et al. Effects of creatine supplementation on body composition, strength, and sprint performance. *Med Sci Sports Exerc* 1998;30(1):73–82.
191. Pritchard NR, Kalra PA. Renal dysfunction accompanying oral creatine supplements. *Lancet* 1998;351:1252–1253.

192. Koshy KM, Griswold E, Schneeberger EE. Interstitial nephritis in a patient taking creatine. *N Engl J Med* 1999;340(10):814–815.
193. Shekelle PG, Hardy ML, Morton SC, et al. Efficacy and safety of ephedra and ephedrine for weight loss and athletic performance: a meta-analysis. *J Am Med Assoc* 2003;289(12):1537–1545.
194. Bent S, Tiedt TN, Odden MC, et al. The relative safety of ephedra compared with other herbal products. *Ann Intern Med* 2003;138(6):468–471.
195. Bell DG, Jacobs I, Zamecnik J. Effects of caffeine, ephedrine and their combination on time to exhaustion during high-intensity exercise. *Eur J Appl Physiol Occup Physiol* 1998;77(5):427–433.
196. Bell DG, Jacobs I. Combined caffeine and ephedrine ingestion improves run times of Canadian Forces Warrior Test. *Aviat Space Environ Med* 1999;70(4):325–329.
197. Bell DG, Jacobs I, McLellan TM, et al. Reducing the dose of combined caffeine and ephedrine preserves the ergogenic effect. *Aviat Space Environ Med* 2000;71(4):415–419.
198. Bell DG, Jacobs I, Ellerington K. Effect of caffeine and ephedrine ingestion on anaerobic exercise performance. *Med Sci Sports Exerc* 2001;33(8):1399–1403.
199. Haller CA, Benowitz NL. Adverse cardiovascular and central nervous system events associated with dietary supplements containing ephedra alkaloids. *N Engl J Med* 2000;343(25):1833–1838.
200. Rezkalla SH, Mesa J, Sharma P, et al. Myocardial infarction temporally related to ephedra—a possible role for the coronary microcirculation. *WMJ* 2002;101(7):64–66.
201. McBride BF, Karapanos AK, Krudysz A, et al. Electrocardiographic and hemodynamic effects of a multicomponent dietary supplement containing ephedra and caffeine: a randomized controlled trial. *JAMA* 2004;291(2):216–221.
202. Kerr JM, Congeni JA. Anabolic-androgenic steroids: Use and abuse in pediatric patients. *Pediatr Clin North Am* 2007;54:771–785.
203. Casavant MJ, Blake K, Griffith J, et al. Consequences of use of anabolic androgenic steroids. *Pediatr Clin North Am* 2007;54:677–690.
204. Smurawa TM, Congeni JA. Testosterone precursors: Use and abuse in pediatric athletes. *Pediatr Clin North Am* 2007;54:787–796.
205. King DS, Sharp RL, Vukovich MD, et al. Effect of oral androstenedione on serum testosterone and adaptations to resistance training in young men: a randomized controlled trial. *J Am Med Assoc* 1999;281(21):2020–2028.
206. Leder BZ, Longcope C, Catlin DH, et al. Oral androstenedione administration and serum testosterone concentrations in young men. *J Am Med Assoc* 2000;283(6):779–782.
207. Grunbaum JA, Kann L, Kinchen SA, et al. Youth risk behavior surveillance—United States, 2001. *MMWR CDC Surveill Summ* 2002;51(4):1–62.
208. Yesalis CE, Barsukiewicz CK, Kopstein AN, et al. Trends in anabolic–androgenic steroid use among adolescents. *Arch Pediatr Adolesc Med* 1997;151(12):1197–1206.
209. Stilger VG, Yesalis CE. Anabolic–androgenic steroid use among high school football players. *J Community Health* 1999;24(2):131–145.
210. Irving LM, Wall M, Neumark-Sztainer D, et al. Steroid use among adolescents: findings from Project EAT. *J Adolesc Health* 2002;30(4):243–252.
211. Catlin DH, Murray TH. Performance-enhancing drugs, fair competition, and Olympic sport. *J Am Med Assoc* 1996;276(3):231–237.
212. Adolescents and anabolic steroids: a subject review. American Academy of Pediatrics. Committee on Sports Medicine and Fitness. *Pediatrics* 1997;99(6):904–908.
213. Elliot DL, Cheong J, Moe EL, et al. Cross-sectional study of female students reporting anabolic steroid use. *Arch Pediatr Adolesc Med* 2007;161:572–577.
214. Goldberg L. Adverse effects of anabolic steroids. *J Am Med Assoc* 1996;276(3):257.
215. Bahrke MS, Yesalis CE, Brower KJ. Anabolic–androgenic steroid abuse and performance-enhancing drugs among adolescents. *Child Adolesc Psychiatr Clin N Am* 1998;7(4):821–838.
216. Dickinson BP, Mylonakis E, Strong LL, et al. Potential infections related to anabolic steroid injection in young adolescents. *Pediatrics* 1999;103(3):694.
217. Daly RC, Su TP, Schmidt PJ, et al. Neuroendocrine and behavioral effects of high-dose anabolic steroid administration in male normal volunteers. *Psychoneuroendocrinology* 2003;28(3):317–331.
218. Friedman IM, Litt IF. Adolescents' compliance with therapeutic regimens. Psychological and social aspects and intervention. *J Adolesc Health Care* 1987;8(1):52–67.
219. Cromer BA, Tarnowski KJ. Noncompliance in adolescents: a review. *J Dev Behav Pediatr* 1989;10(4):207–215.
220. KyngAs HA, Kroll T, Duffy ME. Compliance in adolescents with chronic diseases: a review. *J Adolesc Health* 2000;26(6):379–388.
221. Krupka LR, Vener AM. Drug knowledge (prescription, over-the-counter, social): young adult consumers at risk? *J Drug Educ* 1987;17(2):129–142.
222. Daniel KL, Honein MA, Moore CA. Sharing prescription medication among teenage girls: potential danger to unplanned/undiagnosed pregnancies. *Pediatrics* 2003;111(5, pt 2):1167–1170.
223. Conard LAE, Fortenberry JD, Blythe MJ, et al. Pharmacists' attitudes toward and practices with adolescents. *Arch Pediatr Adolesc Med* 2003;157:361–366.

CHAPTER

26

Victoria Tutag Lehr
Mirjana Lulic Botica
Merene Mathew

Topical Medications

Topical administration represents an important method of delivery of medications for infants and children. Clinicians must remember to inquire about use of topical medications or transdermal or "patch" delivery systems during a medication history. Patients and parents frequently overlook mentioning the use of topical medications during clinical examinations. Topically applied medications may undergo percutaneous absorption, resulting in systemic effects (1–3).

Developmental changes affecting the skin throughout infancy and childhood influence the rate and extent of absorption, metabolism, and bioavailability of topically administered medications (1). The skin is a major body organ for the newborn. Skin accounts for up to 13% of an infant's total body weight compared with only 3% of an average adult's body weight (2). This greater total body surface area ratio to body mass results in a much greater proportion of drug absorbed per kilogram of body weight for infants compared with adults (1–5). Infants are at increased risk for development of toxic drug serum concentrations with topical administration of medications, such as topical anesthetics, corticosteroids, antihistamines, and antiseptics (2–5).

Human skin is composed of two morphologically distinct layers (epithelial and mesenchymal) which originate from two different germ layers during development (2,3). Epithelial structures derived from the ectoderm are the epidermis, pilosebaceous–apocrine unit, eccrine unit, and nails. The ectoderm also generates hair and teeth. The mesoderm generates the mesenchymal structures—collagen, reticular and elastic fibers, blood vessels, muscles, and fat. These form the three layers of human skin: the epidermis, the dermis, and the subcutaneous tissue, which influence the absorption and metabolism of topically administered medications (4).

Epidermal development is markedly influenced by gestation (5,6). Before 30 weeks of gestation, the epidermis is thin, has few cell layers, and a poorly formed stratum corneum (6). This functional superficial layer acts as a barrier, composed of closely packed dead cells undergoing constant exfoliation. Maturation of the epidermis occurs at around 34 weeks of gestation. There is a profound postnatal effect on epidermal development in preterm infants, so histologically the epidermis of the most immature infant resembles that of a term infant by 2 weeks of age. These histological changes parallel development of barrier properties of newborn skin (4,5). Preterm infants younger than 35 weeks of gestation have less well-developed stratum corneum and thinner skin compared with older children and adults. A significant difference in thickness between the stratum corneum of term infants, children, or adults has not been demonstrated (6).

The dermis is beneath the epidermis and contains a rich supply of vascular beds, connective tissue, and lymphatics (6,7). At birth, skin is richly supplied by a disorderly horizontal, capillary network that organizes into the adult papillary loop pattern during the first 2 weeks of life (7). Skin cooling encourages maturation of capillary network loops (7).

Fatty connective tissue is the major component of the subcutaneous layer and starts accumulating around week 14 of gestation (2–4). Fat serves as insulation, cushioning, and an energy source. Fat storage continues to accumulate until birth. The dermis and subcutaneous layer contain sebaceous glands and sweat glands. Sebaceous glands are not fully functional until puberty, while the sweat glands will mature at day 5 of life (3,4).

Percutaneous absorption of a drug requires transfer from skin surface through the stratum corneum to the underlying epidermis and dermis (8–10). Factors contributing to percutaneous absorption of topical medications include physiochemical properties of the drug, concentration of drug in the vehicle, chemical and physical properties of the vehicle, thickness and hydration of the stratum corneum and epidermis, occlusion, and presence of inflamed, diseased, or damaged skin (11).

Passage through the stratum corneum is rate limiting for percutaneous absorption of an exogenous substance (11,12). The stratum corneum is composed of keratinized corneocytes surrounded by a lipid matrix, providing a barrier to percutaneous absorption. Major steps in percutaneous absorption include concentration gradient, the release of the drug from the vehicle into the skin (partition coefficient), and diffusion of the drug through the epidermis (diffusion coefficient) (10–12). The thicker stratum corneum on the palms and soles decreases absorption, whereas thinner skin of the eyelids, face, axillae, and genitals allows for increased absorption.

Percutaneous absorption of topically administered medications in infants differs from that in adults in several clinically significant aspects. Preterm infants have greater cutaneous perfusion and epidermal hydration compared with older infants, children, and adults (2–5). This may result in enhanced percutaneous absorption of topically applied medications, predisposing to systemic drug toxicity (2–5,13).

Hydration enhances permeability of hydrophilic drugs by increasing the diffusion constant (10–12). Although skin thickness is similar in infants and adults, infants have a greater degree of skin hydration and perfusion compared with adults, enhancing skin permeability (1–5). Hydration of the stratum corneum is greatest extent in the axillae, genitals including the diaper area, and the antecubital and popliteal fossae.

Molecular weight and size of drug significantly determine percutaneous absorption (12–15). Solubility of drug in the vehicle and tissue is also integral to drug absorption. In general, the more lipophilic the molecule, the more readily it penetrates the skin (15). The stratum corneum determines the rate of diffusion into the epidermis. The drug may diffuse down along a concentration gradient, bind to sites in the tissue, and undergo vasculature resorption or metabolism by a variety of mixed function monooxygenases or other enzymes (11).

Occlusion with plastic wrap during application of a topical medication will result in increased percutaneous absorption, predisposing to development of toxic serum concentrations of active ingredients or incipients. Occlusive dressings must be used with caution on infants and young children to avoid accumulating toxic serum drug concentrations from enhanced absorption (3).

Infected, broken, or abraded skin allows increased absorption of topical medications. Caution must be taken when applying topical medications to these areas on young infants and children for a prolonged duration of therapy. Monitoring parameters for potential toxicity will ensure safe use of topical medications on skin with an altered barrier.

Type of vehicle affects percutaneous absorption and patient compliance. A review of vehicle pharmacokinetics are discussed in further detail elsewhere (10,11). An ointment is composed of a lipophilic drug in a base such as petrolatum, mineral oil, waxes, or organic alcohols (9,10,13). Ointments impart a relatively high partition coefficient—defined as the relative solubility of a drug in the stratum corneum and vehicle—making them the most efficient vehicle for topical drug delivery (12). Emulsions are mixtures of two immiscible substances. Creams are classified as emulsions of oil in water or water in oil, depending on whether they can be washed off with water or not (9,10,13). An oil-in-water emulsion is more cosmetically acceptable, whereas a water-in-oil emulsion is more occlusive. Foams, emulsions of liquid and gas, may be easily applied to hair-bearing areas. Liquid preparations are divided into monophasic solutions, emulsions, and suspensions. Monophasic solutions include lotions, gels, and oils.

Parents and caregivers require appropriate instructions for safe and effective application of topical creams and ointments. Include a description of the area of application, as well as frequency and duration of use. Indicate whether the product should be rubbed into the skin or applied in a layer of specific thickness. Application of topical medications to large areas of skin of a young infant or child must be avoided secondary to increased skin to body weight ratio, predisposing to increased plasma concentrations of drugs. Caregivers should be instructed to wear a sterile, disposable glove when applying creams or ointments to broken skin. Topical medications should not be shared between patients to avoid cross-contamination.

The site of application should not be covered with an occlusive dressing unless increased absorption is desired. In addition, plastic film occlusive dressings have been associated with bacterial infection in preterm infants (2). Cautions about exposure to sunlight may be appropriate, as phototoxic reactions are possible with a variety of topical medications (16,17).

TOPICAL CORTICOSTEROIDS

Topical corticosteroids have been available since the 1950s and are the cornerstone therapy for inflammatory dermatoses, such as psoriasis, eczema, seborrheic, allergic or atopic dermatitis, insect bites, poison ivy, and other skin irritations (18–20). Large numbers of topical steroids are available in cream, ointment, lotion, gel, solution, and shampoo forms (18,21). Steroid preparations are grouped according to relative anti-inflammatory activity and agents in each group are approximately equivalent (Table 26.1) (18,21). The relative potency of a particular steroid product depends on the characteristics and concentration of the drug and vehicle. In general, ointments and gels are more potent than creams or lotions. However, some products have been formulated to yield comparable potency (22,23).

MECHANISM OF ACTION

Corticosteroids primarily act by binding to cytoplasmic glucocorticoid receptors in the cytosol, followed by translocation of the ligand–receptor complex that enters the nucleus to regulate gene transcription and the inflammatory process (24,25). Other actions of corticosteroids include immunosuppressive, antiproliferative, and vasoconstrictive effects (25,26). Topical corticosteroids are absorbed into skin cells inhibiting inflammatory cells via actions on mediator release and function, inflammatory cell function and release of lysosomal enzymes. The cascade of inflammatory cytokines such as prostaglandins and other inflammatory substances is blocked from release as skin reacts to allergens or irritants, ultimately reducing inflammation and relieving symptoms of pruritus (24–26).

INDICATIONS AND CLINICAL USE

Common conditions responsive to topical corticosteroids include atopic and seborrheic dermatitis; contact, diaper, and irritant dermatitis; neurodermatitis; dyshidrotic eczema; lichen planus; lichen simplex chronicus; nummular dermatitis; pityriasis rosea; psoriasis; and inflammatory phase of xerosis (20,21).

TABLE 26.1 Corticosteroid Preparations

Corticosteroid	*Strength (%)*	*Form*	*Indication and Directions*	*Cost*
Very potent				
Betamethasone dipropionate augmented (Diprolene®) (Diprolene AF®) (Diprosone®)	0.05	C, U	Localized area, resistant thick lesion, palms, soles, scalp	$$$
Clobetasol propionate (Temovate®)	0.05	C, U, G	High potency indications: alopecia areata, atopic dermatitis (resistant), discoid lupus, hyperkeratotic eczema, lichen planus, lichen sclerosus, lichen simplex chronicus, nummular eczema, psoriasis, severe hand eczema (11)	$$$
Halobetasol propionate (Ultravate®)	0.05	C, U		$$$$
Halcinonide (Halog®)	0.1	C, U		$$$$
Diflorasone diacetate (Psorcon®)	0.05	C, U		$$$$
Potent				
Amcinonide (Cyclocort®)	0.1	C, U, L	Localized area, thick lesion, palms, soles, scalp	$$$$
Betamethasone dipropionate (Diprolene®)	0.05	C, U		$$$
Betamethasone valerate (Valisone®)	0.1	U		$$
Desoximetasone (Topicort®)	0.25	C, U		$$$
	0.05	G		$$$
Fluocinolone acetonide (Synalar®, Derma-Smoothe/FS®, Capex®)	0.01	C, S, O, P		$$$$
	0.025	C, U		$$$
Fluocinonide (Lidex®)	0.05	C, U, G, S		$$
Fluticasone propionate (Cutivate®)	0.05	C, L		$$$
	0.005	U		$$$
Triamcinolone acetonide (Aristocort®)	0.5	C, U		$$
Moderately potent				
Betamethasone dipropionate (Diprosone®)	0.05	C, U, L	Moderate potency indications: anal inflammation, asteatotic eczema, atopic dermatitis, lichen sclerosus, nummular eczema, scabies, seborrheic dermatitis, severe dermatitis, severe intertrigo, stasis dermatitis (11)	$$$
Betamethasone valerate (Valisone®)	0.1	C, U, L		$$
	0.05	C		$$
	0.01	C		$$
Clobetasone butyrate (Eumovate®)	0.05	C, U		$$$
Clocortolone pivalate (Cloderm®)	0.1	C		$$$
Desoximetasone (Topicort®)	0.05	C, G		$$$
Fluocinolone acetonide (Lidex®)	0.025	C, U		$$
Flurandrenolide (Cordran®)	0.025	C, U		$$$
	0.05	C, U, L		$$$
	4 $\mu g/cm^2$	Tape		$$$
	0.005	U		$$$
Hydrocortisone buteprate (Pandel®)	0.1	C		$$
Hydrocortisone butyrate (Locoid®)	0.1	C, U, S		$$$
Hydrocortisone valerate (Westcort®)	0.2	C, U		$$
Mometasone furoate (Elocon®)	0.1	C, U, L		$$
Prednicarbate 0.1% (Dermatop®)	0.1	C		$$$
Triamcinolone acetonide (Kenalog®, Aristocort®)	0.1	C, U		$$
	0.025	C, U, L		
Mild				
Aclometasone dipropionate (Aclovate®)	0.05	C, U	Face, folds, genitals, extensive areas of skin	$$$
Desonide (DesOwen®, Tridesilon®)	0.05	C, U, L	Mild potency indications: dermatitis (diaper, face, eyelids), intertrigo, perianal inflammation (11)	$$
Hydrocortisone (Hytone®, Hycort®)	0.5, 1, 2.5	C, U, L		$
Hydrocortisone acetate (Cortef®, Cortaid®)	0.5	C, U		$
	1	C, U		

C, cream; U, ointment; S, solution; G, gel; O, oil; L, lotion; P, shampoo.

PHARMACOKINETICS

Pharmacokinetics of topical corticosteroid use is determined by potency of the corticosteroid, its vehicle, and the skin onto which it is applied (26). Corticosteroid potency is determined in part by its chemical structure and by manipulation of the steroid molecule to produce compounds with greater lipophilicity, fewer mineralocorticoid properties, and higher potency. Corticosteroids can be divided into two classes: fluorinated and nonfluorinated (26). Fluorinated steroids refer to those steroids that have been chemically altered to increase their potency. For example, halogenation at any position increases potency of the steroid. This modification also increases mineralocorticoid effects, enhancing systemic side effects. Other chemical modifications include hydroxylation, addition of double bonds, alteration of functional groups (esterification and methylation), and addition of ketone groups. The altered structure and resulting increase in potency may be due to increased lipophilicity, percutaneous absorption, and/or glucocorticoid receptor binding activity (23–26). The vehicle indirectly affects topical corticosteroid potency by influencing the environment in which the corticosteroid is absorbed. For example, through occlusion, ointments help hydrate the stratum corneum, thereby enhancing penetration of corticosteroids (26–30). In addition, solvents such as propylene glycol and ethanol affect solubility of corticosteroids, enhancing percutaneous absorption. Finally, thickness and integrity of the stratum corneum are inversely proportional to absorption of topical corticosteroids (28,29). Penetration into eyelid skin is therefore better than into palmar skin, and inflamed or diseased skin is more readily penetrated than intact skin (28,31).

THERAPEUTIC GUIDELINES FOR CORTICOSTEROID TREATMENT

Following major principles of steroid use will better guide treatment regimens (22,24,25,28):

1. The risk of adrenal suppression with prolonged or overuse can be decreased by judicious prescribing of initial quantities and limiting number of additional refills.
2. Selection of the specific corticosteroid strength and vehicle depends on location, extent of the skin condition, patient's age, and anticipated duration of treatment.
3. The extent of absorption is based not only on drug potency but rather on the vehicle in which it is formulated. Ointment bases enhance penetration of the drug and may be preferred for thick, lichenified lesions. Creams are preferred for acute and subacute dermatoses. Solutions, lotions, oils, gels, or foams should be prescribed for hair-bearing areas where a non–oil-based vehicle is required.
4. Corticosteroid potency must be considered when prescribing these agents. In general, low-to-medium potency agents should be utilized for treating acute thin inflammatory lesions, whereas, very high potency and high-potency corticosteroids should be reserved for treating chronic hyperkeratotic, lichenified lesions.
5. Low-potency corticosteroids should be used on areas with a thin stratum corneum such as the face, skin folds, and diaper area. Low-potency corticosteroids are preferred for infants and especially low-birth-weight infants who have immature skin with poorly formed epidermal barrier leading to accidental poisoning from percutaneous absorption of chemicals and superficial damage from use of adhesives.
6. Higher-potency corticosteroids may be used if necessary, but for a limited duration and should be reserved for areas with a thick stratum corneum such as the palms and soles of feet. Very potent corticosteroids should not routinely be used for longer than 2 to 3 weeks.
7. Tapering from a more potent to a less potent topical corticosteroid will help prevent a rebound flare. Avoid abrupt discontinuation.
8. Topical corticosteroids should not be used on ulcerated or atrophic skin.
9. Corticosteroid–antifungal combinations should be avoided for treatment of dermatophytoses.
10. Laboratory tests for adrenal suppression should be performed following prolonged treatment particularly over large areas of skin.

ADVERSE EFFECTS

The most common side effects of topical corticosteroids are local: atrophy and striae, both of which may be irreversible (19,20). Other cutaneous side effects include hypopigmentation, telangiectasias, purpura, tinea and scabies incognito, granuloma gluteale infantum, acneiform eruptions, perioral dermatitis, and steroid rosacea. These side effects are more commonly seen with inappropriate use of high-potency fluorinated topical corticosteroids applied for prolonged periods of time on the face and intertriginous areas. Applied periocularly, there is a risk for development of glaucoma or cataracts. Allergic contact dermatitis to corticosteroids should be considered if a patient's condition is unresponsive or made worse with treatment (19,27). Use of combination corticosteroid–antifungal preparations for treatment of dermatophytoses is associated with persistent and recurrent infections (29,30). Tachyphylaxis—diminished response to prolonged application—may develop with prolonged use of topical steroids (22).

The more serious and dreaded complications of topical corticosteroid use are systemic side effects (19). These side effects have been associated with short-term use of high-potency topical steroids and with even short-term use of low-potency formulations. Such effects are identical to those of systemically administered corticosteroids and include suppression of the hypothalamic–pituitary–adrenal axis (HPA), Cushing syndrome, failure to thrive, poor linear growth, hyperglycemia, and glycosuria. Factors augmenting systemic absorption include application of more potent steroids, use over large surface areas, application on skin folds, prolonged use, occlusive dressings, younger age (infants and young children), and liver or renal disease (26,32).

MONITORING PARAMETERS FOR PATIENTS

Parents and caregivers of children and infants initiated on topical corticosteroid therapy should be educated about potential side effects (19,28). Burning, stinging, itching, and redness occur in the affected area with initial application, but dissipate over time as the body adjusts to the medication is a common concern. Patients or caregivers should closely monitor for skin thinning or discoloration. Topical corticosteroids should not be used near the eyes, especially in patients with a history of glaucoma. Treatment durations beyond 2 to 3 weeks for very potent topical corticosteroids should be discouraged. The child's health care provider should be consulted immediately if any vision problems, persistent headaches, increased thirst or urination, unusual weakness or weight loss, and dizziness occur, as these symptoms may indicate HPA suppression from systemic steroid absorption (18,21,24).

TOPICAL IMMUNOMODULATORS

Topical corticosteroids have been the mainstay of therapy for atopic dermatitis, but side effects with higher doses and prolonged application of steroids have limited their use, especially in infants and children (19,33). Atopic dermatitis is a commonly encountered eczematous skin condition presenting in children of all ages. Although the exact etiology of atopic dermatitis is unknown, it may involve genetic and environmental factors as well as defects in skin barrier and immune function (9,33). Among children in whom atopic dermatitis is diagnosed during first 2 years of life, about half develop asthma.

When atopic dermatitis does not improve with conservative measures such as generous use of emollients, alternative therapies should be considered (33–35). Short courses of topical corticosteroids have been traditionally treated disease flares, yet are limited by side effect potential (19,20,33). In the late 1980s, a topical formulation of cyclosporine was developed as an alternative treatment for atopic dermatitis without the corticosteroid side effect profile. However, cyclosporine was found to be ineffective due to large molecular size and poor dermal penetration.

Topical calcineurin inhibitors (TCIs), tacrolimus (Protopic®) and pimecrolimus (Elidel®), are much smaller molecules than cyclosporine and better able to penetrate the skin causing local immunosuppression (33–35). These agents are currently FDA approved for management of atopic dermatitis in patients 2 years of age and older (36–39).

TACROLIMUS AND PIMECROLIMUS (TOPICAL CALCINEURIN INHIBITORS)

Tacrolimus is a macrolide immunosuppressant isolated from the fungus *Streptomyces tsukubaensis* in 1984 (34,35). Pimecrolimus, also a macrolide immunosuppressant, is derived from ascomycin, a natural product of *Streptomyces hygroscopicus* var. *ascomyceticus* (35).

Mechanism of Action

Although the mechanism of action of tacrolimus in atopic dermatitis is not completely understood, in vitro studies reveal that topical tacrolimus binds to specific T-cell receptors resulting in the inhibition of T-lymphocyte activation (Fig. 26.1) (34,40,41). Tacrolimus then forms a complex

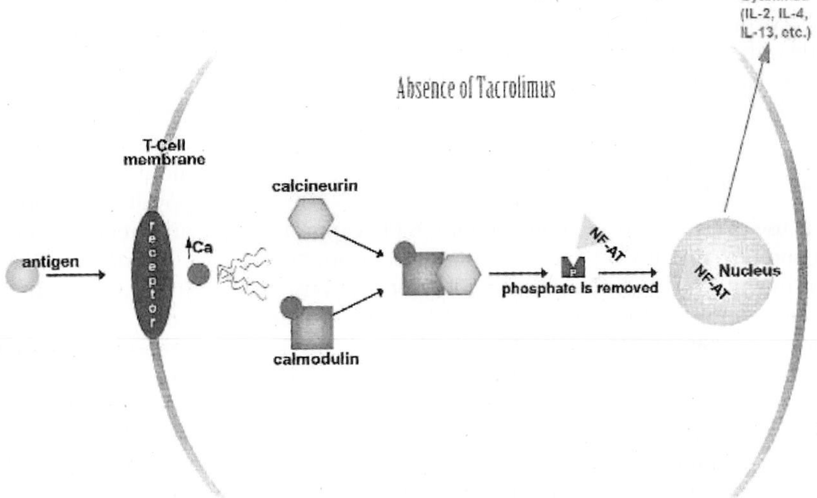

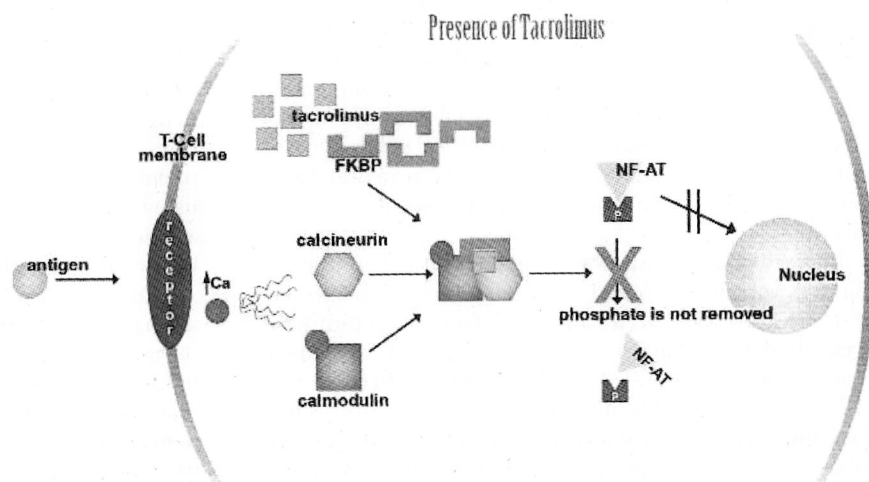

Figure 26.1. Normally, T-cell exposure to an antigen triggers release of calcium (Ca), which binds calmodulin. The Ca–calmodulin complex then binds calcineurin. This calcineurin–calmodulin complex dephosphorylates nuclear factor of activated T cells (NF-AT). The dephosphorylated NF-AT enters the nucleus and activates cytokine transcription. However, in the presence of tacrolimus, this process is inhibited because tacrolimus binds FK-binding protein (FKBP) in the cytoplasm. The tacrolimus–FKBP complex binds to and inhibits the calcineurin–calmodulin complex. NF-AT is thus not dephosphorylated and is unable to enter the nucleus to activate transcription. (From Paller AS. Use of nonsteroidal topical immunomodulators for the treatment of atopic dermatitis in the pediatric population. *J Pediatr* 2001;138:163–168, with permission.)

with FKBP-12, calcium, calmodulin, and calcineurin resulting in the inactivation of the phosphatase activity of calcineurin (34). This results in the prevention of dephosphorylation and translocation of the nuclear factor of activated T cells (NF-AT). NF-AT is a nuclear component that is potentially responsible for initiation of gene transcription for lymphokines such as interleukin 2 (IL-2) and interferon gamma (IFN-γ). Thus, these series of reactions inhibit the transcription of the genes involved in lymphokine formation (34). Tacrolimus also inhibits transcription of genes that encode for the markers involved in the early stages of T-cell activation such as IL-3, IL-4, IL-5, granulocyte-macrophage colony-stimulating factor, and tumor necrosis factor α. Release of preformed mediators from skin mast cells and basophils has also been shown to be inhibited by tacrolimus (34,41).

Pimecrolimus has a mechanism of action similar to tacrolimus (35). The drug binds with increased affinity to macrophilin-12 (FKBP-12) and inhibits T-cell activation by preventing transcription of early cytokines such as IL-2 and IFN-γ (Th1-type) and IL-4 and IL-10 (Th2-type) synthesis from T cells. Pimecrolimus also prevents release of inflammatory cytokines and mediators from mast cells poststimulation with antigen/immunoglobulin E complex in vitro (40,41). Studies demonstrate that pimecrolimus, unlike corticosteroids, interferes with the inflammatory cascade with no effect on keratinocytes, fibroblasts, endothelial cells, langerhans cells, the hypothalamus, or adrenal gland (35).

Indications and Clinical Use

Topical use of tacrolimus and pimecrolimus is FDA approved as second-line therapy for moderate-to-severe atopic dermatitis in children older than 2 years (39). Off-label use of both tacrolimus and pimecrolimus for first-line therapy has been rapidly increasing (36,40–43). This may be due to a perception by clinicians of a better safety profile compared with topical corticosteroids (40). Between June 2003 and May 2004, there were approximately 2 million prescriptions for tacrolimus and pimecrolimus given for children in the United States with approximately half a million of these for children younger than 2 years (40). In reality, long-term safety of these agents is unknown.

Based on concerns of the FDA regarding the increased risk of malignancy associated with systemic immunosuppression with high dose and prolonged therapy with oral calcineurin inhibitors (cyclosporine and tacrolimus), a black-box warning is included in the labeling for use of these agents. This is based on the theoretical risk calculated from animal studies after oral dosing, data from oral use in transplant patients, and rare reported cases of malignancies (39).

Efficacy of tacrolimus was using a randomized, double-blinded, vehicle-controlled study in children 7 to 16 years of age, with 0.03%, 0.1%, and 0.3% tacrolimus ointment prescribed twice-daily treatment compared with vehicle therapy for 23 days (37). Clinical assessment revealed that 67% to 70% of subjects in the three treatment groups had 75% improvement in symptoms compared with 38% of subjects in the vehicle group (37). Furthermore, tacrolimus ointment was shown to be more effective in children with moderate-to-severe atopic dermatitis, with a faster onset of action and similar safety profile compared with pimecrolimus cream (38). Both TCIs have been to treat other inflammatory skin conditions such as psoriasis, lichen planus, seborrheic dermatitis, allergic contact dermatitis, and vitiligo (16,41).

Despite long-term and short-term studies showing efficacy and safety of topical TCIs, it is prudent to prescribe these medications with caution using recommended guidelines (39). When prescribing topical tacrolimus and pimecrolimus, FDA urges health care providers to consider the following: (a) Prescribe only as second line for short-term or intermittent long-term treatment for atopic dermatitis in patients who are not responsive or intolerant to conservative measures and conventional therapies; (b) The effect of these immunomodulator agents on a developing immune system is not known; therefore, avoid their use in children younger than 2 years; (c) Long-term safety profile (>1 year duration of treatment) is unknown, so limit the use of these therapies to short noncontinuous periods of treatment time; (d) Children and adults with compromised immune system should not be prescribed these agents; and (e) Use the minimum amount required to alleviate patient's symptoms (36,39).

TCIs are beneficial for maintenance therapy of atopic dermatitis, once acute control of skin exacerbation is established with topical steroids (40). An open-label study examined combining TCIs with intermittent topical steroids demonstrated greater benefit in long-term atopic dermatitis lesions with combination therapy than with steroids alone (40,43). Tacrolimus and pimecrolimus topical therapy has demonstrated efficacy in management of head and neck dermatitis where steroid use is limited (43).

Pimecrolimus has been used off label for dermatitis in infants (42). During a 6-week double-blind, vehicle-controlled study of 186 infants (3 to 23 months) with mild-to-moderate atopic dermatitis, twice-daily application of pimecrolimus was effective in clearing 54.5% of patients and resulted in improvement in 70% of patients (42). Treatments used in this study included moderately potent topical corticosteroids during flares, pimecrolimus at the first sign of symptoms, and emollients alone for disease-free intervals.

Pharmacokinetics

Tacrolimus, when ingested orally, undergoes hepatic metabolism; however, with topical application, very little drug is systemically absorbed (33,41). Pimecrolimus also does not show any evidence of dermal-mediated drug metabolism (35). In 80% of samples in a study of patients using tacrolimus for the treatment of moderate-to-severe atopic dermatitis, tacrolimus serum concentration was below the detectable concentration (37).

Damaged skin has shown to have a sevenfold increased absorption rate of tacrolimus, but once the integrity of the dermis is restored, the relatively large tacrolimus molecule has limited penetration (33,41). The TCIs show good dermal penetration with minimal systemic absorption as demonstrated by low serum concentrations and may be used safely on the thinner and more sensitive skin of children (37,40). Blood concentrations of topical tacrolimus are typically undetectable or subtherapeutic; the therapeutic range for organ transplant recipients is 5 to 15 ng per mL. Patients in whom the skin barrier function has been significantly compromised are at increased risk for greater absorption from topical tacrolimus. Blood concentrations of topical pimecrolimus are typically less than 2 ng per mL (35,40).

Pimecrolimus is skin selective which makes this agent unique from tacrolimus and corticosteroids. Compared with tacrolimus and corticosteroids, pimecrolimus is more lipophilic and compared with corticosteroids, pimecrolimus has a higher molecular weight (41). Thus, pimecrolimus has a favorable skin penetration–permeation profile and therefore a low degree of dermal absorption, which may be the reason that pimecrolimus is less likely than tacrolimus to induce immunosuppression in animal models (35,38). Pimecrolimus has a high affinity to the dermis due to its highly lipophilic nature but a limited degree of percutaneous penetration due to larger molecular size, making this an ideal therapeutic agent for the treatment of atopic dermatitis without the systemic side effects (40). A study with 22 infants between the ages of 3 and 23 months, even with the application of pimecrolimus on up to 92% of body surface area, resulted in blood concentrations ranging from 0.1 ng per mL to 2.6 ng per mL (37).

Therapeutic Guidelines

Tacrolimus (Protopic) is available as 0.03% and 0.1% ointments (30 and 60 g). The 0.03% ointment (Elidel) is indicated for use in children aged 2 years and older and the 0.1% ointment for patients aged 15 years and older (18,39). Pimecrolimus is available in a 1% cream (30 and 60 g) and approved for use in patients 2 years of age and older. TCIs have a slower onset of action compared with topical corticosteroid therapy; however, they tend to induce a longer remission. Use has been alternated with topical corticosteroids for disease flares (33,41). The TCIs should be used at the first sign of itch or rash, then should be tapered and replaced with a moisturizer for maintenance when symptoms clear (43).

Pimecrolimus, in a cream base, causes less stinging than tacrolimus. Pimecrolimus may be preferred over tacrolimus for facial skin and for daytime use (38,41). Tacrolimus is associated with a high degree of burning sensation and stinging upon application early in therapy. Tacrolimus may be preferred for more severe disease and use on elbows or knees or at nighttime secondary to the ointment base (38,39). Agents should not be applied to areas of skin affected by viral or bacterial infections (35,36,39). Infections should be treated and cleared prior to therapy with a TCI. Avoid use in pregnant and lactating women (39). Tacrolimus is excreted in breast milk (18,34,39).

Adverse Effects

Tacrolimus is well tolerated, with application-site irritation (pruritus and burning sensation) being the most frequently reported adverse event (18,39). Anecdotally, pimecrolimus causes less burning sensation than tacrolimus (38). Duration of symptoms has been reported to last approximately 2 hours for pruritus and less than 15 minutes for burning sensations (16,18). Effects subside as dermatitis improves (37,38,42).

Other significant adverse events, noted more than in vehicle-control groups, include herpes simplex infection, varicella, and nonapplication-site vesiculobullous eruptions (18,39). Interestingly, incidence of cutaneous and noncutaneous infections in patients treated with tacrolimus is lower than what is reported in children with atopic diathesis (18,37,43). There are case reports of patients with lamellar ichthyosis and Netherton syndrome (triad of trichorrhexis invaginata, ichthyosis linearis circumflexa, and atopic dermatitis) with elevated whole-blood tacrolimus concentrations, but without systemic toxicity (36,41). Monitor serum tacrolimus concentrations in patients with congenital abnormalities directly affecting epidermal barrier function. Lymphadenopathy (0.8%) has been reported during clinical trials of tacrolimus and was usually related to infections of the skin (18,39). Rare adverse events include pyrexia and diarrhea. Use an effective method of contraception during therapy with TCIs (pregnancy category C) (18,39).

Monitoring Parameters

If signs and symptoms of atopic dermatitis do not improve after 6 weeks of TCI therapy, reevaluate diagnosis because cutaneous T-cell lymphoma may present as eczema. Monitor area of application for infection. If infection is diagnosed, discontinue TCI application until clinically resolved.

Instructions for Patients and Their Caregivers

Tacrolimus and pimecrolimus should be applied in a thin layer twice daily, rubbing in gently and completely (18,39). Wash hands thoroughly after application. Continue treatment for 1 week after clearing of symptoms. Do not apply tacrolimus ointment to wet skin. Avoid exposure to sunlight and UVA/UVB rays to minimize phototoxicity reactions (18).

Pimecrolimus cream is safe to use on head, neck, and intertriginous areas, applied under clothing and washed off with soap and water. Relief from burning sensation on application may be obtained by chilling medication prior to application. Moisturizers can be applied after application of TCIs, but neither product is approved for use under occlusive dressing.

VITAMIN D_3 ANALOGUES

CALCIPOTRIENE (CALCIPOTRIOL, INN)

Topical application of synthetic vitamin D_3 analogues for treatment of psoriasis began in the 1980s when it was observed that a patient receiving large doses of vitamin D during an osteoporosis study experienced marked improvement in psoriasis lesions (44,45). Large oral doses of vitamin D have been used since the 1930s to control psoriatic lesions (45). Oral vitamin D therapy for psoriasis is limited by low response rate and is often complicated by hypercalcemia. Psoriasis is a life-long inflammatory disorder, which presents in the first or second decade of life for approximately one-third of patients (46). Management of psoriasis may be challenging and calcipotriene offers a "nonsteroidal" alternative (44–46).

Calcipotriene is a synthetic vitamin D_3 analogue approved for treatment of plaque psoriasis for adults in the United States since 1994 (45). Pediatric use is "off label," trials in children aged 2 to 14 years with mild-to-moderate plaque psoriasis involving less than 30% body surface area show the agent to be effective and well tolerated with mild skin irritation at doses up to 50 g/week (45,46). However, careful monitoring for hypercalciuria and hypercalcemia is prudent (47).

Mechanism of Action

Vitamin D analogue is converted in the skin into vitamin D_3 which is subsequently, hepatically and renally, metabolized into the active form, calcitriol (47). Calcitriol regulates intestinal calcium and phosphate absorption, promoting bone formation and mineralization. As a synthetic vitamin D_3 analogue, calcipotriene binds the vitamin D cytoplasmic receptor, subsequently enters the nucleus, and activates gene transcription (48). Although calcipotriene binds the vitamin D receptor with the same affinity as calcitriol, it is 100 times less active on calcium metabolism.

Calcipotriene inhibits keratinocyte proliferation and differentiation reversing the abnormal keratinocyte change in psoriasis. In addition, calcipotriene acts on cytokines involved in immune function. Specifically, decreasing proinflammatory cytokine IL-8 and increasing IL-10, thereby promoting a Th2 response (humoral) and inhibiting the Th1 response (cell mediated), implicated in psoriasis (49,50).

Indications and Clinical Use

Calcipotriene is an effective alternative to topical corticosteroids for managing plaque-type psoriasis (45,48). Improvement usually occurs after 2 weeks of therapy (51–55). Topical vitamin D analogues usually have a slower onset of action compared with topical corticosteroids in the management of psoriasis, yet tend to provide a longer disease-free interval and greater reduction in disease severity index score (48,55). Calcipotriene has the added benefit of not inducing HPA suppression, telangiectasias, tachyphylaxis, or striae like the topical corticosteroids (19,53). When compared with anthralin or 15% of coal tar, calcipotriene was more effective in reducing psoriasis area and severity index score (48,53,55).

Although calcipotriene is effective as monotherapy, combined therapy has proven effective for more resistant psoriasis (51,56). Calcipotriene enhances efficacy of phototherapy, both UVB and psoralen UVA (55,56). Calcipotriene used in combination with betamethasone gives added benefit and may decrease the local irritating effects of calcipotriene. Calcipotriene is chemically unstable and may be degraded in presence of hydrocortisone valerate, ammonium lactate, or salicylic acid (51). Consult a pharmacist for compatibility information (18).

Pharmacokinetics

Systemic absorption of calcipotriene ointment is greater than the cream (53–55). Applying the drug in an ointment base to psoriatic lesions has resulted in systemic absorption of up to 9% of the topically applied dose (18). Absorption of calcipotriene scalp solution can be 1% of the applied dose. Following systemic absorption, the majority of calcipotriene undergoes hepatic metabolism to inactive compounds. Less than 1% of parent drug is recovered in urine and feces.

Therapeutic Guidelines

Calcipotriene is available as 0.005% cream and scalp solution for twice-daily application. The ointment preparation was recently discontinued. Cost (average wholesale price, AWP) for a 60-g tube of 0.005% calcipotriene cream (Dovonex®) is $253.78 and 60 mL of 0.005% scalp solution is $176.00 (57). To decrease site application irritation, calcipotriene is also available in combination with betamethasone dipropionate 0.064% ointment (Taclonex® 0.005%/0.064%), $317.00.

Adverse Effects

Adverse effects include transient irritation of lesions and surrounding skin, photosensitivity, allergic contact dermatitis, and exacerbation of psoriasis lesions. Burning sensation has occurred with application of the cream to the face and flexures (52–55). Hyperpigmentation has been associated with use of the cream but not the solution (18,56). Skin atrophy as well as folliculitis has occurred. Most serious risk is hypercalcemia and hypercalciuria, which usually does not develop with application of less than 100 g of calcipotriene per week for adults or with doses less than 30% of body surface area or 50 g per week for children (52–57).

Monitoring Parameters

Twenty-four hour urine collection for elevated ratios of calcium to creatinine is useful to monitor for hypercalciuria in children receiving applications of calcipotriene to extensive body surface areas (55). Serum calcium concentrations should be drawn and calcipotriene therapy discontinued if hypercalcemia is suspected. Infants and young children are at greater risk compared with adults due to their higher ratio of skin surface area to body mass (1). Hypercalcemia associated with calcipotriene has been reversible upon discontinuation of therapy. Do not use calcipotriene for patients with known or suspected disorders of calcium metabolism or vitamin D toxicity.

Instructions for Patients and Their Caregivers

Calcipotriene cream should be applied in a thin layer to affected area and rubbed in gently (18). Wash hands thoroughly after applying product to avoid spreading the active drug to other areas or risking inadvertent systemic absorption. Do not apply to face or skin folds as these areas are more prone to irritation. Avoid exposing areas of application to sun (natural or artificial) to prevent phototoxicity reactions because of photosensitizing secondary to thinning of the dermis. Apply calcipotriene cream after UVA exposure as the drug is inactivated by UVA (56). Monitor for signs and symptoms of hypercalcemia (fatigue, confusion, loss of appetite, nausea, vomiting, constipation, and increased urination). If these symptoms develop, discontinue use of calcipotriene and contact the prescriber immediately.

TOPICAL ANTIBACTERIALS

Topical antimicrobial agents in some crude form have been used for thousands of years. The dual role of these preparations includes prophylaxis of infections in abrasions, cuts, burns, wounds, and treatment of infections of superficial wounds (58). Topical antimicrobials in primitive societies were derived from animals, minerals, and plants and these crude remedies were used to treat infections, promote healing, reduce pain and inflammation, debride damaged tissue, and mask foul smells (58–64). The 19th century discovery of chemical preservatives and disinfectants improved control of wound infection (5,59,61,65,66).

Today, the majority of the topical antimicrobial use is for the management of mild-to-moderate acne vulgaris (9,67,68). Topical antimicrobials continue to show efficacy for this indication and have antibacterial activity reducing counts of *Propionibacterium* and decreasing the number of inflammatory and noninflammatory lesions (67–73). Topical antimicrobials are available as over-the-counter products and prescription products in many forms (bars, liquids, creams, ointments, gels, shampoos, solutions, wipes, gauzes (18,74–77) for a variety of indications (75–82). These agents must be used cautiously and appropriately to prevent further contribution of the relentless emergence of antibiotic-resistant strains in the presence of limited discovery of new and novel antibiotics (81–85). Dosage forms, indications, and associated common adverse effects for topical antimicrobial agents frequently used for infants and children are summarized in Table 26.2.

TOPICAL ANTIFUNGAL AGENTS

Fungi often infect the skin surface, invading the stratum corneum and are a major cause of superficial skin infections in infants and children (3,86,87). The three species of aerobic fungi collectively known as dermatophytes include *Trichophyton*, *Microsporum* and *Epidermophyton* which require keratin for growth (86). Tinea infections are superficial fungal infections caused by three species of fungi and are commonly named for affected body part, including tinea capitis (scalp), tinea corporis (general skin), tinea cruris (groin), tinea pedis (feet), and tinea unguium (nails) (3,87). Tinea infections are acquired directly from contact with infected humans (anthropophilic organisms) or animals (zoophilic organisms) or indirectly from exposure to contaminated soil or fomites (geophilic organisms). Diagnosis of infection can usually be made with a detailed history and physical examination and potassium hydroxide microscopy. Culture or histological examination is rarely required for diagnosis (78,87–90).

Most tinea infections can be managed with topical therapies; oral treatment is, however, reserved for tinea capitis, severe tinea pedis, and tinea unguium (91–94). Topical therapy with fungicidal allylamines may have slightly higher cure rates and shorter treatment courses than with fungistatic azoles (9,95–97). Antifungal agents may be applied to surface of the skin as creams, ointments, lotions, shampoos, solutions, sprays, foams, powders, and gels, which readily penetrate the stratum corneum (18).

Antifungal agents can kill the fungi (fungicidal agents), or at least render them unable to grow or divide (fungistatic agents). Fungicidal drugs are preferred for treatment of dermatophytic fungal infections (tinea pedis, tinea cruris, tinea corpora, tinea capitis, onychomycosis) (86). Common tinea infections and topical treatments are summarized in Table 26.3.

Azole drugs such as miconazole, clotrimazole, and ketoconazole are fungistatic, limiting fungal growth but depend on epidermal turnover to shed the still-living fungus from skin surface. Allylamines and benzylamines such as terbinafine, naftifine, and butenafine are fungicidal, actually killing fungal organisms. Cure rates are higher and treatment courses are shorter with topical fungicidal allylamines than with fungistatic azoles. Vaginal candida yeast infections respond well to allylamine drugs, but azole drugs are often preferred (95). Onychomycosis is difficult to treat with topical therapies because the nail bed is difficult to penetrate and often requires prolonged systemic treatment (3,94,96,97). Topical antifungal agents used in pediatric practice with their respective mechanism of action, spectrum of activity, indications, common adverse effects, and cost comparison are summarized in Table 26.4.

PEDICULOCIDES

Lice and scabies affect children worldwide. Head lice infestation is one of the most prevalent communicable conditions in the United States, with 12 million cases annually (98). Clinicians caring for infants and children must consider safe, easy to use, and effective treatment options for louse or scabies infestions. Nonpharmacologic treatment such as occlusive agents (petroleum jelly) lack consistent efficacy data (98,99). Gentle cleansers (Cetaphil®) may be successful (100). Pediculocides must be carefully selected for topical use on infants and young children to avoid potential toxicities associated with systemic absorption. Resistance to pediculocides is increasing worldwide as multiple pediculocides are used over time (98,101). Clinicians are advised to review current resistance patterns for their area.

PYRETHRINS AND PERMETHRIN

Pyrethrins are natural insecticides found in the pyrethrum flower, *Chrysanthemum cinerariaefolium*, which has been used for centuries in Iran as an insecticide (102). Permethrin, the generic name for 3-phenoxybenzyl (±)-*cis–trans*-3-(2,2-dichlorovinyl)-2,2-dimethylcyclopropanecarboxylate, is manufactured as a racemic mixture of *cis* and *trans* isomers in a 1:3 ratio for human use (101). Permethrin is a photostable synthetic pyrethroid modeled after the naturally occurring insecticide.

Mechanism of Action

Pyrethrin and permethrin act on the parasite cell membrane ATPases to disrupt sodium transport causing neurotoxicity and paralysis (103).

Indications and Clinical Use

Pyrethrin is available in combination with piperonyl butoxide without a prescription in the United States for

TABLE 26.2 Topical Antimicrobial Preparations (65,69,73,75,77,78,80,83)

Antimicrobial Agent	*Class*	*Mechanism of Action*	*Spectrum of Activity*	*Clinical Use/Therapeutic Guidelines*	*Adverse Effects*	*Cost*
Azelaic acid (20%)	Dietary constituent of whole grain cereals and animal products	Exact mechanism is unknown	*Staphylococcus epidermidis, Propionibacterium acnes*	Acne vulgaris, rosacea (10)	Pruritus, dry skin, dermatitis, hypopigmentation, hypertrichosis, worsening of asthma	$$$
Bacitracin	Isolated in 1943 from a *Bacillus subtilis* strain cultured from an open wound	Inhibits cell wall synthesis by complexing with C55-prenol pyrophosphatase, involved in transfer of polysaccharides, liposaccharides, and peptidoglycans to the cell wall	Bactericidal and has a narrow spectrum of activity directed predominantly against the gram-positive organisms: *Staphylococcus aureus, Streptococcus pneumoniae,* and *Clostridium difficile.* Other susceptible organisms include *Neisseria, Haemophilus influenzae, Treponema pallidum, Actinomyces,* and *Fusobacterium*	To give a broader spectrum of antibacterial coverage, bacitracin is also available in combination with polymyxin and neomycin (Neosporin or triple antibiotic) or with polymyxin alone (Polysporin)	Pruritus and burning at the application site Delayed-type hypersensitivity in patients with chronic stasis dermatitis, conjunctivitis, and keratoconjunctivitis	$
Benzoyl peroxide (2.5%–20%)	Derived from chlorohydroxyquinolin, a byproduct of coal tar	Release of active or free-radical oxygen capable of oxidizing bacterial proteins, removal of excess sebum and mild desquamation	*Propionibacterium acnes*	Acne vulgaris and oily skin (11)	Excessive drying, peeling, erythema, edema	$
Clindamycin (10%)	Derivative of lincomycin, an antibiotic derived from *Streptomyces* species	Binds the 50S subunit of bacterial ribosomes and inhibits protein synthesis Both bacteriostatic and bactericidal in susceptible organisms (6)	Aerobic gram-positive cocci (*Streptococcus* and most *S. aureus,* both of which cause folliculitis) and anaerobic gram-positive and gram-negative organisms, including *Propionibacterium acnes*	Acne vulgaris, folliculitis, erythrasma, rosacea, and Fox–Fordyce disease (15)	Pruritus, burning, erythema, excessive dryness, peeling, and oily skin	$$
Erythromycin (2%)	Fermentation product of *Streptomyces erythreus*	Macrolide antibiotic which irreversibly binds the 50S subunit of bacterial ribosomes, thereby inhibiting protein synthesis	Erythromycin is effective against gram-positive cocci, *Corynebacterium diphtheriae, Haemophilus influenzae, Legionella pneumophila,* Chlamydia organisms, *Treponema pallidum, Mycoplasma pneumoniae, Ureaplasma urealyticum,* and *Propionobacterium acnes*	Acne vulgaris.	Erythema, scaling, tenderness, burning, itching, oiliness, and dryness.	$$

(*continued*)

TABLE 26.2 Topical Antimicrobial Preparations (65,69,73,75,77,78,80,83) (*Continued*)

Antimicrobial Agent	*Class*	*Mechanism of Action*	*Spectrum of Activity*	*Clinical Use/Therapeutic Guidelines*	*Adverse Effects*	*Cost*
Fusidic acid (2%)	Derived from the fungus *Fusidium coccineum*	Inhibits ribosomal translocation which blocks protein synthesis	*Stephylococcal species*, limited activity against *streptococcal* sp., no activity against gram-negative organisms	Acne vulgaris, dermatitis, pyoderma, furuncle, eczema, burns (17)	Rash, pruritus	
Gentamicin (0.1%)	Aminoglycoside derived from *Micromonospora purpurea*	Inhibits the 30S ribosomal subunit, thereby inhibiting protein synthesis	*S. aureus* and gram-negative bacteria such as *Escherichia coli*, *Proteus* organisms, and *Pseudomonas aeruginosa*	Primary skin infections: impetigo contagiosa, superficial folliculitis, ecthyma, furunculosis, sycosis barbae, and pyoderma gangrenosum Secondary skin infections: infectious eczematoid dermatitis, pustular acne, pustular psoriasis, infected seborrheic dermatitis, infected contact dermatitis	Burning, stinging, redness, lacrimation with ophthalmic use Rash, pruritus, erythema with topical use	$$
Metronidazole (0.75%–1%)	Synthetic nitroimidazole derivative	Exact mechanism is unknown Exhibits anti-inflammatory actions	*Bacillus fragilis*, *Bacteroides melaninogenicus*, *Fusobacterium* organisms, *Veillonella* organisms, *Clostridium* organisms, *Peptococcus* organisms, *Peptostreptococcus* organisms, *Entamoeba histolytica*, *Trichomonas vaginalis*, *Giardia lamblia*, and *Balantidium coli*	Acne rosacea Decreases the number of papules and pustules but has no effect on erythema or telangiectasias (19)	Dryness, stinging, burning. Contact allergy has also been reported (31–34)	$$$
Mupirocin (Bactroban®)	Mupirocin is a metabolite of *Pseudomonas fluorescens*	Mupirocin (pseudomonic acid) inhibits bacterial isoleucyl-tRNA synthetase, which in turn leads to impaired synthesis of bacterial RNA, proteins, and cell wall. The concentrations present in topical formulations allow for bactericidal activity	Mupirocin is bactericidal against *S. aureus*, *S. epidermidis*, and *S. pyogenes*. Mupirocin is also active against methicillin-resistant *S. aureus* (MRSA). However, MRSA resistance to mupirocin is gradually increasing. Mupirocin is ineffective against *P. aeruginosa*, *S. faecalis*, *S. faecium*, *S. bovis*, and fungi	Mupirocin is used for treatment of skin infections secondary to staphylococci and streptococci, including impetigo, folliculitis, impetiginized atopic dermatitis, burns, lacerations, and leg ulcers. Intranasal mupirocin may be used to eliminate staphylococci, including MRSA (24)	Adverse events include application-site burning, pain, and itching. Contact allergy is extremely rare, and there have only been two cases reported	$$$

TABLE 26.2 Topical Antimicrobial Preparations (65,69,73,75,77,78,80,83) (*Continued*)

Antimicrobial Agent	*Class*	*Mechanism of Action*	*Spectrum of Activity*	*Clinical Use/Therapeutic Guidelines*	*Adverse Effects*	*Cost*
Neomycin	Neomycin is a bactericidal aminoglycoside first isolated from *Streptomyces fradiae*	Neomycin exerts its effect by binding the bacterial 30S ribosomal subunit and inhibiting protein synthesis	Neomycin has broad gram-negative coverage including *E. coli, Enterobacter aerogenes, Klebsiella pneumoniae,* and *Proteus vulgaris.* Susceptible gram-positive organisms include *S. aureus, Enterobacter faecalis,* and *Mycobacterium tuberculosis.* Neomycin is not active against *P. aeruginosa* and has poor activity against streptococci	Neomycin is widely used for infections of skin and mucous membranes. Used in combination with other topical antibiotics because of resistance to neomycin along with its limited spectrum of activity. Specifically, polymyxin B is added to provide anti-*Pseudomonas* activity, and bacitracin may be added to broaden the gram-positive coverage to include antistreptococcal activity	Contact dermatitis, erythema, rash, urticaria	$
Polymyxin B	Isolated from the aerobic gram-positive rod *Bacillus polymyxa*	The cationic-free amino groups of polymyxin function as a detergent to disrupt the phospholipid bacterial membranes	Polymyxin B is bactericidal in vitro against gram-negative bacteria including *Proteus mirabilis, P. aeruginosa,* and *Serratia marcesscens*	Open wounds, in combination with other topical antibiotics to broaden antibiotic coverage. Bacitracin + polymyxin B is available over the counter as Polysporin® cream. Neomycin + polymyxin B + bacitracin is available over the counter as Neosporin® ointment		$
Silver sulfadiazine (SSD®, Silvadene®)	Derived from the dual mechanisms of its silver and sulfa moieties	Silver ions bind to negatively charged components in proteins and nucleic acids, thereby effecting structural changes in bacterial cell walls, membranes and nucleic acids that affect binding to DNA	Broad spectrum of antimicrobial coverage including gram-positive bacteria, most gram-negative bacteria, and some yeast forms	Adjunct in the prevention and treatment of infection in second- and third-degree burns (6,7)	Significant percutaneous absorption of sulfadiazine can occur especially when applied to extensive burns Not intended for use in premature neonates and infants <2 mo because sulfas may displace bilirubin from protein binding sites and cause kernicterus	$$

(*continued*)

TABLE 26.2 Topical Antimicrobial Preparations (65,69,73,75,77,78,80,83) (*Continued*)

Antimicrobial Agent	*Class*	*Mechanism of Action*	*Spectrum of Activity*	*Clinical Use/Therapeutic Guidelines*	*Adverse Effects*	*Cost*
Sulfacetamide sodium (Sebizon®)	Sulfa derivative	Interferes with bacterial growth; inhibits bacterial folic acid synthesis by a competitive antagonism of para-aminobenzoic acid (PABA)	Bacteriostatic effect against gram-positive and gram-negative bacteria	Seborrheic dermatitis, secondary cutaneous bacterial infections	Rare cases of drug induced systemic lupus erythematous and Stevens–Johnson syndrome have been reported, exfoliative dermatitis, toxic epidermal necrolysis, rash, erythema	$$
Tetracyclines (Topicycline®, Achromycin®)	First isolated from the *Streptomyces species* in the late 1940s	Reversibly bind to the 30S ribosome and inhibit binding of aminoacyl-tRNA to the acceptor site on the 70S ribosome Exact mechanism is unknown for the treatment of acne vulgaris Systemic tetracyclines decrease free fatty acids present in acne lesions	Broad spectrum of activity against gram positive, gram negative, rickettsiae, mycobacterium, and protozoa.	Treatment of acne vulgaris (25)	Yellowing of skin (may be removed by washing off tetracycline)	$$

Notes: Prolonged use of any topical antimicrobial as monotherapy may result in decreased efficacy and antibiotic resistance. Prevent antibiotic resistance by alternating antimicrobials. Combination products are generally more effective than when used alone (84). Combination products may inhibit development of antibiotic resistance (84,85).

treatment of head lice in children older than two years (18,98,102). Brand names of products are summarized in Table 26.5. As the pyrethrins are not ovicidal, retreatment is necessary to kill any newly hatched nymphs.

Permethrin is also available "over the counter" in the United States as a 1% cream rinse for treatment of head lice in children as young as 2 months and is considered first-line treatment secondary to efficacy and safety (18,98,101,102). This agent is safe for use in pregnant women. There is no known cross-reactivity with other pyrethrins. The 5% cream formulation is safe and effective for treatment of scabies and is the treatment of choice in children older than 2 years and pregnant women (104,105). A double-blind, randomized study comparing crotamiton 10% cream with permethrin 5% cream was conducted in children 2 months to 5 years of age, some of whom were lindane treatment failures (105). Four weeks after treatment, 89% of the permethrin-treated group versus 60% of the crotamiton-treated group was cured. Another study compared 5% permethrin cream with 1% lindane lotion for treatment of scabies in patients 2 months to 75 years of age (105). The study demonstrated 91% and 86% cure rates approximately 4 weeks after treatment with permethrin and lindane, respectively. Although permethrin is not FDA approved for treatment in infants younger than 2 months, it was used successfully without side effects in a 23-day-old infant (106). Permethrin 5% cream is also effective in treating head lice, yet is not FDA approved for this indication (18,98,102).

Pharmacokinetics

Both pyrethrin and permethrin demonstrate low dermal absorption (98,102). After application of 5% permethrin cream, mean absorption was less than 1%, and maximum amount absorbed was 2% of the applied dose (102). Pyrethrin and permethrin are metabolized in the skin via ester cleavage, which subsequently allows for rapid urinary excretion of inactive metabolites. Less than 2% of

TABLE 26.3 Therapy for Common Tinea Infections

Infection	Agent	Frequency	Duration (Days)
Tinea corporis, tinea pedis, tinea cruris	Butenafine (Mentax®)	Daily	14
	Clotrimazole (Lotrimin®)	Topical: twice daily	14
		Vaginal: 100 mg/d at bedtime	7
		200 mg/d at bedtime	3
	Econazole (Spectazole®)	Topical: daily	14
			Tinea pedis: 30
	Ketoconazole (Nizoral®)	Topical: once to twice daily	14
	Miconazole (Micatin®, Monistat-Derm® Micatin®)	Twice daily	14
			Tinea pedis/corporis: 30
		Vaginal: 100 mg/d at bedtime	7
		200 mg/d at bedtime	3
	Terbinafine (Lamisil®)	Twice daily	7–30

TABLE 26.4 Topical Antifungal Preparations

Antifungal Agent	Class	Mechanism of Action	Spectrum of Activity	Clinical Use/Therapeutic Guidelines	Adverse Effects	Cost
Amphotericin B (Fungizone®) 3%	Polyene antimycotic derived from *Streptomyces nodosus*	Binds to ergosterol altering cell membrane permeability causing leakage of cell components	*Candida (Monilia) species*	Treatment of cutaneous and mucocutaneous mycotic infections	Erythematic, prorates, burning, drying effect	$
Butenafine (Mentax®) 1%	Benzylamine derivative	Inhibits the epoxidation of squalene and thereby blocking the biosynthesis of ergosterol	*Malassezia furfur, Epidermophyton floccosum, Trichophyton mentagrophytes, Trichophyton rubrum, Trichophyton tonsurans*	Tinea pityriasis versicolor, tinea pedis, tinea corporis, tinea cruris	Burning, stinging, itching	$$$
Ciclopirox (Loprox®, Penlac®) 0.77%, 8%	Synthetic hydroxypiridone derived	Intracellular depletion of essential substrates by inhibiting transmembrane transport decreasing RNA and DNA synthesis	*Trichophyton rubrum, Trichophyton mentagrophytes, E. Floccosum, M. Canis, cutaneous candidiasis due to C. Albicans, Tinea pityriasis due to M. furfur*	Tinea pedis, tinea cruris, tinea corporis, onychomycosis of fingernails and toenails	Burning, erythema	$$$$
Clotrimazole (Lotrimin®) 1%	Imidazole	Inhibit fungal activity by preventing the formation of ergosterol, a molecule required for fungal cell membrane integrity	*Trichophyton rubrum, T. mentagrophytes, E. floccosum, M. canis*	Tinea pedis, tinea cruris, tinea corporis	Erythema, pruritus, urticaria, burning, blistering	$
Econazole nitrate (Spectazole®) 1%	Imidazole	Inhibit fungal activity by preventing the formation of ergosterol, a molecule required for fungal cell membrane integrity	*Trichophyton rubrum, T. mentagrophytes, T. tonsurans, M. canis, M. audouini, M. gypseum, E. floccosum, C. albicans, Malassezia furfur*	Tinea pedis, tinea cruris, tinea corporis, tinea versicolor	Burning, itching, stinging	$$$

(*continued*)

TABLE 26.4 Topical Antifungal Preparations (*Continued*)

Antifungal Agent	*Class*	*Mechanism of Action*	*Spectrum of Activity*	*Clinical Use/Therapeutic Guidelines*	*Adverse Effects*	*Cost*
Gentian violet (1%, 2%)	Antibacterial and antifungal dye	Topical antiseptic/germicide	*Candida, Cryptococcus, Epidermophyton, Trichlophyton*	Topical anti-infective used for treatment of abrasions, minor cuts and superficial fungus infections of the skin	Stains skin and clothing	$
Haloprogin (Halotex®) 1%	Synthetic halogenated phenolic	Unknown mechanism of action but presumed to act on cell wall integrity	*Trichophyton rubrum, T. tonsurans, T. mentagrophytes, Microsporum canis, Epidermophyton floccosum*	Tinea pedis, tinea cruris, tinea corporis, tinea manuum, tinea versicolor	Local irritation, burning, erythema, itching, folliculitis, pruritus	$$$
Iodochlorhydroxyquin (Clioquinol®) 3%	Derivative of chloroquine	Exact mechanism of action is unknown but appears to inhibit DNA structure and function		Tinea pedis, tinea cruris	Burning, skin irritation, skin stain, potential cross-sensitivity with certain antimalarials	$$
Ketoconazole (Nizoral®) 2%	Imidazole	Inhibit fungal activity by preventing the formation of ergosterol, a molecule required for fungal cell membrane integrity	*Trichophyton rubrum, T. mentagrophytes, E. floccosum, M. furfur, Candida* sp, *Microsporum canis, M. audouini, M. gypseum, P. orbiculare*	Tinea corporis, tinea cruris, tinea pedis, tinea versicolor, seborrheic dermatitis	Pruritis, stinging, local irritation	$$
Miconazole (Monistat®, Monistat-Derm®, Micatin®) 2%	Imidazole	Inhibit fungal activity by preventing the formation of ergosterol, a molecule required for fungal cell membrane integrity	*Trichophyton rubrum, T. mentagrophytes, E. floccosum, C Albicans*	Tinea corporis, tinea cruris, tinea pedis, tinea corporis, tinea versicolor, cutaneous candidiasis	Contact dermatitis, burning, local irritation	$
Naftifine (Naftin®) 1%	Synthetic allylamine derivative	Interferes with sterol biosynthesis by inhibiting the enzyme squalene 2,3-epoxidase	*Trichophyton rubrum, T. mentagrophytes, T. tonsurans, Epidermophyton floc. Microsporum canis, M. audouini, M. gypseum, Candida* sp	Tinea pedis, tinea cruris, tinea corporis	Burning, stinging, dryness	$$$
Nystatin (Mycostatin) 100,000 units per gram	Polyene antimycotic derived from *Streptomyces noursei*)	Nystatin irreversibly binds membrane sterols of *Candida* and alters membrane permeability, resulting in loss of essential intracellular components	*C. albicans, C. parapsilosis, C. krusei,* and *C. tropicalis.* Nystatin is, however, ineffective against dermatophytes	Nystatin is effective in the treatment of candidial infections of the skin (intertrigo) and mucous membranes (thrush and vaginal candidiasis)	Contact dermatitis, rash	$
Oxiconazole (Oxistat®) 1%	Imidazole	Inhibit fungal activity by preventing the formation of ergosterol, a molecule required for fungal cell membrane integrity	*Trichophyton rubrum, T. mentagrophytes, Epidermophyton floccosum, Malassezia furfur*	Tinea pedis, tinea cruris, tinea corporis, tinea versicolor	Pruritus, burning, stinging	$$$

TABLE 26.4 Topical Antifungal Preparations (*Continued*)

Antifungal Agent	*Class*	*Mechanism of Action*	*Spectrum of Activity*	*Clinical Use/Therapeutic Guidelines*	*Adverse Effects*	*Cost*
Sulconazole (Exelderm®) 1%	Imidazole	Inhibit fungal activity by preventing the formation of ergosterol, a molecule required for fungal cell membrane integrity	*Trichophyton rubrum, T. mentagrophytes, Epidermophyton floccosum, Malassezia furfur*	Tinea pedis, tinea cruris, tinea corporis	Itching, burning, stinging, redness	$$
Terbinafine (Lamisil®) 1%	Synthetic allylamine derivative	Inhibits squalene epoxidase resulting in deficiency in ergosterol	*E. floccosum, T. mentagrophytes, T. rubrum*	Tinea pedis, tinea cruris, tinea corporis	Local irritation, burning, itching, dryness	$
Terconazole (Terazol®) 0.4%, 0.8%	Triazole	Inhibits fungal activity by preventing the formation of ergosterol, a molecule required for fungal cell membrane integrity	*Candida* sp.	Vaginal yeast infections	Burning, itching	$
Tolnaftate (Tinactin®) 1%	Synthetic allylamine derivative	Inhibits squalene epoxidase resulting in deficiency of ergosterol	*E. floccosum, T. mentagrophytes, T. rubrum*	Tinea pedis, tinea cruris, tinea corporis	Mild irritation	$
Triacetin (Fungoid Tincture®)	Oils derived from plants	Exact mechanism is unknown	*Aureobasidium mansonii, Alternaria solani, Aspergillus niger, C. albicans, Epidermophyton floccosum, Microsporum audouinii, Piedraia hortae, Rhizopus arrhizus*	Onychomycosis, tinea pedis, tinea cruris, tinea corporis, monilial impetigo and dermatitis	Local irritation	$
Undecylenic acid (Cruex®, Fungi-Nail®, Desenex®) 10%–25%	Natural fatty acid derived from castor oil	Fatty acid which slows proliferation of fungus by altering conditions of growth	*E. floccosum, T. mentagrophytes, T. rubrum*	Tinea pedis, tinea cruris	Rash, local irritation, stinging	$

permethrin cream or cream rinse is absorbed into the circulation (102). Permethrin can be detected on hair for up to 10 days after application.

Therapeutic Guidelines

Instructions for use of pyrethrin and permethrin are summarized in Table 26.5. It is recommended that all lice treatments be repeated 7 to 10 days after initial treatment to kill newly hatched nymphs (75,98). Treatment of scabies involves application of permethrin 5% cream from neck to toes for 8 to 12 hours, with particular attention to postauricular areas, web spaces, genitals, and fingernails (104,105). Treatment of scalp and face is recommended for infants younger than 2 years (18). Close contacts should also be treated. In addition, all bedding, towels, and clothing should be washed or at least isolated for 3 days—failure to do so may result in reinfection (98). Parents should be advised that pruritus may persist for up to 3 weeks after treatment. A second treatment at 1 week is particularly important if there is involvement of palms and soles. Treatment of pediculosis (head lice) involves application of permethrin 1% cream rinse for 10 minutes before washing off (98).

Adverse Events

The most common complaints are application-site burning, irritation, and tingling sensation (98,102). Despite permethrin being preserved with formaldehyde, reports of allergic contact dermatitis are rare. Patients allergic to ragweed, chrysanthemum flowers, or plants of the Compositae family may experience contact sensitivity to pyrethrin (102). Children with a history of asthma may experience asthma exacerbations or breathing difficulties during application of pyrethrin.

TABLE 26.5 Summary of Topical Treatments for Head Lice and Scabies

Agent	Brand Name(s)	Formulation	Indication(s)	Directions	Adverse Effects
Pyrethrins	A-200, Licide, Pronto, RID, Tisit, Triple X, and R&C	0.33% shampoo, lotion	Head lice OTC Pregnancy C	Apply to dry hair on day 1, lather, leave on 10 minutes, rinse. Repeat on days 7–10	Local irritation, possible cross-reaction with Compositae plants, asthma exacerbations
Permethrin	Nix, Elimite, Acticin	1% cream rinse, 5% cream	1%: head lice OTC 5%: scabies Prescription Age >2 mo Pregnancy B	For head lice: apply after shampooing, leave on 10 minutes, rinse	Local irritation, burning, tingling at application site
Lindane	NA Kwell withdrawn	1% shampoo, lotion	Head lice Prescription Pregnancy C	Apply to dry hair, leave on 4 minutes, rinse. No retreatment	Central nervous system toxicity, increased seizure risk—not first-line treatment
Malathion	Ovide	0.5% lotion	Head lice Prescription Age >6 yr Pregnancy B	Apply to dry hair, leave on 8–12 hr, rinse. Repeat on days 7–9	Flammable vehicle, scalp irritation
Crotamiton	Eurax	10% cream, lotion	Scabies Off-label: head lice Prescription Limited safety data in children Pregnancy C	For scabies: apply chin to toes Reapply in 24 hr. Leave on for 48 hr, rinse	Local irritation or sensitivity reactions. Severe oral and esophageal, gastric burning and irritation upon ingestion Do not apply to mucus membranes or inflamed skin

NA, not available; OTC, over the counter or available without a prescription in the United States.

LINDANE

Lindane is the gamma isomer of 1,2,3,4,5,6-hexachlorocyclohexane and has been used as an agricultural pesticide for over 50 years (98). This agent has been associated with serious central nervous system toxicities including seizures due to systemic absorption (107). Lindane has a black-box warning secondary to neurotoxicity. Secondary to availability of safer pediculocides, use of lindane has declined. The effectiveness of lindane has declined over the past decade (108–112). Nonetheless, the medication is still available as a generic formulation by prescription in many states in a restricted volume (60 mL) for clinical use (18,98). The brand name product Kwell® has been withdrawn from market. Several states and countries have banned the use of lindane.

Mechanism of Action

Lindane is an organochlorine insecticide that inhibits neurotransmission, resulting in respiratory and muscular paralysis in arthropods via noncompetitive inhibition of γ-aminobutyric acid (GABA) receptor (113). Resistance is due to GABA-receptor mutations (109).

Indications and Clinical Use

The FDA (http://www.fda.gov/cder/drug/infopage/lindane) has outlined specific instructions on lindane use. Lindane 1% lotion is a second-line treatment for scabies and lindane 1% shampoo is a second-line treatment for pediculosis capitis (head lice) or pediculosis pubis (pubic lice) (111). However, lindane should be used only on appropriately selected patients who have failed treatment or cannot tolerate other medications such as permethrin or crotamiton (112).

Pharmacokinetics

Topical application of lindane results in a 10-fold greater absorption than that of permethrin, with serum concentrations 40-fold higher due to difference in metabolism (110,113). Serum concentrations increase with repeated applications. Lindane is widely distributed throughout the body and slowly metabolized and excreted in urine and feces (112). Infants, particularly premature or low-birth-weight infants with reduced body fat concentrations, and young children are at greater risk of elevated lindane concentrations (1).

Therapeutic Guidelines

Lindane 1% lotion may be used for treatment of scabies (18). Patients are instructed to apply a thin layer to the entire body from the neck to toes and wash off completely after 8 hours. Lindane 1% shampoo may be used for pediculosis capitis or pubis (98). Patients are instructed to apply the shampoo to the affected area for 4 minutes before washing off. Applications are restricted to one time, yet lindane is not pediculocidal, and more than one treatment may be required to eradicate lice, leading to possible adverse effects (107,111).

Adverse Events

Common side effects include lindane toxicity, which may result in potentially serious and irreversible central nervous system effects, ranging from headaches to seizures and even death (107). Aplastic anemia has also rarely been reported with use of lindane (107). Lindane is not recommended for use in children younger than 2 years, pregnant or lactating women, patients weighing less than 50 kg, or patients with extensive dermatitis (98).

CROTAMITON

Crotamiton (crotonyl-*N*-ethyl-*O*-toluidine) is a colorless or pale yellow oil used in the treatment of scabies (113). The mechanism of action is unknown. The FDA has approved the agent for treatment of scabies in adults. Crotamiton use is considered safe but is not as effective as permethrin (105). A study of children with scabies showed an eradication rate of 89% after treatment with permethrin cream compared with 60% after treatment with crotamiton (78). Crotamiton is available in a 10% cream or lotion (18,114). Patients are instructed to apply 30 g from neck to toes on 2 consecutive days. Cases of crotamiton-resistant scabies have been reported (115).

PRECIPITATED SULFUR

Sulfur 5% to 10% compounded in cream or ointment has been used for over 150 years in treating scabies (113–115). Mechanism of action is unknown. A recent open-label study used 5% to 10% sulfur in petrolatum to treat scabies in patients 2 months to 6 years of age with a 71% cure rate at 4 weeks posttreatment (116). Mild facial edema was the only significant adverse event. Overall, compounded sulfur preparations are considered safe, with use limited by messiness and offensive odor.

MALATHION

Malathion is an organophosphate acetylcholinesterase inhibitor insecticide indicated for treatment of head lice in children older than 6 years (18,98). Trials using malathion lotion have included children aged 2 to 11 years (100,101). The product was withdrawn from the US market in 1995 and reintroduced in 1999 when more effective pediculocides were needed (98,109,111). Disadvantages of malathion include flammable vehicle, chemical odor, prolonged application time of 8 to 12 hours, and cholinesterase depletion with respiratory depression if accidentally ingested (98,112, 113). Malathion is available by prescription in the United States and is an effective pediculocide (18,98).

RETINOIDS

Retinoids are composed of natural compounds and synthetic derivatives with vitamin A activity. During the 1970s, tretinoin (all-*trans*-retinoic acid) began the era of retinoid therapy for acne vulgaris (117,118). New retinoids are compared with tretinoin efficacy. Newer synthetic retinoids may be more advantageous than tretinoin because of their more specific mechanism of action (119,120). Adapalene, a naphthoic acid derivative, and tazarotene have retinoid and antiinflammatory properties (120–122). Topical retinoids are the foundation of acne treatment for the majority of patients secondary to their comedolytic and anti-inflammatory effects (117,118).

Mechanism of Action

Appreciation of retinoid function requires an understanding of two retinoid receptor families. These two nuclear receptor families include retinoic acid receptors (RARs) and retinoid X receptors (RXRs) (113). Each family is composed of α, β, and γ subtypes. Predominant subtypes in human skin are RAR-α, RAR-γ, RXR-α, and RXR-β. The RARs and RXRs always exist as dimers in vivo, RARs exist as heterodimers complexed with RXR, and RXRs exist as either hetero- or homodimers. These receptors are bound by their ligands, and this receptor–ligand complex binds promoter regions to initiate transcription. Altered gene transcription affects epidermal and follicular keratinocyte growth and differentiation (119). The resultant effect may, in part, explain the comedolytic actions of retinoids. All-*trans*-retinoic acid (tretinoin) is a nonspecific ligand that binds all RAR receptors with high affinity (119). Adapalene, a napthoic acid retinoid, is a synthetic molecule that more specifically binds RAR-β and RAR-γ. Tazarotene, an acetylenic retinoid, is also a synthetic molecule that selectively binds RAR-β and RAR-γ and has no affinity for RXR receptors (120).

Acne lesions are produced by a combination of four primary pathogenic conditions: (a) sebum production by the sebaceous gland; (b) *Propionibacterium acnes* follicular colonization; (c) alteration in the keratinization process; and (c) release of inflammatory mediators into the skin (123). Topical retinoids act on follicular epithelium and loosens comedones, permitting flow of sebum to skin surface (6). Inflammatory changes may also precede hyperkeratinization (123). The topical retinoids with their anti-inflammatory in addition to anticomedone properties (117,118,121–124) are recommended as a foundation in acne therapy except those patients with severe disease (nodule/conglobate) (118).

Indications and Clinical Use

Tretinoin, adapalene, and tazarotene are all effective for treatment of comedogenic acne (117,118). Topical retinoids used in combination with topical or oral antibiotics have been shown to be more effective than either therapy alone (125). Antibiotics reduce the *P. acnes* population and also have direct anti-inflammatory effects, both of which make them effective in treating inflammatory lesions. Overall, topical retinoids will reduce number of acne lesions by 40% to 70% (126). Tazarotene has been shown to be most efficacious (126). Unlike tretinoin, adapalene is not photolabile and may be applied during the daytime and is less irritating to skin compared with tretinoin or tazarotene. Topical steroids are sometimes combined with tazarotene to decrease irritation (121).

Patients should be advised that response to treatment may not be observed for 6 to 8 weeks, and the disease may initially worsen during the first 2 to 4 weeks. Retinoids may also be helpful in treating postinflammatory hyperpigmentation. Retinoids are able to normalize proliferation and differentiation of keratinocytes, giving them usefulness in diseases with abnormal keratinization such as ichthyosis and palmoplantar keratodermas. Other diseases that may be responsive to topical retinoids include Darier disease, flat warts, and oral lichen planus. Tretinoin has demonstrated effectiveness for cosmetic treatment of photoaging and, therefore, may require prior authorization for some prescription plans (127). Tazarotene is effective in psoriasis (56). Bexarotene is a synthetic retinoid used for treatment of stage I cutaneous T-cell lymphoma (mycosis fungoides) (113). Alitretinoin, a naturally occurring endogenous retinoid, is effective for Kaposi sarcoma lesions (113).

Therapeutic Guidelines

Retinoids are not used for spot treatment of individual acne lesions but rather are applied at bedtime to the entire surface of skin prone to development of mild-to-moderate acne (117,118,126). All-*trans*-retinoic acid (tretinoin), vitamin A acid, is marketed as Retin-A, Retin-A-Micro (0.1% sustained release gel, less irritating vehicle), and Avita cream. Concentrations and formulations: 0.025%, 0.05%, and 0.1% cream; 0.01%, 0.025%, 0.04%, and 0.1% gel; and 0.05% solution.

Adapalene (Differin) is available as 0.1% gel, cream, pledgets, and solution. Tazarotene (Tazorac) is available as a 0.05% and 0.1% gel and may be more expensive than other retinoids. Bexarotene (Targretin) is available in a 1% gel for cutaneous T-cell lymphoma. Alitretinoin is available in 0.1% gel for Kaposi sarcoma lesions.

Adverse Events

Erythema, scaling, pruritus, burning, stinging, dryness, increased photosensitivity, and irritation are well-known side effects of topical retinoids, but their occurrence does not necessitate cessation of therapy (124). Sunscreen use and night application should be advised. Spacing out therapy from daily to every other day and to even as much as once weekly may decrease irritation without compromising efficacy. In addition, advising patients that these side effects improve with increased duration of treatment may help to improve compliance. Initiating therapy with a lower concentration of retinoid, then gradually increasing when tolerated, may be an alternative. Several months of treatment may be necessary to achieve desired response.

Tretinoin and adapalene are pregnancy category C, while tazarotene and bexarotene are category X (18). Teratogenic effects of systemic retinoids are well established. Although there are no known reports of teratogenicity with topical retinoids, potential risks warrant their cessation prior to or in event of pregnancy. Patients should be counseled to use an effective form of contraception while using these topical agents. Although risks from retinoid therapy are decreased by administering these agents via the topical route, patient and caregiver education is important to improve outcome and decrease adverse effects of these potent agents in acne therapy.

REFERENCES

1. Kearns GL, Abdel-Rahman SM, Alander SW, et al. Developmental pharmacology—drug disposition, action, and therapy in infants and children. *N Engl J Med* 2003;349(12):1157–1167.
2. Rutter N. The immature skin. *Eur J Pediatr* 1996;155:S18–S20.
3. Campbell JM, Banta-Wright SA. Neonatal skin disorders: a review of selected dermatologic abnormalities. *J Perinatal Neonatal Nurs* 2000;14(1):63–83.
4. Shwayder T, Akland T. Neonatal skin barrier: structure, function, and disorders. *Dermatologic Ther* 2006;18:87–103.
5. Hoath SB, Narendran V. Adhesives and emollients in the preterm infant. *Semin Neonatol* 2000;5:289–296.
6. Fairley JA, Rasmussen JE. Comparison of stratum corneum thickness in children and adults. *J Am Acad Dermatol* 1983;8: 652–654.
7. Genzel-Boroviczeny O, Strotgen J, Harris AG, et al. Orthogonal polarization spectral imaging (OPS): a novel method to measure the microcirculation in term and preterm infants transcutaneously. *Pediatr Res* 2002;51(3):386–391.
8. Rutter N. Percutaneous drug absorption in the newborn: hazards and uses. *Clin Perinatol* 1987;81:911–930.
9. Wolverton S. *Comprehensive dermatologic drug therapy*. Philadelphia, PA: WB Saunders, 2001.
10. Abraham MH, Chandra HS, Mitchell RC. The factors that influence skin penetration of solutes. *J Pharm Pharmacol* 1995;47: 8–16.
11. Bergstrom Kendra G, Strober Bruce E. Principles of topical therapy. In: Wolff K, Goldsmith LA, Katz SI, et al., eds. *Fitzpatrick's dermatology in general medicine*, 7th ed. http://www.accessmedicine.com/content.aspx?aID = 3001636, 2007.
12. Farahmand S, Maibach HI. Estimating skin permeability from physiochemical characteristics of drugs: a comparison between conventional models and an in vivo-based approach. *Int J Pharm* 2009;375:41–47.
13. Ricciatitti-Sibbald D, Sibbald RG. Dermatologic vehicles. *Clin Dermatol* 1988;7(3):11–24.
14. Bronaugh RL, Franz TJ. Vehicle effects on percutaneous absorption: in vivo and in vitro comparisons with human skin. *Br J Dermatol* 1986;115:1–11.
15. Elias PM, Menon GK. Structural and lipid biochemical correlates of the epidermal permeability barrier. *Adv Lipid Res* 1991;24: 1–26.
16. Kunz GD, Zimmermann R, Gross G. Successful treatment of nodular actinic reticuloid with tacrolimus ointment. *Dermatology* 2006;212(4):377–380.
17. Mantle D, Gok MA. Adverse and beneficial effects of plant extracts on skin and skin disorders. *Adverse Drug React Toxicol Rev* 2001;20(2):89–103.
18. Facts and Comparisons® Online 4.0. St Louis, MO: Wolter Kluwer Health, 2009.
19. Hengee UR, Ruzika T, Schwartz RA, et al. Adverse effects of topical corticosteroids. *J Am Acad Dermatol* 2006;54(1):1–15.
20. du Vivier A. Prescribing topical corticosteroids. *Br J Gen Pract* 1993;43(377):491–492.
21. Tadicherla S, Ross K, Shenefelt PD, et al. Topical corticosteroids in dermatology. *J Drugs Dermatol* 2009;8(12):1093–1105.
22. du Vivier A, Stoughton RB. Tachyphylaxis to the action of topically applied corticosteroids. *Arch Dermatol* 1975;111(5):581–583.
23. Jackson DB, Thompson C, McCormack JR, et al. Bioequivalence (bioavailability) of generic topical corticosteroids. *J Am Acad Dermatol* 1989;20(5, pt 1):791–796.
24. Klaus W, Goldsmith L, Katz S, et al. Topical corticosteroids. In: *Fitzpatrick's dermatology in general medicine*, 7th ed.
25. Wolverton SE. *Comprehensive dermatologic drug therapy*. WB Saunders, 2001:562.

26. Goa KL. Clinical pharmacology and pharmacokinetic properties of topically applied corticosteroids. A review. *Drugs* 1998; 36(Suppl 5):51–61.
27. Burden AD, Beck MH. Contact hypersensitivity to topical corticosteroids. *Br J Dermatol* 1992;127(5):497–500.
28. Last AR. Choosing topical corticosteroids. *Am Fam Physician* 2009;79(2):135–140.
29. Wachs GN, Maibach HI. Co-operative double-blind trial of an antibiotic/corticoid combination in impetiginized atopic dermatitis. *Br J Dermatol* 1976;95(3):323–328.
30. Leyden JJ, Kligman AM. The case for steroid–antibiotic combinations. *Br J Dermatol* 1977;96(2):179–187.
31. Stoughton RB. Are generic formulations equivalent to trade name topical glucocorticoids? *Arch Dermatol* 1987;123(10): 1312–1314.
32. Stoughton RB, Wullich K. The same glucocorticoid in brand-name products. Does increasing the concentration result in greater topical biologic activity? *Arch Dermatol* 1989;125(11): 1509–1511.
33. Russell J. Topical tacrolimus: a new therapy for atopic dermatitis. *Am Fam Physician* 2002;66:1899–1902.
34. Bekersky I, Fitzsimmons W, Tanase A, et al. Nonclinical and early clinical development of tacrolimus ointment for the treatment of atopic dermatitis. *J Am Acad Dermatol* 2001;44:S17–S27.
35. Weinberg JM. Formulary review of therapeutic alternatives for atopic dermatitis: focus on pimecrolimus. *J Manag Care Pharm* 2005;11(1):56–64.
36. Leung DM, Boguniewicz M, Broadbent JB, et al. Report of the topical calcineurin inhibitor task force of the American College of Allergy, Asthma and Immunology and the American Academy of Allergy, Asthma and Immunology. *J Allergy Clin Immunol* 2005;115:1249–1253.
37. Boguniewicz M, Fiedler VC, Raimer S, et al. A randomized, vehicle-controlled trial of tacrolimus ointment for treatment of atopic dermatitis in children. *J Allergy Clin Immunol* 1998;102(4, pt 1): 637–644.
38. Paller AS, Lebwohl M, Fleischer AB, et al. Tacrolimus ointment is more effective than pimecrolimus cream with a similar safety profile in the treatment of atopic dermatitis: results from 3 randomized, comparative studies. *J Am Acad Dermatol* 2005;52:810–822.
39. Food and Drug Administration. Elidel (pimecrolimus) cream and protopic (tacrolimus) ointment. April 30, 2009. http://www.fda.gov/Drugs/DrugSafety/PublicHealthAdvisories/ucm051760.htm.
40. Praiser D. Topical corticosteroids and topical calcineurin inhibitors in the treatment of atopic dermatitis: focus on percutaneous absorption. *Am J Ther* 2009;16(3):264–273.
41. Aylin TE, Serap O. Topical calcineurin inhibitors, pimecrolimus and tacrolimus. *Antiinflamm Antiallergy Agents Med Chem* 2007;6: 237–243.
42. Paul C, Cork M, Rossi AB, et al. Safety and tolerability of 1% pimecrolimus cream among infants: experience with 1133 patients treated for up to 2 years. *Pediatrics* 2006;117:e118–e128.
43. Eric L, Simpson MD, Hanifin JM. Atopic dermatitis. *J Acad Dermatol* 2005;53:115–128.
44. Morimoto S, Kumahara Y. A patient with psoriasis caused by 1-α-hydroxyvitamin D_3. *Med J Osaka Univ* 1985;35:51–54.
45. Kragbelle K. Treatment of psoriasis with calcipotriol and with other vitamin D analogues. *J Am Acad Dermatol* 1992;27: 1001–1008.
46. Benoit S, Hamm H. Childhood psoriasis. *Clin Dermatol* 2007; 25:555–562.
47. Pinette KV, Yee YK, Amegadzie BY, et al. Vitamin D receptor as a drug discovery target. *Mini Rev Med Chem* 2003;3(3):193–204.
48. Segaert S, Duvold LB. Calcipotriol cream: a review of its use in the management of psoriasis. *J Dermatolog Treat* 2006;17(6):327–237.
49. Nagpal S, Na S, Rathnachalam R. Noncalcemic actions of vitamin D receptor ligands. *Endocr Rev* 2005;26(5):662–667.
50. Kang S, Yi S, Griffiths CE, et al. Calcipotriene-induced improvement in psoriasis is associated with reduced interleukin-8 and increased interleukin-10 levels within lesions. *Br J Dermatol* 1998; 138:77–83.
51. Patel B, Siskin S, Krazmien R, et al. Compatibility of calcipotriene with other topical medications. *J Am Acad Dermatol* 1998;38: 1010–1011.
52. Lebwohl M, Ortonne JP, Andres P, et al. Calcitriol ointment 3 microg/g is safe and effective over 52 weeks for the treatment of mild to moderate plaque psoriasis. *Cutis* 2009;83(4): 205–212.
53. Darley CR, Cunliffe WJ, Green CM, et al. Safety and efficacy of calcipotriol (Diovenex) in treating children with psoriasis vulgaris. *Br J Dermatol* 1996;135:390–393.
54. Park SB, Suh DH, Youn JI. A pilot study to assess the safety and efficacy of calcipotriol treatment (Diovenex) in treating children with childhood psoriasis. *Pediatr Dermatol* 1999;16: 321–325.
55. Orange AP, Marcoux D, Svensson A, et al. Topical calcipotriol in childhood psoriasis. *J Am Acad Dermatol* 1996;35:203–208.
56. Menter A, Korman NJ, Elmets CA, et al. Guidelines of care for the management of psoriasis and psoriatic arthritis. *J Am Dermatol* 2009;60:643–659.
57. *Red Book: Pharmacy's Fundamental Reference*, 113th ed. Los Angeles, CA: Medical Economics, 2009.
58. Forrest RD. Early history of wound treatment. *J R Soc Med* 1982;75(3):198–205.
59. Hugo WB. A brief history of heat and chemical preservation and disinfection. *J Appl Bacteriol* 1991;71(1):9–18.
60. Mollering RC. Past, present and future of antimicrobial agents. *Am J Med* 1995;99(Suppl 6A):11S–18S.
61. Bowler PG, Duerden BI, Armstrong DG. Wound microbiology and associated approaches to wound management. *Clin Microbiol Rev* 2001;14(2):244–269.
62. Gottardi W. Iodine and iodine compounds. In: Block S, ed. *Disinfectants, sterilisation and preservations*, 3rd ed. Philadelphia, PA: Lea Febinger, 1983.
63. Klasen HJ. Historical review of the use of silver in the treatment of burns. I: Early uses. *Burns* 2000;26(2):117–130.
64. Fox C. Topical therapy and the development of silver sulphadiazine. *Surg Gynecol Obstet* 1968;157:82–88.
65. Geronemus RG, Mertz PM, Eaglstein WH. Wound healing. The effects of topical antimicrobial agents. *Arch Dermatol* 1979; 115(11):1311–1314.
66. O'Meara SM, Cullum NA, Majid M, et al. Systematic review of antimicrobial agents used for chronic wounds. *Br J Surg* 2001; 88(1):4–21.
67. Elsaie ML, Choudhary S. Updates on the pathophysiology and treatment of acne rosacea. *Postgrad Med* 2009;121(5):178–186. Review.
68. Ditre CM. Case-based experience with the simultaneous use of a fixed topical antibiotic/benzoyl peroxide combination and a topical retinoid in the optimization of acne management. *J Drugs Dermatol* 2009;8(12):1127–1131.
69. Pangilinan R, Tice A, Tillotson G. Topical antibiotic treatment for uncomplicated skin and skin structure infections: review of literature. *Expert Rev Anti Infect Ther* 2009;7(8):957–965.
70. McKeage K, Keating GM. Clindamycin/benzoyl peroxide gel (BenzaClin): a review of its use in the management of acne. *Am J Clin Dermatol* 2008;9(3):193–204.
71. Del Rosso JQ. Combination topical therapy in the treatment of acne. *Cutis* 2006;78(2, Suppl 1):5–12.
72. Guay DR. Topical clindamycin in the management of acne vulgaris. *Expert Opin Pharmacother* 2007;8(15):2625–2664.
73. Tan HH. Topical antibacterial treatments for acne vulgaris: comparative review and guide to selection. *Am J Clin Dermatol* 2004;5(2):79–84.
74. Topical fusidic acid. *Nurs Times* 2005;101(3):32.
75. Eekhof JA, Neven AK, Gransjean SP, et al. Minor derm ailments: how good is the evidence for common treatments? *J Fam Pract* 2009;58(9):E2.
76. Paul JC, Pieper BA. Topical metronidazole for the treatment of wound odor: a review of the literature. *Ostomy Wound Manage* 2008;54(3):18–27.
77. Kim B, James W. Postoperative use of topical antimicrobials. *Dermatitis* 2009;20(3):174–180.
78. Moulin F, Quinet B, Raymond J, et al. Managing children skin and soft tissue infections. *Arch Pediatr* 2008;15(suppl 2):S62–S67.
79. Sheth VM, Weitzul S. Postoperative topical antimicrobial use. *Dermatitis* 2008;19(4):181–189.
80. Galmetti C. Local antibiotics in dermatology. *Dermatol Ther* 2008;21(3):187–195.

81. Zeldin Y, Weiler Z, Cohen A, et al. Efficacy of nasal *Staphylococcus aureus* eradication by topical nasal mupirocin in patients with perennial allergic rhinitis. *Ann Allergy Asthma Immunol* 2008;100(6):608–611.
82. Oprica C, Emtestam L, Hagströmer L, et al. Clinical and microbiological comparisons of isotretinoin vs. tetracycline in acne vulgaris. *Acta Derm Venereol* 2007;87(3):246–254.
83. Murata K, Tokura Y. Anti-microbial therapies for acne vulgaris: anti-inflammatory actions of anti-microbial drugs and their effectiveness. *J UOEH* 2007;29(1):63–71.
84. Chalker DK, Shalita A, Smith JG Jr, et al. A double-blind study of the effectiveness of a 3% erythromycin and 5% benzoyl peroxide combination in the treatment of acne vulgaris. *J Am Acad Dermatol* 1983;9:933–936.
85. Eady EA, Farmery MR, Ross JI, et al. Effects of benzoyl peroxide and erythromycin alone and in combination against antibiotic-sensitive and -resistant skin bacteria from acne patients. *Br J Dermatol* 1994;131:331–336.
86. Smith SD, Relman DA. Dermatophytes. In: Wilson WR, Sande MA, eds. *Current diagnosis and treatment in infectious diseases.* New York, NY: McGraw-Hill Professional, 2001:777–778.
87. Hostetter MK. Fungal infections in normal children. In: Gershon AA, Hotez PJ, Katz SL, et al., eds. *Gershon: Krugman's infectious diseases of children,* 11th ed. St. Louis, MO: Mosby, 2004.
88. Noble SL, Forbes RC, Stamm PL. Diagnosis and management of common tinea infections. *Am Fam Physician* 1998;58(1):163–174.
89. Karimzadegan-Nia M, Mir-Amin-Mohammadi A, Bouzari N, et al. Comparison of direct smear, culture and histology for the diagnosis of onychomycosis. *Australas J Dermatol* 2007;48(1):18–21.
90. Hubbard TW. The predictive value of symptoms in diagnosing childhood tinea capitis. *Arch Pediatr Adolesc Med* 1999;153(11): 1150–1153.
91. Fleece D, Gaughan JP, Aronoff SC. Griseofulvin versus terbinafine in the treatment of tinea capitis: a meta-analysis of randomized, clinical trials. *Pediatrics* 2004;114(5):1312–1315.
92. Pickering LK. Tinea capitis. In: Pickering LK, ed. *Red Book: 2006 Report of the Committee on Infectious Diseases.* Elk Grove Village, IL: American Academy of Pediatrics, 2006:654–656.
93. Lamisil (terbinafine). In: *Physician's Desk Reference Red Book 2007.* Oxford, England: Blackwell, 2007:2232.
94. Hart R, Bell-Syer SE, Crawford F, et al. Systematic review of topical treatments for fungal infections of the skin and nails of the feet. *BMJ* 1999;319(7202):79–82.
95. Habif TP. Superficial fungal infections. In: *Clinical dermatology: a color guide to diagnosis and therapy,* 4th ed. New York, NY: Mosby, 2004.
96. Lilly KK, Koshnick RL, Grill JP, et al. Cost-effectiveness of diagnostic tests for toenail onychomycosis: a repeated measure, single-blinded, cross-sectional evaluation of 7 diagnostic tests. *J Am Acad Dermatol* 2006;55(4):620–626.
97. Epstein E. How often does oral treatment of toenail onychomycosis produce a disease-free nail? An analysis of published data. *Arch Dermatol* 1998;134(12):1551–1554.
98. Frankowski BL, Weiner LB; the Committee on School Health; the Committee on Infectious Diseases, American Academy of Pediatrics. Head lice. *Pediatrics* 2002;110:638–643.
99. Burkhart CG, Burkhart CN. Asphyxiation of lice with topical agents, not a reality . . . yet. *J Am Acad Dermatol* 2006;54:721–722.
100. Roberts RJ, Casey D, Morgan DA, et al. Comparison of wet combing with malathion for treatment of head lice in the UK. *Lancet* 2000;356:540–544.
101. Downs AMR, Stafford KA, Harvey I, et al. Evidence for double resistance to permethrin and malathion in head lice. *Br J Dermatol* 1999;141:508–511.
102. Taplin D, Meinking TL. Pyrethrins and pyrethroids in dermatology. *Arch Dermatol* 1990;126:213–221.
103. Kakko I, Toimela T, Tahti H. The synaptosomal membrane bound ATPase as a target for the neurotoxic effects of pyrethroids, permethrin and cypermethrin. *Chemosphere* 2003;51:475–480.
104. Schultz MW, Gomez M, Hansen RC, et al. Comparative study of 5% permethrin cream and 1% lindane lotion for the treatment of scabies. *Arch Dermatol* 1990;126:167–170.
105. Taplin D, Meinking TL, Chen JA, et al. Comparison of crotamiton 10% cream (Eurax) and permethrin 5% cream (Elimite) for the treatment of scabies in children. *Pediatr Dermatol* 1990;7: 67–73.
106. Quarterman MJ, Lesher JL Jr. Neonatal scabies treated with permethrin 5% cream. *Pediatr Dermatol* 1994;11:264–266.
107. Centers for Disease Control and Prevention. Unintentional topical lindane ingestions: United States, 1998–2003. *MMWR Morb Mortal Wkly Rep* 2005;54:533–535.
108. Purvis RS, Tyring SK. An outbreak of lindane-resistant scabies treated successfully with permethrin 5% cream. *J Am Acad Dermatol* 1991;25:1015–1016.
109. Meiking TL, Serrano L, Hard B, et al. Comparative in vitro pediculocidal efficacy of treatments in a resistant head lice population in the United States. *Arch Dermatol* 2002;138:220–224.
110. Meinking TL, Taplin D. Safety of permethrin vs lindane for the treatment of scabies. *Arch Dermatol* 1996;132:959–962.
111. Hansen RC; Working Group on the Treatment of Resistant Pediculosis. Guidelines for the treatment of resistant pediculosis. *Contemp Pediatr* 2000;17(Suppl):1–10.
112. Lebwohl M, Clark L, Levitt J. Therapy for head lice based on life cycle, resistance, and safety considerations. *Pediatrics* 2007;119: 965–974.
113. Hardman JG, Limbird LE. In: *Goodman & Gilman's the pharmacologic basis of therapeutics,* 11th ed. New York, NY: McGraw-Hill, 2006.
114. Paller AS. Scabies in infants and small children. *Semin Dermatol* 1993;12:3–8.
115. Wendel K, Rompalo A. Scabies and pediculosis pubis: an update of treatment regimens and general review. *Clin Infect Dis* 2002;35:S146–S151.
116. Pruksachatkunakorn C, Damrongsak M, Sinthupuan S. Sulfur for scabies outbreaks in orphanages. *Pediatr Dermatol* 2002;19: 448–453.
117. Zaenglein AL, Thiboutot DM. Expert Committee Recommendations for Acne Management. *Pediatrics* 2006;118: 1188–1199.
118. Thiboutot D, Gollnick H; The Steering Committee. New insights into the management of acne: an update from the global alliance to improve outcomes in acne group. *J Am Acad Dermatol* 2009;60;S1–S50.
119. Zheng P, Gendimenico GJ, Mezick JA, et al. Topical all-*trans* retinoic acid rapidly corrects the follicular abnormalities of the rhino mouse. An ultrastructural study. *Acta Derm Venereol* 1993;73:97–101.
120. Shroot B. Pharmacodynamics and pharmacokinetics of topical adapalene. *J Am Acad Dermatol* 1998;39:S17–S24.
121. Lebwohl M, Poulin Y. Tazarotene in combination with topical corticosteroids. *J Am Acad Dermatol* 1998;39:S139–S143.
122. Czernielewski J, Bouclier M, Baker M, et al. Adapalene biochemistry and the evolution of a new topical retinoid for treatment of acne. *J Eur Acad Dermatol Vernereol* 2001;15(Suppl):5–12.
123. Jeremy AH, Holland DB, Leyden JJ. Inflammatory events are involved in acne lesion initiation. *J Invest Dermatol* 2003;121: 20–27.
124. Yentzer BA, McClain RW, Feldman SR. Do topical retinoids cause acne to "flare"? *J Drugs Dermatol* 2009;8(9):799–801.
125. Schlessinger J, Menter A, Gold M, et al. Clinical safety and efficacy studies of a novel formulation combining 1.2% clindamycin phosphate and 0.025% tretinoin for the treatment of acne vulgaris. *J Drugs Dermatol* 2007;6(6):607–615.
126. Haider A, Shaw JC. Treatment of acne vulgaris. *JAMA* 2004;292:726–735.
127. Balkrishnan R, Sansbury JC, Shenolikar RA, et al. Prescribing patterns for topical retinoids within NAMCS data. *J Drugs Dermatol* 2005;4(2):172–179.

CHAPTER

27

John D. Roarty

Ophthalmologic Drugs in Infants and Children

INTRODUCTION

The study of ocular pharmacology in the pediatric population is often limited to case reports and small clinical series. This problem has occurred in many areas of pediatrics. From 1984 through 1989, the Food and Drug Administration (FDA) approved 80% of the drugs without pediatric guidelines (1). The need for inclusion of the child in pharmacologic evaluation has been emphasized by the American Academy of Pediatrics (2).

Written descriptions of the treatment of eye disorders date to the Egyptians (3). Greek and Roman literature describe topical therapy with *collyria*, a substance dissolved in egg white, milk, or water. Up to World War II, few ophthalmic medications were commercially available. The 1950 US Pharmacopeia XIV listed three ophthalmic ointments. The FDA suggested sterility for eye preparations in 1953, with a legal requirement in 1955.

PHARMACOKINETICS

TOPICAL MEDICATIONS

The normal tear volume is 8 to 10 μL. Evaporation accounts for 25% of tear film loss, with 75% discharged into the lacrimal system. The tear turnover rate is about 16%. The volume of most topical preparations is 10 to 25 μL. Excess drug often spills in the nasolacrimal system. It is estimated that only 40% of the medication retained within the lids is present after 1 minute (4). Given the limited amount of drug retained after drop placement and the high washout rate, it is estimated that only 8% of the original medication in the drop is retained after 5 minutes (4).

There are several natural barriers to topically applied drug penetration. The tear film has natural buffers in proteins and bicarbonates. Tears contain approximately 0.7% protein, mostly albumin. The mean pH of the tear films is 7.5, and tears are most effective against acidic compounds (5). The corneal epithelium is five cell layers thick. Cell lipid membranes are hydrophobic. The corneal stroma has a lipid content of about 1% and is hydrophilic. The endothelium is only one cell layer thick and is less significant as a barrier.

Lipophilic drugs are absorbed more readily by the nasal mucosa. Up to 80% of the drug may diffuse into the systemic circulation if it drains into the lacrimal system (6). Methods for decreasing the systemic absorption include punctal occlusion, dilution of drops, and use of microdrops (7). Punctal plugs have improved the efficacy of glaucoma drops in patients with lacrimal insufficiency (8). Local tolerance of topical medication is variable. Ocular concerns include pain on instillation, allergic reactions, delayed healing, punctate keratopathy, disturbances of lacrimal secretion, and disturbances of accommodation (9). Patient comfort is best at a pH of 7.4 (tear film pH). Stability for many topical drugs is a pH as low as 5.0. Thus, choice of the proper pH and buffer capacity is a compromise between drug stability and patient comfort (3).

PERIOCULAR INJECTION

Periocular injection allows for greater intraocular penetration. This is especially true for penetration into the vitreous and the retina. In rabbits, the intraocular concentration was 41 times greater with a retrobulbar application compared with systemic administration. This ratio doubled if the eye was inflamed (10). The eye is supplied by the retinal and choroidal circulation. Systemic access to the vitreous and the retina is restricted by a blood–retina barrier with endothelial tight junctions. The vessels of the choroid allow larger molecules to pass into the choroidal space, but the retinal pigment epithelium, under the retina, and the ciliary nonpigmented epithelium have tight junctions.

DIAGNOSTIC DROPS

Pupil size is determined by sympathetic and parasympathetic influence. The pupil dilator is sympathetic and the constrictor is parasympathetic. The primary sympathetic mydriatic agent is phenylephrine. Phenylephrine is fast acting and of short duration. The 10% solution can cause hypertension, tachycardia, cerebral vascular accidents, and ruptured aneurysms (11,12). Use of topical phenylephrine intraoperatively to effect pupil dilation for surgery has been associated with the development of pulmonary edema (13). A 2.5% preparation is considered safe in the pediatric age group.

Anticholinergic agents such as tropicamide, atropine, and cyclopentolate induce dilation by inhibiting the parasympathetic constrictor muscle and inducing cycloplegia. Tropicamide 0.5% or 1.0% is a short-acting agent with little adverse effect (14). Atropine and cyclopentolate directly inhibit the action of acetylcholine on the smooth muscles in the iris and the ciliary body. They are used to dilate the pupil and to block the accommodative effect of the ciliary muscle. This allows an intraocular examination without pupillary constriction. It also allows determination of the refractive state of the eye without interference from accommodation.

Reported side effects to anticholinergics include angle-closure glaucoma, cardiopulmonary problems, and central nervous system effects. Premature infants and those with neurologic impairments and seizure disorders have a greater risk of systemic side effects. Premature infants are prone to apnea and bradycardia with cyclopentolate. Judicious use in neonates and infants has been recommended. Women, fair children, and children with Down syndrome may be prone to atropine toxicity (15). Systemic anticholinergic toxicity include dry mouth, decreased sweating, hyperthermia, rash, tachycardia, urinary retention, and behavioral changes. Fatal complications have been reported with topical doses no longer available (16). The risk of an adverse effect is greater with the 2% cyclopentolate solution (17). However, a seizure was reported in a 4.5-year-old boy with cerebral palsy and no seizure history with a standard topical instillation of cyclopentolate 1% (18). Topical use of atropine 1% increased the frequency of seizures in a 3-year-old boy (19). A survey of 57 pediatric ophthalmology facilities estimated the risk of severe (monitored in the office a few hours) or very severe (hospital admission) as 2 to 10 episodes per 1.6 million exposures (20).

PRESERVATIVES

Preservatives have been added to drops to prevent microbial contamination. Benzalkonium chloride is the most common. The preservative destabilizes the lipid layer of the tear film and increases the evaporation of the tear film (21). Ocular signs of toxicity can be twice as common with preservative compared with without preservative (22). Ocular signs include stinging, foreign body sensation, tearing, and itching. Superficial punctuate keratitis can occur indicative of epithelial damage. There have been no specific reports of pediatric sensitivity.

OCULAR CONDITIONS

MYOPIA

Myopia is a refractive condition of the eye affecting 80 million children worldwide. Atropine has been suggested to decrease progression of myopia but with significant side effects of hypoaccommodation and photosensitivity. Pirenzepine is an M1-receptor antagonist used to treat dyspepsia in Europe. In United States, a 2-year study of 174 children aged 8 to 12 years treated with topical pirenzepine against placebo showed a 40% reduction in the progression of myopia (23).

OCULAR ALLERGY

Ocular allergy can be treated with vasoconstrictors, antihistamines, mast cell stabilizers, nonsteroidal preparations, and steroids. Routine allergic conjunctivitis can be treated with over-the-counter preparations. Over-the-counter eye drops contain sympathomimetic agents for α-adrenergic vasoconstriction. Accidental oral ingestion of 2 to 3 mL of imidazole in a 2-year-old child resulted in hypothermia, hypoglycemia, central nervous system depression, and respiratory depression (24). Toxicity has been limited to surface discomfort with topical use similar to adults (25).

Many topical agents are multimodal in effect. Ketotifen fumarate 0.025% (Zaditor) and olopatadine HCl 0.1% (Patanol) combine an antihistamine and a mast cell stabilizer effect. Many of these are approved by the FDA for children 3 years and older. The primary complication is surface irritation. No other systemic complications have been reported in the pediatric age group. Finally, topical steroids are used for short times in conjunction with a nonsteroidal anti-inflammatory, antihistamine, or mast cell stabilizer. Long-term use of steroids is problematic, as described in the next subsection.

Vernal conjunctivitis is a less common form of ocular allergy in children and young adults requiring prescription therapy. It presents with severe itching, photophobia, injection of the conjunctiva, and corneal foreign body sensation. Obliteration of the ductules of the lacrimal gland can lead to severe keratitis sicca and corneal ulcer. However, Tabbara reported that the most common cause of loss of sight was steroid related in a small series (26). Twenty-five percent of patients had steroid-induced cataracts and 12% had steroid-induced glaucoma. Topical cyclosporine has been used effectively in pediatric patients with vernal conjunctivitis without complication (27).

Steroids

In the pediatric population, steroids may be used topically for the treatment of external disorders, such as allergic conjunctivitis and keratitis. Intraocular indications include uveitis and postsurgical inflammation. Ocular hypertension secondary to steroid use is well described. Some conditions, such as uveitis and hemangiomas, may require periocular injection of steroids. Systemic cushingoid toxicity can occur with periocular injection of steroids. An 11-year-old boy with severe uveitis was treated with a periocular injection of 80 mg of methylprednisolone every 6 weeks for 6 months. He developed ocular hypertension and a cushingoid habitus (28). Adrenal growth suppression (29) and retinal artery occlusion have occurred after periocular injection for capillary hemangiomas of infancy.

Ocular hypertensive effects have long been described with all methods of delivery. These include oral (30), inhalation (31), nasal, intravenous (32), topical dermatologic (33), periocular (34), and topical drops. Glucocorticoids appear to increase outflow resistance in the trabecular meshwork with no effect on aqueous humor production. Morphologic changes include deposition of amorphous extracellular and fibrillar material in the trabecular beams with long-term use (35).

Steroid-induced ocular hypertension with topical application occurs in up to 30% of patients. A significant pressure rise of 16 mmHg or more can occur in 5% of a normal population (36). In adults, intraocular pressure rises occur after 4 to 6 weeks of steroid use. Intraocular pressures may rise to 50 mmHg (normal 10 to 21 mmHg) and is reversible with cessation of the steroids. In children, reports of ocular hypertensive response with topical therapy vary from 11% (37) to 56% (38). The peak response occurs earlier than in adults, as early as 4 days of continuous use. The younger the patient, the greater is the risk of ocular hypertension (39). The greater sensitivity has been postulated to be secondary to an immature trabecular meshwork and decreased outflow capacity in children as compared with adults (40). Glaucoma and buphthalmos occurred in a 3-week-old infant after only 7 days of topical steroids (41).

Steroid-induced glaucoma may mimic congenital glaucoma with corneal edema, rupture of Descemet's membrane, elevated intraocular pressure, and increased cupping of the optic nerve. This was noted in 73% of 55 eyes in 33 children with a mean age of 7 years (42). Cessation of steroids normalized pressure in only 4 eyes. Trabeculotomy, an angle-opening surgery, was effective in normalizing intraocular pressures in all eyes requiring surgery.

Secondary glaucoma associated with juvenile rheumatoid arthritis and uveitis is particularly difficult to control. Contributing factors are generous steroid use and trabecular changes secondary to the chronic intraocular inflammation. Foster et al. (43) reported an incidence of glaucoma of 42% in their series of 69 patients with juvenile rheumatoid arthritis. Only 17% of the patients were controlled with topical therapy.

The response varies with the type of steroid and method of delivery. Ohji et al. (44) reported a higher risk of ocular hypertension with topical dexamethasone compared with topical fluorometholone. Fluorometholone generated an ocular hypertensive response in one patient. The glucocorticoid receptor is encoded by the GR gene with 24 polymorphisms described. Efforts to delineate the pharmacogenomics have been unsuccessful to date (45).

INFECTION

The etiologic agents of pediatric conjunctivitis are viral and bacterial in 85% of the patients. The primary bacterial agents are *Streptococcus pneumoniae* and *Hemophilus influenzae* (46). A large number of antibiotics are available for the treatment of bacterial conjunctivitis. All of the antibiotics are well tolerated as topical therapy with a few exceptions. Surface irritation is not uncommon, but no more frequent than in the adult population. The antimicrobial spectrum of the antibiotics is the same as in the adult population. Sulfacetamide and neomycin have a particularly high incidence of topical toxicity and hypersensitivity reactions.

Aminoglycosides

Aminoglycosides are effective against a wide range of gram-negative and some gram-positive organisms. They inhibit protein synthesis and interfere with mRNA in the ribosome. There is no systemic toxicity related to topical use. Burning and stinging are common. Hypersensitivity reactions occur in up to 8% of patients using neomycin. The risk of hypersensitivity is less with the other aminoglycosides.

Intraocular and subconjunctival injection of aminoglycosides is used for the treatment of endophthalmitis. Aminoglycosides for prophylaxis after cataract surgery or traumatic ruptured globe repair had been the standard. Gram-negative organisms are common causative agents with endophthalmitis. However, gentamicin, tobramycin, and amikacin have caused macular infarcts with intravitreal or subconjunctival delivery (47). Although a macular infarct is infrequent, it is recommended that aminoglycosides not be used for prophylaxis. It may still be considered if a gram-negative agent is suspected with endophthalmitis. The etiology of the macula infarct is unknown. Infarct may be related to inadvertent perforation of the globe with subconjunctival delivery, sudden changes in the intraocular pressure with injection, or a direct toxic effect due to concentration.

Chloramphenicol

Chloramphenicol is effective against gram-negative and gram-positive aerobic organisms causing conjunctivitis. The first death from aplastic anemia from eye drops was reported in 1955 (48). Chloramphenicol has been reported to cause aplastic anemia after the administration of an ophthalmic ointment in a male adult and recently with drops (49). With systemic application, the risk of aplastic anemia is from 1 in 30,000 to 1 in 50,000 (9). The risk with topical application is estimated at 1 in 100,000 (49,50).

Tetracycline

Tetracycline has a wide range of antimicrobial activity against gram-negative and gram-positive organisms. It inhibits protein synthesis in the ribosome. Tetracycline may be used orally for ocular complications of rosacea. It can cause permanent discoloration of the teeth and depress bone growth by binding with calcium. Enamel dysplasia can occur with exposure from the second trimester to 8 years of age (51).

Quinolones

Nalidixic acid, a quinolone, has been used for gram-negative infections. It inhibits bacterial DNA replication by inhibiting DNA gyrase. Nalidixic acid–induced arthropathy with necrosis of chondrocytes and loss of collagen has been reported in young animals (52). The present generation of the quinolones is considered safer. Systemic administration of fluoroquinolones in adults and children has rarely caused a reversible arthralgia but never arthropathy. Rare adverse events to systemic therapy reported in children include gastrointestinal disturbances, skin rash, green discoloration of the teeth, and anaphylaxis (53). In a large series, topical ophthalmic use for pediatric conjunctivitis has not caused any serious adverse events (54).

Rifabutin

Rifabutin is a semisynthetic antimycobacterial agent similar to rifampin. Uveitis is a known complication in adults. Rifabutin can induce uveitis in the pediatric patient (55). The uveitis may mimic endophthalmitis (56). It may be related to serum levels above therapeutic range. It is recommended that the dosage not exceed 10 mg per kg per day (57).

GLAUCOMA

β-Blockers

Adrenergic blockade may be nonselective, β_1 or β_2. Systemic β-blockers may reduce cardiac output and increase airway resistance in the bronchioles. Topical application results in a reduction in the intraocular pressure. Aqueous production by the ciliary body is decreased. The exact mechanism of this intraocular pressure reduction is unknown. The exacerbation of reactive airway disease has been described with topical application (58). Apnea was induced by topical instillation of timolol 0.25% in an 18-month-old girl (59). The resting heart rate can be reduced with topical instillation, but the inotropic cardiac effect is less. Patients with reactive airway disease and cardiac failure should avoid this class. Cardioselective formulations, such as betaxolol and levobetaxolol, are β_1-blockers. The pressure reduction is similar with less risk of bronchospasm.

Prostaglandin Analogues

Latanoprost 0.005% is a 17-phenyl-substituted prostaglandin analogue for the topical therapy of glaucoma. It works by increasing the uveoscleral outflow. The mechanism is unknown. Associated adult problems include conjunctival hyperemia, punctuate keratopathy, increased iris pigmentation, increased eyelash growth, and cystoid macular edema. The pigmentation effect on the iris and eyelashes has been seen in children. The increase pigmentation is due to increase in the size of mature melanin granules (60). A child with aniridia and glaucoma developed diaphoresis 1 hour after dosing with latanoprost (61). Although latanoprost seems to have few side effects reported in adults or children, Enyedi and Freedman (62) reported little effect on the intraocular pressure in their pediatric population.

α-Agonists

Brimonidine is a selective α-agonist, and reduces aqueous production and increases uveoscleral outflow to control intraocular pressure in glaucoma. In children, it produced a 7% reduction in the pressure. However, Enyedi and Freedman reported that 2 of 32 children, average ages 2.4 and 3.7 years old, respectively, were unarousable and 5 of 32 children demonstrated extreme fatigue secondary to central nervous system depression after topical application (63). Apnea and bradycardia have been reported in the neonatal period.

Apraclonidine hydrochloride is a selective α_2-agonist. It decreases aqueous production by decreasing Na–K ATPase activity in the ciliary body epithelium. As an analogue of clonidine, it has a systemic hypotensive effect. This effect is limited because apraclonidine is hydrophilic. Local side effects include burning and stinging. In adults, systemic and local side effects were significant enough to stop the medication in 23% of patients. Only 2% had severe systemic reactions to topical therapy (64).

Apraclonidine has been used in the diagnosis of Horner syndrome. Cocaine and hydroxyamphetamine drops have been traditionally used to differentiate a pre- from postganglionic lesion. Apraclonidine can be used in lieu of cocaine. However, hypoxia, apnea, and bradycardia have been reported in a 5-month-old infant (65).

Carbonic Anhydrase Inhibitors

Carbonic anhydrase is present in the ciliary body of the eye. Inhibitors suppress aqueous production whether given topically or orally. Limited side effects include burning and stinging. There are no significant systemic effects topically (66).

STRABISMUS

Phospholine iodide 0.125% is a long-acting anticholinesterase and increases tissue acetylcholine. Effects include miosis, increase of outflow of aqueous, decrease in intraocular pressure, and enhanced accommodation. Treatment of glaucoma was the primary indication before development of better medications. Phospholine iodide was used in the past for treatment of accommodative esotropia in children. It is currently used for short-term treatment of consecutive esotropia after surgery for an exotropia. Short-term effects include burning, lacrimation, and headaches. Retinal detachment has been associated with its use. Long-term use may result in the formation of iris cysts, lens opacities, and depression of plasma cholinesterase activity. An acute cholinergic crisis was reported in a 5-year-old girl with unsuspected myasthenia gravis (67).

RETINOPATHY OF PREMATURITY

Antivascular Endothelial Growth Factor

In adults, macular degeneration, diabetic retinopathy, sickle cell retinopathy and vascular occlusion can result in significant abnormal retinal neovascularization. Effective vascular involution has been obtained with intravitreal injection use of anti-vascular endothelial growth factor (VEGF) pharmacotherapies. The majority of the safety and efficacy studies have been for macular degeneration (68). Use for other ocular disorders is being explored such as glaucoma (69). Pegaptanib, a selective VEGF-A antagonist, was approved for intraocular use in 2004. Ranibizumab, a recombinant immunoglobulin G1 isotype antibody fragment, inhibits all isoforms of human VEGF-A. It was approved in 2006. Bevacizumab, a full-length monoclonal antibody, inhibits all forms of VEGF. This agent is FDA approved for colorectal, breast, and lung cancer but not for the eye. These agents have been found to be very effective with the most significant complications related to the delivery. Intraocular inflammation has been reported (70).

Safety in children has not been studied. However, it is being used in advanced retinopathy of prematurity (ROP). Intravitreal use as an adjunct to surgical therapy has been useful in the face of vitreous hemorrhage and early retinal traction in a few reported cases (71,72).

Erythropoietin

Erythropoietin, a renal hormone, stimulates red blood cell production. It has been used to treat neonatal anemia of prematurity with good effect since 1990. Brown et al. (73) demonstrated an increase in active ROP in patients treated with rhEPO. Suk et al. (74) found that the effect on ROP may be related to the gestational age and the dose. Early rhEPO dosing may result retinal vessel stability while later dosing may add to the angiogenic drive.

OPHTHALMOLOGIC EFFECTS WITH SYSTEMIC NONOPHTHALMOLOGIC MEDICATIONS

Transdermal scopolamine has been used to treat nausea and emesis associated with chemotherapy. Unilateral mydriasis with a fixed and dilated pupil occurred with a scopolamine patch in an 11-year-old child with lymphocytic leukemia. Concern for central nervous system disease prompted imaging studies, which were negative (74,75). Transdermal scopolamine was used to control excessive drooling in a 4-year-old child with neurodevelopmental issues. This resulted in a reversible esotropia mimicking a sixth nerve palsy.

Cytosine arabinoside may act by interfering with DNA polymerase and disrupting the S-phase of the cell cycle. It may also be incorporated into DNA and RNA to induce chromosomal breaks. General adverse reactions include fever, bone pain, myalgias, rash, and malaise. There are other rare multisystem effects also. Hemorrhagic conjunctivitis and keratitis are common. This results in severe photophobia, which can be treated with artificial tears and topical steroids (76).

Hydroxychloroquine and *chloroquine sulfate* are used as antimalarial and as anti-inflammatory agents in lupus erythematosus and rheumatoid arthritis. General adverse reactions include headache, gastrointestinal complaints, dermatologic problems, and blood dyscrasias. Ophthalmic effects reported include extraocular muscle palsy, keratitis, corneal deposits, macular edema with a "bull's eye" maculopathy, pigmentary retinopathy resembling retinitis pigmentosa, and visual field defects. Chloroquine, less so hydroxychloroquine, damages lysosomes. This may interfere with phospholipid metabolism and disrupt cell membranes. Degenerative changes are seen in the ganglion cells and photoreceptors. The quinines are metabolized slowly, leading to continued cell damage after the medication is stopped. Adverse effects are dose related, with a cumulative effect. Excessive values exceed 2 mg per kg for chloroquine and 3 mg per kg for hydroxychloroquine.

The reversible corneal deposits can occur within the first 3 weeks of therapy. They clear with cessation of the medication. The retinopathy may persist long term. If discovered early, the retinopathy may be reversed. A central scotoma is detected early by a central visual field test with a red stimulus.

Vigabatrin increases γ-aminobutyric acid (GABA) concentration in the brain by inhibiting GABA transaminase. It has been used for infantile spasm, complex partial seizure, and generalized seizures (77). Color perception was compromised in 32% of adult patients (78). Peripheral visual field loss has been documented in up to 30% of adult patients. The effect was irreversible 6 months after cessation of the drug in one patient. Electroretinogram (ERG) response is reduced to photopic and scotopic stimulation (79). This implies that rod and cone functions are effected. GABA may be involved in phototransduction. It is an inhibitory neurotransmitter in retinal bipolar and amacrine cells. The exact mechanism is unknown. No pediatric visual loss has been reported. However, obtaining visual fields and ERGs is problematic in children.

Topiramate is used in children with generalized and localized seizures. It is a sulfamated monosaccharide D-fructose derivative, and inhibits Na^+ and Ca^{2+} channels, excitatory amino acid receptors, and carbonic anhydrase isozymes. It potentiates GABA-evoked channels (80). In children, adverse central nervous system effects, such as somnolence, behavior changes, and poor concentration, and weight loss appear similar to effects in the adult population. Nephrolithiasis and hepatic toxicity appear less frequently (81). Unusual ocular effects have been reported. Multiple adult case reports of unilateral and bilateral angle-closure glaucoma and induced myopia have been reported. Uveal effusion with anterior displacement of the iris-lens diaphragm has been documented with ultrasound (82,83). A 15-year-old boy developed bilateral retinal striae and myopia with a marked decrease in vision. The visual acuity returned to baseline with cessation of the drug (84). The mechanism of the uveal effusion and retinal edema is unknown. However, uveal effusions have been reported with other sulfa-derived drugs (85).

REFERENCES

1. Center for Drug Evaluation and Research, Food and Drug Administration, Public Health Service. *Offices of Drug Evaluation statistical report* (US Department of Health and Human Services publication 89-233530). Rockville, MD.
2. Guidelines for the ethical conduct of studies to evaluate drugs in pediatric populations. Committee on Drugs. *Pediatrics* 1995;95:286–294.
3. Mullins JD. Ophthalmic preparations. In: Genaro AR, ed. *Remington's pharmaceutical sciences*, 17th ed. Easton, PA: Mack, 1985:1553–1566.
4. Mindel JS. Pharmacokinetics. In: Tasman W, Jaeger EA, eds. *Duane's foundations of clinical ophthalmology*, vol. 3, 6th ed. Philadelphia, PA: Lippincott Williams & Wilkins, 1993:1–17.

5. Carney LG, Mauger TF, Hill RM. Buffering in human tears: pH responses to acid and base challenge. *Invest Ophthalmol Vis Sci* 1989;30:747–754.
6. Hugues FC, le Jeunne C. Systemic and local tolerability of ophthalmic drug formulations. *Drug Saf* 1995;8:365–380.
7. Bhatia SS, Vidyashankar C, Sharma RK, et al. Systemic toxicity with cyclopentolate eye drops. *Indian Pediatr* 2000;37:329–331.
8. Huang TC, Lee DA. Punctal occlusion and topical medications for glaucoma. *Am J Ophthalmol* 1989;107:151–155.
9. Polak BCP. Drugs used in ocular treatment. In: Dukes MNG, Aronson JK, eds. *Meyeler's side effects of drugs. An encyclopedia of adverse reactions and interactions*, 14th ed. Amsterdam: Elsevier, 2000:1636–1648.
10. Levine ND, Aronson SB. Orbital infusion of steroids in the rabbit. *Arch Ophthalmol* 1970;83:599–607.
11. Fraunfelder FW, Fraunfelder FT, Jensvold B. Adverse systemic effect from pledgets of topical ocular phenylephrine 10%. *Am J Ophthalmol* 2002;134:624–625.
12. Apt L. Pharmacology. In: Isenberg SJ, ed. *The eye in infancy*. Chicago, IL: Year Book, 1989:91–99.
13. Baldwin FJ, Morley AP. Intraoperative pulmonary oedema in a child following systemic absorption of phenylephrine eyedrops. *Br J Anaesth* 2002;88:440–442.
14. Chiaviello CT, Bond GR. Dilating the pupil in the pediatric emergency department. *Pediatr Emerg Care* 1994;10:216–218.
15. Lyndon WJ, Hodes T. Possible allergic reactions to cyclopentolate hydrochloride: case reports with literature review of uses and adverse reactions. *Ophthalmic Physiol Opt* 1991;11:16–21.
16. Rengstorff RH, Doughty CB. Mydriatic and cycloplegic drugs: a review of ocular and systemic complications. *Am J Optom Physiol Opt* 1982;59:162–177.
17. Adcock EW. Adverse systemic reactions of topical cyclopentolate hydrochloride. *Ann Ophthalmol* 1976;8:695–698.
18. Fitzgerald DA, Hanson RM, West C, et al. Seizures associated with 1% cyclopentolate eyedrops. *J Paediatr Child Health* 1990;26:106–107.
19. Wright BD. Exacerbation of akinetic seizures by atropine eye drops. *Br J Ophthalmol* 1992;76:179–180.
20. Loewen N, Barry JC. Symposium proceedings. Part I: The use of cycloplegic agents. Results of a 1999 survey of German-speaking centers for pediatric ophthalmology and strabology. *Strabismus* 2000;8:91–99.
21. Willson WS, Duncan AJ, Jay JL. Effect of benzalkonium chloride on the stability of the precorneal tear film in rabbit and man. *Br J Ophthalmol* 1975;59:1083–1088.
22. Pisella PJ, Pouliquen P, Baudouin C. Prevalence of ocular symptoms and sign with preserved and preservative free glaucoma medication. *Br J Ophthalmol* 2002;86:418–423.
23. Siatkowski RM, Cotter SA, Crockett RS, et al. Two-year multicenter, randomized, double-masked, placebo controlled, parallel safety and efficacy study of 2% pirenzepine ophthalmic gel in children with myopia. *J AAPOS* 2008;12:332–339.
24. Tobias JD. Central nervous system depression following accidental ingestion of Visine eye drops. *Clin Pediatr (Phila)* 1996;35:539–540.
25. Mahieu LM, Rooman RP, Goossens E. Imidazoline intoxication in children. *Eur J Pediatr* 1993;152:944–946.
26. Tabbara KF. Ocular complications of vernal keratoconjunctivitis. *Can J Ophthalmol* 1999;34:88–92.
27. Pucci N, Novembre E, Cianferoni A, et al. Efficacy and safety of cyclosporine eyedrops in vernal keratoconjunctivitis. *Ann Allergy Asthma Immunol* 2002;89:298–303.
28. Ozerdem U, Levi L, Cheng L, et al. Systemic toxicity of topical and periocular corticosteroid therapy in an 11-year-old male with posterior uveitis. *Am J Ophthalmol* 2000;130:240–241.
29. Steelman J, Kappy M. Adrenal suppression and growth retardation from ocular corticosteroids. *J Pediatr Ophthalmol Strabismus* 2001;38:177–178.
30. Covell LL. Glaucoma induced by systemic steroid therapy. *Am J Ophthalmol* 1958;45:108–109.
31. Abuekteish F, Kirkpatrick JN, Russell G. Posterior subcapsular cataract and inhaled corticosteroid therapy. *Thorax* 1995;50:674–676.
32. Alfano JE. Changes in the intraocular pressure associated with systemic steroid therapy. *Am J Ophthalmol* 1963;56:245–247.
33. Cubey RB. Glaucoma following the application of corticosteroid to the skin of the eyelids. *Br J Dermatol* 1976;95:207–208.
34. Herschler J. Intractable intraocular hypertension induced by repository triamcinolone acetonide. *Am J Ophthalmol* 1972;74:501–504.
35. Rohen JW, Linner E, Witmer R. Electron microscopic studies on the trabecular meshwork in two cases of corticosteroid-glaucoma. *Exp Eye Res* 1973;17:19–31.
36. Armaly MF. Statistical attributes of the steroid hypertensive response in the clinically normal eye. I. The demonstration of three levels of response. *Invest Ophthalmol* 1963;70:482–491.
37. Biedner BZ, David R, Grudsky A, et al. Intraocular pressure response to corticosteroids in children. *Br J Ophthalmol* 1980;4:198–205.
38. Kwok AK, Lam DS, Ng JS, et al. Ocular-hypertensive response to topical steroids in children. *Ophthalmology* 1997;12:2112–2116.
39. Lam DS, Kwok AD. Accelerated ocular hypertensive response to topical steroids in children. *Br J Ophthalmol* 1997;81:422–423.
40. Lam DS, Kwok AK, Chew S. Accelerated ocular hypertensive response to topical steroids in children. *Br J Ophthalmol* 1997;81:422–423.
41. Hutcheson KA. Steroid-induced glaucoma in an infant. *J AAPOS* 2007;11:522–523.
42. Calixto N, Silva SM, Cronemberger S, et al. Corticosteroid-induced pseudocongenital glaucoma. *Rev Bras Oftalmol* 2000;59: 179–190.
43. Foster CS, Havrlikova K, Baltatzis S, et al. Secondary glaucoma in patients with juvenile rheumatoid arthritis-associated iridocyclitis. *Acta Ophthalmol Scand* 2000;78:576–579.
44. Ohji M, Kinoshita S, Ohmi E, et al. Marked intraocular pressure response to instillation of corticosteroids in children. *Am J Ophthalmol* 1991;112:450–454.
45. Gerzenstein SM, Pletcher MT, Cervino ACL, et al. Glucocorticoid receptor polymorphisms and intraocular pressure response to intravitreal triamcinolone acetonide. *Ophthalmic Genet* 2008;29:166–170.
46. Weiss A, Brinser JH, Nazar-Stewart V. Acute conjunctivitis in children. *J Pediatr* 1993;122:10–14.
47. Compochiaro PA, Conway BP. Aminoglycoside toxicity—a survey of retinal specialists. Implications for ocular use. *Arch Ophthalmol* 1991;109:946–950.
48. Rosenthal RL, Blackman A. Bone marrow hypoplasia following the use of chloramphenicol eye drops. *J Am Med Assoc* 1955;191: 36–37.
49. Wiholm BE, Kelly JP, Kaufman D, et al. Relation of aplastic anaemia to use of choloramphenicol eye drops in two international case reports. *Br Med J* 1998;316:666.
50. Lancaster T, Swart AM, Jick H. Risk of serious hematological toxicity with use of chloramphenicol eye drops in a British general practice database. *Br Med J* 1998;316:667.
51. Witkop CJ, Wolf RO. Hypoplasia and intrinsic staining of enamel following tetracycline therapy. *J Am Med Assoc* 1963;185:100.
52. Burkhardt JE, Hill MA, Carlton WW, et al. Histologic and histochemical changes in articular cartilages of immature beagle dogs dosed with difloxicin, a fluoroquinolone. *Vet Pathol* 1990;27:162–170.
53. Sabella C, Goldfarb J. Fluoroquinolone therapy in pediatrics: where we stand [editorial]. *Clin Pediatr (Phila)* 1997;36: 445–448.
54. Gross RD, Hoffman RO, Lindsay RN. A comparison of ciprofloxacin and tobramycin in bacterial conjunctivitis in children. *Clin Pediatr (Phila)* 1997;36:435–444.
55. Dunn AM, Tizer K, Cervia JS. Rifabutin-associated uveitis in a pediatric patient. *Pediatr Infect Dis J* 1995;14:246–247.
56. Le Saux N, MacDonald N, Dayneka N. Rifabutin ocular toxicity mimicking endophthalmitis. *Pediatr Infect J* 1997;16:716–718.
57. Jewelewicz DA, Schiff WM, Brown S, et al. Rifabutin-associated uveitis in an immunosuppressed pediatric patient without acquired immunodeficiency syndrome. *Am J Ophthalmol* 1998;125:872–873.
58. Jones FL, Ekberg NL. Exacerbation of asthma by timolol. *N Engl J Med* 1979;301:270.
59. Williams T, Ginther WH. Hazard of ophthalmic timolol. *N Engl J Med* 1982;306:1485–1486.
60. Cracknell KPB, Grierson I, Hogg P. Morphometric effects of long-term exposure to latanoprost. *Ophthalmology* 2006;114:938–948.
61. Schmidtborn F. Systemic side-effects of latanoprost in a child with aniridia and glaucoma. *Ophthalmologe* 1998;95:633–634.

62. Enyedi LB, Freedman SF. Latanaprost for the treatment of pediatric glaucoma. *Surv Ophthalmol* 2002;47:S129–S132.
63. Enyedi LB, Freedman SF. Safety and efficacy of brimonidine in children with glaucoma. *J Am Assoc Pediatr Ophthalmol* 2001;5: 281–284.
64. Araujo SV, Bond JB, Wilson RP, et al. Long-term effect of apraclonidine. *Br J Ophthalmol* 1995;79:1098–1101.
65. Watts P, Satterfield D, Lim MK. Adverse effects of apraclonidine used in the diagnosis of Horner syndrome in infants. *J AAPOS* 2007;11:282–283.
66. Whitson JT, Roarty JD, Vijaya L, et al. Efficacy of brinzolamide and levobetaxolol in pediatric glaucomas: a randomized clinical trial. *J AAPOS* 2008;12:239–246.
67. Giles CL, Finkel HP, Nigro MA. Cholinergic crisis induced by phospholine iodide. *Am Orthop J* 1990;40:68–71.
68. Ip MS, Scott IU, Brown GC, et al. Anti-vascular endothelial growth factor pharmacotherapy for age-related macular degeneration: a report by the American Academy of Ophthalmology. *Ophthalmology* 2008;115(10):1837–1846.
69. Grewal DS, Jain R, Kumar H. Evaluation of subconjunctival bevacizumab as an adjunct to trabeculectomy. *Ophthalmology* 2008;115: 2141–2145.
70. Wickremasinghe SS, Michalova K, Gilhotra J, et al. Acute intraocular inflammation after injections of bevacizumab for treatment of age-related macular degeneration. *Ophthalmology* 2008;115:1911–1915.
71. Lalwani GA, Berrocal AM, Murray TG, et al. Off-label use of intravitreal bevacizumab for salvage treatment in progressive threshold retinopathy of prematurity. *Retina* 2008;28(3):S13–S18.
72. Quiroz-Mercado H, Martinez-Castellanos MA, Hernandez-Rojas ML. Antiangiogenic therapy with intravitreal bevacizumab for retinopathy of prematurity. *Retina* 2008;28(3):S19–S25.
73. Brown MS, Baron AE, France ED, et al. Association between higher cumulative doses of recombinant erythropoietin and risk for retinopathy of prematurity. *J AAPOS* 2006;10:143–149.
74. Suk KK, Dunbar JA, Liu A, et al. Human recombinant erythropoietin and the incidence of retinopathy of prematurity. *J AAPOS* 2008;12:233–238.
75. Swartz M. Other diseases: drug toxicity and metabolic and nutritional conditions. In: Ryan SJ, ed. *Retina*, vol. 2. St. Louis, MO: Mosby, 1989:742–744.
76. Itoh M, Aoyama T, Yamamura Y, et al. Effects of the rational use of corticosteroid eye drops for the prevention of ocular toxicity in high dose cytosine arabinoside therapy. *Yakugaku Zasshi* 1999;119: 229–235.
77. Marson AG, Kadir ZA, Hutton JL, et al. The new antiepileptic drugs: a systemic review of their efficacy and tolerability. *Epilepsia* 1997;38:859–880.
78. Nousiainen I, Kalviainen R, Mantyjarvi M. Color vision in epilepsy patients treated with vigabatrin or carbamazepine monotherapy. *Ophthalmology* 2000;107:884–888.
79. Daneshvar H, Racette L, Coupland SG, et al. Symptomatic and asymptomatic visual loss in patients taking vigabatrin. *Ophthalmology* 1999;106:1792–1798.
80. Bourgeois BFD. Pharmacokinetics and pharmacodynamics of topiramate. *J Child Neurol* 2000;15:S27–S30.
81. Levisohn PM. Safety and tolerability of topiramate in children. *J Child Neurol* 2000;15:S22–S26.
82. Rhee DJ, Goldberg MJ, Parrish RK. Bilateral angle-closure glaucoma and ciliary body swelling from topiramate. *Arch Ophthalmol* 2001;119:1721–1723.
83. Sankar PS, Pasquale LR, Grosskreutz CL. Uveal effusion and secondary angle-closure glaucoma associated with topiramate use. *Arch Ophthalmol* 2001;119:1210–1211.
84. Sen HA, O'Halloran HS, Lee WB. Topiramate-induced acute myopia and retinal striae. *Arch Ophthalmol* 2001;119:775–777.
85. Medeiros FA, Zhang XY, Bernd AS, et al. Angle-closure glaucoma associated with ciliary body detachment in patients using topiramate. *Arch Ophthalmol* 2003;121:282–285.

Chokechai Rongkavilit
Nahed Abdel-Haq
Jocelyn Y. Ang
Basim I. Asmar

CHAPTER 28

Sulfonamides

INTRODUCTION

Sulfonamides are some of the most common and the oldest antimicrobial agents used in children. Their mode of action, efficacy, safety, and pharmacologic properties are well known and these drugs remain to be a substantial component of antimicrobial therapies in infants beyond the immediate newborn period and in older children.

MECHANISM OF ACTION

Sulfonamides are synthetic analogues of *para*-aminobenzoic acid (PABA). It contains a benzene ring, with a sulfonamide group and a primary amino group next to the sulfur side chain of the sulfonamide group. The sulfonamides act by preventing the bacterial utilization of PABA for the synthesis of folic acid. PABA is essential for bacterial folic acid biosynthesis and with pteridine, it is incorporated to dihydropteroic acid, the immediate precursor of folic acid by dihydropteroic synthase. Sulfonamides competitively inhibit dihyropteroic synthase. Therefore, those microorganisms that must synthesize their own folic acid are vulnerable to the effect of sulfonamide, and those that can utilize preformed folic acid are not affected by these drugs. Moreover, the bacteriostatic effects of sulfonamides can be counteracted by the use of PABA. The sulfonamides are used often with trimethoprim (TMP), which blocks the conversion of dihydrofolic acid to tetrahydrofolic acid. Mammalian cells are not affected by sulfonamides, since they cannot synthesize folic acid and utilize only preformed folic acid.

SULFAMETHOXAZOLE

Sulfamethoxazole (SMZ) is an intermediate-acting antibacterial sulfonamide that is also available as a component of the trimethoprim–sulfamethoxazole (TMP–SMZ) 5:1 fixed-ratio combination product.

SMZ is rapidly absorbed following oral administration. It undergoes N^4-acetylation and N^4-glucuronide conjugation mainly in the liver. The free form is considered to be the microbiologically active form. The acetylated derivative (major metabolite) is not microbiologically active. Seventy percent of SMZ is bound to plasma proteins; of the unbound portion 80% to 90% is in the nonacetylated form.

Free blood concentrations of 5 to 15 mg per dL are considered therapeutically effective for most infections, with blood concentrations of 12 to 15 mg per dL optimal for serious infections. The maximum blood level of total SMZ should not exceed 20 mg per dL. SMZ is widely distributed into most body tissues. It diffuses into cerebrospinal fluid (CSF) with a peak concentration at 8 hours, reaching about 14% of the simultaneous plasma concentration. The drug diffuses into aqueous humor, vaginal fluid, and middle ear fluid. SMZ crosses the placental barrier and is excreted into breast milk.

SMZ and its metabolites are excreted primarily in the urine. The elimination half-life is 10 hours. The unconjugated forms are excreted by tubular secretion, whereas the acetylated drug is excreted by glomerular filtration. In urine, approximately 20% of SMZ present is unchanged drug, 50% to 70% is acetylated derivative, and 15% to 20% is the glucuronide conjugate. Concentrations of SMZ in urine are approximately 3 times concurrent drug–blood concentrations. The half-life of SMZ is prolonged in patients with renal insufficiency (creatinine clearance less than 20 to 30 mL per minute), and reduced doses should be administered in these patients (1).

CLINICAL USE AND DOSAGE

SMZ is indicated for uncomplicated acute and recurrent urinary tract infections caused by susceptible organisms including *Escherichia coli*, *Klebsiella*, *Enterobacter*, and *Proteus mirabilis*. Currently, the increasing frequency of resistant organisms limits the usefulness of several antibacterial agents including the sulfonamides for the treatment of chronic and recurrent urinary tract infections. The fixed combination TMP–SMZ is preferred over SMZ for most infections (see section on Trimethoprim–Sulfamethoxazole).

Sulfonamides were successfully used, in the past, for the prevention of meningococcal disease in contacts and for the eradication of the chronic meningococcal carrier state. However, because sulfonamide-resistant meningococci are now common, these drugs are usually no longer suitable for these clinical situations. Rifampin, ceftriaxone, or ciprofloxacin are currently recommended as the chemoprophylactic agents for meningococcal infections in United States. In localized epidemics of sulfonamide-sensitive meningococcal disease, chemoprophylaxis with sulfonamides can be used (2).

The recommended oral dose of SMZ in children older than 2 months of age is 50 to 60 mg per kg initially, followed by 25 to 30 mg per kg every 12 hours (maximum, 75 mg per kg per day). SMZ is not indicated in infants younger than 2 months of age, except in the treatment of congenital toxoplasmosis as an adjunct to pyrimethamine.

ADVERSE REACTIONS

SMZ shares the toxic potentials of the sulfonamides. Hemolytic effects include agranulocytosis, aplastic anemia, leukopenia, thrombocytopenia, hemolytic anemia, eosinophilia, and methemoglobinemia. Any sulfonamide may cause hemolysis in patients with glucose 6-phosphate dehydrogenase deficiency. Allergic reactions include anaphylaxis, serum sickness, and conjunctival and scleral injection. Nephrotoxic effects include crystalluria that may cause pain and hematuria. Anuria can occur if the renal pelvis or the ureter becomes completely occluded. Alkalinization of the urine increases solubility as well as enhances the urinary excretion of SMZ and should be used when high doses of SMZ are given. Dermatologic effects include erythema multiforme, Stevens–Johnson syndrome, exfoliative dermatitis, photosensitivity, pruritus, urticaria, and generalized skin eruptions. Gastrointestinal adverse effects include hepatitis, hepatocellular necrosis, pseudomembranous colitis, pancreatitis, nausea, vomiting, diarrhea, anorexia, and abdominal pain. Neurologic complications may include peripheral neuritis, ataxia, vertigo, tinnitus, and headache.

DRUG INTERACTIONS

SMZ may prolong the prothrombin time in patients who are receiving the anticoagulant warfarin. SMZ may inhibit the hepatic metabolism of phenytoin.

TRIMETHOPRIM–SULFAMETHOXAZOLE

CLINICAL PHARMACOKINETICS

The optimal ratio of TMP and SMZ concentrations for synergy has been determined to be 1 part of TMP and 20 parts of SMZ (3). Thus, available preparations are manufactured in a 1:5 fixed ratio of TMP to SMZ. TMP–SMZ is rapidly and well absorbed from the gastrointestinal tract and may be administered without regard to food. Peak serum concentrations of 1 to 2 μg per mL of TMP and 40 to 60 μg per mL of unbound SMZ are reached at 1 to 4 hours after a single dose containing 160 mg of TMP and 800 mg of SMZ. Steady-state peak serum concentrations after multiple-dose administration are usually 50% higher than those obtained after a single dose. The drug is widely distributed in body tissues and fluids, including CSF, middle ear cavity, sputum, bile, and aqueous humor. Half-life is approximately 8 to 14 hours. TMP is excreted mostly unchanged in urine, with approximately 10% to 30% metabolized to an inactive form. SMZ is primarily metabolized in the liver, with approximately 30% excreted unchanged in urine. Because most drug excretion occurs via the kidney, the dosage of TMP–SMZ should be adjusted for a creatinine clearance of less than 30 mL per minute (4).

SPECTRUM OF ACTIVITIES

The combination of TMP–SMZ is usually synergistic and bactericidal (5,6). Both drugs affect bacterial folic acid synthesis. SMZ inhibits dihydropteroate synthase, which catalyses the formation of dihydrofolate from PABA. In the subsequent step of the pathway, TMP inhibits dihydrofolate reductase, which catalyses the formation of tetrahydrofolate from dihydrofolate. By inhibiting tetrahydrofolic acid formation, the active form of folic acid, TMP–SMZ inhibits bacterial thymidine synthesis and results in a bactericidal action. Although these steps follow one another and cause a sequential blockade, this does not necessarily explain the aforementioned synergy. A combination of two drugs that have slightly different bacterial spectrums and different resistance profiles among pathogenic bacteria improves the usefulness of the drug combination.

In general, many *Enterobacteriaceae*, including *E. coli*, *Klebsiella pneumoniae*, and *P. mirabilis*, are susceptible to TMP–SMZ. *Salmonella* and *Shigella* species and enterotoxigenic *E. coli* were previously susceptible to TMP–SMZ. However, the resistant strains have rapidly increased recently worldwide (7–10). TMP–SMZ is active against *Stenotrophomonas maltophilia*, which is typically resistant to other classes of broad-spectrum antibiotics (11). Other nonfermentative organisms, including *Burkholderia cepacia*, *Acinetobacter*, and *Alcaligenes*, which often cause nosocomial infections, are frequently susceptible to TMP–SMZ. However, TMP–SMZ has poor activity against *Pseudomonas aeruginosa*. *Staphylococcus aureus*, the most common skin pathogen, is also susceptible to TMP–SMZ. TMP–SMZ is also active against *Pneumocystis jiroveci* (formerly known as *P. carinii*), *Nocardia*, *Tropheryma whippelii*, *Isospora* species, *Cyclospora* species, and *Toxoplasma gondii*.

MECHANISM OF RESISTANCE

Bacteria may become resistant to TMP–SMZ by several mechanisms, including the development of permeability barriers, efflux pumps, naturally insensitive target enzymes, and genetic alterations in the genes encoding target enzymes. Resistance is transferable. Resistance to SMZ in gram-negative organisms is usually plasmid mediated. Resistance to TMP has been shown to occur by several mechanisms, most often chromosomally mediated, but also involving mutations of bacteria to thymidine-dependent strains, or plasmid-mediated resistance involving altered production or sensitivity of bacterial dihydrofolate reductase. Marked geographic variation in resistance has been demonstrated, with higher incidence typically found in developing countries (12).

ADVERSE REACTIONS

The most frequent adverse effects are gastrointestinal intolerance and cutaneous reactions, each occurring in approximately 3% to 5% of patients. Multiple skin reactions have been described, including a maculopapular rash, urticaria, diffuse erythema, morbilliform rash, erythema multiforme, purpura, and photosensitivity (13,14). These reactions tend to be mild, dose-related, and reversible, and can occasionally be obviated by reduction in dosage without discontinuation of therapy. Fatal hypersensitivity reaction, including Stevens–Johnson syndrome and toxic epidermal necrolysis, rarely occurs. A drug fever with delayed (1 to 2 weeks) onset, often accompanied by a morbilliform rash, may occur. The more severe form of this with multisystem involvement has sometimes been termed the DRESS (drug rash with eosinophilia and systemic symptoms) syndrome. The frequency of adverse effects is substantially higher in immunocompromised patients, particularly in HIV-infected individuals. The rate of adverse reactions to TMP–SMZ in HIV-infected children is approximately 15% (15). Although this is higher than the rate seen in uninfected children, it is substantially lower than the rate seen in HIV-infected adults. The exact mechanisms of increased risk for adverse reactions in this population have not been determined.

TMP–SMZ may decrease the tubular secretion of creatinine and cause a mild elevation of serum creatinine at standard doses without decreasing the glomerular filtration rate (16,17). This is reversible with drug discontinuation. TMP–SMZ has only rarely been associated with direct nephrotoxicity. Hyperkalemia has been observed in patients taking high-dose TMP–SMZ or in patients with preexisting renal insufficiency taking standard TMP–SMZ dosages (18–20). The mechanism could be explained by TMP-induced alteration of transepithelial voltage in distal renal tubule, which results in decreased potassium excretion (21). Hematologic adverse events including anemia, granulocytopenia, megaloblastosis, agranulocytosis, and thrombocytopenia have been reported in children (22,23). Recovery is gradual after the drug is discontinued.

DRUG INTERACTION

SMZ in general can inhibit metabolism of many drugs including warfarin, phenytoin, and sulfonylureas, and it can compete with these agents for binding sites on albumin. Clinically significant exaggeration of anticoagulant effect, CNS toxicity of phenytoin, and hypoglycemia can occur. SMZ use is associated with the increased nephrotoxicity of cyclosporin despite reduction of serum cyclosporin concentrations. SMZ increases the free serum methotrexate fraction. TMP increases serum levels and increases elimination half-life of phenytoin and digoxin.

CLINICAL USE

TMP–SMZ is used as empiric treatment and prophylaxis for urinary tract infection in children. However, the recent use of antibiotics, hospitalization, and immunosuppression has been implicated as factors contributing to increasing TMP–SMZ resistance among urinary tract isolates in adults (24–26). The prevalence of TMP–SMZ resistance among urinary tract isolates in children varies depending on geographic locations. However, limited data indicated an increasing trend of TMP–SMZ resistance up to more than 30% in children with community-acquired urinary tract infection (27–29).

Community-associated methicillin-resistant *S. aureus* (CA-MRSA) has emerged rapidly as a commonly identified cause of skin and soft tissue infections. This has led to consideration for the use of TMP–SMZ in the treatment of CA-MRSA infection. TMP–SMZ is rapidly bactericidal against CA-MRSA in vitro when compared with other orally available antimicrobials (30). The efficacy of TMP–SMZ therapy for CA-MRSA skin and soft tissue infection was reported in a retrospective study (31). It must be emphasized, however, that incision and drainage remains the mainstay treatment of skin and soft tissue infections. In addition, TMP–SMZ is not active against *Streptococcus pyogenes*, another common cause of skin and soft tissue infections. Given the inability to differentiate microbiologic causes reliably on clinical grounds, monotherapy with TMP–SMZ is not recommended empirically unless CA-MRSA is proven by the culture.

Previously, TMP–SMZ was an effective treatment for otitis media, sinusitis, and community-acquired pneumonia. Emerging resistance among respiratory pathogens, especially *S. pneumoniae*, has raised serious concerns regarding the use of TMP–SMZ in respiratory tract infections (32). Thus, the use of TMP–SMZ for respiratory tract infections in children requires consideration of local resistance patterns and individual patient factors such as severity of disease and risk for resistance.

TMP–SMZ is useful in the treatment of gastroenteritis caused by *Shigella*, *Salmonella typhi*, and traveler's diarrhea due to enterotoxigenic *E. coli*. However, it may not be effective in some parts of the world where resistant strains of these organisms are common. *Yersinia enterocolitica*, *Vibrio cholerae*, and *Aeromonas hydrophila* remain susceptible to TMP–SMZ.

TMP–SMZ is the agent of choice for treatment and prophylaxis for *P. jiroveci* infection in children with malignancy, defects in cell-mediated immunity, and HIV infection. Mutations in the *P. jiroveci* dihydropteroate synthase gene have been identified in patients taking TMP–SMZ prophylaxis, and this may play a major role in TMP–SMZ treatment failure (33).

Prophylactic use of TMP–SMZ to prevent recurrent bacterial infections in patients with chronic granulomatous disease and other neutrophil-associated immunodeficiencies has been well documented in children (34,35). Selected patients with Wegener granulomatosis may benefit from TMP–SMZ, although the mechanism of action and degree of clinical efficacy in these patients are uncertain (36).

PEDIATRIC DOSAGE

The pediatric recommended dose is 8 to 12 mg per kg per day of TMP component, or 40 to 60 mg per kg per day of SMZ component, in two divided doses. The daily adult dose is 320 mg of TMP or 1,600 mg of SMZ. For *P. jiroveci* treatment, the dose should be increased to 20 mg per kg per day of TMP component, or 100 mg per kg per day of SMZ component, in four doses intravenously for 21 days. For prophylaxis in immunocompromised patients, the recommended dose is 5 mg of TMP and 25 mg of SMZ per kg per day in two divided doses.

For prophylaxis against *P. jiroveci*, the recommended regimen is 150 mg per m^2 per day of TMP with 750 mg per m^2 per day of SMZ orally, in two divided doses, three times per week on consecutive days (37). The maximum daily dose is 160 mg of TMP and 800 mg of SMZ. The drug may also be given as:

- a single daily dose, three times per week on consecutive days,
- two divided doses, 7 days per week, or
- two divided doses, three times per week on alternate days.

SPECIAL CONSIDERATIONS

The indications for *P. jiroveci* chemoprophylaxis in HIV-infected children are (a) all HIV-infected children younger than 12 months of age regardless of their immunologic status, (b) HIV-infected children older than 12 months of age with severe immune suppression (CDC classification 3), and (c) prior *P. jiroveci* infection (37). This prophylactic regimen may provide additional protection against toxoplasmosis and recurrent bacterial infections, which are common among HIV-infected individuals with severe immune suppression.

Both TMP and SMZ cross placenta and appear in breast milk, with detectable concentrations found in fetal serum in patients taking the drug. TMP–SMZ is listed in Pregnancy Category C by the US Food and Drug Administration.

SULFASALAZINE

PHARMACOKINETICS

Following oral administration, small intestinal absorption accounts for an absolute sulfasalazine bioavailability of 15%. This fraction is highly protein bound and is subsequently excreted in the urine. However, the majority of an orally administered sulfasalazine dose reaches the colon, where it is metabolized by intestinal flora to sulfapyridine and 5-aminosalicylic acid (5-ASA) or mesalazine (38,39). Plasma concentrations of sulfapyridine and 5-ASA peak at about 10 hours after dosing. The long time to peak concentrations is a function of the transit time to the lower intestine. Sulfapyridine is relatively well absorbed from the colon with bioavailability of 60%. Absorbed sulfapyridine undergoes extensive metabolism in the liver via acetylation, hydroxylation, and glucuronidation. Peak concentrations of sulfapyridine depend on the acetylator status of the patient with slow acetylators having higher concentrations and increased likelihood of adverse events (39). In contrast, 5-ASA is less well absorbed with bioavailability of 10% to 30%. 5-ASA is metabolized by the liver and the intestine to *N*-acetyl-5-aminosalicylic acid. Acetylation is phenotype independent. Sulfapyridine and 5-ASA and their metabolites are excreted in the urine (38). However, because the majority of 5-ASA stays in the colon, excretion is primarily in the feces as unchanged 5-ASA or as acetyl-5-ASA (40).

CLINICAL USE

In adults, sulfasalazine is indicated for the treatment of mild to moderate ulcerative colitis and is effective in maintaining disease remission. In addition, it is used as adjunctive therapy with corticosteroids for treatment of severe ulcerative colitis (41). Sulfasalazine may also be active in treating Crohn's disease of the colon, although it is not effective in maintaining remission. Sulfasalazine has also been used to treat adults with collagenous colitis (42).

Sulfasalazine is considered a disease-modifying antirheumatic drug for rheumatoid arthritis. Sulfasalazine is also used in the treatment of rheumatoid arthritis in patients who fail or are unable to tolerate an adequate trial of nonsteroidal anti-inflammatory drugs (43).

In children younger than 2 years of age, the safety and efficacy of sulfasalazine have not been established. Sulfasalazine is used as a second-line treatment of pauciarticular and polyarticular juvenile rheumatoid arthritis in children (44,45). The use of sulfasalazine in the treatment of patients with systemic-onset juvenile rheumatoid arthritis has been associated with increased incidence of adverse effects, particularly serum sickness. Therefore, sulfasalazine use for those patients should be avoided (45).

Sulfasalazine has also been found to produce a significantly greater clinical improvement than placebo in adult patients with plaque type psoriasis and psoriatic arthritis (46). However, other studies have failed to demonstrate significant clinical or radiologic improvement with use of sulfasalazine in psoriatic arthritis (47).

MECHANISM OF ACTION

Sulfasalazine and its two metabolites, sulfapyridine and 5-ASA, have anti-inflammatory and immunomodulatory properties. The mode of action of sulfasalazine is not completely elucidated but may be related to the anti-inflammatory effects of 5-ASA. This has been shown in studies in patients with ulcerative colitis who were given rectal sulfasalazine, sulfapyridine, and 5-ASA, and the results suggest that the therapeutic effects are related to 5-ASA (48).

ADVERSE REACTIONS

Sulfasalazine is metabolized to sulfapyridine and 5-ASA. The adverse effects are more likely to be due to the sulfapyridine moiety and are similar to those with other sulfonamides. These effects are likely to occur among patients who are slow acetylators and when serum concentrations exceed 50 μg per mL. The most frequent adverse effects are gastrointestinal symptoms such as abdominal pain, nausea, and vomiting as well as headache, fever, and skin rash. Hematological adverse events, mainly blood dyscrasias due to bone marrow suppression, have been reported among patients receiving sulfasalazine. These include leukopenia, neutropenia, aplastic anemia, and thrombocytopenia. The hematological side effects appear to be more common among patients receiving sulfasalazine for rheumatoid arthritis than those with inflammatory bowel disease. Hematological reaction may be caused by either the sulfapyridine or the 5-ASA moiety. Although folate deficiency has been reported among patients who received sulfasalazine, cytopenia and megaloblastic anemia have been reported rarely among those patients. Folate deficiency may result from decreased folate absorption and metabolism as well as increased folate requirement secondary to hemolysis of red blood cells (49,50).

Cardiovascular side effects of sulfasalazine include case reports of Raynaud's phenomenon and myocarditis (51,52). Other rarely reported adverse effects of sulfasalazine include exacerbation of episodes of ulcerative colitis, metallic mouth taste, intestinal villous atrophy, pancreatitis, and hair loss (53–55). Rare renal side effects include nephritic syndrome and interstitial nephritis (56). Pulmonary complications have been reported rarely among patients receiving sulfasalazine. Most of these complications are reversible and include cough, dyspnea, fever, pulmonary infiltrates, and eosinophilia. Rarely, fibrosing alveolitis has been reported with sulfasalazine use (57).

Male infertility is a known complication among adults treated with sulfasalazine. Infertility is due to direct toxic effects on the developing spermatozoa and is possibly induced by the sulfapyridine moiety. Infertility is caused by reduced sperm motility and oligospermia (58). The effects are reversible within 2 to 3 months of withdrawal of sulfasalazine treatment (59).

Sulfasalazine-induced lupus has been reported among patients who have a slow acetylator genotype or HLA-haplotype associated with idiopathic SLE (60). Drug-induced lupus has also been reported with 5-ASA (mesalazine) (61). Sulfasalazine may provoke acute porphyric attacks and should not be used in porphyric patients (62). Sulfasalazine may provoke hemolysis in patients with glucose 6-phosphate dehydrogenase deficiency (63). Sulfasalazine may cause reversible yellow-orange discoloration of the urine or skin.

Sulfasalazine use in children with inflammatory bowel disease has been rarely associated with immune-mediated hepatitis and fulminant hepatic failure. The sulfapyridine moiety is believed to be the cause of the reaction. Development of severe sulfasalazine-induced hepatotoxicity requires prompt discontinuation of sulfasalazine and the use of high-dose steroid therapy (64). Hepatitis has also been reported with 5-ASA use (65). Sulfasalazine is contraindicated in patients with hypersensitivity to sulfonamides. It is also contraindicated in children younger than 2 months of age because of the risk of kernicterus.

DRUG INTERACTIONS

Sulfasalazine is converted to active metabolites by the colonic bacterial flora. Concomitant administration of other antibiotics may reduce the efficacy of sulfasalazine by reducing the production of active metabolites. Sulfasalazine may decrease the bioavailability of digoxin and folic acid (66). Sulfasalazine may increase the toxicity of thiopurine antineoplastic agents by inhibition of their metabolism (67).

DOSAGE

Sulfasalazine is administered to children with ulcerative colitis who are 6 years and older at a dose of 40 to 60 mg per kg per day divided into three to six doses. Following clinical improvement the dose may be reduced to 30 mg per kg per day divided into four doses. In children with polyarticular juvenile rheumatoid arthritis, sulfasalazine is administered at a dose of 30 to 50 mg per kg per day into two evenly divided doses. The maximum daily dose is 2 g. Because of the increased frequency of gastrointestinal side effects associated with sulfasalazine, it is advisable to start with a quarter of the maintenance dose with weekly increases to the full maintenance dose in 1 month.

SULFISOXAZOLE

Sulfisoxazole is a short-acting sulfonamide. It is N^1-(3,4-dimethyl-5-isoxazolyl) sulfanilamide and has a molecular weight of 267.30. It is odorless, appears as white to slightly yellowish, slightly bitter, crystalline powder. It is soluble in alcohol and very slightly soluble in water.

Acetyl sulfisoxazole is the tasteless and more palatable form of sulfisoxazole. It is N^1-acetyl sulfisoxazole and has a molecular weight of 309.34. It should be differentiated from N^4-acetyl sulfisoxazole, which is a metabolite of sulfisoxazole. Acetyl sulfisoxazole appears as white or slightly yellow, crystalline powder. It is slightly soluble in alcohol and practically insoluble in water.

CLINICAL PHARMACOKINETICS

Absorption

Sulfisoxazole is absorbed from the GI tract without difficulty. After oral administration, sulfisoxazole is rapidly and completely absorbed; the major site of absorption is the small intestine but some absorption occurs in the stomach. Following a single 2 to 4 g oral dose of sulfisoxazole to healthy adult volunteers, peak plasma concentrations of sulfisoxazole range from 110 to 250 μg per mL. The time of peak plasma concentration ranges from 1 to 4 hours. In the blood sulfisoxazole exits in unbound, protein-bound, and conjugated forms. It is metabolized primarily by acetylation and oxidation in the liver and is absorbed as the free sulfonamide. The free sulfonamide is considered to be the therapeutically active form. Approximately 85% of sulfisoxazole is bound to plasma proteins (primarily to albumin); of the unbound portion, 65% to 72% is in the nonacetylated form and approximately 28% to 35% in blood and urine is acetylated at the N^4 position. In healthy volunteers after multiple oral administration of sulfisoxazole 500 mg four times a day, the average steady-state plasma concentrations of intact sulfisoxazole range from 49.9 to 88.8 μg per mL (mean, 63.4 μg per mL).

N^1-acetyl sulfisoxazole is metabolized to sulfisoxazole in the gastrointestinal tract by digestive enzymes and is absorbed as sulfisoxazole. This process is thought to be responsible for slower absorption and lower peak blood concentrations compared to those attained following administration of a similar oral dose of sulfisoxazole. With persistent administration of acetyl sulfisoxazole, blood concentrations approximate those of sulfisoxazole. The maximum plasma concentrations of sulfisoxazole after a single 4-g dose of acetyl sulfisoxazole to healthy volunteers range from 122 to 282 μg per mL (mean, 181 μg per mL) for the pediatric suspension and from 101 to 202 μg per mL (mean, 144 μg per mL) for the syrup. The peak plasma concentration occurs between 2 and 6 hours post-administration.

Following the same doses of a sulfonamide, variation in blood levels may result. Therefore, blood levels should be measured in patients receiving sulfonamides at the higher recommended doses or those being treated for serious infections. For most infections, free sulfonamide blood levels of 50 to 150 μg per mL may be considered therapeutic, whereas blood levels of 120 to 150 μg per mL may be optimal for serious infections. Adverse reactions occur more frequently when the maximum sulfonamide level exceeds 200 μg per mL.

Distribution

Sulfisoxazole differs from other sulfonamide in that it is distributed only in the body's extracellular space. It is excreted in human milk. It crosses the placenta readily and enters into fetal circulation and also crosses the blood–brain barrier. In healthy individuals, CSF concentrations of sulfisoxazole range from 8% to 57% of blood concentrations; however, in patients with meningitis, CSF concentrations as high as 94 μg per mL have been reported.

Elimination

Sulfisoxazole and its acetylated metabolites are excreted predominantly by the kidneys through glomerular filtration. Following single oral administration of sulfisoxazole, approximately 97% is excreted in the urine within 48 hours; 52% is intact drug, and the remaining is the N^4-acetylated metabolite. After administration of acetyl sulfisoxazole, about 58% is excreted in the urine as total drug within 72 hours.

The half-life of elimination of sulfisoxazole ranges from 4.6 to 7.8 hours after oral administration, whereas for N^1-acetyl sulfisoxazole, the half-lives of elimination from plasma range from 5.4 to 7.4 hours for the pediatric suspension. The elimination of sulfisoxazole has been shown to correlate with creatinine clearance; for instance, in the elderly subjects aged 63 to 75 years with decreased renal function (creatinine clearance, 37 to 68 mL per minute), the elimination of sulfisoxazole has been reported to be slower. Sulfisoxazole is removed by hemodialysis, whereas N^4-acetyl sulfisoxazole seems to be less readily removed.

SPECTRUM OF ACTIVITY

Sulfisoxazole is bacteriostatic and its antibacterial spectrum of sulfisoxazole is similar to other sulfonamides. It inhibits bacterial synthesis by interfering with microbial folic acid synthesis. Specifically, they are competitive inhibitors of dihydropteroate synthetase, which is the enzyme responsible for the incorporation of PABA into dihydropteroic acid.

The following organisms may be susceptible in vitro to sulfonamides: *S. pyogenes*, *S. pneumoniae*, *Haemophilus influenzae*, *H. ducreyi*, *Nocardia*, *Actinomyces*, *Calymmatobacterium granulomatis*, *Chlamydia trachomatis*, *E. coli*, *Neisseria meningitidis*, and *Shigella*. Malarial parasites may also be susceptible to sulfonamides.

MECHANISM OF RESISTANCE

Resistance to sulfonamides is prevalent and common. Different mechanisms of resistance to sulfonamides have been implicated. Resistance in *Enterobacteriaceae* is due to the alteration of dihydropteroate synthetase with reduced affinity for sulfonamides. For staphylococci, pneumococci and gonococci, resistance to sulfonamide may be due to the production of increased quantities of PABA. Plasmid-mediated resistance may be due to the production of drug-resistance enzyme dihydropteroate synthetase or due to decreased bacterial cell permeability to sulfonamides.

ADVERSE REACTION

There are numerous adverse reactions reported similar to other sulfonamides. Anaphylaxis, erythema multiforme (Stevens–Johnson syndrome), toxic epidermal necrolysis, exfoliative dermatitis, angioedema, arteritis and vasculitis, allergic myocarditis, serum sickness, rash, urticaria, pruritus, photosensitivity, conjunctival and scleral injection, generalized allergic reactions, and generalized skin eruptions may occur. Sulfonamides bear certain chemical similarities to some goitrogens, diuretics (acetazolamide and thiazides), and oral hypoglycemia agents. Cross-sensitivity may exist with these agents. Developments of goiter, diuresis, and hypoglycemia have occurred rarely in patients receiving sulfonamides. Crystalluria, hematuria, blood urea nitrogen and creatinine elevations, nephritis, and toxic nephrosis with oliguria and anuria have been reported. The frequency of renal complications is lower in patients receiving sulfisoxazole than other sulfonamides. Hematologic adverse effects include leukopenia, agranulocytosis, aplastic anemia, thrombocytopenia, purpura, hemolytic anemia, anemia, eosinophilia, and clotting disorders. Some may experience headache, dizziness, peripheral neuritis, paresthesia, convulsions, tinnitus, vertigo, ataxia, and increased intracranial hypertension, psychosis, and hallucination.

DRUG INTERACTIONS

Sulfisoxazole may displace the anticoagulant warfarin from albumin-binding sites and prolong the prothrombin time. Sulfisoxazole may also displace thiopental from its binding sites and patients receiving sulfisoxazole may require less thiopental required for anesthesia. Sulfonamides can also displace methotrexate from its protein-binding sides thus increasing methotrexate toxicity. Sulfisoxazole can also potentiate the hypoglycemic effects of sulfonylureas or cause hypoglycemia by itself.

CLINICAL USE

Sulfisoxazole and sulfisoxazole acetyl can be used for treatment of urinary tract infections due to susceptible organisms. They may be useful for meningococcal meningitis prophylaxis with known sulfonamide-sensitive group A strains (not yet proven to be useful for groups B or C strains) and for the treatment of lymphogranuloma venereum. Sulfisoxazole may also be used as chemoprophylaxis for recurrences of rheumatic fever. In children, the sulfisoxazole acetyl and erythromycin ethylsuccinate combination product can be used for treatment of acute otitis media caused by susceptible strains of *H. influenzae*. At present, because of the increasing frequency of resistant organisms, the use of sulfisoxazole and its derivatives is limited only to susceptible organisms with careful and close follow-up.

PREPARATIONS AND DOSAGES

Sulfisoxazole and its derivatives are administered orally; all dosages are expressed in terms of sulfisoxazole. Sulfisoxazole is available in 500-mg tablets. It is also available in combination with 50 mg of phenazopyridine. Sulfisoxazole acetate is available in oral suspension of 500 mg of sulfisoxazole per 5 mL. Sulfisoxazole acetate is also available in combination with erythromycin ethylsuccinate (600 mg of sulfisoxazole and 200 mg of erythromycin per 5 mL of suspension).

The usual dose of sulfisoxazole for adults is 2 to 4 g initially, then followed by maintenance dose of 4 to 8 g daily divided in four to six equal doses. Sulfonamides are contraindicated in infants 2 months of age and younger. For children older than 2 months of age, the usual dose is 75 mg per kg or 2 g per m^2 initially, then followed by 150 mg per kg or 4 g per m^2 daily given in four to six equal doses. The total daily pediatric dosage of sulfisoxazole should not exceed 6 g.

SPECIAL CONSIDERATIONS

Sulfisoxazole is contraindicated in patients with known hypersensitivity to sulfonamides, in infants younger than 2 months of age, pregnant women at term, and nursing mothers of infants younger than 2 months of age because sulfonamide may cause kernicterus by displacing bilirubin from its binding sites.

SULFADIAZINE

Sulfadiazine is well absorbed from the gastrointestinal tract. Peak blood concentration is attained 3 to 6 hours after an oral dose. Sulfadiazine is metabolized in the liver to the acetylated form. Approximately 10% to 40% of the drug in plasma is in the acetylated form. Plasma protein binding is 38% to 48%. The free form is considered to be therapeutically active. Sulfadiazine is distributed into most body tissues and diffuses into the CSF. CSF concentrations are 40% to 60% of those in the blood and are achieved within 4 hours of administration. CSF concentrations are higher when the meninges are inflamed.

Sulfadiazine is eliminated primarily through the kidneys. Drug urine concentration is 10 to 25 times greater than serum levels. Approximately 30% to 44% of the drug is excreted unchanged in the urine and 15% to 40% is eliminated as the acetylated form. The half-life of sulfadiazine ranges from 7 to 12 hours and that of the acetylated metabolite from 8 to 12 hours (68). Sulfadiazine is excreted in breast milk.

CLINICAL USE

The usual adult dosage in adults is 2 to 4 g initially, followed by 2 to 4 g daily administered in three to six equally divided doses. In children older than 2 months of age, the dose is 75 mg per kg initially, followed by 150 mg per kg administered in four to six equally divided doses. The maximum daily dose is 6 g.

Sulfadiazine shares the actions and uses of other sulfonamides. It has been used in the treatment of nocardiosis, toxoplasmosis (combined with pyrimethamine), prophylaxis of rheumatic fever, and treatment of meningococcal carriers.

Nocardiosis

Sulfonamides remain one of the drugs of choice for the treatment of *Nocardia* infections. Sulfadiazine given at 100 mg per kg per day divided every 6 hours, to achieve peak blood levels of 100 to 150 μg per mL, is standard treatment. Treatment is given for a minimum of 6 weeks and often continued for 6 to 12 months. TMP–SMZ has also been used for therapy especially when intravenous route is needed. Patients unable to tolerate sulfonamides may receive minocycline, ampicillin, or erythromycin. Other useful drugs include the third-generation cephalosporin, cefotaxime, or ceftriaxone and imipenem.

Toxoplasmosis

Most cases of acquired toxoplasmosis do not require specific antimicrobial therapy. When indicated (e.g., chorioretinitis or significant organ damage) for symptomatic and asymptomatic congenital toxoplasmosis, sulfadiazine combined with pyrimethamine (supplemented with folinic acid) is recommended. The combination is synergistic against *T. gondii* and is the most widely accepted regimen for treatment of children and adults with acute symptomatic toxoplasmosis.

Rheumatic Fever Prophylaxis

Oral sulfadiazine is as effective as oral penicillin for secondary prophylaxis of rheumatic fever. Sulfonamides have been used for rheumatic fever prophylaxis as alternatives to penicillin for penicillin-allergic patients; however, erythromycin is probably a better alternative. The American Heart Association recommends sulfadiazine 0.5 g once a day for patients weighing 27 kg or less and 1.0 g once a day for patients weighing more than 27 kg (69).

Meningococcal Carriers

Formerly, sulfonamides were extensively and successfully used for the treatment of meningococcal meningitis and septicemia, for prevention of meningococcal disease in contacts, and for the eradication of the chronic meningococcal carrier state. Because sulfonamide-resistant meningococci are now common, these drugs are usually no longer suitable for these clinical situations. Rifampin, ceftriaxone, or ciprofloxacin is currently recommended as the chemoprophylactic agent for meningococcal infections in the United States. In localized epidemics of serogroup B sulfonamide-sensitive meningococcal disease chemoprophylaxis with sulfonamides can be used (2). The dose of sulfadiazine for chemoprophylaxis is 1 g twice daily for adults, 0.5 g twice daily for children 1 to 12 years of age, and 0.5 g once daily for children younger than 1 year of age.

ADVERSE REACTIONS

Hemolytic effects include leukopenia, thrombocytopenia, hemolytic anemia, agranulocytosis, and aplastic anemia. Leukopenia usually occurs within 2 to 4 days of starting sulfadiazine with an estimated frequency of 3% to 5% (70). Thrombocytopenia is a rare complication of sulfonamide therapy (71). Acute hemolytic anemia, a rare complication, can occur as a result of prior sensitization with sulfonamides (72). Sulfonamides can induce hemolysis in patients with glucose-6-phosphate dehydrogenase–deficient red blood cells, producing intravascular hemolysis and hemoglobinuria. Agranulocytosis is rare with the currently used sulfonamides.

Genitourinary Effects

Crystalluria and acute renal failure have been described with the use of high dose-sulfadiazine for a number of conditions including the treatment of toxoplasma encephalitis in patients with AIDS (72,73). Crystalluria occurs because the drug and its acetyl conjugate are excreted in the urine in high concentrations and are highly insoluble. Crystalluria may cause pain and hematuria, and anuria can occur if the renal pelvis or the ureter becomes completely occluded. Crystalluria may be avoided by adequate hydration and alkalinizing the urine to a pH greater than 7.15 without necessarily discontinuing sulfadiazine therapy (72).

Gastrointestinal Effects

Adverse gastrointestinal effects that have been reported with sulfadiazine use include nausea, vomiting, anorexia, diarrhea and abdominal pain, stomatitis, hepatitis, and pancreatitis.

Jaundice in the newborn: Sulfonamides compete with a number of substances, including bilirubin, for albumin-binding sites. Infants born to mothers treated with sulfonamides can develop jaundice with high free serum bilirubin levels or even kernicterus, especially if there is hemolysis. The same can also occur in newborn or premature infants who receive treatment with sulfonamides.

Allergic rashes are fairly frequent complications of sulfonamide therapy. Usually these occur after 1 to 2 weeks of treatment but may appear earlier with prior sensitization. Maculopapular and urticarial rashes are the most common but erythema nodosum, exfoliative dermatitis, and rarely Stevens–Johnson syndrome may occur. Photosensitivity and serum sickness-like illness may also occur.

SILVER SULFADIAZINE (SILVADENE CREAM)

Silver sulfadiazine is formed by combining the weak acid sulfadiazine with silver nitrate to form a white, slightly soluble complex silver salt. Silver sulfadiazine complex does not precipitate chlorides in the body fluids as silver nitrate does. Silver sulfadiazine is nonstaining and odorless.

Sufficient data indicate that silver sulfadiazine inhibits bacteria that are resistant to other antimicrobial agents and that the compound is superior to sulfadiazine. Silver sulfadiazine exerts its antibacterial effect by binding to cell membranes, and to a lesser extent, the bacterial cell wall rather than by interacting with cellular DNA. It has bactericidal activity against many gram-positive and gram-negative organisms, including *P. aeruginosa*, *E. coli*, *Proteus* species, staphylococci, streptococci, and yeast. The topical use of silver sulfadiazine has been very effective for the prevention and treatment of sepsis in burn wounds (74,75). Although silver is not appreciably absorbed systemically, sulfadiazine may be absorbed into the blood especially when the drug is applied to large areas and/or over prolonged periods of time (76,77). During prolonged treatment of wounds involving extensive areas of the body, serum sulfonamide levels may approach therapeutic levels of 8 to 12 mg per dL. If renal function is sufficiently impaired, accumulation of sulfadiazine may occur, particularly if the patient is dehydrated. In patients with extensive burns, it is recommended that serum sulfa levels be monitored during prolonged use of the drug.

CLINICAL USAGE AND ADMINISTRATION

Silver sulfadiazine 1% cream is a topical antimicrobial agent that is indicated as an adjunct for the prevention and treatment of wound sepsis in patients with second- and third-degree burns (74,75).

After burn wounds are cleansed and debrided, silver sulfadiazine cream is applied under sterile conditions. It should be applied with sterile, gloved hand to the burn surface once or twice daily to a thickness approximately 1/16th of an inch. Treatment should be continued until satisfactory healing has occurred or until the burn site is ready for grafting.

ADVERSE REACTIONS

Transient leukopenia has been reported in patients receiving silver sulfadiazine therapy (78,79). White blood cell depression occurs within 2 to 4 days of initiation of therapy. Rebound to normal counts follows onset within 2 to 3 days. Recovery is not influenced by continuation of silver sulfadiazine therapy.

Other infrequent adverse events include skin necrosis, erythema multiforme skin discoloration, burning sensation, and rashes. Because absorption of silver sulfadiazine varies depending on body surface area, it is possible that adverse reactions may occur such as associated thrombocytopenia, dermatologic reactions including Stevens–Johnson syndrome, and exfoliative dermatitis as well as hepatitis and toxic nephrosis.

DAPSONE (4,4′-DIAMINODIPHENYLSULFONE)

CLINICAL PHARMACOKINETICS

Dapsone has excellent oral bioavailability and, despite plasma protein binding of 50% to 90%, penetrates into various tissues well. The predominant route of elimination of dapsone is metabolism, with only 5% to 15% of an administered dose found in urine as unchanged drug (80). Dapsone is extensively metabolized by both oxidative and conjugative processes, forming dapsone hydroxylamine and the *N*-acetylated metabolites MADDS and hydroxymonoacetyldapsone, respectively (81). Deacetylation of the acetylated metabolites also takes place, and an equilibrium between acetylation and deacetylation is reached within a few hours after dapsone administration, resulting in a relatively constant acetylation ratio. N-hydroxylation, mediated by enzymes of the cytochrome P-450 3A4 subfamily, plays a central role in dapsone elimination. Increased cytochrome P-450 3A4 activity in young children explains the more rapid clearance in the patients younger than 2 years of age compared with those older than 2 years of age (82–84). Clinical importance of different dapsone deposition in various age groups is currently unknown.

SPECTRUM OF ACTIVITY

Dapsone is active in vitro against *Mycobacterium leprae* and several other species of *Mycobacterium*. It is also active against *P. jiroveci* (formerly known as *P. carinii*) and *Plasmodium* species.

MECHANISM OF RESISTANCE

Resistance appears slowly, as in up to 10% of patients with lepromatous leprosy who receive dapsone for many years. Resistance has been reported to occur as long as 24 years after the initiation of therapy and most frequently when the drug is given at a low dosage or intermittently. Initial resistance of *M. leprae* to dapsone is increasing. Cross-resistance between dapsone and clofazimine has not been reported in *Mycobacterium* species so far.

ADVERSE REACTIONS

Fatal agranulocytosis has occurred rarely when dapsone is administered in combination with pyrimethamine. Less severe granulocytopenia has occurred with dapsone in combination with chloroquine and primaquine. Severe hemolytic anemia can occur in association with large doses of dapsone (300 to 400 mg daily) or in patients with glucose-6-phosphate dehydrogenase deficiency. Overdose of dapsone may result in methemoglobinemia; its usual features include dyspnea, fatigue, cyanosis, deceptively high pulse oximetry, and chocolate-colored blood. The treatment of dapsone intoxication is intravenous methylene blue for symptomatic methemoglobinemia, gastric decontamination, and early administration of activated charcoal. Dapsone also has neurotoxicity, including peripheral neuropathy. Hypersensitivity reaction can occur 3 to 6 weeks after initiating dapsone. It is more likely to occur in patients with similar adverse reaction to other sulfonamides. A rare adverse effect called sulfone syndrome consists of fever, malaise, exfoliative dermatitis, hepatic necrosis, lymphadenopathy, anemia, and methemoglobinemia.

DRUG INTERACTIONS

Dapsone is a substrate of cytochrome P-450 3A4. Therefore, cytochrome P-450 3A4 inducers, including rifamycins, will increase the hepatic biotransformation of dapsone. By contrast, when dapsone is combined with TMP–SMZ, methemoglobinemia has resulted as a manifestation of dapsone toxicity caused presumably by decreased metabolism of dapsone.

CLINICAL USE

Dapsone is currently used in children with HIV infection who are intolerant of TMP–SMZ for chemoprophylaxis against *P. jiroveci* (85). Dapsone is also used to treat *M. avium* complex infection, in combination with azithromycin and other active antimicrobial agents. It is also effective against other mycobacteria such as *M. ulcerans*, the cause of Buruli ulcer disease (86). Dapsone is also used in combination with other active agents to treat children with leprosy and in some cases of multidrug-resistant tuberculosis. The combination of chlorproguanil–dapsone has good potency against certain malaria strains with borderline responsiveness to sulfadoxine–pyrimethamine (87,88).

PEDIATRIC DOSAGE

The recommended dosage in pediatrics is 2 mg per kg once daily, with the maximum dose of 100 mg. The pharmacokinetic data confirmed that the 2-mg per kg dose achieves the concentrations in serum comparable to those achieved with standard adult dose of 100 mg daily (83).

SPECIAL CONSIDERATIONS

The indications for *P. jiroveci* chemoprophylaxis in HIV-infected children are (a) all HIV-infected children younger than 12 months of age regardless of their immunologic status, (b) HIV-infected children older than 12 months of age with severe immune suppression (CDC classification 3), and (c) prior *P. jiroveci* infection (37). TMP–SMZ is the first drug of choice. Dapsone should be considered only in those with TMP–SMZ intolerance.

REFERENCES

1. Appel GB, Neu HC. Antimicrobial agents in patients with renal disease. *Med Times* 1977;195(9):109–112, 129.
2. Jacobson JA, Chester TJ, Fraser DW. An epidemic disease due to serogroup B Neisseria meningitidis in Alabama: report of an investigation and community-wide prophylaxis with a sulfonamide. *J Infect Dis* 1977;136:104.
3. Bushby SRM. Trimethoprim-sulfamethoxazole: in vitro microbiological aspects. *J Infect Dis* 1978;128(Suppl):S442–S462.
4. Smilack JD. Trimethoprim-sulfamethoxazole. *Mayo Clin Proc* 1999; 74:730–734.
5. Darrell JH, Garrod LP, Waterworth PM. Trimethoprim: laboratory an clinical studies *J Clin Pathol* 1968;21:202–209.
6. Bushby SRM, Hitchings GH. Trimethoprim, a sulfonamide potentiator. *Br J Pharmacol* 1968;33:72–90.
7. Lester SC, del Pilar PM, Wang F, et al. The carriage of Escherichia coli resistant to antimicrobial agents by healthy children in Boston, in Caracas, Venezuela, and in Qin Pu, China. *N Engl J Med* 1990;323:285–289.
8. Hoge CW, Gambel JM, Srijan A, et al. Trends in antibiotic resistance among diarrheal pathogens isolated in Thailand over 15 years. *Clin Infect Dis* 1998;26:341–345.

9. Reploge ML, Fleming DW, Cieslak PR. Emergence of antimicrobial-resistant shigellosis in Oregon. *Clin Infect Dis* 2000;30:515–519.
10. Ackers ML, Puhr ND, Tauxe RV, et al. Laboratory-based surveillance of Salmonella serotype Typhi infections in the United States: antimicrobial resistance in the rise. *JAMA* 2000;283:2668–2673.
11. Muder RR, Harris AP, Muller S, et al. Bacteremia due to Stenotrophomonas (Xanthomonas) maltophilia: a prospective, multicenter study of 91 episodes. *Clin Infect Dis* 1996;22:508–512.
12. Huovinen P, Sundström L, Swedberg G, et al. Trimethoprim and sulfonamide resistance. *Antimicrob Agents Chemother* 1995;39: 279–289.
13. Lawson D, Jick H. Adverse reaction to cotrimoxazole in hospitalized medical patients. *Am J Med Sci* 1978;275:53–57.
14. Jick H. Adverse reactions to trimethoprim-sulfamethoxazole in hospitalized patients. *Rev Infect Dis* 1982;4:426–428.
15. Hunter JM, Cooper DM, Colin AA. Pneumocystis carinii pneumonia: a pediatric prospective. *Ped AIDS HIV Infect* 1995;6: 262–270.
16. Berglund F, Killander J, Pompeius R. Effect of trimethoprim-sulfamethoxazole on the renal excretion of creatinine in man. *J Urol* 1975;114:802–808.
17. Shouval D, Ligumsky M, Ben-Ishay D. Effect of co-trimoxazole on normal creatinine clearance. *Lancet* 1978;1:244–245.
18. Ducharme M, Smythe M, Strohs G. Drug-induced alterations in serum creatinine concentrations. *Ann Pharmacother* 1993;27: 622–633.
19. Choi MJ, Fernandez PC, Patnaik A, et al. Trimethoprim-induced hyperkalemia in patients with AIDS. *N Engl J Med* 1993;328: 703–706.
20. Marinella M. Trimethoprim-induced hyperkalemia: an analysis of reported cases. *Gerontology* 1999;45:209–212.
21. Valazquez H, Perazella M, Wright F, et al. Renal mechanism of trimethoprim-induced hyperkalemia. *Ann Intern Med* 1993;119: 296–301.
22. Asmar BI, Maqbool S, Dajani AS. Hematologic abnormalities after oral trimethoprim-sulfamethoxazole therapy in children. *Am J Dis Child* 1981;135:1100–1103.
23. Bose W, Linzenmeier G, Karama A, et al. Controlled trial of co-trimoxazole in children with urinary-tract infection: bacteriologic efficacy and haematological toxicity. *Lancet* 1974;2:614–616.
24. Lepelletier D, Caroff N, Reynaud A, et al. Escherichia coli: epidemiology and analysis of risk factors for infections caused by resistant strains. *Clin Infect Dis* 1999;29:548–552.
25. Steinke DT, Seaton RA, Phillips G, et al. Factors associated with trimethoprim-resistant bacteria isolated from urine samples. *J Antimicrob Chemother* 1999;43:841–843.
26. Wright SW, Wrenn KD, Haynes ML. Trimethoprim-sulfamethoxazole resistance among urinary coliform isolates. *J Gen Intern Med* 1999;14:606–609.
27. Ladhani S, Gransden W. Increasing antibiotic resistance among urinary tract isolates. *Arch Dis Child* 2003;88:444–445.
28. McLoughlin TG, Joseph MM. Antibiotic resistance patterns of uropathogens in pediatric emergency department patients. *Acad Emerg Med* 2003;10:347–351.
29. Prais D, Straussberg R, Avitzur Y, et al. Bacterial susceptibility to oral antibiotics in community acquired urinary tract infection. *Arch Dis Child* 2003;88:215–218.
30. Kaka AS, Rueda AM, Shelburne SA III, et al. Bactericidal activity of orally available agents against methicillin-resistant Staphylococcus aureus. *J Antimicrob Chemother* 2006;58:680–683.
31. Szumowski JD, Cohen DE, Kanaya F, et al. Treatment and outcomes of infections by methicillin-resistant Staphylococcus aureus at an ambulatory clinic. *Antimicrob Agents Chemother* 2007;51: 423–428.
32. Hoban DJ, Doern GV, Fluit AC, et al. Worldwide prevalence of antimicrobial resistance in Streptococcus pneumoniae, Haemophilus influenzae, and Morexella catarrhalis in the SENTRY Antimicrobial Surveillance Program, 1997–1999. *Clin Infect Dis* 2001;32(Suppl):S81–S93.
33. Kazanjian P, Locke AB, Hossler PA, et al. Pneumocystis carinii mutations associated with sulfa and sulfone prophylaxis failure in AIDS patients. *AIDS* 1998;12:873–878.
34. Weening RS, Kabel P, Pijman P, et al. Continuous therapy with sulfamethoxazole-trimethoprim in patients with chronic granulomatous disease. *J Pediatr* 1983;103:127–130.
35. Mouy R, Fischer A, Vilmer E, et al. Incidence, severity, and prevention of infections in chronic granulomatous disease. *J Pediatr* 1989;114:555–560.
36. Stegeman CA, Tervaert JW, de Jong PE, et al. Trimethoprim-sulfamethoxazole (co-trimoxazole) for the prevention of relapses of Wegener's granulomatosis. *N Engl J Med* 1996;335: 16–20.
37. Centers for Disease Control and Prevention. 2002 USPHS/IDSA guidelines for preventing opportunistic infections among HIV-infected persons—2002. Recommendations of the US Public Health Service and the Infectious Diseases Society of America. *MMWR Recomm Rep* 2002;51(RR-8):1–46.
38. Klotz U. Clinical pharmacokinetics of sulphasalazine, its metabolites and other prodrugs of 5-aminosalicylic acid. *Clin Pharmacokinet* 1985;10(4):285–302.
39. Das KM, Dubin R. Clinical pharmacokinetics of sulphasalazine. *Clin Pharmacokinet* 1976;1(6):406–425.
40. Rijk MC, van Schaik A, van Tongeren JH. Disposition of 5-aminosalicylic acid by 5-aminosalicylic acid-delivering compounds. *Scand J Gastroenterol* 1988;23(1):107–112.
41. Schroeder KW. Role of mesalazine in acute and long-term treatment of ulcerative colitis and its complications. *Scand J Gastroenterol Suppl* 2002;(236):42–47.
42. Bohr J, Tysk C, Eriksson S, et al. Collagenous colitis: a retrospective study of clinical presentation and treatment in 163 patients. *Gut* 1996;39(96):846–851.
43. Fleischmann R. Safety and efficacy of disease-modifying antirheumatic agents in rheumatoid arthritis and juvenile rheumatoid arthritis. *Expert Opin Drug Saf* 2003;2(4):347–365.
44. Huang JL, Chen LC. Sulphasalazine in the treatment of children with chronic arthritis. *Clin Rheumatol* 1998;17(5): 359–363.
45. Brooks CD. Sulfasalazine for the management of juvenile rheumatoid arthritis. *J Rheumatol* 2001;28(4):845–853.
46. Gupta AK, Ellis CN, Siegel MT, et al. Sulfasalazine improves psoriasis. A double-blind analysis. *Arch Dermatol* 1990;126(4): 487–493.
47. Rahman P, Gladman DD, Cook RJ, et al. The use of sulfasalazine in psoriatic arthritis: a clinic experience. *J Rheumatol* 1998; 25(10):1957–1961.
48. Tromm A, Griga T, May B. Oral mesalazine for the treatment of Crohn's disease: clinical efficacy with respect to pharmacokinetic properties. *Hepatogastroenterology* 1999;46(30):3124–3135.
49. Swinson CM, Perry J, Lumb M, et al. Role of sulphasalazine in the aetiology of folate deficiency in ulcerative colitis. *Gut* 1981;22(6): 456–461.
50. Logan EC, Williamson LM, Ryrie DR. Sulphasalazine associated pancytopenia may be caused by acute folate deficiency. *Gut* 1986;27(7):868–872.
51. Reid J, Holt S, Housley E, et al. Raynaud's phenomenon induced by sulphasalazine. *Postgrad Med J* 1980;56(652):106–107.
52. Kristensen KS, Hoegholm A, Bohr L, et al. Fatal myocarditis associated with mesalazine. *Lancet* 1990;335(8689):605.
53. Schwartz AG, Targan SR, Saxon A, et al. Sulfasalazine-induced exacerbation of ulcerative colitis. *N Engl J Med* 1982;306(7): 409–412.
54. Garau P, Orenstein SR, Neigut DA, et al. Pancreatitis associated with olsalazine and sulfasalazine in children with ulcerative colitis. *J Pediatr Gastroenterol Nutr* 1994;18(4):481–485.
55. Fich A, Eliakim R. Does sulfasalazine induce alopecia? *J Clin Gastroenterol* 1988;10(4):466.
56. Corrigan G, Stevens PE. Review article: interstitial nephritis associated with the use of mesalazine in inflammatory bowel disease. *Aliment Pharmacol Ther* 2000;14(1):1–6.
57. Wang KK, Bowyer BA, Fleming CR, et al. Pulmonary infiltrates and eosinophilia associated with sulfasalazine. *Mayo Clin Proc* 1984;59(5):343–346.
58. Birnie GG, McLeod TI, Watkinson G. Incidence of sulphasalazine-induced male infertility. *Gut* 1981;22(6):452–455.
59. Cann PA, Holdsworth CD. Reversal of male infertility on changing treatment from sulphasalazine to 5-aminosalicylic acid. *Lancet* 1984;1(8386):1119.
60. Gunnarsson I, Kanerud L, Pettersson E, et al. Predisposing factors in sulphasalazine-induced systemic lupus erythematosus. *Br J Rheumatol* 1997;36(10):1089–1094.

61. Kirkpatrick AW, Bookman AA, Habal F. Lupus-like syndrome caused by 5-aminosalicylic acid in patients with inflammatory bowel disease. *Can J Gastroenterol* 1999;13(2):159–162.
62. Sieg I, Beckh K, Kersten U, et al. Manifestation of acute intermittent porphyria in patients with chronic inflammatory bowel disease. *Z Gastroenterol* 1991;29(11):602–605.
63. Peppercorn MA. Sulfasalazine. Pharmacology, clinical use, toxicity, and related new drug development. *Ann Intern Med* 1984; 101(3):377–386.
64. Boyer DL, Li BU, Fyda JN, et al. Sulfasalazine-induced hepatotoxicity in children with inflammatory bowel disease. *J Pediatr Gastroenterol Nutr* 1989;8(4):528–532.
65. Deltenre P, Berson A, Marcellin P, et al. Mesalazine (5-aminosalicylic acid) induced chronic hepatitis. *Gut* 1999;44(6): 886–888.
66. Shaffer JL, Houston JB. The effect of rifampicin on sulphapyridine plasma concentrations following sulphasalazine administration. *Br J Clin Pharmacol* 1985;19(4):526–528.
67. Lennard L. Clinical implications of thiopurine methyltransferase–optimization of drug dosage and potential drug interactions. *Ther Drug Monit* 1998;20(5):527–531.
68. Vree TB, O'Reilly WJ, Hekster YA, et al. Determination of the acetylator phenotype and pharmacokinetics of some sulfonamides in man. *Clin Pharmacokinet* 1980;5:274–294.
69. Dajani A, Taubert K, Ferrieri P, et al. Treatment of acute streptococcal pharyngitis and prevention of rheumatic fever: a statement for the health professionals. Committee on Rheumatic Fever, Endocarditis, and Kawasaki Disease of the Council on Cardiovascular Disease in the Young, the American Heart Association. *Pediatrics* 1995;96:758–764.
70. Fraser GL, Beaulieu JT. Leukopenia secondary to sulfadiazine silver. *JAMA* 1979;241:1928.
71. Weinstein L, Madoff MA, Samet CM. The sulfonamides. *N Engl J Med* 1960;263:793, 842, 900, 952.
72. Simon DI, Brosius F, Rothstein DM. Sulfadiazine crystalluria revisited. The treatment of Toxoplasma encephalitis in patients with acquired immunodeficiency syndrome. *Arch Intern Med* 1990;150:2379–2384.
73. Ventura MG, Wybran J, Farber CM. Sulfadiazine revisited. *J Infect Dis* 1989;160:556–557.
74. Monafo WW, West MA. Current treatment recommendations for topical burn therapy. *Drugs* 1990;40(3):364–373.
75. Sawhney CP, Sharma RK, Rao KR, et al. Long-term experience with 1 per cent topical silver sulphadiazine cream in the management of burn wounds. *Burns* 1989;15(6):403–406.
76. Akahane T, Tsukada S. Electron-microscopic observation on silver deposition in burn wounds treated with silver sulphadiazine cream. *Burns Incl Therm Inj* 1982;8(4):271–273.
77. Ballin JC. Evaluation of a new topical agent for burn therapy. Silver sulfadiazine (silvadene). *JAMA* 1974;230(8):1184–1185.
78. Caffee F, Bingham H. Leukopenia and silver sulfadiazine. *J Trauma* 1982;22:586–587.
79. Kiker RG, Carvajal HF, Micak RP, et al. A controlled study of the effects of silver sulfadiazine on white blood cell counts in burned children. *J Trauma* 1977;17(11):835–836.
80. Zuidema J, Hilbers-Modderman E, Merkus F. Clinical pharmacokinetics of dapsone. *Clin Pharmacokinet* 1986;11:299–315.
81. May DG, Proter JA, Uetrectt JP, et al. The contribution of N-hydroxylation and acetylation to dapsone pharmacokinetics in normal subjects. *Clin Pharmacol Ther* 1990;48:619–627.
82. Leeder JS, Kearns GL. Pharmacogenetics in pediatrics: implications for practice. *Pediatr Clin North Am* 1997;44:55–77.
83. Mirochnick M, Cooper E, McIntosh K, et al. Pharmacokinetics of dapsone administered daily and weekly in human immunodeficiency virus-infected children. *Antimicrob Agents Chemother* 1999; 43:2586–2591.
84. Mirochnick M, Cooper E, Capparelli E, et al. Population pharmacokinetics of dapsone in children with human immunodeficiency virus infection. *Clin Pharmacol Ther* 2001; 70:24–32.
85. McIntosh K, Cooper E, Xu J, et al. Toxicity and efficacy of daily vs. weekly dapsone for prevention of Pneumocystis carinii pneumonia in children infected with human immunodeficiency virus. *Pediatr Infect Dis J* 1999;18:432–439.
86. Espey DK, Djomand G, Diomande I, et al. A pilot study of treatment of Buruli ulcer with rifampin and dapsone. *Int J Infect Dis* 2002;6:60–65.
87. Mutabingwa T, Nzila A, Mberu E, et al. Chlorproguanil-dapsone for treatment of drug-resistant falciparum malaria in Tanzania. *Lancet* 2001;358:1218–1223.
88. Sulo J, Chimpeni P, Hatcher J, et al. Chlorproguanil-dapsone versus sulfadoxine-pyrimethamine for sequential episodes of uncomplicated falciparum malaria in Kenya and Malawi: a randomised clinical trial. *Lancet* 2002;360:1136–1143.

CHAPTER

29

Sumathi Nambiar
William J. Rodriguez

Penicillins, Cephalosporins, and Other β-Lactams

THE PENICILLINS

INTRODUCTION

Alexander Fleming discovered penicillin in 1928 (1). In the 1940s, penicillin became available for use in clinical practice. Batchelor and coworkers (2) isolated the 6-aminopenicillanic acid nucleus from *Penicillium chrysogenum,* which served as the basis for the development of semisynthetic penicillins. Subsequently, penicillins with expanded spectrum of activity including some gram-negative organisms were developed (Table 29.1).

NATURAL PENICILLINS

Structure–Activity Relationship

All penicillins contain the 6-aminopenicillanic acid nucleus, which is composed of a β-lactam ring and a five-member thiazolidine ring to which is attached a side chain. The penicillin nucleus is the chief structural requirement for biologic activity. The side chain determines many of the antibacterial and pharmacologic characteristics of a particular type of penicillin (3). Penicillins generally exist as sodium or potassium salts.

Mechanism of Action

Penicillins exert bactericidal action against penicillin-susceptible microorganisms during the stage of active replication. Penicillin interferes with bacterial cell wall synthesis by reacting with one or more penicillin-binding proteins (PBPs). The PBPs, such as transpeptidases, carboxypeptidases, and endopeptidases, are bacterial enzymes involved in cell wall synthesis. Bacteria produce four types of PBPs, and they structurally resemble serine proteases (4). The transpeptidase activity of PBPs is essential for cross-linking adjacent peptidoglycan, and the carboxypeptidases are important for the modification of peptidoglycan. PBPs account for approximately 1% of membrane proteins. They vary in the amounts present, in their role in cell wall assembly, and in their affinity for binding to β-lactam antibiotics (5).

Resistance

Penicillin resistance is mediated mainly through production of β-lactamase, which covalently binds to the β-lactam bond to form an acyl enzyme intermediate, which undergoes rapid hydrolysis, thus destroying the activity of the drug. Gram-positive β-lactamases, such as the staphylococcal penicillinase, are exoenzymes that destroy penicillins before they reach the target PBPs. The β-lactamases of gram-negative bacteria are cell associated and are located in the periplasmic space between the cytoplasmic membrane and the lipopolysaccharide outer membrane. Alteration of PBPs accounts for penicillin resistance among pneumococci, some strains of *Haemophilus influenzae,* and some *Neisseria* spp.

Pharmacokinetics

Metabolism and disposition vary significantly among the various penicillins and also vary with the age of the patients. They are not well absorbed from the gastrointestinal tract, with the exception of phenoxymethyl penicillin (penicillin V) and amoxicillin. Penicillin V is acid stable and is available only for oral use. Penicillin G is not acid stable and hence is generally used parenterally. Penicillins bind to serum proteins, mainly albumin. Penicillins are primarily excreted in the urine in the unchanged form. Tubular secretion accounts for most of the urinary penicillin, and glomerular filtration accounts for only a small fraction. Penicillin does not penetrate well into the cerebrospinal fluid (CSF) in the absence of meningeal inflammation. Repository penicillins such as procaine penicillin or benzathine penicillin provide tissue depots. Procaine penicillin is absorbed over several hours and benzathine penicillin over several days.

Spectrum of Activity

Gram-Positive Cocci

Includes most streptococci, and susceptible strains of staphylococci, enterococci, and pneumococci. Tolerance to penicillin among group B streptococcal isolates has

TABLE 29.1 Types of Penicillins

Natural Penicillins	*Aminopenicillins*	*Penicillinase-Resistant Penicillins*	*Extended-Spectrum Penicillins*
Penicillin G	Amoxicillin	Cloxacillin	Carbenicillin
Penicillin V	Ampicillin	Dicloxacillin	Ticarcillin
Penicillin G procaine		Oxacillin	Piperacillin
Penicillin G benzathine		Nafcillin	Mezlocillin
		Methicillin	Azlocillin

been reported (6,7). Penicillin acts synergistically with gentamicin or tobramycin against many strains of enterococci.

Gram-Positive Bacilli
Corynebacterium diphtheriae, Bacillus anthracis, Actinomyces, Erysipelothrix rhusiopathiae, and *Listeria monocytogenes.*

Gram-Negative Bacteria
Non-β-lactamase-producing strains of *Neisseria gonorrhoeae,* and *H. influenzae, Neisseria meningitidis, Streptobacillus moniliformis,* and *Pasteurella multocida.*

Anaerobic Bacteria
Clostridia spp., *Peptostreptococcus,* and *Propionibacteria.*

Spirochetes
Treponema pallidum, Borrelia burgdorferi, and *Spirillum minus.*

Clinical Uses

Penicillin is effective in the treatment of infections caused by group A streptococci, group B streptococci, meningococci, *Actinomyces,* and *T. pallidum* (Tables 29.2 to 29.4) (8,9). It is also the treatment of choice for infections due to susceptible *Streptococcus pneumoniae,* enterococci, and gonococci. Infections other than meningitis that are due to penicillin-resistant *S. pneumoniae* may not be associated with a less favorable clinical outcome or increased mortality compared with those for penicillin-susceptible infections when treated with high-dose penicillin (10). The breakpoints for penicillin in the treatment of pneumococcal pneumonia were recently updated, whereas the breakpoint for meningitis remains unchanged (11). Infections due to anaerobic mouth flora are generally susceptible to penicillin G. Penicillin V is the drug of choice for prophylaxis against rheumatic carditis and against infections in patients with anatomic or functional asplenia. In patients with poor compliance, intramuscular benzathine penicillin can be used every 3 to 4 weeks. Benzathine penicillin is the drug of choice for primary, secondary, and early or late latent syphilis (except neurosyphilis). For infants with congenital syphilis, penicillin G or procaine penicillin is recommended (12).

Adverse Reactions

Allergic reactions are the major side effects associated with the penicillins. Severe and occasionally fatal anaphylaxis has also occurred. This relates to the ability of penicillins to act as haptens and combine with proteins. The most important antigenic component of the penicillins is the penicilloyl determinant produced by opening of the β-lactam ring. Anaphylactic reactions are estimated to occur in 0.01% to 0.05% of persons receiving penicillins. In patients with a history of life-threatening reactions to penicillin it may be prudent to avoid other β-lactam agents. However, if no other options are available, a trial of desensitization may be attempted. The following hypersensitivity reactions have been described: skin rashes ranging from maculopapular eruptions to exfoliative dermatitis, urticaria, and reactions resembling serum sickness, including chills, fever, edema, arthralgia, and prostration. The Jarisch–Herxheimer reaction has been reported in patients treated for syphilis.

Hematologic toxicity including Coombs-positive hemolytic anemia, leukopenia, and thrombocytopenia has been reported with penicillin use. Penicillins bind to the adenosine diphosphate receptor site in platelets and thereby

TABLE 29.2 Pharmacokinetic Properties of Selected Penicillins (5,8)

Generic Name	*Half-Life (hr)*	*Protein Binding (%)*	*Route of Excretion*
Penicillin G	0.5–1.2	55–65	Renal
Penicillin V	1	80	Renal
Oxacillin	0.5–1.2	90–95	Renal, hepatic
Cloxacillin	0.5	90–95	Renal, hepatic
Dicloxacillin	0.8–1	96–98	Renal, hepatic
Nafcillin	0.5	87–90	Hepatic, renal
Ampicillin	1	15–25	Renal
Amoxicillin	1	17–20	Renal
Ticarcillin	1.0–1.2	45–65	Renal
Piperacillin	0.5–1.3	22	Renal

TABLE 29.3 Penicillin Dosing Recommendations: Neonates (mg/kg/dose or u/kg/dose) (9)

		Infants 0–4 wk of Age	*Infants <1 wk of Age*		*Infants ≥1 wk of Age*	
Antibiotic	*Route*	*BW<1,200 g*	*BW 1,200–2,000 g*	*BW>2,000 g*	*BW 1,200–2,000 g*	*BW>2,000 g*
Penicillin G[a], aqueous	i.v., i.m.	25,000–50,000 q12 h	25,000–50,000 q12 h	25,000–50,000 q8 h	25,000–50,000 q8 h	25,000–50,000 q6 h
Ampicillin (mg/kg)[a]	i.v., i.m.	25–50 q12 h	25–50 q12 h	25–50 q8 h	25–50 q8 h	25–50 q6 h
Procaine penicillin (u)	i.m.	. . .	50,000 q24 h	50,000 q24 h	50,000 q24 h	50,000 q24 h
Ticarcillin (mg/kg)	i.v., i.m.	75 q12 h	75 q12 h	75 q8 h	75 q8 h	100 q8 h
Nafcillin (mg/kg)	i.v., i.m.	25 q12 h	25 q12 h	25 q8 h	25 q8 h	25–35 q6 h
Oxacillin (mg/kg)	i.v., i.m.	25 q12 h	25–50 q12 h	25–50 q8 h	25–50 q8 h	25–50 q6 h

BW, Body weight; i.m., Intramuscular; i.v., intravenous; q6 h, every 6 hr; q8 h, every 8 hr; q12 h, every 12 hr; q24 h, every 24 hr; u, units.
[a]For meningitis, larger dosage is recommended.

interfere with platelet aggregation. Clinically significant bleeding is not common.

Sodium overload and hypokalemia can occur with massive doses of penicillin secondary to the large dose of nonreabsorbable anion in the distal renal tubules. Patients given continuous intravenous therapy with penicillin G potassium in high dosage (10 million to 100 million units daily) may suffer severe or even fatal potassium poisoning, particularly if renal insufficiency is present.

Neurologic toxicity in the form of seizures has been reported following the use of massive doses of penicillin.

Drug Interactions

Concurrent administration of bacteriostatic antibiotics (e.g., erythromycin and tetracycline) may diminish the bactericidal effects of penicillins by slowing the rate of bacterial growth. The clinical significance of this interaction is

TABLE 29.4 Penicillin Dosing Recommendations: Pediatric Patients Excluding Neonates (mg/kg/day or u/kg/day) (9)

		Daily Dose		
Antibiotic	*Route*	*Mild–Moderate Infections*	*Severe Infections*	*Frequency of Administration (i.e., in Divided Doses)*
Penicillin G	i.m., i.v.	25,000–50,000 U	250,000–400,000 U	q4–6 h
Penicillin V	p.o.	25,000–50,000 U	Inappropriate	q6–8 h
Penicillin G, benzathine	i.m.	<27.3 kg (60 lb): 600,000 U ≥27.3 kg: 1,200,000 U	Inappropriate	q1–3 wk
Penicillin G, procaine	i.m.	25,000–50,000 U (max. adult dose 48,000,000 u/24 hr)	Inappropriate	q12–24 h
Oxacillin	i.m., i.v.	100–150 mg/kg	150–200 mg/kg	q4–6 h
Dicloxacillin	p.o.	25–50 mg/kg	Inappropriate	q6 h
Nafcillin	i.m., i.v.	50–100 mg/kg	100–150 mg/kg	q6 h
Ampicillin	i.m., i.v.	100–150 mg/kg	200–400 mg/kg	q6 h
	p.o.	50–100 mg/kg	Inappropriate	q4–6 h
Amoxicillin	p.o.	25–50 mg/kg	Inappropriate	q8 h
Ticarcillin	i.m., i.v.	100–200 mg/kg	200–300 mg/kg	q4–6 h
Piperacillin	i.m., i.v.	100–150 mg/kg	200–300 mg/kg	q4–6 h
Amoxicillin–clavulanic acid[a]	p.o.	90 mg/kg	Inappropriate	q12 h
Ticarcillin–clavulanic acid[b]	i.m., i.v.	100–200 mg/kg	200–300 mg/kg	q6 h
Piperacillin–tazobactam[b]	i.m., i.v.	100 mg piperacillin/12.5 mg tazobactam/kg[c]	240 mg	q8 h
Ampicillin–sulbactam[b]	i.m., i.v.	100–150 mg/kg	200–400 mg/kg	q6 h

i.m., Intramuscular; i.v., intravenous; p.o., oral; q1–3 wk, every 1–3 weeks; q4–6 hr, every 4–6 hr; q6 h, every 6 hr; q6–8 h, every 6–8 hr; q8 h, every 8 hr; q12 h, every 12 hr; q12–24 h, every 12–24 hr.
[a]Amoxicillin:clavulanate 14:1, approved for infants and children ≥3 mo.
[b]Based on the penicillin component.
[c]For 2–9 month old, 80 mg piperacillin/10 mg tazobactam/kg/day in three divided doses (Product label, http://dailymed.nlm.nih.gov/dailymed/drugInfo).

not well documented. Penicillin blood levels may be prolonged by concurrent administration of probenecid, which blocks the renal tubular secretion of penicillins. Penicillins can interact with oral contraceptives (13,14).

AMINOPENICILLINS

Structure–Activity Relationship

Aminopenicillins have a free amino group at the alpha position on the β-lactam ring of the penicillin nucleus, thereby increasing their ability to penetrate the outer membranes of gram-negative organisms.

Mechanism of Action

The mechanism of action is similar to that of penicillins.

Resistance

Aminopenicillins are inactivated by the β-lactamases produced by either gram-positive or gram-negative bacteria.

Pharmacokinetics

Aminopenicillins are cleared by the kidney. Ampicillin achieves therapeutic concentrations in most body fluids including CSF pleural, joint, and peritoneal fluids after parenteral administration. Amoxicillin has better absorption and bioavailability and hence is the preferred oral aminopenicillin. The absorption of amoxicillin is not affected by food.

Spectrum

Compared with penicillin G, ampicillin has increased in vitro efficacy against most strains of enterococci and *L. monocytogenes* as well as against some gram-negative pathogens, such as non-β-lactamase producing strains of *H. influenzae* and *N. gonorrhoeae.* Some strains of *Escherichia coli, Shigella sonnei,* and *Salmonella* including strains of *S. typhi* are resistant.

Clinical Uses

Amoxicillin is the drug of choice for acute otitis media (15,16) (Tables 29.2 to 29.4). Oral amoxicillin is also the drug of choice for treatment of some clinical manifestations of Lyme disease like erythema migrans, isolated facial palsy, and arthritis (17). Parenteral ampicillin is widely used in neonates with sepsis because of its activity against *Listeria.* Amoxicillin is used in combination with clarithromycin and a proton pump inhibitor like omeprazole or lansoprazole for the treatment of *Helicobacter pylori* infections (18,19). A report from the Food and Drug Administration (FDA) provides information on the pharmacokinetics and dosing of amoxicillin for use in the prophylaxis of postexposure inhalational anthrax (15 mg per kg per dose given every 8 hours) (20).

Adverse Events

The incidence of hypersensitivity reactions with aminopenicillins is similar to that of natural penicillins. There is a slightly higher incidence of maculopapular rash associated with ampicillin use in patients with intercurrent viral illnesses, especially due to Epstein–Barr virus.

ANTISTAPHYLOCOCCAL PENICILLINS

Structure–Activity Relationship

These are semisynthetic penicillin derivatives synthesized by the acylation of 6-aminopenicillanic acid to prevent the attachment of staphylococcal penicillinases to the β-lactam ring. Methicillin contains a dimethoxyphenyl group on the penicillin nucleus, and nafcillin is a naphthyl analogue of methicillin. Cloxacillin and dicloxacillin contain chlorine atoms, which increase gastrointestinal absorption and antibacterial activity as well as serum half-life and protein binding.

Mechanism

The penicillinase-resistant penicillins also act by binding to PBPs and preventing cell wall synthesis. They are resistant to the action of bacterial penicillinases by steric hindrance of the acyl side chain, thereby preventing opening of the β-lactam ring.

Resistance

Resistance to semisynthetic penicillins among staphylococci is related to the presence of the *mecA* gene, which results in the synthesis of a unique PBP, PBP2a, which has low affinity for methicillin and other β-lactam antibiotics.

Spectrum

This group of penicillins is effective against β-lactamase-producing isolates of *Staphylococcus aureus* and coagulase-negative staphylococci. They retain most of the activity of the penicillins but are much less active compared with penicillin G against penicillin-susceptible organisms, including non–penicillinase-producing staphylococci and streptococci. Enterococci, gram-negative cocci, *L. monocytogenes,* and anaerobes are resistant to these penicillins.

Pharmacokinetics

Unlike the natural penicillins, nafcillin is predominantly excreted through the biliary system, and hence accumulation can occur in jaundiced neonates. Although nafcillin is available in oral formulations, absorption is erratic. The isoxazolyl penicillins oxacillin, cloxacillin, and dicloxacillin are absorbed after oral administration but adversely affected by food. Serum levels after absorption are higher with cloxacillin and dicloxacillin than with oxacillin. They are excreted primarily by the kidneys with some biliary excretion. Cloxacillin and dicloxacillin are highly protein bound.

Clinical Indications

Methicillin is acid labile, is the least active member of this group of penicillins, and is most likely to cause interstitial nephritis, and hence is no longer used. Semisynthetic penicillins are commonly used in the empiric treatment of skin and skin structure infections and bone and joint infections where *S. aureus* is a likely pathogen (Tables 29.2 to 29.4).

Adverse Events

Interstitial nephritis manifesting clinically as fever, rash, eosinophilia, proteinuria, eosinophiluria, and hematuria is more commonly reported with methicillin use. Elevated aspartate aminotransferase levels and cholestasis usually without jaundice have been reported with oxacillin use. Liver enzymes usually return to normal after discontinuation of therapy.

Drug Interactions

Drug interactions involving nafcillin and both cyclosporine and warfarin have been reported (21–24).

EXTENDED-SPECTRUM PENICILLINS

Structure–Activity Relationship

Carbenicillin is an α-carboxypenicillin. It differs from ampicillin in that an α-carboxyl group is substituted for the α-amino group. Indanyl carbenicillin is a α-carboxy ester of carbenicillin. Ticarcillin is the 3-thienyl analogue of carbenicillin. The acylampicillins are semisynthetic penicillins and include ureidopenicillins (mezlocillin and azlocillin) and piperacillin. Mezlocillin and azlocillin are ureidopenicillins and have a ureido group at the α position. Piperacillin is a piperazine analogue of ampicillin.

Resistance

The extended-spectrum penicillins are susceptible to hydrolysis by β-lactamases of both gram-positive and gram-negative bacteria.

Spectrum

The extended-spectrum penicillins have a broader spectrum of activity than natural penicillins and aminopenicillins. Carbenicillin has greater stability against *Pseudomonas* and some β-lactamase-producing Enterobacteriaceae but is less active than ampicillin against *Streptococcus pyogenes, S. pneumoniae,* and *Enterococcus faecalis.* Ticarcillin has similar spectrum of activity as carbenicillin but is more active against *Pseudomonas aeruginosa.* Piperacillin is similar to ampicillin in activity against gram-positive species. It has good activity against anaerobic cocci and bacilli. It also has activity against members of the Enterobacteriaceae family and *P. aeruginosa.* Some extended-spectrum penicillins are less active than natural penicillins and aminopenicillins against anaerobic bacteria. In contrast to carbenicillin and ticarcillin, acylampicillins have activity against enterococci.

Pharmacokinetics

The extended-spectrum penicillins are administered parenterally, with the exception of indanyl carbenicillin. As a sodium ester, indanyl carbenicillin is acid stable. However, serum or tissue levels are not adequate for the treatment of systemic infections and its use was limited to the treatment of uncomplicated urinary tract infections. The extended-spectrum penicillins have minimal CSF penetration. Primary route of elimination is renal via glomerular filtration and tubular secretion. The ureidopenicillins show dose-related nonlinear kinetics.

Clinical Indications

The extended-spectrum penicillins are effective against a variety of gram-negative organisms and in combination with aminoglycosides are synergistic against many gram-negative bacilli (Tables 29.2 to 29.4). They are generally used clinically in combination with a β-lactamase inhibitor.

Adverse Events

Hypersensitivity reactions occur similar to those with natural penicillins. Because these agents are negatively charged ions, hypokalemia can result from leaching of anions in the distal renal tubule. Platelet dysfunction and prolonged bleeding times have been observed with the use of extended-spectrum penicillins. They can inhibit platelet aggregation by binding to the adenosine diphosphate receptor on platelets. Mezlocillin is the least likely to affect bleeding times.

Drug Interactions

Extended-spectrum penicillins can interact with warfarin, thereby decreasing its anticoagulant effects. Piperacillin can potentiate the action of nondepolarizing blocking agents. Some extended-spectrum penicillins have been shown to interact in solution with aminoglycosides, causing degradation of the aminoglycosides. It is recommended that these drugs not be mixed in solution and their administration be separated by 30 to 60 minutes.

β-LACTAMASE INHIBITORS

The β-lactamase inhibitors are compounds that inhibit many β-lactamases and additionally have weak antibacterial activity. They are available as fixed-combination preparations with a β-lactam antibiotic. Clavulanic acid is produced by the fermentation of *Streptomyces clavuligerus.* It is a β-lactam structurally related to the penicillins and cephalosporins. It contains a β-lactam ring attached to an oxazolidine ring. Sulbactam is a synthetic penicillinate sulfone derived from 6-aminopenicillanic acid and contains a β-lactam ring. Tazobactam is a synthetic penicillanic acid sulfone.

MECHANISM OF ACTION

Clavulanic acid, sulbactam, and tazobactam possess the ability to inactivate a wide variety of β-lactamases by irreversibly binding to the active sites of these enzymes. Clavulanic acid is particularly active against the clinically important plasmid-mediated β-lactamases frequently responsible for transferred drug resistance to penicillins and cephalosporins. Clavulanic acid acts by both transient reversible complex formation and irreversible inactivation. Against *E. coli*-derived β-lactamase, reversible complex formation has been shown to proceed at a faster rate than terminal inactivation. In the presence of excess clavulanic acid, all enzymes will accumulate into one of several irreversibly inactivated forms (25,26). The mechanism of action of sulbactam and tazobactam is similar to that of clavulanic acid (27,28).

Clavulanic acid is the most efficient inhibitor of staphylococcal β-lactamase and is also an effective inhibitor of chromosomally mediated β-lactamase liberated by *Klebsiella pneumoniae, Proteus mirabilis, P. vulgaris, Moraxella catarrhalis, Bacteroides fragilis,* and TEM plasmid-mediated β-lactamase. It less readily inhibits chromosomally mediated β-lactamase of *Citrobacter* species, *Enterobacter* species, indole-positive *Proteus* species, and *Serratia marcescens* (29). Overall, sulbactam is the least active of the three agents (30). No significant difference in activity between the inhibitors exists with respect to anaerobes; therefore, they should be considered comparable with respect to extending anaerobic coverage to their partner antibiotic in treating mixed infections (31).

β-lactamase inhibitors can act as inducers of certain β-lactamases, thus rendering organisms that produce the enzyme less susceptible to the partner antibiotic (32). This effect is most pronounced with clavulanic acid and occurs at concentrations at or above those achievable in vivo (23). Tazobactam does not induce chromosomally mediated β-lactamases at tazobactam levels achieved with the recommended dosage regimen (33). β-lactamase inhibitors also have some intrinsic antibacterial activity. Clavulanic acid demonstrates good activity against *B. fragilis, Acinetobacter* species, and *Legionella pneumophilia* (34). Tazobactam has very low-level binding to PBPs and has the least intrinsic antibacterial activity (30).

PHARMACOKINETICS

Clavulanic acid is well absorbed orally and provides adequate inhibitory activity in most body fluids except CSF and sputum (35,36). Sulbactam is available in oral and parenteral formulations. In the United States, it is available only for parenteral use. Tazobactam is also available only in a parenteral formulation.

PENICILLINS AND β-LACTAMASE INHIBITOR COMBINATIONS

Penicillins and β-lactamase inhibitor combinations used clinically include ampicillin + sulbactam, amoxicillin + clavulanic acid, ticarcillin + clavulanic acid, and piperacillin + tazobactam.

PHARMACOKINETICS

Amoxicillin serum concentrations achieved with amoxicillin + clavulanic acid are similar to those produced by the oral administration of equivalent doses of amoxicillin alone. Amoxicillin and clavulanate potassium are well absorbed from the gastrointestinal tract after oral administration. Dosing in the fasted or fed state has minimal effect on the pharmacokinetics of amoxicillin. Ticarcillin can be detected in tissues and interstitial fluid following parenteral administration. Penetration of ticarcillin into bile and pleural fluid has been demonstrated. Penetration of both ampicillin and sulbactam into CSF in the presence of inflamed meninges has been demonstrated after intravenous administration of ampicillin and sulbactam. Piperacillin and tazobactam are widely distributed into tissues and body fluids including intestinal mucosa, gallbladder, lung, female reproductive tissues (uterus, ovary, and fallopian tube), interstitial fluid, and bile. Mean tissue concentrations are generally 50% to 100% of those in plasma. Distribution of piperacillin and tazobactam into CSF is low in individuals with noninflamed meninges, as with other penicillins (33). The protein binding of either piperacillin or tazobactam is unaffected by the presence of the other compound.

CLINICAL USES

Amoxicillin + Clavulanic Acid

Amoxicillin + clavulanic acid is useful in children with acute otitis media and other respiratory tract infections caused by β-lactamase-producing strains of *H. influenzae* and *M. catarrhalis.* It can be used to treat animal or human bites. Various formulations of this combination are available, with the ratio of amoxicillin to clavulanate varying (4:1, 7:1, and 14:1). The 12-hourly regimen is associated with significantly less diarrhea.

It is approved by the FDA for use in pediatric patients for the following infections: lower respiratory tract infections, otitis media, sinusitis, skin and skin structure infections, and urinary tract infections. A different dosing regimen is recommended for patients younger than 3 months of age.

Ampicillin + Sulbactam

The safety and effectiveness of ampicillin + sulbactam have been established for pediatric patients 1 year of age and older for skin and skin structure infections. The safety and effectiveness have not been established for pediatric patients for intra-abdominal infections.

Ticarcillin + Clavulanic Acid

Ticarcillin + clavulanic acid is approved by the FDA for use in patients from 3 months to 16 years of age. It is not approved for the treatment of septicemia and/or infections in the pediatric population where the suspected or proven pathogen is *H. influenzae* type b. It is currently approved for the following indications: septicemia, including bacteremia; lower respiratory infections; bone and joint infections; skin and skin structure infections; urinary tract infections; gynecologic infections; and intra-abdominal infections.

Piperacillin + Tazobactam

Piperacillin + tazobactam is approved for use in pediatric patients 2 months of age or older with appendicitis and/or peritonitis. The dosing regimens vary for children 9 months of age or older, weighing up to 40 kg, and with normal renal function and for those between 2 and 9 months of age (Table 29.4). Pediatric patients weighing more than 40 kg and with normal renal function should receive the adult dose. There are no dosage recommendations for pediatric patients with impaired renal function.

CEPHALOSPORINS

The first source of cephalosporins was *Cephalosporium acremonium,* a fungus isolated in 1948 by G. Brotzu from the sea near a sewer outlet off the Sardinian coast.

STRUCTURE–ACTIVITY RELATIONSHIP

All cephalosporins are semisynthetic derivatives of a 7-aminocephalosporanic acid nucleus. Like penicillins, cephalosporins possess a β-lactam ring. Modifications of the carbon-3 and carbon-7 positions of the 7-aminocephalosporanic acid nucleus have yielded the three generations. Modifications around this nucleus have stabilized the β-lactam ring to hydrolysis by penicillinases. Modifications around the carbon-3 position are associated with changes in the metabolism or improved pharmacokinetics, and modifications around the carbon-7 position affect β-lactamase stability and antimicrobial activity (37–40). The cephamycins are similar to cephalosporins, but have a methoxy group at position 7 of the β-lactam ring of the 7-aminocephalosporanic acid nucleus. The cephamycins will be discussed along with the second-generation cephalosporins.

MECHANISM OF ACTION

Cephalosporins and cephamycins interfere with synthesis of peptidoglycan in the bacterial cell wall. They bind to and inactivate PBPs, which are enzymes responsible for the synthesis of the bacterial cell wall and include transpeptidases, carboxypeptidases, and endopeptidases.

CLASSIFICATION

Cephalosporins are classified into generations on the basis of their spectrum of microbiologic activity (Table 29.5).

TABLE 29.5 Classification of Cephalosporins

First generation	Third generation
Oral	Oral
Cephalexin	Cefixime
Cefadroxil	Cefpodoxime proxetil
Parenteral	Cefdinir
Cefazolin	Ceftibuten
Cephalothin	Parenteral
Cephradine	Cefotaxime
Second generation	Ceftriaxone
Oral	Ceftazidime
Cefuroxime axetil	Cefoperazone
Cefprozil	Fourth generation
Loracarbef	Parenteral
Cefaclor	Cefepime
Parenteral	
Cefuroxime	
Cefamandole	
Cefonicid	
Cefoxitin	
Cefotetan	

This classification reflects increasing stability of the higher generations to various bacterial β-lactamases. None of the cephalosporins are effective against organisms like methicillin-resistant *S. aureus* (MRSA), enterococci, *L. monocytogenes, L. pneumophila, Stenotrophomonas maltophilia, Clostridium difficile, and Campylobacter jejuni.* Their microbiologic activity is summarized in Table 29.6.

The first-generation cephalosporins have good activity against gram-positive cocci and relatively modest activity against many gram-negative bacteria. Most gram-positive cocci excluding MRSA, enterococci, and *S. epidermidis* are susceptible. Most oral anaerobes are susceptible, excluding *B. fragilis.*

The second-generation cephalosporins are more active against gram-negative bacteria, though less so when compared with the third-generation cephalosporins. They have variable activity against gram-positive cocci. They have improved activity against *H. influenzae, M. catarrhalis, N. meningitidis,* and *N. gonorrhoeae.* The cephamycins have inferior activity against staphylococci but are active against some Enterobacteriaceae and *B. fragilis.*

Third-generation cephalosporins are more active against the Enterobacteriaceae, including the β-lactamase-

TABLE 29.6 Microbiologic Activity of Cephalosporins

	Gram-Positive Cocci[a]	*Gram-Negative Cocci*	*Haemophilus Influenzae*	*Pseudomonas*	*Enterobacteriaceae*	*Bacteroides Fragilis*
First generation	3–4[b]	1	0–2	0	2	0
Second generation	2–3	2	2	0	2–3	0–3[c]
Third generation	0–3	4	4	1–3	4	0–2
Fourth generation	3–4	4	4	4[d]	4	2–3

[a]Excludes methicillin-resistant *Staphylococcus aureus.*
[b]Not effective against penicillin-resistant *Streptococcus pneumoniae.*
[c]The cephamycins have good activity against *Bacteroides* spp.
[d]Ceftazidime and cefoperazone have antipseudomonal activity.

producing strains. They are also active against *S. pneumoniae* (including those with relative penicillin resistance), *S. pyogenes,* and, with the exception of ceftazidime, have clinically useful activity against *S. aureus.* They also have excellent activity against *H. influenzae, M. catarrhalis, N. meningitidis,* and *N. gonorrhoeae.* Ceftazidime and cefoperazone have good antipseudomonal activity.

Fourth-generation cephalosporins have a greater spectrum of activity than the third-generation agents. They are stable against the chromosomally mediated AmpC β-lactamases (41). They are active against the Enterobacteriaceae, *P. aeruginosa, H. influenzae,* and *Neisseria* species (42). They are also effective against gram-positive cocci including methicillin-susceptible *S. aureus, S. pneumoniae,* and other streptococci.

BACTERIAL RESISTANCE

Three mechanisms of resistance to cephalosporins that have been described include inactivation by bacterial β-lactamases, alteration of PBPs, and alteration of bacterial permeability to cephalosporins.

Production of β-lactamases is the most common mechanism of resistance among the gram-negative bacteria. These enzymes are encoded either chromosomally or extrachromosomally through plasmids or transposons. The susceptibility to β-lactamases, however, varies among the different agents. Cefoxitin, cefuroxime, and the third-generation cephalosporins are more resistant to hydrolysis by the β-lactamases produced by gram-negative bacteria than the first-generation agents. The third-generation agents are susceptible to hydrolysis by the inducible, chromosomally encoded β-lactamases and the plasmid extended-spectrum β-lactamases. The fourth-generation agents are poor inducers of type I β-lactamases and less susceptible to hydrolysis by these enzymes compared with the third-generation agents. Altered permeability is more important among gram-negative bacteria than gram-positive bacteria due to the differences in the nature of their cell walls. However, it is unlikely that altered porin permeability alone accounts for resistance among gram-negative bacteria (43). Decreased affinity of PBPs for cephalosporins is the mechanism by which some strains of *N. gonorrhoeae, H. influenzae,* and *S. pneumoniae* have developed resistance to cephalosporins.

PHARMACOKINETICS

Cephalosporins are primarily excreted via the kidneys mainly by glomerular filtration. Dosage should be adjusted in patients with renal insufficiency. However, cefoperazone is excreted predominantly in bile, and ceftriaxone also has significant biliary excretion. Protein binding varies from 10% for cephalexin to 90% for cefoperazone. Table 29.7 provides the important pharmacokinetic features of some of the more commonly used cephalosporins.

Most cephalosporins have good penetration into tissues and fluid compartments. Cephalosporins that can achieve adequate levels in the CSF include cefuroxime, cefotaxime, ceftriaxone, cefepime, and ceftizoxime. Cefuroxime is not indicated, however, for the treatment of meningitis because of reports of delayed CSF sterilization (44). Use of ceftriaxone in the first month of life is avoided because of the high degree of protein binding and hence likelihood of bilirubin displacement. Oral first- and second-generation agents are well absorbed from the gastrointestinal tract. Some cephalosporins, such as cefuroxime and cefpodoxime, are formulated as esters to facilitate absorption. After oral administration they are rapidly hydrolyzed by nonspecific esterases in the intestinal mucosa and blood. The oral third-generation cephalosporins, such as cefixime, are not as well absorbed but achieve adequate systemic concentration to treat infections of the respiratory tract and urinary tract. Coadministration with lidocaine can reduce the discomfort associated with intramuscular cephalosporin administration.

TABLE 29.7 Pharmacokinetic Properties of Cephalosporins

Generic Name	*Half-Life (hr)*	*Protein Binding (%)*	*Route of Excretion*
First generation			
Cefazolin	1.4	86	Renal
Cephalexin	1.2	14	Renal
Cefadroxil	1.3	15	Renal
Second generation			
Cefuroxime axetil	1.4	33	Renal
Cefoxitin	0.8	73	Renal
Cefotetan	3.5	88	Renal
Third generation			
Cefotaxime	1	38	Renal
Ceftriaxone	6–8	90	Renal 65%; biliary 35%
Ceftazidime	1.9	20	Renal
Cefixime	3.8	69	Renal 50%; ? other
Cefpodoxime	2.2	40	Renal
Cefoperazone	1.5–2.5	90–93	Biliary 70%; renal 20%–30%
Fourth generation			
Cefepime	1.5–1.7	19	Renal

CLINICAL USE

First- and second-generation cephalosporins are used in the treatment of a variety of infections in pediatrics. They are used commonly for the treatment of skin and respiratory tract infections. Third-generation cephalosporins are commonly used for the empiric treatment of hospitalized infants and children. The fourth-generation agents, such as cefepime, are used more commonly in the treatment of patients with febrile neutropenia and nosocomial infections.

First-Generation Agents

Members of this class are widely used in the treatment of skin and soft tissue infections. Cefazolin is used commonly for preoperative prophylaxis for surgical procedures involving foreign body implantation and clean and clean-contaminated procedures in which there is a high risk of infection (45,46). The general dosing schedules for oral and parenteral preparations published in the literature are shown in Tables 29.8 to 29.10 (9,47,48).

TABLE 29.8 Dosing of Oral Cephalosporins (Excluding Neonates) (9,47)

Generic Name	*Dose (mg/kg/d)*	*Frequency*[a]
First generation		
Cephalexin	25–50	q6 h
Cefadroxil	30	q12 h
Second generation		
Cefuroxime axetil	20–40	q12 h
Cefprozil	15–30	q12 h
Loracarbef	15–30	q12 h
Cefaclor	20–40	q8–12 h
Third generation		
Cefixime	8	q12h/24 h
Cefpodoxime proxetil	10	q12 h
Cefdinir	14	q12–24 h
Ceftibuten	9	q24 h

q6 h, every 6 hr; q8–12 h, every 8–12 hr; q12 h, every 12 hr; q12 h/24 h, every 12 hr/24 hr; q12–24 h, every 12–24 hr; q24 h, every 24 hr.

Second-Generation Agents

Oral second-generation agents are commonly used for the treatment of respiratory infections including community-acquired pneumonia, sinusitis, and otitis media. Cefuroxime is a commonly used second-generation cephalosporin in pediatrics. It is more stable against the β-lactamases of *H. influenzae, N. gonorrhoeae,* and some Enterobacteriaceae than are the first-generation cephalosporins. It is also more active against *S. pneumoniae* and *S. pyogenes* than are the first-generation agents (49,50). It is recommended as a second-line agent for the treatment of acute otitis media in children (15). Shorter courses of oral second-generation cephalosporins have been shown to be as effective as or superior to penicillin in the treatment of group A streptococcal pharyngitis (51). Cefuroxime is also used in the treatment of Lyme disease in penicillin-allergic patients (52).

Cephamycins such as cefoxitin and cefotetan are used in the treatment of intra-abdominal infections, pelvic inflammatory disease, infected decubitus ulcers, and mixed aerobic–anaerobic soft tissue infections where gram-negative bacteria and anaerobes are likely to be involved. They should not be used for the treatment of life-threatening

TABLE 29.9 Dosing of Parenteral Cephalosporins (Excluding Neonates) (9,47)

	Dose (mg/kg/d)		
Generic Name	*Mild-Moderate Infections*	*Severe Infections*	*Frequency*
First generation			
Cefazolin	25–50	50–100	q8 h
Cephalothin	80–100	100–150	q4–6 h
Second generation			
Cefuroxime	75–100	100–150	q8 h
Cefoxitin	80–100	80–160	q4–6 h
Cefotetan		40–80[a]	q12 h
Third generation			
Cefotaxime	75–100	150–200	q6–8 h[b,c]
Ceftriaxone	50–75	80–100	q12–24 h
Ceftazidime	75–100	125–150	q8 h
Cefoperazone	100–150		q8–12 h
Fourth generation			
Cefepime[d]	100–150	150	q8 h

q4–6 h, every 4–6 hr; q6–8 h, every 6–8 hr; q8 h, every 8 hr; q8–12 h, every 8–12 hr; q12 h, every 12 hr; q12–24 h, every 12–24 hr.

[a]Not approved for pediatric use.

[b]75 mg/kg every 6 hr for treatment of meningitis.

[c]Dosing as high as 300 mg/kg/day divided into three to four doses has been recommended for meningitis (9).

[d]Not approved for meningitis.

TABLE 29.10 Dosing of Cephalosporins in Neonates (9,48)

		Dosage (mg/kg/d) and Frequency of Administration				
		0–4 wk	<1 wk		≥1 wk	
Antibiotic	*Route*	*<1,200 g*	*1,200–2,000 g*	*>2,000 g*	*1,200–2,000 g*	*>2,000 g*
Cefazolin	i.v., i.m.	20 q12 h	20 q12 h	20 q12 h	20 q12 h	20 q8 h
Cefotaxime	i.v., i.m.	50 q12 h	50 q12 h	50 q8–12 h	50 q8 h	50 q6–8 h
Ceftazidime	i.v., i.m.	50 q12 h	50 q12 h	50 q8–12 h	50 q8 h	50 q8 h
Ceftriaxone[a]	i.v., i.m.	50 q24 h	50 q24 h	50 q24 h	50 q24 h	50–75 q24 h

i.m., Intramuscular; i.v., intravenous; q6–8 h, every 6–8 hr; q8 h, every 8 hr; q8–12 h, every 8–12 hr; q12 h, every 12 hr; q24 h, every 24 hr.
[a]Should not be used in hyperbilirubinemic neonates, especially preterm.

B. fragilis infections in the absence of susceptibility information, as up to 15% of *B. fragilis* may be resistant to cephamycins (53). Cephamycins are also recommended as systemic prophylaxis for gastrointestinal surgery and for selected gynecologic procedures (54).

Third-Generation Agents

Cefotaxime and ceftriaxone have similar antibacterial activity. Because of its protein binding, ceftriaxone can be used once daily for most infections except meningitis, which should be treated with a 12-hourly regimen. Ceftriaxone has been used for the outpatient management of infants with fever without a known source. It is also used for the treatment of otitis media (15). Ceftriaxone and cefotaxime are effective in the treatment of bacterial meningitis caused by *S. pneumoniae, H. influenzae,* and *N. meningitidis.* Vancomycin is given in addition to cefotaxime or ceftriaxone for the empiric therapy of meningitis in children to cover for pneumococci with penicillin resistance (minimum inhibitory concentration ≤2 μg per mL) (55,56). Third-generation cephalosporins are also useful in the treatment of nosocomial infections caused by susceptible gram-negative bacilli, including pneumonia, wound infections, and complicated urinary tract infections (57,58). Ceftriaxone is the recommended therapy for all forms of gonorrheal disease (59). Cefixime as a single 400 mg dose is recommended by the Centers for Disease Control and Prevention for the treatment of uncomplicated gonococcal infections of the cervix, urethra, and rectum. Other single-dose cephalosporin therapies that are considered alternative treatment regimens for uncomplicated urogenital and anorectal gonococcal infections include ceftizoxime 500 mg IM, cefoxitin 2 g IM, administered with probenecid 1 g orally, or cefotaxime 500 mg IM. Cefpodoxime 400 mg and cefuroxime axetil 1 g might be oral alternatives (60). Ceftriaxone is also effective in the treatment of Lyme disease (17,61). Because of its antipseudomonal activity, use of ceftazidime should be restricted to the treatment of infections due to *P. aeruginosa.* Ceftazidime has been used in combination with aminoglycosides in the treatment of febrile neutropenia (62). Ceftazidime has been used for the treatment of meningitis caused by *P. aeruginosa* (63). As a single agent ceftazidime is often used for the treatment of acute exacerbation of chronic pulmonary disease in patients with cystic fibrosis (64).

Fourth-Generation Agents

The safety and effectiveness of cefepime have been established in the age groups of 2 months to 16 years in the treatment of uncomplicated and complicated urinary tract infections, uncomplicated skin and skin structure infections, and pneumonia, and as empiric therapy for febrile neutropenic patients. Safety and effectiveness in pediatric patients below the age of 2 months have not been established. Comparative clinical trials have shown that cefepime is comparable to some of the third-generation cephalosporins, including ceftazidime, cefotaxime, and ceftriaxone (65,66). In the treatment of febrile neutropenia, cefepime was comparable to piperacillin–gentamicin (67). In the treatment of acute bacterial meningitis in children, cefepime and cefotaxime were comparable (68). The use of fourth-generation cephalosporins should be limited to the empiric treatment of nosocomial infections in which an increased frequency of AmpC β-lactamase-producing organisms are the likely pathogens (69). Cefepime is used for the treatment of nosocomial infections when extended-spectrum β-lactamase or chromosomally induced β-lactamase resistance is present. *Enterobacter* species with reduced susceptibility or resistance to ceftazidime has shown a favorable response to cefepime (70).

ADVERSE REACTIONS

Maculopapular or morbilliform skin eruptions, drug fever, and a positive Coombs test are common adverse reactions to cephalosporins (71). The frequency of cephalosporin-induced skin rashes varies from 1% to 3% (72). In children treated with cefaclor, a serum sickness-like reaction manifesting as rash and arthritis has been described (73). Reactions like anaphylaxis have been reported. Frequency of anaphylactic reactions to cephalosporins varies from 0.0001% to 0.1% (74,75). Patients who are allergic to penicillins may develop allergic reactions when they receive cephalosporins. The risk in such patients may be up to eight times as for those with no history of penicillin allergy. Patients with a history of allergy to penicillin but with negative skin tests are not at increased risk for cephalosporin allergy (71). Granulocytopenia has also been reported with cephalosporin use. Cephalosporins can inhibit adenosine diphosphate–induced platelet aggregation. This effect is slowly reversible after discontinuation of drug (76).

Immune-mediated thrombocytopenia has been associated with the administration of cephalothin, cefazolin, cefamandole, cefoxitin, and cefaclor (77). Moxalactam, cefamandole, and cefoperazone can interfere with the production of vitamin K-dependent factors. This is believed to be related to the presence of the *N*-methylthiotetrazole side chain, which appears capable of interfering with hepatic vitamin K metabolism (77). Renal toxicity can occur with cephalosporin use. Interstitial nephritis and acute tubular necrosis can occur rarely in association with cephalosporin use. Cephalosporins have been associated with disulfiram-like reaction related to accumulation of acetaldehyde secondary to inhibition of acetaldehyde dehydrogenase by the *N*-methylthiotetrazole ring. Moxalactam, cefamandole, and cefoperazone have been associated with this syndrome, characterized by nausea, flushing, sweating, vomiting, tachycardia, headache, and hypertension. Based on reports of fatal cases in neonates, there has been some recent concern about a potential interaction when ceftriaxone and calcium are coadministered (78). Several cephalosporins have been implicated in triggering seizures, particularly in patients with renal impairment when the dosage was not reduced (33).

NEWER CEPHALOSPORINS

Ceftobiprole and ceftaroline are examples of some new cephalosporins that have activity against MRSA. They are in varying phases of drug development and neither of these products have been approved for use by the FDA (79–81).

CARBAPENEMS

The carbapenems are derivatives of thienamycin, a compound produced by the soil organism *S. cattleya* (82). The basic structure of the carbapenems is similar to the structure of penicillins and cephalosporins. The five-member ring system in the carbapenems is unsaturated and contains a carbon atom instead of a sulfur atom at position 1 (3,83). Carbapenems are stable to most β-lactamases including AmpC β-lactamases and extended-spectrum β-lactamases. Resistance to carbapenems develops when bacteria acquire or develop structural changes within their PBPs, when they acquire metallo-β-lactamases, or when loss of specific outer membrane porins causes changes in membrane permeability (84).

IMIPENEM

Structure

Imipenem is the *N*-formimidoyl derivative of thienamycin. In addition to the structural characteristics of carbapenems, the side chain of imipenem is different from that of penicillins and cephalosporins. Instead of the acylamino side chain, imipenem has a hydroxyethyl side chain, and unlike the other β-lactams, where the side chain is in a *cis* configuration, the side chain of imipenem is in a *trans* configuration. The *trans* conformation is responsible for the stability of imipenem against β-lactamases (85).

Spectrum of Activity

Gram-Positive Organisms

Streptococci including penicillin-resistant *S. pneumoniae*, methicillin-susceptible *S. aureus*, and penicillin-susceptible strains of *E. faecalis* are susceptible to imipenem. Like penicillins, imipenem is bacteriostatic and not bactericidal against enterococci. *Listeria* and *Bacillus* species are also susceptible to imipenem. *E. faecium* and non–β-lactamase-producing strains of enterococci are resistant to imipenem.

Gram-Negative Organisms

Members of the Enterobacteriaceae family including the extended-spectrum β-lactamase producers are susceptible to imipenem. β-Lactamase-producing strains of *H. influenzae* and *N. gonorrhoeae* are also susceptible to imipenem. *P. aeruginosa*, including strains resistant to antipseudomonal penicillins and cephalosporins, and most strains of *Acinetobacter* are susceptible to imipenem. *S. maltophilia* and some strains of *Burkholderia cepacia* are resistant.

Anaerobes

Most anaerobes, including *Peptococcus*, *Peptostreptococcus*, *B. fragilis*, *Fusobacterium*, *Actinomyces*, and *Clostridium* species excluding *C. difficile*, are susceptible to imipenem.

Others

Nocardia asteroides, some *Legionella* species, and *Mycobacterium avium-intracellulare* are inhibited by imipenem.

Mechanism of Action

Imipenem binds with high affinity to PBPs of both gram-positive and gram-negative organisms. Unlike the penicillins and cephalosporins, imipenem binds with high affinity to PBP2 and less avidly to PBP1 in gram-negative bacteria. It is not hydrolyzed by most β-lactamases, penicillinases, cephalosporinases (plasmid or chromosomal) of *S. aureus*, several enteric gram-negative organisms, *P. aeruginosa*, *B. cepacia*, and *B. fragilis*. It is hydrolyzed by a *S. maltophilia* β-lactamase, as well as some *Bacillus* and *Bacteroides* enzymes (85). Carbapenems show a postantibiotic effect, which varies by organism and species (86,87).

Resistance

S. maltophilia and some strains of *B. cepacia* produce β-lactamases that hydrolyze imipenem and other carbapenems. Resistance in *P. aeruginosa* is due to absence or loss of an outer membrane protein or due to the presence of efflux pump systems (88).

Pharmacokinetics

Imipenem is not absorbed orally. In the kidney it is hydrolyzed by the renal peptidase, dehydropeptidase-1 located on the brush border of the proximal renal tubules (89). Thus, imipenem is combined with cilastatin, a dehydropeptidase inhibitor. Cilastatin has no antibacterial activity and does not interfere with the activity of imipenem. Combination with cilastatin also reduces the nephrotoxicity of imipenem (90). Imipenem is widely distributed to different body tissues. In the absence of meningeal inflammation, levels in the CSF are low.

Adverse Reactions

Nausea and vomiting are the two most common adverse events reported. Elevation of liver enzymes and leukopenia have also been reported. Imipenem can cause seizures especially in patients with underlying central nervous system (CNS) defects and in those with decreased renal function when dose adjustment has not been made (91,92). Treatment of infants with bacterial meningitis with imipenem has been associated with drug-related seizure activity (93). Patients who are allergic to other β-lactam antibiotics can have hypersensitivity reactions to imipenem.

Clinical Use

Imipenem is useful in the treatment of infections due to cephalosporin-resistant Enterobacteriaceae, particularly *Citrobacter freundii* and *Enterobacter* species, and in the empiric therapy of serious infections in patients who have previously received multiple antibiotics (85). Imipenem is effective as a single agent in the therapy of febrile neutropenia (94). Imipenem has also been used as a single agent for the treatment of acute pulmonary exacerbations in patients with cystic fibrosis. *P. aeruginosa* can develop resistance during therapy.

Imipenem is approved by the FDA for treatment of the following infections: lower respiratory tract infections, urinary tract infections (complicated and uncomplicated), intra-abdominal infections, gynecologic infections, bacterial septicemia, bone and joint infections, skin and skin structure infections, endocarditis (*S. aureus*), and polymicrobic infections. It is not indicated in patients with meningitis because safety and efficacy have not been established. Imipenem is approved for use in patients from birth through 16 years of age.

Dosage

For patients 3 months of age or older, the recommended regimen for non-CNS infections is 15 to 25 mg per kg per dose administered every 6 hours. Imipenem is not approved in children with CNS infections or in children with impaired renal function who weigh less than 30 kg. For patients 3 months of age or younger who weigh at least 1,500 g, the following dosage schedule is recommended for non-CNS infections (33):

Less than 1 week of age: 25 mg per kg every 12 hours
One to four weeks of age: 25 mg per kg every 8 hours
Four weeks to 3 months of age: 25 mg per kg every 6 hours

MEROPENEM

Structure

Meropenem has a dimethylcarbamoyl pyrolidiolidyn derivative on position 2 of the ring, unlike the *N*-formidyl group in imipenem. This makes it stable to dehydropeptidase-1.

Mechanism of Action

Meropenem acts by binding to the PBPs of bacteria, thereby interfering with cell wall synthesis. Its strongest affinities are toward PBP 2, 3, and 4 of *E. coli* and *P. aeruginosa* and PBP 1, 2, and 4 of *S. aureus*.

Spectrum of Activity

Meropenem is slightly less active against gram-positive bacteria than imipenem and more active against gram-negative bacteria, including some *P. aeruginosa* resistant to imipenem (95). It penetrates membranes of gram-negative organisms better than imipenem (96). Meropenem has a postantibiotic effect similar to that of imipenem.

Resistance

Like imipenem, meropenem is not hydrolyzed by most β-lactamases, penicillinases, or cephalosporinases. Meropenem is hydrolyzed by the β-lactamases of *S. maltophilia*. Meropenem does not bind to the PBPs of *E. faecium*. Because it is more rapidly transported through the porins of gram-negative organisms, resistance due to decreased permeability is uncommon.

Pharmacokinetics

Unlike imipenem, meropenem is not hydrolyzed by the renal dehydropeptidase. Its pharmacology is similar to that of imipenem in other respects.

Clinical Use

Meropenem has been shown to be safe and effective in the treatment of meningitis in children with no increase in drug-related seizure activity (97–99). Studies suggest that meropenem is therapeutically equivalent to imipenem (100,101). Meropenem has been used as a single agent in the treatment of pulmonary exacerbations in patients with cystic fibrosis. Development of resistance has been uncommon (47). Meropenem is currently approved by the FDA for pediatric patients 3 months of age or older for the treatment of intra-abdominal infections like complicated appendicitis and peritonitis and for the treatment of bacterial meningitis in children 3 months of age or older.

Adverse Events

Seizures and other CNS adverse experiences have been reported during treatment with meropenem. These experiences have occurred most commonly in patients with CNS disorders or with bacterial meningitis and/or compromised renal function. Meropenem may be less epileptogenic than imipenem (102,103). In the pediatric clinical trials in patients without meningitis, the most common adverse events reported were diarrhea, rash, nausea, and vomiting. In clinical trials in patients with meningitis, the most common adverse events reported included diarrhea, moniliasis, and glossitis.

Dosage

For pediatric patients 3 months of age or older, the recommended dosage is as follows (104):

10 mg per kg every 8 hours (complicated skin and skin structure infections)
20 mg per kg every 8 hours (intra-abdominal infections)
40 mg per kg every 8 hours (meningitis)

There is no experience in pediatric patients with renal impairment.

ERTAPENEM

Ertapenem has broad-spectrum in vitro activity against most commonly encountered gram-positive and gram-negative bacterial pathogens with the notable exceptions of enterococci, MRSA, *P. aeruginosa,* and *Acinetobacter* (105,106). Its high level of protein binding and serum half-life of 4 hours allow it to be dosed once daily. Ertapenem may be administered intravenously or intramuscularly. Ertapenem is approved by the FDA for the treatment of adults with complicated intra-abdominal infections, complicated urinary tract and complicated skin and skin structure infections, acute pelvic infections, and community-acquired pneumonia. Dosage adjustment is needed in patients with renal impairment. It is also approved for use in children 3 months to 17 years of age for the same indications as in adults. The dose in patients 13 years of age and older is 1 g given once a day. The dose in patients 3 months to 12 years of age is 15 mg per kg twice daily (not to exceed 1 g per day). The product label also states that ertapenem is not recommended for the treatment of meningitis in the pediatric population due to lack of sufficient CSF penetration (107).

DORIPENEM

Doripenem is a new carbapenem that was approved by the FDA in October 2007. It is approved for use in adults with complicated urinary tract infections and complicated intra-abdominal infections. It is not yet approved for use in children.

MONOBACTAMS

AZTREONAM

Aztreonam is a monocyclic β-lactam compound originally isolated from *Chromobacterium violaceum* (108). It differs from other β-lactams structurally in its unique monocyclic β-lactam nucleus. Aztreonam is the only available synthetic monobactam antibiotic.

Mechanism of Action

The bactericidal action of aztreonam results from the inhibition of bacterial cell wall synthesis due to a high affinity of aztreonam for PBP3 present in gram-negative bacteria.

Spectrum of Activity

Aztreonam exhibits potent and specific activity in vitro against a wide spectrum of gram-negative pathogens including members of the Enterobacteriaceae family and *P. aeruginosa.* It is, however, less active than ceftazidime or imipenem against most strains of *P. aeruginosa* (85). Limited activity has been noted against *Acinetobacter* species, *Alcaligenes* species, *B. cepacia,* and *S. maltophilia.* Aztreonam acts synergistically with aminoglycosides against gram-negative bacilli (109). Aztreonam has no significant antibacterial activity against gram-positive organisms or anaerobes.

Resistance

Unlike the majority of β-lactam antibiotics, aztreonam does not induce β-lactamase activity. Its molecular structure confers a high degree of resistance to hydrolysis by β-lactamases produced by most gram-negative and gram-positive pathogens, although it is affected by some β-lactamases produced by *Klebsiella* species and some pseudomonads, resulting in aztreonam resistance (110). Aztreonam resistance may also be related to alterations in outer membrane porin proteins (85).

Pharmacokinetics

In healthy subjects, aztreonam is removed from the body primarily by the kidney, by both active tubular secretion and glomerular filtration. In patients with impaired renal function, the serum half-life and serum concentration of aztreonam are prolonged. The half-life is only slightly prolonged in patients with hepatic impairment. Aztreonam is distributed readily to most body tissues and fluids (111). It enters the CSF after intravenous administration (112). Aztreonam is removed by hemodialysis (113,114).

Clinical Use

Patients who are allergic to penicillins or cephalosporins appear not to react to aztreonam (115). Aztreonam can be used in the treatment of a variety of gram-negative infections including urinary tract, lower respiratory tract, skin and skin structure, intra-abdominal, and gynecologic infections including endometritis and pelvic cellulitis. Aztreonam has been used in the treatment of gram-negative meningitis (116). As its spectrum of activity is limited to gram-negative organisms, aztreonam should not be used as a single agent for empiric therapy in seriously ill patients if gram-positive or anaerobic infections are a possibility. Aztreonam has been used in combination with clindamycin, erythromycin, metronidazole, penicillins, and vancomycin (91). Studies have been conducted evaluating the use of inhaled aztreonam in patients with cystic fibrosis (11,117). Inhaled aztreonam is FDA approved for use in cystic fibrosis patients with P. aeruginosa.

The FDA has approved aztreonam for the following indications: complicated and uncomplicated urinary tract infections, lower respiratory tract infections, septicemia, skin and skin structure infections, intra-abdominal infections, and gynecologic infections, including endometritis and pelvic cellulitis. The FDA has approved aztreonam for use in children 9 months to 16 years of age. Sufficient data are not available for pediatric patients less than 9 months of age or for the following treatment indications/pathogens: septicemia and skin and skin-structure infections (where the skin infection is believed or known to be due to *H. influenzae* type b).

Dosage

Mild to moderate infections: 30 mg per kg every 8 hours.

Moderate to severe infections: 30 mg per kg every 6 to 8 hours.

Maximum recommended dose: 120 mg per kg per day. In pediatric patients with cystic fibrosis, higher doses may be needed. Insufficient data are available regarding dosing in pediatric patients with renal impairment (33).

Adverse Reactions

Adverse reactions described in adults include skin rashes, nausea, and diarrhea. In pediatric clinical trials the common adverse events included rash, diarrhea, and fever. The following laboratory adverse events were noted during clinical trials: increased eosinophils, increased platelets, neutropenia, increased aspartate aminotransferase, increased alanine aminotransferase, and increased serum creatinine. Aztreonam contains 780 mg of arginine per gram of antibiotic, and hence arginine-induced hypoglycemia has been raised as a possible adverse effect (118,119).

ACKNOWLEDGMENT

The views expressed in this chapter represent those of the authors. No official support or endorsement by the U.S. Food and Drug Administration is provided or should be inferred.

REFERENCES

1. Fleming A. On the antibacterial action of cultures of a penicillium, with special reference to their use in the isolation of *B. influenzae. Br J Exp Pathol* 1929;10:226.
2. Batchelor FR, Doyle FP, Naylor JHC, et al. Synthesis of penicillin: 6-aminopenicillanic acid in penicillin fermentations. *Nature* 1959;183:257–258.
3. Petri WA Jr. Antimicrobial agents penicillins, cephalosporins, and other lactam antibiotics. In: Hardman JG, Limbird LE, Gilman AG, eds. *Goodman and Gillman's the pharmacological basis of therapeutics,* 10th ed. New York, NY: McGraw-Hill, 2001:1189–1218.
4. Ghuysen JM. Serine beta lactamases and penicillin-binding proteins. *Annu Rev Microbiol* 1991;45:37–67.
5. Chambers HF. Penicillins. In: Mandell GL, Bennett JE, Dolin R, eds. *Mandell, Douglas, and Bennett's principles and practice of infectious diseases,* 5th ed. Philadelphia, PA: Churchill Livingstone, 2000:261–274.
6. Siegel JD, Shannon KM, DePasse BM. Recurrent infection associated with penicillin tolerant group B streptococci: a report of two cases. *J Pediatr* 1981;99(6):920–924.
7. Betriu C, Gomez M, Sanchez A, et al. Antibiotic resistance and penicillin tolerance in clinical isolates of group B streptococci. *Antimicrob Agents Chemother* 1994;38(9):2183–2186.
8. Reed MD, Blumer JL. Anti-infective therapy. In: Jenson HB, Baltimore RS, eds. *Pediatric infectious diseases,* 2nd ed. Philadelphia, PA: WB Saunders, 2002:147–211.
9. American Academy of Pediatrics. Tables of antibacterial drug doses. In: Pickering LK, ed. *2006 Red book: report of the Committee on Infectious Diseases,* 27th ed. Elk Grove Village, IL: American Academy of Pediatrics, 2006:750–765.
10. Choi EH, Lee NJ. Clinical outcome of invasive infections caused by penicillin-resistant *Streptococcus pneumoniae* in Korean children. *Clin Infect Dis* 1998;26:1346–1354.
11. http://www.accessdata.fda.gov/drugsatfda_docs/label/2008/050638s012lbl.pdf. Accessed March 30, 2010.
12. American Academy of Pediatrics. Syphillis. In: Pickering LK, ed. *2000 Red book: report of the Committee on Infectious Diseases,* 25th ed. Elk Grove Village, IL: American Academy of Pediatrics, 2000: 547–559.
13. True RJ. Interactions between antibiotics and oral contraceptives. *J Am Med Assoc* 1982;247:1408.
14. Dickinson BD, Altman RD, Nielsen NH, et al. Drug interactions between oral contraceptives and antibiotics. *Obstet Gynecol* 2001; 98:853–860.
15. Dowell SF, Butler JC, Giebink GS, et al. Acute otitis media: management and surveillance in an era of pneumococcal resistance—a report from the Drug-resistant *Streptococcus pneumoniae* Therapeutic Working Group. *Pediatr Infect Dis J* 1999;18(1):1–9.
16. American Academy of Pediatrics and American Academy of Family Physicians Clinical Practice Guideline. Subcommittee on Management of Acute Otitis Media. Diagnosis and management of acute otitis media. http://aappolicy.aappublications.org/cgi/reprint/pediatrics;113/5/1451.pdf. Accessed August 5, 2008.
17. American Academy of Pediatrics. Lyme disease. In: Pickering LK, ed. *2006 Red book: report of the Committee on Infectious Diseases,* 27th ed. Elk Grove Village, IL: American Academy of Pediatrics, 2006:428–433.
18. Hassall E. Peptic ulcer disease and current approaches to *Helicobacter pylori. J Pediatr* 2001;138(4):462–468.
19. Malaty HM. *Helicobacter pylori* infection and eradication in paediatric patients. *Paediatr Drugs* 2000;2(5):357–365.
20. http://www.fda.gov/Drugs/EmergencyPreparedness/BioterrorismandDrugPreparedness/ucm072106.htm. Accessed March 30, 2010.
21. Jahansouz F, Kriett JM, Smith CM, et al. Potentiation of cyclosporine nephrotoxicity by nafcillin in lung transplant recipients. *Transplantation* 1993;55(5):1045–1048.
22. Veremis SA, Maddux MS, Pollak R, et al. Subtherapeutic cyclosporine concentrations during nafcillin therapy. *Transplantation* 1987;43(6):913–915.
23. Taylor AT, Pritchard DC, Goldstein AO, et al. Continuation of warfarin–nafcillin interaction during dicloxacillin therapy. *J Fam Pract* 1994;39(2):182–185.
24. Davis RL, Berman W Jr, Wernly JA, et al. Warfarin–nafcillin interaction. *J Pediatr* 1991;118(2):300–303.
25. Fisher J, Charnas RL, Knowles JR. Kinetic studies on the inactivation of *Escherichia coli* RTEM beta-lactamase by clavulanic acid. *Biochemistry* 1978;17:2180–2184.
26. Charnas RL, Fisher J, Knowles JR. Chemical studies on the inactivation of *Escherichia coli* RTEM beta-lactamase by clavulanic acid. *Biochemistry* 1978;17:2185–2189.
27. Labia R, Morand A, Lelievre V, et al. Sulbactam: biochemical factors involved in its synergy with ampicillin. *Rev Infect Dis* 1986; 8(Suppl 5):S496–S502.
28. Fu KP, Neu HC. Comparative inhibition of beta-lactamases by novel beta-lactam compounds. *Antimicrob Agents Chemother* 1979; 15:171–176.
29. Sutherland R. Beta-lactamase inhibitors and reversal of antibiotic resistance. *Trends Pharmacol Sci* 1991;12:227–232.
30. Abdel-Rahman SM, Gregory LK. The beta-lactamase inhibitors: clinical pharmacology and rational application to combination antibiotic therapy. *Pediatr Infect Dis* 1998;17:1185–1194.
31. Appelbaum PC, Jacobs MR, Spangler SK, et al. Comparative activity of beta-lactamase inhibitors YTR 830, clavulanate, and sulbactam combined with beta-lactams against beta-lactamase-producing anaerobes. *Antimicrob Agents Chemother* 1986;30:789–791.
32. Rolinson GH. Evolution of beta-lactamase inhibitors. *Rev Infect Dis* 1991;13(Suppl 9):S727–S732.
33. Primaxin® product label. http://www.fda.gov/cder/foi/label/2008/050587s065,050630s028lbl.pdf. Accessed August 5, 2008.
34. Williams JD. Beta-lactamase inhibition and *in vitro* activity of sulbactam and sulbactam/cefoperazone. *Clin Infect Dis* 1997;24:494–497.
35. Hampel B, Lode H, Bruckner G, et al. Comparative pharmacokinetics of sulbactam/ampicillin and clavulanic acid/amoxycillin in human volunteers. *Drugs* 1988;35(Suppl 7):29–33.
36. Hoffken G, Tetzel P, Lode H. The pharmacokinetics of ticarcillin, clavulanic acid and their combination. *J Antimicrob Chemother* 1986;17(Suppl C):45–55.
37. Abraham EP, Loder PB. Cephalosporin C. In: Flynn A, ed. *Cephalosporins and penicillin chemistry and biology.* New York, NY: Academic Press, 1972:2–26.

38. Neu HC. Structural relationships affecting *in vitro* activity and pharmacologic properties. *Rev Infect Dis* 1986;8:237–259.
39. Neu HC. Relations of structural properties of beta-lactam antibiotics to antibacterial activity. *Am J Med* 1985;79:2–13.
40. Thornsberry C. Review of *in vitro* activity of third-generation cephalosporins and other newer beta-lactam antibiotics against clinically important bacteria. *Am J Med* 1985;79:14–20.
41. Sanders CC. Cefepime. *Clin Infect Dis* 1993;17:369–379.
42. Garau J, Wilson W, Wood M, et al. Fourth generation cephalosporins: a review of *in vitro* activity, pharmacokinetics, pharmacodynamics, and clinical utility. *Clin Microbiol Infect* 1997; 3(Suppl 1):S87–S101.
43. Nikaido H. Outer membrane barrier as a mechanism of antimicrobial resistance. *Antimicrob Agents Chemother* 1989;33(11):1831–1836.
44. Schaad UB, Suter S, Gianella-Borradori A, et al. A comparison of ceftriaxone and cefuroxime for the treatment of bacterial meningitis in children. *N Engl J Med* 1990;322:141–147.
45. Kaiser AB. Antimicrobial prophylaxis in surgery. *N Engl J Med* 1986;315:1129–1138.
46. Antimicrobial prophylaxis in surgery. *Med Lett* 1993;35: 91–94.
47. Philips JL, Abdel-Rahman S, Farrar HC, et al. Antimicrobial agents. In: Long SS, Pickering LK, Prober CG, eds. *Principles and practice of pediatric infectious diseases*, 2nd ed. New York, NY: Churchill Livingstone, 2003:1458–1510.
48. Saez-llorens X, McCracken GH Jr. Clinical pharmacology of antibacterial agents. In: Remington JS, Klein JO, eds. *Infectious diseases of the fetus and newborn infant*, 5th ed. Philadelphia, PA: WB Saunders, 2001:1419–1466.
49. O'Callaghan CH, Sykes RB, Griffith A, et al. Cefuroxime, a new cephalosporin antibiotic: activity *in vitro*. *Antimicrob Agents Chemother* 1976;9:511–519.
50. Neu HC, Fu KP. Cefuroxime, a β-lactamase-resistant cephalosporin with a broad spectrum of gram-positive and gram-negative activity. *Antimicrob Agents Chemother* 1978;13:657–664.
51. Pichichero ME. Evidence for copathogenicity as a mechanism for bacterial resistance. *Infect Dis Clin Pract* 1998;7(Suppl 4): S248–S253.
52. Nadelman RB, Luger SW, Frank E, et al. Comparison of cefuroxime axetil and doxyxycline in the treatment of early Lyme disease. *Ann Intern Med* 1992;117:273–280.
53. Cuchural GH Jr, Tally FP, Jacobus NV, et al. Comparative activities of newer β-lactam agents against members of the *Bacteroides fragilis* group. *Antimicrob Agents Chemother* 1990;34:479–480.
54. Gorbach SL. The role of cephalosporins in surgical prophylaxis. *J Antimicrob Chemother* 1989;23(Suppl D):61–70.
55. Quagliarello VJ, Scheld WM. Treatment of bacterial meningitis. *N Engl J Med* 1997;336:708–716.
56. Committee on Infectious Diseases. Therapy for children with invasive pneumococcal infections. *Pediatrics* 1997;99:289–299.
57. Young JPW, Husson JM, Bruch K, et al. The evaluation of efficacy and safety of cefotaxime: a review of 2500 cases. *J Antimicrob Chemother* 1980;6(Suppl A):293–300.
58. Eron LJ, Park CH, Goldenberg RI, et al. Ceftriaxone therapy of serious bacterial infections. *J Antimicrob Chemother* 1983;12:65–78.
59. Centers for Disease Control and Prevention. 1998 guidelines for treatment of sexually transmitted diseases. *MMWR Morb Mortal Wkly Rep* 1998;47(RR-1):1–111.
60. Updated recommended treatment regimens for gonococcal infections and associated conditions—United States, April 2007. http://www.cdc.gov/std/treatment/2006/updated-regimens.htm. Accessed August 5, 2008.
61. Dattwyler RJ, Halperin JJ, Volkman DJ, et al. Treatment of late Lyme borreliosis—randomized comparison of ceftriaxone and penicillin. *Lancet* 1988;1:1191–1194.
62. Hughes WT, Armstrong D, Bodey GP, et al. Guidelines for the use of antimicrobial agents in neutropenic patients with unexplained fever. *J Infect Dis* 1990;161:381–396.
63. Rodriguez WJ, Khan WN, Cocchetto DM, et al. Treatment of *Pseudomonas meningitis* with ceftazidime with or without concurrent therapy. *Pediatr Infect Dis J* 1990;9(2):83–87.
64. Padoan R, Cambisano W, Costantini D, et al. Ceftazidime monotherapy vs. combined therapy in *Pseudomonas* pulmonary infections in cystic fibrosis. *Pediatr Infect Dis J* 1987;6(7):648–653.
65. Hoepelman AI, Kieft H, Aoun M, et al. International comparative study of cefepime and ceftazidime in the treatment of serious bacterial infections. *J Antimicrob Chemother* 1993;32(Suppl B): 175–186.
66. Zervos M, Nelson M. Cefepime Study Group. Cefepime versus ceftriaxone for empiric treatment of hospitalized patients with community-acquired pneumonia. *Antimicrob Agents Chemother* 1998;42:729–733.
67. Yamamura D, Gucalp R, Carlisle P, et al. Open randomized study of cefepime versus piperacillin–gentamicin for treatment of febrile neutropenic cancer patients. *Antimicrob Agents Chemother* 1997;41:1704–1708.
68. Saez-Llorens X, Castano E, Garcia R, et al. Prospective randomized treatment of cefepime and cefotaxime for treatment of bacterial meningitis in infants and children. *Antimicrob Agents Chemother* 1995;39:937–940.
69. Karchmer AW. Cephalosporins. In: Mandell GL, Douglas JE, Dolin R, eds. *Mandell, Douglas, and Bennett's principles and practice of infectious diseases*, 5th ed. Philadelphia, PA: Churchill Livingstone, 2000:274–291.
70. Sanders WE Jr, Tenney JH, Kessler RE. Efficacy of cefepime in the treatment of infections due to multiply resistant *Enterobacter* species. *Clin Infect Dis* 1996;23:454–461.
71. Kelkar SP, Li JT. Cephalosporin allergy. *N Engl J Med* 2001; 345(11):804–809.
72. Norrby SR. Side effects of cephalosporins. *Drugs* 1987;34(Suppl 2): 105–120.
73. Murray DL, Singer DA, Singer AB, et al. Cefaclor—a cluster of adverse reactions. *N Engl J Med* 1980;303:1003.
74. Meyers BR. Comparative toxicities of third-generation cephalosporins. *Am J Med* 1985;79:96–103.
75. Lin RY. A perspective on penicillin allergy. *Arch Intern Med* 1992; 152:930–937.
76. Johnson GJ. Antibiotic-induced hemostatic abnormalities. In: Peterson PK, Verhoef J, eds. *The antimicrobial agents annual*. Amsterdam: Elsevier, 1986:408–419.
77. Bang NU, Kammer RB. Hematologic complications associated with β-lactam antibiotics. *Rev Infect Dis* 1982;4:S546–S554.
78. http://www.fda.gov/Drugs/DrugSafety/PostmarketDrugSafetyInformationforPatientsandProviders/ucm109103.htm. Accessed March 30, 2010.
79. Anderson SD, Gums JG. Ceftobiprole: an extended-spectrum anti-methicillin-resistant Staphylococcus aureus cephalosporin. *Ann Pharmacother* 2008;42(6):806–816.
80. Moreillon P. New and emerging treatment of Staphylococcus aureus infections in the hospital setting. *Clin Microbiol Infect* 2008;14(Suppl 3):32–41.
81. Talbot GH, Thye D, Das A, et al. Phase 2 study of ceftaroline versus standard therapy in treatment of complicated skin and skin structure infections. *Antimicrob Agents Chemother* 2007;51(10): 3612–3616.
82. Kahan JS, Kahan FM, Goegleman R, et al. Thienamycin, a new beta-lactam antibiotic. I. Discovery, taxonomy, isolation and physical properties. *J Antibiot (Tokyo)* 1979;32:1–12.
83. Blumer JL. Pharmacokinetic determinants of carbapenem therapy in neonates and children. *Pediatr Infect Dis J* 1996;15:733–737.
84. Zhanel GG, Wiebe R, Dilay L, et al. Comparative review of the carbapenems. *Drugs* 2007;67(7):1027–1052.
85. Chambers HF. Other β-lactam antibiotics. In: Mandell GL, Bennett JE, Dolin R, eds. *Mandell, Douglas, and Bennett's principles and practice of infectious diseases*, 5th ed. Philadelphia, PA: Churchill Livingstone, 2000:291–299.
86. Baquero F, Culebras E, Patron C, et al. Postantibiotic effect of imipenem on gram-positive and gram-negative micro-organisms. *J Antimicrob Chemother* 1986;18(Suppl E):47–59.
87. Nadler HL, Pitkin DH, Sheikh W. The postantibiotic effect of meropenem and imipenem on selected bacteria. *J Antimicrob Chemother* 1989;24(Suppl A):225–231.
88. Okamoto K, Gotoh N, Nishino T. *Pseudomonas aeruginosa* reveals high intrinsic resistance to penem antibiotics: penem resistance mechanisms and their interplay. *Antimicrob Agents Chemother* 2001; 45(7):1964–1971.
89. Kropp H, Sundelof JG, Hajdu R, et al. Metabolism of thienamycin and related carbapenem antibiotics by the renal dipeptidase, dehydropeptidase. *Antimicrob Agents Chemother* 1982;22(1):62–70.
90. Kahan FM, Kropp H, Sundelof JG, et al. Thienamycin: development of imipenem–cilastatin. *J Antimicrob Chemother* 1983;12 (Suppl D):1–35.

91. Calandra G, Lydick E, Carrigan J, et al. Factors predisposing to seizures in seriously ill infected patients receiving antibiotics: experience with imipenem/cilastatin. *Am J Med* 1988;84(5): 911–918.
92. Calandra GB, Brown KR, Grad LC, et al. Review of adverse experiences and tolerability in the first 2,516 patients treated with imipenem/cilastatin. *Am J Med* 1985;78(6A):73–78.
93. Wong VK, Wright HT Jr, Ross LA, et al. Imipenem/cilastatin treatment of bacterial meningitis in children. *Pediatr Infect Dis J* 1991;10(2):122–125.
94. Bodey GP, Alvarez ME, Jones PG, et al. Imipenem/cilastatin as initial therapy for febrile cancer patients. *Antmicrob Agents Chemother* 1986;30:211–214.
95. Iaconis JP, Pitkin DH, Sheikh W, et al. Comparison of antibacterial activities of meropenem and six other antimicrobials against *Pseudomonas aeruginosa* isolates from North American studies and clinical trials. *Clin Infect Dis* 1997;24(Suppl 2): S191–S196.
96. Satake S, Yoshihara E, Nakae T. Diffusion of beta-lactam antibiotics through liposome membranes reconstituted from purified porins of the outer membrane of *Pseudomonas aeruginosa. Antimicrob Agents Chemother* 1990;34(5):685–690.
97. Klugman KP, Dagan R; Meropenem Meningitis Study Group. Randomized comparison of meropenem with cefotaxime for treatment of bacterial meningitis. *Antimicrob Agents Chemother* 1995;39:1140–1146.
98. Odio CM, Puig JR, Feris JM, et al. Prospective, randomized, investigator-blinded study of the efficacy and safety of meropenem vs. cefotaxime therapy in bacterial meningitis in children. Meropenem Meningitis Study Group. *Pediatr Infect Dis J* 1999;18(7):581–590.
99. Bradley JS. Meropenem: a new, extremely broad spectrum beta-lactam antibiotic for serious infections in pediatrics. *Pediatr Infect Dis J* 1997;16(3):263–268.
100. Garau J, Blanquer J, Cobo L, et al. Prospective, randomised, multicentre study of meropenem versus imipenem/cilastatin as empiric monotherapy in severe nosocomial infections. *Eur J Clin Microbiol Infect Dis* 1997;16(11):789–796.
101. Colardyn F, Faulkner KL. Intravenous meropenem versus imipenem/cilastatin in the treatment of serious bacterial infections in hospitalized patients. Meropenem Serious Infection Study Group. *J Antimicrob Chemother* 1996;38(3):523–537.
102. Norrby SR. Neurotoxicity of carbapenem antibacterials. *Drug Saf* 1996;15:87–90.
103. Fujii R; Pediatric Study Group of Meropenem. Pharmacokinetic and clinical studies with meropenem in the pediatric field. *Jpn J Antibiot* 1992;45:697–717.
104. Merrem product label. http://www.accessdata.fda.gov/drugsatfda_docs/label/2009/050706s025lblpdf. Accessed March 30, 2010.
105. Fuchs PC, Barry AL, Brown SD. *In vitro* activities of ertapenem (MK-0826) against clinical bacterial isolates from 11 North American medical centers. *Antimicrob Agents Chemother* 2001;45: 1915–1918.
106. Kohler J, Dorso KL, Young K, et al. *In vitro* activities of the potent, broad-spectrum carbapenem MK-0826 (L-749,345) against broad-spectrum beta-lactamase-and extended-spectrum beta-lactamase producing *Klebsiella pneumoniae* and *Escherichia coli* clinical isolates. *Antimicrob Agents Chemother* 1999;43(5):1170–1176.
107. Product label for Invanz. http://www.accessdata.fda.gov/drugsatfda_docs/label/2009/021337s030lbl.pdf. Accessed March 30, 2010.
108. Sykes RB, Cimarusti CM, Bonner DP, et al. Monocyclic beta-lactam antibiotics produced by bacteria. *Nature* 1981;291:489–491.
109. Giamarellou H. Aminoglycosides plus beta-lactams against gram-negative organisms. Evaluation of *in vitro* synergy and chemical interactions. *Am J Med* 1986;80(6B):126–137.
110. Johnson DH, Cunha BA. Aztreonam. *Med Clin North Am* 1995; 79:733–743.
111. Swabb EA. Review of the clinical pharmacology of the monobactam antibiotic aztreonam. *Am J Med* 1985;78:11–18.
112. Duma RJ, Berry AJ, Smith SM, et al. Penetration of aztreonam into the cerebrospinal fluid of patients with and without inflamed meninges. *Antimicrob Agents Chemother* 1984;26:730–733.
113. Fillastre JP, Leroy A, Baudoin C, et al. Pharmacokinetics in patients with chronic renal failure. *Clin Pharmacokinet* 1985;10:91–100.
114. Gerig JS, Bolton ND, Swabb EA, et al. Effect of hemodialysis and peritoneal dialysis on aztreonam pharmacokinetics. *Kidney Int* 1984;26:308–318.
115. Saxon A, Hassner A, Swabb EA, et al. Lack of cross-reactivity between aztreonam, a monobactam antibiotic, and penicillin in penicillin-allergic subjects. *J Infect Dis* 1984;149:16–22.
116. Kilpatrick M, Girgis N, Farid Z, et al. Aztreonam for treating meningitis caused by gram-negative rods. *Scand J Infect Dis* 1991; 23(1):125–126.
117. Retsch-Bogart GZ, Burns JL, Otto KL, et al. AZLI Phase II Study Group. A phase 2 study of aztreonam lysine for inhalation to treat patients with cystic fibrosis and Pseudomonas aeruginosa infection. *Pediatr Pulmonol* 2008;43(1):47–58.
118. Umana MA, Odio CM, Castro E, et al. Evaluation of aztreonam and ampicillin vs. amikacin and ampicillin for treatment of neonatal bacterial infections. *Pediatr Infect Dis J* 1990;9(3):175–180.
119. Uauy R, Mize C, Argyle C, et al. Metabolic tolerance to arginine: implications for the safe use of arginine salt–aztreonam combination in the neonatal period. *J Pediatr* 1991;118(6):965–970.

CHAPTER

30

Matthijs de Hoog
John N. van den Anker

Aminoglycosides and Glycopeptides

AMINOGLYCOSIDES

GENERAL ASPECTS OF AMINOGLYCOSIDES

Aminoglycosides have played a major role in antimicrobial therapy since their discovery in the 1940s (1). Their bactericidal efficacy in gram-negative infections, synergism with β-lactam antibiotics, limited bacterial resistance, and low cost have given these agents a firm place in antimicrobial treatment. However, the successful use of streptomycin (1944), gentamicin (1963), tobramycin (1967), amikacin (1972), and netilmicin (1976) has been complicated by nephrotoxicity and ototoxicity in a significant number of treated patients.

STRUCTURE AND CHEMICAL PROPERTIES

Aminoglycosides comprise two or more amino sugars attached via glycosidic bonds to an aminocyclitol nucleus and have a molecular weight of 445 to 600 daltons. Aminoglycosides can be divided into chemical families with related structures. The relation between the structure of aminoglycosides and their activity is incompletely understood. Aminoglycosides are water-soluble, cationic at normal pH, and are distributed in plasma water. Protein binding is minimal. They have a stable structure over a wide range of temperature and pH (2,3).

Aminoglycosides are inactivated in vitro by concomitant use of β-lactam antibiotics (4–6). Tobramycin seems to be more easily inactivated than netilmicin or amikacin. Aminoglycosides act by altering the integrity of the bacterial cell membrane in growing bacteria by way of disturbing protein synthesis through binding to prokaryotic ribosomes (7,8). These cationic antibiotics bind rapidly and passively to the negatively charged parts of phospholipids and other proteins in the bacterial cell membrane and enter the bacterial cell by way of a self-promoted uptake process (9). The uptake process is related to the concentration of aminoglycoside and can be inhibited by low pH, anaerobic conditions, and hyperosmolarity (10,11).

Although inhibition of protein synthesis plays a major part in bacterial cell death, it is not the sole explanation for the bactericidal effect of aminoglycosides. Other antibiotics that inhibit protein synthesis, like chloramphenicol, are only bacteriostatic. Binding of aminoglycosides to the bacterial cell membrane itself may play a role in rapid bacterial cell death (12).

IN VITRO ACTIVITY

Aminoglycosides have a concentration-dependent bactericidal spectrum encompassing aerobic and gram-negative bacteria like Enterobacteriacae, *Escherichia coli*, *Pseudomonas* species, and *Haemophilus* species. The susceptibility of most gram-negative bacteria to gentamicin, tobramycin, netilmicin, and amikacin is relatively similar (13). Although susceptibility to amikacin is three- to fourfold less than that to the other aminoglycosides, this is compensated by its lower toxicity and therefore higher allowable dose. Gentamicin and tobramycin are comparable in activity, although tobramycin is slightly more active against *Pseudomonas aeruginosa*. They are susceptible to the same modifying enzymes and resistance rates are therefore very similar. In contrast, amikacin is resistant to many of these enzymes, and therefore is often an alternative if strains are resistant to tobramycin or gentamicin. Netilmicin susceptibility is comparable to that of gentamicin and tobramycin, although netilmicin is resistant to some of the gentamicin-inactivating enzymes, and thus in some cases is a good alternative.

The antimicrobial activity of aminoglycosides has four distinct and clinically important aspects: (a) concentration-dependent killing, (b) a postantibiotic effect (PAE), (c) adaptive resistance, and (d) synergism with other antibiotics. In vivo and in vitro studies have shown that the aminoglycoside-induced rate of bacterial killing as well as induction of resistance is peak concentration dependent (14–18). Other in vitro investigations, mimicking in vivo fluctuations of drug concentrations, have shown a single bolus of aminoglycoside to be superior in rate and total amount of bacterial killing to the same dose in a multiple daily-dosing regimen in nonneutropenic animals (19,20).

Aminoglycosides are often reported to have a PAE, meaning that there is suppression of bacterial growth for several hours after antibiotic serum concentrations have dropped below the minimal inhibitory concentration (MIC) (21–23). There are discrepancies between in vivo and in vitro studies on this effect, and studies have indicated that PAE is partly determined by diminished regrowth of bacteria at sub-MICs (21). The clinical relevance of the PAE is unclear, and the emphasis on this effect in discussions on extending dose intervals of aminoglycosides is questionable. Synergy of aminoglycosides with other cell-wall-active antibiotics, like penicillins and cephalosporins, has been established (24,25). This synergy is the basis of the clinical choice for combination therapy of aminoglycosides with penicillins or cephalosporins. Issues of toxicity, which will be discussed later, concentration-dependent killing, a PAE (although doubtful), as well as adaptive resistance constitute the rationale for the change to extended-interval dosing of aminoglycosides (26–28).

DRUG RESISTANCE AND SUSCEPTIBILITY

Resistance to aminoglycosides can occur by three mechanisms: ribosomal resistance, decreased uptake and/or accumulation, and enzymatic modification. Ribosomal resistance will not be discussed because it is only pertinent to streptomycin.

Decreased Uptake and/or Accumulation

A decrease in drug uptake is a clinically significant aspect of aminoglycoside resistance. The underlying mechanism, though probably related to membrane impermeability, is not really known (29). It pertains to all aminoglycosides and is a stable characteristic resulting in a moderate level of resistance (30).

Another important phenomenon in aerobic gram-negative bacteria is called adaptive resistance, defined as a reduced antimicrobial killing in originally susceptible bacterial populations after initial incubation with an aminoglycoside (31). It has clinical relevance especially for immunocompromised patients and in serious infections with gram-negative bacteria. Adaptive resistance is probably related to membrane protein changes and altered expression of regulatory genes of the anaerobic respiratory pathway (32). It can be overcome by higher peak serum concentrations of aminoglycosides, which underscores the need for extended dose intervals (33).

Enzymatic Modification

Aminoglycosides can be modified with subsequent loss of antimicrobial activity by enzymes produced by bacterial pathogens (25). The genetic code for these enzymes is largely contained in plasmids, thereby rendering the resistance easily transferable. In addition, it is important to realize that all susceptible positions in aminoglycosides can be modified by several enzymes and that several inactivating genes can easily develop from a common ancestor, implying that it will be unlikely that making aminoglycosides resistant to inactivation by a specific enzyme will be a worthwhile effort (30).

INDICATIONS

Aminoglycosides are mainly used for treating serious gram-negative infections caused by enteric bacilli. Aminoglycosides are synergistic with cephalosporins and penicillins in the setting of gram-negative infections and are thus often combined with these cell-wall-active antibiotics (25). They are also used in combination treatment with vancomycin for *Staphylococcus aureus* (both methicillin-sensitive and methicillin-resistant strains), *S. epidermidis*, and enterococcal infections (34,35). Oral administration of paromomycin has been successfully used for treating cryptosporidiosis in patients with acquired immune deficiency syndrome (36). In case of empiric treatment with aminoglycosides, local susceptibility patterns have to be taken into account. There are many indications for use of aminoglycosides that are beyond the scope of this chapter. Three conditions will be addressed in more detail: neonatal sepsis, cystic fibrosis (CF), and urinary tract infections.

Neonatal Sepsis

Among major pathogens responsible for bacterial infections during the first month of life, gram-negative bacteria like *E. coli*, *Klebsiella* species, *Enterobacter* species, and *Pseudomonas* species play an increasing role, possibly related to the increased prenatal administration of antibiotics and use of percutaneous central venous catheters in the neonatal intensive care unit (NICU) (37–40). Aminoglycosides are effective against most nosocomial-acquired gram-negative infections in term and preterm infants and are synergistic with β-lactam antibiotics in treating group B streptococcal and coagulase-negative staphylococcal infections. They play an important role in the initial empiric treatment of neonatal septicemia (37–40). Initial treatment combining amoxicillin with gentamicin may be more effective than a combination with cefotaxime (41). After penicillins, aminoglycosides are the most commonly used drugs in the NICU (42). In general, emergence of aminoglycoside-resistant strains other than coagulase-negative streptococci is relatively slow, which is a definite advantage over third-generation cephalosporins (43,44).

Cystic Fibrosis

Acute pulmonary exacerbations of CF are often caused by pseudomonal microorganisms (45). Standard treatment consists of a combination of an aminoglycoside with a β-lactam antibiotic (e.g., ticarcillin) or a quinolone antibiotic and leads to a longer clinical remission than use of a β-lactam alone (46,47). Sequential intravenous/oral ciprofloxacin monotherapy offers a safe and efficacious alternative (48). Higher doses, up to 9 mg per kg per day, are needed because of a higher aminoglycoside clearance in patients with CF (49,50). The safety and efficacy of aerosolized tobramycin maintenance therapy for patients with CF colonized with *P. aeruginosa* has been demonstrated in several studies (51). Dose advice for inhaled tobramycin is 300 mg twice daily for a period of 28 days (52). Systemic bioavailability is approximately 12% and monitoring serum concentrations in patients with renal failure is indicated (53). Once-daily and three times daily dosing in pediatric patients with CF is equally effective and less nephrotoxic (54).

Urinary Tract Infections

Aminoglycosides are excreted by way of glomerular filtration and are partly actively reabsorbed, leading to high parenchymal as well as urine concentrations. This makes these drugs useful in treating acute pyelonephritis and cystitis. Even single doses lead to prolonged periods of adequate concentrations in urine (55,56). Once-daily dosing (ODD) of gentamicin is effective in treating urinary tract infections in children (57).

PHARMACOKINETICS

Aminoglycosides have a pharmacokinetic profile consisting of a rapid distribution phase ($t_{1/2\alpha}$), an elimination phase ($t_{1/2\beta}$), and a second elimination phase ($t_{1/2\gamma}$). The gamma phase can only be determined after discontinuation of the drug. Distribution half-life is 5 to 10 minutes in adults but has never been measured in newborns. The gamma phase in infants is long. Netilmicin was detectable in blood and urine 11 and 14 days after discontinuation, with a $t_{1/2\gamma}$ of 62.4 hours (58). The tissue half-life in renal cortex is 4 to 5 days (59). In general, the serum concentrations and pharmacokinetic data determined in most studies are derived from the elimination phase, which is adequately described by a one-compartment model. There are, however, some studies that have shown a two-compartment model to be superior in predicting serum $t_{1/2\beta}$ and serum concentrations (60–63).

Because aminoglycosides are distributed over extracellular water, there are age-related changes in volume of distribution (V_d) dependent on the decrease of total body water with age. The largest V_d is encountered in premature neonates. Tables 30.1 and 30.2 display age-related pharmacokinetic parameters for aminoglycosides in neonates, infants, and children.

PHARMACOKINETICS IN NEONATES

Many studies in neonates have been performed, and therefore only larger studies in this age group are included. In larger studies V_d of gentamicin ranges from 0.70 L per kg in neonates with a gestational age (GA) less than 32 weeks to 0.32 L per kg in children aged 11 to 18 years (64–66).

The V_d of most drugs is larger in neonates, especially in prematures, primarily due to a higher percentage of extracellular water (67,68). As can be seen in Table 30.1, this also holds true for aminoglycosides. There is a consistently higher V_d for prematures, especially in the group with very low birth weight (VLBW)/GA less than 30 weeks. Most authors have found birth weight (BW) to be the best predictor of V_d (62,69–72), although some have found V_d to be independent of GA (66,73). In practice, this means that prematures will end up having lower peak serum concentrations. The interpatient variability of V_d in these groups is greater, and therefore serum concentrations are difficult to predict in the individual premature infant. Total body clearance (*CL*), associated with GA (62,69,74) and BW (62,69,70,72), is lower, and $t_{1/2\beta}$ is longer, in preterm infants, leading to higher serum trough concentrations in this group. This can be explained by the significant increase of glomerular filtration rate (GFR) with GA and BW described in recent studies (75,76). *CL* and $t_{1/2}$ are also highly variable in VLBW infants. Substantial effort has been put into developing equations, mostly based on population pharmacokinetic studies, which potentially will lead to better prediction of serum concentrations in individual patients (70,72,73). In practice, these equations are not able to adequately predict variability and subsequent serum concentrations in the same patient (64).

Diminishing extracellular fluid in the neonatal period (77) leads to a corresponding decrease in V_d with increasing postnatal age (PNA), again especially in the VLBW group. Recent data have shown a significant postnatal increase in GFR (75,76). A concomitant change in *CL* and $t_{1/2}$ has been shown for amikacin (78), gentamicin (73,74,79–81), netilmicin (58,62), and tobramycin (82), but this result has been refuted by others (71,83).

Patent ductus arteriosus (PDA) as well as postnatal exposure to indomethacin or other nonsteroidal anti-inflammatory drugs alters the rapid postnatal increase in GFR (84,85), possibly through decreased renal blood flow, leading to an increase in V_d and a reduction of *CL*. Increase in V_d of gentamicin is found in infants with PDA (66,86). In this patient group fluid overload is common. Closure of PDA leads to significant decrease in V_d of more than 30% (86,87). Dosage adjustments, based on therapeutic drug monitoring (TDM), should be made in patients with PDA. The effect of indomethacin, used for closure of PDA, as well as surgical closure itself necessitates TDM. Information on gentamicin disposition in infants on extracorporeal membrane oxygenation (ECMO) is scarce. Two small studies (63,88) showed V_d to be increased. Serum half-life in patients on ECMO was 9.55 and 9.24 hours, respectively, and decreased to 3.87 hours in the same patients off ECMO in the study by Dodge et al. (88). On the basis of these data, dosage adjustments should be made in this group of infants. Prenatal exposure to corticosteroids, which is seen increasingly in the VLBW group, leads to increased intrauterine maturation of kidney function, possibly through direct vasodilation mediated by glucocorticoid receptors (76,89). Although this point has not been investigated, it might have a significant effect on pharmacokinetic parameters in this group of infants. These studies indicate that extra TDM is warranted in patients who are on ECMO, have an open ductus Botalli, or are exposed to indomethacin. Aminoglycosides are eliminated from the body by way of glomerular filtration; it is therefore predictable that a relation between GFR and serum concentrations exists. The link between GFR and aminoglycoside pharmacokinetics is often (58,71,73,74,80,90–92), but not consistently (62,80,93,94), described in neonates. Furthermore, in adults it has been shown that aminoglycoside concentrations can change without concomitant change of serum creatinine (95). Keyes et al. (93) showed that serum trough concentrations could not be reliably predicted in newborns with serum creatinine. In conclusion, these studies suggest that, though there is a relation, serum creatinine in the first week of life cannot be accurately used to predict aminoglycoside *CL*.

PHARMACOKINETICS IN INFANTS AND CHILDREN

There are also age-related differences in aminoglycoside pharmacokinetics in infants and older children. Figure 30.1 shows that V_d (for amikacin) decreases with increasing

TABLE 30.1 Results of Pharmacokinetic Studies of Aminoglycosides in Neonates

Aminoglycoside (Reference)	*N*	*GA (wk)*	*PNA (d)*	*Weight (g)*	*CL (mL/min/kg)*	V_d *(L/kg)*	$t_{1/2}$ *(hr)*
Amikacin (360)	32	32 ± 3.6		1,740 ± 810	1.08 ± 0.51	0.655 ± 0.414	7.6 ± 4.4
Amikacin (157)	28	30.5 ± 2.86		1,380 ± 170	0.83 ± 0.28	0.57 ± 0.11	8.4
Amikacin (157)	6	32–40	1–3	1,500–3,400	1.05 ± 0.30	0.70 ± 0.27	2
	5	36–40	5–8	2,100–3,600	1.08 ± 0.42	0.49 ± 0.11	5.6
	11	32–38	>8	1,900–4,600	1.78 ± 0.53	0.73 ± 0.13	5.1
Amikacin (361)	43	25–41	1–29	865–3,860	1.50[a] ± 8.6%[b]	1.07[c] ± 5.9%[b]	
Gentamicin (362)	19		1	<1,500	0.75 ± 0.60	0.72 ± 0.45	13
	18		1	≥1,500	0.97 ± 0.23	0.78 ± 0.39	13.8
	20		4	<1,500	0.50 ± 0.18	0.60 ± 0.26	10.9
	28		4	≥1,500	0.72 ± 0.10	0.50 ± 0.18	8.1
Gentamicin (79)	15	<33	<7	<1,500	0.38 ± 0.15	0.53 ± 0.10	11.1
	15	<33	8–30	<1,500	0.45 ± 0.17	0.50 ± 0.11	10.8
	6	<33	>31	<1,500	1.18 ± 0.45	0.50 ± 0.11	4.4
Gentamicin (363)	12		1.8	<1,000	0.52 ± 0.08	0.35 ± 0.07	7.9
	36		1.8	≥1,000	0.65 ± 0.13	0.38 ± 0.13	6.5
	20	≤30	1.8		0.58 ± 0.12		7.4
	28	>30	1.8		0.63 ± 0.13		6.5
Gentamicin (69)	11	28–33	2–30		1.00	0.597	6.53
		35–38	2–30		1.22	0.538	4.95
	55	39–43	2–30		1.15	0.542	5.17
Gentamicin (66)	216	32.39 ± 2.83	?	1,850 ± 670	0.75 ± 0.25	0.54 ± 0.13	8.98 ± 2.86
	106 (PDA)	29.02 ± 2.92	?	1,160 ± 530	0.67 ± 0.28	0.61 ± 0.15	12.24 ± 7.43
Gentamicin (86)	24 (PDA)	?	<1,500	0.93 ± 0.33	0.64 ± 0.20	8.49 ± 2.69	
	16		?	<1,500	0.83 ± 0.4	0.41 ± 0.08	6.23 ± 1.92
Gentamicin (364)	11	26–33	1–10				13
	6	34–40	1–10				6
Gentamicin (156)							
Control	16	30.6 ± 0.86	<12 hr	1,600 ± 154		0.57 ± 0.03	10.2 ± 0.89
Loading	18	29.2 ± 0.81	<12 hr	1,294 ± 145		0.58 ± 0.02	12.0 ± 0.84
Gentamicin (63)	10 ECMO	36–43	<7		2.78 ± 1.55	0.51 ± 0.11	9.55 ± 4.38
Gentamicin (71)	113	>34 + AS5 ≥ 7	0–50	500–4,500	0.88	0.47	
		≤34 + AS5 < 7			0.73		
		≤34 + AS5 ≥ 7			0.6		
Gentamicin (365)	165	37 ± 4.5	7.8 ± 11.7	2,432 ± 952		0.64 ± 0.22	8.2 ± 4.8
Gentamicin (74)	15	<37	0–2		1.03 ± 0.37		
	27	≥37	0–2		1.40 ± 0.47		
	8	<37	3–7		1.78 ± 0.63		
	16	≥37	3–7		1.78 ± 0.38		
	1	<37	8–28		1.67		
	14	≥37	8–28		1.97 ± 0.43		
Gentamicin (366)	79	27–40	3–7	920–3,550	0.7 (0.68–0.72)[d]	0.47 (0.43–0.52)	8 (7.7–8.3)[d]
Netilmicin (367)	22	27–40	<16	800–3,400	1.07 ± 0.28	0.34 ± 0.11	9.6
Netilmicin (368)	12	28–33	<28	770–2,050	0.83 ± 0.27	0.63 ± 0.24	8.6
Netilmicin (58)	16		<7	<2,000		0.609	4.7
3 mg/kg	8		≥7	<2,000		0.599	4.1
	9		<7	>2,000		0.472	3.4
	23		<7	>2,000		0.617	4.4
4 mg/kg	4		≥7	>2,000		0.510	3.8
Tobramycin (82)	19	29–40	2–4	1,000–3,555	1.15 (0.70–1.83)	0.82 (0.54–1.76)	8.6 (3.5–14.1)
	8		4–7	1,000–3,555	1.14 (0.62–1.56)	0.68 (0.40–1.06)	7.1 (4.6–11.6)
			2–4	1,000–1,500	1.09 (0.74–1.15)	1.04 (0.64–1.36)	11.1 (6.6–14.1)
			4–7	1,000–1,500	1.02 (0.62–1.55)	0.73 (0.46–1.06)	8.7 (5.7–11.6)
Tobramycin (369)	9	28–30	2–6		1.04 ± 0.22	0.84 ± 0.31	9.3 ± 2.8
	11	30–34	2–6		1.13 ± 0.35	0.81 ± 0.20	8.9 ± 3.0
	6	34–40	2–6		1.28 ± 0.31	0.61 ± 0.14	5.6 ± 1.2
	7		2–6	1,000–1,250	1.05 ± 0.20	1.02 ± 0.27	11.3 ± 3.0
	6		2–6	1,260–1,500	1.12 ± 0.39	0.74 ± 0.16	8.2 ± 2.0
	7		2–6	1,500–2,000	1.10 ± 0.32	0.69 ±0.16	7.5 ± 1.6
	6		2–6	2,100–3,500	1.28 ± 0.31	0.61 ± 0.14	5.6 ± 1.2
Tobramycin (370)	8	24–30	3–5	<1,000	0.69 ± 0.10	0.59 ± 0.10	9.9 ± 1.5

AS5, 5′ Apgar score; *CL*, total body clearance; ECMO, extracorporeal membrane oxygenation; GA, gestational age; *N*, Number of patients in study; PDA, patent ductus arteriosus; PNA, postnatal age; $t_{1/2}$, serum half-life; V_d, volume of distribution.

[a]mL/min.

[b]Standard error of estimate.

[c]L.

[d]95% confidence interval.

TABLE 30.2 Results of Pharmacokinetic Studies of Aminoglycosides in Infants and Children

Aminoglycoside (Reference)	*Patient Group*	*N*	*Age*	*CL (mL/min/kg)*	*V_d (L/kg)*	*$t_{1/2}$ (hr)*
Amikacin (371)			<3 yr		0.40 ± 0.07	
Amikacin (109)	PICU patients	13	6.8 yr			2.02 ± 0.64
Amikacin (372)		30	6–12 mo	1.13 (0.3–2.15)	0.50 (0.22–0.73)[a]	2.86 (0.63–6.28)
Amikacin (372)		30	<6 mo	1.05 (0.6–1.8)	0.58 (0.32–0.98)	5.02 (1.46–11.89)
Tobramycin (373)		19	2–8 yr	123.5 ± 10.2[b]	0.49 ± 0.06	2 ± 0.17
Tobramycin (373)		22	11–18 yr	195.0 ± 16[b]	0.40 ± 0.04	1.4 ± 0.10
Gentamicin (169)		44	2.2 ± 3.5 yr	2.05 ± 068	0.424 ± 0.116	2.6 ± 1.0
Gentamicin (130) (ODD)		8	0.5–4 yr		0.43 ± 0.02	0.31 ± 0.01[c]
		11	5–10 yr		0.35 ± 0.01	0.37 ± 0.01
		12	11–18 yr		0.32 ± 0.01	0.37 ± 0.01
Gentamicin/ tobramycin (374)	Bone marrow transplants	33	9 mo–15 yr	1.71 ± 0.53	0.32 ± 0.07	2.32 ± 0.65
Amikacin (375)	Normal renal function	8	3–11 yr	3.0 ± 1.25	0.208 ± 0.11	1.19 ± 0.19

CL, Total body clearance; ODD, once-daily dosing; PICU, pediatric intensive care unit; $t_{1/2}$, serum half-life; V_d, volume of distribution.
[a]V_d = total V_d.
[b]mL/min/1.73 m^2.
[c]Elimination rate constant K_e.

PNA and *CL* decreases with increasing PNA (96). Changes in both V_d and *CL* are most pronounced in the first 2 weeks of life. V_d decreases by one-third when comparing patients younger and older than 3 months (97). A concomitant change in peak serum concentrations with age is seen (98). It is questionable whether these changes are clinically relevant for dose or dose interval in pediatric patients beyond the neonatal age.

V_d and total plasma *CL* for aminoglycosides are increased in patients with CF, necessitating larger doses in this patient group (46,49,50).

A relation between GFR and aminoglycoside *CL* in pediatric patients has been established, and aminoglycoside dosing has to be adjusted according to creatinine *CL* (99,100).

EFFICACY

Efficacy of aminoglycosides is related to both the peak serum concentration-to-MIC ratio (peak/MIC) and the area under the time-versus-concentration curve (AUC/MIC) in clinical and experimental studies (14,17,101). Peak/MIC ratios of 5 to 10 are desirable for clinical efficacy. In the neonatal

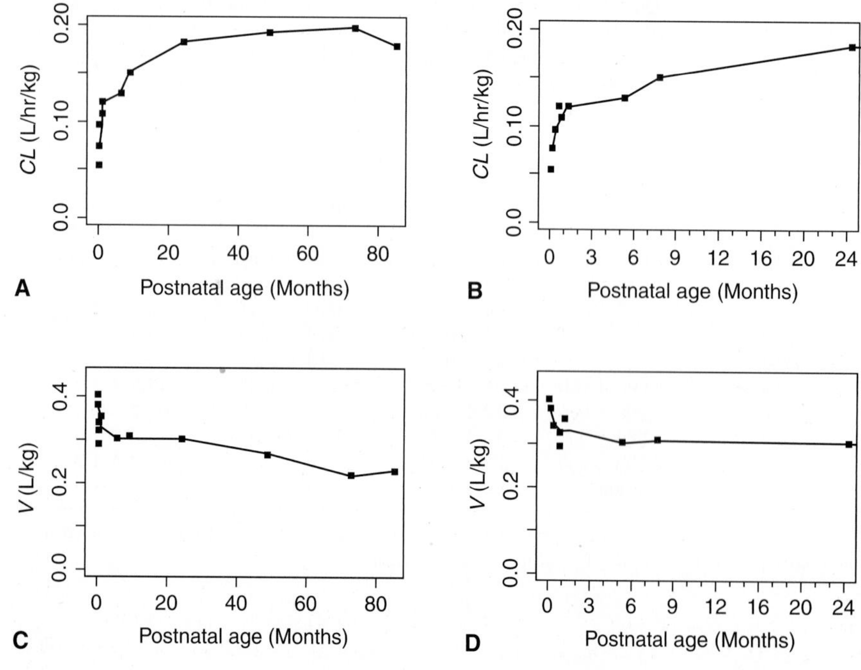

Figure 30.1. Age-dependent differences in amikacin pharmacokinetics in children. Change of mean clearance (*CL*) with increasing postnatal age for all children (**A**) and for neonates and infants only (**B**). Change of volume of distribution (*V*) with increasing postnatal age for all children (**C**) and for neonates and infants only (**D**). In every plot, each dot represents a point estimate of the mean clearance or volume of distribution for a given value of postnatal age. Solid lines correspond to the smoothed data. (Adapted from Treluyer JM, Merle Y, Tonnelier S, et al. Nonparametric population pharmacokinetic analysis of amikacin in neonates, infants, and children. *Antimicrob Agents Chemother* 2002;46:1381–1387, with permission.)

period aminoglycosides are administered in combination treatment of suspected neonatal sepsis. Monitoring the efficacy of antibiotic treatment in neonates is difficult. Culture-proven early-onset sepsis occurs in approximately 2% of VLBW infants, but there are limitations to blood cultures in neonates, and single blood cultures can be false negative (102,103). Furthermore, increasing prenatal treatment of mothers with antibiotics obscures culture results in newborns. Early detection of neonatal sepsis remains difficult. Laboratory tests are unspecific and clinical signs can be ambiguous. Neonatal sepsis is suspected in many VLBW infants on clinical grounds, and antibiotic treatment is frequently started and discontinued after 48 to 72 hours when blood cultures and results of other tests remain negative (104). Given the infrequent occurrence of positive blood cultures, these cannot be used as a marker for antibiotic efficacy. Laboratory data, including C-reactive protein, complete blood cell count, and ratio of immature to total neutrophils, lack sufficient sensitivity to detect neonatal sepsis and can therefore not be used to evaluate efficacy (105). The same counts for clinical features (e.g., respiratory rate, skin color), which either cannot be quantified or lack a clearly defined relation between predictor and outcome.

In recent years aminoglycoside dosing in children has changed to ODD. Although theoretically this should lead to an increase of efficacy and a decrease of toxicity, this has not been clearly demonstrated in adults and has not been extensively studied in infants and children. Most studies did not address dose–response effect; some studies compared ODD to multiple daily doses (MDD) (106,107). In these studies both efficacy and toxicity were comparable. Urinary tract infections were effectively treated with ODD or thrice-daily dosing (TDD) of gentamicin in 179 pediatric patients (106). Severe bacterial infections in 52 pediatric patients were equally effectively treated with ODD and TDD of gentamicin in combination with a β-lactam antibiotic. Fever as well as C-reactive protein decreased comparably in both groups (107). ODD treatment of febrile children undergoing stem cell transplantation showed a tendency for less nephrotoxicity and more efficacy (108). The combination of amikacin with a β-lactam antibiotic showed satisfactory clinical results in 98% of severe bacterial infections in 56 infants and children (109).

TOXICITY

The major specific side effects of aminoglycosides are nephrotoxicity and ototoxicity. Neurotoxicity by way of blockade of neuromuscular synapses with prolonged muscle weakness after the use of muscle relaxants has not been described in infants. The delayed-type hypersensitivity reaction of the skin is mostly seen after use of topical application of neomycin or framycetin and has not been described in neonates. Nephro- and ototoxicity will be described in further detail.

Nephrotoxicity

Aminoglycoside nephrotoxicity is induced by way of proximal tubular injury leading to cell necrosis. The mechanisms of toxicity have been mostly studied in animals, where it was shown to induce glomerular and tubular damage both pre- and postnatally (110). Less than 5% of filtered aminoglycosides binds to the brush-border membrane of proximal tubular cells and is actively reabsorbed, finally causing cell death. The degree of nephrotoxicity is determined by the quantity of aminoglycosides stored in the proximal tubular cell and the intrinsic potency of the drug to damage subcellular structures (111). In several large meta-analytical studies toxicity seems to be related to high trough concentrations, indicating that these concentrations are not low long enough to prevent renal accumulation. Nephrotoxicity related to ODD as compared with MDD was found to be equal or less in these studies (26,27,112–114). A recent prospective study in adults showed that both probability and time of occurrence of nephrotoxicity are negatively influenced by MDD (115). There is no clear distinction in level of nephrotoxicity among the four aminoglycosides in studies in adults (59).

The incidence of aminoglycoside nephrotoxicity in neonates is not well known but seems to be considerably lower than in adults. Enduring glomerular filtration impairment has not been conclusively shown in prospective studies (116–119). No difference in renal function was found between ODD and MDD for amikacin and gentamicin (117,120).

Reversible tubular dysfunction has been shown in many studies involving neonates (116,118,119,121–125) and is more pronounced in term infants than in preterm newborns (117,118,124), which is possibly explained by maturity-dependent blood supply differences of the outer parts of the kidney and lower binding constants in the immature kidney (126). In infants with a GA greater than 34 weeks no difference in proximal tubular damage was found between ODD and MDD of amikacin (117). Urinary electrolyte loss is higher at peak serum concentrations (116,121). In the ill term and especially preterm infant, who is already at risk for electrolyte disturbances, the increased loss during aminoglycoside therapy might be clinically relevant and warrants extra monitoring (127).

Incidence of nephrotoxicity in children is not well known but seems to be more uncommon than in adults (109,128,129). No difference in nephrotoxicity between ODD and MDD has been demonstrated in most studies in children (106,107,130), except for CF, were ODD showed less toxicity (54).

Ototoxicity

Aminoglycosides are potentially cochleo- and vestibulotoxic. They accumulate in the lymphatic fluid of the inner ear, from which they are only slowly eliminated (24 to 36 hours) (131). There is evidence for saturable uptake in animals (132). Certain gene mutations lead to a familial increased risk of aminoglycoside-induced sensorineural hearing loss (133). Sequentially outer hair cells, inner hair cells, and spiral ganglional neurons are damaged. Aminoglycosides seem to give a polyamine-like enhancement of glutamate *N*-methyl-D-aspartate receptor activity, resulting in excessive entry of sodium and calcium, which leads to excitotoxic cell death (134). Hearing loss is usually bilateral, symmetrical, and permanent, and can also have a delayed onset of months (131). Most authors suggest that ototoxicity is related to total dose and duration of therapy rather than to serum aminoglycoside serum concentrations, but the relation to aminoglycoside serum concentrations remains unclear. This form of toxicity usually occurs in patients who have received either long or repeated courses of aminoglycosides (135). No difference in incidence between ODD and MDD could be demonstrated (112,115). In experimental studies, amikacin appears to be more cochleotoxic than do gentamicin and tobramycin. Netilmicin is probably the least ototoxic aminoglycoside (129). Although vestibulotoxicity is a disabling side effect in adults, it has not been shown in neonates.

There are many pitfalls in relating use of aminoglycosides to loss of hearing in infants. Hearing loss in neonates occurs in 0.1% to 0.3% of cases (136). Numerous risk factors for neonatal hearing loss have been identified. Perinatal infections, meningitis, prematurity, hyperbilirubinemia, BW less than 1,500 g, asphyxia, respiratory distress syndrome, mechanical ventilation, antibiotics, and diuretics have all been incriminated (137). Even though some studies show a relation to administration of aminoglycosides, it remains difficult to separate the effect of aminoglycoside use from concomitant factors (136).

Ototoxicity is an infrequent occurrence in neonatal studies. Many studies did not find any aminoglycoside-related toxicity. In some studies delayed onset of hearing loss has been described (138,139). Several studies found a transient hearing loss (140,141). Some studies found a relation with duration (137,142) and total dose (137,143). Recently, the relation between exposure to tobramycin and the risk of detecting hearing loss with hearing screening was studied (144). Exposure to tobramycin in terms of treatment duration, total dose, or serum concentrations was not related to a failure to pass hearing screening. Cotreatment with vancomycin or loop diuretics was not associated with an increased chance of hearing loss in this study as in other studies (117,129,144,145). The results lead us to conclude that aminoglycoside-related hearing loss in infants is infrequent, possibly transient, and might be late in appearing. No clear relation was found to peak and trough concentrations. Ototoxicity in infants and children is infrequent as well, although it was not often explicitly studied. Recent studies investigating ODD and MDD of aminoglycosides did not detect any ototoxicity (107,109,130). Other studies only found transient hearing loss (146,147). In contrast, hearing loss was demonstrated in pediatric patients with CF exposed to prolonged and/or repeated aminoglycoside treatment, also with inhalation therapy (53,148,149).

AMINOGLYCOSIDE THERAPEUTIC DRUG MONITORING AND DOSING

Dose and dosing interval are determined by the desired therapeutic range and pharmacokinetic as well as pharmacodynamic properties of a drug. It is difficult to define the desired therapeutic range for aminoglycosides. Peak concentrations of greater than 4 to 5 mg per L are generally accepted as necessary for antibacterial efficacy when dosing thrice daily (17,95,150,151). Efficacy of aminoglycosides is related to the ratio of peak serum concentration to the MIC of the infecting microorganism and the AUC. In vitro ratios of 10:1 prevent emergence of aminoglycoside-resistant pathogens (14,17). Commonly accepted trough concentration goals in adults are less than 2 mg per L, but when dosing once a day, most authors keep less than 1 mg per L as a safe limit (28,152,153). Based on the aminoglycoside susceptibility of gram-negative pathogens involved in neonatal septicemia, a reasonable target range for neonates would therefore be peak serum concentrations of 5 to 10 mg per L for gentamicin, netilmicin, and tobramycin and 15 to 30 mg per L for amikacin. Trough concentration goals are less than 2 mg per L when dosing thrice daily and less than 0.5 to 1.0 mg per L for ODD in gentamicin, netilmicin, and tobramycin and 1.5 to 3 mg per L for amikacin.

Neonates

Aminoglycoside dosing in newborns has been revised toward larger doses at extended intervals (1,12). A substantial reduction in inter- and intraindividual variation of serum concentrations can be achieved with the use of dedicated pediatric vials as has been demonstrated for amikacin (154). Recent studies have demonstrated that serum concentrations as described in the foregoing can be reached with doses of 3.5 to 5 mg per kg (gentamicin, tobramycin, netilmicin) and 7.5 to 20 mg per kg (amikacin) (81,85, 120,155–161). From the viewpoint of efficacy it is important to obtain an adequate peak serum concentration after the first dose, which has led several authors to advise a loading dose of aminoglycosides (87,153,160,162). This goal can also be reached without loading doses (64,155). Dosing intervals range from 12 to 48 hours, depending on GA and PNA.

Dosing charts for neonates of varying GAs and PNAs have been developed as well (163,164).

Routine TDM for aminoglycosides is normally performed around the third or fourth dose and is based on the assumption that steady state is more or less attained. For several reasons this assumption is not valid in neonates in the first week of life. Antibiotic courses in neonates are often discontinued after a few days when blood cultures and other tests remain negative. Because extended-interval (24 to 48 hours, depending on GA) dosing of aminoglycosides is now a general practice, steady state would not be reached before discontinuation of the drug, and TDM would therefore not be performed in time to be of use. Using population pharmacokinetic principles and Bayesian feedback it was postulated that two serum samples after the first dose (1 hour and 12 to 18 hours) could help optimize TDM, but this still needs to be validated (165). Efficacy and toxicity have not been clearly related to peak or trough serum concentrations with extended dose intervals, and clinically important nephro- and ototoxicity are rare in neonates in courses shorter than 7 days. Furthermore, subsequent serum concentrations cannot be adequately predicted in this age group (15,64). The importance of routine TDM in the first week of life for efficacy and toxicity reasons has therefore been questioned. An exception should be made for neonatal patients with renal failure, patients with obvious neonatal asphyxia (e.g., 5′ Apgar score of <5 at 5 minutes), and patients exposed to drugs or situations that are known to significantly alter pharmacokinetic behavior (e.g., indomethacin, ECMO). In these difficult-to-manage patients use of a population model with feedback of repeated serum concentrations as well as repeated serum creatinine might be useful in guiding therapy.

Infants and Children

Aminoglycoside dosing in infants and children has changed toward ODD over the last decade. A number of studies have evaluated ODD versus TDD, with daily doses varying from 4.5 to 7.5 mg per kg (106,130,146,166). These studies contain a heterogeneous patient population of serious gram-negative infections and urinary tract infections. Mean peak concentrations obtained with ODD were 9.8 to 20.4 mg per L and sufficient for most microorganisms to obtain a peak/MIC ratio of greater than 10. Mean trough concentrations range from 0.18 to 0.5 mg per L. A meta-analysis has shown similar results in efficacy and toxicity for ODD versus TDD (167).

Routine TDM is normally performed around the third or fourth dose. Predicting future serum concentrations in a pediatric population with the help of a Bayesian feedback model is possible (168,169). The necessity of routine TDM in pediatric patients with normal renal function and receiving short courses (<10 days) is still questionable (170,171).

GLYCOPEPTIDES

GENERAL ASPECTS OF GLYCOPEPTIDE ANTIBIOTICS

Glycopeptide antibiotics are a group of antibiotics with related structure and similar antimicrobial activity. The two major clinically important compounds in this group are vancomycin and teicoplanin. Vancomycin is an antibiotic first isolated from an Indonesian jungle soil sample in 1956, and was the first of the class of glycopeptide antibiotics. It was largely supplanted by methicillin sodium, introduced in 1960, because of the frequent occurrence of side effects associated with vancomycin use, including generalized skin eruptions, phlebitis, fever, and, more importantly, deafness and renal failure (172,173). Reduction of impurities and a concomitant decrease in incidence of side effects as well as the emergence of methicillin-resistant staphylococci have led to a resurgence of vancomycin use (174–176). Teicoplanin was introduced in 1982.

Despite the emergence of vancomycin-resistant enterococci, vancomycin still is the most widely used glycopeptide antibiotic and is a cornerstone in antibiotic treatment of gram-positive infections in adults, children, and neonates.

Structure and Chemical Properties

Vancomycin and teicoplanin are the commonly used glycopeptide antibiotics and are unrelated to other antibiotics. They are complex soluble glycopeptides, consisting of a seven-membered peptide chain, in the form of three large rings. Five of the seven amino acid residues are common to all glycopeptides (177–179). A disaccharide, composed of glucose and vancosamine, is also present but is not part of the cyclic structure. The molecular weight of vancomycin is 1,448 daltons (180).

Vancomycin is hydrophobic but less so than teicoplanin (179). It has a moderate protein binding in adults (10% to 55%) and exerts its activity over a wide pH range of 6.5 to 8 (181,182). Protein binding in neonates is higher (72% to 81%), but binding to bilirubin is not concentration dependent indicating a low possibility of an increase in free bilirubin (183). Vancomycin can be inactivated by heparin in high concentrations (184). Teicoplanin can be added to parenteral solutions (185).

Method of Action

The bactericidal activity of glycopeptide antibiotics is based on the inhibition of bacterial cell wall synthesis. Vancomycin as well as teicoplanin complex, by way of hydrogen binding, to the D-alanyl-D-alanine portion of peptides found only in bacterial cell walls. The binding of this large molecule to the peptide side chain shields the substrate from the enzyme peptidoglycan synthetase (186). This interferes with cross-linking of cell wall peptidoglycans, and therefore bacterial cell wall rigidity cannot be achieved (179,180,187). The mechanism of action implies that vancomycin can only exert its effect on growing bacteria. Other, less important modes of action are alteration of the permeability of cytoplasmic membranes and selective inhibition of RNA synthesis (188,189).

In Vitro Antimicrobial Activity

Glycopeptides are bactericidal for a host of aerobic and anaerobic gram-positive bacteria. Strains of *S. epidermidis* and *S. aureus* are susceptible, although emergence of vancomycin-intermediate-resistant strains is a growing concern, which will be discussed later (190).

Normal MICs are in the range of 1 to 5 mg per L (187). For teicoplanin there is no simple relationship between serum levels and efficacy (191). The MIC_{90} for *S. aureus* is less than 1 mg per L (in 90% of cases), as it is for *Enterococcus faecalis* and *E. faecium*. The MIC_{90} is 4 to 6 mg per L for *S. epidermidis*. Vancomycin is bacteriostatic for enterococci (181). Teicoplanin is active against vancomycin-resistant *S. aureus* and *Enterococcus* species.

Important aspects of the antimicrobial activity of vancomycin for clinical practice are (a) lack of concentration-dependent killing, (b) a PAE, and (c) synergism with other antibiotics.

Lack of Concentration-Dependent Killing

Several recent studies have shown that the extent of bacterial killing is not related to peak serum concentrations but is related to the time the antibiotic concentration is maintained above the MIC (192–194). This may, however, be dependent on time of exposition. An in vivo study showed that in the first 12 hours the MIC was the most important factor, whereas for the total first 24 hours the AUC was more important (192–195). There are conflicting conclusions in the translation of in vitro and in vivo results to vancomycin dosing. Most authors advocate 12-hour intervals in adults. Some give continuous infusion and others dose once daily (196–198). Treatment failures due to ODD have been described (199,200). Continuous infusion of vancomycin was proven to be as effective as intermittent dosing (196,201). For teicoplanin, which has a longer serum half-life, ODD is commonly used.

Postantibiotic Effect

Vancomycin shows an in vitro PAE against *S. aureus, S. epidermidis,* and enterococcal species, lasting 1 to 6 hours (193,202–204). The PAE for teicoplanin against *S. aureus* is 2.4 to 4.1 hours (205).

As with aminoglycosides, PAE should be studied under conditions simulating time-versus-concentration curves seen in clinical practice. The duration of PAE seems to be far longer when bacteria remain exposed to vancomycin concentrations of 0.1 to 0.3 mg per L, indicating a sub-MIC effect (193). In vivo experiments relating PAE to vancomycin concentrations are scarce. A definite conclusion on the clinical importance of the PAE of vancomycin cannot be drawn.

Synergy with Other Antibiotics

Combination of vancomycin with an aminoglycoside or rifampicin is synergistic for *S. aureus* (both methicillin-sensitive and methicillin-resistant strains) and *S. epidermidis* and enterococcal infections (34,35). Teicoplanin and rifampicin are antagonistic (206). In enterococcal infections synergy can be achieved in most cases by adding an aminoglycoside as well (207).

DRUG RESISTANCE

Clinically important resistance to glycopeptides is seen in enterococci, *S. aureus,* and *S. epidermidis.* An unsettling increase of vancomycin-resistant enterococci has been noted in the United States, related to selection pressure by indiscriminate use of vancomycin (208,209). Resistance in enterococci has been linked to at least four genes and types of resistance, Van A, Van B, Van C, and Van D. Van A and Van B resistance can be transferred by way of plasmid conjugation to other enterococci (197,210). Van A leads to vancomycin and teicoplanin resistance and Van B resistance retains susceptibility to teicoplanin (181). The Van C phenotype shows low-level vancomycin resistance but remains susceptible to teicoplanin (197,211,212). There is an increasing number of reports on intermediate resistance in *S. aureus* and *S. epidermidis* (190). MIC values as high as 16 mg per L with minimal bactericidal concentrations of 64 mg per L have been reported for *S. epidermidis,* with a concomitant resistance to teicoplanin (213). The emergence of vancomycin-intermediate-resistant strains of *S. aureus* (VIRSA) is of concern (190,214). Resistance is related to thickened and aggregated cell walls (215). There is cross-resistance to teicoplanin. Infection with VIRSA is associated with treatment failure of vancomycin (216).

An important mechanical factor in clinical resistance of *S. epidermidis* infections to vancomycin is the production of a biofilm by the bacteria, which shields it from the antibiotic, with a consequent reduction of antibiotic efficacy (217,218). Furthermore, glycopeptides are large molecules, which inhibit diffusion into localized infection sites like endocarditis.

INDICATIONS

Glycopeptide antibiotics are the drugs of choice for methicillin-resistant strains of staphylococcal infections. They are an alternative, though less effective, for patients with methicillin-susceptible organisms who are allergic to penicillins or cephalosporins. In case of prosthetic-device-related *S. epidermidis* infections they should be combined with an aminoglycoside or rifampicin to enhance efficacy (34). In serious enterococcal infections they should be combined with an aminoglycoside as well. They are also used for the treatment of penicillin-resistant streptococci and enterococci. Use in possible or proven pneumococcal meningitis should be considered given the increase of penicillin resistance. One indication is described in more detail in the next subsection.

Line-Related Infections in Neonates and Children

Vancomycin and teicoplanin are widely used as empiric antibiotics for the treatment of line-related infections in neonates, especially due to the increase of coagulase-negative staphylococci as a cause of late-onset neonatal sepsis (219,220). Late-onset neonatal septicemia has significant impact on outcome and length of hospital stay (221–223). In this setting, the continuous use of low-dose vancomycin or teicoplanin added to parenteral nutrition has been advocated (224–229). Although a reduction in number of catheter-related gram-positive infections in preterm infants has been shown, no decrease in mortality or length of stay has been proven (230,231). In these studies an increase in vancomycin resistant organisms has not been demonstrated (231,232). Still, given the concerns about development of resistance by overuse of vancomycin, routine prophylaxis with low-dose vancomycin should not be given (230,233,234). Line-related infections in children are also primarily treated with a glycopeptide antibiotic combined with a third-generation cephalosporin. In neutropenic children the combination of ceftazidime with aminoglycoside with addition of a glycopeptide is often used as initial empiric treatment. Prevention of central venous catheter-related infections in immunocompromised children with use of a vancomycin/ciprofloxacin/heparin flush has been suggested (235). Prophylactic treatment with teicoplanin in neutropenic patients has been advocated as well (236). However, as in neonates, development of resistance is of primary concern (233).

PHARMACOKINETICS

Glycopeptides have a pharmacokinetic profile consisting of a distribution phase ($t_{1/2\alpha}$), which is longer than in aminoglycosides, and an elimination phase ($t_{1/2\beta}$). They are eliminated from the body primarily by way of glomerular filtration. After 24 hours, 80% to 90% of an administered dose of vancomycin can be recovered from urine in adults (197). A small amount is eliminated by nonrenal mechanisms of unknown origin (237). Glycopeptide pharmacokinetics in pediatric patients has been described using a model-independent, one- or two-compartment model. A one-compartment model seems to be a valid tool in predicting serum concentrations in the postdistribution phase (237,238). Because in most studies peak serum concentrations 1 hour after a 1-hour infusion are considered, this is very likely the case. Earlier, serum sampling in the distribution phase might lead to an underestimation of the apparent volume of distribution (V_d). Tables 30.3 and 30.4

TABLE 30.3 Results of Pharmacokinetic Studies of Glycopeptides in Neonates

Antibiotic/ Patient Group	*N*	*GA (wk)*	*PNA (d)*	*PCA (wk)*	*BW (g)*	*CL (mL/min/kg)*	V_d *(L/kg)*	$t_{1/2}$ *(hr)*	*Reference*
Vancomycin									
Dose 10 mg/kg	7	32	3.3		1,230	15[a]	0.74[b]	9.8	240
Dose 15 mg/kg	7	34	4.7		1,570	27[a]	0.71[b]	5.9	240
Dose 15 mg/kg	7	40	2.6		3,070	30[a]	0.69[b]	6.7	240
Weight ≤ 1 kg	3		29[c]	30[c]	830[c]	1.099 ± 0.293	0.97 ± 0.43[b]	9.92 ± 2.59	256
Weight > 1 kg	6		40[c]	32.7[c]	1,378[c]	1.030 ± 0.22	0.65 ± 0.36[b]	5.35 ± 0.77	256
No means available	11	27–40	27	29–41	850–4,380			3.5–9.6	242
PCA < 41 wk	14	26–40	8–66	32–41		1.34 ± 0.46	0.48 ± 0.17	4.87	260
PCA > 43 wk	6	31	90–210	54.2		1.67 ± 0.61	0.38 ± 0.04	3.04	260
	20	26.5		36.4	1,300		0.69 ± 0.15		264
First dose	15	28.4	21	31.4	1,069	1.22 ±0.7[d]	0.53 ± 0.13	6.0 ± 2.0	248
Steady state	12					1.16 ± 0.6[d]	0.52 ± 0.1	6.6 ± 2.1	248
	13	29.8[c]	30[c]	38[c]	1,375[c]	1.44 ± 0.89[c]	0.47 ± 0.15[c]	5.1 ± 3.0[c]	259
	15	29.0	29	33.2	1,297	1.07 ± 0.34	0.48 ± 0.09	5.6 ± 1.6	258
	11		10[c]	30.9[c]	1,262[c]	0.74 ± 0.20[c]	0.51 ± 0.03[b,c]	8.5 ± 2.8[c]	257
	29	31.2	18	33.4	1,860	1.01 ± 0.37	0.55 ± 0.21		266
PCA 27–30 wk	16	26.6	18	29.4	972	1.00 ± 0.07	0.55 ± 0.02	6.63 ± 0.35	220
PCA 31–36 wk	15	29.4	23	32.9	1,379	1.17 ± 0.08	0.56 ± 0.02	5.59 ± 0.36	220
PCA ≥37 wk	13	35.9	24	39.2	2,616	1.33 ± 0.08	0.57 ± 0.02	4.90 ± 0.39	220
Day 2	15		90		6,400	1.5 ± 0.5	0.81 ± 0.6	5.3 ± 3.2	262
Day 8	15		90		6,400	1.2 ± 0.4	0.44 ± 0.19	3.4 ± 1.2	255
	11	30.8	18	33.4	1,186	0.63 ± 0.18	0.48 ± 0.13		241
Standard dose	24	29.2	30	33.5	1,500	1.19 ± 0.55			198
Adjusted dose	29	30.5	24	33.9	1,800	0.99 ± 0.41	0.61 ± 0.39		198
Development algorithm	72	29.4	26	32.9		1.26 ± 0.55	0.65 ± 0.34	6.9 ± 4.5	254
Testing algorithm	17	28.4	39	32.0		1.40 ± 0.67	0.67 ± 0.28	6.5 ± 3.3	254
Exposed to indomethacin	4	26	18	28.5	810	0.6 ± 0.17	0.57 ± 0.06	11.9 ± 3.7	274
No indomethacin	19	29.3	34	34.2	1,780	1.2 ± 0.53	0.52 ± 0.08	5.6 ± 1.6	274
PDA + indomethacin	6		7	29.0		0.38 ± 0.15	0.71 ± 0.36	24.6 ± 12.4	261
No PDA controls	5		15	32.0		0.90 ± 0.57	0.48 ± 0.17	7.0 ± 1.8	261
ECMO	12	39	2[e]		3,300	0.78 ± 0.19	1.06 ± 0.45	16.9 ± 9.5	281
ECMO	15	38.8	13		3,100	0.65 ± 0.28	0.45 ± 0.18	8.29 ± 2.23	282
No ECMO	15	39.7	8		3,400	0.79 ± 0.41	0.39 ± 0.12	6.53 ± 2.05	282
NONMEM[f] Two-compartment	192	29.6	15		1,480		0.76 ± 54.1%[g]		238
NONMEM[f] One-compartment	30	27.6	16		1,305		0.50 ± 19.3%[g]		238
NONMEM analysis[f]	59	29	19	32	1,520		0.67 ± 18%[g]		263
NONMEM analysis[f]	108	28.9	14		1,045	0.95 ± 31%[g]	0.43 ± 25%[g]	6 ± 34%[g]	376
NONMEM analysis[f]	37	33.5	70		2,820				
NONMEM analysis[f]	59	24–34	11.9		1,300				279
		24				0.9 ±1 9%[g,h]	39 ± 19%[g,h]		279
		34				2.0 ± 19%[g,h]	39 ± 19%[g,h]		279
Teicoplanin									
NICU	4	Term	3–25		3,260	0.26 ± 0.05	0.61 ± 0.08	30.3 ± 6.3	245
5 mg/kg ODD	34	VLBW					0.25 ± 0.07	29.2 ± 27.9	
3 mg/kg TDD	15	VLBW					0.31 ± 0.12	43.2 ± 29.8	227

BW, Body weight; *CL*, clearance; ECMO, extracorporeal membrane oxygenation; GA, gestational age, mean value; *N*, number of patients; NICU, neonatal intensive care unit; NONMEM, nonlinear mixed-effects modeling; ODD, once-daily dosing; PCA, postconception age; PDA, patent ductus arteriosus; PNA, postnatal age; $t_{1/2}$, serum half-life; TDD, thrice-daily dosing; V_d, volume of distribution; VLBW, very low birth weight.

[a] mL/min/1.73 m^2.

[b] Apparent volume of distribution of β-phase.

[c] Calculated from individual values for patients.

[d] mL/min.

[e] Age when put on ECMO.

[f] Population analysis.

[g] Population mean ± interindividual variability.

[h] *CL* in L/hr/70 kg, V_d in L/70 kg.

TABLE 30.4 Results of Pharmacokinetic Studies of Glycopeptides in Infants and Children

Antibiotic/ Patient Group	*N*	*Age*	*CL (mL/min/kg)*	V_d *(L/kg)*	$t_{1/2}$ *(h)*	*Reference*
Vancomycin						
Cancer patients	28	4.0 ± 3.3 yr	2.55 ± 0.55	0.63 ± 0.08	3.0 ± 0.5	345
Cancer patients	33	5.7 ± 4.1 yr	2.48 ± 0.47	0.64 ± 0.08	3.1 ± 0.6	301
Infants and children	31	4.2 ± 5.1 yr	1.90 ± 0.52	0.62 ± 0.10	4.0 ± 0.9	301
CSF shunt placement	8	8.3 ± 7.0 yr	1.83 ± 0.83[a]	0.54 ± 0.15[b]	4.8 ± 4.0	291
Cancer patients	30	6.0 ± 4.7 yr	1.83 ± 1.67	0.62 ± 0.3	10.5 ± 7.9	302
Controls	8	5.4 ± 4.1 yr	1.0 ± 1.0	1.3 ± 0.6	14.9 ± 9.1	302
General pediatric, population model	78		1.72 ± 45%[c]	0.43 ± 43%[c]	3.9 ± 57%[c]	358
MRSA	49			0.52 (0.44–0.60)[d]		377
	12	3.1 mo	50[e]	0.60	4.1	240
	4	4.3 mo	81[e]	0.96	4.1	240
	5	3.9 yr	163[e]	0.82	2.4	240
	7	5.58 yr	131[e]	0.76	3.0	240
	6	7.58 yr	134[e]	0.54	2.2	240
Teicoplanin						
Urinary infection	6	7 yr	0.47 ± 0.1	0.54 ± 0.17	20.5 ± 5.5	262
Bone marrow transplant	21	5.2 ± 3.5 yr	0.48 ± 0.16[a]	0.69 ± 0.30[b]	21.4 ± 4.9	335
Prophylaxis	21		0.83 ± 0.08[f]	0.83 ± 0.08[f,g]	51.8 ± 2.7[f]	275
PICU (no renal failure) day 1	12	6 ± 3.1 yr	0.66 ± 0.04	0.46 ± 0.04	11.3 ± 1.0	299
PICU (no renal failure) day 5	12	6 ± 3.1 yr	0.61 ± 0.04	0.56 ± 0.09	16.1 ± 3.4	299
	6	4–12 yr	0.47	0.54	20.5	378
PICU (no renal failure)	21	7 d–12 yr	0.75	1.02	17.4	284

N, Number of patients in study; *CL*, clearance; V_d, volume of distribution; $t_{1/2}$, serum half-life; CSF, cerebrospinal fluid; MRSA, methicillin-resistant *Staphylococcus aureus*; PICU, pediatric intensive care unit.
[a]Two-compartment model, overall clearance.
[b]Two-compartment model, total distribution volume.
[c]Population mean ± interindividual variability.
[d]Population mean ± 95% confidence interval.
[e]mL/min/1.73 m^2.
[f]Mean ± SE.
[g]Volume of distribution at steady state.

display age-related pharmacokinetic parameters for glycopeptides in neonates, infants, and children.

Pharmacokinetics in Neonates

Pharmacokinetic parameters of vancomycin in neonates are different from those in adults. These differences are largely determined by the change in amount of body water and maturation of renal function in the first weeks of life, both in term and preterm newborn infants. This means that neonates and especially prematures have a larger V_d and decreased *CL* than do infants, children, and adults. These changes also result in higher interindividual differences in neonates than in adults.

Vancomycin is mostly used intravenously in neonates. Distribution half-life ($t_{1/2\alpha}$) is approximately 0.5 to 1 hour in adults (239). In neonates and infants it ranges from 0.05 to 0.49 hour but has only been determined explicitly in one study in which data for infants and neonates were pooled (240). Others have suggested that $t_{1/2\alpha}$ might be longer, even up to 4 hours (238,241,242). Average V_d in the steady state (V_{ss}) in term neonates for vancomycin as well as teicoplanin ranges from 0.57 to 0.69 L per kg, although very few studies, totaling only 31 patients, have specifically looked at this age group. For neonates of various GAs, V_{ss} ranges from 0.38 to 0.97 L per kg. Surprisingly, for VLBW on teicoplanin a low V_d was found in one study (0.25 to 0.31 L per kg) (227). In special subgroups, especially neonates on ECMO, V_{ss} is even higher. The overall V_{ss} range is comparable to values described in adults (239). As mentioned by Rodvold et al. (243), V_d studied after a single dose or calculated with the elimination $t_{1/2\beta}$ was often larger than V_{ss}. Distribution correlates well with several clinical parameters, as shown in Table 30.3.

Because meningitis often accompanies sepsis in neonates, penetration of vancomycin in cerebrospinal fluid (CSF) is of possible concern. Vancomycin dosing leads to CSF concentrations of 7% to 21% of the serum concentration in adults (197). The initial study in infants found a similar percentage (240). Later reports mentioned CSF concentrations ranging from 0.2 to 17.3 mg per L, with vancomycin CSF penetration ranging from 7.1% to 68% (244–247). No clear relation of CSF concentration to serum concentration was found. As in adults, there is a significant correlation between CSF concentration and markers for meningeal inflammation (181,244). Data on this subject are scarce, however, and vancomycin cannot be relied on to adequately treat gram-positive meningitis when given as a single antibiotic.

There are no data on pharmacokinetics of intraventricular administration of vancomycin in neonates.

In neonates 44% of vancomycin was recovered unchanged in urine after 8 hours (248). Factors that have to be considered in excretion are *CL*, mainly determined by renal function, and serum half-life, which is dependent on the elimination rate constant (K_e). There are several important clinical features, discussed in what follows, that influence pharmacokinetic behavior in neonates.

Mean *CL* of vancomycin in adults (0.71 to 1.31 mL per kg per minute) is often higher than that reported in neonates and infants, although ranges are similar (249–252).

In neonates, vancomycin *CL* ranges from 0.63 to 1.5 mL per kg per minute, depending on GA and/or post conceptional age (PCA) (Table 30.3). Teicoplanin *CL* is lower, at 0.26 mL per kg per minute. Vancomycin $t_{1/2\beta}$ in adults ranges from 4 to 8 hours in patients with normal renal function. Mean $t_{1/2\beta}$ in neonates of varying gestational and postconceptional ages ranges from 3.5 to 10 hours (220,240,248, 253–261) for vancomycin and from 29.2 to 43.2 hours for teicoplanin (227,262).

Given the route of elimination, an association between GFR and excretion is logical. Serum creatinine and creatinine *CL* in neonates have been correlated to *CL* of vancomycin in several studies (198,242,257,258,263–267). In population pharmacokinetic studies the importance of creatinine *CL* as a covariate differs. Three studies found creatinine and creatinine *CL* to be an important covariate (263,268,269), but two others did not (238,267). One study did not include creatinine or creatinine *CL* as a covariate in the model (238). In the case of terminal renal failure, vancomycin *CL* by way of hemodialysis and/or peritoneal dialysis is slow, with a single dose of 15 mg per kg leading to trough serum concentrations of greater than 4 to 5 mg per L after 7 days in adults (270). In neonates with terminal renal failure, a dosing regimen of 15 mg per kg once a week seems justified. In neonates with renal failure, vancomycin *CL* can be significantly increased by using venovenous hemodiafiltration with a high-flux membrane (271).

Taken together, the published evidence strongly favors a clear relation between renal function in terms of serum creatinine or creatinine *CL* and the *CL* of vancomycin.

Several clinical features are important for pharmacokinetic behavior in neonates. Gestational age, PNA, and postconceptional age can all be expected to alter pharmacokinetics of vancomycin, and all three age-related factors have been related to vancomycin pharmacokinetics in neonates.

The V_d of most drugs is larger in neonates than in adults, especially in prematures and is primarily due to a higher percentage of extracellular water (67,68). Creatinine *CL* (mL per minute) shows a positive correlation with GA (272,273). On the basis of GA, premature neonates are expected to have a longer $t_{1/2\beta}$ due to both a larger V_d and a decreased *CL*. In most studies both unstandardized vancomycin *CL* and V_{ss} demonstrate a relation to GA, but significance disappears when these parameters are normalized for weight (258,266,267). This implies that if weight is incorporated in the model description, GA is not an important determinant of vancomycin V_{ss} or *CL*.

The postnatal increase in GFR seen in neonates and the reduction of extracellular fluid (75–77) imply that $t_{1/2\beta}$ for vancomycin should decrease with increasing PNA. This is an inconsistent finding in studies (220,242,248,257–260, 266,267,274). V_{ss} (L), but not standardized V_{ss} (L per kg), has been related to PNA (258,266). Postconceptional age has been well described in relation to pharmacokinetic parameters for vancomycin. As might be expected on the basis of both the influence of GA as well as PNA, there is also a positive relation between postconceptional age and development of renal function (272). Clearance (mL per minute) as well as standardized *CL* (mL per kg per minute) has been related to PCA with a concomitant change in $t_{1/2\beta}$ (198,220,242,248,258–260,264–268,274). PCA is strongly correlated with weight, partly explaining the relation of weight to pharmacokinetic parameters in several studies (238,242,267–269,274). As with PNA, only unstandardized V_{ss} (L) has a significant correlation with PCA (220,248, 258,266,274).

Overall, PCA has a stronger influence on vancomycin pharmacokinetics than GA or PNA. The diminished influence of GA and PNA can be explained by several factors. The combined effects of GA and PNA are integrated in PCA. Also, prenatal exposure to corticosteroids seems to increase maturation of renal function prenatally and therefore limit the effect of GA on *CL* (76). Furthermore, postnatal increase of GFR seems to be higher than intrauterine increase (275). At the same PCA, this might imply that the effect of slower maturation of kidney function in prematures is canceled out by the difference in intra- and extrauterine development of GFR. A third and maybe more important factor is that vancomycin is seldom given in the first week of life. Because a large increase of kidney function in neonates takes place in this period, the dynamics of these changes and their influence on vancomycin pharmacokinetics are not seen in the studies mentioned here. These data suggest that *CL* in relation to postconceptional age is the main determinant in the pharmacokinetic profile of vancomycin in neonates.

Prenatal as well as postnatal exposure to indomethacin has been shown to negatively affect increase of kidney function in neonates (76,276,277). A PDA can increase V_{ss} and decrease *CL* in neonates (275,278). Several studies have addressed the effect of indomethacin or ibuprofen treatment of PDA on vancomycin pharmacokinetics in newborns (261,267,274,279). Although a definite conclusion cannot be drawn on the grounds of these studies, they suggest that indomethacin treatment of PDA leads to an increase of V_d and a decrease of *CL*, warranting extra TDM in these patients.

ECMO influences pharmacokinetic behavior of drugs in neonates. Clearance of vancomycin is decreased, V_d is higher, and serum half-life is longer in most studies (280–283). Although these studies were relatively small and results were somewhat obscured by differences in renal function, a longer serum half-life in vancomycin-treated neonates on ECMO is likely.

Pharmacokinetics in Infants and Children

Distribution half-life ($t_{1/2\alpha}$) in pediatric studies ranges from 0.04 to 1.11 hours for vancomycin and 0.79 to 2.0 hours for teicoplanin (240,284–286). Volume of distribution of vancomycin as well as teicoplanin appears to be smaller than in adults. Teicoplanin is distributed mainly to a third compartment in neonates; in children a bicompartmental model may suffice (248,286). Surprisingly, in children younger than 1 year V_d and *CL* are threefold lower than in children older than 1 year leading to a larger percentage of expected subtherapeutic serum concentrations in older children (286).

Continuous intraperitoneal treatment of peritonitis in children on dialysis with either vancomycin 30 mg per L or teicoplanin 20 mg per L of dialysate leads to serum concentrations of approximately 20 mg per L after 1 week for both antibiotics (287). The bioavailability of vancomycin during intraperitoneal administration is 70% (288). Intermittent (once a week treatment) with vancomycin (30 mg per kg) or teicoplanin (15 mg per kg) results in trough serum concentrations after 1 week of 8 to 10 mg per L (287). As in neonates, distribution to CSF is of interest. Intravenous administration of vancomycin leads to an average vancomycin CSF concentration of 10% of the serum concentration, without a significant correlation in individual patients with ventricular shunt infections (244). In children, Spears and Koch (289) reported CSF concentrations of less than 0.8 mg per L in seven samples 1 to 12 hours after the vancomycin dose. In pediatric patients with meningitis a CSF-to-serum ratio of 0.14 to 0.28 was found (290). However, penetration is only 0.77% to 18% in patients without meningeal or ventricular inflammation (291,292).

Daily intrathecal administration of 10 mg of teicoplanin or 20 mg of vancomycin led to trough CSF concentrations of 3.3 to 4.8 and 14.5 to 193 mg per L, respectively, in single patient and showed wide variability in patients exposed to combined intravenous and intrathecal treatment, warranting TDM (293–296).

Vancomycin showed prolonged elimination from CSF in an accidental case of intraventricular administration (295). Teicoplanin concentrations in pus range from 37% to 110% of serum concentrations (297).

On cardiopulmonary bypass vancomycin and teicoplanin concentrations drop by 77% and 53%, respectively (298).

Vancomycin and teicoplanin *CL* depends mainly on renal function. Clearance of glycopeptide antibiotics is more rapid in children than in adults, though reasons for this phenomenon are not clear (240,299). As with distribution, age-related differences in *CL* are not well known, though *CL* of vancomycin seems to peak at 1 year and then decrease (274). For teicoplanin there is no age-related difference in elimination half-life (300). Clearance in pediatric oncology as well as pediatric intensive care patients is higher (284,299,301,302). Initiation of cardiopulmonary bypass abruptly decreases vancomycin concentrations by 44.5% (303). Clearance on ECMO is dependent on the duration of use of the membrane (304). Clearance with peritoneal dialysis depends on the time of indwelling fluid and accounts for 25% to 32% of total body clearance (288).

MICROBIOLOGIC AND CLINICAL EFFICACY AND RESISTANCE

Vancomycin is bactericidal for a host of aerobic and anaerobic gram-positive bacteria. Strains of *S. epidermidis* and *S. aureus* are susceptible to vancomycin, although emergence of vancomycin-intermediate-resistant strains is a growing concern (190). Vancomycin is bacteriostatic for enterococci (181).

Based on in vitro studies, vancomycin trough concentrations should exceed 4 to 5 mg per L (305). Vancomycin CSF concentrations of 5 to 10 mg per L are needed for the treatment of CNS infections (306).

Vancomycin is still widely used as the first-choice antibiotic for the treatment of CNS infections in neonates (307). This choice is mostly based on the in vitro activity of this antibiotic. A second reason is that vancomycin-resistant gram-positive pathogens are still uncommon in the NICU and have not seemed to increase over recent years. Vancomycin is also used for the treatment of methicillin-resistant *S. aureus* in the NICU, but no studies on efficacy in this patient group have been performed.

Data on clinical efficacy of vancomycin in adults are scarce. No correlation has been shown between serum vancomycin concentrations and clinical cure. Regimens associated with peak and trough concentrations ranging from 18 to 47 and from 2 to 13 μg per mL, respectively, showed acceptable rates of effectiveness, but failures in these treatment groups had the same serum concentrations (308). Serum bactericidal titers of greater than 1:8 are related to treatment success and high minimal bactericidal titer-to-MIC ratios to treatment failure, but exact information pertaining to efficacy does not exist (309,310). Data on efficacy in pediatric patients are scarce. Vancomycin was effectively used in neonates and infants of varying GAs and dosing regimens (247,260,289,311). Vancomycin had a clinical success rate of 89% of children and 77% of neonates with various gram-positive infections (311,312). A relation to serum bactericidal titers of 1:8 was observed with vancomycin peak concentrations of 12 mg per L or more (247). Continuous infusion of vancomycin was effective in 13 documented invasive infections with concentrations ranging from 3 to 37.6 mg per L (198). Intermittent as well as continuous vancomycin or teicoplanin is effective in treating peritoneal dialysis-associated peritonitis. For vancomycin there are no definitive data relating serum concentrations to effect. These studies, with relative few numbers of patients, show that a wide range of vancomycin peak and trough concentrations is effective against gram-positive infections, especially coagulase negative staphylococci, in neonates and infants. These results, however, do not validate the presently used therapeutic range of peak concentrations of 20 to 40 mg per L and trough concentrations of 5 to 10 mg per L.

Teicoplanin dosage regimens were based on the need to obtain trough serum concentrations above the MIC. Research in adults has indicated the need to give higher doses for deep-seated infections. Serum trough concentrations greater than 10 mg per L are associated with higher success rates in adults (313). Teicoplanin is effective in treating late-onset neonatal sepsis with median trough serum concentrations of 12.3 mg per L and 32% of troughs less than 10 mg per L (314). Clinical and bacteriologic response in neonates with daily doses of 8 to 10 mg per kg after a loading dose of 10 to 20 mg per kg ranges from 80% to 100% (315). Daily doses of 10 mg per kg in children and 6 mg per kg in neonates appear to be sufficient for efficacy (315,316). A dose of 8 mg per kg per 12 hours is recommended in pediatric intensive care unit patients to achieve serum trough concentrations greater than 1 mg per L. In febrile neutropenic children maintenance doses of 20 mg per kg are needed to obtain trough serum concentrations greater than 10 mg per L. In this patient group teicoplanin 10 mg per kg (with loading doses) is effective in combination treatment with other antibiotics (317,318). As with vancomycin, no clear relation between serum concentrations and effect has been demonstrated in the pediatric population.

TOXICITY

Toxicity related to glycopeptides, mainly vancomycin use, has been the subject of numerous reports. Toxicity can be divided into infusion-related adverse effects and drug-related toxicity. The most frequent problem encountered was the "red man" syndrome, a histamine-mediated rash of the face, neck, upper trunk, back, and arms. This phenomenon, extremely uncommon with teicoplanin, is associated with pruritus, tingling, flushing, tachycardia, and shock, and is related to the rate of infusion (187). It has been described in neonates and children, related to an infusion duration of less than 1 hour, and in 7 of 20 patients with infusion duration of 1 hour or more (240,245). Three cases of cardiac arrest (two fatal) associated with rapid infusion of vancomycin have been described (289,319,320). The incidence of most of these side effects decreased enormously with the removal of impurities from early preparations in the 1960s. Reported drug-related toxicity includes neutropenia, thrombocytopenia, eosinophilia, trombophlebitis, chills, fever, rash, nephrotoxicity, and ototoxicity. Nephro- and ototoxicity are described in more detail in what follows.

Nephrotoxicity

Vancomycin can cause reversible nephrotoxicity in humans and has been studied extensively. Animal models have failed to demonstrate significant nephrotoxicity when vancomycin was given alone (294,295). Vancomycin, in contrast to teicoplanin, can enhance aminoglycoside-induced renal toxicity in animals and possibly in humans (175,321,322). The incidence mentioned in adults varies from 5% to 18%. Vancomycin toxicity has been related to trough concentrations greater than 10 mg per L, but in most studies it remains unclear whether elevated serum trough concentrations are the cause or consequence of renal failure (323,324).

Teicoplanin nephrotoxicity is more common in prolonged or high-dose therapy. Teicoplanin is associated with lower nephrotoxicity rates in children than is vancomycin (325).

Vancomycin nephrotoxicity has been studied in several groups of neonates, though seldom explicitly. Many studies could not detect any nephrotoxicity, either defined as a rise in serum creatinine or as clinical or biochemical signs of renal failure (240,242,247,257,260,326).

Some studies found a reversible rise in serum creatinine (198,255,265). In most cases, patients were exposed to aminoglycosides as well, though cotreatment is not a clear risk factor in neonates and children (327). Renal toxicity is not related to either peak serum concentrations greater than 40 mg per L or trough serum concentrations greater than 10 mg per L (328). Large overdoses without renal consequences have been described (329). High peak or trough serum concentrations were seen only in patients in whom a serum creatinine rise was seen during treatment. This implies that the high serum vancomycin concentration is not the cause, but the result, of renal dysfunction, as is often thought in clinical practice.

It has to be noted that there are no long-term data on nephrotoxicity in neonates. This is an issue that will have to be addressed in prospective follow-up studies.

Vancomycin nephrotoxicity in infants and children is also rare. Most studies have not found evidence for vancomycin-induced nephrotoxicity (240,247). Acute tubular necrosis as a result of vancomycin toxicity has been described (330,331). Most children with a rise in serum creatinine were simultaneously exposed to an aminoglycoside and did not show a relationship to serum concentration. In a limited number of studies vancomycin does not enhance aminoglycoside-induced tubulopathy in children (327,332,333). Renal dysfunction is often reversible, with or without discontinuation of treatment (325,333,334).

The overall conclusion from this information is that vancomycin-induced nephrotoxicity in neonates, infants, and children is rare and reversible, and there is no clear relation to serum concentrations.

Studies of teicoplanin use in neonates, infants, and children have not demonstrated significant nephrotoxicity (284,299,314,335). Teicoplanin nephrotoxicity was not seen in a neonate with an accidental overdose (336).

Ototoxicity

Information on glycopeptide ototoxicity is scarce. Vancomycin is said to be potentially vestibulo- and cochleotoxic (337). Tinnitus seems to precede hearing loss. As with aminoglycosides, hearing loss is more pronounced in the high-frequency range (8 to 16 kHz) (321). There are animal studies relating ototoxicity to vancomycin in combination with an aminoglycoside, but there is little evidence for ototoxicity of vancomycin alone (338,339). The first report of vancomycin-related ototoxicity in humans was in 1958 (182). Reported incidence of ototoxicity in adults is less than 2% (308). Reports on ototoxicity are fraught with methodologic problems. Most studies were retrospective and included patients who had been exposed to other ototoxic medication, mainly aminoglycosides (337).

A relation between vancomycin-related ototoxicity and serum concentrations could not be demonstrated from available literature (321). A confounding factor, as in nephrotoxicity, is that the time of serum sampling in relation to dose is not always mentioned, which clouds interpretation of these serum concentrations. Data on vancomycin ototoxicity in neonates, infants, and children are scarce. Neonates born to mothers who received vancomycin in the second or third trimester of pregnancy did not show hearing loss (340). Brain stem evoked response audiometry and behavioral audiometry did not demonstrate any ototoxicity in 12 neonates and children (247). Large accidental overdoses in infants, with serum concentrations exceeding 300 mg per L, did not result in hearing loss (329,341). Vancomycin ototoxicity in neonates is not related to duration of treatment or abnormal peak/trough serum concentrations (144).

Pediatric burn patients exposed to a number of ototoxic medications showed hearing loss in 22% of cases, possibly related to total dose of vancomycin (342). Intraperitoneal treatment of peritoneal dialysis-associated peritonitis with either vancomycin or teicoplanin showed one case of vancomycin-related hearing loss (287). Early vancomycin administration in pneumococcal meningitis may increase the risk of hearing loss (343). Teicoplanin is reported to be less ototoxic than vancomycin (322). Teicoplanin-related ototoxicity has not been described in pediatric patients.

In summary, glycopeptide-related hearing loss in infants and children is sporadic, and no clear relation to serum concentrations or patterns of underlying illness can be detected. The usefulness of TDM of vancomycin for that aspect is thus doubtful.

GLYCOPEPTIDE DOSING AND DOSE INTERVAL

As in other drugs, vancomycin dose and dosing interval are determined by its desired therapeutic range and pharmacokinetic properties. Historically, vancomycin dosing has been titrated to obtain peak serum concentrations between 20 and 40 mg per L and serum trough concentrations of 5 to 10 mg per L. There is little scientific evidence for both ranges. The upper limit of 40 mg per L is based on the fact that the earliest study, describing ototoxicity with peak concentrations greater than 80 mg per L, suggested that peaks should not exceed 50 mg per L (182). As described before, there is no clear relation between oto- or nephrotoxicity and serum concentrations. Also, there is no microbiologic or clinical evidence for increased effectiveness of vancomycin at advised peak concentrations. The lower limit of the range for trough concentrations seems to be reasonable. Susceptibility of most microorganisms for which vancomycin is used is less than 1 to 2 mg per L. With a maximal protein binding of 50%, this means that vancomycin trough concentrations will have to exceed 4 mg per L to remain above the MIC during the whole dosing interval (305). Although there are some reports relating nephrotoxicity to trough serum concentrations greater than 10 mg per L, there is insufficient evidence to rigidly adhere to this goal (323).

Nevertheless, these desired ranges of concentrations still are the goal of dosing regimens advised for neonates and infants. Many dosing strategies for neonates, related to PNA, PCA, body weight, or serum creatinine, have been defined, with dose intervals ranging from continuous dosing to every 48 hours. Recently published dosing strategies are listed in Table 30.5. Although an extension of dose interval to more than 8 hours has been suggested, especially in VLBW infants, trough serum concentrations less than 5 mg per L found in several studies should lead to caution (220,257,259,263,265,344). Current dosing advice in children is 10 mg per kg every 6 hours. Pediatric oncology patients need higher doses of both vancomycin (up to 75 mg per kg per 24 hours) and teicoplanin (up to 20 mg per kg per 24 hours) (335,345,346). A single dose of vancomycin 15 mg per kg is sufficient to maintain adequate trough serum concentrations during cardiopulmonary bypass.

Once-daily dosing for teicoplanin in neonates is advised at 8 to 10 mg per kg after a loading dose of 15 to 20 mg per kg (315). For children a daily dose of 10 mg per kg after loading of 20 mg per kg is generally sufficient. In pediatric intensive care unit patients, this dosing regimen leads to insufficient trough serum concentrations, and doses of 8 mg per kg every 12 hours are advised (284,299). For deep-seated infections or endocarditis higher doses might be needed.

THERAPEUTIC DRUG MONITORING

Therapeutic drug monitoring of vancomycin is mostly performed at steady state, with serum concentrations taken just before and 1 hour after completion of the intravenous infusion. Target concentrations are peaks between 20 and 40 mg per L and troughs of 5 to 10 mg per L. Peak serum concentrations depend on the timing of sampling, and since there is a wide variety in sampling time in relation to dose, this should be taken into account when setting goals in therapy (347,348). Strangely enough, despite these differences in timing, most authors adhere to the same peak level goals. Vancomycin serum concentrations are mainly determined by fluorescence polarization immunoassay (FPIA), though the enzyme-multiplied immunologic technique and radioimmunoassay are also used in clinical practice. It has been reported that FPIA can overestimate vancomycin serum concentrations in adult patients with renal failure as well as in neonates younger than 30 weeks based on a cross-reactivity with an inactive vancomycin-degradation product (CDP-1) (349,350). This could lead to errors in calculating pharmacokinetic parameters (243). The new modified FPIA assay does not show the same disadvantage (351). For teicoplanin high-performance liquid chromatography and FPIA are mainly used. The available bioassay is affected by use of other antimicrobials.

Routine TDM for teicoplanin is not performed in pediatric patients. There is no clear relation between serum concentrations and clinical efficacy and toxicity, which has a substantially lower incidence than with vancomycin (315). TDM should be reserved for special patient categories with difficult-to-predict serum concentrations (such as renal failure), patients not responding to therapy, or infections that require higher serum concentrations (such as endocarditis).

The rationale for routine TDM of vancomycin in the pediatric setting is dubious. Neither efficacy nor toxicity shows a clear relation to serum concentrations, and this is especially true for peak values. There is a large interindividual variation, especially between neonates and infants with different PCAs, with a concomitant effect on obtained peak and trough serum concentrations. Several studies have shown that vancomycin concentrations can be below the therapeutic range with standard dosing (253,352). There is, however, no clear relation of peak concentration to toxicity and effect, so the clinical importance of this interindividual variation is doubtful. Furthermore, it has been shown in neonates and adults that peak serum concentrations greater than 40 mg per L are seldom seen with trough concentrations below 10 to 15 mg per L in patients without overt renal failure (353–355). Given these considerations, routine monitoring of peak serum concentrations is questionable. A case can be made for monitoring trough concentrations only, although this is also debatable. Based on in vitro studies, vancomycin trough concentrations should exceed 4 to 5 mg per L (305). Acceptable cure rates with trough concentrations ranging

TABLE 30.5 Currently Recommended Vancomycin Dosing Regimen in Neonates and Infants

PCA (wk)	*BW (g)*	*Serum Creatinine (μmol/L)*	*Target Peak/ Trough (mg/L)*	*Dose (mg/kg)*	*Interval (hr)*	*Reference*
<27	<800		25–35/5–10	18	36	220
27–30	800–1,200		25–35/5–10	18	24	
31–36	1,200–2,000		25–35/5–10	18	18	
>36	>2,000		25–35/5–10	15	12	
≤32[a]				12.5	12	267
≤32[b]				10	12	
>32[a]				10	8	
>32[b]				7.5	8	
25–26				7 LD, 10	Continuous	198
27–28				7 LD, 12	Continuous	
29–30				7 LD, 15	Continuous	
31–32				7 LD, 18	Continuous	
33–34				7 LD, 20	Continuous	
35–36				7 LD, 23	Continuous	
37–38				7 LD, 26	Continuous	
39–40				7 LD, 29	Continuous	
41–42				7 LD, 31	Continuous	
43–44				7 LD, 34	Continuous	
>45				7 LD, 40	Continuous	
		20–29		20	8	263
		30–39		20	12	
		40–49			15	12
		50–59		12	12	
		60–79		15	18	
		80–100		15	24	
		>100		15	Depending on trough	
All				10	8	253
		≥1.7[c]		15	48	269
		1.3–1.6[c]		10	24	
		1.0–1.2[c]		15	24	
		0.7–0.9[c]		20	24	
		≤0.6[c]		15	12	
All		>90 μmol/L		20	Continuous	201
		<90 μmol/L		30	Continuous	201

BW, Body weight; LD, loading dose; PCA, postconceptional age.
[a]No indomethacin and/or mechanical ventilation.
[b]Indomethacin and/or mechanical ventilation.
[c]Serum creatinine in mg/dL.

from 2 to 18.8 mg per L have been described in neonates and children (247,259,260). Except for endocarditis, there are no clinical studies in neonates, children, or adults that have substantiated the clinical need for higher serum concentrations (181). Several dosing regimens discussed before, especially those with dose intervals exceeding 8 hours, have shown that trough serum concentrations can be lower than 5 mg per L, indicating a need for trough-level monitoring (220,255,257,259,263,265,344). Trough-level monitoring should thus be aimed at ascertaining that serum concentrations remain greater than 5 mg per L.

Several studies have investigated the predictive performance of TDM with vancomycin in the neonatal setting (238,241,254,257,266,352,353,355). Controlling dose and/or dose interval with TDM can be performed using first-order elimination kinetics, as proposed by Sawchuk and Zaske (356), or with a Bayesian method. In adults, Bayesian feedback (357) is associated with a better predictive performance than the method of Sawchuk and Zaske. The neonatal dosing interval can be estimated by obtaining two serum samples (257). In neonates and infants, without renal failure additional feedback concentrations are needed approximately every 14 days (266). Several population pharmacokinetic models incorporating clinical denominators have shown the capability of adequately predicting serum concentrations (238,253,274,358,359). These models might also help in obviating the need for routine TDM.

REFERENCES

1. Waksman SA, Bugie E, Schatz A. Isolation of antibiotic substances from soil microorganisms with special reference to streptothricin and streptomycin. *Proc Staff Meet Mayo Clin* 1944;19:537–548.

2. Gilbert DN, Kohlhepp SJ. New sodium hydroxide digestion method for measurement of renal tobramycin concentrations. *Antimicrob Agents Chemother* 1986;30(3):361–365.
3. Weinstein MJ, Wagman GH, Oden EM, et al. Biological activity of the antibiotic components of the gentamicin complex. *J Bacteriol* 1967;94(3):789–790.
4. Pickering LK, Rutherford I. Effect of concentration and time upon inactivation of tobramycin, gentamicin, netilmicin and amikacin by azlocillin, carbenicillin, mecillinam, mezlocillin and piperacillin. *J Pharmacol Exp Ther* 1981;217(2):345–349.
5. McLaughlin JE, Reeves DS. Clinical and laboratory evidence for inactivation of gentamicin by carbenicillin. *Lancet* 1971;1(7693):261–264.
6. Walterspiel JN, Feldman S, Van R, et al. Comparative inactivation of isepamicin, amikacin, and gentamicin by nine beta-lactams and two beta-lactamase inhibitors, cilastatin and heparin. *Antimicrob Agents Chemother* 1991;35(9):1875–1878.
7. Hancock RE. Aminoglycoside uptake and mode of action–with special reference to streptomycin and gentamicin. I. Antagonists and mutants. *J Antimicrob Chemother* 1981;8(4):249–276.
8. Hancock RE, Farmer SW, Li ZS, et al. Interaction of aminoglycosides with the outer membranes and purified lipopolysaccharide and OmpF porin of Escherichia coli. *Antimicrob Agents Chemother* 1991;35(7):1309–1314.
9. Taber HW, Mueller JP, Miller PF, et al. Bacterial uptake of aminoglycoside antibiotics. *Microbiol Rev* 1987;51(4):439–457.
10. Damper PD, Epstein W. Role of the membrane potential in bacterial resistance to aminoglycoside antibiotics. *Antimicrob Agents Chemother* 1981;20(6):803–808.
11. Mates SM, Patel L, Kaback HR, et al. Membrane potential in anaerobically growing Staphylococcus aureus and its relationship to gentamicin uptake. *Antimicrob Agents Chemother* 1983;23(4):526–530.
12. Kadurugamuwa JL, Lam JS, Beveridge TJ. Interaction of gentamicin with the A band and B band lipopolysaccharides of Pseudomonas aeruginosa and its possible lethal effect. *Antimicrob Agents Chemother* 1993;37(4):715–721.
13. Sanders CC, Sanders WE, Goering RV. In vitro studies with Sch 21420 and Sch 22591: activity in comparison with six other aminoglycosides and synergy with penicillin against enterococci. *Antimicrob Agents Chemother* 1978;14:178.
14. Blaser J, Stone BB, Groner MC, et al. Comparative study with enoxacin and netilmicin in a pharmacodynamic model to determine importance of ratio of antibiotic peak concentration to MIC for bacterial activity and emergence of resistance. *Antimicrob Agents Chemother* 1987;31:1054–1060.
15. Gerber AU, Feller-Segessenmann C. In-vivo assessment of in-vitro killing patterns of Pseudomonas aeruginosa. *J Antimicrob Chemother* 1985;15(Suppl A):201–206.
16. Kapusnik JE, Hackbarth CJ, Chambers HF, et al. Single, large, daily dosing versus intermittent dosing of tobramycin for treating experimental pseudomonas pneumonia [published erratum appears in *J Infect Dis* 1988;158(4):911]. *J Infect Dis* 1988;158(1):7–12.
17. Moore RD, Lietman PS, Smith CR. Clinical response to aminoglycoside therapy: importance of the ratio of peak concentration to minimal inhibitory concentration. *J Infect Dis* 1987;155(1):93–99.
18. Vogelman B, Craig WA. Kinetics of antimicrobial activity. *J Pediatr* 1986;108(5 pt 2):835–840.
19. Blaser J, Stone BB, Zinner SH. Efficacy of intermittent versus continuous administration of netilmicin in a two-compartment in vitro model. *Antimicrob Agents Chemother* 1985;27(3):343–349.
20. Dudley MN, Zinner SH. Single daily dosing of amikacin in an in-vitro model. *J Antimicrob Chemother* 1991;27(Suppl C):15–19.
21. Fantin B, Ebert S, Leggett J, et al. Factors affecting duration of in-vivo postantibiotic effect for aminoglycosides against gram-negative bacilli. *J Antimicrob Chemother* 1991;27(6):829–836.
22. Schlaeffer F, Blaser J, Laxon J, et al. Enhancement of leucocyte killing of resistant bacteria selected during exposure to aminoglycosides or quinolones. *J Antimicrob Chemother* 1990;25(6):941–948.
23. Vogelman B, Gudmundsson S, Turnidge J, et al. In vivo postantibiotic effect in a thigh infection in neutropenic mice. *J Infect Dis* 1988;157(2):287–298.
24. Giamarellou H. Aminoglycosides plus beta-lactams against gram-negative organisms. Evaluation of in vitro synergy and chemical interactions. *Am J Med* 1986;80(6B):126–137.
25. Gilbert D. Aminoglycosides. In: Mandell G, Bennett J, Dolin R, eds. *Principles and practice of infectious diseases*, 5th ed. Philadelphia, PA: Churchill Livingstone, 2000;307–335.
26. Barza M, Ioannidis J, Cappeleri J, et al. Single or multiple daily doses of aminoglycosides: a meta-analysis. *BMJ* 1996;312:338–344.
27. Blaser J, Konig C. Once-daily dosing of aminoglycosides. *Eur J Clin Microbiol Infect Dis* 1996;14:1029–1038.
28. Nicolau DP, Freeman CD, Belliveau PP, et al. Experience with a once-daily aminoglycoside program administered to 2,184 adult patients. *Antimicrob Agents Chemother* 1995;39(3):650–655.
29. Chambers HF, Sande MA. Antimicrobial agents: the aminoglycosides. In: Goodman L, Gilman A, Limbird L, eds. *The pharmacological basis of therapeutics*, 9th ed. New York, NY: McGraw-Hill, 1995:1103–1121.
30. Mingeot-Leclercq MP, Glupczynski Y, Tulkens PM. Aminoglycosides: activity and resistance. *Antimicrob Agents Chemother* 1999;43(4):727–737.
31. Karlowsky JA, Zelenitsky SA, Zhanel GG. Aminoglycoside adaptive resistance. *Pharmacotherapy* 1997;17(3):549–555.
32. Karlowsky JA, Hoban DJ, Zelenitsky SA, et al. Altered denA and anr gene expression in aminoglycoside adaptive resistance in Pseudomonas aeruginosa. *J Antimicrob Chemother* 1997;40(3):371–376.
33. Xiong YQ, Caillon J, Kergueris MF, et al. Adaptive resistance of Pseudomonas aeruginosa induced by aminoglycosides and killing kinetics in a rabbit endocarditis model. *Antimicrob Agents Chemother* 1997;41(4):823–826.
34. Karchmer AW, Archer GL, Dismukes WE. Staphylococcus epidermidis causing prosthetic valve endocarditis: microbiologic and clinical observations as guides to therapy. *Ann Intern Med* 1983;98(4):447–455.
35. Watanakunakorn C, Tisone JC. Synergism between vancomycin and gentamicin or tobramycin for methicillin-susceptible and methicillin-resistant Staphylococcus aureus strains. *Antimicrob Agents Chemother* 1982;22(5):903–905.
36. Fichtenbaum CJ, Ritchie DJ, Powderly WG. Use of paromomycin for treatment of cryptosporidiosis in patients with AIDS. *Clin Infect Dis* 1993;16(2):298–300.
37. Baker CJ. Antibiotic therapy in neonates whose mothers have received intrapartum group B streptococcal chemoprophylaxis. *Pediatr Infect Dis J* 1990;9(2):149–150.
38. Fanaroff AA, Korones SB, Wright LL. A controlled trial of intravenous immune globulin to reduce nosocomial infections in very-low-birth-weight infants. *N Engl J Med* 1994;330:1107–1113.
39. Gladstone IM, Ehrenkranz RA, Edberg SC, et al. A ten-year review of neonatal sepsis and comparison with the previous fifty-year experience. *Pediatr Infect Dis J* 1990;9(11):819–825.
40. Shah SS, Ehrenkranz RA, Gallagher PG. Increasing incidence of gram-negative rod bacteremia in a newborn intensive care unit. *Pediatr Infect Dis J* 1999;18(7):591–595.
41. Clark RH, Bloom BT, Spitzer AR, et al. Empiric use of ampicillin and cefotaxime, compared with ampicillin and gentamicin, for neonates at risk for sepsis is associated with an increased risk of neonatal death. *Pediatrics* 2006;117(1):67–74.
42. Anonymous. Early neonatal drug utilization in preterm newborns in neonatal intensive care units. Italian Collaborative Group on Preterm Delivery. *Dev Pharmacol Ther* 1988;11:1–7.
43. Bryan CS, John JF Jr., Pai MS, et al. Gentamicin vs cefotaxime for therapy of neonatal sepsis. Relationship to drug resistance. *Am J Dis Child* 1985;139(11):1086–1089.
44. de Man P, Verhoeven BA, Verbrugh HA, et al. An antibiotic policy to prevent emergence of resistant bacilli. *Lancet* 2000;355(9208):973–978.
45. Webb AK. The treatment of pulmonary infection in cystic fibrosis. *Scand J Infect Dis Suppl* 1995;96:24–27.
46. Kearns GL, Hilman BC, Wilson JT. Dosing implications of altered gentamicin disposition in patients with cystic fibrosis. *J Pediatr* 1982;100(2):312–318.
47. Smith AL, Doershuk C, Goldmann D, et al. Comparison of a beta-lactam alone versus beta-lactam and an aminoglycoside for pulmonary exacerbation in cystic fibrosis. *J Pediatr* 1999;134(4):413–421.

48. Church DA, Kanga JF, Kuhn RJ, et al. Sequential ciprofloxacin therapy in pediatric cystic fibrosis: comparative study vs. ceftazidime/tobramycin in the treatment of acute pulmonary exacerbations. The Cystic Fibrosis Study Group. *Pediatr Infect Dis J* 1997;16(1):97–105; discussion 123–126.
49. Touw DJ, Knox AJ, Smyth A. Population pharmacokinetics of tobramycin administered thrice daily and once daily in children and adults with cystic fibrosis. *J Cyst Fibros* 2007;6(5):327–333.
50. Lam W, Tjon J, Seto W, et al. Pharmacokinetic modelling of a once-daily dosing regimen for intravenous tobramycin in paediatric cystic fibrosis patients. *J Antimicrob Chemother* 2007;59(6): 1135–1140.
51. Gibson RL, Emerson J, McNamara S, et al. Significant microbiological effect of inhaled tobramycin in young children with cystic fibrosis. *Am J Respir Crit Care Med* 2003;167(6):841–849.
52. Pai VB, Nahata MC. Efficacy and safety of aerosolized tobramycin in cystic fibrosis. *Pediatr Pulmonol* 2001;32(4):314–327.
53. Patatanian L. Inhaled tobramycin-associated hearing loss in an adolescent with renal failure. *Pediatr Infect Dis J* 2006;25(3):276–278.
54. Smyth A, Tan KH, Hyman-Taylor P, et al. Once versus three-times daily regimens of tobramycin treatment for pulmonary exacerbations of cystic fibrosis—the TOPIC study: a randomised controlled trial. *Lancet* 2005;365(9459):573–578.
55. Khan AJ, Kumar K, Evans HE. Single-dose gentamicin therapy of recurrent urinary tract infection in patients with normal urinary tracts. *J Pediatr* 1987;110(1):131–135.
56. Wallen L, Zeller WP, Goessler M, et al. Single-dose amikacin treatment of first childhood E. coli lower urinary tract infections. *J Pediatr* 1983;103(2):316–319.
57. Hodson EM, Willis NS, Craig JC. Antibiotics for acute pyelonephritis in children. *Cochrane Database Syst Rev* 2007;(4): CD003772.
58. Siegel JD, McCracken GH Jr., Thomas ML, et al. Pharmacokinetic properties of netilmicin in newborn infants. *Antimicrob Agents Chemother* 1979;15(2):246–253.
59. Swan SK. Aminoglycoside nephrotoxicity. *Semin Nephrol* 1997; 17(1):27–33.
60. Garcia B, Barcia E, Perez F, et al. Population pharmacokinetics of gentamicin in premature newborns. *J Antimicrob Chemother* 2006;58(2):372–379.
61. Evans WE, Feldman S, Barker LF, et al. Use of gentamicin serum levels to individualise therapy in children. *J Pediatr* 1978;93: 133–137.
62. Fattinger K, Vozeh S, Olafsson A, et al. Netilmicin in the neonate: population pharmacokinetic analysis and dosing recommendations. *Clin Pharmacol Ther* 1991;50(1):55–65.
63. Southgate WM, DiPiro JT, Robertson AF. Pharmacokinetics of gentamicin in neonates on extracorporeal membrane oxygenation. *Antimicrob Agents Chemother* 1989;33(6):817–819.
64. de Hoog M, Mouton JW, Schoemaker RC, et al. Extended-interval dosing of tobramycin in neonates: implications for therapeutic drug monitoring. *Clin Pharmacol Ther* 2002;71(5):349–358.
65. Miron D. Once daily dosing of gentamicin in infants and children. *Pediatr Infect Dis J* 2001;20(12):1169–1173.
66. Williams BS, Ransom JL, Gal P, et al. Gentamicin pharmacokinetics in neonates with patent ductus arteriosus. *Crit Care Med* 1997;25(2):273–275.
67. Miranda JC, Schimmel MM, James LS, et al. Gentamicin kinetics in the neonate. *Pediatr Pharmacol (New York)* 1985;5(1):57–61.
68. van den Anker JN. Pharmacokinetics and renal function in preterm infants. *Acta Paediatr* 1996;85:1393–1399.
69. Izquierdo M, Lanao JM, Cervero L, et al. Population pharmacokinetics of gentamicin in premature infants. *Ther Drug Monit* 1992;14(3):177–183.
70. Jensen PD, Edgren BE, Brundage RC. Population pharmacokinetics of gentamicin in neonates using a nonlinear, mixed-effects model. *Pharmacotherapy* 1992;12(3):178–182.
71. Thomson AH, Way S, Bryson SM, et al. Population pharmacokinetics of gentamicin in neonates. *Dev Pharmacol Ther* 1988;11(3): 173–179.
72. Weber W, Kewitz G, Rost KL, et al. Population kinetics of gentamicin in neonates. *Eur J Clin Pharmacol* 1993;44(Suppl 1):S23–S25.
73. Brion LP, Fleischman AR, Schwartz GJ. Gentamicin interval in newborn infants as determined by renal function and postconceptional age. *Pediatr Nephrol* 1991;5(6):675–679.
74. Pons G, d'Athis P, Rey E, et al. Gentamicin monitoring in neonates. *Ther Drug Monit* 1988;10(4):421–427.
75. Bueva A, Guignard JP. Renal function in preterm neonates. *Pediatr Res* 1994;36:572–577.
76. van den Anker JN, Hop WC, de Groot R, et al. Effects of prenatal exposure to betamethasone and indomethacin on the glomerular filtration rate in the preterm infant. *Pediatr Res* 1994;36(5):578–581.
77. Bidiwala KS, Lorenz JM, Kleinman LI. Renal function correlates of postnatal diuresis in preterm infants. *Pediatrics* 1988;82:50–58.
78. Sardemann H, Colding H, Hendel J, et al. Kinetics and dose calculations of amikacin in the newborn. *Clin Pharmacol Ther* 1976; 20(1):59–66.
79. Kildoo C, Modanlou HD, Komatsu G, et al. Developmental pattern of gentamicin kinetics in very low birth weight (VLBW) sick infants. *Dev Pharmacol Ther* 1984;7(6):345–356.
80. Rodvold KA, Gentry CA, Plank GS, et al. Prediction of gentamicin concentrations in neonates and infants using a Bayesian pharmacokinetic model. *Dev Pharmacol Ther* 1993;20(3–4):211–219.
81. Vervelde ML, Rademaker CM, Krediet TG, et al. Population pharmacokinetics of gentamicin in preterm neonates: evaluation of a once-daily dosage regimen. *Ther Drug Monit* 1999;21(5): 514–519.
82. Nahata MC, Powell DA, Durrell DE, et al. Intrapatient variation in tobramycin kinetics in low birth weight infants during first postnatal week. *Eur J Clin Pharmacol* 1984;26(5):647–649.
83. Faura CC, Garcia MR, Horga JF. Changes in gentamicin serum levels and pharmacokinetic parameters in the newborn in the course of treatment with aminoglycoside. *Ther Drug Monit* 1991; 13(3):277–280.
84. Allegaert K, Cossey V, Langhendries JP, et al. Effects of co-administration of ibuprofen-lysine on the pharmacokinetics of amikacin in preterm infants during the first days of life. *Biol Neonate* 2004;86(3):207–211.
85. Allegaert K, Anderson BJ, Cossey V, et al. Limited predictability of amikacin clearance in extreme premature neonates at birth. *Br J Clin Pharmacol* 2006;61(1):39–48.
86. Watterberg KL, Kelly HW, Johnson JD, et al. Effect of patent ductus arteriosus on gentamicin pharmacokinetics in very low birth weight (less than 1,500 g) babies. *Dev Pharmacol Ther* 1987; 10(2):107–117.
87. Gal P, Ransom JL, Weaver RL. Gentamicin in neonates: the need for loading doses. *Am J Perinatol* 1990;7(3):254–257.
88. Dodge WF, Jelliffe RW, Zwischenberger JB, et al. Population pharmacokinetic models: effect of explicit versus assumed constant serum concentration assay error patterns upon parameter values of gentamicin in infants on and off extracorporeal membrane oxygenation. *Ther Drug Monit* 1994;16(6):552–559.
89. Celsi G, Nishi A, Akusjarvi G, et al. Abundance of Na(+)-K(+)-ATPase mRNA is regulated by glucocorticoid hormones in infant rat kidneys. *Am J Physiol* 1991;260(2 pt 2):F192–F197.
90. Koren G, James A, Perlman M. A simple method for the estimation of glomerular filtration rate by gentamicin pharmacokinetics during routine drug monitoring in the newborn. *Clin Pharmacol Ther* 1985;38(6):680–685.
91. McCracken GH Jr., Chrane DF, Thomas ML. Pharmacologic evaluation of gentamicin in newborn infants. *J Infect Dis* 1971; 124(Suppl 124):214–219.
92. McCracken GH, West NR, Horton LJ. Urinary excretion of gentamicin in the neonatal period. *J Infect Dis* 1971;123(3):257–262.
93. Keyes PS, Johnson CK, Rawlins TD. Predictors of trough serum gentamicin concentrations in neonates. *Am J Dis Child* 1989; 143(12):1419–1423.
94. Paap CM, Nahata MC. Clinical pharmacokinetics of antibacterial drugs in neonates. *Clin Pharmacokinet* 1990;19(4):280–318.
95. McGowan JE Jr., Terry PM, Huang TS, et al. Nosocomial infections with gentamicin-resistant Staphylococcus aureus: plasmid analysis as an epidemiologic tool. *J Infect Dis* 1979;140(6): 864–872.
96. Treluyer JM, Merle Y, Tonnelier S, et al. Nonparametric population pharmacokinetic analysis of amikacin in neonates, infants, and children. *Antimicrob Agents Chemother* 2002;46(5):1381–1387.
97. Kelman AW, Thomson AH, Whiting B, et al. Estimation of gentamicin clearance and volume of distribution in neonates and young children. *Br J Clin Pharmacol* 1984;18(5):685–692.

98. Echeverria P, Siber GR, Paisley J, et al. Age-dependent dose response to gentamicin. *J Pediatr* 1975;87(5):805–808.
99. Hickey S, McCracken G. Antibacterial therapeutic agents. In: Feigin R, Cherry J, eds. *Textbook of pediatric infectious diseases.* Philadelphia, PA: WB Saunders Company, 1998:2614–2648.
100. Lanao JM, Dominguez-Gil AA, Dominguez-Gil A, et al. Pharmacokinetics of amikacin in children with normal and impaired renal function. *Kidney Int* 1981;20(1):115–121.
101. Craig WA, Redington J, Ebert SC. Pharmacodynamics of amikacin in vitro and in mouse thigh and lung infections. *J Antimicrob Chemother* 1991;27(Suppl C):29–40.
102. Schelonka RL, Chai MK, Yoder BA, et al. Volume of blood required to detect common neonatal pathogens. *J Pediatr* 1996; 129(2):275–278.
103. Stoll BJ, Gordon T, Korones SB, et al. Early-onset sepsis in very low birth weight neonates: a report from the national institute of child health and human development neonatal research network. *J Pediatr* 1996;129(1):72–80.
104. Klein JO, Michael Marcy S. Bacterial sepsis and meningitis. In: Remington JS, Klein JO, eds. *Infectious diseases of the fetus and newborn infant*, 4th ed. Philadelphia, PA: WB Saunders Company, 1995:836.
105. Arnon S, Litmanovitz I. Diagnostic tests in neonatal sepsis. *Curr Opin Infect Dis* 2008;21(3):223–227.
106. Carapetis JR, Jaquiery AL, Buttery JP, et al. Randomized, controlled trial comparing once daily and three times daily gentamicin in children with urinary tract infections. *Pediatr Infect Dis J* 2001;20(3):240–246.
107. Uijtendaal EV, Rademaker CM, Schobben AF, et al. Once-daily versus multiple-daily gentamicin in infants and children. *Ther Drug Monit* 2001;23(5):506–513.
108. Sung L, Dupuis LL, Bliss B, et al. Randomized controlled trial of once- versus thrice-daily tobramycin in febrile neutropenic children undergoing stem cell transplantation. *J Natl Cancer Inst* 2003; 95(24):1869–1877.
109. Kafetzis DA, Sianidou L, Vlachos E, et al. Clinical and pharmacokinetic study of a single daily dose of amikacin in paediatric patients with severe gram-negative infections. *J Antimicrob Chemother* 1991;27(Suppl C):105–112.
110. Kent AL, Maxwell LE, Koina ME, et al. Renal glomeruli and tubular injury following indomethacin, ibuprofen, and gentamicin exposure in a neonatal rat model. *Pediatr Res* 2007;62(3):307–312.
111. Kaloyanides GJ, Pastoriza-Munoz E. Aminoglycoside nephrotoxicity. *Kidney Int* 1980;18:571–582.
112. Ali MZ, Goetz MB. A meta-analysis of the relative efficacy and toxicity of single daily dosing versus multiple daily dosing of aminoglycosides [see comments]. *Clin Infect Dis* 1997;24(5):796–809.
113. MacGowan A, Reeves D. Serum aminoglycoside concentrations: the case for routine monitoring. *J Antimicrob Chemother* 1994;34(5): 829–837.
114. Munckhof WJ, Grayson ML, Turnidge JD. A meta-analysis of studies on the safety and efficacy of aminoglycosides given either once daily or as divided doses. *J Antimicrob Chemother* 1996;37: 645–663.
115. Rybak MJ, Abate BJ, Kang L, et al. Prospective evaluation of the effect of an aminoglycoside dosing regimen on rates of observed nephrotoxicity and ototoxicity. *Antimicrob Agents Chemother* 1999; 43(7):1549–1555.
116. Giapros VI, Andronikou S, Cholevas VI, et al. Renal function in premature infants during aminoglycoside therapy. *Pediatr Nephrol* 1995;9(2):163–166.
117. Langhendries JP, Battisti O, Bertrand JM, et al. Once-a-day administration of amikacin in neonates: assessment of nephrotoxicity and ototoxicity. *Dev Pharmacol Ther* 1993;20(3–4):220–230.
118. Leititis JU, Zimmerhackl LB, Burghard R, et al. Evaluation of local renal function in newborn infants under tobramycin therapy. *Dev Pharmacol Ther* 1991;17(3–4):154–160.
119. Parini R, Rusconi F, Cavanna G, et al. Evaluation of the renal and auditory function of neonates treated with amikacin. *Dev Pharmacol Ther* 1982;5(1–2):33–46.
120. Lundergan FS, Glasscock GF, Kim EH, et al. Once-daily gentamicin dosing in newborn infants. *Pediatrics* 1999;103(6 pt 1): 1228–1234.
121. Andronikou S, Giapros VI, Cholevas VI, et al. Effect of aminoglycoside therapy on renal function in full-term infants. *Pediatr Nephrol* 1996;10(6):766–768.
122. Giacoia GP, Schentag JJ. Pharmacokinetics and nephrotoxicity of continuous intravenous infusion of gentamicin in low birth weight infants. *J Pediatr* 1986;109(4):715–719.
123. Gordjani N, Burghard R, Muller D, et al. Urinary excretion of adenosine deaminase binding protein in neonates treated with tobramycin. *Pediatr Nephrol* 1995;9(4):419–422.
124. Gouyon JB, Aujard Y, Abisror A, et al. Urinary excretion of N-acetyl-glucosaminidase and beta-2-microglobulin as early markers of gentamicin nephrotoxicity in neonates. *Dev Pharmacol Ther* 1987;10(2):145–152.
125. Rajchgot P, Prober CG, Soldin S, et al. Aminoglycoside-related nephrotoxicity in the premature newborn. *Clin Pharmacol Ther* 1984;35(3):394–401.
126. Williams PD, Bennett DB, Gleason CR, et al. Correlation between renal membrane binding and nephrotoxicity of aminoglycosides. *Antimicrob Agents Chemother* 1987;31:570–574.
127. Chiruvolu A, Engle WD, Sendelbach D, et al. Serum calcium values in term and late-preterm neonates receiving gentamicin. *Pediatr Nephrol* 2008;23(4):569–574.
128. Kraus DM, Pai MP, Rodvold KA. Efficacy and tolerability of extended-interval aminoglycoside administration in pediatric patients. *Paediatr Drugs* 2002;4(7):469–484.
129. McCracken GH Jr. Aminoglycoside toxicity in infants and children. *Am J Med* 1986;80(6B):172–178.
130. Bass KD, Larkin SE, Paap C, et al. Pharmacokinetics of once-daily gentamicin dosing in pediatric patients. *J Pediatr Surg* 1998; 33(7):1104–1107.
131. Stringer SP, Meyerhoff WL, Wright CG. Ototoxicity. In: Paparella MM, Gluckmann JL, Meyerhoff WL, eds. *Otolaryngology.* Philadelphia, PA: WB Saunders Company, 1991:1653–1669.
132. Preston SL, Briceland LL. Single daily dosing of aminoglycosides. *Pharmacotherapy* 1995;15:297–316.
133. Estivill X, Govea N, Barcelo E, et al. Familial progressive sensorineural deafness is mainly due to the mtDNA A1555G mutation and is enhanced by treatment of aminoglycosides. *Am J Hum Genet* 1998;62(1):27–35.
134. Ernfors P, Canlon B. Aminoglycoside excitement silences hearing [news; comment]. *Nat Med* 1996;2(12):1313–1314.
135. McCormack JP, Jewesson PJ. A critical reevaluation of the "therapeutic range" of aminoglycosides. *Clin Infect Dis* 1992;14(1): 320–339.
136. Hess M, Finckh-Kramer U, Bartsch M, et al. Hearing screening in at-risk neonate cohort. *Int J Pediatr Otorhinolaryng* 1998;46: 81–89.
137. Borradori C, Fawer CL, Buclin T, et al. Risk factors of sensorineural hearing loss in preterm infants. *Biol Neonate* 1997; 71(1):1–10.
138. Kawashiro N, Tsuchihashi N, Koga K, et al. Delayed post-neonatal intensive care unit hearing disturbance. *Int J Pediatr Otorhinolaryngol* 1996;34(1–2):35–43.
139. Nield TA, Schrier S, Ramos AD, et al. Unexpected hearing loss in high-risk infants. *Pediatrics* 1986;78(3):417–422.
140. Finitzo-Hieber T, McCracken GH Jr., Brown KC. Prospective controlled evaluation of auditory function in neonates given netilmicin or amikacin. *J Pediatr* 1985;106(1):129–136.
141. Tsai CH, Tsai FJ. Auditory brainstem responses in term neonates treated with gentamicin. *Acta Paediatr Sin* 1992;33(6):417–422.
142. Chayasirisobhon S, Yu L, Griggs L, et al. Recording of brainstem evoked potentials and their association with gentamicin in neonates. *Pediatr Neurol* 1996;14(4):277–280.
143. Bernard PA. Freedom from ototoxicity in aminoglycoside treated neonates: a mistaken notion. *Laryngoscope* 1981;91(12): 1985–1994.
144. de Hoog M, van Zanten BA, Hop WC, et al. Newborn hearing screening: tobramycin and vancomycin are not risk factors for hearing loss. *J Pediatr* 2003;142(1):41–46.
145. Salamy A, Eldredge L, Tooley WH. Neonatal status and hearing loss in high-risk infants [see comments]. *J Pediatr* 1989;114(5): 847–852.
146. Elhanan K, Siplovich L, Raz R. Gentamicin once-daily versus thrice-daily in children. *J Antimicrob Chemother* 1995;35(2): 327–332.
147. Vigano A, Principi N, Brivio L, et al. Comparison of 5 milligrams of netilmicin per kilogram of body weight once daily versus 2 milligrams per kilogram thrice daily for treatment of gram-negative

pyelonephritis in children. *Antimicrob Agents Chemother* 1992; 36(7):1499–1503.

148. Katbamna B, Homnick DN, Marks JH. Effects of chronic tobramycin treatment on distortion product otoacoustic emissions. *Ear Hear* 1999;20(5):393–402.
149. Stavroulaki P, Vossinakis IC, Dinopoulou D, et al. Otoacoustic emissions for monitoring aminoglycoside-induced ototoxicity in children with cystic fibrosis. *Arch Otolaryngol Head Neck Surg* 2002;128(2):150–155.
150. Mattie H, Craig WA, Pechere JC. Determinants of efficacy and toxicity of aminoglycosides [see comments]. *J Antimicrob Chemother* 1989;24(3):281–293.
151. Moore RD, Smith CR, Lietman PS. The association of aminoglycoside plasma levels with mortality in patients with gram-negative bacteremia. *J Infect Dis* 1984;149:443–448.
152. Prins JM, Weverling GJ, de Blok K, et al. Validation and nephrotoxicity of a simplified once-daily aminoglycoside dosing schedule and guidelines for monitoring therapy. *Antimicrob Agents Chemother* 1996;40(11):2494–2499.
153. Semchuk W, Borgmann J, Bowman L. Determination of a gentamicin loading dose in neonates and infants. *Ther Drug Monit* 1993;15(1):47–51.
154. Allegaert K, Anderson BJ. Interindividual variability of aminoglycoside pharmacokinetics in preterm neonates at birth. *Eur J Clin Pharmacol* 2006;62(12):1011–1012.
155. de Hoog M, Schoemaker RC, Mouton JW, et al. Tobramycin population pharmacokinetics in neonates. *Clin Pharmacol Ther* 1997;62(4):392–399.
156. Isemann BT, Kotagal UR, Mashni SM, et al. Optimal gentamicin therapy in preterm neonates includes loading doses and early monitoring. *Ther Drug Monit* 1996;18(5):549–555.
157. Kenyon CF, Knoppert DC, Lee SK, et al. Amikacin pharmacokinetics and suggested dosage modifications for the preterm infant. *Antimicrob Agents Chemother* 1990;34(2):265–268.
158. Kotze A, Bartel PR, Sommers DK. Once versus twice daily amikacin in neonates: prospective study on toxicity. *J Paediatr Child Health* 1999;35(3):283–286.
159. Petersen PO, Wells TG, Kearns GL. Amikacin dosing in neonates: evaluation of a dosing chart based on population pharmacokinetic data. *Dev Pharmacol Ther* 1991;16(4):203–211.
160. Semchuk W, Shevchuk YM, Sankaran K, et al. Prospective, randomized, controlled evaluation of a gentamicin loading dose in neonates. *Biol Neonate* 1995;67(1):13–20.
161. Thingvoll ES, Guillet R, Caserta M, et al. Observational trial of a 48-hour gentamicin dosing regimen derived from Monte Carlo simulations in infants born at less than 28 weeks' gestation. *J Pediatr* 2008;153(4):530–534.
162. Watterberg KL, Kelly HW, Angelus P, et al. The need for a loading dose of gentamicin in neonates. *Ther Drug Monit* 1989;11(1): 16–20.
163. Labaune JM, Bleyzac N, Maire P, et al. Once-a-day individualized amikacin dosing for suspected infection at birth based on population pharmacokinetic models. *Biol Neonate* 2001;80(2): 142–147.
164. Langhendries JP, Battisti O, Bertrand JM, et al. Adaptation in neonatology of the once-daily concept of aminoglycoside administration: evaluation of a dosing chart for amikacin in an intensive care unit. *Biol Neonate* 1998;74(5):351–362.
165. Touw DJ, Westerman EM, Sprij AJ. Therapeutic drug monitoring of aminoglycosides in neonates. *Clin Pharmacokinet* 2009; 48(2):71–88.
166. Postovsky S, Ben Arush MW, Kassis E, et al. Pharmacokinetic analysis of gentamicin thrice and single daily dosage in pediatric cancer patients. *Pediatr Hematol Oncol* 1997;14(6):547–554.
167. Contopoulos-Ioannidis DG, Giotis ND, Baliatsa DV, et al. Extended-interval aminoglycoside administration for children: a meta-analysis. *Pediatrics* 2004;114(1):e111–e118.
168. Carlstedt BC, Uaamnuichai M, Day RB, et al. Aminoglycoside dosing in pediatric patients. *Ther Drug Monit* 1989;11(1):38–43.
169. Kraus DM, Dusik CM, Rodvold KA, et al. Bayesian forecasting of gentamicin pharmacokinetics in pediatric intensive care unit patients. *Pediatr Infect Dis J* 1993;12(9):713–718.
170. Logsdon BA, Phelps SJ. Routine monitoring of gentamicin serum concentrations in pediatric patients with normal renal function is unnecessary. *Ann Pharmacother* 1997;31(12):1514–1518.
171. Massey KL, Hendeles L, Neims A. Identification of children for whom routine monitoring of aminoglycoside serum concentrations is not cost effective. *J Pediatr* 1986;109(5):897–901.
172. Esposito AL, Gleckman RA. Vancomycin. A second look. *JAMA* 1977;238(16):1756–1757.
173. Waisbren B, Kleinerman L, Skemp J. Comparative clinical effectiveness and toxicity of vancomycin, ristocetin and kanamycin. *Arch Intern Med* 1960;106:179–193.
174. Appel GB, Neu HC. The nephrotoxicity of antimicrobial agents (second of three parts). *N Engl J Med* 1977;296(13):722–728.
175. Bailie GR, Neal D. Vancomycin ototoxicity and nephrotoxicity. A review. *Med Toxicol Adverse Drug Exp* 1988;3(5):376–386.
176. Newsom SW. Vancomycin. *J Antimicrob Chemother* 1982;10(4): 257–259.
177. Barna JC, Williams DH. The structure and mode of action of glycopeptide antibiotics of the vancomycin group. *Annu Rev Microbiol* 1984;38:339–357.
178. Perkins HR, Nieto M. The chemical basis for the action of the vancomycin group of antibiotics. *Ann N Y Acad Sci* 1974;235(0): 348–363.
179. Reynolds PE. Structure, biochemistry and mechanism of action of glycopeptide antibiotics. *Eur J Clin Microbiol Infect Dis* 1989; 8(11):943–950.
180. Pfeiffer RR. Structural features of vancomycin. *Rev Infect Dis* 1981;3(Suppl):S205–S209.
181. Fekety R. Vancomycin, teicoplanin and the streptogramins: quinupristin and dalfopristin. In: Mandell GL, Bennet JE, Dolin R, eds. *Mandell, Douglas, and Bennett's principles & practice of infectious diseases*, 5th ed. Philadelphia, PA: Churchill Livingstone, 2000:382–392.
182. Geraci JE, Heilman FR, Nichols DR. Antibiotic therapy of bacterial endocarditis. VII. Vancomycin for acute micrococcal endocarditis. *Proc Staff Meet Mayo Clin* 1958;33:172–181.
183. Sando M, Sato Y, Iwata S, et al. In vitro protein binding of teicoplanin to neonatal serum. *J Infect Chemother* 2004;10(5): 280–283.
184. Barg NL, Supena RB, Fekety R. Persistent staphylococcal bacteremia in an intravenous drug abuser. *Antimicrob Agents Chemother* 1986;29(2):209–211.
185. Tounian P, Jehl F, Pauliat S, et al. Stability and compatibility of teicoplanin in parenteral nutrition solutions used in pediatrics. *Clin Nutr* 1999;18(3):159–165.
186. Watanakunakorn C. The antibacterial action of vancomycin. *Rev Infect Dis* 1981;3(Suppl):S210–S215.
187. Wilhelm MP. Vancomycin. *Mayo Clin Proc* 1991;66(11):1165–1170.
188. Jordan D, Innis W. Selective inhibition of ribonucleic acid synthesis in Staphylococcus aureus by vancomycin. *Nature* 1959; 184:1894.
189. Jordan D, Mallory H. Site of action of vancomycin on Staphylococcus aureus. *Antimicrob Agents Chemother* 1964;4:489.
190. Smith TL, Pearson ML, Wilcox KR, et al. Emergence of vancomycin resistance in Staphylococcus aureus. Glycopeptide-Intermediate Staphylococcus aureus Working Group. *N Engl J Med* 1999;340(7):493–501.
191. Chambers HF, Kennedy S. Effects of dosage, peak and trough concentrations in serum, protein binding, and bactericidal rate on efficacy of teicoplanin in a rabbit model of endocarditis. *Antimicrob Agents Chemother* 1990;34(4):510–514.
192. Duffull SB, Begg EJ, Chambers ST, et al. Efficacies of different vancomycin dosing regimens against Staphylococcus aureus determined with a dynamic in vitro model. *Antimicrob Agents Chemother* 1994;38(10):2480–2482.
193. Lowdin E, Odenholt I, Cars O. In vitro studies of pharmacodynamic properties of vancomycin against Staphylococcus aureus and Staphylococcus epidermidis. *Antimicrob Agents Chemother* 1998;42(10):2739–2744.
194. Peetermans WE, Hoogeterp JJ, Hazekamp-van Dokkum AM, et al. Antistaphylococcal activities of teicoplanin and vancomycin in vitro and in an experimental infection. *Antimicrob Agents Chemother* 1990;34(10):1869–1874.
195. Mouton JW. *Vancomycin killing kinetics.* Presented at the International Conference on Antimicrobial Agents and Chemotherapy, San Diego, CA, September 28–October 1, 1997.
196. James JK, Palmer SM, Levine DP, et al. Comparison of conventional dosing versus continuous-infusion vancomycin therapy

for patients with suspected or documented gram-positive infections. *Antimicrob Agents Chemother* 1996;40(3):696–700.
197. Lundstrom TS, Sobel JD. Antibiotics for gram-positive bacterial infections. Vancomycin, teicoplanin, quinupristin/dalfopristin, and linezolid. *Infect Dis Clin North Am* 2000;14(2):463–474.
198. Pawlotsky F, Thomas A, Kergueris MF, et al. Constant rate infusion of vancomycin in premature neonates: a new dosage schedule. *Br J Clin Pharmacol* 1998;46:163–167.
199. Marik PE. The failure of a once-daily vancomycin dosing regimen in patients with normal renal function. *J Antimicrob Chemother* 1997;40(5):745–746.
200. Marik PE. Failure of once-daily vancomycin for staphylococcal endocarditis. *Pharmacotherapy* 1998;18(3):650–652.
201. Plan O, Cambonie G, Barbotte E, et al. Continuous-infusion vancomycin therapy for preterm neonates with suspected or documented Gram-positive infections: a new dosage schedule. *Arch Dis Child Fetal Neonatal Ed* 2008;93(6):F418–F421.
202. Cooper MA, Jin YF, Ashby JP, et al. In-vitro comparison of the post-antibiotic effect of vancomycin and teicoplanin. *J Antimicrob Chemother* 1990;26(2):203–207.
203. Hanberger H, Nilsson LE, Maller R, et al. Pharmacodynamics of daptomycin and vancomycin on Enterococcus faecalis and Staphylococcus aureus demonstrated by studies of initial killing and postantibiotic effect and influence of Ca2+ and albumin on these drugs. *Antimicrob Agents Chemother* 1991;35(9): 1710–1716.
204. Rybak MJ, Cappelletty DM, Moldovan T, et al. Comparative in vitro activities and postantibiotic effects of the oxazolidinone compounds eperezolid (PNU-100592) and linezolid (PNU-100766) versus vancomycin against Staphylococcus aureus, coagulase-negative staphylococci, Enterococcus faecalis, and Enterococcus faecium. *Antimicrob Agents Chemother* 1998;42(3):721–724.
205. Drabu YJ, Blakemore PH. The post-antibiotic effect of teicoplanin: monotherapy and combination studies. *J Antimicrob Chemother* 1991;27(Suppl B):1–7.
206. Schaad HJ, Chuard C, Vaudaux P, et al. Teicoplanin alone or combined with rifampin compared with vancomycin for prophylaxis and treatment of experimental foreign body infection by methicillin-resistant Staphylococcus aureus. *Antimicrob Agents Chemother* 1994;38(8):1703–1710.
207. Watanakunakorn C, Bakie C. Synergism of vancomycin-gentamicin and vancomycin-streptomycin against enterococci. *Antimicrob Agents Chemother* 1973;4(2):120–124.
208. Centers for Disease Control and Prevention. Nosocomial enterococci resistant to vancomycin–United States, 1989–1993. *MMWR Morb Mortal Wkly Rep* 1993;42(30):597–599.
209. Frieden TR, Munsiff SS, Low DE, et al. Emergence of vancomycin-resistant enterococci in New York City. *Lancet* 1993; 342(8863): 76–79.
210. Leclercq R, Derlot E, Weber M, et al. Transferable vancomycin and teicoplanin resistance in Enterococcus faecium. *Antimicrob Agents Chemother* 1989;33(1):10–15.
211. Shlaes DM, Etter L, Gutmann L. Synergistic killing of vancomycin-resistant enterococci of classes A, B, and C by combinations of vancomycin, penicillin, and gentamicin. *Antimicrob Agents Chemother* 1991;35(4):776–779.
212. Vincent S, Minkler P, Bincziewski B, et al. Vancomycin resistance in Enterococcus gallinarum. *Antimicrob Agents Chemother* 1992; 36(7):1392–1399.
213. Herwaldt L, Boyken L, Pfaller M. In vitro selection of resistance to vancomycin in bloodstream isolates of Staphylococcus haemolyticus and Staphylococcus epidermidis. *Eur J Clin Microbiol Infect Dis* 1991;10(12):1007–1012.
214. Hiramatsu K, Hanaki H, Ino T, et al. Methicillin-resistant Staphylococcus aureus clinical strain with reduced vancomycin susceptibility. *J Antimicrob Chemother* 1997;40(1):135–136.
215. Cui L, Ma X, Sato K, et al. Cell wall thickening is a common feature of vancomycin resistance in Staphylococcus aureus. *J Clin Microbiol* 2003;41(1):5–14.
216. Sieradzki K, Roberts RB, Haber SW, et al. The development of vancomycin resistance in a patient with methicillin-resistant Staphylococcus aureus infection. *N Engl J Med* 1999;340(7): 517–523.
217. Blaser J, Vergeres P, Widmer AF, et al. In vivo verification of in vitro model of antibiotic treatment of device-related infection. *Antimicrob Agents Chemother* 1995;39(5):1134–1139.
218. Evans RC, Holmes CJ. Effect of vancomycin hydrochloride on Staphylococcus epidermidis biofilm associated with silicone elastomer. *Antimicrob Agents Chemother* 1987;31(6):889–894.
219. Kallman J, Kihlstrom E, Sjoberg L, et al. Increase of staphylococci in neonatal septicaemia: a fourteen-year study. *Acta Paediatr* 1997;86(5):533–538.
220. McDougal A, Ling EW, Levine M. Vancomycin pharmacokinetics and dosing in premature neonates. *Ther Drug Monit* 1995;17(4): 319–326.
221. Freeman J, Epstein MF, Smith NE, et al. Extra hospital stay and antibiotic usage with nosocomial coagulase-negative staphylococcal bacteremia in two neonatal intensive care unit populations. *Am J Dis Child* 1990;144(3):324–329.
222. Gray JE, Richardson DK, McCormick MC, et al. Coagulase-negative staphylococcal bacteremia among very low birth weight infants: relation to admission illness severity, resource use, and outcome. *Pediatrics* 1995;95(2):225–230.
223. Stoll BJ, Gordon T, Korones SB, et al. Late-onset sepsis in very low birth weight neonates: a report from the National Institute of Child Health and Human Development Neonatal Research Network. *J Pediatr* 1996;129(1):63–71.
224. Baier RJ, Bocchini JA Jr., Brown EG. Selective use of vancomycin to prevent coagulase-negative staphylococcal nosocomial bacteremia in high risk very low birth weight infants. *Pediatr Infect Dis J* 1998;17(3):179–183.
225. Kacica MA, Horgan MJ, Ochoa L, et al. Prevention of gram-positive sepsis in neonates weighing less than 1500 grams. *J Pediatr* 1994;125(2):253–258.
226. Moller JC, Nachtrodt G, Richter A, et al. Prophylactic vancomycin to prevent staphylococcal septicaemia in very-low-birth-weight infants [letter]. *Lancet* 1992;340(8816):424.
227. Moller JC, Nelskamp I, Jensen R, et al. Teicoplanin pharmacology in prophylaxis for coagulase-negative staphylococcal sepsis of very low birthweight infants. *Acta Paediatr* 1996;85(5): 638–639.
228. Moller JC, Rossa M, Nachtrodt G, et al. Preventive antibiotic administration for prevention of nosocomial septicemia in very small premature infants (VLBW infants)—preventive vancomycin administration against infections with coagulase negative streptococci—prevention of translocation with oral cefixime therapy in intestinal colonization with pathogenic gram-negative pathogens. *Klin Padiatr* 1993;205(3):140–144.
229. Spafford PS, Sinkin RA, Cox C, et al. Prevention of central venous catheter-related coagulase-negative staphylococcal sepsis in neonates. *J Pediatr* 1994;125(2):259–263.
230. Craft AP, Finer NN, Barrington KJ. Vancomycin for prophylaxis against sepsis in preterm neonates. *Cochrane Database Syst Rev* 2000;2.
231. Garland JS, Alex CP, Henrickson KJ, et al. A vancomycin-heparin lock solution for prevention of nosocomial bloodstream infection in critically ill neonates with peripherally inserted central venous catheters: a prospective, randomized trial. *Pediatrics* 2005; 116(2):e198–e205.
232. Safdar N, Maki DG. Use of vancomycin-containing lock or flush solutions for prevention of bloodstream infection associated with central venous access devices: a meta-analysis of prospective, randomized trials. *Clin Infect Dis* 2006;43(4):474–484.
233. O'Grady NP, Alexander M, Dellinger EP, et al. Guidelines for the prevention of intravascular catheter-related infections. Centers for Disease Control and Prevention. *MMWR Recomm Rep* 2002;51(RR-10):1–29.
234. Vermont CL, Hartwig NG, Fleer A, et al. Persistence of clones of coagulase-negative staphylococci among premature neonates in neonatal intensive care units: two-center study of bacterial genotyping and patient risk factors. *J Clin Microbiol* 1998;36(9): 2485–2490.
235. Henrickson KJ, Axtell RA, Hoover SM, et al. Prevention of central venous catheter-related infections and thrombotic events in immunocompromised children by the use of vancomycin/ciprofloxacin/heparin flush solution: a randomized, multicenter, double-blind trial. *J Clin Oncol* 2000;18(6):1269–1278.
236. Schaison G, Baruchel A, Arlet G. Prevention of gram-positive and Candida albicans infections using teicoplanin and fluconazole: a randomized study in neutropenic children. *Br J Haematol* 1990;76(Suppl 2):24–26.

237. Golper TA, Noonan HM, Elzinga L, et al. Vancomycin pharmacokinetics, renal handling, and nonrenal clearances in normal human subjects. *Clin Pharmacol Ther* 1988;43(5):565–570.
238. Seay RE, Brundage RC, Jensen PD, et al. Population pharmacokinetics of vancomycin in neonates [published erratum appears in *Clin Pharmacol Ther* 1995;58(2):142]. *Clin Pharmacol Ther* 1994; 56(2):169–175.
239. Matzke GR, Zhanel GG, Guay DR. Clinical pharmacokinetics of vancomycin. *Clin Pharmacokinet* 1986;11(4):257–282.
240. Schaad UB, McCracken GH Jr., Nelson JD. Clinical pharmacology and efficacy of vancomycin in pediatric patients. *J Pediatr* 1980;96(1):119–126.
241. Burstein AH, Gal P, Forrest A. Evaluation of a sparse sampling strategy for determining vancomycin pharmacokinetics in preterm neonates: application of optimal sampling theory. *Ann Pharmacother* 1997;31(9):980–983.
242. Schaible DH, Rocci ML Jr., Alpert GA, et al. Vancomycin pharmacokinetics in infants: relationships to indices of maturation. *Pediatr Infect Dis* 1986;5(3):304–308.
243. Rodvold KA, Everett JA, Pryka RD, et al. Pharmacokinetics and administration regimens of vancomycin in neonates, infants and children. *Clin Pharmacokinet* 1997;33(1):32–51.
244. McGee SM, Kaplan SL, Mason EO Jr. Ventricular fluid concentrations of vancomycin in children after intravenous and intraventricular administration. *Pediatr Infect Dis J* 1990;9(2):138–139.
245. Odio C, Mohs E, Sklar FH, et al. Adverse reactions to vancomycin used as prophylaxis for CSF shunt procedures. *Am J Dis Child* 1984;138(1):17–19.
246. Reiter PD, Doron MW. Vancomycin cerebrospinal fluid concentrations after intravenous administration in premature infants. *J Perinatol* 1996;16(5):331–335.
247. Schaad UB, Nelson JD, McCracken GH Jr. Pharmacology and efficacy of vancomycin for staphylococcal infections in children. *Rev Infect Dis* 1981;3(Suppl):S282–S288.
248. Reed MD, Kliegman RM, Weiner JS, et al. The clinical pharmacology of vancomycin in seriously ill preterm infants. *Pediatr Res* 1987;22(3):360–363.
249. Guay DR, Vance-Bryan K, Gilliland S, et al. Comparison of vancomycin pharmacokinetics in hospitalized elderly and young patients using a Bayesian forecaster. *J Clin Pharmacol* 1993; 33(10):918–922.
250. Le Normand Y, Milpied N, Kergueris MF, et al. Pharmacokinetic parameters of vancomycin for therapeutic regimens in neutropenic adult patients. *Int J Biomed Comput* 1994;36(1–2):121–125.
251. Pou L, Rosell M, Lopez R, et al. Changes in vancomycin pharmacokinetics during treatment. *Ther Drug Monit* 1996;18(2): 149–153.
252. Rodvold KA, Blum RA, Fischer JH, et al. Vancomycin pharmacokinetics in patients with various degrees of renal function. *Antimicrob Agents Chemother* 1988;32(6):848–852.
253. de Hoog M, Schoemaker RC, Mouton JW, et al. Vancomycin population pharmacokinetics in neonates. *Clin Pharmacol Ther* 2000;67(4):360–367.
254. Fofah OO, Karmen A, Piscitelli J, et al. Failure of prediction of peak serum vancomycin concentrations from trough values in neonates. *Pediatr Infect Dis J* 1999;18(3):299–300.
255. Gous AG, Dance MD, Lipman J, et al. Changes in vancomycin pharmacokinetics in critically ill infants. *Anaesth Intensive Care* 1995;23(6):678–682.
256. Gross JR, Kaplan SL, Kramer WG, et al. Vancomycin pharmacokinetics in premature infants. *Pediatr Pharmacol (New York)* 1985; 5(1):17–22.
257. Jarrett RV, Marinkovich GA, Gayle EL, et al. Individualized pharmacokinetic profiles to compute vancomycin dosage and dosing interval in preterm infants [see comments]. *Pediatr Infect Dis J* 1993;12(2):156–157.
258. Kildoo CW, Lin LM, Gabriel MH, et al. Vancomycin pharmacokinetics in infants: relationship to postconceptional age and serum creatinine. *Dev Pharmacol Ther* 1989;14(2):77–83.
259. Lisby-Sutch SM, Nahata MC. Dosage guidelines for the use of vancomycin based on its pharmacokinetics in infants. *Eur J Clin Pharmacol* 1988;35(6):637–642.
260. Naqvi SH, Keenan WJ, Reichley RM, et al. Vancomycin pharmacokinetics in small, seriously ill infants. *Am J Dis Child* 1986; 140(2):107–110.
261. Spivey JM, Gal P. Vancomycin pharmacokinetics in neonates. *Am J Dis Child* 1986;140(9):859.
262. Tarral E, Jehl F, Tarral A, et al. Pharmacokinetics of teicoplanin in children. *J Antimicrob Chemother* 1988;21(Suppl A):47–51.
263. Grimsley C, Thomson AH. Pharmacokinetics and dose requirements of vancomycin in neonates. *Arch Dis Child Fetal Neonatal Ed* 1999;81(3):F221–F227.
264. James A, Koren G, Milliken J, et al. Vancomycin pharmacokinetics and dose recommendations for preterm infants. *Antimicrob Agents Chemother* 1987;31(1):52–54.
265. Leonard MB, Koren G, Stevenson DK, et al. Vancomycin pharmacokinetics in very low birth weight neonates. *Pediatr Infect Dis J* 1989;8(5):282–286.
266. Rodvold KA, Gentry CA, Plank GS, et al. Bayesian forecasting of serum vancomycin concentrations in neonates and infants. *Ther Drug Monit* 1995;17(3):239–246.
267. Silva R, Reis E, Bispo MA, et al. The kinetic profile of vancomycin in neonates. *J Pharm Pharmacol* 1998;50(11):1255–1260.
268. Kimura T, Sunakawa K, Matsuura N, et al. Population pharmacokinetics of arbekacin, vancomycin, and panipenem in neonates. *Antimicrob Agents Chemother* 2004;48(4):1159–1167.
269. Capparelli EV, Lane JR, Romanowski GL, et al. The influences of renal function and maturation on vancomycin elimination in newborns and infants. *J Clin Pharmacol* 2001;41(9):927–934.
270. Cantu TG, Yamanaka-Yuen NA, Lietman PS. Serum vancomycin concentrations: reappraisal of their clinical value [see comments]. *Clin Infect Dis* 1994;18(4):533–543.
271. Goebel J, Ananth M, Lewy JE. Hemodiafiltration for vancomycin overdose in a neonate with end-stage renal failure. *Pediatr Nephrol* 1999;13(5):423–425.
272. Leake RD, Trygstad CW, Oh W. Inulin clearance in the newborn infant: relationship to gestational and postnatal age. *Pediatr Res* 1976;10(8):759–762.
273. van den Anker JN, de Groot R, Broerse HM, et al. Assessment of glomerular filtration rate in preterm infants by serum creatinine: comparison with inulin clearance. *Pediatrics* 1995;96(6): 1156–1158.
274. Asbury WH, Darsey EH, Rose WB, et al. Vancomycin pharmacokinetics in neonates and infants: a retrospective evaluation. *Ann Pharmacother* 1993;27(4):490–496.
275. van den Anker JN, Hop WC, Schoemaker RC, et al. Ceftazidime pharmacokinetics in preterm infants: effect of postnatal age and postnatal exposure to indomethacin. *Br J Clin Pharmacol* 1995; 40(5):439–443.
276. Gleason CA. Prostaglandins and the developing kidney. *Semin Perinatol* 1987;11(1):12–21.
277. Guignard JP, Gouyon JB. Adverse effects of drugs on the immature kidney. *Biol Neonate* 1988;53(4):243–252.
278. Gal P, Gilman JT. Drug disposition in neonates with patent ductus arteriosus. *Ann Pharmacother* 1993;27(11):1383–1388.
279. Anderson BJ, Allegaert K, Van den Anker JN, et al. Vancomycin pharmacokinetics in preterm neonates and the prediction of adult clearance. *Br J Clin Pharmacol* 2007;63(1):75–84.
280. Mulla H, Pooboni S. Population pharmacokinetics of vancomycin in patients receiving extracorporeal membrane oxygenation. *Br J Clin Pharmacol* 2005;60(3):265–275.
281. Amaker RD, DiPiro JT, Bhatia J. Pharmacokinetics of vancomycin in critically ill infants undergoing extracorporeal membrane oxygenation. *Antimicrob Agents Chemother* 1996;40(5): 1139–1142.
282. Buck ML. Vancomycin pharmacokinetics in neonates receiving extracorporeal membrane oxygenation. *Pharmacotherapy* 1998; 18(5):1082–1086.
283. Hoie EB, Swigart SA, Leuschen MP, et al. Vancomycin pharmacokinetics in infants undergoing extracorporeal membrane oxygenation. *Clin Pharm* 1990;9(9):711–715.
284. Sanchez A, Lopez-Herce J, Cueto E, et al. Teicoplanin pharmacokinetics in critically ill paediatric patients. *J Antimicrob Chemother* 1999;44(3):407–409.
285. Wrishko RE, Levine M, Khoo D, et al. Vancomycin pharmacokinetics and Bayesian estimation in pediatric patients. *Ther Drug Monit* 2000;22(5):522–531.
286. Lukas JC, Karikas G, Gazouli M, et al. Pharmacokinetics of teicoplanin in an ICU population of children and infants. *Pharm Res* 2004;21(11):2064–2071.

287. Schaefer F, Klaus G, Muller-Wiefel DE, et al. Intermittent versus continuous intraperitoneal glycopeptide/ceftazidime treatment in children with peritoneal dialysis-associated peritonitis. The Mid-European Pediatric Peritoneal Dialysis Study Group (MEPPS). *J Am Soc Nephrol* 1999;10(1):136–145.
288. Blowey DL, Warady BA, Abdel-Rahman S, et al. Vancomycin disposition following intraperitoneal administration in children receiving peritoneal dialysis. *Perit Dial Int* 2007;27(1):79–85.
289. Spears RL, Koch R. The use of vancomycin in pediatrics. *Antibiot Annu* 1959–1960;7:798–803.
290. Klugman KP, Friedland IR, Bradley JS. Bactericidal activity against cephalosporin-resistant Streptococcus pneumoniae in cerebrospinal fluid of children with acute bacterial meningitis. *Antimicrob Agents Chemother* 1995;39(9):1988–1992.
291. Fan-Havard P, Nahata MC, Bartkowski MH, et al. Pharmacokinetics and cerebrospinal fluid (CSF) concentrations of vancomycin in pediatric patients undergoing CSF shunt placement. *Chemotherapy* 1990;36(2):103–108.
292. Jorgenson L, Reiter PD, Freeman JE, et al. Vancomycin disposition and penetration into ventricular fluid of the central nervous system following intravenous therapy in patients with cerebrospinal devices. *Pediatr Neurosurg* 2007;43(6):449–455.
293. Jacobs F, Deleluse F, Raftopoulos C, et al. Intraventricular vancomycin in CSF shunt infections. *Neurosurgery* 1987;21(1):112–113.
294. Losonsky GA, Wolf A, Schwalbe RS, et al. Successful treatment of meningitis due to multiply resistant Enterococcus faecium with a combination of intrathecal teicoplanin and intravenous antimicrobial agents. *Clin Infect Dis* 1994;19(1):163–165.
295. Pau AK, Smego RA Jr., Fisher MA. Intraventricular vancomycin: observations of tolerance and pharmacokinetics in two infants with ventricular shunt infections. *Pediatr Infect Dis* 1986;5(1):93–96.
296. Bafeltowska JJ, Buszman E, Mandat KM, et al. Therapeutic vancomycin monitoring in children with hydrocephalus during treatment of shunt infections. *Surg Neurol* 2004;62(2):142–150; discussion 50.
297. Dagan R, Einhorn M, Howard C, et al. Outpatient and inpatient teicoplanin treatment for serious Gram-positive infections in children. *Pediatr Infect Dis J* 1993;12(6):S17–S20.
298. Shime N, Kato Y, Kosaka T, et al. Glycopeptide pharmacokinetics in current paediatric cardiac surgery practice. *Eur J Cardiothorac Surg* 2007;32(4):577–581.
299. Reed MD, Yamashita TS, Myers CM, et al. The pharmacokinetics of teicoplanin in infants and children. *J Antimicrob Chemother* 1997;39(6):789–796.
300. Terragna A, Ferrea G, Loy A, et al. Pharmacokinetics of teicoplanin in pediatric patients. *Antimicrob Agents Chemother* 1988;32(8):1223–1226.
301. Chang D. Influence of malignancy on the pharmacokinetics of vancomycin in infants and children. *Pediatr Infect Dis J* 1995;14(8):667–673.
302. Krivoy N, Peleg S, Postovsky S, et al. Pharmacokinetic analysis of vancomycin in steady state in pediatric cancer patients. *Pediatr Hematol Oncol* 1998;15(4):333–338.
303. Hatzopoulos FK, Stile-Calligaro IL, Rodvold KA, et al. Pharmacokinetics of intravenous vancomycin in pediatric cardiopulmonary bypass surgery. *Pediatr Infect Dis J* 1993;12(4):300–304.
304. Dagan O, Klein J, Gruenwald C, et al. Preliminary studies of the effects of extracorporeal membrane oxygenator on the disposition of common pediatric drugs. *Ther Drug Monit* 1993;15(4):263–266.
305. Begg EJ, Barclay ML, Kirkpatrick CJ. The therapeutic monitoring of antimicrobial agents. *Br J Clin Pharmacol* 1999;47(1):23–30.
306. Nagl M, Neher C, Hager J, et al. Bactericidal activity of vancomycin in cerebrospinal fluid. *Antimicrob Agents Chemother* 1999;43(8):1932–1934.
307. Rubin LG, Sanchez PJ, Siegel J, et al. Evaluation and treatment of neonates with suspected late-onset sepsis: a survey of neonatologists' practices. *Pediatrics* 2002;110(4):e42.
308. Leader WG, Chandler MH, Castiglia M. Pharmacokinetic optimisation of vancomycin therapy. *Clin Pharmacokinet* 1995;28(4):327–342.
309. Louria D, Kaminski T, Buchman J. Vancomycin in severe staphylococcal infections. *Arch Intern Med* 1961;107:225–240.
310. Sorrell TC, Packham DR, Shanker S, et al. Vancomycin therapy for methicillin-resistant Staphylococcus aureus. *Ann Intern Med* 1982;97(3):344–350.
311. Kaplan EL. Vancomycin in infants and children: a review of pharmacology and indications for therapy and prophylaxis. *J Antimicrob Chemother* 1984;14(Suppl D):59–66.
312. Deville JG, Adler S, Azimi PH, et al. Linezolid versus vancomycin in the treatment of known or suspected resistant gram-positive infections in neonates. *Pediatr Infect Dis J* 2003;22(9 Suppl):S158–S163.
313. Wilson AP. Clinical pharmacokinetics of teicoplanin. *Clin Pharmacokinet* 2000;39(3):167–183.
314. Degraeuwe PL, Beuman GH, van Tiel FH, et al. Use of teicoplanin in preterm neonates with staphylococcal late-onset neonatal sepsis. *Biol Neonate* 1998;73(5):287–294.
315. Fanos V, Kacet N, Mosconi G. A review of teicoplanin in the treatment of serious neonatal infections. *Eur J Pediatr* 1997;156(6):423–427.
316. Bassetti D, Cruciani M. Teicoplanin therapy in children: a review. *Scand J Infect Dis Suppl* 1990;72:35–37.
317. Bernig T, Weigel S, Mukodzi S, et al. Antibiotic sequential therapy for febrile neutropenia in pediatric patients with malignancy. *Pediatr Hematol Oncol* 2000;17(1):93–98.
318. Lehrnbecher T, Stanescu A, Kuhl J. Short courses of intravenous empirical antibiotic treatment in selected febrile neutropenic children with cancer. *Infection* 2002;30(1):17–21.
319. Best CJ, Ewart M, Sumner E. Perioperative complications following the use of vancomycin in children: a report of two cases. *Br J Anaesth* 1989;62(5):576–577.
320. Boussemart T, Cardona J, Berthier M, et al. Cardiac arrest associated with vancomycin in a neonate [letter]. *Arch Dis Child Fetal Neonatal Ed* 1995;73(2):F123.
321. Duffull SB, Begg EJ. Vancomycin toxicity. What is the evidence for dose dependency? *Adverse Drug React Toxicol Rev* 1994;13(2):103–114.
322. Wood MJ. The comparative efficacy and safety of teicoplanin and vancomycin [see comments]. *J Antimicrob Chemother* 1996;37(2):209–222.
323. Rybak MJ, Albrecht LM, Boike SC, et al. Nephrotoxicity of vancomycin, alone and with an aminoglycoside. *J Antimicrob Chemother* 1990;25(4):679–687.
324. Schumacher GE, Barr JT. Using population-based serum drug concentration cutoff values to predict toxicity: test performance and limitations compared with Bayesian interpretation. *Clin Pharm* 1990;9(10):788–796.
325. Sidi V, Roilides E, Bibashi E, et al. Comparison of efficacy and safety of teicoplanin and vancomycin in children with antineoplastic therapy-associated febrile neutropenia and gram-positive bacteremia. *J Chemother* 2000;12(4):326–331.
326. Sakata H, Maruyama S, Ishioka T, et al. Change of renal function during vancomycin therapy in extremely low birthweight infants. *Acta Paediatr Jpn* 1996;38(6):619–621.
327. Nahata MC. Lack of nephrotoxicity in pediatric patients receiving concurrent vancomycin and aminoglycoside therapy. *Chemotherapy* 1987;33(4):302–304.
328. Bhatt-Mehta V, Schumacher RE, Faix RG, et al. Lack of vancomycin-associated nephrotoxicity in newborn infants: a case-control study. *Pediatrics* 1999;103(4):e48.
329. Miner LJ, Faix RG. Large vancomycin overdose in two premature infants with minimal toxicity. *Am J Perinatol* 2004;21(8):433–438.
330. Wicklow BA, Ogborn MR, Gibson IW, et al. Biopsy-proven acute tubular necrosis in a child attributed to vancomycin intoxication. *Pediatr Nephrol* 2006;21(8):1194–1196.
331. Wu CY, Wang JS, Chiou YH, et al. Biopsy proven acute tubular necrosis associated with vancomycin in a child: case report and literature review. *Ren Fail* 2007;29(8):1059–1061.
332. Goren MP, Baker DK Jr., Shenep JL. Vancomycin does not enhance amikacin-induced tubular nephrotoxicity in children. *Pediatr Infect Dis J* 1989;8(5):278–282.
333. Odio C, McCracken GH, Nelson JD. Nephrotoxicity associated with vancomycin-aminoglycoside therapy in four children. *J Pediatr* 1984;105:491–493.
334. Dean RP, Wagner DJ, Tolpin MD. Vancomycin/aminoglycoside nephrotoxicity [letter]. *J Pediatr* 1985;106(5):861–862.
335. Dufort G, Ventura C, Olive T, et al. Teicoplanin pharmacokinetics in pediatric patients. *Pediatr Infect Dis J* 1996;15(6):494–498.

336. Fanos V, Mussap M, Khoory BJ, et al. Renal tolerability of teicoplanin in a case of neonatal overdose. *J Chemother* 1998; 10(5):381–384.
337. Brummett RE. Ototoxicity of vancomycin and analogues. *Otolaryngol Clin North Am* 1993;26(5):821–828.
338. Brummett RE, Fox KE, Jacobs F, et al. Augmented gentamicin ototoxicity induced by vancomycin in guinea pigs. *Arch Otolaryngol Head Neck Surg* 1990;116(1):61–64.
339. Lutz H, Lenarz T, Weidauer H, et al. Ototoxicity of vancomycin: an experimental study in guinea pigs. *ORL J Otorhinolaryngol Relat Spec* 1991;53(5):273–278.
340. Reyes MP, Ostrea EM Jr., Cabinian AE, et al. Vancomycin during pregnancy: does it cause hearing loss or nephrotoxicity in the infant? [see comments]. *Am J Obstet Gynecol* 1989;161(4): 977–981.
341. Burkhart KK, Metcalf S, Shurnas E, et al. Exchange transfusion and multidose activated charcoal following vancomycin overdose. *J Toxicol Clin Toxicol* 1992;30(2):285–294.
342. Hall JW III, Herndon DN, Gary LB, et al. Auditory brainstem response in young burn-wound patients treated with ototoxic drugs. *Int J Pediatr Otorhinolaryngol* 1986;12(2):187–203.
343. Buckingham SC, McCullers JA, Lujan-Zilbermann J, et al. Early vancomycin therapy and adverse outcomes in children with pneumococcal meningitis. *Pediatrics* 2006;117(5):1688–1694.
344. Koren G, James A. Vancomycin dosing in preterm infants: prospective verification of new recommendations. *J Pediatr* 1987; 110(5):797–798.
345. Chang D, Liem L, Malogolowkin M. A prospective study of vancomycin pharmacokinetics and dosage requirements in pediatric cancer patients. *Pediatr Infect Dis J* 1994;13(11):969–974.
346. Piro CC, Crossno CL, Collier A, et al. Initial vancomycin dosing in pediatric oncology and stem cell transplant patients. *J Pediatr Hematol Oncol* 2009;31(1):3–7.
347. Duffull SB, Chambers ST, Begg EJ. How vancomycin is used in Australasia—a survey. *Aust N Z J Med* 1993;23(6):662–666.
348. Fitzsimmons WE, Postelnick MJ, Tortorice PV. Survey of vancomycin monitoring guidelines in Illinois hospitals. *Drug Intell Clin Pharm* 1988;22(7–8):598–600.
349. Anne L, Hu M, Chan K, et al. Potential problem with fluorescence polarization immunoassay cross-reactivity to vancomycin degradation product CDP-1: its detection in sera of renally impaired patients. *Ther Drug Monit* 1989;11(5):585–591.
350. Sym D, Smith C, Meenan G, et al. Fluorescence polarization immunoassay: can it result in an overestimation of vancomycin in patients not suffering from renal failure? *Ther Drug Monit* 2001;23(4):441–444.
351. Smith PF, Petros WP, Soucie MP, et al. New modified fluorescence polarization immunoassay does not falsely elevate vancomycin concentrations in patients with end-stage renal disease. *Ther Drug Monit* 1998;20(2):231–235.
352. Miles MV, Li L, Lakkis H, et al. Special considerations for monitoring vancomycin concentrations in pediatric patients. *Ther Drug Monit* 1997;19(3):265–270.
353. de Hoog M, Mouton JW, van den Anker JN. Why monitor peak vancomycin concentrations? [letter]. *Lancet* 1995;345:646.
354. Saunders NJ. Why monitor peak vancomycin concentrations? *Lancet* 1994;344:1748–1750.
355. Shackley F, Roberts P, Heath P, et al. Trough-only monitoring of serum vancomycin concentrations in neonates. *J Antimicrob Chemother* 1998;41:141–142.
356. Sawchuk R, Zaske D. Pharmacokinetic dosage regimens which utilize multiple intravenous infusions: gentamicin in burn patients. *J Pharmacokinet Biopharm* 1976;4:183–195.
357. Pryka RD, Rodvold KA, Erdman SM. An updated comparison of drug dosing methods. Part IV: vancomycin. *Clin Pharmacokinet* 1991;20(6):463–476.
358. Lamarre P, Lebel D, Ducharme MP. A population pharmacokinetic model for vancomycin in pediatric patients and its predictive value in a naive population. *Antimicrob Agents Chemother* 2000;44(2):278–282.
359. Ohnishi A, Yano Y, Ishibashi T, et al. Evaluation of Bayesian predictability of vancomycin concentration using population pharmacokinetic parameters in pediatric patients. *Drug Metab Pharmacokinet* 2005;20(6):415–422.
360. Padovani EM, Pistolesi C, Fanos V, et al. Pharmacokinetics of amikacin in neonates. *Dev Pharmacol Ther* 1993;20(3–4):167–173.
361. Allegaert K, Scheers I, Adams E, et al. Cerebrospinal fluid compartmental pharmacokinetics of amikacin in neonates. *Antimicrob Agents Chemother* 2008;52(6):1934–1939.
362. Nakae S, Yamada M, Ito T, et al. Gentamicin dosing and pharmacokinetics in low birth weight infants. *Tohoku J Exp Med* 1988;155(3):213–223.
363. Koren G, Leeder S, Harding E, et al. Optimization of gentamicin therapy in very low birth weight infants. *Pediatr Pharmacol (New York)* 1985;5(1):79–87.
364. Dahl LB, Melby K, Gutteberg TJ, et al. Serum levels of ampicillin and gentamicin in neonates of varying gestational age. *Eur J Pediatr* 1986;145(3):218–221.
365. Faura CC, Feret MA, Horga JF. Monitoring serum levels of gentamicin to develop a new regimen for gentamicin dosage in newborns. *Ther Drug Monit* 1991;13(3):268–276.
366. Botha JH, du Preez MJ, Adhikari M. Population pharmacokinetics of gentamicin in South African newborns. *Eur J Clin Pharmacol* 2003;59(10):755–759.
367. Granati B, Assael BM, Chung M, et al. Clinical pharmacology of netilmicin in preterm and term newborn infants. *J Pediatr* 1985; 106(4):664–669.
368. Kuhn RJ, Nahata MC, Powell DA, et al. Pharmacokinetics of netilmicin in premature infants. *Eur J Clin Pharmacol* 1986;29: 635–637.
369. Nahata MC, Powell DA, Durrell DE, et al. Effect of gestational age and birth weight on tobramycin kinetics in newborn infants. *J Antimicrob Chemother* 1984;14(1):59–65.
370. Nahata MC, Powell DA, Gregoire RP, et al. Tobramycin kinetics in newborn infants. *J Pediatr* 1983;103(1):136–138.
371. Bressolle F, Gouby A, Martinez JM, et al. Population pharmacokinetics of amikacin in critically ill patients. *Antimicrob Agents Chemother* 1996;40(7):1682–1689.
372. Marik PE, Havlik I, Monteagudo FS, et al. The pharmacokinetic of amikacin in critically ill adult and paediatric patients: comparison of once- versus twice-daily dosing regimens. *J Antimicrob Chemother* 1991;27(Suppl C):81–89.
373. Hoecker JL, Pickering LK, Swaney J, et al. Clinical pharmacology of tobramycin in children. *J Infect Dis* 1978;137(5):592–596.
374. Jacobson PA, West NJ, Price J, et al. Gentamicin and tobramycin pharmacokinetics in pediatric bone marrow transplant patients. *Ann Pharmacother* 1997;31(10):1127–1131.
375. Lanao JM, Berrocal A, Calvo MV, et al. Population pharmacokinetic study of gentamicin and a Bayesian approach in patients with renal impairment. *J Clin Pharm Ther* 1989;14(3): 213–223.
376. de Hoog M, Mouton JW, van den Anker JN. Vancomycin: pharmacokinetics and administration regimens in neonates. *Clin Pharmacokinet* 2004;43(7):417–440.
377. Yasuhara M, Iga T, Zenda H, et al. Population pharmacokinetics of vancomycin in Japanese pediatric patients. *Ther Drug Monit* 1998;20(6):612–618.
378. Lemerle S, de La Rocque F, Lamy R, et al. Teicoplanin in combination therapy for febrile episodes in neutropenic and non-neutropenic paediatric patients. *J Antimicrob Chemother* 1988; 21(Suppl A):113–116.

CHAPTER

31

Urs B. Schaad

Fluoroquinolones

BACKGROUND

Despite class label warnings against use in children, prescriptions for quinolone antibiotics to treat infections in children have become increasingly prevalent. Many of the characteristics of the contemporary fluoroquinolones, the derivatives of the first quinolone antibiotic, nalidixic acid, are particularly appealing for certain pediatric populations. The fluoroquinolones are rapidly bactericidal and have an extended antimicrobial spectrum that includes *Pseudomonas*, gram-positive cocci, and intracellular pathogens. They have advantageous pharmacokinetic properties, such as absorption from the gastrointestinal tract, excellent penetration into many tissues, and good intracellular diffusion. These antimicrobials have been effective in the treatment or prevention of a variety of bacterial infections in adults, including infections of the respiratory and urinary tracts, skin and soft tissue, bone and joint, and eye and ear. Overall, fluoroquinolones are generally well tolerated; the most frequent adverse events during treatment are gastrointestinal disturbances, reactions of the central nervous system, and skin reactions (1,2).

The use of fluoroquinolones in children has been limited because of their potential to induce arthropathy in juvenile animals (3–5). This extraordinary form of age-related drug toxicity has been shown with all the fluoroquinolones tested so far and has led to important restrictions: Their use has been considered to be contraindicated in children, in growing adolescents, and in women during pregnancy and lactation. Since the mid-1980s, many children have received treatment with fluoroquinolones, however, because they are the only oral antimicrobials with potential activity against such multiple resistant and difficult-to-treat infections as *Pseudomonas aeruginosa* infections in children with cystic fibrosis, complicated urinary tract infections, and enteric infections in developing countries. Results of these trials indicate that prolonged therapy with the fluoroquinolones is effective and well tolerated in pediatric patients, with no significant evidence of arthropathy, bone abnormalities, or other serious adverse events (6). Besides feared arthrotoxicity, the second major concern regarding use of fluoroquinolones in children is the potential impact on bacterial resistance development (6).

MECHANISM OF ACTION AND ANTIBACTERIAL SPECTRUM

Quinolones inhibit bacterial DNA synthesis by targeting the enzymatic activities of DNA gyrase and topoisomerase IV (7). All quinolones have excellent activity against gram-negative bacteria, particularly Enterobacteriaceae, *Haemophilus* spp., *Moraxella catarrhalis*, and *Neisseria* spp. They also have activity against many strains of *P. aeruginosa* and methicillin-susceptible *Staphylococcus aureus* but weak activity against methicillin-resistant *S. aureus* and coagulase-negative staphylococci. Ciprofloxacin is the most potent available fluoroquinolone against gram-negative pathogens. Levofloxacin, gatifloxacin, moxifloxacin, and gemifloxacin are more active against gram-positive organisms, including *Streptococcus pneumoniae*. Atypical pathogens, including *Mycoplasma* spp., *Chlamydia* spp., *Legionella* spp. and *Ureaplasma urealyticum*, are susceptible to fluoroquinolones. The early fluoroquinolones had limited activity against anaerobes; however, the new compounds (e.g., moxifloxacin and gatifloxacin) have improved anaerobic activity. They also have activity against mycobacteria and excellent intracellular penetration.

Concentrations of fluoroquinolones in bile, lung, and urine are higher than in serum, whereas concentrations in saliva, bone, and cerebrospinal fluid are usually lower than in serum. However, cerebrospinal fluid concentrations are clinically useful for treatment of meningitis.

QUINOLONE ARTHROPATHY

HISTORY

Soon after the marketing of nalidixic acid in 1962, a child with soreness in one wrist during therapy for urinary tract infection was described (8). Nalidixic acid was not initially contraindicated in children but approved for use in children with urinary tract infections in March 1964. Eight years later, another report described a 22-year-old woman who developed severe polyarthritis during a second course of nalidixic acid (9). These "incapacitating" cases of arthralgia/arthritis were considered as allergic manifestations. Data on file of the manufacturers were cited to contain "about a dozen

TABLE 31.1 Retrospective Matched Control Search for Cartilage Toxicity in Nalidixic Acid–Treated Pediatric Patients: Details of Patients and Therapies

Investigator, Country	*Year of Report*	*No. of Patient Pairs*	*Age at Therapy (yr)*[a]	*Duration of Nalidixic Acid Therapy (d)*[a]	*Follow-Up Time (yr)*[a]
Schaad and Wedgwood-Krucko, Switzerland (12)	1987	11	0.3–9.6 (1.4)	9–600 (17)	3–12 (8)
Rumler and von Rodhden, Germany (13)	1987	201	1–7.2 (6.5)	27–1,689 (168)	≥2
Adam, Germany (14)	1989	50	0.1–11 (4.8)	10–815 (118)	≥2
Nuutinen et al., Finland (15)	1994	39	0.3–10.1 (5.3)	6–570 (86)	15–25 (20)

[a]Ranges (mean value).

such reports." These clinical observations with nalidixic acid prompted experimental exposure of laboratory animals to quinolone compounds. The first observations of quinolone-induced cartilage toxicity made with nalidixic, oxolinic, and pipemidic acid administration to young beagle dogs were reported by Ingham et al. in 1977 (10), Tatsumi et al. in 1978 (11), and Gough et al. in 1979 (3).

USE OF NALIDIXIC ACID IN CHILDREN

Four groups performed retrospective matched control search for cartilage toxicity in pediatric patients who had received nalidixic acid therapy, in most cases for acute or recurrent urinary tract infections (12–15). Details of patients and therapies are shown in Table 31.1. History for symptoms and clinical/radiological examinations compatible with possible arthropathies were recorded, and at follow-up examination growth curves and functional and radiological joint findings were obtained. The results were similar in the index and control cases. All reports concluded that nalidixic acid does not cause arthropathy in children, even after long-term and high-dose therapy.

ANIMAL EXPERIMENTS

All quinolones tested, including the older compounds and the newer derivatives, have been shown to induce changes in immature cartilage of weight-bearing joints in all laboratory animals tested (mice, rats, dogs, marmosets, guinea pigs, rabbits, and ferrets) (2,4,5,16). Quinolone-induced arthropathy is limited to juvenile animals, except when pefloxacin has been used. Juvenile dogs are generally more sensitive to the arthropathic effects of quinolones than are other species. Healing of quinolone-induced arthropathy is incomplete even after complete clinical recovery; structural changes are at least in part irreversible.

Typical histopathological lesions after quinolone exposure include fluid-filled blisters, fissures, erosions, and clustering of chondrocytes, usually accompanied by noninflammatory joint effusion. Under the electron microscope, necrosis of the chondrocytes and swelling of the mitochondria are observed initially, followed by disruption of extracellular matrix (17). Loss of collagen and glycosaminoglycan is an early sequela to the degeneration of chondrocytes (18). When clinically manifested, the quinolone-induced joint lesions present as acute arthritis, including limping and swelling. The specific mechanism(s) responsible for the initiation of quinolone-induced arthropathy has not been determined. At present, inhibition of mitochondrial DNA replication (19) and the role of magnesium deficiency (20,21) are the most discussed hypotheses.

Neither pharmacokinetic nor pharmacodynamic data can explain the variable arthropathic "power" of different compounds. There is also no clear effect of the molecular structure of the given compound regarding its cartilage toxicity (e.g., quinolones that are fluorinated versus quinolones that are not fluorinated).

POSSIBLE MONITORING FOR QUINOLONE-INDUCED CARTILAGE TOXICITY IN PATIENTS

The available methods for monitoring for quinolone-induced cartilage toxicity are the following:

- Histopathology—the gold standard (22).
- MRI—the parameters are surface, thickness, and structure of cartilage; presence of effusion (especially recessus suprapatellaris); and bone/cartilage integrity (23–25). Predictive value of MRI has been shown in studies with rabbits, pigs, and dogs (26).
- Sonography—measurement includes presence/absence of effusion and thickness and surface of cartilage (24–27).
- Clinical examination—indicating symptoms and signs would be arthralgia, limping, and joint swelling and for long-term follow-up growth rate; in many animal experiments, cartilage toxicity was documented without any clinical manifestation.

REVIEW OF PUBLISHED DATA

A comprehensive review of published reports including monitoring for quinolone-induced cartilage toxicity in patients was performed (28–35). The reviewed studies included all case reports of suspected quinolone-associated arthralgia/arthropathy in children and adolescents and all multipatient studies on the use of quinolone compounds in skeletally immature patients (open-label and controlled trials) in which there were data on safety, especially regarding potential arthropathy. Most of the data were based on clinical findings—musculoskeletal complaints and joint examination. Such findings do not allow one to distinguish between coincidental joint problems and quinolone-induced arthropathy. Only rarely MRI, ultrasonography, and growth curve have been used for either short-term or long-term evaluation. With the exception of the findings in two cystic fibrosis patients (22), the gold standard parameter "histopathology" is lacking. There are four conclusions:

1. To date, there is no unequivocal documentation of quinolone-induced arthropathy in patients as described in juvenile animals; quinolone arthropathy remains an experimental laboratory phenomenon in juvenile animals.
2. Clinical observations temporally related to quinolone use are reversible episodes of arthralgia, with and without effusions that do not lead to long-term sequelae when treatment with the agents is discontinued.
3. Most joint complaints associated with quinolone use are coincidental and do not represent adverse effects. Possible coincidental conditions include arthropathy and hypertrophic pulmonary osteoarthropathy associated with cystic fibrosis (36) and reactive, traumatic, and rheumatic joint diseases.
4. It is postulated that the so-called allergic arthritis initially described in nalidixic acid-treated patients does exist but is not the same as the quinolone-induced arthropathy in animals. These adverse events are always transient arthralgic or arthritic manifestations, usually involving large joints and occurring during the first and second week of therapy. The overall incidence is 1% to 3% (−18%) depending on the studied patient group and quinolone compound.

TENDINOPATHY

Other musculoskeletal adverse effects of quinolones are tendinitis and tendon rupture. Review of the literature on fluoroquinolone-associated tendinopathy (37–40) reveals the following. The incidence in a healthy population is very low, especially in children (39). In most cases, the Achilles tendon is affected with symptoms compatible with painful tendinitis or with rupture—usually occurring during the second week of treatment. Fluoroquinolone-associated tendinopathy increases in patients who have renal dysfunction (hemodialysis, after renal transplantation). There is a correlation between long-term cortical steroid therapy and age 60 years or older; the male-to-female ratio is approximately 2:1.

DEVELOPMENT OF BACTERIAL RESISTANCE

As mentioned before, there is great concern regarding the potential impact of widespread fluoroquinolone use in children on bacterial resistance development (6,16,31,41,42). Historically, antimicrobial use has led to the development of drug resistance. The relevant drivers are overuse (volume of antibiotic used in humans and in animals), misuse (inappropriate use), clonal spread (global travel, hygiene, hospital, daycare, family, switch of serotypes), and type of antibiotic. Overuse (e.g., for viral infection, as prophylaxis, many veterinarian indications) reflects inadequate knowledge of the prescribing physician and unavailability of diagnostic methods. Appropriate use (avoidance of misuse) includes not only selection of an optimal antibiotic but also individual optimization of dosage and duration of therapy. Well-defined antibiotic policies, good hygiene measures, and strong infection control programs represent key points for limiting the spread of antibiotic resistance.

Bacteria can become resistant to quinolones by mutations in the target molecules (gyrase protein, topoisomerase) or by active drug efflux. With regard to quinolone resistance, great variations exist among bacterial species, clinical settings, and local epidemiology. Resistance is the phenotypic expression corresponding to genetic changes caused by either mutation or acquisition of new genetic information. In some cases, multidrug resistance occurs. *S. pneumonia* is one of the most important respiratory pathogens, playing a major role in upper and lower respiratory tract infections. Pneumococcal resistance to antimicrobials may be acquired by means of horizontal transfer followed by homologous recombination of genetic material from the normal flora of the human oral cavity or by means of mutation. Resistance in pneumococci to penicillins and macrolides has been increasing for some time, but more recently fluoroquinolone resistance has become an issue as well (43,44). Fluoroquinolone resistance is not limited to *S. pneumoniae* and has been documented in other pathogens, including those responsible for urinary, respiratory, and gastrointestinal tract infections; skin and soft-tissue and bone and joint infections; sexually transmitted diseases; and ulcers (41,42).

Evidence is accumulating that multidrug resistance in pneumococci is related to prescription of antimicrobial agents to a crucial reservoir of these organisms—children. This multidrug resistance likely occurs because children, more often than adults, are colonized with high-density populations of pneumococci in the nasopharynx, which increases the potential for resistance development (41). Supporting this concern are studies of daycare centers and pediatric long-term care centers that have found a very high prevalence of nasopharyngeal carriage of drug-resistant strains of *S. pneumoniae* (45,46). Overcrowding facilitates the transmission of resistance strains from colonized to susceptible infants and children, who serve as a source for further transmission to family members and ultimately to the general population (47).

A new concern about widespread use of fluoroquinolones to treat children and adults is the recognition of horizontal transfer of fluoroquinolone resistance from viridans group streptococci (e.g., *S. oralis* and *S. mitis*) to *S. pneumoniae* (48,49). When resistance mutations develop in these naturally commensal organisms as a result o fluoroquinolone exposure (even in the absence of pathogenic pneumococci), any subsequent pneumococcal infection carries the risk that the infecting strain of *S. pneumoniae* will readily acquire fluoroquinolone resistance-determining DNA regions when antimicrobial therapies are instituted. These fluoroquinolone-resistant *S. pneumoniae* can be spread easily from child to parent, followed by widespread dissemination to the adult population. The dangerous triad of antibiotic overuse and misuse, a reservoir of resistant genes, and a closed-space pneumococcal infection (e.g., otitis media) could come together with widespread, uncontrolled use of fluoroquinolones in the pediatric patients (41).

PHARMACOLOGY

The pharmacokinetic data on fluoroquinolones in pediatric patients are limited, and for neonatal patients, the data are anecdotal only (50–54). The results of available studies, most of which were conducted in cystic fibrosis patients, indicate that systemic clearance is increased in young children; this has led to recommendations for relatively high doses. In general, fluoroquinolones are absorbed rapidly from the gastrointestinal tract. The range for bioavailability is vast, however, with norfloxacin being 10% to 30% and ofloxacin 80% to 90%. All of the newer compounds except norfloxacin have excellent tissue and intracellular penetration at the recommended therapeutic doses. Quinolones generally are excreted either predominantly in the urine (often as parent compound) or through the bile, in which some undergo enterohepatic recirculation.

POTENTIAL INDICATIONS

ESTABLISHED USE

Since the mid-1980s, fluoroquinolones have been used in pediatric patients primarily in circumstances in which they were the only antimicrobial choice for infections caused by multiple-resistant organisms (6,16,31). These included pseudomonal infections in children with cystic fibrosis (24,27,32,54,55), complicated urinary tract infections (56, 57), enteric infections in developing countries (28,58,59), and chronic ear infections (60). Results of controlled clinical trials in patients with these four indications have shown comparable efficacy of the fluoroquinolones and conventional regimens.

Preliminary experience in pediatric patients also indicates that the fluoroquinolones are effective and safe for the prevention or therapy for infections in neutropenic cancer patients (61,62) and for the eradication of nasopharyngeal carriage of meningococci (63). Fluoroquinolones also have been used successfully when severe infections, including meningitis during the neonatal period, are due to enterobacteria resistance to standard treatment (33,34,64).

FUTURE USE

Research on chemical modifications of the quinolones has been aimed at (a) more potent derivatives, (b) less frequent resistance, (c) better penetration into cerebrospinal fluid, and (d) improved patient tolerability. Some of the newer compounds have achieved many of these goals.

Of major interest for pediatricians are the effective cerebrospinal fluid penetration and the excellent in vitro activity of the new fluoroquinolones against the pathogens that commonly cause bacterial meningitis in children older than 3 months, including strains of *S. pneumoniae* resistant to β-lactams and to other antibiotics. Based on efficacy data in experimental animals and good cerebrospinal fluid penetration data in humans, a large multicenter, randomized, clinical trial was conducted in children with bacterial meningitis to compare the safety and efficacy of trovafloxacin with that of ceftriaxone with or without vancomycin therapy (65). This study was terminated earlier than planned because of concerns regarding potential, life-threatening liver toxicity associated with the use of trovafloxacin in adults with severe infections. Of the initially planned 284 children to be examined, only 203 (71%) were available for analysis at the time of trial closure. Although optimal statistical power required to draw firm conclusions was not reached, study results suggested that trovafloxacin is therapeutically equivalent to ceftriaxone with or without vancomycin for the management of bacterial meningitis in infants and children. Rates of bacterial eradication, cure, severe sequelae, and death were similar for both treatment groups at the end of treatment and at follow-up assessments. Future trials with other new fluoroquinolone compounds are warranted in pediatric patients with meningitis, but they will be difficult to conduct in view of the risk of rare side effects and possible treatment delays, which are a more important factor than resistance in the occurrence of sequelae.

Other potential future uses of newer fluoroquinolone compounds include childhood otitis media (66). Increased resistance of pneumococci and other pathogens to available antibiotics raises concerns about bacteriologic and clinical failure in children with acute otitis media. Few therapeutic options exist for patients with recurrent infections or recent treatment failure. The good efficacies of the fluoroquinolones gatifloxacin and levofloxacin in pediatric patients with refractory acute otitis media were shown in two trials each (67–70). For recurrent otitis media and otitis media treatment failure, the new fluoroquinolones seem to fill an unmet need. Nevertheless, an application for gatifloxacin licensure for pediatric use was withdrawn, because the Food and Drug Administration proposed risk management procedures that precluded reasonable pediatric use (71).

SUMMARY

The two major concerns regarding use of fluoroquinolones in children are development of bacterial resistance and cartilage toxicity as described in juvenile animals. The risk for rapid emergence of resistance among pneumococci and other common bacterial pathogens, associated with widespread, uncontrolled use of fluoroquinolones in pediatric patients, is a realistic threat. Cartilage toxicity with fluoroquinolones is a laboratory phenomenon in juvenile animals, and no arthropathy has been documented unequivocally in the large numbers of children treated with these agents. Nevertheless, expectant observation is warranted for any new quinolone use in pediatrics.

Based on available data showing the safety and efficacy of the fluoroquinolones, selected pediatric patients should not be deprived of the therapeutic advantages that these agents have to offer. The quinolones should never be used in pediatrics for routine treatment, however, when alternative safe and effective antimicrobials are known. To date, established pediatric indications for the fluoroquinolones include bronchopulmonary exacerbation in cystic fibrosis, complicated urinary tract infection, invasive gastrointestinal infection, and chronic ear infection. Potential pediatric indications are bacterial meningitis and refractory acute otitis media.

In most countries, fluoroquinolones so far are approved for use only in pediatric patients with cystic fibrosis and complicated urinary tract infection. Authorization for broader use of new fluoroquinolones in children must combine efforts of experts in microbiology and infectious diseases, regulatory authorities, and pharmaceutical manufacturers. Postmarketing surveillance must include an adequate risk management plan feasible for patients, parents, and drug companies.

Will fluoroquinolone ever be recommended for common infections in children (72)? The triad of feared arthrotoxicity, potential resistance explosion, and enormous requirements regarding adequate study and postmarketing control suggests that the answer is no. Therefore, these antimicrobials will continue to serve mainly for second-line use in children, only after failure of an earlier treatment and when other antibiotics approved for pediatrics cannot be used.

REFERENCES

1. Stahlmann R. Safety profile of the quinolones. *J Antimicrob Chemother* 1990;26(Suppl D):31–44.
2. Stahlmann R, Lode H. The quinolones—safety overview: toxicity, adverse events, and drug interactions. In: Andriole VT, ed. *The quinolones.* London: Academic Press, 1988:201–203.
3. Gough A, Barsoum NJ, Mitchell L, et al. Juvenile canine drug-induced arthropathy: clinicopathological studies on articular lesions caused by oxolinic and pipemidic acids. *Toxicol Appl Pharmacol* 1979;51:177–187.
4. Christ W, Lehnert T, Ulbrich B. Specific toxicologic aspects of the quinolones. *Rev Infect Dis* 1988;10(Suppl 1):141–146.
5. Schluter G. Ciprofloxacin: toxicologic evaluation of additional safety data. *Am J Med* 1989;87(Suppl 5A):37–39.
6. Schaad UB, Salam MA, Aujard Y, et al. Use of fluoroquinolones in pediatrics: consensus report of an International Society of Chemotherapy commission. *Pediatr Infect Dis J* 1995;14:1–9.
7. Gootz TD, Brighty KE. Fluoroquinolone antibacterials: SAR, mechanism of action, resistance and clinical aspects. *Med Res Rev* 1996; 16:433–486.
8. McDonald DF, Short HB. Usefulness of nalidixic acid in treatment of urinary tract infections. *Antimicrob Agents Chemother* 1964; 64:628–631.
9. Bailey RR, Natale R, Linton AL. Nalidixic acid arthralgia. *Can Med Assoc J* 1972;107:604–607.
10. Ingham B, Brentnall DW, Dale EA, et al. Arthropathy induced by anti-bacterial fused n-alkyl-4-pyrodoine-3-carboxylic acids. *Toxicol Lett* 1977;1:21–26.
11. Tatsumi H, Senda H, Yatera S, et al. Toxicological studies on pipemidic acid. V. Effect on diarthrodial joints of experimental animals. *J Toxicol Sci* 1978;3:357–367.
12. Schaad UB, Wedgwood-Krucko J. Nalidixic acid in children: retrospective matched controlled study for cartilage toxicity. *Infection* 1987;15:165–168.
13. Rumler W, von Rodhden L. Does nalidixic acid produce joint toxicity in childhood? In: Book of abstracts of the 15th International Congress of Chemotherapy, Istanbul, Turkey, 1987:1029–1031.
14. Adam D. Use of quinolone in pediatric patients. *Rev Infect Dis* 1989;11(Suppl 5):S1113–S1116.
15. Nuutinen M, Turtinen J, Uhari M. Growth and joint symptoms in children treated with nalidixic acid. *Pediatr Infect Dis J* 1994;13: 798–800.
16. Schaad UB. Use of the quinolones in pediatrics. In: Andriole VT, ed. *The quinolones,* 3rd ed. San Diego: Academic Press, 2000: 455–475.
17. Stahlmann R, Merker HJ, Hinz N, et al. Ofloxacin in juvenile non-human primates and rats: arthropathia and drug plasma concentrations. *Arch Toxicol* 1990;64:193–204.
18. Burkhardt JE, Hill MA, Carlton WW. Morphologic and biochemical changes in articular cartilages of immature beagle dogs dosed with difloxacin. *Toxicol Pathol* 1992;20:246–252.
19. Kato M, Takada S, Ogawara S, et al. Effect of levofloxacin on glycosaminoglycan and DNA synthesis of cultured rabbit chondrocytes at concentrations inducing cartilage lesions in vivo. *Antimicrob Agents Chemother* 1995;39:1979–1983.
20. Forster C, Kociok K, Shakibaei M, et al. Integrins on joint cartilage chondrocytes and alterations by ofloxacin or magnesium deficiency in immature rats. *Arch Toxicol* 1996;70:261–270.
21. Vormann J, Forster C, Zippel U, et al. Effects of magnesium deficiency on magnesium calcium content in bone and cartilage in developing rats in correlation to chondrotoxicity. *Calcif Tissue Int* 1997;61:230–238.
22. Schaad UB, Sander E, Wedgwood J, et al. Morphologic studies for skeletal toxicity after prolonged ciprofloxacin therapy in two juvenile cystic fibrosis patients. *Pediatr Infect Dis J* 1992;11:1047–1049.
23. Schaad UB, Stoupis C, Wedgwood J, et al. Clinical, radiologic and magnetic resonance monitoring for skeletal toxicity in pediatric patients with cystic fibrosis receiving a three-month course of ciprofloxacin. *Pediatr Infect Dis J* 1991;10:723–729.
24. Richard DA, Nousia-Arvanitakis S, Sollich V, et al; Cystic Fibrosis Study Group. Oral ciprofloxacin versus intravenous ceftazidime plus tobramycin in pediatric cystic fibrosis patients: comparison of antipseudomonas efficacy and assessment of safety using ultrasonography and magnetic resonance imaging. *Pediatr Infect Dis J* 1997;16:572–578.
25. Arico M, Bossi G, Caselli D, et al. Long-term magnetic resonance survey of cartilage damage in leukemic children treated with fluoroquinolones. *Pediatr Infect Dis* 1995;14:713–714.
26. Gylys-Morin VM, Hajek PC, Sartoris DJ, et al. Articular cartilage defects: detectability in cadaver knees with MR. *Am J Radiol* 1987; 148:1153–1157.
27. Church DA, Kanga JF, Kuhn RF, et al. Sequential ciprofloxacin therapy in pediatric cystic fibrosis: comparative study vs. ceftazidime/tobramycin in the treatment of acute pulmonary exacerbations. *Pediatr Infect Dis J* 1997;16:97–105.
28. Pradhan KM, Arora NK, Jena A, et al. Safety of ciprofloxacin therapy in children: magnetic resonance images, body fluid levels of fluoride and linear growth. *Acta Paediatr* 1995;84:555–560.
29. Bethell DB, Hien TT, Phi LT, et al. Effects on growth of single short courses of fluoroquinolones. *Arch Dis Child* 1996;74:44–46.
30. Burkhardt JE, Walterspiel JN, Schaad UB. Quinolone arthropathy in animals versus children. *Clin Infect Dis* 1997;25:1196–1204.
31. Gendrel D, Chalumeau M, Moulin F, et al. Fluoroquinolones in paediatrics: a risk for the patient or for the community? *Lancet Infect Dis* 2003;3:537–546.
32. Chalumeau M, Tonnelier S, D'Athis P, et al. Fluoroquinolone safety in pediatric patients: a prospective, multicenter, comparative cohort study in France. *Pediatrics* 2003;111:e714–e719.
33. Drossou-Agakidou V, Roilides E, Papakyriakidou-Koliouska P, et al. Use of ciprofloxacin in neonatal sepsis: lack of adverse effects up to one year. *Pediatr Infect Dis J* 2004;23:346–349.
34. Ahmed ASMNU, Khan NZ, Saha SK, et al. Ciprofloxacin treatment in preterm neonates in Bangladesh. Lack of effects on growth and development. *Pediatr Infect Dis J* 2006;25:1137–1141.
35. Noel GJ, Bradley JS, Kauffmann RE, et al. Comparative safety profile of levofloxacin in 2523 children with a focus on four musculoskeletal disorders. *Pediatr Infect Dis J* 2007;26:879–891.
36. Phillips BB, David T. Pathogenesis and management of arthropathy in cystic fibrosis. *J R Soc Med* 1996;79(Suppl 12):44–50.
37. van der Linden PD, van de Lei J, Nab HW, et al. Achilles tendinitis associated with fluoroquinolones. *Br J Clin Pharmacol* 1999;48: 433–437.
38. van der Linden PD, Sturkenboom MCJM, Herings RMC, et al. Fluoroquinolones and risk of Achilles tendon disorders: case-control study. *BMJ* 2002;324:1306–1307.
39. Yee CL, Duffy C, Gerbino PG, et al. Tendon or joint disorders in children after treatment with fluoroquinolones or azithromycin. *Pediatr Infect Dis J* 2002;21:525–529.

40. Khaliq Y, Zhanel GG. Fluoroquinolone-associated tendinopathy: a critical review of the literature. *Clin Infect Dis* 2003;36:1404–1410.
41. Mandell LA, Peterson LR, Wise R, et al. The battle against emerging antibiotic resistance: should fluoroquinolones be used to treat children? *Clin Infect Dis* 2002;35:721–727.
42. Hooper DC. New uses for new and old quinolones and the challenge of resistance. *Clin Infect Dis* 2000;30:243–254.
43. Chen DK, McGeer A, De Azavedo JC, et al. Decreased susceptibility of Streptococcus pneumoniae to fluoroquinolones in Canada. *N Engl J Med* 1999;341:233–239.
44. Ho PL, Yung RW, Tsang DN, et al. Increasing resistance of Streptococcus pneumoniae to fluoroquinolones: results of a Hong Kong multicentre study in 2000. *J Antimicrob Chemother* 2001;48:659–665.
45. Yagupsky P, Porat N, Fraser D, et al. Acquisition, carriage, and transmission of pneumococci with decreased antibiotic susceptibility in young children attending a day care facility in southern Israel. *J Infect Dis* 1998;177:1003–1012.
46. Mannheimer SB, Riley LW, Roberts RB. Association of penicillin-resistant pneumococci with residence in a pediatric chronic care facility. *J Infect Dis* 1996;174:513–519.
47. Kronenberger CB, Hoffmann RE, Lezotte DC, et al. Invasive penicillin-resistant pneumococcal infections: a prevalence and historical cohort study. *Emerg Infect Dis* 1996;2:121–124.
48. Gonzales J, Georgiou M, Alcaide F, et al. Fluoroquinolone resistance mutations in the parC, parE, and gyrA genes of clinical isolates of viridans group streptococci. *Antimicrob Agents Chemother* 1998;42:2792–2798.
49. Ferrandiz MJ, Fernoll A, Linares J, et al. Horizontal transfer of parC and gyrA in fluoroquinolone-resistant clinical isolates of Streptococcus pneumoniae. *Antimicrob Agents Chemother* 2000;44: 840–847.
50. Blumer JL, Stern RC, Myers CM, et al. Pharmacokinetics and pharmacodynamics of ciprofloxacin in cystic fibrosis. In: Abstracts of 14th International Congress on Chemotherapy, Kyoto, 1985;112.
51. Stutman HR, Shalit I, Marks MI, et al. Pharmacokinetics of two dosage regimens of ciprofloxacin during a two-week-therapeutic trial in patients with cystic fibrosis. *Am J Med* 1987;82 (Suppl 4A): 142–145.
52. Peltola H, Vaarala M, Renkonen O, et al. Pharmacokinetics of single dose of oral ciprofloxacin in infants and small children. *Antimicrob Agents Chemother* 1992;36:1086–1090.
53. Schaeffer HG, Strass H, Wedgwood J, et al. Pharmacokinetics of ciprofloxacin in pediatric cystic fibrosis patients. *Antimicrob Agents Chemother* 1996;40:29–34.
54. Rubio TT, Miles MV, Lettiere JT, et al. Pharmacokinetic disposition of sequential intravenous/oral ciprofloxacin in pediatric cystic fibrosis patients with acute pulmonary exacerbation. *Pediatr Infect Dis J* 1997;16:112–117.
55. Schaad UB, Wedgwood J, Ruedeberg A, et al. Ciprofloxacin as antipseudomonal treatment in patients with cystic fibrosis. *Pediatr Infect Dis J* 1997;16:106–111.
56. Fujii R. The use of norfloxacin in children in Japan. *Adv Antineopl Chemother* 1992;11:219–232.
57. Koyle MA, Barqawi A, Wild J, et al. Pediatric urinary tract infections: the role of fluoroquinolones. *Pediatr Infect Dis J* 2003;22: 1133–1137.
58. Green S, Tillotson G. Use of ciprofloxacin in developing countries. *Pediatr Infect Dis J* 1997;16:150–159.
59. Salam MA, Dhar U, Khan WA, et al. Randomised comparison of ciprofloxacin suspension and pivmecillinam for childhood shigellosis. *Lancet* 1998;352:522–527.
60. Lang R, Goshen S, Raas-Rothschild A. Oral ciprofloxacin in the management of chronic suppurative otitis media without cholesteatoma in children. *Pediatr Infect Dis J* 1992;11:925–929.
61. Freifeld A, Pizzo P. Use of fluoroquinolones for empirical management of febrile neutropenia in pediatric cancer patients. *Pediatr Infect Dis J* 1997;16:140–146.
62. Patrick CC. Use of fluoroquinolones as prophylaxis agents in patients with neutropenia. *Pediatr Infect Dis J* 1997;16:135–139.
63. Cuevas LE, Kazembe P, Mughogho GK, et al. Eradication of nasopharyngeal carriage of Neisseria meningitidis in children and adult in rural Africa: a comparison of ciprofloxacin and rifampicin. *J Infect Dis* 1995;171:728–731.
64. Krcmery V, Filka J, Uher J, et al. Ciprofloxacin in treatment of nosocomial meningitis in neonates and in infants: report of 12 cases and review. *Diagn Microbiol Infect Dis* 1999;35:75–80.
65. Saez-Llorens X, Mccoig C, Feris JM, et al. Quinolone treatment for pediatric bacterial meningitis: a comparative study of trovafloxacin and ceftriaxone with or without vancomycin. *Pediatr Infect Dis J* 2002;21:14–22.
66. Dagan R, Arguedas A, Schaad UB. Potential role of fluoroquinolone therapy in childhood otitis media. *Pediatr Infect Dis J* 2004;23:390–398.
67. Leibovitz E, Piglansky L, Raiz S, et al. Bacteriologic and clinical efficacy of oral gatifloxacin for the treatment of recurrent/ nonresponsive acute otitis media: an open label, noncomparative, double tympanocentesis study. *Pediatr Infect Dis J* 2003;22: 943–949.
68. Arguedas A, Sher L, Lopez E, et al. Open label, multicenter study of gatifloxacin treatment of recurrent otitis media and acute otitis media treatment failure. *Pediatr Infect Dis J* 2003;22:949–955.
69. Pichichero ME, Arguedas A, Dagan R, et al. Safety and efficacy of gatifloxacin therapy for children with recurrent acute otitis media (AOM) and/or AOM treatment failure. *Clin Infect Dis* 2005;41:470–478.
70. Arguedas A, Dagan R, Pichichero M, et al. An open-label, double tympanocentesis study of levofloxacin therapy in children with, or at high risk for, recurrent or persistent acute otitis media. *Pediatr Infect Dis J* 2006;25:1102–1109.
71. Marchant CD. Gatifloxacin therapy for children. *Clin Infect Dis* 2005;41:479–480.
72. Schaad UB. Will fluoroquinolones ever be recommended for common infections in children? *Pediatr Infect Dis J* 2007;26:865–867.

CHAPTER

32

Basim I. Asmar
Nahed M. Abdel-Haq

Macrolides, Chloramphenicol, and Tetracyclines

MACROLIDES

ERYTHROMYCIN

Erythromycin is the prototype of the macrolides. It has been one of the main antibiotics used in the treatment of pediatric infections since 1952. Erythromycin is a broad-spectrum antibiotic that has been primarily used to treat respiratory and skin and soft tissue infections (SSTIs) in children who are allergic to penicillin as well as infections due to penicillin-resistant organisms. Erythromycin is derived from *Streptomyces erythreus*, originally obtained from a soil sample in the Philippines (1).

Chemical Structure

Erythromycin consists of a 14-membered macrocyclic lactone ring with two appended deoxy sugar moieties, deconamine and cladinose, at positions 5 and 3 of the ring. Erythromycin base is poorly soluble in water and easily degraded by gastric acid. Because it is a large molecule, erythromycin diffuses through membranes slowly. This results in unpredictable erythromycin levels in serum and tissue following oral administration (Fig. 32.1) (2).

Mechanism of Action/Mechanism of Antibacterial Resistance

Erythromycin and other macrolides inhibit bacterial pathogens by binding to the peptidyltransferase region of the 50S subunit of bacterial 70S ribosomes causing inhibition of bacterial protein synthesis. Macrolides are bacteriostatic. Erythromycin and other macrolides appear to inhibit the translocation step during bacterial protein synthesis rather than peptide bond formation. The translocation step involves movement of the peptidyl tRNA molecule from the acceptor site of the ribosome to the donor site (3,4).

Acquired bacterial resistance to macrolides involves one of three mechanisms: (a) alteration of the ribosomal binding site, (b) decreased accumulation of the drug due to an active efflux pump, or (c) macrolide inactivation by esterases or by phosphorylation or glycosylation at the 2′-position (5). Modification of the ribosomal binding site by methylation is the most common clinically significant resistance mechanism in gram-positive bacteria. Methylase enzyme production may be inducible or constitutive and is mediated by *erm* genes (*ermA, ermB, ermC*). The MLSB phenotype is conferred by *erm* genes, indicating resistance to macrolides, lincosamides, and type B streptogramins, which share the same ribosomal binding site. MLSB resistance is due to modification of the 23S rRNA binding site at adenine 2058 by methylation (6,7). Resistance to the 14- or 15-membered macrolides may be the result of efflux pumps encoded by genes such as *mefE* in *Streptococcus pneumoniae*, *mrsA* in *Staphylococcus aureus*, and *mefA* in group A beta hemolytic *Streptococcus* (GABHS) (8–10). Chromosomal mutation involving the 50S ribosomal protein is another mechanism of resistance to macrolides in gram-positive cocci (6).

In Vitro Efficacy

In vitro activity of erythromycin and other macrolides has been shown to be greater in alkaline media possibly due to increased penetration of the bacterial cell wall. The spectrum of activity of erythromycin includes gram-positive cocci such as *S. pneumoniae*, *Streptococcus pyogenes*, and *S. aureus* as well as atypical and intracellular pathogens such as *Chlamydia pneumoniae*, *Chlamydia trachomatis*, *Mycoplasma pneumoniae*, and *Ureaplasma urealyticum* (11,12). Erythromycin is active in vitro against gram-positive bacilli such as *Bacillus anthracis*, *Clostridium* species, and *Corynebacterium* species. Erythromycin also has excellent activity against *Legionella pneumophila*, *Bordetella pertussis*, and *Campylobacter jejuni*. Less activity has been shown against *Eikenella*, *Haemophilus influenzae*, *Pasteurella*, and *Brucella*. Most *Treponema* species, *Rickettsia rickettsiae*, and to a lesser extent *Borrelia burgdorferi* and *Helicobacter pylori* are inhibited by erythromycin (13,14).

Clinical Indications

Erythromycin is considered the drug of choice for a number of pediatric infections. It is also considered an alternative to penicillin in patients with penicillin allergy. Erythromycin

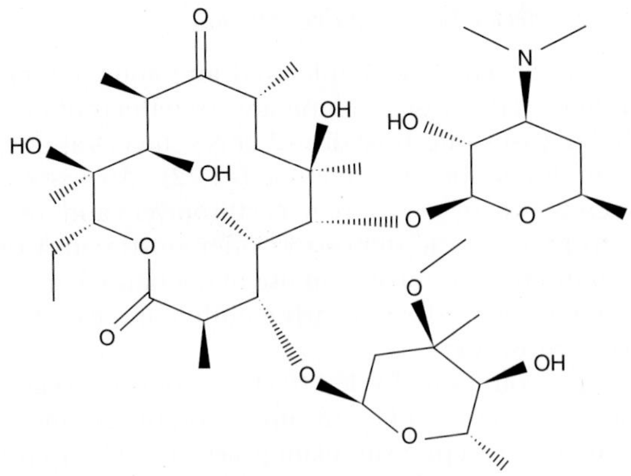

Figure 32.1. Structure of erythromycin.

is active against *B. pertussis.* In addition to eradicating nasopharyngeal carriage and preventing infection with *B. pertussis,* erythromycin may shorten the clinical course of illness if started during the catarrhal or early paroxysmal phase of pertussis. Erythromycin is indicated in the early treatment of pertussis as well as prophylaxis of close contacts (15). Following identification of *M. pneumoniae* as a frequent cause of pneumonia in school-age children, adolescents, and young adults, erythromycin became an important component of antibiotic treatment of pneumonia among these patients. Erythromycin has been shown to shorten the duration of clinical illness and time to radiologic clearance in patients with *Mycoplasma* pneumonia (16). In the 1970s, *C. trachomatis* was identified as an important cause of pneumonia in neonates and young infants. *C. trachomatis* causes pneumonia in infants 3 weeks to 4 months of age and ophthalmia neonatorum in infants younger than 30 days. Treatment with erythromycin has been shown to eradicate nasopharyngeal carriage of the organism and hasten recovery of conjunctivitis and pneumonia (17). The recommended treatment for both infections is erythromycin 50 mg per kg per day in four divided doses for 14 days. In addition, nongonococcal urethritis caused by *C. trachomatis* usually responds to a 7-day course of oral erythromycin, although doxycycline is probably more effective. The newer agents, azithromycin and ofloxacin, are also effective (18). Erythromycin is an alternative to tetracycline for treatment of *C. trachomatis* infection during pregnancy (19). For nongonococcal urethritis caused by *U. urealyticum,* doxycycline is the drug of choice, but erythromycin is also effective. This organism can also cause bacteremia, pneumonia, or meningitis in the neonate and should be treated with intravenous erythromycin (20). Erythromycin has also been found to be effective in the treatment of pneumonia caused by *Chlamydophila pneumoniae, L. pneumophilia,* and *Legionella micdadei* as well as in the treatment of Legionnaires disease (21,22). Erythromycin remains the drug of choice for *Legionella* pneumonia. Mild infections may be treated by oral erythromycin, whereas moderate and severe infections should be treated by intravenous erythromycin. Erythromycin in combination with rifampin should be used for very ill patients and for those not responding to erythromycin (23). Erythromycin is considered the drug of choice for treating diarrhea caused by *C. jejuni* when clinically indicated (24). Although the effect of erythromycin on the course of illness is controversial, erythromycin may be given to patients who have fever, bloody stools, or symptoms persisting for longer than 1 week.

Erythromycin is an alternative to penicillin for the treatment of GABHS pharyngitis in patients who are allergic to penicillin. However, increased rates of infection with macrolide-resistant GABHS have been reported in areas of the world where macrolides are excessively used (such as Finland and Japan) resulting in treatment failures (25). Erythromycin is an effective alternative to penicillin G for treatment of pneumococcal pneumonia. It is also an alternative antibiotic for treatment of other pneumococcal infections outside the central nervous system (CNS) that are caused by susceptible strains. Similarly, erythromycin may be used as an alternative treatment for infections caused by susceptible strains of *B. anthracis* and *Eikenella corrodens.* Erythromycin in combination with sulfa drugs is effective against *H. influenzae* and *Moraxella catarrhalis* (26).

Although erythromycin may show in vitro susceptibility against *Treponema,* it is inferior to penicillin for treatment of syphilis. Erythromycin is not indicated in neurosyphilis and is no longer considered acceptable alternative therapy for penicillin-allergic pregnant women (27). It usually results in cure of the mother, but because placental transfer of the drug is inconsistent, the fetus may remain infected.

Erythromycin is considered an alternative treatment to amoxicillin for early-localized Lyme disease in children younger than 8 years who are allergic to penicillin (28).

For endocarditis chemoprophylaxis, oral erythromycin given 2 hours before the dental procedure and 6 hours later is recommended for standard-risk penicillin-allergic patients. Erythromycin is a suitable alternative to penicillin for prophylaxis against rheumatic fever.

Pharmacokinetic Properties

Degradation of erythromycin base by gastric acid results in reduced oral bioavailability. Food increases gastrointestinal acidity and may delay absorption. Thus, erythromycin base is administered as enteric-coated tablets or as capsules containing enteric-coated pellets that dissolve in the duodenum. Esters of the erythromycin base (stearate, estolate, and ethylsuccinate) have been formulated to improve acid stability and facilitate absorption. Erythromycin stearate is less readily destroyed in the stomach and is dissociated in the duodenum liberating erythromycin, which is absorbed. Erythromycin estolate is also less susceptible to acid than is the base and hence is better absorbed. Its bioavailability is not affected by food. It is absorbed mainly as ester, and then hydrolyzed in serum to active erythromycin. Erythromycin ethylsuccinate is also well absorbed after oral administration. Food increases its bioavailability (29). After absorption, erythromycin ethylsuccinate is hydrolyzed into active erythromycin.

Satisfactory serum concentrations are achieved following intravenous administration of erythromycin. Peak concentrations attained 1 hour after intravenous infusion are usually 4- to 10-fold greater than those attained after oral erythromycin (30). After intravenous administration of erythromycin lactobionate to preterm neonates at either 25 or 40 mg per kg per day divided into four doses every

6 hours, peak serum levels were 3.05 to 3.69 μg per mL and 1.92 to 2.9 μg per mL for the 40 and 25 mg per kg per day groups, respectively (31). Erythromycin diffuses well into intracellular fluids and body tissues except the cerebrospinal fluid (CSF) and the CNS. Middle ear fluid concentration is about 50% of serum concentration. This concentration may be sufficient to inhibit the highly sensitive *S. pyogenes* and *S. pneumoniae* but may be too low for treatment of otitis media caused by *H. influenzae* (32). Tonsillar concentrations are adequate after oral administration (33). Children with chlamydial conjunctivitis treated with erythromycin have tear fluid concentration of erythromycin approximately equal to simultaneous serum concentration. Erythromycin is concentrated in human polymorphonuclear leukocytes (34). Significant intracellular penetration occurs resulting in activity against intracellular pathogens (35).

Studies of single 10 mg per kg oral doses of erythromycin estolate and ethylsuccinate in infants younger than 4 months with *C. trachomatis* infection have shown similar peak serum concentrations (C_{max}) of erythromycin (36). Similar findings were noted after repeat dosing to steady state. Single-dose studies also showed similar time to C_{max} (T_{max}) for both formulations. However, multiple-dose studies in infants 3 to 48 months of age showed that T_{max} was longer for the estolate formulation, resulting in larger area of activity under the curve (AUC) at steady state (36). In neonates, absorption of erythromycin appears to be delayed and bioavailability is not influenced by feeding (37).

The majority of macrolides including erythromycin are eliminated via hepatic metabolism and/or biliary excretion. Erythromycin is excreted as the active form in the bile. Macrolides are substrates of the hepatic enzyme cytochrome P450 3A4. Reduction in the activity of this enzyme secondary to disease or immaturity can result in elevated levels of macrolides. At therapeutic concentrations, 80% to 90% of erythromycin in the blood is protein bound. Erythromycin crosses the placenta, but fetal plasma drug concentrations are considerably lower and less predictable than those in the mother (38). Erythromycin is partly excreted in the urine: about 2.5% of orally administered dose and 15% of parenterally administered dose. A considerable proportion of erythromycin is excreted in the bile. In general, renal or hepatic dysfunction has little effect on the pharmacokinetics of macrolides including erythromycin, and dosage adjustment is not necessary in most occasions (39,40).

Dose/Regimens

The usual dosage of erythromycin base in children is 30 to 50 mg per kg per day administered in two to four equally divided doses. The maximum daily dose is 4 g. Erythromycin is available in base form, stearate, ethyl succinate, and estolate preparations. In severe infections, erythromycin may be administered by the intravenous route at a dosage of 15 to 50 mg per kg per day in four equally divided doses. The intravenous dose should be given by slow infusion over at least 1 hour to minimize the risk of cardiac arrhythmias. For newborns, oral erythromycin is administered at a dose of 10 mg per kg given every 12 hours for those younger than 1 week and every 8 hours for those 1 week of age and older.

Adverse Effects/Toxicity/Precautions

Erythromycin is the least-tolerated antibiotic among the macrolides. The most common adverse effects of erythromycin are gastrointestinal disturbances such as abdominal pain or discomfort and nausea (41,42). An association between very early exposure to erythromycin and infantile hypertrophic pyloric stenosis was demonstrated. Cooper et al. found that erythromycin use in neonates 3 to 13 days of life was associated with nearly eightfold increased risk of pyloric stenosis (43).

The gastrointestinal side effects are possibly related to the prokinetic action of erythromycin on the gut mediated by its motilin-receptor-stimulating activity (44). Reported allergic reactions include fever, rashes, joint pain, generalized pruritus, and Stevens–Johnson syndrome. Reversible hepatic dysfunction and liver enzyme abnormalities have been reported 10 to 14 days following erythromycin use. These include colicky abdominal pain, cholestasis, elevated transaminase levels, jaundice, and eosinophilia (41,42). Cholestatic hepatitis has been reported mainly with the estolate formulation and only rarely with the other derivatives. It may represent a hypersensitivity reaction to the estolate ester (42). Reversible neurosensory hearing loss affecting all hearing frequencies has been reported mostly in association with use of high doses in patients with impaired renal function (45). Thrombophlebitis and venous irritation have been reported with intravenous erythromycin infusions. The incidence and severity of these infusion reactions can be reduced by slowing of the rate of infusion and/or reducing the concentration of erythromycin in the infusate (42). Intravenous administration of erythromycin to infants and children has been associated with cardiotoxicity manifested by bradycardia, hypotension, torsades de pointes (polymorphous ventricular tachycardia), and cardiac arrest (30).

Drug Interactions

Macrolides interact with a variety of drugs by inhibiting the metabolism of the drugs via the cytochrome P450 (CYP) hepatic microsomal enzymes (46). Significant drug interactions occur with concomitant administration of erythromycin with antihistamines, cisapride, carbamazepine, valproate, theophylline, cyclosporine, digoxin, warfarin, and benzodiazepines (46–50). The interaction occurs via the induction of the CYP enzymes, which subsequently convert the macrolide to a nitrosoalkane metabolite forming an inactive complex with the iron of CYP.

Concomitant administration of erythromycin and theophylline can result in increased concentrations of theophylline. This is believed to be due to decreased clearance of theophylline by erythromycin. The reduction in clearance is variable (5% to 40%) and is related to type of erythromycin formulation, type of patient, and dose and duration of erythromycin therapy (40). Concomitant administration of erythromycin and cyclosporine results in increased concentrations of cyclosporine. The increase is in the range of 75% to 215% in cyclosporine AUC and is possibly due to decreased cyclosporine clearance, increased bioavailability, or both (49). The interaction with digoxin is also believed to be via increasing the bioavailability of digoxin secondary to inhibition of the metabolizing bacteria, particularly *Eubacterium lentum*, in the large bowel. The interaction occurs in a small percentage of patients (10%) and is less likely to occur with the capsule preparations of digoxin (50).

AZITHROMYCIN

Erythromycin has long been considered one of the main antibiotics for treating pediatric infections. Erythromycin has been characterized by a number of drawbacks, however, which resulted in the search for newer macrolides. Among these drawbacks are the narrow spectrum of activity, the poor oral tolerance, and the unfavorable pharmacokinetic properties. Azithromycin is a long-acting macrolide that has been synthesized to overcome the drawbacks of erythromycin.

Chemical Structure

Azithromycin is synthesized by incorporation of a 6-methyl-substituted nitrogen atom into position 9a of the 14-member macrolide ring (Fig. 32.2). This results in the expansion of the ring to 15 members, and accordingly azithromycin is classified as an azalide rather than a macrolide. The modification at the 9a position also results in a compound with more stability to degradation by gastric acid, improved oral absorption, and improved adverse effect profile (51).

Mechanism of Action/Mechanism of Antibacterial Resistance

Similar to other macrolide antibiotics, azithromycin inhibits protein synthesis by binding to the 50S ribosomal subunit, resulting in inhibition of peptide translocation. The mechanisms of resistance to azithromycin are similar to those of erythromycin and other macrolides.

In Vitro Efficacy

In general, azithromycin is more active than erythromycin against gram-negative organisms but provides no advantage over erythromycin in activity against gram-positive organisms (52). Many of the organisms that are resistant to erythromycin are also resistant to azithromycin (53). Improved in vitro activity compared with that of erythromycin has been shown against *Haemophilus* species, *M. catarrhalis*, *Legionella* species, *Pasteurella multocida*, *B. burgdorferi*, *Mycoplasma* species, *Neisseria gonorrhea*, *C. trachomatis*, and *Campylobacter* species. Azithromycin has appreciable activity against *Mycobacterium avium* complex (MAC) and *Bartonella* species (54,55). Azithromycin is active against *S. pneumoniae*, *S. pyogenes*, and methicillin-susceptible *S. aureus* (56). Macrolide resistance is common among staphylococci (*S. aureus* and coagulase-negative staphylococci). Resistance has also been increasingly reported among *S. pneumoniae* strains and *S. pyogenes* (57,58). Methicillin-resistant staphylococci are also resistant to erythromycin. Streptococci and staphylococci that are resistant to erythromycin are also resistant to azithromycin and clarithromycin. Penicillin-resistant *S. pneumoniae* strains are usually resistant to azithromycin. The prevalence of resistance to macrolides is related to geographical variation, antibiotic usage patterns, and subsequent antibiotic selection pressure. Azithromycin has similar in vitro activity to erythromycin against *C. pneumoniae* and *B. pertussis* (59,60). Azithromycin has been shown to exhibit postantibiotic effect against respiratory tract pathogens such as *S. pneumoniae*, *H. influenzae*, and *S. pyogenes* (61). This effect together with the host immune defenses can contribute to clinical efficacy of azithromycin at sites of infection when serum levels fall below the minimal inhibitory concentration (MIC) of the organism. Azithromycin is also active in vitro against *Toxoplasma gondii*.

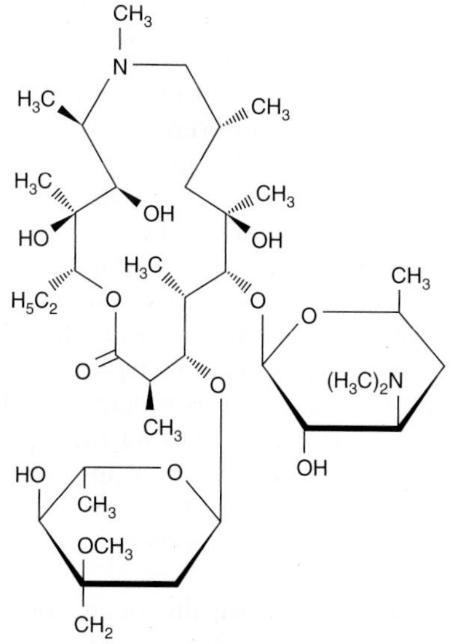

Figure 32.2. Structure of azithromycin.

Clinical Indications

Antibiotic treatment is indicated for treatment of acute GABHS pharyngitis to decrease the duration of symptoms and to prevent the spread to others and the subsequent development of rheumatic fever. Although oral penicillin V remains the drug of choice, a shorter course of oral azithromycin may result in better compliance. Treatment of GABHS pharyngitis using azithromycin 10 mg per kg on the first day followed by 5 mg per kg once daily for the next 4 days has not been shown to be effective. Two large double-blind, multicenter trials that compared azithromycin given at a dose of 12 mg per kg once a day for 5 days with penicillin V for 10 days for treatment of GABHS pharyngitis showed higher clinical responses and higher GABHS eradication rates in the azithromycin-treated groups (62). As a result, the Food and Drug Administration (FDA) approved the use of azithromycin at 12 mg per kg once daily for treatment of GABHS pharyngitis among children 2 years of age and older. Studies with shorter courses of azithromycin for 3 days produced variable results (63,64). This short course of azithromycin is not currently recommended. Azithromycin 12 mg per kg once daily for 5 days may be used as an alternative to penicillin V for treatment of GABHS pharyngitis in areas of low incidence of GABHS macrolide resistance.

Acute otitis media (AOM) is one of the most frequent infections in children. The most common bacterial pathogens are *S. pneumoniae*, non-typeable *H. influenzae*, and *M. catarrhalis.* Choice of antibiotic treatment for AOM depends on the likelihood of bacterial resistance and on compliance-related factors such as frequency, palatability, and cost of the antibiotic. In clinical trials comparing azithromycin with other drugs and in which tympanocentesis was performed at baseline, rates of clinical efficacy were variable. In a study comparing azithromycin with amoxicillin–clavulanate, Dagan et al. (65) showed that azithromycin was less likely to eradicate all bacterial pathogens from middle ear fluid in 136 evaluable patients. Bacteriologic outcomes for *S. pneumoniae* correlated with National Committee for Clinical Laboratory Standards (NCCLS) breakpoints and bacteriologic failures correlated with clinical failures. In this study, bacteriologic failures in AOM caused by *S. pneumoniae* were higher with azithromycin than with amoxicillin–clavulanate, although the difference was not statistically significant (65). Decreased bacteriologic efficacy of azithromycin was subsequently demonstrated in another study (66). These findings suggest that although azithromycin may be an acceptable second-line antibiotic for AOM, its routine use in such a common pediatric infection may lead to increased resistance rates not only to macrolides but also to other antibiotics.

Azithromycin and other macrolides may be used as first-line treatment for respiratory tract infections caused by atypical organisms such as *M. pneumoniae* and *C. pneumoniae.* Azithromycin for 5 days or erythromycin for 14 days is used to treat *C. trachomatis* pneumonia in young infants caused by maternal vertical transmission (67).

Azithromycin (10 mg per kg on day 1 followed by 5 mg per kg on days 2 through 5) may be considered for treatment of community-acquired pneumonia (CAP) in children older than 5 years and adolescents who are candidates for outpatient therapy. Harris et al. (68) studied the role of azithromycin in CAP in children. In a double-blind trial, azithromycin was compared with either amoxicillin–clavulanate in children 6 months to 5 years of age or erythromycin in children older than 5 years (68). Although therapeutic outcomes were satisfactory and similar in the two treatment groups, there were differences in pathogens and failure rates between age groups independent of treatment assignment. A significantly higher clinical failure rate was found in younger children than in older ones. However, the role of viral infections in younger patients was not addressed. Azithromycin and other macrolides should not be considered as the first choice for treatment of pneumonia in children younger than 5 years because broad-spectrum activity against atypical organisms is not considered important in this age group.

Treatment of SSTIs with macrolides including azithromycin depends on the local rate of resistance among *S. pyogenes* and *S. aureus* strains. The efficacy of azithromycin in treatment of SSTIs has been shown in adults and children (69). In areas where the prevalence of macrolide-resistant *S. aureus* is high, a child with SSTI should be treated with an antibiotic that is active against β-lactamase-producing strains of *S. aureus.* In recent years, community-acquired methicillin resistant *S. aureus* (CA-MRSA) has emerged as a major pathogen causing SSTIs. These strains may be susceptible to clindamycin, trimethoprim–sulfamethoxazole, linezolid, or quinolones but are almost always resistant to macrolides. Clinicians should therefore avoid the use of macrolide for treatment of SSTI in areas of high CA-MRSA prevalence (70).

Macrolides including erythromycin, azithromycin, and clarithromycin are recommended for the treatment and prevention of pertussis (71).

Erythromycin prevents transmission but not the course of illness. The standard treatment and prevention regimen of pertussis remains erythromycin given at a 40 to 50 mg per kg daily for 14 days. However, compliance with this regimen may be affected by the long duration of therapy, the four-times-daily dosing, and the gastrointestinal side effects. *B. pertussis* is susceptible in vitro to erythromycin, clarithromycin, and azithromycin (72). One study showed that azithromycin given at a dose of 10 mg per kg once daily for 5 days was effective in eradicating *B. pertussis* from the nasopharynx in eight of eight children after 1 week of treatment (73). In another study, azithromycin given at 10 mg per kg on day 1 followed by 5 mg per kg daily for 4 days was as effective as 10 mg per kg daily for 3 days in eradicating *B. pertussis* from the upper respiratory tract in infants and young children (74). Because of concerns for pyloric stenosis in young infants due to erythromycin use in the neonatal period, azithromycin is the recommended macrolide for prevention and treatment of pertussis in infants younger than one month (71).

Azithromycin and clarithromycin have also been used in the treatment and prophylaxis of MAC infections. Patients with acquired immune deficiency syndrome (AIDS) are at risk of disseminated MAC. Prophylaxis with either azithromycin or clarithromycin is indicated in all human immunodeficiency virus (HIV)-infected patients with CD4 cell count less than 50 per mL (75). Although macrolide resistance has been identified among some patients receiving prophylaxis, the overall effectiveness remains high (65). MAC has also been identified as a cause of cervical lymphadenitis in children (76,77). The definite treatment of nontuberculous mycobacterial lymphadenitis including MAC is surgical excision. However, if the patient is at high risk of surgical complications or if complete surgical excision is difficult, azithromycin or clarithromycin can be given as an alternative treatment (78).

Azithromycin has been used in treatment of lymphadenitis caused by *Bartonella henselae,* the agent causing cat scratch disease (CSD). *B. henselae* has been shown to be susceptible in vitro to different antibiotics. Reports of clinical improvement of CSD with different antibiotics in addition to macrolides included rifampin, trimethoprim–sulfamethoxazole, fluoroquinolones, and gentamicin (79). In a double-blind study, Bass et al. found that azithromycin given as a 5-day course (10 mg per kg on day 1 followed by 5 mg per kg for 4 consecutive days) accelerated the resolution of lymphadenitis caused by typical, uncomplicated CSD within the first month of treatment (80). The efficacy of azithromycin in treatment of other or atypical manifestations of CSD is not clear. However, in normal children, most clinical manifestations of CSD are benign and self-limited, and the majority of infections do not require antibiotic therapy (81).

Erythromycin has historically been the most commonly used drug for treatment of Legionnaires disease. However, the newer macrolides, especially azithromycin, have excellent in vitro activity, fewer adverse events, and greater intracellular and lung tissue distribution. Thus, the newer macrolides, particularly azithromycin, have become the oral drugs of choice for treatment of Legionnaires disease (82). In critically ill adults with legionellosis, intravenous azithromycin with or without levofloxacin has been recommended (83). The safety and efficacy of intravenous azithromycin in children younger than 16 years have not yet been established.

For treatment of uncomplicated chlamydia cervicitis and nongonococcal urethritis, a single 2-g dose of azithromycin has been shown to be as effective as the traditional 7-day course of oral doxycycline (84).

Azithromycin has been used to treat *Cryptosporidium parvum* infections in immunocompromised adults and children. *C. parvum* causes an asymptomatic or self-limiting gastroenteritis in otherwise healthy people. However, in immunocompromised patients, *C. parvum* may cause severe intestinal fluid losses with dehydration or chronic diarrhea and wasting. Different antimicrobial regimens have been used in adults with inconsistent results (85,86). No specific treatment regimen has produced consistent beneficial effects in children. Azithromycin had been used in nine children aged 14 months to 15 years with cryptosporidiosis associated with AIDS or cancer. The dosages varied from 10 to 40 mg per kg per day for 10 to 31 days. Clinical improvement had been documented early in the course of treatment in some patients (87,88). Some relapses have also occurred. The role of azithromycin in clinical resolution of cryptosporidiosis remains to be clarified.

Azithromycin may also offer an alternative treatment for controlling trachoma. Trachoma is an infectious keratoconjunctivitis caused by *C. trachomatis.* It is considered the most common cause of preventable blindness worldwide (89). Public health programs have focused on the use of ocular ointments of sulfonamides, tetracyclines, and erythromycin derivatives to control trachoma (90). However, these regimens may be confounded by lack of compliance and frequent side effects. Clinical trials compared oral azithromycin with the standard use of tetracycline or oxytetracycline ointments for treating trachoma in children. In two trials, a single azithromycin dose of 20 mg per kg was as effective as standard ointment therapy (91,92). A third trial showed that three different regimens of azithromycin were as effective as oxytetracycline/polymyxin B ointment (93).

Azithromycin has also been shown to have activity against enteric pathogens including *Salmonella typhi* (94). Preliminary studies have shown that azithromycin is effective in treating uncomplicated typhoid fever in adults and children (95,96). A study of 64 Egyptian children age 4 to 17 years compared azithromycin suspension given at 10 mg per kg per day for 7 days with intramuscular ceftriaxone given at 75 mg per kg per day for 7 days. Cure was achieved in 91% of the azithromycin group and 97% of the ceftriaxone group (96). None of the children in the azithromycin group had relapses, compared with 14% of those in the ceftriaxone group. Larger studies are needed including children living in areas with significant prevalence of multidrug-resistant *S. typhi.*

Pharmacokinetic Properties

When administered to children at the regimen of 10 mg per kg once followed by 5 mg per kg per day on days 2 through 5, azithromycin exhibits pharmacokinetic properties similar to those in adults (97). Food intake significantly decreases the bioavailability of the capsule and the powdered suspension of azithromycin. Therefore, azithromycin should be administered 1 hour before or 2 hours after intake of food or antacid. However, the tablet form of azithromycin may be taken without regard to food (98). Peak plasma concentrations are achieved 2 hours after a dose (97). Azithromycin distributes well into tissues including tonsils and adenoid tissues and into middle ear fluid (99,100). Clinically effective levels are achieved in these tissues and middle ear fluid long after the last dose of azithromycin is administered (99). Tissue concentrations as high as twice the serum concentrations may be achieved. Good intracellular penetration of azithromycin contributes to its efficacy in management of infections caused by intracellular organisms such as *Chlamydia* species and MAC. Tissue delivery is further enhanced by neutrophil and macrophage uptake of azithromycin to sites of infection (101). Despite its fairly rapid absorption and high tissue bioavailability, when azithromycin is given at the recommended dosage regimen, achievable serum concentrations are detected far below the minimum inhibitory concentration of some pediatric pathogens (0.026 to 0.043 μg per mL). This should be taken into consideration during management of potentially bacteremic organisms such as *S. pneumoniae, H. influenzae,* and *S. pyogenes* (29). Azithromycin is slowly eliminated. The elimination half-life of azithromycin in children is 32 to 64 hours. This allows once-daily dosing of azithromycin (53). Therapeutically significant concentrations of azithromycin may persist in tissues for additional 5 days after a 5-day course. Plasma protein binding of azithromycin is saturable, ranging from 50% at a concentration of 20 to 50 μg per L to 7% at 1,000 μg per L (56). Azithromycin is largely eliminated unchanged in the urine and stools (98). Significant renal impairment (creatinine clearance of <30 mL per minute) reduces the rate of urinary clearance of azithromycin (98). Azithromycin, like erythromycin, increases the rate of gastric emptying and thus may alter the absorption of azithromycin or other drugs (102).

Dose/Regimens

In most pediatric infections including otitis media and pneumonia, azithromycin is administered in single daily doses at 10 mg per kg on the first day of treatment followed by 5 mg per kg per day on days 2 through 5. The regimen for GABHS pharyngitis is 12 mg per kg per day for 5 days. The maximum daily dose is 500 mg. Azithromycin may be administered as a 3-day course of 10 mg per kg per day or as a single dose of 30 mg per kg for AOM or pneumonia. However, there are no current approved clinical indications for these regimens in pediatric infections. For adolescents and adults with uncomplicated *C. trachomatis* genital tract infection, azithromycin may be administered as a single 1-g oral dose (67).

For treatment and postexposure prophylaxis of pertussis in children younger than 6 months including neonates, the recommended dose is 10 mg per kg once daily for 5 days.

For children 6 months of age or older, the dose is 10 mg per kg on first day followed by 5 mg per kg once daily for the next 4 days (71).

Intravenous azithromycin is given to adults at a dose of 500 mg once daily. There are no current approved indications for use of intravenous azithromycin in children due to lack of sufficient data. However, a single-daily dose of 10 mg per kg (maximum 500) given to children 6 months to 16 years of age was tolerated with no serious adverse events and showed comparable pharmacokinetic properties among study patients (103).

Adverse Effects/Toxicity/Precautions

Azithromycin is more tolerable than erythromycin. Azithromycin oral suspension has demonstrated an excellent safety and tolerability profile in children treated for different infections. Comparative trials with pooled tolerability results have shown overall better tolerability of azithromycin than other oral comparator agents. Adverse events with azithromycin are usually mild, infrequent, of short duration, and reversible. In children, adverse events also appear to be dose related. They were reported in 7.6% of patients receiving 30 mg per kg and 16.6% of those receiving 60 mg per kg total dose (both given once daily for 5 days). The most prevalent adverse events were gastrointestinal events such as diarrhea (3.1%), vomiting (2.5%), abdominal pain (1.9%), and loose stools (1.0%). Transient elevation of hepatic transaminases has been reported. Dermatologic complications (mainly rash) occurred in 1.5% of patients and neurologic side effects (mainly headache) occurred in 0.6% of patients (104). Children allergic to erythromycin may have cross-hypersensitivity reactions to azithromycin. Azithromycin is contraindicated in children who are allergic to erythromycin or any other macrolide antibiotics.

Drug Interactions

Food, antacids, and H_2-blockers reduce the absorption of azithromycin by 50%. Azithromycin reportedly has no significant interactions with carbamazepine, cimetidine, methylprednisolone, terfenadine, or midazolam. Known or potential interactions with other drugs such as cyclosporine, digoxin, theophylline, and warfarin may occur. Levels of these medications should be monitored with concomitant azithromycin use. Azithromycin should not be administered with ergot alkaloids (55).

CLARITHROMYCIN

Clarithromycin is a broad-spectrum macrolide that has activity against pathogens causing respiratory tract infections in children. Although clarithromycin has similar in vitro activity to erythromycin, it has the advantage of additional activity against selected pathogens, a longer half-life, enhanced lipophilicity, and increased concentrations in cells and tissues (105).

Chemical Structure

Clarithromycin is a 6-methoxy-erythromycin. The addition of a methoxy group at the 6 position of the macrolide ring results in a compound that is less resistant to acid hydrolysis and therefore has fewer gastrointestinal side effects (106). Clarithromycin is metabolized to an active 14-hydroxy-clarithromycin, a metabolite that has antibacterial activity similar to the parent compound. Thus, the clinical efficacy of clarithromycin and its metabolite against organisms may be higher than that suggested by in vitro susceptibility tests (Fig. 32.3) (107).

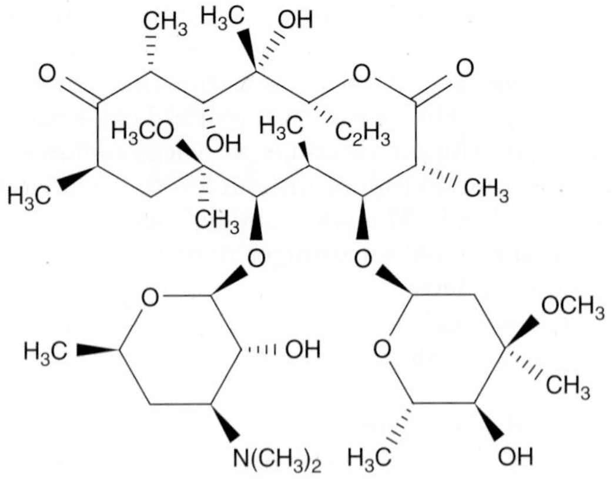

CH_3 H_3C OH O O O H_3CO OH H_3C C_2H_3 H_3C CH_3 CH_3 O O O OCH_3 H_3C OH O CH_3 $N(CH_3)_2$ H_3C OH

Figure 32.3. Structure of clarithromycin.

Mechanism of Action/Mechanism of Antibacterial Resistance

Similar to other macrolide antibiotics, clarithromycin inhibits protein synthesis by binding to the 50S ribosomal subunit and inhibiting peptide translocation (98). Like other macrolides, the most clinically significant acquired resistance to clarithromycin is of the MLS type and indicates cross-resistance to other macrolides. This resistance is mediated by production of methylases promoted by *erm* genes (6).

In Vitro Efficacy

Clarithromycin is active against a wide range of gram-positive and gram-negative bacteria, pathogens causing atypical pneumonia (*M. pneumoniae*, *C. pneumoniae*, and *Legionella* species), mycobacteria, and protozoa. Clarithromycin has similar activity to other macrolides against *S. pneumoniae*, *S. pyogenes*, *S. aureus*, and *M. catarrhalis*. Streptococci and staphylococci that are resistant to erythromycin are also resistant to clarithromycin. Penicillin-resistant *S. pneumoniae* strains are usually resistant to clarithromycin. Anaerobes are variably susceptible to clarithromycin. Gram-positive anaerobes tend to be more susceptible to clarithromycin than gram-negative anaerobes. Clarithromycin is more active in vitro than erythromycin against *C. trachomatis*, *C. pneumoniae*, *M. pneumoniae*, *L. pneumophilia*, *B. burgdorferi*, and *B. pertussis* (60,106,107). Clarithromycin is ineffective against gram-negative enteric bacteria and methicillin-resistant staphylococci (29,108). *H. influenzae* is susceptible or intermediately susceptible to clarithromycin alone. However, the antimicrobially active metabolite is approximately twice as active against *H. influenzae*. Clarithromycin has excellent activity against *Haemophilus ducreyi*. Clarithromycin is more active than azithromycin against nontuberculous mycobacteria. Clarithromycin is particularly active against MAC and has activity against other mycobacteria such as *Mycobacterium chelonei* and some subspecies of *Mycobacterium fortuitum*. Clarithromycin is also effective against *Mycobacterium leprae* (29,54). *Mycobacterium tuberculosis* is less susceptible to clarithromycin than nontuberculous mycobacteria. Clarithromycin has been shown to have inhibitory activity against *T. gondii* (109).

Clinical Indications

Clarithromycin has been shown to be an effective alternative to penicillin in treatment of GABHS pharyngitis. Clarithromycin was found to have comparable clinical success rates to penicillin V. It was also associated with higher GABHS eradication rates than penicillin V in one study (110). Clarithromycin has also been shown to be an effective and safe alternative treatment of AOM in children. Following multiple doses of clarithromycin suspension, sustained concentrations of clarithromycin and its 14-hydroxy metabolite were above the MIC of most pathogens causing AOM. Clarithromycin has been shown to have a similar safety and efficacy profile as amoxicillin in treatment of AOM in children (111). In a comparative study of clarithromycin and amoxicillin–clavulanate in treatment of AOM and in which tympanocentesis was performed in 175 of 180 patients, Aspin et al. (112) found that a 10-day course of clarithromycin at 15 mg per kg per day produced similar improvement and cure rates to amoxicillin–clavulanate at 40 mg per kg per day given for 10 days. Recurrence of infection and rates of persistence in middle ear fluid were similar in both groups. However, gastrointestinal side effects were reported less frequently among patients receiving clarithromycin (112). A 10-day course of clarithromycin has also been shown to be as effective and safe as a 3-day azithromycin course in treatment of AOM in children (113). Good clinical response and convenient dosing suggest clarithromycin as an attractive alternative therapy in AOM (114). However, similar to azithromycin, caution should be exercised in routinely prescribing clarithromycin as a first-line treatment in such a common pediatric infection.

Clarithromycin has been found to be effective in the treatment of pneumonia caused by atypical organisms such as *M. pneumoniae* and *C. pneumoniae*. Clarithromycin may be used orally in patients with CAP who do not require hospitalization (115). Clarithromycin is active in vitro against *B. pertussis* but has not been routinely recommended for routine treatment and prophylaxis of pertussis (105).

Clarithromycin is part of the combination therapy for *H. pylori*-induced peptic ulcer disease (116). Clarithromycin is also part of the multidrug regimen therapy of disseminated MAC infection, which may also include rifampin, isoniazid, ethambutol, and clofazimine (117). Clarithromycin, in combination with other antibiotics, is used for treatment of other nontuberculous mycobacterial infections (118).

Pharmacokinetic Properties

Clarithromycin is well absorbed from the gastrointestinal tract; absorption is not affected by food intake. The oral bioavailability is 52% to 55%. First-pass metabolism results in the appearance of the active 14-hydroxy metabolite (107). Clarithromycin is not extensively protein bound. The major route of elimination is biliary excretion. Approximately 30% to 40% of the administered dose is excreted in urine. Elimination half-life of clarithromycin and its 14-hydroxy metabolite is 5 and 7 hours, respectively (107). Dosage adjustments are required for patients with severe renal failure (creatinine clearance <30 mL per minute). Clarithromycin's long half-life allows for twice-daily administration. Clarithromycin is concentrated in cells and tissues including lungs, nasal mucosa, and tonsils and in MEF. Clarithromycin and its metabolite concentrate in lungs and middle ear fluid (MEF) at higher levels than in plasma (99). Clarithromycin concentration in respiratory tract exceeds that of plasma by ratios of up to 8.82:1 in MEF, 3.1:1 in bronchial secretions, and 28.7:1 in lung tissue (119–121).

Dose/Regimens

The usual dose of clarithromycin in children is 7.5 mg per kg (up to 500 mg per dose) given twice daily. The duration of treatment of AOM and pneumonia in children is 10 days.

Adverse Effects/Toxicity/Precautions

Clarithromycin has fewer gastrointestinal adverse events than erythromycin. The most frequently reported adverse events among children receiving clarithromycin suspension were diarrhea (6.6%), vomiting (6.3%), abdominal pain (2.4%), and headache (1.6%). Adverse events requiring withdrawal of clarithromycin occurred in less than 2% of treated children (29,122). Hypersensitivity reactions range from mild skin rashes and urticaria to anaphylactic reactions and Stevens–Johnson syndrome. Other adverse events include stomatitis, glossitis, oral candidiasis, and dizziness. Unusual reactions reported among adults with underlying conditions include hepatic failure, cholestatic hepatitis, leukocytoclastic vasculitis, thrombocytopenic purpura, and visual hallucinations. Reversible hearing loss has been reported rarely among adults receiving clarithromycin 1,000 mg twice daily for MAC infection (117). The risk of long-term hearing impairment among children taking long-term clarithromycin therapy is unclear.

Drug Interactions

Clarithromycin interacts with other drugs via inhibition of the cytochrome P450 enzyme system, particularly CYP3A (123). In general, clarithromycin exhibits fewer drug interactions than erythromycin. However, clinically significant interactions have been reported with theophylline, digoxin, carbamazepine, cyclosporine, and tacrolimus. These agents require drug level monitoring and appropriate dose adjustment when used concomitantly with clarithromycin. Significant interactions also occur when clarithromycin is concomitantly used with rifampin and rifabutin. Both rifampin and rifabutin induce the metabolism of clarithromycin (124).

ROXITHROMYCIN

Roxithromycin is another macrolide antibiotic related to erythromycin.

Mechanism of Action/Mechanism of Antibacterial Resistance

Similar to erythromycin and other macrolides, roxithromycin interferes with protein synthesis by attachment to the 50S rRNA subunit of the bacterial ribosome (125). Roxithromycin has the ability to penetrate cellular walls and concentrate in lymphocytes and macrophages at concentrations that can exceed the plasma concentration. This explains the ability of roxithromycin to treat intracellular organisms (125). In addition, roxithromycin enhances the chemotactic activity of neutrophils. In vitro studies have also shown that roxithromycin may enhance neutrophil apoptosis with resultant decrease in the inflammatory response at sites of tissue infection and inflammation (126,127).

The mechanisms of resistance are similar to other macrolides.

In Vitro Activity

The in vitro activity of roxithromycin is similar to that of erythromycin. Roxithromycin is active against streptococci including viridans streptococci; GABHS; group B, C, F, and G streptococci; and *S. pneumoniae.* Roxithromycin is also active against atypical and intracellular organisms such as *M. pneumoniae, C. trachomatis, B. pertussis, L. pneumophilia,* and *U. urealyticum.* Other in vitro susceptible strains include *H. influenzae, H. ducreyi, M. catarrhalis,* methicillin-susceptible strains of *S. aureus, P. multocida,* and *Listeria monocytogenes.* Although activity against anaerobes including *Bacteroides oralis* is generally poor, roxithromycin is active against *Actinomyces* species, *Bacteroides urealyticus, Bacteroides melaninogenicus, Peptostreptococcus* species, and *Propionibacterium acnes.* Roxithromycin is not active against the Enterobacteriaceae group as well as the non-fermentative gram-negative bacilli such as *Pseudomonas aeruginosa* (29,125).

Clinical Indications

Despite the superior pharmacokinetic profile of roxithromycin over erythromycin, roxithromycin has been shown to be equivalent to erythromycin in treatment of different infections. Roxithromycin is effective in treatment of streptococcal pharyngitis, otitis media, SSTIs caused by susceptible organisms, infections in the upper and lower respiratory tract, Lyme disease, isosporiasis, and nongonococcal urethritis (128,129).

Pharmacokinetic Properties

Roxithromycin is rapidly absorbed after oral intake, and absorption is minimally affected by food (130). Peak serum levels (C_{max}) are achieved in 2 hours (125). After an initial oral dose of 2.5 mg per kg, serum concentration of roxithromycin remains above the minimum inhibitory concentration for about 12 hours. Steady-state levels in children are reached after 6 days; C_{max} of 8 to 10 μg per mL can be reached after a dose of 2.5 mg per kg every 12 hours for 6 days. Approximately 86% to 96% of roxithromycin in serum is protein bound (131,132,133). Roxithromycin has good distribution in various body fluids and tissues including tonsils, adenoids, and middle ear fluid. High levels have been achieved in respiratory tissues and fluids as well as in the male and female genital tracts. Distribution into the CSF and the CNS is poor (134). The distribution half-life of roxithromycin is approximately 4 hours. Because of the higher volume of distribution in children compared with adults, elimination half-life is 20 hours compared with 12 hours in adults (132). Roxithromycin is not extensively metabolized. Approximately 53% of roxithromycin dose is excreted in feces and 10% is excreted in the urine (134). The elimination half-life is increased in patients with hepatic or renal insufficiency, and dosage adjustments may be needed (134).

Dose/Regimen

The dose in children for most clinical indications is 2.5 to 5 mg per kg every 12 hours. The duration of treatment depends on the severity and type of infection. The usual adult dose is 150 to 300 mg twice daily.

Adverse Effects/Toxicity/Precautions

The most common adverse events associated with roxithromycin use are gastrointestinal events, occurring in 5% of patients. These include anorexia, abdominal cramps, nausea, vomiting, and diarrhea (135). Other mild adverse events are headache and itching, and have been reported in 1% to 5% of patients receiving roxithromycin (136). Asymptomatic elevation of liver enzymes has been reported in patients receiving roxithromycin. Individual case reports of substantial liver enzyme elevation and fulminant hepatitis have also been reported (137). Other rarely reported adverse events include transient eosinophilia and thrombocytosis, pancreatitis, hyperglycemia, and nail discoloration. However, a causal relationship with roxithromycin therapy has not been established (138–140).

Drug Interactions

Although roxithromycin has a less inhibitory effect on cytochrome P450 enzymes than does erythromycin, some reports suggest that roxithromycin can interact with other medications leading to potentially significant clinical interaction. Similar to other macrolide antibiotics, roxithromycin may decrease the metabolism of other medications such as benzodiazepines, causing elevated plasma concentrations of these medications (141). Concomitant administration of roxithromycin and carbamazepine was not found to affect the pharmacokinetics of carbamazepine (142). Potential decreased intestinal degradation of digoxin by roxithromycin can cause an increase in digoxin serum concentration (143). Like erythromycin, roxithromycin has the potential to exacerbate the cardiac toxic effects of astemizole and pimozide when roxithromycin is concomitantly administered with either drug

(144). Roxithromycin does not appear to interfere with the efficacy of oral contraceptives (145). Coadministration of proton pump inhibitors and roxithromycin does not alter the bioavailability of either medication. The interaction potential of roxithromycin with theophylline or warfarin is controversial (146–148).

CHLORAMPHENICOL

Chloramphenicol is an antibiotic that was first isolated in 1947 from the soil bacterium *Streptomyces venezuelae* (149). After its relatively simple structure was determined, it was prepared synthetically, and by 1948 chloramphenicol became available for general use. Chloramphenicol was considered the first "broad-spectrum" antibiotic because of its activity against many gram-positive and gram-negative bacteria, anaerobic bacteria, as well as rickettsiae.

By 1950, chloramphenicol was incriminated as a cause of serious and fatal blood dyscrasias. In 1958, a unique toxic effect of chloramphenicol on the newborn infants known as "gray baby syndrome" was recognized, which resulted in further uncertainty regarding chloramphenicol use. For these reasons, chloramphenicol is reserved as alternative therapy in patients with serious infections such as meningitis, typhoid fever, and typhus who cannot be treated with other, safer drugs because of resistance or allergy.

CHEMICAL STRUCTURE

The chloramphenicol molecule contains a nitrobenzene moiety and is a derivative of dichloroacetic acid. Its structural formula is shown in Figure 32.4.

MECHANISM OF ACTION/MECHANISM OF ANTIBACTERIAL RESISTANCE

Chloramphenicol inhibits bacterial protein synthesis by binding reversibly to the 50S ribosomal subunit. This prevents the attachment of the amino acid–containing end of the aminoacyl-tRNA to the acceptor site on the 50S ribosomal subunit. As a result the interaction between peptidyltransferase and its amino acid substrate cannot occur, and the peptide bond formation is prevented (150). This results in the block of protein synthesis, producing static inhibition of most sensitive microorganisms. Mammalian mitochondria contain 70S ribosomes that also bind chloramphenicol, leading to inhibition of mitochondrial protein synthesis in mammalian cells. The effect of chloramphenicol against these cells has been suggested as the cause of the dose-related bone marrow suppression of the drug (151).

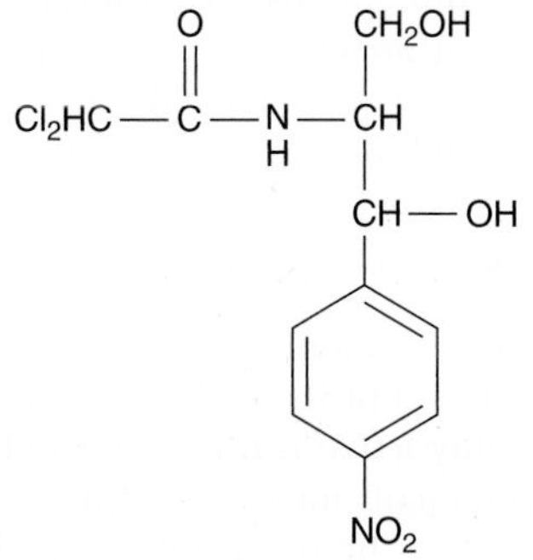

Figure 32.4. Structure of chloramphenicol.

Resistance to chloramphenicol is primarily due to production of the enzyme acetyltransferase, which acetylates the antibiotic to an inactive diacetyl derivative (152). The acetylated derivative fails to bind to bacterial ribosomes. The production of acetyltransferase is plasmid (R factor) mediated and has been responsible for epidemics of chloramphenicol-resistant typhoid fever and *Shigella* dysentery (153–155). The unrestricted over-the-counter sales of chloramphenicol in certain developing countries may have contributed to the emergence of resistant *Salmonella* strains (155,156). In the United States, chloramphenicol resistance in *Salmonella* has been linked to the use of chloramphenicol on dairy farms (157).

Nonenzymatic resistance due to bacterial impermeability to the antibiotic and mutation in the bacterial 50S ribosome have been described but are rare.

INDICATIONS/THERAPEUTIC USES

Chloramphenicol has a wide spectrum of antimicrobial activity, which includes aerobic and anaerobic bacteria, rickettsiae, mycoplasma, and chlamydiae. Bacterial strains are considered susceptible if they are inhibited by concentration of 8 μg per mL or less. Most of the susceptible gram-positive and gram-negative bacteria are inhibited by concentrations easily achievable in serum. However, more active or less toxic therapeutic agents are available for treatment of infections caused by these pathogens.

Although chloramphenicol is classified as a bacteriostatic agent, it may be bactericidal against certain species such as *H. influenzae, Neisseria meningitidis,* and *S. pneumoniae.*

Gram-Negative Aerobic Bacteria

Most *Escherichia coli* and *Klebsiella pneumoniae* strains and many *Proteus* species are usually susceptible to chloramphenicol. However, resistant strains have emerged as a result of the clinical use of chloramphenicol. For example, the routine use of chloramphenicol for treating neonatal sepsis resulted in the emergence of chloramphenicol resistance in up to 50% of *E. coli* or *Klebsiella* in one neonatal unit (158). The combination of chloramphenicol and gentamicin may exhibit an antagonistic effect against some enteric gram-negative organisms such as *E. coli* and *Klebsiella.* Chloramphenicol appears to suppress the bactericidal action of gentamicin against these organisms (159). In vitro studies have also shown that chloramphenicol antagonizes cefotaxime and ceftriaxone bactericidal activity against *E. coli* and group B streptococci (160).

Salmonella strains including *S. typhi* are generally susceptible to chloramphenicol. Resistant *Salmonella* strains have been occasionally recovered in the United States, but imported *Salmonella* strains may be highly resistant. Chloramphenicol-resistant *S. typhi* isolates have been detected in several countries. In India, occasional strains of *S. typhi* resistant to chloramphenicol have been isolated since 1962, but since 1972, multiple antibiotic-resistant strains of *S. typhi* and of other salmonellae have been encountered increasingly (161). Of 241 *S. typhi* isolates recovered in Peru during 1981 to 1983, 71 (29.9%) were resistant to chloramphenicol. These strains were susceptible to ceftriaxone, imipenem, ampicillin–clavulanate, norfloxacin, and ciprofloxacin. More recently, in Pakistan 20% of cases of typhoid fever were caused by strains of *S. typhi* resistant to ampicillin, chloramphenicol, and co-trimoxazole (162). Other recent reports of multiresistant *Salmonella* were from India (163) and Bangladesh (164). Acquired resistance of *S. typhi* can occur during treatment by acquisition of resistance gene(s) on a plasmid or transposon from other intestinal organisms (165).

Most other gram-negative bacteria are susceptible to chloramphenicol. *Neisseria meningitides* and *Neisseria gonorrhoeae* are very sensitive. Resistant strains of *N. meningitides* have been reported but are rare. *N. gonorrhoeae* strains including β-lactamase producers are almost always susceptible to chloramphenicol. *H. influenzae* and *Haemophilus parainfluenzae* are also very sensitive. Chloramphenicol-resistant but ampicillin-susceptible strains of *H. influenzae* b have been isolated in the United States (166) and England (167) from children with meningitis. Strains of *H. influenzae* b resistant to chloramphenicol and ampicillin were also isolated from patients with meningitis or bacteremia in the United States (168,169), England (170–172), Australia (173,174), Spain (175), and the Dominican Republic (176). Three children who died of meningitis due to *H. influenzae* b resistant to chloramphenicol and ampicillin in Bangkok were reported in 1980 (177). On the other hand, in a study from Pakistan, 47.5% of *H. influenzae* strains were resistant to co-trimoxazole, 5.1% to ampicillin, but none to chloramphenicol (178). Nonencapsulated *H. influenzae* resistant to chloramphenicol and ampicillin has also been reported from Holland (179) and the United Kingdom (180,181). Overall, chloramphenicol-resistant *Haemophilus* species remain relatively rare in developed countries. In the United States, the resistance rate of *H. influenzae* b is less than 1% (176,182). Similar results of surveys in United Kingdom have been reported. Data from developing countries are not available.

Brucella species, *B. pertussis*, *P. multocida*, *Vibrio cholera*, and *Vibrio parahaemolyticus* are susceptible to chloramphenicol. Rare resistant strains of *V. cholera* have been detected (183). The *Moraxella* species are susceptible, as is *H. pylori* (184), and most strains of *Aeromonas* species (185) are also sensitive. *P. aeruginosa* has always been completely resistant and this is due to an active efflux pump, which removes chloramphenicol from the bacterial cell (186). *Burkholderia cepacia* (187) and *Flavobacteria* (188) are also resistant.

Gram-Positive Cocci

S. pneumoniae, *S. pyogenes*, group B streptococci, and α-hemolytic streptococci (viridans streptococci) are usually sensitive to chloramphenicol. *S. aureus* strains tend to be less susceptible, with MIC greater than 8 μg per mL. Methicillin-resistant strains of *S. aureus* are usually resistant to chloramphenicol, and this is due to inactivation of the drug by plasmid-mediated chloramphenicol acetyltransferase (189). Chloramphenicol-resistant *S. pyogenes* have been detected in Japan (190) but appear to be rare elsewhere. Although chloramphenicol-resistant pneumococci have been detected in several countries including France, Britain, West Africa, Australia, and the United States, they are also considered to be rare. Resistance in these strains is due to plasmid-mediated chloramphenicol acetyltransferase. Pneumococci resistant to multiple drugs including penicillin G and chloramphenicol detected in South Africa were associated with serious infections (191,192). Pneumococci resistant to penicillin and chloramphenicol have also been reported in Spain, Pakistan (178), and Korea (193). Chloramphenicol-resistant *Enterococcus faecalis* strains are not uncommon.

Anaerobic Bacteria

Aerobic gram-positive cocci including *Peptococcus* and *Peptostreptococcus* species are susceptible to chloramphenicol (194). Among the anaerobic gram-positive bacilli, most *Clostridium* species including *C. tetani* and *C. perfringens* are susceptible. However, many strains of *C. difficile* are resistant (195). The gram-negative anaerobic bacilli *Bacteroides*, including *B. fragilis* (159), *Fusobacterium*, *Prevotella*, and *Veillona* species, are very susceptible to chloramphenicol (196). Chloramphenicol is also active against mycoplasmas, leptospira, and *Treponema pallidum*. *Chlamydia* species including those that cause pneumonia, conjunctivitis, psittacosis, and lymphogranuloma venereum are sensitive. Rickettsiae that cause Rocky Mountain spotted fever and various typhus fevers are susceptible to chloramphenicol. Chloramphenicol is also active against *Coxiella burnetii*, the agent that causes Q fever.

Historically, chloramphenicol had a prominent role in the treatment of children with serious infections, including meningitis. Factors that favored its use included its excellent diffusion into all body fluids such as CSF, vitreous humor, and joint fluid. This made it useful in the treatment of meningitis, bacterial ophthalmitis, and septic arthritis. Chloramphenicol concentrations in CSF average 0.5 to 0.66 of serum concentration (197). Chloramphenicol also penetrates into leukocytes and tissues, making it useful in the treatment of typhoid fever and infections in patients with chronic granulomatous disease. The diffusion of chloramphenicol into the CNS tissue fluid is superior to that of any other antibiotic because of its high lipid solubility. Brain tissue levels are about nine times the simultaneous serum level (198). This and the knowledge that anaerobic bacteria are almost always present in brain abscesses made chloramphenicol an ideal antimicrobial for the treatment of brain abscesses.

INDICATIONS FOR USE

Chloramphenicol is no longer the drug of choice for any specific infection except for typhoid fever in areas where cost and availability make it the drug of choice. Therapy with chloramphenicol must be limited to conditions where the benefit of the drug outweighs the risks of the potential toxicities.

Typhoid Fever

Chloramphenicol remains an excellent drug for treatment of typhoid fever and other types of systemic *Salmonella* infections; however, safer drugs are available, including ampicillin, co-trimoxazole, and third-generation cephalosporins. Third-generation cephalosporins are the drugs of choice for treatment of such infections.

Typhoid fever is usually treated by chloramphenicol for a period of 2 weeks (199). Chloramphenicol is of no value for the eradication of *Salmonella* carrier state. In addition, treatment of patients with acute *Salmonella* gastroenteritis with chloramphenicol usually prolongs the period of excretion of *Salmonella* after clinical recovery (200).

Bacterial Meningitis

Chloramphenicol is very effective for the treatment of meningitis due to *H. influenzae* type b (201). Since the widespread occurrence of strains of *H. influenzae* resistant to ampicillin, chloramphenicol has become the preferred drug for serious infections due to this organism. However, either one of the third-generation cephalosporins, cefotaxime or ceftriaxone, is used by clinicians in developed countries for both the initial and continuation treatment of *H. influenzae* meningitis. Chloramphenicol remains an alternative effective drug for treatment of meningitis in patients who have severe allergy to β-lactams. Chloramphenicol is a good alternative agent for treatment of meningococcal meningitis (202). Treatment of *S. pneumoniae* meningitis with chloramphenicol may be unsatisfactory at times because some strains are inhibited but not killed. In addition, penicillin-resistant *S. pneumoniae* strains are frequently resistant to chloramphenicol. Third-generation cephalosporins are very effective for the treatment of these infections. The use of chloramphenicol in gram-negative bacillary meningitis has been disappointing both in neonates and in adults (203). This is probably due to lack of bactericidal activity against gram-negative bacilli at concentrations achieved in the CSF.

Anaerobic Infections

Chloramphenicol is very active against most anaerobic bacteria, including *Bacteroides fragilis*. The drug is effective for the treatment of brain abscesses and intra-abdominal infections, which are frequently caused by anaerobic organisms. However, other equally effective and less toxic drugs are available for treatment of such infections, including metronidazole for brain abscesses and clindamycin, cefoxitin, cefotetan, and ampicillin/sulbactam for intra-abdominal infections.

Rickettsial Infections

Chloramphenicol is effective in the treatment of Rocky Mountain spotted fever, epidemic typhus, scrub typhus, murine typhus, and Mediterranean fever (204,205). Tetracyclines are equally effective and less toxic and are usually used in moderate cases. Chloramphenicol is preferred by some when parenteral therapy is required for very ill patients, during pregnancy, and for young children younger than 8 years. Moreover, tetracycline cannot be used in the presence of renal failure.

Gram-Negative Aerobic Enteric Infections

Chloramphenicol is effective in many infections caused by these organisms except *P. aeruginosa*. However, aminoglycosides such as gentamicin or tobramycin or a third-generation cephalosporin are usually preferred. Chloramphenicol should not be used for treatment of urinary tract infections because other effective and safer drugs are available.

Enterococcal Infections

Strains of *Enterococcus faecium* have become resistant to penicillin, ampicillin, and vancomycin. Some of these strains may be susceptible to chloramphenicol, and the drug has been shown to be effective in the treatment of some serious vancomycin-resistant enterococcal infections (206). Other effective and less toxic agents are available for treatment of these infections such as linezolid and quinupristin–dalfopristin (207).

PHARMACOKINETIC PROPERTIES

Chloramphenicol is very lipid soluble but is minimally water soluble. Water solubility is achieved by attaching a polar group to the chloramphenicol molecule by an ester linkage. The palmitate ester is available in liquid preparation for oral use, and the succinate ester is provided for intravenous use. Both ester forms are biologically inactive and must be hydrolyzed after administration to release the active free chloramphenicol. Chloramphenicol palmitate, taken orally, is hydrolyzed in the proximal small intestine by pancreatic enzymes, which results in the release of free chloramphenicol, which is absorbed as the active compound. The crystalline form of chloramphenicol (in capsule form) is well absorbed from the gastrointestinal tract after oral administration.

Chloramphenicol succinate is rapidly hydrolyzed within the body following intravenous administration into the biologically active chloramphenicol. The mechanism of in vivo hydrolysis is not clear, but esterases of the liver, kidneys, and lungs may be involved. The disappearance of chloramphenicol succinate from serum of infants and children is highly variable and unpredictable. In 14 infants younger than 1 month, the mean unhydrolyzed serum chloramphenicol succinate measured at 6 hours after administration was 11% compared with a mean of 1.4% in 11 children 1 to 16 years of age (208). Therefore, infants during the first month of life appear to hydrolyze the succinate ester less efficiently than older infants. Chloramphenicol succinate also is subject to renal elimination from plasma before hydrolysis. The renal clearance of the "prodrug" in infants and children is highly variable and therefore affects the bioavailability of chloramphenicol. In 45 hospitalized infants and children 3 days to 16 years old who were receiving chloramphenicol succinate, only 51% of peak serum concentrations were within the "therapeutic" range, defined as 10 to 25 μg per mL. Seven of 45 had "subtherapeutic" concentrations, and 15 of 45 had chloramphenicol concentrations above 25 μg per mL.

A substantial but variable fraction of chloramphenicol succinate was excreted unchanged in urine. A mean of 33% (range 6% to 60%) of the administered dose was recovered unhydrolyzed in the urine. A mean of 18% of the dose was excreted as chloramphenicol glucuronide and 14% as free chloramphenicol (208).

The variation in the hydrolysis rate and the variable renal elimination of chloramphenicol succinate following intravenous administration markedly influence the achievable serum concentrations of active chloramphenicol. The succinate ester that persists in the body also acts as "prodrug" reservoir, which releases chloramphenicol continuously and results in lower and delayed serum peaks.

Nonesterified active chloramphenicol is metabolized primarily in the liver, where it is conjugated into water-soluble glucuronide and then is excreted in this inactive form by the kidneys. Eighty-five percent to 90% of the dose is excreted as glucuronide and 10% to 15% as chloramphenicol base. The partial renal elimination of unhydrolyzed chloramphenicol succinate results in an unusual bioavailability problem because this excreted fraction of the drug is quite variable and it is impossible to compensate for it by increasing the dose by a predetermined percentage.

The high variation in hydrolysis and renal excretion of chloramphenicol succinate contributes substantially to the wide variability in its apparent half-life and body clearance. Reported apparent half-lives range from 2.1 to 8.3 hours (mean 3.98 hours) (209) and 1.7 to 12 hours (mean 5.1 hours) (208). Body clearance of chloramphenicol also ranges from 0.122 to 0.429 L per kg per hour (209).

Chloramphenicol palmitate taken orally is hydrolyzed in the small intestine by pancreatic esterases yielding free chloramphenicol. The bioavailability of chloramphenicol is approximately 80% when administered as a suspension of chloramphenicol palmitate. Peak serum chloramphenicol concentrations are generally observed between 2 and 3 hours following oral administration (210,211).

Distribution

Chloramphenicol is extensively distributed to many tissues and body fluids. Various concentrations have been detected in the brain, heart, lung, kidney, liver, and spleen. Chloramphenicol also diffuses into vitreous humor (212), CSF (197,210,211,213,214), pleural fluid (215), synovial fluid (216), and saliva (217) and crosses the placenta. Chloramphenicol crosses the blood–brain barrier into CSF in children and adults with normal and inflamed meninges. CSF concentration is approximately 50% of simultaneous serum concentration but may range from 20% to 99% of serum concentration (210,211,213,214). Only minor fluctuations were noted during a dosing interval, in contrast to the respective serum concentration.

PROTEIN BINDING

Protein binding of chloramphenicol is about 53% in serum and 66% in plasma of adults (218). Binding occurs primarily with albumin. Bilirubin does not appear to displace chloramphenicol from bilirubin-binding sites and does not alter serum protein binding of chloramphenicol (219). In general, the unbound drug is considered to be the active entity. The percentage of unbound chloramphenicol increases as serum albumin concentration decreases (218). The percentage of unbound chloramphenicol may increase in other body fluids with less protein content than plasma such as CSF.

DOSAGE

Most chloramphenicol-susceptible organisms are inhibited by a concentration of 10 μg per mL or less. Chloramphenicol dose-dependent toxicity is very unlikely at serum concentration less than 25 μg per mL. Therefore, a dose of chloramphenicol that provides serum concentration of 10 to 25 μg per mL would be generally effective and safe for treatment of serious infections. A calculated dose that can theoretically provide a serum concentration within this therapeutic range is not always feasible because of the wide variability in the metabolism and excretion of chloramphenicol.

Chloramphenicol palmitate suspension given orally produces more predictable serum levels than those obtained after the succinate ester is given intravenously. Oral doses of 60 to 75 mg per kg per day result in serum concentrations between 15 and 25 μg per mL (220). A dose of 75 mg per kg per day is recommended as a starting dose for most patients beyond the newborn period. The total daily dose is administered in four daily doses given every 6 hours. This dose may subsequently be adjusted contingent on serum concentrations.

Recommended doses for the intravenous chloramphenicol succinate are 25 mg per kg per day for premature infants and term infants younger than 2 weeks and 50 mg per kg per day for older term infants and children. For serious infections, 75 to 100 mg per kg per day is suggested for infants older than 2 weeks and for older children. The total daily dose is given in four daily doses every 6 hours. These doses, however, frequently result in serum concentrations outside the therapeutic range. In one study of 107 infants receiving recommended doses of chloramphenicol, 33% had serum concentrations between 10 and 20 μg per mL, 50% above 20 μg per mL, and 11% below 10 μg per mL (221). In another study of 45 infants and children receiving intravenous chloramphenicol succinate, only 51% of peak serum concentration was within the "therapeutic" range of 10 to 25 μg per mL. Seven of 45 had "subtherapeutic" levels and 15 of 45 had chloramphenicol concentration above 25 μg per mL (208).

Because of the narrow therapeutic range of chloramphenicol concentrations and the lack of correlation between dose and serum concentration, it is recommended that serum concentrations be monitored during therapy if at all possible (197,208,213,221). Active chloramphenicol does not accumulate in patients with renal failure and therefore the drug may be given in the usual recommended dose. Inactive chloramphenicol metabolites accumulate in the serum of patients with renal failure but have not been associated with known toxicity.

Because chloramphenicol is metabolized in the liver, its body clearance is reduced in patients with liver dysfunction. When used in these patients, chloramphenicol serum levels should be monitored.

TOXICITY

The most important toxic effects of chloramphenicol occur in the bone marrow. These effects are of two types. The first is a reversible erythroid suppression of the bone marrow probably due to chloramphenicol inhibition of mitochondrial protein synthesis, which in turn impairs iron incorporation into heme. Suppression of erythropoiesis occurs if excessive concentrations of the drug are maintained for a sufficient length of time (222). This effect is dose related and usually reversible. Bone marrow suppression tends to occur when peak chloramphenicol concentrations consistently exceed 25 μg per mL or concentrations at 6 hours after a dose that exceed 15 μg per mL (223). Early signs reflect arrest of erythropoiesis and include reticulocytopenia, increased serum iron, and eventually a decrease in erythrocyte count. With continued use of the drug at sufficient doses, thrombocytopenia and neutropenia may occur within 2 to 3 weeks. The risk of this dose-related toxicity can be minimized by maintaining serum chloramphenicol concentration less than 25 μg per mL and by limiting the duration of drug administration to the minimum required for adequate treatment.

The second type of toxicity is a rare, but usually fatal, idiosyncratic response frequently manifested as aplastic anemia. It is not dose related, and a genetic predisposition is suggested by the occurrence of pancytopenia in identical twins. It is rare and is estimated to occur once in every 24,500 to 40,000 patients (0.004% to 0.0025%) who receive the antibiotic (224). All blood cell lines are affected, resulting in pancytopenia, which is frequently irreversible. This toxicity most commonly occurs after therapy is discontinued. The fatality rate is high when bone marrow aplasia is complete. Although several theories have been advanced, the mechanism of this aplastic anemia associated with chloramphenicol administration is unknown. Although most cases have been reported after oral therapy, a number of cases of aplastic anemia from parenteral chloramphenicol and even after the administration of eye drops have also been reported (225,226).

Gray Baby Syndrome

Fatal chloramphenicol toxicity may develop in neonates, especially premature babies, when they are exposed to high doses of chloramphenicol. The illness, the gray baby syndrome, has been reported in infants who were receiving chloramphenicol doses of 100 to 200 mg per kg per day and had serum chloramphenicol serum concentrations of 70 to 250 μg per mL, which are 10 times the therapeutic blood concentrations (227). The illness usually begins 2 to 9 days after treatment is started and manifests as vomiting, refusal to suck, irregular and rapid breathing, abdominal distention, and periods of cyanosis and passage of loose green stools. In the subsequent 24 hours, affected infants become flaccid, turn ashen gray in color, and become hypothermic. Death can occur within 2 days of onset of symptoms. Chloramphenicol toxicity in neonates results from (a) failure of drug conjugation because of inadequate hepatic glucuronyl transferase during first 3 to 4 weeks of life and (b) inadequate renal excretion of unconjugated chloramphenicol in the newborn (228). In premature infants and neonates, chloramphenicol should be reduced to 25 mg per kg per day and antibiotic blood levels should be monitored. This syndrome has also been reported in toddlers (229) and after accidental overdoses in adults (230). Impaired myocardial contractility due to interference in myocardial tissue respiration and oxidative phosphorylation contribute to the clinical picture (231). It is generally associated with serum chloramphenicol of greater than 50 μg per mL and unexplained acidosis (232).

Chloramphenicol is removed to a small extent by peritoneal dialysis or hemodialysis. Exchange transfusion or charcoal hemoperfusion have been used to accelerate drug removal (233,234).

Decreased visual acuity due to optic neuritis has been described in patients who received prolonged chloramphenicol treatment. Although this effect is generally reversible, loss of vision has occurred in some cases (235). Other neurologic sequelae that have been described include peripheral neuritis, headache, depression, and mental confusion. Adverse effects involving the gastrointestinal tract include nausea, vomiting and diarrhea, and stomatitis. Prolonged chloramphenicol administration can result in bleeding due to decreased vitamin K synthesis.

Drug Interactions

Chloramphenicol inhibits hepatic microsomal cytochrome P450 enzymes, which results in prolongation of half-lives of drugs metabolized by this system (236). This includes tolbutamide, phenytoin, dicoumarol, chlorpropamide, antiretroviral protease inhibitors, and rifabutin. Toxicity due to these drugs may occur if they are given in their usual doses to patients who are receiving chloramphenicol (237,238). Conversely, concurrent administration of phenytoin and chloramphenicol succinate results in elevated chloramphenicol peak and trough serum levels. This may be the result of competition for binding sites rather than induction of hepatic enzymes. Concurrent administration of chloramphenicol succinate and phenobarbital shortens the half-life of the antibiotic, causing reduction of the peak and trough serum levels of chloramphenicol (239). Chloramphenicol is primarily bacteriostatic and will antagonize the bactericidal activity of penicillins, cephalosporins, and aminoglycosides. In vitro growth kinetic assays have demonstrated inhibition of the early bactericidal activity of ampicillin against group B streptococci by chloramphenicol (240). In vitro time kill curves have also shown the antagonistic effect of chloramphenicol on the bactericidal activity of cefotaxime and ceftriaxone against *E. coli* and group B streptococci (160). Chloramphenicol also appears to suppress the bactericidal action of gentamicin against *E. coli* and *Klebsiella* (159).

TETRACYCLINES

Tetracyclines were introduced soon after penicillin G and the sulfonamides. They were discovered by screening soil specimens for antibiotic-producing microorganisms. The first compound, chlortetracycline, was introduced in 1948 (241), and subsequently many tetracyclines have been developed. Tetracyclines were known as "broad-spectrum"

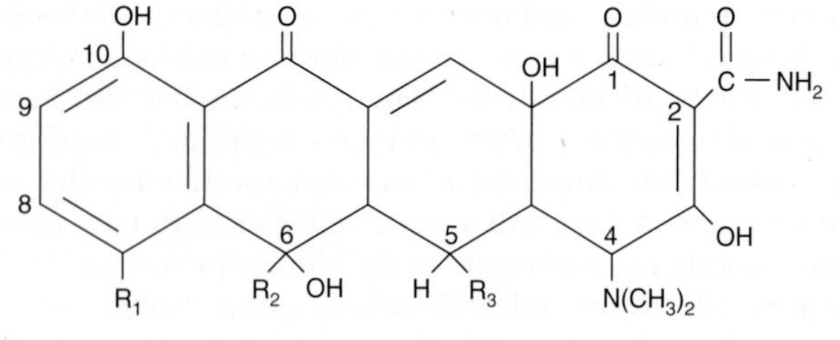

Tetracycline nucleus

Figure 32.5. Structure of tetracycline nucleus.

antibiotics because of their activity against a number of gram-positive and gram-negative bacteria as well as rickettsiae and chlamydiae. As a result of their broad in vitro activity and proven clinical effectiveness, they became widely used therapeutic agents.

Chlortetracycline was the first natural tetracycline, isolated from *Streptomyces aureofaciens* in 1948, and oxytetracycline was later derived from *Streptomyces rimosus* in 1950. Tetracycline was first produced semisynthetically from chlortetracycline in 1953. Demeclocycline was derived from a mutant strain of *S. aureofaciens.* The two long-acting compounds doxycycline and minocycline were derived semisynthetically in 1966 and 1967, respectively. Those currently marketed include tetracycline, oxytetracycline, and demeclocycline and the newer semisynthetic compounds doxycycline and minocycline.

CHEMICAL STRUCTURE

The basic tetracycline structure consists of a hydronaphthacene nucleus with four fused rings. Tetracycline analogues differ from each other by substituent variations at carbon 5, 6, or 7 of the basic structure (Fig. 32.5).

MECHANISM OF ACTION/MECHANISM OF BACTERIAL RESISTANCE

Tetracyclines are bacteriostatic agents that inhibit bacterial protein synthesis. They reversibly bind to the 30S subunits of bacterial ribosomes. Tetracyclines inhibit the binding of the enzyme aminoacyl-tRNA to the ribosomal acceptor site on the mRNA–ribosome complex (242,243). This prevents the addition of new amino acids into the growing peptide chain. Studies of tetracycline in *E. coli* show that tetracycline passively diffuses through outer membrane porins and then traverses the cytoplasmic membrane by energy-independent and energy-dependent mechanisms (244). In higher concentrations, tetracyclines also inhibit mammalian protein synthesis particularly in mitochondrial ribosomes (245). Although these ribosomes are not present in sufficient concentration within these structures to produce severe toxicity, this antianabolic effect can aggravate preexisting renal function impairment (246).

Resistance to tetracyclines is predominantly due to decreased accumulation of antibiotic within the cell. The genes encoding for resistance are called *tet,* or tetracycline resistance determinants. They are most often carried on plasmids but can be chromosomal. Resistance is achieved by increasing ability of the cell to efflux the antibiotic (150). The *tet* genes encode for membrane proteins that mediate energy-dependent efflux. Efflux has been demonstrated in enterobacteriaceae, enterococci, staphylococci, *V. cholera,* and *Bacteroides.* Resistance to one tetracycline usually implies resistance to all tetracyclines. However, partial cross-resistance occurs, and many tetracycline-resistant bacteria are susceptible to doxycycline and minocycline. A second but less common mechanism of resistance is due to altered ribosomal targets (encoded by different *tet* genes). This results in the inability of tetracyclines to prevent attachment of aminoacyl-tRNA to the ribosomal receptor site. This has been described in some organisms including *N. gonorrhoeae* and *Mycoplasma.* A third mechanism of resistance, enzymatic inactivation of tetracyclines, encoded for by another *tet* gene, has been demonstrated in vitro in *E. coli,* but its clinical significance is not known (247).

EVIDENCE OF EFFICACY/THERAPEUTIC USES

Tetracyclines have a broad spectrum of activity, which includes aerobic and anaerobic gram-positive and gram-negative bacteria, chlamydiae, rickettsiae, mycoplasma, *Ureaplasma,* and spirochetes. In general, the lipophilic analogues have better antibacterial activity by weight than the more hydrophilic ones. Therefore, it follows that minocycline and doxycycline are more active at lower concentration against susceptible organisms than the other tetracyclines. Despite these differences, for cost reasons it is recommended that tetracycline be used in the clinical microbiology laboratory to determine susceptibility for all analogues (248). Organisms inhibited by 1 μg per mL or less are considered highly susceptible, those inhibited by 1 to 5 μg per mL are intermediately susceptible, whereas those not inhibited by 5 μg per mL are resistant. Bacterial resistance to any one member of the class usually results in cross-resistance to the other tetracyclines.

Tetracyclines are in general active against gram-positive microorganisms; however, problems of resistance and the availability of more effective agents limit their use for treatment of infections caused by many gram-positive bacteria. Tetracyclines are active against staphylococci; however, many strains, especially those recovered in hospitals, readily develop resistance. Both doxycycline and minocycline are more active against *S. aureus* than tetracycline. Therefore, in vitro susceptibility testing should be performed if these drugs are to be used for treatment of staphylococcal infections (249,250).

Resistance to tetracyclines among group A streptococci has varied from 5% to 35% in Europe and in the United States (251,252). Group B streptococci are frequently resistant to tetracyclines (253).

Most *S. pneumoniae* strains are susceptible to tetracycline and doxycycline; however, penicillin-resistant strains are often resistant to them (254). Tetracycline- and penicillin-resistant pneumococci are very prevalent in some European countries (255). In the United States, some penicillin-resistant pneumococci are also tetracycline resistant (256). Most enterococci are resistant to tetracycline.

Minocycline has excellent activity against *Nocardia* species, especially *N. asteroides.* Other tetracyclines are less active (257).

Tetracyclines are considered effective against several gram-negative bacteria; however, their activity has been limited by the emergence of resistant strains.

Most *P. aeruginosa* and many *Salmonella* and *Shigella* strains are resistant. *Serratia marcescens* and *Proteus* species are usually resistant.

Gonococci and meningococci are very susceptible; however, gonococci resistant to penicillin tend to be resistant to tetracycline (258).

Most strains of *C. jejuni* and *Campylobacter fetus* are susceptible to tetracyclines (259). *H. pylori* is susceptible to tetracyclines and also to penicillins, erythromycin, cephalosporins, clindamycin, and rifampicin and usually metronidazole (260). Tetracyclines are active against *Aeromonas hydrophila* and *Plesiomonas shigelloides* (185). *Brucella* species are uniformly susceptible to tetracycline (261,262).

V. cholera, both classical and El Tor biotypes, which cause gastroenteritis, *Vibrio vulnificus*, which is associated with septicemia or cellulites, and other vibrios (*V. parahaemolyticus*, *V. alginolyticus*), which cause food-borne gastroenteritis, are susceptible to tetracyclines (263,264). Some strains of enterotoxigenic *E. coli* are also susceptible (265). Most *Yersinia enterocolitica* and *Yersinia pseudotuberculosis* are susceptible to tetracycline, aminoglycosides, third-generation cephalosporins, trimethoprim–sulfamethoxazole, and chloramphenicol (266). *Yersinia pestis*, the etiologic agent of plague, is susceptible in vitro to tetracycline, streptomycin, gentamicin, and chloramphenicol (267).

B. henselae, the etiologic agent of CSD, and *Bartonella quintana*, which causes louse trench fever, are susceptible to tetracycline (268,269). *L. pneumophila* is quite susceptible to doxycycline and minocycline (270). *Burkholderia* (*Pseudomonas*) *pseudomallei* (melioidosis) is usually susceptible to tetracycline and minocycline (271).

Tetracyclines are active against many anaerobic bacteria (272). Of the gram-negative anaerobes, *Fusobacterium* and *Prevotella* are frequently susceptible. A variable number of *Bacteroides* species are susceptible to doxycycline; however, clindamycin, chloramphenicol, and metronidazole are more active and are the preferred drugs for treatment of infections caused by *B. fragilis*. Gram-positive anaerobes also have variable susceptibility. The activity of tetracyclines against *Actinomyces* is especially clinically relevant. *Propionibacterium* is frequently susceptible, whereas *Peptococcus* is frequently resistant.

M. pneumoniae is susceptible to all tetracyclines (273,274). *Mycoplasma hominis* is usually susceptible, but some resistant strains have been recently noted (275).

Tetracyclines are effective against *U. urealyticum*; however, resistant strains have been reported to naturally exist (276,277) and shown to be induced in vitro (272).

C. trachomatis, the cause of trachoma, genital infections, and perinatally acquired respiratory infections in young infants, is susceptible to tetracyclines, especially doxycycline and minocycline. The MIC of doxycycline against this organism is 0.06 μg per mL or less (278). Occasional resistant strains have been encountered (279,280). *C. pneumoniae* (respiratory pathogen) is susceptible to tetracyclines (281,282). *Chlamydia psittaci*, which causes psittacosis, is also susceptible to tetracyclines (283).

Many pathogenic spirochetes are susceptible to tetracyclines. *B. burgdorferi*, the etiologic agent of Lyme disease, is highly susceptible to tetracyclines and is also susceptible to ampicillin, ceftriaxone, and imipenem (284). *T. pallidum* is susceptible to tetracycline; however, its MIC (0.2 μg per mL) against this organism is much higher than that of penicillin G (0.0005 μg per mL) (285). The leptospira are susceptible to tetracycline.

Tetracyclines are very effective against the rickettsiae, which cause a variety of spotted fevers and typhus fevers. Rocky Mountain spotted fever is caused by *R. rickettsiae* and Mediterranean spotted fever by *Rickettsia conorii*. Murine typhus is caused by *Rickettsia typhi*, epidemic typhus by *Rickettsia prowazekii*, and scrub typhus by *Rickettsia tsutsugamushi*. Tetracyclines are active against all these rickettsiae (MIC = 0.25 μg per mL), with doxycycline being the most active (MIC = 0.1 μg per mL) (205). *C. burnetii*, the etiologic agent of Q fever, is also susceptible (205).

Ehrlichia species, which are obligate intracellular bacteria, are susceptible to tetracyclines (286). Tetracyclines, especially doxycycline, are effective against malarial parasites, including chloroquine-resistant *Plasmodium falciparum* (287,288).

THERAPEUTIC USES

The extensive use of tetracyclines for treatment of infections and as an additive to animal feeds (to facilitate growth) has led to a dramatic increase in bacterial resistance, and as a result their use has declined. However, tetracyclines remain the drugs of choice or are the effective alternative therapy for a variety of bacterial infections. They are especially useful for the treatment of infections caused by rickettsiae, mycoplasma, and chlamydiae.

The use of tetracyclines during the tooth development period (last half of pregnancy, infancy, and childhood to age 8 years) may cause permanent discoloration of the teeth. Therefore, tetracycline drugs should not be used in this age group unless other treatment is not likely to be effective or if alternative therapy is contraindicated.

Rickettsial Infections

Tetracyclines are very effective in the treatment of rickettsial infections including Rocky Mountain spotted fever, Q fever, rickettsialpox, epidemic typhus (Brill disease), murine typhus, and scrub typhus (289,290). In almost all clinical situations, doxycycline is the drug of choice. Chloramphenicol is also effective for these diseases and is sometimes preferred for very severe infections. For adults and children weighing more than 45 kg, the recommended doxycycline treatment is 100 mg orally every 12 hours. For children weighing less than 45 kg, doxycycline 2.2 mg per kg per day is given every 12 hours for 7 to 10 days. Patients with severe disease who require hospitalization, are vomiting, or are comatose should receive parenteral therapy at a dose of 100 mg intravenously every 12 hours (291).

Mycoplasma pneumoniae Infections

The drugs of choice in pneumonia due to *M. pneumoniae* are either erythromycins or tetracyclines. The two drugs are equally effective in shortening the duration of illness

(273). Erythromycin is the drug of choice in children because of the adverse effects of tetracyclines on teeth. The regimen of tetracycline or erythromycin in children with *M. pneumoniae* pneumonia is 40 to 50 mg per kg per 24 hour administered every 6 hours for 10 days. For adolescents and adults, the dose is 2 g per 24 hour divided every 6 hours.

Mycoplasma hominis Infections

M. hominis is an inhabitant of the genitourinary tract and has been implicated as a cause of salpingitis and postpartum septicemia. Illness due to *M. hominis* infection is rare in children. This organism should be considered as an etiologic possibility in neonates with meningitis and with abscesses in whom routine cultures are negative (292,293). Therapy with doxycycline is usually successful (294).

Ureaplasma urealyticum

U. urealyticum and *Chlamydia* species are the major cause of nongonococcal urethritis. Tetracyclines are usually effective against infections caused by both organisms (295). However, resistant strains have been reported (296). Patients with nongonococcal urethritis should be treated with tetracycline 40 mg per kg per 24 hour every 6 hours; patients weighing more than 50 kg should receive 500 mg every 6 hours for 10 days (297). *Ureaplasma* and *Chlamydia* are also susceptible to erythromycin, which is a useful alternative for patients in whom tetracycline is contraindicated.

Chlamydia Infections

Tetracyclines are effective for the treatment of *Chlamydia* infections. Lymphogranuloma venereum, caused by *C. trachomatis* serovars L1, L2, L3, responds to tetracycline treatment (298). Recommended treatment is doxycycline 100 mg twice daily for 3 weeks. Alternative treatment is erythromycin.

For uncomplicated *C. trachomatis* genital tract infection in adolescents and adults, oral doxycycline 100 mg twice daily for 7 days is effective; however, azithromycin 1 g given as a single dose is also effective and preferred because of better compliance (299). Because coinfection with *N. gonorrhoeae* and *C. trachomatis* is common, doxycycline or azithromycin should be administered empirically in addition to the other agent used for treatment of gonorrhea (18).

C. trachomatis frequently is a coexistent pathogen in acute pelvic inflammatory disease. Recommended treatment is doxycycline, 100 mg intravenously twice daily, for at least 48 hours after clinical improvement followed by oral therapy at the same dosage to complete 14 days (18).

Respiratory infections due to *C. pneumoniae* in older children and adults are commonly treated with doxycycline 100 mg twice daily for 14 to 21 days. Erythromycin, azithromycin, and clarithromycin are also effective. For children, either erythromycin (for 10 to 14 days) or clarithromycin (for 10 days) can be used (282).

The most widely used therapy for trachoma is topical treatment with tetracycline, erythromycin, or sulfacetamide ointment twice a day for 2 months or oral erythromycin or doxycycline for 40 days if the infection is severe. Azithromycin 20 mg per kg (maximum 1 g once per week) for 3 weeks is also effective (299).

Penicillin G is the best drug for treatment of syphilis. Nonpregnant, penicillin-allergic patients who have primary, secondary, or latent syphilis can be treated with a tetracycline (500 mg four times daily for 14 days) or doxycycline (100 mg orally twice daily for 2 weeks). However, pregnant patients, children and adults with neurosyphilis, and patients allergic to penicillin should be treated whenever possible with penicillin G after desensitization (18).

EHRLICHIOSIS

This is a tick-borne infection caused by obligate intracellular bacteria of the genus *Ehrlichia*. Infection causes undifferentiated fever with leukopenia, thrombocytopenia, and elevations in serum aminotransferase levels. Rash is an infrequent sign. The treatment of choice for human monocytic ehrlichiosis (*Ehrlichia chaffeensis*) and human granulocytic ehrlichiosis (*Ehrlichia equi*) is either tetracycline or doxycycline usually administered for 7 days (286).

LYME DISEASE

B. burgdorferi, the etiologic agent of Lyme disease, is highly sensitive to tetracycline (300). It is also susceptible to ampicillin, ceftriaxone, and imipenem. Erythromycin appears to be active in vitro but may be less so in vivo. Tetracycline is considered the most effective treatment for early manifestations, such as erythema migrans, of this disease. Recommendation for treatment of early disease is tetracycline orally four times per day, or doxycycline 100 mg twice daily for 20 to 30 days for adults and children older than 8 years. In younger children, amoxicillin or cefuroxime are alternative agents. Lyme arthritis can also be treated successfully with a 1-month course of oral doxycycline (301). Although doxycycline has been successful in treatment of Lyme meningitis in some patients, ceftriaxone is superior (302).

BRUCELLOSIS

Tetracyclines are effective in the treatment of acute and chronic infections caused by *Brucella melitensis, Brucella suis,* and *Brucella abortus.* Because brucellae are intracellular pathogens, it is believed that penetration into the cells is a requirement for effective therapy. Tetracyclines are very effective agents for treating brucellosis and have a mean MIC of less than 1 μg per mL. The regimen of choice is tetracycline 30 to 40 mg per kg per 24 hour, maximum daily dose 2 g per 24 hour, divided into four oral doses for 4 to 6 weeks (or doxycycline 5 mg per kg per 24 hour, maximum daily dose 200 mg, divided twice a day) in combination with streptomycin 15 to 30 mg per kg per 24 hour, maximum daily dose 1 g, divided into two intramuscular doses for 2 to 3 weeks (or gentamicin 5 mg per kg per 24 hour divided twice daily for 5 days) (303). For children younger than 8 years, recommended treatment is a combination of trimethoprim and sulfamethoxazole

(10/50 mg per kg per 24 hour) given twice daily for 3 weeks plus gentamicin (5 mg per kg per 24 hour) twice daily for the first 5 days (304) or trimethoprim–sulfamethoxazole plus rifampin (20 mg per kg per 24 hour) for 8 to 12 weeks (305).

CHOLERA

Correction of dehydration associated with cholera is the most important treatment measure. Oral tetracyclines have been shown to be effective in eradicating vibrio organisms from stools and shortening the volume and duration of diarrhea. Tetracycline-resistant strains of *V. cholera* are uncommon. Oral tetracycline is given as 50 mg per kg per 24 hour, divided into four doses every 6 hours for 3 days (maximum dose 2 g per day) or as a single dose of 25 mg per kg (maximum dose 1 g). Oral doxycycline is given as two doses of 2 mg per kg on day 1 followed by single dose of 2 mg per kg on days 2 and 3 (maximum single dose 100 mg) or a single dose of 7 mg per kg (maximum dose 300 mg) (306). Because tetracyclines can cause discoloration of deciduous and permanent teeth, they have not been routinely used to treat children, even though the risk is small with such relatively short courses. Furazolidone has been the agent used routinely in children to treat cholera (5 mg per kg per day divided into four doses for 3 days, maximum dose 400 mg; or a single dose of 7 mg per kg, maximum dose 300 mg) (307).

MALARIA

Tetracyclines have been used for treatment of chloroquine-resistant *Malaria falciparum*. The response to tetracycline alone is slow, and a regimen of quinine sulfate combined with tetracycline is more successful. Tetracycline 6.25 mg per kg every 6 hours (maximum 250 mg daily) or doxycycline 2 mg per kg every 12 hours (maximum 100 mg every 12 hours) given for 7 days, in addition to a full course of quinine sulfate 25 mg per kg per 24 hour orally in divided doses every 8 hours (maximum 650 mg every 8 hours) for 3 to 7 days. For prevention of chloroquine-resistant *Malaria falciparum* infection, doxycycline 2 mg per kg daily, up to 100 mg, is given (beginning 1 to 2 days before travel, continuing for the duration of stay, and for 4 weeks after leaving) (308).

ACNE

Topical keratolytic agents may be effective for mild disease; however, for severe acne the addition of antibiotics may be of benefit. Tetracyclines often given in an oral dose of 250 mg twice daily may be continued for months or even years. Tetracyclines may act by inhibiting the anaerobic *P. acnes* organisms that colonize the sebaceous follicles. These organisms metabolize lipids into free fatty acids, which cause inflammation in the follicular wall. They also produce chemotactic agents that attract polymorphonuclear cells into the follicular wall. Long-term use of tetracyclines seems to be well tolerated with few side effects because of the low dose used and the age of the patients. Erythromycin or trimethoprim–sulfamethoxazole were also shown to be effective oral agents.

TABLE 32.1 Pharmacokinetic Properties of Tetracyclines (309–312)

Antibiotic	*Gastrointestinal Absorption (%)*	*Half-life (hr)*	*Protein Binding (%)*
Short acting			
Oxytetracycline	58	9	35
Tetracycline	77	8	65
Intermediate			
Demeclocycline	66	12	91
Long acting			
Doxycycline	93	18	93
Minocycline	95	16	76

PHARMACOKINETIC PROPERTIES: ABSORPTION, METABOLISM, ELIMINATION

Tetracycline compounds can be divided into three groups according to their different half-lives. The short-acting group includes chlortetracycline, oxytetracycline, and tetracycline; demeclocycline is an intermediate-acting compound; and long-acting agents include doxycycline and minocycline. Some pharmacokinetic properties of these compounds are shown in Table 32.1.

Oral administration is the preferred route because of the thrombophlebitis associated with the intravenous route and pain with the intramuscular injection. Absorption of most tetracyclines from the gastrointestinal tract, primarily in the proximal small bowel, is incomplete. Tetracyclines form insoluble complexes with aluminum, calcium, iron, magnesium, zinc, and other bivalent and trivalent cations. Therefore, concurrent ingestion of milk and other dairy products, antacids, calcium or iron supplements, bismuth subsalicylate, and other agents can impair tetracycline absorption.

Plasma concentrations of the tetracyclines achieved following oral administration vary among individuals due to the variability of their absorption. Oxytetracycline and tetracycline are incompletely absorbed (58% to 77%). Their peak plasma concentration is achieved 2 to 4 hours after an oral dose. Their half-lives range from 8 to 9 hours. These drugs are given every 6 hours. Peak plasma concentrations of 2 to 2.5 μg per mL are achieved after 250 mg oral dose. Demeclocycline is also incompletely absorbed (66%) and has a half-life of about 12 hours, resulting in effective plasma concentration for 24 to 48 hours. Therefore, this drug is administered in lower daily doses than oxytetracycline and tetracycline.

Doxycycline and minocycline are absorbed almost completely (93% to 95%) and have the longest half-lives, 16 to 18 hours. Thus, high serum levels are achieved with relatively small doses. Because of its long half-life, therapeutic plasma levels of doxycycline can be maintained with a single daily dose, although twice-daily dosing is usually recommended (309).

Following an oral dose of 200 mg of doxycycline, a plasma concentration of 3 μg per mL is achieved at 2 hours and a sustained concentration of 1 μg per mL for 8 to 12 hours. The plasma concentrations of doxycycline are equivalent following oral and parenteral routes. The absorption of doxycycline or minocycline is not affected by food. The half-lives of these compounds are mainly determined by their rate of renal excretion. Chlortetracycline is an exception; it has a short half-life despite having a slow rate of renal clearance due to its instability both in vitro and in vivo (310). Adequate therapeutic concentrations in the urine are achieved by all tetracyclines, with the exception of chlortetracycline and minocycline, for the treatment of urinary tract infections by susceptible bacteria. Serum protein binding of these compounds varies but tends to be higher for the intermediate- and long-acting compounds (Table 32.1) (311,312). This is a possible contributing factor to their slow rate of renal excretion.

Tetracyclines are distributed widely throughout the body. They can be found in many tissues and body fluids including lung, liver, kidney, brain, sputum, and mucosal secretions. They accumulate in the liver, spleen, bone marrow, bone, dentine, and the enamel, including the enamel of nonerupted teeth. Levels of tetracycline in CSF are about 10% to 26% of blood levels (313,314). Inflammation of the meninges is not a requirement for penetration into CSF. Concentrations in synovial fluid and sinus mucosa approach that in blood (315,316). Tetracyclines concentrate in bile at levels 5 to 20 times those in serum. Minocycline and, to a lesser extent, doxycycline are more lipophilic than the other tetracyclines. This is the likely reason why these two agents attain higher concentrations in saliva and tears (317). Tetracyclines cross the placenta and enter fetal circulation and amniotic fluid. They accumulate in fetal bone and teeth, and therefore should not be given during pregnancy (318). Relatively high concentrations of tetracyclines are detected in breast milk (319). Most tetracyclines, with the exception of doxycycline, are eliminated primarily by the kidneys. Although they are concentrated in the liver and then excreted by way of bile into the intestines, they are partially reabsorbed via the enterohepatic circulation. Even when given parenterally, these drugs are excreted into the intestinal tract as a result of excretion into bile. Clearance of these drugs in the kidneys is by glomerular filtration. Therefore, their renal excretion is significantly affected by the renal function status of the patient. The tetracyclines should not be used in patients with renal failure. Doxycycline is the only exception, because it is excreted in the gastrointestinal tract mostly as an inactive conjugate and does not accumulate significantly in patients with renal failure. Decreased hepatic function or biliary tract obstruction decreases biliary excretion of these drugs and results in higher plasma concentration and longer half-life. Minocycline is significantly metabolized in the liver and is recovered in much lower concentration from both urine and feces than the other tetracyclines. Its renal clearance is also low and it persists in the body after its administration is stopped because of its retention in fatty tissues. Minocycline half-life is not prolonged in patients with hepatic failure. All tetracyclines are slowly removed from blood by hemodialysis, but the rate of removal by peritoneal dialysis is poor (320,321).

DOSES AND ROUTES

Tetracyclines are available in different forms for oral, parenteral, and topical administration. For oral administration, the recommended oral dose of tetracyclines varies with the severity and nature of the infection being treated. Oral tetracycline dose ranges from 1 to 2 g per day in adults; for children older than 8 years, the regimen is 25 to 50 mg per kg daily in four divided doses. The regimen of doxycycline for adults is 100 mg every 12 hours for the first 24 hours, followed by 100 mg once a day, or twice daily when severe infection is present. For children older than 8 years, the doxycycline regimen is 4 to 5 mg per kg per day divided into two doses given every 12 hours for the first day, followed by 2 to 2.5 mg per day given as a single daily dose.

The regimen of minocycline for adults is 200 mg on day 1, then 100 mg every 12 hours after that; for children older than 8 years, minocycline is given at 4 mg per kg on the first day, then 2 mg per kg every 12 hours.

Parenteral Administration

The preferred parenteral tetracycline is doxycycline. It is used for treatment of severe infections, or in patients who cannot ingest the oral preparation or have associated nausea or vomiting. For adults, the intravenous regimen of doxycycline is 200 mg given in one or two doses on the first day, followed by 100 to 200 mg daily thereafter. The dosage for children is 4 mg per kg given in two equal doses on the first day, followed by 2.2 mg per kg single-daily maintenance dose. Minocycline intravenous dosing for adults is an initial loading dose of 200 mg, followed by 100 mg every 12 hours. In children older than 8 years, the initial dose is 4 mg per kg, followed by 2 mg per kg every 12 hours.

Parenteral preparations of tetracycline are no longer available in the United States. Where available, the usual adult daily dose is 500 mg to 1 g, administered in equally divided doses every 6 to 12 hours. In severe infections, a maximum dose of 2 g per day may be given.

Local Application

Topical use of tetracyclines is not recommended except for local use in the eye. Ophthalmic ointments and suspensions of tetracycline hydrochloride, chlortetracycline hydrochloride, and oxytetracycline hydrochloride are available.

ADVERSE EFFECTS

Gastrointestinal Effects

All tetracyclines may produce gastrointestinal irritation to varying degrees especially when given orally. Gastric distress, abdominal discomfort, nausea, and vomiting may occur. Gastrointestinal symptoms usually subside quickly when the tetracycline is stopped. Tetracyclines may also cause antibiotic-associated colitis. Gastric distress can be reduced by administering the drug with food. However, tetracyclines should not be given with dairy products.

Hepatic Toxicity

Rarely, hepatitis-like illness may develop during oral treatment with tetracycline, doxycycline, or minocycline or following intravenous administration of doxycycline. The hepatitis can occasionally be severe but usually resolves after discontinuation of the drug. The risk of such complication has been estimated to be 1.56 cases per 1 million (322). Overdosage of intravenous tetracycline can be particularly dangerous during pregnancy and has been associated with symptoms of nausea, fever, and vomiting followed by jaundice. In severe cases, the disease can be associated with hematemesis, renal failure with acidosis, and, in fatal cases, coma and terminal hypotension (323).

Hypersensitivity Reactions

These are uncommon and usually manifest as urticaria, facial swelling, or bronchospasm. Rarely, anaphylaxis may occur. The Jarisch–Herxheimer reaction may occur when tetracyclines are used to treat a spirochetal infection such as *B. burgdorferi* infection (Lyme disease) or other infections such as brucellosis or tularemia.

Photosensitivity

Patients treated with doxycycline, and less often other tetracyclines, may develop mild-to-severe photosensitivity reactions when exposed to sunlight (324). Minocycline is less likely to cause this side effect.

Effects on Teeth

Tetracyclines are deposited in calcifying areas of bones and teeth and may cause permanent yellow or brown discoloration of the teeth. This is purely a cosmetic disadvantage of these agents. Tetracyclines may deposit in the deciduous teeth if administered to children early in life or given to their mother during pregnancy because they cross the placenta (325). Risk is highest when tetracycline is given to neonates and babies prior to first dentition. Pigmentation of permanent teeth may occur if the drug is given between 2 months and 5 years of age when the teeth are being calcified. However, children up to 8 years may be susceptible to this complication. The type of discoloration may vary according to the particular tetracycline used. Chlortetracycline produces gray-brown teeth, whereas tetracycline and oxytetracycline cause yellow discoloration. The degree of discoloration depends on the amount of tetracycline administered. Discoloration becomes obvious in children who have several courses of the drug.

Nephrotoxicity

Tetracyclines may cause further rise in blood urea and serum creatinine in patients with renal disease. This is probably due to inhibition of protein synthesis by the drug, which results in a catabolic effect (326).

Neurotoxic Effects

An uncommon complication of bulging anterior fontanel may occur in infants receiving usual doses of tetracycline. The condition is characterized by irritability, vomiting, and tense bulging fontanel associated with elevated CSF pressure, normal number of cells, and normal glucose and protein content. Rapid resolution occurs when the drug is discontinued (327). Benign increased intracranial hypertension caused by tetracycline and minocycline has been reported in both adults and children (328,329). Clinical manifestations include severe headache and blurring of vision associated with papilledema. Most cases have occurred in young adults and some children, and the majority had been taking tetracycline for acne for periods of days to months.

Minocycline, but not other tetracyclines, has been associated with reversible vestibular disturbance manifesting as dizziness, ataxia, vertigo, tinnitus with weakness, nausea, and vomiting. Minocycline has also been associated with lightheadedness and feeling of dissociation (330).

DRUG INTERACTIONS

Tetracyclines form insoluble complexes with bivalent and trivalent cations including aluminum, calcium, iron, magnesium, and zinc. Therefore, concurrent ingestion of antacids, calcium, iron supplements, or bismuth subsalicylate as well as milk and other dairy products can impair tetracycline absorption. Therefore, administration of the drugs should be spaced by 2 hours (331,332).

Carbamazepine, diphenylhydantoin, and barbiturates increase the hepatic metabolism of doxycycline, causing a decrease in the normal half-life of the drug by almost one-half (333,334). Digoxin is inactivated by gastrointestinal bacteria in some patients, and a course of tetracycline might reduce that. Therefore, antibiotic administration to such patients may cause a rise in serum digoxin level (335).

REFERENCES

1. Weber JM, Wierman CK, Hutchinson CR. Genetic analysis of erythromycin production in *Streptomyces erythreus*. *J Bacteriol* 1985;164(1):425–433.
2. Klein JO. History of macrolide use in pediatrics. *Pediatr Infect Dis J* 1997;16(4):427–431.
3. Mazzei T, Mini E, Novelli A, et al. Chemistry and mode of action of macrolides. *J Antimicrob Chemother* 1993;31(Suppl C):1–9.
4. Brittain DC. Erythromycin. *Med Clin North Am* 1987;71(6):1147–1154.
5. Weisblum B. Inducible resistance to macrolides, lincosamides and streptogramin type B antibiotics: the resistance phenotype, its biological diversity, and structural elements that regulate expression—a review. *J Antimicrob Chemother* 1985;16(Suppl A):63–90.
6. Horaud T, Le Bouguenec C, Pepper K. Molecular genetics of resistance to macrolides, lincosamides, and streptogramin B (MLS) in streptococci. *J Antimicrob Chemother* 1985;16(Suppl A):111–135.
7. Novick RP, Murphy E. MLS-resistance determinants in *Staphylococcus* and their molecular evolution. *J Antimicrob Chemother* 1985;16(Suppl A):101–110.
8. Tait-Kamradt A, Clancy J, Cronan M, et al. *mefE* is necessary for the erythromycin-resistant M phenotype in *Streptococcus pneumoniae*. *Antimicrob Agents Chemother* 1997;41(10):2251–2255.
9. Eady EA, Ross JI, Tipper JL, et al. Distribution of genes encoding erythromycin ribosomal methylases and an erythromycin efflux pump in epidemiologically distinct groups of staphylococci. *J Antimicrob Chemother* 1993;31(2):211–217.
10. Clancy J, Petitpas J, Dib-Hajj F, et al. Molecular cloning and functional analysis of a novel macrolide-resistance determinant, *mefA*, from *Streptococcus pyogenes*. *Mol Microbiol* 1996;22(5):867–879.
11. Washington JA II, Wilson WR. Erythromycin: a microbial and clinical perspective after 30 years of clinical use (1). *Mayo Clin Proc* 1985;60(3):189–203.

12. Roblin PM, Montalban G, Hammerschlag MR. Susceptibilities to clarithromycin and erythromycin of isolates of *Chlamydia pneumoniae* from children with pneumonia. *Antimicrob Agents Chemother* 1994;38(7):1588–1589.
13. Kirst HA. New macrolides: expanded horizons for an old class of antibiotics. *J Antimicrob Chemother* 1991;28(6):787–790.
14. Shendurnikar N. Erythromycin. *Indian Pediatr* 1988;25(8):780–783.
15. American Academy of Pediatrics. Pertussis. In: Pickering LK, ed. *Red book: 2003 report of the Committee of Infectious Diseases*, 26th ed. Elk Grove Village, IL: American Academy of Pediatrics, 2003:472–486.
16. Atmar RL, Greenberg SB. Pneumonia caused by *Mycoplasma pneumoniae* and the TWAR agent. *Semin Respir Infect* 1989;9(1): 19–31.
17. Bell TA. *Chlamydia trachomatis, Mycoplasma hominis,* and *Ureaplasma urealyticum* infections of infants. *Semin Perinatol* 1985;4(1):19–31.
18. Centers for Disease Control and Prevention. Sexually transmitted diseases treatment guidelines 2002. *MMWR Recomm Rep* 2002;51(RR-6):1–78.
19. Toomey KE, Barnes RC. Treatment of *Chlamydia trachomatis* genital infection. *Rev Infect Dis* 1990;12(Suppl 6):S645–S655.
20. Waites KB, Crouse DT, Cassell GH. Antibiotic susceptibilities and therapeutic options for *Ureaplasma urealyticum* infections in neonates. *Pediatr Infect Dis J* 1992;11:23–29.
21. Rettig PJ. Chlamydial infections in pediatrics: diagnostic and therapeutic considerations. *Pediatr Infect Dis* 1986;5(1):158–162.
22. Keys TF. Therapeutic considerations in the treatment of *Legionella* infections. *Semin Respir Infect* 1987;2(4):270–273.
23. Edelstein PH. Legionnaires disease. *Clin Infect Dis* 1993;16: 741–747.
24. Ramaswamy K, Jacobson K. Infectious diarrhea in children. *Gastroenterol Clin North Am* 2001;30(3):611–624.
25. Gerber MA. Antibiotic resistance in group A streptococci. *Pediatr Clin North Am* 1995;42(3):539–551.
26. Wald ER. Antimicrobial therapy of pediatric patients with sinusitis. *J Allergy Clin Immunol* 1992;90(3, pt 2):469–473.
27. American Academy of Pediatrics. Syphilis. In: Pickering LK, ed. *Red book: 2003 report of the Committee of Infectious Diseases*, 26th ed. Elk Grove Village, IL: American Academy of Pediatrics, 2003: 595–607.
28. Berger BW. Lyme disease. *Semin Dermatol* 1993;12(4):357–362.
29. Guay DR. Macrolide antibiotics in paediatric infectious diseases. *Drugs* 1996;51(4):515–536.
30. Farrar HC, Walsh-Sukys MC, Kyllonen K, et al. Cardiac toxicity associated with intravenous erythromycin lactobionate: two case reports and a review of the literature. *Pediatr Infect Dis J* 1993; 2:688–691.
31. Waites KB, Sims PJ, Crouse DT, et al. Serum concentrations of erythromycin after intravenous infusion in preterm neonates treated for *Ureaplasma urealyticum* infection. *Pediatr Infect Dis J* 1994;13:287–293.
32. Bass JW, Steele RW, Wiebe RA, et al. Erythromycin concentrations in middle ear exudates. *Pediatrics* 1971;48:417–422.
33. Ginsburg CM, McCracken GH Jr, Culberston MC. Concentrations of erythromycin in serum and tonsil: comparison of the estolate and ethyl succinate suspensions. *J Pediatr* 1976;89:1011–1013.
34. Ishiguro M, Koga H, Kohno S, et al. Penetration of macrolides into human polymorphonuclear leukocytes. *J Antimicrob Chemother* 1989;24:719–729.
35. van den Broek PJ. Antimicrobial drugs, microorganisms, and phagocytes. *Rev Infect Dis* 1989;11(2):213–245.
36. Butler DR, Kuhn RJ, Chandler MH. Pharmacokinetics of anti-infective agents in paediatric patients. *Clin Pharmacokinet* 1994; 26(5):374–395.
37. Paap CM, Nahata MC. Clinical pharmacokinetics of antibacterial drugs in neonates. *Clin Pharmacokinet* 1990;19(4):280–318.
38. Philipson A, Sabath LD, Charles D. Transplacental passage of erythromycin and clindamycin. *N Engl J Med* 1973;288: 1219–1221.
39. Kirst HA, Sides GD. New directions for macrolide antibiotics: pharmacokinetics and clinical efficacy. *Antimicrob Agents Chemother* 1989;33(9):1419–1422.
40. Nilsen OG. Comparative pharmacokinetics of macrolides. *J Antimicrob Chemother* 1987;20(Suppl B):81–88.
41. Eichenwald HF. Adverse reactions to erythromycin. *Pediatr Infect Dis* 1986;5(1):147–150.
42. Periti P, Mazzei T, Mini E, et al. Adverse effects of macrolide antibacterials. *Drug Saf* 1993;9(5):346–364.
43. Cooper WO, Griffin MR, Arbogast P, et al. Very early exposure to erythromycin and infantile hypertrophic pyloric stenosis. *Arch Pediatr Adolesc Med* 2002;156(7):647–650.
44. Itoh Z. Motilin and clinical application. *Peptides* 1997;18(4): 593–608.
45. Brummett RE. Ototoxic liability of erythromycin and analogues. *Otolaryngol Clin North Am* 1993;26(5):811–819.
46. Ludden TM. Pharmacokinetic interactions of the macrolide antibiotics. *Clin Pharmacokinet* 1985;10(1):63–79.
47. Honig PK, Smith JE, Wortham DC, et al. Population variability in the pharmacokinetics of terfenadine: the case for a pseudo-polymorphism with clinical implications. *Drug Metabol Drug Interact* 1994;11(2):161–168.
48. Upton RA. Pharmacokinetic interactions between theophylline and other medication (Part I). *Clin Pharmacokinet* 1991;20 (1):66–80.
49. Yee GC, McGuire TR. Pharmacokinetic drug interactions with cyclosporin (Part I). *Clin Pharmacokinet* 1990;19(4):319–332.
50. Rodin SM, Johnson BF. Pharmacokinetic interactions with digoxin. *Clin Pharmacokinet* 1988;15(4):227–244.
51. Rodvold KA, Piscitelli SC. New oral macrolide and fluoroquinolone antibiotics: an overview of pharmacokinetics, interactions, and safety. *Clin Infect Dis* 1993;17(Suppl 1):S192–S199.
52. Hammerschlag MR. Azithromycin and clarithromycin. *Pediatr Ann* 1993;22(3):160–166.
53. Langtry HD, Balfour JA. Azithromycin. A review of its use in paediatric infectious diseases. *Drugs* 1998;56(2):273–297.
54. Peters DH, Friedel HA, McTavish D. Azithromycin. Review of its antimicrobial activity, pharmacokinetic properties and clinical efficacy. *Drugs* 1992;44(5):750–799.
55. Wondrack L, Massa M, Yang BV, et al. Clinical strain of *Staphylococcus aureus* inactivates and causes efflux of macrolides. *Antimicrob Agents Chemother* 1996;40(4):992–998.
56. Alos JI, Aracil B, Oteo J, et al. Significant increase in the prevalence of erythromycin-resistant, clindamycin- and miocamycin-susceptible (M phenotype) *Streptococcus pyogenes* in Spain. *J Antimicrob Chemother* 2003;51(2):333–337.
57. Neu HC. Clinical microbiology of azithromycin. *Am J Med* 1991;91(3 A):12S–18S.
58. Hammerschlag MR, Qumei KK, Roblin PM. *In vitro* activities of azithromycin, clarithromycin, L-ofloxacin, and other antibiotics against *Chlamydia pneumoniae. Antimicrob Agents Chemother* 1992;36(7):1573–1574.
59. Brown BA, Wallace RJ Jr, Onyi GO, et al. Activities of four macrolides, including clarithromycin, against *Mycobacterium fortuitum, Mycobacterium chelonae,* and *M. chelonae*-like organisms. *Antimicrob Agents Chemother* 1992;36(1):180–184.
60. Wolfson C, Branley J, Gottlieb T. The Etest for antimicrobial susceptibility testing of *Bartonella henselae. J Antimicrob Chemother* 1996;38(6):963–968.
61. Bergman KL, Olsen KM, Peddicord TE, et al. Antimicrobial activities and postantibiotic effects of clarithromycin, 14-hydroxy-clarithromycin, and azithromycin in epithelial cell lining fluid against clinical isolates of *Haemophilus influenzae* and *Streptococcus pneumoniae. Antimicrob Agents Chemother* 1999;43(5):1291–1293.
62. Still JG. Management of pediatric patients with group A beta hemolytic *Streptococcus* infection: treatment options. *Pediatr Infect Dis J* 1995;14:S57–S61.
63. Pacifico L, Scopetti F, Ranucci A, et al. Comparative efficacy and safety of 3-day azithromycin and 10-day penicillin V treatment of group A beta-hemolytic streptococcal pharyngitis in children. *Antimicrob Agents Chemother* 1996;40(4):1005–1008.
64. O'Doherty B. Azithromycin versus penicillin V in the treatment of paediatric patients with acute streptococcal pharyngitis/tonsillitis. Paediatric Azithromycin Study Group. *Eur J Clin Microbiol Infect Dis* 1996;15(9):718–724.
65. Dagan R, Johnson CE, McLinn S, et al. Bacteriologic and clinical efficacy of amoxicillin/clavulanate vs. azithromycin in acute otitis media. *Pediatr Infect Dis J* 2000;19(2):95–104.
66. Dagan R, Leibovitz E, Fliss DM, et al. Bacteriologic efficacies of oral azithromycin and oral cefaclor in treatment of acute otitis media in infants and young children. *Antimicrob Agents Chemother* 2000;44(1):43–50.

67. American Academy of Pediatrics. *Chlamydia trachomatis.* In: Pickering LK, ed. *Red book: 2009 report of the Committee of Infectious Diseases*, 28th ed. Elk Grove Village, IL: American Academy of Pediatrics, 2009:255–259.
68. Harris JA, Kolokathis A, Campbell M, et al. Safety and efficacy of azithromycin in the treatment of community-acquired pneumonia in children. *Pediatr Infect Dis J* 1998;17(10):865–871.
69. Montero L. A comparative study of the efficacy, safety and tolerability of azithromycin and cefaclor in the treatment of children with acute skin and/or soft tissue infections. *J Antimicrob Chemother* 1996;37(Suppl C):125–131.
70. Abdel-Haq N, Al-Tatari H, Chearskul P, et al. Methicillin-resistant *Staphylococcus aureus* (MRSA) in hospitalized children: correlation of molecular analysis with clinical presentation and antimicrobial susceptibility (ABST) results. *Eur J Clin Microbiol Infect Dis* 2009;28:547–551.
71. American Academy of Pediatrics. Pertussis (whooping cough). In: Pickering LK, ed. *Red book: 2009 report of the Committee of Infectious Diseases*, 28th ed. Elk Grove Village, IL: American Academy of Pediatrics, 2009:504–519.
72. Hoppe JE, Bryskier A. *In vitro* susceptibilities of *Bordetella pertussis* and *Bordetella parapertussis* to two ketolides (HMR 3004 and HMR 3647), four macrolides (azithromycin, clarithromycin, erythromycin A, and roxithromycin), and two ansamycins (rifampin and rifapentine). *Antimicrob Agents Chemother* 1998;42(4):965–966.
73. Aoyama T, Sunakawa K, Iwata S, et al. Efficacy of short-term treatment of pertussis with clarithromycin and azithromycin. *J Pediatr* 1996;129(5):761–764.
74. Bace A, Zrnic T, Begovac J, et al. Short-term treatment of pertussis with azithromycin in infants and young children. *Eur J Clin Microbiol Infect Dis* 1999;18(4):296–298.
75. Centers for Disease Control and Prevention. USPHS/IDSA guidelines for prevention of opportunistic infections in persons with human immunodeficiency virus. *Morb Mortal Wkly Rep* 2002;51:1-RR8.
76. Griffith DE. Risk–benefit assessment of therapies for *Mycobacterium avium* complex infections. *Drug Saf* 1999;21(2):137–152.
77. Wolinsky E. Mycobacterial lymphadenitis in children: a prospective study of 105 nontuberculous cases with long-term follow-up. *Clin Infect Dis* 1995;20(4):954–963.
78. Pacifico L. Azithromycin in children: a critical review of the evidence. *Curr Ther Res Clin Exp* 2002;63(1):54–76.
79. Margileth AM. Antibiotic therapy for cat-scratch disease: clinical study of therapeutic outcome in 268 patients and a review of the literature. *Pediatr Infect Dis J* 1992;11(6):474–478.
80. Bass JW, Freitas BC, Freitas AD, et al. Prospective randomized double blind placebo-controlled evaluation of azithromycin for treatment of cat-scratch disease. *Pediatr Infect Dis J* 1998;17(6):447–452.
81. Conrad DA. Treatment of cat-scratch disease. *Curr Opin Pediatr* 2001;13(1):56–59.
82. Edelstein PH. Antimicrobial chemotherapy for Legionnaire's disease: a review. *Clin Infect Dis* 1995;21(Suppl 3):S265–S276.
83. Klein NC, Cunha BA. Treatment of Legionnaire's disease. *Semin Respir Infect* 1998;13(2):140–146.
84. Martin DH, Mroczkowski TF, Dalu ZA, et al. A controlled trial of a single dose of azithromycin for the treatment of chlamydial urethritis and cervicitis. The Azithromycin for Chlamydial Infections Study Group. *N Engl J Med* 1992;327(13):921–925.
85. Dionisio D, Orsi A, Sterrantino G, et al. Chronic cryptosporidiosis in patients with AIDS: stable remission and possible eradication after long-term, low dose azithromycin. *J Clin Pathol* 1998;51(2):138–142.
86. Blanshard C, Shanson DC, Gazzard BG. Pilot studies of azithromycin, letrazuril and paromomycin in the treatment of cryptosporidiosis. *Int J STD AIDS* 1997;8(2):124–129.
87. Vargas SL, Shenep JL, Flynn PM, et al. Azithromycin for treatment of severe *Cryptosporidium* diarrhea in two children with cancer. *J Pediatr* 1993;123(1):154–156.
88. Hicks P, Zwiener RJ, Squires J, et al. Azithromycin therapy for *Cryptosporidium parvum* infection in four children infected with human immunodeficiency virus. *J Pediatr* 1996;129(2):297–300.
89. Thylefors B, Negrel AD, Pararajasegaram R, et al. Global data on blindness. *Bull World Health Organ* 1995;73(1):115–121.
90. Dawson CR, Schachter J. Strategies for treatment and control of blinding trachoma: cost-effectiveness of topical or systemic antibiotics. *Rev Infect Dis* 1985;7(6):768–773.
91. Bailey RL, Arullendran P, Whittle HC, et al. Randomised controlled trial of single-dose azithromycin in treatment of trachoma. *Lancet* 1993;342(8869):453–456.
92. Tabbara KF, Abu-el-Asrar A, al-Omar O, et al. Single-dose azithromycin in the treatment of trachoma. A randomized, controlled study. *Ophthalmology* 1996;103(5):842–846.
93. Dawson CR, Schachter J, Sallam S, et al. A comparison of oral azithromycin with topical oxytetracycline/polymyxin for the treatment of trachoma in children. *Clin Infect Dis* 1997;24(3):363–368.
94. Gordillo ME, Singh KV, Murrah BE. *In vitro* activity of azithromycin against bacterial enteric pathogens. *Antimicrob Agents Chemother* 1993;24(3):363–368.
95. Girgis NI, Butler T, Frenck RW, et al. Azithromycin versus ciprofloxacin for treatment of uncomplicated typhoid fever in a randomized trial in Egypt that included patients with multidrug resistance. *Antimicrob Agents Chemother* 1999;43(6):1441–1444.
96. Frenck RW Jr, Nakhla I, Sultan Y, et al. Azithromycin versus ceftriaxone for the treatment of uncomplicated typhoid fever in children. *Clin Infect Dis* 2000;31(5):1134–1148.
97. Nahata MC, Koranyi KI, Luke DR, et al. Pharmacokinetics of azithromycin in pediatric patients with acute otitis media. *Antimicrob Agents Chemother* 1995;39(8):1875–1877.
98. Nightingale CH. Pharmacokinetics and pharmacodynamics of newer macrolides. *Pediatr Infect Dis J* 1997;16(4):438–443.
99. Pukander J, Rautianen M. Penetration of azithromycin into middle ear effusions in acute and secretory otitis media in children. *J Antimicrob Chemother* 1996;37(Suppl C):53–61.
100. Vaudaux BP, Cherpillod J, Dayer P. Concentrations of azithromycin in tonsillar and/or adenoid tissue from paediatric patients. *J Antimicrob Chemother* 1996;37(Suppl C):53–61.
101. Gladue RP, Bright GM, Isaacson RE, et al. *In vitro* and *in vivo* uptake of azithromycin (CP-62,993) by phagocytic cells: possible mechanism of delivery and release at sites of infection. *Antimicrob Agents Chemother* 1989;33(3):277–282.
102. Sifrim D, Matsuo H, Janssens J, et al. Comparison of the effects of midecamycin acetate and azithromycin on gastrointestinal motility in man. *Drugs Exp Clin Res* 1994;20(3):121–126.
103. Jacobs RF, Maples HD, Aranda JV, et al. Pharmacokinetics of intravenously administered azithromycin in pediatric patients. *Pediatr Infect Dis J* 2005;24(1):34–39.
104. Treadway G, Pontani D. Paediatric safety of azithromycin: worldwide experience. *J Antimicrob Chemother* 1996;37(Suppl C):143–149.
105. Klein JO. Clarithromycin: where do we go from here? *Pediatr Infect Dis J* 1993;12(12, Suppl 3):S148–S151.
106. Neu HC. The development of macrolides: clarithromycin in perspective. *J Antimicrob Chemother* 1991;27(Suppl A):1–9.
107. Ferrero JL, Bopp BA, Marsh KC, et al. Metabolism and disposition of clarithromycin in man. *Drug Metab Dispos* 1990;18(4):441–446.
108. Peters DH, Clissold SP. Clarithromycin. A review of its antimicrobial activity, pharmacokinetic properties and therapeutic potential. *Drugs* 1992;44(1):117–164.
109. Derouin F, Chastang C. Activity *in vitro* against *Toxoplasma gondii* of azithromycin and clarithromycin alone and with pyrimethamine. *J Antimicrob Chemother* 1990;25(4):708–711.
110. Still JG, Hubbard WC, Poole JM, et al. Comparison of clarithromycin and penicillin VK suspensions in the treatment of children with streptococcal pharyngitis and review of currently available alternative antibiotic therapies. *Pediatr Infect Dis J* 1993;12(12, Suppl 3):S134–S141.
111. Pukander JS, Jero JP, Kaprio EA, et al. Clarithromycin vs. amoxicillin suspensions in the treatment of pediatric patients with acute otitis media. *Pediatr Infect Dis J* 1993;12(12, Suppl 3):S118–S121.
112. Aspin MM, Hoberman A, McCarty J, et al. Comparative study of the safety and efficacy of clarithromycin and amoxicillin–clavulanate in the treatment of acute otitis media in children. *J Pediatr* 1994;125(1):136–141.
113. Arguedas A, Loaiza C, Rodriguez F, et al. Comparative trial of 3 days of azithromycin versus 10 days of clarithromycin in the treatment of children with acute otitis media with effusion. *J Chemother* 1997;9(1):44–50.

114. Gooch WM III, Gan VN, Corder WT, et al. Clarithromycin and cefaclor suspensions in the treatment of acute otitis media in children. *Pediatr Infect Dis J* 1993;12(Suppl 3):S128–S133.
115. Block S, Hedrick J, Hammerschlag MR, et al. *Mycoplasma pneumoniae* and *Chlamydia pneumoniae* in pediatric community-acquired pneumonia: comparative efficacy and safety of clarithromycin vs. erythromycin ethylsuccinate. *Pediatr Infect Dis J* 1995;14(6):471–477.
116. Kiyota K, Habu Y, Sugano Y, et al. Comparison of 1-week and 2-week triple therapy with omeprazole, amoxicillin, and clarithromycin in peptic ulcer patients with *Helicobacter pylori* infection: results of a randomized controlled trial. *J Gastroenterol* 1999;34(Suppl 11):76–79.
117. Dautzenberg B, Truffot C, Legris S, et al. Activity of clarithromycin against *Mycobacterium avium* infection in patients with the acquired immune deficiency syndrome. A controlled clinical trial. *Am Rev Respir Dis* 1991;144(3, pt 1):564–569.
118. Griffith DE, Aksamit T, Brown-Elliott BA, et al. An official ATS/IDSA statement: diagnosis, treatment, and prevention of nontuberculous mycobacterial diseases. *Am J Respir Crit Care Med* 2007;175(4):367–416.
119. Gan VN, McCarty JM, Chu SY, et al. Penetration of clarithromycin into middle ear fluid of children with acute otitis media. *Pediatr Infect Dis J* 1997;16(1):39–43.
120. Fraschini F, Scaglione F, Pintrucci G, et al. The diffusion of clarithromycin and roxithromycin into nasal mucosa, tonsil and lung in humans. *J Antimicrob Chemother* 1991;27(Suppl A): 61–65.
121. Fish DN, Gotfried MH, Danziger LH, et al. Penetration of clarithromycin into lung tissues from patients undergoing lung resection. *Antimicrob Agents Chemother* 1994;38(4):876–878.
122. Craft JC, Siepman N. Overview of the safety profile of clarithromycin suspension in pediatric patients. *Pediatr Infect Dis J* 1993;12(Suppl 3):S142–S147.
123. Tinel M, Descatoire V, Larrey D, et al. Effects of clarithromycin on cytochrome P-450. Comparison with other macrolides. *J Pharmacol Exp Ther* 1989;250(2):746–751.
124. Wallace RJ Jr, Brown BA, Griffith DE, et al. Reduced serum levels of clarithromycin in patients treated with multidrug regimens including rifampin or rifabutin for *Mycobacterium avium–M. intracellulare* infection. *J Infect Dis* 1995;171(3):747–750.
125. Young RA, Gonzalez JP, Sorkin EM, Roxithromycin. A review of its antibacterial activity, pharmacokinetic properties and clinical efficacy. *Drugs* 1989;37(1):8–41.
126. Kawashima M, Yatsunami J, Fukuno Y, et al. Inhibitory effects of 14-membered ring macrolide antibiotics on bleomycin-induced acute lung injury. *Lung* 2002;180(2):73–89.
127. Neu HC. Roxithromycin—an overview. *Br J Clin Pract* 1988;42 (Suppl 55):1–3.
128. Grassi C, Bartucci F, Chumdermpadetsuk S, et al. Roxithromycin in the treatment of pediatric tract infections. *Br J Clin Pract* 1988;42(Suppl 55):104–106.
129. Bazet MC, Blanc F, Chumdermpadetsuk S, et al. Roxithromycin in the treatment of pediatric infections. *Br J Clin Pract* 1988;42 (Suppl 55):117–118.
130. Segre G, Bianchi E, Zanolo G, et al. Influence of food on the bioavailability of roxithromycin versus erythromycin stearate. *Br J Clin Pract* 1988;42(Suppl 55):55–57.
131. Kafetzis DA, Krotsi-Laskari M, Tremblay D, et al. Multiple dose pharmacokinetics in infants and children treated with roxithromycin. *Br J Clin Pract* 1988;42(Suppl 55):58.
132. Demotes-Mainard FM, Vincon GA, Albin HC. Pharmacokinetics of a new macrolide, roxithromycin, in infants and children. *J Clin Pharmacol* 1989;29(8):752–756.
133. Zini R, Fournet MP, Barre J, et al. *In vitro* study of roxithromycin binding to serum proteins and erythrocytes in humans. *Br J Clin Pract* 1988;42(Suppl 55):54.
134. Puri SK, Lassman HB. Roxithromycin: a pharmacokinetic review of a macrolide. *J Antimicrob Chemother* 1987;20(Suppl B): 89–100.
135. Melcher GP, Hadfield TL, Gaines JK, et al. Comparative efficacy and toxicity of roxithromycin and erythromycin ethylsuccinate in the treatment of streptococcal pharyngitis in adults. *J Antimicrob Chemother* 1988;22(4):549–556.
136. Worm AM, Hoff G, Kroon S, et al. Roxithromycin compared with erythromycin against genitourinary chlamydial infections. *Genitourin Med* 1989;65(1):35–38.
137. Poirier R. Comparative study of clarithromycin and roxithromycin in the treatment of community-acquired pneumonia. *J Antimicrob Chemother* 1991;27(Suppl A):109–116.
138. Agache P, Amblard P, Moulin G, et al. Roxithromycin in skin and soft tissue infections. *J Antimicrob Chemother* 1987;20(Suppl B):153–156.
139. Souweine B, Fialip J, Ruivard M, et al. Acute pancreatitis associated with roxithromycin therapy. *DICP* 1991;25(10):1137.
140. Dawn G, Kanwar AJ, Dhar S. Nail pigmentation due to roxithromycin. *Dermatology* 1995;191(4):342–343.
141. Hiller A, Olkkola KT, Isohanni P, et al. Unconsciousness associated with midazolam and erythromycin. *Br J Anaesth* 1990;65(6): 826–828.
142. Saint-Salvi B, Tremblay D, Surjus A, et al. A study of the interaction of roxithromycin with theophylline and carbamazepine. *J Antimicrob Chemother* 1987;20(Suppl B):121–129.
143. Corallo CE, Rogers IR. Roxithromycin-induced digoxin toxicity. *Med J Aust* 1996;165(8):433–434.
144. Hoppu K, Tikanoja T, Tapanainen P, et al. Accidental astemizole overdose in young children. *Lancet* 1991;338(8766):538–540.
145. Meyer B, Muller F, Wessels P, et al. A model to detect interactions between roxithromycin and oral contraceptives. *Clin Pharmacol Ther* 1990;47(6):671–674.
146. Ghose K, Ashton J, Rohan A. Possible interaction of roxithromycin with warfarin. *Clin Drug Investig* 1995;10:302–309.
147. Paulsen O, Nilsson LG, Saint-Salvi B, et al. No effect of roxithromycin on pharmacokinetic or pharmacodynamic properties of warfarin and its enantiomers. *Pharmacol Toxicol* 1988;63 (4):215–220.
148. Hashiguchi K, Niki Y, Soejima R. Roxithromycin does not raise serum theophylline levels. *Chest* 1992;102(2):653–654.
149. Bartz QR. Isolation and characterization of chloromycetin. *J Biol Chem* 1948;172(2):445–450.
150. Yamaguchi A, Onmori H, Kaneko-Ohdera M, et al. pH-dependent accumulation of tetracycline in *Escherichia coli. Antimicrob Agents Chemother* 1991;35:53.
151. Roodyn DB, Wilkie D. The biogenesis of mitochondria. *Science* 11, October 1968;162:251–253.
152. Okkamoto S, Mizuno D. Mechanisms of chloramphenicol and tetracycline resistance in *Escherichia coli. J Gen Microbiol* 1964;35: 125–133.
153. Gangarosa EJ, Bennett JV, Wyatt C, et al. An epidemic-associated episome? *J Infect Dis* 1972;126:215–218.
154. Butler T, Linh NN, Arnold K, et al. Chloramphenicol-resistant typhoid fever in Vietnam associated with R-factor. *Lancet* 1973; 2:983–985.
155. Halder KK, Dalal BS, Ghose E, et al. Chloramphenicol-resistant *Salmonella typhi*: the cause of recent outbreak of enteric fever in Calcutta. *Indian J Pathol Microbiol* 1992;35(1):11–17.
156. Drug resistance in salmonellas [editorial]. *Lancet* 1982;1: 1391–1392.
157. Spika JS, Waterman SH, Soo Hoo GW, et al. Chloramphenicol-resistant *Salmonella newport* traced through hamburger to dairy farms. *N Engl J Med* 1987;316:565–570.
158. Prober CG, Rajchgot P, Bannatyne RM, et al. Impact of chloramphenicol use on bacterial resistance in neonatal intensive care unit. *Lancet* 1983;2(8342):158.
159. Klastersky K, Husson M. Bactericidal activity of the combinations of gentamicin with clindamycin or chloramphenicol against species of *Escherichia coli* and *Bacteroides fragilis. Antimicrob Agents Chemother* 1977;12(2):135–138.
160. Asmar BI, Pranito M, Dajani AS. Antagonistic effect of chloramphenicol in combination with cefotaxime or ceftriaxone. *Antimicrob Agents Chemother* 1988;32(9):1375–1378.
161. Sharma KB, Bhat MB, Pasricha A, et al. Multiple antibiotic resistance among *Salmonella* in India. *J Antimicrob Chemother* 1979;5 (1):15–21.
162. Bhutta ZA, Naqvi SH, Razzaq RA, et al. Multidrug-resistant typhoid in children: presentation and clinical features. *Rev Infect Dis* 1991;13(5):832–836.
163. Jesudasan MJ, John TJ. Multiresistant *Salmonella typhi* in India. *Lancet* 1990;336:252.

164. Albert MJ, Haider K, Nahar S, et al. Multiresistant *Salmonella typhi* in Bangladesh. *J Antimicrob Chemother* 1991;27:554–545.
165. Datta N, Richards H, Datta C. *Salmonella typhi in vivo* acquires resistance to both chloramphenicol and co-trimoxazole. *Lancet* 1981;1(8231):1181–1183.
166. Barrett FF, Taber LH, Morris CR, et al. A 12 year review of the antibiotic management of *Haemophilus influenzae* meningitis. *J Pediatr* 1972;81:370–377.
167. Kinmouth AL, Storrs CN, Mitchell RG. Meningitis due to chloramphenicol-resistant *Haemophilus influenzae* type b. *Br Med J* 1978; 1:694.
168. Mendelman PM, Doroshow CA, Gandy SL, et al. Plasmid-mediated resistance in multiply resistant *Haemophilus influenzae* type b causing meningitis: molecular characterization of one strain and review of the literature. *J Infect Dis* 1984;150:30–39.
169. Doern GV, Jorgensen JH, Thornsberry C, et al. National collaborative study of the prevalence of antimicrobial resistance among clinical isolates of *Haemophilus influenzae. Antimicrob Agents Chemother* 1988;32:180–185.
170. Garvey RJ, McMullin GP. Meningitis due to beta lactamase producing type b *Haemophilus influenzae* resistant to chloramphenicol. *Br Med J* 1983;287:1183–1184.
171. Powell M, Price EH. Invasive infections due to *Haemophilus influenzae* type b resistant to ampicillin and chloramphenicol. *J Antimicrob Chemother* 1990;26:149–151.
172. Dimopoulo ID, Kraak WA, Anderson EC, et al. Molecular epidemiology of unrelated cluster of multiresistant strains of *Haemophilus influenzae. J Infect Dis* 1992;165:1069–1075.
173. Wild BE, Pearman JW, Richardson CJ, et al. Multiple-antibiotic resistant *Haemophilus influenzae* type b meningitis in Western Australia. *Med J Aust* 1986;144:666–667.
174. Collignon PJ, Bell JM, MacInnes SJ, et al. A national collaborative study of resistance to antimicrobial agents in *Haemophilus influenzae* in Australia hospitals. *J Antimicrob Chemother* 1992;30:153–163.
175. Catry MA, Vaz Pato MV. *Haemophilus influenzae* type b resistant to ampicillin and chloramphenicol. *Br Med J* 1983;287:1471.
176. Centers for Disease Control. Ampicillin and chloramphenicol resistance to systemic *Haemophilus influenzae* disease. *MMWR Morb Mortal Wkly Rep* 1984;35–37.
177. Simasathien S, Duangmani C, Escheverria P. *Haemophilus influenzae* type b resistant to ampicillin and chloramphenicol in an orphanage in Thailand. *Lancet* 1980;2(8206):1214–1217.
178. Mastro TD, Nomani NK, Ishaq Z, et al. Use of nasopharyngeal isolates of *Streptococcus pneumoniae* and *Haemophilus influenzae* from children in Pakistan for surveillance for antimicrobial resistance. *Pediatr Infect Dis J* 1993;12(10):824–830.
179. Manten A, van Klingeren B, Dessens-Kroon M. Chloramphenicol resistance in *Haemophilus influenzae. Lancet* 1976;1(7961):702.
180. Heymann CS, Turk DC, Rotimi VO. Multiple antibiotic resistance in *Haemophilus influenzae. Lancet* 1981;1:553.
181. Sills JA, McMahon P, Hall E, et al. *Haemophilus influenzae* type b resistant to chloramphenicol and ampicillin. *Br Med J* 1983; 286:722.
182. Jorgensen JH. Update on mechanisms and prevalence of antimicrobial resistance in *Haemophilus influenzae. Clin Infect Dis* 1992; 14:1119–1123.
183. Mhalu FS, Mmari PW, Ijumba J. Rapid emergence of El Tor *Vibrio cholera* epidemic in Tanzania. *Lancet* 1979;1(8112):345–347.
184. Goodwin CS, Blake P, Blincow E. The minimum inhibitory and bactericidal concentrations of antibiotics and anti-ulcer agents against *Campylobacter pyloridis. J Antimicrob Chemother* 1986;17(3): 309–314.
185. Janda JM, Guthertz LS, Kokka RP, et al. *Aeromonas* species in septicemia: laboratory characteristics and clinical observations. *Clin Infect Dis* 1994;19(1):77–83.
186. Li XZ, Livermore DM, Nikaido H. Role of efflux pump(s) in intrinsic resistance of *Pseudomonas aeruginosa*: active efflux as a contributing factor to beta-lactam resistance. *Antimicrob Agents Chemother* 1994;38(8):1742–1752.
187. Burns JL, Hedin LA, Lien DM. Chloramphenicol resistance in *Pseudomonas cepacia* because of decreased permeability. *Antimicrob Agents Chemother* 1989;33(2):136–141.
188. Aber RC, Wennersten C, Moellering RC Jr. Antimicrobial susceptibility of flavobacteria. *Antimicrob Agents Chemother* 1978;14(3): 483–487.
189. Schwarz S, Cardoso M. Nucleotide sequence and phylogeny of chloramphenicol acetyltransferase encoded by plasmid p SCS7 from *Saphylococcus aureus. Antimicrob Agents Chemother* 1991;35: 1551–1556.
190. Nakae M, Murai T, Kaneko Y, et al. Drug-resistance in *Streptococcus pyogenes* strains have been reported in Japan (1974–1975). *Antimicrob Agents Chemother* 1977;12:427–428.
191. Oppenheim B, Koornhof HJ, Austrian R. Antibiotic-resistant pneumococcal disease in children at Baragwanth Hospital, Johannesburg. *Pediatr Infect Dis* 1986;5(5):520–524.
192. Klugman KP, Koornhof HJ. Drug resistance patterns and serogroups or serotypes of pneumococcal isolates, from cerebrospinal fluid or blood, 1979–1986. *J Infect Dis* 1988;158(5): 956–964.
193. Lee HJ, Park YJ, Jang SH, et al. High incidence of resistance to multiple antimicrobials in clinical isolates of *Streptococcus pneumoniae* from a university hospital in Korea. *Clin Infect Dis* 1995;20:826–835.
194. Ohm-Smith MJ, Hadley WK, Sweet RL. *In vitro* activity of new beta-lactam antibiotics and other antimicrobial drugs against anaerobic isolates from obstetric and gynecological infections. *Antimicrob Agents Chemother* 1982;22(4):711–714.
195. Delmee M, Avesani V. Correlation between serogroup and susceptibility to chloramphenicol, clindamycin, erythromycin, rifampicin and tetracycline among 308 isolates of *Clostridium difficile. J Antimicrob Chemother* 1988;22(3):325–331.
196. George WL, Kirby BD, Sutter VL, et al. Gram-negative anaerobic bacilli; their role in infection and patterns of susceptibility to antimicrobial agents. II. Little known *Fusobacterium* species and miscellaneous genera. *Rev Infect Dis* 1981;3(3):599–626.
197. Friedman CA, Lovejoy FC, Smith AL. Chloramphenicol disposition in infants and children. *J Pediatr* 1979;95:1071–1078.
198. Kramer PW, Griffith RS, Campbell RL. Antibiotic penetration of the brain: comparative study. *J Neurosurg* 1968;31:295–302.
199. Snyder MJ, Perroni J, Gonzalez O, et al. Comparative efficacy of chloramphenicol, ampicillin and co-trimoxazole in the treatment of typhoid fever. *Lancet* 1976;2:1155–1157.
200. Aserkoff B, Bennet JV. Effect of antibiotic therapy in acute salmonellosis on the fecal excretion of salmonellae. *N Engl J Med* 1969;281:636–640.
201. Koskiniemi M, Pettay O, Raivio M, et al. *Haemophilus influenzae* meningitis. A comparison between chloramphenicol and ampicillin therapy with special reference to impaired hearing. *Acta Paediatr Scand* 1978;67:17–24.
202. Halstensen A, Vollset SE, Haneberg B, et al. Antimicrobial therapy and case fatality in meningococcal disease. *Scand J Infect Dis* 1987;19(4):403–407.
203. Cherubin CE, Corrado ML, Nair SR, et al. Treatment of gram-negative bacillary meningitis: the role of the new cephalosporins. *Rev Infect Dis* 1982;(Suppl):S453–S464.
204. Snyder MJ, Woodward TE. The clinical use of chloramphenicol. *Med Clin North Am* 1970;54:1187–1197.
205. Raoult D, Drancourt M. Antimicrobial therapy of rickettsial diseases. *Antimicrob Agents Chemother* 1991;35:2457.
206. Norris AH, Reill JP, Edelstein PH, et al. Chloramphenicol for the treatment of vancomycin-resistant enterococcal infections. *Clin Infect Dis* 1995;20:1137–1144.
207. Shrestha NK, Chua JD, Tuohy MJ, et al. Antimicrobial susceptibility of vancomycin-resistant *Enterococcus faecium*; potential utility of fosfomycin. *Scand J Infect Dis* 2003;35(10):12–14.
208. Kauffman RE, Miceli JN, Strebel L, et al. Pharmacokinetics of chloramphenicol and chloramphenicol succinate in infants and children. *J Pediatr* 1981;98:315–320.
209. Sack CM, Koup JR, Smith AL. Chloramphenicol pharmacokinetics in infants and young children. *Pediatrics* 1980;66(4): 579–840.
210. Pickering LK, Hoecker JL, Kramer, et al. Clinical pharmacology of two chloramphenicol preparations in children: sodium succinate (iv) and palmitate (oral) esters. *J Pediatr* 1980;96(4):757–761.
211. Yogev R, Kolling WM, Williams T. Pharmacokinetic comparison of intravenous and oral chloramphenicol in patients with *Haemophilus influenzae* meningitis. *Pediatrics* 1981;67(5):656–660.
212. Abraham RK, Burnett HH. Tetracycline and chloramphenicol studies on rabbit and human eyes. *Arch Ophthalmol* 1955;54: 641–659.

213. Black SB, Levine P, Shinefield HR. The necessity for monitoring chloramphenicol levels when treating neonatal meningitis. *J Pediatr* 1978;92;235–236.
214. Dunkle LM. Central nervous system chloramphenicol concentration in premature infants. *Antimicrob Agents Chemother* 1978;13:427–429.
215. Woodward TE, Wisseman CL. *Chloromycetin (chloramphenicol)*. New York: Medical Encyclopedia, 1958;24–28.
216. Rapp GF, Griffith RS, Hebble WM. The permeability of traumatically inflamed synovial membrane to commonly used antibiotics. *J Bone Joint Surg* 1966;48:1534–1540.
217. Koup JR, Lau AH, Brodsky B, et al. Relationship between serum and saliva chloramphenicol concentrations. *Antimicrob Agents Chemother* 1979;15:658–661.
218. Kurz H, Mauser-Ganshorn A, Stickel HH. Differences in the binding of drugs to plasma proteins from newborn and adult man. I. *Eur J Clin Pharmacol* 1977;11(6):463–467.
219. Koup JR, Lau AH, Brodsky B, et al. Chloramphenicol pharmacokinetics in hospitalized patients. *Antimicrob Agents Chemother* 1979;15(5):651–657.
220. Kauffman RE, Thirumoorthi MC, Buckley JA, et al. Relative bioavailability of intravenous chloramphenicol succinate and oral chloramphenicol palmitate in infants and children. *J Pediatr* 1981;99:963–967.
221. Lietman PS. Chloramphenicol and the neonate—1979 review. *Clin Perinatol* 1979;6(1):151–162.
222. Oski FA. Hematologic consequences of chloramphenicol therapy. *J Pediatr* 1979;94:515–516.
223. O'Gorman Hughes DW. Studies on chloramphenicol. II. Possible determinants and progress of haematopoietic toxicity during chloramphenicol therapy. *Med J Aust* 1973;2:1142–1146.
224. Wallerstein RO, Condit PK, Kasper CK, et al. Statewide study of chloramphenicol treatment and fatal aplastic anemia. *J Am Med Assoc* 1969;208;2045–2051.
225. Plaut ME, Best WR. Aplastic anemia after parenteral chloramphenicol: warning renewed. *N Engl J Med* 1982;306:1486.
226. Daum RS, Cohen DL, Smith AL. Fatal aplastic anemia following apparent "dose-related" chloramphenicol toxicity. *J Pediatr* 1979; 94:403–406.
227. Lietman PS, White TJ, Shaw WV. Chloramphenicol: an enzymological microassay. *Antimicrob Agents Chemother* 1976;10:347–353.
228. Burns LE, Hodgman JE, Cass AB. Fatal circulatory collapse in premature infants receiving chloramphenicol. *N Engl J Med* 1959;261:1318–1321.
229. Craft AW, Brocklebank JT, Hey EN, et al. The "grey toddler." Chloramphenicol toxicity. *Arch Dis Child* 1974;49:235–237.
230. Thompson WL, Anderson SE, Lipsky JJ, et al. Overdoses of chloramphenicol. *J Am Med Assoc* 1975;234:149–150.
231. Fripp RR, Carter MC, Werner JC, et al. Cardiac function and acute chloramphenicol toxicity. *J Pediatr* 1983;103:487–490.
232. Evans LS, Kleiman MB. Acidosis as a presenting feature of chloramphenicol toxicity. *J Pediatr* 1986;108:475–477.
233. Freundlick M, Cynamon H, Tamer A, et al. Management of chloramphenicol intoxication in infancy by charcoal hemoperfusion. *J Pediatr* 1983;103:485–487.
234. Stevens DC, Kleinman MB, Lietman PS, et al. Exchange transfusion in acute chloramphenicol toxicity. *J Pediatr* 1981;99: 651–653.
235. Chloramphenicol blindness [editorial]. *Br Med J* 1965;1:1511.
236. Halpert J. Further studies of the suicide inactivation of purified rat liver cytochrome P-450 by chloramphenicol. *Mol Pharmacol* 1982;21:166–172.
237. Christensen LK, Skovsted L. Inhibition of drug metabolism by chloramphenicol. *Lancet* 1969;2:1397–1399.
238. Rose JQ, Choi HK, Schentag JJ, et al. Intoxication caused by interaction of chloramphenicol and phenytoin. *J Am Med Assoc* 1977;237:2630–2631.
239. Krasinski K, Kusmiesz H, Nelson JD. Pharmacologic interactions among chloramphenicol, phenytoin and phenobarbital. *Pediatr Infect Dis* 1982;1(4):232–235.
240. Weeks JL, Mason EO, Baker CJ. Antagonism of ampicillin and chloramphenicol for meningeal isolates of group B streptococci. *Antimicrob Agents Chemother* 1981;20(3):281–285.
241. Finland M. Twenty-fifth anniversary of the discovery of Aureomycin: the place of tetracyclines in antimicrobial therapy. *Clin Pharmacol Ther* 1974;15:3–8.
242. Cundliff E, McQuillen K. Bacterial protein synthesis: the effects of antibiotics. *J Mol Biol* 1967;30:137–146.
243. Craven GR, Gavin R, Fanning T. The transfer RNA binding site of the 30 S ribosome and the site of tetracycline inhibition. *Cold Spring Harb Symp Quant Biol* 1969;34:129–137.
244. Chopra I, Hawkey PM, Hintin M. Tetracyclines, molecular and clinical aspects. *J Antimicrob Chemother* 1992;29:245–277.
245. Beard NS Jr, Armentrout SA, Weisberger AS. Inhibition of mammalian protein synthesis by antibiotics. *Pharmacol Rev* 1969;21: 213–245.
246. Shils ME. Renal disease and the metabolic effects of tetracycline. *Ann Intern Med* 1963;58:389–408.
247. Beveniste R, Davies J. Mechanisms of antibiotic resistance in bacteria. *Annu Rev Biochem* 1973;42:471–506.
248. National Committee for Clinical Laboratory Standards. *Methods for dilution antimicrobial susceptibility tests for bacteria that grow aerobically*. Approved standard (NCCLS Publication M7-A). Villanova, PA: National Committee for Clinical Laboratory Standards, 1985.
249. WHO. Surveillance of the resistance of *Staphylococcus aureus* to antibiotics. *Wkly Epidemiol Rec* 1982;57:265.
250. Ayliffe CA, Lilly HA, Lowbury EJ. Decline of hospital *Staphylococcus*? Incidence of multiresistant *Staph aureus* in three Birmingham hospitals. *Lancet* 1979;1:538–541.
251. Report of an Ad Hoc Study Group on Antibiotic Resistance. Tetracycline resistance in pneumococci and group A streptococci. *Br Med J* 1977;1:131–133.
252. Bourbeau P, Campos M. Current antibiotic susceptibility of group A beta-hemolytic streptococci. *J Infect Dis* 1982;145(6): 916–918.
253. Baker CJ, Webb BJ, Barrett FF. Antimicrobial susceptibility of group B streptococci isolated from a variety of clinical sources. *Antimicrob Agents Chemother* 1976;10(1):128–131.
254. Doern GV, Pfaller MA, Kugler K, et al. Prevalence of antimicrobial resistance among respiratory tract isolates of *S. pneumoniae* in North America: 1997 results from the ENTRY antimicrobial surveillance program. *Clin Infect Dis* 1998;27:764–770.
255. Hryniewicz W. Bacterial resistance in Eastern Europe—selected problems. *Scand J Infect Dis* 1994;93:33–39.
256. Moreno F, Crisp C, Jorgensen JH, et al. The clinical and molecular epidemiology of bacteremias at a university hospital caused by pneumococci not susceptible to penicillin. *J Infect Dis* 1995; 172(2):427–432.
257. Gutman L, Goldstein FW, Kitzis MD, et al. Susceptibility of *Nocardia asteroids* to 46 antibiotics including 22 beta-lactams. *Antimicrob Agents Chemother* 1983;23:248–251.
258. Centers for Disease Control. Antibiotic-resistant strains of *Neisseria gonorrhoeae*. *MMWR Morb Mortal Wkly Rep* 1987;36(Suppl 55):1–18.
259. Vanhoof R, Vanderlinden MP, Dierickx K, et al. Susceptibility of *Campylobacter fetus* subsp. *jejuni* to twenty-nine antimicrobial agents. *Antimicrob Agents Chemother* 1978;14:553–556.
260. Fennerty MB. *Helicobacter pylori*. *Arch Int Med* 1994;154:721–727.
261. Farrell ID, Hinchliffe PM, Robertson L. Sensitivity of *Brucella* spp to tetracycline and its analogues. *J Clin Pathol* 1976;29: 1097–1100.
262. Rubenstein E, Lang R, Shasha B, et al. *In vitro* susceptibility of *Brucella melitensis* to antibiotics. *Antimicrob Agents Chemother* 1991; 35:1925–1927.
263. Morris JG Jr, Black RE. Cholera and other vibrioses in the United States. *N Engl J Med* 1985;312(6):342–350.
264. Midani S, Rathore MH. *Vibrio* species infection of a catfish spine puncture wound. *Pediatr Infect Dis* 1994;13:333–334.
265. Sack DA, Kaminsky DC, Sack RB, et al. Prophylactic doxycycline for travelers' diarrhea. Results of prospective double-blind study of Peace Corps Volunteers in Kenya. *N Engl J Med* 1978;298: 758–763.
266. Abdel-Haq NM, Asmar BI, Abuhammour WM, et al. *Yersinia enterocolitica* infection in children. *Pediatr Infect Dis J* 2000;19:954–959.
267. The choice of antimicrobial drugs. The Medical Letter on Drugs and Therapeutics, 2000. http://medicalletter.org/.
268. Regnery R, Tappero J. Unraveling mysteries associated with cat scratch disease, bacillary angiomatosis, and related syndromes. *Emerg Infect Dis* 1995;1(1):16–21.
269. Maurin M, Gasquet S, Ducco C, et al. MICs of 28 antibiotic compounds for 14 *Bartonella* (formerly *Rochalimaea*) isolates. *Antimicrob Agents Chemother* 1995;39(11):2387–2391.

270. Thornsberry C, Baker CN, Kirven LA. *In vitro* activity of antimicrobial agents on Legionnaire's disease bacterium. *Antimicrob Agents Chemother* 1978;13(1):78–80.
271. Eickoff TC, Bennet JV, Hayes PS, et al. *Pseudomonas pseudomallei* susceptibility to chemotherapeutic agents. *J Infect Dis* 1970;121: 95–102.
272. Sutter VL, Finegold SM. Susceptibility of anaerobic bacteria to 23 antimicrobial agents. *Antimicrob Agents Chemother* 1976;10: 736–752.
273. McCormack WM. Susceptibility of mycoplasmas to antimicrobial agents: clinical implications. *Clin Infect Dis* 1993;17(Suppl 1): 200–201.
274. Rylander M, Hallander HO. *In vitro* comparison of the activity of doxycycline, tetracycline, erythromycin and a new macrolide, CP 62993, against *Mycoplasma pneumoniae, Mycoplasma homonis,* and *Ureaplasma urealyticum. Scand J Infect Dis* 1988;53:12–17.
275. Roberts MC, Koutsky LA, Holms KK, et al. Tetracycline-resistant *Mycoplasma hominis* strains contain streptococci *tet M* sequences. *Antimicrob Agents Chemother* 1985;28(1):141–143.
276. Taylor-Robinson D, Furr PM. Clinical antibiotic resistance of *Ureaplasma urealyticum. Pediatr Infect Dis* 1986;5(6 Suppl): S335–S337.
277. Robertson JA, Stemke GW, Maclellan SG, et al. Characterization of tetracycline-resistant strains of *Ureaplasma urealyticum. J Antimicrob Chemother* 1988;21(3):319–332.
278. Rice RJ, Bhullar V, Mitchell SH, et al. Susceptibilities of *Chlamydia trachomatis* isolates causing uncomplicated female genital tract infections and pelvic inflammatory disease. *Antimicrob Agents Chemother* 1995;39(3):760–762.
279. Stimson JB, Hale J, Bowie WR, et al. Tetracycline-resistant *Ureaplasma urealyticum*: a cause of persistent nongonococcal urethritis. *Ann Intern Med* 1981;94(2):192–194.
280. Jones RB, Van der Pol B, Martin DH, et al. Partial characterization of *Chlamydia trachomatis* isolates resistant to multiple antibiotics. *J Infect Dis* 1990;162(6):1309–1315.
281. Grayston JT, Campbell LA, Kuo CC, et al. A new respiratory tract pathogen. *Chlamydiae pneumoniae strain* TWAR. *J Infect Dis* 1990; 161(4):618–625.
282. Hammerschlag MR. Antimicrobial susceptibility and therapy of infections caused by *Chlamydiae pneumoniae. Antimicrob Agents Chemother* 1994;38(9):1873–1878.
283. Khatib R, Thirumoorthi MC, Kelly B, et al. Severe psittacosis during pregnancy and suppression of antibody response with early therapy. *Scand J Infect Dis* 1995;27(5):519–521.
284. Johnson SE, Klein GP, Schmid GP, et al. Susceptibility of the Lyme disease spirochete to seven antimicrobial agents. *Yale J Biol Med* 1984;57:549–553.
285. Norris SJ, Edmondson DG. *In vitro* culture system to determine MICs and MBCs of antimicrobial agents against *Treponema pallidum* subsp. *pallidum* (Nichols strain). *Antimicrob Agents Chemother* 1988;32:68–74.
286. Dumler JS, Bakken JS. Ehrlichial diseases of humans: emerging tick-borne infections. *Clin Infect Dis* 1995;20(5):1102–1110.
287. Clyde DF, Miller RM, DuPont HL, et al. Antimalarial effects of tetracyclines in man. *J Trop Med Hyg* 1971;74(11):238–242.
288. Colwell EJ, Hickman RL, Kosakal S. Tetracycline treatment of chloroquine-resistant falciparum malaria in Thailand. *J Am Med Assoc* 1972;220(5):684–686.
289. Ming-Yuan F, Walker DH, Shu-rong Y, et al. Epidemiology and ecology of rickettsial diseases in the Peoples Republic of China. *Rev Infect Dis* 1987;9:823–840.
290. Perine PL, Chandler BP, Krause DK. A clinico-epidemiological study of epidemic typhus in Africa. *Clin Infect Dis* 1992;14: 1149–1158.
291. American Academy of Pediatrics. Rocky Mountain spotted fever. In: Pickering LK, ed. *Red book: 2003 report of the Committee on Infectious Diseases,* 26th ed. Elk Grove Village, IL: American Academy of Pediatrics, 2003:532–534.
292. Valencia GB, Banzon F, Cummings M, et al. *Mycoplasma hominis* and *Ureaplasma urealyticum* in neonates with suspected infection. *Pediatr Infect Dis J* 1993;12(7):571–573.
293. Abdel-Haq N, Asmar B, Brown W. *Mycoplasma hominis* scalp abscess in the newborn. *Pediatr Infect Dis J* 2002;21(12): 1171–1173.
294. Spencer RC, Brown CB. Septicaemia in a renal transplant patient due to *Mycoplasma hominis. J Infect* 1983;6:267–268.
295. Bowie WR, Alexander ER, Stimson JB, et al. Therapy of nongonococcal urethritis. Double-blind randomized comparison of two doses and two durations of minocycline. *Ann Intern Med* 1981;95:306–311.
296. Prentice MJ, Taylor-Robinson D, Csonka GW. Non-specific urethritis. A placebo-controlled trial of minocycline in conjunction with laboratory investigations. *Br J Vener Dis* 1976;52: 269–275.
297. Handsfield HH. Gonorrhea and nongonococcal urethritis. Recent advances. *Med Clin North Am* 1978;62(5):925–943.
298. Jawetz E. Chemotherapy of chlamydial infections. *Adv Pharmacol Chemother* 1969;7:253–282.
299. American Academy of Pediatrics. *Chlamydia trachomatis.* In: Pickering LK, ed. *Red book: 2003 report of the Committee on Infectious Diseases,* 26th ed. Elk Grove Village, IL: American Academy of Pediatrics, 2003:238–243.
300. Johnson RC, Kodner C, Russel M. *In vitro* and *in vivo* susceptibility of the Lyme disease spirochete, *Borrelia burgdorferi,* to four antimicrobial agents. *Antimicrob Agents Chemother* 1987;31: 164–167.
301. Steere AC. Musculoskeletal manifestations of Lyme disease. *Am J Med* 1995;98(Suppl 4 A):44–48.
302. Pachner AR. Early disseminated Lyme disease: Lyme meningitis. *Am J Med* 1995;98(Suppl 4 A):30–37.
303. Hall WH. Modern therapy for brucellosis in humans. *Rev Infect Dis* 1990;12:1060–1099.
304. Lubani MM, Dudin KL, Sharda DC, et al. A multicenter therapeutic of 1100 children with brucellosis. *Pediatr Infect Dis J* 1989;8:75–78.
305. Al-Eissa YA, Kambal AM, Al-Nasser MN, et al. Childhood brucellosis: a study of 102 cases. *Pediatr Infect Dis J* 1990;9:74–79.
306. Anonymous. Cholera in 1994: part 1. *Wkly Epidemiol Rec* 1994;70: 201–208.
307. Rabbani GH, Butler T, Shahrier M, et al. Efficacy of a single dose of furazolidone for treatment of cholera in children. *Antimicrob Agents Chemother* 1991;35:1864–1867.
308. American Academy of Pediatrics. Malaria. In: Pickering LK, ed. *Red book: 2003 report of the Committee on Infectious Diseases,* 26th ed. Elk Grove Village, IL: American Academy of Pediatrics, 2003: 414–419.
309. Fabre J, Milek E, Kalfopoulos P, et al. The kinetics of tetracycline in man: digestive absorption and serum concentrations. In: *Doxycycline (Vibramycin): a compendium of clinical evaluation.* New York: Pfizer Laboratories, 1973:13–18.
310. Kunin CM, Dornbush AC, Finland M. Distribution and excretion of four tetracycline analogues in normal young men. *J Clin Invest* 1959;38:1950.
311. Bennet JV, Mickwait JS, Barrett JE, et al. Comparative serum binding of four tetracyclines under simulated *in vivo* conditions. *Antimicrob Agents Chemother* 1965;5:180–182.
312. McDonald H, Kelley RG, Allen ES, et al. Pharmacokinetic studies on minocycline in man. *Clin Pharmacol Ther* 1973;14: 852–861.
313. Wood WS, Kipnis GP. The concentrations of tetracycline, chlortetracycline, and oxytetracycline in the cerebrospinal fluid after intravenous administration. In: Welch H, Marti-Ibanez F, eds. *Antibiotics annual, 1953–1954.* New York: Medical Encyclopedia, 1953:98–101.
314. Yim CW, Flynn NM, Fitzgerald FT. Penetration of oral doxycycline into the cerebrospinal fluid in patients with latent or neurosyphilis. *Antimicrob Agents Chemother* 1985;28:347–348.
315. Parker RH, Schmid F. Antimicrobial activity of synovial fluid during therapy of septic arthritis. *Arthritis Rheum* 1971;14:96–104.
316. Lundberg C, Malmburg A, Ivemark BI. Antibiotic concentrations in relation to structural changes in maxillary sinus mucosa following intramuscular or peroral treatment. *Scand J Infect Dis* 1974;6:187–195.
317. Hoeprich PD, Warshauer DM. Entry of four tetracyclines into saliva and tears. *Antimicrob Agents Chemother* 1974;5:330–336.
318. LeBlanc AL, Perry JE. Transfer of tetracycline across the human placenta. *Tex Rep Biol Med* 1967;25:541–545.
319. Briggs GG, Freeman RK, Yaffe SJ. *Drugs in pregnancy and lactation,* 4th ed. Baltimore, MD: Williams & Wilkins, 1994: 808–811.
320. Greenberg PA, Sanford JP. Removal and absorption of antibiotics in patients with renal failure undergoing peritoneal dialysis:

tetracycline, chloramphenicol, kanamycin and colistimethate. *Ann Intern Med* 1967;66:465–470.

321. Whelton A, Schach von Wittenau M, Twomey TM, et al. Doxycycline pharmacokinetics in the absence of renal function. *Kidney Int* 1974;5:365–371.
322. Carson JL, Strom BL, Duff A, et al. Acute liver disease associated with erythromycins, sulfonamides, and tetracyclines. *Ann Intern Med* 1993;119:576–583.
323. Schultz JC, Adamson JS Jr, Workman WW, et al. Fatal liver disease after administration of tetracycline in high doses. *N Engl J Med* 1963;269:999–1004.
324. Glette J, Sandberg S, Haneberg B, et al. Effect of tetracyclines and UV light on oxygen consumption by human leukocytes. *Antimicrob Agents Chemother* 1984;26(4):489–492.
325. Kline AH, Blattner RJ, Lunin M. Transplacental effect of tetracyclines on teeth. *J Am Med Assoc* 1964;188:178–180.
326. Lew HT, French SW. Tetracycline nephrotoxicity and nonoliguric acute renal failure. *Arch Intern Med* 1966;118:123–128.
327. Mull MM. The tetracyclines, a critical reappraisal. *Am J Dis Child* 1966;112:483–493.
328. Maroon JC, Mealy J Jr. Benign intracranial hypertension. Sequel to tetracycline therapy in a child. *J Am Med Assoc* 1971;216(9): 1479–1480.
329. Walters BN, Gubbay SS. Tetracycline and benign intracranial hypertension: report of five cases. *Br Med J* 1981;282(6257):19–20.
330. Fanning WL, Gump DW, Sofferman RA. Side effects of minocycline: a double-blind study. *Antimicrob Agents Chemother* 1977;11 (4):712–717.
331. Neuvonen PJ, Gothoni G, Hackman R, et al. Interference of iron with the absorption of tetracycline in man. *Br Med J* 1970;4: 532–534.
332. Gugler R, Allgayer H. Effects of antacids on the clinical pharmacokinetics of drugs: an update. *Clin Pharmacokinet* 1990;18:210–219.
333. Pentitila O, Neuvonen PJ, Lehtovaara R. Interaction between doxycycline and some antiepileptic drugs. *Br Med J* 1974;2:470–472.
334. Neuvonen PJ, Pentitila O. Interactions between doxycycline and barbiturates. *Br Med J* 1974;1(907):535–536.
335. Lindenbaum J, Rund DG, Butler VP Jr, et al. Inactivation of digoxin by the gut flora: reversal by antibiotic therapy. *N Engl J Med* 1981;305(14):789–794.

CHAPTER

33

David J. Diemert

Anthelminthic Drugs in Children

INTRODUCTION

Worldwide, some of the most common childhood infections are caused by helminths. Of these, schistosomiasis and the soil-transmitted helminths (STHs) which include roundworm (*Ascaris lumbricoides*), whipworm (*Trichuris trichiura*), and the hookworms *Ancylostoma duodenale* and *Necator americanus*, are the most prevalent. According to the World Health Organization (WHO), more than 400 million preschool children (aged 1 to 4 years) and more than 1 billion school children (aged 5 to 14 years) live in areas that put them at risk of being infected with one or more of the STHs or schistosomes (1). School-aged children living in the rural, resource-limited areas of the tropics are at particular risk of helminth infections due to the STHs and schistosomes, as has been demonstrated by numerous epidemiologic studies. This age group often suffers from the highest worm burdens and in turn, the related complications such as iron deficiency anemia due to hookworm, intestinal or biliary tract obstruction due to *A. lumbricoides*, dysentery syndrome or rectal prolapse due to *T. trichiura*, and hepatobiliary or urinary schistosomiasis (2). However, considerably greater numbers of children develop more insidious disease from chronic infections due to these parasites, such as malnutrition and impaired physical fitness and development (3,4). In addition, chronic infection with STHs and schistosomes impairs childhood intellectual and cognitive development, thus adversely affecting both learning capacity and school attendance (5,6).

Because of the negative impact on childhood growth and development of the STHs and schistosomiasis, the WHO, United Nations Children's Fund, and the World Bank have encouraged and funded programs that provide anthelminthic medications to children living in endemic areas through periodic mass administration campaigns in elementary schools and through child health days. In these mass drug administration (MDA) programs, children receive a single dose of a benzimidazole drug such as albendazole or mebendazole once or twice a year in regions with high prevalence of STHs, whereas those living in areas endemic for schistosomiasis receive a single dose of praziquantel at the same interval. Both drugs are administered simultaneously in areas such as many parts of sub-Saharan Africa and Brazil, where the infections are coendemic. MDA has been shown in prospective studies to result in catch-up growth or in growth that is faster than that of children who remain infected with helminths (7).

Although the logistics of administering hundreds of millions of doses of anthelminthic drugs annually throughout the developing world are daunting, the potential benefits are evident. However, a major drawback to this approach is that children remain susceptible to STH and schistosome infections following treatment, and in areas of intense transmission reinfection can occur rapidly within months (8). Therefore, in many parts of the developing world, administration of anthelminthics would have to be conducted on a twice- or thrice-yearly basis to have a substantial impact, which is difficult to sustain (9). Furthermore, although school-aged children typically experience the highest *Ascaris*, *Trichuris*, and schistosome worm burdens, adults can also be infected so that school-based interventions might miss an important reservoir and therefore not interrupt the transmission cycle within a community (10). Another potentially critical problem with current MDA programs is that widespread benzimidazole drug resistance might develop in the STHs. Such resistance has already been documented in intestinal nematodes that infect sheep and cattle throughout the southern hemisphere, where these drugs have been used indiscriminately (11). There is concern that widespread use of the benzimidazoles in humans could similarly lead to the development of resistance in the STHs. The same concern exists for praziquantel in the case of schistosomiasis. Given the lack of alternative medications that are effective against the major STHs or schistosomiasis, such a scenario could be potentially devastating.

Unfortunately, the situation is compounded by the fact that there are relatively few new anthelminthic drugs that are currently under development. Interestingly, some medications that have been developed for nonhelminth infections have been found to have effects on some widespread helminth infections and could potentially make up for the dearth of alternative anthelminthics to the current first-line therapies. For example, the artemisinins such as artesunate and artemether, although originally developed as antimalarials, have been shown to be active against the early liver stages of schistosomes (12). Although not beneficial as monotherapy due to stage-specific activity, combination with existing drugs such as praziquantel is being explored to improve efficacy. Similarly, the antibacterials doxycycline and rifampin have both shown efficacy in the control of lymphatic filariasis and onchocerciasis (13). For both of these agents, the mechanism of action is by targeting the *Wolbachia* endosymbionts present in most human filariae except *Loa loa* and which are essential for worm fertility and survival. Treatment with several weeks of doxycycline or rifampin has been shown to sterilize adult female filarial worms and even lead to their death; amelioration of symptomatic disease has also been observed in clinical trials. The use of the artemisinins and doxycycline or rifampin in the treatment of schistosomiasis and filariasis, respectively, represents exciting new developments in the field of anthelminthic drug research; however, these drugs are covered in separate chapters of this book given that their primary indications are for infections other than helminths.

This chapter will give special attention to the benzimidazoles and praziquantel due to their widespread use throughout the world to treat the STHs and schistosomiasis, respectively. In children living in the United States, these helminthiases are seen predominantly in those who have immigrated from endemic areas. Of the endemically transmitted helminths, the nematode infection caused by *Toxocara canis* (dog roundworm) has emerged as one of the most common helminthiases in the United States, especially in urban areas with large numbers of Hispanic children (14,15). Albendazole is the treatment of choice for toxocariasis. Finally, cysticercosis caused by infection with the larval stage of the pork tapeworm *Taenia solium* has emerged as a leading cause of childhood seizures in American cities bordering Mexico such as Los Angeles, San Diego, Tucson, and San Antonio (16). Both albendazole and praziquantel are first-line agents for treating active cysticercal lesions (Table 33.1).

BENZIMIDAZOLE COMPOUNDS

This class of drugs includes some of the most commonly used anthelminthics in the world, such as albendazole, mebendazole, thiabendazole, and triclabendazole. Albendazole and mebendazole, in particular, are widely used and have been proven to be extremely effective in the WHO's global deworming programs. Because of their broad spectrum of activities, albendazole and mebendazole are the cornerstone medications for treating intestinal helminths, although currently only albendazole is commercially available in the United States. Globally, however, they are the two major drugs used to treat the pediatric STH infections trichuriasis, ascariasis, and hookworm, which together are estimated to affect more than 1 billion children worldwide (2). In addition, albendazole is now used together with diethylcarbamazine (DEC) or ivermectin for the control of lymphatic filariasis in MDA programs conducted in endemic regions (17).

MECHANISM OF ACTION

All of the benzimidazole derivatives act by binding irreversibly to intracellular tubulin in nematodes and platyhelminths, thereby inhibiting its polymerization and assembly into microtubules. The loss of cytoplasmic microtubule formation results in impaired uptake of glucose by the adult and larval stages of susceptible helminths (18). The inhibition of glucose uptake results in the depletion of glycogen stores and in the reduced production of adenosine triphosphate (19). Death of the helminth is probably achieved because of this disruption of energy production, which results in starvation of the parasite (18,20).

ALBENDAZOLE

Albendazole is a broad-spectrum, synthetic, oral benzimidazole-derivative anthelminthic agent. It was originally introduced in Australia in 1977 as an anthelminthic for sheep, and in the early 1980s it was licensed for human use. Albendazole is comparable in efficacy to mebendazole but offers two distinct advantages over it. First, for most intestinal nematode infections, albendazole requires only a single administration to be effective. This offers an obvious advantage in ensuring patient compliance, especially in the pediatric population. For MDA programs in endemic regions, albendazole is often preferred to mebendazole due to its greater efficacy and ease of use. Another advantage offered by albendazole is that it has an active metabolite, albendazole sulphoxide, which undergoes slower elimination than the parent drug and likely accounts for most of the activity. For systemic helminthic infections, albendazole can be used in moderate doses to achieve the same effect as high doses of mebendazole. Along with mebendazole, albendazole is currently one of the main drugs used to treat intestinal nematode infections, although it should be noted that in the United States, albendazole is not licensed for this indication.

Indications

Albendazole is currently licensed for the treatment of cystic hydatid disease (echinococcosis) of the liver, lung, and peritoneum caused by the larval form of the dog tapeworm *Echinococcus granulosus* (21). However, for this disease, albendazole is most often used as an adjunct to surgical excision or percutaneous drainage of hydatid cysts, both pre- and postoperatively, to reduce the risk of recurrence due to spillage of scolices during surgery (22–27). The efficacy of albendazole in the treatment of alveolar hydatid disease due to *E. multilocularis* has not been clearly demonstrated but may be considered in unresectable cases (28).

The other label indication for albendazole is for treatment of parenchymal neurocysticercosis due to active lesions caused by the larval forms of the pork tapeworm *T. solium*. In neurocysticercosis, the larval form of *T. solium* localizes in the brain of the human host where it can remain encysted for years. Albendazole, along with praziquantel, is one of the chemotherapeutic agents used as part of the management of this clinical syndrome (29–34). The role of larvicidal medications such as albendazole in the treatment of neurocysticercosis is complicated and far from straightforward. Albendazole appears to be most effective in symptomatic patients with viable cysts within

TABLE 33.1 Recommended Drugs for Treatment of Pediatric Helminthic Infections

Helminth	*Drug of Choice*
Nematodes	
Ascaris *lumbricoides* (roundworm)	Albendazole 400 mg × 1 d Mebendazole 500 mg × 1 d or 100 mg bid × 3 d Pyrantel pamoate 11 mg/kg base × 1 d (not to exceed 1 g) Ivermectin 150–200 μg/kg × 1 d levamisole 2.5 mg/kg × 1 d
Trichuris trichiura (whipworm)	Mebendazole 500 mg × 1 d or 100 mg bid × 3 d Albendazole 400 mg/d × 1–3 d
Hookworm	
Necator americanus *Ancylostoma duodenale*	Albendazole 400 mg × 1 d Mebendazole 500 mg × 1 d or 100 mg bid × 3 d Pyrantel pamoate 11 mg/kg/d base × 3 d (not to exceed 1 g/d)
Cutaneous larva migrans (dog and cat hookworm)	Albendazole 400 mg qd × 3 d Ivermectin 200 μg/kg/d × 1–2 d Thiabendazole 50 mg/kg/d × 2–4 d
Enterobius vermicularis (pinworm)	Pyrantel pamoate 11 mg/kg base × 1 d (not to exceed 1 g), repeat treatment in 2 wk Albendazole 400 mg × 1 d, repeat in 2 wk Mebendazole 100 mg × 1 d, repeat in 2 wk (all family members or persons in close contact with the patient should also be treated)
Strongyloides stercoralis	Ivermectin 200 μg/kg/d × 1–2 d Thiabendazole 50 mg/kg/d divided into two doses × 2–4 d (longer treatment may be required in hyperinfection or disseminated disease)
Capillaria philippinensis	Albendazole 400 mg qd × 10 d Mebendazole 200 mg bid × 20 d
Toxocara canis (visceral/ocular larva migrans)	Albendazole 400 mg bid × 5 d Mebendazole 200 mg bid × 5 d (optimal duration of treatment unknown. For severe disease or ocular involvement, consider corticosteroids)
Trichinella spiralis	Albendazole 400 mg bid × 8–14 d Mebendazole 200–400 mg tid × 3 d, then 400–500 mg tid × 10 d (consider corticosteroids for severe disease)
Trichostrongylus spp.	Pyrantel pamoate 11 mg/kg base × 1 d (not to exceed 1 g) Albendazole 400 mg × 1 d Mebendazole 100 mg tid × 3 d
Gnathostoma spinigerum	Albendazole 400 mg bid × 21 d Ivermectin 200 μg/kg/d × 2 d
Filarial nematodes	
Lymphatic filariasis *(Wuchereria bancrofti, Brugia malayi, B. timori), Loa loa*	Diethylcarbamazine 1 mg/kg × 1 d on day 1, 3 mg/kg/d divided into three doses on day 2, 3–6 mg/kg/d divided into three doses on day 3, then 6 mg/kg/d divided into three doses on days 4–14
Onchocerca volvulus	Ivermectin 150 μg/kg × 1 d every 6–12 mo[a]
Mansonella ozzardi	Ivermectin 200 μg/kg × 1[a] d
M. perstans	Albendazole 400 mg bid × 10 d Mebendazole 100 mg bid × 30 d
M. streptocerca	Diethylcarbamazine 6 mg/kg/d × 14 d Ivermectin 150 μg/kg × 1[a] d
Cestodes	
Taenia saginata, T. solium, Diphyllobothrium latum, Dipylidium caninum	Praziquantel 10 mg/kg × 1 d
Hymenolepsis nana	Praziquantel 25 mg/kg × 1 d
T. solium (cysticerosis)	Albendazole 15 mg/kg/d (maximum 800 mg) divided into two doses for 8–30 d Praziquantel 100 mg/kg/d divided into three doses × 1 d, then 50 mg/kg/d divided into three doses × 29 d (consider corticosteroids and anticonvulsants during administration of larvicidal therapy)
Echinococcus granulosis (hydatid disease)	Albendazole 15 mg/kg/d (maximum 800 mg) bid × 1–6 mo (chemotherapy is usually an adjunct to surgery or percutaneous cyst drainage)
Trematodes	
Schistosoma haematobium, S. mansoni, S. intercalatum	Praziquantel 40 mg/kg/d in 1–2 doses × 1 d
S. japonicum, S. mekongki	Praziquantel 60 mg/kg/d in 1–3 doses × 1 d
Fasciola hepatica	Triclabendazole 10 mg/kg × 1 d
Clonorchis sinensis, Opisthorchis viverrini	Praziquantel 75 mg/kg/d divided into three doses × 2 d
Metorchis conjunctus, Fasciolopsis buski, Heterophyes heterophyes, Metagonimus yokogawai	Praziquantel 75 mg/kg/d divided into three doses × 1 d
Nanophyetus salmincola	Praziquantel 60 mg/kg/d divided into three doses × 1 d
Paragonimus westermani (lung fluke)	Praziquantel 75 mg/kg/d divided into three doses × 2 d Triclabendazole 10 mg/kg × 1–2 doses

bid, twice daily; d, day; mo, month; qd, daily; tid, thrice daily.
[a]Not macrofilaricidal but temporarily decreases blood or skin microfilaria count.
Source: The Medical Letter, Inc. In: Abramowicz M, ed. *Drugs for parasitic infections*, 1st ed. New Rochelle, NY: The Medical Letter, 2007.

the cerebral parenchyma and in the rapidly progressive form of cysticercosis (33). However, since cysts that appear calcified on imaging represent old cysticerci that have died, patients with these will not benefit from treatment with albendazole. Furthermore, a single ring-enhancing lesion with surrounding edema likely represents a dying cyst, for which albendazole will also not be useful. Patients with intraventricular or meningeal cysts may be treated with albendazole as part of a multidisciplinary approach that often involves measures to reduce intracranial pressure, and surgery. It is extremely important to note that the use of larvicidal chemotherapy in neurocysticercosis may result in an intense inflammatory response that can induce seizures and life-threatening increases in intracranial pressure. Therefore, concurrent administration of systemic corticosteroids and anticonvulsants together with careful monitoring for intracranial hypertension should always be considered in symptomatic neurocysticercosis patients who receive albendazole (34). In addition, before initiating albendazole therapy for neurocysticercosis, patients should be examined for ocular cysticerci. If these are seen, the benefits of larvicidal drugs should be weighed against the possibility of permanent visual loss caused by albendazole-induced changes to existing lesions (21).

Besides these approved indications, the most common use of albendazole in practice is to treat the intestinal STH infections due to *A. lumbricoides, T. trichuris,* and hookworm, even though these do not appear on the product label. Furthermore, although also not listed on the product label, albendazole has been used to successfully treat cutaneous larva migrans caused by *A. braziliense* or *A. caninum* (dog and cat hookworm) and enterobiasis (35,36). When used to treat pinworm infection due to *Enterobius vermicularis,* single-dose treatment should be repeated 2 weeks later to kill worms that have developed from eggs that were not affected by the initial treatment; also, since this infection is highly contagious and other family members are frequently infected, treatment of the entire household is recommended (36).

Other off-label uses of albendazole include as an alternative agent for treating infection with *Strongyloides stercoralis, Capillaria philippinensis,* and *Trichostrongylus.* Albendazole is also used as an alternative treatment of taeniasis caused by adult *T. solium* or *T. saginata* (beef tapeworm) (37,38). Even though praziquantel is superior for the treatment of taeniasis, albendazole is often used in endemic countries because it is cheaper and has a broader spectrum of anthelminthic activity.

In visceral larva migrans due to infection with *T. canis* or *T. cati,* the use of chemotherapy is warranted only when the disease is severe or when there is ocular involvement; as with neurocysticercosis, treatment is usually combined with a corticosteroid to reduce the inflammatory response to dying parasites (39). Albendazole is also used in the treatment of trichinosis (trichinellosis) caused by *Trichinella spiralis* (40). Administration of the drug is most effective if given early in the course of infection and works by acting on adult worms within the intestinal mucosa before they produce larvae that then penetrate muscle. Systemic corticosteroids are commonly used concurrently, especially in patients with severe symptoms, to minimize potential inflammatory reactions to dying larvae.

Finally, albendazole has recently been used in combination with either DEC or ivermectin for the control of filarial infections (17). MDA programs for the reduction of morbidity due to *Wuchereria bancrofti* or *Brugia malayi* (lymphatic filariasis) and *Onchocerca volvulus* (river blindness) are the current strategies for these diseases; annual or biannual administration of the drug combinations leads to reduction in microfilaremia which reduces both the clinical manifestations of infection and transmission within affected communities.

Pharmacokinetics

Albendazole is poorly and erratically absorbed from the gastrointestinal tract because of its low aqueous solubility (18,21). However, absorption of albendazole is greatly increased (up to fivefold) if the medication is taken with food containing relatively high-fat content (18). Albendazole is rapidly metabolized by the liver mostly to its active metabolite albendazole sulphoxide, which undergoes slower elimination than the parent drug, which is therefore detectable in only negligible amounts in the plasma. Albendazole sulphoxide is mostly protein-bound and is widely distributed throughout the body (as opposed to mebendazole) and can be detected in cerebrospinal fluid, urine, bile, hydatid cyst fluid, cyst wall, and liver (18,21,41,42). Urinary excretion of albendazole sulphoxide is minimal whereas concentrations in bile are similar to those achieved in plasma. Albendazole sulphoxide is also further metabolized to albendazole sulfone and other oxidative metabolites.

Pediatric Considerations

Albendazole has been found to be teratogenic (embryotoxicity and skeletal malformations) in pregnant rats and rabbits (18,21,43,44). Teratogenicity occurred in rats given oral daily doses of 10 and 30 mg per kg during gestation days 6 to 15 and in rabbits given oral doses of 30 mg per kg daily during gestation days 7 to 19. In the rabbit study, maternal toxicity (33% mortality) was noted at 30 mg per kg daily. Teratogenicity in humans has not been observed, and a recent study of more than 800 women treated with albendazole during the second and third trimesters demonstrated no adverse effects (45). Use in the first trimester, however, is still not recommended.

Limited studies on the relationship of age to the effects of albendazole have been performed in children younger than 6 years. Although hydatid disease is uncommon in infants and young children, no pediatric-specific problems have been documented in infants and young children who were treated with albendazole for this infection. In addition, five studies involving children as young as 1 year treated with albendazole for neurocysticercosis, which occurs more frequently than hydatid disease in children, did not document pediatric-specific problems (21). Given the limited available safety information, albendazole use in children younger than 2 years, like that of mebendazole, is not recommended in the prescribing information given by the manufacturer.

Since the 1990s, however, albendazole has been used safely in treating populations of entire communities irrespective of age, sex, or infection status as part of MDA programs. As the result of albendazole's widespread use and the lack of observed pediatric-specific problems, the WHO has developed a different recommendation than the manufacturers', and now recommends that it can be used safely in a single, reduced dose of 200 mg in children older than 12 months and younger than 24 months (46).

Drug–Drug Interactions

Cimetidine

Cimetidine decreases the oral bioavailability of albendazole, either by reducing gastric acid production or by inhibiting cytochrome P450 (CYP)-mediated metabolism of albendazole to its active metabolite (47).

Corticosteroids

Concurrent use of albendazole with corticosteroids (such as in the treatment of neurocysticercosis) has been shown to increase the steady-state plasma concentration of albendazole sulphoxide, possibly by reducing the rate of elimination (21,29,30,48,49). However, no modification of the dose of albendazole is recommended in this situation.

Praziquantel

Praziquantel increases the mean maximum plasma concentration and area under the plasma concentration–time curve of albendazole sulphoxide by approximately 50% but does not require modification of albendazole dosing (21).

Theophylline

Although the pharmacodynamics of theophylline were unchanged after a single dose of albendazole when tested in six healthy subjects, this drug has been shown to induce CYP 1A activity in hepatoma cells in vitro (21). Since theophylline is a substrate for this enzyme, plasma concentrations should be monitored during and following treatment with albendazole.

Precautions

Patients with Biliary Obstruction

Patients with extrahepatic biliary obstruction have reduced elimination of albendazole and increased plasma concentrations of albendazole sulphoxide, potentially increasing the incidence of toxicities such as bone marrow suppression, although no specific dosing modification is recommended by the manufacturer (21).

Side Effects

Albendazole is generally very well tolerated. The most common reported side effects include abdominal pain, nausea, vomiting, and headache (20,21,29,37,50–52). Much less common are hypersensitivity reactions including rash and urticaria and reversible alopecia and leukopenia (21,53). Rarely, agranulocytosis can occur. With prolonged therapy such as for hydatid disease, mild to moderate elevations of hepatic enzymes can occur that resolve upon discontinuation of the drug, although acute hepatic failure and hepatitis have been reported (54). Hepatic transaminases should be measured every 2 weeks while on extended therapy.

Pediatric Dosage

Albendazole is available only as a chewable oral tablet: for younger children, tablets should be crushed or chewed and swallowed. Information on the use of albendazole in children younger than 12 months is limited. If used for extended periods at high doses such as for hydatid disease, complete blood cell counts with leukocyte differential and hepatic transaminases should be performed every 2 weeks due to the risk of blood dyscrasias and hepatitis, respectively.

- *Ascariasis, trichuriasis,* and *hookworm:* 400 mg as a single dose. For trichuriasis, three daily doses may be required.
- *Hydatid disease:* 15 mg per kg per day (maximum 800 mg) in two divided doses for 1 to 6 months. Given in 28-day cycles with 14-day albendazole-free intervals. When used as an adjunct to surgery or percutaneous drainage, it should be started at least 1 week prior to drainage and for up to 3 months after.
- *Neurocysticercosis:* 15 mg per kg per day (maximum 800 mg) in two divided doses for 8 to 30 days. May be repeated if necessary.
- *Cutaneous larva migrans:* 400 mg daily for 3 days.
- *Toxocariasis (visceral larval migrans)*: 400 mg twice daily for 5 days.
- *Capillariasis:* 400 mg daily for 10 days.
- *Enterobiasis:* 400 mg as a single dose; repeat in 2 weeks.
- *Trichinosis:* 400 mg twice daily for 8 to 14 days.

WHO Recommendation

In community MDA programs for intestinal helminthiases, a single 200 mg dose of albendazole has been shown to be both safe and effective in children older than 12 months and younger than 24 months (17). Children older than 24 months should receive the full 400 mg dose during MDA programs.

MEBENDAZOLE

Mebendazole is an orally administered, synthetic benzimidazole that has a broad spectrum of anthelminthic activity and a low incidence of adverse effects. It was used for decades in the United States since licensure by the Food and Drug Administration (FDA) in 1974 but is no longer marketed in this country. It is structurally similar to albendazole, and, like albendazole, it is particularly effective against susceptible intestinal nematodes such as *A. lumbricoides, T. trichiura, E. vermicularis,* and hookworm. Together with pyrantel pamoate, albendazole, and levamisole, mebendazole is one of the four essential broad-spectrum anthelminthics recommended by the WHO for the treatment of intestinal nematode infections.

Indications

Mebendazole is used to treat intestinal nematodes and is effective in eliminating ascariasis, enterobiasis, trichuriasis, and hookworm infections (*A. duodenale* and *N. americanus*) (55–57). Together with albendazole, it is one of the most common drugs used in MDA programs worldwide for the control of intestinal nematode infections. Although this drug was never specifically licensed for these indications, mebendazole has also been used to treat infections caused by *C. philippinensis* and *Gnathostoma spinigerum* (19,58).

However, since mebendazole is poorly adsorbed from the gastrointestinal tract it is not a recommended first-line treatment of tissue-dwelling helminth infections such as cysticercosis and hydatid disease. Although mebendazole has been used in the past as an adjunct treatment of hydatid and alveolar echinococcosis, it has since been replaced by albendazole for these infections due to its superior and more consistent systemic absorption from the gastrointestinal tract.

Mebendazole is also used as an alternative to albendazole in the treatment of trichinosis (40). As with albendazole, treatment is most effective if given early in the course of infection and concomitant administration of systemic corticosteroids reduces the likelihood of complications due to inflammatory reactions to dying parasites.

Pharmacokinetics

Mebendazole has limited solubility in water and therefore is poorly absorbed (approximately 5% to 10%) from the gastrointestinal tract (59). However, absorption is increased when it is ingested with fatty foods, although even then the amount absorbed shows remarkable interindividual variability (18). Given its poor absorption, mebendazole is poorly effective in treating systemic helminth infections. Whatever is absorbed undergoes rapid first-pass metabolism in the liver to multiple different protein-bound metabolites. Clearance is predominantly as metabolites in urine and bile, although the majority is found unchanged in the feces because of lack of absorption (18).

Pediatric Considerations

Mebendazole crosses the placenta, and studies in rats given single oral doses as low as 10 mg per kg have shown it to be teratogenic and embryotoxic. However, a postmarketing survey in pregnant women who inadvertently took mebendazole during the first trimester did not show an incidence of spontaneous abortion or malformation greater than that of the general population. In 170 deliveries at term, mebendazole has not been shown to be teratogenic in humans (56). In addition, studies in which pregnant women were specifically treated with mebendazole have shown no increase in spontaneous abortions or congenital defects (60). Because of the important impact of hookworm infection and other STHs during pregnancy, the WHO now recommends the use of mebendazole during the second and third trimesters of pregnancy.

Although the use of mebendazole in children younger than 2 years has traditionally not been recommended, this was solely on the basis of a lack of adequate safety information in this age group. However, several large studies have recently shown the anthelminthic efficacy of this drug in this age group without significant adverse effects (61). Accordingly, the WHO now recommends that mebendazole can be safely used in children between the ages of 12 and 24 months in addition to older children (46).

Drug–Drug Interactions

Carbamazepine

Carbamazepine has been shown to lower mebendazole plasma concentrations by induction of hepatic microsomal enzymes and to impair the therapeutic response. Adjustment of dosage may be required (62).

Metronidazole

Stevens–Johnson syndrome has been reported when mebendazole was used in combination with metronidazole (63). Therefore, this combination should be avoided.

Precautions

Patients with Inflammatory Bowel Disease

Patients with inflammatory bowel disease (Crohn's disease or ulcerative colitis) may experience increased absorption and toxicity of mebendazole, especially if given in high doses (64).

Patients with Hepatic Impairment

Patients with impaired hepatic function may experience increased incidence of side effects because of reduced metabolism of the drug. Accordingly, the dose may need to be decreased.

Side Effects

Mebendazole is very well tolerated, likely due to its poor absorption so that systemic side effects are rare. Reported side effects include gastrointestinal disturbances such as abdominal pain, diarrhea, nausea, and vomiting; headache and dizziness; and hypersensitivity reactions such as fever, skin rash, and pruritis (18,41,56). Transient increases in serum levels of hepatic transaminases, alkaline phosphatase, and blood urea nitrogen may be seen following prolonged periods of use (41). Similarly, although not commonly used now for this indication, high-dose therapy for hydatid disease has been associated with development of alopecia and reversible neutropenia and lymphopenia (41).

Pediatric Dosage

In countries where it is available, mebendazole is supplied as a chewable tablet or suspension for oral administration. Because of the lack of safety information in children younger than 12 months, use of mebendazole in the age group should be avoided.

- *Ascariasis, trichuriasis,* and *hookworm:* 500 mg as a single dose or 100 mg twice daily for 3 days.
- *Enterobiasis:* 100 mg as a single dose. Repeat in 2 to 3 weeks.
- *Capillariasis:* 200 mg twice daily for 20 days.
- *Trichinosis:* 200 to 400 mg three times daily for 3 days, then 400 to 500 mg three times daily for 10 days.

WHO Recommendation

For the treatment of intestinal nematodes, mebendazole can be safely used in children between 12 and 24 months when given at the same dose as for older children (46).

THIABENDAZOLE

Thiabendazole was the first benzimidazole anthelminthic to be developed and was licensed for human use by the FDA in 1967. Although it is one of the most potent anthelminthic drugs, thiabendazole is also one of the least tolerated given its association with a high incidence of side effects such as gastrointestinal upset. Accordingly, thiabendazole has largely been replaced by the newer benzimidazoles such as albendazole and mebendazole. However, it is still marketed as a first-line treatment of infection with *S. stercoralis* and *T. spiralis*, as well as of cutaneous and visceral larva migrans. Because of the toxicity associated with oral administration, off-label topical application of the oral suspension has been used in treating localized cutaneous larva migrans, although this is not an approved use of the drug.

Indications

With the development of less toxic anthelminthics such as mebendazole, albendazole, and ivermectin, oral thiabendazole is now uncommonly used for the treatment of helminth infections. In the past, a topical formulation of thiabendazole was marketed for the treatment of cutaneous larva migrans. Unfortunately, this form of the drug is no longer commercially available in North America, although the oral tablet or suspension of thiabendazole remains a treatment option for cutaneous larva migrans (65,66).

Oral thiabendazole may be used to treat infections with *S. stercoralis*, including the hyperinfection syndrome, in both immunosuppressed and immunocompetent patients. However, ivermectin has effectively supplanted its use for this indication because of possible greater efficacy (although results of comparative studies are mixed) and lower incidence of side effects (67,68). Combination therapy with ivermectin has been suggested by some experts, especially for disseminated strongyloidiasis, although results from clinical trials are lacking (69). Thiabendazole is also indicated for the treatment of visceral larva migrans and trichinosis; when used during the invasion stage of infection with *T. spiralis*, thiabendazole has been associated with improvement in symptoms and fever as well as reduction in eosinophilia (70). Although not listed on the product label, thiabendazole has also been successfully used to treat capillariasis and trichostrongyliasis.

Given its relatively higher toxicity and lower effectiveness, thiabendazole should not be considered as a first-line treatment of ascariasis, enterobiasis, trichuriasis, or hookworm infection, although it may be used if more effective and less toxic drugs are unavailable or their use is contraindicated.

Pharmacokinetics

Thiabendazole is rapidly and well absorbed from the gastrointestinal tract and reaches peak plasma concentrations within 1 to 2 hours (65). Thiabendazole differs from both mebendazole and albendazole in that it undergoes both hepatic and renal elimination. Following absorption, it is rapidly metabolized by the liver to inactive 5-hydroxythiabendazole, which is further metabolized into glucuronide and sulfate conjugates that are eliminated in the urine within 48 hours after an oral dose (65).

Pediatric Considerations

Since data on the safety and effectiveness of thiabendazole in children weighing less than 13.6 kg (30 lb) are limited, use of this medication in such children is not recommended by the manufacturer (65). Reproduction studies in rabbits given doses of up to 15 times the usual human dose and in rats given doses equivalent to the usual human have not resulted in teratogenic effects. However, in another study in mice given 10 times the usual human dose in olive oil (but not in aqueous suspension), cleft palate and axial skeletal defects were observed (65). Because of this, use of thiabendazole is not recommended during pregnancy. Furthermore, since it is not known whether thiabendazole is excreted in breast milk, the drug should not be administered to nursing mothers.

Drug–Drug Interactions

Theophylline

Thiabendazole may compete with theophylline for sites of hepatic metabolism and reduce its clearance by more than 50%, raising its serum levels to potentially toxic concentrations (71,72). Blood levels of theophylline should therefore be monitored carefully when these drugs are administered together.

Precautions

Hepatic and Renal Impairment

Thiabendazole levels can be increased in patients with renal or hepatic impairment and dosage may need to be adjusted (73).

Side Effects

Thiabendazole is one of the more poorly tolerated anthelminthics. Among the more common side effects are gastrointestinal reactions such as anorexia, diarrhea, nausea, abdominal pain, and vomiting which may sometimes be severe, and neurologic reactions such as dizziness, fatigue, headache, irritability, and numbness or tingling of the hands and feet (65). Less commonly, hypersensitivity reactions may be observed, including skin rashes, erythema multiforme, and rarely, fatal Stevens–Johnson syndrome (74). Intrahepatic cholestasis, jaundice, and parenchymal liver damage have been reported in patients treated with thiabendazole and in some cases, hepatic damage has been severe and irreversible.

Rarely, ocular symptoms (blurred vision and abnormal sensation in the eyes), drying of the mucous membranes, and sicca syndrome have been reported, sometimes lasting for prolonged periods after use of thiabendazole (75). In some patients, neuropsychiatric toxicity can be severe and includes seizures, tinnitus, delirium, confusion, and hallucinations. An interesting yet harmless effect has been reported by some patients who excrete a metabolite that imparts an asparagus-like or other unusual odor to the urine.

Pediatric Usage

Thiabendazole is supplied as chewable tablets or an oral suspension (100 mg per mL). Experience with thiabendazole in children weighing less than 13.6 kg (30 lb) is limited.

- *Strongyloidiasis:* 50 mg per kg daily divided into two doses, for 2 days. For hyperinfection syndrome: 50 mg per kg daily divided into two doses, for 5 to 7 days. May be repeated if required.
- *Cutaneous larva migrans:* 50 mg per kg daily divided into two doses for 2 to 4 days.
- *Visceral larva migrans* and *trichinosis:* 50 mg per kg daily divided into two doses for 2 to 4 days.

TRICLABENDAZOLE

Triclabendazole is a benzimidazole compound that differs from others in this class in that it lacks activity against nematodes. However, it has been widely used since coming onto the market in 1983 for the treatment of fascioliasis in livestock, for which it is very effective. The first reported use of triclabendazole to treat fascioliasis in humans was in 1986 (76). Although it has been on the WHO's list of essential medicines since 1997, it has not been licensed in the United States or Canada and is therefore not commercially available in these countries.

Fascioliasis is an infection of livestock such as cattle and sheep, but humans can be infected by eating raw or undercooked aquatic vegetables such as watercress that are contaminated with encysted larvae. Fascioliasis has become a food-borne infection of significant importance in several areas of the world such as the Andean highlands of Bolivia, Ecuador, and Peru, the Nile delta of Egypt, and northern Iran. Because praziquantel is not generally efficacious for the treatment of fascioliasis, triclabendazole is an important drug in the treatment and control of this infection.

Indications

Triclabendazole is the first-line treatment of infections caused by *Fasciola hepatica* (sheep liver fluke) and *F. gigantica* (giant liver fluke). It is active against both adult *Fasciola* worms present in the biliary ducts and the immature larval stages that migrate through the hepatic parenchyma (76–78). Triclabendazole is also used as an alternative agent in the treatment of infections caused by *Paragonimus westermani* (lung fluke) (79,80).

Pharmacokinetics

Following oral administration, absorption of triclabendazole from the gastrointestinal tract is increased two- to threefold when taken after a fatty meal (78,79). The drug undergoes extensive first-pass metabolism in the liver, where it is oxidized to active sulphoxide and sulphone metabolites that are highly protein-bound (81). Triclabendazole and its metabolites are further hydroxylated by the liver and secreted into the biliary tract. Approximately 95% of orally administered triclabendazole (unchanged or as metabolites) is secreted in bile.

Pediatric Considerations

Safety data on the use of triclabendazole in children are limited (78,79). However, children in fascioliasis- and paragonimiasis-endemic regions have been successfully treated with triclabendazole without pediatric-specific adverse reactions being reported.

Side Effects

Treatment with triclabendazole is generally well tolerated. Mild and transient abdominal pain, biliary colic, nausea, vomiting, fever, and hepatomegaly, as well as transient increases in hepatic enzymes, are likely related to self-limited biliary obstruction caused by the dying liver flukes (76,78,79,82).

Pediatric Usage

Triclabendazole is supplied as chewable tablets.

- *Fascioliasis:* 10 mg per kg as a single dose. Treatment may be repeated after 2 weeks or 6 months if necessary. The WHO recommends 20 mg per kg in two doses given 12 hours apart for severe cases of fascioliasis.
- *Paragonimiasis:* 10 mg per kg as a single dose or twice in 1 day.

OTHER ANTINEMATODE AGENTS

PYRANTEL PAMOATE

Pyrantel pamoate is a tetrahydropyrimidine-derived anthelminthic agent first developed for veterinarian use in 1966. In 1971, it was approved by the FDA for the treatment of pinworm (*E. vermicularis*) infections but it is now sold over the counter for this indication and is no longer a regulated product. It is listed by the WHO as one of the four essential broad-spectrum drugs for intestinal helminth infections and has been extensively used in helminth control programs, especially in Latin America and Southeast Asia.

Indications

In the United States, pyrantel has been primarily used for the treatment of pinworm. However, it is also very effective against the intestinal nematodes *A. lumbricoides* and *Trichostrongylus* (55,83,84). It is moderately effective against both species of hookworm but less so against *N. americanus* than *A. duodenale* (55). It is not very effective in treating either trichuriasis or strongyloidiasis.

Mechanism of Action

Pyrantel pamoate binds to an ion channel that forms a nicotinic acetylcholine receptor on the body muscle of nematodes (85). Binding to the recognition site of this excitatory receptor induces entry of calcium which in turn leads to depolarization and spastic paralysis of the nematode muscle that can result in passive expulsion of the worm from the host's gastrointestinal tract (86). Because pyrantel causes paralysis of the worms prior to expulsion, they are typically expelled intact, which makes it useful as a tool for identifying the morphologic features of adult parasites. Such information may be useful for epidemiologic and clinical investigations.

Pharmacokinetics

Pyrantel is poorly and incompletely absorbed from the gastrointestinal tract, with a time to peak concentration of between 1 and 3 hours (83,84). The drug is partially metabolized in the liver and a small percentage is excreted in the urine while the majority is eliminated unchanged in the feces (83,84).

Pediatric Considerations

Studies in animals have not shown that pyrantel causes adverse effects in the fetus. Adequate and well-controlled studies in humans have not been done. The use of pyrantel in the first trimester of pregnancy is not recommended.

As with albendazole and mebendazole, children younger than 2 years who are infected with helminths are excluded from treatment with pyrantel on the basis of the information given by the manufacturers of the drugs. However, this recommendation is made solely on the basis of a lack of information on the treatment of this age group, rather than studies documenting adverse effects. Furthermore, the WHO has been using pyrantel as a single dose for the treatment of STH infections in endemic communities for years, and no age-specific adverse effects have been reported.

Drug–Drug Interactions

Piperazine, an older-generation anthelminthic that is now rarely used, may antagonize the anthelminthic effects of pyrantel and therefore these should not be used in combination.

Precautions

In a single case report, a patient with myasthenia gravis had worsening of symptoms after use of pyrantel (87). Although a cause-and-effect relationship was not established, caution should be exercised when prescribing pyrantel to patients with this autoimmune disorder.

Side Effects

Side effects of pyrantel are generally mild and transient and include diarrhea, abdominal pain, nausea, vomiting, and headache. Less common neurological effects such as dizziness, drowsiness, irritability, and insomnia may also occur. In some individuals, skin hypersensitivity reactions such as rash and pruritis have also been reported (83,84). Transient mild elevations in serum hepatic transaminases have been detected in up to 2% of patients after a single dose (84).

Pediatric Dosage

Pyrantel pamoate is supplied as either chewable tablets or an oral suspension (50 mg per mL). Children younger than 2 years and those weighing less than 11 kg (24.2 lb) should not be treated with pyrantel pamoate. For children older than 2 years the maximum daily dosage should not exceed 1 g (46,83).

- *Ascariasis, trichostrongyliasis,* and *enterobiasis:* 11 mg per kg base as a single dose. For enterobiasis, repeat in 2 weeks.
- *Hookworm:* 11 mg per kg base once a day for 3 days.

WHO Recommendation

Pyrantel pamoate is one of the four drugs recommended by the WHO as essential medications for the treatment of soil-transmitted helminthiases. For the treatment of *Ascaris, Trichuris,* and hookworm infections in MDA programs, pyrantel pamoate is given as a single 10 mg per kg dose, regardless of age.

LEVAMISOLE

Levamisole hydrochloride is a synthetic imidazothiazole derivative with both broad-spectrum anthelminthic and immunomodulating activities. It was first marketed as a veterinary anthelminthic in Belgium in 1965 but was licensed for human use in Brazil in 1966. However, the drug was never approved in the United States as an anthelminthic but rather as an adjunct therapy with 5-fluorouracil after surgical resection in patients with Dukes stage C colon cancer. Since it was withdrawn from the market by the manufacturer in 2001, the drug is no longer commercially available in the United States or in many other countries. Nonetheless, it remains one of the four broad-spectrum anthelminthics recommended by the WHO for treatment of intestinal nematodes together with albendazole, mebendazole, and pyrantel pamoate.

Indications

Although no longer available in the United States, levamisole is still commonly used in helminth control programs throughout the world. In several clinical trials conducted in endemic areas, levamisole has been shown to be very effective in treating *A. lumbricoides* and *Trichostrongylus,* although it has shown considerably less activity against hookworm, *T. trichiura, S. stercoralis,* and *E. vermicularis* (55).

Mechanism of Action

Levamisole binds to an ion channel that forms a nicotinic acetylcholine receptor on the body muscle of nematodes (85). Binding to the recognition site of this excitatory receptor induces entry of calcium which in turn leads to depolarization and spastic paralysis of the nematode muscle that can result in passive expulsion of the worm from the host's gastrointestinal tract (86).

Pharmacokinetics

The drug is rapidly and almost completely absorbed from the gastrointestinal tract, after which it is metabolized in the liver and then eliminated in the urine largely as metabolites within 2 days of ingestion (88,89).

Pediatric Considerations

Levamisole has been widely administered as single-dose treatments in global helminth control programs. No specific adverse effects in children have been reported. Levamisole is excreted in breast milk and treatment of nursing mothers is not recommended (90).

Side Effects

When used as a single-dose treatment for nematode infections, levamisole is generally well tolerated. Although blood dyscrasias including agranulocytosis and leukopenia have been reported following prolonged high-dose adjuvant treatment of colon cancer, these have not been observed when used as an anthelminthic. Mostly mild and transient side effects have been reported, including nausea, vomiting, abdominal pain, dizziness, and headache (90,91). However, a rare encephalitic syndrome following single-dose administration has been reported from a large cohort study in China (92).

Pediatric Dosage

Levamisole is supplied as chewable tablets for oral administration: *Ascariasis, Trichostrongylus:* 2.5 mg per kg as a single dose.

ANTIFILARIAL ANTHELMINTHICS

The medications ivermectin and diethylcarbamazine have traditionally formed this class of anthelminthics, although albendazole has been shown to have antifilarial properties and is now used in combination with both of these drugs as part of MDA programs in endemic areas.

IVERMECTIN

Ivermectin is a semisynthetic, oral macrocyclic lactone derived from the avermectins, a class of broad-spectrum antiparasitic agents produced naturally by *Streptomyces avermitilis.* The drug was originally developed as a veterinary product but was approved for human use by the FDA in 1996. Worldwide, it has been used primarily for the treatment of filarial infections: the WHO officially lists ivermectin as a core essential antifilarial drug and recommends its use for the treatment of onchocerciasis, or river blindness. In the United States, the drug is also licensed for the treatment of *S. stercoralis* intestinal infections.

Mechanism of Action

Ivermectin has specific microfilaricidal actions. It binds selectively and with high affinity to glutamate-gated chloride ion channels in invertebrate muscle and nerve cells of the microfilaria. This binding causes an increase in the permeability of the cell membrane to chloride ions and results in hyperpolarization of the cell, leading to paralysis and death of the parasite. It is also believed to act as an agonist of the neurotransmitter gamma-aminobutyric acid, thereby disrupting gamma-aminobutyric acid–mediated neurosynaptic transmission in the CNS (93,94).

Although not macrofilaricidal (i.e., does not kill adult worms), ivermectin may also impair normal intrauterine development of *O. volvulus* microfilariae and may inhibit their release from the uteri of gravid female worms.

Indications

Ivermectin is licensed for the treatment of onchocerciasis and intestinal strongyloidiasis. For the management and control of river blindness caused by *O. volvulus,* it is the drug of choice (13,93,95). The drug has no effect on adult *O. volvulus* worms; rather, the microfilariae are targeted. Since it is the host reaction to microfilaria that results in most of the pathology due to this infection, repeated episodic treatment with ivermectin has been shown to reduce levels of microfilaria in the skin and the cornea and thus prevent morbidity (96). In endemic regions, it is suggested that annual treatment with 150 μg per kg can effectively and drastically reduce the incidence of river blindness (17). Although not licensed for this use, ivermectin is also used for the treatment of several other filarial parasites, including *W. bancrofti, B. malayi, Mansonella ozzardi,* and *L. loa* (13,95,97,98).

Besides onchocerciasis, the other primary indication for ivermectin is in the treatment of strongyloidiasis. Ivermectin has become the treatment of choice for both intestinal and disseminated strongyloidiasis because of the favorable side effect profile compared with thiabendazole, although the manufacturer lists only the nondisseminated form of the infection as an approved indication (68,93,99,100). For uncomplicated disease, treatment for 1 to 2 days is recommended; in the case of immunocompromised patients, treatment should be repeated 2 to 3 weeks after the first course to ensure eradication of the infection. For hyperinfection and/or disseminated infection, daily treatment should be continued until resolution of symptoms and larvae have not been detected in the feces for at least 2 weeks (i.e., the duration of one autoinfection cycle). Some authors recommend continuing ivermectin in individuals with a history of hyperinfection for prolonged periods given the possibility of relapse that has been documented following treatment and apparent clearance of the parasite, especially if a state of immunocompromise continues (101).

Ivermectin has been shown to be highly effective in treating cutaneous larva migrans and is generally considered to be the treatment of choice for this condition (66,102). Single-dose treatment is usually effective, although in some cases, one or two supplemental doses may be necessary. Although not usually used for treating ascariasis, ivermectin does have good activity against this nematode infection although its efficacy for treating hookworm or *T. trichiura* is much poorer (55).

Besides being an effective anthelminthic, single-dose ivermectin is also very effective in treating scabies.

Pharmacokinetics

Ivermectin is absorbed from the gastrointestinal tract into the blood following oral administration and reaches peak plasma levels in 4 hours (93,94,103). It is metabolized by the liver and is excreted in the feces over an estimated period of 12 days, with less than 1% of the dose excreted in the urine. The drug does not cross the blood–brain barrier.

Pediatric Considerations

Given the lack of well-controlled safety and efficacy studies in young children, the use of ivermectin is not recommended in children weighing less than 15 kg (33 lb) (93). Similarly, adequate studies have not been conducted in pregnant women. However, studies of mothers who had been inadvertently treated with ivermectin during pregnancy have reported no significant increase in the rate of spontaneous abortion, stillbirth, or major congenital malformations (104).

Precautions

Some patients who are coinfected with *O. volvulus* and *L. loa* and who have received ivermectin as part of MDA programs have suffered from serious encephalopathy following treatment (105). The etiology of this adverse effect is not well understood, but it has been shown to correlate with the density of *L. loa* microfilaremia (106).

Side Effects

Ivermectin is generally well tolerated. The most common side effects are mild abdominal pain, abdominal distention, nausea, diarrhea, dizziness, and pruritis. When used in the treatment of onchocerciasis, multiple adverse reactions have been reported, although most of these are likely due to the body's reaction to the dying microfilaria than to direct effects of the drug. These are more common in patients with advanced disease and high microfilariae counts in the eye. They include limbitis, punctate opacity, conjunctivitis, and eyelid edema (eye or eyelid irritation, pain, redness, or swelling). These side effects usually resolve without corticosteroid treatment. Other side effects reported during the treatment of onchocerciasis include arthralgia, myalgia, facial and peripheral edema, headache, fever, lymphadenopathy, pruritis, and tachycardia. Many of these side effects can be effectively treated. For instance, systemic corticosteroids may be administered either concurrently with ivermectin or with the onset of severe reactions. Antihistamines and analgesics may also be used to alleviate some of the side effects, which usually peak around the second or third day following ivermectin administration.

Patients taking ivermectin for the treatment of strongyloidiasis and other helminthiases report a different set of side effects, which include diarrhea, dizziness, skin rash, postural hypotension, anorexia, somnolence, and tremor (93).

Pediatric Dosage

Ivermectin is indicated only for children weighing 15 kg (33 lb) or more because of lack of safety information in smaller children. The drug is supplied as oral tablets that should be taken on an empty stomach with liquids.

- *Onchocerciasis:* 150 μg per kg as a single dose; may be repeated every 6 to 12 months, depending on the recurrence of symptoms and/or microfilariae in the skin.
- *Strongyloidiasis:* 200 μg per kg as a single dose. In general, additional doses are not necessary except in select patients with hyperinfection syndrome or disseminated disease. Follow-up fecal examination should be performed to verify clearance of infection.
- *Cutaneous larva migrans:* 200 μg per kg daily for 1 to 2 days.

WHO Recommendation

The WHO recommends community-wide annual or biannual treatment with a single oral dose of ivermectin (150 μg per kg) in regions where onchocerciasis is endemic (17). In areas where lymphatic filariasis is coendemic with onchocerciasis (and therefore diethylcarbamazine is contraindicated), ivermectin should be administered in combination with a single dose of albendazole (17). However, if *L. loa* is coendemic, caution should be exercised and active surveillance for ivermectin-associated encephalopathy should be instituted before initiating MDA campaigns with ivermectin.

DIETHYLCARBAMAZINE

DEC citrate, a synthetic derivative of piperazine, is a highly effective antifilarial drug that has been in use since the 1940s. It is the drug of choice in the treatment of systemic lymphatic filariasis, loiasis, and tropical pulmonary eosinophilia. In contrast to ivermectin, DEC has both macrofilaricidal (against the adult worm) and microfilaricidal (against the larvae) properties (107). Unfortunately, manufacturing and marketing of DEC was discontinued in the United States in 2007 due to the paucity of filariasis cases in this country, in addition to its decreasing use in the veterinary field due to the availability of newer drugs. Although it is not commercially available in the United States, the drug can still be obtained from the Drug Service of the Centers for Disease Control and Prevention on a compassionate use basis.

However, in regions of the world where lymphatic filariasis is endemic such as India, sub-Saharan Africa, and Southeast Asia, DEC is available through the auspices of the WHO for control programs in which annual community-wide single-dose administration has been shown to drastically reduce transmission and over time, the number of filarial-infected individuals in the community. In China, for example, where during the 1950s there were more than 30 million cases of lymphatic filariasis, the widespread use of DEC has resulted in the elimination of transmission.

Indications

DEC remains a mainstay for both the curative and suppressive therapy for systemic lymphatic filariasis caused by *W. bancrofti*, *B. malayi*, and *B. timori* and loiasis caused by *L. loa* (107,108). Although DEC has in the past been used for the treatment of ascariasis, the availability of newer, safer, and more effective anthelminthics has supplanted its use for this indication.

Although administration of multiday courses of DEC can be curative for lymphatic filariasis and loiasis, worldwide the most common use of DEC is in community-wide filariasis control programs in endemic regions, where the goal is suppression of microfilaremia to interrupt the transmission cycle. Once-yearly single-dose administration of the drug, either alone or in combination with albendazole or ivermectin, reduces blood microfilaria levels by greater than 90% for a full year and is highly effective in reducing the number of new infections in these communities over time (109). Although evidence is mixed, some studies have shown an improved effect on microfilaremia when DEC is administered in combination with albendazole over DEC alone, which has led the WHO to recommend this strategy as part of lymphatic filariasis elimination programs (110). Interestingly, in the past, DEC-fortified salt has been used in areas such as parts of China to eliminate lymphatic filariasis, although currently this strategy is not being pursued (111).

Mechanism of Action

DEC has primarily microfilaricidal actions, but it also has some activity against adult *W. bancrofti, B. malayi,* and *B. timori* worms (112). Despite more than 60 years of use, the mechanism of action remains unclear, although it likely involves both direct effects against the worm and indirect effects on the host. Pharmacological studies have shown that DEC interferes with the synthesis of cyclooxygenase products such as prostacyclin and prostaglandin-E2 by microfilariae (113). Recently, evidence has emerged that DEC can induce fragmentation of nuclear DNA in microfilariae, leading to induction of apoptosis. In addition, DEC may alter the host–parasite interface at the level of the immune system by inducing host mechanisms that lead to the degeneration of the parasite (114).

Pharmacokinetics

DEC is rapidly absorbed following oral administration and widely distributed in nonfatty tissues. It undergoes primarily hepatic metabolism to diethylcarbamazine *N*-oxide (115). Peak serum concentrations are reached in 1 to 2 hours and it is excreted, largely as urinary metabolites, within 48 hours.

Pediatric Considerations

Although no specific safety studies of DEC have been performed in children, experience from many years of use in filariasis eradication programs in endemic areas has not indicated any pediatric-specific problems (116,117). Accordingly, the WHO recommends use of DEC as part of lymphatic filariasis control programs in endemic areas in all children older than 2 years (17). Use of DEC in children younger than 2 years is not recommended.

Drug–Drug Interactions

Any substance that alkalinizes the urine, such as sodium bicarbonate, may reduce renal clearance of the drug and its metabolites and therefore increase the incidence of side effects.

Precautions

Renal Impairment

In instances of significant renal impairment (e.g., glomerular filtration rate <50 mL per minute), dose reduction should be considered, although no specific recommendations exist.

Side Effects

DEC is generally well tolerated, although arthralgia, headache, malaise, dizziness, nausea, and vomiting have all been reported. In individuals who are heavily infected, more severe reactions may be observed which are most likely due to a host immunologic reaction to disintegrating worms (118). In the case of lymphatic filariasis, these effects may include fever, myalgia, transient hematuria, urticaria, bronchospasm, transient lymphangitis and lymphadenitis, and exacerbation of lymphedema. In patients with high levels of microfilaremia due to *L. loa,* encephalopathy and retinal hemorrhage may occur following treatment with DEC.

Severe allergic reactions may occur following a single dose of DEC in patients coinfected with *O. volvulus.* Termed the Mazzotti reaction, it is an acute inflammatory response characterized by fever, hypotension, and an ocular reaction that results from the death of microfilariae and can be fatal or cause permanent vision loss. For this reason, treatment with DEC in coinfected patients or in regions endemic for onchocerciasis is contraindicated.

Pediatric Dosage

DEC is supplied as tablets for oral administration. Use in children younger than 2 years is not recommended; *lymphatic filariasis or loiasis*: 1 mg per kg as a single dose on the first day, 3 mg per kg divided into three doses on the second day, 3 to 6 mg per kg divided into three doses on the third day, and then 6 mg per kg per day divided into three doses on days 4 to 14.

WHO Recommendation

For suppression of microfilaremia in MDA programs in regions where lymphatic filariasis is endemic but onchocerciasis is not coendemic, the WHO recommends community-wide annual treatment with a single dose, 6 mg per kg, of DEC orally, in combination with a single dose of albendazole (17).

ANTICESTODE AND ANTITREMATODE ANTHELMINTHICS

PRAZIQUANTEL

Praziquantel is a synthetic isoquinoline–pyrazine derivative that has a broad spectrum of anthelminthic activities. It is effective in the treatment of infections due to all species of *Schistosoma* and most other trematodes (flukes) and cestodes (tapeworms). The drug's safety and effectiveness when administered as a single oral dose have also lent it to easy incorporation into MDA programs for control of several infections but most importantly, for schistosomiasis (17). Because praziquantel is the only medication that is effective against all species of *Schistosoma*, there is growing concern that resistance to praziquantel may develop given its increasing usage (119). Worryingly, there have been reports of low cure rates using praziquantel to treat schistosomiasis in regions of Africa, particularly in Senegal (120), although this finding has been attributed by some authors to the intense transmission in these regions, leading to rapid reinfection with the parasite (121).

Although praziquantel is effective and widely used in treating most trematode and cestode infections, it is *not* effective against *F. hepatica* or in hydatid disease.

Indications

Praziquantel is highly effective in treating most cestode and trematode infections. According to the label, it is indicated for the treatment of infections due to all species of *Schistosoma*, including *Schistosoma mansoni*, *S. haematobium*, *S. mekongi*, *S. japonicum*, and *S. intercalatum*, as well as infections due to the liver flukes *Clonorchis sinensis* (Chinese or Oriental liver fluke) and *Opisthorchis viverrini* (122,123).

Although not listed on the manufacturer's label, there is also wide experience in using praziquantel in the treatment of *Diphyllobothrium latum*, *Dipylidium caninum*, *Hymenolepis nana* (dwarf tapeworm), *Metagonimus yokogawai* (intestinal fluke), *P. westermani* (oriental lung fluke) and other *Paragonimus* species, and taeniasis caused by *T. solium* (pork tapeworm) or *T. saginata* (beef tapeworm) (122,124).

Praziquantel is also one of the first-line treatments for neurocysticercosis. As with albendazole, corticosteroids should be administered concurrently in most cases to control inflammation, edema, and/or other reactions due to dying cysticerci. Praziquantel should not be administered if ocular cysticerci are present because of the risk of permanent loss of vision resulting from the inflammatory response against dying parasites.

In addition, despite its otherwise broad-spectrum anthelminthic effects, praziquantel is not very effective in treating infections caused by *Echinococcus* species or *F. hepatica* (sheep liver fluke).

Mechanism of Action

Although the precise mechanism of action for praziquantel is unknown, studies suggest that the drug increases cell membrane permeability in susceptible worms, which leads to tegumental damage and paralytic muscular contraction, leading to worm death and elimination (125,126). The muscular contraction and paralysis may be due to a specific action on calcium ion channels leading to an influx into the parasite. The anthelminthic effect of praziquantel has been well documented using *S. mansoni* as a model in several studies. After exposure to praziquantel, the tegument in the neck region of adult helminths develops blebs as well as intense vacuolization at several sites that ultimately results in its disintegration, leading to exposure or release of concealed antigens that serve as targets to the host immune system. This is followed by attachment of phagocytes to the parasite and ultimately, death of the worm (125). A functioning host immune system is therefore critical in inducing parasite death.

Praziquantel is manufactured as a 1:1 racemate mixture, with only the levo enantiomer having antischistosomal properties (127). Therefore, half of a praziquantel tablet consists of an inactive ingredient, and recent evidence suggests that the inactive form accounts for the drug's bitter taste (128). To reduce the amount of drug needed to treat infections, the WHO's Special Programme for Research and Training in Tropical Diseases has prioritized the low-cost production of pure levo-praziquantel, although this has not yet been achieved.

Pharmacokinetics

Praziquantel is rapidly absorbed (>75%) from the gastrointestinal tract following oral administration, and absorption is increased if taken with a carbohydrate-rich meal (129). Maximum serum concentrations are achieved between 1 and 3 hours following an oral dose (130). It undergoes extensive first-pass hepatic metabolism mostly into mono- and di-hydroxylated derivatives that lack anthelminthic activity, with only a small amount of active drug reaching the systemic circulation (122,123). Concentrations of the drug in cerebrospinal fluid are between 15% and 20% that in serum. Praziquantel and its metabolites are also found in breast milk at levels approximately 25% those of maternal serum. Elimination is through the kidneys and occurs rapidly, with greater than 70% excreted within 24 hours; small amounts are eliminated in the feces (122).

Pediatric Considerations

Praziquantel has not been found to have adverse effects on fertility or to be teratogenic in animal reproductive toxicity studies conducted in rats and rabbits given up to 300 mg per kg per day (46). In addition, several cases of inadvertent use during pregnancy have not resulted in adverse pregnancy outcomes. However, since no well-controlled studies in pregnant women have been performed, the manufacturer recommends use of praziquantel during pregnancy only if clearly needed (123). Despite this, the WHO has issued a recommendation that, given the morbidity related to schistosomiasis and the beneficial effect of praziquantel treatment, pregnant women with schistosomiasis should be offered treatment (46). In particular, they should not be excluded from MDA programs in regions of high prevalence of schistosomiasis.

Similarly, although the manufacturer recommends withholding nursing on the day of praziquantel treatment and for the subsequent 72 hours because the drug is excreted in breast milk, the WHO regards the use of praziquantel during lactation as safe (46).

Finally, adequate safety studies of praziquantel have not been performed in children younger than 4 years, so use of the drug in this pediatric population is not recommended by the manufacturers (123).

Drug–Drug Interactions

Carbamazepine and Phenytoin
In a small controlled study, it was found that patients taking carbamazepine or phenytoin chronically for seizure disorders attained significantly lower plasma concentrations following a single dose of praziquantel (7.9% and 24% of the control group, respectively) (131). This effect is thought to be due to induction of the cytochrome P-450 microsomal enzyme system by the anticonvulsant medications. Accordingly, patients on carbamazepine or phenytoin may require a larger dose of praziquantel.

Cimetidine
Cimetidine increases the plasma concentration of praziquantel by twofold when the two medications are taken together (132).

Corticosteroids
Concurrent administration of dexamethasone with praziquantel has been shown to reduce praziquantel plasma concentrations by approximately half (133). However, the clinical implications of this finding have not been determined and an increase in the dose of praziquantel when used with corticosteroids to treat neurocysticercosis has not been recommended.

Precautions

Hepatic Dysfunction
In patients with moderate to severe hepatic dysfunction due to chronic *S. mansoni* infection (Child-Pugh class B or C), significant increases in praziquantel half-life and maximum plasma concentrations have been observed (134). Use of praziquantel in this population should be exercised with caution.

Neurocysticercosis
For parenchymal neurocysticercosis with viable cysts, treatment with praziquantel leads to more rapid resolution of cysts and some studies have demonstrated a reduced likelihood of seizures. Treatment of single or few enhancing lesions (i.e., dying cysts) is less clear, although some experts recommend treatment; multiple enhancing lesions generally warrant treatment. However, for patients with only calcified lesions, treatment is not indicated, as the cysts are already dead. The management of ventricular, subarachnoid and spinal cysts is often complicated and may involve surgical resection, placement of ventricular shunts (in the presence of raised intracranial pressure), anticonvulsants, and corticosteroids, with or without specific antiparasitic medication.

If praziquantel is used in the treatment of neurocysticercosis, concurrent administration of a systemic corticosteroid is often recommended, especially if there are multiple cysts, to reduce the inflammatory reaction to dying cysts that may result in seizures or raised intracranial pressure. The use of praziquantel is absolutely contraindicated in the presence of ocular cysticercosis because the destruction of parasites in the eye may result in irreversible loss of vision. A thorough ophthalmologic examination for ocular cysticerci should be conducted before starting treatment with praziquantel.

Side Effects

Praziquantel is generally considered to be a very safe drug. Side effects are usually mild and transient and may include dizziness, drowsiness, headache, and malaise, as well as gastrointestinal effects such as abdominal cramps or pain and loss of appetite, although all of these can also be associated with schistosomiasis, the most common indication for its use. These side effects are more common and may be more severe in patients with heavy worm burdens and likely result from the body's response to the dying worms. Less common side effects include nausea, vomiting, loose stools, urticaria, arthralgia, myalgia, and low-grade fever. The drug has a bitter taste which can make it unpalatable, especially to younger children.

Pediatric Dosage

The use of praziquantel is not recommended in children younger than 4 years due to a lack of adequate safety information in young children (123). The WHO has developed and validated a "dose pole" that calculates the amount of drug to be administered by measurement of a child's height (by having them stand next to it) (135). Tablets of praziquantel should be washed down unchewed with liquids during a meal. If administered in divided doses, intervals of not less than 4 hours and not more than 6 hours should be used.

- *S. haematobium, S. intercalatum,* and *S. mansoni:* 40 mg per kg per day in a single or divided dose, for 1 day.
- *S. japonicum* and *S. mekongi:* 60 mg per kg per day in a single or divided dose, for 1 day.
- *Clonorchiasis* and *opisthorchiasis:* 75 mg per kg per day in three divided doses, for 2 days.
- *Cysticercosis:* 100 mg per kg in three divided doses for 1 day, then 50 mg per kg per day in three divided doses, for 29 days.
- *Fasciolopsis buski, Heterophyes heterophyes, M. yokogawai,* and *Metorchis conjunctus:* 75 mg per kg per day in three divided doses, for 1 day.
- *Paragonimiasis:* 75 mg per kg per day in three divided doses, for 2 days.
- *Tapeworms: D. latum, T. saginata, T. solium,* and *D. caninum:* 10 mg per kg as a single dose.
- *Hymenolepis nana:* 25 mg per kg as a single dose. Heavy infections may require repeated therapy after 10 days.

FUTURE DEVELOPMENTS

Unfortunately, given the fact that helminth infections affect predominantly the rural poor living in the tropics and subtropics (136), investment in developing new anthelminthic medications has been limited, and in fact, several of the existing medications have significant availability problems. Should resistance develop to the currently used medications such as the benzimidazoles in the case of nematode infections or praziquantel in the case of schistosomiasis, the consequences in terms of global health would be devastating given the lack of alternative medications that are active against these parasites.

Several strategies are being developed to either delay or deal with the likelihood of drug resistance developing in helminths. First, the option of using existing anthelminthics in combination—similar to the current strategies targeting treatment of malaria and human immunodeficiency virus infections—is being explored as a strategy for reducing the possibility of resistance developing to any single anthelminthic drug. MDA programs are already administering the combination of DEC or ivermectin with albendazole for the control of lymphatic filariasis (17). Although not currently being used in control programs, studies conducted so far suggest that a combination of mebendazole and levamisole is much more effective than either drug alone against hookworm and *T. trichuris* infections (8,137). Similarly, the combination of ivermectin and albendazole increased the cure rate of *T. trichuris* infections over that of either drug (138). For schistosomiasis, the combination of praziquantel with artemisinins, such as artesunate or artemether that have activity against the early liver stage of infection, is currently being studied, although the evidence so far is inconclusive (139).

Second, although small in number, there are some new drugs that are being developed for use in humans. As with current anthelminthics such as ivermectin and triclabendazole, drugs from the veterinary field are being considered for crossover use in humans. One of the leading such candidates is moxidectin, a macrocyclic lactone of similar structure to ivermectin. Currently registered worldwide to treat canine heartworm and parasitic infections of livestock, moxidectin is now being assessed in clinical trials for the treatment of onchocerciasis (140). Like ivermectin, its exact mechanism of action is unknown but it binds to glutamate-gated chloride channels in the parasites, resulting in muscle contraction, paralysis, and eventual death of the worms. Of note, blood levels of moxidectin are maintained for considerably longer periods of time than ivermectin, so that the possibility exists that it may even have macrofilaricidal effects, although this remains to be demonstrated in clinical trials.

For the intestinal nematodes, the anthelminthic tribendimidine is most likely to be licensed in the near future. Although first developed in the early 1980s in China, where it is currently licensed for human use, it has not been licensed elsewhere and further clinical trials will likely be required before registration can occur outside of China. Tribendimidine is a synthetic derivative of amidantel and has been shown in both animal models and human studies to be highly active against *A. lumbricoides* and hookworm infections due to either *N. americanus* or *A. duodenale*; activity against *T. trichuris* and *E. vermicularis* appears to be less impressive (141). Of interest, efficacy against hookworm infections due to *N. americanus* appears to be improved over that of albendazole. The mechanism of action of this drug is currently unknown.

Lastly, for several reasons, including the possibility of drug resistance developing in existing anthelminthics, the lack of alternative anthelminthics, and the fact that in highly endemic areas, reinfection following treatment occurs frequently and rapidly for several of the helminth infections described in this chapter such as the STHs and schistosomiasis, control measures other than anthelminthic medications are being developed. High on the list of such alternative control tools are new vaccines targeting infections such as hookworm, schistosomiasis, and onchocerciasis (142–144). Hopefully, if widespread drug resistance in these parasites does develop, new vaccines will be ready by the time this occurs.

REFERENCES

1. World Health Organization. Soil-transmitted helminthiasis. Progress report on number of children treated with anthelminthic drugs: an update towards the 2010 global target. *Wkly Epidemiol Rec* 2008;82(27/28):237–252.
2. Bethony J, Brooker S, Albonico M, et al. Soil-transmitted helminth infections: ascariasis, trichuriasis, and hookworm. *Lancet* 2006; 367(9521):1521–1532.
3. McGarvey ST. Schistosomiasis: impact on childhood and adolescent growth, malnutrition, and morbidity. *Semin Pediatr Infect Dis* 2000;11:269–274.
4. de Silva NR. Impact of mass chemotherapy on the morbidity due to soil-transmitted nematodes. *Acta Trop* 2003;86(2–3): 197–214.
5. Drake LJ, Jukes MCH, Sternberg RJ, et al. Geohelminth infections (ascariasis, trichuriasis, and hookworms): cognitive and developmental impacts. *Semin Pediatr Infect Dis* 2000;11: 245–251.
6. Jardim-Botelho A, Raff S, Rodrigues R, et al. Hookworm, *Ascaris lumbricoides* infection and polyparasitism associated with poor cognitive performance in Brazilian schoolchildren. *Trop Med Int Health* 2008;13(8):994–1004.
7. Sur D, Saha DR, Manna B, et al. Periodic deworming with albendazole and its impact on growth status and diarrhoeal incidence among children in an urban slum of India. *Trans R Soc Trop Med Hyg* 2005;99(4):261–267.
8. Albonico M, Bickle Q, Ramsan M, et al. Efficacy of mebendazole and levamisole alone or in combination against intestinal nematode infections after repeated targeted mebendazole treatment in Zanzibar. *Bull World Health Organ* 2003;81(5):343–352.
9. Albonico M, Smith PG, Ercole E, et al. Rate of reinfection with intestinal nematodes after treatment of children with mebendazole or albendazole in a highly endemic area. *Trans R Soc Trop Med Hyg* 1995;89:538–541.
10. Bethony J, Chen JZ, Lin SX, et al. Emerging patterns in hookworm infection: peak prevalence and intensity of Necator infection among the elderly, Hainan Province, Peoples Republic of China. *Clin Infect Dis* 2002;35:1336–1344.
11. Conder GA, Campbell WC. Chemotherapy of nematode infections of veterinary importance, with special reference to drug resistance. *Adv Parasitol* 1995;35:1–84.
12. Utzinger J, Xiao SH, Tanner M, et al. Artemisinins for schistosomiasis and beyond. *Curr Opin Investig Drugs* 2007;8(2):105–116.
13. Hoerauf A. Filariasis: new drugs and new opportunities for lymphatic filariasis and onchocerciasis. *Curr Opin Infect Dis* 2008;21(6): 673–681.
14. Hotez PJ, Wilkins PP. Toxocariasis: America's most common neglected infection of poverty and a helminthiasis of global importance? *PLoS Negl Trop Dis* 2009;3(3):e400.
15. Sharghi N, Schantz PM, Caramico L, et al. Environmental exposure to *Toxocara* as a possible risk factor for asthma: a clinic-based case-control study. *Clin Infect Dis* 2001;32(7):e111–e116.
16. Wallin MT, Kurtzke JF. Neurocysticercosis in the United States: review of an important emerging infection. *Neurology* 2004;63(9): 1559–1564.
17. World Health Organization. *Preventive chemotherapy in human helminthiasis.* Geneva, Switzerland: World Health Organization, 2006.
18. Dayan AD. Albendazole, mebendazole and praziquantel. Review of non-clinical toxicity and pharmacokinetics. *Acta Trop* 2003;86: 141–159.
19. Keystone JS, Murdoch JK. Mebendazole. *Ann Intern Med* 1979; 91(4):582–586.
20. Horton J. Albendazole: a broad spectrum anthelminthic for treatment of individuals and populations. *Curr Opin Infect Dis* 2002;15(6):599–608.

21. GlaxoSmithKline. Albenza (albendazole) prescribing information. Research Triangle Park, NC:GlaxoSmithKline, Inc; Issued: August 2007.
22. The Medical Letter, Inc. Echinococcosis. In: Abramowicz M, ed. *Drugs for parasitic infections*, 1st ed. New Rochelle, NY: The Medical Letter, 2007:53–54.
23. Aygun E, Sahin M, Odev K, et al. The management of liver hydatid cysts by percutaneous drainage. *Can J Surg* 2001;44(3): 203–209.
24. Teggi A, Lastilla MG, DeRosa F. Therapy of human hyatid disease with mebendazole and albendazole. *Antimicrob Agents Chemother* 1993;37(8):1679–1684.
25. Todorov T, Vutova K, Mechkov G, et al. Chemotherapy of human cystic echinococcosis: comparative efficacy of mebendazole and albendazole. *Ann Trop Med Parasitol* 1992;86(1):59–66.
26. Horton RJ. Chemotherapy of echinococcus infection in man with albendazole. *Trans R Soc Trop Med Hyg* 1989;83(1):97–102.
27. Junghanss T, da Silva AM, Horton J, et al. Clinical management of cystic echinococcosis: state of the art, problems, and perspectives. *Am J Trop Med Hyg* 2008;79(3):301–311.
28. Lidove O, Chauveheid MP, Papo T, et al. Echinococcus multilocularis massive pericardial infection: late and dramatic improvement under albendazole therapy. *Am J Med* 2005;118(2): 195–197.
29. Takanayagui OM, Jardim E. Therapy for neurocysticercosis: comparison between albendazole and praziquantel. *Arch Neurol* 1992;49(3):290–294.
30. Del Brutto OH, Sotelo J, Aguirre R, et al. Albendazole therapy for giant subarachnoid cysticerci. *Arch Neurol* 1992;49(5):535–538.
31. Cruz M, Cruz I, Horton J. Clinical evaluation of albendazole and praziquantel in the treatment of cerebral cysticercosis. *Trans R Soc Trop Med Hyg* 1991;85:244–247.
32. Botero D, Uribe CS, Sanchez JL, et al. Short course albendazole treatment for neurocysticercosis in Colombia. *Trans R Soc Trop Med Hyg* 1993;87(5):576–577.
33. García HH, Evans CA, Nash TE, et al. Current consensus guidelines for treatment of neurocysticercosis. *Clin Microbiol Rev* 2002; 15:747–756.
34. Garcia HH, Del Brutto OH. Cysticercosis Working Group in Peru. Neurocysticercosis: updated concepts about an old disease. *Lancet Neurol* 2005;4:653–661.
35. Davies HD, Sakuls P, Keystone JS. Creeping eruption. A review of clinical presentation and management of 60 cases presenting to a tropical disease unit. *Arch Dermatol* 1993;129(5):588–591.
36. St Georgiev V. Chemotherapy of enterobiasis (oxyuriasis). *Expert Opin Pharmacother* 2001;2(2):267–275.
37. Zhong HL, Cao WJ, Rossignol JF, et al. Albendazole in nematode, cestode, trematode and protozoan (Giardia) infections. *Chin Med J (Engl)* 1986;99(11):912–915.
38. de Kaminsky RG. Albendazole treatment in human taeniasis. *Trans R Soc Trop Med Hyg* 1991;85:648–650.
39. Despommier D. Toxocariasis: clinical aspects, epidemiology, medical ecology, and molecular aspects. *Clin Microbiol Rev* 2003;16(2): 265–272.
40. Gottstein B, Pozio E, Nöckler K. Epidemiology, diagnosis, treatment, and control of trichinellosis. *Clin Microbiol Rev* 2009;22(1): 127–145.
41. Reynolds JEF, ed. *Martindale, the extra pharmacopeia*, 29th ed. London: Pharmaceutical Press, 1989:47–48, 57–59.
42. De Rosa F, Teggi A. Treatment of *Echinococcus granulosus* hydatid disease with albendazole. *Ann Trop Med Parasitol* 1990;84(5): 467–472.
43. Liu YH, Wang XG, Gao P, et al. Experimental and clinical trial of albendazole in the treatment of Clonorchiasis sinensis. *Chin Med J (Engl)* 1991;104(1):27–31.
44. Ramalingam S, Sinniah B, Krishnan U. Albendazole, an effective single dose, broad spectrum anthelminthic drug. *Am J Trop Med Hyg* 1982;31(2):263–266.
45. Ndyomugyenyi R, Kabatereine N, Olsen A, et al. Efficacy of ivermectin and albendazole alone and in combination for treatment of soil-transmitted helminths in pregnancy and adverse events: a randomized open label controlled intervention trial in Masindi district, western Uganda. *Am J Trop Med Hyg* 2008;79(6): 856–863.
46. World Health Organization. *Report of the WHO informal consultation on the use of praziquantel during pregnancy/lactation and albendazole/mebendazole in children under 24 months.* Geneva, Switzerland: World Health Organization, 2002.
47. Nagy J, Schipper HG, Koopmans RP, et al. Effect of grapefruit juice or cimetidine coadministration on albendazole bioavailability. *Am J Trop Med Hyg* 2002;66(3):260–263.
48. Takayanagui OM, Lanchote VL, Marques MP, et al. Therapy for neurocysticercosis: pharmacokinetic interaction of albendazole sulfoxide with dexamethasone. *Ther Drug Monit* 1997;19(1): 51–55.
49. Jung H, Hurtado M, Medina MT, et al. Dexamethasone increases plasma levels of albendazole. *J Neurol* 1990;237:279–280.
50. Pene P, Mojon M, Garin JP, et al. Albendazole: a new broad spectrum anthelminthic. Double-blind multi-center clinical trial. *Am J Trop Med Hyg* 1982;31(2):263–266.
51. Macedo NA, Pineyro MI, Carmona C. Contact urticaria and contact dermatitis from albendazole. *Contact Dermatitis* 1991;25(1): 73–75.
52. Rossignol JF, Maisonneuve H. Albendazole: placebo-controlled study in 870 patients with intestinal helminthiasis. *Trans R Soc Trop Med Hyg* 1983;77(5):707–711.
53. Steiger U, Cotting J, Reichen J. Albendazole treatment of echinococcosis in humans: effects on microsomal metabolism and drug tolerance. *Clin Pharmacol Ther* 1990;47(3):347–353.
54. Choi GY, Yang HW, Cho SH, et al. Acute drug-induced hepatitis caused by albendazole. *J Korean Med Sci* 2008;23(5):903–905.
55. Keiser J, Utzinger J. Efficacy of current drugs against soil-transmitted helminth infections: systematic review and meta-analysis. *JAMA* 2008;299(16):1937–1948.
56. Vermox (Janssen). In: *PDR Physician's desk reference*, 49th ed. Montvale, NJ: Medical Economics, 1995:1203–1204.
57. Albonico M, Smith PG, Hall A, et al. A randomized controlled trial comparing mebendazole and albendazole against *Ascaris*, *Trichuris*, and hookworm infections. *Trans R Soc Trop Med Hyg* 1994;88(5):585–589.
58. The Medical Letter, Inc. Capillariasis and gnathostomiasis. In: Abramowicz M, ed. *Drugs for parasitic infections*, 1st ed. New Rochelle, NY: The Medical Letter, 2007:12, 25.
59. Dollery CT. Mebendazole. In: *Therapeutic drugs*, vol 2, 2nd ed. Edinburgh, UK: Churchill Livingstone, 1999:M12–M15.
60. Gyorkos TW, Larocque R, Casapia M, et al. Lack of risk of adverse outcomes after deworming in pregnant women. *Pediatr Infect Dis J* 2006;25:791–794.
61. Montresor A, Awasthi S, Crompton DWT. Use of benzimidazoles in children younger than 24 months for the treatment of soil-transmitted helminthiasis. *Acta Trop* 2003;86:223–232.
62. Luder PJ, Siffert B, Witassek F, et al. Treatment of hydatid disease with high oral doses of mebendazole. *Eur J Clin Pharmacol* 1986;31(4):443–448.
63. Chen KT, Twu SJ, Chang HJ, et al. Outbreak of Stevens–Johnson syndrome/toxic epidermal necrolysis associated with mebendazole and metronidazole use among Filipino laborers in Taiwan. *Am J Public Health* 2003;93(3):489–492.
64. Braithwaite PA, Roberts MS, Allan RJ, et al. Clinical pharmacokinetics of high dose mebendazole in patients treated for cystic hydatid disease. *Eur J Clin Pharmacol* 1982;22:161–169.
65. Merck and Co, Inc. Mintezol (thiabendazole) [package insert]. Whitehouse Station, NJ: Merck and Co, Inc; Issued: June 2003.
66. Heukelbach J, Feldmeier H. Epidemiological and clinical characteristics of hookworm-related cutaneous larva migrans. *Lancet Infect Dis* 2008;8(5):302–309.
67. Igual-Adell R, Oltra-Alcaraz C, Soler-Company E, et al. Efficacy and safety of ivermectin and thiabendazole in the treatment of strongyloidiasis. *Expert Opin Pharmacother* 2004;5(12):2615–2619.
68. Gann PH, Neva FA, Gam AA. A randomized trial of single- and two-dose ivermectin versus thiabendazole for treatment of strongyloidiasis. *J Infect Dis* 1994;169(5):1076–1079.
69. Lim S, Katz K, Krajden S, et al. Complicated and fatal Strongyloides infection in Canadians: risk factors, diagnosis and management. *CMAJ* 2004;171(5):479–484.
70. Watt G, Saisorn S, Jongsakul K, et al. Blinded, placebo-controlled trial of antiparasitic drugs for trichinosis myositis. *J Infect Dis* 2000;182(1):371–374.

71. Sugar AM, Kearns PJ Jr, Haulk AA, et al. Possible thiabendazole-induced theophylline toxicity. *Am Rev Respir Dis* 1980;122(3):501–503.
72. Lew G, Murray WE, Lane JR, et al. Theophylline–thiabendazole drug interaction. *Clin Pharm* 1989;8:225–227.
73. Bauer LA, Raisys VA, Watts MT, et al. The pharmacokinetics of thiabendazole and its metabolites in an anephric patient undergoing hemodialysis and hemoperfusion. *J Clin Pharmacol* 1982;22:276–280.
74. Johnson-Reagan L, Bahna SL. Severe drug rashes in three siblings simultaneously. *Allergy* 2003;58(5):445–447.
75. Bion E, Pariente EA, Maitre F. Severe cholestasis and sicca syndrome after thiabendazole. *J Hepatol* 1995;23(6):762–763.
76. Keiser J, Utzinger J. Food-borne trematodiasis: current chemotherapy and advances with artemisinins and synthetic trioxolanes. *Trends Parasitol* 2007;23(11):555–562.
77. Bennett JL, Kohler P. *Fasciola hepatica*: action in vitro of triclabendazole on immature and adult stages. *Exp Parasitol* 1987;63(1):49–57.
78. Apt W, Aguilera X, Vega F, et al. Treatment of human chronic fascioliasis with triclabendazole: drug efficacy and serologic response. *Am J Trop Med Hyg* 1995;52:532–535.
79. Keiser J, Engels D, Büscher G, Utzinger J. Triclabendazole for the treatment of fascioliasis and paragonimiasis. *Expert Opin Investig Drugs* 2005;14(12):1513–1526.
80. Calvopiña M, Guderian RH, Paredes W, et al. Comparison of two single-day regimens of triclabendazole for the treatment of human pulmonary paragonimiasis. *Trans R Soc Trop Med Hyg* 2003;97(4):451–454.
81. Fairweather I. Triclabendazole: new skills to unravel an old(ish) enigma. *J Helminthol* 2005;79(3):227–234.
82. Belgraier AH. Common bile duct obstruction due to *Fasciola hepatica*. *N Y State J Med* 1976;76:936–937.
83. Product Information: Combantrin (pyrantel pamoate), Pfizer Canada, Quebec, Canada. In: Repchinkski C, ed. *Compendium of pharmaceuticals and specialties*, 36th ed. Ottawa, Canada: Canadian Pharmacists Association, 2001:336–337.
84. Pitts NE, Migliardi JR. Antiminth (pyrantel pamoate). *Clin Pediatr (Phila)* 1974;13(1):87–94.
85. Köhler P. The biochemical basis of anthelmintic action and resistance. *Int J Parasitol* 2001;31(4):336–345.
86. Martin RJ, Robertson AP. Mode of action of levamisole and pyrantel, anthelmintic resistance, E153 and Q57. *Parasitology* 2007;134(pt 8):1093–1104.
87. Bescansa E, Nicolas M, Aguado C, et al. Myasthenia gravis aggravated by pyrantel pamoate. *J Neurol Neurosurg Psychiatry* 1991;54(6):563.
88. Renoux G. The general immunopharmacology of levamisole. *Drugs* 1980;19:89–99.
89. Kouassi E, Caillé G, Léry L, et al. Novel assay and pharmacokinetics of levamisole and p-hydroxylevamisole in human plasma and urine. *Biopharm Drug Dispos* 1986;7(1):71–89.
90. World Health Organization. Levamisole. *WHO essential medicines library*. http://apps.who.int/emlib/MedicineDisplay.aspx?Language=EN&MedIDName=384%40levamisole. Accessed May 27, 2009.
91. Awadzi K, Edwards G, Opoku NO, et al. The safety, tolerability and pharmacokinetics of levamisole alone, levamisole plus ivermectin, and levamisole plus albendazole, and their efficacy against *Onchocerca volvulus*. *Ann Trop Med Parasitol* 2004;98(6):595–614.
92. Zheng RY, Jiang ZC, Zhang X. Relationship between levamisole and encephalitis syndrome. *Zhonghua Nei Ke Za Zhi* 1992;31(9):530–532, 585.
93. Merck and Co, Inc. Stromectol (ivermectin) [package insert]. Whitehouse Station, NJ: Merck and Co, Inc; Issued: February 2009.
94. Gyatt H, de Silva N, Bundy D. Anthelminthics: a comparative review of their clinical pharmacology. *Drugs* 1997;53(5):769–788.
95. Udall DN. Recent updates on onchocerciasis: diagnosis and treatment. *Clin Infect Dis* 2007;44(1):53–60.
96. Boussinesq M, Chippaux JP, Ernould JC, et al. Effect of repeated treatments with ivermectin on the incidence of onchocerciasis in northern Cameroon. *Am J Trop Med Hyg* 1995;53:63–67.
97. Kumaraswami V, Ottesen EA, Vijayasekaran V, et al. Ivermectin for the treatment of *Wuchereria bancrofti* filariasis. Efficacy and adverse reactions. *JAMA* 1988;259(21):3150–3153.
98. Ottesen EA, Vijayasekaran V, Kumaraswami V, et al. A controlled trial of ivermectin and diethylcarbamazine in lymphatic filariasis. *N Engl J Med* 1990;322(16):1113–1117.
99. Marti H, Haji HJ, Savioli L, et al. A comparative trial of a single-dose ivermectin versus three days of albendazole for treatment of *Strongyloides stercoralis* and other soil-transmitted helminth infections in children. *Am J Trop Med Hyg* 1996;55(5):477–481.
100. Torres JR, Isturiz R, Murillo J, et al. Efficacy of ivermectin in the treatment of strongyloidiasis complicating AIDS. *Clin Infect Dis* 1993;17(5):900–902.
101. Keiser PB, Nutman TB. *Strongyloides stercoralis* in the immunocompromised population. *Clin Microbiol Rev* 2004;17(1):208–217.
102. Bouchaud O, Houzé S, Schiemann R, et al. Cutaneous larva migrans in travelers: a prospective study, with assessment of therapy with ivermectin. *Clin Infect Dis* 2000;31(2):493–498.
103. Edwards G, Dingsdale A, Helsby N, et al. The relative systemic availability of ivermectin after administration as capsule, tablet, and oral solution. *Eur J Clin Pharmacol* 1988;35:681–684.
104. Gyapong JO, Chinbuah MA, Gyapong M. Inadvertent exposure of pregnant women to ivermectin and albendazole during mass drug administration for lymphatic filariasis. *Trop Med Int Health* 2003;8(12):1093–1101.
105. Scientific Working Group on Serious Adverse Events in *Loa loa* endemic areas. Report of a Scientific Working Group on Serious Adverse Events following Mectizan(R) treatment of onchocerciasis in *Loa loa* endemic areas. *Filaria J* 2003;2(Suppl 1):S2.
106. Gardon J, Gardon-Wendel N, Demanga-Ngangue, et al. Serious reactions after mass treatment of onchocerciasis with ivermectin in an area endemic for *Loa loa* infection. *Lancet* 1997;350(9070):18–22.
107. Ottesen EA. Lymphatic filariasis: treatment, control and elimination. *Adv Parasitol* 2006;61:395–441.
108. Partono F, Purnomo Oemijati S, Soewarta A. The long term effects of repeated diethylcarbamazine administration with special reference to microfilaraemia and elephantiasis. *Acta Trop* 1981;38:217–225.
109. Ottesen EA, Duke BO, Karam M, et al. Strategies and tools for the control/elimination of lymphatic filariasis. *Bull World Health Organ* 1997;75(6):491–503.
110. Critchley J, Addiss D, Gamble C, et al. Albendazole for lymphatic filariasis. *Cochrane Database Syst Rev* 2005;(4):CD003753.
111. Gelband H. Diethylcarbamazine salt in the control of lymphatic filariasis. *Am J Trop Med Hyg* 1994;50(6):655–662.
112. Noroes J, Dreyer G, Santos A, et al. Assessment of the efficacy of diethylcarbamazine on adult *Wuchereria bancrofti* in vivo. *Trans R Soc Trop Med Hyg* 1997;9(1):78–81.
113. Kanesa-thasan N, Douglas JG, Kazura JW. Diethylcarbamazine inhibits endothelial and microfilarial prostanoid metabolism in vitro. *Mol Biochem Parasitol* 1991;49(1):11–19.
114. Maizels RM, Denham DA. Diethylcarbamazine (DEC): immunopharmacological interactions of an anti-filarial drug. *Parasitology* 1992;105(Suppl):S49–S60.
115. Edwards G, Awadzi K, Breckenridge AM, et al. Diethylcarbamazine disposition in patients with onchocerciasis. *Clin Pharmacol Ther* 1981;30(4):551–557.
116. Pani S, Subramanyam Reddy G, Das L, et al. Tolerability and efficacy of single dose albendazole, diethylcarbamazine citrate (DEC) or co-administration of albendazole with DEC in the clearance of *Wuchereria bancrofti* in asymptomatic microfilaraemic volunteers in Pondicherry, South India: a hospital-based study. *Filaria J* 2002;1(1):1.
117. Fox LM, Furness BW, Haser JK, et al. Tolerance and efficacy of combined diethylcarbamazine and albendazole for treatment of *Wuchereria bancrofti* and intestinal helminth infections in Haitian children. *Am J Trop Med Hyg* 2005;73(1):115–121.
118. Addiss D, Dreyer G. Treatment of lymphatic filariasis. In: Nutman BT, ed. *Lymphatic filariasis*. London, UK: Imperial College Press, 2000:151–199.
119. Doenhoff MJ, Cioli D, Utzinger J. Praziquantel: mechanisms of action, resistance and new derivatives for schistosomiasis. *Curr Opin Infect Dis* 2008;21(6):659–667.

120. Gryseels B, Mbaye A, De Vlas SJ, et al. Are poor responses to praziquantel for the treatment of *Schistosoma mansoni* infections in Senegal due to resistance? An overview of the evidence. *Trop Med Int Health* 2001;6(11):864–873.
121. King CH, Muchiri EM, Ouma JH. Evidence against rapid emergence of praziquantel resistance in *Schistosoma haematobium,* Kenya. *Emerg Infect Dis* 2001;7(6):1069–1070.
122. King CH, Mahmoud AAF. Drugs five years later: praziquantel. *Ann Intern Med* 1989;110(4):290–296.
123. Bayer Healthcare. Biltricide (praziquantel) [package insert]. Wayne, NJ: Bayer Healthcare; Issued: August 2007.
124. The Medical Letter, Inc. Tapeworm infection. In: Abramowicz M, ed. *Drugs for parasitic infections,* 1st ed. New Rochelle, NY: The Medical Letter, 2007:53–54.
125. Brindley PJ, Sher A. The chemotherapeutic effect of praziquantel against *Schistosoma mansoni* is dependent on host antibody response. *J Immunol* 1987;139:215–220.
126. Dollery CT. Praziquantel. In: *Therapeutic drugs,* vol 2, 2nd ed. Edinburgh, UK: Churchill Livingstone, 1999:184–188.
127. Fenwick A, Savioli L, Engels D, et al. Drugs for the control of parasitic diseases: current status and development in schistosomiasis. *Trends Parasitol* 2003;19(11):509–515.
128. Meyer T, Sekljic H, Fuchs S, et al. Taste, a new incentive to switch to (R)-praziquantel in schistosomiasis treatment. *PLoS Negl Trop Dis* 2009;3(1):e357.
129. Mandour ME, el Turabi H, Homeida MM, et al. Pharmacokinetics of praziquantel in healthy volunteers and patients with schistosomiasis. *Trans R Soc Trop Med Hyg* 1990;84(3):389–393.
130. Watt G, White NJ, Padre L, et al. Praziquantel pharmacokinetics and side effects in *Schistosoma japonicum*-infected patients with liver disease. *J Infect Dis* 1988;157(3):530–535.
131. Bittencourt PR, Gracia CM, Martins R, et al. Phenytoin and carbamazepine decrease oral bioavailability of praziquantel. *Neurology* 1992;42:492–496.
132. Jung H, Medina R, Castro N, et al. Pharmacokinetic study of praziquantel administered alone and in combination with cimetidine in a single-day therapeutic regimen. *Antimicrob Agents Chemother* 1997;41:1256–1259.
133. Vazquez ML, Jung H, Sotelo J. Plasma levels of praziquantel decrease when dexamethasone is given simultaneously. *Neurology* 1987;37:1561–1562.
134. el Guiniady MA, el Touny MA, Abdel-Bary MA, et al. Clinical and pharmacokinetic study of praziquantel in Egyptian schistosomiasis patients with and without liver cell failure. *Am J Trop Med Hyg* 1994;51(6):809–818.
135. Montresor A, Odermatt P, Muth S, et al. The WHO dose pole for the administration of praziquantel is also accurate in non-African populations. *Trans R Soc Trop Med Hyg* 2005;99(1):78–81.
136. Hotez PJ, Fenwick A, Savioli L, et al. Rescuing the bottom billion through control of neglected tropical diseases. *Lancet* 2009; 373(9674):1570–1575.
137. Zu LQ, Jiang ZX, Yu SH, et al. Treatment of soil-transmitted helminth infections by anthelmintics in current use. *Zhongguo Ji Sheng Chong Xue Yu Ji Sheng Chong Bing Za Zhi* 1992;10(2): 95–99.
138. Olsen A. Efficacy and safety of drug combinations in the treatment of schistosomiasis, soil-transmitted helminthiasis, lymphatic filariasis and onchocerciasis. *Trans R Soc Trop Med Hyg* 2007;101(8): 747–758.
139. Danso-Appiah A, Utzinger J, Liu J, et al. Drugs for treating urinary schistosomiasis. *Cochrane Database Syst Rev* 2008;(3): CD000053.
140. Cotreau MM, Warren S, Ryan JL, et al. The antiparasitic moxidectin: safety, tolerability, and pharmacokinetics in humans. *J Clin Pharmacol* 2003;43(10):1108–1115.
141. Xiao SH, Hui-Ming W, Tanner M, et al. Tribendimidine: a promising, safe and broad-spectrum anthelmintic agent from China. *Acta Trop* 2005;94(1):1–14.
142. Diemert DJ, Bethony JM, Hotez PJ. Hookworm vaccines. *Clin Infect Dis* 2008;46:282–288.
143. Hotez PJ, Bethony JM, Oliveira SC, et al. Multivalent anthelminthic vaccine to prevent hookworm and schistosomiasis. *Expert Rev Vaccines* 2008;7(6):745–752.
144. Lustigman S, James ER, Tawe W, et al. Towards a recombinant antigen vaccine against *Onchocerca volvulus. Trends Parasitol* 2002; 18(3):135–141.

CHAPTER

34

Alexander O. Tuazon
Cecilia C. Maramba-Lazarte

Antituberculosis Drugs

Tuberculosis remains a major global health problem, though the incidence per capita, prevalence, and death rates for tuberculosis are falling. Current challenges include the difficulty in correctly prescribing and adhering to complex and lengthy treatment protocols, emergence of *Mycobacterium tuberculosis* strains resistant to multiple drugs, and human immunodeficiency virus (HIV) infection (1). An estimated 1.7 million died due to tuberculosis in 2006. Of an estimated 14.4 million prevalent cases in the same year, 9.2 million or 64% were new cases of which 8% were HIV-positive (2). Of new cases, about 11% occur in children younger than 15 years, with countries reporting 3% to 25% of all cases (3).

Children are commonly infected through exposure to an infectious adult. The majority of infected children remain well and the only evidence of infection may be a positive tuberculin skin test, termed latent tuberculosis infection (LTBI). Progression to disease usually occurs within 2 years following exposure and infection. Infants and children younger than 5 years and the immunocompromised are at particular risk of developing disease. A small proportion of children, who are generally older, develop postprimary tuberculosis either due to reactivation or by reinfection (3,4).

Childhood tuberculosis is usually extrapulmonary in location. Severe and disseminated tuberculosis, such as tuberculous meningitis and miliary tuberculosis, may occasionally occur especially in children younger than 3 years (3). It is commonly primary, which has a much smaller bacterial load than adult-type tuberculosis with cavitation and sputum production. Bacterial confirmation of tuberculosis therefore will be difficult in children, and the choice of drugs will usually depend on results from the index case. On the other hand, failure, relapse, and development of resistance to antituberculosis drugs are of lesser concern (3,5,6).

Management guidelines are available (Table 34.1) for both resource-poor (3,5) and affluent areas (6). Central to these recommendations are short-course drug regimens administered by directly observed therapy (DOT), which involves providing the antituberculosis drugs directly to the patient and watching as he or she swallows the medications. While bacillary load and the type of disease may influence the effectiveness of treatment regimens, treatment outcomes in children are generally good, even in young and immunocompromised children, provided that treatment starts promptly. There is a low risk of adverse events associated with use of the recommended treatment regimens (3).

For LTBI in children, isoniazid administered for 6 to 12 months is the preferred treatment. It has also been shown to be effective as prophylaxis (7,8) but poor adherence is observed, especially with unsupervised treatment (9–11). An alternative treatment regimen of 3 to 4 months isoniazid plus rifampicin for the treatment of LTBI showed similar efficacy to 9 months isoniazid treatment with improved adherence (11,12). On the other hand, preventive therapy with rifampicin plus pyrazinamide causes severe hepatotoxicity and should generally not be offered to treat LTBI (13–16).

For an asymptomatic infant born into a household with an infectious tuberculosis patient, daily isoniazid is administered for 6 months or up to at least 3 months following cessation of relevant exposure, at which time a tuberculin test is done. If the tuberculin test is positive, treatment is continued as for LTBI, otherwise if the test is negative isoniazid is discontinued. Prophylactic treatment should be adjusted if the index case has a drug-resistant strain.

The principles of treatment of tuberculosis disease in infants and children are similar to that in adults, while keeping in mind pharmacokinetic differences and possibility of adverse effects (3,6,17,18). Published studies of treatment of children with tuberculosis (19–31) caused by organisms known or presumed to be susceptible to the first-line drugs have shown excellent results for pulmonary and lymph node tuberculosis, but less so for meningitis. For tuberculous meningitis, the higher end of the daily doses is recommended. Also, recent pharmacokinetic studies of isoniazid, pyrazinamide, and ethambutol have shown lower plasma drug levels in children than in adults suggesting that dosages per kilogram body weight need to be higher for children (32–34).

Short-course treatments are administered in two phases. An initial intensive phase, typically 2 months, employs a combination of drugs that is effective in rapidly eliminating the organism and in minimizing the chance for the development of resistance. Four drugs, usually isoniazid, rifampicin, pyrazinamide and ethambutol, are recommended when there is

TABLE 34.1 Recommended Treatment Regimens for Tuberculosis in Children

	WHO (3)		*IUALTD (5)*		*ATS/CDC/IDSA (6)*	
Clinical Presentation	*Intensive Phase*	*Continuation Phase*	*Intensive Phase*	*Continuation Phase*	*Intensive Phase*	*Continuation Phase*
New smear (+) PTB	2HRZE	4HR or 6HE	2HRZE 2 HRZE	4HR or 4(HR) 3 or 2 6TH or 6HE	2HRZE or 2(HRZE)5 2w(HRZE)7 or 5 then 6w (HRZE)2 2(HRZE)3 2HRE or 2(HRE)5	4HR or 4(HR)5 4HR 2× weekly for 6 wk 4(HR)3 7HR or 7(HR)5
New smear (−) w/extensive parenchymal involvement	2HRZE	4HR or 6HE	2HRZE	4HR or 4(HR) 3 or 2	2HRZE	4HR
New severe EPTB (disseminated, pericardiac, bone, abdominal, spinal)	2HRZE	4HR or 6HE	2HRZE	4HR or 4(HR) 3 or 2	2HRZE	4–7HR
TB meningitis	2HRZS	4HR	2HRZE	4HR or 4(HR) 3 or 2	2HRZE	7–10HR
New smear (−) pulmonary TB (primary)	2HRZ	4HR	2HRZE (?)	4HR or 4(HR) 3 or 2	2HRZ	4HR
Previously treated smear (+) TB (relapse, treatment after interruption, treatment failure)	2HRZES/ 1HRZE	5HRE	2 HRZES/ 1HRZE[a] (daily)	5HRE[a] (3× weekly)	Combined HRZE< FQ, IA (with or without another second-line drug)[a]	
MDR-TB	Individualized regimen[a]		None		Individualized regimen[a]	

ATS, American Thoracic Society; CDC, Centers for Disease Control and Prevention; E, ethambutol; EPTB, extrapulmonary tuberculosis; FQ, fluoroquinolone; H, isoniazid; IA, injectable agent (streptomycin, kanamycin, amikacin); IDSA, Infectious Diseases Society of America; IUATLD, International Union Against Tuberculosis and Lung Diseases; MDR-TB, multidrug-resistant tuberculosis; PTB, pulmonary tuberculosis; R, rifampicin; S, streptomycin; T, thioacetazone; WHO, World Health Organization; Z, pyrazinamide.
The number before a phase is the duration in months (w, weeks). A number after a letter is the number of doses per week. If there is no number after a letter, then treatment with that drug is daily. Note: 5 days DOT = daily.
[a]Treatment is expert-supervised; susceptibility-guided DOT, directly observed therapy.

risk of resistance, or when children and adolescents develop adult-type pulmonary tuberculosis. However, when the infecting strain is fully susceptible, or the likelihood of failure is low as in primary tuberculosis commonly seen in children, an initial phase combination of isoniazid, rifampicin, and pyrazinamide may be used (6). In the subsequent continuation phase, less number of drugs are administered but for at least 4 months to ensure that the patient is completely cured and does not relapse after completion of therapy (5,35,36).

Children with HIV infection and confirmed or presumptive tuberculosis disease are treated with the 6-month regimen with good response as in HIV-uninfected children. Cotrimoxazole as prophylaxis for other infections is administered and initiation of antiretroviral therapy should be carefully evaluated. Tuberculosis treatment failure can be due to noncompliance with therapy, poor drug absorption, drug resistance, and alternative diagnoses (3).

Resistance to isoniazid and/or rifampicin is the most important, as these two drugs form the mainstay of current chemotherapy. For cases with monoresistance to isoniazid, ethambutol is added to the intensive phase. For patients with more extensive disease, consideration should be given to the addition of a fluoroquinolone and to prolonging treatment to a minimum of 9 months. Monoresistance to rifampicin should be treated with isoniazid, ethambutol, and a fluoroquinolone for at least 12 to 18 months, with the addition of pyrazinamide for at least the first 2 months (3).

Multidrug resistant tuberculosis (MDR-TB) is resistant to at least both isoniazid and rifampicin and accounts for 4.3% of all tuberculosis cases (37). Mainly transmitted from an adult source case with MDR-TB, it is often not suspected unless a history of contact with an adult case is known. Children with MDR-TB should be treated with at least four drugs to which the bacterial strain, or that of its source case, is susceptible. Treatment should be given daily and preferably under DOT. Duration of treatment is usually 18 months or more. With correct dosing, few long-term adverse events are seen with any of the more toxic second-line drugs in children. Treatment, however, is difficult and a referral to a specialist is advised (3).

ISONIAZID

Isoniazid, a hydrazide derivative of isonicotinic acid, is the most widely used first-line drug for tuberculosis. Isoniazid inhibits synthesis of long-chain mycolic acids, which are constituents of mycobacterial cell walls. It has the most potent early bactericidal activity against actively dividing *M. tuberculosis* (17) but is bacteriostatic against nondividing tubercle bacilli. Isoniazid-resistant strains demonstrate a reduced catalase-peroxidase activity, which has been associated with deletions or point mutations in the *katG* gene (38–40).

Isoniazid as single-drug therapy is indicated only for the prophylaxis of contacts of sputum smear-positive or culture-positive tuberculosis cases and for the treatment of LTBI. It is used in combination with other drugs for active disease (Table 34.1). In both, susceptibility of the bacilli to isoniazid should be established or confidently assumed. Isoniazid is administered orally at 5 mg per kg (range 4 to 15 mg per kg, maximum 300 mg) daily (3,5,6), or intermittently at 10 mg per kg (range 8 to 12 mg per kg) thrice weekly (3,5), or 20 to 30 mg per kg (maximum 900 mg) twice weekly (6). It may be administered intramuscularly.

EFFICACY DATA IN CHILDREN

In children who received isoniazid prophylaxis for 6 months, only 1.9% developed active tuberculosis within a 10-year follow-up period (7). In another study, development of active disease was low among tuberculin-positive children who received isoniazid. A morbidity rate of 4.2 per 1,000 children was observed after a mean observation period of 6.1 years (41). Efficacy studies of isoniazid combined with other first-line drugs in short-course treatments in children with active tuberculosis showed excellent results approaching at least 95% efficacy in pulmonary and lymph node tuberculosis (19–28). The efficacy against tuberculous meningitis, however, is less, with increased mortality and sequelae for survivors (29–31).

The pharmacokinetic profile is dependent on N-acetylation capacity, which is trimodally distributed into slow, intermediate, or rapid phenotypes in accordance with the genotype of the polymorphic *N*-acetyltransferase (42,43). Peoples of European origin are predominantly slow acetylators, whereas Asian peoples are predominantly rapid acetylators (44,45). The lower plasma concentration seen in rapid acetylators becomes significant only in a once weekly dosing regimen, where a poorer response is observed (44).

Absorption of isoniazid is rapid and complete but is reduced by food. The effect of antacids on absorption is less clear (46–48). Peak plasma concentrations are reached in 1 to 2 hours (18,46–48). Isoniazid is distributed in all body fluids and tissues, (18,49,50), with excellent penetration into the cerebrospinal fluid (CSF) (51–53). The apparent volume of distribution is 0.62 to 0.83 L per kg with no significant difference between slow and rapid acetylators (54).

Isoniazid undergoes extensive presystemic metabolism. Isoniazid is acetylated by the liver to metabolites, which are excreted in the urine. Acetylisoniazid is further hydrolyzed to isonicotinic acid and monoacetylhydrazine. Isonicotinic acid is conjugated with glycine to form isonicotinylglycine, whereas monoacetylhydrazine is further acetylated to diacetylhydrazine. All metabolites are essentially devoid of antituberculosis activity. Hepatotoxicity is associated with an incompletely acetylated hydrazide group found in monoacetylhydrazine and isoniazid (44).

Half-life in adults is 0.7 to 2 hours for rapid acetylators and 2.3 to 3.5 hours for slow acetylators (44,48,55). Isoniazid is largely excreted in the urine within 24 hours, mostly as inactive metabolites. Renal excretion is independent of acetylator status.

PHARMACOKINETIC DATA IN CHILDREN

Isoniazid levels expected in children is basically similar to adults. Excellent penetration into the CSF of children with tuberculous meningitis has been demonstrated (53). A trimodal pharmacokinetic profile is also evident in children. Clearance is 3.83 and 6.88 mL per minute per kg and half-life is 2.91 and 1.36 hours in slow and rapid acetylators, respectively. Apparent volume of distribution is 0.83 L per kg, and as in adults is not affected by acetylator phenotype (54). Younger children eliminate isoniazid faster than older children in all three genotypes. As a group, children eliminate isoniazid faster and achieve significantly less serum concentrations than adults who receive the same milligram per kilogram body weight dose. An isoniazid dose of at least 10 mg per kg might be more appropriate to rapid acetylators to achieve the recommended serum concentration of 1.5 mg per L (32).

Genetically slow acetylators are more at risk for various isoniazid-related toxicities. Acute poisoning is associated with significant toxicity and mortality, with slow acetylators at risk. Nausea, vomiting, hypotension, leukocytosis, hyperpyrexia, respiratory distress, seizures, and coma are seen in children. Metabolic acidosis, ketonuria, hyperglycemia, mild hyperkalemia, increased urinary excretion of pyridoxine, impaired liver function, and rhabdomyolysis have been observed (56–60).

The induction of seizures by isoniazid has been attributed to its lowering effect on pyridoxine levels, which may affect formation and catabolism of gamma-aminobutyric acid. Gram-for-gram treatment with vitamin B_6 is recommended, and high-dose intravenous pyridoxine terminates seizures and may awake patients from coma (57,61). Niacinamide has also been shown to be effective in reversing isoniazid-induced hyperkinesis, suggesting interference by isoniazid of nicotinamide adenine dinucleotide–catalyzed reactions (56).

Dose-dependent peripheral neuropathies occur more in slow acetylators (62). It is uncommon and rare in children, except in malnourished patients whose vitamin B_6 deficiency may result from or be aggravated by loss of pyridoxal hydrazone of isoniazid. Symptoms include tingling, numbness, tenderness, weakness, and stiffness in the extremities. It can be prevented by daily administration of supplementary vitamin B_6 (18,63).

There is an appreciable but low risk of hepatotoxicity with isoniazid at current recommended dosing regimens. Elevations of liver enzymes are usually transient and normalize with continued therapy. Slow acetylators are possibly at increased risk (45).

HEPATOTOXICITY IN CHILDREN

Asymptomatic liver dysfunction to frank liver disease can occur with isoniazid administration in children. Risk factors include severe tuberculous disease, higher isoniazid doses, and coadministration with rifampicin. With isoniazid alone, the occurrence is 0.18% to 0.5%, which is much less common than in adults (64–67).

Reported hematologic adverse effects include agranulocytosis, hemolytic anemia, sideroblastic anemia, aplastic anemia, thrombocytopenia, eosinophilia, red cell aplasia, and disseminated intravascular coagulation (68–70). Anorexia and nausea (69), gynecomastia (71), hyperthermia (72), pancreatitis (73,74), rheumatoid-like and lupus-like arthritis (69), and rhabdomyolysis (59,60) have been reported. Dermatologic side effects and hypersensitivity are uncommon (25,69).

Caution must be observed in the presence of liver disease and regular monitoring of liver enzymes is recommended. A full dose may still be given in impaired renal function (75). Isoniazid may increase pyridoxine requirements in children (63,76). Serum vitamin D concentrations are low when isoniazid is taken but rise to normal after discontinuance of isoniazid (77–79).

Isoniazid inhibits microsomal enzymes. Metabolism may thus be impaired leading to increased serum concentration and potentiation of the effects of warfarin, theophylline, triazolam (17), diazepam (80), and antiepileptics such as carbamazepine (81), phenytoin (82,83), and valproic acid (84). On the other hand, concomitant administration of isoniazid leads to decreased effectiveness of methoxyflurane, isoflurane, sevoflurane, and enflurane (85).

Concentrations of isoniazid increase with concomitant administration of aminosalicylic acid (17) or ethionamide (46), which may lead to toxic manifestations. On the other hand, its concentration decreases with antacid (47), prednisone, and prednisolone (17). Isoniazid may act as a monoamine oxidase inhibitor and may lead to excessive responses to pressor amines (17,86). Increased risk of hepatotoxicity has been observed with administration of isoniazid with paracetamol (17) and rifampicin.

Isoniazid is readily transmitted across the placenta but is not associated with a detectable increase in birth defects (87). It is excreted in breast milk, but the reported relative infant dose, about 1.2% of the weight adjusted maternal dose, is below the 10% notional level of concern for nursing infants (50,88).

RIFAMPICIN

Rifampicin (rifampin) is a semisynthetic derivative of the natural antibiotic rifamycin B and belongs to the class of naphthalenic rifamycins (17,89). It has a wide spectrum of activity against bacteria, including some strains of atypical mycobacteria. Only its role in the treatment of tuberculosis will be discussed.

Rifampicin binds to the β-subunit of bacterial RNA polymerase, thereby inhibiting transcription of DNA to RNA. It specifically inhibits transition from synthesis of short oligoribonucleotides to full-length transcripts. Rifampicin is bactericidal for both intracellular and extracellular mycobacteria (18). Bacilli dormant much of the time but occasionally metabolizing for short periods are killed more rapidly by rifampicin than by isoniazid during short-course chemotherapy (90). Most resistant isolates have missense mutations, deletions, or insertions within the region of the RNA polymerase β-subunit gene (*rpoB*) (91,92).

Rifampicin is rapidly and completely absorbed from the gastrointestinal tract, though the suspension is only 50% absorbed by pediatric patients (93). Food may delay and reduce peak serum concentrations (89,94). The bentonite excipient in certain *p*-aminosalicylic acid preparations may impede gastrointestinal absorption of rifampicin (89,95). Peak concentrations of 4 to 32 μg per mL are reached in 1 to 4 hours (46,47), well above levels for tuberculosis.

Rifampicin distributes widely, including exudates in tuberculous lung cavities, bronchial secretions, and alveolar macrophages (89,96). Protein binding is 70% to 75% and the volume of distribution is 55 L (46). CSF penetration is slow (51), but therapeutic levels may be achieved with inflamed meninges (52,97). There is little presystemic metabolism, but repeated administration induces hepatic endoplasmic reticular enzymes, with consequent reduction in serum half-life and area under the curve (89).

Rifampicin is desacetylated to a biologically active metabolite, 25-*O*-desacetylrifampicin, and hydrolyzed to 3-formylrifamycin. Part of rifampicin may be conjugated with glucuronic acid during hepatic metabolism. Desacetylrifampicin is a more polar compound with increased capacity for biliary excretion. Unchanged rifampicin is reabsorbed, creating enterohepatic circulation, whereas 25-*O*-desacetylrifampicin is poorly absorbed, facilitating elimination. Enzyme induction increases the metabolism of rifampicin and the biliary excretion of desacetylrifampicin (89).

Dose-dependent half-life is 2.3 to 5.1 hours but decreases subsequently to 2 to 3 hours because of increased hepatic metabolism (46,48,89). The principal excretion pathway is bile, with urine as secondary pathway. Urinary concentration increases with doses above 450 mg, when biliary excretion is more saturated. Impaired hepatic function or biliary excretion, but not impaired renal function, may require modification of dosage and careful monitoring.

PHARMACOKINETIC DATA IN CHILDREN

In children older than 1 year, metabolism of rifampicin is similar to that in adults. In single dose studies, peak serum concentrations of 3.5 to 15 μg per mL were reached 2 to 4 hours after preprandial administration of 10 mg per kg body weight of rifampicin. Half-life and urinary excretion are the same as in adults. In infants, serum peak levels are delayed and elimination is comparatively slow. Furthermore, because hepatic mechanisms and biliary excretion are less fully developed, more rifampicin is excreted in the urine and there is less change with time because induction is low at this age (89).

Rifampicin is an essential drug in the treatment of tuberculosis with susceptible bacilli (see Table 34.1 for use in treatment regimens). It should be given by DOT combined with other effective antimycobacterial agents to avoid emergence of resistance (3,6). Rifampicin is administered orally at 10 mg per kg (range 8 to 20 mg per kg, maximum 600 mg) daily (3,5,6), or intermittently at 10 mg per kg (range 8 to 12 mg per kg) thrice weekly (3,5), or at 10 to 20 mg per kg (maximum 600 mg) twice weekly (6). It may be administered intravascularly.

Gastrointestinal adverse reactions include anorexia, nausea, vomiting, and abdominal discomfort. Diarrhea is less frequently reported (69). Severe adverse effects are not common but are usually related to sensitization or to its effects on other drugs through enzyme induction. Sensitivity is more common with intermittent therapy, which may result in the flu syndrome, shock, hemolytic anemia, and renal failure (69,98). If purpura occurs, discontinuation of rifampicin is recommended and the drug should not be reintroduced.

Hepatic reactions occur with rifampicin in chronic liver disease and patients need careful monitoring. Combination with drugs such as isoniazid and pyrazinamide may aggravate the situation (99,100). The rise in liver enzymes is usually transient (101). Unless liver function tests continue to deteriorate, these changes are not an indication for discontinuing treatment.

Other adverse effects reported include cutaneous pigmentation, or the red man syndrome (102), cutaneous vasculitis (103), hyperglycemia which is probably due to increased glucose absorption (104), thrombocytopenia (105), lupus syndrome (106), ulcerative colitis (107), and venous thrombosis (108). Urine becomes highly colored (red, orange, pink) and tears turn pink (69).

HEPATOTOXICITY IN CHILDREN

In children treated with rifampicin and isoniazid, 3.3% developed jaundice in the first 10 weeks of treatment. Limiting the dose of isoniazid to 10 mg per kg and rifampicin to 15 mg per kg may minimize hepatotoxicity (66).

Contraindications include hypersensitivity, jaundice, and severe hepatic disease. Treatment dosages should be adjusted in severe liver impairment and significant renal failure and deferred in patients with jaundice.

Rifampicin induces hepatic microsomal enzymes, including CYP3A4 (109). Serum concentrations of drugs metabolized by these liver enzymes may be decreased by the coadministration of rifampicin. Examples of drugs relevant to children include corticosteroids (110), diazepam (111), digoxin (112), midazolam (113), narcotics and analgesics (methadone, morphine, phenobarbitone) (69), theophylline (114), and vitamin D (78,79). On the other hand, serum concentrations of rifampicin are decreased by ethambutol, *p*-aminosalicylic acid, ketoconazole, and phenobarbital. The effect of these interactions on the clinical efficacy of rifampicin needs to be studied (115).

Serum concentrations at birth range from 12% to 33% of maternal serum (87,89). While rifampicin is dysmorphogenic in rats and mice, there has been no evidence of teratogenicity in infants (69,116). It is excreted in breast milk but not in amounts likely to cause harm (50).

PYRAZINAMIDE

Pyrazinamide is a synthetic pyrazine analog of nicotinamide. It is an essential drug and one of the cornerstones of short-course tuberculosis therapy. Pyrazinamide is bactericidal to *M. tuberculosis* at acidic pH values found inside cells. To be bactericidal, it requires an enzyme, pyrazinamidase, to produce active pyrazinoic acid (117). Like rifampicin, pyrazinamide kills best the slowly or intermittently metabolizing semidormant bacilli within macrophages (118). It acts by disruption of membrane transport and energy depletion (119).

Pyrazinamide increases the efficacy of other antituberculosis drugs. Its use in combination with other drugs as part of short course-regimens has shown excellent results. Resistance is rapid if used solely. Table 34.1 shows recommended treatment regimens with pyrazinamide. It is administered orally at 25 mg per kg (range 15 to 30 mg per kg, maximum 2 g) daily (3,5,6), or intermittently at 35 mg per kg (range 30 to 40 mg per kg) thrice weekly (3,5), or 50 mg per kg (maximum 2 g) twice weekly (6).

Absorption of pyrazinamide after oral administration is rapid and nearly complete (46). Peak plasma concentrations are observed within 1 to 2 hours (49,120–122). Pyrazinamide is widely distributed in tissues and fluids, including CSF (52). The volume of distribution is 0.75 to 1.65 L per kg (121). Pyrazinamide is hydrolyzed in the liver to the major active metabolite, pyrazinoic acid, by a microsomal deamidase. Pyrazinoic acid is hydroxylated to the main excretory product, 5-hydroxypyrazinoic acid, by xanthine oxidase (122,123). Alternatively, pyrazinamide may be converted to 5-hydroxy-pyrazinamide by xanthine oxidase and further to 5-hydroxy-pyrazinoic acid by deamidase. Of the dose, 30% to 40% is excreted in urine as pyrazinoic acid and 2% to 4% as unchanged pyrazinamide (46,120,121,123). Half-life is between 2 and 24 hours and prolonged with impaired hepatic and renal function (48,120–122). Clearance is 61 mL per minute (122).

PHARMACOKINETIC DATA IN CHILDREN

Estimates of pyrazinamide concentrations indicate linear pharmacokinetics in children with tuberculosis. After administration of pyrazinamide, incomplete or delayed absorption and greater volume of distribution are seen in children compared with adults. However, reported half-life and clearance estimates in children have been varied (33).

The principal adverse effect is dose-related liver toxicity, which is usually asymptomatic but may appear anytime during therapy. Rapid elevation of liver enzymes occurs but is transient. Hyperuricemia occurs but is usually asymptomatic (69). Monitoring of liver enzymes and uric acid is recommended. Pyrazinamide should be promptly discontinued with rising liver enzymes, evidence of clinical hepatotoxicity, or joint pains. Other common adverse effects include flushing, mild anorexia, nausea, and myalgia (69,124). Hypersensitivity, photosensitization, and rash are rarely observed (24,125). Sideroblastic anemia is rare and reversible (69).

SAFETY IN CHILDREN

In 114 children with pulmonary tuberculosis, clinical adverse effects to pyrazinamide were uncommon and mild. Slight elevation in liver enzymes was observed in 20% with none exhibiting clinical hepatitis. Serum uric acid increased above normal in 10% of children, but none had signs of gout or arthralgia. Abdominal pain was seen in 1.8% and vomiting with anorexia in 2.6%. In no case was treatment interrupted (27).

There are no data on safety and teratogenicity in pregnancy (126). There is minimal transfer in breast milk (50).

ETHAMBUTOL

Ethambutol is the dextrorotatory isomer of the synthetic compound 2,2′-ethylenediimino-di-1-butanol dihydrochloride. It is bacteriostatic against *M. tuberculosis.* At higher doses of 50 mg per kg, it exhibits bactericidal activity (127). Ethambutol produces detrimental alteration of cell wall structure (128,129). Missense changes in *embB* codon 306 are associated with resistance in *M. tuberculosis* isolates (130,131).

Ethambutol is used primarily to prevent emergence of resistance to first-line drugs. In the treatment of MDR-TB, ethambutol becomes a first-line agent (Table 34.1). It demonstrates synergism by enhancing penetration of the other drugs, especially ciprofloxacin (132).

Oral absorption of ethambutol is approximately 80% (46). Peak concentrations are reached in 2 to 4 hours (18) but are lower following a meal than when fasting (133). Protein binding is 6% and the volume of distribution is 18.9 to 21.2 L (46). Ethambutol concentrates in erythrocytes, which act as a deposit from which the drug slowly reenters plasma.

Tissue concentrations are higher than in serum or plasma, except for the central nervous system (133) where it penetrates poorly. CSF levels rise with meningeal inflammation but only to levels below inhibitory concentration (18,46). About 10% to 20% of the drug undergoes hepatic metabolism. The metabolite ethambutol aldehyde is inactive (46). Approximately 50% to 70% of an oral dose is excreted unchanged in the urine. Half-life is 3.53 to 4.59 hours. In impaired renal function, the dose must be reduced (18,46,69,134).

PHARMACOKINETIC DATA IN CHILDREN

Slow and incomplete absorption of ethambutol is common in children (34). Ethambutol serum levels reached after oral administration increase with age, with serum levels lower in younger children than in older children (135). Pharmacokinetic estimates in children with tuberculosis when compared with adults showed that elimination is faster while half-life is shorter. Furthermore, apparent volume of distribution and clearance are lower, though weight-normalized clearance is higher. Studies of ethambutol in children have found plasma drug levels lower than typical minimum inhibitory concentration values. In almost all cases, maximal serum concentration, C_{max}, failed to reach minimum inhibitory concentration and higher dosages per kilogram body weight compared with that for adults have been suggested for children (34,136). Results suggest not only lower serum concentrations but also a shortened period of maximum serum concentrations in young children as compared with adults (137).

Table 34.1 shows recommended regimens using ethambutol. Ethambutol should not to be used in children too young to undergo visual acuity testing, unless it is used to treat drug-resistant tuberculosis. Based on recent studies that raised concern on low drug levels achieved in children, a daily dose of 20 mg per kg (15 to 25 mg per kg) is recommended. At this dose, effective therapeutic concentration (defined as >2 μg per mL) is approached and balances compensation for deficiency of serum concentration and risk of ocular toxicity (133,138). A dose of 30 mg per kg (25–35) is recommended when given three times weekly (138). Higher doses may be preferred in HIV-positive patients, who tend to have lower ethambutol concentrations and in patients to whom ethambutol is especially important to the regimen as when isoniazid- or rifampicin-resistant *M. tuberculosis* isolates are documented or suspected (34).

Ethambutol is generally well tolerated. Mild hyperuricemia and gouty arthritis have been reported infrequently (69). Rare adverse effects include hypersensitivity, hepatitis (69), thrombocytopenia (139), neutropenia, and eosinophilia (140). The most serious adverse effect is retrobulbar optic neuritis (69,141), which can lead to decrease in visual acuity and even loss of ability to discriminate colors red and green. It is fairly common with high doses of 50 mg per kg per day and is also related to duration and renal insufficiency. However, a review of the literature did not reveal major ocular side effects among children treated with ethambutol. Only 2 of 3,811 children (0.05%) who received ethambutol developed possible ocular toxicity (142). Based on recent data, however, it has been suggested that the rare ethambutol toxicity is due to the considerably lower serum concentrations reached in children (133).

Ethambutol has been successfully used in pregnancy. Transplacental transfer has been documented to be at least 75% of that of maternal serum concentrations. This was associated with a normal infant (87). Ethambutol is excreted in trace amounts in breast milk (49), which should be safely ingested by an infant (50).

STREPTOMYCIN

Streptomycin is an aminoglycoside antibiotic derived from *Streptomyces griseus.* It is active against a broad spectrum of bacteria, including mycobacteria. Only its role in the treatment of tuberculosis will be discussed. Streptomycin inhibits protein synthesis of extracellular bacilli. Binding to a specific protein on the 30S subunit of the microbial ribosome, streptomycin causes misreading of the messenger RNA leading to production of nonfunctional peptide chains (143). It is bactericidal in vitro but bacteriostatic in vivo. Resistance occurs, and the incidence increases with longer therapy (18).

Streptomycin is not absorbed from the gut and must be given parenterally. After intramuscular administration, peak serum concentrations are reached in 1 hour (46). Protein binding is 19% to 34% (46,144). With a dose of 15 mg per kg, the peak concentration is in the range of 40 μg per mL (18). Streptomycin distributes into body fluids and bronchial secretions (96). CSF penetration is poor, even when it increases slightly with meningeal inflammation (51,52). The volume of distribution is 76 to 115 L (46). Metabolites have not been identified. About 30% to 80% is recovered unchanged in urine. Elimination half-life is 2 to 3 hours and is longer in newborns, in adults more than 40 years (46,69,144), and in those with renal impairment (144).

Streptomycin is used during the intensive phase as a fourth drug in the treatment of tuberculosis if ethambutol is not available or cannot be used (see Table 34.1). The efficacy of streptomycin is approximately equal to that of ethambutol in the initial phase of tuberculosis therapy. However, it is interchangeable with ethambutol only if the tubercle bacillus is susceptible to streptomycin or if resistance is unlikely (6). The usual dose for children is 15 mg per kg per day (range 12 to 40 mg per kg per day, maximum 1 g per day), and the drug must be administered by deep intramuscular injection or intravascularly (3,5,6). Dosage need not be adjusted with hepatic insufficiency but must be reduced with impaired renal function. Audiometry and renal profile monitoring is recommended (6).

Hypersensitivity reactions to streptomycin are common and can be severe (25). Streptomycin produces a dose-related neuromuscular blockade. Ototoxicity occurs, with

TABLE 34.2 Alternative Drugs for the Treatment of Drug-Resistant Tuberculosis (3,6,119,145,146)

Drug, Route	*Mechanism of Action*	*Target Site*	*Daily Dose (mg/kg)*	*Maximum Daily Dose*	*Pharmacology*	*Adverse Effects*	*Precautions*
Aminoglycosides i.v., i.m.	Inhibition of protein synthesis	16S rRNA			Bactericidal; low CSF levels; used for streptomycin resistance; kanamycin and amikacin cross-resistance; resistant to amikacin may be susceptible to capreomycin	Ototoxic, nephrotoxic, neuromuscular blockade	Avoid in pregnancy; [b]renal dosing
Kanamycin			15–30	1 g			
Amikacin			15–22.5	1 g			
Capreomycin[a]			15–30	1 g			
Cycloserine p.o.	Inhibition of peptidoglycan synthesis	D-alanine racemase	10–20	1 g	Bacteriostatic; excellent CSF penetration; no cross resistance with other agents; interferes with phenytoin elimination	Psychiatric, neurological; pyridoxine used for prevention	Avoid in pregnancy; [b]renal dosing
Ethionamide or protionamide p.o.	Inhibition of mycolic acid synthesis	Acyl carrier protein reductase	15–20	1 g	Bactericidal; significant CSF concentration; hepatic metabolism; renal elimination	Vomiting, GI irritation, hypothyroidism, malabsorption	Teratogenic; contraindicated in pregnancy
Fluoroquinolones p.o., i.v.	Inhibition of DNA synthesis	DNA gyrase			Bactericidal; poor to moderate CSF penetration; cross resistance within the class; prolongs half-life of theophylline	GI irritation, concern with arthropathy and arthritis in children	Avoid in pregnancy; [b]renal dosing
Ciprofloxacin			20–40[c]	2 g			
Ofloxacin			15–20[c]	800 mg			
Gatifloxacin			7.5–10	400 mg			
Levofloxacin			7.5–10	750 mg			
Moxifloxacin			7.5–10	400 mg			
Para-aminosalicylic acid p.o., i.v.	Inhibition of folic acid and iron metabolism	Unknown	150	12 g	Bacteriostatic; low CSF levels; acetylated in the liver	Vomiting, GI irritation; hepatotoxic, hypersensitivity reactions	Teratogenic in animals; avoid in pregnancy; [b]renal dosing

CSF, Cerebrospinal fluid; GI, gastrointestinal; i.m., intramuscular; i.v., intravenous; p.o., oral.
[a]A polypeptide, acts similarly as an aminoglycoside.
[b]Adjust dose in renal impairment.
[c]Give in two divided doses.

vestibular damage more common than auditory, though both can occur. It is nephrotoxic but least among aminoglycosides (69). Ototoxicity and nephrotoxicity are related both to cumulative dose and to peak serum concentration (18). Caution must be exercised with concomitant administration of neuromuscular blockers ototoxic and nephrotoxic drugs. Vestibular depression is an indication for discontinuation of streptomycin therapy.

Streptomycin is the only antituberculosis agent contraindicated in pregnancy due to its harmful effects on the fetus. Approximately one in six newborns develop some degree of hearing loss or vestibular defects (87). Appearance in breast milk does not appear to be significant (49,50).

THIOACETAZONE

Thioacetazone is a derivative of thiosemicarbazone shown to be bacteriostatic against the tubercle bacilli. It is inexpensive and thus used in many developing countries. However, the high rate of adverse events limits its use. The usual dosage in children is 2 to 2.5 mg per kg given daily (5). The mechanism of action is unknown. Thioacetazone is rapidly absorbed from the gastrointestinal tract. Peak plasma concentrations are reached in 2 to 6 hours. It is almost completely eliminated from serum within 24 hours. Geographic variability in susceptibility of *M. tuberculosis* to thioacetazone and in adverse effects has been observed. Patients in East Africa tolerate the drug better than Asians. Gastrointestinal (weight loss, nausea, vomiting) and neurologic (headache, blurred vision, perioral numbness, mental symptoms, and peripheral nerve symptoms) adverse events are most frequent, followed by cutaneous adverse events. Idiosyncratic toxic epidermolysis may occur in HIV patients and is contraindicated in this population (17). Thioacetazone may also potentiate the vestibular toxicity of streptomycin (18).

ALTERNATIVE DRUGS

For the treatment of tuberculosis with strains resistant to the first-line drugs, second-line drugs should be used in combination with first-line drugs to which the infecting pathogen may still be sensitive (Table 34.2). Resistant cases are difficult to treat, thus a referral to a specialist is recommended. When drug susceptibility tests are available it should be utilized to direct therapy. For treatment of these cases, at least four drugs which are likely to be effective are administered, including a fluoroquinolone and an injectable agent for at least 6 months in the intensive phase. Daily dosing, rather than intermittent, is preferred and DOT is necessary. The duration of treatment should be at least 18 months after culture conversion. Since antituberculosis medication is dosed according to body weight, monthly monitoring of body weight should be done and dosage adjustments should be made accordingly. Experience with the use of second-line drugs in children is not too extensive, but so far, few long-term adverse effects have been documented including the use of fluoroquinolones. Clinical trials are underway which attempt to shorten present chemotherapy of newly diagnosed cases using fluoroquinolones in combination with other agents (3,119,145).

REFERENCES

1. Laurenzi M, Ginsberg A, Spigelman M. Challenges associated with current and future TB treatment. *Infect Disord Drug Targets* 2007;7:105–119.
2. World Health Organization. *Global tuberculosis control: surveillance, planning, financing: WHO report 2008.* WHO/HTM/TB/2008.393.
3. World Health Organization. *Guidance for national tuberculosis programmes on the management of tuberculosis in children.* WHO/HTM/TB/2006. 371. Geneva, Switzerland: World Health Organization, 2006.
4. Marais BJ, Gie RP, Schaaf HS, et al. The natural history of childhood intra-thoracic tuberculosis—a critical review of the prechemotherapy literature. *Int J Tuberc Lung Dis* 2004;8:392–402.
5. Caminero Luna J. *A tuberculosis guide for specialist physicians* [English translation]. Paris, France: International Union Against Tuberculosis and Lung Diseases, 2005.
6. American Thoracic Society, Centers for Disease Control and Prevention, Infectious Disease Society of America. Treatment of tuberculosis. *Am J Respir Crit Care Med* 2003;167:603–662.
7. Comstock GW, Hammes LM, Pio A. Isoniazid prophylaxis in Alaskan boarding schools. A comparison of two doses. *Am Rev Respir Dis* 1969;100:773–779.
8. International Union Against Tuberculosis Committee on Prophylaxis. Efficacy of various durations of isoniazid preventive therapy for tuberculosis: five years of follow-up in the IUAT trial. *Bull World Health Organ* 1982;60:555–564.
9. Marais BJ, van Zyl S, Schaaf HS, et al. Adherence to isoniazid preventive chemotherapy in children: a prospective community based study. *Arch Dis Child* 2006;91:762–765.
10. Smieja MJ, Marchetti CA, Cook DJ, et al. Isoniazid for preventing tuberculosis in non-HIV infected persons. *Cochrane Libr* 1999;4:1–12.
11. Van Zyl S, Marais BJ, Hesseling AC, et al. Adherence to antituberculosis chemoprophylaxis and treatment in children. *Int J Tuberc Lung Dis* 2006;10:13–18.
12. Spyridis NP, Spyridis PG, Gelesme A, et al. The effectiveness of a 9-month regimen of isoniazid alone versus 3 and 4-month regimens of isoniazid plus rifampin for treatment of latent tuberculosis infection in children: results of an 11-year randomized study. *Clin Infect Dis* 2007;45:715–722.
13. Van Hest R, Baars H, Kik S, et al. Hepatotoxicity of rifampicin-pyrazinamide and isoniazid preventive therapy and tuberculosis treatment. *Clin Infect Dis* 2004;39:488–496.
14. Centers for Disease Control and Prevention. Update: adverse event data and revise American Thoracic Society/CDC recommendations against the use of rifampin and pyrazinamide for treatment of latent tuberculosis infection—United States, 2003. *MMWR Morb Mortal Wkly Rep* 2003;52:735–739.
15. Jasmer RM, Saukkonen JJ, Blumberg HM, et al. Short-course rifampin and pyrazinamide compared with isoniazid for latent tuberculosis infection: a multicenter clinical trial. *Ann Intern Med* 2002;137:640–647.
16. McNeill L, Allen M, Estrada C, et al. Pyrazinamide and rifampin vs isoniazid for the treatment of latent tuberculosis: improved completion rates but more hepatotoxicity. *Chest* 2003;123:102–106.
17. Rieder HL. *Interventions for tuberculosis control and elimination.* France: International Union Against Tuberculosis and Lung Disease (IUATLD), 2002.
18. Bass JBJ, Farer LS, Hopewell PC, et al. Treatment of tuberculosis and tuberculosis infection in adults and children. American Thoracic Society and The Centers for Disease Control and Prevention. *Am J Respir Crit Care Med* 1994;149:1359–1374.
19. Reis FJC, Bedran MBM, Moura JAR, et al. Six-month isoniazid-rifampin treatment for pulmonary tuberculosis in children. *Am Rev Respir Dis* 1990;142:996–999.
20. Abernathy RS, Dutt AK, Stead WW, et al. Short course chemotherapy for tuberculosis in children. *Pediatrics* 1983;72:801–806.

21. Gocmen A, Ozcelic U, Kiper N, et al. Short course intermittent chemotherapy in childhood tuberculosis [abstract]. *Infection* 1993;21:324–327.
22. Al-Dossary FS, Ong LT, Correa AG, et al. Treatment of childhood tuberculosis with a six month directly observed regimen of only two weeks of daily therapy. *Pediatr Infect Dis J* 2002;21:91–97.
23. Tsakalidis D, Pratsidou P, Hitoglou-Makedou A, et al. Intensive short course chemotherapy for treatment of Greek children with tuberculosis. *Pediatr Infect Dis J* 1992;11:1036–1042.
24. Pelosi F, Budani H, Rubenstein C, et al. Isoniazid, rifampin and pyrazinamide in the treatment of childhood tuberculosis with duration adjusted to the clinical status. *Am Rev Respir Dis* 1985;131(Suppl):A229.
25. Biddulph J. Short course chemotherapy for childhood tuberculosis. *Pediatr Infect Dis J* 1990;9:794–801.
26. Te Water Naude JM, Donald PR, Hussey GD, et al. Twice weekly vs daily chemotherapy for childhood tuberculosis. *Pediatr Infect Dis J* 2000;19:405–410.
27. Kumar L, Dhand R, Singhi PD, et al. A randomized trial of fully intermittent vs. daily followed by intermittent short course chemotherapy for childhood tuberculosis. *Pediatr Infect Dis J* 1990;9:802–806.
28. Sanchez-Albisua I, Vidal, ML, Joya-Verde G, et al. Tolerance of pyrazinamide in short course chemotherapy for pulmonary tuberculosis in children. *Pediatr Infect Dis J* 1997;16:760–763.
29. Jawahar MS, Sivasubramanian S, Vijayan VK, et al. Short course chemotherapy for tuberculous lymphadenitis in children. *Br Med J* 1990;301:359–362.
30. Visudhiphan P, Chiemchanya S. Evaluation of rifampicin in the treatment of tuberculous meningitis in children. *J Pediatr* 1975; 87:983–986.
31. Ramachandran P, Duraipandian M, Nagarajan M, et al. Three chemotherapy studies of tuberculous meningitis in children. *Tubercle* 1986;67:17–29.
32. Schaaf HS, Parkin DP, Seifart HI, et al. Isoniazid pharmacokinetics in children treated for pulmonary tuberculosis. *Arch Dis Child* 2005;90:614–618.
33. Zhu M, Starke JR, Burman WJ, et al. Population pharmacokinetic modeling of pyrazinamide in children and adults with tuberculosis. *Pharmacotherapy* 2002;22:686–695.
34. Zhu M, Burman WJ, Starke JR, et al. Pharmacokinetics of ethambutol in children and adults with tuberculosis. *Int J Tuberc Lung Dis* 2004;8:1360–1367.
35. Rieder HL, Arnadottir T, Trebucq A, et al. Tuberculosis treatment: dangerous regimens? *Int J Tuberc Lung Dis* 2001;5:1–3.
36. Jacobs RF, Abernathy RS. The treatment of tuberculosis in children. *Pediatr Infect Dis* 1985;4:513–517.
37. Zignol M, Hosseini MS, Wright A, et al. Global incidence of multidrug resistant tuberculosis. *J Infect Dis* 2006;194:479–485.
38. Van Soolingen D, de Haas PEW, van Doorn HR, et al. Mutations at amino acid position 315 of the *katG* gene are associated with high-level resistance to isoniazid, other drug resistance, and successful transmission of Mycobacterium tuberculosis in the Netherlands. *J Infect Dis* 2000;182:1788–1790.
39. Wengenack NL, Uhl JR, St Amand AL, et al. Recombinant Mycobacterium tuberculosis KatG(S315 T) is a competent catalase-peroxidase with reduced activity toward Isoniazid. *J Infect Dis* 1997;176:722–727.
40. Ramaswamy S, Musser JM. Molecular genetic basis of antimicrobial agent resistance in Mycobacterium tuberculosis: 1998 update. *Tuberc Lung Dis* 1998;79:3–29.
41. Hsu KHK. Thirty years after isoniazid. Its impact on tuberculosis in children and adolescents. *JAMA* 1984;251:1283–1285.
42. Deguchi T, Mashimo M, Suzuki T. Correlation between acetylator phenotypes and genotypes of polymorphic arylamine *N*-acetyltransferase in human liver. *J Biol Chem* 1990;265:12757–12760.
43. Parkin DP, Vandenplas S, Botha FJH, et al. Trimodality of isoniazid elimination. Phenotype and genotype in patients with tuberculosis. *Am J Respir Crit Care Med* 1997;155:1717–1722.
44. Ellard GA. The potential clinical significance of the isoniazid acetylator phenotype in the treatment of pulmonary tuberculosis. *Tubercle* 1984;65:211–227.
45. Weber WW, Hein DW. N-acetylation pharmacogenetics. *Pharmacol Rev* 1985;37:26–79.
46. Holdiness MR. Clinical pharmacokinetics of the antituberculosis drugs. *Clin Pharmacokinet* 1984;9:511–544.
47. Hurwitz A, Scholzman DI. Effects of antacids on gastrointestinal absorption of isoniazid in rat and man. *Am Rev Respir Dis* 1974;109:41–47.
48. Peloquin CA, Namdar R, Dodge AA, et al. Pharmacokinetics of isoniazid under fasting conditions, with food, and with antacids. *Int J Tuberc Lung Dis* 1999;3:703–710.
49. Chaplin S, Sanders GL, Smith JM. Drug excretion in human breast milk. *Adv Drug React Ac Pois Rev* 1982;1:255–287.
50. Snider DE, Powell KE. Should women taking antituberculosis drugs breastfeed? *Arch Intern Med* 1984;144:589–590.
51. Ellard GA, Humphries MJ, Allen BW. Cerebrospinal fluid drug concentrations and the treatment of tuberculous meningitis. *Am Rev Respir Dis* 1993;148:650–655.
52. Holdiness MR. Cerebrospinal fluid pharmacokinetics of the antituberculosis drugs. *Clin Pharmacokinet* 1985;10:532–534.
53. Donald PR, Gent WL, Seifart HI, et al. Cerebrospinal fluid isoniazid concentrations in children with tuberculous meningitis: the influence of dosage and acetylation status. *Pediatrics* 1992; 89:247–250.
54. Kergueris MF, Bourin M, Larousse C. Pharmacokinetics of isoniazid: influence of age. *Eur J Clin Pharmacol* 1986;30:335–340.
55. Acocella G, Bonollo L, Garimold M, et al. Kinetics of rifampicin and isoniazid administered alone and in combination to normal subjects and patients with liver disease. *Gut* 1972;13:47–53.
56. Brown CV. Acute isoniazid poisoning. *Am Rev Respir Dis* 1972;105:206–216.
57. Miller J, Robinson A, Percy AK. Acute isoniazid poisoning in childhood. *Am J Dis Child* 1980;134:290–292.
58. Shah BR, Santucci K, Sinert R, et al. Acute isoniazid neurotoxicity in an urban hospital. *Pediatrics* 1995;95:700–704.
59. Blowey DL, Johnson D, Verjee Z. Isoniazid-associated rhabdomyolysis. *Am J Emerg Med* 1995;13:543–544.
60. Panganiban LR, Makalinao IR, Cortes-Maramba NP. Rhabdomyolysis in isoniazid poisoning. *Clin Toxicol* 2001;39: 143–151.
61. Brent J, Vo N, Kulig K, et al. Reversal of prolonged isoniazid-induced coma by pyridoxine. *Arch Int Med* 1990;150:1751–1753.
62. Tuberculosis Chemotherapy Centre, Madras. The prevention and treatment of isoniazid toxicity in the therapy of pulmonary tuberculosis. 1. An assessment of two vitamin B preparations and glutamic acid. *Bull World Health Organ* 1963;28:455–475.
63. Krishnamurthy DV, Selkon JB, Ramachandran K, et al. Effect of pyridoxine on vitamin B6 concentrations and glutamic oxaloacetate transaminase activity in whole blood of tuberculous patients receiving high-dosage isoniazid. *Bull World Health Organ* 1967;36:853–870.
64. Beaudry PH, Brickman HF, Wise MB, et al. Liver enzyme disturbance during isoniazid chemoprophylaxis in children. *Am Rev Respir Dis* 1974;110:581–584.
65. Bailey WC, Weill H, DeRouen TA, et al. The effect of isoniazid on transaminase levels. *Ann Intern Med* 1974;81:200–202.
66. O'Brien RJ, Long MW, Cross FS, et al. Hepatotoxicity from isoniazid and rifampin among children treated for tuberculosis. *Pediatrics* 1983;72:491–499.
67. Nakajo MM, Rao M, Steiner P. Incidence of hepatotoxicity in children receiving isoniazid chemoprophylaxis. *Pediatr Infec Dis J* 1989;8:649–650.
68. Stuart JJ, Roberts HR. Isoniazid and disseminated intravascular coagulation. *Ann Intern Med* 1976;84:490.
69. Girling DJ. Adverse effects of antituberculosis drugs. *Drugs* 1982;23:56–74.
70. Veale KS, Huff ES, Nelson BK, et al. Pure red cell aplasia and hepatitis in a child receiving isoniazid therapy. *J Pediatr* 1992; 120:146–148.
71. Braunstein GD. Gynecomastia. *New Engl J Med* 1993;328: 490–495.
72. Lopez-Contreras J, Ruiz D, Domingo P. Isoniazid-induced toxic fever. *Rev Infect Dis* 1991;13:775.
73. Rabassa TG, Shukla U, Samo T, et al. Isoniazid-induced acute pancreatitis. *Ann Intern Med* 1994;121:433–434.
74. Chan KL, Chan HS, Lui SF, et al. Recurrent acute pancreatitis induced by isoniazid. *Tubercle Lung Dis* 1994;75:383–385.
75. Bowersox DW, Winerbaur RH, Stewart GL, et al. Isoniazid dosage in patients with renal failure. *N Engl J Med* 1973;289: 84–87.

76. Pellock JM, Howell J, Kendig EL, et al. Pyridoxine deficiency in children treated with isoniazid. *Chest* 1985;87:658–661.
77. Brodie MJ, Boobis AR, Hillyard CJ, et al. Effect of isoniazid on vitamin D metabolism and hepatic monoxygenase activity. *Clin Pharmacol Ther* 1981;30:363–367.
78. Brodie MJ, Boobis AR, Hillyard CJ, et al. Effect of rifampicin and isoniazid on vitamin D metabolism. *Clin Pharmacol Ther* 1982;32:525–530.
79. Davies PDO, Brown RC, Church HA, et al. The effect of antituberculous chemotherapy on vitamin D and calcium metabolism. *Tubercle* 1987;68:261–266.
80. Ochs HR, Greenblatt DJ, Roberts GM. Diazepam interaction with antituberculosis drugs. *Clin Pharmacol Ther* 1981;29:671–678.
81. Block SH. Carbamazapine–isoniazid interaction. *Pediatrics* 1982;69:494–495.
82. Miller RR, Porter J, Greenblatt DJ. Clinical importance of the interaction of phenytoin and isoniazid. *Chest* 1979;75:356–358.
83. Kutt H, Brennan R, DeHeija H, et al. Diphenylhydantoin intoxication. A complication of isoniazid therapy. *Am Rev Respir Dis* 1970;101:377–383.
84. Dockweiler U. Isoniazid-induced valproic acid toxicity, or vice versa [letter]. *Lancet* 1987;2:152.
85. Mazze RI, Woodruff RE, Heerdt ME. Isoniazid-induced enflurane defluorination in humans. *Anesthesiology* 1982;57:5–8.
86. Gannon R, Pearsall W, Rowley R. Isoniazid, meperidine, and hypotension [letter]. *Ann Intern Med* 1983;99:415.
87. Holdiness MR. Transplacental pharmacokinetics of the antituberculosis drugs. *Clin Pharmacokinet* 1987;13:123–129.
88. Singh N, Golani A, Patel Z, et al. Transfer of isoniazid from circulation to breast milk in lactating women on chronic therapy for tuberculosis. *Br J Clin Pharmacol* 2007;65:418–422.
89. Kenny MT, Strates B. Metabolism and pharmacokinetics of the antibiotic rifampin. *Drug Metab Rev* 1981;12:159–218.
90. Dickinson JM, Mitchison DA. Experimental models to explain the high sterilizing activity of rifampin in the chemotherapy of tuberculosis. *Am Rev Respir Dis* 1981;123:367–371.
91. Telenti A, Imboden P, Marchesi F, et al. Detection of rifampicin-resistance mutations in Mycobacterium tuberculosis. *Lancet* 1993;341:647–650.
92. Donnabella V, Martiniuk F, Kinney D, et al. Isolation of the gene for the beta subunit of RNA polymerase from rifampicin-resistant Mycobacterium tuberculosis and identification of new mutations. *Am J Respir Cell Mol Biol* 1994;11:639–643.
93. Koup JR, Williams-Warren J, Viswanathan CT, et al. Pharmacokinetics of rifampin in children. II. Oral bioavailability. *Ther Drug Monit* 1986;8:17–22.
94. Siegler DI, Bryant M, Burley DM, et al. Effect of meals on rifampicin absorption. *Lancet* 1974;ii:197–198.
95. Boman G, Hannegren A, Malmborg A, et al. Drug interaction: decreased serum concentrations of rifampicin when given with PAS. *Lancet* 1971;i:800.
96. Braga PC. Antibiotic penetrability into bronchial mucus: pharmacokinetics and clinical considerations. *Curr Ther Res* 1991;49: 300–327.
97. D'Oliveira JJG. Cerebrospinal fluid concentrations of rifampin in meningeal tuberculosis. *Am Rev Respir Dis* 1972;106:432–437.
98. Cohn JR, Fye DL, Sills JM, et al. Rifampin-induced renal failure. *Tubercle* 1985;66:289–293.
99. Girling DJ. The hepatic toxicity of antituberculous regimens containing isoniazid, rifampicin and pyrazinamide. *Tubercle* 1978;59:13–32.
100. Lees AW, Alan GW, Smith J, et al. Toxicity from rifampicin plus isoniazid and rifampicin plus ethambutol therapy. *Tubercle* 1971;52:182–190.
101. Baron DN, Bell JL. Serum enzyme changes in patients receiving antituberculosis therapy with rifampicin or para-amino-salicylic acid, plus isoniazid and streptomycin. *Tubercle* 1964;55:115–120.
102. Holdiness MR. A review of the redman syndrome and rifampicin overdosage [abstract]. *Med Toxicol Adverse Drug Exp* 1989;4: 444–451.
103. Iredale J, Sankeran R, Wathen CG. Cutaneous vasculitis associated with rifampicin therapy. *Chest* 1989;96:215–216.
104. Takasu N, Yamada T, Miura H, et al. Rifampicin-induced early phase hyperglycemia in humans. *Am Rev Respir Dis* 1982;125: 23–27.
105. Blajchman MA, Lowry RC, Pettit JE, et al. Rifampicin-induced immune thrombocytopenia. *Br Med J* 1970;3:24–26.
106. Berning SE, Iseman MD. Rifamycin-induced lupus syndrome. *Lancet* 1997;349:1521–1522.
107. Tajima A, Mine T, Ogata E. Rifampicin-associated ulcerative colitis. *Ann Intern Med* 1992;116:778–779.
108. White NW. Venous thrombosis and rifampicin. *Lancet* 1989;ii: 434–435.
109. Adedoyin A, Mauro K, Dubisty C, et al. Chronic modulation of CYP2D6 and CYP3A4 activities by quinidine and rifampicin respectively. *Clin Pharmacol Ther* 1995;57:210.
110. Lee KH, Shin JG, Chong WS, et al. Time course of the changes in prednisolone pharmacokinetics after co-administration or discontinuation of rifampin. *Eur J Clin Pharmacol* 1993;45:287–289.
111. Ohnhaus EE, Brockmeyer N, Dylewicz P, et al. The effect of antipyrine and rifampin on the metabolism of diazepam. *Clin Pharmacol Ther* 1987;42:148–156.
112. Rodin SM, Johnson BF. Pharmacokinetic interactions with digoxin. *Clin Pharmacokinet* 1988;15:227–244.
113. Backman JT, Olkkola KT, Neuvonen PJ. Rifampin drastically reduces plasma concentrations and effects of oral midazolam. *Clin Pharmacol Ther* 1996;59:7–13.
114. Powell-Jackson PR, Jamieson AP, Gray BJ, et al. Effect of rifampin on theophylline pharmacokinetics in humans. *Am Rev Respir Dis* 1985;131:939–940.
115. Venkatesan K. Pharmacokinetic drug interactions with rifampicin. *Clin Pharmacokinet* 1992;22:47–65.
116. Steen JS, Staintin-Ellis DM. Rifampicin in pregnancy. *Lancet* 1977;ii:604–605.
117. Konno K, Feldmann FM, McDermott W. Pyrazinamide susceptibility and amidase activity of tubercle bacilli. *Am Rev Respir Dis* 1967;95:461–469.
118. Crowle AJ, Sbarbaro JA, May MH. Inhibition by pyrazinamide of tubercle bacilli within cultured human macrophages. *Am Rev Respir Dis* 1986;134:1052–1055.
119. Zhang Y. The magic bullets and tuberculosis drug targets. *Annu Rev Pharmacol Toxicol* 2005;45:529–564.
120. Ellard GA. Absorption, metabolism and excretion of pyrazinamide in man. *Tubercle* 1969;50:144–158.
121. Bareggi SR, Cerutti R, Pirola R, et al. Clinical pharmacokinetics and metabolism of pyrazinamide in healthy volunteers. *Drug Res* 1987;37:849–854.
122. Lacroix C, Phan Hoang T, Nouveau J, et al. Pharmacokinetics of pyrazinamide and its metabolites in healthy subjects. *Eur J Clin Pharmacol* 1989;36:395–400.
123. Ellard GA, Haslam RM. Observations on the reduction of the renal elimination of urate in man caused by the administration of pyrazinamide. *Tubercle* 1976;57:97–103.
124. Zierski M, Bek E. Side effects of drug regimens used in short-course chemotherapy for pulmonary tuberculosis. A controlled clinical study. *Tubercle* 1980;61:41–49.
125. Maurya V, Panjabi C, Shah A. Pyrazinamide induced photoallergy. *Int J Tuberc Lung Dis* 2001;5:1075–1076.
126. Snider DE, Layde RM, Johnson MW, et al. Treatment of tuberculosis during pregnancy. *Am Rev Respir Dis* 1980;122:65–69.
127. Jindani A, Aber VR, Edwards EA, et al. The early bactericidal activity of drugs in patients with pulmonary tuberculosis. *Am Rev Respir Dis* 1980;121:939–949.
128. Deng L, Mikusova K, Robuck KG, et al. Recognition of multiple effects of ethambutol on metabolism of mycobacterial cell envelope. *Antimicrob Agents Chemother* 1995;39:694–701.
129. Mikusova K, Slayden RA, Besra GS, et al. Biogenesis of the mycobacterial cell wall and the site of action of ethambutol. *Antimicrob Agents Cheother* 1995;39:2484–2489.
130. Telenti A, Philipp WJ, Sreevatsan S, et al. The *emb* operon, a gene cluster of *Mycobacterium tuberculosis* involved in resistance to ethambutol. *Nat Med* 1997;3:567–570.
131. Sreevatsan S, Stockbauer KE, Pan X, et al. Ethambutol resistance in *Mycobacterium tuberculosis*: critical role of *embB* mutations. *Antimicrob Agents Chemother* 1997;41:1677–1681.
132. Hoffner SE, Kratz M, Olsson-Liljequist B, et al. In-vitro synergistic activity between ethambutol and fluorinated quinolones against Mycobacterium avium complex. *J Antimicrob Chemother* 1989;24: 317–324.

133. Donald PR, Maher D, Mariitz JS, et al. Ethambutol dosage for the treatment of children: literature review and recommendations. *Int J Tuberc Lung Dis* 2006;10:1318–1330.
134. Jenne JW, Beggs WH. Correlation of in vitro and in vivo kinetics with clinical use of isoniazid, ethambutol, and rifampin. *Am Rev Respir Dis* 1973;107:1013–1021.
135. Hussels H, Kroening U, Magdorf K. Ethambutol and rifampicin serum levels in children: second report on combined administration of ethambutol and rifampicin. *Pneumonologie* 1973;149:31–38.
136. Graham SM, Bell DJ, Nyirongo S, et al. Low levels of pyrazinamide and ethambutol in children with tuberculosis and impact of age, nutritional status, and human immunodeficiency virus infection. *Antimicrob Agents Chemother* 2006;50:407–413.
137. Thee S, Detjen A, Quarcoo D, et al. Ethambutol in paediatric tuberculosis: aspects of ethambutol serum concentration, efficacy and toxicity in children. *Int J Tuberc Lung Dis* 2007;11(9): 965–971.
138. World Health Organization. *Implementing the WHO Stop TB Strategy: a Handbook for National Tuberculosis Programmes.* WHO/HTM/TB/2008.401.
139. Rabinovitz M, Pitlik SD, Halevy J, et al. Ethambutol-induced thrombocytopenia. *Chest* 1982;81:765–766.
140. Wong CF, Yew WW. Ethambutol-induced neutropenia and eosinophilia. *Chest* 1994;106:1638–1639.
141. Kahana LM. Toxic ocular effect of ethambutol [abstract]. *Can Med Assoc J* 1987;137:213–216.
142. Trebucq A. Should ethambutol be recommended for routine treatment of tuberculosis in children? A review of the literature. *Int J Tuberc Lung Dis* 1997;1:12–15.
143. Kogut M, Prizant E. Effect of dihydrostreptomycin on ribosome function in vivo. *Antimicrob Agent Chemother* 1975;7:341–348.
144. Kunin CM. A guide to use of antibiotics in patients with renal disease. *Ann Intern Med* 1967;67:151–158.
145. Rich M, Cegielski P, Jaramillo E, Lambregts K, eds. *Guidelines for the programmatic management of drug-resistant tuberculosis.* Geneva, Switzerland: World Health Organization, 2009 (WHO/HTM/TB/2006/361).
146. Brunton L, ed. *Goodman & Gilman's the pharmacologic basis of therapeutics*, 11th ed. New York, NY: The McGraw-Hill Companies, 2006.

CHAPTER

35

Michael Cohen-Wolkowiez
William J. Steinbach
Daniel K. Benjamin Jr.*

Antifungal Agents

Because of advances in aggressive chemotherapeutic agents and frequent use of organ transplantation, fungal pathogens are an expanding complication in immunocompromised patients (1). Fortunately, the therapeutic armamentarium for invasive fungal infections has markedly increased in the last decade and more importantly both regulatory agencies and industry have worked cohesively to evaluate the use of these agents in the pediatric population. We will review the major systemic antifungal agents in clinical use or advanced testing (Table 35.1), excluding those antifungal agents that presently remain in the early stages of development (i.e., sordarins, pradimicins, or benanomycins).

POLYENES

AMPHOTERICIN B

Mechanism of Action

The oldest antifungal class is the polyene macrolides, amphotericin B and nystatin. Since its initial approval for use in 1958, amphotericin B remains the "gold standard" for invasive fungal infection treatment as well as the standard of comparison for all newer antifungal agents. However, the fact that amphotericin B remained at such a post was not solely by virtue of its effectiveness but rather due to the lack of alternatives until recent studies (2). Amphotericins A and B are natural fermentation products of a soil actinomycete collected in Venezuela in 1953, but although each has antifungal properties, amphotericin A was not developed (3). Amphotericin B is so named because it is amphoteric, forming soluble salts in both acidic and basic environments (4). However, because of its insolubility in water, amphotericin B for clinical use is actually amphotericin B mixed with the detergent deoxycholate in a 3:7 mixture (4,5).

The polyenes bind to ergosterol, the major sterol found in fungal cytoplasmic membranes. The lipophilic amphotericin B acts by preferential binding to fungal membrane ergosterols, creating transmembrane channels, which result in an increased permeability to monovalent cations. The fungicidal activity is believed to be due to a damaged barrier and subsequent cell death through leakage of essential nutrients from the fungal cell. Amphotericin B also has oxidant activity that disrupts cellular metabolism (6), inhibits proton adenosine triphosphatase (ATPase) pumps, depletes cellular energy reserves, and promotes lipid peroxidation to result in an increase in membrane fragility and ionized calcium leakage (5,7,8).

Pharmacology

Amphotericin B is released from its carrier and distributes very efficiently (>90%) with lipoproteins, taken up preferentially by organs of the reticuloendothelial system, and follows a three-compartment distribution model. There is an initial 24- to 48-hour distributional half-life reflecting uptake by host lipids, very slow release and excretion into urine and bile, and a subsequent terminal elimination half-life of up to 15 days (9). In a small series (n = 13) evaluating the pharmacokinetics of amphotericin B among premature infants (27.4 ± 5 weeks), 9 subjects showed elimination of amphotericin B at steady state with an estimated elimination half-life of 14.8 hours (5 to 82). The rest of the infants, however, showed minimal drug elimination during the dosing interval suggesting substantial drug accumulation and interindividual variability (10).

Experimental in vitro and in vivo studies support concentration-dependent killing with a prolonged postantifungal effect, suggesting that large daily doses will be most effective and achieving optimal peak concentrations is important (11). Peak levels are achieved 1 hour after a 4-hour infusion and reach a plateau at the third consecutive day of a constant dose (4). There is a relationship between total dose administered and tissue concentrations, suggesting a progressive accumulation with continued drug administration (12). However, there is no evidence of a clinical dose effect (13) to support higher doses (>1 mg per kg per day) of amphotericin B (14). In adults, cerebrospinal fluid (CSF) values are only 2% to 4% of serum

*Dr. Benjamin receives support from the United States Government for his work in pediatric and neonatal clinical pharmacology (1R01HD057956-02, 1R01FD003519-01, 1U10-HD45962-06, 1K24HD 058735-01, and Government Contract HHSN267200700051C), the non profit organization Thrasher Research Foundation for his work in neonatal candidiasis (http://www.thrasherresearch.org), and from industry for neonatal and pediatric drug development (http://www.dcri.duke.edu/research/coi.jsp).

TABLE 35.1 Formulations of Selected Systemic Antifungal Agents

Drug Class	*Drug Name (Brand/Investigational Name)*	*Formulation*
Pyrimidine analogue	5-Fluorocytosine (Ancoban)	p.o.
Polyene	Amphotericin B deoxycholate (Fungizone)	i.v.
	Amphotericin B lipid complex (Abelcet)	i.v.
	Amphotericin B colloidal dispersion (Amphocil; Amphotec)	i.v.
	Liposomal amphotericin B (AmBisome)	i.v.
Triazole	Fluconazole (Diflucan)	p.o., i.v.
	Itraconazole (Sporanox)	p.o., i.v.
	Voriconazole (VFend)	p.o., i.v.
	Posaconazole (Noxafil)	p.o.
	Ravuconazole (BMS-207147; ER-30346)	p.o.
Echinocandin	Caspofungin (Cancidas)	i.v.
	Anidulafungin (Eraxis)	i.v.
	Micafungin (Mycamine)	i.v.

i.v., Intravenous; p.o., oral.

concentrations and sometimes difficult to detect (15). In a small series of premature infants born at 27.4 (±5) weeks' gestational age ($n = 5$), however, CSF amphotericin B concentrations were 40% to 90% of serum concentrations obtained simultaneously (10).

In addition to conventional amphotericin B deoxycholate, three fundamentally different lipid-associated formulations have been developed that offer the advantage of an increased daily dose of the parent drug, better delivery to the primary reticuloendothelial organs (lungs, liver, spleen) (16,17), and reduced toxicity. The US Food and Drug Administration (FDA) approved amphotericin B lipid complex (ABLC) in December 1995, amphotericin B colloidal dispersion (ABCD) in December 1996, and liposomal amphotericin B (L-amphotericin B) in August 1997 (18).

ABLC (Abelcet, Enzon Corporation, Bridgewater, NJ) is a tightly-packed ribbon-like structure of a bilayered membrane formed by combining dimyristoyl phosphatidylcholine, dimyrisotyl phosphatidylglycerol and amphotericin B in a ratio of 7:3:3. ABCD (Amphocil, AstraZeneca, London; or Amphotec, Intermune Pharmaceuticals, Brisbane, CA) is composed of disk-like structures of cholesteryl sulfate complexed with amphotericin B in an equimolar ratio. L-amphotericin B (AmBisome, Fujisawa Healthcare, Inc., Deerfield, IL), the only "true liposomal" product, consists of small uniformly sized unilamellar vesicles of a lipid bilayer of hydrogenated soy phosphatidylcholine-distcaryl phosphatidylglycerol-cholesterol-amphotericin B in the ratio 2:0.8:1:0.4 (19,20).

Lipid formulations of amphotericin B generally have a slower onset of action and are less active than amphotericin B in time-kill studies, presumably due to the required disassociation of free amphotericin B from the lipid vehicle (21). It is postulated that activated monocytes/macrophages take up drug-laden lipid formulations and transport them to the site of infection where phospholipases release the free drug (18,22). The different pharmacokinetics and toxicities of the lipid formulations are reflected in the dosing recommendations: ABLC is recommended at 5 mg per kg per day, ABCD at 3 to 5 mg per kg per day, and L-amphotericin B at 1 to 5 mg per kg per day. However, most clinical data have been obtained with the use of these preparations at 5 mg per kg per day. Animal studies clearly indicate that on a similar dosing schedule the lipid products are almost always not as potent as amphotericin B, but that the ability to safely administer higher daily doses of the parent drug improves their efficacy (15) and they compare favorably with the amphotericin B deoxycholate preparation with less toxicity. A multicenter maximum tolerated dose study of L-amphotericin B using doses from 7.5 to 15 mg per kg per day

TABLE 35.2 Spectrum of Activity of Selected Antifungal Agents

Drug	*Important Clinical Uses*
Amphotericin B	*Blastomyces dermatitidis, Coccidioides immitis, Cryptococcus neoformans, Histoplasma capsulatum, Paracoccidioides brasiliensis, Sporotrix schenckii, most Candida species, Aspergillus, Zygomycetes* (NOT: *Candida lusitaniae, Scedosporium, Fusarium, Trichosporon)*
5-Fluorocytosine	Only in combination therapy for *Candida, C. neoformans,* dematiaceous molds
Fluconazole	Most *Candida, C. neoformans, B. dermatitidis, H. capsulatum, C. immitis, P. brasiliensis* (NOT: *C. krusei, C. glabrata, Aspergillus)*
Itraconazole	*Candida, Aspergillus, B. dermatitidis, H. capsulatum, C. immitis, P. brasiliensis*
Voriconazole	*Candida, Aspergillus, Fusarium, B. dermatitidis, H. capsulatum, C. immitis, Malassezia* species, *Scedosporium,* dematiaceous molds (NOT: *Zygomycetes*)
Posaconazole	*Candida, Aspergillus, Fusarium, H. capsulatum, C. immitis, Zygomycetes,* dematiaceous molds
Caspofungin	*Candida, Aspergillus* (NOT: *C. neoformans, Fusarium, Zygomycetes*)
Micafungin	*Candida, Aspergillus* (NOT: *C. neoformans, Fusarium, Zygomycetes*)
Anidulafungin	*Candida, Aspergillus* (NOT: *C. neoformans, Fusarium, Zygomycetes*)

found a nonlinear plasma pharmacokinetic profile with a maximal concentration at 10 mg per kg per day and no demonstrable dose-limiting nephrotoxicity or infusion-related toxicity (23).

Lipid formulations have the added benefit of increased tissue concentration compared with conventional amphotericin B, specifically the liver, lungs, and spleen. However, it is not entirely clear whether these higher concentrations in tissue are truly available to the microfoci of infection. L-amphotericin B has a comparatively higher peak plasma level and prolonged circulation in plasma (19), whereas ABCD has a lower plasma level than amphotericin B after infusion but a longer half-life and larger volume of distribution (24).

Several reviews have focused on amphotericin B pharmacokinetics in children. In one study of five premature infants and five older children the volume of distribution was smaller and the elimination clearance more rapid than previously reported in adults. Serum levels were approximately half of those in adults with comparable doses, and interpatient variability was marked in the premature infants (25). Other studies have confirmed interpatient variability in pediatric patients including lower serum levels in smaller children with higher total clearance, indicating perhaps that they received too low of a dose. In addition, older, heavier children with a relatively higher exposure to amphotericin B may be overdosed and at greater risk for toxicity (26,27). One study examined ABLC in six children with hepatosplenic candidiasis and showed that steady state was reached in 7 days with continued resolution of lesions even after drug discontinuation (28). A population PK analysis of 39 pediatric patients with cancer aged an average of 6.5 years (0.17 to 17) weighing an average of 21.1 kg (6.1 to 84.1) receiving 0.8 to 5.9 mg per kg of body weight per day of L-amphotericin B found that body weight exhibits a significant influence in its pharmacokinetic parameters. The estimated clearance and volume of distribution in the central compartment in this population was 0.44 L per hour and 3.12 L, respectively. Through simulations of doses ranging from 1 to 12.5 mg per kg per day it was found that infants weighing less than 20 kg may require higher doses than heavier children (29). Weight was also the most influential predictor of population pharmacokinetic parameters among neonates [median weight 1.06 kg (0.48 to 4.9); median gestational age, 27 weeks (24 to 41)] with invasive candidiasis treated with ABLC at 2.5 to 5 mg per kg of body weight for a median of 21 days (4 to 47 days). In this population, postnatal and gestational age did not influence clearance or volume of distribution of ABLC (30).

Toxicities, Side Effects, and Drug Interactions

Tolerance to amphotericin B deoxycholate is limited by its acute and chronic toxicities. In addition to fungal ergosterol the drug also interacts with cholesterol in human cell membranes, which likely accounts for its toxicity (31). Up to 80% of patients receiving amphotericin B develop either infusion-related toxicity or nephrotoxicity (4), especially with concomitant therapy with nephrotoxic drugs such as aminoglycosides, vancomycin, cyclosporine, or tacrolimus (32,33). Amphotericin B also has a constrictive effect on the afferent and efferent renal arterioles, leading to a reduction in the glomerular filtration rate (34).

Renal function usually returns to normal after cessation of amphotericin B, although permanent renal impairment is common after larger doses (2). Amphotericin B nephrotoxicity is generally less severe in infants and children than in adults, likely due to the more rapid clearance of the drug in children. Lipid formulations appear to stabilize amphotericin B in a self-associated state so that it is not available to interact with the cholesterol of human cellular membranes (19,35). Another theory for the decreased nephrotoxicity of lipid formulations is the preferential binding of its amphotericin B to serum high-density lipoproteins compared with amphotericin B's binding to low-density lipoproteins (36). The high-density lipoprotein-bound amphotericin B appears to be released to the kidney more slowly, or to a lesser degree. For infusion-related toxicity there is a general agreement that L-amphotericin B has less toxicity than ABLC whereas ABCD appears closer in toxicity to conventional amphotericin B (37,38).

Clinical Studies

The recommended dose of amphotericin B is 1.0 to 1.5 mg per kg per day and optimal duration of therapy is unknown but largely dependent on underlying disease, extent of the patient's fungal infection, resolution of any neutropenia, lessening immunosuppression, and the return of graft function following bone marrow or organ transplantation (39,40). There is no total dose of amphotericin B recommended, and the key to success has been suggested to give high doses in the initial phase of therapy and reduce the dose if toxicity develops (41). According to the FDA, all three lipid formulations are currently indicated for patients with systemic mycoses, primarily invasive aspergillosis, who are intolerant of or refractory to conventional amphotericin B. In addition, L-amphotericin B is approved as empiric therapy for the neutropenic patient with persistent fever, despite broad-spectrum antibiotic therapy (17). Many experts also suggest possible initial therapy with lipid amphotericin B formulations in patients with marginal renal function or those receiving nephrotoxic drugs.

There are no data or consensus opinions among authorities indicating improved efficacy of any new amphotericin B lipid formulation over conventional amphotericin B (17,18,34,38,42). One exception is that L-amphotericin B has shown less frequent infusion-related adverse events than the other lipid formulations and conventional amphotericin B (18). This fact leaves the clearest indication for a lipid formulation over amphotericin B to be reducing nephrotoxicity, which is an important clinical feature in complex patients with invasive mycoses.

Pediatric Clinical Studies

Because amphotericin B is the oldest commonly used systemic antifungal, there are the most pediatric data for this agent. The first review of pediatric antifungal therapy was in 1969 (43) and covered the nephrotoxicity of amphotericin B in 39 pediatric patients. An open-label study of 111 treatment episodes with ABLC in pediatric patients revealed a well-tolerated drug with generally stable renal function over 6 weeks of therapy. There was a complete or partial therapeutic response in 70% of patients, including 56% for aspergillosis and 81% for candidiasis (44). A retrospective study of 46 pediatric patients who received ABLC confirmed the minimal decline in renal function and reported an overall response rate of 83%, including 78% against aspergillosis and 89% against candidiasis (45).

In a prospective, randomized controlled trial of 49 children who received ABCD versus amphotericin B there was significantly less renal toxicity in the ABCD group (12%) versus the amphotericin B group (52.4%). Although not statistically significant, a greater proportion of children who received ABCD (69%) versus amphotericin B (41%) also had a successful outcome (46). A retrospective analysis of 30 children found that a short course of 7 to 14 days of amphotericin B after the last positive blood culture for *Candida* species was adequate for treatment in children (47). Prophylactic liposomal amphotericin B administered for the first 100 days post–allogeneic stem cell transplantation in children reduced the incidence of invasive mold infections in a retrospective single center study (48). From 1996 to 2000 the safety and efficacy of ABLC injection was assessed in 548 children with cancer (0 to 20 years of age) who were enrolled in the Collaborative Exchange of Antifungal Research registry. Response data for 89% (255/285) of patients with documented pathogens showed that a complete or partial response was achieved in 54.9% of patients. Among patients with proven *Aspergillus* infection, the response rates were 37.5% to 40.5%. In this report, elevations in serum creatinine of more than 1.5 and more than 2.5 times baseline values were seen in 24.8% and 8.8% of all patients, respectively. The use of ABLC in pediatric patients with cancer intolerant of or refractory to conventional antifungal therapy is recommended (49).

There is very limited published experience in neonates despite extensive use, and one review of L-amphotericin B in neonates showed that the agent is well tolerated, and renal function previously diminished while on conventional amphotericin B improved while on the liposomal formulation (50).

PYRIMIDINE ANALOGUES

5-FLUOROCYTOSINE

Mechanism of Action

5-Fluorocytosine (5-FC; Ancoban, ICN Pharmaceuticals, Costa Mesa, CA) is a fluorinated analogue of cytosine first synthesized in 1957 as a potential antitumor agent (51), first used to treat human disease in 1968 (52), and initially approved for use in 1972 (17). Unfortunately, 5-FC has little inherent anti-*Aspergillus* activity (53) and most reports detail clinical failure with monotherapy for yeast infections (54). Its antimycotic activity results from the rapid conversion of 5-FC into 5-fluorouracil (5-FU) within susceptible fungal cells (55,56). The two mechanisms of action of 5-FU are incorporation into fungal RNA in place of uridylic acid to inhibit fungal protein synthesis and inhibition of thymidylate synthetase to inhibit fungal DNA synthesis (55). The latter appears to be the dominant mechanism. Clinical and microbiologic antifungal resistance appears to develop quickly to 5-FC monotherapy, so clinicians have reserved it for combination approaches to augment other more potent antifungals.

Pharmacology

Fungistatic 5-FC is thought to enhance the antifungal activity of amphotericin B, especially in anatomical sites where amphotericin B penetration is often suboptimal such as CSF, heart valves, and the vitreal body (13). 5-FC penetrates well into most body sites because it is small, highly water-soluble, and not bound by serum proteins to any great extent (55). One explanation for the synergism detected with amphotericin B + 5-FC is that the membrane-permeabilizing effects of low concentrations of amphotericin B facilitate penetration of 5-FC to the cell interior (3). Using a *Candida albicans* model, Beggs and Sarosi suggested that synergism actually results from sequential and not combined action, with amphotericin B acting alone until its gradual oxidation results in its depletion, at which point 5-FC acts on surviving fungal cells' RNA and DNA synthesis (3,57). 5-FC is available only as an oral formulation in the United States, and the correct dose is 150 mg per kg per day in four divided doses.

Toxicities, Side Effects, and Drug Interactions

The toxicity of 5-FC is hypothesized to be due to its conversion to 5-FU, with reports of patients receiving 5-FC for antifungal treatment having serum 5-FU levels in the range found after chemotherapeutic doses (58). However, a pilot study of six patients found undetectable levels of 5-FU in patients receiving 5-FC therapy, suggesting it unlikely that 5-FC toxicity is indeed caused by 5-FU exposure, as originally hypothesized. However, the patients in this study received 5-FC intravenously, and thereby bypassed the conversion of oral 5-FC to 5-FU by the human intestinal microflora (59).

5-FC may exacerbate myelosuppression in patients with neutropenia and toxic levels may develop when in combination with amphotericin B due to nephrotoxicity of the amphotericin B and the decreased renal clearance of 5-FC (39). Routine serum 5-FC level monitoring is warranted in high-risk patients, since peak serum concentrations of 100 μg per mL or greater (2 hours postdose) are associated with bone marrow aplasia. In a review of a multicenter trial of 194 patients who received amphotericin B + 5-FC for cryptococcal meningitis, one or more toxic drug reactions (including azotemia, renal tubular acidosis, leukopenia, thrombocytopenia) developed in 103 patients (60). Toxicity appeared in the first 2 weeks of therapy in 56% of patients and in the first 4 weeks of therapy in 87% of patients. In a study involving 33 neonates in the United Kingdom treated with intravenous or oral 5-FC who underwent therapeutic drug monitoring, drug concentrations were low (trough, <20 mg per L or peak, <50 mg per L) in 40.5%; undetectable in 5.1%; high (trough level >40 mg per L or peak >80 mg per L) in 38.9%; and potentially toxic (>100 mg per L) in 9.9% (61). Given the narrow therapeutic range, the need for therapeutic drug monitoring and oral administration in the United States, this drug is seldom used in neonates.

Clinical Studies

Nearly all clinical studies involving 5-FC are combination antifungal protocols for cryptococcal meningitis, due to the inherently rather weak antifungal activity of 5-FC monotherapy. The first comparative clinical cryptococcal meningitis study with amphotericin B + 5-FC was in 1979 (62) and found a benefit to the combination over amphotericin B alone. One multicenter study of 194 patients with cryptococcal meningitis concluded that 4 weeks of amphotericin B + 5-FC should be reserved for patients without neurologic complications or immunosuppressive therapy, but in a more high-risk population 6 weeks of combination therapy resulted in less relapses (63). Further studies included a multicenter trial that found similar results with consolidation therapy using either itraconazole or fluconazole for 8 weeks after 2 weeks of initial amphotericin B + 5-FC therapy (64).

While other studies have evaluated different combinations for cryptococcal meningitis (65–67), amphotericin B + 5-FC is currently recommended as initial therapy for cryptococcal meningitis after substantial study, and it is also suggested for use in candidal meningitis (68). 5-FC fills an important role in conjunction with amphotericin B, as 5-FC will penetrate into the CSF much better compared with amphotericin B's poor penetration, and 5-FC treated patients had less relapses compared with those receiving only amphotericin B.

Pediatric Clinical Studies

The use of 5-FC in premature neonates is discouraged. A study evaluating risk factors and mortality of neonatal candidiasis among extremely premature infants showed that infants with *Candida* meningitis who received amphotericin B in combination with 5-FC had a prolonged time to sterilize the CSF compared with those receiving amphotericin B monotherapy (median of 17.5 vs. 6 days, respectively) (69).

AZOLES

The azoles are subdivided into imidazoles and triazoles on the basis of the number of nitrogens in the azole ring (7), with the structural differences resulting in different binding affinities for the cytochrome P450 (CYP) enzyme system. With the exception of ketoconazole, the imidazoles have been limited to treatment of superficial mycoses and none, including ketoconazole, have activity against the mold *Aspergillus.* Of the older first-generation triazoles, fluconazole is also ineffective against *Aspergillus,* but itraconazole does possess activity against *Aspergillus.* Newer second-generation triazoles (voriconazole, posaconazole, and ravuconazole) are modifications of prior triazoles with an expanded antifungal spectrum of activity and generally lower minimum inhibitory concentration values compared to the older compounds (70).

MECHANISM OF ACTION

The azole antifungals are heterocyclic synthetic compounds that inhibit the fungal cytochrome $P450_{14DM}$ (also known as lanosterol 14α-demethylase), which catalyzes a late step in ergosterol biosynthesis. The drugs bind to the heme group in the target protein and block demethylation of the C-14 of lanosterol, leading to substitution of methylated sterols in the membrane and depletion of ergosterol. The result is an accumulation of precursors with abnormalities in fungal membrane permeability, membrane-bound enzyme activity, and lack of coordination of chitin synthesis (71,72).

FLUCONAZOLE

Pharmacology

Fluconazole (Diflucan, Pfizer Inc., New York, NY) is a bis-triazole that was discovered in 1982 and approved by the FDA for use in treating cryptococcosis and *Candida* infections in 1990. An in vitro time–kill study showed that the rate of fluconazole fungistatic activity was not influenced by concentration once the maximal fungistatic concentration was surpassed (concentration-independent), which is in contrast to the concentration-dependent fungicidal activity of amphotericin B (71) or caspofungin (73). Fluconazole is well absorbed from the gastrointestinal tract and is cleared predominantly by the renal route as unchanged drug, whereas metabolism accounts for only a minor proportion of fluconazole clearance (74). Binding to plasma proteins is low (12%) (75). Gastric absorption of oral fluconazole is virtually unaffected by pH or the presence of food in the stomach.

Fluconazole is available as either an oral or an intravenous form, and oral fluconazole has a high bioavailability of approximately 90% relative to its intravenous administration. Fluconazole passes into tissues and fluids very rapidly, probably due to its relatively low lipophilicity and limited degree of binding to plasma proteins. Concentrations of fluconazole are 10- to 20-fold higher in the urine than in blood, and drug concentrations in the CSF and vitreous humor of the eye are approximately 80% of those found simultaneously in blood (75). The concentrations of fluconazole in body fluids such as vaginal secretions, breast milk, saliva, and sputum are also similar to those in blood, and the fluid:blood ratio remains stable after multiple doses. There is a linear plasma concentration–dose relationship.

It is clear that simple conversion of the corresponding adult dosage of fluconazole on a weight basis is inappropriate for pediatric patients. A review of five separate fluconazole pharmacokinetic studies in 113 pediatric patients, including 12 premature neonates (74) showed that with the exception of neonates, fluconazole clearance is generally more rapid in children than in adults, with a mean plasma half-life of approximately 20 hours compared with approximately 30 hours in adult patients. Therefore, to achieve comparable exposure in pediatric patients, the daily fluconazole dose needs to be essentially doubled for children older than 3 months. Correct pediatric fluconazole doses should be proportionately higher than adult doses, generally 10 to 12 mg per kg per day.

In neonates the volume of distribution is significantly greater and more variable than in infants and children, and doubling the dose for neonatal patients is necessary to achieve comparable plasma concentrations. The increased volume of distribution is thought to be due to the larger amount of body water found in the total body volume of neonates. However, there is also a slow elimination of fluconazole, with a mean half-life of 88.6 hours at birth, decreasing to approximately 55 hours at 2 weeks of age. This is due to the reduced activity of hepatic enzymes for biotransformation as well as reduced glomerular filtration for the first month of life. As renal function continues to develop, the fluconazole plasma half-life decreases (74); however, a recent population pharmacokinetic study in premature infants suggests that maintenance fluconazole doses of 12 mg per kg per day are necessary to achieve exposures similar to older children and adults (76). In addition, a loading dose of 25 mg per kg would achieve steady-state concentrations sooner than the traditional dosing scheme (77). This strategy is currently being evaluated in a phase I clinical trial.

Children with human immunodeficiency virus (HIV) infection who receive oral fluconazole achieve similar serum concentrations to intravenous dosing and this indicates a nearly complete degree of absorption (78). In fact, there have also been comparable concentrations after either oral or intravenous administration in children younger than 3 months (79). The bioavailability of enteral fluconazole is adequate in even critically ill surgical patients (79). The peritoneal bioavailability of fluconazole is also excellent for treating dialysis patients with peritonitis. A prospective study of 17 children on dialysis found that fluconazole was excreted almost solely through the dialysate and the terminal half-life was significantly longer in the children requiring peritoneal dialysis (80). Finally, there is a theoretical advantage to the oral suspension fluconazole over capsules for oral thrush, as in one study of health volunteers the peak saliva levels of fluconazole were higher in those flushing their mouth for 2 minutes with the oral suspension than in those who swallowed the capsule (81).

Toxicities, Side Effects, and Drug Interactions

Side effects of fluconazole are uncommon. In one study of 24 immunocompromised children, elevated transaminases were observed in only two cases (82). A large review of 78 reports that used fluconazole in a total of 726 children younger than the age of 1 year showed that it was generally well tolerated and reaffirmed the guidelines to increase the interval between doses due to the prolonged elimination during the first month of life (83). Another review of 562 children from 12 clinical studies confirmed that pediatric results mirror the excellent safety profile seen in adults. The most common side effects were gastrointestinal upset (7.7%) (vomiting, diarrhea, nausea) and a skin rash (1.2%) (84). Fluconazole affects the metabolism of cyclosporine, leading to its increased concentration when used together (76).

Clinical Studies

A review of two randomized clinical trials showed that patients who received fluconazole versus placebo for prophylaxis against candidiasis while undergoing allogeneic bone marrow transplantation had lower rates of candidal infection and gut graft-versus-host disease (85). Additional studies revealed that either fluconazole (200 mg per day) versus low-dose amphotericin B (0.2 mg per kg per day) or high dose (400 mg per day) versus low-dose (200 mg per day) fluconazole prophylaxis showed any difference in incidence of fungal infections or survival (86,87).

For treatment of invasive candidiasis, a multicenter trial of 236 patients found that those treated with fluconazole + amphotercin B versus fluconazole alone trended toward better success and more rapid resolution of *Candida* fungemia with the combination (88). In another randomized trial for treatment of fungal infections using medical and surgical intensive care unit patients, there was a significant decrease in *Candida* species infections in the group that received fluconazole versus placebo (89).

Unlike itraconazole or ketoconazole, fluconazole is particularly appropriate for urinary tract infections due to its concentrating effect in the bladder. Fluconazole is also effective for superficial skin infections, since the stratum corneum: serum ratio is 37 (90).

Pediatric Clinical Studies

An open, prospective, randomized pilot study in 50 children undergoing remission induction or consolidation chemotherapy showed that those patients who received either fluconazole or nystatin prophylaxis for *Candida* infections had similar rates of success (91). A study of 40 young infants (aged 2 days to 3 months) with either nonresponse or contraindication to standard antifungal therapy treated with fluconazole showed a 97% clinical and mycological response rate (92). In a prospective, randomized double-blind trial over a 30-month period of 100 infants with birth weights less than 1,000 g, those infants who received fluconazole for 6 weeks had a decrease in fungal colonization (22% vs. 60%) as well as a decrease in the development of invasive fungal infection compared with placebo (0% vs. 20%) (93). A larger prospective, randomized double-blind, controlled trial conducted in nine neonatal intensive care units in Italy among 322 infants with birth weight less than 1500 g showed that a fluconazole prophylaxis regimen of 3 to 6 mg per kg several times per week for 4 to 6 weeks reduced the incidence of *Candida* colonization [9.8% in the 6 mg group, 7.7% in the 3 mg group, and 29.2% in the placebo group ($p < .001$)] and invasive fungal infections [2.7% in the 6 mg group ($p = .005$), 3.8% in the 3 mg group ($p = .02$), and 13.2% in the placebo group] (94). A retrospective study evaluating the incidence of invasive candidiasis and *Candida*-related mortality among infants with birth weights less than 1,000 g who received fluconazole prophylaxis (3 mg per kg several times per week) for 6 weeks showed that the incidence of invasive candidiasis and *Candida*-associated mortality decreased. In the group receiving fluconazole, no increase in fluconazole resistant *Candida* strains was observed (95). Similarly, another report demonstrated that the use of fluconazole prophylaxis for 4 to 6 weeks in infants with birth weights less than 1500 g did not increase the incidence of fungal colonization and infections caused by natively fluconazole-resistant *Candida* species (96). Results of fluconazole prophylaxis studies in premature infants are encouraging; however, the universal implementation of such strategy across nurseries is discouraged because (a) the rate of *Candida* infections varies greatly among centers (97) and (b) there is insufficient neurodevelopmental follow-up data in these infants to justify prophylaxis (98). A multicenter international trial is underway to answer questions regarding the most appropriate prophylaxis regimen and the need of prophylaxis based on individual nursery systemic *Candida* infection rates.

ITRACONAZOLE

First publicly described in 1983 (99,100) and available for clinical use in 1990, itraconazole (Sporanox, Janssen Pharmaceuticals, Titusville, NJ) adopted a triazole nucleus with higher specificity for the fungal CYP enzyme system than the older imidazoles (101). Itraconazole's fungicidal activity is not as efficient as that of amphotericin B because inhibition of sterol synthesis takes longer than directly creating channels within the cell membrane (102). Historically there had been several constraints with itraconazole: no parenteral formulation, erratic oral absorption in high-risk patients, and significant drug interactions. These pharmacokinetic concerns have been addressed with both an intravenous formulation and a better absorbed oral preparation.

Pharmacology

Itraconazole has a high volume of distribution and accumulates in tissues, and the tissue-bound levels are probably more clinically relevant to infection treatment than serum levels (72). Itraconazole is poorly water-soluble, not reliably absorbed from the gastrointestinal tract in its capsule formulation, and has high protein binding (11). It has a relatively long half-life of 25 to 50 hours, which allows for once-daily dosing (103).

Dissolution and absorption of itraconazole are affected by gastric pH. Patients with achlorhydria or H_2-receptor antagonist use may demonstrate impaired absorption, whereas coadministration of the capsule with acidic beverages such as colas or cranberry juice may enhance its absorption (104). Administering a dose with food significantly increases the absorption of the capsule formulation, but the new oral suspension with a cyclodextrin base is better absorbed on an empty stomach (15). Elimination of itraconazole is primarily hepatic, so there is no need for dosage adjustment in renal failure (72).

To overcome problems with variable absorption, itraconazole has now been solubilized in cyclodextrin, with its substantial improvement in absorption of drug as an oral solution (72,105). This allows itraconazole to be available as an oral capsule, oral solution, and intravenous formulation. Cyclodextrins are naturally occurring doughnut-shaped glucose oligomers produced by enzymatic degradation of starch that have been chemically modified for medical use. The external face of the molecule is hydrophilic to facilitate solubilization of the complex in water and shield a lipophilic guest molecule (106). Once itraconazole is released from the host cyclodextrin it follows its standard pharmacokinetics, with steady-state concentration reached in the second week of daily dosing.

A new intravenous formulation of itraconazole was approved by the FDA for pulmonary and extrapulmonary aspergillosis in patients who are intolerant of or refractory to amphotericin B (107). The intravenous formulation can rapidly achieve high steady-state plasma concentrations (108,109) as opposed to the 7- to 10-day period needed for the capsule or oral formulation (110). In children, itraconazole oral solution produces a maximum concentration lower than in adults which could potentially justify higher dosing in younger children, whereas other pharmacokinetic properties such as half-life are similar to values in adults (111). The intravenous preparation is not recommended for patients with reduced renal clearance because the impact or toxicity of the cyclodextrin is not known. In a single dose (2.5 mg per kg) pharmacokinetic study of itraconazole in children aged 7 months to 17 years ($n = 33$), pharmacokinetic parameters of itraconazole were highly variable across age groups and, therefore, no age dependence was observed in drug disposition. Overall, the estimated C_{max} was 1,015 (±692) ng per mL, systemic clearance was 702.8 (±499.4) mL per hour per kg, and half-life was 20.2 (±12.8) hours (112). Pediatric dosing for itraconazole is not exact, but generally felt to be higher than adult doses and approximately 3 to 10 mg per kg per day.

Toxicities, Side Effects, and Drug Interactions

Side effects are relatively few and include nausea and vomiting (10%), elevated transaminases (5%), (113) and peripheral edema. Although it has not been shown in children, there have been reports of development of cardiomyopathy while receiving this azole. As a potent inhibitor of the fungal CYP3A4 enzyme, itraconazole also has affinity for the human enzyme, and this produces important drug interactions. Prior or concurrent use of rifampin, phenytoin, carbamazepine, and phenobarbital should be avoided. Any drug handled by this cytochrome pathway with normally low bioavailability, extensive first-pass metabolism, or a narrow therapeutic window may be especially vulnerable (114).

Patients receiving cyclosporine who are treated with a triazole should have an immediate dose reduction of cyclosporine followed by frequent monitoring of serum levels. In one study there was an increase in tacrolimus or cyclosporine levels 48 hours after completing an intravenous itraconazole loading dose, so a 50% tacrolimus or cyclosporine dose reduction is recommended after an intravenous itraconazole loading dose (115). Furthermore, the azoles may also increase serum levels and intracellular levels of cytotoxic drugs such as vincristine and anthracyclines (31) or protease inhibitors (116). Azole–drug interactions may also lead to decreased plasma concentration of the azole, related to either decreased absorption or increased metabolism (17).

Although the theoretical concern of polyene–azole antagonism due to ergosterol mechanisms of action exists, combination with amphotericin B does appear safe in a recent survey of clinical practice of 93 invasive-aspergillosis patients treated with this sequential therapy (117).

Clinical Studies

Itraconazole has roles in the therapy of numerous fungal infections. A multicenter open-label study was performed in 31 patients with pulmonary invasive aspergillosis who received 14 days of intravenous itraconazole followed by 12 weeks of capsules. The intravenous form was well tolerated and target therapeutic concentrations were obtained within 2 days in 91% of patients and in all patients within 1 week of intravenous treatment. These levels were also maintained after switching to oral therapy, and a complete or partial response was seen in 48% (15/31) of patients (108).

A randomized controlled trial comparing itraconazole oral solution versus fluconazole suspension for prevention of fungal infections in 445 hematological malignancy patients revealed that more proven fungal infections occurred in the fluconazole arm and more of these were fatal (118). In addition, there were no cases of invasive aspergillosis in the itraconazole arm, there were significantly more cases of aspergillosis in the fluconazole arm, and most were fatal. This study reinforces that while itraconazole and fluconazole provide effective prophylaxis against *Candida* infections, itraconazole offers additional protection against aspergillosis. Similarly, in a randomized trial of liver transplant recipients, those patients treated with oral itraconazole developed less proven fungal infections than did those receiving fluconazole for the same time period (119).

A double-blind trial of 63 patients with HIV infection in Thailand with itraconazole versus placebo showed that development of systemic fungal infection decreased from 16.7% of patients given placebo versus 1.6% taking itraconazole, with only one infection with *Penicillium marneffei* in the itraconazole treatment arm (120).

Pediatric Clinical Studies

A phase I study in 26 HIV-infected children showed that the cyclodextrin itraconazole solution was well tolerated and efficacious against oropharyngeal candidiasis, including responses in all patients with fluconazole-resistant isolates (121). Although not standardized, a commonly used dose of itraconazole for pediatric patients is 3 to 5 mg per kg per day once daily, with doses used up to 10 mg per kg per day. Itraconazole (10 mg per kg per day loading dose and 5 mg per kg per day maintenance dose) administered to 53 pediatric patients for 100 days following hematological stem cell transplantation to prevent invasive fungal infections was well tolerated. In this cohort, one patient suffered from invasive candidiasis; 21% (11/53) discontinued the medication mostly to prolonged fever ($n = 7$); and 19% (10/53) had doubling of aspartate aminotransferase baseline values (122). The use of itraconazole over fluconazole in this population is attractive because of its antimold properties; however, given the metabolic profile of itraconazole, high potential for drug interactions, and high exposure variability in pediatric patients, newer triazole agents (i.e., voriconazole) continue to be the first line of therapy against invasive mold infections.

VORICONAZOLE

Voriconazole (VFend; Pfizer Inc., New York, NY) is a new second-generation triazole and a synthetic derivative of fluconazole. First introduced in 1995, it was developed as part of a program to enhance the potency and antifungal spectrum of fluconazole largely through the addition of a methyl group to fluconazole's propyl backbone and the substitution of a triazole moiety with a fluoropyrimidine group (123). Voriconazole generally has the spectrum of activity of itraconazole, yet the bioavailability of fluconazole. Importantly, it has both fungicidal and fungistatic activity against *Aspergillus* (123–125).

Pharmacology

Voriconazole is extensively metabolized by the liver and shows approximately 90% oral bioavailability. It appears that CYP2C19 plays a major role in the metabolism of voriconazole, and this enzyme exhibits genetic polymorphism, dividing the population into poor and extensive metabolizers as a result of a point mutation in the gene encoding the protein of CYP2C19 (126). About 5% to 7% of the White population has a deficiency in expressing this enzyme, so genotype plays a key role in the pharmacokinetics of voriconazole (127). As many as 20% of non-Indian Asians have low CYP2C19 activity and can achieve voriconazole levels as much as fourfold greater than those homozygous subjects who metabolize the drug more extensively (128). Even though most of the voriconazole metabolism occurs through the cytochrome P-450 enzymatic system, recent animal models suggest that 25% of the remaining metabolism is mediated by the flavin-containing monooxygenase pathway (129).

Voriconazole is available as an oral tablet or an intravenous solution. Voriconazole is 44% to 67% plasma bound, in adults it exhibits nonlinear pharmacokinetics, has a variable half-life of approximately 6 hours (130) with large interpatient variation in blood levels (131), and has good CSF penetration (70,101,132–135). Time–kill studies against *Candida* species and *Cryptococcus neoformans* revealed in vitro nonconcentration-dependent fungistatic activity, similar to that of fluconazole (136).

Oral absorption is nonlinear and rapid, with an approximately fivefold accumulation over 14 days in one study of hematologic malignancy patients (135). In a study assessing voriconazole levels after intravenous-to-oral switching, mean voriconazole levels did fall following oral administration compared to intravenous administration, but most subjects achieved steady state 4 days after dosing began. Maximum plasma voriconazole levels occurred at the end of the 1-hour intravenous infusion and between 1.4 and 1.8 hours after oral administration (127). A pharmacokinetic study in six patients with cirrhosis demonstrated that hepatic-impaired patients should receive the same oral loading dose, but half the maintenance dose (137). In contrast to adults, elimination of voriconazole is linear in children. A multicenter safety, population pharmacokinetic study of single (3 to 4 mg per kg) and multiple

(12 mg per kg per day loading dose, 6 to 8 mg per kg per day maintenance dose) intravenous voriconazole doses in immunocompromised pediatric patients (n = 35, 2 to 11 years of age) showed that body weight was more influential than age in accounting for the observed variability in voriconazole pharmacokinetics and elimination capacity correlated with CYP2C19 genotype. Exposures were similar at 4 mg per kg every 12 hours in children (median area under the concentration–time curve 14,227 ng per hour per mL) and 3 mg per kg in adults [median area under the curve (AUC), 13,855 ng per hour per mL]. Visual disturbances occurred in 13% of the patients (138).

Toxicities, Side Effects, and Drug Interactions

Voriconazole's main side effects include reversible dose-dependent visual disturbances (increased brightness, blurred vision) (139) in as many as one-third of treated patients, elevated hepatic transaminases with increasing doses (140,141), and occasional skin reactions likely due to photosensitization (101,123,142).

As with other azoles the potential exists to modify the metabolism of other drugs, including a contraindication for concomitant use with sirolimus. In one study coadministration of voriconazole and tacrolimus elevated trough tacrolimus levels in one liver transplant patient nearly 10-fold (143), and in another study tacrolimus levels were significantly increased 2.2-fold when coadministered with voriconazole (144). In a study of renal transplant patients, concomitant administration of voriconazole with cyclosporine also resulted in a 1.7-fold increase in the geometric mean for cyclosporine area under the plasma concentration–time curve, so it is recommended that the cyclosporine dose be halved and levels monitored frequently (145). However, voriconazole does not affect mycophenolic acid (146).

Clinical Studies

The largest prospective clinical trial of voriconazole as primary therapy for invasive aspergillosis involved 392 patients at 92 centers in 19 countries over 3 years and compared initial randomized therapy with voriconazole versus amphotericin B followed by conventional therapy. Patients who initially received voriconazole had statistically significantly better complete or partial response (53%) versus those initially receiving amphotericin B (32%). Survival also improved to 71% for voriconazole versus 58% for those initially receiving amphotericin B (147). Analysis in an open, noncomparative multicenter study of 116 patients, treated with voriconazole as primary therapy (60 patients) or salvage therapy (56 patients) also yielded encouraging results: 14% had a complete, 34% had a partial, and 21% had a stable response to voriconazole, whereas 31% failed to respond to therapy (131). These data forged the way for FDA approval of voriconazole for initial therapy for invasive aspergillosis in May 2002.

A multicenter trial of voriconazole versus fluconazole in treating esophageal candidiasis in 391 immunocompromised patients showed similar success rates with voriconazole (98.3%) and fluconazole (95.1%) (148). Although overall safety and tolerability of both antifungals was acceptable, fewer patients discontinued voriconazole due to poor clinical response, but more patients discontinued voriconazole than fluconazole because of laboratory abnormalities or adverse events.

Pediatric Clinical Studies

Voriconazole has been studied in an open-label evaluation of 58 children with a proven or probable invasive fungal infection who received voriconazole on a compassionate basis if they were refractory or intolerant of conventional antifungal therapy (149). Most patients (72%) had aspergillosis, but the group also included scedosporiosis (14%), candidiasis (7%), and others. At the end of therapy (median duration 93 days), a total of 45% of children had a complete or partial response, and only 7% were discontinued from voriconazole because of intolerance. Stratifying outcome by pathogen revealed a complete or partial response of 43% against aspergillosis, 50% against candidemia, and 63% against scedosporiosis. The most commonly reported adverse events in these children included elevation in hepatic transaminases, skin rash and photosensitivity reaction, and abnormal vision. Intravenously administered voriconazole has been used successfully in preterm infants of very low birth weight with primary cutaneous aspergillosis (150).

POSACONAZOLE

In September 2006 the FDA approved posaconazole (Noxafil, Schering Corporation, Kenilworth, NJ) for the prophylaxis and treatment of disseminated candidiasis and aspergillosis in severely immunocompromised patients and for the treatment of oropharyngeal candidiasis. Posaconazole is a second-generation triazole antifungal agent available as a suspension for oral administration. The antimicrobial spectrum of posaconazole is similar to that of voriconazole; however, the former is active against zygomycetes.

Pharmacology

Posaconazole reaches maximum plasma concentrations 3 to 5 hours after ingestion. Dose proportional increases in plasma exposure (AUC) to posaconazole were observed following single oral doses from 50 to 800 mg and following multiple dose administration from 50 mg BID to 400 mg BID. Steady-state plasma concentrations are attained at 7 to 10 days following multiple-dose administration (151). When administered with a nonfat and high-fat diet posaconazole exposure and maximum concentration are 3 to 4 times higher than the fasting state (152). In addition, posaconazole exposure is maximized with acidic beverages, administration in divided doses, and absence of proton pump inhibitors (153). Posaconazole distributes well into tissues, is 98% protein bound, and is not a substrate for the cytochrome P-450 enzymatic system. However, about 20% of the parent drug is glucoronidated by phase 2 enzymes. Posaconazole is eliminated with a mean half-life of 25 hours (19 to 31 hours) with a total body clearance (CL/F) of 4.1 to 6.6 mL per minute per kg (154); it is predominantly eliminated in the feces with renal clearance playing a minor role. Therefore, no dose adjustment is necessary in mild to moderate renal insufficiency. Posaconazole is fungicidal in vitro with likely time-dependent killing (11).

Toxicities, Side Effects, and Drug Interactions

Posaconazole is primarily metabolized via uridine diphosphate (UDP) glucuronidation (phase 2 enzymes) and is a substrate for P-glycoprotein (P-gp) efflux. Therefore, inhibitors or inducers (i.e., rifabutin, phenytoin) of these clearance pathways may affect posaconazole plasma concentrations (155). Posaconazole is also a CYP34A inhibitor and, therefore, coadministration results in increased plasma concentrations of the following products: cyclosporine (75% dose reduction required) (155), tacrolimus (60% dose reduction required), rifabutin, midazolam, and phenytoin (155). Posaconazole causes transient hepatic reactions including mild to moderate elevations in alanine aminotransferase, aspartate aminotransferase, alkaline phosphatase, and total bilirubin (155).

Clinical Studies

In a multicenter randomized, single-blinded study of posaconazole ($n = 304$) versus fluconazole or itraconazole ($n = 298$) in neutropenic patients undergoing chemotherapy for acute myelogenous leukemia or myelodysplastic syndromes, posaconazole was superior in preventing invasive fungal infections (156). Proven or probable invasive fungal infections were reported in 2% in the posaconazole group versus 8% in the fluconazole or itraconazole group (absolute reduction in the posaconazole group, −6%; 95% CI, −9.7 to −2.5%; $p < .001$). Fewer patients in the posaconazole group had invasive aspergillosis (1 vs. 7%, $p < .001$) and survival was significantly longer among recipients of posaconazole than among recipients of fluconazole or itraconazole ($p = .04$). Serious adverse events (i.e., torsades de pointes) possibly or probably related to posaconazole were higher when compared with fluconazole or itraconazole (6 vs. 2%, $p = .01$) (156). Another multiple site, randomized, double-blinded study in patients with allogeneic hematopoietic stem cell transplantation and graft versus hosts disease showed that posaconazole was not inferior to fluconazole in the prevention of invasive fungal infections (157). Posaconazole has also been used successfully in the treatment of six adult patients who received salvage treatment (800 mg per day) for 6 to 34 weeks for severe forms of histoplasmosis ($n = 1$, pulmonary; $n = 5$, disseminated disease) (158).

Pediatric Clinical Studies

In a study of eight patients (seven pediatric patients 9 to 18 years of age) with chronic granulomatous disease and proven invasive mold infection refractory to standard therapy, posaconazole ($n = 6$,400 mg orally twice per day; $n = 1$,200 mg orally three times per day) was well tolerated (159). Another report including data from 24 patients with active zygomycosis who were enrolled in two open-label, nonrandomized, multicentered compassionate trials that evaluated oral posaconazole as salvage therapy for invasive fungal infections showed that two children aged 7 and 17 years had partial response to posaconazole (160).

RAVUCONAZOLE

Ravuconazole (Bristol-Myers Squibb Company, Princeton, NJ) is structurally more similar to fluconazole and voriconazole, containing a thiazole instead of a second triazole. It is often fungicidal (161,162), has 47% to 74% bioavailability with linear pharmacokinetics (101), and a long half-life of approximately 100 hours (163). The drug is well absorbed following oral administration, and its absorption is enhanced by food (162). Penetration of ravuconazole into healthy rat tissue showed that concentration of drug in the lungs was two to six times higher than the corresponding blood concentration (164). Ravuconazole has not been approved by the FDA.

Pharmacology

Ravuconazole is well tolerated, with headache a main side effect, and urine studies suggest no CYP isoenzyme induction (70). Ravuconazole was also well tolerated in healthy human subjects in single (163) and multiple doses (165). Ravuconazole and coadministration with simvastatin was well tolerated in 20 health subjects and showed that ravuconazole was a less potent inhibitor of the CYP3A4 enzyme than other triazole antifungals (166). Ravuconazole did not affect nelfinavir in 14 healthy volunteers (167).

Clinical Studies

A randomized trial of 76 patients with ravuconazole cured 76% of esophageal candidiasis patients 7 days after administration, with a safety profile similar to fluconazole (168). A substudy analysis of HIV-positive patients with oropharyngeal candidiasis showed a 95% response rate after 5 days of therapy (169). Ravuconazole was evaluated in a multicenter, phase I/II randomized, double-blind, placebo controlled trial, dose-ranging study of toenail onychomycosis. For 12 weeks participants ($n = 151$) received one of the following dosing regimens: 200 mg per day; 100 mg per week; 400 mg per week; or placebo. Clinical, microbiological cure and clinical response were reportedly greater in those who received ravuconazole 200 mg per day (170).

Pediatric Clinical Studies

There are no clinical trials of ravuconazole in children.

ECHINOCANDINS

MECHANISM OF ACTION

For years, most development of new systemic antifungals focused on chemically modifying existing classes (171). An entirely new class of antifungals, the echinocandins and the amino-containing pneumocandin analogues, are cyclic hexapeptide agents that interfere with cell wall biosynthesis by noncompetitive inhibition of 1,3-β-D-glucan synthase, an enzyme present in fungi but absent in mammalian cells (70,101). This 1,3-β-D-glucan, an essential cell wall polysaccharide, forms a fibril of three helically entwined linear polysaccharides and provides structural integrity for the fungal cell wall (172,173).

Echinocandins inhibit hyphal tip growth, converting the mycelium to small clumps of cells, but the older septated cells with little glucan synthesis are not killed (171). Therefore, the echinocandin activity end point is morphological change, not in vitro medium clearing. Echinocandins are generally fungicidal in vitro against *Candida* species, although not as rapidly as amphotericin B (11,101), but appear to be fungistatic against *Aspergillus* (40). As a class these agents are not metabolized through the CYP enzyme system but through a presumed O-methyl-transferase, lessening some of the drug interactions and side effects seen with the azole class. The echinocandins appear to have a prolonged and dose-dependent fungicidal antifungal effect on *C. albicans*, compared with the fungistatic fluconazole (174).

Although echinocandin B was first described in 1974 as a natural product of *Aspergillus nidulans* (175), drug development in this class has only recently expanded. Cilofungin, the first echinocandin B, was developed for *Candida* infections but clinical investigation was discontinued due to possible toxicity of the vehicle, polyethylene glycol (176). Three compounds in this class (caspofungin, micafungin, and anidulafungin) are FDA-approved for use in adults.

Few studies have evaluated the use of echinocandins in children; most constitute early phase I/II safety and pharmacokinetic studies. Because neonates with candidemia often suffer from disseminated disease in the central nervous system, which is associated with neurodevelopmental impairment, dosing of antifungal agents in this population should target the central nervous system.

An experimental rabbit model of hematogenous *Candida* meningoencephalitis in which micafungin was used as a prototype echinocandin suggests that doses of 8 mg per kg per day are necessary to achieve maximal microbicidal activity in the central nervous system parenchyma of rabbits (177). When these data are extrapolated to the neonatal population using simulation techniques, the lowest fungal burden in the neonatal central nervous system parenchyma is achieved with micafungin doses of 10 to 15 mg per kg per day (177).

CASPOFUNGIN

Pharmacology

Caspofungin (Cancidas; Merck Co., Whitehouse Station, NJ) is a fungicidal, water-soluble semisynthetic derivative of the natural product pneumocandin B_0 (178). It has linear pharmacokinetics (179), is hepatically excreted with a β-phase half-life of 9 to 10 hours (180), and has uncommon adverse effects (181–183). Parenteral administration is preferred due to the low bioavailability when administered orally (182,183). It is not metabolized by the CYP isoenzyme system (184) and the rate of killing for caspofungin in time–kill studies is greater than that of amphotericin B, which does not require cell growth for activity (173).

The usual course is to begin with a loading dose followed by a daily maintenance dose (171), usually 70 mg followed by 50 mg daily in adults. Pharmacokinetics in healthy volunteers revealed linear pharmacokinetics and dose-proportional AUC concentration data. Much of the dose accumulation is achieved in the first week of dosing, and renal insufficiency has little effect on the pharmacokinetics of caspofungin (185,186). Caspofungin has been evaluated at double the recommended dose (100 mg in adults) with an approximately 2.5-fold AUC (187). Two pharmacokinetic studies of mild to moderate hepatic insufficiency resulted in elevations of caspofungin plasma concentrations observed in patients with mild hepatic insufficiency, and a dose reduction from 50 to 35 mg daily following the standard 70-mg loading dose was recommended in this setting (185).

Pharmacokinetics are different in children: levels are lower in smaller children and the half-life is reduced. A study evaluated the pharmacokinetics of caspofungin in 39 children (2 to 17 years) with neutropenia and showed that in patients receiving 50 mg per m^2 per day (maximum, 70 mg per day), the AUC_{0-24} was similar to that for the exposure in adults receiving 50 mg per day and was consistent across age ranges. In this study, weight-based dosing (1 mg per kg per day) was suboptimal when compared with body surface area regimens and adult dosing (188).

Toxicities, Side Effects, and Drug Interactions

1,3-β-glucan is a selective target present only in fungal cell walls and not in mammalian cells; therefore, the drug mechanism–based toxicity for the echinocandins are limited (173). Plasma concentrations of tacrolimus are reduced by about 20% with coadministration of caspofungin, necessitating the close monitoring of tacrolimus levels, but tacrolimus does not alter the pharmacokinetics of caspofungin (141). Cyclosporine increased the AUC of caspofungin by about 35%, although plasma concentrations of cyclosporine were not altered by coadministration of caspofungin (189). Mycophenolate and caspofungin have no relevant interactions (186). There appears to be no apparent myelotoxicity or nephrotoxicity with the agent (186).

Clinical Studies

Caspofungin was approved by the FDA in February 2001 for refractory aspergillosis or intolerance to other therapies, and in January 2003, it was approved for candidemia and various other sites of invasive *Candida* infections. In the pivotal clinical study leading to FDA approval, 56 patients with acute invasive aspergillosis underwent "salvage" therapy after failing (45 patients) primary therapy for more than a week or developing significant nephrotoxicity. Recipients had a 41% (22/54) favorable response with caspofungin (167) and follow-up on all 90 patients enrolled in that trial revealed that 45% had a complete or partial response (190). A Spanish study before licensure revealed a 67% (8/12) favorable response rate among patients with proven or probable invasive aspergillosis (191).

There have been several clinical trials evaluating caspofungin in esophageal candidiasis. One study of 128 patients found an 89% clinical success rate, compared with 63% in those patients receiving amphotericin B. In addition, therapy was stopped only in 7% of caspofungin patients, compared with 24% of amphotericin B patients (192,193). A study comparing daily caspofungin with fluconazole showed favorable similar response rates (81% vs. 85%), but symptoms recurred 4 weeks after stopping therapy in 28% of patients who received caspofungin versus 17% of those who received fluconazole (194). Another study evaluated patients with clinically fluconazole-resistant esophageal candidiasis and found that 7/11 (64%) patients had favorable responses to caspofungin, including patients with isolates showing in vitro fluconazole resistance (195).

In a multicenter trial of 239 patients with invasive candidiasis, 73.4% of patients who received caspofungin had a favorable response at the end of therapy, compared with 61.7% in the amphotericin B group (196). There was a comparable outcome for both candidemia and intra-abdominal candidiasis. Mortality was similar in both groups, and the proportion of patients with drug-related adverse events was significantly higher in the amphotericin B group. Caspofungin was evaluated against liposomal amphotericin B in the empirical treatment of patients with persistent fever and neutropenia. Caspofungin was not inferior to liposomal amphotericin B in 1,095 subjects (including 11 children) with overall success rates of 34% for caspofungin and for liposomal amphotericin B (95.2 CI for the difference, −5.6 to 6.0%). Among patients with baseline fungal infections, a higher proportion of those treated with caspofungin had a successful outcome (52% vs. 26%, $p = .04$). Patients who received caspofungin sustained fewer renal and infusion-related events than those treated with the comparator (197). Caspofungin also had similar success rates as itraconazole in an open-label, randomized study of antifungal prophylaxis in patients undergoing induction chemotherapy for acute myelogenous leukemia or myelodysplastic syndrome (198).

Pediatric Clinical Studies

In children, the use of caspofungin has been limited to refractory cases of invasive candidiasis, as salvage or combination therapy in other invasive fungal infections including aspergillosis (199,200) and in cases of patients with fever and neutropenia. A single center, retrospective review of 56 children (median age, 8 years; range 1 to 17 years) who received caspofungin as empirical therapy for fever and neutropenia during 2005 to 2006 showed that 79% of caspofungin courses resulted in an overall favorable response; 15% of courses experienced an adverse drug-related event that was probably or possibly attributable to caspofungin; and 1 of 19 children receiving caspofungin and cyclosporine concurrently developed hepatotoxicity possibly related to caspofungin (201).

Caspofungin in newborns has been used off-label as single or adjuvant therapy for refractory cases of disseminated candidiasis. A study from Costa Rica reported the use of caspofungin (0.5 to 1 mg per kg per day for the first 2 to 3 days and 1 to 2 mg per kg per day for the remaining of the course) among 10 neonates (mean gestational age 33.5 ± 1.77) with refractory disseminated candidiasis; all patients had a sterile blood culture within 3 to 7 days of starting caspofungin and the drug was well tolerated (202). Through a retrospective chart review, another center identified 13 cases of neonates [median gestational age 27 weeks (range, 24 to 28)] treated with caspofungin (1 to 1.5 mg per kg per day) for refractory disseminated candidiasis; 11 of the infants achieved blood sterilization within a median of 3 days (range, 1 to 21). However, all but three patients had their intravascular lines removed prior to the onset of caspofungin therapy (203). In this cohort, two patients died within 2 days of starting caspofungin; one patient developed severe thrombophlebitis after the initial dose; two patients had hypokalemia while on caspofungin; and four patients had a greater than threefold elevation of alanine aminotransferase and aspartate aminotransferase (203).

Additional studies of caspofungin in the pediatric population are necessary to assess its efficacy. In addition, pharmacokinetic studies in neonates are needed prior to the widespread use of this antifungal agent in the nursery.

MICAFUNGIN

Pharmacology

Micafungin (Fujisawa Healthcare, Inc., Deerfield, IL) is an echinocandin lipopeptide compound (101,204,205) with a half-life of approximately 12 hours, and similar to other echinocandins is fungistatic in vitro versus *Aspergillus* (206). A population pharmacokinetic analysis of micafungin administered to adults after stem cell transplantation revealed that a two-compartment model with zero-order input and first-order elimination best described micafungin disposition. Estimated population pharmacokinetic parameters included volume of distribution at the central compartment of 10.4 L (±5.60) and systemic clearance of 1.165 L per hour (±0.38). Weight was a significant predictor of micafungin clearance suggesting that patients with weights of 66.3 kg or more require higher micafungin doses (150 mg daily) to achieve similar exposures as in patients of lower body weight receiving 100 mg daily of micafungin (207).

There are dose-independent linear plasma pharmacokinetics with the highest drug concentrations detected in the lung, followed by the liver, spleen, and kidney. Micafungin was undetectable in the CSF (208), but levels were detected in the brain tissue, choroidal layer, meninges, and cerebellum in an experimental rabbit animal model (177). Time–kill study of micafungin against *Candida* species demonstrated potent fungicidal activity against most isolates, including a concentration-dependent postantifungal effect (209).

The pharmacokinetics of micafungin have been evaluated in children and young infants. A phase I, dose escalation study evaluated the pharmacokinetics of micafungin in 77 children (2 to 17 years of age) with fever and neutropenia. Within the dosing range of 0.5 to 4 mg per kg per day micafungin demonstrated linear pharmacokinetics; clearance, volume of distribution, and half-life remained relatively constant over the dose range and did not change with repeated administration; and an inverse relation between age and clearance was observed. Mean systemic clearance (0.385 ± 0.15 vs. 0.285 ± 0.12 mL per minute per kg for 2 to 8 years and 9 to 17 years, respectively) was significantly greater and mean half-life (11.6 ± 2.8 vs. 13.3 ± 4.3 hours) was significantly shorter in patients aged 2 to 8 years compared with those of 9 to 17 years (210). A follow-up population pharmacokinetic study using the same data showed that weight was a significant predictor of micafungin clearance in pediatric patients. To achieve micafungin exposures equivalent to adults receiving 100, 150, and 200 mg daily, as evidenced by simulation profiles, children require dosages higher than 3 mg per kg (211). Another population pharmacokinetic study of micafungin administered to a Japanese population (including children) also showed that weight was the most significant predictor of micafungin clearance in pediatric patients (212).

A phase I, sequential and single-dose (0.75, 1.5, and 3.0 mg per kg) study of intravenous micafungin in 18 premature infants (mean gestational age 26.4 ± 2.4 weeks) weighing more than 1,000 g showed that micafungin pharmacokinetics in preterm infants was linear; premature infants displayed a shorter half-life (8 hours) and a more rapid rate of clearance (approximately 39 mL per hour per kg) compared with published data in older children and adults (213). In this study, an additional four infants weighing less than 1,000 g received 0.75 mg per kg per day of micafungin and demonstrated shorter mean half-life (5.5 hours) and more rapid mean clearance per body weight (79.3 ± 12.5 mL per hour per kg) when compared with the heavier infants (213). These results suggest that young infants may require higher micafungin doses when compared with older children and adults. Preliminary data in 12 premature infants (mean birth weight and gestational age 851 g and 27 weeks, respectively) suggest that a micafungin dose of 15 mg per kg per day achieves similar exposures [mean area under the curve 437.5 (± 99.4) mg per hour per L] to adults receiving 5 mg per kg per day (214). Micafungin doses of 7 to 10 mg per kg per day administered to 13 premature infants (mean birth weight and gestational age 1449 (±1211) g 27.3 (±4.68) weeks, respectively) provided adequate exposure (median area under the curve of 258.1 to 291.2 mg per hour per L) to achieve levels thought to be needed to treat central nervous system candidiasis (215).

Toxicities, Side Effects, and Drug Interactions

The safety profile of micafungin is optimal when compared with other antifungal agents. In clinical trials including those of micafungin used for treatment of localized and invasive candidiasis as well as prophylaxis studies in patients post–stem cell transplantation have demonstrated fewer adverse events than liposomal amphotericin B and fluconazole. Overall, the safety of micafungin was assessed in 3,083 patients and 501 volunteers in 41 clinical studies, who received single or multiple doses of the drug, ranging from 12.5 mg to 150 or more mg per day. The most common adverse events experienced by these patients were related to the gastrointestinal tract (i.e., nausea, diarrhea). Hypersensitivity reactions associated with micafungin have been reported and 5% of patients receiving the product may develop liver enzyme elevation (216). Hyperbilirubinemia, renal impairment, and hemolytic anemia related to micafungin use have also been identified in postmarketing surveillance of the drug. The most common adverse events in a phase I micafungin study of 77 children (2 to 17 years of age) with fever and neutropenia were diarrhea (19.5%), epistaxis (18.2%), abdominal pain (16.9%), and headache (16.9%) (210). Micafungin has very few drug interactions; however, when administered simultaneously it increases overall exposure (AUC) of sirolimus (21%), nifedipine (18%), and itraconazole (22%) (216).

Clinical Studies

In a study of 20 patients micafungin was well tolerated with no severe adverse events and a maximum tolerated dose was not reached at 4 mg per kg per day (217). In an open-label, multicenter study of micafungin monotherapy against invasive fungal infections, overall clinical response was 60% with no safety-related issues (218). A recent study of micafungin combined with an existing antifungal agent in pediatric and adult bone marrow transplant patients with invasive aspergillosis revealed an overall complete or partial response of 39%, including 40% specifically in allogeneic transplant patients (219). A study comparing prophylaxis of 882 stem cell transplant patients found that micafungin had greater success for preventing yeast and mold infections (80%) versus fluconazole prophylaxis (73.5%), with a comparable safety profile (220). An open-label, noncomparative, multinational study in adult and pediatric patients with a variety of diagnoses (i.e., Hematopoietic stem cell transplantation [HSCT], hematologic malignancies) conducted from 1998 to 2002 evaluated the use of micafungin monotherapy and combination therapy in 225 patients with invasive aspergillosis (221). A favorable response at the end of therapy was seen in 36% of patients. Of those treated only with micafungin, favorable responses were seen in 50% of the primary and 41% of the salvage therapy group (221).

Micafungin has been evaluated in the treatment of immunocompromised patients with candidiasis. A randomized, double-blind, dose-response study of 245 patients with acquired immunodeficiency syndrome/human immunodeficiency virus infection and esophageal candidiasis showed that the endoscopic cure rate was dose-dependent with 50 mg [16.3 (±4.2) days duration], 100 mg [13.4 (±4.5) days duration], and 150 mg [14.0 (±3.5) days duration] of micafungin per day at 68.8%, 77.4%, and 89.8%, respectively (222). The endoscopic cure rate for 100 and 150 mg of micafungin per day (83.5%) was comparable to that for 200 mg of fluconazole [14.0 (±3.3) days duration] per day (86.7%; 95% CI for the difference in endoscopic cure rate, −14.0% to 7.7%). Clinical and severity secondary end points were also comparable between the two products; however, after discontinuation of therapy, nine patients receiving micafungin had a worsening of severity score or had relapsed disease versus none of the patients in the fluconazole group (222). More recently, micafungin (100 mg per day, $n = 202$) was evaluated in a phase III, randomized, double-blind study against liposomal amphotericin B (3 mg per kg per day, $n = 190$)

for candidemia and invasive candidiasis. Treatment success was observed for 89.6% of patients treated with micafungin versus 89.5% of patients treated with liposomal amphotericin B, meeting noninferiority criteria (223). There were fewer treatment-related adverse events with micafungin than there were with liposomal amphotericin B (223). Micafungin at doses of 100 and 150 mg daily was also noninferior to caspofungin in an international, randomized, double-blinded study of adults (n = 595) with candidemia or invasive candidiasis (224), and in a phase III randomized study it was found to be superior to fluconazole in the prevention of invasive fungal infections among adults (n = 882) undergoing hematopoietic stem cell transplantation (225).

Pediatric Studies

Of the three drugs within the echinocandin class, micafungin has been the one most extensively studied in children including several pharmacokinetic studies in neonates. A pediatric substudy (n = 106, ages 0 to 16 years including 14 neonates) was conducted between 2003 and 2005 as part of a double-blind, randomized, multinational trial comparing micafungin (2 mg per kg per day) with liposomal amphotericin B (3 mg per kg per day) as first-line treatment for invasive candidiasis (226). Treatment success was defined as clinical and mycologic response at the end of therapy. The median duration of study drug administration was 15 days for micafungin (range, 3 to 42 days) and 14.5 days for liposomal amphotericin B (range, 2 to 34 days). In a modified intent-to-treat analysis the rate of overall treatment success was similar for micafungin (72.9%, 35/48) when compared with liposomal amphotericin B (76.0%, 38/50), with an adjusted difference between treatment groups of −2.4 (95% CI 20.1, 15.3) when stratified by neutropenic status. However, when stratified by age group, liposomal amphotericin B outperformed micafungin in all age groups except for the neonatal group (226). This observation could be related to the low micafungin dose used in this trial. In general, micafungin was better tolerated than liposomal amphotericin B as evidenced by the fewer adverse events that led to discontinuation of therapy (226).

ANIDULAFUNGIN

Pharmacology

Anidulafungin (Pfizer Inc, New York, NY) is a semisynthetic terphenyl-substituted antifungal derived from echinocandin B, a lipopeptide fungal product (227). It has linear pharmacokinetics with the longest half-life of all the echinocandins (approximately 18 hours) (228) and has shown fungistatic or fungicidal activity in different settings (229). Pharmacokinetic analysis in healthy rabbits revealed linear pharmacokinetics with dose-proportional increases in AUC (230). Neither end-stage renal impairment, dialysis, nor mild to moderate hepatic failure changes the pharmacokinetics of anidulafungin in patients (231).

Anidulafungin fits a three-compartment open pharmacokinetic model, with a terminal elimination half-life of up to 30 hours (230). Tissue concentrations after multiple dosing were highest in lung and liver, followed by spleen and kidney, with measurable concentrations in the brain tissue. The pharmacokinetics showed approximately sixfold lower mean peak concentrations in plasma and twofold lower AUC values compared to values with similar doses of caspofungin and micafungin.

There is only one study evaluating the pharmacokinetics of anidulafungin in pediatric patients (232). Twenty-five children aged 2 to 17 years with neutropenia were given anidulafungin (1.5 to 3 mg per kg loading dose, 0.75 to 1.5 mg per kg per day maintenance dose) for a mean duration of 8.7 days (range, 1 to 23 days). Exposure to anidulafungin increased in a manner consistent with dose proportionality within all age cohorts. Maximum anidulafungin plasma concentrations occurred immediately after administration and steady-state plasma concentrations were achieved after administration of the loading dose. At steady state the mean half-life, systemic clearance, and area under the curve within a dosing interval were 23.1 (±9.0) and 19.9 (±4.3) hours, 0.0175 (±0.0077) and 0.0159 (±0.0063) L per hour per kg, and 48.6 (±15.7) and 99.5 (±33.5) mg per hour per L for children receiving 0.75 mg per kg per day and 1.5 mg per kg per day, respectively (232). The concentration profiles at those maintenance doses of anidulafungin in pediatric patients aged 2 to 17 years were similar to those of adult patients receiving 50 or 100 mg per day, respectively. The current anidulafungin formulation requires reconstitution with 20% dehydrated alcohol; therefore, its safety and pharmacokinetic profile in infants younger than 2 years is being evaluated in a new formulation that does not contain alcohol.

Toxicities, Side Effects, and Drug Interactions

A phase I study reported anidulafungin to be well tolerated in 29 healthy volunteers, with the highest dose cohort experiencing transient liver function test elevations that exceeded twice the upper limit of normal (233). In a separate study, 12 subjects with mild or moderate hepatic impairment did not cause clinically significant changes in the pharmacokinetic parameters of anidulafungin (234). However, in patients with severe hepatic impairment the plasma concentrations of anidulafungin are decreased and plasma clearance increased (235). In vitro testing in human hepatic microsomes showed that anidulafungin did not affect cyclosporine, (236) nor tacrolimus (237), but there was a small (21%) increase in anidulafungin concentration when coadministered with cyclosporine (238). In a study of 25 neutropenic children receiving anidulafungin as empirical therapy, four patients in the group receiving 0.75 mg per kg per day experienced adverse events considered by the investigator to be possibly or probably related to anidulafungin. These events included feeling abnormal, facial erythema and rash, elevation in serum blood urea nitrogen, and fever and hypotension (232).

Clinical Studies

In a phase II, open label, dose range study, adult patients (n = 120) with candidemia and/or candidiasis were randomized to receive 50, 75, or 100 mg of intravenous anidulafungin daily (after a loading dose on day 1) until 2 weeks after clinical cure or improvement (and eradication or presumed eradication of *Candida*). Of the 68 patients available at follow-up, eradication showed a dose-related trend with 74, 85, and 89% success at 50, 75, and 100 mg per day of anidulafungin (239). In this study, no correlation was found between in vitro *Candida* minimum inhibitory concentration and anidulafungin eradication. Another phase II study showed clinical and endoscopic success in 95% and 92% of patients, respectively, with azole-refractory mucosal candidiasis and sustained clinical success in 47% of patients after discontinuation of anidulafungin (100 mg loading, 50 mg maintenance dose) therapy (240).

A phase III, randomized, double-blind study in adult patients ($n = 245$, 97% without neutropenia) with invasive candidiasis (89% with candidemia) showed that anidulafungin was not inferior to fluconazole in the treatment of invasive candidiasis (241). In this study, the frequency and types of adverse events were similar in the two groups and all-cause mortality was 31% in the fluconazole group and 23% in the anidulafungin group ($p = .13$) (241).

Pediatric Studies

No clinical studies of anidulafungin in children have been published aside from the PK and safety study conducted in 25 neutropenic children (232).

ALLYLAMINES

The allylamine class of antifungals (242), which includes terbinafine, inhibits the enzyme squalene epoxidase in the fungal biosynthesis of ergosterol and is currently indicated for the treatment of superficial dermatophyte and yeast infections. Since its introduction into clinical practice in 1991, clinicians have used oral terbinafine (Lamisil; Novartis Research Institute, Vienna, Austria) mainly for dermatophyte infections of the skin and nails (243). There is no available intravenous formulation. Terbinafine is well tolerated (244), has a bioavailability after oral administration of 70% to 80%, and is highly lipophilic with a terminal half-life of up to 3 weeks (245). The metabolism of terbinafine is not dependent on the CYP system but metabolism takes place extensively in the liver (15), with subsequent excretion in the urine (243). Terbinafine is rapidly absorbed following oral administration in humans (246).

The lipophilic terbinafine concentrates highest in the sebum and hair with quantifiable concentrations 56 to 90 days after a final oral dose and a slow redistribution from the peripheral sites back to the central plasma compartment. Tissue distribution in rats using high-performance liquid chromatography after a 6 mg per kg intravenous dose revealed a slow uptake and efflux of terbinafine in the skin, with an estimated redistribution half-life from the skin of 1.6 days. Approximately 60% and 28% of the apparent volume of distribution of terbinafine was to the skin and adipose tissue, respectively (247). Further analysis of terbinafine distribution in human blood shows a higher affinity for plasma proteins than blood cells in a concentration-independent manner (248). There have been reports of side effects with terbinafine, including hepatitis (249,250), pancytopenia (249,251), hair loss (252), and drug interaction with tricyclic antidepressants (253,254). Pharmacokinetic modeling indicated that at steady state almost all of the terbinafine (94%) in the human body resides in adipose and skin tissues, with only 0.4% in the lung (255), which might theoretically lead to difficulty in treating systemic fungal infections with terbinafine (256).

FUTURE DIRECTIONS

Over the last 3 decades, amphotericin B deoxycholate has been the preferred antifungal agent used in children and adults; however, its clinical use was hampered by the nephrotoxicity and infusion-related toxicity. Lipid formulations of amphotericin B have improved its side effects profile, but over the last 5 years the antifungal armamentarium has increased. Most of these new therapies, including second-generation triazoles and the echinocandins, have an excellent safety profile and in adults have proven efficacious in phase II and III studies.

The number of antifungal studies conducted in children is limited and is mainly related to phase I/II safety and pharmacokinetic studies. While there have been many phase III antifungal clinical trials in adults, there has never been a large phase III antifungal clinical trial dedicated to children. Consequently, most information for the pediatrician has been extrapolated from adults.

REFERENCES

1. Groll AH, Shah PM, Mentzel C, et al. Trends in postmortem epidemiology of invasive fungal infections at a university hospital. *J Infect* 1996;33:23–32.
2. Kullberg BJ, de Pauw BE. Therapy of invasive fungal infections. *Neth J Med* 1999;55:118–127.
3. Warnock DW. Amphotericin B: an introduction. *J Antimicrob Chemother* 1991;28:27–38.
4. Gallis HA, Drew RH, Pickard WW. Amphotericin B: 30 years of clinical experience. *Rev Infect Dis* 1990;12:308–329.
5. Latge JP. *Aspergillus fumigatus* and aspergillosis. *Clin Microbiol Rev* 1999;12:310–350.
6. Brajtburg J, Powderly WG, Kobayashi GS, et al. Amphotericin B: current understanding of mechanisms of action. *Antimicrob Agents Chemother* 1990;34:183–188.
7. Meis JFM, Verweij PE. Current management of fungal infections. *Drugs* 2001;61:13–25.
8. Manavathu EK, Dimmock JR, Vashishtha SC, et al. In-vitro and in-vivo susceptibility of Aspergillus fumigatus to a novel conjugated styryl ketone. *J Antimicrob Chemother* 1998;42:585–590.
9. Atkinson AJ Jr, Bennett JE. Amphotericin B pharmacokinetics in humans. *Antimicrob Agents Chemother* 1978;13:271–276.
10. Baley JE, Meyers C, Kliegman RM, et al. Pharmacokinetics, outcome of treatment, and toxic effects of amphotericin B and 5-fluorocytosine in neonates. *J Pediatr* 1990;116:791–797.
11. Groll AH, Piscitelli SC, Walsh TJ. Antifungal pharmacodynamics: concentration-effect relationships in vitro and in vivo. *Pharmacotherapy* 2001;21:133S–148S.
12. Christensen KJ, Bernard EM, Gold JWM, et al. Distribution and activity of amphotericin B in humans. *J Infect Dis* 1985;152:1037–1043.
13. Denning DW, Stevens DA. Antifungal and surgical treatment of invasive aspergillosis: review of 2,121 published cases. *Rev Infect Dis* 1990;12:1147–1200.

14. Ellis M. Amphotericin B preparations: a maximum tolerated dose in severe invasive fungal infections? *Transpl Infect Dis* 2000; 2:51–61.
15. Luna B, Drew RH, Perfect JR. Agents for treatment of invasive fungal infections. *Otolaryngol Clin North Am* 2000;33:277–299.
16. Proffitt RT, Satorius A, Chiang SM, et al. Pharmacology and toxicology of a liposomal formulation of amphotericin B (AmBisome) in rodents. *J Antimicrob Chemother* 1991;28:49–61.
17. Dismukes WE. Introduction to antifungal agents. *Clin Infect Dis* 2000;30:653–657.
18. Wong-Beringer A, Jacobs RA, Guglielmo BJ. Lipid formulations of amphotericin B: Clinical efficacy and toxicities. *Clin Infect Dis* 1998;27:603–618.
19. Hiemenz JW, Walsh TJ. Lipid formulations of amphotericin B: recent progress and future directions. *Clin Infect Dis* 1996;22: S133–S144.
20. Brajtburg J, Bolard J. Carrier effects on biological activity of amphotericin B. *Clin Microbiol Rev* 1996;9:512–531.
21. Ralph ED, Khazindar AM, Barber KR, et al. Comparative in vitro effects of liposomal amphotericin B, amphotericin B-deoxycholate, and free amphotericin B against fungal strains determined by using MIC and minimal lethal concentration susceptibility studies and time–kill curves. *Antimicrob Agents Chemother* 1991;35: 188–191.
22. Luke RG, Boyle JA. Renal effects of amphotericin B lipid complex. *Am J Kidney Dis* 1998;31:780–785.
23. Walsh TJ, Goodman JL, Pappas P, et al. Safety, tolerance, and pharmacokinetics of high-dose liposomal amphotericin B (AmBisome) in patients infected with Aspergillus species and other filamentous fungi: maximum tolerate dose study. *Antimicrob Agents Chemother* 2001;45:3487–3496.
24. Fielding RM, Smith PC, Wang LH, et al. Comparative pharmacokinetics of amphotericin B after administration of a novel colloidal delivery system, ABCD, and a conventional formulation to rats. *Antimicrob Agents Chemother* 1991;35:1208–1213.
25. Starke JR, Mason EOJ, Kramer WG, et al. Pharmacokinetics of amphotericin B in infants and children. *J Infect Dis* 1987;155: 766–774.
26. Nath CE, McLachlan AJ, Shaw PJ, et al. Population pharmacokinetics of amphotericin B in children with malignant diseases. *Br J Clin Pharmacol* 2001;52:671–680.
27. Benson JM, Nahata MC. Pharmacokinetics of amphotericin B in children. *Antimicrob Agents Chemother* 1989;33:1989–1993.
28. Walsh TJ, Whitcomb T, Piscitelli S, et al. Safety, tolerance, and pharmacokinetics of amphotericin B lipid complex in children with hepatosplenic candidiasis. *Antimicrob Agents Chemother* 1997; 41:1944–1948.
29. Hong Y, Shaw PJ, Nath CE, et al. Population pharmacokinetics of liposomal amphotericin B in pediatric patients with malignant diseases. *Antimicrob Agents Chemother* 2006;50:935–942.
30. Wurthwein G, Groll AH, Hempel G, et al. Population pharmacokinetics of amphotericin B lipid complex in neonates. *Antimicrob Agents Chemother* 2005;49:5092–5098.
31. de Pauw BE. New antifungal agents and preparations. *Int J Antimicrob Agents* 2000;16:147–150.
32. Patterson DL, Singh N. Interactions between tacrolimus and antimicrobial agents. *Clin Infect Dis* 1997;21:430–435.
33. Finquelievich JL, Odds FC, Queiroz-Telles F, et al. New advances in antifungal treatment. *Med Mycol* 2000;38:317–322.
34. Walsh TJ, Hiemenz JW, Seibel NL, et al. Amphotericin B lipid complex for invasive fungal infections: analysis of safety and efficacy in 556 cases. *Clin Infect Dis* 1998;26:1383–1396.
35. Schmitt HJ. New methods of delivery of amphotericin B. *Clin Infect Dis* 1993;17:S501–S506.
36. Wasan KM, Rosenblum MG, Cheung L, et al. Influence of lipoproteins on renal cytotoxicity and antifungal activity of amphotericin B. *Antimicrob Agents Chemother* 1994;38:223–227.
37. Ringden O, Jonsson V, Hansen M, et al. Severe and common side-effects of amphotericin B lipid complex (Abelcet). *Bone Marrow Transplant* 1998;22:733–734.
38. Graybill JR, Tollemar J, Torres-Rodriguez JM, et al. Antifungal compounds: controversies, queries and conclusions. *Med Mycol* 2000;38:323–333.
39. Stevens DA, Kan VL, Judson MA, et al. Practice guidelines for diseases caused by *Aspergillus*. *Clin Infect Dis* 2000;30:696–709.
40. Kontoyiannis DP. A clinical perspective for the management of invasive fungal infections: focus on IDSA guidelines. *Pharmacotherapy* 2001;21:175S–187S.
41. Denning DW. Invasive aspergillosis. *Clin Infect Dis* 1998;26: 781–805.
42. Dix SP, Andriole VT. Lipid formulations of amphotericin B. *Curr Clin Top Infect Dis* 2000;20:1–23.
43. Cherry JD, Lloyd CA, Quilty JF, et al. Amphotericin B therapy in children. A review of the literature and a case report. *J Pediatr* 1969;75:1063–1069.
44. Walsh TJ, Seibel NL, Arndt C, et al. Amphotericin B lipid complex in pediatric patients with invasive fungal infections. *Pediatr Infect Dis J* 1998;18:702–708.
45. Herbrecht R, Auvrignon A, Andres E, et al. Efficacy of amphotericin B lipid complex in the treatment of invasive fungal infections in immunocompromised paediatric patients. *Eur J Clin Microbiol Infect Dis* 2001;20:77–82.
46. Sandler ES, Mustafa MM, Tkaczewski I, et al. Use of amphotericin B colloidal dispersion in children. *J Pediatr Hematol Oncol* 2000;22:242–246.
47. Donowitz LG, Hendley JO. Short-course amphotericin B therapy for candidemia in pediatric patients. *Pediatrics* 1995;95: 888–891.
48. Roman E, Osunkwo I, Militano O, et al. Liposomal amphotericin B prophylaxis of invasive mold infections in children post allogeneic stem cell transplantation. *Pediatr Blood Cancer* 2008;50:325–330.
49. Wiley JM, Seibel NL, Walsh TJ. Efficacy and safety of amphotericin B lipid complex in 548 children and adolescents with invasive fungal infections. *Pediatr Infect Dis J* 2005;24:167–174.
50. Al Arishi H, Frayha HH, Kalloghlian A, et al. Liposomal amphotericin B in neonates with invasive candidiasis. *Am J Perinatol* 1998;15:643–648.
51. Duschinsky R, Pleven E, Heidelberger C. The synthesis of 5-fluoropyrimidines. *J Am Chem Soc* 1957;79:4559–4560.
52. Benson JM, Nahata MC. Clinical use of systemic antifungal agents. *Clin Pharm* 1988;7:424–438.
53. Firkin FC. Therapy of deep-seated fungal infections with 5-fluorocytosine. *Aust N Z J Med* 1974;4:462–467.
54. Young RC, Bennett JE, Vogel CL, et al. Aspergillosis: the spectrum of the disease in 98 patients. *Medicine* 1970;49:147–173.
55. Vermes A, Guchelaar H-J, Dankert J. Flucytosine: a review of its pharmacology, clinical indications, pharmacokinetics, toxicity and drug interactions. *J Antimicrob Chemother* 2000;46:171–179.
56. Bennett JE. Flucytosine. *Ann Intern Med* 1977;86:319–321.
57. Beggs WH, Sarosi GA. Further evidence for sequential action of amphotericin B and 5-fluorocytosine against *C. albicans*. *Chemotherapy* 1982;28:341–344.
58. Diasio RB, Lakings DE, Bennett JE. Evidence for conversion of 5-fluorocytosine to 5-fluorouracil in humans: possible factor in 5-fluorocytosine clinical toxicity. *Antimicrob Agents Chemother* 1978; 14:903–908.
59. Vermes A, Guchelaar H-J, van Kuilenburg AB, et al. 5-fluorocytosine-related bone-marrow depression and conversion to fluorouracil: a pilot study. *Fundam Clin Pharmacol* 2002;16:39–47.
60. Stamm AM, Diasio RB, Dismukes WE, et al. Toxicity of amphotericin B plus flucytosine in 194 patients with cryptococcal meningitis. *Am J Med* 1987;83:236–242.
61. Pasqualotto AC, Howard SJ, Moore CB, et al. Flucytosine therapeutic monitoring: 15 years experience from the UK. *J Antimicrob Chemother* 2007;59:791–793.
62. Bennett JE, Dismukes WE, Duma RJ, et al. A comparison of amphotericin B alone and combined with flucytosine in the treatment of cryptococcal meningitis. *N Engl J Med* 1979;301: 126–128.
63. Dismukes WE, Cloud G, Gallis HA, et al. Treatment of cryptococcal meningitis with combination amphotericin B and flucytosine for four as compared with six weeks. *N Engl J Med* 1987; 317:334–341.
64. van der Horst CM, Saag MS, Cloud GA, et al. Treatment of cryptococcal meningitis associated with the acquired immunodeficiency syndrome. National Institute of Allergy and Infectious Diseases Mycoses Study Group and AIDS Clinical Trials Group. *N Engl J Med* 1997;337:15–21.

65. Mayanja-Kizza H, Oishi K, Mitarai S, et al. Combination therapy with fluconazole and flucytosine for cryptococcal meningitis in Ugandan patients with AIDS. *Clin Infect Dis* 1998;26:1362–1366.
66. Larsen RA, Bozzette SA, Jones BE, et al. Fluconazole combined with flucytosine for treatment of cryptococcal meningitis in patients with AIDS. *Clin Infect Dis* 1994;19:741–745.
67. Chotmongkol V, Sukeepaisarncharoen W, Thavornpitak Y. Comparison of amphotericin B, flucytosine and itraconazole with amphotericin B and flucytosine in the treatment of cryptococcal meningitis in AIDS. *J Med Assoc Thai* 1997;80:416–425.
68. Rex JH, Walsh TJ, Sobel JD, et al. Practice guidelines for the treatment of candidiasis. *Clin Infect Dis* 2000;30:662–678.
69. Benjamin DKJ, Stoll BJ, Fanaroff AA, et al. Neonatal candidiasis among extremely low birth weight infants: risk factors, mortality rates, and neurodevelopmental outcomes at 18 to 22 months. *Pediatrics* 2006;117:84–92.
70. Ernst EJ. Investigational antifungal agents. *Pharmacotherapy* 2001; 21:165S–175S.
71. Klepser ME, Wolfe EJ, Jones RN, et al. Antifungal pharmacodynamic characteristics of fluconazole and amphotericin B tested against *Candida albicans. Antimicrob Agents Chemother* 1997;41: 1392–1395.
72. De Beule K, Van Gestel J. Pharmacology of itraconazole. *Drugs* 2001;61:27–37.
73. Ernst EJ, Klepser ME, Ernst ME, et al. In vitro pharmacodynamic properties of MK-0991 determined by time–kill methods. *Diagn Microbiol Infect Dis* 1999;33:75–80.
74. Brammer KW, Coates PE. Pharmacokinetics of fluconazole in pediatric patients. *Eur J Clin Microbiol Infect Dis* 1994;13:325–329.
75. Wildfeuer A, Laufen H, Schmalreck AF, et al. Fluconazole: comparison of pharmacokinetics, therapy, and in vitro susceptibility. *Mycoses* 1997;40:259–265.
76. Wade KC, Wu D, Kaufman DA, et al. Population pharmacokinetics of fluconazole in young infants. *Antimicrob Agents Chemother* 2008;52:4043–4049.
77. Debruyne D. Clinical pharmacokinetics of fluconazole in superficial and systemic mycoses. *Clin Pharmacokinet* 1997;33:52–77.
78. Nahata MC, Brady MT. Pharmacokinetics of fluconazole after oral administration in children with human immunodeficiency virus infection. *Eur J Clin Pharmacol* 1995;48:291–293.
79. Buijk SLCE, Gyssens IC, Mouton JW, et al. Pharmacokinetics of sequential intravenous and enteral fluconazole in critically ill surgical patients with invasive mycoses and compromised gastrointestinal function. *Intensive Care Med* 2001;27:115–121.
80. Wong S-F, Leung MP, Chan M-Y. Pharmacokinetics of fluconazole in children requiring peritoneal dialysis. *Clin Ther* 1997;19: 1039–1047.
81. Koks CHW, Meenhorst PL, Hillebrand MJX, et al. Pharmacokinetics of fluconazole in saliva and plasma after administration of an oral suspension and capsules. *Antimicrob Agents Chemother* 1996;40:1935–1937.
82. Vscoli CE, Castagnola M, Fioredda B, et al. Fluconazole in the treatment of candidiasis in immunocompromised children. *Antimicrob Agents Chemother* 1991;35:365–367.
83. Schwarze R, Penk A, Pittrow L. Administration of fluconazole in children below 1 year of age. *Mycoses* 1999;42:3–16.
84. Novelli V, Holzel H. Safety and tolerability of fluconazole in children. *Antimicrob Agents Chemother* 1999;43:1955–1960.
85. Marr KA, Seidel K, Slavin MA, et al. Prolonged fluconazole prophylaxis is associated with persistent protection against candidiasis-related death in allogeneic marrow transplant recipients: long-term follow-up of a randomized, placebo-controlled trial. *Blood* 2000;96:2055–2061.
86. MacMillan ML, Goodman JL, DeFor TE, et al. Fluconazole to prevent yeast infections in bone marrow transplantation patients: a randomized trial of high versus reduced dose, and determination of the value of maintenance therapy. *Am J Med* 2002;112:369–379.
87. Koh LP, Kurup A, Goh YT, et al. Randomized trial of fluconazole versus low-dose amphotericin B in prophylaxis against fungal infections in patients undergoing hematopoietic stem cell transplantation. *Am J Hematol* 2002;71:260–267.
88. Rex JH, Pappas PG, Karchmer AW, et al. A randomized and blinded multicenter trial of high-dose fluconazole + placebo vs. fluconazole + amphotericin B as treatment of candidemia in non-neutropenic patients. In: Microbiology ASf, ed. *Program and abstracts of the 41st Interscience Conference on Antimicrobial Agents and Chemotherapy*; 2001; Chicago, IL. Washington, DC: American Society for Microbiology, 2001.
89. Garbino J, Lew DP, Romand J-A, et al. Prevention of severe *Candida* infections in nonneutropenic, high-risk, critically ill patients: a randomized, double-blind, placebo-controlled trial in patients treated by selective digestive decontamination. *Intensive Care Med* 2002;28:1708–1717.
90. Faergemann J, Laufen H. Levels of fluconazole in serum, stratum corneum, epidermis-dermis (without stratum corneum) and eccrine sweat. *Clin Exp Dermatol* 1993;18:102–106.
91. Groll AH, Just-Nuebling G, Kurz M, et al. Fluconazole versus nystatin in the prevention of *Candida* infections in children and adolescents undergoing remission induction or consolidation chemotherapy for cancer. *J Antimicrob Chemother* 1997;40:855–862.
92. Fasano C, O'Keeffe J, Gibbs D. Fluconazole treatment of neonates and infants with severe fungal infections not treatable with conventional agents. *Eur J Clin Microbiol Infect Dis* 1994;13: 325–354.
93. Kaufman D, Boyle R, Hazen KC, et al. Fluconazole prophylaxis against fungal colonization and infection in preterm infants. *N Engl J Med* 2001;345:1660–1666.
94. Manzoni P, Stolfi I, Pugni L, et al. A multicenter, randomized trial of prophylactic fluconazole in preterm neonates. *N Engl J Med* 2007;356:2483–2495.
95. Healy CM, Campbell JR, Zaccaria E, et al. Fluconazole prophylaxis in extremely low birth weight neonates reduces invasive candidiasis mortality rates without emergence of fluconazole-resistant Candida species. *Pediatrics* 2008;121:703–710.
96. Manzoni P, Leonessa M, Galletto P, et al. Routine use of fluconazole prophylaxis in a neonatal intensive care unit does not select natively fluconazole-resistant Candida subspecies. *Pediatr Infect Dis J* 2008;27:731–737.
97. Cotten CM, McDonald S, Stoll B, et al. The association of third-generation cephalosporin use and invasive candidiasis in extremely low birth-weight infants. *Pediatrics* 2006;118:717–722.
98. Benjamin DK Jr. First, do no harm. *Pediatrics* 2008;121:831–832.
99. Van Cutsem J, Van Gerven F, Van de Ven M-A, et al. Itraconazole, a new triazole that is orally active against *Aspergillus. Antimicrob Agents Chemother* 1984;26:527–534.
100. Borgers M, Van de Ven M-A, Willemsens G, et al. Morphologic evaluation of R 51211, a new antimycotic. In: Program and abstracts of the 13th Annual International Congress on Chemotherapy Proceedings part 61, SE 48/2–13;1983; Vienna, Austria; 1983.
101. Walsh TJ, Viviani MA, Arathoon E, et al. New targets and delivery systems for antifungal therapy. *Med Mycol* 2000;38:335–347.
102. Manavathu EK, Cutright JL, Chandrasekar PH. Organism-dependent fungicidal activity of azoles. *Antimicrob Agents Chemother* 1998;42:3018–3021.
103. Heykants J, Van de Valde V, Van Rooy P. The clinical pharmacokinetics of itraconazole: an overview. *Mycoses* 1989;32:67–87.
104. Anonymous. Itraconazole. *Med Lett Drugs Ther* 1993;35:7–9.
105. Barone JA, Moskovitz BL, Guarnieri J, et al. Enhanced bioavailability of itraconazole in hydroxypropyl-beta-cyclodextrin solution versus capsules in healthy volunteers. *Antimicrob Agents Chemother* 1998;42:1862–1865.
106. Stevens DA. Itraconazole in cyclodextrin solution. *Pharmacotherapy* 1999;19:603–611.
107. Slain D, Rogers PD, Cleary JD, et al. Intravenous itraconazole. *Ann Pharmacother* 2001;35:720–729.
108. Caillot D, Bassaris H, McGeer A, et al. Intravenous itraconazole followed by oral itraconazole in the treatment of invasive pulmonary aspergillosis in patients with hematologic malignancies, chronic granulomatous disease, or AIDS. *Clin Infect Dis* 2001; 33:e83–e90.
109. Boogaerts M, Maertens J. Clinical experience with itraconazole in systemic fungal infections. *Drugs* 2001;61:39–47.
110. Chiller TM, Stevens DA. Treatment strategies for Aspergillus infections. *Drug Resist Updat* 2000;3:89–97.
111. de Repentigny L, Ratelle J, Leclerc J-M, et al. Repeated-dose pharmacokinetic of an oral solution of itraconazole in infants and children. *Antimicrob Agents Chemother* 1998;42:404–408.

112. Abdel-Rahman SM, Jacobs RF, Massarella J, et al. Single-dose pharmacokinetics of intravenous itraconazole and hydroxypropyl-beta-cyclodextrin in infants, children, and adolescents. *Antimicrob Agents Chemother* 2007;51:2668–2673.
113. Tucker RM, Haq Y, Denning DW, et al. Adverse events associated with itraconazole in 189 patients on chronic therapy. *J Antimicrob Chemother* 1990;26:561–566.
114. Katz HI. Drug interactions of the newer oral antifungal agents. *Br J Dermatol* 1999;141:26–32.
115. Leather HL, Wingard JR. Characterizing the pharmacokinetic drug interaction between intravenous itraconazole and intravenous tacrolimus or intravenous cyclosporine in allogenic bone marrow transplant patients. In: Microbiology ASf, ed. *Program and abstracts of the 41st Interscience Conference on Antimicrobial Agents and Chemotherapy*; December 16–19, 2001; Chicago, IL. Washington, DC: American Society for Microbiology, 2001.
116. MacKenzie-Wood AR, Whitfield MJ, Ray JE. Itraconazole and HIV protease inhibitors: an important interaction. *Med J Aust* 1999;170:46–47.
117. Patterson TF, Kirkpatrick WR, White M, et al. Invasive aspergillosis: disease spectrum, treatment practices, and outcomes. *Medicine* 2000;79:250–260.
118. Morgenstern GR, Prentice AG, Prentice HG, et al. A randomized controlled trial of itraconazole versus fluconazole for the prevention of fungal infections in patients with haematological malignancies. *Br J Haematol* 1999;105:901–911.
119. Winston DJ, Busuttil RW. Randomized controlled trial of oral itraconazole solution versus intravenous/oral fluconazole for prevention of fungal infections in liver transplant recipients. *Transplantation* 2002;74:688–694.
120. Chariyalertsak S, Supparatpinyo K, Sirisanthana T, et al. A controlled trial of itraconazole as primary prophylaxis for systemic fungal infections in patients with advanced human immunodeficiency virus infection in Thailand. *Clin Infect Dis* 2002;34:277–284.
121. Groll AH, Wood L, Roden M, et al. Safety, pharmacokinetics, and pharmacodynamics of cyclodextrin itraconazole in pediatric patients with oropharyngeal candidiasis. *Antimicrob Agents Chemother* 2002;46:2554–2563.
122. Grigull L, Kuehlke O, Beilken A, et al. Intravenous and oral sequential itraconazole antifungal prophylaxis in paediatric stem cell transplantation recipients: a pilot study for evaluation of safety and efficacy. *Pediatr Transplant* 2007;11:261–266.
123. Sabo JA, Abdel-Rahman SM. Voriconazole: a new triazole antifungal. *Ann Pharmacother* 2000;34:1032–1043.
124. Manavathu EK, Cutright JL, Chandrasekar PH. In vitro susceptibility of itraconazole-resistant isolates of Aspergillus fumigatus to voriconazole. *Clin Microbiol Infect* 1997;3:81.
125. Johnson EM, Szekely A, Warnock DW. In-vitro activity of voriconazole, itraconazole and amphotericin B against filamentous fungi. *J Antimicrob Chemother* 1998;42:741–745.
126. Goldstein JA, deMorais SMF. Biochemistry and molecular biology of the human CYP2 C subfamily. *Pharmacogenetics* 1994;4:285–299.
127. Purkins L, Wood N, Ghahramani P, et al. Pharmacokinetics and safety of voriconazole following intravenous- to oral-dose escalation regimens. *Antimicrob Agents Chemother* 2002;46:2546–2553.
128. Johnson LB, Kauffman CA. Voriconazole: a new triazole antifungal agent. *Clin Infect Dis* 2003;36:630–637.
129. Yanni SB, Annaert PP, Augustijns P, et al. Role of flavin-containing monooxygenase in oxidative metabolism of voriconazole by human liver microsomes. *Drug Metab Dispos* 2008;36:1119–1125.
130. Ghannoum MA, Kuhn DM. Voriconazole—better chances for patients with invasive mycoses. *Eur J Med Res* 2002;7:242–256.
131. Denning DW, Ribaud P, Milpied N, et al. Efficacy and safety of voriconazole in the treatment of acute invasive aspergillosis. *Clin Infect Dis* 2002;34:563–571.
132. Sheehan DJ, Hitchcock CA, Sibley CM. Current and emerging azole antifungal agents. *Clin Microbiol Rev* 1999;12:40–79.
133. Clancy C, Nguyen N. In vitro efficacy and fungicidal activity of voriconazole against *Aspergillus* and *Fusarium* species. *Eur J Clin Microbiol Infect Dis* 1998;17:573–575.
134. Chiou CC, Groll AH, Walsh TJ. New drugs and novel targets for treatment of invasive fungal infections in patients with cancer. *Oncologist* 2000;5:120–135.
135. Blummer JL, Yanovitch S, Schlamm H, et al. Pharmacokinetics and safety of oral voriconazole in patients at risk of fungal infections: a dose escalation study. In: Microbiology ASf, ed. *Program and abstracts of the 41st Interscience Conference on Antimicrobial Agents and Chemotherapy*; December 16–19, 2001; Chicago, IL. Washington, DC: American Society for Microbiology, 2001.
136. Klepser ME, Malone D, Lewis RE, et al. Evaluation of voriconazole pharmacodynamics using time-kill methodology. *Antimicrob Agents Chemother* 2000;44:1917–1920.
137. Tan KKC, Wood N, Weil A. Multiple-dose pharmacokinetics of voriconazole in chronic hepatic impairment. In: Microbiology ASf, ed. *Program and abstracts of the 41st Interscience Conference on Antimicrobial Agents and Chemotherapy*; December 16–19, 2001; Chicago, IL.Washington, DC: American Society for Microbiology, 2001.
138. Walsh TJ, Karlsson MO, Driscoll T, et al. Pharmacokinetics and safety of intravenous voriconazole in children after single- or multiple-dose administration. *Antimicrob Agents Chemother* 2004;48:2166–2172.
139. Lazarus HM, Blummer JL, Yanovich S, et al. Safety and pharmacokinetics of oral voriconazole in patients at risk of fungal infection: a dose escalation study. *J Clin Pharmacol* 2002;42:395–402.
140. Tan KKC, Brayshaw N, Oakes M. Investigation of the relationship between plasma voriconazole concentrations and liver function test abnormalities in therapeutic trials. In: Microbiology ASf, ed. *Program and abstracts of the 41st Annual Interscience Conference on Antimicrobial Agents and Chemotherapy*; December 16–19, 2001; Chicago, IL. Washington, DC: American Society for Microbiology, 2001.
141. Stone J, Holland S, Wickersham P, et al. Drug interactions between caspofungin and tacrolimus. In: Microbiology ASf, ed. *Program and abstracts of the 41st Interscience Conference on Antimicrobial Agents and Chemotherapy*; 2001; Chicago, IL. Washington, DC: American Society for Microbiology, 2001.
142. Denning DW, Griffiths CEM. Muco-cutaneous retinoid-effects and facial erythema related to the novel triazole antifungal agent voriconazole. *Clinical Dermatology* 2001;26:648–653.
143. Venkataramanan R, Zang S, Gayowski T, et al. Voriconazole inhibition of the metabolism of tacrolimus in a liver transplant recipient and in human liver microsomes. *Antimicrob Agents Chemother* 2002;46:3091–3093.
144. Wood N, Tan K, Allan R, et al. Effect of voriconazole on pharmacokinetics of tacrolimus. In: Microbiology ASf, ed. *Program and abstracts of the 41st Interscience Conference on Antimicrobial Agents and Chemotherapy*; 2001; Chicago, IL. Washington, DC: American Society for Microbiology, 2001.
145. Romero A, Le Pogamp P, Nilsson L-G, et al. Effect of voriconazole on the pharmacokinetics of cyclosporine in renal transplant patients. *Clin Pharmacol Ther* 2002;71:226–234.
146. Wood N, Abel S, Fielding A, et al. Voriconazole does not affect the pharmacokinetics of mycophenolic acid. In: Microbiology ASf, ed. *Program and abstracts of the 41st Interscience Conference on Antimicrobial Agents and Chemotherapy*; 2001; Chicago, IL. Washington, DC: American Society for Microbiology, 2001.
147. Herbrecht R, Denning DW, Patterson TF, et al. Voriconazole versus amphotericin B for primary therapy of invasive aspergillosis. *N Engl J Med* 2002;347:408–415.
148. Ally R, Schurmann D, Kreisel W, et al. A randomized, double-blind, double-dummy, multicenter trial of voriconazole and fluconazole in the treatment of esophageal candidiasis in immunocompromised patients. *Clin Infect Dis* 2001;33:1447–1454.
149. Walsh TJ, Lutsar I, Driscoll T, et al. Voriconazole in the treatment of aspergillosis, scedosporiosis and other invasive fungal infections in children. *Pediatr Infect Dis J* 2002;21:240–248.
150. Frankenbusch K, Eifinger F, Kribs A, et al. Severe primary cutaneous aspergillosis refractory to amphotericin B and the successful treatment with systemic voriconazole in two premature infants with extremely low birth weight. *J Perinatol* 2006;26:511–514.
151. Courtney R, Pai S, Laughlin M, et al. Pharmacokinetics, safety, and tolerability of oral posaconazole administered in single and multiple doses in healthy adults. *Antimicrob Agents Chemother* 2003;47:2788–2795.

152. Courtney R, Wexler D, Radwanski E, et al. Effect of food on the relative bioavailability of two oral formulations of posaconazole in healthy adults. *Br J Clin Pharmacol* 2004;57:218–222.
153. Krishna G, Moton A, Ma L, et al. The pharmacokinetics and absorption of posaconazole oral suspension under various gastric conditions in healthy volunteers. *Antimicrob Agents Chemother* 2009;53(3):958–66. Epub December 15, 2008.
154. Courtney R, Sansone A, Smith W, et al. Posaconazole pharmacokinetics, safety, and tolerability in subjects with varying degrees of chronic renal disease. *J Clin Pharmacol* 2005;45: 185–192.
155. Schiller DS, Fung HB. Posaconazole: an extended-spectrum triazole antifungal agent. *Clin Ther* 2007;29:1862–1886.
156. Cornely OA, Maertens J, Winston DJ, et al. Posaconazole vs. fluconazole or itraconazole prophylaxis in patients with neutropenia. *N Engl J Med* 2007;356:348–359.
157. Ullmann AJ, Lipton JH, Vesole DH, et al. Posaconazole or fluconazole for prophylaxis in severe graft-versus-host disease. *N Engl J Med* 2007;356:335–347.
158. Restrepo A, Tobon A, Clark B, et al. Salvage treatment of histoplasmosis with posaconazole. *J Infect* 2007;54:319–327.
159. Segal BH, Barnhart LA, Anderson VL, et al. Posaconazole as salvage therapy in patients with chronic granulomatous disease and invasive filamentous fungal infection. *Clin Infect Dis* 2005;40: 1684–1688.
160. Greenberg RN, Mullane K, van Burik JA, et al. Posaconazole as salvage therapy for zygomycosis. *Antimicrob Agents Chemother* 2006;50:126–133.
161. Moore CB, Walls CM, Denning DW. In vitro activity of the new triazole BMS-207147 against *Aspergillus* species in comparison with itraconazole and amphotericin B. *Antimicrob Agents Chemother* 2000;44:441–443.
162. Arikan S, Rex JH. Ravuconazole. *Curr Opin Investig Drugs* 2002;3:555–561.
163. Olsen SJ, Mummaneni V, Rolan P, et al. Ravuconazole single ascending oral dose study in healthy subjects. In: Microbiology ASf, ed. *Program and abstracts of the 40th Interscience Conference on Antimicrobial Agents and Chemotherapy*; September 17–20, 2000; Toronto, Ontario, Canada. Washington, DC: American Society for Microbiology, 2000.
164. Mikamo H, Yin XH, Hayasaki Y, et al. Penetration of ravuconazole, a new triazole antifungal, into rat tissues. *Chemotherapy* 2002;48:7–9.
165. Grasela DM, Olsen SJ, Mummaneni V, et al. Ravuconazole multiple ascending oral dose study in healthy subjects. In: Microbiology ASf, ed. *Program and abstracts for the 40th Interscience Conference on Antimicrobial Agents and Chemotherapy*; September 17–20, 2000; Toronto, Ontario, Canada. Washington, DC: American Society for Microbiology, 2000.
166. Mummaneni V, Geraldes M, Hadjilambris OW, et al. Effect of ravuconazole on the pharmacokinetics of simvastatin in healthy subjects. In: Microbiology ASf, ed. *Program and abstracts of the 40th Interscience Conference on Antimicrobial Agents and Chemotherapy*; September 17–20, 2000; Toronto, Ontario, Canada. Washington, DC: American Society for Microbiology, 2000.
167. Mummaneni V, Hadjilambris OW, Nichola P, et al. Ravuconazole does not affect the pharmacokinetics of nelfinavir. In: Microbiology ASf, ed. *Program and abstracts of the 41st Interscience Conference on Antimicrobial Agents and Chemotherapy*; December 16–19; 2001; Chicago, IL. Washington, DC: American Society for Microbiology, 2001.
168. Beale M, Queiroz-Telles F, Banhegyi D, et al. Randomized, double-blind study of the safety and antifungal activity of ravuconazole relative to fluconazole in esophageal candidiasis. In: Microbiology ASf, ed. *Program and abstracts of the 41st Interscience Conference on Antimicrobial Agents and Chemotherapy*; 2001; Chicago, IL. Washington, DC: American Society for Microbiology, 2001.
169. Marino M, Mummaneni V, Norton J, et al. Ravuconazole exposure-response relationship in HIV+ patients with oropharyngeal candidiasis. In: Microbiology ASf, ed. *Program and abstracts of the 41st Interscience Conference on Antimicrobial Agents and Chemotherapy*; 2001; Chicago, IL. Washington, DC: American Society for Microbiology, 2001.
170. Gupta AK, Leonardi C, Stoltz RR, et al. A phase I/II randomized, double-blind, placebo-controlled, dose-ranging study evaluating the efficacy, safety and pharmacokinetics of ravuconazole in the treatment of onychomycosis. *J Eur Acad Dermatol Venereol* 2005;19:437–443.
171. Graybill JR. The echinocandins, first novel class of antifungals in two decades: will they live up to their promise? *Int J Clin Pract* 2001;55:633–638.
172. Kurtz MB, Douglas CM. Lipopeptide inhibitors of fungal glucan synthase. *J Med Vet Mycol* 1997;35:79–86.
173. Bartizal K, Gill CJ, Abruzzo GK, et al. In vitro preclinical evaluation studies with the echinocandin antifungal MK-0991 (L-743,872). *Antimicrob Agents Chemother* 1997;41:2326–2332.
174. Ernst EJ, Klepser ME, Pfaller MA. Postantifungal effects of echinocandin, azole, and polyene antifungal agents against Candida albicans and Cryptococcus neoformans. *Antimicrob Agents Chemother* 2000;44:1108–1111.
175. Benz F, Knuessel F, Nuesch J, et al. Echinocandin B, ein neuartiges polypeptid antibioticum aus *Aspergillus nidulans* var echinulatus: isolierung and baudsteine. *Helv Chim Acta* 1974;57: 2459– 2477.
176. Arathoon E. Clinical efficacy of echinocandin antifungals. *Curr Opin Infect Dis* 2001;14:685–691.
177. Hope WW, Mickiene D, Petraitis V, et al. The pharmacokinetics and pharmacodynamics of micafungin in experimental hematogenous Candida meningoencephalitis: implications for echinocandin therapy in neonates. *J Infect Dis* 2008;197:163–171.
178. Chiller T, Farrokhshad K, Brummer E, et al. Influence of human sera on the *in vitro* activity of the echinocandin caspofungin (MK-0991) against *Aspergillus fumigatus*. *Antimicrob Agents Chemother* 2000;44(12):3302–3305.
179. Groll AH, Gullick BM, Petraitiene R, et al. Compartmental pharmacokinetics of the antifungal echinocandin caspofungin (MK-0991) in rabbits. *Antimicrob Agents Chemother* 2001;45:596–600.
180. Stone JA, Holland SD, Wickersham PJ, et al. Single- and multiple-dose pharmacokinetics of caspofungin in healthy men. *Antimicrob Agents Chemother* 2002;46:739–745.
181. Stone EA, Fung HB, Kirschenbaum HL. Caspofungin: an echinocandin antifungal agent. *Clin Ther* 2002;24:351–377.
182. Hajdu R, Thompson R, Sundelof JG, et al. Preliminary animal pharmacokinetics of the parenteral antifungal agent MK-0991 (L-743,872). *Antimicrob Agents Chemother* 1997;41:2339–2344.
183. Abruzzo GK, Flattery AM, Gill CJ, et al. Evaluation of the echinocandin antifungal MK-0991 (L-743,872): efficacies in mouse models of disseminated aspergillosis, candidiasis, and cryptococcosis. *Antimicrob Agents Chemother* 1997;41:2333–2338.
184. Hoang A. Caspofungin acetate: an antifungal agent. *Am J Health Syst Pharm* 2001;58:1206–1214.
185. Stone J, Holland S, Li S, et al. Effect of hepatic insufficiency on the pharmacokinetics of caspofungin. In: Microbiology ASf, ed. *Program and abstracts of the 41st Interscience Conference on Antimicrobial Agents and Chemotherapy*; December 16–19, 2001; Chicago, IL. Washington, DC: American Society for Microbiology, 2001.
186. Sable CA, Nguyen B-YT, Chodakewitz JA, et al. Safety and tolerability of caspofungin acetate in the treatment of fungal infections. *Transpl Infect Dis* 2002;4:25–30.
187. Stone J, Migoya E, Li S, et al. Safety and pharmacokinetics of higher doses of caspofungin. In: Microbiology ASf, ed. *Program and abstracts of the 42nd Annual Interscience Conference on Antimicrobial Agents and Chemotherapy*; 2002; San Diego. Washington, DC: American Society for Microbiology, 2002.
188. Walsh TJ, Adamson PC, Seibel NL, et al. Pharmacokinetics, safety, and tolerability of caspofungin in children and adolescents. *Antimicrob Agents Chemother* 2005;49:4536–4545.
189. Keating GM, Jarvis B. Caspofungin. *Drugs* 2001;61:1121–1129.
190. Maertens J, Raad I, Petrikkos G, et al. Update on the multicenter noncomparative study of caspofungin in adults with invasive aspergillosis refractory or intolerant to other antifungal agents: analysis of 90 patients. In: Microbiology ASf, ed. *Program and abstracts of the 42nd Interscience Conference on Antimicrobial Agents and Chemotherapy*; September 27–30, 2002; San Diego, CA. Washington, DC: American Society for Microbiology, 2002.
191. Sanz-Rodriguez C, Aguado JM, Cisneros JM, et al. Caspofungin therapy in documented fungal infections: Spanish experience before licensure of the drug. In: Microbiology ASf, ed. *Program and abstracts of the 42nd Interscience Conference on Antimicrobial Agents and Chemotherapy*; September 27–30, 2002; San Diego,

CA. Washington, DC: American Society for Microbiology, 2002.

192. Villaneuva A, Arathoon EG, Gotuzzo E, et al. A randomized double-blind study of caspofungin versus amphotericin for the treatment of candidal esophagitis. *Clin Infect Dis* 2001;33:1529–1535.
193. Arathoon E, Gotuzzo E, Noriega LM, et al. Randomized, double-blind multicenter study of caspofungin versus amphotericin B for treatment of oropharyngeal and esophageal candidiasis. *Antimicrob Agents Chemother* 2002;46:451–457.
194. Villaneuva A, Gotuzzo E, Arathoon E, et al. A randomized double-blind study of caspofungin versus fluconazole for the treatment of esophageal candidiasis. *Am J Med* 2002;113:294–299.
195. Kartsonis N, DiNubile MJ, Bartizal K, et al. Efficacy of caspofungin in the treatment of esophageal candidiasis resistant to fluconazole. *J Acquir Immune Defic Syndr* 2002;31:183–187.
196. Mora-Duarte J, Betts R, Rotstein C, et al. Comparison of caspofungin and amphotericin B for invasive candidiasis. *N Engl J Med* 2002;347:2020–2029.
197. Walsh TJ, Teppler H, Donowitz GR, et al. Caspofungin versus liposomal amphotericin B for empirical antifungal therapy in patients with persistent fever and neutropenia. *N Engl J Med* 2004;351:1391–1402.
198. Mattiuzzi GN, Alvarado G, Giles FJ, et al. Open-label, randomized comparison of itraconazole versus caspofungin for prophylaxis in patients with hematologic malignancies. *Antimicrob Agents Chemother* 2006;50:143–147.
199. Merlin E, Galambrun C, Ribaud P, et al. Efficacy and safety of caspofungin therapy in children with invasive fungal infections. *Pediatr Infect Dis J* 2006;25:1186–1188.
200. Cesaro S, Giacchino M, Locatelli F, et al. Safety and efficacy of a caspofungin-based combination therapy for treatment of proven or probable aspergillosis in pediatric hematological patients. *BMC Infect Dis* 2007;7:28.
201. Koo A, Sung L, Allen U, et al. Efficacy and safety of caspofungin for the empiric management of fever in neutropenic children. *Pediatr Infect Dis J* 2007;26:854–856.
202. Odio CM, Araya R, Pinto LE, et al. Caspofungin therapy of neonates with invasive candidiasis. *Pediatr Infect Dis J* 2004;23:1093–1097.
203. Natarajan G, Lulic-Botica M, Rongkavilit C, et al. Experience with caspofungin in the treatment of persistent fungemia in neonates. *J Perinatol* 2005;25:770–777.
204. Mikamo H, Sato Y, Tamaya T. *In vitro* antifungal activity of FK463, a new water-soluble echinocandin-like lipopeptide. *J Antimicrob Chemother* 2000;46:485–487.
205. Hatano K, Morishita Y, Nakai T, et al. Antifungal mechanism of FK463 against Candida albicans and Aspergillus fumigatus. *J Antibiot (Tokyo)* 2002;55:219–222.
206. Tawara S, Ikeda F, Maki K, et al. *In vitro* activities of a new lipopeptide antifungal agent, FK463, against a variety of clinically important fungi. *Antimicrob Agents Chemother* 2000;44:57–62.
207. Gumbo T, Hiemenz J, Ma L, et al. Population pharmacokinetics of micafungin in adult patients. *Diagn Microbiol Infect Dis* 2008;60:329–331.
208. Okugawa S, Ota Y, Tatsuno K, et al. A case of invasive central nervous system aspergillosis treated with micafungin with monitoring of micafungin concentrations in the cerebrospinal fluid. *Scand J Infect Dis* 2007;39:344–346.
209. Ernst EJ, Roling EE, Petzold CR, et al. In vitro activity of micafungin (FK-463) against *Candida* spp.: microdilution, time–kill, and postantifungal-effect studies. *Antimicrob Agents Chemother* 2002;46:3846–3853.
210. Seibel NL, Schwartz C, Arrieta A, et al. Safety, tolerability, and pharmacokinetics of micafungin (FK463) in febrile neutropenic pediatric patients. *Antimicrob Agents Chemother* 2005;49:3317–3324.
211. Hope WW, Seibel NL, Schwartz CL, et al. Population pharmacokinetics of micafungin in pediatric patients and implications for antifungal dosing. *Antimicrob Agents Chemother* 2007;51:3714–3719.
212. Tabata K, Katashima M, Kawamura A, et al. Linear pharmacokinetics of micafungin and its active metabolites in Japanese pediatric patients with fungal infections. *Biol Pharm Bull* 2006;29:1706–1711.
213. Heresi GP, Gerstmann DR, Reed MD, et al. The pharmacokinetics and safety of micafungin, a novel echinocandin, in premature infants. *Pediatr Infect Dis J* 2006;25:1110–1115.
214. Smith P, Walsh T, Hope W, et al. Pharmacokinetics of an elevated dosage of micafungin in premature neonates. In: Research SfP, ed. *Program and abstracts of the Annual Pediatric Academic Societies Meeting*; May 5–9, 2008; Society for Pediatric Research Honolulu, Hawaii, 2008.
215. Benjamin DK Jr, Smith P, Arrieta A, et al. Safety and pharmacokinetics of repeat-dose micafungin in neonates. In: Microbiology ASf, ed. *Program and abstracts of the 48th Annual Interscience Conference on Antimicrobial Agents and Chemotherapy*; 2008; Washington, DC: American Society for Microbiology, 2008.
216. Micafungin FDA label. In: Food and Drug Administration. www.fda.gov. Published 2005.
217. Powles R, Sirohi B, Chopra R, et al. Assessment of maximum tolerated dose of FK463 in cancer patients undergoing haematopoetic stem cell transplantation. In: Microbiology ASf, ed. *Program and abstracts of the 41st Interscience Conference on Antimicrobial Agents and Chemotherapy*; December 16–19, 2001; 2002; Chicago, IL. Washington, DC: American Society for Microbiology, 2001.
218. Kohno S, Masaoka T, Yamaguchi H. A multicenter, open-label clinical study of FK463 in patients with deep mycoses in Japan. In: Microbiology ASf, ed. *Program and abstracts of the 41st Interscience Conference on Antimicrobial Agents and Chemotherapy*; December 16–19, 2001; Chicago, IL. Washington, DC: American Society for Microbiology, 2001.
219. Ratanatharathorn V, Flynn P, Van Burik JA, et al. Micafungin in combination with systemic antifungal agents in the treatment of refractory aspergillosis in bone marrow transplant patients. In: Hematology ASo, ed. *Program and abstracts of the American Society of Hematology 44th Annual Meeting*; December 6–10, 2002; Philadelphia, PA. Washington, DC: American Society of Hematology, 2002.
220. Van Burik J, Ratanatharathorn V, Lipton J, et al. Randomized, double-blind trial of micafungin versus fluconazole for prophylaxis of invasive fungal infections in patients undergoing hematopoietic stem cell transplant, NIAID/BAMSG protocol 46. In: Microbiology ASf, ed. *Program and abstracts of the 42nd Interscience Conference on Antimicrobial Agents and Chemotherapy*; September 27–30, 2002; San Diego, CA. Washington, DC: American Society for Microbiology, 2002.
221. Denning DW, Marr KA, Lau WM, et al. Micafungin (FK463), alone or in combination with other systemic antifungal agents, for the treatment of acute invasive aspergillosis. *J Infect* 2006;53:337–349.
222. de Wet N, Llanos-Cuentas A, Suleiman J, et al. A randomized, double-blind, parallel-group, dose-response study of micafungin compared with fluconazole for the treatment of esophageal candidiasis in HIV-positive patients. *Clin Infect Dis* 2004;39:842–849.
223. Kuse ER, Chetchotisakd P, da Cunha CA, et al. Micafungin versus liposomal amphotericin B for candidaemia and invasive candidosis: a phase III randomised double-blind trial. *Lancet* 2007;369:1519–1527.
224. Pappas PG, Rotstein CM, Betts RF, et al. Micafungin versus caspofungin for treatment of candidemia and other forms of invasive candidiasis. *Clin Infect Dis* 2007;45:883–893.
225. van Burik JA, Ratanatharathorn V, Stepan DE, et al. Micafungin versus fluconazole for prophylaxis against invasive fungal infections during neutropenia in patients undergoing hematopoietic stem cell transplantation. *Clin Infect Dis* 2004;39:1407–1416.
226. Queiroz-Telles F, Berezin E, Leverger G, et al. Micafungin versus liposomal amphotericin B for pediatric patients with invasive candidiasis: substudy of a randomized double-blind trial. *Pediatr Infect Dis J* 2008;27:820–826.
227. Zhanel GG, Karlowsky JA, Harding GA, et al. *In vitro* activity of a new semisynthetic echinocandin, LY-303366, against systemic isolates of *Candida* species, *Cryptococcus neoformans*, *Blastomyces dermatitidis*, and *Aspergillus* species. *Antimicrob Agents Chemother* 1997;41:863–865.
228. Lucas R, De Sante K, Hatcher B, et al. LY303366 single dose pharmacokinetics and safety in healthy volunteers. In: Microbiology ASf, ed. *Program and abstracts of the 36th Annual Interscience Conference on Antimicrobial Agents and Chemotherapy*; 1996; New Orleans. Washington, DC: American Society for Microbiology, 1996.

229. Petraitis V, Petraitiene R, Groll AH, et al. Antifungal efficacy, safety, and single-dose pharmacokinetics of LY303366, a novel echinocandin B, in experimental pulmonary aspergillosis in persistently neutropenic rabbits. *Antimicrob Agents Chemother* 1998;42:2898–2905.
230. Groll AH, Mickiene D, Petraitiene R, et al. Pharmacokinetic and pharmacodynamic modeling of anidulafungin (LY303366): reappraisal of its efficacy in neutropenic animal models of opportunistic mycoses using optimal plasma sampling. *Antimicrob Agents Chemother* 2001;45:2845–2855.
231. Dowell JA, Stogniew M, Krause D, et al. Anidulafungin does not require dosage adjustment in subjects with varying degrees of hepatic or renal impairment. *J Clin Pharmacol* 2007;47:461–470.
232. Benjamin DKJ, Driscoll T, Seibel NL, et al. Safety and pharmacokinetics of intravenous anidulafungin in children with neutropenia at high risk for invasive fungal infections. *Antimicrob Agents Chemother* 2006;50:632–638.
233. Thye D, Shepherd B, White RJ, et al. Anidulafungin: a phase 1 study to identify the maximum tolerated dose in healthy volunteers. In: Microbiology ASf, ed. *Program and abstracts of the 41st Interscience Conference on Antimicrobial Agents and Chemotherapy*; December 16–19, 2001; Chicago, IL. Washington, DC: American Society for Microbiology, 2001.
234. Thye D, Kilfoil T, White RJ, et al. Anidulafungin: pharmacokinetics in subjects with mild and moderate hepatic impairment. In: Microbiology ASf, ed. *Program and abstracts of the 41st Interscience Conference on Antimicrobial Agents and Chemotherapy*; December 16–19, 2001; Chicago, IL. Washington, DC: American Society for Microbiology, 2001.
235. Thye D, Kilfoil T, Kilfoil G, et al. Anidulafungin: pharmacokinetics in subjects with severe hepatic impairment. In: Microbiology ASf, ed. *Program and abstracts of the 42nd Annual Interscience Conference on Antimicrobial Agents and Chemotherapy*; 2002; San Diego, CA: Washington, DC: American Society for Microbiology, 2002.
236. White RJ, Thye D. Anidulafungin does not affect the metabolism of cyclosporine by human hepatic microsomes. In: Microbiology ASf, ed. *Program and abstracts of the 41st Interscience Conference on Antimicrobial Agents and Chemotherapy*; 2001; Chicago, IL. Washington, DC: American Society for Microbiology, 2001.
237. Dowell JA, Stogniew M, Krause D, et al. Lack of pharmacokinetic interaction between anidulafungin and tacrolimus. *J Clin Pharmacol* 2007;47:305–314.
238. Thye D, Kilfoil T, Kilfoil G, et al. Anidulafungin: safety and pharmacokinetics in subjects receiving concomitant cyclosporine. In: Microbiology ASf, ed. *Program and abstracts of the 42nd Annual Interscience Conference on Antimicrobial Agents and Chemotherapy*; 2002; San Diego, CA. Washington, DC: American Society for Microbiology, 2002.
239. Pfaller MA, Diekema DJ, Boyken L, et al. Effectiveness of anidulafungin in eradicating Candida species in invasive candidiasis. *Antimicrob Agents Chemother* 2005;49:4795–4797.
240. Vazquez JA, Schranz JA, Clark K, et al. A phase 2, open-label study of the safety and efficacy of intravenous anidulafungin as a treatment for azole-refractory mucosal candidiasis. *J Acquir Immune Defic Syndr* 2008;48:304–309.
241. Reboli AC, Rotstein C, Pappas PG, et al. Anidulafungin versus fluconazole for invasive candidiasis. *N Engl J Med* 2007;356:2472–2482.
242. Petranyi G, Ryder NS, Stutz A. Allylamine derivatives: new class of synthetic antifungal agents inhibiting fungal squalene epoxidase. *Science* 1984;224:1239–1241.
243. Perez A. Terbinafine: broad new spectrum of indications in several subcutaneous and systemic and parasitic diseases. *Mycoses* 1999;42:111–114.
244. Harrari S. Current strategies in the treatment of invasive *Aspergillus* infections in immunocompromised patients. *Drugs* 1999;58:621–631.
245. Balfour JA, Faulds D. Terbinafine, a review of its pharmacodynamic and pharmacokinetic properties, and therapeutic potential in superficial mycoses. *Drugs* 1992;43:259–284.
246. Kovarik JM, Kirkessell S, Humbert H, et al. Dose-proportional pharmacokinetics of terbinafine and its N-demethylated metabolite in healthy volunteers. *Br J Dermatol* 1992;126:8–13.
247. Hosseini-Yeganeh M, McLachlan AJ. Tissue distribution of terbinafine in rats. *J Pharm Sci* 2001;90:1817–1828.
248. Hosseini-Yeganeh M, McLachlan AJ. In-vitro distribution of terbinafine in rat and human blood. *J Pharm Pharmacol* 2002;54: 277–281.
249. Conjeevaram G, Vongthavaravat V, Sumner R, et al. Terbinafine-induced hepatitis and pancytopenia. *Dig Dis Sci* 2001;46:1714–1716.
250. Anania FA, Rabin L. Terbinafine hepatotoxicity resulting in chronic biliary ductopenia and portal fibrosis. *Am J Med* 2002;112: 741–742.
251. Aguilar C, Mueller KK. Reversible agranulocytosis associated with oral terbinafine in a pediatric patient. *J Am Acad Dermatol* 2001;45:632–634.
252. Richert B, Uhoda I, De la Brassinne M. Hair loss after terbinafine treatment. *Br J Dermatol* 2001;145:842.
253. Teitelbaum ML, Pearson VE. Imipramine toxicity and terbinafine. *Am J Psychiatry* 2001;158:2086.
254. O'Reardon JP, Hetznecker JM, Rynn MA, et al. Desipramine toxicity with terbinafine. *Am J Psychiatry* 2002;159:492.
255. Hosseini-Yeganeh M, McLachlan AJ. Physiologically based pharmacokinetic model for terbinafine in rats and humans. *Antimicrob Agents Chemother* 2002;46:2219–2228.
256. Kovarik JM, Mueller EA, Zehender H, et al. Multiple-dose pharmacokinetics and distribution in tissue of terbinafine and metabolites. *Antimicrob Agents Chemother* 1995;39:2738–2741.

CHAPTER

36

Richard J. Whitley
Edward P. Acosta
David W. Kimberlin

Antiviral Drugs: Treatment of the Fetus and Newborn

INTRODUCTION

Parenteral therapy of viral infections of the newborn and infant became a reality with the introduction of vidarabine (adenine arabinoside) for the treatment of neonatal herpes simplex virus (HSV) infections in the early 1980s. Since then, acyclovir has become the treatment of choice for neonatal HSV infections, as well as a number of other herpesvirus infections. Similarly, ganciclovir has been established as beneficial for the treatment of congenital cytomegalovirus (CMV) infections that involve the central nervous system (CNS). Although other viruses can infect the newborn, including rubella and parvovirus, this chapter will review the lessons learned from treating neonatal and congenital infections and will consider therapies for respiratory virus infections of infants. Although the natural history of these diseases is reviewed elsewhere in this textbook, a brief summary will precede a detailed discussion of established and alternative therapeutics. The reader is referred to more extensive reviews of antiviral therapy in children and adults (1).

THERAPY OF HERPES SIMPLEX VIRUS INFECTIONS

Neonatal HSV infections occur in approximately 1 in 3,200 deliveries in the USA (2) and of these, approximately two-thirds develop some form of CNS disease (3). The majority of cases are caused by HSV-2 (4). The risk of transmission is increased with primary maternal infection during the third trimester and can be decreased by cesarean delivery if HSV has been isolated from the cervix or external genitalia near the time of delivery (2). As reviewed by Kimberlin, 85% of neonatal HSV cases occur due to peripartum transmission, 10% occur via postnatal transmission, and only 5% are due to transmission in utero (5).

Infants with intrauterine HSV infection are characterized by the triad of cutaneous (active lesions, scarring), neurologic (microcephaly, hydranencephaly), and eye findings (chorioretinitis, microphthalmia) present at birth. Intrauterine HSV infection has been found to occur with both primary and recurrent maternal HSV infections (6), although the risk from a recurrent infection is less.

HSV infection acquired in the peripartum or postpartum period can be categorized as skin, eye, and/or mouth (SEM) disease, CNS disease, or disseminated disease. By definition, SEM disease does not involve the CNS. Disseminated disease may involve the CNS along with multiple other organ systems including the liver, adrenals, gastrointestinal tract, and the skin, eyes, or mouth. CNS disease may have skin involvement but does not involve other visceral systems. Of all infants with neonatal HSV infections, approximately 33% have CNS disease, while about 25% have disseminated disease (7). Of infants with disseminated disease, approximately 60% to 75% will have CNS involvement (8). Therefore, by combining these statistics, it can be approximated that 50% of infants with neonatal HSV infection will have CNS involvement.

The pathogenesis of CNS involvement in neonatal HSV infections differs depending on whether or not the infection is disseminated. Encephalitis associated with dissemination is due to hematogenous spread, whereas isolated encephalitis or encephalitis associated with only skin involvement likely occurs because of retrograde intraneuronal transport of HSV (3). This corresponds to the clinical presentations of disseminated versus CNS disease in that the blood-borne spread of disseminated disease presents earlier (9 to 11 days of life on average) and causes more diffuse brain involvement with multiple areas of hemorrhagic necrosis, while CNS disease occurring via slower axonal transport presents later (around 16 to 17 days of life) and typically causes more focal CNS involvement (9).

In the pre-antiviral era, infants with neonatal HSV infections had significant morbidity and mortality. Infants with disseminated disease had an 85% mortality by 1 year of age, and only 50% of survivors had normal neurodevelopmental outcomes; likewise, infants with CNS disease had a mortality rate of 50% by 1 year of age with only 33% of survivors having normal neurodevelopmental outcomes (10). The early era of antiviral therapy for neonatal HSV infection was marked by improved mortality with intravenous vidarabine as well as with standard dose (SD) intravenous acyclovir (30 mg per kg per day in three divided doses). The 1 year mortality for disseminated disease improved to 50% with vidarabine and 61% with SD acyclovir, whereas the 1 year mortality for CNS disease dropped to 14% for both vidarabine and SD acyclovir (11). More recently, high-dose (HD) acyclovir has been shown to further improve upon these mortality figures. Using HD intravenous acyclovir (60 mg per kg per day in three divided doses for 21 days), Kimberlin demonstrated 1 year mortality rates of 29% and 4% for disseminated and CNS diseases, respectively (12). This study also showed that HD acyclovir improves morbidity for infants with disseminated disease (83% of survivors had normal neurodevelopmental outcomes) but not for infants with CNS disease (31% of survivors had normal neurodevelopmental outcomes).

Babies with SEM involvement have the best prognosis and, as noted below, require only 14 days of HD intravenous acyclovir therapy. Importantly, health care providers must exclude an asymptomatic or subclinical CNS infection at presentation by determining whether the cerebrospinal fluid (CSF) is negative for HSV DNA by polymerase chain reaction. With skin recurrences, the management (intravenous vs. oral therapy) of these children must be individualized according to the nature of their illness at the time of recurrence.

Infants can also experience primary gingivostomatitis secondary to HSV-1. Limited controlled clinical trial data are available to define efficacy of therapy, but most experts would recommend treatment, either intravenous or oral, depending upon the severity of illness.

THERAPY OF NEONATAL VARICELLA ZOSTER VIRUS INFECTIONS

Women who experience primary varicella zoster virus (VZV) infections within 48 hours of delivery have children at risk for the development of chickenpox within the first 3 weeks of life. Newborns delivered to these women traditionally receive zoster immune globulin (ZIG) to prevent disease. However, with sporadic shortages of ZIG, some newborns may experience neonatal disease. Although no controlled clinical trials have evaluated acyclovir therapy of this disease, experts would recommend this drug for the treatment of neonatal VZV disease.

AVAILABLE THERAPIES FOR HSV AND VZV INFECTIONS

ACYCLOVIR (ACYCLOGUANOSINE, ZOVIRAX, ACV)

Acyclovir is the most frequently prescribed antiviral agent for the management of HSV infections of the newborn and infant. It has been available for clinical use for nearly three decades and has demonstrated remarkable safety and efficacy against mild to severe infections caused by HSV and VZV in both normal and immunocompromised patients, including the newborn.

Chemistry and Mechanism of Action

Acyclovir is a deoxyguanosine analogue. After preferential uptake by viral-infected cells, acyclovir is phosphorylated by virus-encoded thymidine kinase (TK). Subsequent di- and triphosphorylation are catalyzed by host cell enzymes. Acyclovir triphosphate prevents viral DNA synthesis by inhibiting viral DNA polymerase (13).

Spectrum and Resistance

Acyclovir is most active against HSV; activity against VZV is also substantial but approximately 10-fold less. Although not related to the therapy of the newborn, Epstein Barr virus (EBV) is only moderately susceptible to acyclovir because EBV has minimal TK activity. Activity against CMV is poor because CMV does not have TK activity and CMV DNA polymerase is poorly inhibited by acyclovir triphosphate (13).

Resistance of HSV and VZV to acyclovir has become an important clinical problem, especially among immunocompromised patients exposed to long-term therapy (14). Resistance has not been considered a problem in the therapy of newborn infections at this time, although it has been reported (15). Viral resistance to acyclovir usually results from mutations in the viral TK gene, although mutations in the viral DNA polymerase gene can also rarely occur. Resistant isolates can cause severe, progressive, debilitating mucosal disease and, rarely, visceral dissemination (16,17). Isolates of HSV resistant to acyclovir have also been reported in normal hosts, most commonly in patients with frequently recurrent genital infection who have been treated with chronic acyclovir (18).

Indications

Acyclovir is effective for the treatment of infections caused by HSV and VZV in both immunocompetent and immunocompromised hosts, including the newborn. For the treatment of neonatal HSV infections, the recommended dose is 20 mg per kg every 8 hours intravenously. The duration of therapy for SEM disease is 14 days, while for those babies with either CNS or disseminated disease, therapy should be extended for 21 days. Several studies are investigating the application of end of treatment polymerase chain reaction detection of viral DNA at the completion of antiviral therapy. If the CSF is positive for HSV DNA, most experts recommend continuing therapy until the CSF is cleared of viral DNA.

Pharmacokinetics

After intravenous doses of 2.5 to 15 mg per kg, steady-state concentrations of acyclovir range from 6.7 to 20.6 μg per mL. Acyclovir is widely distributed; high concentrations are attained in kidneys, lung, liver, heart, and skin vesicles; concentrations in the CSF are about 50% of those in the plasma (19). Acyclovir crosses the placenta and accumulates in breast milk. Protein binding ranges from 9% to 33%, and less than 20% of drug is metabolized to biologically inactive metabolites.

In the absence of compromised renal function, the half-life of acyclovir is 2 to 3 hours in older children and adults and 2.5 to 5 hours in neonates with normal creatinine clearance. More than 60% of administered drug is excreted in the urine (19). Elimination is prolonged in patients with renal dysfunction; the half-life is approximately 20 hours in persons with end-stage renal disease, necessitating dose modifications for those with creatinine clearance less than 50 mL per minute per 1.73 m^2 (20). Acyclovir is effectively removed by hemodialysis but not by continuous ambulatory peritoneal dialysis (13,21).

Adverse Effects

Acyclovir generally is a safe drug. Oral acyclovir sometimes causes mild gastrointestinal upset, rash, and headache. If it extravasates, intravenous acyclovir can cause severe inflammation, phlebitis, and sometimes a vesicular eruption leading to cutaneous necrosis at the injection site. Also, if given by rapid intravenous infusion or to poorly hydrated patients or those with preexisting renal compromise, intravenous acyclovir can cause reversible nephrotoxicity. Renal dysfunction results from obstructive nephropathy caused by the formation of acyclovir crystals precipitating in renal tubules. Occasionally administration of acyclovir by the intravenous route is associated with rash, sweating, nausea, headache, hematuria, and hypotension. High doses of intravenous acyclovir (60 mg per kg per day) in neonates and the prolonged use of oral acyclovir following neonatal disease have been associated with neutropenia in uncontrolled trials (15,12).

The most serious side effect of acyclovir is neurotoxicity, which usually occurs in subjects with compromised renal function who attain high serum concentrations of drug (22). Neurotoxicity is manifest as lethargy, confusion, hallucinations, tremors, myoclonus, seizures, extrapyramidal signs, and changes in state of consciousness developing within the first few days of initiating therapy. These signs and symptoms usually resolve spontaneously within several days of discontinuing acyclovir.

Although acyclovir is mutagenic at high concentrations in some in vitro assays, it is not teratogenic in animals. Limited human data suggest that acyclovir use in pregnant women is not associated with congenital defects or other adverse pregnancy outcomes.

Drug Interactions

Somnolence and lethargy may occur in subjects being treated with both zidovudine and acyclovir. The likelihood of renal toxicity of acyclovir is increased when administered with nephrotoxic drugs such as cyclosporine or amphotericin B. Concomitant administration of probenecid prolongs acyclovir's half-life, whereas acyclovir can decrease the clearance and prolong the half-life of drugs such as methotrexate that are eliminated by active renal secretion (13).

UNTESTED THERAPY FOR NEONATAL HSV AND VZV INFECTIONS

VALACYCLOVIR (VALTREX)

Valacyclovir has been available for a decade in a tablet formulation. It has a safety and efficacy profile similar to that of acyclovir but offers potential pharmacokinetic advantages. A pediatric liquid formulation has been evaluated (23).

Chemistry, Mechanism of Action, Spectrum, and Resistance

Valacyclovir is a prodrug of acyclovir and as such has the same mechanism of action, antiviral spectrum, and potential for development of resistance (1,13).

Indications

Valacyclovir has the same indications as acyclovir. Although data from controlled clinical trials are limited, because of greater bioavailability, valacyclovir may be advantageous in treating infections caused by viruses relatively less sensitive to acyclovir than HSV (e.g., VZV and CMV). Pharmacokinetics in neonates and very young infants do not support the use of valacyclovir liquid formulation in these populations.

Pharmacokinetics

In contrast to the low bioavailability of acyclovir, the bioavailability of valacyclovir exceeds 50% (13,24). Peak serum concentrations ranging from 0.8 to 8.5 μg per mL following doses of 100 to 2,000 mg are attained about 1.5 hours after a dose. Oral valacyclovir provides plasma acyclovir concentrations comparable to those following a comparable dose of intravenous acyclovir. All other pharmacokinetic characteristics are similar to those of acyclovir (25).

Adverse Effects

The profiles of adverse effects observed with valacyclovir therapy are the same as those observed with acyclovir. In addition, manifestations resembling thrombotic microangiopathy have been described in patients with AIDS receiving high doses of valacyclovir, although the causal relationship to valacyclovir is not absolutely established (26).

Dosage

Valacyclovir dosages in children older than 2 years have recently been approved by the Food and Drug Administration (FDA) as 20 mg per kg administered two to three times daily (27). Adults are treated with 500 to 100 mg per dose, two to three times per day. The higher dose is for the treatment of herpes zoster and the lower dose for the treatment of genital herpes. Suppression of recurrent oral and genital herpes infections has been accomplished with single daily doses of 500 mg and 1,000 mg, respectively.

FAMCICLOVIR (FAMVIR)

Chemistry and Mechanism of Action

Famciclovir is the prodrug of penciclovir. Like acyclovir, penciclovir is a guanosine analogue that has activity against HSV-1, HSV-2, and VZV in vitro. It is similarly phosphorylated by viral TK and subsequently converted to its active form, penciclovir triphosphate. However, its mechanism of action differs from acyclovir in that, while a competitive inhibitor of DNA polymerase, it does not cause chain termination. Penciclovir has minimal oral bioavailability. Famciclovir is the diacetyl ester prodrug of penciclovir and confers 70% bioavailability (1,13). At the present time, no formulation exists for newborns and infants.

Spectrum and Resistance

The spectrum of activity of the parent drug, penciclovir, is identical to acyclovir. Resistance occurs in a fashion identical to that of acyclovir, as well, with mutation of the viral TK being the most common (1,13).

Indications

Famciclovir is indicated for treatment of herpes zoster infections as well as genital herpes and has similar efficacy to valacyclovir. There have been no studies of famciclovir in the neonate. However, if a pediatric formulation became available, there would be an option for the treatment of neonatal HSV infection involving the skin, eye, and mouth.

Pharmacokinetics

Famciclovir is excreted by the kidney and thus requires dose adjustment in patients with renal insufficiency (13).

Adverse Effects

Famciclovir is tolerated well with minimal side effects with headache and gastrointestinal upset being most common.

THERAPY OF CONGENITAL CYTOMEGALOVIRUS INFECTION

CMV commonly infects humans worldwide, with a seroprevalence of approximately 40% in adolescents and approaching 90% in adults with poor socioeconomic status (28,29). Congenital CMV infection is the most common congenital infection in the developed world and occurs in about 1% of liveborn infants in the United States (30). Congenital CMV infections most commonly occur via intrauterine transmission, but since the virus is shed in body fluids, transmission can also be acquired perinatally during delivery or postnatally through breast milk.

Of all infants born with congenital CMV infection, approximately 7% to 10% have clinically evident disease at birth (31). Clinical characteristics of intrauterine infection include intrauterine growth restriction, hepatosplenomegaly, jaundice, thrombocytopenia, microcephaly, periventricular calcifications, and chorioretinitis. As reviewed by Dollard, true mortality rates are difficult to obtain and have been reported to be as high as 30% for symptomatic infants (32), but more likely average about 5% to 10% (33). Death usually is due to non-CNS manifestations of the infection, such as hepatic dysfunction or bleeding. An estimated 40% to 58% of infants with symptomatic congenital CMV infection have permanent sequelae, whereas infants who are asymptomatic at birth suffer permanent sequelae nearly 14% of the time (32). Sensorineural hearing loss (SNHL), mental retardation, seizures, psychomotor and speech delays, learning disabilities, chorioretinitis, optic nerve atrophy, and defects in dentition are the most common long-term consequences (34). As opposed to intrauterine infections, perinatally acquired CMV infections are not typically associated with long-term sequelae, though acute illness has been reported in premature very low-birth-weight infants (35). In full-term infants, perinatal infections are commonly asymptomatic, but may present with pneumonitis within the first few months of life (36).

Congenital CMV infection is the consequence of maternal-fetal infection, with most symptomatic congenital cases occurring because of asymptomatic maternal infection. The pathogenesis of CNS involvement in congenital CMV infection begins with disseminated viremic spread, including the endothelial cells of the brain and epithelial cells of the choroid plexus. From the endothelial cells of the brain, the virus spreads to contiguous astrocytes. From the choroid plexus, the virus spreads to the ependymal surfaces via the CSF. Once these cells are infected, the virus undergoes continuous replication, which leads to characteristic intranuclear inclusion bodies and cell death. As antibodies are produced in the face of continuous viral replication, immune complexes form as well, leading to further immune-mediated damage (34). Although the specific pathogenesis of CMV-mediated SNHL has not been elucidated, histology has shown evidence of infection in the cells of both the cochlear and vestibular endolabyrinth (37). CMV has also been isolated from the cochlear perilymph upon autopsy of infants with congenital CMV infection (38).

Recent studies of ganciclovir treatment of congenital CMV infections involving the CNS have been promising. Using ganciclovir at doses of 12 mg per kg per day divided every 12 hours for a duration of 6 weeks, improved hearing outcomes were demonstrated in neonates with symptomatic congenital CMV infections involving the CNS (as evidenced by microcephaly, intracranial calcifications, abnormal CSF for age, chorioretinitis, and/or hearing deficits) (39). The primary endpoint was improved brainstem-evoked response (BSER) between baseline and 6-month follow-up (or no deterioration at the 6-month follow-up if the baseline BSER was normal). For total evaluable ears, 69% of patients who received ganciclovir met the primary endpoint as opposed to 39% of the control group. No patients receiving ganciclovir had worsening of their hearing between baseline and 6 months. Ganciclovir recipients also had more rapid resolution of alanine aminotransferase (ALT) abnormalities than did the control group, though they were significantly more likely to become neutropenic. Additional analyses of this randomized controlled trail suggest that ganciclovir may also reduce neurodevelopment delays (40). Improvement of mortality has not yet been shown with ganciclovir therapy.

TREATMENT OF CMV INFECTIONS

GANCICLOVIR (CYTOVENE)

Ganciclovir was the first antiviral available for the therapy and prevention of infections caused by CMV. It has proved to be a very valuable drug for immunocompromised patients, particularly hematopoietic stem cell transplant recipients, who suffer substantial morbidity and mortality from CMV infections and, more recently, in children with congenital CMV infection, albeit it is not yet approved by US FDA.

Chemistry and Mechanism of Action

Ganciclovir is structurally similar to acyclovir except for a hydroxymethyl group on its acyclic side chain. The initial phosphorylation step is carried out by pUL97, which is a viral protein kinase. Cellular kinases then phosphorylate the agent two additional times to convert it into its triphosphate derivative, which is able to inhibit the CMV DNA polymerase encoded by *UL97* as well as incorporate into and terminate viral DNA.

Ganciclovir triphosphate is a competitive inhibitor of herpesviral DNA polymerases, resulting in cessation of DNA chain elongation (1,13).

Spectrum and Resistance

Ganciclovir has similar activity to acyclovir against HSV-1, HSV-2, and VZV, but, in contrast with acyclovir, its greatest activity is against CMV. Resistance of CMV isolates usually results from mutations in the *UL97* gene (41). Mutations in the CMV DNA polymerase gene occur less often.

Indications

Ganciclovir is licensed for several indications outside of the newborn. Reviews summarize these clinical outcomes (42). For the treatment of neonates congenitally infected with CMV, a controlled trial has been performed (39). As noted above, compared with no treatment, ganciclovir therapy prevented hearing deterioration at 2 years, although about two-thirds of treated infants developed neutropenia, often requiring dose modification.

Pharmacokinetics

Oral bioavailability of ganciclovir is poor, with less than 10% of drug being absorbed following oral administration (43,44). The oral formulation of ganciclovir is no longer marketed. Peak serum concentrations of ganciclovir after 6 mg per kg (newborn dose) of intravenously administered drug range from 8 to 11 μg per mL, with concentrations sufficient to inhibit sensitive strains of CMV in aqueous humor, subretinal fluid, CSF, and brain tissue (1). The elimination half-life of ganciclovir is 2 to 3 hours, and most of the drug is eliminated unchanged in the urine. The pharmacokinetics of ganciclovir in the neonatal population is similar to those of adults (45,46). Dose reduction, proportional to the degree of reduction in creatinine clearance, is necessary for persons with impaired renal function. A supplemental dose is recommended after dialysis because it is efficiently removed by hemodialysis (47).

Adverse Effects

Myelosuppression is the most common adverse effect of ganciclovir; dose-related neutropenia (<1,000 WBC per μL) is the most consistent hematologic aberration, with an incidence of about 40% (44). Neutropenia is dose limiting in about one of seven courses and reverses after drug is stopped. Neutropenia is less frequent following oral administration of ganciclovir. Thrombocytopenia (<50,000 platelets per μL) occurs in approximately 20% and anemia in about 2% of ganciclovir recipients. Two percent to 5% of ganciclovir recipients experience headache, confusion, altered mental status, hallucinations, nightmares, anxiety, ataxia, tremors, seizures, fever, rash, and abnormal levels of serum hepatic enzymes, either singly or in some combination.

Dosage

The dose of ganciclovir for therapy of symptomatic congenital CMV infection is 12 mg per kg per day, given by intravenous infusion in two divided daily doses for 6 weeks.

VALGANCICLOVIR (VALCYTE)

Valganciclovir was approved by the FDA in March, 2001, for the treatment of CMV retinitis. Because it is well absorbed after oral administration, it may represent a favorable option to intravenously administered ganciclovir for the treatment of congenital CMV infection. Currently, it is licensed for the treatment of CMV infections in selected transplant populations and for CMV retinitis in patients with HIV/AIDS.

Chemistry, Mechanism of Action, Spectrum, and Resistance

Valganciclovir is the L-valine ester prodrug of ganciclovir and as such has the same mechanism of action, antiviral spectrum, and potential for development of resistance as ganciclovir (1,13).

Indications

Valganciclovir has similar indications to ganciclovir. However, based upon limited controlled trials published to date, it currently is approved for the induction and maintenance therapy of CMV retinitis and select transplant populations (48). It is currently under investigation for the treatment of congenital CMV infection. This randomized controlled trial, being performed by the National Institute of Allergy and Infectious Diseases (NIAID) Collaborative Antiviral Study Group (CASG), employs SNHL as its primary endpoint with safety and neurodevelopment outcomes as secondary endpoints.

Pharmacokinetics

Valganciclovir is rapidly converted to ganciclovir, with a mean plasma half-life of about 30 minutes (48). The absolute bioavailability of valganciclovir exceeds 60% and actually is enhanced by about 30% with concomitant administration of food (49). The area under the curve of ganciclovir after oral administration of valganciclovir is one-third to one-half of that attained after intravenous administration of ganciclovir. Patients with impaired renal function require dosage reduction that is roughly proportional to their reduction in creatinine clearance.

The pharmacokinetics of valganciclovir in the newborn is different from older children and adults. Following an average single dose of 16 mg per kg valganciclovir in 19 neonates, mean ganciclovir oral clearance was 9.3 mL per minute per kg and distribution volume was 2.2 L per kg (50). In a healthy adult population receiving a single 900 mg valganciclovir dose ($n = 12$), these same ganciclovir parameters were 5.4 mL per minute per kg and 1.6 L per kg, respectively (51). Other pharmacokinetic parameters were similar, but the decreased neonatal clearance is consistent with age-related changes in ganciclovir disposition.

Adverse Effects

The most common side effects associated with valganciclovir therapy in adult populations include diarrhea (41%), nausea (30%), neutropenia (27%), anemia (26%), and headache (22%) (48). Only a limited number of newborns have received valganciclovir therapy. The only significant finding was that of neutropenia in 34% of patients (50).

Dosage

The dose of valganciclovir is tailored to the patient's age and renal function. At this time, the drug is not approved for administration to newborns with congenital CMV infection.

UNPROVEN AND UNTESTED THERAPIES FOR NEONATAL HSV, VZV, AND CONGENITAL CMV INFECTIONS

The following two medications are utilized to treat HSV, VZV, and CMV infections in older children and adults. Data on these medications are provided should antiviral resistance occur with either HSV or CMV infections of the newborn. Neither drug has been evaluated in proof of principle studies in the newborn and both are associated with significant toxicity.

CIDOFOVIR (HPMPC, VISTIDE)

Cidofovir was first approved for use in the United States for the therapy of AIDS-associated retinitis caused by CMV. This remains the main indication for this antiviral.

Chemistry and Mechanism of Action

Cidofovir is a novel acyclic phosphonate nucleoside analogue with a mechanism of action similar to that of other nucleoside analogues. In contrast to acyclovir, viral enzymes are not required for initial phosphorylation because native cidofovir has a single phosphate group already attached. Following diphosphorylation by cellular kinases, cidofovir competitively inhibits DNA polymerase (52). The active form of cidofovir exhibits a 25- to 50-fold greater affinity for viral DNA polymerase compared with the cellular DNA polymerase (13).

Spectrum and Resistance

Cidofovir is active against HSV and CMV, including acyclovir- and foscarnet-resistant HSV isolates and ganciclovir- and foscarnet-resistant CMV mutants (53). It is also active in vitro against VZV, EBV, human herpesvirus-6, human herpesvirus-8, polyomaviruses, adenovirus, and human HPV.

A small number of cidofovir-resistant CMV isolates that are also resistant to ganciclovir on the basis of mutations within the DNA polymerase gene have been described (54). A CMV mutant resistant to ganciclovir, foscarnet, and cidofovir has also been reported (55).

Indications

Cidofovir delays retinal disease progression in patients with AIDS (56,57). Cidofovir has also been useful in the management of disease caused by acyclovir-resistant HSV isolates (58). Anecdotal reports of improvement of laryngeal papillomatosis following intralesional injection of cidofovir have been published, but a definitive conclusions regarding efficacy is not possible based upon this limited experience (59,60).

Pharmacokinetics

Only 2% to 26% of cidofovir is absorbed after oral administration, therefore it is given intravenously. The plasma half-life of cidofovir is 2.6 hours, but active intracellular metabolites of cidofovir have half-lives of 17 to 48 hours (61). Ninety percent of the drug is excreted in the urine, primarily by renal tubular secretion (62). Importantly, the drug does not cross the blood–brain barrier and, therefore, should not be used to treat CNS infections.

Adverse Effects

Because cidofovir concentrates in renal cells in amounts 100 times greater than in other tissues, nephrotoxicity is the main adverse effect, especially if hydration is not well maintained (61,62). Manifestations of renal toxicity include proteinuria and glycosuria. Aggressive intravenous prehydration, coadministration of probenecid, and avoidance of other nephrotoxic agents reduce the likelihood of toxicity. Cidofovir is contraindicated in patients with a serum creatinine of more than 1.5 mg per dL, a calculated creatinine clearance of 55 mL per minute or less, or a urine protein of 100 mg per dL and drug should be discontinued if serum creatinine increases to 0.5 mg per dL or more above baseline.

Dosage

Cidofovir is administered intravenously to older children and adults as a 5 mg per kg dose once per week with probenecid. Patients with compromised renal (calculated creatinine clearance <55 mL per minute) are treated every 2 weeks. The dose should be reduced from 5 mg per kg to 3 mg per kg if serum creatinine increases to more than 0.3 mg per dL above baseline. There are no data for dosing the newborn with cidofovir.

FOSCARNET (PFA, FOSCAVIR)

Foscarnet is the only antiherpes drug that is not a nucleoside analogue. It is not a first-line drug but is useful for the treatment of infections caused by resistant herpesviruses.

Chemistry and Mechanism of Action

Foscarnet is an inorganic pyrophosphate analogue that directly inhibits DNA polymerase by blocking the pyrophosphate binding site (13,63).

Spectrum and Resistance

Foscarnet inhibits all known human herpesviruses, including most ganciclovir-resistant CMV isolates and acyclovir-resistant HSV and VZV strains. It is also active against HIV. Resistance occurs as a result of DNA polymerase mutations. Strains of CMV, HSV, and VZV with reduced sensitivity to foscarnet have been reported (63,64).

Indications

Foscarnet is as effective as ganciclovir for therapy of sight-threatening chorioretinitis caused by CMV in adult patients with AIDS (65). Because of its inherent activity against HIV, it may even offer a survival advantage for treated patients (66). Refractory cases of chorioretinitis may respond to a combination of foscarnet and ganciclovir. Foscarnet is also effective in the therapy of CMV infections caused by ganciclovir-resistant strains of virus (66). Limited data also suggest that foscarnet may be of benefit when administered to patients with AIDS who have gastrointestinal and pulmonary infections caused by CMV.

Infections caused by acyclovir-resistant strains of HSV and VZV have been successfully controlled with foscarnet (67,68).

Pharmacokinetics

Only about 20% of foscarnet is absorbed after oral administration. Maximum serum concentration attained after an intravenous dose of 60 mg per kg is approximately 500 μmol per L (63). CSF concentrations are about two-thirds of those in serum. The half-life of foscarnet is about 48 hours, and 80% of an administered dose is eliminated unchanged in the urine. Dose reduction, proportional to reduction in creatinine clearance, is necessary. Hemodialysis efficiently eliminates foscarnet and therefore a supplemental dose is recommended after dialysis (69). There are no data on the use of foscarnet in the newborn.

Adverse Effects

The most common adverse effects of foscarnet are nephrotoxicity and metabolic derangements. Evidence of nephrotoxicity includes azotemia, proteinuria, acute tubular necrosis, crystalluria, and interstitial nephritis. Serum creatinine concentrations increase in up to 50% of patients. Fortunately, renal function returns to normal within 2 to 4 weeks of discontinuing therapy. Preexisting renal disease, concurrent use of other nephrotoxic drugs, dehydration, rapid injection, or continuous intravenous infusion of drug are risk factors for developing renal dysfunction (70).

Metabolic disturbances associated with foscarnet therapy include hypo- and hypercalcemia and hypo- and hyperphosphatemia (71). Hypocalcemia can be associated with paresthesias, tetany, seizures, and arrhythmias. Metabolic disturbances are minimized if foscarnet is administered by slow infusion. CNS symptoms associated with foscarnet therapy include headache, tremor, irritability, seizures, and hallucinations. Fever, nausea, vomiting, abnormal serum hepatic enzymes, anemia, granulocytopenia, and genital ulcerations have also been reported.

Drug Interactions

Concomitant use of amphotericin B, cyclosporine, gentamicin, and other nephrotoxic drugs increases the likelihood of renal dysfunction. Coadministration of pentamidine increases the risk of hypocalcemia. Anemia and neutropenia are more common when patients also are receiving zidovudine.

Dosage

The usual dose of foscarnet for CMV infection is 180 mg per kg per day in three divided doses for 14 to 21 days, followed by a daily maintenance dose of 90 to 120 mg per kg. The dosage of foscarnet used for infections caused by acyclovir-resistant HSV and VZV infections is 120 mg per kg per day in three divided doses.

THERAPY OF RESPIRATORY VIRUS INFECTIONS

Although numerous viral infections cause pulmonary disease in the newborn and infant, licensed therapies exist for only two diseases: influenza and respiratory syncytial virus (RSV) infection. For a more comprehensive review of the etiology of lung disease in pediatric and adult patients, the reader is referred to excellent reviews (13,72).

INFLUENZA

There are three influenza viruses (A, B, and C) which are members of the orthomyxovirus family. These viruses have segmented negative-sense RNA genomes, an envelope derived from the host cell, and characteristic surface glycoproteins that are involved in the entry and release of the virus from host cells. Influenza C causes only minor illness that does not usually require therapy. Influenza A and B, however, can both cause seasonal epidemics with significant morbidity and mortality. Influenza A is also the source of occasional pandemics.

Recognizing that vaccination against the influenza virus is a more effective measure in reducing the burden of disease (16), specific antiviral agents are useful in the prophylaxis and treatment of infection. Two specific viral proteins are targets for current therapies: the M2 protein, which is an ion channel in the viral membrane of influenza A, and neuraminidase, which is a surface glycoprotein common to both influenza A and B.

Over the past several years, there has been increasing concern for an influenza pandemic, recognizing the severe disease encountered in Asia and the Middle Ease secondary to H5N1. To date, H5N1 infections, while associated with significant mortality, remain localized and are not easily secondarily transmitted. However, because recently there has been global spread of novel influenza A H1N1 (swine influenza), emergency use authorization (EUA) was granted by the FDA, Centers for Disease Control and Prevention (CDC), and the World Health Organization for the use of oseltamivir in babies younger than 1 year (73,74). Importantly, there have been thousands of cases globally, including disease on three continents, and over 100 deaths (74,75).

The available therapies are summarized below.

AMANTADINE (SYMMETREL) AND RIMANTADINE (FLUMADINE)

Amantadine and rimantadine are closely related antiviral agents and were approved for use in the United States in 1966 and 1993, respectively. Although they are useful for the prevention and treatment of infections caused by influenza A virus, vaccination against influenza is a more cost-effective means of reducing disease burden. As noted below, their utility has been limited by the development of antiviral resistance.

Chemistry and Mechanism of Action

Amantadine and rimantadine are structurally related symmetric tricyclic amines. The influenza virus M2 protein, which forms a channel that spans the viral membrane, is the target for both of these antivirals. Blocking this channel limits the penetration of hydrogen ions, and the concurrent drop in pH, in the interstices of the viral particle (76). Viral replication is inhibited because a drop in pH is required for dissociation of the M1 protein from the ribonucleoprotein complexes, a process that is necessary to initiate replication (77).

Spectrum and Resistance

Amantadine and rimantadine are active only against susceptible influenza A viruses (and not influenza B); rimantadine is 4- to 10-fold more active than amantadine (78).

Resistance to these drugs, which typically appears in the treated patient within 2 to 3 days of initiating therapy, results from a mutation in the RNA sequence encoding for the M2 protein transmembrane domain (79). More than 25% of treated patients shed resistant strains by the day 5 of treatment (80). Although the clinical significance of isolating resistant strains from treated patients is not clear, transmission of resistant strains to household contacts can occur, and failure of drug prophylaxis can result (79). Currently, virtually all H3N2 strains of influenza circulating worldwide are resistant to these drugs.

Indications

Amantadine and rimantadine are useful for the prevention and treatment of infections caused by influenza type-A virus, specifically H1N1. Prophylaxis with either drug prevents more than 50% of infections and about 80% of clinical illnesses caused by type-A influenza H1N1 virus (81,82). Although vaccine administration would be more effective, prophylaxis of high-risk hosts is recommended for those who cannot tolerate vaccine because of toxicity or allergies and in those for whom vaccine is unlikely to induce protective immunity because of immunosuppression (83). Prophylaxis is also indicated for 2 weeks following vaccination if influenza A is already circulating in the community (83). Amantadine and rimantadine have been used to control outbreaks of infection occurring within households, schools, nursing homes, and hospitals (84).

Amantadine and rimantadine are effective in the treatment of influenza A H1N1 infections in adults and children if treatment is initiated within 2 days of the onset of symptoms (85,86). Drug therapy results in reduced duration of viral excretion, fever, and other systemic complaints. Compared with placebo, the duration of illness is shortened by about 1 day.

Pharmacokinetics

Amantadine and rimantadine are well absorbed after oral administration; food does not interfere with absorption of either drug (87,88). After 100-mg doses, peak serum concentrations of both drugs range from 0.4 to 0.8 μg per mL. Concentrations of both antivirals in nasal secretions exceed 50% of serum concentrations. The half-life of amantadine (12 to 18 hours) is about half that of rimantadine (24 to 36 hours). Although more than 90% of amantadine is excreted unchanged in the urine, rimantadine is metabolized extensively with less than 15% excreted unchanged in the urine. As a result, substantial dose adjustments of amantadine are necessary in persons with creatinine clearances of less than 80 mL per minute per 1.73 m^2, but dose adjustments for rimantadine are not necessary unless creatinine clearance is less than 10 mL per minute per 1.73 m^2 (89).

Adverse Effects

In general, side effects are less frequent and less severe with rimantadine. The most common complaints associated with the administration of both drugs are dose-related gastrointestinal and CNS symptoms (90). Common gastrointestinal complaints include nausea, vomiting, and dyspepsia. Common CNS disturbances, evident in about 10% of amantadine and 2% of rimantadine recipients, include anxiety, depression, insomnia, difficulty in concentration, and confusion; hallucinations and seizures occur less often. Long-term amantadine therapy has been associated with vision loss, hypotension, urinary retention, peripheral edema, and congestive heart failure. In children, the incidence of side effects in rimantadine recipients is similar to that observed in placebo recipients (91).

Dosage

The usual regimen of amantadine in children is 5 mg per kg per day given in one to two divided doses. The regimen of rimantadine is also 5 mg per kg per day, but it usually is administered as a single-daily dosing. The dosing of both drugs for adults is 100 to 200 mg per day.

OSELTAMIVIR AND ZANAMIVIR

Oseltamivir and zanamivir are licensed antiviral agents that are active against both influenza A and B viral strains. Both drugs have been approved by the FDA for use in children; however, there is limited clinical experience with these drugs in children. As noted below, studies performed by the NIAID CASG are expanding knowledge on the use of oseltamivir in infants younger than 1 year.

OSELTAMIVIR (TAMIFLU)

Chemistry and Mechanism of Action

Oseltamivir is an ethyl ester prodrug, hydrolyzed by hepatic esterases to biologically active oseltamivir carboxylate. Its biologic action results from inhibition of influenza neuraminidase. Inhibition of neuraminidase prevents penetration of the virus to the cell surface, and because neuraminidase is required for optimal release of progeny virus from infected cells, inhibition of this enzyme decreases the spread of virus and intensity of infection.

Spectrum and Resistance

Because neuraminidase is a highly conserved enzyme in influenza viruses, oseltamivir is active against all strains of influenza type-A and influenza type-B viruses. Resistance can develop as a result of a mutation in the active site of the neuraminidase molecule. Initial studies of resistance indicated a very low probability, namely 1.5% (92); however, over the past two influenza seasons, H1N1 has become virtually 100% resistant to oseltamivir worldwide. Resistance develops at H274Y (73). Importantly, novel H1N1 (swine influenza) remains susceptible to oseltamivir.

Indications

Oseltamivir is effective in the prevention and therapy of infections caused by either influenza A or influenza B viruses. Because of the global development of resistance of H1N1 seasonal influenza, treatment recommendations issued by the CDC for the 2008–2009 influenza season require the coadministration of an adamantine and a neuraminidase inhibitor. Administration of oseltamivir for 6 weeks during the peak of influenza season has been shown to decrease the rate of infection by approximately 50% and the rate of illness by more than 80%, if the circulating strain is susceptible (93). However, this approach has never been studied in infants. Prevention of transmission of influenza infection among family members exposed to influenza in their households has also been demonstrated (94). In addition, oseltamivir is effective in treating influenza infections if initiated within 1 to 2 days of the onset of symptoms. Duration of illness among both adult and pediatric drug recipients is reduced by 1 to 1.5 days compared with duration of illness among placebo recipients (95–97). The frequency of physician-diagnosed secondary complications leading to antibiotic prescriptions also appears to be reduced by oseltamivir therapy (96,97). Retrospective reviews of hospital databases support the benefit of oseltamivir therapy in the reduction of cardiac events as well. Until recently, it was licensed only for patients older than 2 years; however, with the introduction of novel H1N1, an EUA allows for therapy of patients of all ages (73).

Pharmacokinetics

The bioavailability of oseltamivir is about 75%; coadministration with food does not affect absorption. More than 90% of oseltamivir (prodrug) is metabolized to oseltamivir carboxylate, the active metabolite. Peak plasma concentration of active compound following multiple, 75-mg doses administered twice a day is approximately 350 ng per mL. The half-life of oseltamivir carboxylate is 6 to 10 hours; it is eliminated by glomerular filtration and tubular secretion (97). Dose adjustment is recommended for patients with a creatinine clearance of less than 30 mL per minute, as oseltamivir carboxylate exposure is inversely proportional to declining renal function. The pharmacokinetics of oseltamivir in pediatric patients older than 12 years is similar to those in adult patients, but younger patients (3 to 12 years) showed more rapid clearances of the prodrug and carboxylate, resulting in lower exposures. As age increases, oral clearance of the carboxylate decreases in a linear fashion. Carboxylate exposure in older patients (65 to 78 years) is 25% to 35% higher compared with younger adults, but no dose change is recommended in this population.

Adverse Effects

About 10% of patients treated with oseltamivir experience nausea without vomiting, and an additional 10% have nausea with vomiting. These side effects generally are mild and usually occur on the first 2 days of therapy. Insomnia and vertigo also occasionally occur in oseltamivir recipients. Importantly, while an initial concern in Japan, CNS toxicity has neither been found in a retrospective study performed by the NIAID CASG nor a prospective pharmacokinetic/pharmacodynamic study (98).

Dosage

The pediatric dose of oseltamivir suspension is 2 mg per kg administered twice daily. The recommended adult dose is 75 mg given twice daily.

ZANAMIVIR (RELENZA)

Chemistry and Mechanism of Action

Zanamivir is structurally similar to oseltamivir, and it also interferes with the function of the influenza neuraminidase enzyme.

Spectrum and Resistance

The in vitro activity of zanamivir against influenza A and influenza B strains is similar to that of oseltamivir. Decreased susceptibility to zanamivir, resulting from mutations in both the viral hemagglutinin and neuraminidase, has been described in an immunocompromised patient infected with influenza B (99).

Indications

Inhaled zanamivir, either administered for 4 weeks as seasonal prophylaxis or for 5 days, following presumed exposure to influenza in the community, has been shown to reduce the likelihood of influenza infection and disease (100,101). Short-term prophylaxis within households, begun within 24 hours of the index case becoming ill, also is effective (102).

Zanamivir is effective in the treatment of influenza A and influenza B virus infections occurring in adults (103,104) and children older than 20 years (105). On average, zanamivir-treated patients improve 1.0 to 2.5 days faster than placebo recipients (106). Zanamivir therapy also appears to reduce the frequency of antibiotic prescriptions for secondary respiratory complications of influenza infections.

Zanamivir resistance to seasonal influenza as well as novel H1N1 (swine influenza) has not been reported.

Pharmacokinetics

Zanamivir is administered by oral inhalation because it has poor oral bioavailability. Less than 15% of an inhaled dose of zanamivir is distributed to the airways and lungs; most is deposited in the oropharynx (107). Nonetheless, concentrations of drug exceed 1,000 ng per mL in sputum for 6 hours after inhalation, greatly exceeding the amount needed to inhibit influenza A and B viruses. About 10% of an inhaled dose of zanamivir is absorbed; peak serum concentrations range from 17 to 142 ng per mL after a 10-mg dose(107). The plasma half-life of zanamivir ranges from 2.5 to 5 hours; drug is excreted unchanged in the urine. No adjustment in dosing is necessary for renal insufficiency because of the limited amount of systemically absorbed drug.

Adverse Effects

Zanamivir is very well tolerated. A decline in pulmonary function and bronchospasm has been reported in some patients with underlying airway disease (108).

Dosage

The recommended dose of zanamivir for children and adults is 10 mg (given in two inhalations of 5 mg each), administered twice daily for 5 days.

RESPIRATORY SYNCYTIAL VIRUS

RSV is a nonsegmented, single-stranded negative sense RNA virus that is a member of the paramyxoviridae family. RSV is a major cause of lower respiratory infection in children and is also associated with significant morbidity and mortality in immunocompromised hosts. Small molecule therapeutics for the treatment of RSV remain a significant unmet medical need.

RIBAVIRIN (VIRAZOLE; REBETRON COMBINATION THERAPY)

Ribavirin is available for inhaled use for the therapy of severe lower respiratory tract infection. It is also available as an oral and intravenous formulation (compassionate plea release from the FDA) for the therapy of Lassa fever. It is also available as a mainstay in the treatment of hepatitis C virus infection when coadministered with pegylated interferon.

Chemistry and Mechanism of Action

Ribavirin is a synthetic nucleoside analogue, and most closely resembles guanosine in structure. The 5′-phosphate derivatives and the deribosylated base of ribavirin interfere with the capping and elongation of messenger RNA (109).

Spectrum and Resistance

Ribavirin is active against a wide range of both RNA and DNA viruses, including myxo-, paramyxo-, arena-, bunya-, herpes-, adeno-, pox-, and retroviruses (110). It has also been considered a therapeutic for influenza virus; however, the data are extremely limited. Activity against RNA viruses is greater than that against DNA viruses; concentrations of drug required to inhibit replication of influenza, parainfluenza, and RSV range from 3 to 10 μg per mL (111). Viral resistance to ribavirin has not been observed.

Indications

Ribavirin aerosol is approved for the therapy of lower respiratory tract infections caused by RSV, but considerable controversy exists over the circumstances under which its use is indicated in spontaneously breathing infants. Although multiple placebo-controlled trials have demonstrated that ribavirin improved respiratory signs and symptoms and increased oxygenation, differences in critical endpoints such as number of days the patient received oxygen therapy and duration of hospitalization were not observed (112–114). Controversy also exists regarding the use of aerosol ribavirin in the management of children being mechanically ventilated for RSV infection. One randomized, placebo-controlled trial demonstrated benefit (115), but subsequent trials demonstrated lack of efficacy (116) or even prolongation of intensive care unit stay and/or hospitalization associated with this therapy (117).

Intravenously administered ribavirin is effective in the management of life-threatening infections caused by Lassa fever and hemorrhagic fever with renal syndrome (118). Oral ribavirin has been recommended for prophylaxis against Lassa fever in exposed contacts (119). Although there are many anecdotal reports of ribavirin therapy for other infections, including those caused by influenza, parainfluenza, and measles virus, efficacy against these infections is not established. As noted above, ribavirin in combination with interferon-α (Rebetron) is useful in the management of infections caused by hepatitis C virus (120,121).

Pharmacokinetics

The aerosolized formulation of ribavirin (Virazole) and the oral formulation in combination with pegylated interferon-α (Rebetron) are approved for use in the United States. Aerosolized delivery of ribavirin is accomplished with a small-particle aerosol generator (SPAG), which delivers a steady flow of small particles (median mass diameter of 1.3 mm). When 20 mg per mL of drug is instilled into the SPAG reservoir, an estimated 1.8 mg per kg per hour of ribavirin is deposited in the respiratory tract; the precise amount of drug delivered to the respiratory tract depends on the child's ventilation and lung pathology (122). A small amount of ribavirin is absorbed systemically following aerosolized delivery, but the concentration of drug in the respiratory tract is much higher than that in plasma. Levels in respiratory secretions often exceed 1,000 μg per mL, and mean plasma concentration is 1.10 μg per mL after 8 hours of aerosolization (123). The half-life of ribavirin in tracheal secretions ranges from 1.4 to 2.5 hours.

The oral bioavailability of ribavirin is about 40%; peak plasma concentrations range from 1.3 to 3.2 μg per mL after doses of 600 to 2,400 mg (124). Peak concentrations following intravenous therapy are approximately 10-fold greater. Levels of ribavirin in CSF are approximately 70% of plasma concentrations of the drug (125). The half-life of ribavirin is 18 to 36 hours; less than one-third of systemically administered drug is recovered unchanged in urine, and an additional one-third is excreted as metabolites (124).

Adverse Effects

Ribavirin is concentrated in red blood cells, and high concentrations of the drug are associated with reversible anemia (124). Increases in serum bilirubin, iron, and uric acid may also result from systemic therapy.

Aerosolized ribavirin occasionally is associated with mild conjunctival irritation and rash. Transient wheezing may accompany therapy. Unless careful attention is paid to modifying the circuitry and frequently changing in-line filters, ribavirin can precipitate, plugging the ventilator valves and tubing, when used in mechanically ventilated infants (126).

Health care personnel caring for children receiving aerosolized ribavirin may be exposed inadvertently to the drug. However, only 1 of 29 health care workers evaluated in two studies in which drug was being administered to children by ventilator, oxygen tent, or oxygen hood had detectable drug in red blood cells, and none had drug detected in urine or serum samples (127,128).

Dosage

The usual dosage of aerosolized ribavirin is 20 mg per mL of drug instilled in the SPAG reservoir and administered for 12 to 22 hour per day for 3 to 6 days. A dose of 60 mg per mL administered for 2-hour periods three times a day also is well tolerated and results in less environmental exposure of health care personnel without compromising efficacy. The usual intravenous regimen of ribavirin is 4 g per day in adults; 15 to 30 mg per kg per day may be appropriate for children (129).

SUMMARY

Clearly, therapeutic advances have been achieved in the treatment of herpesvirus infections, most notably HSV, VZV, and CMV. With the treatment of influenza, the neuraminidase inhibitors offer new therapeutic opportunities. However, the propensity for the rapid appearance of resistance poses significant challenges for both the utilization of current therapies as well as the need to develop improved treatments. Unfortunately, drugs with alternative mechanisms of action are only approaching clinical trials. In addition, the unmet medical need for safe and efficacious therapies of other respiratory pathogens, particularly RSV, must be emphasized.

ACKNOWLEDGMENT

Work reported in this review was supported by a contract NO-1-AI- 30025 and a grant from the State of Alabama.

REFERENCES

1. Kimberlin D. Antiviral agents. In: Long S, Pickering L, Prober C, eds. *Principles and practice of pediatric infectious diseases*, 3rd ed. New York: Elsevier, 2008:1470–1488.
2. Brown ZA, Wald A, Morrow RM, et al. Effect of serologic status and cesarean delivery on transmission rates of herpes simplex virus from mother to infant. *JAMA* 2003;289:203–209.
3. Whitley RJ. Herpes simplex virus. In: Scheld WM, Mara C, Whitley RJ, eds. *Infections of the central nervous system,* 3rd ed. Philadelphia, PA: Lippincott Williams & Wilkins, 2004:123–144.
4. Kimberlin DW, Lin C-Y, Jacobs RF, et al. Natural history of neonatal herpes simplex virus infections in the acyclovir era. *Pediatrics* 2001;108:223–229.
5. Kimberlin DW. Management of HSV encephalitis in adults and neonates: diagnosis, prognosis and treatment. *Herpes* 2007;14(1):11–16.
6. Hutto C, Arvin A, Jacobs R, et al. Intrauterine herpes simplex virus infections. *J Pediatr* 1987;110(1):97–101.
7. Whitley RJ, Corey L, Arvin A, et al. Changing presentation of herpes simplex virus infection in neonates. *J Infect Dis* 1988;158(1):109–116.
8. Whitley RJ. Herpes simplex virus infections. In: Remington JS, Klein JO, eds. *Infectious diseases of the fetus and newborn infants*, 3rd ed. Philadelphia, PA: W.B. Saunders Company, 1990:282–305.
9. Whitley RJ, Roizman B. Herpes simplex viruses. In: Richman DD, Whitley RJ, Hayden FG, eds. *Clinical virology*, 2nd ed. Washington, DC: ASM Press, 2004:375–401.
10. Whitley RJ, Nahmias AJ, Soong SJ, et al. Vidarabine therapy of neonatal herpes simplex virus infection. *Pediatrics* 1980;66(4):495–501.
11. Whitley R, Arvin A, Prober C, et al. A controlled trial comparing vidarabine with acyclovir in neonatal herpes simplex virus infection. *N Engl J Med* 1991;324(7):444–449.
12. Kimberlin DW, Lin CY, Jacobs RF, et al. Safety and efficacy of high-dose intravenous acyclovir in the management of neonatal herpes simplex virus infections. *Pediatrics* 2001;108(2):230–238.
13. Yin M, Brust J, Tieu H, et al. Anti-hepatitis virus and anti-respiratory virus agents. In: Richman D, Whitley R, Hayden F, eds. *Clinical virology*. Washington, DC: ASM Press, 2009:217–264.
14. Englund JA, Zimmerman ME, Swierkosz EU, et al. Herpes simplex virus resistant to acyclovir. A study in a tertiary care center. *Ann Intern Med* 1990;112:416–422.

15. Kimberlin D, Powell D, Gruber W, et al. Administration of oral acyclovir suppressive therapy following neonatal herpes simplex virus disease limited to the skin, eyes, and mouth: results of a Phase I/II trial. *Pediatr Infect Dis J* 1996;15:247–254.
16. Field AK, Biron KK. "The end of innocence" revisited: resistance of herpesviruses to antiviral drugs. *Clin Microbiol Rev* 1994;7(1): 1–13.
17. Lyall EG, Ogilvie MM, Smith NM, et al. Acyclovir resistant varicella zoster and HIV infection. *Arch Dis Child* 1994;70(2):133–135.
18. Morfin F, Thouvenot D. Herpes simplex virus resistance to antiviral drugs. *J Clin Virol* 2003;26(1):29–37.
19. Wagstaff AJ, Faulds D, Goa KL. Aciclovir. A reappraisal of its antiviral activity, pharmacokinetic properties and therapeutic efficacy. *Drugs* 1994;47:153–205.
20. Laskin OL, Longstreth JA, Whelton A, et al. Effect of renal failure on the pharmacokinetics of acyclovir. *Am J Med* 1982;73(1A): 197–201.
21. Krasny HC, Liao SH, de Miranda P, et al. Influence of hemodialysis on acyclovir pharmacokinetics in patients with chronic renal failure. *Am J Med* 1982;73(1A):202–204.
22. Revankar SG, Applegate AL, Markovitz DM. Delirium associated with acyclovir treatment in a patient with renal failure. *Clin Infect Dis* 1995;21(2):435–436.
23. Kimberlin DW, Jacobs RF, Weller S, et al. Pharmacokinetics and safety of extemporaneously compounded valacyclovir oral suspension in pediatric patients from 1 month to 12 years of age. *Clin Infect Dis* 2010;50:221–228.
24. Jacobson MA. Valaciclovir (BW256U87): the L-valyl ester of acyclovir. *J Med Virol* 1993;(Suppl 1):150–153.
25. Soul-Lawton J, Seaber E, On N, et al. Absolute bioavailability and metabolic disposition of valaciclovir, the L-valyl ester of acyclovir, following oral administration to humans. *Antimicrob Agents Chemother* 1995;39:2759–2764.
26. Bell WR, Chulay JD, Feinberg JE. Manifestations resembling thrombotic microangiopathy in patients with advanced HIV disease in a cytomegalovirus disease prophylaxis trial (ACT6204). *Medicine (Baltimore)* 1997;76:369–380.
27. Valtrex package insert, 2008. http://us.gsk.com/products/assets/us_valtrex.pdf. Accessed June 15, 2009.
28. Griffiths PD, Emery VC. Cytomegalovirus. In: Richman DD, Whitley RJ, Hayden FG, eds. *Clinical virology*, 2nd ed. Washington, DC: ASM Press, 2002:433–461.
29. Staras SA, Dollard SC, Radford KW, et al. Seroprevalence of cytomegalovirus infection in the United States, 1988–1994. *Clin Infect Dis* 2006;43(9):1143–1151.
30. Demmler GJ. Infectious Diseases Society of America and Centers for Disease Control. Summary of a workshop on surveillance for congenital cytomegalovirus disease. *Rev Infect Dis* 1991;13(2):315–329.
31. Conboy TJ, Pass RF, Stagno S, et al. Early clinical manifestations and intellectual outcome in children with symptomatic congenital cytomegalovirus infection. *J Pediatr* 1987;111(3):343–348.
32. Dollard SC, Grosse SD, Ross DS. New estimates of the prevalence of neurological and sensory sequelae and mortality associated with congenital cytomegalovirus infection. *Rev Med Virol* 2007;17(5):355–363.
33. Ross SA, Boppana SB. Congenital cytomegalovirus infection: outcome and diagnosis. *Semin Pediatr Infect Dis* 2005;16(1):44–49.
34. Griffiths PD, McLaughlin JE. Cytomegalovirus. In: Scheld WM, Whitley RJ, Marra CM, eds. *Infections of the central nervous system.* Philadelphia, PA: Lippincott Williams & Wilkins, 2004:159–173.
35. Maschmann J, Hamprecht K, Dietz K, et al. Cytomegalovirus infection of extremely low-birth weight infants via breast milk. *Clin Infect Dis* 2001;33(12):1998–2003.
36. Brasfield DM, Stagno S, Whitley RJ, et al. Infant pneumonitis associated with cytomegalovirus, chlamydia, pneumocystis, and ureaplasma. *Pediatrics* 1987;79:76–83.
37. Strauss M. Human cytomegalovirus labyrinthitis. *Am J Otolaryngol* 1990;11(5):292–298.
38. Davis LE, Johnsson LG, Kornfeld M. Cytomegalovirus labyrinthitis in an infant: morphological, virological, and immunofluorescent studies. *J Neuropathol Exp Neurol* 1981;40(1):9–19.
39. Kimberlin DW, Lin CY, Sanchez PJ, et al. Effect of ganciclovir therapy on hearing in symptomatic congenital cytomegalovirus disease involving the central nervous system: a randomized, controlled trial. *J Pediatr* 2003;143(1):16–25.
40. Oliver SE, Cloud GA, Sánchez PJ, et al. Neurodevelopmental outcomes following ganciclovir therapy in symptomatic congenital cytomegalovirus infections involving the central nervous system. *J Clin Virol* 2009;46(S):S22–S26.
41. Markham A, Faulds D. Ganciclovir: an update of its therapeutic use in cytomegalovirus infection. *Drugs* 1994;48:455.
42. Rha B, Kimberlin DW, Whitley R. Antiviral drugs. In: Jerome K, ed. *Laboratory diagnosis of viral infections*, 3rd ed. New York: Informa Healthcare, 2009.
43. Reddy V, Hao Y, Lipton J, et al. Management of allogeneic bone marrow transplant recipients at risk for cytomegalovirus disease using a surveillance bronchoscopy and prolonged pre-emptive ganciclovir therapy. *J Clin Virol* 1999;13(3):149–159.
44. Jacobson MA, Gambertoglio JG, Aweeka FT, et al. Foscarnet-induced hypocalcemia and effects of foscarnet on calcium metabolism. *J Clin Endocrinol Metab* 1991;72(5):1130–1135.
45. Frenkel LM, Capparelli EV, Dankner WM, et al. Oral ganciclovir in children: pharmacokinetics, safety, tolerance, and antiviral effects. The Pediatric AIDS Clinical Trials Group. *J Infect Dis* 2000;182(6):1616–1624.
46. Trang JM, Kidd L, Gruber W, et al. Linear single-dose pharmacokinetics of ganciclovir in newborns with congenital cytomegalovirus infections. *Clin Pharmacol Ther* 1993;53:15–21.
47. Swan SK, Munar MY, Wigger MA, et al. Pharmacokinetics of ganciclovir in a patient undergoing hemodialysis. *Am J Kidney Dis* 1991;17(1):69–72.
48. Cocohoba JM, McNicholl IR. Valganciclovir: an advance in cytomegalovirus therapeutics. *Ann Pharmacother* 2002;36(6): 1075–1079.
49. Jung D, Dorr A. Single-dose pharmacokinetics of valganciclovir in HIV- and CMV-seropositive subjects. *J Clin Pharmacol* 1999; 39(8):800–804.
50. Kimberlin DW, Acosta EP, Sanchez PJ, et al. A pharmacokinetic and pharmacodynamic assessment of oral valganciclovir in the treatment of symptomatic congenital cytomegalovirus disease. *J Infect Dis* 2008;197(6):836–845.
51. Czock D, Scholle C, Rasche FM, et al. Pharmacokinetics of valganciclovir and ganciclovir in renal impairment. *Clin Pharmacol Ther* 2002;72(2):142–150.
52. Ho HT, Woods KL, Bronson JJ, et al. Intracellular metabolism of the antiherpes agents (s)-1-{3-hydroxy-2-(phosphonylmethoxy) propyl}cytosine. *Mol Pharmacol* 1992;41:197–202.
53. Safrin S, Cherrington J, Jaffe HS. Clinical uses of cidofovir. *Rev Med Virol* 1997;7(3):145–156.
54. Lurain N, Spafford LE, Thompson KD. Mutation in the UL97 open reading frame of human cytomegalovirus strains resistant to ganciclovir. *J Virol* 1994;68:4427–4431.
55. Cherrington JM, Miner R, Allen SJW, et al. *Sensitivities of human cytomegalovirus (HCMV) clinical isolates to cidofovir.* In: Eight International Conference on Antiviral Research, Santa Fe, NM, April 23–28, 1995.
56. The Studies of Ocular Complications of AIDS Research Group in collaboration with the AIDS Clinical Trials Group. Cidofovir (HPMPC) for the treatment of cytomegalovirus retinitis in patients with AIDS: the HPMPC Peripheral Cytomegalovirus Retinitis Trial. *Ann Intern Med* 1997;126:264–274.
57. Lalezari JP, Staagg RJ, Kuppermann BD, et al. Intravenous cidofovir for peripheral cytomegalovirus retinitis in patients with AIDS: a randomized, controlled trial. *Ann Intern Med.* 1997;126: 257–263.
58. Lalezari JP, Drew WL, Glutzer E, et al. Treatment with intravenous (S)-1-[3-hydroxy-2-(phosphonylmethoxy)propyl)-cytosine of acyclovir-resistant mucocutaneous infection with herpes simplex virus in a patient with AIDS. *J Infect Dis* 1994;170: 570–572.
59. Kimberlin DW, Malis DJ. Juvenile onset recurrent respiratory papillomatosis: possibilities for successful antiviral therapy. *Antiviral Res* 2000;45(2):83–93.
60. Pransky SM, Magit AE, Kearns DB, et al. Intralesional cidofovir for recurrent respiratory papillomatosis in children. *Arch Otolaryngol Head Neck Surg* 1999;125(10):1143–1148.
61. Cundy KC, Petty BG, Flaherty J, et al. Clinical pharmacokinetics of cidofovir in human immunodeficiency virus-infected patients. *Antimicrob Agents Chemother* 1995;39:1247–1252.
62. Lalezari JP, Drew WL, Glutzer E, et al. (S)-1{3-hydroxy-2-(phosphonylmethoxy)propyl}cytosine (cidofovir): results of a phase

I/II study of a novel antiviral nucleotide analogue. *J Infect Dis* 1995;171:788–796.
63. Wagstaff AJ, Bryson HM. Foscarnet: a reappraisal of its antiviral activity, pharmacokinetic properties and therapeutic use in immunocompromised patients with viral infectious. *Drugs* 1994;48:199–226.
64. Safrin S, Kemmerly S, Plotkin B, et al. Foscarnet-resistant herpes simplex virus infection in patients with AIDS. *J Infect Dis* 1994; 169:193–196.
65. Snoeck R, Andrei G, Gerard M, et al. Successful treatment of progressive mucocutaneous infection due to acyclovir- and foscarnet-resistant herpes simplex virus with (S)-1-(3-hydroxy-2-phosphonylmethoxypropyl)cytosine (HPMPC). *Clin Infect Dis* 1994;18(4):570–578.
66. Jacobson MA, Drew WL, Feinberg J, et al. Foscarnet therapy for ganciclovir-resistant cytomegalovirus retinitis in patients with AIDS. *J Infect Dis* 1991;163:1348–1351.
67. Safrin S, Berger TG, Gilson I. Foscarnet therapy in five patients with AIDS and acyclovir-resistant varicella zoster virus infection. *Ann Intern Med* 1991;115:19–21.
68. Studies of Ocular Complications of AIDS Research Group. Mortality in patients with the acquired immunodeficiency syndrome treated with either foscarnet or ganciclovir for cytomegalovirus retinitis. *N Engl J Med* 1992;326:213–220.
69. Safrin S, Crumpacker C, Chatis P, et al. A controlled trial comparing foscarnet with vidarabine for acyclovir-resistant mucocutaneous herpes simplex in the acquired immunodeficiency syndrome. The AIDS Clinical Trials Group. *N Engl J Med* 1991; 325(8):551–555.
70. MacGregor RR, Graziani AL, Weiss R, et al. Successful foscarnet therapy for cytomegalovirus retinitis in an AIDS patient undergoing hemodialysis: rationale for empiric dosing and plasma level monitoring. *J Infect Dis* 1991;164(4):785–787.
71. Deray G, Martinez F, Katlama C, et al. Foscarnet nephrotoxicity: mechanism, incidence and prevention. *Am J Nephrol* 1989;9(4): 316–321.
72. Hayden F, Palese P. Influenza virus. In: Richman D, Whitley R, Hayden F, eds. *Clinical virology*. Washington, DC: ASM Press, 2009:943–976.
73. Centers for Disease Control. Emergency use authorization of Tamiflu, 2009. http://www.cdc.gov/h1n1flu/eua/tamiflu.htm. Accessed June 16, 2009.
74. Kimberlin D, Acosta E, Sanchez P, et al. *Oseltamivir pharmacokinetics (PK) in infants: interim results from multicenter trial*. In: 47th Annual Meeting of the Infectious Diseases Society of America (IDSA), Philadelphia, PA, 2009.
75. World Health Organization. Influenza A (H1N1): epidemic and pandemic alert and response, 2009. http://www.who.int/csr/disease/swineflu/en/index.html. Accessed June 16, 2009.
76. Pinto LH, Holsinger LJ, Lamb RA. Influenza virus M2 protein has ion channel activity. *Cell* 1992;69(3):517–528.
77. Bui M, Whittaker G, Helenius A. Effect of M1 protein and low pH on nuclear transport of influenza virus ribonucleoproteins. *J Virol* 1996;70(12):8391–8401.
78. Valette M, Allard JP, Aymard M, et al. Susceptibilities to rimantadine of influenza A/H1N1 and A/H3N2 viruses isolated during the epidemics of 1988 to 1989 and 1989 to 1990. *Antimicrob Agents Chemother* 1993;37(10):2239–2240.
79. Hayden F, Couch R. Clinical and epidemiologic importance of influenza A viruses resistant to amantadine and rimantadine. *Rev Med Virol* 1992;2:89–96.
80. Hayden FG, Belshe RB, Clover RD, et al. Emergence and apparent transmission of rimantadine-resistant influenza A virus in families. *N Engl J Med* 1989;321:1696–1702.
81. Demicheli V, Jefferson T, Rivetti D, et al. Prevention and early treatment of influenza in healthy adults. *Vaccine* 2000;18(11–12): 957–1030.
82. Couch RB. Prevention and treatment of influenza. *N Engl J Med* 2000;343:1778–1787.
83. Prevention and control of influenza. Recommendations of the Immunization Practices Advisory Committee (ACIP). *MMWR Recomm Rep* 1992;41(RR-9):1–17.
84. Douglas RG, Jr. Drug therapy: prophylaxis and treatment of influenza. *N Engl J Med* 1990;322:443–450.
85. Hall CB, Dolin R, Gala CL, et al. Children with influenza A infection: treatment with rimantadine. *Pediatrics* 1987;80:275–282.
86. van Voris LP, Betts RF, Hayden FG, et al. Successful treatment of naturally occurring influenza A/USSR/77 H1N1. *JAMA* 1981;245: 1128–1131.
87. Aoki FY, Sitar DS. Clinical pharmacokinetics of amantadine hydrochloride. *Clin Pharmacokinet* 1988;14(1):35–51.
88. Capparelli EV, Stevens RC, Chow MS, et al. Rimantadine pharmacokinetics in healthy subjects and patients with end-stage renal failure. *Clin Pharmacol Ther* 1988;43(5):536–541.
89. Horadam VW, Sharp JG, Smilack JD, et al. Pharmacokinetics of amantadine hydrochloride in subjects with normal and impaired renal function. *Ann Intern Med* 1981;94(4, pt 1):454–458.
90. Dolin R, Reichman RC, Madore HP, et al. A controlled trial of amantadine and rimantadine in the prophylaxis of influenza A infection. *N Engl J Med* 1982;307(10):580–584.
91. Clover RD, Crawford SA, Abell TD, et al. Effectiveness of rimantadine prophylaxis of children within families. *Am J Dis Child* 1986;140(7):706–709.
92. Covington E, Mendel D, Escarpe P, et al. *Phenotypic and genotypic assay of influenza virus neuraminidase indicates a low incidence of viral drug resistance during treatment with oseltamivir.* In: 11th International Symposium on Influenza and Other Respiratory Viruses, Grand Cayman, 1999.
93. Hayden FG, Atmar RL, Schilling M, et al. Use of the selective oral neuraminidase inhibitor oseltamivir to prevent influenza. *N Engl J Med* 1999;341:1336–1343.
94. Munoz FM, Galasso GJ, Gwaltney JM, et al. Current research on influenza and other respiratory viruses: II international symposium. *Antiviral Res* 2000;46(2):91–124.
95. Treanor JJ, Hayden FG, Vrooman PS, et al. Efficacy and safety of the oral neuraminidase inhibitor oseltamivir in treating acute influenza. *JAMA* 2000;283:1016–1024.
96. Nicholson KG, Aoki FY, Osterhause A, et al. Treatment of acute influenza: efficacy and safety of the oral neuraminidase inhibitor oseltamivir. *Lancet* 2000;355:1845–1850.
97. Wood N, Aitken M, Sharp S, et al. *Tolerability and pharmacokinetics of the influenza neuraminidase inhibitor RO-64-0802 (GS4071) following oral administration of the prodrug Ro-64-0796 (GS4104) to healthy male volunteers.* In: 37th Interscience Conference on Antimicrobial Agents and Chemotherapy, Toronto, 1997.
98. Shalabi M, Abughali N, Abzug M, et al. *Safety of oseltamivir vs. amantadine or rimantadine in children under 1 year of age.* IDSA Annual Meeting, 2007.
99. Gubareva LV, Matrosovich MN, Brenner MK, et al. Evidence for zanamivir resistance in an immunocompromised child infected with influenza B virus. *J Infect Dis* 1998;178(5):1257–1262.
100. Monto AS, Robinson DP, Herlocher ML, et al. Zanamivir in the prevention of influenza among healthy adults: a randomized controlled trial. *JAMA* 1999;282:31–35.
101. Kaiser L, Henry D, Flack NP, et al. Short-term treatment with zanamivir to prevent influenza: results of a placebo-controlled study. *Clin Infect Dis* 2000;30(3):587–589.
102. Hayden FG, Gubareva LV, Monto AS, et al. Inhaled zanamivir for the prevention of influenza in families. *N Engl J Med* 2000; 343:1282–1289.
103. Randomised trial of efficacy and safety of inhaled zanamivir in treatment of influenza A and B virus infections. The MIST (Management of Influenza in the Southern Hemisphere Trialists) Study Group. *Lancet* 1998;352(9144):1877–1881.
104. Makela MJ, Pauksens K, Rostila T, et al. Clinical efficacy and safety of the orally inhaled neuraminidase inhibitor zanamivir in the treatment of influenza: a randomized, double-blind, placebo-controlled European study. *J Infect* 2000;40(1):42–48.
105. Hedrick JA, Barzilai A, Behre U, et al. Zanamivir for treatment of symptomatic influenza A and B infection in children five to twelve years of age: a randomized controlled trial. *Pediatr Infect Dis J* 2000;19(5):410–417.
106. Gubareva LV, Kaiser L, Hayden FG. Influenza virus neuraminidase inhibitors. *Lancet* 2000;355:827–835.
107. Cass LM, Brown J, Pickford M, et al. Pharmacoscintigraphic evaluation of lung deposition of inhaled zanamivir in healthy volunteers. *Clin Pharmacokinet* 1999;36(Suppl 1):21–31.
108. Cass LM, Gunawardena KA, Macmahon MM, et al. Pulmonary function and airway responsiveness in mild to moderate asthmatics given repeated inhaled doses of zanamivir. *Respir Med* 2000;94(2):166–173.

109. Sidwell RW, Robins RK, Hillyard IW. Ribavirin: an antiviral agent. *Pharmacol Ther* 1979;6:123–146.
110. Huggins JW. Prospects for treatment of viral hemorrhagic fevers with ribavirin, a broad-spectrum antiviral drug. *Rev Infect Dis* 1989;11:750–761.
111. Gilbert BE, Knight V. Biochemistry and clinical applications of ribavirin. *Antimicrob Agents Chemother* 1986;30(2):201–205.
112. Hall CB, McBride JT, Walsh EE, et al. Aerosolized ribavirin treatment of infants with respiratory syncytial viral infection: a randomized double-blind study. *N Engl J Med* 1983;308:1443–1447.
113. Groothuis JR, Woodin KA, Katz R, et al. Early ribavirin treatment of respiratory syncytial viral infection in high-risk children. *J Pediatr* 1990;117(5):792–798.
114. Conrad DA, Christenson JC, Waner JL, et al. Aerosolized ribavirin treatment of respiratory syncytial virus infection in infants hospitalized during an epidemic. *Pediatr Infect Dis J* 1987;6: 152–158.
115. Smith DW, Frankel LR, Mathers LH, et al. A controlled trial of aerosolized ribavirin in infants receiving mechanical ventilation for severe respiratory syncytial virus infection. *N Engl J Med* 1991;325:24–29.
116. Moler FW, Steinhart CM, Ohmit SE, et al. Effectiveness of ribavirin in otherwise well infants with respiratory syncytial virus-associated respiratory failure. Pediatric Critical Study Group. *J Pediatr* 1996;128(3):422–428.
117. Law BJ, Wang EE, MacDonald N, et al. Does ribavirin impact on the hospital course of children with respiratory syncytial virus (RSV) infection? An analysis using the pediatric investigators collaborative network on infections in Canada (PICNIC) RSV database. *Pediatrics* 1997;99(3):E7.
118. McCormick JB, King IJ, Webb PA, et al. Lassa fever: effective therapy with ribavirin. *N Engl J Med* 1986;314:20–26.
119. Holmes GP, McCormick JB, Trock SC, et al. Lassa fever in the United States. Investigation of a case and new guidelines for management. *N Engl J Med* 1990;323(16):1120–1123.
120. McHutchison JG, Gordon SC, Schiff ER, et al. Interferon alfa-2b alone or in combination with ribavirin as initial treatment for chronic hepatitis C. Hepatitis Interventional Therapy Group. *N Engl J Med* 1998;339:1485–1492.
121. Poynard T, Marcellin P, Lee SS, et al. Randomised trial of interferon alpha2b plus ribavirin for 48 weeks or for 24 weeks versus interferon alpha2b plus placebo for 48 weeks for treatment of chronic infection with hepatitis C virus. International Hepatitis Interventional Therapy Group (IHIT). *Lancet* 1998;352(9138): 1426–1432.
122. Knight V, Yu CP, Gilbert BE, et al. Estimating the dosage of ribavirin aerosol according to age and other variables. *J Infect Dis.* 1988;158(2):443–448.
123. Connor JD, Hintz M, Van Dyke R, et al. Ribavirin pharmacokinetics in children and adults during therapeutic trials. In: Smith RA, Knight V, Smith JAD, eds. *Clinical applications of ribavirin.* Orlando, FL: Academic Press, 1984:107–123.
124. Laskin OL, Longstreth JA, Hart CC, et al. Ribavirin disposition in high-risk patients for acquired immunodeficiency syndrome. *Clin Pharmacol Ther* 1987;41:546–555.
125. Connor E, Morrison S, Lane J, et al. Safety, tolerance, and pharmacokinetics of systemic ribavirin in children with human immunodeficiency virus infection. *Antimicrob Agents Chemother* 1993;37(3):532–539.
126. Frankel LR, Wilson CW, Demers RR, et al. A technique for the administration of ribavirin to mechanically ventilated infants with severe respiratory syncytial virus infection. *Crit Care Med* 1987;15(11):1051–1054.
127. Harrison R, Bellows J, Rempel D, et al. Assessing exposures of health-care personnel to aerosols of ribavirin—California. *MMWR Morb Mortal Wkly Rep* 1988;37:560–563.
128. Rodriguez WJ, Bui RH, Connor JD, et al. Environmental exposure of primary care personnel to ribavirin aerosol when supervising treatment of infants with respiratory syncytial virus infections. *Antimicrob Agents Chemother* 1987;31(7):1143–1146.
129. McCarthy AJ, Bergin M, De Silva LM, et al. Intravenous ribavirin therapy for disseminated adenovirus infection. *Pediatr Infect Dis J* 1995;14(11):1003–1004.

CHAPTER

37

Victoria Tutag Lehr
Merene Mathew
Harry T. Chugani
Jacob V. Aranda

Anticonvulsants

Epilepsy during infancy and childhood represents a therapeutic challenge because as many as 30% of children continue to have seizures refractory to treatment (1). Antiepileptic drugs (AEDs) remain the primary treatment modality for seizures (2–5). Multidrug regimens are often necessary to maximize seizure control and minimize adverse effects. During the past 20 years, numerous second- and third-generation AEDs have been approved in the United States (2–5). These AEDs include felbamate, gabapentin, lamotrigine, topiramate, tiagabine (TIG), levetiracetam (LEV), oxcarbazepine (OXC), zonisamide (ZNS), pregabalin, lacosamide, and rufinamide (2,3,5). Overall, these newer agents have shown more favorable side effect profiles, fewer drug–drug interactions, and less complex monitoring requirements compared with older AEDs (5–7). Pediatric clinicians (non-epileptologists) have been slow to replace older agents with new AEDs for many reasons, including long experience with older AEDs, insufficient postmarketing experience assessing relative efficacy, tolerability, and safety in infants and children, and increased relative cost (7). Many of the new AEDs are broad spectrum in mechanism of action offering improved seizure control with fewer adverse effects, particularly for those pediatric patients with intractable seizure disorders.

There is a paucity of data from well-designed clinical trials of the newer AEDs in infants and children. Extrapolation of data from trials in adults to pediatric patients is questionable, given age-related differences in pharmacokinetics, seizure types, and seizure etiology (8–10). In addition, children frequently have comorbidities such as mental retardation and behavioral disorders. Adverse effects and the variable pharmacokinetics of an AED, as a child undergoes maturational changes from birth to adolescence, with or without the presence of comorbidities, complicate anticonvulsant therapy (8–13). Pharmacokinetic differences may be partially responsible for age-related differences in the incidence of adverse effects observed with AEDs (12,13).

Interactions of AEDs with other agents are common; therefore, it is important to anticipate and minimize the risks of interactions to avoid loss of seizure control or development of toxicity (13–15). The newer AEDs such as lacosamide, LEV, and topiramate do not extensively induce metabolism of other AEDs, thereby offering an advantage over older agents (5,6,15). The risk–benefit ratio of AEDs must be considered when developing medication regimens.

In January 2008, the US Food and Drug Administration (FDA) issued an alert about a possible increased risk for suicidality associated with use of AEDs when prescribed for epilepsy (16–19). The relationship between suicidality and epilepsy is a complex, multifactorial issue (16). The contribution of AEDs to suicidality is unclear in view of confounders such as concomitant drug therapy, mental health diagnoses, effects of chronic epilepsy, and severity of epilepsy. Parents, caregivers, and patients must be reassured and counseled about the risks of withdrawing or discontinuing AED therapy without clinician supervision or approval. However, it is prudent that all patients with epilepsy be routinely evaluated for depression, anxiety, and suicidality, especially during periods of AED dosage adjustment (16,18,19).

INITIATION OF ANTICONVULSANT THERAPY

Initial anticonvulsant therapy is selected on the basis of seizure type and findings on the electroencephalogram (20). Additional factors influencing the selection of AED therapy include patient age, gender, history of drug reactions, concomitant disease states and medications, ease of administration, cost, and clinician familiarity with the individual AED.

PHENYTOIN

Phenytoin continues to be used in pediatrics for status epilepticus, generalized tonic–clonic seizures, and partial seizures with or without secondary generalization (21,22). This hydantoin is often administered as a second-line agent for status epilepticus after administration of benzodiazepines have failed to control seizures (23).

Phenytoin continues to be considered second-line therapy for managing neonatal seizures after phenobarbital has failed (24–27). However, in a randomized, clinical trial by Painter et al. in 59 neonates with seizures, phenytoin and phenobarbital were equally, but incompletely, effective in controlling neonatal seizures (25). When either of these medications was administered as single therapy, fewer than half of the babies had control of their seizures (26). Phenytoin and phenobarbital continue to be used in the management of neonatal seizures, although newer agents such as LEV are gaining popularity (27). In a large multicenter retrospective study (n = 6,099 infants) of neonatal seizure management, phenytoin was the second most frequently administered nonbenzodiazepine (27).

Phenytoin's primary anticonvulsant effect at therapeutic concentrations is related to use-dependent blockade of voltage-sensitive sodium channels, thus inhibiting repetitive neuronal firing (4). Additional actions include alteration of Na^+, K^+, and Ca^{2+} conduction; membrane potentials; and concentrations of amino acids, norepinephrine, acetylcholine, and γ-aminobutyric acid (GABA).

The major route of phenytoin metabolism is hepatic oxidation by cytochrome P450 (CYP450) enzymes CYP2C9 and CYP2C19 to the inactive metabolite 5-(*p*-hydroxyphenyl)-5-phenylhydantoin (28). This metabolic pathway is capacity limited and therefore saturable. As phenytoin serum concentrations increase, the fraction of drug eliminated per unit time decreases. Small increases in dose can result in disproportionately large increases in phenytoin serum concentration. These nonlinear kinetics occur in adults as well as in children of all ages and is described by Michaelis–Menten equations (29). Therefore, smaller incremental dose increases are recommended, as therapeutic phenytoin serum concentrations are approached.

Initial phenytoin dosing for neonates is 15 to 20 mg per kg intravenous or oral as a loading dose, followed by 4 to 7 mg per kg per day in divided doses every 12 hours as a maintenance dose. To avoid cardiac toxicity, bradyarrhythmias, and hypotension associated with the propylene glycol and ethanol constituents of parenteral formulations, the maximum rate of phenytoin intravenous infusion is 0.5 mg per kg per minute. Phenytoin injection is compatible only with normal saline. Oral phenytoin loading doses need to be administered in two to three divided doses and administered every 2 hours to optimize absorption. The maintenance dose is initiated 12 hours after administration of the loading dose (30).

Phenytoin dosage must be slowly adjusted according to the individual patient's requirements, clinical response, and serum concentrations (30). Because of nonlinear kinetics, it is prudent to initiate therapy with the lower end of the dosing range and increase incrementally until clinical response, assessing for toxicity. Initial maintenance dosages are based on age and weight: neonates (<4 weeks), 3 to 5 mg per kg per day; infants (4 weeks to <1 year), 4 to 8 mg per kg per day; children (1 to <12 years), 4 to 10 mg per kg per day; adolescents (12 to <18 years), 4 to 8 mg per kg per day; adults (18 years and older), 4 to 7 mg per kg per day.

Caution is advised when changing dosage forms of phenytoin, as these vary in phenytoin content. For example, the parenteral form, phenytoin sodium, contains 92% phenytoin and the oral suspension is free phenytoin acid. As the phenytoin dose is increased and the therapeutic range is approached, the difference in phenytoin content between the dose formulations becomes critical to avoid toxicity secondary to a disproportionate increase in serum concentration (29).

Phenytoin has a narrow therapeutic range for the general population of 10 to 20 μg per mL for total drug concentration and 1 to 2 μg per mL for unbound or free drug (31). Free phenytoin serum determinations are essential in the setting of hypoalbuminemia, azotemia, or reduced binding because the free fraction of the drug determines therapeutic effect and toxicity. Secondary to reduced plasma protein binding and decreased metabolic capacity, the therapeutic range is lower during the neonatal period, 8 to 15 μg per mL (32). Phenytoin binding at approximately 3 months of age resembles that of adults.

Infants exposed to phenytoin in utero or to phenobarbital therapy prior to phenytoin will have increased phenytoin elimination secondary to hepatic enzyme induction (33). There is considerable variability in correlation of clinical response with serum concentration in cases of decreased plasma protein binding, hypoalbuminemia, uremia, renal dysfunction, and hyperbilirubinemia. During the first 2 weeks of life, the infant's metabolic capacity increases significantly, resulting in increased phenytoin dose requirements. In general, infants have the highest phenytoin metabolic capacity, which generally results in dose requirements up to four times that of adults. During childhood, phenytoin metabolism decreases and approaches that of adults at around 10 years of age (29) (Fig. 37.1).

Therapeutic drug monitoring (TDM) is recommended for phenytoin to optimize therapeutic effect and minimize risk of toxicity. Frequency of serum sampling for phenytoin depends on the clinical situation. After administration of a phenytoin-loading dose, serum sampling is often performed to ascertain achievement of therapeutic serum concentrations. Samples must not be drawn within 1-hour postend phenytoin infusion to allow for drug distribution.

For oral and intravenous maintenance therapy, trough serum concentrations are usually drawn just prior to the morning dose. On initiating a maintenance regimen, phenytoin concentrations are drawn within 3 to 4 days starting therapy. This is not a steady-state determination; however, subtherapeutic or supratherapeutic concentrations may be detected at this time, thus avoiding breakthrough seizures or toxicity. Once a stable phenytoin regimen is achieved, serum sampling is performed every 1 to 2 weeks in hospital or every 1 to 6 months in outpatients. Sampling is indicated when a change in clinical status occurs, when a drug with potential for interacting with phenytoin is added to or deleted from the regimen, when changing phenytoin dosage forms or dosage, or to verify absorption of the dose or compliance. Significant variations in the pharmacokinetics occur during the neonatal period with intravenous and oral phenytoin therapy (34,35). Controversy exists regarding whether neonates have the ability to absorb oral formulations of phenytoin (36). However, oral phenytoin therapy has been documented to achieve predicted serum concentrations in a study of premature infants (25). In addition to the rapidly changing elimination kinetics, concomitant therapy with potent enzyme inducers, such as phenobarbital and carbamazepine (CBZ), may result in unpredictable fluctuations in phenytoin serum concentration (28).

Numerous clinically significant pharmacokinetic and pharmacodynamic drug interactions involving phenytoin have been described (6,14,15,37,38). Agents with potential for interacting with phenytoin are too numerous to list here as new drugs are developed and practice evolves. Clinicians

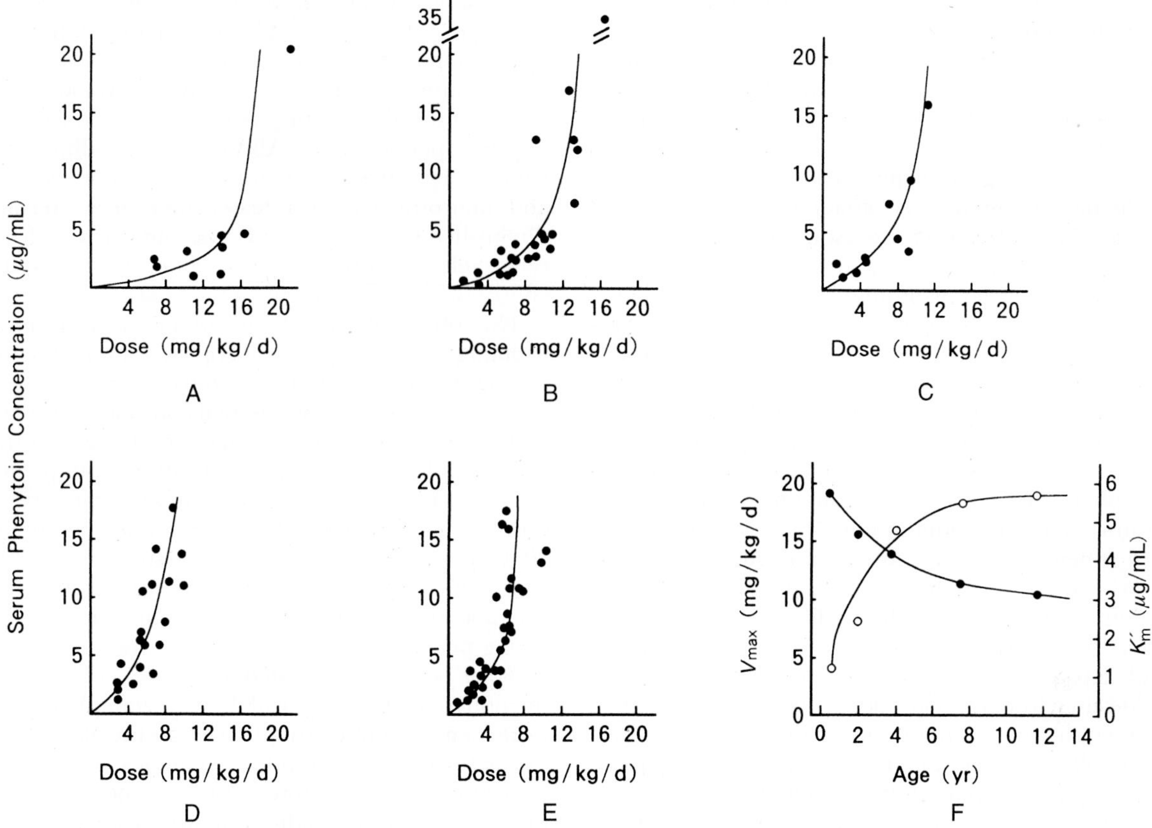

Figure 37.1. (A–E) Phenytoin dose and serum concentration in different age groups. (F) Change of V_{max} (•) and K'_m (○) with increasing age. (Modified from Nishihara K, Kohda Y, Saitoh Y, et al., lgaku-No-Ayumki 1978;107:512–515, with permission.)

are encouraged to consult with pharmacists and to review the current drug interaction literature when prescribing phenytoin therapy for their patients. Phenytoin serum concentrations may be increased by zidovudine and reduced by continuous nasogastric feedings (37). Concomitant therapy with valproic acid (VPA) significantly increases the free fraction of phenytoin. Interactions with other AEDs and phenytoin are prevalent and may be significant (14,15).

Phenytoin may decrease serum concentrations and the effectiveness of lamotrigine, VPA, felbamate, ethosuximide, primidone, potentially resulting in loss of seizure control. A consideration for adolescents receiving phenytoin therapy with oral contraceptives is the potential for phenytoin to lower estrogen and progestin serum concentrations, resulting in contraceptive failure. Higher dose oral contraceptives in addition to barrier methods are recommended for these patients (6,38). The potential for precipitating drug interactions must be evaluated whenever another agent is added to or removed from a therapeutic regimen containing phenytoin.

FOSPHENYTOIN

Fosphenytoin sodium (Cerebryx), 5,5-diphenyl-3-(phosphonooxy) methyl-2,4-imidazolidine-dione disodium, is the phosphorylated prodrug of phenytoin (39). Fosphenytoin is supplied as a 75-mg per mL parenteral injection, which is equivalent to 50 mg phenytoin sodium per mL. Fosphenytoin must be prescribed in terms of phenytoin equivalents (PEs), with 1 mg PE equal to 1.5 mg fosphenytoin. Phenytoin toxicity may result from misinterpretation of fosphenytoin dosage. Advantages over phenytoin include aqueous solution without propylene glycol and a more neutral pH of 8.6. Fosphenytoin is compatible with dextrose 5% water or normal saline, and also may be administered via intramuscular injection. Cardiac toxicity during intravenous infusion and local reactions at the site of injection occur less frequently with fosphenytoin than with phenytoin. Transient parethesias, burning, and pruritis have occurred during intravenous infusion of fosphenytoin. The rate of intravenous infusion for fosphenytoin is three times faster than that of phenytoin infusion, providing an advantage for rapid loading in status epilepticus.

Fosphenytoin is cleaved to phenytoin by nonspecific phosphatases in red blood cells and in hepatic and other tissues. Conversion half-life is 8 to 15 minutes and may be prolonged in renal or hepatic insufficiency (40). Fosphenytoin displaces phenytoin from plasma proteins, resulting in increased free phenytoin concentrations until the conversion is complete. Phenytoin serum concentrations should not be drawn until the conversion to phenytoin is complete, approximately 2 hours post-end infusion of fosphenytoin or 4 hours after intramuscular administration. It has been postulated that the increased free fraction may be cleared rapidly in infants, resulting in difficulty in maintaining therapeutic serum concentrations.

Fosphenytoin is approximately 10 times the cost of phenytoin injection; therefore, cost–benefit analysis is indicated. Restricting fosphenytoin use to patients without intravenous access or with prior local reactions to phenytoin administration, or for cases of status epilepticus, has been recommended (41,42). There is no apparent therapeutic benefit in using fosphenytoin over phenytoin that justifies the higher cost in other situations (43).

There are limited data on the use of fosphenytoin in the newborn (44–46). Fosphenytoin was administered to two extremely low-birth-weight infants with apparent adequate conversion to phenytoin and no adverse effects (44). Takeoka et al. reported seizure control in four infants ranging in age from 34 weeks to 1 year treated with fosphenytoin; however, doses of up to 10 mg PE per kg per day were required to maintain therapeutic phenytoin serum concentrations (45). Three of the infants had been receiving phenobarbital therapy at the time of fosphenytoin administration. In addition to probable induction of CYP450 by phenobarbital, the investigators suggested that the infants may have had an enhanced phenytoin rate of elimination. There was no significant difference in conversion rate of fosphenytoin to phenytoin in two multicenter studies of 78 patients ranging in age from 1 day to 16 years. Subjects received fosphenytoin loading doses of 18 to 20 mg PE per kg per minute via intravenous infusion (62/78) or 12 to 20 mg PE per kg per minute via intramuscular injection (16/78). Mean fosphenytoin-to-phenytoin conversion half-life was 8.3 minutes (2.5 to 18.5 minutes), which is similar to adult values (7.9 minutes). There was no significant difference in conversion half-life across age groups. Total and free phenytoin serum concentrations were similar to those in adults. There were no documented cases of toxicity or serious adverse effects. Infants and children in status epilepticus are at high risk for site reactions from phenytoin intravenous infusions. Fosphenytoin provides an effective, well-tolerated alternative to phenytoin in infants and children where venous access is not available and/or rapid loading is desirable (46).

PHENOBARBITAL

Phenobarbital, the 5-ethyl-5-phenyl-substituted barbiturate, remains first-line management for neonatal seizures (24,27,47). However, it is frequently ineffective in achieving complete seizure control in neonatal seizures (47). A retrospective study of infants with neonatal seizures ($n = 146$) showed no benefit of phenobarbital treatment after discharge home with respect to preventing seizure recurrence or long-term disability compared with no treatment in a multicenter retrospective study (48). Although clinical trials are needed, newer agents such as LEV and topiramate may develop a role in the management of neonatal seizures as experience is gained with their use in the NICU population (49,50).

Other indications are generalized tonic–clonic seizures, partial seizures, and prolonged febrile convulsions. Advantages of phenobarbital include a wide spectrum of seizure activity, wide therapeutic range, availability of parenteral and oral dose forms, low cost, and extensive experience of use in pediatrics. Disadvantages include respiratory depression, sedation, physical dependence, negative cognitive effects, hyperactivity, and potential adverse effects on developing neuronal cells (51,52).

The anticonvulsant effect of phenobarbital is related to potentiation of inhibitory neurotransmission by prolonging the open state of GABA-mediated sodium channels. Glutamate-induced excitatory transmission is decreased and neurotransmitter release from nerve terminals is diminished via blocking of L-type and N-type calcium currents. Selective suppression of abnormal neurons may also contribute to its therapeutic effect (52).

Phenobarbital has a large volume of distribution, distributing into all tissues, with approximately 50% bound to plasma protein. Volume of distribution decreases with increasing gestational age as total body water decreases and body fat increases. These changes in volume of distribution may result in high (interpatient) variability in phenobarbital serum concentrations achieved after standard loading doses. In general, initial dosing recommendations for 10 to 20 mg per kg assume a volume of distribution of 1.0 L per kg to achieve serum concentrations of 15 to 20 mg per mL. Therapeutic phenobarbital serum concentrations are 10 to 30 mg per mL. Reduced binding on the order of 20% to 25% has been demonstrated in neonates (53,54). Because phenobarbital is a weak acid, lower serum pH will enhance tissue penetration. Distribution across the blood–brain barrier is relatively slow (15 to 20 minutes after peak serum concentrations); therefore, dosing protocols need to allow for equilibration after administration. Wide interindividual variability in volume of distribution and elimination among neonates makes it necessary to measure phenobarbital serum concentrations (54,55).

The primary route of elimination for phenobarbital is metabolism via hepatic microsomal CYP450 enzymes and NADPH–cytochrome c reductase. Dosing reduction is advised in hepatic insufficiency. Phenobarbital clearance does not appear to undergo significant changes due to autoinduction, although it is a potent inducer of other hepatically metabolized agents such as theophylline, CBZ, phenytoin, cimetidine, and digoxin (14). Serum concentrations of phenobarbital may be increased by VPA or, in some instances, phenytoin. Serum concentration monitoring of phenobarbital is indicated when potentially interacting agents are added to or removed from therapeutic regimens. Clinicians are encouraged to consult with pharmacists and review the current literature and labeling when prescribing medications for patients taking phenobarbital to avoid precipitating a drug or drug–disease state interaction.

Phenobarbital has a long elimination half-life, with newborns demonstrating the slowest clearance (average 100 to 200 hours). Premature neonates may have unexpectedly increased clearance of phenobarbital, possibly secondary to increased liver size compared to body weight. Touw et al. reported that total body clearance of phenobarbital per kilogram of body weight tends to increase with increasing fetal maturity (55). Therefore, extremely premature infants would have not yet undergone the decrease in liver size relative to increasing body weight that occurs during the final weeks of gestation. During the first weeks of life, considerable variability occurs in phenobarbital elimination as hepatic enzymes mature or as a result of enzyme reduction from exposure to other drugs (53,54). Phenobarbital clearance rapidly increases during the first 2 weeks of life, peaking between 6 months and 12 months of age.

The loading dose of phenobarbital for the management of neonatal seizures is 20 mg per kg intravenous (24). The goal is to achieve a phenobarbital serum concentration of 15 to 40 μg per mL. Serum concentrations above 40 to 50 μg per mL may produce respiratory depression and coma, with 80 μg per mL associated with respiratory depression and death. There are reports of neonates tolerating phenobarbital serum concentrations of 60 to 80 μg per mL with respiratory support; however, bradycardia is frequently associated with serum concentrations greater than 50 μg per mL.

Additional doses of 5 to 10 mg per kg administered at 30-minute to 1-hour intervals may be required if seizures persist. Maintenance doses of 6 mg per kg per day are administered every 12 hours in divided doses. The long half-life of phenobarbital precludes the need for continuous infusions. However, continuous administration of daily doses of 5 mg per kg per day or more may result in accumulation of phenobarbital during the first weeks of life; therefore, doses of 2 to 4 mg per kg per day may be more appropriate for neonates younger than 2 weeks.

Studies have demonstrated that infants may require up to 40 mg per kg total loading dose (53,55). Effective seizure control has been related to phenobarbital dose, with 70% control with doses of 40 mg per kg (24). Neonates receiving extracorporeal membrane oxygenation may require larger phenobarbital doses to achieve effective serum concentrations secondary to a larger volume of distribution (56). Older studies report efficacy rates between 32% and 36% with standard dosing (57–59).

Children 1 to 18 years of age usually require phenobarbital loading doses of 10 to 20 mg per kg. The rate of administration is 2 mg per kg per minute for children weighing less than 40 kg, and not more than 100 mg per minute for children weighing more than 40 kg; the rate is 60 mg per minute for adults. Maintenance doses are 3 to 5 mg per kg per day for children 1 to 15 years of age, and 2 mg per kg per day for adults.

An initial phenobarbital serum concentration may be drawn 2 to 3 hours after administration of a loading dose to verify serum concentration (60–62). Secondary to a long half-life, steady-state serum concentrations may not be achieved for 2 to 4 weeks in neonates and infants. Serum concentration sampling may be repeated after 3 to 4 days of maintenance dosing to determine if dose titration is necessary; however, this does not reflect the steady-state phenobarbital serum concentration. Documentation of steady-state serum concentration should be performed after 3 to 4 weeks of therapy. Indications for phenobarbital serum concentration sampling include loss of seizure control, possible toxicity, dosage changes, and addition or deletion of potentially interacting agents.

CARBAMAZEPINE

Carbamazepine, CBZ, an iminodibenzyl derivative (iminostilbene) with a tricyclic antidepressant structure, has been used in adults and children as anticonvulsant for older than 30 years (63–65). This drug remains one of first-line treatments for partial motor, partial complex, and secondarily generalized tonic–clonic seizures. CBZ is not recommended for first-line management of primary generalized seizures due to possible exacerbation of these seizures (66). There is increasing use of CBZ for management of neonatal seizures (67–69). Advantages over other older AEDs include less sedation and a mood stabilization effect (70,71). Serious, although rare, aplastic anemia and agranulocytosis have been associated with CBZ therapy (72). Leukopenia and thrombocytopenia may occur, requiring hematologic monitoring (73). Rash, hypersensitivity reactions, including Stevens–Johnson syndrome, and toxic epidermal necrolysis are possible (74). CBZ has also been associated with significant weight gain (75).

Carbamazepine is available as a liquid suspension (Tegretol, 50 mg per mL), chewable tablets (Tegretol, 100 mg per mL), regular tablets (Tegretol and generic, 200 mg), sustained-release granules (Carbitrol, 200, 400 mg), and controlled-release formulation (Tegretol XR, 100, 200, 400 mg). There is no parenteral dosage form of CBZ. There may be considerable variability in rate of absorption of generic CBZ formulations compared with Tegretol, and therefore changing formulations must be performed with caution and close monitoring (76).

Carbamazepine's mechanism of action is similar to that of phenytoin, that is, use-dependent blockade of voltage-sensitive sodium channels, resulting in neuronal membrane stabilization and inhibition of repetitive firing of neurons (63). Other anticonvulsant effects include presynaptic decrease of synaptic transmission and possibly potentiation of postsynaptic effects of GABA.

The primary elimination pathway of CBZ is metabolism via the CYP3A4 and CYP1A2/2C8 isozymes (75). Half-lives of CBZ in adults are 12 to 17 hours, with shorter values in children and infants. Neonates exposed to CBZ in utero have been reported to show half-lives of 8.2 to 48.0 hours. An active metabolite, CBZ-10,11-epoxide, is formed in a 0.1:0.2 ratio, and is inactivated via epoxide hydrolysis. CBZ induces its own metabolism (autoinduction) in a dose-dependent manner, resulting in decreased half-life and increased dose requirements several weeks after initiating or adjusting dosing. As a result, CBZ is prone to interactions with other drugs metabolized by the CYP450 enzyme system (77–79). Common drug interactions between CBZ and drugs commonly prescribed in the newborn include phenytoin (variable effect, phenytoin serum concentrations may increase, decrease, or remain unchanged, or CBZ concentrations may decrease) and phenobarbital (decreased CBZ serum concentrations) (6,14,77). As CBZ is approximately 75% bound to albumin (and CBZ-10,11-epoxide is approximately 50% albumin bound), there is potential for drug interactions that involve binding (14,38,78). Valproate will increase the unbound fraction of CBZ-10,11-epoxide, possibly resulting in increased neurotoxicity; however, for many patients, this interaction may not be clinically significant. Concomitant therapy with LEV may potentiate adverse central nervous system (CNS) effects of CBZ (79).

Carbamazepine has been used for controlling neonatal seizures as primary or second- or third-line therapy after phenobarbital and phenytoin (67–69). Loading doses of 10 mg per kg via nasogastric tube followed by maintenance doses of 7 to 23 mg per kg daily in two to three divided doses have been reported to be safe and effective in neonates, including preterm infants (gestational age <30 weeks, weight <1,000 g). Apparent adequate absorption of CBZ occurs even in the smallest, critically ill neonates, as therapeutic CBZ serum concentrations were achieved in these studies. Further investigation is needed to determine the safety and efficacy of CBZ in neonates, as this agent offers another therapeutic option for management of neonatal seizures. CBZ requires serum concentration monitoring for optimal therapeutic benefit in view of interpatient variability in pharmacokinetics and narrow therapeutic range (80,81).

OXCARBAZEPINE

Oxcarbazepine (Trileptal) is the 10-ketocogener of CBZ and requires hepatic metabolism to 10-monohydroxycarbazepine, which is primarily responsible for its pharmacologic effects (82–84). Monohydroxy-CBZ is eliminated 96% by the kidneys. There is a lower potential for drug interactions due to reduced plasma protein binding and less potent induction of hepatic enzymes (83).

Oxcarbazepine was approved for use in the United States in 2000, but this agent has been used in Europe for several years (82,85). A recent review of European practice reveals OXC initial monotherapy as a treatment of choice for complex partial seizures in children (64). Indications for treatment of partial seizures as monotherapy in children aged 4 years or older through adulthood or as add-on therapy in partial seizures with or without secondary generalization for children 2 years of age through adulthood with partial seizures (85). Dose forms are an oral suspension, Trileptal, 300 mg per 5 mL (of OXC), and 150-mg, 300-mg, and 600-mg tablets. The oral tablets and suspension are interchangeable on a milligram-to-milligram equivalent basis. This is an important consideration when converting from one dosage form to another as a child matures and the tablet form may be preferred.

Oxcarbazepine has been referred to as a "cleaner" version of CBZ due to lack of autoinduction and less fewer CNS and hematologic adverse effects (82). However, there is an increased potential for hyponatremia with OXC compared with CBZ. This may be significant, as a serum sodium of less than 125 mEq per L has been reported in 2.5% of patients receiving OXC. Skin rashes and serious dermatologic manifestations such as Steven–Johnson syndrome and toxic necrolysis have developed during therapy with OXC (84). Cross reactivity with CBZ is possible; therefore, switching between these agents requires close monitoring in the event of a potential adverse reaction (74). As an inducer of hepatic microsomal enzymes, OXC is prone to drug interactions, although to a lesser extent than CBZ. OXC may inhibit hepatic metabolism of phenytoin and phenobarbital resulting potentially supratherapeutic concentrations of these agents. When adding or removing OXC from a patient's drug regimen, close monitoring for potential drug–drug interactions is advised (6,14,15,38).

In a blinded, randomized, parallel-group study of infants and young children (1 month to <4 years of age, $n = 128$), with inadequately controlled partial seizures, OXC oral suspension was administered in low dose (10 mg per kg per d) or high dose (60 mg per kg per d) regimens as add-on therapy (86). Overall, high-dose OXC was significantly ($p < .05$) more effective than low dose in controlling partial seizures as measured by during continuous video-EEG monitoring. Adverse effects associated with OXC study treatment (>10% patients) were primarily mild somnolence and temperature elevation.

There are limited data on OXC in neonates, with the exception of reports of OXC PK-PD in newborns acquiring the drug transplacentally (87,88). Further investigation is needed to define the role and dosage of this agent in the management of seizures in the neonate and young infant.

VALPROIC ACID AND SODIUM VALPROATE

Valproic acid (2-propylvaleric dipropyl acetic acid), the free acid form of sodium valproate, has been approved for anticonvulsant use in the United States for over 30 years (89). This agent is available as oral and parenteral formulations. The active form in plasma is the valproate ion; therefore, all dose forms in this discussion will be referred to as VPA.

Dose forms are valproate sodium for intravenous injection, 100 mg (of VPA) per mL (Depacon), and valproate sodium oral solution (Depakene) 250 mg per 5 mL. Other formulations are VPA liquid-filled capsules (Depakene) 250 mg; divalproex sodium capsules containing coated particles to mix with food (Depakote Sprinkle) 125 mg VPA equivalent; enteric-coated delayed-release tablets (Depakote) containing 125-, 250-, and 500-mg VPA equivalent; and extended-release tablets (Depakote ER) containing 250- and 500-mg VPA equivalent. The rate of gastric absorption of VPA is dose-form dependent; overall bioavailability is 80% to 90%. Food slows down the rate but not the extent of absorption. Peak serum VPA concentrations are achieved approximately 2 hours after oral administration of syrup or uncoated tablets, 3 to 5 hours after single-dose administration of the enteric-coated divalproex sodium tablet, and 7 to 13 hours after multiple dosing. Parenteral valproate sodium is indicated for situations when therapeutic serum concentrations need to be achieved rapidly, such as in status epilepticus, neonatal seizures, or following surgery when the patient cannot be given oral medications.

Valproic acid is effective for many seizure types including myoclonic, tonic, atonic, absence, generalized tonic–clonic seizures, and partial-onset seizures (89,90). Many clinicians consider this agent to be the drug of choice for absence or atypical absence seizures. VPA has been used in the management of neonatal seizures, usually as a second- or third-line alternative after failure with phenobarbital and phenytoin (91–93). There is some evidence that VPA may be effective in the management of Lennox–Gastaut syndrome and infantile spasms (IS) (94–97). VPA therapy is a strategy for the management of IS resistant to treatment with adrenocorticotropic hormone (ACTH), vigabatrin (VGB), or prednisone (97).

The broad spectrum of anticonvulsant activity of VPA has not been fully elucidated. Mechanisms of action include (a) use-dependent blockade of voltage-sensitive sodium channels, resulting in neuronal membrane stabilization and inhibition of repetitive firing of neurons; (b) increased brain concentrations of GABA possibly secondary to increased synthesis via glutamic acid decarboxylase;

(c) increasing GABA concentrations by inhibition of GABA transporter GAT-1, therefore blocking conversion of GABA to succinic semialdehyde; and (d) increased membrane potassium conduction (89).

Valproic acid is highly plasma protein bound in a concentration-dependent manner, with the free fraction increasing with increasing serum concentration. Binding is reduced in renal or hepatic disease, in uremia, or in the presence of other highly plasma-protein-bound drugs.

Valproic acid undergoes hepatic biotransformation via glucuronidation, beta and omega oxidation, hydroxylation, ketone formation, and desaturation (90). Glucuronidation with urinary excretion of the β-glucuronidation is the most important pathway. There are two metabolites with anticonvulsant activity, 2-ene VPA and 4-ene VPA. Hepatotoxicity and embryotoxicity are most likely associated with the 4-ene VPA metabolite. This serious adverse effect of VPA is more frequent in children younger than 2 years and anticonvulsant polytherapy and received a black box warning in the United States. Side effects frequently encountered during VPA therapy include weight gain, nausea, easy bruising secondary to thrombocytopenia, and tremor. Weight gain secondary to VPA therapy may be a major concern among clinicians, parents, and patients. A recent retrospective review of 94 patients aged 2 to 20 years taking VPA suggests that children may be less likely to gain significant amounts of weight while taking this medication compared with adult patients (98). These results must be documented in larger, prospective trials. The longer-acting VPA preparations have been reported to be associated with less weight gain when administered once daily (99).

The metabolism of VPA is sensitive to enzyme induction and inhibits the metabolism of other drugs (6,14,15,38). Therefore, patients receiving phenobarbital, CBZ, or primidone may have increased VPA dose requirements (100). Doses of phenobarbital or primidone may need to be reduced by 20% to 40% when VPA is added to a regimen containing these agents. VPA also inhibits the metabolism of ethosuximide and lamotrigine. Phenytoin serum concentrations may be decreased by the addition of VPA, or free fractions of phenytoin may be increased by binding displacement as described previously. It is prudent to monitor serum concentrations of concomitantly administered anticonvulsants as well as clinical signs and symptoms of toxicity whenever VPA therapy is initiated or discontinued.

Clearance of VPA follows first-order kinetics with half-lives ranging from 5 to 20 hours in adults, and 9 hours in adults receiving multiple AEDs (90,100). Wide interpatient differences in clearance have been reported. Variables affecting VPA clearance include age, VPA serum concentration, length of treatment, dose, free fraction, and current enzyme-inducing AED polytherapy. Age has been reported to be one of the most important variables affecting intrapatient variability of VPA elimination, and polytherapy is the most important effect on interpatient variability (90,100). Premature newborns have the slowest clearance, but gestational age does not appear to influence clearance after 10 days of age. Neonates have half-lives of 15 to 65 hours for VPA. Clearance increases over the first months of life, with adult values achieved at around 14 years of age.

Initial oral doses of VPA are 20 to 30 mg per kg for premature infants, 40 mg per kg for term neonates younger than 10 days, and 50 mg per kg for infants older than 10 days. Initial doses in children are 10 to 20 mg per kg per day, but they may require 30 to 100 mg per kg per day to achieve adequate serum concentrations. For neonatal seizures, the oral dose is 20 mg per kg, followed by 10 mg per kg every 12 hours (92).

Therapeutic drug monitoring is of limited use for VPA therapy because of its wide therapeutic index, high intrapatient variability, poor correlation between clinical response and serum concentration, serum concentration-dependent binding, and short half-life. The clinical effect of VPA can lag behind its therapeutic concentration. In addition, there is a nonlinear relationship between dose and plasma concentration. Thus, free serum concentrations can increase without increase in total concentration. One needs to draw "trough" serum concentrations at set times during the dosing regimen for useful interpretation. However, serum monitoring of VPA concentrations can be valuable but has to be interpreted cautiously. Therapeutic range is 40 to 100 μg per mL. Toxicity usually occurs at serum concentrations more than 80 to 100 μg per mL, although some patients may tolerate VPA serum concentrations up to 150 μg per mL. Serum concentrations are frequently drawn prior to the morning dose (trough concentration). Because of diurnal variation in VPA serum concentration, sampling times relative to dose administration must be consistent when serum concentrations are compared (100).

ETHOSUXIMIDE

Ethosuximide (2-ethyl-2-methyl succinimide) is one of the drugs of choice for absence seizures (101,102). This agent is ineffective for partial seizures or tonic–clonic seizures. The mechanism of action is reduction of low-threshold T-type calcium currents, blocking synchronized firing of pacemaker neurons responsible for generating an absence seizure. Ethosuximide is administered in combination with phenobarbital or phenytoin for management of absence seizures in patients with tonic–clonic seizures to avoid exacerbation of generalized tonic–clonic seizures. Generalized tonic–clonic seizures were demonstrated to be rare in children with absence seizures receiving ethosuximide (103). This retrospective study (n = 238) reported that children receiving valproate and ethosuximide monotherapy had the same low risk of generalized tonic–clonic seizures. Prospective trials are necessary to further evaluate the role of ethosuximide in this seizure type.

The drug is available as 250-mg capsules (Zarontin) and 250 mg per 5 mL oral solution. The oral solution may contain sodium benzoate which displaces bilirubin and is a metabolite of benzyl alcohol; therefore, this product should be administered with cautious monitoring to neonates.

Ethosuximide is rapidly absorbed and not plasma protein bound (100). Metabolism is hepatic hydroxylation to inactive metabolites, with 10% to 20% of dose excreted unchanged in the urine. Clearance is increased in children, with half-lives of 30 hours compared with 40 to 60 hours in adults. Steady-state serum concentrations are not achieved for 7 to 10 days. VPA may inhibit the metabolism of ethosuximide, resulting in increased serum concentrations.

Initial pediatric ethosuximide dosing is 20 to 30 mg per kg per day. To improve tolerance and avoid gastrointestinal adverse effects of nausea, vomiting, and diarrhea, it is best to administer one-third of the total daily dose after evening meal for 5 days, then administer one-third after lunch for 5 days, then finally add the remaining one-third after breakfast (102).

The therapeutic range for ethosuximide is 40 to 100 μg per mL (100). Wide variability due to apparent nonlinearity in the relationship between dose per kilogram and respective plasma concentration makes pharmacokinetic adjustment of this agent difficult. Serum ethosuximide concentrations are useful in verification of therapeutic range during initiation of therapy, ruling out toxicity, noncompliance, or to identify high-dose requirements.

LAMOTRIGINE

Lamotrigine, 3,5-diamino-6-(2,3-dichlorapenyl)-1,2,4-triazine, was approved for use in the United States in 1994. This broad-spectrum AED is indicated as adjunctive therapy for management of partial seizures in adults, and as monotherapy in patients converting from VPA or a hepatic enzyme inducing AED (CBZ, phenytoin, phenobarbital, or primidone) (104,105). Lamotrigine is also effective as adjunctive therapy for generalized seizures in Lennox–Gastaut syndrome in adults and children (95,106).

Lamotrigine has become widely used in children for typical and atypical absence, atonic, myoclonic and tonic seizures, Rett syndrome, and IS (97,101,104). Advantages over CBZ and phenytoin include minimal cognitive side effects and improved behavior (104,105).

Lamotrigine (Lamictal) is available for oral administration as tablets in 25-, 100-, 150-, and 200-mg forms. Chewable/dispersible tablets are available in 2-, 5-, and 25-mg strengths. Dispersible tablets can be dissolved in a small amount of water or juice, by waiting 1 minute, swirling to disperse the drug, and immediately administering. Extemporaneous oral preparations of 1 mg per mL with short-term stability may be compounded from tablets (107). Clinicians are advised to consult with their institution's pharmacist.

The complete mechanism of action for lamotrigine has not been fully described. The inhibition of voltage- and use-dependent sodium channels in a manner similar to CBZ and phenytoin does not explain lamotrigine's efficacy in absence seizures or in other generalized seizures. Proposed mechanisms of action include modulation of excitatory amino acid neurotransmission and voltage-activated Ca^{2+} channels (104,106).

Lamotrigine is metabolized via glucuronidation to 2-*N*-glucuronide (104,108,109). Average lamotrigine half-life in adults was 24.1 to 35 hours in patients receiving lamotrigine monotherapy, and was decreased to 14 hours (6.4 to 32.2 hours) by concurrent treatment with enzyme-inducing AEDs. Increased clearance of lamotrigine in infants younger than 2 months has been reported by Mikati et al. (105). Age-related decreases in clearance occur during the first year of life (110). Children aged 5 to 11 years have significantly longer lamotrigine half-lives than younger children; however, concurrent therapy with enzyme induction agents decreases apparent clearance of lamotrigine at any age. Considerable intraindividual variation in lamotrigine half-life has been reported for all age groups (111).

Valproic acid may reduce clearance of lamotrigine by 40% to 60% via inhibition of glucuronidation (112). This is independent of the presence of enzyme-inducing agents. Concurrent therapy with VPA increases the risk for development of lamotrigine rash (105,110). Rash is the most severe adverse effect associated with lamotrigine therapy and more frequent in children compared with adults. Rash usually occurs within the first 8 weeks of therapy and may progress to life-threatening Steven–Johnson syndrome or toxic epidermal necrolysis. The rash is considered to be a generalized hypersensitivity reaction. The risk of rash may be minimized by slow dose titration during initiation of lamotrigine therapy. The estimated risk of developing a potentially life-threatening rash with lamotrigine is 1 in 1,000 for adults and from 1 in 100 to 1 in 200 for children (113). The risk of rash is described in a US boxed warning for the drug.

The dosage for lamotrigine depends on the patient's concomitant medications such as VPA and the enzyme inducing AEDs (phenytoin, phenobarbital, CBZ, or primidone) (112–114). Clinicians are advised to consult the current package labeling and literature for stepwise dosing guidelines when initiating lamotrigine therapy for their patients.

1. Patients older than 16 years receiving enzyme-inducing AEDs without VPA should receive 50 mg once daily for 2 weeks, increasing to 100 mg daily divided into two doses for 2 weeks, titrating by 100 mg daily every 1 to 2 weeks to an effective maintenance dose of 300 to 500 mg per day.
2. For patients taking VPA, the initial lamotrigine dose is 25 mg every other day for 2 weeks, then 25 mg daily for 2 weeks, then titrating upward by 25 to 50 mg daily every 1 to 2 weeks until effective response is achieved (usually 100 to 150 mg per day in two divided doses).
3. For children 2 to 12 years of age receiving enzyme-inducing AEDs without VPA, the regimen is 0.6 mg per kg per day in two divided doses, increasing by 1.2 mg per kg per day every 1 to 2 weeks to effective response, usually at 5 to 15 mg per kg per day. Younger children may require three daily doses due to increased apparent clearances.
4. For children 2 to 12 years of age receiving VPA, the regimen is 0.2 per mg per kg per day for 2 weeks, increasing to 0.5 mg per kg per day and 1 mg per kg per day at 2-week intervals (maximum recommended dose of 5 mg per kg per day). Because of tablet size, dose should be rounded down to the nearest whole tablet size.
5. Limited experience exists with lamotrigine dosing in the newborn; however, doses of 2 to 10 mg per kg per day have been used in infants ranging in age from 2 weeks to 1 year for the management of intractable partial seizures (IS and/or partial seizures) (96).

Serum lamotrigine concentrations are not routinely monitored due to the lack of reliable concentration response data. Reported serum concentrations associated with efficacy are 2 to 4 μg per mL and 1 to 5 μg per mL (115). Patients receiving lamotrigine should be instructed to inform all clinicians involved in their care when adding or stopping any medications as this agent participates in many drug interactions, especially with oral contraceptives (6,14,15). Lamotrigine may cause photosensitivity reactions; therefore, it is imperative that the prescriber and pharmacist instruct the patient in appropriate use of physical sunscreen protection methods and use of sunblock.

FELBAMATE

Felbamate, a derivative of the sedative meprobamate, was approved in the United States in 1993 for the management of partial seizures, with or without secondary generalization, in adults and in children with Lennox–Gastaut syndrome (116–119). This agent has demonstrated effectiveness in treatment of refractory IS (120). Felbamate is administered orally as Felbatol suspension 600 mg per 5 mL and tablets 400 and 600 mg. Tablets are scored for dosing flexibility.

Felbamate is not a first-line AED. Aplastic anemia and acute hepatic failure associated with felbamate therapy have limited its use to cases of severe seizures that are refractory to alternative AEDs (121–124). The risk of aplastic anemia associated with felbamate has been estimated by the manufacturer to be in the range of 1 patient in 2,000. Risk factors may be female gender, age older than 17 years, prior AED hypersensitivity, AED polytherapy, and prior immune disease or cytopenia.

Proposed mechanisms of action for felbamate are via *N*-methyl-D-aspartate receptor antagonism at glycine-binding sites, and possibly a direct effect on ion channels. The primary route of elimination is hepatic hydroxylation (<20%) via CYP3A4/2E1, 10% glucuronidation, and 25% hydrolysis, with approximately 50% eliminated unchanged in the urine. Metabolites do not appear to contribute to anticonvulsant effect, but a reactive metabolite, atropaldehyde, may be related to cytotoxicity (124).

Felbamate clearance is inversely correlated with age, and therefore children (half-life 16 hours) require higher doses per kilogram compared with adults (half-life 16 to 23 hours) (108).

As felbamate participates in some clinically important interactions with other AEDs, it is imperative to review all medications the patient may be taking prior to prescribing this agent (21–23). For example, felbamate increases serum concentrations of phenytoin in a dose-dependent manner, and therefore it is recommended that phenytoin dose be decreased by 20% to 30% when felbamate is added to the regimen. Felbamate clearance may also be induced by phenytoin. Felbamate may increase phenobarbital serum concentrations, and, conversely, phenobarbital may increase the clearance of felbamate (6,14). The effectiveness of oral contraceptives may be decreased via induction of metabolism by felbamate (38).

Dosage recommendations for felbamate in children 2 to 14 years of age are 15 mg per kg per day in three to four divided doses, increasing at weekly intervals to a maximum of 45 mg per kg per day in divided doses or 3,600 mg per day whichever is less (125). For children older than 14 years and adults, initial dose is 1.2 g daily in divided doses, increasing in 1.2 g daily increments at weekly intervals to a maximum daily dose of 3.6 g in three to four divided doses. Caution must be used when adding felbamate to regimens of enzyme-inducing AEDs, in which case doses of the other agents must be decreased by 20% to 30% to prevent related toxicities (108,126). There are limited data on the use of felbamate in children younger than 2 years. Serum felbamate monitoring has not been established for routine use (124). Dose is titrated to clinical efficacy; however, a therapeutic range of 30 to 100 μg per mL has been used (108). Monitoring for toxicities using complete blood cell count with differential and platelet count and hepatic function tests at baseline and at regular intervals during therapy and in the immediate period after discontinuation is recommended. Patients, their parents, and caregivers must receive instruction on self-monitoring for signs and symptoms of toxicities including rash, tendency to bruising, bleeding, sore throat, yellow tinged skin, gastrointestinal symptoms, unusual fatigue, loss of appetite, and dark urine. If these signs of possible felbamate toxicity are noticed, the patient should be instructed to contact their physician immediately.

TOPIRAMATE

Topiramate (TPM), 2,3:4,5-bis-*O*-(1-methylethylidene)-(beta)-D-fructopyranose sulfamate, was originally synthesized during an effort to develop a gluconeogenesis-blocking agent (2,3,5,21). This agent is approved for use as initial monotherapy for primary generalized tonic–clonic seizures or partial onset seizures in children 10 years of age or older through adulthood. TPM is used as adjunctive treatment of primary generalized tonic–clonic seizures or partial onset seizures in children 2 to 16 years of age and in adults (76,91,127). The drug is considered first-line therapy in myoclonic and generalized tonic–clonic seizures after VPA and first-line monotherapy in symptomatic generalized tonic–clonic seizures in healthy infants. Efficacy has been demonstrated in Lennox–Gastaut syndrome in combination with other AEDs in children and adults, as well as for IS (95,97,128,129). Formulations of TPM are Topamax Sprinkle capsules 15 and 25 mg, and tablets 25, 100, and 200 mg. Generic formulations have recently become available in the United States at a lower cost. An extemporaneous oral topiramate 6 mg per mL suspension may be prepared using 100 mg tablets (130).

TPM has several mechanisms of anticonvulsant activity: (a) blockade of neuronal membrane sodium channels, (b) enhancement of GABA inhibition via modulation of a nonbenzodiazepine-type receptor, (c) blockade of kainate-evoked currents at the glutamate receptor, and (d) selective inhibition of central carbonic anhydrase isozymes II and IV (131). This AED is also a weak carbonic anhydrase inhibitor.

Renal clearance is the primary route of elimination for TPM, with minimal hepatic oxidation via CYP3 A. In the absence of hepatic enzyme induction, 50% to 80% of a dose is excreted unchanged in the urine (131). Age significantly correlates with TPM clearance (132). Mean elimination half-life is 19 to 23 hours in adults and 15.4 hours in children, and TPM serum concentrations are usually 33% lower in children than in adults. In the presence of concomitant therapy with enzyme-inducing AEDs, TPM clearance is increased and the half-life is reduced to 12 to 15 hours in adults and 7.5 hours in children. There are limited data on the clearance of TPM in the newborn. Infants receiving

TPM therapy for management of refractory IS demonstrated slightly higher mean clearances than children and adolescents (12). When combined with phenytoin, CBZ, phenobarbital, and OXC, TPM serum concentrations are significantly lower compared with TPM monotherapy (12,14,15). VPA and lamotrigine have no significant effect on TPM metabolism. TPM may decrease the effectiveness of hormonal contraceptives, reducing serum concentrations of ethinyl estradiol by up to 50% (38). As with other AEDs, caution and a careful review of the patient's current medications is warranted when prescribing topiramate (or discontinuing this agent) from a therapeutic regimen.

Adverse effects associated with TPM are primarily CNS related and most frequently are somnolence, fatigue, and difficulty with concentration, word-finding disturbance, nervousness, headache, ataxia, and anorexia, with or without weight loss. Weight loss associated with a decrease in appetite may be a concern for young children undergoing rapid growth and development. In addition, language problems, speech disorders, and aggressive behavior have been reported. Somnolence and fatigue occur early in therapy and may affect up to 30% of patients receiving TPM, and occur more frequently early during therapy and at higher doses.

An increased incidence of nephrolithiasis, metabolic acidosis (133), and acute myopia associated with secondary angle-closure glaucoma has been reported in children and in adults receiving TPM (134). The ocular syndrome usually develops within 1 month of initiating TPM therapy with symptoms of a sudden decrease in visual acuity with or without eye pain. Risk factors associated with the development of metabolic acidosis and nephrolithiasis are concomitant use of another carbonic anhydrase inhibitor and cotreatment with the ketogenic diet. Maintenance of adequate fluid intake and acid–base monitoring are recommended for patients receiving TPM. Serum bicarbonate concentrations should be obtained at baseline prior to initiation of therapy and periodically throughout treatment to detect hyperchloremic metabolic acidosis prior to the development of clinical signs and symptoms of hyperventilation, arrhythmias, fatigue, altered consciousness.

Oligohydrosis and hyperthermia have been observed in patients, the majority of whom are children, receiving TPM therapy (133). Cases were associated with warm environments and/or vigorous activity. The mechanism for this adverse effect is unknown.

The use of TPM is limited primarily by CNS-related adverse effects. Therefore, the manufacturer recommends a slower initial dose titration schedule based on clinical experience demonstrating improved tolerability and reduced rate of discontinuation. Initial TPM dosage as add-on therapy for the management of partial seizures with or without secondary generalization, primary generalized tonic–clonic seizures, or seizures associated with Lennox–Gastaut syndrome in children aged 2 to 16 years is 5 to 9 mg per kg per day in two divided doses (initial dose should be 25 mg or less, using a range of 1 to 3 mg per kg per day) administered at night for 1 week. On the basis of clinical response and tolerability, dose is increased every 1 to 2 weeks by 1 to 3 mg per kg in two divided doses. Initial daily doses of 0.5 to 1 mg per kg may be followed by increases of 0.5 to 1 mg weekly or 1 to 3 mg every other week. Young children (<5 years of age) may require daily doses of 15 to 20 mg per kg, and infants may require up to 30 mg per kg per day divided into three daily doses. The usual adult (17 years of age and older) dose for TPM is 400 mg daily divided into two daily doses.

Therapeutic drug monitoring of TPM is not routinely performed secondary to lack of a clinically defined therapeutic range, wide interpatient variability in dose–serum concentration relationship, and overlap of serum concentrations related to toxicity and nonresponse.

GABAPENTIN

Gabapentin (GBP; Neurontin) is an amino acid analogue of GABA that was developed during a search for a spasmolytic (21,22,135,136). This agent was approved for use in the United States in 1994 (135). Indications include add-on management of partial seizures with or without secondary generalization in adults and children aged 12 years and older, and partial seizures in children 3 to 12 years of age (136). GBP is not effective for myoclonic or absence seizures. Dose forms of GBP (Neurontin) are capsules 100, 300, and 400 mg; solution 250 mg per 5 mL; and tablets 100, 300, 400, 600, and 800 mg. Generic formulations are available.

The exact mechanism of action for GBP is unknown. Contrary to its GABA-like structure, this agent is not a GABA mimetic. However, this AED modifies the synaptic or nonsynaptic release of GABA in the brain, as patients receiving GBP have been shown to increase concentrations of brain GABA (137). GBP may modulate neurotransmission through binding with the α_2-δ voltage-dependent calcium subunit (137). GBP decreases the glutamate release on reduced presynaptic entry on calcium via voltage-activated channels.

Gabapentin demonstrates dose-related, saturable, oral bioavailability, which is not significant with three-times-daily administration at usual doses. Doses more than 4,800 mg daily, four-times-daily dosing may increase bioavailability (138).

Gabapentin is not metabolized, so it does not induce hepatic metabolism and is primarily excreted unchanged by the kidneys, and therefore clearance correlates with creatinine clearance (2,3,135). The half-life in adults with normal renal function is 5 to 7 hours. Higher clearances are observed in children younger than 5 years, with variable clearances in infants. Infants younger than 1 year may require up to 30% higher daily doses of GBP than older children. Dosage adjustment is indicated for patients with renal insufficiency. GBP is water soluble, widely distributed, and binds minimally (<3%) to plasma protein.

Significant drug interactions do not occur with GBP (6,14,15,38). Aluminum hydroxide and magnesium hydroxide combination antacids may reduce the oral bioavailability of GBP by 20%, and therefore separating doses of GBP and antacid by more than 2 hours is recommended (14). The absence of effect on hepatic enzymes and protein binding enhance this agent's role as add-on therapy with other AEDs.

Overall, GBP is well tolerated, with the most frequent adverse effects consisting of somnolence, dizziness, ataxia, fatigue, tremor, and headache. In children 3 to 12 years of age, viral infection, fever, nausea, somnolence, and behavioral disturbances have been associated with GBP therapy (135). Behavioral disturbances may be dose related and an exacerbation of preexisting conditions (developmental delays, attention deficit hyperactivity disorder) (139).

The regimen of GBP as an add-on therapy for the treatment of partial seizures in adults and children older than 12 years is 900 to 1,800 mg daily, initiating with 300 mg three times daily. Some patients have tolerated daily GBP doses of 3,600 mg (140). The short half-life of GBP requires that doses must be administered three times daily, not exceeding 12 hours between doses. For children 3 to 4 years of age, 40 mg per kg daily administered in three divided doses is the usual recommendation, with therapy initiated at 10 to 15 mg per kg per day, increasing in weekly increments. Children 5 years of age and older usually require 25 to 35 mg per kg per day. Children 3 to 12 years of age have tolerated daily doses up to 50 mg per kg. There are no data on GBP dosing in premature infants. Dosage guidelines are established for adjustment of GBP dose in renal impairment (140).

Serum concentration monitoring is not routinely performed for GBP; however, the linear kinetics and apparent therapeutic effect of this agent reveal that the therapeutic range is 2 to 6 μg per mL. Currently, doses are adjusted on the basis of clinical response and adverse effects (135).

LEVETIRACETAM

Levetiracetam (LEV; Keppra), (S)-α-ethyl-2-oxo-1-pyrrolidine acetamide, was approved in 1999 as add-on therapy for the treatment of partial onset seizures in adult and adolescents (16 years of age and older) (2,8,21,141). Recently, LEV has been used as an alternative to phenobarbital in the management of neonatal seizures (27). The mechanism of action of LEV may be counteraction of kindling acquisition evoked by $GABA_A$-receptor antagonism (142,143). LEV binds to synaptic vesicle protein affecting neuronal GABA and glycine-gated currents, as well as voltage-dependent potassium currents (143).

Dosage forms of LEV are scored tablets (Keppra); 250, 500, 750, or 1,000 mg tablets; oral solution 100 mg per mL, or solution for intravenous infusion 100 mg per mL (144). The parenteral form must be diluted with 100 mL of an appropriate intravenous solution prior to injection and is for intravenous infusion only, not direct intravenous or intramuscular injection. Generic forms of the drug are available.

Oral absorption of LEV is rapid and complete. LEV undergoes minimal metabolism, with approximately 24% undergoing hydrolysis of the acetamide group to an inactive carboxylic acid metabolite, independent of CYP450 isozymes (143). The remainder of the dose is excreted unchanged in the urine. With only 10% plasma protein binding, and a low-affinity substrate for inhibitor of isozymes, significant drug interactions are rare (6,14,15,38). LEV may increase adverse effects of CBZ or topiramate requiring a dosage reduction in these drugs.

Levetiracetam has a linear pharmacokinetic profile. The apparent clearance of LEV correlates with glomerular filtration. The half-life of LEV in adults is 7 to 8 hours, compared with 6 hours in children. Children may require higher LEV doses on a milligram per kilogram per day basis compared with adults (143). Increased renal clearance for LEV in children compared with adults has been documented (145,146).

The dose of LEV for adolescents 16 years of age and older and adults as adjunct therapy for management of partial seizures is 500 mg twice daily, increasing by 1,000 mg daily at weekly intervals based on response, to a maximum of 3,000 mg daily (144). Data on LEV dosage for younger children and infants are limited (147,148). Daily doses of 20 and 60 mg per kg have been reported in children (143,144). Initial doses are 10 to 15 mg per kg per day in two divided doses, increasing by 10 to 20 mg per kg per day every 1 to 2 weeks to effective response, or a maximum dose of 60 mg per kg per day. A rapid titration schedule over a mean period of 10 days in a small number of patients ($n = 8$) has been used (149). Dosage must be adjusted in renal insufficiency (144).

Levetiracetam was administered in doses of 8 to 10 mg per day to children ($n = 200$), aged 0.3 to 19 years (median age 9 years), for the management of intractable epilepsy (147). A small ($n = 28$) retrospective study of children younger than 2 years (mean age 12.5 months, range 2 weeks to 22 months) showed that LEV was associated with seizure reduction in 54% of patients. Efficacy was highest in patients with generalized epilepsy compared with focal epilepsy. Overall adverse events were minimal (148).

Adverse effects with LEV therapy are dose related and include somnolence, fatigue, ataxia, headache, and behavioral changes (agitation, hostility, aggression, irritability). Behavioral effects including depression, emotional liability, nervousness, and agitation associated with LEV usually appear within the first 5 months of therapy and are usually not severe enough to require discontinuation of LEV (145). Suicidal ideation and attempted suicide is rare in children taking this agent. Overall, adverse effects associated with LEV have been mild to moderate, dose related, and occur within the first month of therapy. LEV may have fewer cognitive effects than other AEDs (146,150,151). As with other newer AEDs, the role of TDM of LEV therapy has not been established for LEV. A therapeutic range of 6 to 20 μg per mL has been suggested.

TIAGABINE

Tiagabine (TIG; Gabitril), a GABA reuptake inhibitor, was approved in 1997 for adjunctive treatment of partial seizures in adolescents and adults (152). Efficacy has been demonstrated in young children with refractory complex partial seizures, with poor response reported for myoclonic seizures and IS (153). There is insufficient evidence to recommend TIG as first-line therapy for partial seizures in pediatric patients.

Tiagabine preferentially inhibits GABA transporter isoform-1 (GAT-1) in neurons and glia, and increases extracellular GABA concentrations in the forebrain and hippocampus, thus prolonging inhibitory effects on receptors of postsynaptic cells (152). Dose forms of TIG are (Gabitril) 2-, 4-, 12-, and 16-mg tablets. Generic formulations are now available. Extemporaneously prepared oral solutions can be compounded for young children unable to swallow tablets (154).

Tiagabine is highly (96%) plasma protein bound and undergoes extensive metabolism via CYP3A4 isozymes, with less than 2% of a dose excreted unchanged in the urine. TIG does not appear to induce or inhibit hepatic microsomal enzymes; however, concomitant therapy with enzyme-inducing AEDs will decrease its elimination half-life from 7 to 9 hours to 4 to 7 hours (6). In children aged 3 to 10 years, TIG half-life is 3 hours with concomitant enzyme-inducing AED therapy (153). Dosage does not need to be adjusted in renal impairment; however, hepatic impairment requires lower doses administered at longer intervals as clearance of unbound drug may be decreased by as much as 60%.

Clinically important drug interactions with TIG increase dose requirements secondary to increased clearance with concomitant therapy with enzyme-inducing AEDs (6,14,15). Concomitant therapy with CBZ, phenytoin, primidone, and phenobarbital may increase TIG clearance by as much as 60%. TIG dose reductions may be necessary when the concomitant AED is discontinued or dose is decreased. Because macrolides are inhibitors of CYP3A4, concomitant therapy with erythromycin, troleandomycin, or clarithromycin may increase TIG plasma concentrations. There is potential for displacement from plasma proteins by TIG of other highly bound agents such as VPA, salicylates, and naproxen resulting in increased free TIG concentrations (14,15).

The adult regimen of TIG for adjunctive therapy in the management of partial seizures is 4 mg once daily for the first week, increased by 4 to 8 mg (administered as two to four daily doses) at weekly intervals to reach a daily dose of 32 to 56 mg (155). For adolescents 12 to 18 years of age, initial TIG dosing is 4 mg once daily for the first week of therapy, followed by 4 mg twice daily, increasing by 4 to 8 mg daily (in two to four divided doses) weekly, until a daily dose of 32 mg is reached if necessary. TIG dose needs to be reduced in hepatic insufficiency, but there are no data on specific recommendations. There are insufficient data for routine TDM with TIG.

Dose-related adverse effects of TIG are dizziness, difficulty with concentration, irritability, and paresthesia. Less common are ataxia and depression. Overall, TIG has been well tolerated in children.

VIGABATRIN

Vigabatrin (VGB; Sabril, Canada), a structural GABA analogue, has demonstrated efficacy in adults and children as adjunctive therapy for the management of refractory partial seizures, with or without generalization, and as monotherapy for the treatment of IS (97,156,157). VGB appears to be very effective in reducing seizures caused by tuberous sclerosis (158). This agent exacerbates typical absence and myoclonic seizures, and therefore should not be used for idiopathic generalized seizures. Experience with VGB in the treatment of Lennox–Gastaut syndrome is limited, particularly in cases with predominately myoclonic type seizures. VGB is administered as the racemic mixture, although only the S(+)-enantiomer is active. Dose formulations of VGB (Sabril) are 500-mg tablets and 500-mg powder sachets for dissolution in 10 mL of water, juice, milk, or infant formula.

Since 1989, VGB has been used in many countries, but approved for use in the United States only in 2009. Peripheral visual field defects may occur in up to one-third of patients receiving VGB (158). Since 1997 when visual field defects associated with VGB exposure were first published, observational studies have investigated the prevalence of this adverse effect (159–161). Guidelines for screening patients for the visual side effects of VIG have been published (161).

As with TIG, VGB exerts its anticonvulsive activity by decreasing the inactivation of GABA. VGB increases brain concentrations of GABA by acting as a surrogate substrate for GABA-transaminase (GABA-T) (162). This agent binds irreversibly to GABA-T, permanently inactivating the enzyme. Upon withdrawal of VGB, normal GABA-T activity may take several days to be restored. A ceiling effect has been demonstrated with VGB dosing beyond which there is no more therapeutic effect, only more adverse effects. This plateau for VGB may be related to a negative feedback inhibition of GABA synthesis, secondary to high GABA concentrations. Therefore, the pharmacodynamic effect does not correlate with the VGB half-life.

Vigabatrin is primarily eliminated via the kidneys, with up to 70% of the drug eliminated unchanged in the urine. Elimination half-life for adults is 5 to 7 hours, and oral absorption is rapid and complete, with minimal plasma protein binding. VGB does not appear to induce CYP450 enzymes, but concomitant therapy with enzyme-inducing agents decreases its elimination half-life (163). There have been no significant differences in pharmacokinetic parameters of the biologically active enantiomer between young children (5 months to 2 years) and older children (4 to 14 years), and therefore a weight-based dose adjustment is not recommended for these age ranges (164).

Drug interactions with VGB are an increase in the clearance of CBZ, phenytoin, phenobarbital, and primidone (6,163–165). When VGB is added to a regimen containing one of these agents, monitoring of patient response and serum concentrations of the other AED is recommended.

The initial adult daily dose of VGB is 1,000 mg divided in one to two doses, increasing by 250- to 500-mg increments weekly to total daily dose of 2,000 to 4,000 mg (165). Slow titration may improve tolerance of somnolence and mood effects.

Petroff and Rothman, using magnetic resonance spectroscopy, measured the increase in GABA associated with VGB in the human brain and cerebrospinal fluid (166). A plateau in GABA concentrations was achieved with a daily VGB dose of 3,000 mg. Therefore, on the basis of this dose–response curve, there is no need to increase VGB dose above 3,000 mg daily. Doses of up to 6,000 mg daily have been used; however, there are data that higher doses may be associated with more adverse effects without therapeutic benefit.

Considerable variation in response has been demonstrated with some patients between doses of 1 and 4 g. A ceiling effect and tachyphylaxis may also occur (167). Responses from placebo-controlled clinical trials of VGB 2 and 3 g daily as add-on therapy in adults with refractory partial seizures have demonstrated a 50% or greater reduction in frequency in seizures (168). VGB is not effective as monotherapy in adults.

The initial VGB dosing for children with refractory epilepsy is 40 mg per day administered in one or two doses, titrating, based on response, to 100 mg per kg per day. Efficacy in children has been similar to that observed in adults.

For infants with IS, initial dose of VGB is 50 to 100 mg per kg per day, administered in two divided doses, titrating up to 150 mg per kg per day. VGB doses of up to 400 mg per kg daily have been reported (169). Similar efficacy has been reported in studies comparing VGB and ACTH for IS. However, VGB is far better tolerated than ACTH.

Adverse effects of VGB are fatigue, somnolence, dizziness, blurred vision, nystagmus, ataxia, weight gain, abdominal pain, diarrhea, and depression. Infants and young children may also exhibit hypo- or hypertonia, hyperexcitability, and insomnia. Mania, depression, and psychosis have been associated with VGB therapy. Ophthalmic evaluation is recommended prior to the initiation of VGB in view of the risk of peripheral visual field deficit and irreversible vision loss (169,170).

Although a tentative target range of 6 to 278 μmol per L for VGB serum concentrations has been identified, a recent investigation was unable to demonstrate a significant difference in VGB serum concentrations among responders to therapy and nonresponders (7). Considering the unique mechanism of action of VGB, a correlation between serum concentration and clinical effect may not be possible. Therefore, TDM may be limited with several other newer AEDs, to excluding toxicity, malabsorption, or noncompliance in specific cases (7).

ZONISAMIDE

Zonisamide (ZNS; Zonegran), 1,2-benzisoxazole-3 methanesulfonamide, was approved for use in the United States in 2000 for adjunctive therapy in the management of partial seizures in adolescents 16 years of age and older (4,171). Presently, ZNS lacks an indication for general pediatric use in the United States, although the drug has been available in Japan and South Korea since 1989 as Excegran (172). Clinical experience and open-label trials suggest efficacy in children with partial and generalized onset epilepsies, IS, and West syndrome (171–175).

A sulfonamide derivative, ZNS is contraindicated in patients with sulfonamide hypersensitivity. Dosage forms are Zonegran capsules 100 mg (United States) and Excegran tablets 100 mg, 200 mg per g powder formulation (Japan).

The mechanism of action of ZNS is related to the blocking of sodium channel recovery and T-type calcium channel current and binding to GABA-receptor chloride channels. Inhibition of dopamine turnover and increased dopamine synthesis may also contribute to its anticonvulsant activity (176). ZNS, such as topiramate, is a weak inhibitor of carbonic anhydrase, an effect that may be responsible for the propensity of these agents to induce oligohidrosis (177–179).

Zonisamide is well absorbed after oral administration with 85% bioavailability and has been administered as a rectal suppository (179a). Approximately 40% to 60% is plasma protein bound. Similar to other sulfonamide derivatives, ZNS demonstrates saturable binding to erythrocytes, achieving concentrations two to eight times higher than in plasma.

Zonisamide undergoes hepatic acetylation to *N*-acetyl ZNS and reduction primarily via CYP3A4 to inactive 2-sulfamoylacetyl phenol and subsequent glucuronide formation. Approximately 15% of a dose is eliminated unchanged in the urine. Elimination half-life is 24 to 60 hours. The clearance of ZNS is linear and then follows first-order kinetics in children with daily doses of more than 10 mg per kg. A meta-analysis from Japan has suggested increased clearance in children compared with adults (177).

Zonisamide does not appear to inhibit P450 isoenzymes and has no significant effect on steady-state serum concentrations of phenytoin, VPA, phenobarbital, or CBZ. However, ZNS inhibits metabolism of CBZ to 10,11-epoxide. The metabolism of ZNS is subject to induction by other AEDs (6,14,15,38). Plasma concentrations of ZNS may be decreased by phenytoin, phenobarbital, and CBZ, possibly increasing ZNS dose requirements. Caution must be used when adding or removing ZNS to or from a patient's therapeutic regimen.

Serum concentration monitoring of ZNS is not routinely performed in the United States, but there are some data to suggest that its efficacy is associated with serum concentrations of 10 to 40 μg per mL (179). Adverse CNS effects are more frequent with serum concentrations greater than 30 μg per mL.

Initial ZNS dose for adults and adolescents older than 16 years as adjunctive therapy for partial seizures is 100 mg daily, increasing after 2 weeks to 200 mg daily for 2 weeks (180). ZNS may be administered as a single daily dose secondary to a long half-life. Dose may be further increased to 300 and 400 mg daily at 2-week intervals, allowing serum concentrations to reach steady state at each dose level. Because of long half-life (63 hours), steady state may not be achieved for 2 to 3 weeks. Increasing the ZNS dose at 3-week intervals may allow for improved tolerance of drug-related drowsiness, headache, or mental slowing. Usual adult dose range is 100 to 600 mg daily, with increased incidence of adverse effects at doses above 300 mg daily.

Zonisamide dosing for infants and children is 1 to 2 mg per kg per day administered in two to three divided doses, increasing on the basis of response and tolerance of adverse effects by increments of 1 to 2 mg per kg per day every 2 weeks to a maximum of 12 mg per kg per day (179). Effective dose ranges have been reported to be 2 to 12 mg per kg per day. Low-dose ZNS monotherapy (3 to 5 mg per kg per day) was reported to be effective and well tolerated in infants with IS (181). Dosage reduction is indicated in renal and hepatic disease (180). ZNS should not be used in patients with creatinine clearances less than 50 mL per minute.

Adverse effects associated with ZNS include fatigue, somnolence, dizziness, ataxia, headache, nystagmus, paresthesia, confusion, difficulty concentrating, impaired memory, mental slowing, loss of spontaneity, agitation, irritability, depression, anorexia, diarrhea, abdominal pain, anorexia, and rash (177–181). The true incidence of adverse effects related to ZNS monotherapy is difficult to ascertain because ZNS is frequently administered with other AEDs. Mania in children and psychosis in adults have been associated with ZNS.

Oligohydrosis and hyperthermia, similar to effects seen with topiramate, have been reported in children receiving

ZNS therapy (178,179). Cases of ZNS-associated oligohydrosis and/or fever, the majority in children, have been reported in the United States (178). Parents and caregivers must be instructed to maintain adequate hydration and avoid overheated conditions for children receiving ZNS, particularly in hot climates or during warm weather. However, in comparison with other newer AEDs, ZNS appears to be well tolerated. Clinical trials comparing ZNS to other AEDs in children and infants are needed.

LACOSAMIDE

Lacosamide (Vimpat) is a new compound with analgesic and anticonvulsant activity approved in the United States during late 2008 as add-on treatment for partial seizures in adults (182). The approval was based on three randomized controlled trials as add-on therapy compared with placebo in management of partial onset seizures (5,8,183–185). This agent is used off label for the management of refractory seizures for children. Data from lacosamide use in infants and children are accumulating; however, controlled clinical trials are needed.

The mechanism of action is a unique interaction with slow sodium channel inactivation without affecting fast inactivation (186). In contrast to AEDs, such as phenytoin and lamotrigine that block sodium channels when activated, lacosamide facilitates slow inactivation of sodium channels in terms of kinetics and voltage dependency (186). The effect may be selective for those neurons participating in seizure activity. Repeatedly depolarized neurons have persistent sodium activity which promotes neuronal excitation.

Drug interactions to date include agents prolonging the PR interval such as calcium channel blockers and β-blockers (183–186). Despite metabolism via microsomal CYP2C19, no drug–drug interactions with microsomal inducers, such as CBZ or inhibitors, or substrates, such as omeprazole, have been reported to date (5,8,186). Head to head trials are necessary to advantages of lacosamide over other new AEDs. No clear advantage of lacosamide over LEV has been observed to date. Side effects include dizziness, headache, double vision, ataxia, multi-organ hypersensitivity reaction, PR interval prolongation, and heart block. Euphoria associated with lacosamide administration giving a Schedule V Controlled substance status in the United States initial adult doses are 50 mg oral/intravenous twice daily with a maximum of 200 mg per day (186). Lacosamide is available in oral and parenteral dosage forms. Secondary to the high oral bioavailability, there is no advantage to using the intravenous lacosamide in patients with intact oral routes (187).

PREGABALIN

Pregabalin (Lyrica) was the first AED with controlled substance status in the United States secondary to the side effect of euphoria and somnolence (188). This AED was approved by the FDA for adjunctive therapy in adults with refractory partial onset seizures (188,189). Pregabalin is similar to gabapentin in that it is a structural, not a functional, analogue of the neurotransmitter GABA (189). Pregabalin is a specific ligand that potently binds to the α_2-δ type 1 and 2 subunits, a protein associated with voltage-gated calcium channels in the CNS. This agent is hydrophilic but readily crosses the blood–brain barrier decreasing depolarization-induced calcium influx in nerve terminals. The reduction in the inward calcium currents reduces the release of glutamate, noradrenaline, and substance P in the brain. Pregabalin, although structurally related to GABA, does not effect GABA uptake or degradation and is not active at GABA-A and GABA-B receptor sites (189).

Pregabalin is available as 25, 50, 75, 100, 200, and 300 mg capsules. Elimination follows linear pharmacokinetics. Absorption from the gut is rapid with approximately 90% bioavailability and peak plasma concentration is achieved in 1 hour (188). Half-life ranges from 5.8 to 6.3 hours. Pregabalin undergoes minimal metabolism (<2%) and is not protein bound. Like gabapentin, approximately 98% of pregabalin is eliminated unchanged through renal excretion. Pregabalin does not induce or inhibit enzyme activity.

Pregabalin is similar to gabapentin or LEV in that it is currently being evaluated as an add-on therapy in patients with partial-onset seizures (188,190). Dosing guidelines for pediatric patients have not been established. Adult anticonvulsant pregabalin doses are 150 to 600 mg per day administered in two divided doses (188,189). A small (n = 19) open-label study of the drug in children aged 4 to 15 years with resistant seizures used 150 to 300 mg per day with good results and minimal adverse effects (190). Common adverse effects were somnolence and weight gain as well as a worsening of myoclonic seizures.

Pregabalin and AED combinations are generally well tolerated, and may be used concomitantly with VPA, lamotrigine, phenytoin, and CBZ without concern for drug–drug interactions (191). Therapeutic ranges for pregabalin of 2.8 to 8.2 μg per mL have been established, yet secondary to variability in correlation of response for a wide range of patients, serum concentrations are not routinely monitored (7,192). This agent may be more expensive per dose than older AEDs; however, cost and inconvenience of laboratory monitoring for TDM and toxicity with the older agents must be considered.

RUFINAMIDE

Rufinamide (Banzel), a triazole derivative (1-[2,6-difluorobenzyl]-1 H-1,2,3-triazole-4-carboxamide), received FDA approval in 2008 for the adjunctive treatment of seizures associated with Lennox–Gastaut syndrome in patients 4 years of age and older (193). Approval was based on the results of a single, multicenter, double-blind study of 138 male and females with refractory seizures between the ages of 4 and 30 years, which compared rufinamide with placebo (194). The patients in the study had 90 or more seizures per months while receiving three AEDs. Severity of seizures decreased in 53.4% of patients.

As rufinamide is currently approved for children who are 4 years of age and older, there is a paucity of information for pediatric dosing (195). Doses used for children have been 10 mg per kg per day with a maximum dose of 45 mg per kg per day (195). The oral adult dose is 400 to 800 mg per day to a daily maximum dose of 3,200 mg.

Rufinamide exhibits its anticonvulsant effects through limiting neuronal sodium-dependent action potential firing. The drug may prolong the recovery phase of the inactivated neuronal sodium channel and exert a membrane stabilizing effect (196,197). Rufinamide is well absorbed, greater than 85%, and in the lower dosage range is better absorbed in the fed state. Rufinamide is not a CYP450 substrate but is extensively metabolized by the liver through hydrolysis by carboxylesterases to carboxylic acid derivative (pharmacologically inactive) which is then excreted in the urine. Impaired renal function does not affect rufinamide pharmacokinetics (197,198). Steady-state serum concentrations are achieved in 2 days with repeated dosing which is consistent with the elimination half-life of 6 to 10 hours (198). Plasma protein binding of rufinamide is not extensive with the apparent volume of distribution and apparent oral clearance relating to body surface area. Population modeling shows a positive correlation between a reduction in seizure frequency and steady-state plasma rufinamide concentrations using data from placebo-controlled trials. In the absence of interacting concomitant medication, population pharmacokinetic modeling indicates the oral clearance of rufinamide may be higher in children than in adults, although the potential differences between children and adult rufinamide pharmacokinetics have not been explored in formal clinical trials (198).

In humans, rufinamide may have some enzyme-inducing potential. This AED appears to be a mild CYP3A4 inducer. Population pharmacokinetic modeling suggests that rufinamide does not alter the oral clearance of topiramate or VPA, but may slightly increase the oral clearance of CBZ and lamotrigine and slightly decrease the clearance of phenobarbital and phenytoin (the predicted changes were <20%) (198). With the exception of phenytoin in which a dosage reduction may be required if given concomitantly with rufinamide, it is unlikely necessary to make similar changes in the dosages of the other AEDs described above. Lamotrigine, topiramate, or benzodiazepines do not affect the pharmacokinetics of rufinamide based on population-based pharmacokinetic modeling. However, VPA may increase plasma rufinamide concentrations. Plasma concentrations of rufinamide may be increased by as much as 70% (14,15,195). Conversely, concomitant use of CBZ, VGB, phenytoin, phenobarbital, and primidone was associated with a −13.7% to −46.3% range decrease in plasma rufinamide concentrations. The minimum of 13.7% decrease was seen in female children comedicated with VGB, and the maximum of 46.3% decrease was seen in female adults who were concomitantly taking phenytoin, phenobarbital, or primidone (198).

In a 2009 study aimed to explore the effectiveness and tolerability of rufinamide in a study population consisting of 45 children and 15 adults (age range 1 to 50 years), the highest response rate was observed in patients with Lennox–Gastaut syndrome (54.8%) while the lowest was observed in patients with partial epilepsy (23.5%). Rufinamide was well tolerated in patients, with most frequently occurring adverse events being fatigue (18.3%), vomiting (13.3%), and loss of appetite (10.0%) (195). The risk of adverse effects is concentration related (198), possibly suggesting a future role for TDM.

Overall, rufinamide provides an additional AED option for add-on therapy in refractory conditions. To date, this agent appears to be well tolerated, easily titrated, and has manageable drug–drug interactions.

POTENTIAL ANTIEPILEPTIC DRUGS IN CLINICAL DEVELOPMENT

Current AED regimens provide adequate seizure control in fewer than 50% of patients (3). Research continues in an effort to develop more effective, less toxic AEDs (5). Agents under development include retigabine, safinamide, talampanel, valrocemide, remacemide, and losigamone. As AED development continues, it is imperative to conduct appropriately designed controlled trials in infants and children. The effect of AEDs on behavior and cognitive development must be considered as outcomes in appropriately designed clinical trials for infants and children. Age and developmentally specific pharmacodynamic, pharmacokinetic, and safety data will optimize management of AED therapy in this vulnerable population.

REFERENCES

1. Cockerell OC, Johnson AL, Sander JW, et al. Remission of epilepsy: results from the national general practice study of epilepsy. *Lancet* 1995;346:140–144.
2. Verdu P. New drugs for pediatric epilepsy. *Acta Neurol Scand Suppl* 2005;181:17–20.
3. Bialer M. New antiepileptic drugs that are second generation to existing antiepileptic drugs. *Expert Opin Investig Drugs* 2006;15(6): 637–647.
4. Holland KD. Efficacy, pharmacology, and adverse effects of antiepileptic drugs. *Neurol Clin* 2001;19(2):313–345.
5. Luszczki JJ. Third-generation antiepileptic drugs: mechanisms of action, pharmacokinetics and interactions. *Pharmacol Rep* 2009;61(2):197–216.
6. Perucca E. Clinically relevant drug interactions with antiepileptic drugs. *Br J Clin Pharmacol* 2006;61(3):246–255.
7. Johannessen SI, Tomson T. Pharmacokinetic variability of newer antiepileptic drugs: when is monitoring needed? *Clin Pharmacokinet* 2006;45(11):1061–1075.
8. Hwang H, Kim KJ. New antiepileptic drugs for pediatric epilepsy. *Brain Dev* 2008;30(9):549–555.
9. Bartelink IH, Rademaker CM, Schobben AF, et al. Guidelines on paediatric dosing on the basis of developmental physiology and pharmacokinetic considerations. *Clin Pharmacokinet* 2006;45(11): 1077–1097.
10. Kearns GL, Abel-Rahman SM, Alander SW, et al. Developmental pharmacology-drug disposition, action, and therapy in infants and children. *N Engl J Med* 2003:349(12):1157–1167.
11. Anderson GD. Children versus adults: pharmacokinetic and adverse-effect differences. *Epilepsia* 2002;43(Suppl 3):S53–S59.
12. May TW, Rambeck B, Jurgens U. Serum concentrations of topiramate in patients with epilepsy: influence of dose, age, and comedication. *Ther Drug Monit* 2002;24:366–374.
13. Dodson WE. Pharmacokinetic principles of antiepileptic therapy in children. In: Pellock JM, Dodson WE, Branter-Inthaler S, eds. *Pediatric epilepsy: diagnosis and therapy.* New York: Demos Medical Publishing, 2001:317–327.
14. Riva R, Albani F, Contin M, et al. Pharmacokinetic interactions between antiepileptic drugs: clinical considerations. *Clin Pharmacokinet* 1996;31(6):470–493.
15. Patsalos PN, Perucca E. Clinically important drug interactions in epilepsy: general features and interactions between antiepileptic drugs. *Lancet Neurol* 2003;2(6):347–356.
16. Bell GS, Mula M, Sander JW. Suicidality in people taking antiepileptic drugs: what is the risk? *CNS Drugs* 2009;23(4):281–292.
17. Dr. Katz memo and briefing document to PCNS and PD Advisory Committees (2008) Briefing document for the July 10,

2008 Advisory Committees to discuss antiepileptic drugs (AEDs) and suicidality. http://www.fda.gov/ohrms/dockets/ac/08/briefing/2008–4372b1–01-FDA-Katz.pdf.

18. US Department of Health and Human Services, Food and Drug Administration, Center for Drug Evaluation and Research, Office of Translational Sciences, Office of Biostatistics. Statistical review and evaluation: antiepileptic drugs and suicidality. May 21, 2008.
19. Hesfdorffer DC, Kanner AM. FDA alert on suicide: fire or false alarm? *Epilepsia* 2009;50(5):978–986.
20. Azar NJ, Aboul-Khali NW. Considerations in choice of antiepileptic for treatment of epilepsy. *Semin Neurol* 2008;28(3):305–316.
21. Perucca E. Current trends in antiepileptic drug therapy. *Epilepsia* 2003;44(Suppl 4):S41–S47.
22. Sicca F, Contaldo A, Rey E, et al. Phenytoin administration in the newborn and infant. *Brain Dev* 2000;22(1):35–40.
23. Kalviainen R, Eriksson K, Parviainen I. Refractory generalized convulsive status epilepticus: a guide to treatment. *CNS Drugs* 2005;19(90):759–768.
24. Evans D, Levene M. Neonatal seizures. *Arch Dis Child Fetal Neonatal Ed* 1998;78(1):F70–F75.
25. Painter MJ, Scher MS, Stein AD, et al. Phenobarbital compared with phenytoin for the treatment of neonatal seizures. *N Engl J Med* 1999;341(7):485–489.
26. Levene M. The clinical conundrum of neonatal seizures. *Arch Dis Child Fetal Neonatal Ed* 2002;86(2):F75–F77.
27. Blume HK, Garrison MM, Christakis DA. Neonatal seizures: treatment and treatment in 31 United States pediatric hospitals. *J Child Neurol* 2009;24(2):148–154.
28. Levy RH. Cytochrome P450 isozymes and antiepileptic drug interactions. *Epilepsia* 1995;36(Suppl 5):S8–S13.
29. Dodson WE. The nonlinear kinetics of phenytoin in children. *Neurology* 1982;32:42–48.
30. Biglin K, Holzhauzen K, Szof C, Lulic-Botica M. Drug Formulary for the Newborn. Neonatal Intensive Care Units and Department of Pharmacy, 2003, Children's Hospital of Michigan.
31. Ahn JE, Cloyd JC, Brundage RC, et al. Phenytoin half-life and clearance during maintenance therapy in adults and elderly patients with epilepsy. *Neurology* 2008;71(1):38–43.
32. Lougham PM, Greenwald A, Purton WW, et al. Pharmacokinetic observations of phenytoin disposition in the newborn and young infant. *Arch Dis Child* 1977;52:302–309.
33. Rane A. Urinary excretion of diphenylhydantoin metabolites in newborn infants. *J Pediatr* 1974;85:534–535.
34. Rane CT, Gogtay NJ, Kadam VS, et al. Subtherapeutic levels of phenytoin with standard doses in infants: need to review dosage schedule. *Br J Clin Pharmacol* 1999;48(3):465–466.
35. Painter MJ, Pippenger MB, MacDonald H, et al. Phenobarbital and diphenylhydantoin levels in neonates with seizures. *J Pediatr* 1978;92:315–319.
36. Diaz RA, Sandro J, Serratosa J. Clinically significant interactions with phenytoin. *Neurologist* 2008;14(6, Suppl 1):S55–S65.
37. Williams NT. Medication administration through enteral feeding tubes. *Am J Health Syst Pharm* 2008;65(24):2347–2357.
38. Sabers A. Pharmacokinetic interactions between contraceptives and antiepileptic drugs. *Seizure* 2008;17(2):141–144.
39. Browne TR, Kugler AR, Eldon MA. Pharmacology and pharmacokinetics of fosphenytoin. *Neurology* 1996;46(Suppl 1):S3–S7.
40. Aweeka FT, Gottwald MD, Maher RW. Pharmacokinetics of fosphenytoin in a patient with hepatic or renal disease. *Epilepsia* 1999; 40:777–782.
41. Touchette DR, Rhoney DR. Cost-minimization analysis of phenytoin and fosphenytoin in the emergency department. *Pharmacotherapy* 2000;20(8):908–916.
42. Johnson J, Wrenn K. Inappropriate fosphenytoin use in the ED. *Am J Emerg Med* 2001;19(4):293–294.
43. Kai E, Tapani K, Reetta K. Fosphenytoin. *Expert Opin Drug Metab Toxicol* 2009;5(6)695–701.
44. Kriel RL, Cifuentes RF. Fosphenytoin in infants of extremely low birth weight. *Pediatr Neurol* 2001;24:219–221.
45. Takeoka M, Krishnamoorthy S, Soman T, et al. Fosphenytoin in infants. *J Child Neurol* 1998;13:537–540.
46. Morton LD. Clinical experience with fosphenytoin in children. *J Child Neurol* 1998;13(Suppl 1):S19–S22.
47. Gilman TJ, Gal P, Duchowny MS, et al. Rapid sequential phenobarbital treatment of neonatal seizures. *Pediatrics* 1989;83: 674–678.
48. Guillet R, Kwon J. Seizure recurrence and developmental disabilities after neonatal seizures: outcomes are unrelated to use of phenobarbital prophylaxis. *J Child Neurol* 2007;22(4):389–339.
49. Silverstein FS, Ferriero DM. Off-label use of antiepileptic drugs for the treatment of neonatal seizures. *Pediatr Neurol* 2008;39(2): 77–79.
50. Shoemaker MT, Rotenberg JS. Levetiracetam for the treatment of neonatal seizures. *J Child Neurol* 2007;22(1):95–98.
51. Diaz J, Schain RJ, Bailey BG. Phenobarbital induced brain growth retardation in artificially reared rat pups. *Biol Neonate* 1977;32: 77–82.
52. Farwell JR, Lee YJ, Hintz DG. Phenobarbital for febrile seizures: effects on intelligence and seizure recurrence. *N Engl J Med* 1990; 322:364–369.
53. Gilman ME, Toback JW, Gal P, et al. Individualizing phenobarbital dosing in neonates. *Clin Pharmacol* 1983;2:258–262.
54. Fischer JH, Lockman LA, Zaske D, et al. Phenobarbital maintenance dose requirements in treating neonatal seizures. *Neurology* 1981;31:1042–1044.
55. Touw DJ, Graafland O, Cranendonk A, et al. Clinical pharmacokinetics of phenobarbital in neonates. *Eur J Pharm Sci* 2000; 12(2):111–116.
56. Elliot ES, Buck ML. Phenobarbital dosing and pharmacokinetics in a neonate receiving extracorporeal membrane oxygenation. *Ann Pharmacother* 1999;33(4):419–422.
57. Pitlick W, Painter M, Pippenger C. Phenobarbital pharmacokinetics in neonates. *Clin Pharmacol Ther* 1978;23:346–349.
58. Van Orman CB, Darwish HZ. Efficacy of phenobarbitone in neonatal seizures. *Can J Neurol Sci* 1985;12:95–99.
59. Painter MJ, Pippenger C, Wasterlain CG. Phenobarbital and phenytoin in neonatal seizures: metabolism and tissue distribution. *Neurology* 1981;31:1107–1112.
60. Dodson WE, Rust RS. Phenobarbital: absorption, distribution and excretion. In: Levy RH, Mattson RH, Meldrum BS, eds. *Antiepileptic drugs*, 4th ed. New York: Raven Press, 1995:293–304.
61. Painter MJ. Phenobarbital: clinical use. In: Levy RH, Mattson RH, Meldrum BS, eds. *Antiepileptic drugs*, 4th ed. New York: Raven Press, 1995:329–340.
62. Anderson DM. Phenobarbital. In: Murphy JE, ed. *Clinical pharmacokinetics*. Bethesda, MD: American Society of Hospital Pharmacists, 1993:2103–2104.
63. Livingston S, Villamatar C, Sakata Y, et al. Use of carbamazepine in epilepsy. *J Am Med Assoc* 1967;200:116–119.
64. Wheless JW, Clarke DF, Arzimanoglou, et al. Treatment of pediatric epilepsy: European expert opinion, 2007. *Epileptic Disord* 2007;9(4):353–412.
65. Mattson RH, Cramer JA, Collins JF. Comparison of carbamazepine, phenobarbital, phenytoin, primidone, in partial and secondarily generalized tonic clonic seizures. *N Engl J Med* 1985; 313:145–151.
66. Sachdeo RC, Chokroverty S. Enhancement of absences with carbamazepine. *Epilepsia* 1985;26:534.
67. Singh B, Singh P, al Hifizi I, et al. Treatment of neonatal seizures with carbamazepine. *J Child Neurol* 1996;11(5):378–382.
68. Hoppen T, Elger CE, Bartmann P. Carbamazepine in phenobarbital-non responders: experience with ten preterm infants. *Eur J Pediatr* 2001;160(7):444–447.
69. MacKintosh DA, Baird-Lampert J, Buchanan N. Is carbamazepine an alternative maintenance for neonatal seizures? *Dev Pharmacol Ther* 1987;10(2):100–106.
70. Herranz JL, Armijo JA, Arteaga R. Clinical side effects of phenobarbital, primidone, phenytoin, carbamazepine, and valproate during monotherapy in children. *Epilepsia* 1988;29:794–804.
71. Tohen M, Castillo J, Baldessarini RJ, et al. Blood dyscrasias with carbamazepine and valproate: a pharmacoepidemiological study of 2,228 patients at risk. *Am J Psychiatry* 1995;152:413–418.
72. Bowden CL. Introduction: the role of anticonvulsants as mood stabilizers. *J Clin Psychiatry* 2001;62(Suppl 14):3–4.
73. Silverstein FS, Boxer Johnston MV. Hematological monitoring during therapy with carbamazepine in children. *Ann Neurol* 1983; 13:685–686.
74. Troost RJ, Van Parys JA, Hooijkaas H, et al. Allergy to carbamazepine: parallel in vivo and in vitro detection. *Epilepsia* 2006; 37(11):1093–1099.
75. Ness-Abramof R, Apovian CM, Drug-induced weight gain. *Drugs Today* 2005;41(8):547–555.

76. Wheless JW, Venkataraman V. New formulations of drugs in epilepsy. *Expert Opin Pharmacother* 1999;1:49–60.
77. Morselli PL. Carbamazepine: absorption, distribution, and excretion. In: Levy RH, Mattson RH, Meldrum BS, eds. *Epileptic drugs*, 4th ed. New York: Raven Press, 1995:473–490.
78. Spina E, Pisani F, Perucca E. Clinically significant drug interactions with carbamazepine: an update. *Clin Pharmacokinet* 1996; 31(3):198–214.
79. Patsalos SN. The pharmacokinetic characteristics of levetiracetam. *Methods Find Exp Clin Pharmacol* 2003;25:123–129.
80. Garnett RH. Carbamazepine. In: Murphy JE, ed. *Clinical pharmacokinetics*. Bethesda, MD: American Society of Hospital Pharmacists, 1993:21–34.
81. Levy RH, Wilensky AJ, Anderson GD. Carbamazepine, valproic acid, phenobarbital, and ethosuximide. In: Evans WE, Schetag JJ, Jusko WJ, eds. *Applied pharmacokinetics: principles of therapeutic drug monitoring*. Vancouver, Canada: Applied Therapeutics, 1992: 26-1–26-9.
82. Glauser TA. Oxcarbazepine in the treatment of epilepsy. *Pharmacotherapy* 2001;21(8):904–919.
83. Dickinson RG, Hooper WD, Dunstan PR, et al. First dose and steady state pharmacokinetics of oxcarbazepine and its 10-hydroxymetabolite. *Eur J Clin Pharmacol* 1989;37:69–74.
84. Wellington K, Goa KL. Oxcarbazepine: an update of its efficacy in the management of epilepsy. *CNS Drugs* 2001;15(21):137–163.
85. Dam M, Ekberg R, Loyning Y. A double-blind study comparing oxcarbazepine and carbamazepine in patients with newly diagnosed previously untreated epilepsy. *Epilepsy Res* 1989;3:70–76.
86. Pina-Garza JE, Espinoza R, Nordli D, et al. Oxcarbazepine adjunctive therapy in infants and young children with partial seizures. *Neurology* 2005;65(9):1370–1375.
87. Bulau P, Paar WD, von Unruh GE. Pharmacokinetics of oxcarbazepine and 10-hydroxy carbazepine in a newborn child of an oxcarbazepine treated mother. *Eur J Clin Pharmacol* 1988;34(3): 311–313.
88. Cetinkaya M, Ozkan H, Koksal N. Unilateral radius aplasia due to lamotrigine and oxcarbazepine use in pregnancy. *J Matern Fetal Neonatal Med* 2009;21(12):927–930.
89. Loscher W. Basic pharmacology of valproate: a review after 35 years of clinical use for the treatment of epilepsy. *CNS Drugs* 2002;16:669–673.
90. Bourgeois BFD. Valproic acid: clinical use. In: Levy RH, Mattson RH, Meldrum BS, eds. *Antiepileptic drugs*, 4th ed. New York: Raven Press, 1995:633–639.
91. Glauser TA. Expanding first-line therapy options for children with partial seizures. *Neurology* 2000;55(Suppl 1):S30–S37.
92. Gal P, Oles KS, Gilman JT, et al. Valproic acid efficacy, toxicity, and pharmacokinetics in neonates with intractable seizures. *Neurology* 1988;38:467–471.
93. Alfonso I, Alvarez LA, Gilman J, et al. Intravenous valproate dosing in neonates. *J Child Neurol* 2000;15(12):827–829.
94. Ito M, Okuno T, Hattori H, et al. Vitamin B6 and valproic acid in treatment of infantile spasms. *Pediatr Neurol* 1991;7(2):91–96.
95. Wheless JW, Cornair J. Lennox–Gastaut syndrome. *Pediatr Neurol* 1997;17:203–211.
96. Prats JM, Garaizar C, Rua MJ. Infantile spasms treated with high doses of sodium valproate: initial response and follow-up. *Dev Med Child Neurol* 1991;33:617–625.
97. Tsao CY. Current trends in the treatment of infantile spasms. *Neuropsychiatr Dis Treat* 2009;5:289–299.
98. Sharpe C, Wolfson T, Trauner DA. Weight gain in children treated with valproate. *J Child Neurology* 2009;338:24:338–341.
99. Smith MC, Centrorino F, Welge JA, et al. Clinical comparison of extended-release divalproex versus delayed-release divalproex: pooled data analyses from nine trials. *Epilepsy Behav* 2004;5: 746–751.
100. Battino D, Estienne M, Avanzini G. Clinical pharmacokinetics of antiepileptic drugs in paediatric patients. Part I: Phenobarbital, primidone, valproic acid, ethosuximide, and mesuximide. *Clin Pharmacokinet* 1995;29(4):257–286.
101. Panayiotopoulos CP. Treatment of typical absence seizures and related epileptic syndromes. *Paediatr Drugs* 2001;3(5):379–403.
102. Schneider S. Clinical use of ethosuximide, methsuximide, and trimethadione. In: Pellock HM, Dodson WE, Bourgeois BFD, eds. *Pediatric epilepsy*, 2nd ed. New York: Demos Medical Publishing, 2001:447–452.
103. Schmitt B, Korvacevic-Preradovic T, Critelli H, et al. Is ethosuximide a risk factor for generalized tonic–clonic seizures in absence epilepsy? *Neuropediatrics* 2007;38(2):83–87.
104. Willmore LJ. Lamotrigine. *Expert Rev Neurother* 2001;1:33–39.
105. Mikati MA, Fayad M, Koleilat M, et al. Efficacy, tolerability, and kinetics of lamotrigine in infants. *J Pediatr* 2002;141(1):31–35.
106. Fitton A, Goa KL. Lamotrigine: an update of its pharmacology and therapeutic use in epilepsy. *Drugs* 1995;50:691–713.
107. Nahatta MC, Morosco RS, Hipple RT. Stability of lamotrigine in two extemporaneously prepared suspensions at 4 C and 25 C. *Am J Health Syst Pharm* 1999;56(93):240–242.
108. Battino D, Estienne M, Avanzini G. Clinical pharmacokinetics of antiepileptic drugs in paediatric patients. Part II: Phenytoin, carbamazepine, sulthiame, lamotrigine, vigabatrin, oxcarbazepine, and felbamate. *Clin Pharmacokinet* 1995;29(5):341–369.
109. Culy CR, Goa KL. Lamotrigine. A review of its use in childhood epilepsy. *Paediatr Drugs* 2000;2(4):299–330.
110. Meador KJ, Baker GA. Behavioral and cognitive effects of lamotrigine. *J Child Neurol* 1997;12(Suppl 1):S44–S47.
111. Messenheimer J. Efficacy and safety of lamotrigine in pediatric patients. *J Child Neurol* 2002;17:2S34–2S42.
112. Eriksson AS, Hoppu K, Nergardh A. Pharmacokinetic interactions between lamotrigine and other antiepileptic drugs in children with intractable epilepsy. *Epilepsia* 1996;37:769–773.
113. Guberman AH, Besag FM, Brodie MJ. Lamotrigine induced rash: risk/benefit considerations in adults and children. *Epilepsia* 1999;40:985–991.
114 Lamotrigine In*: Lexicomp's pediatric dosage handbook*. 15th ed. Hudson, OH: American Pharmacists Association, 2008:1011–1016.
115. Granett WR. Lamotrigine: pharmacokinetics. *J Child Neurol* 1997;12(Suppl 1):S10–S15.
116. Pellock JM. Felbamate. *Epilepsia* 1999;40(Suppl 5):S57–S62.
117. Pellock JM, Fraught E, Leppik IE, et al. Felbamate: concensus of current clinical experience. *Epilepsy Res* 2006;71:89–101.
118. Leppik IE, Dreifuss FE, Pledger GW, et al. Felbamate for partial seizures: a double-blind, placebo controlled study. *Neurology* 1991; 41:1785–1789.
119. Carmant L, Holmes GL, Sawyer S, et al. Efficacy of felbamate in therapy for partial epilepsy in children. *J Pediatr* 1994;125:481–486.
120. Hosain S, Nagarajan L, Carson D, et al. Felbamate for refractory infantile spasms. *J Child Neurol* 1997;12(7):466–468.
121. Cilio MR, Kartashov AI, Vigevano F. The long term use of felbamate in children with severe refractory epilepsy. *Epilepsy Res* 2001;47:1–7.
122. Zupanc ML, Werner R, Arentz L. Efficacy of felbamate in the treatment of medically refractory epilepsy in children. *Epilepsia* 2003;4:273.
123. Kaufman DW, Kelly JP, Anderson T, et al. Evaluation of cases of aplastic anemia among patients treated with felbamate. *Epilepsia* 1997;38:1265–1269.
124. Pellock JM. Felbamate in epilepsy therapy: evaluating the risks. *Drug Saf* 1999;21:225–239.
125. Felbamate. In: *Lexicomp's pediatric dosage handbook*, 15th ed. Hudson, OH: American Pharmacists Association, 2008:718–721.
126. Glue P, Banfield CR, Perhach JL, et al. Pharmacokinetic interactions with felbamate. *Clinical Pharmacokinetics* 1997;33:214–224.
127. Sachedo RC, Reife RA, Lim P, et al. Topiramate monotherapy for partial onset seizures. *Epilepsia* 1997;38:294–300.
128. Sachedo RC, Glauser TA, Ritter F, et al. A double-blind, randomized trial of topiramate in Lennox–Gastaut syndrome. Topiramte YL Study Group. *Neurology* 1999;52:1330–1337.
129. Glauser TA, Clark PO, Strawsburg R. A pilot study of topiramate in the treatment of infantile spasms. *Epilepsia* 1998;39:1324–1328.
130. Nahata MC. Topiramate. In: Nahata MC, Pai VB, Hipple TF, eds. *Pediatric Drug formulations*, 5th ed. Cincinnati, OH: Harvey Whitney Books, Co., 2004;1–7.
131. Shank RP, Gardocki JF, Streeter AJ. An overview of the pre-clinical aspects of topiramate: pharmacology, pharmacokinetics, and mechanism of action. *Epilepsia* 2000;41(Suppl 1):S3–S9.
132. Glauser TA, Miles MV, Tang P, et al. Topiramate pharmacokinetics in infants. *Epilepsia* 1999;40:788–791.
133. Philippi H, Boor R, Reitter B. Topiramate and metabolic acidosis in infants and toddlers. *Epilepsia* 2002;43(7):744–747.
134. Thambi L, Kapcala LP, Chambers W, et al. Topiramate-associated secondary angle-closure glaucoma: a case series. *Arch Ophthalmol* 2002;120(8):1108.

135. McLean MJ. Gabapentin. *Epilepsia* 1995;36(Suppl 2):S73–S86.
136. Anhut H, Ashman P, Feuerstein TJ, et al. Gabapentin as add-on therapy in patients with seizures: a double-blind, placebo-controlled study. *Epilepsia* 1994;35:795–801.
137. Maneuf YP, Gonzales MI, Sutton KS, et al. Cellular and molecular action of the putative GABA-mimetic, gabapentin. *Cell Mol Life Sci* 2003;60(4):742–750.
138. Gidal BE, DeCerce J, Brockbrader HN. Gabapentin bioavailability: effect of dose and frequency of administration in adult patients with epilepsy. *Epilepsy Res* 1998;31:91–99.
139. Lee DO, Steingard RJ, Cesena M. Behavioral side effects of gabapentin in children. *Epilepsia* 1996;37:501–502.
140. Gabapentin. In: *Lexicomp's pediatric dosage handbook*, 15th ed. Hudson, OH: American Pharmacists Association, 2008:808–811.
141. Gorji A, Hohling JM, Madeja M, et al. Effect of levetiracetam on epileptiform discharge in human neocortical slices. *Epilepsia* 2002;43(12):1480–1487.
142. Stratton SC, Large CH, Cox B, et al. Effects of lamotrigine and levetiracetam on seizure development in a rat amygdala kindling model. *Epilepsy Res* 2003;53(1–2):95–106.
143. Pellock JM, Glauser RA, Bebin EM, et al. Pharmacokinetic study of levetiracetam in children. *Epilepsia* 2001;42(12):1574–1579.
144. Levetiracetam. In: *Lexicomp's pediatric dosage handbook*, 15th ed. Hudson, OH: American Pharmacists Association, 2008:1028–1031.
145. Grosso S, Franzoni E, Coppola G, et al. Efficacy and safety of levetiracetam in children: with refractory epilepsy. *Seizure* 2005; 14(4);248–253.
146 Vigevano F. Levetiracetam in pediatrics. *J Child Neurol* 2005; 20(2):87–93.
147. Perry MS, Benatar M. Efficacy and tolerability of levetiracetam in children less than 4 years old: a retrospective review. *Epilepsia* 2007;48(6);1123–1127.
148. Krief P, Li Kan, Maytal J. Efficacy of levetiracetam in children with epilepsy younger than 2 years of age. *J Child Neurol* 2008; 23(5):582–584.
149. Vaisleib II, Neff RA. Rapid dosage titration of levetiracetam in children. *Pharmacotherapy* 2008;28(3):393–396.
150. Cramer JA, Arrigo C, Van Hammer G. Effect of levetiracetam on epilepsy-related quality of life. N132 Study Group. *Epilepsia* 2000; 42(7):868–874.
151. Lagae L, Buyse G, Deconink A, et al. Effect of levetiracetam in refractory childhood epilepsy syndromes. *Eur J Paediatr Neurol* 2003;7(3):123–128.
152. Sills GJ. Pre-clinical studies with the GABAergic compounds vigabatrin and tiagabine. *Epileptic Disord* 2003;5(1):51–56.
153. Pellock JM. Tiagabine (Gabitril) experience in children. *Epilepsia* 2001;42(Suppl 3):49–51.
154. Nahata MC, Morosco RS. Stability of tiagabine in two oral liquid vehicles. *Am J Health Syst Pharm* 2003;60(1):75–77.
155. Tiagabine. In: *Lexicomp's pediatric dosage handbook*, 15th ed. Hudson, OH: American Pharmacists Association, 2008:1696–1699.
156. Richens A. Pharmacology and clinical pharmacology of vigabatrin. *J Child Neurol* 1991;6(Suppl 2):S7–S10.
157. Elterman RD, Shields WD, Mansfield KA, et al. Infantile spasms vigabatrin study group. Randomized trial of vigabatrin in patients with infantile spasms. *Neurology* 2001;57(8):1416–1421.
158. Curatolo P, Verdecchia M, Bombardierie R. Vigabatrin for tuberous sclerosis complex. *Brain Dev* 2001;23:649–653.
159. Wild JM, Ahn HS, Baulac M, et al. Vigabatrin and epilepsy: lessons learned. *Epilepsia* 2007;48:1318–1327.
160. Nicholson A, Leach JP, Chadwick CW, et al. The legacy of vigabatrin in a regional epilepsy clinic. *J Neurol, Neurosurg Psychiatry* 2002;73:327–329.
161. Chacko KR, Ganesh A, Bulusu S, et al. Vigabatrin associated retinal dysfunction in children with epilepsy. *Arch Dis Child* 2001; 85(6):469–473.
162. Patsalos PN, Duncan JS. The pharmacology and pharmacokinetics of vigabatrin. *Rev Contemp Pharmacother* 1995;6:447–456.
163. Sanchez-Alcaraz A, Quintana MB, Lopez E, et al. Effect of vigabatrin on the pharmacokinetics of carbamazepine. *J Clin Pharmacol Ther* 2002;27(6):427–430.
164. Dalla Bernadina B, Fontana E, Vigevano F. Efficacy and tolerability of vigabatrin in children with refractory partial seizures: a single-blind dose-increasing study. *Epilepsia* 1995;36:687–691.
165. Hoechst Marion Roussel Ltd. Vigabatrin data sheet. In: *ABPI data sheet compendium*. London: Association of the British Pharmaceutical Industry, 1999.
166. Petroff OA, Rothman DL. Measuring human brain GABA *in vivo*: effects of GABA-transaminase inhibition with vigabatrin. *Mol Neurobiol* 1998;16(1):97–121.
167. Michelucci R, Veri L, Passarelli D. Long-term follow-up study of vigabatrin in the treatment of refractory epilepsy. *J Epilepsy* 1994; 7:88–93.
168. Beran RG, Berkovic SF, Buchanan N. A double-blind, placebo controlled crossover study of vigabatrin 2 g/day and 3 g/day in uncontrolled partial seizures. *Seizure* 1996;5:259–265.
169. Aicardi J, Mumford J, Dumas C, et al. Vigabatrin as initial therapy for infantile spasms: a European retrospective survey. Sabril IS Investigator and Peer Review Groups. *Epilepsia* 1996;37:638–642.
170. Revised guideline for prescribing vigabatrin in children. Vigabatrin Pediatric Advisory Group. *Br Med J* 2000;320(7246): 1404–1405.
171. Oommen KJ, Mathews S. Zonisamide: a new epileptic drug. *Clin Neuropharmacol* 1999;33(4):192–200.
172. Glauser TA, Pellock JM. Zonisamide in pediatric epilepsy: review of the Japanese experience. *J Child Neurol* 2002;17(2):87–96.
173. Yanai S, Hanai T, Narazaki O. Treatment of infantile spasms with zonisamide. *Brain Dev* 1999;21(3):157–161.
174. Suzuki Y. Zonisamide in West syndrome. *Brain Dev* 2001;23(7): 658–661.
175. Suzuki Y, Inmai K, Toribe Y, et al. Long-term response to zonisamide in patients with West syndrome. *Neurology* 2002;58(10): 1556–1559.
176. Okada M, Kaneko S, Hirano T, et al. Effects of zonisamide on dopaminergic system. *Epilepsy Res* 1995;22(3):193–205.
177. Chung AM, Ehand LS. Experience with zonisamide in children: results from a meta-analysis. *Paediatr Drugs* 2008;10(4):217–254.
178. Knudsen JF, Thambi LR, Kapcala LP, et al. Oligohydrosis and fever in pediatric patients treated with zonisamide. *Pediatr Neurol* 2003;28(3):184–189.
179. Low PA, Steven J, Peschel T, et al. Zonisamide and associated oligohidrosis and hyperthermia. *Epilepsy Res* 2004;(62):27–34.
179a. Mimaki T. Clinical pharmacology and therapeutic drug monitoring of zonisamide. *Ther Drug Monit* 1998;20:593–596.
180. Zonisamide. In: *Lexicomp's pediatric dosage handbook*, 15th ed. Hudson, OH: American Pharmacists Association, 2008: 1813–1816.
181. Suzuki Y, Nagai T, Ono J, et al. Zonisamide monotherapy in newly diagnosed infantile spasms. *Epilepsia* 1997;38(9):1035–1038.
182. Curia G, Biagini G, Perucca E, et al. Lacosamide: a new approach to target voltage-gated sodium currents in epileptic disorders. *CNS Drugs* 2009;23(7):555–568.
183. Ben-Machachem E, Biton V, Jatuzis D, et al. Efficacy and safety of lacosoamide as adjunctive therapy in adults with partial-onset seizures. *Epilepsia* 2007;48:1308–1317.
184. Halusz P, Kavisinen R, Mazurkiewicz-Beldzinska M et al. Adjunctive lacosamide for partial onset seizures: efficacy and safety results from a randomized controlled trial. *Epilepsia* 2009; 50(3):443–455.
185. Cross SA, Curran SA. Lacosamide: in partial-onset seizures. *Drugs* 2009;64(4):449–459.
186. Biagini G. Lacosamide pharmacology, mechanism of action and pooled efficacy and safety data in partial onset seizures. *Expert Rev Neurother* 2009;9(1):33–43.
187. Biton V, Rosenfeld WE, Whitesides J, et al. Intravenous lacosamide as a replacement for oral lacosamide in patients with partial-onset seizures. *Epilepsia* 2008;(49):418–424.
188. Hamandi K, Sander JW. Pregabalin: a new antiepileptic drug for refractory epilepsy. *Seizure* 2006;15(2):73–78.
189. Ben-Machachem E. Pregabalin pharmacology and its relevance to clinical practice. *Epilepsia* 2004;45(Suppl 6):S13–S18.
190. Jan MM, Zuberi SA, Alsaihati BA. Pregablin: preliminary experience in intractable childhood epilepsy. *Pediatric Neurology* 2009; 40(5):347–350.
191. Berry D, Milligan C. Analysis of pregabalin as therapeutic concentrations in human plasma/serum by reversed phase HPLC. *Ther Drug Monit* 2005;27:451–456.
192. Brodie MJ, Wilson EA, Wesche DI, et al. Pregabalin drug interaction studies: lack of effect on the pharmacokinetics of

carbamazepine, pheytoin, lamotrigine, and valproate in patients with partial epilepsy. *Epilepsia* 2005;46:1407–1413.

193. Saneto RP, Anderson GD. Onset of action and seizure control in Lennox–Gaustaut syndrome: focus on rufinamide. *Ther Clin Risk Manag* 2009;5(2):271–280.
194. Glauser T, Kluger G, Sachdeo R, et al. Rufinamide for generalized seizures associated with Lennox-Gastaut syndrome. *Neurology* 2008;70(21):1950–1958.
195. Kluger G, Kurlemann G, Haberlandt E, et al. Effectiveness and tolerability of rufinamide in children and adults with refractory epilepsy: first European experience. *Epilepsy Behav* 2009;14(3): 491–495.
196. Deeks ED, Scott LJ. Rufinamide. *CNS Drugs* 2006;20(9): 751–760.
197. Hakimian S, Cheng-Hakimian A, Anderson GD, et al. Rufinamide: a new anti-epileptic medication. *Expert Opin Pharmacother* 2007; 8(12):1931–1940.
198. Perucca E, Cloyd J, Critchley D, et al. Rufinamide: clinical pharmacokinetics and concentration-response relationships in patients with epilepsy. *Epilepsia* 2008;49(7):1123–1141.

CHAPTER

38

Adelaide Robb

Psychopharmacology in Children and Adolescents

Treatment of psychiatric disorders in children and adolescents must happen after several important events have occurred. The clinician must take an accurate history, family history, and cognitive and mental status examination. This chapter covers the common psychiatric disorders that begin early in childhood such as ADHD and autism, disorders that present in middle childhood such as anxiety and depression, and adult psychiatric disorders that have their onset in adolescence such as bipolar disorder and schizophrenia. It is important to interview the parent, child, and collateral sources including teachers and other caregivers when assessing for childhood psychiatric disorders.

One needs to have baseline levels of physical symptoms such as appetite, sleep, movement disorders (tics, dystonia, etc.), and somatic complaints prior to initiation of pharmacotherapy, so preexisting symptoms are not captured as treatment emergent adverse events. It is also important to have baseline laboratories, electrocardiogram, vital signs, and height and weight, as treatments may alter any or all of these parameters.

CLINICAL PHARMACOLOGY: GENERAL CONSIDERATIONS

Key aspects of clinical pharmacology will affect the overall outcome of psychotropic drug use in children and adolescents. These include absorption and bioavailability, distribution, metabolism, pharmacogenetics, drug interactions, and elimination. Dosing considerations are particularly important for children. Because clearance rates per kilogram of body weight in children can be faster for some, but not all, drugs, such as paroxetine (1), it is evident that optimal dosing in children cannot be achieved solely by reduction in adult dosage on the basis of weight. Renwick showed that clearance of drugs adjusted for body weight can be twice as high in children as in adults (2). This could be because in children, clearing organs, such as liver and kidney, represent a higher fraction of body weight (3). According to Edwards (3), the average drug concentration with chronic administration under steady-state conditions is given by the following equation:

$$C_{ss,av} = \frac{F \times \text{dose}}{\text{Cl} \times \Upsilon}$$

where Cl is clearance and Υ is the dosing interval. In the pediatric literature, there is, however, a paucity of information on the relationship between drug concentration and effect. When only bioavailability is taken into consideration, the following formula can contribute to guide dosing in children:

$$\text{dose}_{\text{child}} = \text{dose}_{\text{adult}} \times \frac{\text{Cl}_{\text{child}}}{\text{Cl}_{\text{adult}}}$$

These formulas, however, cannot be precise indicators of treatment, as clearance rates for specific drugs and dose/effect relationships in children are often not known. In view of the limitations of available data on polymorphic metabolism, drug interactions, clearance, and defined target plasma concentration, children treated with psychoactive medication should be closely monitored (3). With the advent of BPCA (Best Pharmaceuticals for Children Act), FDAMA (FDA Modernization Act), and the Pediatric Rule, more studies on medications including psychotropic medications have been performed in children and adolescents. One such study of the pharmacokinetics of aripiprazole shows that in this trial the pharmacokinetics were linear and close to that of adults (4).

ATTENTION-DEFICIT HYPERACTIVITY DISORDER

Attention-deficit hyperactivity disorder (ADHD) is a neurodevelopmental disorder characterized by impairments in attention and concentration with or without hyperactivity and impulsivity (5). Current diagnostic regimens require onset of symptoms before the age of 7 and impairment in two of three settings, home, school/work, and social (6).

The rates of ADHD vary across the life span with elementary school children ranging from 6% to 10%, adolescents

4% to 6%, and adults up to 4.4% (5,7). In childhood, ADHD seems to be more common in boys, but as one passes through adolescence and into adulthood, the ratio becomes closer to 1:1 (5,7). Long-term consequences of ADHD include school and occupational failure, substance abuse, divorce, car accidents, legal problems, and a variety of comorbid psychiatric disorders (8,9). Despite these grim statistics, a recent study of young men with ADHD treated with stimulants compared with those without stimulant treatment showed that treatment reduced the rates of comorbid psychiatric disorders and grade retention at 10-year follow-up, meaning that treatment had short- and long-term consequences on quality of life and psychiatric sequelae (10).

First-line treatment is now primarily the long-acting agents in stimulant and nonstimulant categories (5). Positive trials for a variety of long-acting stimulants (methylphenidate and amphetamine) and the norepinephrine reuptake inhibitor atomoxetine have led to labeling for pediatric and adolescent use, and all three categories can be used as first-line treatment (11). It should be noted that atomoxetine carries a black box labeling for suicidality at rates lower than those seen in the antidepressants. Other agents have been seen as superior to placebo in clinical trials but not FDA approved due to issues around safety including modafinil (Stevens–Johnson syndrome) and bupropion (seizures and suicidality) (12,13). The latest agents studied have been the α-adrenergic agents clonidine in a NINDS trial and long-acting guanfacine in several industry-sponsored trials that led to FDA approval and labeling in 2009 (14,15).

Having this selection of agents stimulants, norepinephrine reuptake inhibitors, and α agonists makes it unlikely that one would need to go to combination therapy or nonlabeled medications, but both options may be necessary if a child fails FDA-approved medications (11). Even with the lack of systemic long-term trials, there is some prospective information on long-term effects on growth with both stimulants and atomoxetine (16,17). Concerns about cardiovascular issues with stimulants have led to a variety of warnings and scared clinicians away from using these medications (18,19).

AUTISM

Autism is a pervasive developmental disorder with an onset by the age of 3 years, characterized by impairments in reciprocal social interactions and communications and by unusually restricted, repetitive, and stereotyped patterns of behaviors and interests (6). The sex ratio is 4:1 male to female, and the prevalence of autism spectrum disorders (ASD) is as high as 60 per 10,000 births and full symptom autism at 10 to 20 per 10,000 live births (20). For many families, there seems to be a genetic aspect to the disorder and an increased risk of developing autism with increasing paternal age and presence of a sibling with the disorder (21). A variety of etiologies and genetic causes seem to exist for those with ASD.

To date, no medications have been found to correct the underlying deficits in communication seen in children with autism. Pharmacologic agents are used to target the comorbid psychiatric disorders including ADHD, anxiety, and depression that can impair a child's functioning in the classroom and are discussed in other sections of this chapter. This section on autism will focus on the treatment of irritability and aggression seen in youth with autism that frequently disrupts school and home placements, leading to hospitalizations or placements in residential settings. The best evidence for the use of pharmacologic agents to treat aggression and irritability in children with autism and ASD is seen with risperidone and aripiprazole (22–25). Risperidone is currently FDA approved for the indication, and aripiprazole submitted two large positive trials and is FDA approved for the irritability autism indication. Other antipsychotics and mood stabilizers have been studied in smaller open-label trials for the treatment of aggression and irritability in autism (26). At low doses, these medications can reduce irritability and lead to improved attention and concentration, decrease stereotypies, and improve academic and social functioning.

Other interventions that have been tried for the treatment of autism are gluten and/or casein-free diets, chelation, secretin, and avoidance of childhood immunizations. None have been proven in double-blind trials to improve functioning and all may lead to health difficulties. Parents and clinicians should stay with proven treatments.

ANXIETY AND DEPRESSION

Anxiety disorders affect 10% to 20% of youth throughout childhood and adolescence (27,28). The practice parameters for the treatment of anxiety recommend the use of multimodal treatment, which includes psychotherapy, especially cognitive behavioral therapy (CBT), and pharmacotherapy (27). The anxiety disorders include simple phobia, generalized anxiety disorder, panic disorder, separation anxiety disorder, posttraumatic stress disorder, and obsessive-compulsive disorder (OCD). The best-studied therapy modality for anxiety disorders is CBT for all of anxiety disorders with some benefit from desensitization or more simple behavioral therapy proving effective in simple phobias. Two large groupings of trials have examined the treatment of anxiety disorders in children and adolescents. The first group is monotherapy industry-funded trials and the second group is the NIH-funded medication monotherapy and combination trials.

For the treatment of OCD, several medications are FDA approved in pediatrics including clomipramine, fluoxetine, fluvoxamine, and sertraline (29–32). Studies in paroxetine were also positive but not FDA approved (33). Positive treatment trials for generalized anxiety disorder and social phobia were also done with venlafaxine, paroxetine, and sertraline, however, these trials while providing efficacy and safety information did not lead to additional FDA labeling (34–37). The largest trial for posttraumatic stress disorder with sertraline did not lead to FDA labeling because the medication arm did not separate from placebo in the trial (38). The two National Institute of Mental Health (NIMH) trials of pediatric anxiety disorders examined a trio of anxiety disorders frequently seen together in children—generalized anxiety disorder, separation anxiety disorder, and social phobia. The first trial showed that fluvoxamine was superior to placebo in the reduction of anxiety symptoms (39). In the more recent trial of these three anxiety disorders, the investigators showed that a combination of sertraline plus manualized CBT produced the greatest reduction in anxiety symptoms followed by sertraline and CBT which were both superior to placebo (40). The NIMH combination trial for OCD showed that combining sertraline and CBT produced the largest reduction in OCD symptoms followed by CBT then sertraline which were both superior to placebo (41). The main finding from the NIMH multimodal trials in anxiety was that combining medication and CBT led to larger reductions in symptoms than placebo and CBT or medication monotherapy. Risk–benefit analysis of the antidepressant trials for anxiety showed that the number needed to treat (NNT) for improvement was 6 for OCD and 3 for non-OCD anxiety disorders and the number needed to harm (NNH) regarding suicidality was 200 for OCD and 143 for non-OCD anxiety (42). This meta-analysis clearly outlines the superiority of benefit over risk in the FDA anxiety registration trials.

Major depressive disorder is a recurrent disorder that affects as many as 2% to 4% of children and teenagers with 20% cumulative risk by the end of adolescence (43). Pediatric depression must meet all of the adult criteria except that children may fail to gain the expected weight and more frequently present with an irritable mood (6,43). Symptoms may include more difficulty with anhedonia, complaints of boredom, and loss of interaction with friends. Younger children may also exhibit more somatic symptoms than adults. The male-to-female ratio of depression in children is 1:1, whereas in adolescents and adults the ratio is 1:2.

Treatment for depression in children and adolescents may include medication, psychotherapy with dialectical behavioral therapy and CBT as the most effective or a combination of both. The older antidepressants including monoamine oxidase inhibitors and tricyclics have a history of failed pediatric trials and are not FDA approved for treatment of adolescent depression. The serotonin-norepinephrine reuptake inhibitor (SNRI) venlafaxine also had two failed trials. Although the adolescent subset of subjects did show improvement, FDA labeling was not pursued, in part, due to a high suicidality signal (44). Only two selective serotonin reuptake inhibitors (SSRIs) have had consistent separation from placebo in double-blind trials of depression in youth. Fluoxetine had been FDA approved in pediatric and adolescent depression, based on one single-site and one multi-site trial (45,46). The second agent approved for adolescent depression was in 2009 with escitalopram after a positive trial of citalopram in children and teens, a negative trial of escitalopram in children and teens (although the adolescent subgroup did separate from placebo), and a third positive adolescent trial of escitalopram (47–49). All the other SSRIs and the SNRI venlafaxine have been tried in pediatric depression but have not been labeled for use in depression either due to side effect burden or lack of efficacy usually as a function of elevated placebo response rate (50–52). The meta-analysis of the antidepressants for pediatric depression shows that the NNT of 10 still outweighs the NNH for suicidality of 112 (42). A further examination of the same trials revealed that the high placebo response rate in pediatric antidepressant trials was directly related to the number of study sites in a trial while the antidepressant response rate did not vary with the number of study sites (53).

In the two large NIMH trials of adolescent depression, two main questions are asked and answered. In TADS (treatment of adolescent depression study), the group shows that combination treatment of CBT plus fluoxetine leads to improvement in 71% of those in the trial, blinded fluoxetine is second best with a response rate of 60.6%, and CBT and placebo are equivalent in treatment response rates at week 12 in the trial (54). Those individuals on CBT arms have lower rates of suicidality in the trial as well. In a second trial of adolescents who have failed at least one trial of an SSRI TORDIA (Treatment of Resistant Depression in Adolescents), the investigators ask two questions. Should you try a second SSRI or switch to an SNRI? Does adding CBT to a medication switch improve response rates? In this trial, switching to either group leads to a 40.5% response rate, while adding CBT improves response rates to 54.8% (55). The use of CBT in TORDIA did not reduce suicidality in the participants.

Suicidal ideation and attempts in clinical registration trials led to the black box labeling of all antidepressants in individuals younger than 18 years and later younger than 25 years for increased risk of ideation and attempts. Large epidemiologic studies have not shown increases in suicide associated with treatment in young people (56). This label change has led to restrictions in antidepressant use, decreased rates of depression diagnosis, and possible increases in rates of completed suicide in those individuals younger than 21 years (57–59). As we have seen dramatic changes in diagnosis, treatment, and rates of completed suicides in those younger than 18 years, the FDA and therapeutic community may wish to reconsider the need for a black box warning on all antidepressants.

BIPOLAR DISORDER

Adult bipolar disorder has FDA-approved medications in a variety of categories including mood stabilizers (lithium), antiepileptic drugs, and atypical antipsychotics. Pediatric bipolar disorder has been complicated by controversy over diagnosis and treatment. Many children and adolescents with bipolar disorder have a rapidly fluctuating course and more frequent psychotic symptoms than adults (60). Treatment in children must include close monitoring of symptoms and response to treatment in a multimodal setting to include pharmacotherapy, psychoeducation about illness and course, educational interventions, and psychotherapy including individual, family, and group therapy.

Some of the adult treatments are less effective or less well studied in children and adolescents. Lithium has been successfully used in several small trials of bipolar disorder and is FDA approved for bipolar disorder in children aged 12 years and older (61). Two other federally funded trials of pediatric bipolar disorder have examined lithium—CoLT (Collaborative Lithium Trial) and TEAM (Treatment of Early Age Mania). TEAM is finished but results are not available in this head-to-head comparison of lithium, risperidone, and valproic acid. CoLT, a lithium versus placebo trial, is finished with stage one and the larger double-blind lithium trial is about to start enrollment. Several double-blind trials of anticonvulsants have failed to show superiority of drug over placebo including oxcarbazepine, valproic acid, and topiramate (62–64). Lamotrigine is currently being tested as an adjunctive mood stabilizer in children aged 10 to 17 years who are partial responders to one or two other mood stabilizers.

The medications with the highest rate of positive trials in pediatric bipolar disorder for mixed and manic episodes are the atypical antipsychotics (65–67). Two atypical antipsychotics are already FDA approved and labeled for pediatric bipolar disorder, aripiprazole and risperidone. Three more have been approved pending final labeling for bipolar: quetiapine as a first-line agent and olanzapine and ziprasidone as second-line agents due to weight and cardiac issues (68).

SCHIZOPHRENIA

Schizophrenia can present in adolescence in 39% of males often having more severe cognitive impairments and poorer outcomes (69). In the last 6 years, a variety of registration trials and an NIMH-funded trial have examined the use of atypical antipsychotics in the treatment of adolescent schizophrenia. The practice parameters for adolescent schizophrenia have stressed the importance of multimodal treatment including psychopharmacology as a key part of treatment. Other important aspects of the treatment plan for schizophrenia include educational interventions including vocational and special education settings, psychoeducation about the disorder, family, individual, and group therapies (69). Double-blind trials with atypical antipsychotics have been positive with aripiprazole, clozapine, olanzapine, risperidone, and quetiapine (68,70–73). A trial of ziprasidone was stopped for lack of efficacy (74). A trial of paliperidone was recently completed but study results are not yet available. The largest NIMH trial TEOSS (Treatment of Early Onset Schizophrenia Spectrum study) compared two atypical antipsychotics (risperidone and olanzapine) with a typical antipsychotic (molindone) (75). Although all of the atypical antipsychotics, except ziprasidone, are effective in the treatment of schizophrenia, they do not come without a large set of side effects, including elevated prolactin, changes in lipid profile, weight gain, glucose and insulin changes, and even the development of diabetes in some individuals (76). These side effects must be monitored, and future treatments for schizophrenia need to improve positive and negative symptoms of the disorder without adding to other health burdens in the cardiovascular and endocrine systems.

CONCLUSIONS

In the last 10 years, the field of pediatric psychopharmacology has expanded rapidly, in part, due to BPCA and has led to extensive testing and labeling of medications for the treatment of psychiatric disorders in children. With the most recent reauthorization of the bill, even medications that do not show efficacy compared with placebo will still contain safety labeling about adverse events from the clinical trials. Treating psychiatric disorders in children and adolescents requires safe and effective treatments with further information about long-term safety. As personalized medicine advances, we will continue to discover and test new medications for mental illnesses in children. Some of the future challenges in this arena will include examining duration of treatment, long-term adverse events, and minimizing poor cardiovascular outcomes with medications.

ACKNOWLEDGMENTS

The author has been supported by grants from Forest, Glaxo Smith Kline, Janssen, Pfizer, Sepracor, and Supernus. She has a subcontract from NICHD.

REFERENCES

1. Findling RL, Reed MD, Myers C, et al. Paroxetine pharmacokinetics in depressed children and adolescents. *J Am Acad Child Adolesc Psychiatry* 1999;38:952–959.
2. Renwick AG. Toxicokinetics in infants and children in relation to the ADI and TDI. *Food Addit Contam* 1998;15(Suppl):17–35.
3. Edwards DJ. Clinical pharmacology of psychoactive drugs. In: Rosenberg DR, Davanzo PA, Gershon S, eds. *Pharmacotherapy for child and adolescent psychiatric disorders*. New York: Marcel Dekker, 2002:71–85.
4. Findling RL, Kauffman RE, Sallee FR, et al. Tolerability and pharmacokinetics of aripiprazole in children and adolescents with psychiatric disorders: an open-label, dose-escalation study. *J Clin Psychopharmacol* 2008;28(4):441–446.
5. Pliszka S, AACAP Work Group on Quality Issues. Practice parameter for the assessment and treatment of children and adolescents with attention-deficit/hyperactivity disorder. *J Am Acad Child Adolesc Psychiatry* 2007;46(7):894–921.
6. American Psychiatric Association. *Diagnostic and statistical manual of mental disorders*, 4th ed., text rev. (DSM-IV-TR). Washington, DC: American Psychiatric Association, 2000.
7. Kessler RC, Chiu WT, Demler O, et al. Prevalence, severity, and comorbidity of 12-month DSM-IV disorders in the National Comorbidity Survey Replication. *Arch Gen Psychiatry* 2005;62: 617–627.
8. Hansen C, Weiss D, Last CG. ADHD boys in young adulthood: psychosocial adjustment. *J Am Acad Child Adolesc Psychiatry* 1999; 38:165–171.
9. Mannuzza S, Klein RG, Bessler A, et al. Educational and occupational outcome of hyperactive boys grown up. *J Am Acad Child Adolesc Psychiatry* 1997;36(9):1222–1227.
10. Biederman J, Monuteaux MC, Spencer T, et al. Do stimulants protect against psychiatric disorders in youth with ADHD? A 10-year follow-up study. *Pediatrics* 2009;124(1):71–78.
11. Pliszka SR, Crismon ML, Hughes CW, et al. The Texas Children's Medication Algorithm Project: revision of the algorithm for pharmacotherapy of attention-deficit/hyperactivity disorder. *J Am Acad Child Adolesc Psychiatry* 2006;45(6):642–657.
12. Biederman J, Pliszka SR. Modafinil improves symptoms of attention-deficit/hyperactivity disorder across subtypes in children and adolescents. *J Pediatr* 2008;152(3):394–399.
13. Monuteaux MC, Spencer TJ, Faraone SV, et al. A randomized, placebo-controlled clinical trial of bupropion for the prevention of smoking in children and adolescents with attention-deficit/hyperactivity disorder. *J Clin Psychiatry* 2007;68(7):1094–1101.
14. Palumbo DR, Sallee FR, Pelham WE Jr, et al. Clonidine for attention-deficit/hyperactivity disorder: I. Efficacy and tolerability outcomes. *J Am Acad Child Adolesc Psychiatry* 2008;47(2):180–188.
15. Sallee F, McGough J, Wigal T, et al. Guanfacine extended release in children and adolescents with attention-deficit/hyperactivity disorder: a placebo-controlled trial [published online ahead of print December 20, 2008]. *J Am Acad Child Adolesc Psychiatry* 2009; 48(2):155–165.
16. Pliszka SR, Matthews TL, Braslow KJ, et al. Comparative effects of methylphenidate and mixed salts amphetamine on height and weight in children with attention-deficit/hyperactivity disorder. *J Am Acad Child Adolesc Psychiatry* 2006;45(5):520–526.

17. Spencer TJ, Kratochvil CJ, Sangal RB, et al. Effects of atomoxetine on growth in children with attention-deficit/hyperactivity disorder following up to five years of treatment. *J Child Adolesc Psychopharmacol* 2007;17(5):689–700.
18. Warren AE, Hamilton RM, Bélanger SA, et al. Cardiac risk assessment before the use of stimulant medications in children and youth: a joint position statement by the Canadian Paediatric Society, the Canadian Cardiovascular Society, and the Canadian Academy of Child and Adolescent Psychiatry. *Can J Cardiol* 2009; 25(11):625–630.
19. Perrin JM, Friedman RA, Knilans TK; Black Box Working Group; Section on Cardiology and Cardiac Surgery. Cardiovascular monitoring and stimulant drugs for attention-deficit/hyperactivity disorder. *Pediatrics* 2008;122(2):451–453.
20. Newschaffer CJ, Croen LA, Daniels J, et al. The epidemiology of autism spectrum disorders. *Annu Rev Public Health* 2007;28:235–258.
21. Bill BR, Geschwind DH. Genetic advances in autism: heterogeneity and convergence on shared pathways. *Curr Opin Genet Dev* 2009; 19(3):271–278.
22. Research Unit on Pediatric Psychopharmacology Autism Network. Risperidone in children with autism and serious behavioral problems. *N Engl J Med* 2002;347(5):314–321.
23. Shea S, Turgay A, Carroll A, et al. Risperidone in the treatment of disruptive behavioral symptoms in children with autistic and other pervasive developmental disorders [published online ahead of print October 18, 2004]. *Pediatrics* 2004;114(5):e634–e641.
24. Marcus RN, Owen R, Kamen L, et al. A placebo-controlled, fixed-dose study of aripiprazole in children and adolescents with irritability associated with autistic disorder. *J Am Acad Child Adolesc Psychiatry* 2009;48(11):1110–1119.
25. Owen R Sikich L, et al. A multicenter, double-blind, randomized, placebo-controlled, flexible-dose, parallel-group study of aripiprazole in the treatment of irritability in children and adolescents (6–17 years) with autistic disorder. *Pediatrics* 2009;124(6): 1533–1540.
26. Stigler KA, McDougle CJ. Pharmacotherapy of irritability in pervasive developmental disorders. *Child Adolesc Psychiatr Clin N Am* 2008;17(4):739–752.
27. Connolly SD, Bernstein GA; Work Group on Quality Issues. Practice parameter for the assessment and treatment of children and adolescents with anxiety disorders. *J Am Acad Child Adolesc Psychiatry* 2007;46(2):267–283.
28. Benjamin RS, Costello EJ, Warren M. Anxiety disorders in a pediatric sample. *J Anxiety Disord* 1990;4:293–316.
29. DeVeaugh-Geiss J, Moroz G, Biederman J, et al. Clomipramine hydrochloride in childhood and adolescent obsessive-compulsive disorder—a multicenter trial. *J Am Acad Child Adolesc Psychiatry* 1992;31:45–49.
30. Geller DA, Hoog SL, Heiligenstein JH, et al. Fluoxetine treatment for obsessive-compulsive disorder in children and adolescents: a placebo-controlled clinical trial. *J Am Acad Child Adolesc Psychiatry* 2001;40(7):773–779.
31. Riddle MA, Reeve EA, Yaryura-Tobias JA, et al. Fluvoxamine for children and adolescents with obsessive-compulsive disorder: a randomized, controlled, multicenter trial. *J Am Acad Child Adolesc Psychiatry* 2001;40(2):222–229.
32. March JS, Biederman J, Wolkow R, et al. Sertraline in children and adolescents with obsessive-compulsive disorder: a multicenter randomized controlled trial. *JAMA* 1998;280:1752–1756.
33. Geller DA, Wagner KD, Emslie G, et al. Paroxetine treatment in children and adolescents with obsessive-compulsive disorder: a randomized, multicenter, double-blind, placebo-controlled trial. *J Am Acad Child Adolesc Psychiatry* 2004;43:1387–1396.
34. Wagner KD, Berard R, Stein MB, et al. A multicenter, randomized, double-blind, placebo-controlled trial of paroxetine in children and adolescents with social anxiety disorder. *Arch Gen Psychiatry* 2004a;61:1153–1162.
35. Rynn MA, Siqueland L, Rickels K. Placebo-controlled trial of sertraline in the treatment of children with generalized anxiety disorder. *Am J Psychiatry* 2001;158:2008–2014.
36. March JS, Entusah AR, Rynn M, et al. A randomized controlled trial of venlafaxine ER versus placebo in pediatric social anxiety disorder. *Biol Psychiatry* 2007;62:1149–1154.
37. Rynn MA, Riddle MA, Yeung PP, et al. Efficacy and safety of extended-release venlafaxine in the treatment of generalized anxiety disorder in children and adolescents: two placebo-controlled trials. *Am J Psychiatry* 2007;164(2):290–300.
38. Robb AS, Cueva JE, Sporn J, et al. Sertraline treatment of children and adolescents with posttraumatic stress disorder: a double-blind, placebo-controlled trial. Under review.
39. Research Units on Pediatric Psychopharmacology Anxiety Study Group (RUPP). Fluvoxamine for the treatment of anxiety disorders in children and adolescents. *N Engl J Med* 2001;344:1279–1285.
40. Walkup JT, Albano AM, Piacentini J, et al. Cognitive behavioral therapy, sertraline, or a combination in childhood anxiety. *N Engl J Med* 2008;359:2753–2766.
41. Pediatric OCD Treatment Study (POTS) Team. Cognitive-behavior therapy, sertraline, and their combination for children and adolescents with obsessive-compulsive disorder: the Pediatric OCD Treatment Study (POTS) randomized controlled trial. *JAMA* 2004;292(16):1969–1976.
42. Bridge JA, Iyengar S, Salary CB, et al. Clinical response and risk for reported suicidal ideation and suicide attempts in pediatric antidepressant treatment: a meta-analysis of randomized controlled trials. *JAMA* 2007;297(15):1683–1696.
43. Birmaher B, Brent D; Workgroup on Quality Issues. Practice parameter for the assessment and treatment of children and adolescents with depressive disorders. *J Am Acad Child Adolesc Psychiatry* 2007;46(11):1503–1526.
44. Emslie GJ, Findling RL, Yeung PP, et al. Venlafaxine ER for the treatment of pediatric subjects with depression: results of two placebo-controlled trials. *J Am Acad Child Adolesc Psychiatry* 2007; 6(4):479–488.
45. Emslie GJ, Rush AJ, Weinberg WA, et al. A double-blind, randomized, placebo-controlled trial of fluoxetine in children and adolescents with depression. *Arch Gen Psychiatry* 1997;54:1031–1037.
46. Emslie GJ, Heiligenstein JH, Wagner KD, et al. Fluoxetine for acute treatment of depression in children and adolescents: a placebo-controlled, randomized clinical trial. *J Am Acad Child Adolesc Psychiatry* 2002;41:1205–1215.
47. Wagner KD, Jonas J, Findling RL, et al. A double-blind, randomized, placebo-controlled trial of escitalopram in the treatment of pediatric depression. *J Am Acad Child Adolesc Psychiatry* 2006; 45(3):280–288.
48. Wagner KD, Robb AS, Findling RL, et al. A randomized, placebo-controlled trial of citalopram for the treatment of major depression in children and adolescents. *Am J Psychiatry* 2004;161(6): 1079–1083.
49. Emslie GJ, Ventura D, Korotzer A, et al. Escitalopram in the treatment of adolescent depression: a randomized placebo-controlled multisite trial. *J Am Acad Child Adolesc Psychiatry* 2009;48(7): 721–729.
50. Wagner KD, Ambrosini P, Rynn M, et al. Efficacy of sertraline in the treatment of children and adolescents with major depressive disorder: two randomized controlled trials. *J Am Med Assoc* 2003; 290:1033–1041.
51. Emslie GJ, Wagner KD, Kutcher S. Paroxetine treatment in children and adolescents with major depressive disorder: a randomized, multicenter, double-blind, placebo-controlled trial. *J Am Acad Child Adolesc Psychiatry* 2006;45(6):709–719.
52. Emslie GJ, Findling RL, Yeung PP, et al. Venlafaxine ER for the treatment of pediatric subjects with depression: results of two placebo-controlled trials. *J Am Acad Child Adolesc Psychiatry* 2007; 46:479–488.
53. Bridge JA, Birmaher B, Iyengar S, et al. Placebo response in randomized controlled trials of antidepressants for pediatric major depressive disorder. *Am J Psychiatry* 2009;166(1):42–49.
54. March J, Silva S, Petrycki S, et al. Fluoxetine, cognitive behavioral therapy, and their combination for adolescents with depression: Treatment for Adolescents With Depression Study (TADS) randomized controlled trial. *JAMA* 2004;292:807–820.
55. Brent DA, Emslie G, Clarke G, et al. Switching to another SSRI or to venlafaxine with or without cognitive behavioral therapy for adolescents with SSRI-resistant depression: the TORDIA randomized controlled trial. *JAMA* 2008;299(8):901–913.
56. Jick H, Kaye JA, Jick SS. Antidepressants and the risk of suicidal behaviors. *JAMA* 2004;292(3):338–343.
57. Bridge JA, Greenhouse JB, Weldon AH, et al. Suicide trends among youths aged 10–19 years in the United States, 1996–2005. *JAMA* 2008;300(9):1025–1026.

58. Gibbons, RD, Hur K, Bhaumik DK, et al. The relationship between antidepressant prescription rates and rate of early adolescent suicide. *Am J Psychiatry* 2006;163(11):1898–1904.
59. Libby AM, Brent DA, Morrato EH, et al. Decline in treatment of pediatric depression after FDA advisory on risk of suicidality with SSRIs. *Am J Psychiatry* 2007;164(6):884–891.
60. McClellan J, Kowatch R, Findling RL, et al. Practice parameter for the assessment and treatment of children and adolescents with bipolar disorder. *J Am Acad Child Adolesc Psychiatry* 2007; 46(1):107–125.
61. Geller B, Cooper TB, Sun K, et al. Double-blind and placebo-controlled study of lithium for adolescent bipolar disorders with secondary substance dependency. *J Am Acad Child Adolesc Psychiatry* 1998;37:171–178.
62. Wagner KD, Kowatch RA, Emslie GJ, et al. A double-blind, randomized, placebo-controlled trial of oxcarbazepine in the treatment of bipolar disorder in children and adolescents. *Am J Psychiatry* 2006;163(7):1179–1186.
63. Wagner KD, Redden L, Kowatch RA, et al. A double-blind, randomized, placebo-controlled trial of divalproex extended-release in the treatment of bipolar disorder in children and adolescents. *J Am Acad Child Adolesc Psychiatry* 2009;48(5):519–532.
64. Delbello MP, Findling RL, Kushner S, et al. A pilot controlled trial of topiramate for mania in children and adolescents with bipolar disorder. *J Am Acad Child Adolesc Psychiatry* 2005;44(6):539–547.
65. Findling RL, Nyilas M, Forbes RA, et al. Acute treatment of pediatric bipolar I disorder, manic or mixed episode, with aripiprazole: a randomized, double-blind, placebo-controlled study. *J Clin Psychiatry* 2009;70(10):1441–1451.
66. Haas M, Delbello MP, Pandina G, et al. Risperidone for the treatment of acute mania in children and adolescents with bipolar disorder: a randomized, double-blind, placebo-controlled study. *Bipolar Disord* 2009;11(7):687–700.
67. Tohen M, Kryzhanovskaya L, Carlson G, et al. Olanzapine versus placebo in the treatment of adolescents with bipolar mania. *Am J Psychiatry* 2007;164(10):1547–1556.
68. Kuehn BM. FDA panel OKs 3 antipsychotic drugs for pediatric use, cautions against overuse. *JAMA* 2009;302(8):833–834.
69. American Academy of Child and Adolescent Psychiatry. Practice parameter for the assessment and treatment of children and adolescents with schizophrenia. *J Am Acad Child Adolesc Psychiatry* 2001;40(7 Suppl):4S–23S.
70. Findling RL, Robb AS, Nyilas M, et al. A multiple-center, randomized, double-blind, placebo-controlled study of oral aripiprazole for treatment of adolescents with schizophrenia. *Am J Psychiatry* 2008;165(11):1432–1441.
71. Kumra S, Frazier JA, Jacobsen LK, et al. Childhood-onset schizophrenia. A double-blind clozapine–haloperidol comparison. *Arch Gen Psychiatry* 1996;53:1090–1097.
72. Kryzhanovskaya L, Schulz SC, McDougle C, et al. Olanzapine versus placebo in adolescents with schizophrenia: a 6-week, randomized, double-blind, placebo-controlled trial. *J Am Acad Child Adolesc Psychiatry* 2009;48(1):60–70.
73. Haas M, Eerdekens M, Kushner S, et al. Efficacy, safety and tolerability of two dosing regimens in adolescent schizophrenia: double-blind study. *Br J Psychiatry* 2009;194(2):158–164.
74. www.clinicaltrials.gov/ct2/show/NCT00265382 trial ending communicated as of March 24, 2009.
75. Sikich L, Frazier JA, McClellan J, et al. Double-blind comparison of first- and second-generation antipsychotics in early-onset schizophrenia and schizo-affective disorder: findings from the treatment of early-onset schizophrenia spectrum disorders (TEOSS) study. *Am J Psychiatry* 2008;165(11):1420–1431.
76. Correl CU, Manu P, Olshanskiy V, et al. Cardiometabolic risk of second-generation antipsychotic medications during first-time use in children and adolescents. *JAMA* 2009;302(16):1765–1773.

CHAPTER

39

Yesim Yilmaz-Demirdag
Sanaa A. Mahmoud
Sami L. Bahna

Antihistamine Drugs

Antihistamines are among the most frequently used medications worldwide. As a body chemical, histamine has a role in health as well as in a variety of diseases. This chapter describes the physiologic role and the pathologic consequences of histamine release. The histamine receptors and their various functions are reviewed, and the clinical pharmacology and therapeutic uses of H_1 antihistamines are summarized. Antagonists to H_2 and H_3 receptors as well as the H_4 receptors are briefly discussed.

HISTORICAL BACKGROUND

Histamine, initially called β-aminoethylimidazole, was first discovered as a constituent of ergot and then was chemically synthesized in 1907 (1). Soon after, Dale and Laidlaw (2,3) discovered that histamine stimulated a host of smooth muscle cells and had an intense vasodilator action. In their experiments, they found that histamine induced shock-like syndrome in frogs and mammals. Histamine caused bronchospasm, myocardial contraction, and cardiac and pulmonary vasoconstriction. It also caused a fall in the systemic blood pressure due to capillary dilation resulting in pooling of blood in the capillary bed and a substantial extravascular loss of plasma.

In 1927, Best and coworkers (4) isolated histamine from fresh samples of liver and lung establishing that this amine is a natural constituent of the body. Demonstration of its presence in a variety of other tissues soon followed, hence its name after the Greek word "histos" for tissues. In the same year, Lewis (5) further expanded on the vascular effects of histamine, which suggested that this mediator could be released from cells in the skin on stimulation with appropriate trauma causing the "wheal-and-flare response," which is also known as "the triple wheal-and-flare response." This reaction includes an immediate local reddening due to vasodilatation, a wheal due to increased vascular permeability and a flare response due to indirect vasodilatation secondary to axonal reflex. In 1952, Riley and West (6) discovered that the mast cell is the major source for histamine. Later they showed a correlation between the number of mast cells and the histamine content in a variety of animal tissues as well as in urticaria pigmentosa lesions in humans (7). They also found histamine in the circulating basophils. In 1953, Mongar and Schild (8) published the first series of studies concerning the mechanism of histamine release from mast cells. Subsequent studies focused on the role of calcium in histamine release by antigens and other ligands (9).

HISTAMINE

SYNTHESIS, STORAGE, AND METABOLISM OF HISTAMINE

Histamine is a hydrophilic molecule comprising an imidazole ring and an amino group connected by two methylene groups (10). Histamine occurs in plants as well as in animal tissues and is a component of some venoms and a variety of insect secretions. It is synthesized in the Golgi apparatus of mast cells and basophils by decarboxylation of a semi-essential amino acid L-histidine, a reaction catalyzed by the enzyme histamine decarboxylase. Once formed, histamine is either stored in the cytoplasmic granules of mast cells (and basophils) or rapidly inactivated. Histamine is mostly (70%) metabolized through methylation by *N*-methyltransferase to *N*-methyl histamine and partly (30%) through oxidation by diamine oxidase to imidazole acetic acid (11). A very small amount of released histamine (2% to 3%) is excreted in the urine unchanged. The turnover of histamine in the mast cell secretory granules is slow. When histamine is depleted from its stores, it may take weeks before its concentration returns to normal levels. Histamine metabolites have little or no activity and are excreted in the urine.

The main site of histamine storage in most tissues is the mast cell. The latter is found in the loose connective tissue of all organs, especially around blood vessels, nerves, and lymphatics. It is most abundant in the shock organs of allergic diseases, namely the skin and the mucosa of the respiratory and the gastrointestinal tracts (12). The human heart contains large numbers of mast cells, localized primarily in the wall of the right atrium (13). In addition to mast cells and basophils, histamine is present in the epidermis, enterochromaffin cells of the fundus of the stomach, and neurons within the central nervous system (CNS) (10,14).

HISTAMINE RECEPTORS

To date, four distinct types of receptors have been demonstrated. The existence of more than one type of histamine receptor was suggested in 1966 by Ash and Schild (15) who noted that the classic antihistamine mepyramine could block histamine-induced contractions of guinea pig ileum but not histamine-induced gastric acid secretion. The effects of histamine on H_1, H_2, H_3, and H_4 receptors and their distributions in humans are presented in Table 39.1. Human H_1 receptors have approximately 45% homology with muscarinic receptors (16).

The H_3 receptor was identified in 1983 (17) and its gene was cloned in 1999 (18). It acts as a presynaptic autoreceptor and is expressed in the central and peripheral nervous systems where it modulates neurotransmission. It has been recently shown that H_3 receptors are involved in the blood–brain barrier function and may play a favorable role in neuroinflammation (19). H_3 agonists (e.g., imetit and immepip) decrease histamine release and thus might be useful in the treatment of a variety of gastrointestinal, cardiac, and neurologic disorders (e.g., migraine and schizophrenia) (20).

The H_4 receptor was described in 2000 and its structure showed about 40% similarity to H_3 receptor (21). The H_4-receptor gene was mapped to chromosome 18 (22). H_4 receptors may have a significant role in the inflammatory process in atopic dermatitis and asthma (23).

EFFECTS OF HISTAMINE

Cardiovascular

Injection of histamine in human causes a decrease in blood pressure and an increase in the heart rate. The blood pressure drops because of the direct vasodilator action on the arterioles and precapillary sphincters. The increase in heart rate results from a direct stimulatory action on the myocardium, mainly through the H_2 receptors, as well as through a reflex-compensatory tachycardia secondary to hypotension (14). Both H_1 and H_2 receptors seem to be involved in these responses; hence, a combination of H_1 and H_2 antihistamines is often more effective in preventing the cardiovascular effects of histamine than either alone.

Stimulation of H_1 receptors in the atrioventricular node slows down the heart rate by decreasing atrioventricular nodal conduction (24). Cardiac H_1 receptors are also found in epicardial coronary vessels where they mediate vasoconstriction (25). H_2 receptors are found in the coronary

TABLE 39.1 Histamine Receptor Types

	H_1 Receptor	*H_2 Receptor*	*H_3 Receptor*	*H_4 Receptor*
Chromosome	3p25	5q35.2	20q13.33	18q11.2
Amino acids	487	359	445	390
Signal transduction	↑PLC, IP3, DAG, Ca^{2+}	↑cAMP	↓cAMP, ↑Ca^{2+}, MAPK	↓cAMP, ↑Ca^{++}, MAPK
Tissues/cells	Lung, CNS, CVS, adrenals, epithelial cells, neutrophils, eosinophils, monocytes/macrophages, DC, T cells, B cells, hepatocytes	Heart, stomach, CNS, airway and vascular smooth muscle, endothelial cells, epithelial cells, neutrophils, eosinophils, monocytes	CNS, peripheral nervous system, eosinophils, DC, monocytes	Eosinophils, neutrophils, DC, T cells, basophils, mast cells, neurons
Functions	Pruritus, pain, flushing, headache, cough, sleep/wakefulness, decreased appetite, body temperature, hypotension, tachycardia, vascular permeability, decreased AV node conduction, bronchial smooth muscle constriction, prostaglandin secretion, recruitment of inflammatory cells, release of inflammatory mediators	Flushing, headache, hypotension, gastric acidity, vascular permeability, chronotropic, inotropic, bronchial smooth muscle relaxation, airway mucus secretion, stimulation of T-suppressor cells, decreased neutrophil and basophil chemotaxis, inhibition of natural killer cells, reduced lymphocyte cytotoxicity and proliferation	Prevention of excessive bronchoconstriction, inhibition of gastric acidity, sleep, cognition, inhibition of histamine synthesis, and neurotransmitter release (histamine, dopamine, serotonin, norepinephrine, acetylcholine)	Pruritus, bronchoconstriction, chemotaxis

AV node, atrioventricular node; cAMP, cyclic adenosine monophosphate; CNS, central nervous system; CVS, cardiovascular system; DAG, diacylglycerol; DC, dendritic cells; IP3, inositol triphosphate; MAPK, mitogen-activated protein kinase; PLC, phospholipase C.
Adapted from Simons FE. Advances in H_1-antihistamines. *N Engl J Med* 2004;351:2203–2217 and Huang JF, Thurmond RL. The new biology of histamine receptors. *Curr Allergy Asthma Rep* 2008;8:21–27.

vasculature, where their vasodilator action opposes that of H_1 receptors (25). H_2 receptors are also widely distributed throughout the myocardium and nodal tissue where they exert positive inotropic and chronotropic effects, respectively (24,25). H_3 receptors in the heart are present in the presynaptic postganglionic sympathetic fibers and are autoinhibitory to presynaptic norepinephrine release (26,27). The widespread distribution of histamine receptors throughout the myocardium, nodal tissue, and coronary vasculature suggests a significant role in the physiologic regulation of the normal healthy heart. Nault and coworkers (28) reported that H_1 antihistamines (loratadine) in young healthy subjects did not alter the autonomic cardiovascular control. However, an H_2 antihistamine (ranitidine) altered cardiac sympathovagal balance when administered alone. Such a finding indicates a shift toward sympathetic predominance in heart rate regulation, with a potential of inducing arrhythmias.

Histamine-induced vasodilation causes transudation of fluid and even large molecules such as proteins into the perivascular tissue resulting in skin hives or mucosal edema associated with allergic reactions. The vasodilator effect of histamine is mediated by both H_1 and H_2 receptors located on different cell types in the vascular bed: H_1 receptors on the vascular endothelium and both H_1 and H_2 receptors on the smooth muscle cells (10).

Activation of H_1 receptors leads to increased intracellular Ca^{2+}, activation of phospholipase A_2, and the local production of nitric oxide, an endothelium-derived relaxing factor (29). Nitric oxide diffuses to the smooth muscle cell, where it activates a soluble guanylyl cyclase and causes accumulation of cyclic guanosine monophosphate (cGMP). The cGMP-dependent protein kinase release and a decrease in intracellular Ca^{2+} seem to be involved in the smooth muscle relaxation caused by this cyclic nucleotide.

Nonvascular Smooth Muscle

Histamine-induced bronchospasm has been demonstrated in both humans and guinea pigs. Although some H_2 receptors are present in human bronchial smooth muscle, their dilator effect is much dominated by the spasmogenic influence of H_1 receptors. In asthma, histamine-induced bronchospasm may involve an additional reflex component that arises from irritation of afferent vagal nerve endings (10).

Histamine has lesser effects on nonbronchial smooth muscle. It causes various degrees of uterine muscle contraction, but such an effect is negligible on the human uterus, gravid or not. The response of the intestinal muscle varies according to the species and region but is primarily contraction. The effect on other smooth muscles (e.g., urinary bladder, ureter, gall bladder, and iris) is minimal or inconsistent.

Gastric Acid Secretion

Histamine stimulates gastric acid secretion by the parietal cells through H_2 receptors as well as stimulation of vagal reflex and gastrin release (30). It also increases the output of pepsin and the intrinsic factor. The activation of H_2 receptors on the parietal cells leads to increase in adenyl cyclase activity, cyclic adenosine monophosphate (cAMP) concentration, and intracellular Ca^{2+}.

Central Nervous System

Histaminergic neurons have been identified in some areas of the brain. H_1 receptors are found throughout the CNS and are densely concentrated in the hypothalamus. Histamine acts as a neurotransmitter along with the other biogenic amines, serotonin, dopamine, norepinephrine, and acetylcholine (31). Histamine increases wakefulness and inhibits appetite through H_1 receptors. Neuronal histamine is involved in arousal, learning, memory, locomotor activity, food intake, and other physiologic processes.

Presynaptic H_3 receptors play important role in inhibiting the synthesis and release of histamine in the histaminergic neurones in the CNS. H_3-receptor agonists (e.g., (R)-α-methylhistamine, imetit, and immepip) reduce the release of several amines in various areas of the brain, including histamine, norepinephrine, dopamine, 5-hydroxytryptamine, and possibly acetylcholine (14).

Immune System and Inflammatory Response

A recent review on the role of histamine in immunologic and allergic inflammation has been published (32). Many inflammatory cells express H_1, H_2, and H_4 receptors. The H_4 receptor is found more on the dendritic cells, mast cells, eosinophils, monocytes, basophils, and T cells. In general, H_1 receptors stimulate proinflammatory activity through increased cell migration to areas of inflammation, whereas H_2 receptors act as a potent suppressor of inflammatory and effector functions. Histamine also facilitates several proinflammatory activities through H_4 receptors. Most ligands that target H_1 and H_2 receptors have little affinity for H_4 receptors. The H_4 receptor may play a role in chemotaxis of mast cells, eosinophils, and dendritic cells. The role of the H_4 receptor in inflammatory and pruritic response has been verified in vivo (33–35).

Allergy Response

Histamine release occurs when allergen binds to the specific immunoglobulin E (IgE) molecule on the mast cells and basophils in previously sensitized individuals. Histamine release from these cells depends on the rise in intracellular Ca^{2+} (10). Although histamine was the first identified mediator of allergic inflammation, numerous other mediators exist. They are either preformed in the granules (e.g., serotonin, tryptase, chymases, carboxypeptidases, acid hydrolases, oxidative enzymes, chemotactic factors, and proteoglycans such as heparin and chondroitin sulfate) or newly formed from the mast cell membrane (e.g., prostaglandin D_2 and leukotrienes).

Elevated plasma histamine levels are present in conditions associated with increased mast cell number (e.g., mastocytosis) or activation (e.g., anaphylaxis or other allergic diseases) (36). Increased histamine levels have also been noted in the skin and plasma of patients with atopic dermatitis and in chronic urticaria (37–39). Recently, it was demonstrated that a special type of dendritic cells (the inflammatory dendritic epidermal cells), express H_4 receptors in skin lesions of atopic dermatitis (23). Increased levels of histamine have been found in bronchoalveolar lavage fluid in patients with asthma (40). However, H_1 and H_2 blockers have minimal therapeutic effect in asthma, suggesting a possible role of H_4 receptors.

EXTRINSIC FACTORS CAUSING DIRECT HISTAMINE RELEASE

A large number of agents cause direct histamine release from mast cells without prior sensitization or involvement of specific antibodies. These include peptides that contain basic amino acids (arginine and/or lysine), complement derivatives (C3a, C4a, and C5a), substance P, hymenoptera venom constituents such as melittin, and chemicals and therapeutic agents such as morphine, codeine, dextrans, blood substitutes, polymyxin B, radiocontrast media, quaternary ammonium compounds, pyridinium compounds, piperidines, alkaloids, and plasma expanders. Basically, pathways that result in a decrease in cAMP or pathways that result in an increase in cGMP will cause histamine release. The flushing and hypotension (the red-man syndrome) that often occurs during vancomycin infusion is probably due to direct histamine release (41). Various degrees of direct histamine release may also occur in certain individuals in response to particular foods (e.g., tomatoes, strawberries) or physical agents (e.g., dermographism) (42).

ANTIHISTAMINE PREPARATIONS

Development of antihistamines for allergy, gastric ulcers, motion sickness, and insomnia has utilized the diverse actions of histamine. These drugs have been so successful and widely used that the term "antihistamine" has become commonplace and mostly refer to H_1 antihistamines. In general, an antihistamine to a particular type of histamine receptor is not effective against the others. Since allergic reactions are primarily mediated through the activation of H_1 receptors, emphasis in this chapter will be given to H_1 antihistamines more than to the other types of antihistamines.

For years it was believed that H_1 antihistamines acted through competition with histamine for the receptors. Recent research showed that H_1 receptors exist in both active and inactive isoforms that are in equilibrium on the cellular surface and respond to the agonist (histamine) and inverse agonists (antihistamines), respectively (43). In other words, antihistamines act as inverse agonists that bind and stabilize the inactive form of the receptor shifting the equilibrium to the inactive state. This new understanding is rather important.

H_1 ANTIHISTAMINES

The first H_1 antihistamine, compound F929, was discovered in 1937 by Staub and Bovet (44). Shortly afterwards, Halpern in 1942 developed the first antihistamine for human use, phenbenzamine (*Antergan*) (45). Later diphenhydramine and numerous other preparations became available. Most H_1 antihistamines are stable, water-soluble salts and have similar pharmacologic actions and therapeutic applications. In general, the molecular structure of H_1 antihistamines comprises a double-aromatic unit linked by a two- or three-atom chain attached to a tertiary amino basic group. The histamine molecule has similar structure but differs from antihistamines (i.e., inverse agonists) in possessing only one aromatic (imidazole) unit and in being levorotatory, whereas antihistamines are dextrorotatory.

H_1 antihistamines have been traditionally classified into six groups: the ethanolamines, ethylenediamines, alkylamines, piperazines, piperidines, and phenothiazines. With the development of newer "nonsedating" preparations, they are generally classified as first- and second-generation antihistamines (Table 39.2). Some of the second-generation preparations are active metabolites of first-generation compounds; for example, fexofenadine, levocetirizine, and desloratadine are active metabolites of terfenadine, cetirizine, and loratadine, respectively.

TABLE 39.2 Chemical and Functional Classifications of H_1 Antihistamines

	Functional Classification	
Chemical Classification	*First Generation*	*Second Generation*
Alkylamines	Brompheniramine, chlorpheniramine, pheniramine	Acrivastine
Ethanolamines	Carbinoxamine, dimenhydrinate, diphenhydramine, doxylamine, phenyltoloxamine	
Ethylenediamines	Antazoline, pyrilamine, tripelennamine	
Phenothiazines	Methdilazine, promethazine	
Piperazines	Hydroxyzine, meclizine, oxatomide	Cetirizine, levocetirizine
Piperidines	Cyproheptadine, diphenylpyraline, ketotifen	Astemizole,[a] terfenadine,[a] fexofenadine, loratadine, desloratadine, ebastine, levocabastine, mizolastine, olopatadine
Phenothiazines	Methdilazine, promethazine	
Others	Doxepin[b]	Azelastine, emedastine, epinastine

[a]These antihistamines have been discontinued due to cardiotoxicity.
[b]Doxepin is classified as a tricyclic antidepressant and has H_1- and H_2-antihistamine effects.
Adapted from Simons FE. Advances in H_1-antihistamines. *N Engl J Med* 2004;351:2203–2217.

PHARMACOLOGIC PROPERTIES OF H_1 ANTIHISTAMINES

In general, first-generation H_1 antihistamines are rapidly absorbed and metabolized. Their binding to the receptors is readily reversible by spontaneous dissociation or by high levels of histamine. Most first-generation antihistamines have a short duration of action and optimally may need to be administered every 4 to 6 hours. Because of their lipophilicity and low molecular weight, they easily cross the blood–brain barrier, bind to the H_1 receptors, and create their CNS side effects (Table 39.3), primarily sedation, but in certain subjects CNS stimulation may occur.

The second-generation H_1 antihistamines are lipophobic and have high molecular weights and thus do not easily cross the blood–brain barrier, with minimal CNS adverse effects (16,46). They have longer duration of action (12 to 24 hours) because they strongly bind to the receptors and dissociate slowly (47). To date, at least 11 second-generation anti-H_1 preparations were studied in double-blind, placebo-controlled studies in children.

Almost all first-generation H_1 preparations have some antimuscarinic effect. Even at usual doses, they often cause dryness of the mucous membranes and sometimes urinary retention or blurred vision. Certain first-generation H_1 antihistamines, particularly promethazine, have α-adrenergic blocking ability (14). Others may exhibit antiserotonin activity (e.g., cyproheptadine) (14) or antidopamine effect (e.g., phenothiazines) (48). In high concentrations, some H_1 antihistamines, particularly promethazine, have a local anesthetic effect that can be more potent than procaine (10). Some CNS effects can be of therapeutic value, for example, dimenhydrinate and diphenhydramine for motion sickness and diphenhydramine in decreasing drug-induced extrapyramidal symptoms. Over the last two decades, some H_1-antihistamines have been found to have antiallergic, anti-inflammatory properties apart from their action on H_1 receptors (49,50). They downregulate allergic inflammation either by direct activation of H_1 receptors or indirectly through nuclear factor κB by suppressing antigen presentation, expression of proinflammatory cytokines and cell adhesion molecules, and chemotaxis. These antiallergic properties are believed to be due to their suppression of mast cell and basophil activity (51,52).

In addition to variation in their H_1-blocking activity and anti-inflammatory properties, the effect of H_1 antihistamines on various target organs varies widely, probably due to differences in their tissue deposition capacity. Moreover, it seems that the response, in terms of clinical efficacy and side effects, to any particular anti-H_1 medication varies from one patient to another (53). Such heterogeneity in response can be due to gene abnormalities in the synthetic and/or metabolic pathways or in the receptors (54,55). Polymorphisms of the enzymes in the metabolic pathway could enhance or delay their degradation. For example, one single nucleotide polymorphism for histamine *N*-methyltransferase, C314 T, results in decrease in enzyme activity and is found in 5% to 10% of the general population (56).

Desloratadine has better pharmacokinetics and lesser drug–drug interactions than its parent drug loratadine. Also, levocetirizine has better receptor affinity and selectivity than cetirizine.

TABLE 39.3 Mechanism of Common Side Effects of H_1 Antihistamines

Through H_1 receptor
Increased sedation
Decreased cognitive and psychomotor performance
Increased appetite
Through muscarinic receptor
Dry mouth
Urinary retention
Sinus tachycardia
Through α-adrenergic receptor
Hypotension
Dizziness
Reflex tachycardia
Through serotonin receptor
Increased appetite
K^+ and other cardiac ion-channels
Prolonged QT intervals

Adapted from Simons FE. New H_1-receptor antagonists: clinical pharmacology. *Clin Exp Allergy* 1990;20(Suppl 2):19–24.

PHARMACOKINETICS OF H_1 ANTIHISTAMINES

Comparative pharmacology of H_1 antihistamines has been reviewed recently (57). For most first-generation H_1 antihistamines, the pharmacokinetics (absorption, distribution, metabolism, and eliminations) has not been optimally investigated. Pharmacodynamic studies (correlations between drug concentrations and activity) were carried out for only a few preparations. Furthermore, first-generation H_1 antihistamines have not been investigated in young children or in patients with renal or hepatic insufficiency. Also, there are only a few studies regarding drug–drug and drug–food interactions (Table 39.4).

Most antihistamines are well absorbed from the gastrointestinal tract, achieving peak plasma concentration generally in 1 to 3 hours, with a therapeutic effect usually for 4 to 6 hours, and may last up to 24 hours for the newer preparations (10). The clinical effect persists even though the serum concentration of the parent compound has declined to the lowest limit of analytical detection, which suggests a continued action by active metabolites in the tissues. For some antihistamines, such as fexofenadine, bioavailability can be affected by the coadministration of foods such as grapefruit or bitter orange juice (58) or of other drugs such as verapamil, probenecid, and cimetidine (59).

Drug clearance is a measure of elimination. It is the volume of plasma that is completely cleared of the drug within a given period of time and is expressed as volume/time. The total body clearance of H_1 antihistamines is the sum of clearance from all organs and includes both hepatic and renal clearances. The clearance rate and plasma half-life vary widely from one preparation to another. The half-life is a measure of the time during which the drug plasma concentration decreases by 50%. H_1 antihistamines have half-life ranging from less than 24 hours up

TABLE 39.4 Pharmacokinetics, Formulations, and Pediatric Doses of H_1 Antihistamines

Generic Name	*Proprietary Name*	*Form (mg)*	t_{max} *(hr)*	$t_{1/2}$ *(hr)*	*Main Elimination Route*	*Drug–Drug Interaction*	*Pediatric Dose*
First Generation							
Astemizole	Hismanal	L: 10/5 mL T: 10	0.5	11 d	NA	Yes	0.2 mg/kg/d ≥12 yr: 10 mg q24 hr
Brompheniramine maleate	Alacol[a]	L: 2/5 mL D: 0.4/1 mL	NA	NA	NA	NA	2–5 yr:1 mg q4 hr 6–11 yr: 2 mg q4 hr ≥12 yr: 4 mg q4 hr
Carbinoxamine maleate	Palgic, Carbinox	L: 4/5 mL T: 4	NA	NA	NA	NA	1–17 mo: 0.5–2 mg q6 hr 2–3 yr: 2 mg q6–8 hr 3–6 yr: 2–4 mg q6–8 hr ≥6 yr: 4–6 mg q6–8 hr
Chlorpheniramine maleate	Chlortrimeton	L: 2/5 mL, 4/5 mL T: 4, 8[b], 12[b]	2.8	27.9	NA	Possible	6–11 yr: 2 mg q4–6 hr ≥12 yr: 4 mg q4–6 hr
Cyproheptadine hydrochloride	Periactin	L: 2/5 mL T: 4	NA	NA	NA	NA	2–6 yr: 0.25 mg/kg/d (q8–12 hr) 7–14 yr: 4 mg/d (q8–12 hr)
Dimenhydrinate	Dramamine	L: 12.5/5 mL 12.5/4 mL T: 50	NA	NA	NA	NA	2–5 yr: 12.5–25 mg q6–8 hr 6–11 yr: 25 mg q6–8 hr ≥12 yr: 50–100 mg q4–6 hr
Diphenhydramine hydrochloride	Benadryl	L: 12.5/5 mL T: 12.5, 25 C: 12.5, 25, 50 I: 50/mL S: 12.5, 25	1.7	9.2	NA	Possible	5 mg/kg/d (q6 hr) p.o., i.m., i.v. (max dose: 300 mg/d)
Hydroxyzine hydrochloride	Atarax Vistaril	L: 10/5 mL T: 10, 25, 50 I: 25, 50/mL	2.1	20	NA	Possible	<6 yr: 50 mg/d (q6–8 hr p.o.) ≥6 yr: 50–100 mg/d (q6–8 hr p.o.) or 0.5–1 mg/kg/dose q4–6 hr i.m.
Promethazine	Phenergan	L: 6.25/5 mL T: 12.5, 25, 50 Supp: 12.5, 25, 50 I: 25, 50/mL	NA	NA	NA	NA	≥2 yr: 6.25–12.5 mg q8 hr (0.1 mg/kg/dose, max: 12.5 mg/dose q6 hr for anti allergic action) >2 yr: 0.25–1 mg/kg/dose q4–6 hr p.o., i.m., i.v., p.r. for nausea/vomiting max: 25 mg/dose
Second Generation							
Acrivastine[c]	Semprex	C: 8	1.4	1.7	Renal	Unlikely	≥12 yr: 8 mg q6 hr
Cetirizine hydrochloride[c,d]	Zyrtec	L: 5/5 mL T: 5, 10	1	7.4	Renal	Unlikely	6 mo–<2 yr: 2.5 mg/d 2–5 yr: 2.5–5 mg/d ≥6–11 yr: 5–10 mg/d
Desloratadine[e]	Clarinex	L: 0.5/mL T: 5	1.5	24	Renal	Unlikely	6 mo–<1 yr: 1 mg q24 hr 1–5 yr: 1.25 mg q24 hr 6–11 yr: 2.5 mg q24 hr ≥12 yr: 5 mg q24 hr
Ebastine	Ebastel	T: 10	2.6	10	Renal	NA	NA
Fexofenadine[e]	Allegra	L: 30/5 mL T: 30, 60, 180	1–3	14.4	Bile	Unlikely	6 mo–<2 yr: 15 mg q12 hr 2–11 yr: 30 mg q12 hr ≥12 yr: 60 mg q12 hr
Ketotifen[c]	Zaditen	L: 1/5 mL T: 1.2	3.6	18.3	Renal	NA	>3 yr: 1 mg q12 hr

(*continued*)

TABLE 39.4 Pharmacokinetics, Formulations, and Pediatric Doses of H_1 Antihistamines (*Continued*)

Generic Name	*Proprietary Name*	*Form (mg)*	t_{max} *(hr)*	$t_{1/2}$ *(hr)*	*Main Elimination Route*	*Drug–Drug Interaction*	*Pediatric Dose*
Levocetirizine	Xyzal	L: 2.5/5 mL T: 5	0.8	7	Renal	Unlikely	6–11 yr: 2.5 mg q24 hr ≥12 yr: 5 mg q24 hr
Loratadine[e]	Claritin	L: 5/5 mL T: 10	1.2	7.8	Renal	Unlikely	2–5 yr: 5 mg q24 hr ≥6 yr: 10 mg q24 hr
Mizolastine	Mizollen	T: 10	1.5	12.9	Renal	NA	NA
Rupatadine	Rupafin, Rupax	T: 10	0.75	5.9	Bile	NA	≥12 yr: 10 mg q24 hr
Olopatadine	Patanase Pataday	N: 0.4%, 0.6%			NA		≥12 yr: 2 squirts q12 hr
Azelastine	Astelin	N: 1%	4–5	22	Bile	Unlikely	5–11 yr: 1 squirt q12 hr ≥12 yr: 2 squirts q12 hr

C, capsule or caplet; D, dropper; L, liquid; N, nasal; S, strips orally disintegrated; p.o., oral; Supp, suppository; T, tablet; i.v., intravenous; i.m., intramuscular; NA, data not available; t_{max}, average time from oral intake to peak plasma drug concentration; $t_{1/2}$, average terminal elimination half-life.

[a]Commercial preparation contains other medications.

[b]Sustained release.

[c]Mild sedative effect.

[d]Dose may be increased for children aged 12–23 mo to a max of 2.5 mg p.o. q12 hr, for children aged 2–5 yr to a max of 5 mg/24 hr.

[e]No sedative effect.

to a few days in children (60,61) and up to several days in adults (62,63) (Table 39.4).

The volume of distribution is a proportionality factor that relates the drug plasma concentration to its total amount in the body. Hence, the higher the degree of the drug's tissue distribution and binding, the lower is its concentration in the plasma. The volume of distribution of H_1 antihistamines varies widely, for example, 0.33 L per kg for levocabastine but exceeds 100 L per kg for loratadine and ebastine (10,14).

All first-generation H_1 antihistamines and most of the second-generation are metabolized by the hepatic cytochrome P450 (CYP450) system (64). Consequently, their metabolism can be affected by competition for the CYP enzymes by other drugs (e.g., ketoconazole and macrolide antibiotics) (60). Certain metabolites of two specific preparations, namely astemizole and terfenadine, can cause cardiac arrhythmia (torsades de pointes) if administered in high doses or in association with drugs that compete with the CYP system, or in the presence of liver or heart disease. This led to the withdrawal of terfenadine from the US market in 1998 and of astemizole in 1999 (10). Such arrhythmias have not been reported in association with loratadine, cetirizine, azelastine, or fexofenadine (the active metabolite of terfenadine) (14). The latter has slow and limited absorption by the oral route, minimal hepatic metabolism, with bioavailability around 30%, and a half-life around 14.4 hours (65).

Cetirizine and loratadine are primarily excreted into the urine, whereas fexofenadine and azelastine are mostly excreted in feces (14,66,67) (Table 39.4). It is worth noting that when combined with pseudoephedrine, the pharmacokinetics of loratadine or cetirizine does not change (68). Unlike other H_1 antihistamines, cetirizine is not metabolized by the CYP system and 70% of the drug excreted unchanged in the urine within 72 hours (61,62). The suppressive effect of antihistamines on the wheal-and-flare response to the percutaneous application of histamine or specific allergens varies from one preparation to another (64). Before allergy skin testing or bronchial challenge, it is generally recommended to discontinue first-generation H_1 antihistamines for 2 to 3 days and second-generation preparations for 7 to 10 days (69).

CLINICAL USES OF H_1 ANTIHISTAMINES

H_1 antihistamines are primarily used in the treatment of allergic diseases, particularly of the skin and the upper respiratory tract. First-generation preparations have not been optimally studied in allergic disorders. On the other hand, second-generation preparations have been adequately investigated in seasonal and perennial allergic rhinoconjunctivitis and chronic urticaria especially in adults. In fact, they are the first choice in the treatment of allergic rhinitis, allergic conjunctivitis, and chronic urticaria (16,46,70,71). Studies on these drugs in children are limited in number and are mostly for short durations (72).

In general, H_1 antihistamines are most effective to control allergy symptoms when taken on a regular basis rather than as needed (73), development of tolerance is rare (74). A recent study on respiratory allergies demonstrated that during the offending pollen season, the as needed use of desloratadine was as effective as regular intake in relieving nasal symptoms. However, the lower airway symptoms were better controlled on daily treatment (75).

Allergic Rhinoconjunctivitis

Histamine is one of the principle mediators released during nasal and ocular allergic inflammation causing itching,

TABLE 39.5 Ocular Antihistamine Preparations

Drug	*Action*	*Proprietary Name*	*Dosage*	*Side Effects*
Levocabastine	H_1 antihistamine	Livostin	>12 yr: 1 drop q6–12 hr	Ocular stinging, burning, headache
Olopatadine	H_1 antihistamine, mast cell stabilizer	Patanol	>3 yr: 1–2 drops q6–12 hr	Headache
Emedastine	H_1 antihistamine, inhibits eosinophil chemotaxis	Emadine	>3 yr: 1 drop q6 hr	Headache
Ketotifen	H_1 antihistamine, mast cell stabilizer, inhibits PAF, inhibits eosinophils	Zaditor	>3 yr: 1 drop q8–12 hr	Conjunctival injection, headache
Azelastine	H_1 antihistamine, mast cell stabilizer	Optivar	>3 yr: 1 drop q12 hr	Ocular burning, headache, bitter taste
Epinastine	H_1 and H_2 antihistamine, mast cell stabilizer, anti-inflammatory	Elestat	>3 yr: 1 drop q12 hr	Upper respiratory tract infection

sneezing, rhinorrhea, and lacrimation. Histamine-induced nasal obstruction is due to increased mucosal blood flow, enhanced nasal vascular permeability, and plasma protein exudation from fenestrated superficial capillaries.

The efficacy of H_1 antihistamines in allergic rhinitis has been well documented (76). Several studies have shown the efficacy and safety of H_1 antihistamines in children 4 to 12 years of age with seasonal allergic rhinitis (72,76). Using nasal airflow measurement, fexofenadine and desloratadine significantly reduced the nasal airway resistance (77,78). Antihistamines are most effective if started before the peak of pollination (63). Studies on children showed that all nasal symptoms and quality of life significantly improved on desloratadine 5 mg daily (79) or fexofenadine 30 mg twice daily (80). Also levocetirizine 5 mg per day was highly effective in improving nasal symptoms in school-age children with seasonal or perennial allergic rhinitis and in adolescents with perennial allergic rhinitis (81,82). To increase the relief of nasal blockage, α-adrenergic agonist decongestants, such as pseudoephedrine or phenylpropanolamine, may be added. In fact, the combination significantly improves other allergic rhinitis symptoms better than either drug alone (83).

In general, topical H_1 antihistamines have a more rapid onset of action than oral formulations. However, topical formulations require administration more than once a day (84). For example, both azelastine nasal preparation and levocabastine nasal and ocular preparations have rapid onset of action (10 to 15 minutes) and duration of effect for up to 12 hours (85,86). Because only a small quantity reaches the systemic circulation after topical application of these two antihistamines, the sedative effect is minimal. In a randomized, controlled study, azelastine nasal spray was found to be as effective as oral cetirizine in inhibiting allergen-induced mediator release from nasal mucosal mast cells (87). The choice of a particular antihistamine preparation would depend on the patient's preference for route of administration, dose regimen, as well as on potential benefits and side effects.

Likewise, ophthalmic preparations provide faster and superior relief than systemic antihistamines. Most of the ophthalmic H_1-antihistamines have multiple actions such as mast cell stabilization, inhibition of eosinophil chemotaxis, and H_2 antihistamine properties (88). Table 39.5 presents the common preparations, recommended dosage, mechanism of action, and side effects.

Asthma

Histamine is among several mediators of asthma, though not a major one. Multiple studies showed that the intake of antihistamines by patients with allergic rhinitis and asthma lead to improvement in symptoms, reduced need for bronchodilators, and modest, yet significant, increase in FEV_1 (89,90).

The differential effect of H_1 antihistamines on the early- versus late-phase bronchial responses is not clear (91). A prospective large multicenter study showed that cetirizine delays or, in some cases, prevents the development of asthma in infants with atopic dermatitis sensitized to grass pollen and, to a lesser extent, house dust mite during the 18-month treatment period and for the following 18-month duration (92).

Skin

H_1 antihistamines are the mainstay in the treatment of urticaria, with more striking benefit in acute than in chronic cases. Their action on the afferent C nerve fibers of the skin reduces the itching, on the axonic reflexes reduces the erythema, and on the endothelium of the postcapillary venules reduces extravasation and wheal formation (93). In chronic urticaria, fexofenadine in a dose of 120 mg per day was superior to diphenhydramine 50 mg per day (94), and of 180 mg per day was superior to chlorpheniramine 8 mg per day (93). Cetirizine 10 mg once daily was as effective as hydroxyzine 25 mg three times a day in reducing the frequency of exacerbation and average size of skin wheals (95). In some cases, the combination of H_1 and H_2 antihistamines results in better effect (96). Doxepin (a strong H_1 and H_2 antihistamine) is frequently used, particularly in severe cases, with good results (97). Cetirizine has been found to relieve delayed-pressure urticaria (98). In addition to clinical improvement, ketotifen reduced the plasma histamine levels in some patients with physical urticaria (99). The regular, long-term intake of levocetirizine, 0.125 mg per kg per day, was effective in preventing and treating urticaria in atopic young children (100).

In atopic dermatitis, itching is a major symptom, and histamine is one of its multiple mediators. First-generation antihistamines are commonly used in alleviating itching. It is debatable whether such effect is through blocking H_1 receptors in the skin or through inducing central sedation. In a study on children with atopic dermatitis, the antipruritic effect of a single dose of hydroxyzine was maintained for up to 24 hours when the drug's plasma concentration had become negligible (101). Some studies showed that loratadine and cetirizine can relieve atopic dermatitis symptoms in doses higher than those used for rhinitis (102,103). In addition, long-term regular treatment with levocetirizine prevented and treated urticaria in young children with atopic dermatitis (100).

In addition to the above conditions, antihistamines are useful in alleviating the symptoms of various cutaneous adverse drug reactions, including serum sickness. They are effective in preventing reactions secondary to direct histamine releasers, such as vancomycin (red-man syndrome) (10). They also induce marked relief of local reactions to insect stings or bites (104), and to various degrees in cases of mastocytosis (105).

Anaphylaxis

In systemic anaphylaxis, where the initial treatment must include epinephrine, H_1 antihistamines may be useful in reversing or limiting the progress of most anaphylaxis components. For rapid onset, parenteral administration is preferable over the oral route.

For maximal inhibition of flushing, headaches, hypotension, and tachycardia, a combination of H_1 and H_2 antihistamines is required (106). The additional administration of H_2 antihistamines is useful in the treatment or prophylaxis of acute systemic hypersensitivity reactions to radiocontrast media (107). In cases of idiopathic or exercise-induced anaphylaxis, the daily administration of oral H_1 antihistamines is often recommended.

Other

Upper Respiratory Tract Infections

H_1 antihistamines, alone or in combination with other medications, are commonly used to alleviate the symptoms of upper respiratory tract infections. Such a practice is not well supported by well-controlled studies. In most studies on children with viral upper respiratory infections, the administration of H_1 antihistamines resulted in the same rate of improvement in symptoms as placebo did (108). A meta-analysis (109) concluded that antihistamines as monotherapy did not significantly alleviate the symptoms of common cold in adults or children. However, when combined with decongestants, a modest beneficial effect was noted in older children and adults but not in young children.

Otitis Media

In otitis media, viral or bacterial, increased histamine levels can be seen in the middle ear fluid (110). However, the clinical effect of H_1 antihistamines in this condition was not statistically significant (111). A recent meta-analysis (112) found that the routine use of antihistamines for treating acute otitis media in children cannot be recommended. Nevertheless, the persistence rate at 2 weeks was lower when an antihistamine–decongestant combination was used.

Sedation

First-generation antihistamines, particularly diphenhydramine, are commonly used to improve sleep problems in children. This empiric use has been challenged by a recent study (113).

In addition to the above effects, certain H_1 antihistamines, such as diphenhydramine, hydroxyzine, and promethazine, have analgesic action. It is possible that this action is not due to histamine receptor binding but rather due to some other pharmacologic properties of these preparations (114).

Adverse Effects

The common mechanisms of side effects of H_1 antihistamines are summarized in Table 39.3. Sedation is the most frequently encountered side effect of the first-generation group and varies widely from one preparation to another and from one person to another. However, this effect may be desirable in cases of severe itching, such as in urticaria and atopic dermatitis. Sedation is less with the concomitant use of α-adrenergic decongestants. Concurrent ingestion of alcohol or other CNS suppressants markedly enhances the CNS side effects (115).

On the other hand, most second-generation H_1 antihistamines have no or minimal sedative effect and can be administered with alcohol, sedatives, hypnotics, antidepressants, or other CNS-active substances (116,117). The sedative effect of cetirizine is reported by 6% of patients (118).

Diphenhydramine in the recommended doses is relatively safe. However, toxicity has been reported, particularly from higher doses. First-generation H_1 antihistamines may have paradoxical CNS stimulatory effect in infants and young children resulting in irritability, nervousness, excitation, insomnia, and even seizures (16,119,120). There was some concern about apnea in infants and even sudden infant death syndrome related to the administration of first-generation antihistamines (121). The Food and Drug Administration (FDA) added a warning black box to the label of promethazine, including a contraindication for use in children younger than 2 years because of reported serious adverse events, such as respiratory depression and CNS reactions, including seizures (122).

It has been reported that school performance is worsened by the intake of diphenhydramine but not by loratadine (123), which may be attributed to the improvement of rhinitis rather than to the lack of its sedative effect. However, such finding was not reported by another study (124). In spite of its slight sedative effect, cetirizine long-term intake by children with atopic dermatitis showed no adverse effects on learning (125).

The antimuscarinic effect of first-generation antihistamines can cause dry mouth, dysfunctional urine voiding, and sinus tachycardia. Through α-adrenergic suppression, some antihistamines cause hypotension, dizziness, and reflex tachycardia (16).

Gastrointestinal adverse effects of antihistamines are seen in 1.4% to 10.1% of patients and include loss of appetite, nausea, vomiting, dyspepsia, and constipation or diarrhea (118). Their occurrence can be reduced by taking the drug with meals. Cyproheptadine, however, causes appetite stimulation, which is believed to be secondary to antiserotonin effect (126). Ketotifen may cause some weight gain as well (127). Patients taking intranasal azelastine often complain of a bitter taste.

Cardiac arrhythmias have been a main concern in treatment with antihistamines. They are not class effects but rather are related to particular preparations. Terfenadine and astemizole have been abandoned because of their increased risk of causing serious arrhythmias particularly in patients with heart disease, hypokalemia, or concomitant intake of medications metabolized by the CYP450 system (128,129). Arrhythmias are very rarely associated with the intake of cyproheptadine, diphenhydramine, hydroxyzine, or tricyclic antidepressants (130). At least in the recommended doses, acrivastine, azelastine, cetirizine, ebastine, fexofenadine, loratadine, and mizolastine have not been reported to cause any electrocardiographic changes (131–133).

Other rare adverse effects that have been reported include hypersensitivity reactions that can be in the form of drug fever (10), pruritic exanthema (134), urticaria (135), dermatitis (136), photosensitization (137), and even anaphylaxis (138). Hematologic adverse reactions are rare and can be in the form of leukopenia, agranulocytosis, or hemolytic anemia (10).

Overdosage

Toxicity usually results from the administration of a quantity several fold the recommended dose or occurs in patients with renal or hepatic disease. Most reported toxicities have been related to the first-generation antihistamines—brompheniramine, chlorpheniramine, cyproheptadine, dimenhydrinate, diphenhydramine, doxylamine, hydroxyzine, and promethazine. These preparations are also implicated in suicide attempts and in infant homicides (119,139). Symptoms of overdose usually occur within 15 to 30 minutes after ingestion and are mostly related to the CNS. Although adults and older children usually develop drowsiness and lethargy, young children often develop stimulation such as hallucination, excitation, ataxia, incoordination, athetosis, and convulsions (10).

The antimuscarinic effect is manifested as dry mouth, flushed face, fever, pupillary dilation, urinary retention, decreased gastrointestinal motility, hypotension, and tachycardia. In patients overdosed with a first-generation antihistamine, dose-dependent cardiac toxicity, including prolonged QTc interval and torsade de pointes, may occur. The patient should be monitored until QTc interval normalizes. Torsade de pointes requires cardioversion and pacing. In such instances, it would be prudent to avoid the antiarrhythmic medications—quinidine, flecainide, amiodarone, and sotalol, as they may further prolong the QTc interval (130). Severe cases may end up in cardiorespiratory collapse, coma, and even death (140). Because there are no specific antidotes for H_1 antihistamine, treatment consists of appropriate symptomatic and supportive measures. Some cases might need hemodialysis. Activated charcoal is helpful in reducing the absorption of the drug (141). Because of the CNS suppressive effect of antihistamines, ipecac is usually ineffective in inducing emesis in such patients.

Second-generation H_1 antihistamines rarely cause significant toxicity, and the treatment is primarily supportive and symptomatic because most such preparations are not dialyzable (142).

Use during Pregnancy and Lactation

H_1 antihistamines can cross the placenta to various degrees. According to the FDA drug classification safety during pregnancy (Table 39.6), category B includes chlorpheniramine, diphenhydramine, cetirizine, levocetirizine, loratadine, and topical emedastine, epinastine, and olopatadine and category C includes azatadine, hydroxyzine, fexofenadine, azelastine, levocabastine, and olopatadine.

No teratogenic effect was demonstrated for cetirizine (143) and loratadine (144). A recent study found that none of the 14 antihistamines taken during early pregnancy by 738 women was linked to any of 26 isolated major birth defects (145). Another study found no significant difference in the rate of congenital anomalies in the offspring of pregnant women who took loratadine or other antihistamines, compared with those who took nonteratogenic medications (146). Nevertheless, the administration

TABLE 39.6 Food and Drug Administration Pregnancy Risk Categories

Category	*Animal Studies*	*Teratogenicity*[a] *Human Studies*	*Benefit May Outweigh the Risk*
A	Negative	Negative	Yes
B	Negative	Not done	Yes
B	Positive	Negative	Yes
C	Positive	Not done	Yes
C	Not done	Not done	Yes
D	Positive or negative	Positive	Yes
X[a]	Positive	Reports positive	No

[a]Drug is contraindicated during pregnancy.

of a large therapeutic dose of a first-generation H_1 antihistamine such as hydroxyzine or diphenhydramine shortly before delivery was associated with withdrawal symptoms (tremulousness and irritability) in the newborn (147,148).

In lactating mothers receiving first-generation H_1 antihistamines, irritability or drowsiness has been reported in their nursing infants (149). Second-generation H_1 antihistamines are also excreted in breast milk (e.g., 0.03% of the total maternal loratadine dose) (150); however, they have not been reported to cause symptoms in the nursing neonate.

INTERACTIONS WITH OTHER MEDICATIONS AND FOODS

For H_1 antihistamines that cause sedation, the addition of other drugs that suppress the CNS (e.g., tricyclic antidepressants, barbiturates, hypnotics, sedatives, tranquilizers, and alcohol) would impose danger, particularly while the patient is driving or operating machinery. Similarly, the autonomic blocking effects of conventional antihistamines are additional to the antimuscarinic and α-adrenergic-blocking effects. Monoamine oxidase inhibitors were found to prolong and intensify the antimuscarinic effects of antihistamines (14).

All first-generation H_1 antihistamines and some second-generation preparations such as desloratadine and loratadine are metabolized by the hepatic CYP450 system in the liver. The activity of this enzyme can be altered by other drugs. Therefore, plasma concentration of H_1 antihistamines decreases with the concomitant intake of drugs that stimulate the CYP450 enzyme system, for example, benzodiazepines. The opposite would occur as a result of coadministration of macrolides, antifungals, or calcium antagonists, which compete for the CYP450 system.

The coadministration of fexofenadine and ketoconazole or erythromycin increases the plasma level of fexofenadine but does not affect the pharmacokinetics of ketoconazole or erythromycin. The fexofenadine absorption is decreased by approximately 40% if administered within 15 minutes of taking aluminum- and magnesium-containing antacid (151).

Fexofenadine is absorbed via an active transport system in the intestine. The ingestion of grapefruit juice with fexofenadine lowers the peak plasma drug concentration to 58% and mean area under the curve (plasma drug concentration–time) to 53% by inhibiting an organic anion transporting polypeptide (58).

H_2 ANTIHISTAMINES

H_2 antihistamines have been widely used in gastric peptic disease (Chapter 50) and in a variety of conditions that are briefly mentioned below.

CHEMISTRY AND PHARMACOKINETICS

In the United States, at present there are four preparations of H_2 antihistamines: cimetidine, famotidine, nizatidine, and ranitidine (Table 39.7). They differ mainly in their pharmacokinetics and propensity to cause drug interactions. H_2 antihistamines do not bind to other histamine receptor subtypes.

H_2 antihistamines are rapidly absorbed after oral administration, with peak plasma concentrations at 1 to 3 hours. Their volume of distribution ranges from 0.8 to 1.18 L per kg and binding to plasma proteins from 15% to 35% (152). Absorption may be enhanced by food or decreased by antacids, but these effects probably are not clinically significant. Therapeutic levels are achieved rapidly after intravenous administration and are maintained for 4 to 5 hours for cimetidine, 6 to 8 hours for ranitidine, and 10 to 12 hours for famotidine. Only small quantities are metabolized by the liver. The half-life of H_2 antihistamines ranges from 1.3 to 4 hours. Their excretion is mainly by the kidney; hence, the dose should be reduced in patients with renal disease (152,153). Neither hemodialysis nor peritoneal dialysis clears significant amounts.

USES IN ALLERGIC AND IMMUNOLOGIC DISORDERS

Allergic Rhinitis and Asthma

H_1 antihistamines administered simultaneously with H_2 antihistamines were found to be significantly more effective in decreasing nasal airflow resistance induced by histamine or allergen challenge than either alone (154). However, H_2 antihistamines have no primary role in the treatment of allergic rhinitis or asthma, but they could be useful in patients with concomitant gastroesophageal reflux (155).

Skin

As mentioned earlier, some patients with chronic urticaria or dermographism experience more improvement by adding H_2 antihistamines to anti-H_1 preparations (96). Some tricyclic antidepressants, such as doxepin, have potent H_1- and H_2-antihistamine properties (156). As an H_1 antihistamine, doxepin is 800 times more potent than diphenhydramine and 50 times more potent than hydroxyzine, and as an H_2 antihistamine, it is 6 times more potent than cimetidine (157).

The combination of oral H_2 antihistamine (ranitidine) and topical corticosteroid was shown to be more effective than the latter alone in atopic dermatitis (158). Doxepin ointment has shown marked relief of pruritus associated with atopic dermatitis, though in some patients causes burning sensation and occasionally sensitization (159).

Anaphylaxis

In anaphylaxis, increased histamine release results in a variety of responses, including vasodilation and hypotension. As mentioned earlier, combination of H_1 and H_2 antihistamines is more effective than H_1 alone to treat these symptoms. However, the rapid intravenous administration of cimetidine can induce hypotension, bradycardia, and even asystole (160).

Immunomodulation

A few studies have demonstrated a role for H_2 antihistamines as potential immunomodulators. Cimetidine 30 to 40 mg per kg of body weight daily for 3 to 6 months resulted in resolution of warts in some patients (161). It is also useful in

TABLE 39.7 H_2 Antihistamines

Drug (Proprietary)	*Formulation (mg)*	*Bioavailability (Oral) (%)*	V_d *(L/kg)*	$t_{1/2}$ *(hr)*	*Pediatric Dosage*
Cimetidine (Tagamet)	T: 100,[a] 200, 300, 400, 800 L: 300/5 mL I: 150/mL	30–80	0.8–1.2	1.5–2.3	**Neonate:** p.o./i.m./i.v. 5–20 mg/kg/24 hr q6–12 hr **Infant:** p.o./i.m./i.v. 10–20 mg/kg/24 hr q6–12 hr **Child:** p.o./i.m./i.v. 20–40 mg/kg/24 hr q6 hr
Famotidine (Pepcid)	T: 10,[a] 20, 40 L: 40/5 mL I: 10/mL	37–45	1.1 - 1.4	2.5–4	**Neonate:** i.v. 0.5 mg/kg q24 hr **≥3 mo–1 yr (GERD):** p.o. 0.5 mg/kg q12 hr **Child:** i.v. initial: 0.6–0.8 mg/kg/24 hr q8–12 hr (max: 40 mg/d) p.o. initial: 1–1.2 mg/kg/24 hr q8–12 hr (max: 40 mg/d) Peptic ulcer: p.o. 0.5 mg/kg/24 hr q.h.s. or q12 hr (max: 40 mg/d) GERD: p.o. 1 mg/kg/24 hr q12 hr (max: 80 mg/d) **Adolescent:** Duodenal ulcer: p.o. 20 mg q12 hr or 40 mg q.h.s. × 4–8 wk, then 20 mg q.h.s.; i.v. 20 mg q12 hr Esophagitis and GERD: p.o. 20 mg q12 hr
Nizatidine (Axid)	C: 75, 150, 300	75–100	1.2–1.6	1.1–1.6	Not established
Ranitidine (Zantac)	T: 75,[a] 150, 300 L: 15/mL I: 25/mL	30–88	1.2–1.9	1.6–2.4	**Neonate:** p.o. 2–4 mg/kg/24 hr q8–12 hr i.v. 2 mg/kg/24 hr q6–8 hr **>1 mo–16 yr:** Duodenal/gastric ulcer: p.o./i.m./i.v. 2–4 mg/kg/d q12 hr (max: 150 mg/d) GERD/erosive esophagitis: p.o. 5–10 mg/kg/d q12 hr (GERD max: 300 mg/d; erosive esophagitis max: 600 mg/d) i.m./i.v. 5–10 mg/kg/d q6–8 hr (max: 150 mg/d)

C, capsule; GERD, gastroesophageal reflux disease; i.m., intramuscular; I, injectable; i.v., intravenous; L, liquid; max, maximum; p.o., oral; q, every; q.h.s., every night; T, tablet; $t_{1/2}$, terminal elimination half-life; V_d, volume of distribution.
[a]Over-the-counter preparation.

improving the symptoms of PFAPA syndrome (periodic fever, cervical adenitis, pharyngitis, aphthous stomatitis) in a dose of 150 mg once or twice a day or 20 to 40 mg per kg daily (162). Cimetidine has shown an immunomodulator effect in patients with acquired immune deficiency syndrome (163). It also prolonged survival of patients with resectable gastric and colorectal cancer and caused significant melanoma regression (164). In renal transplant patients, cimetidine contributed to the allograft maintenance. H_2 antihistamines may also have immunomodulatory functions in patients with autoimmune disorders, such as sclerosing panencephalomyelitis or psoriasis (165,166).

Use during Pregnancy and Lactation

The intake of H_2 antihistamines during the first trimester does not seem to have a teratogenic risk (167). Nevertheless, its use during pregnancy should be limited to cases when the anticipated benefits outweigh the unknown fetal risks. Although H_2 antihistamines are excreted in breast milk (168), the quantity seems to be too small to constitute a risk to the nursing infant.

ADVERSE EFFECTS OF H_2 ANTIHISTAMINES

H_2 antihistamines rarely cause side effects (10). Less than 3% of patients receiving cimetidine and less than 1% of those receiving ranitidine, famotidine, or nizatidine develop side effects, mainly gastrointestinal (diarrhea or constipation) or CNS (headache, somnolence, or confusion). Prolonged use of cimetidine in high doses may cause reversible gynecomastia, breast tenderness, or impotence in men, possibly because it displaces endogenous androgens from their receptor sites.

INTERACTIONS WITH OTHER MEDICATIONS

Cimetidine reduces the hepatic metabolism of certain drugs including warfarin, phenytoin, propranolol, nifedipine, chlordiazepoxide, diazepam, certain tricyclic antidepressants, lidocaine, theophylline, and metronidazole (169) especially in the presence of hepatic dysfunction or in the elderly (153). Drugs that are best absorbed in acidic environment (e.g., ketoconazole and itraconazole) should be given at least 2 hours before H_2 antihistamines (170). The gastrointestinal absorption of cimetidine is reduced if administered with certain antacids (10).

In recommended doses, ranitidine does not inhibit the CYP450 enzymes in the liver, though it may affect the bioavailability of certain drugs (e.g., triazolam). On the other hand, famotidine and nizatidine do not bind to the CYP450 system, and no drug interactions have been identified with these two drugs (14).

H_3 ANTIHISTAMINES

H_3 antihistamines stimulate histamine production and enhance the release of other neurotransmitters such as serotonin, acetylcholine, norepinephrine, dopamine, and *N*-methyl-D-aspartate. Hence, their potential in the management of obesity, depression, seizures, cognitive dysfunction, and attention-deficit hyperactivity disorder in children (171).

Because the stimulation of H_3 receptors inhibits norepinephrine release which is involved in reversing the hypotension in anaphylaxis, blockade of H_3 receptor may have a beneficial effect as demonstrated in canine model of anaphylaxis (172). Some H_3 agonists and inverse agonists are currently in phase II clinical trials and their application might be in the near future (171).

H_4 ANTIHISTAMINES

H_4 receptor has the highest sequence homology with the H_3 receptor and can bind to H_3 antihistamines, though with lower affinity (54). It is expressed primarily on cells of hematopoietic origin (notably mast cells, basophils, and eosinophils) and to a lesser extent on the intestinal mucosal epithelium (54,173,174), suggesting a possible role in inflammatory conditions. A newly developed selective H_4 antihistamine (JNJ7777120) has demonstrated a high potency in blocking H_4-mediated responses (175). H_4 antihistamines are promising therapy for certain inflammatory conditions that involve mast cells and eosinophils, such as allergic rhinitis, asthma, and rheumatoid arthritis (176).

REFERENCES

1. Windaus A, Vogt W. Synthèse des imidazolyllathylamins. *Ber Deutsch Chem Ges* 1907;3:3691–3695.
2. Dale HH, Laidlaw PP. Further observations on the action of beta-iminazolylethylamine. *J Physiol* 1911;43:182–195.
3. Dale HH, Laidlaw PP. The physiological action of beta-iminazolylethylamine. *J Physiol* 1910;41:318–344.
4. Best CH, Dale HH, Dudley HW, et al. The nature of the vasodilator constituents of certain tissue extracts. *J Physiol* 1927;62:397–417.
5. Lewis T. *The blood vessels of human skin and their responses.* London, UK: Shaw & Son, 1927.
6. Riley JF, West GB. Histamine in tissue mast cells. *J Physiol* 1952;117:72–73.
7. Riley JF, West GB. The occurrence of histamine in mast cells. In: Silva RE, ed. *Handbook of experimental pharmacology: histamine and antihistamines,* vol. XVIII, Part I. New York: Springer-Verlag, 1966:116–135.
8. Mongar JL, Schild HO. Quantitative measurement of the histamine-releasing activity of a series of mono-alkyl-amines using minced guinea pig lung. *Br J Pharmacol Chemother* 1953;8:103–109.
9. Foreman J, Mongar JL. The control of secretion from mast cells. In: Pepys J, Edwards AM, eds. *The mast cell in health and disease.* England: Pitman Medical, 1980:30–37.
10. Skidgel RA, Erdos EG. Histamine, bradykinin, and their antagonists. In: Brunton LL, Lazo JS, Parker KL eds. *Goodman & Gilman's The pharmacological basis of therapeutics,* 11th ed. New York: McGraw-Hill Companies Inc., 2006.
11. Kapeller-Adler R. Histamine catabolism in vitro and in vivo. *Fed Proc* 1965;24:757–765.
12. Metcalfe DD. Effector cell heterogeneity in immediate hypersensitivity reactions. *Clin Rev Allergy* 1983;1:311–325.
13. McNeill JH. Histamine and the heart. *Can J Physiol Pharmacol* 1984;62:720–726.
14. Katzung BG. Histamine, serotonin, & the ergot alkaloids. In: Katzung BG, ed. *Basic & clinical pharmacology,* 10th ed. New York: McGraw-Hill Companies Inc., 2007.
15. Ash AS, Schild HO. Receptors mediating some actions of histamine. *Br J Pharmacol Chemother* 1966;27:427–439.
16. Simons FE. Advances in H_1-antihistamines. *N Engl J Med* 2004;351:2203–2217.
17. Arrang JM, Garbarg M, Schwartz JC. Auto-inhibition of brain histamine release mediated by a novel class (H_3) of histamine receptor. *Nature* 1983;302:832–837.
18. Lovenberg TW, Roland BL, Wilson SJ, et al. Cloning and functional expression of the human histamine H_3 receptor. *Mol Pharmacol* 1999;55:1101–1107.
19. Teuscher C, Subramanian M, Noubade R, et al. Central histamine H_3 receptor signaling negatively regulates susceptibility to autoimmune inflammatory disease of the CNS. *Proc Natl Acad Sci U S A* 2007;104:10146–10151.
20. Leurs R, Hoffmann M, Wieland K, et al. H_3 receptor gene is cloned at last. *Trends Pharmacol Sci* 2000;21:11–12.
21. Nakamura T, Itadani H, Hidaka Y, et al. Molecular cloning and characterization of a new human histamine receptor, HH4R. *Biochem Biophys Res Commun* 2000;279:615–620.
22. Nguyen T, Shapiro DA, George SR, et al. Discovery of a novel member of the histamine receptor family. *Mol Pharmacol* 2001;59:427–433.
23. Dijkstra D, Stark H, Chazot PL, et al. Human inflammatory dendritic epidermal cells express a functional histamine H_4 receptor. *J Invest Dermatol* 2008;128:1696–1703.
24. Hattori Y. Cardiac histamine receptors: their pharmacological consequences and signal transduction pathways. *Methods Find Exp Clin Pharmacol* 1999;21:123–131.
25. Bristow MR, Ginsburg R, Harrison DC. Histamine and the human heart: the other receptor system. *Am J Cardiol* 1982;49:249–251.
26. Imamura M, Poli E, Omoniyi AT, et al. Unmasking of activated histamine H_3-receptors in myocardial ischemia: their role as regulators of exocytotic norepinephrine release. *J Pharmacol Exp Ther* 1994;271:1259–1266.
27. Malinowska B, Godlewski G, Schlicker E. Histamine H_3 receptors—general characterization and their function in the cardiovascular system. *J Physiol Pharmacol* 1998;49:191–211.
28. Nault MA, Milne B, Parlow JL. Effects of the selective H_1 and H_2 histamine receptor antagonists loratadine and ranitidine on autonomic control of the heart. *Anesthesiology* 2002;96:336–341.
29. Palmer RM, Ferrige AG, Moncada S. Nitric oxide release accounts for the biological activity of endothelium-derived relaxing factor. *Nature* 1987;327:524–526.

30. Bechi P, Romagnoli P, Panula P, et al. Gastric mucosal histamine storing cells. Evidence for different roles of mast cells and enterochromaffin-like cells in humans. *Dig Dis Sci* 1995;40:2207–2213.
31. Panula P, Airaksinen MS, Pirvola U, et al. A histamine-containing neuronal system in human brain. *Neuroscience* 1990;34:127–132.
32. Thurmond RL, Gelfand EW, Dunford PJ. The role of histamine H_1 and H_4 receptors in allergic inflammation: the search for new antihistamines. *Nat Rev Drug Discov* 2008;7:41–53.
33. Varga C, Horvath K, Berko A, et al. Inhibitory effects of histamine H_4 receptor antagonists on experimental colitis in the rat. *Eur J Pharmacol* 2005;522:130–138.
34. Dunford PJ, O'Donnell N, Riley JP, et al. The histamine H_4 receptor mediates allergic airway inflammation by regulating the activation of CD4+ T cells. *J Immunol* 2006;176:7062–7070.
35. Dunford PJ, Williams KN, Desai PJ, et al. Histamine H_4 receptor antagonists are superior to traditional antihistamines in the attenuation of experimental pruritus. *J Allergy Clin Immunol* 2007; 119:176–183.
36. Serafin WE, Austen KF. Mediators of immediate hypersensitivity reactions. *N Engl J Med* 1987;317:30–34.
37. Johnson HH Jr, Deoreo GA, Lascheid WP, et al. Skin histamine levels in chronic atopic dermatitis. *J Invest Dermatol* 1960;34: 237–238.
38. Juhlin L. Localization and content of histamine in normal and diseased skin. *Acta Derm Venereol* 1967;47:383–391.
39. Kaplan AP, Horakova Z, Katz SI. Assessment of tissue fluid histamine levels in patients with urticaria. *J Allergy Clin Immunol* 1978;61:350–354.
40. Wenzel SE, Fowler AA III, Schwartz LB. Activation of pulmonary mast cells by bronchoalveolar allergen challenge. In vivo release of histamine and tryptase in atopic subjects with and without asthma. *Am Rev Respir Dis* 1988;137:1002–1008.
41. Levy JH, Kettlekamp N, Goertz P, et al. Histamine release by vancomycin: a mechanism for hypotension in man. *Anesthesiology* 1987;67:122–125.
42. de Weck AL. Pathophysiologic mechanisms of allergic and pseudo-allergic reactions to foods, food additives and drugs. *Ann Allergy* 1984;53:583–586.
43. Leurs R, Church MK, Taglialatela M. H_1-antihistamines: inverse agonism, anti-inflammatory actions and cardiac effects. *Clin Exp Allergy* 2002;32:489–498.
44. Staub AM, Bovet D. Action de la thymoxyethyl-diethylamine (929F) et des ethers phenoliques sur le choc anaphylactique du cobaye. *CRS Soc Biol* 1937;125:818.
45. Halpern BN. Les antihistaminiques de synthèse: essai de chimiothérapie des etas allergiques. *Arch Int Pharmacodyn Ther* 1942;68: 339–408.
46. Holgate ST, Canonica GW, Simons FE, et al. Consensus Group on New-Generation Antihistamines (CONGA): present status and recommendations. *Clin Exp Allergy* 2003;33:1305–1324.
47. Simons FE. New H_1-receptor antagonists: clinical pharmacology. *Clin Exp Allergy* 1990;20(Suppl 2):19–24.
48. Campbell M, Bateman DN. Pharmacokinetic optimisation of antiemetic therapy. *Clin Pharmacokinet* 1992;23:147–160.
49. Church MK, Gradidge CF. Inhibition of histamine release from human lung in vitro by antihistamines and related drugs. *Br J Pharmacol* 1980;69:663–667.
50. Vena GA, Cassano N, Buquicchio R, et al. Antiinflammatory effects of H_1-antihistamines: clinical and immunological relevance. *Curr Pharm Des* 2008;14:2902–2911.
51. Agrawal DK. Anti-inflammatory properties of desloratadine. *Clin Exp Allergy* 2004;34:1342–1348.
52. Wu P, Mitchell S, Walsh GM. A new antihistamine levocetirizine inhibits eosinophil adhesion to vascular cell adhesion molecule-1 under flow conditions. *Clin Exp Allergy* 2005;35:1073–1079.
53. Carlsen KH, Kramer J, Fagertun HE, et al. Loratadine and terfenadine in perennial allergic rhinitis. Treatment of nonresponders to the one drug with the other drug. *Allergy* 1993;48: 431–436.
54. Hough LB. Genomics meets histamine receptors: new subtypes, new receptors. *Mol Pharmacol* 2001;59:415–419.
55. Tsai YJ, Hoyme HE. Pharmacogenomics: the future of drug therapy. *Clin Genet* 2002;62:257–264.
56. Igaz P, Fitzimons CP, Szalai C, et al. Histamine genomics in silico: polymorphisms of the human genes involved in the synthesis, action and degradation of histamine. *Am J Pharmacogenomics* 2002;2:67–72.
57. Simons FE, Simons KJ. H_1 antihistamines: current status and future directions. *World Allergy Organiz J* 2008;1:145–155.
58. Dresser GK, Kim RB, Bailey DG. Effect of grapefruit juice volume on the reduction of fexofenadine bioavailability: possible role of organic anion transporting polypeptides. *Clin Pharmacol Ther* 2005;77:170–177.
59. Yasui-Furukori N, Uno T, Sugawara K, et al. Different effects of three transporting inhibitors, verapamil, cimetidine, and probenecid, on fexofenadine pharmacokinetics. *Clin Pharmacol Ther* 2005;77:17–23.
60. Simons FE, Bergman JN, Watson WT, et al. The clinical pharmacology of fexofenadine in children. *J Allergy Clin Immunol* 1996; 98:1062–1064.
61. Watson WT, Simons KJ, Chen XY, et al. Cetirizine: a pharmacokinetic and pharmacodynamic evaluation in children with seasonal allergic rhinitis. *J Allergy Clin Immunol* 1989;84:457–464.
62. Simons FE, Simons KJ. H_1 receptor antagonists: clinical pharmacology and use in allergic disease. *Pediatr Clin North Am* 1983;30: 899–914.
63. Wood SG, John BA, Chasseaud LF, et al. The metabolism and pharmacokinetics of 14 C-cetirizine in humans. *Ann Allergy* 1987; 59:31–34.
64. Simons FE, Simons KJ. The pharmacology and use of H_1-receptor-antagonist drugs. *N Engl J Med* 1994;330:1663–1670.
65. Chen C. Some pharmacokinetic aspects of the lipophilic terfenadine and zwitterionic fexofenadine in humans. *Drugs R D* 2007; 8:301–314.
66. Spencer CM, Faulds D, Peters DH. Cetirizine. A reappraisal of its pharmacological properties and therapeutic use in selected allergic disorders. *Drugs* 1993;46:1055–1080.
67. Russell T, Stoltz M, Weir S. Pharmacokinetics, pharmacodynamics, and tolerance of single- and multiple-dose fexofenadine hydrochloride in healthy male volunteers. *Clin Pharmacol Ther* 1998;64:612–621.
68. Wellington K, Jarvis B. Cetirizine/pseudoephedrine. *Drugs* 2001; 61:2231–2240; discussion 2241–2242.
69. Bernstein IL, Li JT, Bernstein DI, et al. Allergy diagnostic testing: an updated practice parameter. *Ann Allergy Asthma Immunol* 2008;100:S1–148.
70. Plaut M, Valentine MD. Clinical practice. Allergic rhinitis. *N Engl J Med* 2005;353:1934–1944.
71. Hair PI, Scott LJ. Levocetirizine: a review of its use in the management of allergic rhinitis and skin allergies. *Drugs* 2006;66: 973–996.
72. de Benedictis FM, de Benedictis D, Canonica GW. New oral H_1 antihistamines in children: facts and unmeet needs. *Allergy* 2008;63:1395–1404.
73. Ciprandi G, Ricca V, Tosca M, et al. Continuous antihistamine treatment controls allergic inflammation and reduces respiratory morbidity in children with mite allergy. *Allergy* 1999;54:358–365.
74. Bachert C, Bousquet J, Canonica GW, et al. Levocetirizine improves quality of life and reduces costs in long-term management of persistent allergic rhinitis. *J Allergy Clin Immunol* 2004; 114:838–844.
75. Dizdar EA, Sekerel BE, Keskin O, et al. The effect of regular versus on-demand desloratadine treatment in children with allergic rhinitis. *Int J Pediatr Otorhinolaryngol* 2007;71:843–849.
76. Carr WW. Pediatric allergic rhinitis: current and future state of the art. *Allergy Asthma Proc* 2008;29:14–23.
77. Horak F, Stubner UP, Zieglmayer R, et al. Effect of desloratadine versus placebo on nasal airflow and subjective measures of nasal obstruction in subjects with grass pollen-induced allergic rhinitis in an allergen-exposure unit. *J Allergy Clin Immunol* 2002;109: 956–961.
78. Wilson AM, Haggart K, Sims EJ, et al. Effects of fexofenadine and desloratadine on subjective and objective measures of nasal congestion in seasonal allergic rhinitis. *Clin Exp Allergy* 2002;32: 1504–1509.
79. Kim K, Sussman G, Hebert J, et al. Desloratadine therapy for symptoms associated with perennial allergic rhinitis. *Ann Allergy Asthma Immunol* 2006;96:460–465.
80. Meltzer EO, Scheinmann P, Rosado Pinto JE, et al. Safety and efficacy of oral fexofenadine in children with seasonal allergic

rhinitis—a pooled analysis of three studies. *Pediatr Allergy Immunol* 2004;15:253–260.
81. Potter PC. Levocetirizine is effective for symptom relief including nasal congestion in adolescent and adult (PAR) sensitized to house dust mites. *Allergy* 2003;58:893–899.
82. Potter PC. Efficacy and safety of levocetirizine on symptoms and health-related quality of life of children with perennial allergic rhinitis: a double-blind, placebo-controlled randomized clinical trial. *Ann Allergy Asthma Immunol* 2005;95:175–180.
83. Sussman GL, Mason J, Compton D, et al. The efficacy and safety of fexofenadine HCl and pseudoephedrine, alone and in combination, in seasonal allergic rhinitis. *J Allergy Clin Immunol* 1999;104: 100–106.
84. Horak F, Zieglmayer UP, Zieglmayer R, et al. Azelastine nasal spray and desloratadine tablets in pollen-induced seasonal allergic rhinitis: a pharmacodynamic study of onset of action and efficacy. *Curr Med Res Opin* 2006;22:151–157.
85. McTavish D, Sorkin EM. Azelastine. A review of its pharmacodynamic and pharmacokinetic properties, and therapeutic potential. *Drugs* 1989;38:778–800.
86. Dechant KL, Goa KL. Levocabastine. A review of its pharmacological properties and therapeutic potential as a topical antihistamine in allergic rhinitis and conjunctivitis. *Drugs* 1991;41: 202–224.
87. Jacobi HH, Skov PS, Poulsen LK, et al. Histamine and tryptase in nasal lavage fluid after allergen challenge: effect of 1 week of pretreatment with intranasal azelastine or systemic cetirizine. *J Allergy Clin Immunol* 1999;103:768–772.
88. Bielory L, Lien KW, Bigelsen S. Efficacy and tolerability of newer antihistamines in the treatment of allergic conjunctivitis. *Drugs* 2005;65:215–228.
89. Grant JA, Nicodemus CF, Findlay SR, et al. Cetirizine in patients with seasonal rhinitis and concomitant asthma: prospective, randomized, placebo-controlled trial. *J Allergy Clin Immunol* 1995;95: 923–932.
90. Baena-Cagnani CE, Berger WE, DuBuske LM, et al. Comparative effects of desloratadine versus montelukast on asthma symptoms and use of beta 2-agonists in patients with seasonal allergic rhinitis and asthma. *Int Arch Allergy Immunol* 2003;130:307–313.
91. Jutel M, Blaser K, Akdis CA. Histamine in allergic inflammation and immune modulation. *Int Arch Allergy Immunol* 2005;137:82–92.
92. Warner JO. A double-blinded, randomized, placebo-controlled trial of cetirizine in preventing the onset of asthma in children with atopic dermatitis: 18 months' treatment and 18 months' posttreatment follow-up. *J Allergy Clin Immunol* 2001;108:929–937.
93. Simons FE, Silver NA, Gu X, et al. Clinical pharmacology of H_1-antihistamines in the skin. *J Allergy Clin Immunol* 2002;110: 777–783.
94. Simons FE, Johnston L, Gu X, et al. Suppression of the early and late cutaneous allergic responses using fexofenadine and montelukast. *Ann Allergy Asthma Immunol* 2001;86:44–50.
95. Breneman DL. Cetirizine versus hydroxyzine and placebo in chronic idiopathic urticaria. *Ann Pharmacother* 1996;30:1075–1079.
96. Bleehen SS, Thomas SE, Greaves MW, et al. Cimetidine and chlorpheniramine in the treatment of chronic idiopathic urticaria: a multi-centre randomized double-blind study. *Br J Dermatol* 1987;117:81–88.
97. Greene SL, Reed CE, Schroeter AL. Double-blind crossover study comparing doxepin with diphenhydramine for the treatment of chronic urticaria. *J Am Acad Dermatol* 1985;12:669–675.
98. Kontou-Fili K, Maniatakou G, Demaka P, et al. Therapeutic effects of cetirizine in delayed pressure urticaria: clinicopathologic findings. *J Am Acad Dermatol* 1991;24:1090–1093.
99. Huston DP, Bressler RB, Kaliner M, et al. Prevention of mast-cell degranulation by ketotifen in patients with physical urticarias. *Ann Intern Med* 1986;104:507–510.
100. Simons FE. H_1-antihistamine treatment in young atopic children: effect on urticaria. *Ann Allergy Asthma Immunol* 2007;99: 261–266.
101. Simons FE, Simons KJ, Becker AB, et al. Pharmacokinetics and antipruritic effects of hydroxyzine in children with atopic dermatitis. *J Pediatr* 1984;104:123–127.
102. Juhlin L, Arendt C. Treatment of chronic urticaria with cetirizine dihydrochloride a non-sedating antihistamine. *Br J Dermatol* 1988;119:67–71.
103. Monroe EW. Relative efficacy and safety of loratadine, hydroxyzine, and placebo in chronic idiopathic urticaria and atopic dermatitis. *Clin Ther* 1992;14:17–21.
104. Karppinen A, Kautiainen H, Petman L, et al. Comparison of cetirizine, ebastine and loratadine in the treatment of immediate mosquito-bite allergy. *Allergy* 2002;57:534–537.
105. Friedman BS, Santiago ML, Berkebile C, et al. Comparison of azelastine and chlorpheniramine in the treatment of mastocytosis. *J Allergy Clin Immunol* 1993;92:520–526.
106. Lieberman P. The use of antihistamines in the prevention and treatment of anaphylaxis and anaphylactoid reactions. *J Allergy Clin Immunol* 1990;86:684–686.
107. Winbery SL, Lieberman PL. Histamine and antihistamines in anaphylaxis. *Clin Allergy Immunol* 2002;17:287–317.
108. Smith MB, Feldman W. Over-the-counter cold medications. A critical review of clinical trials between 1950 and 1991. *JAMA* 1993;269:2258–2263.
109. Sutter AI, Lemiengre M, Campbell H, et al. Antihistamines for the common cold. *Cochrane Database Syst Rev* 2003:CD001267.
110. Chonmaitree T, Patel JA, Lett-Brown MA, et al. Virus and bacteria enhance histamine production in middle ear fluids of children with acute otitis media. *J Infect Dis* 1994;169:1265–1270.
111. Cantekin EI, Mandel EM, Bluestone CD, et al. Lack of efficacy of a decongestant–antihistamine combination for otitis media with effusion ("secretory" otitis media) in children. Results of a double-blind, randomized trial. *N Engl J Med* 1983;308:297–301.
112. Coleman C, Moore M. Decongestants and antihistamines for acute otitis media in children. *Cochrane Database Syst Rev* 2008: CD001727.
113. Merenstein D, Diener-West M, Halbower AC, et al. The trial of infant response to diphenhydramine: the TIRED study—a randomized, controlled, patient-oriented trial. *Arch Pediatr Adolesc Med* 2006;160:707–712.
114. Raffa RB. Antihistamines as analgesics. *J Clin Pharm Ther* 2001; 26:81–85.
115. Roehrs T, Zwyghuizen-Doorenbos A, Roth T. Sedative effects and plasma concentrations following single doses of triazolam, diphenhydramine, ethanol and placebo. *Sleep* 1993;16:301–305.
116. Patat A, Stubbs D, Dunmore C, et al. Lack of interaction between two antihistamines, mizolastine and cetirizine, and ethanol in psychomotor and driving performance in healthy subjects. *Eur J Clin Pharmacol* 1995;48:143–150.
117. Hindmarch I, Bhatti JZ. Psychomotor effects of astemizole and chlorpheniramine, alone and in combination with alcohol. *Int Clin Psychopharmacol* 1987;2:117–119.
118. Kalivas J, Breneman D, Tharp M, et al. Urticaria: clinical efficacy of cetirizine in comparison with hydroxyzine and placebo. *J Allergy Clin Immunol* 1990;86:1014–1018.
119. Baker AM, Johnson DG, Levisky JA, et al. Fatal diphenhydramine intoxication in infants. *J Forensic Sci* 2003;48:425–428.
120. Wyngaarden JB, Seevers MH. The toxic effects of antihistaminic drugs. *J Am Med Assoc* 1951;145:277–282.
121. Cantu TG. Phenothiazines and sudden infant death syndrome. *DICP* 1989;23:795–796.
122. Starke PR, Weaver J, Chowdhury BA. Boxed warning added to promethazine labeling for pediatric use. *N Engl J Med* 2005;352: 2653.
123. Vuurman EF, van Veggel LM, Uiterwijk MM, et al. Seasonal allergic rhinitis and antihistamine effects on children's learning. *Ann Allergy* 1993;71:121–126.
124. Bender BG, McCormick DR, Milgrom H. Children's school performance is not impaired by short-term administration of diphenhydramine or loratadine. *J Pediatr* 2001;138:656–660.
125. Stevenson J, Cornah D, Evrard P, et al. Long-term evaluation of the impact of the h_1-receptor antagonist cetirizine on the behavioral, cognitive, and psychomotor development of very young children with atopic dermatitis. *Pediatr Res* 2002;52:251–257.
126. Arisaka O, Shimura N, Nakayama Y, et al. Cyproheptadine and growth. *Am J Dis Child* 1988;142:914–915.
127. Schwarzer G, Bassler D, Mitra A, et al. Ketotifen alone or as additional medication for long-term control of asthma and wheeze in children. *Cochrane Database Syst Rev* 2004:CD001384.
128. Monahan BP, Ferguson CL, Killeavy ES, et al. Torsades de pointes occurring in association with terfenadine use. *JAMA* 1990; 264:2788–2790.

129. Woosley RL, Sale M. QT interval: a measure of drug action. *Am J Cardiol* 1993;72:36B–43B.
130. Woosley RL. Cardiac actions of antihistamines. *Annu Rev Pharmacol Toxicol* 1996;36:233–252.
131. Sale ME, Barbey JT, Woosley RL, et al. The electrocardiographic effects of cetirizine in normal subjects. *Clin Pharmacol Ther* 1994;56:295–301.
132. Craig-McFeely PM, Acharya NV, Shakir SA. Evaluation of the safety of fexofenadine from experience gained in general practice use in England in 1997. *Eur J Clin Pharmacol* 2001;57:313–320.
133. Ten Eick AP, Blumer JL, Reed MD. Safety of antihistamines in children. *Drug Saf* 2001;24:119–147.
134. Demoly P, Messaad D, Benahmed S, et al. Hypersensitivity to H_1-antihistamines. *Allergy* 2000;55:679–680.
135. Tella R, Gaig P, Bartra J, et al. Urticaria to cetirizine. *J Investig Allergol Clin Immunol* 2002;12:136–137.
136. Epstein E. Dermatitis due to antihistaminic agents. *J Invest Dermatol* 1949;12:151.
137. Horio T. Allergic and photoallergic dermatitis from diphenhydramine. *Arch Dermatol* 1976;112:1124–1126.
138. Barranco P, Lopez-Serrano MC, Moreno-Ancillo A. Anaphylactic reaction due to diphenhydramine. *Allergy* 1998;53:814.
139. Bockholdt B, Klug E, Schneider V. Suicide through doxylamine poisoning. *Forensic Sci Int* 2001;119:138–140.
140. Hestand HE, Teske DW. Diphenhydramine hydrochloride intoxication. *J Pediatr* 1977;90:1017–1018.
141. Guay DR, Meatherall RC, Macaulay PA, et al. Activated charcoal adsorption of diphenhydramine. *Int J Clin Pharmacol Ther Toxicol* 1984;22:395–400.
142. Awni WM, Yeh J, Halstenson CE, et al. Effect of haemodialysis on the pharmacokinetics of cetirizine. *Eur J Clin Pharmacol* 1990;38: 67–69.
143. Einarson A, Bailey B, Jung G, et al. Prospective controlled study of hydroxyzine and cetirizine in pregnancy. *Ann Allergy Asthma Immunol* 1997;78:183–186.
144. Moretti ME, Caprara D, Coutinho CJ, et al. Fetal safety of loratadine use in the first trimester of pregnancy: a multicenter study. *J Allergy Clin Immunol* 2003;111:479–483.
145. Gilboa SM, Strickland MJ, Olshan AF, et al. Use of antihistamine medications during early pregnancy and isolated major malformations. *Birth Defects Res A Clin Mol Teratol* 2009;85:137–150.
146. Diav-Citrin O, Shechtman S, Aharonovich A, et al. Pregnancy outcome after gestational exposure to loratadine or antihistamines: a prospective controlled cohort study. *J Allergy Clin Immunol* 2003;111:1239–1243.
147. Parkin DE. Probable Benadryl withdrawal manifestations in a newborn infant. *J Pediatr* 1974;85:580.
148. Prenner BM. Neonatal withdrawal syndrome associated with hydroxyzine hydrochloride. *Am J Dis Child* 1977;131:529–530.
149. Ito S, Blajchman A, Stephenson M, et al. Prospective follow-up of adverse reactions in breast-fed infants exposed to maternal medication. *Am J Obstet Gynecol* 1993;168:1393–1399.
150. Hilbert J, Radwanski E, Affrime MB, et al. Excretion of loratadine in human breast milk. *J Clin Pharmacol* 1988;28:234–239.
151. PDR. Physicians' Desk Reference. 63rd edition; 2009:2684–2687.
152. Lin JH. Pharmacokinetic and pharmacodynamic properties of histamine H_2-receptor antagonists. Relationship between intrinsic potency and effective plasma concentrations. *Clin Pharmacokinet* 1991;20:218–236.
153. Gladziwa U, Koltz U. Pharmacokinetic optimisation of the treatment of peptic ulcer in patients with renal failure. *Clin Pharmacokinet* 1994;27:393–408.
154. Wang D, Clement P, Smitz J. Effect of H_1 and H_2 antagonists on nasal symptoms and mediator release in atopic patients after nasal allergen challenge during the pollen season. *Acta Otolaryngol* 1996;116:91–96.
155. Gustafsson PM, Kjellman NI, Tibbling L. A trial of ranitidine in asthmatic children and adolescents with or without pathological gastro-oesophageal reflux. *Eur Respir J* 1992;5:201–206.
156. Goldsobel AB, Rohr AS, Siegel SC, et al. Efficacy of doxepin in the treatment of chronic idiopathic urticaria. *J Allergy Clin Immunol* 1986;78:867–873.
157. Richelson E. Tricyclic antidepressants and histamine H_1 receptors. *Mayo Clin Proc* 1979;54:669–674.
159. Veien NK, Kaaber K, Larsen PO, et al. Ranitidine treatment of hand eczema in patients with atopic dermatitis: a double-blind, placebo-controlled trial. *J Am Acad Dermatol* 1995;32:1056–1057.
159. Shelley WB, Shelley ED, Talanin NY. Self-potentiating allergic contact dermatitis caused by doxepin hydrochloride cream. *J Am Acad Dermatol* 1996;34:143–144.
160. Coursin DB, Farin-Rusk C, Springman SR, et al. The hemodynamic effects of intravenous cimetidine versus ranitidine in intensive care unit patients: a double-blind, prospective, cross-over study. *Anesthesiology* 1988;69:975–978.
161. Gooptu C, Higgins CR, James MP. Treatment of viral warts with cimetidine: an open-label study. *Clin Exp Dermatol* 2000;25: 183–185.
162. Femiano F, Lanza A, Buonaiuto C, et al. Oral aphthous-like lesions, PFAPA syndrome: a review. *J Oral Pathol Med* 2008;37:319–323.
163. Bourinbaiar AS, Jirathitikal V. Low-cost anti-HIV compounds: potential application for AIDS therapy in developing countries. *Curr Pharm Des* 2003;9:1419–1431.
164. Nielsen HJ. Histamine-2 receptor antagonists as immunomodulators: new therapeutic views? *Ann Med* 1996;28:107–113.
165. Anlar B, Gucuyener K, Imir T, et al. Cimetidine as an immunomodulator in subacute sclerosing panencephalitis: a double blind, placebo-controlled study. *Pediatr Infect Dis J* 1993; 12:578–581.
166. Kristensen JK, Petersen LJ, Hansen U, et al. Systemic high-dose ranitidine in the treatment of psoriasis: an open prospective clinical trial. *Br J Dermatol* 1995;133:905–908.
167. Magee LA, Inocencion G, Kamboj L, et al. Safety of first trimester exposure to histamine H_2 blockers. A prospective cohort study. *Dig Dis Sci* 1996;41:1145–1149.
168. Obermeyer BD, Bergstrom RF, Callaghan JT, et al. Secretion of nizatidine into human breast milk after single and multiple doses. *Clin Pharmacol Ther* 1990;47:724–730.
169. Shapiro LE, Shear NH. Drug interactions: proteins, pumps, and P-450s. *J Am Acad Dermatol* 2002;47:467–484; quiz 485–468.
170. Bodey GP. Azole antifungal agents. *Clin Infect Dis* 1992;14(Suppl 1): S161–S169.
171. Sander K, Kottke T, Stark H. Histamine H_3 receptor antagonists go to clinics. *Biol Pharm Bull* 2008;31:2163–2181.
172. Chrusch C, Sharma S, Unruh H, et al. Histamine H_3 receptor blockade improves cardiac function in canine anaphylaxis. *Am J Respir Crit Care Med* 1999;160:1142–1149.
173. Oda T, Morikawa N, Saito Y, et al. Molecular cloning and characterization of a novel type of histamine receptor preferentially expressed in leukocytes. *J Biol Chem* 2000;275:36781–36786.
174. Hofstra CL, Desai PJ, Thurmond RL, et al. Histamine H_4 receptor mediates chemotaxis and calcium mobilization of mast cells. *J Pharmacol Exp Ther* 2003;305:1212–1221.
175. Thurmond RL, Desai PJ, Dunford PJ, et al. A potent and selective histamine H_4 receptor antagonist with anti-inflammatory properties. *J Pharmacol Exp Ther* 2004;309:404–413.
176. Fung-Leung WP, Thurmond RL, Ling P, et al. Histamine H_4 receptor antagonists: the new antihistamines? *Curr Opin Investig Drugs* 2004;5:1174–1183.
177. Huang JF, Thurmond RL. The new biology of histamine receptors. *Curr Allergy Asthma Rep* 2008;8:21–27.

CHAPTER

40

Hengameh H. Raissy
H. William Kelly
Stanley J. Szefler

Antiasthmatics

INTRODUCTION

Asthma is the most common chronic disease among children in the United States affecting about 9 million children younger than 18 years (1). In 2005, 8.95% of children had a current diagnosis of asthma, and an asthma attack was reported by about 4 million children in the previous year (1). Twenty-five percent of emergency room visits are for asthma (2) and children will account for 44% of the asthma hospitalizations (3). The prevalence rate of asthma is highest in children 5 to 17 years old at 9.6% (4) and resulted in 12.8 million missed schooldays by this age group in 2003 (5). Although the rate of asthma is greater in boys than in girls younger than 11 years old, it is about equal during puberty (4). The prevalence of asthma is higher in African Americans, 20%, compared with whites in 2006 (6). In addition, the rate of hospitalization in African Americans is three times higher and they are 2.5 times more likely to die because of asthma (4).

The rate of asthma in children younger than 5 years has increased more than 160% in years 1980 to 1994 (7), and it has been estimated that the number of patients with asthma will increase to more than 100 million by 2025 (8). In spite of increased prevalence of asthma in the United States, hospital admission and mortality of asthma have slightly decreased in the last few years (4). However, 80% to 90% of the asthma deaths can be prevented (9).

Asthma is a multifactorial and complex disease. The National Asthma Education and Prevention Program's Expert Panel Report 3 (EPR3): Guidelines for the Diagnosis and Management of Asthma defines asthma as "a common chronic disorder of the airways that is complex and characterized by variable and recurring symptoms, airflow obstruction, bronchial hyperresponsiveness, and an underlying inflammation." The airways inflammation has been demonstrated in the central and peripheral airways, and it involves activation of all airway cells including eosinophils, T lymphocytes, macrophages, mast cells, bronchial smooth muscle, epithelial cells, and fibroblasts (9). These activated cells further regulate airway inflammation and release cytokines and growth factors leading to chronic inflammation, airway remodeling, airflow obstruction, bronchial hyperresponsiveness, and increased risk of asthma exacerbations. Although the exact etiology of the inflammatory process leading to asthma is not well defined, innate immunity (the balance between Th-1 and Th-2 cytokine response), genetics, and environmental factors seem to interact for different asthma phenotypic expressions (10).

The developing immune system begins in the early weeks of gestation, going through several steps of maturation up until and beyond birth. However, because of this immaturity and continual development of the immune system, asthma per se is not observed in the neonate. Approximately 80% of childhood asthma develops before the age of 6 years (10), and may present differently among children. The asthma phenotype differentiates between transient wheezers and persistent wheezers. Transient wheezers (wheezing only at <3 years old) are not at an increased risk for developing asthma later in life; persistent wheezers or late onset wheezers (wheezing only between 3 and 6 years old) are at greater risk for development of asthma later in life (11). Interestingly, longitudinal studies have shown that a decline in lung function growth occurs by age of 6 with the most deficits in children with the onset of symptoms before age of 3 (11). Recently, a positive asthma predictive index has been developed to identify children younger than 3 years with high risk of developing persistent asthma later in life. The risk factors are either one of the following—parental history of asthma, a physician diagnosis of atopic dermatitis, or evidence of sensitization to aeroallergens—or two of the following: evidence of sensitization to foods, 4% or more peripheral blood eosinophilia, or wheezing apart from colds (9,12). In general, a decline in lung growth has not been noted in children, 5 to 12 years of age with mild or moderate persistent asthma through 11 to 17 years of age except for a subset of children (13).

Asthma begins early in life and what determines the severity of asthma or its persistent versus intermittent characteristics remains yet to be determined. It has consistently been shown that asthma is a chronic inflammatory disease regardless of its severity, and the therapy has been focused on the prevention and suppression of inflammation. The current therapeutic options are use of long-term controller medications to manage underlying inflammation and use of rescue medications to manage acute exacerbations (9). The EPR3 provides recommendations for assessment of severity and control, which require assessing both impairment and risk domains in children aged 0 to 4 years and 5 to 11 years (Table 40.1) (9). The EPR3 also provides guidance on classifying severity based on the level of therapy required to control asthma (Table 40.2) (9). The steps of therapy recommended by EPR3 for infants and young children are provided in Figure 40.1 (9). Adolescents are treated as adults and not presented here (9). This chapter will provide the pharmacologic basis for those recommendations.

AEROSOL DELIVERY IN CHILDREN

The most effective antiasthmatics are delivered as aerosols, and delivery of the aerosols into the airways of children is the primary determinant of dose, but like all dosage forms, aerosol delivery presents many unique challenges depending on the age of the child (9). There are three systems of aerosol delivery in clinical practice: (1) nebulizers that generate aerosol clouds by forcing air and fluid up through adjacent open-ended tubes that strike a baffle at high speed creating the aerosol (jet nebulizer) and ultrasonic nebulizers that produce an aerosol by vibrating liquid above a transducer; (2) metered-dose inhalers (MDIs) that force a propellant and solution or micronized suspension of drug stored in a pressurized canister out through a small orifice by opening a stem valve creating an aerosol of particles that diminish in size as the propellant evaporates; and (3) breath-activated, dry-powder inhalers (DPIs) that contain either individually packed micronized doses of drug plus excipients such as lactose or a compact bulk of drug from which micronized doses are shaven off prior to inhalation (they are called "breath activated" because inhalation by the patient creates the aerosol) (14). Because of these differing mechanisms for aerosol production, each device creates different challenges in children.

DEVICE-SPECIFIC ISSUES

The primary determinant of potential delivered dose from each of the systems is particle size generated. All devices produce heterodispersed aerosol clouds that are characterized by their mass median aerodynamic diameter (MMAD). In spontaneously breathing adults, particles greater than 10 μm deposit in the oropharynx, those between 5 and 10 μm deposit in the trachea and large bronchi, particles 1 to 5 μm deposit in the lower airways (often called "the respirable fraction"), and particles smaller than 0.5 μm act as a gas and can be exhaled (14). Very few of the delivery devices generate aerosols with the same MMAD, thus significant differences in the percentage of drug dose delivered to the lung occur both across devices (i.e., jet nebulizer vs. DPI) and within devices (MDI vs. MDI) across the manufacturers. The labeling of doses is also dependent on the type of device but is not dependent on actual dose delivered to the lung. The dosing for nebulizers is based upon the amount of drug put into the nebulizer. The dose for MDIs is based upon the amount of drug that reaches the patient's mouth (leaves the actuator) following actuation in the United States and the amount that exits the canister in most of the rest of the world. The dose of a DPI is that dose that is available for inhalation following activation of the dose (puncturing the blister, breaking the capsule, or shaving off the dose).

The most frequently prescribed delivery device is the MDI due to its portability and convenience. Recently, the MDI has undergone significant changes due to the Montreal Protocol to eventually end the use of ozone depleting chlorofluorocarbons (9). The introduction of hydrofluoroalkanes (HFAs) as the propellant has been associated with reformulation of some of the inhaled corticosteroids (ICSs) as solutions instead of micronized suspensions (14,15). The reformulation in concert with valve stem and actuator redesign has resulted in products with significantly reduced MMADs markedly improving lung delivery. For example, HFA-propelled beclomethasone dipropionate has a lung delivery in adults of 50% to 60% versus 4% to 10% delivery for the older chlorofluorocarbon-propelled preparations (16). However, other HFA-MDIs such as albuterol, fluticasone propionate, and budesonide/formoterol combination are still formulated as micronized suspensions and deliver 10% to 25% of the actuated dose (9).

The MDI is the most complicated system to use for patients. It requires multiple steps and good coordination of actuation during a slow deep inhalation. Many patients have significant difficulty coordinating actuation and inhalation reducing delivery of drug from MDIs (9,14). Spacer devices, particularly valved holding chambers (VHCs), have been developed to overcome the inability to coordinate actuation and inhalation. The VHCs are attached to the mouthpiece of an MDI, and the valve allows flow out of the VHC during inhalation and not into the VHC during exhalation (14). This allows young patients to breathe normally through a mouthpiece or a snug fitting face mask while an adult actuates the MDI. Although this method of delivery has proven to be efficacious in numerous clinical trials, it is noteworthy that currently no MDI + VHC combination has been approved by the US Food and Drug Administration (FDA) (12,17,18). The various VHCs also produce significant differences in delivery of drug that is drug and device dependent. For example, a VHC may improve delivery from one MDI product and decrease delivery from another MDI product, or two different VHCs may result in significantly different deliveries from the same MDI product (14,19). When using VHCs, it is important to actuate the inhaler only once before taking the inhalation, as actuating multiple times into the device reduces delivery due to coalescence of the particles (14,20). Last, the older plastic VHCs could develop static electricity on the walls over time resulting in attraction of the smaller respirable particles decreasing drug availability (20). This could be reduced by rinsing the devices with dilute home dishwashing detergent weekly or by using the newer VHCs with antistatic lining (21).

The DPIs were developed in response to the Montreal Protocol, but the FDA has determined that they are not considered an alternative to chlorofluorocarbon MDIs. However, they continue to be developed and are probably the easiest to teach patients to use and are associated with fewer mistakes by patients (14). The DPIs require a different inhalation technique that is rapid and deep and most produce optimal delivery at inspiratory flows 60 L per minute or more (14). The rapid deep inhalation, while not optimal for delivery of drug into peripheral airways, helps to break up the larger drug particle aggregates. The effect of inspiratory flow is dependent upon the DPI. For

TABLE 40.1 Assessing Asthma Control and Adjusting Therapy in Children (9)

Components of Control		Assessing Asthma Control and Adjusting Therapy in Children					
		Well Controlled		**Not Well Controlled**		**Very Poorly Controlled**	
		Ages 0–4	**Ages 5–11**	**Ages 0–4**	**Ages 5–11**	**Ages 0–4**	**Ages 5–11**
Impairment	Symptoms	≤2 d/wk but not more than once on each day		>2 d/wk or multiple times on ≤2 d/wk		Throughout the day	
	Nighttime awakenings	≤1x/month		>1x/month	≥2x/month	>1x/wk	≥2x/wk
	Interference with normal activity	None		Some limitation		Extremely limited	
	Short-acting β_2-agonist use for symptom control (not prevention of EIB)	≤2 d/wk		>2 d/wk		Several times per day	
	Lung function • FEV_1 (predicted) or peak flow personal best • FEV_1/FVC	N/A	>80% >80%	N/A	60–80% 75–80%	N/A	<60% <75%
Risk	Exacerbations requiring oral systemic corticosteroids	0–1x/yr		2–3x/yr	≥2x/yr	>3x/yr	≥2x/yr
	Reduction in lung growth	N/A	Requires long-term followup	N/A		N/A	
	Treatment-related adverse effects	Medication side effects can vary in intensity from none to very troublesome and worrisome. The level of intensity does not correlate to specific levels of control but should be considered in the overall assessment of risk.					
Recommended Action for Treatment **(See "Fig. 40.1" for treatment steps.)** **The stepwise approach is meant to assist, not replace, clinical decisionmaking required to meet individual patient needs.**		• Maintain current step. • Regular followup every 1–6 months. • Consider step down if well controlled for at least 3 months.		Step up 1 step	Step up at least 1 step	• Consider short course of oral systemic corticosteroids, • Step up 1–2 steps	
				• **Before step up:** Review adherence to medication, inhaler technique, and environmental control. If alternative treatment was used, discontinue it and use preferred treatment for that step. • **Reevaluate the level of asthma control in 2–6 weeks to achieve control; every 1–6 months to maintain control.** **Children 0–4 years old:** If no clear benefit is observed in 4–6 weeks, consider alternative diagnoses or adjusting therapy. **Children 5–11 years old:** Adjust therapy accordingly. • **For side effects,** consider alternative treatment options.			

EIB, exercise-induced bronchospasm, FEV_1, forced expiratory volume in 1 second; FVC, forced vital capacity; ICU, intensive care unit; N/A, not applicable

Notes:

- The level of control is based on the most severe impairment or risk category. Assess impairment domain by patient's or caregiver's recall of previous 2–4 weeks. Symptom assessment for longer periods should reflect a global assessment, such as whether the patient's asthma is better or worse since the last visit.
- At present, there are inadequate data to correspond frequencies of exacerbations with different levels of asthma control. In general, more frequent and intense exacerbations (e.g., requiring urgent, unscheduled care, hospitalization, or ICU admission) indicate poorer disease control.

TABLE 40.2 Classifying Asthma Severity and Initiating Therapy in Children (9)

Classifying Asthma Severity and Initiating Therapy in Children

Components of Severity		Intermittent		Persistent: Mild		Persistent: Moderate		Persistent: Severe	
		Ages 0–4	Ages 5–11	Ages 0–4	Ages 5–11	Ages 0–4	Ages 5–11	Ages 0–4	Ages 5–11
Impairment	Symptoms	≤2 d/wk		>2 d/wk but not daily		Daily		Throughout the day	
	Nighttime awakenings	0	≤2x/mo	1–2x/mo	3–4x/mo	3–4x/mo	>1x/wk but not nightly	>1x/wk	Often 7x/wk
	Short-acting β_2-agonist use for symptom control	≤2 d/wk		>2 d/wk but not daily		Daily		Several times per day	
	Interference with normal activity	None		Minor limitation		Some limitation		Extremely limited	
	Lung function		Normal FEV_1 between exacerbations						
	• FEV_1 (predicted) or peak flow (personal best)	N/A	>80%	N/A	>80%	N/A	60%–80%	N/A	<60%
	• FEV_1/FVC		>85%		>80%		75%–80%		<75%
Risk	Exacerbations requiring oral systemic corticosteroids (consider severity and interval since last exacerbation)	0–1/yr (see notes)		≥2 exacerbations in 6 months requiring oral systemic corticosteroids, or ≥4 wheezing episodes/1 year lasting >1 day AND risk factors for persistent asthma	≥2x/year (see notes) Relative annual risk may be related to FEV_1				
Recommended Step for Initiating Therapy (See "Fig. 40.1" for treatment steps.) The stepwise approach is meant to assist, not replace, the clinical decisionmaking required to meet individual patient needs.		Step 1 (for both age groups)		Step 2 (for both age groups)		Step 3 and consider short course of oral systemic corticosteroids	Step 3: medium-dose ICS option and consider short course of oral systemic corticosteroids	Step 3 and consider short course of oral systemic corticosteroids	Step 3: medium-dose ICS option OR step 4 and consider short course of oral systemic corticosteroids

Notes: In 2–6 weeks, depending on severity, evaluate level of asthma control that is achieved.
- Children 0–4 years old: If no clear benefit is observed in 4–6 weeks, stop treatment and consider alternative diagnoses or adjusting therapy.
- Children 5–11 years old: Adjust therapy accordingly.

Step up if needed (first check inhaler technique, adherence, environmental control, and comorbid conditions)

Assess control

Step down if possible (and asthma is well controlled at least 3 months)

Children 0–4 Years of Age

	Step 1	Step 2	Step 3	Step 4	Step 5	Step 6
	Intermittent Asthma	Persistent Asthma: Daily Medication Consult with asthma specialist if step 3 care or higher is required. Consider consultation at step 2.				
Preferred	SABA PRN	Low-dose ICS	Medium-dose ICS	Medium-dose ICS + LABA *or* Montelukast	High-dose ICS + LABA *or* Montelukast	High-dose ICS + LABA *or* Montelukas + Oral corticosteroids
Alternative		Cromolyn *or* Montelukast				
	Each step: Patient Education and Environmental Control					
Quick-Relief Medication	• SABA as needed for symptoms. Intensity of treatment depends on severity of symptoms. • With viral respiratory symptoms: SABA q4–6 hours up to 24 hours (longer with physician consult). Consider short course of oral systemic corticosteroids if exacerbation is severe or patient has history of previous severe exacerbations. Caution: Frequent use of SABA may indicate the need to step up treatment. See text for recommendations on initiating daily long-term-control therapy.					

Notes

- The stepwise approach is meant to assist, not replace, the clinical decisionmaking required to meet individual patient needs.
- If an alternative treatment is used and response is inadequate, discontinue it and use the preferred treatment before stepping up.
- If clear benefit is not observed within 4–6 weeks, and patient's/family's medication technique and adherence are satisfactory, consider adjusting therapy or an alternative diagnosis.
- Studies on children 0–4 years of age are limited. Step 2 preferred therapy is based on Evidence A. All other recommendations are based on expert opinion and extrapolation from studies in older children.
- Clinicians who administer immunotherapy should be prepared and equipped to identify and treat anaphylaxis that may occur.

Key: Alphabetical listing is used when more than one treatment option is listed within either preferred or alternative therapy. ICS, inhaled corticosteroid; LABA, inhaled long-acting beta$_2$-agonist; LTRA, leukotriene receptor antagonist; oral corticosteroids, oral systemic corticosteroids; SABA, inhaled short-acting beta$_2$-agonist

Children 5–11 Years of Age

	Step 1	Step 2	Step 3	Step 4	Step 5	Step 6
	Intermittent Asthma	Persistent Asthma: Daily Medication Consult with asthma specialist if step 4 care or higher is required. Consider consultation at step 3.				
Preferred	SABA PRN	Low-dose ICS	Low-dose ICS + LABA, LTRA, *or* Theophylline *OR*	Medium-dose ICS + LABA	High-dose ICS + LABA	High-dose ICS + LABA + Oral corticosteroids
Alternative		Cromolyn, LTRA, Nedocromil, *or* Theophylline	Medium-dose ICS	Medium-dose ICS + LTRA *or* Theophylline	High-dose ICS + LTRA *or* Theophylline	High-dose ICS + LTRA *or* Theophylline + oral corticosteroids
	Each step: Patient Education, Environmental Control, and Management of Comorbidities Steps 2–4: Consider subcutaneous allergen immunotherapy for patients who have persistent, allergic asthma.					
Quick-Relief Medication	• SABA as needed for symptoms. Intensity of treatment depends on severity of symptoms: up to 3 treatments at 20-minute intervals as needed. Short course of oral systemic corticosteroids may be needed. Caution: Increasing use of SABA or use >2 days a week for symptom relief (not prevention of EIB) generally indicates inadequate control and the need to step up treatment.					

Notes

- The stepwise approach is meant to assist, not replace, the clinical decisionmaking required to meet individual patient needs.
- If an alternative treatment is used and response is inadequate, discontinue it and use the preferred treatment before stepping up.
- Theophylline is a less desirable alternative due to the need to monitor serum concentration levels.
- Step 1 and step 2 medications are based on Evidence A. Step 3 ICS and ICS plus adjunctive therapy are based on Evidence B for efficacy of each treatment and extrapolation from comparator trials in older children and adults—comparator trials are not available for this age group; steps 4–6 are based on expert opinion and extrapolation from studies in older children and adults.
- Immunotherapy for steps 2–4 is based on Evidence B for house-dust mites, animal danders, and pollens; evidence is weak or lacking for molds and cockroaches. Evidence is strongest for immunotherapy with single allergens. The role of allergy in asthma is greater in children than adults.
- Clinicians who administer immunotherapy should be prepared and equipped to identify and treat anaphylaxis that may occur.

Key: Alphabetical listing is used when more than one treatment option is listed within either preferred or alternative therapy. ICS, inhaled corticosteroid; LABA, inhaled long-acting β_2-agonist; LTRA, leukotriene receptor antagonist; SABA, inhaled short-acting β_2-agonist

Figure 40.1. The stepwise approach for management of asthma in children (9).

example, the Pulmicort® Flexhaler™, with a higher internal resistance, has a reduction in respirable particles of 50% at an inspiratory flow of 30 L per minute compared with that of 60 L per minute, whereas with the Asmanex® Twisthaler™, the amount of drug emitted from the device was constant at inspiratory flows of 30 to 70 L per minute (22,23).

Nebulizers are approved as medical devices and so do not have as stringent criteria for approval as generic drugs. They only need to be as good as any product that is already marketed (14). Jet nebulizers require a source of compressed air and so are not as portable as either an MDI or DPI. Each nebulizer has optimal operating conditions but in general an airflow of 5 to 12 L per minute produces aerosol clouds with an MMAD of 4 to 8 μm (14,17). Ultrasonic nebulizers produce similar delivery as jet nebulizers with the exception of micronized suspensions for which they are ineffective (14). Once nebulizers are set up, they are the simplest for the patient, as they require only normal tidal breathing and so are often favored for young infants who use them with a face mask.

PATIENT-SPECIFIC ISSUES

Infants and young children clearly have significant differences in airway geometry so that data from normal adults do not necessarily apply, but because of logistical and ethical considerations, radiolabeled aerosol studies are rare in children. However, the adult values for respirable particles are used as a measuring stick for the development of aerosol delivery devices, all of which are designed for adults and then used in children. Many children 5 years of age or younger cannot coordinate inhalation and actuation with MDIs, and children 4 years of age or younger often require the use of a face mask for delivery from both nebulizers and MDI + VHC (14,17,18). The use of a face mask reduces delivery to about one-half that of a mouthpiece as infants are obligate nose breathers, and part of the dose is filtered out by the nose (24). Infants also have lower tidal volumes (tidal volume is a relatively constant 7 to 10 mL per kg throughout life). Infants weighing less than 15 kg will not necessarily be able to completely empty the VHC; however, they may receive higher μg per kg doses based on lack of air entrainment on inhalation (25). So there are a number of factors that can have potentially offsetting effects on aerosol delivery in infants compared with older children. For example, in in vitro models, tidal volumes for those 2 years or younger versus those for 4- to 5-year-olds show higher microgram per kilogram doses delivered to those aged 2 years or younger (26–28). However, a wait time between actuation and inhalation of 5 seconds decreases delivery by 30% to 50% (20,27). Finally, the child should be breathing quietly and not crying as delivery by both nebulizer and MDI + VHC in the crying infant reduces delivery by as much as 80% (24). Unfortunately, if infants and young children resist the use of a face mask, parents and caregivers revert to a "blow-by" method, where they hold the mask or end of the tube connected to the nebulizer close to the infants' mouth and nose. However, studies have shown that holding the mask 1 cm from the face can reduce delivery 50% to 60% and at 2 cm as much as 85% (25). In clinical trials, superiority has not been established for MDI + VHC over nebulization (17,18).

Unfortunately, many children aged 5 years or younger cannot attain a peak inspiratory flow of 60 L per minute (14). The internal resistance of the DPI can also affect the ability of children to generate flow through the device. In one study, 78% of 4-year-olds could generate an inspiratory flow of at least 30 L per minute through a Diskus™, 89% through an Aerolizer™, but only 56% through a Turbuhaler™ (29). The use of DPIs should be reserved for children aged 4 years or older.

INHALED CORTICOSTEROIDS

MECHANISM OF ACTION

Corticosteroids are the most potent anti-inflammatory agents available for management of asthma. They have a broad array of anti-inflammatory effects. The glucocorticoid receptor (GR) resides in the cytoplasm of cells and is ubiquitous in tissues and cells throughout the body explaining its myriad effects. The corticosteroid enters the cell cytoplasm via passive diffusion across the cell membrane and binds with the inactive GR complex, dissociating the GR complex from heat shock proteins and immunophilin (30). Then the activated GR translocates into the nucleus where it binds to DNA at specific sequences called glucocorticoid response elements where it promotes the production of anti-inflammatory proteins such as lipocortin-1, β_2-adrenergic receptor (β_2-AR), secretory leukocyte inhibitory protein, and IκB-α (31). In addition, it inhibits transcription activation of many proinflammatory cytokines that are activated through tumor necrosis factor-α and nuclear factor-κB (i.e., interleukins 1–6, 8, 11, 12, 13; chemokines; matrix metalloproteinase-9; adhesion molecules; inducible nitric oxide synthase; endothelin-1) (30,31). Although there is a single gene encoding the human GR, splice variants have been identified and one, the GRβ isoform, although usually inactive, has been reported to be increased in corticosteroid-resistant patients (30).

The effects of corticosteroids are cell and tissue specific which explain many of their clinical effects. Corticosteroids reduce mucus secretion, produce vasoconstriction reducing airway mucosal blood flow and endothelial cell leaking (31,32). These latter effects, along with reduction in nitric oxide production, decrease vascular and tissue edema that contribute to airways obstruction. It has been posited that the vascular effects of corticosteroids contribute to the acute improvement following frequent high doses of inhaled corticosteroids (ICSs) in patients presenting to the emergency department (33). Corticosteroids inhibit cytokine release from respiratory epithelial cells, macrophages, and T lymphocytes (31). Corticosteroids increase the number of β_2-ARs in airway smooth muscle attenuating or modulating tolerance due to chronic β_2-agonist stimulation but not completely reversing it (34). Corticosteroids decrease the number of dendritic cells and eosinophils in the airways by inducing apoptosis and reduce the number of circulating eosinophils and reduce the number and activation of T lymphocytes. Corticosteroids do not inhibit the release of soluble mediators from tissue mast cells (histamine and leukotrienes) but reduce their number and influx into airway smooth muscle cells (31). This explains

TABLE 40.3 Adverse Effects of Glucocorticoid Administration (35)

Aseptic necrosis of bone
Cataracts
Central redistribution of fat
Glaucoma
Hypertension
Hypokalemia
Hyperglycemia
HPA axis suppression
Impaired wound healing
Moon face
Osteoporosis (bone fracture)
Pseudotumor cerebri
Psychiatric disorders
Pancreatitis
Skin striae
Subcutaneous tissue atrophy
Sodium and water retention
Myopathy (skeletal muscle)

why acute administration of a corticosteroid has no effect on the early asthmatic response to inhaled allergen or exercise but that chronic administration results in significant attenuation of these responses. As the GR is found throughout all cells and tissues, a potential for significant adverse effects listed in Table 40.3 exists (35). Therefore, corticosteroids with high topical activity with pharmacokinetic properties that limit systemic activity that can be administered by inhalation were developed.

The ICSs are considered the preferred long-term controller medications for all levels of persistent asthma due to their consistent efficacy resulting in reduction in bronchial hyperresponsiveness and asthma exacerbations and improvement in lung function. The current ICSs approved for use in the United States and their recommended doses for children are listed in Table 40.4 that is modified from the EPR3 (9,14). Chemical modifications of the corticosteroids produce different binding affinities (potency) for the GR (Table 40.5) that can simply be overcome by giving equipotent doses (14,35). Thus, when assessing "clinical comparable doses," lung delivery from various delivery devices as well as potency need to be taken into account. Table 40.4 also presents the clinically comparable doses for children established by comparative clinical trials (9,15). There are relatively little data in children aged 4 years or younger where delivery issues become even more variable. Although it has been postulated that the newer HFA-MDI ICSs formulated to deliver ultrafine particle may have greater efficacy due to penetration into the small airways, clinical trials do not support a difference other than that produced by total lung delivery (15).

PHARMACOKINETICS

Differences in the molecular structures of ICSs result in altered pharmacokinetic properties of these agents (Table 40.5), which are the primary determinants of the topical to systemic activity (therapeutic index) (15). Figure 40.2 provides a schematic of where each of the pharmacokinetic variables can affect the therapeutic index (9,14,35). The inhaled route of administration has the advantage of delivering drug to the site of action, but only 5% to 60% of the inhaled dose is delivered to the lung; about 50% to 80% of the drug deposits in the oropharynx and swallowed while the rest is exhaled or left in the device (14,15). Topical selectivity of the ICSs can be improved by decreasing oral bioavailability, increasing systemic clearance, and prolonging residence time in the lung (15,35,36). Systemic

TABLE 40.4 Current ICS Available for Children and their Clinically Comparable Doses (9,14)

Agent	*Low Daily Dose (μg)*	*Medium Daily Dose (μg)*	*High Daily Dose (μg)*
Beclomethasone dipropionate HFA MDI, Qvar® (40 and 80 μg/actuation)	80–160	>160–320	>320
Budesonide DPI (Turbuhaler® 50 μg/dose, Flexhaler® 90 and 180 μg/dose)	180–400	>400–800	>800
Nebulizer solution, Pulmicort Respules® (250, 500, 1,000 μg/2 mL)	500	1,000	2,000
Dose for children 0–4 years old	250–500	>500	>1,000
Ciclesonide[a] HFA MDI, Alvesco® (80 and 160 μg/actuation)	80–160	>160–320	>320
Flunisolide CFC MDI Aerobid® (250 μg/actuation)	500–750	1,000–1,250	>1,250
HFA MDI, Aerospan® (80 μg/actuation)	160	320	≥640
Fluticasone propionate HFA MDI, Fovent® (44, 110, 220 μg/actuation)	88–176	>176–352	>352
Dose for children 0–4 years old[b]	176	>176–352	>352
DPI, Flovent Diskus® (50 μg/dose)	100–200	>200–400	>400
Mometasone furoate DPI, Asmanex Twisthaler® (200 and 400 μg/dose)	110	220–440	>440

[a]Not approved for children <12 years old.
[b]Not FDA approved for the age group.

TABLE 40.5 Receptor Binding Affinities and Pharmacokinetic Properties of the ICS (14,35)

ICS (%)	Binding Affinity[a]	Systemic Clearance (L/hr)	Oral Bioavailability (%)	Lung Delivery
Beclomethasone dipropionate	0.4	150	20	50–60
Budesonide	9.4	84	11	15–30
Ciclesonide	0.12	152	<1	50
Flunisolide	1.8	58	20	68
Fluticasone propionate	18	66	≥1	20
Mometasone furoate	23	53	<1	11
Triamcinolone acetonide	3.6	45–69	23	22

[a]Receptor binding affinities of ICS relative to dexamethasone equal to 1.

bioavailability of ICSs depends on the oral bioavailability and the amount of drug which enters the systemic circulation via lungs. Oral bioavailability can be altered by oral absorption, increased first-pass intestinal wall and hepatic metabolism mediated by the cytochrome P450 3A4 (CYP3A4) isozymes, and decreasing oropharyngeal deposition by using a VHC with MDI for compounds with significant oral absorption such as beclomethasone dipropionate (15,35,36). However, for compounds with very high first-pass metabolism such as fluticasone propionate, using a VHC with an MDI may actually increase systemic exposure by increasing lung delivery (19,35). This can adversely affect the therapeutic index (35,37). Although children aged 2 years or younger can theoretically receive higher milligram per kilogram doses of ICSs than do older children as discussed above, there is insufficient data to determine whether they are at greater risk for adverse systemic effects.

Systemic clearance is the primary determinant other than dose for steady-state serum concentrations with chronic dosing. Most of the ICSs undergo unrestrictive hepatic extraction and metabolism by CYP3A4 so that their clearances approach liver blood flow (≈90 L per hour) (15,36). The exceptions are the active metabolites of beclomethasone dipropionate (beclomethasone 17-monopropionate) and ciclesonide (desisobutyryl-ciclesonide) that apparently undergo extrahepatic metabolism possibly via blood esterases (15). Retention in the lung allows ongoing exposure to the GRs and exposes the systemic circulation to lower concentrations. It occurs with more lipophilic compounds such as fluticasone propionate and is evidenced by a longer elimination half-life for inhaled than intravenous administration (15). Some of the ICSs undergo intracellular fatty acid esterification at the free hydroxyl group at the carbon 21 position (i.e., budesonide, triamcinolone acetonide

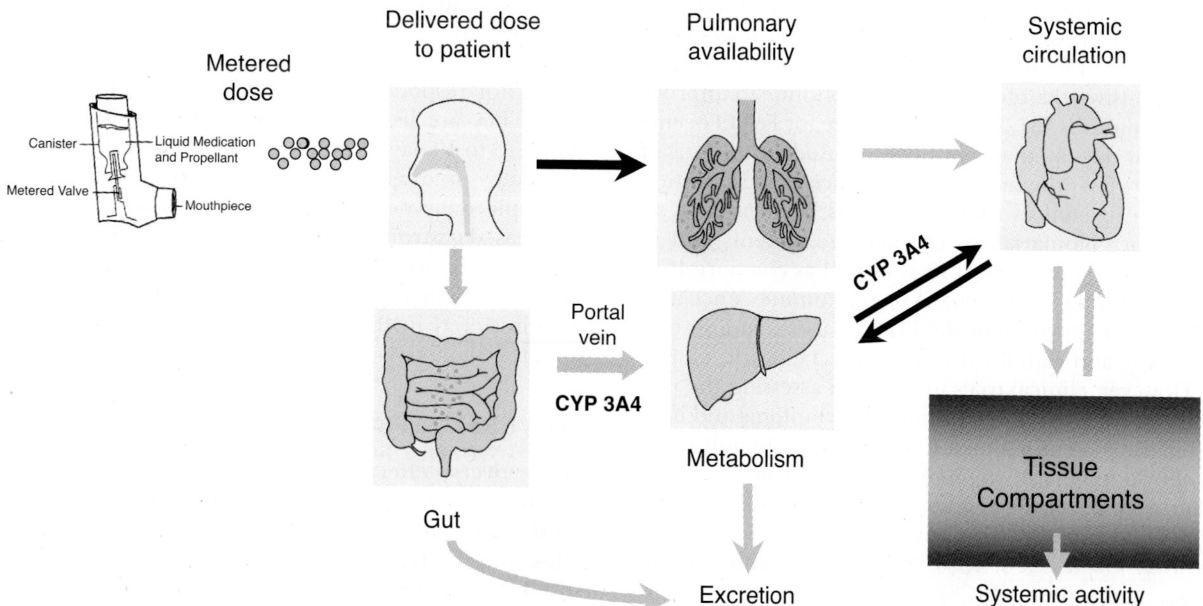

Figure 40.2. Effects of various factors on systemic activity of ICS (9,14,35).

and desisobutyryl-ciclesonide), which maintains a depot of drug in the cell (15,36). However, this property has not been established to confer an improved therapeutic index or prolonged duration of effect over agents that do not undergo esterification.

CLINICAL USE

Figure 40.1 presents the current EPR3 recommendations that, regardless of age, ICSs are the preferred agents for persistent asthma and the dose should be based on the severity and control of the disease. The ICSs are the only agents demonstrated to reduce the risk of dying from asthma (9). Furthermore, low-medium doses of ICSs have consistently been shown to improve lung function, decrease bronchial hyperresponsiveness and asthma exacerbations, and reduce the need for as needed rescue with short-acting β_2-agonists and oral corticosteroids (9,12,38,39). In addition, ICSs reduce sputum eosinophils and fraction of exhaled nitric oxide (FeNO), a downstream end product of eosinophilic inflammation. Comparative clinical trials in children aged 5 to 11 years show that they are more effective than all alternative long-term controllers (9,38,40–45). In addition, studies in children younger than 5 years have shown fluticasone propionate by MDI + VHC and budesonide nebulization suspension to be more efficacious than cromolyn and budesonide nebulization to be more effective than montelukast (46–48). Chronic administration of ICSs reduces the degree of bronchial hyperresponsiveness in children, including exercise-induced bronchospasm (EIB) (38,49). They reduce EIB more effectively and consistently than does montelukast (50). Despite their activity in preventing exacerbations and reducing symptoms and airway responsiveness, ICS therapy does not prevent loss of lung function, does not prevent development of asthma in high-risk infants, and does not enhance the lung growth in children with asthma (12,13,38,51).

The clinical response to ICSs varies among patients, but most asthma symptoms will improve in 1 to 2 weeks, with maximum improvement in 1 to 2 months. Maximum improvement in lung function requires 3 to 6 weeks of treatment and at least 1 to 3 months to improve bronchial hyperresponsiveness, although it may continue to improve over many months (31,38). The response for FeNO occurs within a few days so that it has been touted as a means of monitoring ICS therapy for adherence and adjusting doses (52). In clinical trials, FeNO has been used as an inflammatory biomarker to characterize patients and to compare relative potency of ICSs as well as compare ICSs to other therapies (43,52–54). A chemoluminescence analyzer has been approved by the FDA for use in monitoring ICS therapy and handheld devices are being developed (52). However, clinical trials in children assessing the utility of monitoring FeNO in addition to symptoms and lung function have obtained mixed results; so, although it has been shown to be able to predict future exacerbations, its routine use is uncertain and requires further study (55,56).

For those patients who have not achieved adequate control on low doses of ICSs, the EPR3 recommends an increase in the dose of ICSs or add an adjunct therapy such as a leukotriene-receptor antagonist (LTRA) or an inhaled long-acting β_2-agonist (LABA) (9). The preferred recommendations vary with age primarily because no adjunctive therapy to ICSs has been evaluated in children younger than 5 years, and minimal studies have compared adjunctive therapy to increased ICS in children aged 5 to 11 years and only recently have adjunctive therapies been directly compared (56b). In addition, dose–response studies for ICSs in children are few. The ICSs are considered to have a relatively flat dose–response curve. In children 4 to 14 years old, the response to fluticasone propionate tends to plateau between 100 and 200 μg daily in most patients with some further benefit in more severe patients obtained at 400 μg daily (57). A dose–response study of budesonide between 200, 400, and 800 μg daily, which is one-half as potent as fluticasone propionate, confirms these findings (58). In adults with relatively moderate-to-severe asthma, doubling the dose of ICS does not decrease asthma exacerbations but quadrupling the dose does despite minimal effect on lung function (59,60). Similar studies have not been carried out in children, but in general, a doubling of the dose of ICS does not significantly increase benefit (15,57,58). In young children and infants, the data are even less clear. One study comparing fluticasone propionate 100 and 200 μg daily by MDI + VHC and face mask in 237 infants 12 to 47 months old reported a dose response for decreased exacerbations; however, the decrease in exacerbations for the 100 μg daily was not significantly different from placebo (39). In addition, the pivotal trials for budesonide nebulizer suspension failed to demonstrate a dose–response for 500 to 1,000 μg daily after the dose exceeded 250 μg once daily which was not consistently more effective than placebo across studies (61).

The issue of once-daily administration of the ICSs to improve compliance is often raised. Although only budesonide and mometasone furoate currently have once-daily FDA approved labeling, most mild persistent patients controlled on low to medium dose ICS can be adequately controlled with once-daily administration with all the ICSs. None of the ICSs have specific pharmacokinetic properties that allow for once-daily dosing and they all work more effectively in moderate-to-severe asthma with twice-daily dosing (15).

Oral corticosteroids are indicated for asthma exacerbations not responding to inhaled short-acting β_2-agonists (9). They are usually administered as a short course or burst (3 to 10 days) at the equivalent dose of 1 to 2 mg per kg daily prednisolone equivalent once or twice daily. Multiple daily dosing may provide superior activity and decreased gastrointestinal effects. The number of oral corticosteroid bursts is used to determine both risk and the level of control (Table 40.2) (9). Oral corticosteroids administered in the emergency department and continued for 3 to 7 days reduce the risk of relapse (9).

ADVERSE EFFECTS

The adverse effects of ICSs are dose related (35). The degree of systemic exposure depends on the inhaler design, patient's technique, physical property of the particles, and the pharmacokinetics. All of the ICSs have relatively few adverse effects at the low-medium doses and when they are used properly. Although there are potential differences based upon pharmacokinetics, patients are at risk of experiencing systemic effects at high doses of the ICSs and should be monitored appropriately.

Deposition of the ICSs in the oropharynx may lead to dysphonia and hoarseness, oral candidiasis, and cough at the time of inhalation. Dysphonia and hoarseness are dose-related side effects with an incidence of 5% to 50% and may be due to the myopathy of the laryngeal muscles (31,62). Oral candidiasis is also dose related with an incidence of less than 5%, and may be prevented by rinsing the mouth with water after the dose (62). In infants using either nebulized ICS or MDI + VHC with a face mask, the nose and mouth should be washed off after each treatment. Cough is mainly due to local irritation and may be resolved by changing the delivery device, the rate of inhalation, or using a VHC.

The systemic side effects of the ICSs include suppression of the hypothalamus–pituitary–adrenal (HPA) axis, adrenal insufficiency, Cushing syndrome, osteoporosis, skin thinning and ecchymoses, cataracts, and growth retardation in children. Suppression of HPA axis is a rare event and is usually clinically insignificant (35,63). Nonetheless, adrenal insufficiency has been reported in children when high doses have been used (64,65). A recent large survey in France found 46 cases of adrenal insufficiency, 24 of which were associated with ICS use, 14 of which were children 0.3 to 14 years old (median 9.5 years old) (65). Seven were with fluticasone propionate, five with budesonide, and two with beclomethasone dipropionate. All patients received a daily dose of 500 μg or more beclomethasone equivalent ($\geq$250 μg daily fluticasone propionate). Of the total 24 cases, 12 were associated with potential drug interactions (6 ritonavir and 6 itraconazole) with fluticasone propionate and budesonide (see discussion later). There are several methods for assessing the integrity of the HPA axis, ranging from testing for basal production of the adrenal glands to reserve capacity. Tests of basal production include spot morning serum cortisol, serial overnight (12-hour) or 24-hour area under the curve serum cortisol (AUC_{0-24}), and 12-hour (overnight) and 24-hour urine free cortisol (UFC) (corrected for creatinine to normalize data) concentration testing (35,66,67). Serum cortisol AUC_{0-24} and 24-hour UFC are the most sensitive, and UFC has the advantage of not requiring blood draws in children; however, they do not assess the ability of the HPA axis to respond to stress (35,66). The gold standards for assessing full integrity of the HPA axis are the insulin tolerance test and metyrapone tests, which are relatively invasive and difficult to perform; therefore, adrenocorticotropic hormone (ACTH) cortisol stimulation test is performed as the standard. Low-dose slow infusion of ACTH is being touted as more sensitive, as it gives a dose of ACTH similar to that seen during stress as opposed to the supraphysiologic doses used with the standard ACTH stimulation that may give false negative results (66). However, the results of low-dose ACTH tests have not been completely validated and may produce false-positive results in patients without clinically relevant suppression (35,66). There does not appear to be a chronic cumulative effect of medium dose ICSs on the HPA axis as measured over 3 years in children receiving budesonide 400 μg daily (68). Four or less oral courses of prednisone per year is not associated with adrenal suppression, and significant adrenal suppression does not occur following individual short courses less than 10 days (9).

High-dose ICSs can reduce bone mineral density and increase the risk of fracture in older patients at risk; however, the data in children are less clear (35). Bone mineral density does not seem to be altered with low to medium doses of the ICSs (38); however, a recent prospective study over a median of 7 years in children 5 to 12 years old reported a decrease in bone mineral accretion with medium dose ICS in boys but not girls that did not result in an increased risk of osteopenia or fractures (69). An epidemiologic study of 97,387 children 4 to 17 years old receiving ICSs in the United Kingdom reported an increased crude risk of fracture in those receiving greater than 200 μg per day beclomethasone dipropionate equivalent, but when adjusted for measures of asthma severity, the increased risk disappeared (70). A nested case-control analysis using the same UK database also failed to demonstrate a significant increase in fracture risk from current ICS use or current long-term exposure ($\geq$20 prescriptions) (71). However, short courses of oral prednisone have been associated with a dose-dependent decrease in bone mineral accretion and an increased risk of osteopenia (at least two bursts per year) and fractures (four or more bursts per year) (69,72).

A more relevant potential adverse event and a great concern of some parents is the effect of the ICSs on growth. Long-term prospective studies in prepubertal children on low-medium doses of the ICSs have shown a reduction in growth velocity in the first 6 months to year of therapy that then returns to normal (12,31,35,38,47,51) The overall effect on height is 1 to 2 cm, and currently all studies suggest that children are expected to achieve their predicted adult height (35,38,73). Differences on growth have been detected between the ICSs as would be predicted by their differences in delivery and pharmacokinetics (35,37). Fluticasone dipropionate by DPI produced less effect on growth than equivalent doses of either budesonide or beclomethasone dipropionate by DPI (74,75), but produced similar effect to budesonide when administered by MDI + VHC which enhances systemic availability of fluticasone propionate (76). Of note fluticasone propionate by DPI at 100 and 200 μg daily did not produce a decrease in growth in children down to 4 years old but did produce a significant reduction of 1.1 cm over 2 years in infants 1 to 3 years of age receiving 176 μg daily by MDI + VHC and face mask (12,35). Monitoring the linear growth in all children on ICSs is recommended by the EPR3 (9).

Cataracts are uncommon in children and have not been reported in children on ICSs (31). Other suspected adverse reactions with ICSs reported from pharmacovigilance reporting systems are psychiatric symptoms and abnormalities of teeth (77). The association with ICSs is not clear, but various psychiatric symptoms have been reported for systemic corticosteroids.

DRUG INTERACTIONS

Some of the ICSs including budesonide, fluticasone propionate, and mometasone undergo hepatic and intestinal metabolism by cytochrome CYP3A4 isoenzymes (15,78). As a result, ICSs should be used cautiously with potent inhibitors of CYP3A4 such as protease inhibitors, macrolides, ketoconazole, and itraconazole (78). Clinically significant Cushing syndrome and adrenal suppression and deaths have been reported (65,79,80). Systemic corticosteroids will also have decreased clearance and prolonged half-lives when coadministered with CYP3A4 inhibitors.

β_2-AGONISTS

The β_2-agonists are the most effective bronchodilators for asthma and they are classified as either short- or long-acting β_2-agonists. Short-acting β_2-agonists have about 3 to 8 hours duration of action depending on how it is measured, and they include albuterol, levalbuterol, pirbuterol, terbutaline, and epinephrine which is the only one available over the counter. The LABAs have a duration of action of 12 hours or more and are primarily used in combination with ICSs. Available LABAs are formoterol, salmeterol, and arformoterol.

MECHANISM OF ACTION

All of the β_2-agonists work through binding of the β_2-AR, a G-protein coupled receptor on cell surfaces (81). Infants are born with fully functional airway smooth muscles (both neural network and functional receptors) whose mass relative to airway size is fully developed by 25 weeks' gestation (82). In the body, the β_2-ARs are in a state of equilibrium between the active and inactive isoforms and binding by an agonist results in a shift of the equilibrium favoring the activated isoform (81). Activation results in adenylate cyclase producing cyclic adenosine monophosphate to increase protein kinase A resulting in a decrease in unbound calcium to produce smooth muscle relaxation (81,83). Pharmacologically, β_2-agonists are functional antagonists because they reverse smooth muscle constriction regardless of the mechanism (83). As the β_2-AR is designed to accommodate endogenous catecholamines (dopamine, L-epinephrine and norepinephrine), the chemical modifications designed to produce greater selectivity for the β_2-AR produce compounds less efficient for shifting the equilibrium (81). Thus, all synthetic β_2-agonists exhibit less efficacy for increasing cyclic adenosine monophosphate levels and are considered partial agonists. Each drug exhibits a different level of partial agonism with salmeterol having the most followed by albuterol, terbutaline, and pirbuterol with formoterol having greater efficacy though less than the full agonists epinephrine and isoproterenol (34). Partial agonism is less important in tissue with large numbers of β_2-ARs (bronchial smooth muscle) than tissues with low numbers (cardiac tissue, mast cells, and inflammatory cells). The β_2-agonists are selective by virtue of having even less efficacy for other adrenergic receptors (i.e., α_1, α_2, and β_1). Their relative selectivity for adrenergic receptors is illustrated in Table 40.6 with salmeterol and formoterol equivalent with greater selectivity than albuterol, pirbuterol, and terbutaline that are equivalent (34). Aerosol administration makes them all more bronchoselective and the selectivity of all these agents diminishes at high doses.

TABLE 40.6 Relative Selectivity and Potency of β-Agonists for Adrenergic Receptors (34)

	β_1-Receptor	*β_2-Receptor*	*β_2 Potency*
Albuterol	+	+++	2
Formoterol	+	++++	0.12
Isoproterenol	++++	++++	1
Metaproterenol	+++	+++	15
Pirbuterol	+	+++	5
Salmeterol	+	++++	0.5
Terbutaline	+	+++	4

Unlike the endogenously produced catecholamines, the synthetic β_2-agonists have a chiral carbon and exist as a 1:1 racemic mixture of enantiomers except for levalbuterol and arformoterol (34,84). Formoterol has two chiral carbons (84). As biological systems are stereoselective, one of the enantiomers provides a better fit and greater efficacy at the β_2-AR, and for β_2-agonists, the R-enantiomers are the most active component with higher affinities ranging from 100- to 1,000-fold for the β_2-AR (34,84). Intact animal models and in vitro studies with isolated tracheal and bronchial strips reported that [S]-isoproterenol and [S]-albuterol resulted in increased responsiveness of bronchial smooth muscle and other proinflammatory effects (85,86). This led to the development and eventual FDA approval of levalbuterol, the single [R]-enantiomer of albuterol, and more recently arformoterol, the [R,R]-enantiomer of formoterol (84,86). However, similar studies with [S]-terbutaline and [S,S]-formoterol have not demonstrated an increase in responsiveness (85). Standard bronchodilator dose–response studies have established that all of the bronchodilation and systemic β_2-adrenergic effects reside in the [R]-enantiomers so that when administered in equivalent [R]-enantiomeric doses, racemic albuterol and formoterol do not differ from levalbuterol and arformoterol, respectively (87,88). The effect of the [S]-enantiomer of albuterol on airway responsiveness in humans has been inconsistent (89–91). If it does enhance airways responsiveness, the effect is small and easily overcome by the bronchodilating properties of the [R]-enantiomer (91). Some have suggested that high concentrations of [S]-albuterol may act as an inverse agonist (86), limiting the bronchodilator effectiveness of the [R]-enantiomer, but a study exploring this hypothesis found no such effect (91).

The β_2-AR genes are located on the long arm of chromosome 5q31-q32 coding for a protein containing 413 amino acids (84). The amino acid sequence of the receptor can be altered producing polymorphisms. The most common polymorphisms of the β_2-AR are single amino acid substitutions called single nucleotide polymorphisms (SNPs). Genetic variation may explain some of the interindividual differences in response to a β_2-agonist (92–94). A total of nine different polymorphisms have been identified and three common ones have been studied in detail due to functional differences found in vitro: amino acid at positions 16, encoding either arginine [Arg] or glycine [Gly]; position 27, encoding either glutamine [Gln] or glutamic acid [Glu]; and position 164, encoding either isoleucine

(Ile) or threonine (Thr) (84,92). Individuals may be heterozygous or homozygous for each polymorphism, and there are differences between races in allele frequency as well as haplotype structure (paired SNPs) that represent linkage disequilibrium (SNP pairs that occur more frequently together in populations than by chance alone, i.e., 94% of Arg/Arg is found with Gln/Gln) (84,93). The homozygous Gly/Gly 16 β_2-AR downregulates to a greater extent than Gly/Arg followed by Arg/Arg (92). The homozygous Glu/Glu at position 27 of the receptor protects against downregulation compared with homozygous Gln/Gln; however, when Glu/Glu and Gly/Gly are combined, the effect of Gly/Gly is more dominant and the protection against downregulation diminishes (92). Substitution of Ile for Thr in position 164 can decrease the binding affinity of the receptor by as much as four times and the homozygous Ile appears to be lethal (92). Clinical studies in asthma have been inconsistent, with some showing greater bronchodilation for Arg/Arg patients and with other studies not showing that effect (5,14). In addition, tolerance has been demonstrated across all genotypes (84). Newer investigations are assessing haplotypes as well as expanding haplotypes to include polymorphisms into other areas of the β_2-AR gene. Additional studies are exploring alternate genes that may determine response such as the receptors for the signal transduction that activate adenylyl cyclase (93).

Continuous stimulation of the β_2-AR will result in diminished response or tolerance. Tolerance to the β_2-agonists can occur within a week of regular administration as a result of downregulation of the receptors as well as a decrease in binding affinity to the receptors (uncoupling) (80,82). Tolerance levels off after a few weeks and does not worsen over time. Because tolerance develops at the receptor level, cross tolerance to other β_2-agonists occurs. There is no relationship between potency or efficacy and the induction of tolerance and clinical trials demonstrate tolerance from all of the β_2-agonists (34,83,84). Because of the large number of β_2-ARs in bronchial smooth muscle, tolerance is more easily detected in other cells with a lower density of receptors (i.e., cardiac, vascular, mast cells, epithelium, lymphocytes) (81). Bronchoprovocation studies using bronchoconstriction (exercise, methacholine, or histamine) challenges more readily detect tolerance in patients than bronchodilation studies (95–99). Unlike the decreased bronchodilation that can easily be overcome with an additional dose of β_2-agonist (95,96), the decrease in bronchoprotection cannot be easily overcome by an increased dose (34). Agonist-induced tolerance of the β_2-ARs can be at least partially overcome by the administration of systemic corticosteroids and partially prevented by coadministration of ICSs (34,83,100). Although the time required for a clinical response differs among patients, β_2-receptors density increases within 4 hours after administration of systemic steroid and response to β_2-agonist occurs within 2 to 12 hours depending on the severity of the acute asthma exacerbation (34,81,83).

In addition to tolerance from continuous stimulation, severe airway inflammation, particularly that induced by viral infections, reduces the efficacy of β_2-agonists by producing uncoupling with the receptors (34,83). The uncoupling is felt to be produced, at least in part, by interleukin-1β and tumor necrosis factor-α (34). Increased concentrations of bronchoconstrictive functional antagonists (i.e., cysteinyl leukotrienes, histamine, acetylcholine, or substance P) produce a right movement and flattening of the dose–response curve reducing both the apparent potency and efficacy of the β_2-agonists. This effect is partially mediated through cross-talk of these mediators with G-inhibitory receptors that can impair accumulation of cyclic AMP (34). In theory, the weaker partial agonists would be the most affected but that has not been shown clinically. These factors probably all come into play during severe asthma exacerbations where patients do not respond to the usual low doses of short-acting β_2-agonists (34,81,83).

PHARMACOKINETICS

The short-acting β_2-agonists are hydrophilic and relatively rapidly absorbed orally and from lung tissue which limits their duration when taken as aerosols. The short-acting β_2-agonists do not partition into the plasmalemma lipid bilayer of airway smooth muscle and so readily diffuse into the microcirculation away from the β_2-ARs (101). Albuterol, pirbuterol, and terbutaline are well absorbed orally but undergo first-pass sulfate conjugation in the gut and liver so their systemic bioavailability varies ($\approx$50% albuterol and $\approx$20% terbutaline) (102). However, metabolism is stereoselective and [R]-albuterol is preferentially metabolized over its [S]-enantiomer, whereas [S]-terbutaline is preferentially metabolized over its [R]-enantiomer so that with repeated dosing there tends to be accumulation of [S]-albuterol (85). This potential accumulation and evidence for greater lung retention of [S]-albuterol have been used as explanations why the patients receiving high doses of albuterol with acute exacerbations may not respond as well to racemic albuterol as levalbuterol (86). The short-acting β_2-agonists are eliminated unchanged renally and through hepatic sulfate conjugation and have widely varying elimination half-lives: albuterol 3.2 to 6 hours, pirbuterol 2.5 hours, and terbutaline 20 hours (102). A study in children 8 to 15 years old reported a slightly greater clearance and shorter terminal half-life of 12 hours for terbutaline (102).

LABAs are highly lipophilic, which accounts for their longer lung retention and greater duration of action (101,103). Following inhalation, the LABAs partition into the lipid bilayer where they then slowly leak into the aqueous biophase to attach to the receptor (101,103). Formoterol has about a 10-fold lower lipophilicity and an amphiphilic component compared with salmeterol so that its onset of action is similar to short-acting β_2-agonists (34,84,103). On the other hand, salmeterol has a longer duration and slower offset (101). A newer LABA in phase 3 clinical trials, indacaterol, has been reported to have a rapid onset of action with a bronchodilatory effect lasting over 24 hours that is dose dependent (104,105). Formoterol is about 50% to 60% orally available and 10% excreted unchanged and the rest metabolized by glucuronide conjugation and to a minor extent *O*-demethylation involving CYP2D6, CYP2C19, CYP2C9, and CYP2A6 (106). Following oral administration, it has a terminal half-life of 3.4 hours and following inhalation 10 hours indicating lung retention as the rate-limiting step (107,108). Pharmacokinetic data on salmeterol are extremely limited due to low systemic concentrations achieved with usual doses. It appears to have 25% oral bioavailability due to extensive first-pass metabolism by gut and hepatic CYP3A4 isozymes, and it is primarily eliminated by CYP3A4 hydroxylation with an elimination half-life of 5.5 hours (109).

CLINICAL USE

The short-acting inhaled β_2-agonists are indicated for the management of bronchospasm manifested by cough, dyspnea, shortness of breath, and wheezing on an as needed basis. Regular use of short-acting β_2-agonists is not indicated because it does not improve outcomes (110,111). Regular use of short-acting β_2-agonists can result in an increase in bronchial hyperresponsiveness (84,112). By using short-acting β_2-agonists only as rescue, their use is also a monitoring tool to assess control of asthma, patients who need to use their rescue medication more than 2 days per week are considered not well controlled and need to be evaluated further (9). Patients using 2 or more canisters per month are at an increased risk of severe life-threatening asthma exacerbations. The short-acting β_2-agonists are the most effective therapy for the prevention of EIB used 5 to 15 minutes before exercise (113,114). They provide complete protection against EIB to 95% or more of patients even if the patients have been taking regular β_2-agonists and have tolerance (97,114). Although available as syrups for young children, oral short-acting β_2-agonists are not recommended due to their poor efficacy, longer duration until effect, greater toxicity, and inability to prevent EIB (9). Other than delivery device, there are no specific age-related issues involving short-acting β_2-agonists in children. Infants have fully functional smooth muscle and β_2-ARs throughout their bronchioles, and comparisons of MDIs + VHCs versus nebulization show that they are equally effective for acute bronchospasm (18,115).

The LABAs are currently indicated as an adjunct therapy with ICSs in patients who are not controlled with low to medium doses of ICSs (Fig. 40.1) (9). Currently, LABAs are not approved by FDA in children younger than 4 years nor have they been assessed in clinical trials for this age group. The LABAs are also approved for protection against EIB in children 5 to 11 years old. After single doses, they effectively block EIB for up to 8 to 9 hours postdose; however, regular use leads to tolerance and decreases the duration of protection to 4 to 6 hours, and therefore not much better than the short-acting β_2-agonists (98,99).

Use of LABAs for the management of asthma remains controversial. Early long-term trials in children clearly demonstrated that LABAs were inferior to ICS therapy (116,117). More recently, the Pediatrics and Pulmonary-Allergy Drugs Advisory Committees to the FDA voted to remove the indication for asthma in children for LABA monotherapy but to maintain the indication for combination ICS/LABA therapy (118). Because of the lack of any clinically relevant anti-inflammatory activity, the national guidelines have always stated that LABAs are not indicated for monotherapy (9). LABAs have been shown to improve lung function, decrease symptoms, and use of rescue medication in children when added to ICSs (116,117,119,120). However, until recently, combination ICS/LABA therapy had not produced a reduction in risk of exacerbation and has been associated with an increased risk of severe exacerbations resulting in hospitalization (56b,121,122). The increased risk of severe exacerbations in children is driven by 1-year-long trial of the addition of formoterol or placebo to usual therapy (123). The children were required to take ICS (75%) or cromolyn or nedocromil (25%) at baseline and still not well controlled. As the anti-inflammatory was not a study drug, it was not provided and adherence was simply monitored by patient report. Patients in the formoterol group had significantly greater number of hospitalizations for asthma; however, it was not greater when discontinuation due to asthma worsening was added to the placebo group. Two more recent large 1-year-long randomized clinical trials in children have shown a decrease or no change in risk of asthma exacerbation when combination therapy was compared with higher dose of ICSs (124,125). However, study design peculiarities preclude these trials from being definitive. In the first study showing no difference in exacerbations, the dose of the ICS, fluticasone propionate, was not only reduced in half but administered once daily with salmeterol administered twice daily while in the high dose ICS arm, fluticasone propionate was administered twice daily (124). The approved labeling for fluticasone propionate in children is twice daily. The second study compared budesonide, 320 μg once daily plus terbutaline for rescue, to budesonide/formoterol, 80/4.5 μg once daily plus the same dose as needed for rescue (125). Although budesonide is indicated once daily, as needed use of the combination is not, and the FDA-approved labeling for combination is twice daily and it specifically states that it is not to be used as needed for rescue (126). Therefore, more appropriate long-term trials of combination therapy are required in children.

The mechanism by which LABAs may increase the risk of serious asthma exacerbations is not clear. Although chronic use produces tolerance, patients receiving LABAs respond as well to the short-acting inhaled β_2-agonists they receive in the emergency department as those who did not receive LABAs (127). A review of exacerbations in a large long-term trial found no difference in the characteristics of worsening of lung function (rapidity and severity of drop) or response to treatment (128). The worsening of peak flow and increased exacerbations associated with regular administration of short-acting β_2-agonists to patients with Arg/Arg genotype is not seen with LABAs (129–131). In fact, increasing bronchial hyperresponsiveness is not seen with regular use of LABAs in adults or children (132,133). Although the combination of ICS/LABA has been shown to be superior to the addition of a leukotriene modifier to ICS therapy in adults, no comparison studies have been performed in children (134).

ADVERSE EVENTS

Paradoxical bronchospasm has been reported with use of β_2-agonists, but this is a relatively rare phenomenon. The β_2-ARs are ubiquitous throughout the body; in cardiac tissue they affect conductance to increase heart rate as well as prolong QTc interval and produce ST segment depression but have not been associated with torsades de pointes. The vascular effects of β_2 stimulation include vasodilation leading to lower diastolic blood pressure and decreased microvascular leakage, the former contributes to the reflex increase in heart rate (135). The metabolic effects include gluconeogenesis, sodium/potassium ATPase stimulation, and increased lactate production resulting in hypokalemia, hyperglycemia, and lactic acidosis at high doses (135). Skeletal muscle and neuromuscular transmission is enhanced leading to fine tremor that usually disappears with chronic administration. In general, these agents should be used with caution in patients with cardiovascular disorders, convulsive disorders, diabetes mellitus, hyperthyroidism, and hypokalemia, as the adverse events of β_2-agonists may potentiate the underlying disease or they may interact with other medications. As these adverse effects are all mediated by β_2-AR stimulation, they occur similarly for the single enantiomer drugs as for the racemic mixtures when given in equipotent doses (84,87,88). Because of their greater retention in the lung, the LABAs produce fewer systemic effects than the short-acting β_2-agonists with a fourfold or greater increase over recommended dose to produce significant changes in heart rate, serum potassium, glucose, or QTc interval (135,136). In a crossover study of 20 children aged 6 to 11 years with asthma, administered cumulative doses of formoterol 45 μg and terbutaline 5,000 μg (equipotent) over a 2.5-hour time period, formoterol produced significantly less hypokalemia, hyperglycemia, QTc prolongation, blood pressure effect, and increased lactate (137). Values fell out of the normal range more frequently with the terbutaline than formoterol, and the duration of abnormalities was not significantly longer for formoterol. Comparisons of formoterol and salmeterol administered by DPIs in adults and children indicate a four- to fivefold difference in potency for both bronchodilation and systemic activity (135,138).

DRUG INTERACTIONS

Potential physiologic drug interactions with β_2-agonists include nonselective β-antagonists, thiazide and loop diuretics, digoxin, theophylline, and other drugs that prolong QTc interval. The product label for all β_2-agonists includes the statement that coadministration of monoamine oxidase inhibitors or tricyclic antidepressants with β_2-agonists may potentiate the cardiovascular effect of these agents. However, this is a holdover from the potential hypertensive crisis mediated by the coadministration of ephedrine, the indirect acting drug that causes the release of endogenous catecholamines from nerve terminals as well as administration of epinephrine. The β_2-agonists do not induce the release of endogenous catecholamines nor do they produce vasoconstriction and there is a paucity of data supporting these interactions.

There are few pharmacokinetic interactions with the β_2-agonists. Serum digoxin has decreased by 16% and 22% after a single dose of intravenous and oral albuterol, respectively, in patients who have been on digoxin for at least 10 days. Coadministration of salmeterol with strong CYP3A4 inhibitors such as ketoconazole, ritonavir, atazanavir, clarithromycin, indinavir, itraconazole, nefazodone, nelfinavir, saquinavir, and telithromycin may increase the risk of cardiovascular adverse events due to increased oral bioavailability of salmeterol. Ketoconazole 400 mg daily for 7 days resulted in a 16-fold increase in plasma salmeterol area under the curve in 20 healthy subjects, 3 were withdrawn from the study because of cardiovascular side effects (109). Coadministration of erythromycin and salmeterol has resulted in a 40% increase in salmeterol serum concentration at steady state.

CHROMONES

MECHANISM OF ACTION

The chromones include cromolyn sodium and nedocromil with anti-inflammatory activity used in the treatment of asthma. They are only active by inhalation. The chromones prevent the mast cell activation and degranulation possibly by inhibiting chloride transport and protein kinase C (139). Administered just prior to allergen exposure, they prevent both the early and late asthma response including eosinophil activation and mediator release (139). They both inhibit EIB administered prior to exercise (140). In addition, they inhibit bronchoconstriction induced by sulfur dioxide and bradykinin presumably by inhibiting afferent C-fiber stimulation (139). This mechanism may be responsible for their activity in reducing cough in asthma as well as angiotensin-converting enzyme-induced cough.

PHARMACOKINETICS

Both cromolyn and nedocromil are highly ionized water-soluble compounds at physiologic pH, so do not enter cells and cross membranes and are poorly absorbed orally (<1%) so only effective by inhalation (139). They are rapidly eliminated unchanged in the urine or biliary tract. Intravenous cromolyn has a terminal half-life of 11 to 22 minutes so inhaled cromolyn exhibits an absorption rate limited half-life of less than 2 hours (141). They are rapidly absorbed from the lung so require multiple daily dosing (four times daily for cromolyn and two to four times daily for nedocromil) for optimal benefit. Lack of absorption across cell membranes probably accounts for the lack of significant adverse effects from the chromones (139,141).

CLINICAL USE

Cromolyn sodium by nebulizer solution is indicated as an alternative to ICSs for treatment of mild persistent asthma (9). Several clinical trials have shown that chromones are not as effective as ICSs for controlling asthma symptoms, improving lung function, and preventing exacerbations (38,44,46,47,142). The few comparative trials with other controllers (theophylline and montelukast) have failed to demonstrate significant differences in controlling asthma (141,143). However, parents preferred once-daily montelukast to three times daily cromolyn (143). A meta-analysis has suggested that there is insufficient evidence to support the use of cromolyn in young children (142). However, the study providing the largest population that drove the results of this meta-analysis administered the cromolyn by actuating multiple puffs from an MDI into a VHC with a face mask while the patients breathed for 30 seconds (144). This dosage and delivery method for patients aged

1 to 4 years is an unproven method (more than one puff in a VHC at a time reduces delivery) (20). In addition, numerous studies in the meta-analysis used different dosage forms and various age ranges; thus, it is unclear that it was even appropriate to combine the studies. Studies of cromolyn nebulizer solution administered four times daily have demonstrated beneficial effects, and cromolyn nebulizer solution has gained regulatory label approval in the United States and in other countries for children younger than 2 years. In addition, retrospective studies of large integrated medical/pharmacy databases suggest that dispensing of cromolyn reduces the risk of emergency department visits and hospitalizations at least for children (145,146).

Pretreatment with the chromones prior to exercise is effective for preventing EIB (114,140). Cromolyn and nedocromil were equally effective when administered by either MDI or DPI (140). The chromones were less effective than short-acting inhaled β_2-agonists but more effective than the attenuating effect of anticholinergics providing complete protection in 73% of patients versus 56% of patients receiving anticholinergics (114). They have not been directly compared with LTRAs but they appear to be more effective, as LTRAs generally produce attenuation and only produce complete blocking in 40% to 55% of children (113,147).

Except for cough with cromolyn and bad taste with nedocromil, these drugs have a strong safety profile (140).

LEUKOTRIENE MODIFIERS

MECHANISM OF ACTION

The leukotriene modifiers are the first drugs inhibiting a specific pathway or mediator in the vast array of inflammatory pathways that have established efficacy in asthma. Leukotrienes (LTs) are eicosanoids derived from arachidonic acid via the 5-lipoxygenase pathway and are produced in eosinophils, mast cells, and alveolar macrophages (148). The synthesis can lead to the production of LTB4 that is involved with the chemotaxis of neutrophils and/or to the production of the cysteinyl leukotrienes (CysLTs) LTC4, LTD4, and LTE4. These stimulate the CysLT1 receptor in airway smooth muscle to cause constriction and the CysLT2 receptor in the vascular smooth muscle to produce constriction and promote chemotaxis (149). LTD4 and LTC4 are approximately 1,000 times more potent than histamine in producing bronchoconstriction (150). The CysLT1 receptor is most highly expressed in spleen, peripheral blood leukocytes including eosinophils, and lung smooth muscle cells and interstitial lung macrophages (149). The rank potency of agonist activation for the CysLT1 receptor is LTD4 > LTC4 > LTE4 and for the CysLT2 receptor is LTC4 = LTD4 > LTE4 (149). Although less potent, LTE4 is the more stable compound and excreted in the urine and has been used as a marker for leukotriene production. The cysteinyl leukotrienes produce bronchoconstriction, tissue edema, and increased mucus secretion. The leukotriene modifiers currently consist of a 5-lipoxygenase inhibitor, zileuton, and two selective CystLT1 receptor antagonists, montelukast, and zafirlukast (148). The relative localization of CysLT1 receptors accounts for their selectivity for the lungs and peripheral eosinophils and relative lack of systemic effects so that it is unnecessary to give them as aerosols.

PHARMACOKINETICS

Zileuton is only available as extended-release tablets for twice daily dosing in children 12 years old and adults and is recommended to be used with food because food increases its bioavailability (151). Zileuton is metabolized by hepatic CYP1A2, CYP2C9, and CYP3A4. About 94% of the zileuton dose is excreted in the urine and the rest in the feces. Zafirlukast is approved for children younger than 5 years and should be taken 1 hour before or 2 hours after meals because administration with food decreased the bioavailability by 40% (152). Zafirlukast is extensively metabolized by CYP2C9. Following oral administration, 10% of the dose is excreted renally and the rest is excreted in the urine. Montelukast has a mean oral bioavailability of 64% which is not affected by meals. Montelukast is metabolized by CYP3A4 and CYP2C9 (153). Montelukast and its metabolites are extensively excreted via the biliary tract.

CLINICAL USE

No evidence exists for significant differences in efficacy for the various leukotriene modifiers. Differences in dosing and relative safety (see later) do exist that have made montelukast the de facto preferred LTRA in children. The leukotriene modifiers are often considered as anti-inflammatory and they do result in a decrease in FeNO that is considered a marker of airway inflammation, and reduce serum eosinophils and have decreased sputum eosinophils (150). However, they are significantly less effective than low-dose ICSs for improving lung function, controlling asthma symptoms, reducing asthma exacerbations and bronchial hyperresponsiveness, and reducing FeNO (154). They have been used as adjunctive therapy with ICS, as studies have demonstrated that leukotriene production may be relatively resistant to ICS therapy (134). Compared with LABAs as adjunctive therapy, the leukotriene modifiers are less effective for reducing the risk of exacerbations requiring corticosteroids, improving daily symptom scores, night time awakenings, rescue medication use, and lung function (134).

Two recent randomized trials question the significance of the anti-inflammatory activity of the leukotriene modifiers (155,156). In a 24-week comparison of the addition of either theophylline or montelukast to usual therapy in 489 patients with poorly controlled asthma (74% to 79% receiving ICSs across groups), neither theophylline nor montelukast reduced the number of episodes of poor asthma control compared with placebo, although both produced small improvements in lung function (155). In the subset of patients not receiving ICSs, theophylline was more effective than montelukast and placebo at improving asthma symptoms and montelukast was not better than placebo. The second study compared the combination of an LTRA and LABA to low-dose ICS and LABA in 192 patients randomized in the 14-week crossover trial with a 4-week washout between treatments (156). The Data Safety and Monitoring Board terminated the study after only

94 patients completed because of a highly significant greater number of treatment failures, the primary endpoint, in the LTRA plus LABA combination. In addition, measures of airway inflammation [i.e., FeNO, sputum eosinophils, and sputum eosinophil cationic protein (ECP)] all worsened on the leukotriene arm of the study. A crossover trial in 24 children 5 to 12 years old with persistent asthma controlled with ICS therapy comparing 4 weeks of placebo, 5 mg montelukast, and 50 μg fluticasone by DPI confirmed these results (54). Spirometry and FeNO were the primary outcome variables measured at the end of a 2-week run-in period and then at the end of 2 and 4 weeks of each treatment period. Both postbronchodilator forced expiratory volume in 1 second (FEV_1) and FeNO were significantly better on fluticasone than either placebo or montelukast, and montelukast was not better than placebo.

Montelukast is often prescribed for children with persistent asthma because of its lack of adverse effects and ease of administration. However, comparative trials have demonstrated it to be significantly less effective in children 6 to 14 years of age than therapy with low-dose ICSs (40–42,54,157,158). Because of the variability in response to various anti-asthmatics, a crossover trial in 144 children 6 to 17 years old with mild-to-moderate asthma was designed to determine which patients may preferentially respond to montelukast versus ICS (158). Only 5% of patients responded to montelukast only, defined as a 7.5% increase in FEV_1 compared with 23% that responded to only ICSs. Overall 22% of the children had a positive response to montelukast and was associated with higher urinary LTE4 concentrations. Interestingly, this compares to 58% of adults who achieved that level or greater lung function response in a recent large randomized parallel trial comparing montelukast with beclomethasone dipropionate (159). Other evidence that the response to leukotriene modifiers may be age dependent is that montelukast was approved based upon pharmacokinetics and safety and extrapolated efficacy for all of the dosage forms for children younger than 6 years (153). In children 2 to 5 years of age, montelukast improved some asthma outcomes compared with placebo in reducing day and night time symptoms increasing asthma free days and as needed β_2-agonists (160). However, no improvement in any of those same outcomes was seen in a placebo-controlled trial in infants 6 to 24 months of age (161). On the other hand, ICS therapy has been shown to markedly improve the above constellation of symptoms as well as significantly decrease the risk of asthma exacerbations in infants younger than 6 months (39,61).

It has been argued that the "real world" effectiveness of the LTRAs in children is underestimated by randomized clinical trials, as the ease of administration (once daily oral therapy) will improve compliance compared with ICSs and result in similar effectiveness over time (162). However, adherence with long-term therapy in asthma, as in other chronic diseases, is generally poor (40% to 70% as measured by pharmacy refill rates), and studies have demonstrated only marginally greater adherence to montelukast compared with ICSs in children, and the only independently supported study found no difference in adherence in children 3 to 18 years old between montelukast and ICSs (163). In addition, a large retrospective study of a medical/pharmacy integrated database assessing outcomes over 12 months in 3,647 children prescribed either an ICS or montelukast found significantly more treatment failures, hospitalizations for asthma, and a significantly greater annualized cost for asthma care for those receiving montelukast despite significantly greater numbers of dispensing of the montelukast than the ICS (164). These "real world" effectiveness results are consistent with the differences seen in the randomized clinical trials.

Montelukast has FDA-approved labeling for prevention of EIB in patients 15 years and older. LTRAs attenuate but rarely completely protect against EIB. Chronic treatment with montelukast reduces EIB by 20% to 50%; however, up to 50% of patients may not respond (165–167). The onset and the duration of effect on EIB after one dose of montelukast have been evaluated in children (147). Children, 7 to 13 years old, performed an exercise challenge 2, 12, and 24 hours after a single dose of montelukast. Montelukast produced a significant protection against EIB compared with placebo only at 12 hours postdose, percent fall in FEV_1 (9.78 ± 1.85 vs. 18.69 ± 2.83, respectively). A significant difference was seen in the percentage of patients on montelukast (50%) compared with placebo (31%) with EIB protection defined as less than 15% fall in maximum FEV_1 only at 12 hours postdose. These results again suggest more attenuation than complete protection against EIB. More recently, montelukast was compared to standard therapy of two inhalations of albuterol in a crossover study in children 7 to 17 years of age (113). Using 15% drop in FEV_1 as the endpoint, 100% of the patients receiving albuterol and 55% of patients receiving montelukast were protected and the response was independent of the concentration of LTE4 in the exhaled breath condensate. In this study, patients continued to use albuterol as needed so that any tolerance to albuterol would not be washed out and the exercise challenge was performed at 12 hours post montelukast dose, the time of maximum effect.

An area of recent interest for using LTRAs is the prophylaxis against viral-induced asthma exacerbations in patients who are symptom free between exacerbations (168,169). The corticosteroids have not been considered effective for this asthma phenotype in children. A randomized controlled trial of montelukast 4 or 5 mg daily in 549 children aged 2 to 5 years for 12 months reported that exacerbations were reduced to 1.6 per pt/year from 2.34 per pt/year (168). However, exacerbations were defined as any 3 consecutive days of daytime symptoms or two treatments of inhaled β_2-agonists or rescue with corticosteroids or hospitalization. When using standard definition of exacerbation (rescue with oral corticosteroids, hospitalization, unscheduled physician visit), there was no difference from placebo. In addition, based upon review of history at entry would appear that many of the patients would be considered persistent and not intermittent asthma (9). A controlled trial that administered montelukast or placebo to children aged 2 to 14 years who had intermittent asthma at the first sign of a viral infection and continued for 7 days reported a modest decline in health care resource utilization, symptoms, days off from school, and parent time off of work (169). However, again montelukast did not reduce the number of more severe asthma episodes as measured by oral corticosteroid use and hospitalizations.

A recent large clinical trial from the Childhood Asthma Research and Education (CARE) network of the National Institutes of Health (NIH) compared intermittent as needed use of an ICS (budesonide nebulizer suspension 1 mg twice daily) or montelukast 4 mg once daily or placebo for 7 days along with as needed albuterol at the onset of respiratory tract illness in 238 children 1 to 5 years old (170). Although they did not demonstrate a reduction in the number of patients requiring oral corticosteroids or emergency health-care visits, they did report a differential response in that those children with a positive asthma predictive index demonstrated significant reductions in severity of symptoms during exacerbations for both active therapies compared with placebo. Thus, montelukast has not been found to be superior to ICSs in episodic viral wheezing in infants and children.

ADVERSE EVENTS

Elevation of one or more hepatic function enzymes has been reported with zileuton and zafirlukast which may progress, remain unchanged, or resolve within 3 weeks of therapy. Cases of liver failure have been reported with zafirlukast. A baseline ALT measurement followed monthly for the next 3 months and then every 2 to 3 months is recommended for zileuton, whereas signs of liver dysfunction (diarrhea, jaundice) are recommended for zafirlukast with monitoring ALT if these signs occur.

Churg-Strauss syndrome, a vascular inflammation that is accompanied by tissue and blood eosinophilia, and is usually accompanied by severe asthma symptoms, has been reported in patients taking zafirlukast or montelukast (171,172). Although the frequency of this adverse effect is rare and appears primarily as case-reports, it is important to be aware of this possible effect. Although the exact cause of the syndrome is not known, the syndrome has been reported when the dose of oral steroid was reduced and some have suggested that it is merely an unmasking of a disease that was misdiagnosed as asthma initially. However, cases have occurred in patients not receiving oral corticosteroids. Other adverse events reported with zafirlukast include headache, infection, nausea, diarrhea, abdominal pain, asthenia, fever, myalgia, vomiting, and dizziness. The most common side effects of montelukast include fatigue, fever, pain, dyspepsia, headache, dizziness, rash, nasal congestion, cough, influenza, and elevated AST and ALT.

DRUG INTERACTIONS

Zileuton significantly interacts with theophylline, warfarin, and propranolol resulting in an increase in concentration of these medications. Coadministration of these medications with zileuton requires close monitoring and dose adjustment. Coadministration of zafirlukast and warfarin has also lead to an increase in prothrombin time by 35%. Plasma concentration of zafirlukast was decreased by 30% and 40% when coadministered with theophylline or erythromycin and the concentration was increased by 45% when it was used with high doses of aspirin. Studies looking at coadministration of montelukast and theophylline, warfarin or digoxin did not show any significant reaction with these drugs.

METHYLXANTHINES (THEOPHYLLINE)

MECHANISM OF ACTION

Theophylline is a nonselective phosphodiesterase (PDE) inhibitor that prevents degradation of intracellular cyclic AMP and cyclic GMP (173). The PDE isoenzymes currently thought to be important for theophylline's clinical effects are PDE III, predominant in airway smooth muscle, and PDE IV, involved in regulation of the following inflammatory cells mast cells: mast cells, neutrophils, eosinophils, and T lymphocytes (173). In addition, theophylline has been shown to activate histone deacetylase that is involved in the corticosteroid-induced decrease in proinflammatory gene expression (174). Decreased histone deacetylase activity is felt to be involved in the relative resistance to corticosteroids seen in some patients with asthma and in most patients with COPD (175). However, it would appear that the moderate bronchodilation is primarily responsible for the antiasthmatic effect of theophylline. Selective PDE IV inhibitors have not demonstrated significant effects in clinical asthma (174). A recent study testing the hypothesis that low-dose theophylline would be more beneficial in asthma patients receiving ICSs than those not as a result of its activation of histone deacetylase reported just the opposite (155).

PHARMACOKINETICS

The benefit and risks from theophylline relate to serum concentrations. Maximum potential benefit with minimal risk of adverse effects is achieved at peak concentrations of 5 to 15 μg per mL (9). Since concentrations can vary greatly among children receiving the same dose, because of variable rates of metabolism, serum concentrations must be measured to adjust dosage. Outside of the neonatal period, theophylline is principally eliminated by capacity-limited hepatic metabolism that is genetically determined and can be further altered by environmental exposures such as age, febrile viral infections, smoking, and dietary changes (173). Theophylline is predominantly metabolized by CYP1A2 and to a lesser extent CYP3A3 and CYP2E1 isozymes and is about 35% to 40% protein bound (173). In general, children 1 to 6 years old have the greatest systemic clearance and therefore require higher milligram per kilogram maintenance dosing. Theophylline is 95% to 100% absorbed orally and its absorption rate exhibits diurnal variability with slower absorption in the evening (173). Clinically, it is primarily administered as sustained-release preparations to minimize multiple daily dosing and serum concentration fluctuations (173).

CLINICAL USE

Sustained-release theophylline is still considered an alternative, not preferred, maintenance and adjunctive therapy to the ICSs in children 5 to 11 years of age but not in children 0 to 4 years of age (9). Lack of clinical trial data on efficacy and potential for serious adverse effects in young children and infants is why it is no longer recommended in 0- to 4-year-olds (9,45,176). When using theophylline in 5- to 11-year-olds, serum drug concentration monitoring is

TABLE 40.7 Factors Affecting Theophylline Clearance (181)

Decreased Clearance	*Decrease (%)*	*Increased Clearance*
Cimetidine	−25 to −60	Rifampin
Macrolides: Erythromycin,	−25 to −50	Carbamazepine
TAO, clarithromycin		Phenobarbital
		Phenytoin
Allopurinol	−20	Charcoal-broiled meat
Propranolol	−30	
Quinolones:	−20 to −50	High-protein diet
Ciprofloxacin, enoxacin, pefloxacin		Smoking
Interferon	−50	Sulfinpyrazone
Thiabendazole	−65	Moricizine
Ticlopidine	−25	Aminoglutethimide
Zileuton	−35	
Systemic viral illness	−10 to −50	

required to prevent serious toxicity. As a result of the potential for severe toxicity, the moderate bronchodilation produced by theophylline relative to the β_2-agonists, and questionable anti-inflammatory activity, theophylline has been relegated to second-line adjunctive therapy with ICSs. Early trials suggested that theophylline improves lung function slightly in patients not adequately controlled on low-dose ICSs but to an extent similar to doubling the dose of ICSs (177,178). However, the two more recent trials, one in children and one in adults, have questioned the efficacy of adding theophylline to ICSs (155,179). The first study showed no advantage of either montelukast or theophylline when added to usual therapy in adult patients with poorly controlled asthma receiving ICSs, although in the subset of patients not receiving ICSs theophylline, but not montelukast, improved some outcomes (155).

In the second study, investigators added theophylline to baseline ICS therapy in a randomized controlled trial in 36 children 6 to 18 years old for 12 weeks. There was a significant increase in peak expiratory flow but not FEV_1 or specific airway resistance in the theophylline group. There was a reduction in blood ECP but not eosinophils or various subtypes of T lymphocytes and no change in cold air challenge. Comparisons of LABAs with theophylline consistently show LABAs to be superior in efficacy (180). Theophylline has modest dose-related attenuation of EIB (173).

ADVERSE EFFECTS

Theophylline produces significant dose-related toxicity from mild caffeine-like central nervous stimulation, headache, and nausea at high therapeutic concentrations that can be uncomfortable for some patients to serious vomiting, cardiac arrhythmias, seizures, and cerebral ischemia at high concentrations. Some of these toxicities are due to adenosine antagonistic effects of theophylline. Elderly and young children are at particular risk for serious toxicities due to altered metabolism in young children secondary to acute febrile viral illnesses (9,181).

DRUG INTERACTIONS

Theophylline is associated with a number of drug interactions from drugs that inhibit and induce the hepatic cytochrome P450 enzymes. Only those drugs that produce at least a 20% reduction or 50% increase in clearance are likely to produce clinically significant interactions, but there is a significant interpatient variability, so the clinician should use caution with all potentially interacting drugs. These are listed in Table 40.7 (181).

ANTI-IMMUNOGLOBULIN E

MECHANISM OF ACTION

Omalizumab is a recombinant monoclonal anti-immunoglobulin E (IgE) antibody with 5% composition from murine sequences and the rest from human (182). Omalizumab binds to the Fc portion of the IgE antibody and prevents it from binding to the receptor (FcεRI) on mast cells and basophils and also results in a decrease in free IgE serum concentration. This leads to a decrease in the release of inflammatory mediators in response to allergen exposure and a decrease in expression of FcεRI on airway submucosal cells and basophils (182). Omalizumab also induces eosinophil apoptosis in patient with allergic asthma (183).

PHARMACOKINETICS

The dose of omalizumab is based on patient's baseline total serum IgE and body weight and it is administered subcutaneously at 2- or 4-week intervals. Omalizumab has an average absolute bioavailability of 62%. The peak serum concentration after a single dose exceeds 10,000 ng per mL and free IgE drops to 10 ng per mL (184). Total IgE rises as the omalizumab + IgE complex has a slow elimination half-life of 26 days and it is primarily through the reticuloendothelial system (185). Omalizumab reaches steady state at 28 weeks. Target free IgE concentrations are below 50 ng per mL and are usually reached after the first dose and obtained in 95% of patients using the dosing table (184). Despite rapid reduction in IgE, it takes 12 to 16 weeks for maximum therapeutic effect. Following discontinuation of omalizumab, free IgE concentrations are near baseline after about 120 days with the return of symptoms and lung function paralleling the drop after only a few days (184). This represents a hysteresis with onset taking longer than offset.

CLINICAL USE

Omalizumab is recommended to be used as an adjunctive therapy in patients 12 years or older with moderate to severe atopic asthma not adequately controlled with combination ICS/LABA (Fig. 40.1) (9). Although, omalizumab is approved for use in moderate persistent asthma as adjunctive therapy to patients on ICSs, it has not been compared to current adjunctive therapy (LABA, leukotriene modifiers, or theophylline). However, it is the only therapy to demonstrate improved outcomes in those patients poorly controlled on high-dose ICS/LABA including reduction in severe exacerbations (186,187). The effects of omalizumab on baseline lung function as measured by FEV_1 are not consistent and may be explained in part by the design of the studies where a reduction in dose of oral or ICS is an outcome (188–190). Approximately 65% to 80% of patients respond to omalizumab with a 50% or more reduction in corticosteroid dosage compared with 50% to 55% of patients on placebo across clinical trials (182,184,186–190). The only currently published study in 334 children, 6 to 12 years old, omalizumab resulted in 16% more patients able to reduce their ICS dose than those on placebo (65.3% vs. 49.5%), but there were no significant differences in lung function, symptoms, or exacerbations (9). It is unclear how long patients must continue omalizumab if they respond. The potential benefits appear to last only as long as the drug is administered (184,191,192).

A major consideration with use of omalizumab is its high cost. Depending on the dosage, the cost varies between \$6,000 and \$36,000 per year (182,193,194). The cost-effectiveness of omalizumab has been investigated and the results have differed because of differences in clinical trials used for the analysis, and whether cost-effectiveness is based upon a third party payer's versus societal perspective (193–196). A recent analysis did not find omalizumab cost-effective for most patients with severe asthma suggesting clinicians should explore alternative medications before starting omalizumab (196). Omalizumab seems to be cost-effective when used in nonsmoker patients, whom despite maximal asthma therapy they have been hospitalized five or more times or 20 days or longer per year (195). More clinical trials are needed to compare omalizumab to other alternative medications as an adjunct therapy to ICSs. Patients who cannot tolerate medium to high doses of ICSs in combination with LABA may benefit from addition of omalizumab.

ADVERSE EFFECTS

The most common side effects are local reactions at the site of injection, upper respiratory tract infection, viral infection, headache, sinusitis, and pharyngitis. The most serious side effects are malignancies and anaphylaxis reactions. In the clinical trials, the rate of cancer was 0.35% within 1 year; all tumors (except one) were solid (185). Considering the time course of tumor development and the fact that they were solid tumor suggest that they preexisted. Current evidence does not support a causal relationship between omalizumab and development of cancer and there is no difference in incidence of cancer between patients on omalizumab and the general population. However, long-term follow-up studies of greater than 3 years are warranted to investigate the safety of omalizumab.

Serious anaphylaxis and anaphylactoid reactions have been reported in premarketing clinical trials and in post-marketing spontaneous reports which resulted in addition of a boxed warning to the product label. The rate of the reaction is about 0.1% and it can happen after any dose of omalizumab. It usually occurs within 2 hours of injections; however, it may be delayed up to 24 hours (197). Sixty-one percent of reactions occurred after the first three doses. It is recommended that patients be observed up to 2 hours after the first three injections and then up to 30 minutes after subsequent injections and be taught how to recognize symptoms of anaphylaxis (197). Another potential side effect is an increase in incidence or severity of helminthic infection as a result of a decrease in IgE serum concentration. In a 1-year clinical trial in patients at high risk for geohelminthic infections, patients on omalizumab had an odds ratio of 1.96 to have an infection; however, the response to anti-helminth therapy among treatment groups did not differ (198). Monitoring high-risk patients for helminthic infection while on omalizumab is recommended. There are no known drug interactions associated with omalizumab.

SUMMARY

Asthma therapy for children has advanced significantly over the last 40 years with a change in approach to management occurring almost every 10 years. This is primarily based on the introduction of new medications at intervals approximating 10 years. As usual, all medications are initially studied in adults and adolescents, then studies are conducted in children 5 to 11 years of age, and finally studies are conducted for those children younger than 5 years. The steps to studying medications in children have been accelerated in the last 15 years due to FDA directives. For asthma, several long-term control medications including nebulized budesonide and oral montelukast are now approved down to 1 year of age.

With the advances in conducting clinical trials in young children, prompted by studies conducted in the NIH asthma networks and the NICHD Pediatric Pharmacology Research Unit Network, it is anticipated that more medications will continue to be evaluated in children to provide specific product labeling for all age groups. The next significant advance in childhood asthma will be to identify medications designed to prevent the onset and progression of asthma. This might even mean developing a medication that is primarily used for the treatment of emerging asthma in young children.

REFERENCES

1. Akinbami LJ. *The state of childhood asthma, United States, 1980–2005. Advance data from vital and health statistics, no 381.* Hyattsville, MD: National Center for Health Statistics, 2006.
2. New Asthma Estimates: Tracking Prevalence, Health Care and Mortality, NCHS, CDC, 2001.

3. National Hospital Discharge Survey, NCHS, US CDC, 2000.
4. American Lung Association. Trends in asthma morbidity and mortality. American Lung Association Epidemiology & Statistics Unit Research and Program Services. July 2006. http://www.lungusa.org.
5. Akinbami, L. Asthma prevalence, health care use and mortality: United States 2003–2005, CDC National Center for Health Statistics, 2006.
6. American Lung Association. Epidemiology & Statistics Unit, Research and Program Services. Trends in Asthma Morbidity and Mortality, November 2007.
7. Centers for Disease Control. Surveillance for Asthma—United States, 1960–1995, MMWR, 1998;47 (SS-1).
8. Masoli M, Fabian D, Holt S, et al. Global Initiative for Asthma (GINA) Program. The global burden of asthma: executive summary of the GINA Dissemination Committee report. *Allergy* 2004; 59:469–478.
9. National Institutes of Health, National Heart, Lung, and Blood Institute. National Asthma Education and Prevention Program. Full Report of the Expert Panel: Guidelines for the diagnosis and management of asthma (EPR-3) 2007. http://www.nhlbi.nih.gov/guidelines/asthma. Accessed April 28, 2009.
10. Busse WW, Lemanske RF Jr. Asthma. *N Eng J Med* 2001:344: 350–362.
11. Morgan WJ, Stern DA, Sherrill DL, et al. Outcome of asthma and wheezing in the first 6 years of life: follow-up through adolescence. *Am J Respir Crit Care Med* 2005;172:1253–1258.
12. Guilbert TW, Morgan WJ, Zeiger RS, et al. Long-term inhaled corticosteroids in preschool children at high risk for asthma. *N Engl J Med* 2006;354:1985–1997.
13. Covar RA, Spahn JD, Murphy JR, et al. Childhood Asthma Management Program Research Group. Progression of asthma measured by lung function in the childhood asthma management program. *Am J Respir Crit Care Med* 2004;170:234–241.
14. Dolovich MA, MacIntyre NR, Dhand R, et al. Consensus conference on aerosols and delivery devices. *Respir Care* 2000;45:588–776.
15. Kelly HW. Comparison of inhaled corticosteroids: an update. *Ann Pharmacother* 2009;43:519–527.
16. Leach CL, Davidson PJ, Hasselquist BE, et al. Lung deposition of hydrofluoralkane-134a beclomethasone is greater than that of chlorofluorocarbon fluticasone and chlorofluorocarbon beclomethasone: a cross-over study in healthy volunteers. *Chest* 2002;122: 510–516.
17. Dolovich MB, Ahrens RC, Hess DR, et al. Device selection and outcomes of aerosol therapy: evidence-based guidelines. *Chest* 2005; 127:335–371.
18. Raissy HH, Kelly HW. MDI versus nebulizers for acute asthma. *J Pediatr Pharmacol Ther* 2004;9:226–234.
19. Liang J, Asmus MJ, Hochaus G, et al. Differences in inhaled fluticasone bioavailability between holding chambers in children with asthma. *Pharmacotherapy* 2002;22:947–953.
20. Wildhaber JH, Devadason SG, Eber E, et al. Effect of electrostatic charge, flow, delay and multiple actuations on the in vitro delivery of salbutamol from different small volume spacers for infants. *Thorax* 1996;51:985–988.
21. Pierart F, Wildhaber JH, Vrancken I, et al. Washing plastic spacers in household detergent reduces electrostatic charge and greatly improves delivery. *Eur Respir J* 1999;13:673–678.
22. Product information: Pulmicort Flexhaler (R), (budesonide inhalation powder) for oral inhalation. AstraZeneca LP, Wilmington, DE, 2008.
23. Product information: Asmanex Twisthaler (R), (mometasone furoate inhalation powder) for oral inhalation only. Schering-Plough Corporation, Kenilworth, NJ, October 2008.
24. Wildhaber JH, Dore ND, Wilson JM, et al. Inhalation therapy in asthma: nebulizer or pressurized metered-dose inhaler with holding chamber? In vivo comparison of lung deposition in children. *J Pediatr* 1999;135:28–33.
25. Everard ML, Clark AR, Milner AD. Drug delivery from jet nebulisers. *Arch Dis Child* 1992;67:586–591.
26. Janssens HM, De Jongste JC, Hop WC, et al. Extra-fine particles improve lung delivery of inhaled steroids in infants: a study in an upper airway model. *Chest* 2003;123:2083–2088.
27. Finlay WH, Zuberbuhler P. In vitro comparison of beclomethasone and salbutamol metered-dose inhaler aerosols inhaled during pediatric tidal breathing from four valved holding chambers. *Chest* 1998;114:1676–1680.
28. Product information: QVAR (R), (beclomethasone dipropionate HFA) Inhalation Aerosol. Teva Specialty Pharmaceuticals LLC, Horsham, PA, 2008.
29. Raissy HH, Davies L, Marshik P, et al. Inspiratory flow through dry-powder inhalers (DPIs) in asthmatic children 2 to 12 years old. *Pediatr Asthma Allergy Immunol* 2006;19:223–230.
30. Leung DY, Bloom JW. Update on glucocorticoid action and resistance. *J Allergy Clin Immunol* 2003;111:3–22.
31. Barnes PJ, Pedersen S, Busse WW. Efficacy and safety of inhaled corticosteroids: new developments. *Am J Respir Crit Care Med* 1998; 157:S1–S53.
32. Kumar SD, Brieva JL, Danta I, et al. Transient effect of inhaled fluticasone on airway mucosal blood flow in subjects with and without asthma. *Am J Respir Crit Care Med* 2000;161:918–921.
33. McFadden ER Jr. Acute Severe Asthma. *Am J Respir Crit Care Med* 2003;168:740–759.
34. Anderson GP. Interactions between corticosteroids and β-adrenergic agonists in asthma disease induction, progression, and exacerbation. *Am J Respir Crit Care Med* 2000;161:S188–S196.
35. Kelly HW. Potential adverse effects of inhaled corticosteroids. *J Allergy Clin Immunol* 2003;112:469–478.
36. Derendorf H, Nave R, Drollman A, et al. Relevance of pharmacokinetics and pharmacodynamics of inhaled corticosteroids to asthma. *Eur Respir J* 2006;28:1042–1050.
37. Martin RJ, Szefler SJ, Chinchilli VM, et al. Systemic effect comparisons of six inhaled corticosteroid preparations. *Am J Respir Crit Care Med* 2002;165:1377–1383.
38. Childhood Asthma Management Program Research Group. Long-term effects of budesonide or nedocromil in children with asthma. *N Engl J Med* 2000;343:1054–1063.
39. Bisgaard H, Gillies J, Groenewald M, et al. The effect of inhaled fluticasone propionate in the treatment of young asthmatic children. A dose comparison study. *Am J Respir Crit Care Med* 1999; 160:126–131.
40. Garcia Garcia ML, Wahn U, Gilles L, et al. Montelukast, compared with fluticasone, for control of asthma among 6- to 14-year-old patients with mild asthma: the MOSAIC study. *Pediatrics* 2005;116:360–369.
41. Ostrom NK, Decotis BA, Lincourt WR, et al. Comparative efficacy and safety of low-dose fluticasone propionate and montelukast in children with persistent asthma. *J Pediatr* 2005;147:213–220.
42. Verberne AA, Frost C, Roorda RJ, et al. One year treatment with salmeterol compared with beclomethasone in children with asthma. The Dutch Paediatric Asthma Study Group. *Am J Respir Crit Care Med* 1997;156:688–695.
43. Tinkelman DG, Reed CE, Nelson HS, et al. Aerosol beclomethasone dipropionate compared with theophylline as primary treatment of chronic, mild to moderately severe asthma in children. *Pediatrics* 1993;92:64–77.
44. Guevara JP, Ducharme FM, Keren R, et al. Inhaled corticosteroids versus sodium cromoglycate in children and adults with asthma. *Cochrane Database Syst Rev* 2006;2:CD003558.
45. Seddon P, Bara A, Ducharme FM, et al. Oral xanthines as maintenance treatment for asthma in children. *Cochrane Database Syst Rev* 2006;1:CD002885.
46. Bisgaard H, Allen D, Milanowski J, et al. Twelve month safety and efficacy of inhaled fluticasone propionate in children aged 1 to 3 years with recurrent wheezing. *Pediatrics* 2004;113:e87–e94.
47. Leflein JG, Szefler SJ, Murphy KR, et al. Nebulized budesonide inhalation suspension compared with cromolyn sodium nebulizer solution for asthma in young children: results of a randomized outcomes trial. *Pediatrics* 2002;109:866–872.
48. Szefler SJ, Baker JW, Uryniak T, et al. Comparative study of budesonide inhalation suspension and montelukast in young children with mild persistent asthma. *J Allergy Clin Immunol* 2007; 120:1043–1050.
49. Petersen R, Agertoft L, Pedersen S. Treatment of exercise-induced asthma with beclomethasone dipropionate in children with asthma. *Eur Respir J* 2004;24:932–937.
50. Vidal C, Fernández-Ovide E, Piñeiro J, et al. Comparison of montelukast versus budesonide in the treatment of exercise-induced bronchoconstriction. *Ann Allergy Asthma Immunol* 2001; 86:655–658.
51. Pauwels RA, Pedersen S, Busse WW, et al. Early intervention with budesonide in mild persistent asthma: a randomized, double-blind trial. *Lancet* 2003;361:1071–1076.

52. Silkoff PE, Carlson M, Burke T, et al. The Aerocrine exhaled nitric oxide monitoring system NIOX is cleared by the US Food and Drug Administration for monitoring therapy in asthma. *J Allergy Clin Immunol* 2004;114:1241–1256.
53. Raissy HH, Cain H, Crowley M, et al. Comparison of the systemic effects of fluticasone propionate and triamcinolone acetonide administered in equipotent doses in children with asthma. *Pediatr Asthma Allergy Immunol* 2003;16:283–293.
54. Caffey LF, Raissy HH, Marshik P, et al. A crossover comparison of fluticasone propionate and montelukast on inflammatory indices in children with asthma. *Pediatr Asthma Allergy Immunol* 2005;18: 123–130.
55. Szefler SJ, Mitchell H, Sorkness CA, et al. Management of asthma based on exhaled nitric oxide in addition to guideline-based treatment for inner-city adolescents and young adults: a randomised controlled trial. *Lancet* 2008;372:1065–1072.
56. de Jongste JC, Carraro S, Hop WC, et al., CHARISM Study Group. Daily telemonitoring of exhaled nitric oxide and symptoms in the treatment of childhood asthma. *Am J Respir Crit Care Med* 2009;179:93–97.
56b. Lemanske RF Jr, Mauger DT, Sorkness CA, et al. Step-up therapy for children with uncontrolled asthma receiving inhaled corticosteroids. *N Engl J Med* 2010;362:975–985.
57. Masoli M, Weatherall M, Holt S, et al. Systematic review of the dose–response relation of inhaled fluticasone propionate. *Arch Dis Child* 2004;89:902–907.
58. Shapiro G, Bronsky EA, LaForce CF, et al. Dose-related efficacy of budesonide administered via a dry powder inhaler in the treatment of children with moderate to severe persistent asthma. *J Pediatr* 1998;132:976–982.
59. O'Byrne PM, Barnes PJ, Rodriguez-Roisin R, et al. Low dose inhaled budesonide and formoterol in mild persistent asthma: the OPTIMA randomized trial. *Am J Respir Crit Care Med* 2001;164: 1392–1397.
60. Pauwels RA, Lofdahl CG, Postma DS, et al. Effect of inhaled formoterol and budesonide on exacerbations of asthma. Formoterol and corticosteroids establishing therapy (FACET) international study group. *N Engl J Med* 1997;337:1405–1411.
61. Szefler SJ, Eigen H. Budesonide inhalation suspension: a nebulized corticosteroid for persistent asthma. *J Allergy Clin Immunol* 2002;109:730–742.
62. Ronald NJ, Bhalla RK, Earis J. The local side effects of inhaled corticosteroids: current understanding and review of the literature. *Chest* 2004;126:213–219.
63. Zöllner EW. Hypothalamic-pituitary-adrenal axis suppression in asthmatic children on inhaled corticosteroids (Part 2)—the risk as determined by gold standard adrenal function tests: a systematic review. *Pediatr Allergy Immunol* 2007;18:469–474.
64. Sim D, Griffiths A, Armstrong D, et al. Adrenal suppression from high-dose inhaled fluticasone propionate in children with asthma. *Eur Respir J* 2003;21:633–636.
65. Molimard M, Girodet PO, Pollet C, et al. Inhaled corticosteroids and adrenal insufficiency: prevalence and clinical presentation. *Drug Saf* 2008;31:769–774.
66. Zöllner EW. Hypothalamic-pituitary-adrenal axis suppression in asthmatic children on inhaled corticosteroids: Part 1. Which test should be used? *Pediatr Allergy Immunol* 2007;18:401–409.
67. Raissy HH, Marshik PL, Scott S, et al. Urinary free cortisol in hispanic and non-hispanic children with mild asthma and non-asthmatic normals. *Pediatr Asthma Allergy Immunol* 2006;19: 100–105.
68. Bacharier LB, Raissy HH, Wilson L, et al. The long-term effect of budesonide on hypothalamic-pituitary-adrenal axis function in children with mild to moderate asthma. *Pediatrics* 2004;113: 1693–1699.
69. Kelly HW, Van Natta ML, Covar RA, et al. CAMP Research Group. Effect of long-term corticosteroid use on bone mineral density in children: a prospective longitudinal assessment in the Childhood Asthma Management Program (CAMP) study. *Pediatrics* 2008;122:e53–e61.
70. van Staa TP, Bishop N, Leufkens HG, et al. Are inhaled corticosteroids associated with an increased risk of fracture in children? *Osteoporos Int* 2004;15:785–791.
71. Schlienger RG, Jick SS, Meier CR. Inhaled corticosteroids and the risk of fractures in children and adolescents. *Pediatrics* 2004; 469–473.
72. van Staa TP, Cooper C, Leufkens HG, et al. Children and the risk of fractures caused by oral corticosteroids. *J Bone Miner Res* 2003; 18:913–918.
73. Agertoft L, Pedersen S. Effect of long term treatment with budesonide on adult height in children with asthma. *N Engl J Med* 2000;343:1064–1069.
74. Ferguson AC, Van Bever HP, Teper AM, et al. A comparison of the relative growth velocities with budesonide and fluticasone propionate in children with asthma. *Respir Med* 2007;101: 118–129.
75. De Benedictis FM, Teper A, Green RJ, et al. Effects of 2 inhaled corticosteroids on growth: results of a randomized controlled trial. *Arch Pediatr Adolesc Med* 2001;155:1248–1254.
76. Acun C, Tomac N, Ermis B, et al. Effects of inhaled corticosteroids on growth in asthmatic children: a comparison of fluticasone propionate with budesonide. *Allergy Asthma Proc* 2005;26: 204–206.
77. de Vries TW, de Langen-Wourste JJ, van Puijenbroek E, et al. Reported adverse drug reactions during use of inhaled steroids in children with asthma in the Netherlands. *Eur J Clin Pharmacol* 2006;62:343–346.
78. Dresser GK, Spence JD, Bailey DG. Pharmacokinetic–pharmacodynamic consequences and clinical relevance of cytochrome P450 3A4 inhibition. *Clin Pharmacokinet* 2000;38:41–57.
79. Samaras K, Pett S, Gowers A, et al. Iatrogenic Cushing's syndrome with osteoporosis and secondary adrenal failure in human immunodeficiency virus-infected patients receiving inhaled corticosteroids and ritonavir-boosted protease inhibitors: six cases. *J Clin Endocrinol Metab* 2005;90:4394–4398.
80. Bolland MJ, Bagg W, Thomas MG, et al. Cushing's syndrome due to interaction between inhaled corticosteroids and itraconazole. *Ann Pharmacother* 2004;38:46–49.
81. Anderson GP. Current issues with β_2-adrenergic agonists: pharmacology and molecular and cellular mechanisms. *Clin Rev Allergy Immunol* 2006;31(2–3):119–130.
82. Sward-Comunelli SL, Mabry SM, Truog WE, et al. Airway muscle in preterm infants: changes during development. *J Pediatr* 1997; 130:570–576.
83. Jenne JW, Kelly HW. β_2 agonists. In: Murphy S, Kelly HW, eds. *Pediatric asthma (lung biology in health and disease series/126)*. New York: Marcel Dekker, Inc., 1999.
84. Kelly HW. What is new with the β_2 agonists: issues in the management of asthma. *Ann Pharmacother* 2005;39:931–938.
85. Waldeck B. Enantiomers of bronchodilating β_2-adrenoceptor agonists: Is there a cause for concern? *J Allergy Clin Immunol* 1999;103:742–748.
86. Berger WE. Levalbuterol: pharmacologic properties and use in the treatment of pediatric and adult asthma. *Ann Allergy Asthma Immunol* 2003;90:583–592.
87. Lotvall J, Palmqvist M, Arvidsson P, et al. The therapeutic ratio of R-albuterol is comparable with that of RS-albuterol in asthmatic patients. *J Allergy Clin Immunol* 2001;108:726–731.
88. Lötvall J, Palmqvist M, Ankerst J, et al. The effect of formoterol over 24 h in patients with asthma: the role of enantiomers. *Pulm Pharmacol Ther* 2005;18:109–113.
89. Perrin-Fayolle M. Salbutamol in the treatment of asthma. *Lancet* 1995;346:1101.
90. Cockcroft DW, Swystun VA. Effect of single doses of S-salbutamol, R-salbutamol, racemic salbutamol, and placebo on the airway response to methacholine. *Thorax* 1997;52:845–848.
91. Raissy HH, Harkins M, Esparham A, et al. Comparison of the dose–response to levalbuterol with and without pretreatment with S-albuterol after methacholine-induced bronchoconstriction. *Pharmacotherapy* 2007;27:1231–1236.
92. Small KM, McGraw DW, Liggett SB. Pharmacology and physiology of adrenergic receptor polymorphisms. *Annu Rev Pharmacol Toxicol* 2003;43:381–411.
93. Weiss ST, Litonja AA, Lange C, et al. Overview of the pharmacogenetics of asthma treatment. *Pharmacogenomics J* 2006;6: 311–326.
94. Drazen JM, Silverman EK, Lee TH. Heterogeneity of therapeutic responses in asthma. *Br Med Bull* 2000;56:1054–1070.
95. van der Woude HJ, Winter TH, Aalbers R. Decreased bronchodilating effect of salbutamol in relieving methacholine induced moderate bronchoconstriction during high dose treatment with long acting β_2 agonists. *Thorax* 2001;56:529–535.

96. Jones SL, Cowan JO, Flannery EM, et al. Reversing acute bronchoconstriction in asthma: the effect of bronchodilator tolerance after treatment with formoterol. *Eur Respir J* 2001;17:368–373.
97. Inman MD, O'Byrne PM. The effect of regular inhaled albuterol on exercise-induced bronchoconstriction. *Am J Respir Crit Care Med* 1996;153:65–69.
98. Simons FE, Gerstner TV, Cheang MS. Tolerance to the bronchoprotective effect of salmeterol in adolescents with exercise-induced asthma using concurrent inhaled glucocorticoid treatment. *Pediatrics* 1997;99:655–659.
99. Ramage L, Lipworth BJ, Ingram CG, et al. Reduced protection against exercise induced bronchoconstriction after chronic dosing with salmeterol. *Respir Med* 1994;88:363–368.
100. Lipworth BJ, Aziz I. Bronchodilator response to albuterol after regular formoterol and effects of acute corticosteroid administration. *Chest* 2000;117:156–162.
101. Anderson GP, Linden A, Rabe KF. Why are long-acting beta-adrenoceptor agonists long-acting? *Eur Respir J* 1994;7:569–578.
102. Morgan DJ. Clinical pharmacokinetics of beta-agonists. *Clin Pharmacokinet* 1990;18:270–294.
103. Kips JC, Pauwels RA. Long-acting inhaled β_2 agonist therapy in asthma. *Am J Respir Crit Care Med* 2001;164:923–932.
104. LaForce C, Alexander M, Deckelmann R, et al. Indacaterol provides sustained 24 h bronchodilation on once-daily dosing in asthma: a 7-day dose-ranging study. *Allergy* 2008;63:103–111.
105. Pearlman DS, Greos L, LaForce C, et al. Bronchodilator efficacy of indacaterol, a novel once-daily beta2-agonist, in patients with persistent asthma. *Ann Allergy Asthma Immunol* 2008;101:90–95.
106. Formoterol fumarate inhalation powder (Foradil Aerolizer) package insert. Kenilworth, NJ: Schering Corporation, 2002.
107. Lecaillon JB, Kaiser G, Palmisano M, et al. Pharmacokinetics and tolerability of formoterol in healthy volunteers after a single high dose of Foradil dry powder inhalation via Aerolizer. *Eur J Clin Pharmacol* 1999;55(2):131–138.
108. Bartow RA, Brogden RN. Formoterol: an update of its pharmacological properties and therapeutic efficacy in the management of asthma. *Drugs* 1998;56:303–322.
109. Salmeterol inhalation aerosol (Serevent Diskus) package insert. Research Triangle Park, NC: GlaxoSmithKline, 2003.
110. Dennis SM, Sharp SJ, Vickers MR, et al. Regular inhaled salbutamol and asthma control: the TRUST randomised trial. *Lancet* 2000;355:1675–1679.
111. Drazen JM, Israel E, Boushey HA, et al. Comparison of regularly scheduled with as-needed use of albuterol in mild asthma. *N Engl J Med* 1996;335:841–847.
112. van Schayck CP, Graafsma SJ, Visch MB, et al. Increased bronchial hyperresponsiveness after inhaling salbutamol during 1 year is not caused by subsensitization to salbutamol. *J Allergy Clin Immunol* 1990;86:793–800.
113. Raissy HH, Kelly F, Harkins M, et al. Pretreatment with Albuterol vs. Montelukast in Exercise Induced Bronchospasm in Children. *Pharmacotherapy* 2008;28:287–294.
114. Spooner C, Spooner GR, Rowe BH. Mast-cell stabilising agents to prevent exercise-induced bronchoconstriction. *Cochrane Database Syst Rev* 2003;(4):CD0023.
115. Cates CJ, Bara A, Crilley JA, et al. Holding chambers versus nebulizers for beta-agonist treatment of acute asthma. *Cochrane Database Syst Rev* 2003;(2):CD000052.
116. Pohunek P, Kuna P, Jorup C, et al. Budesonide/formoterol improves lung function compared with budesonide alone in children with asthma. *Pediatr Allergy Immunol* 2006;17:458–465.
117. Russell G, Williams DA, Weller P, et al. Salmeterol xinafoate in children on high dose inhaled steroids. *Ann Allergy Asthma Immunol* 1995;75:423–428.
118. Pediatric Advisory Committee. Review of Serevent. US Department of Health and Human Services, Food and Drug Administration. November 28, 2007:3–4. http://www.fda.gov/ohrms/dockets/ac/07/minutes/2007-4325m2_112807.pdf. Last accessed April 24, 2008.
119. Malone R, LaForce C, Nimmagadda S, et al. The safety of twice daily treatment with fluticasone propionate and salmeterol in pediatric patients with persistent asthma. *Ann Allergy Asthma Immunol* 2005;95:66–71.
120. Zimmerman B, D'Urzo A, Berube D. Efficacy and safety of formoterol Turbuhaler® when added to inhaled corticosteroid treatment in children with asthma. *Pediatr Pulmonol* 2004;37:122–127.
121. Bisgaard H. Effect of long-acting β_2 agonists on exacerbation rates of asthma in children. *Pediatr Pulmonol* 2003;36:391–398.
122. Cates CJ, Cates MJ, Lasserson TJ. Regular treatment with formoterol for chronic asthma: serious adverse events. *Cochrane Database Syst Rev* 2008;(4):CD006923.
123. Bensch G, Berger WE, Blokhin BM, et al. One-year efficacy and safety of inhaled formoterol dry powder in children with persistent asthma. *Ann Allergy Asthma Immunol* 2002;89:180–190.
124. Sorkness CA, Lemanske RF, Mauger DT, et al. Long-term comparison of 3 controller regimens for mild-moderate persistent childhood asthma: the Pediatric Asthma Controller Trial. *J Allergy Clin Immunol* 2007;119:64–72.
125. Bisgaard H, Le Roux P, Bjamer D, et al. Budesonide/formoterol maintenance plus reliever therapy: a new strategy in pediatric asthma. *Chest* 2006;130(6):1733–1743.
126. Budesonide and formoterol fumarate dehydrate inhalation aerosol (Symbicort) package insert. Wilmington, DE: AstraZeneca AP, 2009.
127. Korosec M, Novak RD, Myers E, et al. Salmeterol does not compromise the bronchodilator response to albuterol during acute episodes of asthma. *Am J Med* 1999;107:209–213.
128. Tattersfield AE, Postma DS, Barnes PJ, et al. Exacerbations of asthma—a descriptive study of 425 severe exacerbations. *Am J Respir Crit Care Med* 1999;160:594–599.
129. Taylor DR, Drazen JM, Herbison GP, et al. Asthma exacerbations during long term beta agonist use: influence of beta(2) adrenoceptor polymorphism. *Thorax* 2000;55:762–767.
130. Israel E, Chinchilli VM, Ford JG, et al. Regularly scheduled albuterol treatment in asthma: genotype-stratified, randomised, placebo-controlled cross-over trial. *Lancet* 2004;364:1505–1512.
131. Bleecker ER, Yancey SW, Baitinger LA, et al. Salmeterol response is not affected by beta2-adrenergic receptor genotype in subjects with persistent asthma. *J Allergy Clin Immunol* 2006;118: 809–816.
132. Cheung D, Timmers MC, Zwinderman AH, et al. Long-term effects of long-acting β_2-adrenoceptor agonist, salmeterol, on airway hyperresponsiveness in patients with mild asthma. *N Engl J Med* 1992;327:1198–1203.
133. Zarkovic J, Gotz MH, Holgate ST, et al. Effect of long-term regular salmeterol treatment in children with moderate asthma. *Clin Drug Invest* 1998;15:169–175.
134. Ducharme FM, Lasserson TJ, Cates CJ. Long-acting beta2-agonists versus anti-leukotrienes as add-on therapy to inhaled corticosteroids for chronic asthma. *Cochrane Database Syst Rev* 2006;(4):CD003137.
135. Guhan AR, Cooper S, Oborne J, et al. Systemic effects of formoterol and salmeterol: a dose–response comparison in healthy subjects. *Thorax* 2000;55:650–656.
136. Palmqvist M, Ibsen T, Mellén A, et al. Comparison of the relative efficacy of formoterol and salmeterol in asthmatic patients. *Am J Respir Crit Care Med* 1999;160:244–249.
137. Kaae R, Agertoft L, Pedersen S, et al. Cumulative high doses of inhaled formoterol have less systemic effects in asthmatic children 6–11 years-old than cumulative high doses of inhaled terbutaline. *Br J Clin Pharmacol* 2004;58:411–418.
138. Pohunek P, Matulka M, Rybnícek O, et al. Dose-related efficacy and safety of formoterol (Oxis) Turbuhaler compared with salmeterol Diskhaler in children with asthma. *Pediatr Allergy Immunol* 2004;15:32–39.
139. Lowery M, Kelly KJ. Cromolyn and nedocromil. In: Li JT, ed. *Pharmacotherapy of Asthma.* New York, NY: Taylor and Francis, 2006: 195–231.
140. Kelly K, Spooner CH, Rowe BH. Nedocromil sodium versus sodium cromoglycate for preventing exercise-induced bronchoconstriction: a systematic review. *Eur Respir J* 2001;17:39–45.
141. Murphy S, Kelly HW. Cromolyn sodium: A review of mechanisms and clinical use in asthma. *Drug Intell Clin Pharm* 1987; 21:22–35.
142. van der Wouden JC, Tasche MJA, Bernsen RMD, et al. Sodium cromoglycate for asthma in children. *Cochrane Database Syst Rev* 2003;3:D002173.
143. Bukstein DA, Bratton DL, Firriolo KM, et al. Evaluation of parental preference for the treatment of asthmatic children aged 6 to 11 years with oral montelukast or inhaled cromolyn: a randomized, open-label, crossover study. *J Asthma* 2003;40: 475–485.

144. Tasche MJA, van der Wouden JC, Uijen JHJM, et al. Randomised, placebo-controlled trial of inhaled sodium cromoglycate in 1–4-year-old children with moderate asthma. *Lancet* 1997;350: 1060–1064.
145. Donahue JG, Weiss ST, Livingston JM, et al. Inhaled steroids and the risk of hospitalization for asthma. *JAMA* 1997;277:887–891.
146. Adams RJ, Fuhlbrigge A, Finkelstein JA, et al. Impact of inhaled antiinflammatory therapy on hospitalization and emergency department visits for children with asthma. *Pediatrics* 2001;107: 706–711.
147. Peroni DG, Piacentini GL, Ress M, et al. Time efficacy of a single dose of montelukast on exercise-induced asthma in children. *Pediatr Allergy Immunol* 2002;13:434–437.
148. Leff AR. Role of leukotrienes in bronchial hyperresponsiveness and cellular responses in airways. *Am J Respir Crit Care Med* 2000; 161(2, pt 2):S125–S132.
149. Lynch KR, O'Neill GP, Liu Q, et al. Characterization of the human cysteinyl leukotriene CysLT1 receptor. *Nature* 1999;399:789–793.
150. Ducharme FM, Di Salvio F. Anti-leukotriene agents compared to inhaled corticosteroids in the management of recurrent and/or chronic asthma in adults and children. *Cochrane Database Syst Rev* 2004;1:CD002314.
151. Zileuton extended-release oral tablets (Zyflo CR) package insert. Lexington, MA: Critical Therapeutics Inc., 2007.
152. Zafirlukast (Accolate) package insert. Wilmington, DE: Zeneca Pharmaceuticals, 2007.
153. Montelukast sodium (Singulair) package insert. Whitehouse Station, NJ: Merck & Co., Inc., 2008.
154. Ducharme F, Schwartz Z, Kakuma R. Addition of anti-leukotriene agents to inhaled corticosteroids for chronic asthma. *Cochrane Database Syst Rev* 2004;1:CD003133.
155. The American Lung Association Asthma Clinical Research Centers. Clinical trial of low-dose theophylline and montelukast in patients with poorly controlled asthma. *Am J Respir Crit Care Med* 2007;175:235–242.
156. Deykin A, Wechsler ME, Boushey HA, et al. Combination therapy with a long-acting β-agonist and a leukotriene antagonist in moderate asthma. *Am J Respir Crit Care Med* 2007;175:228–234.
157. Peroni D, Bodini A, Del Giudice MM, et al. Effect of budesonide and montelukast in asthmatic children exposed to relevant allergens. *Allergy* 2005;60:206–210.
158. Szefler SJ, Phillips BR, Martinez FD, et al. Characterization of within-subject responses to fluticasone and montelukast in childhood asthma. *J Allergy Clin Immunol* 2005;115:233–242.
159. Israel E, Chervinsky PS, Friedman B, et al. Effects of montelukast and beclomethasone on airway function and asthma control. *J Allergy Clin Immunol* 2002;110:847–854.
160. Knorr B, Franchi LM, Bisgaard H, et al. Montelukast, a leukotriene receptor antagonist, for the treatment of persistent asthma in children aged 2 to 5 years. *Pediatrics* 2001;108(3):E48.
161. van Adelsberg J, Moy J, Wei LX, et al. Safety, tolerability, and exploratory efficacy of montelukast in 6- to 24-month-old patients with asthma. *Curr Med Res Opin* 2005;21:971–979.
162. Bukstein DA, Luskin AT, Bernstein A. "Real world" effectiveness of daily controller medicine in children with mild persistent asthma. *Ann Allergy Asthma Immunol* 2003;90:543–549.
163. Carter ER, Ananthakrishnan M. Adherence to montelukast versus inhaled corticosteroids in children with asthma. *Pediatr Pulmonol* 2003;36:301–304.
164. Stempel DA, Kruzikas DT, Manjunath R. Comparative efficacy and cost of asthma care in children with asthma treated with fluticasone propionate and montelukast. *J Pediatr* 2007;150:162–167.
165. Villaran C, O'Neill SJ, Helbling A, et al. Montelukast versus salmeterol in patients with asthma and exercise-induced bronchoconstriction. *J Allergy Clin Immunol* 1999;104:547–553.
166. Kemp JP, Dockhorn RJ, Shapiro GG, et al. Montelukast once daily inhibits exercise-induced bronchoconstriction in 6–14 year old children with asthma. *J Pediatr* 1998;133:424–428.
167. Leff JA, Busse WW, Pearlman D, et al. Montelukast, a leukotriene-receptor antagonist, for the treatment of mild asthma and exercise-induced bronchoconstriction. *N Engl J Med* 1998;339:147–152.
168. Bisgaard H, Zielen S, Garcia-Garcia ML, et al. Montelukast reduces asthma exacerbations in 2- to 5-year-old children with intermittent asthma. *Am J Respir Crit Care Med* 2005;171:315–322.
169. Robertson CF, Price D, Henry R, et al. Short-course montelukast for intermittent asthma in children: a randomized controlled trial. *Am J Respir Crit Care Med* 2007;175:323–329.
170. Bacharier LB, Phillips BR, Zeiger RS, et al. Episodic use of an inhaled corticosteroid or leukotriene receptor antagonist in preschool children with moderate-to-severe intermittent wheezing. *J Allergy Clin Immunol* 2008;122:1127–1135.
171. Katz RS, Papernick M. Zafirlukast and Churg-Strauss syndrome. *JAMA* 1998;279:1949.
172. Solans R, Bosch JA, Selva A, et al. Montelukast and Churg–Strauss syndrome. *Thorax* 2002;57:183–185.
173. Weinberger M, Hendeles L. Theophylline in asthma. *N Engl J Med* 1996;334:1380–1388.
174. Barnes PJ. Theophylline: new perspectives for an old drug. *Am J Respir Crit Care Med* 2003;167:813–818.
175. Adcock IM, Barnes PJ. Molecular mechanisms of corticosteroid resistance. *Chest* 2008;134:394–401.
176. Kelly HW. Non-corticosteroid therapy for the long-term control of asthma. *Expert Opin Pharmacother* 2007;8:2077–2087.
177. Evans DJ, Taylor DA, Zetterstrom O, et al. A comparison of low-dose inhaled budesonide plus theophylline and high-dose inhaled budesonide for moderate asthma. *N Engl J Med* 1997; 337(20):1412–1418.
178. Lim S, Jatakanon A, Gordon D, et al. Comparison of high dose inhaled steroids, low dose inhaled steroids plus low dose theophylline, and low dose inhaled steroids alone in chronic asthma in general practice. *Thorax* 2000;55:837–841.
179. Suessmuth S, Freihorst J, Gappa M. Low-dose theophylline in childhood asthma: a placebo-controlled, double-blind study. *Pediatr Allergy Immunol* 2003;14:394–400.
180. Davies B, Brooks G, Devoy M. The efficacy and safety of salmeterol compared to theophylline: meta-analysis of nine controlled studies. *Respir Med* 1998;92:256–263.
181. Edwards DJ, Zarowitz BJ, Slaughter RL. Theophylline. In: Evans WE, Schentag JJ, Jusko WJ, eds. *Applied pharmacokinetics: principles of therapeutic drug monitoring*, 3rd ed. Vancouver: Applied Therapeutics Inc., 1992:13-1–13-38.
182. Strunk RC, Bloomberg GR. Omalizumab for asthma. *N Engl J Med* 2006;354:2689–2695.
183. Noga O, Hanf G, Brachmann I, et al. Effect of omalizumab treatment on peripheral eosinophil and T-lymphocyte function in patients with allergic asthma. *J Allergy Clin Immunol* 2006;117: 1493–1499.
184. Slavin RG, Ferioli C, Tannenbaum SJ, et al. Asthma symptom re-emergence after omalizumab withdrawal correlates well with increasing IgE and decreasing pharmacokinetic concentrations. *J Allergy Clin Immunol* 2009;123:107–113.
185. Omalizumab for subcutaneous use (Xolair) package insert. South San Francisco, CA: Genentech, Inc., 2008.
186. Humbert M, Beasley R, Ayres J, et al. Benefits of omalizumab as add-on therapy in patients with severe persistent asthma who are inadequately controlled despite best available therapy (GINA 2002 step 4 treatment): INNOVATE. *Allergy* 2005;60: 309–316.
187. Ayres JG, Higgins B, Chilvers ER, et al. Efficacy and tolerability of anti-immunoglobulin E therapy with omalizumab in patients with poorly controlled (moderate-to-severe) allergic asthma. *Allergy* 2004;59:701–708.
188. Vignola AM, Humbert M, Bousquet J, et al. Efficacy and tolerability of anti-immunoglobulin E therapy with omalizumab in patients with concomitant allergic asthma and persistent allergic rhinitis: SOLAR. *Allergy* 2004;59:709–717.
189. Lanier BQ, Corren J, Lumry W, et al. Omalizumab is effective in the long-term control of severe allergic asthma. *Ann Allergy Asthma Immunol* 2003;91:154–159.
190. Niven R, Chung KF, Panahloo Z, et al. Effectiveness of omalizumab in patients with inadequately controlled severe persistent allergic asthma: an open-label study. *Respir Med* 2008;102: 1371–1378.
191. Saini SS, MacGlashan DW Jr, Sterbinsky SA, et al. Down-regulation of human basophil IgE and FC epsilon RI alpha surface densities and mediator release by anti-IgE-infusions is reversible in vitro and in vivo. *J Immunol* 1999;162(9):5624–5630.
192. Corren J, Shapiro G, Reimann J, et al. Allergen skin tests and free IgE levels during reduction and cessation of omalizumab therapy. *J Allergy Clin Immunol* 2008;121(2):506–511.
193. Marcus P. Practice Management Committee, American College of Chest Physicians. Incorporating anti-IgE (omalizumab) therapy into pulmonary medicine practice: practice management implications. *Chest* 2006;129:466–474.

194. Brown R, Turk F, Dale P, et al. Cost-effectiveness of omalizumab in patients with severe persistent allergic asthma. *Allergy* 2007;62: 149–153.
195. Oba Y, Salzman GA. Cost-effectiveness analysis of omalizumab in adults and adolescents with moderate-to-severe allergic asthma. *J Allergy Clin Immunol* 2004;114:265–269.
196. Wu AC, Paltiel AD, Kuntz KM, et al. Cost-effectiveness of omalizumab in adults with severe asthma: results from the Asthma Policy Model. *J Allergy Clin Immunol* 2007;120:1146–1152.
197. Cox L, Platts-Mills TA, Finegold I, et al. American Academy of Allergy, Asthma & Immunology; American College of Allergy, Asthma and Immunology. American Academy of Allergy, Asthma & Immunology/American College of Allergy, Asthma and Immunology Joint Task Force Report on omalizumab-associated anaphylaxis. *J Allergy Clin Immunol* 2007;120:1373–1377.
198. Cruz AA, Lima F, Sarinho E, et al. Safety of anti-immunoglobulin E therapy with omalizumab in allergic patients at risk of geohelminth infection. *Clin Exp Allergy* 2007;37:197–207.

CHAPTER

41

John T. Wilson
Victoria Tutag Lehr
Erika Crane
Margaret Ann Springer

Antipyretics

INTRODUCTION

Fever has been recognized since antiquity and variously attributed to a myriad of causes from excessive yellow bile to demonic possession. This complex entity has been poorly understood, inconsistently diagnosed, and treated. Fever, or perceived fever, continues to be one of the most common reasons for a child's presentation for medical care (1). However, opinions vary widely among clinicians, parents, and patients regarding the exact definition of fever, its physiology, function, and management. Variability exists in the methods, instruments, and body sites for appropriate assessment of body temperature.

This chapter uses the definition of fever established in 1987 by the International Union of Physiological Sciences Thermal Commission, namely, "a state of elevated core temperature, which is often, but not necessarily, part of the defensive responses of multicellular organisms (host) to the invasion of live (microorganisms) or inanimate matter recognized as pathogenic or alien by the host" (2). Fever as a component of the febrile response involves a cytokine-mediated rise in core temperature, generation of acute-phase reactants, and activation of numerous physiologic, endocrinologic, and immunologic systems (2). It is important to distinguish fever from hyperthermia, an unregulated rise in body temperature that does not involve pyrogenic cytokines and is unresponsive to antipyretics (2). The clinical dilemma "to treat or not to treat," and the clinical pharmacology of antipyretic drugs for use in pediatric patients will be discussed.

PHYSIOLOGY OF FEVER

Understanding fever requires a review of the body's thermoregulatory system, a complex neural network extending from the hypothalamus and limbic system through the lower brain stem and reticular formation into the spinal cord and sympathetic ganglia. Thermosensitive neurons in the preoptic region of the rostral hypothalamus are important in regulation of the thermoregulatory system, which maintains the body's temperature within a narrow range via a central entity termed the "set point." No longer regarded as a single temperature perceived at a single anatomic site, the set point is thought to be a range of temperatures perceived in multiple areas of the hypothalamus. Deviations from the set point can provoke multiple thermoregulatory responses (2). When the preoptic temperature rises above its set point, based on circulation-borne neuronal signals from thermosensors throughout the skin and core areas of the body, physiologic heat-loss responses are triggered. If the temperature falls below the set point, heat-retention and heat-production responses are activated (2,3).

During activities such as exercise, excess heat is generated by normal biochemical processes; the thermoregulatory response is heat loss until body temperature returns within normal range. When the body temperature falls below the normal range, heat conservation processes ensue. In response, pyrogens alter the function of the hypothalamic neurons and raise the set point. The febrile response is stimulated with endogenous mediators of fever activating a series of responses to decrease heat loss and increase heat production. This contrasting phenomenon that produces fever is clinically recognized as "a pyrogen-mediated rise in body temperature above the normal range" (2). Viewed in this context, fever is regarded by many to be an adaptive response, potentially beneficial to the patient.

Cytokines are among the more important pyrogens. These pleiotropic, intensely powerful proteins function singly or in groups to convey information from cell to cell within a complex network. The febrile response is mediated by exogenous and endogenous pyrogens. Exogenous pyrogens are of microbial origin inducing host cells, especially macrophages, to produce endogenous pyrogens. The most common endogenous pyrogenic cytokines are interleukin-1 (IL-1), tumor necrosis factor-α (TNF-α), IL-6, and interferon-γ (IFN-γ). These cytokines interact with receptors in the anterior hypothalamus to activate phospholipase A2, which in turn liberates plasma arachidonic acid as a substrate for the production of prostaglandin E2 (PGE2), catalyzed by cyclooxygenase (COX). Prostaglandin E2 in turn resets the hypothalamic set point and produces fever (see Fig. 41.1). Antipyretic drugs interrupt this pathway producing their pharmacologic effect (2).

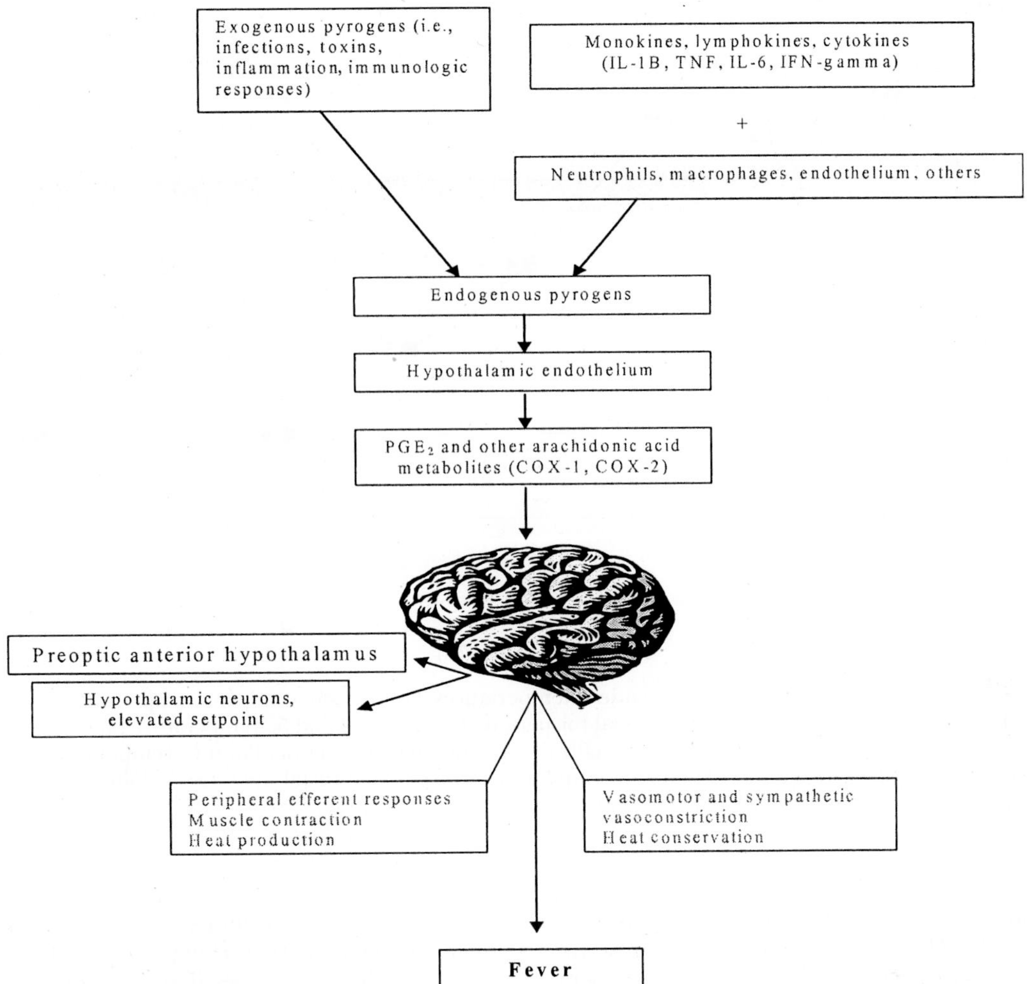

Figure 41.1. Prostaglandin synthesis and febrile responses. COX, cyclooxygenase; IFN, interferon; IL Interleukin; PGE_2, prostaglandin E_2. (Adapted from Powell KR. In: Behrman RM, Kliegman HB, Jenson, eds. *Nelson textbook of pediatrics*, 16th ed. Philadelphia, PA: WB Saunders, 2000:736–738; and Dinarello CA, Cannon JG, Wolff SM. New concepts on the pathogenesis of fever. *Rev Infect Dis* 1988;10:168–189, with permission.)

PITFALLS OF SITE-DEPENDENT MEASUREMENT OF FEVER

Diagnosis of fever in the clinical setting requires precise measurement of body temperature and characterization of that measurement as elevated. This is problematic in pediatric practice because there is no universal definition of "normal" body temperature for children of various ages. Important unresolved issues exist concerning age-related fluctuations in body temperature. In addition, there is lack of consensus on the optimal body site for measuring body temperature or the most appropriate thermometer that should used for this measurement (5). A 1995 survey demonstrated wide variation in perceptions of normal body temperature among physicians, medical students, and graduate students (6). There is long-standing disagreement on the merits of various anatomic sites (rectum, mouth, axilla, tympanic membrane, temporal artery) as accurate reflections of body temperature (5,6). Many types of thermometers are marketed, ranging from oral, rectal, and axillary, to infrared thermometers that measure the arterial blood temperature in the tympanic membrane (7). A recent innovation in thermometry measures the temperature of the temporal artery (8). Supralingual digital pacifier thermometers may provide a convenient method of measuring temperature in children younger than 2 years (9,10). The sensitivity and specificity of the pacifier thermometer has been compared with tympanic and glass mercury thermometers in children younger than 2 years (9). In this small study ($n = 81$), temperature measurements were obtained at supralingual, tympanic, and rectal sites using the mercury thermometer as the standard. Overall, the pacifier thermometer was shown to provide temperature measurements similar to the tympanic device, providing an alternative assessment method for small children. Another smaller investigation ($n = 25$) comparing pacifier and rectal temperatures in children aged 7 days to 24 months in a pediatric hospital reported

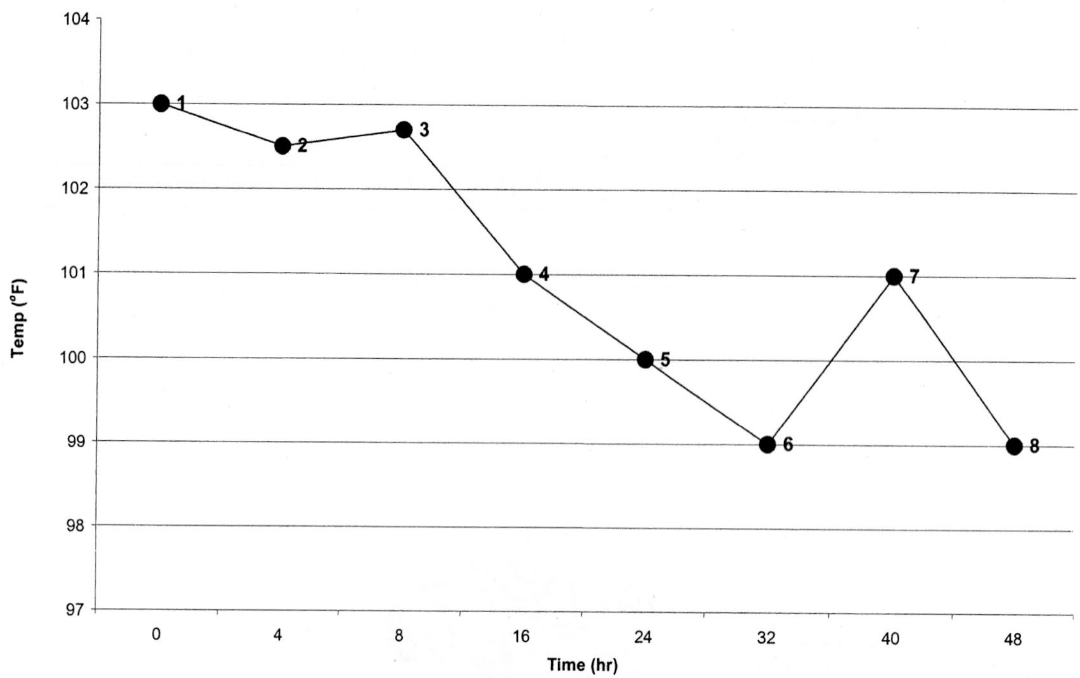

Figure 41.2. Hypothetical site-dependent temperatures. Points 1–3: Admission temperature 103°F and antibiotics started. Site is rectal for periods 1–3. Points 4 and 5: Temperature falls, presumably due to antibiotic action, but actually the site was changed to oral. Point 6: Temperature falls, but axillary site was used. Point 7: Temperature "spike" when rectal site is used. Point 8: Temperature falls as recorded at axillary site.

high correlations between rectal and pacifier temperature measurements (10). These data support the use of this type of device as an alternative method for measuring temperature in young children at home, although the relatively high cost of the device, US $15.00, and long duration (6 minutes) required to obtain a temperature measurement may be a barrier to use in clinical settings and for some parents.

Infrared tympanic thermometers are commonly used for children in emergency departments and clinics secondary to their ease of application in the external auditory canal and rapid, accurate measurement (7,11,12). Tympanic thermometry has been demonstrated to be more accurate than using an electronic axillary thermometer for measuring temperature in febrile and afebrile infants ($n = 106$) in a pediatric emergency department (12). Body temperature was measured using infrared tympanic thermometry, an electronic axillary thermometer and a standard rectal thermometer. For febrile and afebrile infants, tympanic temperature measurements correlated more closely with rectal temperatures than the axillary temperatures. There was also a lower mean difference between the tympanic and rectal temperatures compared with the tympanic and axillary temperatures. This is not unexpected as core temperature can be obtained by direct contact with the tympanic membrane (7). However, the process of obtaining an electronic tympanic temperature was demonstrated to be five times faster than using the axillary method.

When considering thermometers for pediatric use, the optimal device would allow accurate, fast, safe, and convenient measurement of temperature at a reasonable cost. In 1999, the US Environmental Protection Agency recommended that mercury no longer be used for thermometers (13). The agency advises that these devices be replaced with mercury-free alternatives. Children are more sensitive to the effects of mercury toxicity compared with adults; therefore, a broken mercury thermometer is a potential hazard (13). Many hospitals and health care systems have converted to mercury-free medical equipment.

An accepted definition of fever in children is a rectal temperature greater than or equal to 38°C or 100.4°F (14). All too frequently, however, little attention is given to consistency of site or technique for measurement, or to observer error. For example, the rectal site is seldom used in children older than 1 year. Figure 41.2 illustrates some of the many difficulties of temperature measurement and interpretation in a 1-year-old child admitted for suspected sepsis.

These site differences are consistent with the work of Brown and Wilson (5), who found respective mean differences (in degrees Fahrenheit) from rectal temperature of 1.31, 2.23, 4.28, and 5.75 for oral, axillary, abdominal skin, and forehead skin, respectively. A probability nomogram gave the best predictive power for likelihood of differences between sites. These investigators (14) and others (15) also proposed area under-the-curve estimation as a more accurate means of documenting temperature height and fever duration, noting that this method is especially useful when site differences and antipyretic drug efficacy are compared (5,14,16).

Obviously, the data in Figure 41.2 are misleading; using such data without appropriate explanation and interpretation could hinder effective clinical practice. For temperatures

1 to 3, a fever is documented. Because the temperature is lower at temperatures 4 to 6, it is assumed that the prescribed antibiotic regimen was therapeutically appropriate, when the real reason for the perceived drop in temperature is the change of measurement site. Until temperature 7 is measured (rectally), persistence of the fever is not evident. The temperature measured at 8 is axillary, and is a reflection of the site, rather than an actual temperature spike. Alternatively, caregivers could have changed antibiotic treatment at 7 and viewed point 8 (erroneously) as defervescence rather than as a site-selection difference. Similar problems could result from failure to consider the effect of the use of different measuring devices (thermometers, electronic thermocouples, infrared ear devices). It is difficult to discuss fever and its management if methods for temperature measurement are inadequately documented in clinical practice and in the literature.

PERCEPTIONS OF FEVER: MISINFORMATION AND MYTH

Another complicating factor in the diagnosis and management of fever is "fever phobia," first described by Dr. Barton Schmitt in 1980. His study revealed that parents often view fever as a disease rather than a sign or symptom. Schmitt found that many caregivers believed that fever could cause serious side effects, such as brain damage (17). As Crocetti and colleagues reported in 2001, misconceptions about fever and its role in disease process persist in the new millennium (18). In a study of 340 caregivers in an urban setting, 91% reported that they believed that fever could cause brain damage and death, and that a temperature could rise to 110°F if left untreated (17). Both studies documented numerous inaccurate beliefs about what constituted fever, how often it should be checked, and how often it should be treated (17,18). Fever phobia still causes parental anxiety and may lead to excessive fever monitoring (sometimes at intervals of <1 hour), overzealous antipyretic treatment, and inappropriate use of other fever-reducing practices, such as sponging (17). More recently, Crocetti's study was replicated in the United Kingdom with similar results in terms of parental fears, level of parental anxiety, aggressive measurement, and treatment of childhood fever (19).

Factors such as education level, socioeconomic status, and insurance coverage may also influence how a parent perceives and responds to childhood fever (20). Similarly, recent research has focused on similarities and differences in fever perception and management in various ethnic and cultural groups (20). Specifically, the parents' attributed cause of fever as well as use of complementary or alternative therapies to treat fever may vary greatly between ethnic groups (21,22). It is incumbent upon the health care provider to ask parents about their ethnic or cultural practices for handling fever and counsel as appropriate.

Caregivers who do not understand fever physiology may be overanxious to treat their children. However, many health care providers do not define "high" fever or explain its function in the body's defensive response (23). Health care providers who fail to educate themselves, their patients, patient's parents, and caregivers about the nature of fever, its significance, and its appropriate treatment may perpetuate fever phobia and its consequences (18,24). One consequence of fever phobia may be that about 50% of parents make dosing errors when administering acetaminophen (APAP) and ibuprofen (IBU) for fever to their infants and children; more than one-half of the caregivers surveyed in a study administered inappropriate doses of both drugs (25).

CONTROVERSIES OF MANAGEMENT

Provocative articles published since 1992 primarily address management of the febrile child from the standpoint of extent of illness, etiologic evaluation, and treatment (26,27–33). A guideline that emerged was stratification based on fever, as well as age, white blood cell count, and suspected site of infection. Advocated evidence-based approaches neglected prior or concomitant use of antipyretics to alter temperatures observed. Although recent or partial treatment with an antibiotic may modify a pyretic response, less recognized or cited is the role of antipyretics. This issue is exacerbated by approximately 50% of parents giving inaccurate information about use of these drugs (34). Overall evaluation and management of fever must consider confounding by the ubiquitously available APAP or IBU. Indeed, the temperature profile of Figure 41.2 could have been produced by an unrecognized or unreported administration of antipyretics given by nurse or parent on a pro re nata basis, removing a valuable index of disease severity. In children, a delay in initiation of antibiotic therapy occurred in those given an antipyretic (35).

A defensive or beneficial role of fever argues against the use of antipyretic drugs. This issue was summarized recently by Mackowiak and others (36–38). Admonitions in support of treatment are often rooted in fever phobia (39) or the comfort of caregivers who believe that fever per se is noxious. Examples abound that it may not be (36), even at different phylogenetic levels. Elevation of body temperature has enhanced a resistance to some viruses and bacteria in mammals. In humans, a positive correlation between temperature and survival was noted in those with bacterial infection. The adaptive response of fever is suggested by prolongation of viral illnesses in those receiving an antipyretic. Consistent with a beneficial effect is that pyrogenic cytokines were found to have immune-potentiating effects or to enhance resistance. On the other hand, they may enhance physiologic abnormalities associated with serious infection such as a gram-negative sepsis or that provoked artificially by lipopolysaccharide. Brandts and coworkers (40) found evidence for prolongation of APAP-treated-children's response to malaria. APAP was associated with an increased period for lesion crusting in children with varicella (41). In our opinion, altered cytokine release via modulation of fever has of yet an unknown relation to organism, site involved, and severity of infection. More data are needed for antipyretic drug treatment guidelines on this basis alone.

Another point to consider is the danger from a high fever (36,42), which apparently has not been demonstrated at or rarely above 41°C. Of concern, however, are special populations with cardiac or pulmonary disorders where antipyretic treatment may lessen metabolic demands. Mackowiak (36) asserted that this effect on the risk/benefit ratio has not been substantiated, especially from the standpoint of effects on coronary blood flow and loss of fluid with sweating (summarized in reference 43). The recurrence of febrile seizures does not appear to be influenced by antipyretic drugs (44–48).

Another area of controversy is the use of antipyretics to prevent postvaccination febrile responses in children. Currently, the American Academy of Pediatrics (AAP) and the Advisory Committee on Immunization Practices recommend prophylactic postvaccination antipyretic therapy only in children at a higher risk for seizures than the general population. Despite this recommendation, the incidence of postimmunization use of APAP and IBU in pediatric practices is 89% and 56%, respectively (49). A recent meta-analysis found that neither APAP nor IBU reduced the incidence in postimmunization fever in children after administration of the DTaP vaccine (50). This finding was confirmed in a 2008 randomized controlled trial (51). Similarly, rates of postimmunization pain and local skin reactions were also not affected by the use of prophylactic antipyretics (49,52).

Relief of discomfort and controversial effects on the host immune response may be due to anti-inflammatory and analgesic rather than (or in addition to) antipyretic properties of IBU and APAP. These agents effectively relieve pain, arthralgias, and myalgias that often accompany fever producing illnesses (43). Notable is the beneficial effect found with IBU on mortality of hypothermic patients with sepsis (53). However, in another report the multiple effects of IBU, including a lowering of body core temperature, did not affect organ failure or mortality in patients with sepsis (54). Combined relief of symptoms affects drug selection. For fever alone, and not to obscure signs of an underlying inflammatory illness, then APAP is reasonable combined with a opioid (e.g., codeine) if moderate pain relief is needed. IBU provides relief of fever, pain, and inflammation at appropriate doses. Preservation of fever as a sign of disease in those children with pain supports selection of an opioid analgesic without antipyretic properties. Understanding the pathophysiology of fever, pain, and inflammation will likely lead to the development of selective-action drugs. Until then, one must realize that more is being affected, perhaps deleteriously, than fever. The effect of antipyretic drug action on children must be considered if the short-term solution of antipyresis will be exchanged for adverse outcome-altered host response or morbidity as in the case of Reye syndrome associated with aspirin use (55–57).

Modulation of fever by antipyretic drug use failed to be of diagnostic significance (58) for discerning disease severity or its bacteremic nature. This failure may be partly due to the nonlinear pharmacokinetics of these drugs (16,59). Some suggest that nonsteroidal anti-inflammatory drugs (NSAIDs) (naproxen, indomethacin, diclofenac) may be more effective for fever from cancer than from infection (60–62). We are unaware of pediatric studies that have shown this distinction, although it would be important for drug selection.

Ketorolac is the only parenteral NSAID available in the United States that is approved for pain and has been used off-label in the treatment of fever (63–65). This NSAID is frequently used for analgesia in children for the management of sickle cell pain or for postoperative pain (63,64). The parenteral form and rapid onset of action would make this agent an ideal antipyretic in situations in which the oral route is not available provided the patient has no contraindications to NSAID administration. An 11-year-old girl with viral meningitis presented with an oral temperature of 39.8°C of 1-day duration was unable to tolerate oral medication but showed good antipyretic response to a single intravenous dose of 0.5 mg per kg of ketorolac (64). Randomized, controlled trials are needed to determine the efficacy and safety of this NSAID as an antipyretic for pediatric use.

No less controversial than combined or alternating antipyretic drug therapy is fever management by external cooling mechanisms. Axelrod (66) reviewed this issue recently. Vasoconstriction and shivering occur, and discomfort is a notable deterrent for children. The main advantage for tepid-water sponging is an early, usually within 30 minutes, reduction in temperature. When combined with an antipyretic drug, this early reduction was advantageous over drug therapy alone. Later enhancement of the fever reduction by the combination was not consistent from analysis of data from seven studies. One study (67) revealed extreme discomfort in febrile children sponged with ice water or isopropyl alcohol in water, the latter practice is now discouraged (68). Resolution of inconsistent findings for the combination of external cooling and antipyretic drug treatment requires use of one temperature site (preferably ear or rectal) and allocation of children of similar age and initial temperature to a three-arm study (combination, cooling, and antipyretic drug). Exclusion criteria for similar studies should follow recent recommendations (69).

ANTIPYRETIC DRUGS

Detailed characteristics of disposition, safety, and efficacy of ASA and APAP were given in the previous editions of this chapter (70), and IBU and naproxen have been discussed (71). A brief summary follows to provide information useful for topics emphasized in this chapter (also see Table 41.1).

ASPIRIN

Treatment of fever as a clinical entity has been important in the history of medicine for centuries (72). Willow leaves, now known to contain salicylate, were among the earliest known treatments of fever recorded around 1500 B.C.E. Around 1763, willow bark extract was used as an antipyretic. In the mid-1800s salicylic acid was chemically synthesized from willow bark (73). Chemical synthesis of acetylsalicylic acid (ASA, aspirin) in 1853 produced a drug with enhanced oral tolerability, which was used clinically for antipyresis for adults in 1899 and for children in 1901 (59). It is interesting that one-fourth of the adult dose (325 mg), presumably produced by breaking the adult tablet into quarter-sections, was empirically used as the pediatric dose. Pharmacokinetic and pharmacodynamic data and

TABLE 41.1 Disposition and Effect Characteristics of Acetaminophen (APAP) and Ibuprofen (IBU)[a]

	Pharmacokinetics			*Pharmacodynamics*		
	$t_{1/2}$	V_d	*Cl*	T_{onset}	T_{dur}	*Labeled Dose (mg/kg)*
APAP 12.5 mg/kg	1.81	859	277	30 min	4	APAP 10–15 every 4–6 hr
IBU 5 mg/kg	1.65	182	89	1–2 hr	6–8	IBU 5–10 every 6–8 hr
IBU 10 mg/kg	1.48	217	99	1–2 hr	6–8	
IBU 8 mg/kg					6–8	
<1 yr				69 min		
>6 yr				109 min		

APAP, acetaminophen; *Cl*, clearance (mL/kg/hr); IBU, ibuprofen; $t_{1/2}$, half-life (hr); T_{dur}, time of duration (hr); T_{onset}, time of onset; V_d, volume of distribution (mL/kg).
[a]Reference numbers are given in parentheses.
Data from references 4, 16, 59, 77–79.

the plasma concentration range for ASA toxicity and efficacy were described after 80 years of pediatric dosing (59).

Regarded for decades as a mainstay of analgesic and antipyretic therapy, aspirin and other salicylates decrease fever and pain by interrupting the synthesis of prostaglandins, particularly PGE-2. Salicylates are characterized as nonselective inhibitors of both forms of cyclooxygenase (COX-1 and COX-2), the first enzymes in the prostaglandin synthetic pathway (see Fig. 41.1). Because COX-1 is expressed in the stomach, this lack of selectivity is responsible for the gastric side effects frequently associated with aspirin therapy.

Salicylates are absorbed rapidly from the gastrointestinal (GI) tract and achieve peak serum concentrations in approximately 1 hour. Salicylates distribute throughout most body tissues, including the central nervous system, and readily cross the placental barrier. The volume of distribution of aspirin is approximately 170 mL per kg at normal doses. Dose-dependent protein binding and volume of distribution have been demonstrated (74). The apparent plasma half-life ($t_{1/2}$) for salicylic acid ranges from approximately 2.5 hours in low doses to longer than 12 hours at high doses. Consequently, small increases in dose can lead to large increases in plasma levels resulting in toxicity, or salicylism, which can be fatal. Simulated plasma levels for iatrogenic toxicity have been described (59). Aspirin is effective in the treatment of fever, pain, and inflammatory diseases, and is also used as an antiplatelet agent. However, because of the risk of adverse effects, such as GI bleeding, hypersensitivity, and particularly Reye syndrome, aspirin is seldom recommended for the treatment of fever in children.

ACETAMINOPHEN

The antipyretic effect of APAP was also discovered in the latter part of the nineteenth century (59). This drug was used for children in 1956 with early doses based on those for ASA. Pediatric use continued for years without a pharmacokinetic (PK) and pharmacodynamic (PD) basis for APAP dose until plasma concentrations were analyzed in febrile children and PK efficacy simulations performed (59).

As a nonselective COX inhibitor, APAP has analgesic and antipyretic effects similar to those of ASA. However, APAP is only weakly anti-inflammatory. It is rapidly and almost completely absorbed from the GI tract, achieving plasma peak concentration in 30 to 60 minutes, with a half-life of approximately 2 hours at therapeutic doses. APAP is metabolized via hepatic glucuronidation and sulfation and excreted in the urine. The volume of distribution (V_d) is approximately 0.8 to 1 L per kg, with less than 20% plasma protein binding. At therapeutic doses, APAP is well tolerated, causing occasional skin rashes and other allergic reactions. Rarely, APAP use has been associated with neutropenia, thrombocytopenia, and pancytopenia. The most serious effects of APAP are found in acute overdosage, when a dose-dependent, potentially fatal hepatic necrosis is possible. Because of its short half-life, a sustained-release APAP was evaluated in children and found to be similar to 4-hourly doses of the immediate-release preparation, offering no advantage (75).

IBUPROFEN

IBU, another nonselective COX inhibitor, has become a widely accepted effective analgesic, anti-inflammatory, and antipyretic drug in children (16,76). It is rapidly absorbed after oral administration and reaches peak plasma concentrations in 15 to 30 minutes. The plasma half-life is approximately 2 hours. IBU is metabolized in the liver and excreted, along with its metabolites, in the urine. IBU is highly protein bound (>90%) with an average V_d of 0.15 L per kg. Approximately 10% to 15% of patients discontinue the use of IBU because of GI side effects.

PHARMACODYNAMICS

Little doubt exists about the efficacy of antipyretic drugs when used at labeled doses for exogenous or endogenous pyrogen-induced fever. Emerging concepts about their PD provide a rational basis for their clinical application. These are in addition to understanding fundamental mechanisms of action by inhibiting COX to decrease PGE2 in the hypothalamus and to reduce proinflammatory mediators, among other actions (43).

An early study showed a discordant relationship between plasma concentrations and antipyretic response following a single dose of ASA, choline salicylate, APAP, (59) or IBU (16,77–79). A lag period of approximately 2 hours exists,

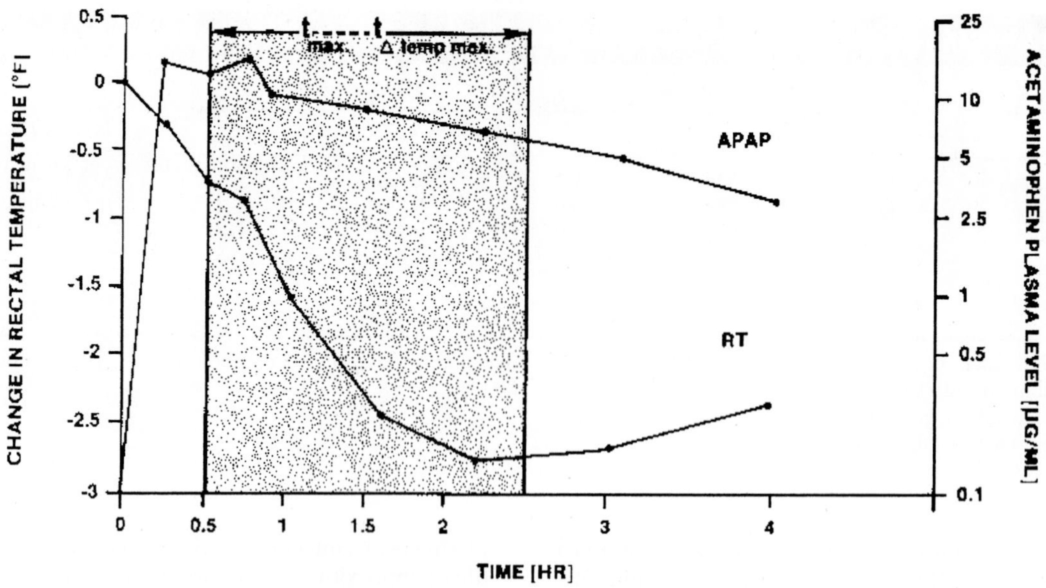

Figure 41.3. Rectal temperature (RT) change and plasma acetaminophen (APAP) levels as defined by an inclusive interval. APAP dose was 12.4 mg/kg. The inclusive interval is depicted by data from and including t_{max} to and including $t_{\Delta temp\ max}$. This interval is diagrammed for population averages. (From Wilson JT, Brown RD, Bocchini JA, et al. Efficacy, disposition, and pharmacodynamics of aspirin, acetaminophen, and choline salicylate in young febrile children. *Ther Drug Monit* 1982;4(2):147–180, with permission.)

as shown for APAP in Figure 41.3, such that peak drug plasma concentration occurs before the maximum reduction in temperature. Time for deep compartment (brain) distribution, inhibition of COX for PGE2 production, and vasodilation for heat dissipation was proposed to explain the lag period. Data from the shaded area of Figure 41.3 gave the best correlation between APAP plasma concentrations and maximum efficacy. Temporal changes for plasma concentration and temperature data of APAP and salicylate were subjected to simulation analyses to produce estimates of a therapeutic plasma concentration range (salicylate, 50 to 100 μg per mL; APAP, 4 to 18 μg per mL). The range was useful for dose estimations, but less so for single-dose response monitoring because of the observed discordance. It may prove useful for plasma concentration monitoring of repeated doses.

Furthermore, for APAP and ASA (16,59) a major confounding response was demonstrated for initial temperature. As seen in Figure 41.4 for ASA and APAP, a nonlinear PD resulted from higher initial temperature, giving a greater reduction in fever following a single dose of antipyretic drug. Design, and hence data interpretation, of antipyretic studies must control for this variable.

Two other variables were identified recently in an extensive study of 178 children given APAP or two IBU dose strengths (80). A slope function and a sigmoidal cyclic function were identified and added to an antipyresis model to achieve satisfactory fits for PD analysis, and a nonlinear PD was again observed for initial temperature. It was hypothesized that the slope function was determined by the etiology of the pyresis and hence would change with the stimulus for fever. The cyclic function was proposed in relation to temperature regulation. Both coexist in the febrile child and confound use of the simple sigmoid E_{max} effect model to explain antipyretic drug effects. Discovery of these two other functions may allow a probe of antipyresis specific for drug (e.g., ASA vs. APAP vs. NSAIDs) or disease (e.g., cancer or infection) as alluded to elsewhere in this chapter.

COMPARATIVE EFFICACY

Multiple studies have demonstrated the efficacy of both APAP and IBU for the management of fever. The two drugs exhibit important differences in pharmacokinetics and efficacy characteristics. For example, one study found that IBU has a shorter half-life than does APAP (118.2 vs. 172.3 minutes) but a longer absorption time (16.3 vs. 5.3 minutes) (79). However, in the same study, APAP reached maximum plasma concentration more quickly than IBU (12.31 vs. 26.67 minutes). Implications for clinicians are that APAP has more rapid onset of effect, but that the antipyretic effect of IBU lasts longer. These findings for this APAP and IBU comparison agree with those of other studies (16,81–84) when a single dose of either drug was used in the range of 5 to 10 mg per kg IBU and 10 to 12 mg per kg APAP. One study (85) found equivalent antipyretic effects for IBU and APAP when similar doses were used. Repeated doses in febrile children showed no difference between these drugs (76,86). Of concern in these comparative studies is the effect of dose. For either APAP (87) or IBU (16,83,84), a higher single dose enhances antipyretic efficacy, but this was not seen with repeated doses (76). The recommended single oral antipyretic dose of APAP is 10 to 15 mg per kg every 4 to 6 hours for infants and

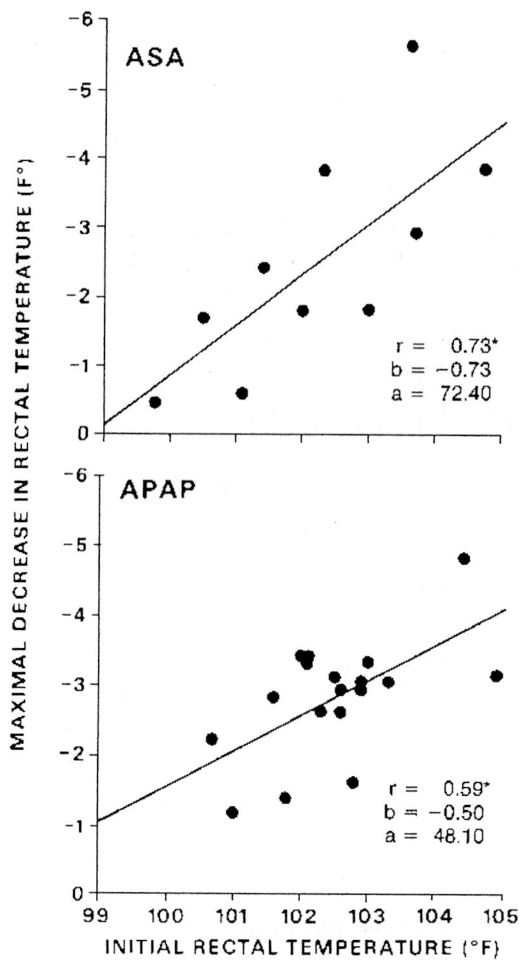

Figure 41.4. Correlation between initial rectal temperature and maximal decrease in rectal temperature for children treated with aspirin (ASA) or acetaminophen (APAP). Initial rectal temperature ($temp_i$) prior to dosing is compared with the maximal decrease in rectal temperature ($\Delta temp_{max}$) as observed in 10 and 18 children given a single oral dose of ASA or APAP, respectively. The data shown for APAP are taken from Groups III and IV. $^*p < .05$ for *r*, Student *t* test and analysis of variance for linearity (*t* and ANOVA not shown). *a*, Intercept; *b*, slope. (From Wilson JT, Brown RD, Bocchini JA, et al. Efficacy, disposition, and pharmacodynamics of aspirin, acetaminophen, and choline salicylate in young febrile children. *Ther Drug Monit* 1982;4(2):147–180, with permission.)

children, and that of IBU is 5 to 10 mg per kg given every 6 to 8 hours (Table 41.1). Use of a higher APAP dose may show efficacy similar to IBU at 10 mg per kg, but, especially with repeated high doses, safety assessment is lacking and is of concern, as discussed later.

Another important issue during the last decade has been that of loading dose. Treluyer and associates (87) reported that an APAP loading dose of 30 mg per kg lowered temperature significantly more than a 15-mg per kg dose.

Onset of fever decrement was shorter and duration longer after the higher APAP dose. The incidence of clinical side effects was similar, but safety of repeated high doses or that assessed by biochemical indices has not been determined.

ALTERNATING OR TWO-DRUG THERAPY

PK–PD analysis provides insights into the use of more than one antipyretic, either alternating or concurrently. This practice can be explained in terms of knowledge of ASA and APAP disposition and the plasma concentration range for antipyretic efficacy that yielded simulations of two-drug treatments (4,59,71). Data and dose labeling of ASA prior to 1979 resulted in a simulated subtherapeutic concentration after the first dose and likely led to doubling the dose to achieve efficacy and also resulted in later toxicity or use of APAP. The short half-life of APAP and its use as the first dose resulted in subtherapeutic serum concentrations for most of the dosing interval. Label doses (for 1981) of APAP alone produced subtherapeutic serum concentrations for the majority for patients. If ASA and APAP were administered in an alternating manner (either one as the first dose), then the subtherapeutic concentration for either drug, especially after first dose, was covered by the other drug (Fig. 41.5). In a similar manner, IBU, with a longer duration of antipyresis, is expected to cover periods of APAP ineffectiveness. Accordingly, alternating regimens seemed to stem from parents or physicians reacting to a minimal antipyretic efficacy, especially following the first dose.

Despite the lack of scientific evidence that this practice is beneficial, the alternating use of IBU and APAP is commonly recommended by pediatricians (88,89). Somewhat disturbingly, one study found that 50% of responders to a survey, all of whom were practicing pediatricians in the United States, advised caregivers to give their children alternating doses of APAP and IBU; 29% of all survey participants made this treatment decision based on recommendations from the AAP (89), which actually urged discretion for alternating doses (90). Two recent studies addressed the antipyretic efficacy and short-term safety of alternating APAP with IBU with varied results (91,92). The study by Sarrell et al. (91) in 2006 was a randomized, double-blinded parallel-group trial, which demonstrated a mean lower temperature, a more rapid reduction in fever, and fewer fever recurrences in the alternating antipyretic group. They also found no serious adverse effects of alternating APAP and IBU within the study period of 14 days. Critiques of this project have focused on the study design (subjects had unusually high temperatures and received a loading dose of an antipyretic prior to maintenance therapy), clinical significance of the fever reduction, and concerns that alternating antipyretic therapy will increase chances for dosing error and promote parental fever phobia (93,94). The labeled dosing schedule differs for each drug (i.e., IBU every 6 to 8 hours and APAP every 4 hours) so that time of dosing may prove awkward for parents, caregiver, and nursing staff to follow. The safety of this practice has not been demonstrated. A randomized, double-blind placebo control study in 2008 demonstrated a significant reduction in fever of less than 1°C between 4 to 5 hours with the alternating of APAP and IBU; however, it was not sustained over the study period (92).

Similarly, safety has not been shown for use of a combined ASA plus APAP treatment that showed a greater decrement in fever for a longer period (95). This is not likely to be studied because of concerns for the relation

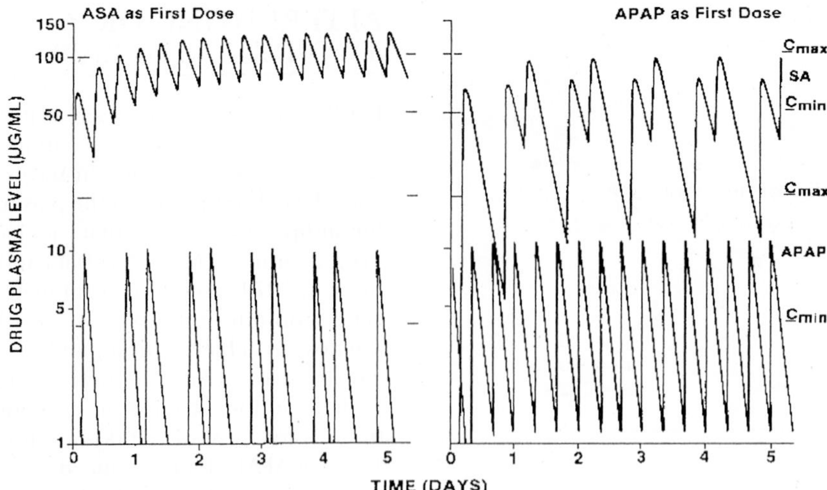

Figure 41.5. Predicted drug plasma levels for alternate dosing with aspirin (ASA) or acetaminophen (APAP) (alternating every 4 hr). Simulation parameters are defined in Wilson et al (59). Label doses of 1981 for age were used: average 13.2 mg/kg for ASA (10.2 mg/kg for salicylate, SA) and 9.9 mg/kg for APAP as Tylenol Elixir, 120 mg/5 mL. One nightly dose was deleted for whichever drug was scheduled for night administration. **Left:** ASA dose was given first, followed by APAP alternating every 4 hr. **Right:** APAP dose was given first, followed by ASA alternating every 4 hr. (From Wilson JT, Brown RD, Bocchini JA, et al. Efficacy, disposition, and pharmacodynamics of aspirin, acetaminophen, and choline salicylate in young febrile children. *Ther Drug Monit* 1982;4(2):147–180, with permission.)

between ASA and Reye syndrome (55–57,96). One study (97) showed an increase in plasma ASA concentrations following simultaneous administration of ASA and APAP. If a similar drug interaction were documented in children receiving alternating treatments of APAP and IBU, then it would pose safety issues. Perhaps a better approach would be to use one drug at the effective dose and dosing interval. This is apparent from an APAP loading dose study (87) but applies only to a single dose and awaits safety information. Effective dosing of only one drug is approximated by current approved labeling for children's APAP and IBU.

TOXICITY

Summaries of antipyretic drug toxicity (98,99), and especially that of APAP (90), contain citations for the major areas to be discussed here. Foremost for risk analysis is short-term use as for fever versus long-term use for other conditions and also whether dose is augmented by over-the-counter products containing the same drug. GI effects are dependent on type of NSAID and range from discomfort to physically evident lesions. These lesions are considered by most to occur less commonly with IBU and APAP. Many GI toxicity reports are from prolonged use by adults and may not apply to intermittent treatment of febrile children. Oliguric renal failure secondary to prostaglandin inhibition in states of dehydration may be pertinent to febrile children who have not consumed adequate liquids for 1 to 2 days or have become dehydrated a result of underlying illness. Sodium and water retention are seen with NSAIDs, and patients with insulin-dependent diabetes may be at risk for hyperkalemia (see reference 100 for pathogenesis). A large office-based study found IBU and APAP to have comparable safety for short-term use (median treatment of 3 days) when examining rates of hospitalization for GI bleeding, anaphylaxis, and acute renal failure (101). Similarly, an inpatient study confirmed the incidence of acute renal failure to be less and comparable between children receiving short-term antipyretic therapy with either APAP or IBU (102).

APAP hepatotoxicity from a single overdose is well known; however, an increased awareness of overdose associated with therapeutic intent in children has been reported (103–105). Unintentional therapeutic error accounted for 25% of fatal cases in a survey. Sustained administration of supratherapeutic doses was a hallmark of cases, about half of whom died (103). Of concern was possible coadministration of over-the-counter products containing APAP. This and use of adult-strength formulations or misinterpretation of dose information for pediatric products were likely contributing causes. Changes in cytochrome P-450 2E, which bioactivates APAP to the toxic intermediate *N*-acetyl-*p*-benzoquinone, resulting from concurrent drugs or diet may be important, as are depletions of glucuronide or sulfate conjugation precursors in a child malnourished secondary to the febrile illness. Oxidative stress and covalent adduct formation were likely contributory, with 3-(cystein-s-yl)–APAP adduct measurements proposed as a surrogate marker of toxicity for the latter. Later studies (106–108) did not demonstrate this in children receiving therapeutic doses of APAP, even in those with liver transaminase elevation or cytochrome P-450-enzyme-inducing drugs, thereby indicating safety of such doses. The APAP–cys adduct was detected in APAP overdose patients and correlated with liver aspartate aminotransferase activity (109). The high-pressure liquid chromatography assay for APAP-cys has improved its clinical utility, and recent studies have demonstrated a role in identifying APAP toxicity in children with acute liver toxicity of otherwise indeterminate etiology (110,111). A role for proinflammatory cytokines was recently indicated by high interleukin-8 levels in those with APAP hepatotoxicity (107). This may offer new insights for detection and treatment.

Recommended dosing guidelines vary in regard to the safe amount of APAP to be ingested by children. It is generally agreed that a single ingestion of greater than 200 mg per kg causes acute toxicity and hepatocellular damage, although this dose may be as low as 120 to 150 mg per kg (90,112). Under greater debate is the total daily dose which is associated with hepatocellular damage. Determining the safe total daily dose is important in preventing unintentional therapeutic error by repeated supratherapeutic doses or use of multiple APAP-containing products. Nelson Textbook of Pediatrics states that repeated doses of APAP at 60 mg per kg per day on consecutive days may be associated with hepatic disease in some children (112). Other sources suggest 75 mg per kg per day to 90 mg per kg per day of APAP as a safe maximum total daily dose in most children (104,113).

The AAP statement (90) on APAP toxicity addresses additional points, including the apparent lower risk of APAP toxicity in children than in adults (114–116) and factors that promote toxicity (117). Variable absorption from rectal administration may lead to excessive and frequent doses of APAP (90). Although one PK study (118) found no accumulation to supratherapeutic levels of APAP given by this route. Recent studies have found no increase in clinical efficacy with rectal versus oral APAP, and no heightened fever reduction with high-dose rectal APAP (119,120). In a table of drugs interacting with APAP (90), a distinction is made for acute versus chronic ingestion of ethanol, with the former reducing and the latter increasing toxicity. Decision to treat APAP hepatotoxicity must consider dose (minimal single toxic dose of 120 to 150 mg per kg of body weight), plasma level versus time of ingestion [see Rumack nomogram (121) for acute ingestion], and interacting effects of drugs, diet, and illness. The high risk of mortality is notable for a child who has serum concentrations in the toxic range after long-term APAP administration. Intoxication follows a 3- to 5-day time course from emesis to right upper quadrant pain to hepatic failure. For detailed clinical signs and guidelines for *n*-acetylcysteine treatment, see the AAP statement (90) and the current one from a regional poison control center. Epidemiologic studies show a good safety profile for APAP and IBU when used for a short period in febrile children (101,116,122) and recent meta-analysis studies reveal a similar safety profile (123–125).

Evaluation of fever in infants and children may be challenging due to the variety of thermometer devices available on the market. It is important to use the same type of device and same body site when comparing multiple temperature measurements. When antipyretic therapy is prescribed, caregivers must be informed of risks of excessive dosing. Clear instructions should include the dose, frequency, duration of therapy, and the specific strength and formulation for the infant or child. Age-appropriate measuring devices such as measuring cups, oral syringes, or dosing spoons should be provided with the formulation to ensure accurate dosing. The pharmacist or physician should be consulted to provide individualized dosing instruction to the parent or the caregiver. As many other medications contain APAP or IBU, the child's other medications should be reviewed to avoid administration of these drugs from multiple sources. Risks from antipyretic drug therapy can be minimized by careful attention to the pediatric label for dose and frequency of administration.

REFERENCES

1. McCarthy PL. Fever. *Pediatr Rev* 1998;19(12):401–407; quiz, 408.
2. Mackowiak PA. Temperature regulation and the pathogenesis of fever. In: Mandell GL, Douglas RG, Bennett JE, eds. *Principles and practice of infectious diseases*, 5th ed. Philadelphia, PA: Churchill Livingstone, 2000:604–622.
3. Dinarello CA, Cannon JG, Wolff SM. New concepts on the pathogenesis of fever. *Rev Infect Dis* 1988;10(1):168–189.
4. Wilson JT. Clinical pharmacology of pediatric antipyretic drugs. *Ther Drug Monit* 1985;7(1):2–11.
5. Brown RD, Wilson JT. Quantification of fever. *Clin Pediatr (Phila)* 1992;31(4):228–229.
6. Mackowiak PA, Wasserman GS. Physicians' perceptions regarding body temperature in health and disease. *South Med J* 1995; 88(9):934–938.
7. Pompei F, Pompei M. *Physicians reference handbook on temperature: vital sign assessment with infrared thermometry*. Watertown, MA: Exergen Corporation, 1996.
8. Greenes DS, Fleisher GR. Accuracy of a non-invasive temporal artery thermometer for use in infants. *Arch Pediatr Adolesc Med* 2001;155(3):376–381.
9. Backstrand RL, Wilshaw R, Moran S, et al. Supralingual temperatures compared to tympanic and rectal temperatures. *Pediatr Nurs* 1996;22(5):436–438.
10. Braun CA. Accuracy of pacifier thermometers in young children. *Pediatr Nurs* 2006;32(5):413–418.
11. Kocoglu H, Goksu S, Tsik M, et al. Infrared tympanic thermometer can accurately measure the body temperature in children in an emergency room setting. *Int J Pediatr Otorhinolaryngol* 2002;65(1):39–43.
12. El-Rhadi S, Patel S. An evaluation of tympanic thermometry in a paediatric emergency department. *Emerg Med J* 2006;23:40–41.
13. U.S. EPA. *Developing a virtual elimination strategy for mercury*. Washington, DC: U.S. Environmental Protection Agency, 1999.
14. Brown RD, Kearns G, Eichler VF, et al. A probability nomogram to predict rectal temperature in children. *Clin Pediatr (Phila)* 1992;31(9):523–531.
15. Anttila M, Himberg JJ, Peltola H. Precise quantification of fever in childhood bacterial meningitis. *Clin Pediatr (Phila)* 1992;31(4): 221–227.
16. Wilson JT, Brown RD, Kearns GL, et al. Single-dose, placebo-controlled comparative study of ibuprofen and acetaminophen antipyresis in children. *J Pediatr* 1991;119(5):803–811.
17. Schmitt BD. Fever phobia: misconceptions of parents about fevers. *Am J Dis Child* 1980;134:176–181.
18. Crocetti M, Moghbeli N, Serwint J. Fever phobia revisited: have parental misconceptions about fever changed in 20 years? *Pediatrics* 2001;107(6):1241–1246.
19. Purssell E. Parental fever phobia and its evolutionary correlates. *J Clin Nurs* 2008;18:210–218.
20. Taveras EM, Durousseau S, Flores G. Parents' beliefs and practices regarding childhood fever. A study of a multiethnic and socioeconomically diverse sample of parents. *Pediatr Emerg Care* 2004;20(9):579–587.
21. Crocetti M, Sabath B, Cranmer L, et al. Knowledge and management of fever among Latino parents. *Clin Pediatr (Phila)* 2009; 48:183–189.
22. Tessler H, Gorodischer R, Press J, et al. Unrealistic concerns about fever in children: the influence of cultural–ethnic and sociodemographic factors. *Isr Med Assoc J* 2008;10:346–349.

23. May A, Bauchner H. Fever phobia: the pediatrician's contribution. *Pediatrics* 1992;90(6):851–854.
24. Karwowska A, Nijessen-Jordan C, Johnson D, et al. Parental and health care provider understanding of childhood fever: a Canadian perspective. *CJEM* 2002;4(6):394–400.
25. Li SF, Lacher B, Crain EF. Acetaminophen and ibuprofen dosing by parents. *Pediatr Emerg Care* 2000;16(6):394–397.
26. Kramer MS, Shapiro ED. Management of the young febrile child: a commentary on recent practice guidelines. *Pediatrics* 1997; 100(1):128–134.
27. Eskerund JR, Laerum E, Fagerthun H, et al. Fever in general practice. I: frequency and diagnosis: *Fam Pract* 1992;9:263–269.
28. Bauchner H, Pelton SI. Management of the young febrile child: a continuing controversy. *Pediatrics* 1997;100(1):137–138.
29. Isaacman DJ, Kaminer K, Veligeti H, et al. Comparative practice patterns of emergency medicine physicians and pediatrics emergency medicine physicians managing fever in young children. *Pediatrics* 2001;108(2):354–358.
30. Young PC. The management of febrile infants by primary-care pediatricians in Utah: comparison with published practice guidelines. *Pediatrics* 1995;95(5):623–627.
31. Baraff LJ, Bass JW, Fleisher GR, et al. Practice guideline for the management of infants and children 0 to 36 months of age with fever without source. Agency for Health Care Policy and Research. *Ann Emerg Med* 1993;22(7):1198–1210.
32. Baraff LJ. Management of infants and children 3 to 36 months of age with fever without source. *Pediatr Ann* 1993;22(8):497–498, 501–504.
33. Baraff LJ, Schriger DL, Bass JW, et al. Management of the young febrile child. Commentary on practice guidelines. *Pediatrics* 1997;100(1):134–136.
34. Wilson JT. Concomitant microanalysis of salicylic acid and acetaminophen in plasma of febrile children. *Ther Drug Monit* 1979;1(4): 459–473.
35. Done AK. Treatment of fever in 1982: a review. *Am J Med* 1983; 74(6A):27–35.
36. Mackowiak PA. Physiological rationale for suppression of fever. *Clin Infect Dis* 2000;31(Suppl 5):S185–S189.
37. Kluger MJ, Kozak W, Conn CA, et al. The adaptive value of fever. *Infect Dis Clin North Am* 1996;10(1):128–134.
38. Kluger MJ, Kozak W, Conn CA, et al. Role of fever in disease. *Ann N Y Acad Sci* 1998;856:224–233.
39. Avner JR, Baker MD. Management of fever in infants and children. *Emerg Med Clin North Am* 2002;20(1):49–67.
40. Brandts CH, Ndjave M, Graninger W, et al. Effect of paracetamol on parasite clearance time in *Plasmodium falciparum* malaria. *Lancet* 1997;350(9079):704–709.
41. Doron TF, DeAngelis C, Baumgardner RA, et al. Acetaminophen: more harm than good for chickenpox? *J Pediatr* 1989;114(6): 1045–1048.
42. Mackowiak PA, Boulant JA. Fever's glass ceiling. *Clin Infect Dis* 1996;22(3):525–536.
43. Aronoff DM, Neilson EG. Antipyretics: mechanisms of action and clinical use in fever suppression. *Am J Med* 2001;111(4): 304–315.
44. Mackowiak PA, Bartlett JG, Borden EC, et al. Concepts of fever: recent advances and lingering dogma. *Clin Infect Dis* 1997;25: 119–138.
45. Rosman NP. Febrile convulsions. In: Mackowiak PA, ed. *Fever: basic mechanisms and management*, 2nd ed. Philadelphia, PA: Lippincott–Raven, 1997:267–277.
46. van Stuijvenberg M, Derksen-Lubsen G, Steyerberg EW, et al. Randomized, controlled trial of ibuprofen syrup administered during febrile illnesses to prevent febrile seizure recurrences. *Pediatrics* 1998;102(5):E51.
47. Schnaiderman D, Lahat E, Sheefer T, et al. Antipyretic effectiveness of acetaminophen in febrile seizures: ongoing prophylaxis versus sporadic usage. *Eur J Pediatr* 1993;152(9):747–749.
48. El-Radhi AS, Barry W. Do antipyretics prevent febrile convulsions? *Arch Dis Child* 2003;88:641–642.
49. Taddio A, Manley J, Potash L, et al. Routine immunization practices: use of topical anesthetics and oral analgesics. *Pediatrics* 2007;120:e637–e643.
50. Manely J, Taddio A. Acetaminophen and ibuprofen for prevention of adverse reactions associated with childhood immunizations. *Ann Pharmacother* 2007;41:1227–1232.
51. Yalcin SS, Gumus A, Yurdakok K. Prophylactic use of acetaminophen in children vaccinated with diphtheria-tetanus-pertussis. *World J Pediatr* 2008;4(2):127–129.
52. Jackson LA, Dunstan M, Starkovich P, et al. Prophylaxis with acetaminophen or ibuprofen for prevention of local reactions to the fifth diphtheria-tetanus toxoids-acellular pertussis vaccination: a randomized, controlled trial. *Pediatrics* 2006;117:620–625.
53. Arons MM, Wheeler AP, Bernard GR, et al. Effects of ibuprofen on the physiology and survival of hypothermic sepsis. Ibuprofen in Sepsis Study Group. *Crit Care Med* 1999;27(4):699–707.
54. Bernard GR, Wheeler AP, Russell JA, et al. The effects of ibuprofen on the physiology and survival of patients with sepsis. The Ibuprofen in Sepsis Study Group. *N Engl J Med* 1997;336(13): 912–918.
55. Starko KM, Ray CG, Dominguez LB, et al. Reye's syndrome and salicylate use. *Pediatrics* 1980;66(6):859–864.
56. Wilson JT, Brown RD. Reye syndrome and aspirin use: the role of prodromal illness severity in the assessment of relative risk. *Pediatrics* 1982;69(6):822–825.
57. Food and Drug Administration. Labeling for oral and rectal over-the-counter drug products containing aspirin and nonaspirin salicylates; Reye's syndrome warning. Final rule. *Fed Regist* 2003; 68(74):18861–18869.
58. Mackowiak PA. Diagnostic implications and clinical consequences of antipyretic therapy. *Clin Infect Dis* 2000;31(Suppl 5): S230–S233.
59. Wilson JT, Brown RD, Bocchini JA Jr, et al. Efficacy, disposition and pharmacodynamics of aspirin, acetaminophen, and choline salicylate in young febrile children. *Ther Drug Monit* 1982;4(2): 147–180.
60. Chang JC, Gross HM. Utility of naproxen in the differential diagnosis of fever of undetermined origin in patients with cancer. *Am J Med* 1984;76(4):597–603.
61. Chang JC. NSAID test to distinguish between infectious and neoplastic fever in cancer patients. *Postgrad Med* 1988;84(8): 71–72.
62. Tsavaris N, Zinelis A, Karabelis A, et al. A randomized trial of the effect of three non-steroid anti-inflammatory agents in ameliorating cancer-induced fever. *J Intern Med* 1990;228(5):451–455.
63. Beiter JL Jr, Simon HK, Chambliss CR, et al. Intravenous ketorolac in the emergency department of sickle cell pain and predictors of its effectiveness. *Arch Pediatr Adolesc Med* 2001;155(4): 496–500.
64. Munro HM, Walton SR, Malviya S, et al. Low-dose ketorolac improves morphine analgesia and reduces morphine requirements following posterior spinal fusion in adolescents. *Can J Anaesth* 2002;49(5):461–466.
65. Gerhardt RT, Gerhardt DM. Intravenous ketorolac in the treatment of fever. *Am J Emerg Med* 2000;18(4):500–501.
66. Axelrod P. External cooling in the management of fever. *Clin Infect Dis* 2000;31(Suppl 5):S224–S229.
67. Steele RW, Tanaka PT, Lara RP, et al. Evaluation of sponging and of oral antipyretic therapy to reduce fever. *J Pediatr* 1970;77(5): 824–829.
68. Arditi M, Kilner MS. Coma following use of rubbing alcohol for fever control. *Am J Dis Child* 1987;141(3):237–238.
69. Wilson JT, Brown RD, Kearns GL; PPRU Network. Clinical trials with antipyretic drugs in febrile children: a position statement on exclusion criteria. *Curr Ther Res* 2000;61(1):31–35.
70. Linakis JG, Lovejoy FH. Antipyretics. In: Yaffe SJ, Aranda JV, eds. *Pediatric pharmacology: therapeutic principles in practice.* Philadelphia, PA: WB Saunders, 1992:335–344.
71. Wilson JT, Springer MA. Antipyretics. In: Yaffee SJ, Aranda JV, eds. *Pediatric pharmacology: therapeutic principles in practice.* Philadelphia, PA: WB Saunders, 2005:563–573.
72. Mackowiak PA. Brief history of antipyretic therapy. *Clin Infect Dis* 2000;31(Suppl 5):S154–S156.
73. Stone E. An account of the success of the bark of the willow in the cure of agues. *Phil Trans R Soc Lond* 1763;53:195–200.
74. Levy G, Yaffe SJ. Relationship between dose and apparent volume of distribution and salicylate in children. *Pediatrics* 1974;54(6): 713–717.
75. Wilson JT, Helms R, Pickering BD, et al. Acetaminophen controlled-release sprinkles versus acetaminophen immediate-release elixir in febrile children. *J Clin Pharmacol* 2000;40(4): 360–369.

76. Walson PD, Galletta G, Chomilo F, et al. Comparison of multidose ibuprofen and acetaminophen therapy in febrile children. *Am J Dis Child* 1992;146(5):626–632.
77. Brown RD, Wilson JT, Kearns GL, et al. Single-dose pharmacokinetics of ibuprofen and acetaminophen in febrile children. *J Clin Pharmacol* 1992;32(3):231–241.
78. Kaufman RE, Nelson MV. Effect of age on ibuprofen pharmacokinetics and antipyretic response. *J Pediatr* 1992;121(6):969–973.
79. Kelley MT, Walson PD, Edge JH, et al. Pharmacokinetics and pharmacodynamics of ibuprofen isomers and acetaminophen in febrile children. *Clin Pharmacol Ther* 1992;52(2):181–189.
80. Brown RD, Kearns GL, Wilson JT. Integrated pharmacokinetic–pharmacodynamic model for acetaminophen, ibuprofen, and placebo antipyresis in children. *J Pharmacokinet Biopharm* 1998; 26(5):559–579.
81. Wong A, Sibbald A, Ferrero F, et al. Antipyretic effects of dipyrone versus ibuprofen versus acetaminophen in children: results of a multinational, randomized, modified double-blind study. *Clin Pediatr* 2001;40(6):313–324.
82. Autret E, Breart G, Jonville AP, et al. Comparative efficacy and tolerance of ibuprofen syrup and acetaminophen syrup in children with pyrexia associated with infectious diseases and treated with antibiotics. *Eur J Clin Pharmacol* 1994;46(3):197–201.
83. Walson PD, Galletta G, Braden NJ, et al. Ibuprofen, acetaminophen, and placebo treatment of febrile children. *Clin Pharmacol Ther* 1989;46(1):9–17.
84. Kaufman RE, Sawyer LA, Scheinbaum ML. Antipyretic efficacy of ibuprofen vs. acetaminophen. *Am J Dis Child* 1992;146(5): 622–625.
85. Vauzelle-Kervroedan F, d'Athis P, Pariente-Khayat A, et al. Equivalent antipyretic activity of ibuprofen and paracetamol in febrile children. *J Pediatr* 1997;131(5):683–687.
86. McIntyre J, Hull D. Comparing efficacy and tolerability of ibuprofen and paracetamol in fever. *Arch Dis Child* 1996;74(2): 164–167.
87. Treluyer JM, Tonnelier S, d'Athis P, et al. Antipyretic efficacy of an initial 30-mg/kg loading dose of acetaminophen versus a 15-mg/kg maintenance dose. *Pediatrics* 2001;108(4):E73.
88. Mayoral CE, Marino RV, Rosenfeld W, et al. Alternating antipyretics: is this an alternative? *Pediatrics* 2000;105(5): 1009–1012.
89. Diez Domingo J, Burgos Ramirez A, Garrido Garcia J, et al. Use of alternating antipyretics in the treatment of fever in Spain. *An Esp Pediatr* 2001;55(6):503–510.
90. American Academy of Pediatrics, Committee on Drugs. Acetaminophen toxicity in children. *Pediatrics* 2001;108(4): 1020–1024.
91. Sarrell EM, Wielunsky E, Cohen HA. Antipyretic treatment in young children with fever: acetaminophen, ibuprofen or both alternating in a randomized, double-blind study. *Arch Pediatr Adolesc Med* 2006;160:197–202.
92. Kramer LC, Richards PA, Thompson AM, et al. Alternating antipyretics: antipyretics efficacy of acetaminophen versus acetaminophen alternated with ibuprofen in children. *Clin Pediatr (Phila)* 2008;47(9):907–911.
93. Fimbres A. Alternating acetaminophen and ibuprofen for fever: the only alternative? *AAP Grand Rounds* 2006;15:67–68.
94. Schmitt BD. Concerns over alternating acetaminophen and ibuprofen for fever. *Arch Pediatr Adolesc Med* 2006;160:157.
95. Steele RW, Young FS, Bass JW, et al. Oral antipyretic therapy. Evaluation of aspirin–acetaminophen combination. *Am J Dis Child* 1972;123(3):204–206.
96. Brown RD, Wilson JT. Aspirin consumption and severity of Reye's syndrome. *Pediatrics* 1983;71(2):293–295.
97. Cotty VF, Sterbenz FJ, Mueller F, et al. Augmentation of human blood acetylsalicylate concentrations by the simultaneous administration of acetaminophen with aspirin. *Toxicol Appl Pharmacol* 1977;41(1):7–13.
98. Plaisance KI. Toxicities of drugs used in the management of fever. *Clin Infect Dis* 2000;31(Suppl 5):S219–S223.
99. Plaisance KI, Mackowiak PA. Antipyretic therapy: physiologic rationale, diagnostic implications, and clinical consequences. *Arch Intern Med* 2000;160(4):449–456.
100. Bleumink GS, Feenstra J, Sturkenboom M, et al. Nonsteroidal antiinflammatory drugs and heart failure. *Drugs* 2003;63(6):525–534.
101. Lesko SM, Mitchell AA. An assessment of the safety of pediatric ibuprofen. A practitioner-based randomized clinical trial. *J Am Med Assoc* 1995;273(12):929–933.
102 Lesko SM, Mitchell AA. Renal function after short-term ibuprofen use in infants and children. *Pediatrics* 1997;100:954–957.
103. Heubi JE, Barbacci MB, Zimmerman HJ. Therapeutic misadventures with acetaminophen: hepatotoxicity after multiple doses in children. *J Pediatr* 1998;132:22–27.
104. Kearns GL, Leeder JS, Wasserman GS. Acetaminophen overdose with therapeutic intent. *J Pediatr* 1998;132(1):5–8.
105. Kearns GL, Leeder JS, Wasserman GS. Acetaminophen intoxication during treatment: what you don't know can hurt you. *Clin Pediatr (Phila)* 2000;39(3):133–144.
106. James LP, Farrar HC, Sullivan JE, et al. Measurement of acetaminophen–protein adducts in children and adolescents with acetaminophen overdoses. *J Clin Pharmacol* 2001;41(8):846–851.
107. James LP, Farrar HC, Darville TL, et al. The Pediatric Pharmacology Research Unit Network NICHD. Elevation of serum interleukin 8 levels in acetaminophen overdose in children and adolescents. *Clin Pharmacol Ther* 2001;70(3):280–286.
108. James LP, Wilson JT, Simar R, et al. The PPRU Network. Evaluation of occult acetaminophen hepatotoxicity in hospitalized children receiving acetaminophen. *Clin Pediatr (Phila)* 2001;40(5): 243–248.
109. Muldrew KL, James LP, Coop L, et al. Determination of acetaminophen–protein adducts in mouse liver and serum and human serum after hepatotoxic doses of acetaminophen using high-performance liquid chromatography with electrochemical detection. *Drug Metab Dispos* 2002;30(4):446–451.
110. James LP, Alonso LS, Hinson JA, et al. Detection of acetaminophen protein adducts in children with acute liver failure of indeterminate cause. *Pediatrics* 2006;118:e676–e681.
111. Davern TJ, James LP, Hinson JA, et al. Measurement of serum acetaminophen-protein adducts in patients with acute liver failure. *Gastroentrology* 2006;130:687–694.
112. Kliegman RM, Behrman RE, Jenson HB, Stanton B. *Nelson Textbook of Pediatrics*, 18th ed. Philadelphia, PA: Saunders Elsevier, 2007.
113. Kozer E, Greenberg R, Zimmerman DR, et al. Repeated supratherapeutic doses of paracetamol in children—a literature review and suggested clinical approach. *Acta Paediatr* 2006;95:1165–1171.
114. Rumack BH, Matthew H. Acetaminophen overdose in young children. Treatment and effects of alcohol and other additional ingestants in 417 cases. *Am J Dis Child* 1984;138(5):428–433.
115. Rumack BH. Acetaminophen overdose in children and adolescents. *Pediatr Clin North Am* 1986;33(3):691–701.
116. Lesko SM, Mitchell AA. The safety of acetaminophen and ibuprofen among children younger than two years old. *Pediatrics* 1999;104(4):E39.
117. Rivera-Penera T, Gugig R, Davis J, et al. Outcome of acetaminophen overdose in pediatric patients and factors contributing to hepatotoxicity. *J Pediatr* 1997;130:300–304.
118. Hahn TW, Henneberg SW, Holm-Knudsen RJ, et al. Pharmacokinetics of rectal paracetamol after repeated dosing in children. *Br J Anaesth* 2000;85(4):512–519.
119. Scolink D, Kozer E, Jacobson S, et al. Comparison of oral versus normal and high-dose rectal acetaminophen in the treatment of febrile children. *Pediatrics* 2002;110:553–556.
120. Goldstein LH, Berlin M, Berkovitch M, et al. Effectiveness of oral vs rectal acetaminophen: a meta-analysis. *Arch Pediatr Adolesc Med* 2008;162(11):1042–1046.
121. Rumack BH, Matthew H. Acetaminophen poisoning and toxicity. *Pediatrics* 1975;55(6):871–876.
122. Lesko SM, Louik C, Vezina RM, et al. Asthma morbidity after the short-term use of ibuprofen in children. *Pediatrics* 2002;109(2):E20.
123. Perrott DA, Piira T, Goodenough B, Champion GD. Efficacy and safety of acetaminophen vs ibuprofen for treating children's pain or fever: a meta-analysis. *Arch Pediatr Adolesc Med.* 2004 June: 158(6):521–6.
124. Southey ER, Soares-Weiser K, Kleijnen J. Systematic review and meta-analysis of the clinical safety and tolerability of ibuprofen compared with paracetamol in paediatric pain and fever. *Curr Med Res Opin.* 2009 Sep; 25(9):2207–22.
125. Pierce CA, Voss B. Efficacy and safety of Ibuprofen and acetaminophen in children and adults: a meta-analysis and qualitative review. *Ann Pharmacother* 2010 Mar; 44(3):489–506. Epub 2010 Feb 11.

CHAPTER

42

Eli Zalzstein
Rafael Gorodischer

Cardiovascular Drugs

DRUGS USED IN THE MANAGEMENT OF CONGESTIVE HEART FAILURE

GENERAL CONSIDERATIONS

Heart failure is defined as the pathophysiologic state wherein the heart is unable to pump adequate volume of blood and oxygen at a rate appropriate to the body's metabolic demands. Heart failure is now considered more a cardiocirculatory disorder than simply a disease of the heart. Typically, it is characterized in hemodynamic terms and is considered to occur when changes take place in one or more of the determinants of cardiac output, including preload, afterload, contractility, and heart rate. Depression of the intrinsic contractile performance of the cardiac muscle is typical for myocardial and for ischemic heart disease. Structural defects of the heart or great vessels result in abnormal loading conditions; they lead to heart failure even when the muscle contractility is normal. Large left-to-right shunts, valvular insufficiency, and atrioventricular (AV) malformations lead to volume overload, whereas obstructive lesions such as severe aortic stenosis may lead to pressure overload and failure. Extracardiac conditions like hyperthyroidism, anemia, and severe malnutrition may result in high cardiac output failure secondary to unbalanced demand supply of the heart.

As a reaction to heart failure the body activates compensatory mechanisms to maintain adequate systemic oxygen delivery. Renal salt and water retention and augmentation of cardiac preload relationship maximize cardiac output through the Frank–Starling law. Catecholamine release is another compensatory mechanism, which augments myocardial contractility and heart rate. Myocardial hypertrophy leads initially to decreased ventricular wall stress but finally may deteriorate to decreased contractility. All these compensatory mechanisms contribute initially to maintain pump function but finally lead to progressive deterioration in cardiac performance and congestive heart failure.

The progressive impairment of ventricular function is the result of structural and conformational changes of the heart, with deleterious remodeling due to hypertrophy and fibrosis. Increased systemic and intracardiac neurohormone concentrations are a main factor in promoting cardiac remodeling. In addition, neurohormones act as growth factors for cardiac myocytes and fibroblasts. This new knowledge has led to the use of agents that block the renin–angiotensin–aldosterone system and the sympathetic nervous system to inhibit, and even reverse, cardiac remodeling (1).

The heart of the young infant responds in a more limited fashion to inotropic agents than that of the older child or adult (2–6). This is due to the biologic immaturity and restricted functional reserve of the young heart as well as the different pathogenesis of cardiac decompensation of the myocardium in infants with left-to-right shunts (7,8), a lower ratio of active myofilaments to noncontractile elements (9), greater stiffness of the ventricle (10,11), underdeveloped cardiac sympathetic nerves (12,13), and higher cardiac output per unit surface area (14). Differences in electrolyte concentration and in a number of metabolic reactions have also been described in the newborn myocardium (15,16).

Traditionally, digitalis glycosides and diuretics have been key drugs in the management of congestive heart failure. Concern with the low therapeutic index of digitalis led to the increased use of natural and synthetic catecholamines in acute situations and to the introduction of novel inotropic agents. The myocardium of many infants with congenital heart defects may already be working at the peak of its contractile force; thus, it may be unable to sustain adequate blood flow because of volume overload (due to left to right shunting in patent ductus arteriosus and ventricular septal defect) or pressure overload (in obstructive lesions) (2,7,8). The use of systemic vasodilators reduces cardiac workload in infants and children in heart failure.

Therapy has shifted from purely hemodynamic manipulation to include neurohumoral modulation. Therapeutic classes that have emerged in the last decades include angiotensin-converting enzyme (ACE) inhibitors, spironolactone, β-blockers, β-type natriuretic peptide (nesiritide), and triiodothyronine.

DIGOXIN

Digoxin is the most commonly used cardiac glycoside, has been studied more than other preparations, and is the glycoside recommended for routine use in pediatric patients. Objective data on its efficacy in the treatment of congestive heart failure have been provided in adults with normal sinus rhythm (17).

The main action of digitalis is to increase the force of myocardial contraction. The positive inotropic effect in a patient with heart failure results in slowing of cardiac rate, disappearance of gallop rhythm, improved tissue perfusion, diuresis, relief of edema, and decreased venous pressure and heart and liver size. Cardiac glycosides also affect the metabolism, conduction, refractory period, excitability, and automaticity of the myocardium. In addition, they have extracardial hemodynamic effects such as arteriolar and venous constriction, both by direct action on vascular smooth muscle and by neural effects.

Mechanism of Action

Digitalis glycosides bind to multiple sites in many cells, including those of the myocardium (18–21). The pharmacologic actions of digitalis on the heart, however, seem to be due to surface interactions in the cardiac sarcolemma and are not correlated with the total tissue uptake of the drug (21–24).

The most specific action of cardiac glycosides seems to be the well-known inhibition of the Na^+, K^+ exchange pump of the cell membrane. Intimately related to the Na^+ pump is the Na^+, K^+-ATPase which is located in the cardiac sarcolemma; it is inhibited by cardiac glycosides. Digitalis is postulated to enhance contraction by increasing the influx of Ca^{2+} as a result of inhibition of the Na^+, K^+-ATPase system.

A large body of evidence supports the hypothesis that the Na^+, K^+-ATPase is the receptor for cardiac glycosides (25). However, some facts do not fit this theory: The positive inotropic effect of cardiac glycosides is terminated by washing, whereas the inhibition of Na^+, K^+-ATPase persists; the kinetics of the inhibition of the Na^+, K^+-ATPase and of the positive inotropic effect are different, and the therapeutic concentrations of free digitalis in plasma are too low to evoke any inhibition of the Na^+ pump in the heart (26,27).

Digitalis glycosides also influence cardiac function indirectly, by their action on the vagal nerve. In addition to improving hemodynamics, digitalis glycosides also have significant neurohormonal modulatory effects and reduce plasma renin and norepinephrine concentrations. Digoxin modulates the increased sympathetic autonomic activity, probably by improving arterial baroreceptor reflexes (28,29).

Absorption

Digoxin is available in both oral and parenteral forms. Gastrointestinal absorption varies from patient to patient and results in a lower serum concentration than does parenteral administration. In some patients, bioavailability of digoxin is affected by intestinal flora (30). P-glycoprotein, present in intestinal cells, pumps digoxin back into the intestinal lumen and thereby limits its absorption (31,32). Drugs such as quinidine, verapamil, spironolactone, and dipyridamole inhibit P-glycoprotein and increase digoxin bioavailability (33,34).

Distribution and Plasma Protein Binding of Digoxin

The affinity of digoxin for plasma proteins is low both in adults and in newborn infants. The apparent volume of distribution of digoxin in infants and in children is much greater than in adults (35–38). The affinity for digoxin varies in different tissues and is greatest in the ventricular myocardium (36,39). A linear relationship exists between myocardium and serum concentration over a wide range of concentrations (37,39,40). Greater myocardial and erythrocyte concentrations have been found in children during digitalization than in the course of chronic administration of digoxin (37,40).

Endogenous Digoxin-Like Substances

Endogenous digoxin-like substances (EDLS) have been determined in the serum of newborn infants, pregnant women, and patients with hypertension or renal and hepatic disease (41–44). EDLS may interfere with the clinical interpretation of serum concentrations during digoxin therapy. Newborn infants not treated with digoxin and not exposed to it in utero may have measurable concentrations of the glycoside within the "therapeutic" range. Concentrations tend to decrease with increasing gestational age.

Most digoxin assays do not have the specificity to fully distinguish EDLS from exogenous digoxin, although EDLS do not possess the same therapeutic properties as the drug. The resultant artificial elevation of a reported digoxin level or a completely factitious level in a patient not taking the drug can have pharmacokinetic and clinical consequences (45,46).

Cross-reactivity with EDLS may be avoided with a high-performance liquid chromatography assay. Although highly specific, the high-performance liquid chromatography assay is not practical for routine clinical use and is less sensitive as compared with the fluorescence polarization immunoassay (47). A microparticle enzyme and the TD_xDigoxin fluorescent polarization immunoassay reportedly minimize EDLS cross-reactivity (48,49).

Renal Excretion

Digoxin is excreted largely unchanged in the urine. A linear relationship exists between the renal clearance of digoxin and creatinine; in adult subjects, these two values are usually identical (50–52). It is subjected to active tubular secretion and to some degree of tubular reabsorption (50,51).

Renal clearance of digoxin is low during the first weeks of life and increases progressively until adult values are attained at about 5 months of age (53). At any given age, however, renal clearance of digoxin in infants is greater than the simultaneously determined creatinine clearance (53,54). The rate of digoxin clearance is age dependent and correlates with renal P-glycoprotein expression (55). Renal excretion of digoxin is impaired in patients with renal failure (56). Diuretics such as furosemide do not significantly affect renal excretion of digoxin (57).

Clinical Efficacy of Digoxin in Fetuses, Infants, and Children

Whereas the efficacy of cardiac glycosides in supraventricular arrhythmias is well established (58), similar evidence for efficacy in congestive heart failure in children has been controversial; inotropic agents may not improve hemodynamics substantially (59–62). Because cardiac failure stems from a congenital malformation in most of these cases (e.g., ventricular septal defect or persistent ductus arteriosus), the already hyperactive and presumably healthy myocardium may not benefit from digitalis.

Most infants and children with congestive heart failure are treated with digoxin, diuretics, and other drugs, which makes it difficult to assess the net effect of the glycoside in a given patient. Only about half of infants with ventricular septal defect alone may benefit from digoxin therapy (60,61,63–66). Studies in adults indicate that digoxin does have a significant salutatory effect in patients with heart failure (17,30,67).

In the treatment of supraventricular tachycardia, digoxin is efficacious because of both direct and indirect (autonomic) effects. It slows the rate of the sinus node through the vagal nerve and increases the refractory period, thus abolishing reentry of supraventricular tachycardia. Because protracted periods of fetal tachyarrhythmias (supraventricular tachycardia, atrial flutter, and atrial fibrillation) may cause congestive heart failure and fetal death, transplacental therapy with digoxin as well as other antiarrhythmics (e.g., quinidine, verapamil, amiodarone) is given. Maternal digitalization appears to be the treatment of choice in such cases, relying on the excellent transplacental distribution of the glycoside. Digoxin is also used in the treatment of fetal congestive heart failure with sinus rhythm (68).

Digoxin Toxicity

A substantial proportion (up to 25%) of hospitalized adults receiving digoxin experience some degree of adverse effects related to the drug (69). Although similar figures are lacking in pediatric patients, there is a clinical impression that toxicity is not as common in children, but large studies in infants and children are not available. Digoxin toxicity in infants is more common with loading ("digitalization") doses than during maintenance therapy. A significant cause of digoxin toxicity is unintentional therapeutic error. The arrhythmias induced by digitalis are more likely to occur and are more severe in patients with cardiac disease. Hypokalemia, hypocalcemia, hypomagnesemia, and hypoxia are likely to increase the risk of toxicity; kaliuretic diuretics, which are often coadministered with digoxin, are a common reason for its toxicity.

The effective antidote for digoxin toxicity is a preparation of Fab fragments from antidigoxin antisera. The neutralizing dose of Fab fragments is based on the digoxin dose or the total body digoxin burden.

Digoxin Dose

Individual response to the drug varies, making it necessary to adjust the dosage according to the patient's response. Digoxin therapy is most effective when the medication is given orally (Table 42.1). A digitalizing dose may be given over the first 24 hours, with one-half of the total digitalizing dose given initially and two one-quarter doses of the total digitalizing dose at 6- to 8-hour intervals following the previous dose. Oral maintenance therapy is usually begun 12 hours after the last digitalizing dose. When early signs of heart failure are present, the maintenance dose may be started without the digitalizing dose, although the full therapeutic effect will not be reached for 4 to 7 days. The advantage of this last approach is that it requires only one dosage calculation and decreases the likelihood of dosage errors or acute toxicity. Patients with inflammatory disease of the myocardium and in the postoperative state often have an enhanced sensitivity to the drug, which requires reducing the administered dose. The parenteral dose is generally calculated to be 25% less than the oral dose. Intravenous digoxin therapy can be used in instances of acute, severe heart failure. However, other forms of parenteral inotropic support are available that maybe more efficacious and safer to use.

TABLE 42.1 Digoxin Dosage Schedule

	Total Digitalizing Dose (μg/kg)	*Maintenance Dose (μg/kg/day)*
Premature infants (<37 wk)	20–25	5
Full-term infant	30	8–10
Infants <2 yr	30–40	8–10
Child 2–10 yr	30–40	8–10
Child >10 yr	10	2–5
Maximum dose	1 mg total	0.025 mg total

Adverse Effects

Common adverse effects of digitalis include the heart (sinus bradycardia, A-V block, ventricular tachycardia, and fibrillation) and other systems: the gastrointestinal (nausea, vomiting, anorexia, diarrhea), the central nervous (dizziness, headache, malaise, pain, alterations in vision, aphasia, delirium), and others (i.e., gynecomastia).

Drug Interactions

Drugs coadministered with digoxin may interfere with the disposition of cardiac glycosides and cause potentially toxic serum concentrations (70). Quinidine, spironolactone, verapamil, amiodarone, and carvedilol (71) may elevate the serum concentration of digoxin and cause toxicity. Those drugs may inhibit the tubular secretion of digoxin, as they decrease its renal clearance without affecting the glomerular filtration rate. Whenever those drugs are coadministered with digoxin, the dose of the cardiac glycoside should be decreased, with careful monitoring of its serum concentrations.

Several drugs known to decrease the glomerular filtration rate (such as indomethacin and cyclosporine) may cause potentially toxic accumulation of digoxin (72,73).

Therapeutic Monitoring of Digoxin Therapy

In principle, digoxin could be a good candidate for monitoring therapy by measuring its serum concentration because it has a low therapeutic index, its effect is not easily measurable during routine therapy, and a poor correlation exists between dose and serum concentration. However, a clear association between serum concentration and toxic and nontoxic effects does not exist, and assays for its measurement are not sufficiently specific. As mentioned, the existence of EDLS in the newborn may lead to spurious elevation of digoxin measurements. Still, serum digoxin concentrations correlate better than digoxin doses with its pharmacologic effect (74). Extremely high or immeasurable levels help in the decision of whether the patient has toxic symptoms.

Most authorities regard the therapeutic range of digoxin to be 0.5 to 2.0 ng per mL. With digoxin concentrations above 2 ng per mL there is an increased risk of digitalis toxicity. However, there is a wide "gray zone" of levels that may be toxic in one individual and nontoxic in another. Even at serum concentrations above 5 ng per mL, about one-third of pediatric patients may not show symptoms or signs of toxicity (75). A variety of clinical conditions, including hypokalemia, hypocalcemia, hypomagnesemia, and chronic heart disease, may increase the risk of toxicity of digitalis glycosides.

Little information exists on the correlation of serum concentrations of digoxin with inotropic effects; more data exist on the relationship between its serum concentrations and its antiarrhythmic effects. Some investigators have observed a good correlation, whereas others have not (76–79).

Optimal hemodynamic, neurohormonal, and clinical effects may be achieved in adults with a dose that results in a plasma concentration of about 0.7 ng per mL; no additional benefits are seen with concentrations above 1 ng per mL (30).

Measurement of serum digoxin concentrations is recommended in cases of suspected toxicity, in suspected accidental or suicidal digoxin ingestion, in high-risk patients (renal failure, following cardiac surgery), and in suspected underdigitalization (lack of compliance, inadequate dose, or gastrointestinal disturbances) (80).

OTHER INOTROPIC AGENTS

Catecholamines

Adrenergic agents exert a positive inotropic effect by acting directly on β_1-adrenergic receptors of the myocardium. They may be used temporarily in the management of congestive heart failure (except in congestive failure due to obstructive lesions) until a more permanent therapy is established. Their clinical use is limited by their positive chronotropic action and tendency to exacerbate cardiac arrhythmias. There is no clear relationship between plasma catecholamine concentration and effect. Their actions in the heart include interaction with plasma membrane G protein, stimulation of adenyl cyclase, increased intracellular concentration of cyclic adenosine monophosphate (AMP), and Ca^{2+} delivery to cardiac contractile proteins, mediated by cyclic AMP-dependent protein kinases (81). The function of adrenergic receptors is affected by catecholamine as well as by tissue perfusion and pH. Clinical use of these agents is summarized in Table 42.2.

Epinephrine

Epinephrine (adrenaline), the major hormone secreted by the adrenal medulla, is a potent stimulator of both α- and β-adrenergic receptors and exerts complex effects on various organs. Following subcutaneous or slow intravenous administration, it increases the force of myocardial contraction and the heart rate, with a resultant increase in cardiac output and systolic pressure; diastolic pressure usually falls because of its effect on β_2-adrenergic receptors of skeletal muscle vasculature. The increased work of the heart is achieved at the expense of greater oxygen consumption and decreased cardiac efficiency. In the kidneys, epinephrine increases vascular resistance and decreases plasma flow. Epinephrine also induces automaticity of the myocardium, and its intravenous administration may cause cardiac arrhythmias.

The effects of epinephrine infusion on regional blood flow are of concern in the management of critically ill children. The pulmonary vascular bed contains α- and β_2

TABLE 42.2 Use of Selected Inotropic Agents

Drug	*Indications*	*Route and Dosage*
Epinephrine (adrenaline)	Cardiac resuscitation	i.v. or intratracheal 0.01–0.03 mg/kg/dose every 3–5 min, as needed
	Cardiac decompensation following cardiac surgery	i.v. 0.1–1.0 μg/kg/min per response
	Anaphylactic shock	s.c. 0.01 mg/kg/dose
Isoproterenol (Isuprel)	Failure of other inotropic agents; bradycardia	i.v. initially 0.05–0.1 μg/kg/min: increase if necessary (heart rate, peripheral perfusion) up to 2 μg/kg/min
Dopamine	Heart failure (asphyxiated neonates, for cardiac surgery), shock (cardiogenic, septic), renal failure	i.v. 1–20 μg/kg/min
Dobutamine	Acute cardiac decompensation	i.v. 2.5–20 μg/kg/min
Inamrinone	Cardiac decompensation when inotropic support and vasodilation are desirable	i.v. 0.75 mg/kg, followed by a maintenance i.v. infusion of 3–5 μg/kg/min (neonates), and 5–10 μg/kg/min (infants and children)

i.v., Intravenous; s.c., subcutaneous.

receptors, and pulmonary vasoconstriction (α stimulation) or vasodilation (β_2 stimulation) can be expected, depending on the infusion rate, the duration of exposure to epinephrine, the presence of failure hypoxia, and the preexisting pulmonary vascular tone (82–87). At low and medium doses (less than 0.5 to 0.8 μg per kg per minute) epinephrine decreases pulmonary vascular resistance (PVR) and increases pulmonary blood flow; ventilation/perfusion mismatch may result. Higher doses appear to raise PVR if the preinfusion PVR was normal. However, even under these circumstances systemic vascular resistance is increased more than PVR, so that in patients with intracardiac defects, epinephrine infusion would favor left-to-right shunting. Conversely, if the preinfusion PVR was elevated by either hypoxia or sepsis, even high-dose epinephrine administration (1 to 3.5 μg per kg per minute) may yield predominantly β-adrenergic stimulation and pulmonary vasodilation (88–90).

Few data exist on the pharmacokinetics of epinephrine in children (88). Plasma elimination half-life is very short (around 2 minutes).

Whereas noncatecholamine sympathomimetic amines act indirectly in the heart (through release of norepinephrine), epinephrine directly stimulates β_1-adrenergic receptors of cardiac muscles and pacemaker and conductive tissue.

Epinephrine is administered only parenterally. After oral administration it is readily metabolized in the gut and the liver. It is readily absorbed by mucosa of the tracheobronceal tree, a route employed in cardiac resuscitation. It was shown to be safe as inhaled form in limited conditions as transient tachypnea of the new born (91). Epinephrine is rapidly inactivated by catecholamine-*O*-methyltransferase (COMT) and monoaminooxidase of the liver and other tissues, and its metabolites are excreted in the urine.

Toxic effects include restlessness, anxiety, fear, headache, tremor, pallor, dizziness, and palpitation. The major life-threatening toxic effect is the induction of ventricular arrhythmias. Interaction between epinephrine and halogenated hydrocarbon anesthetics may result in ventricular fibrillation. Tissue ischemia can occur as a consequence of peripheral vasoconstriction, especially with high rates of infusion.

Epinephrine for injection is a sterile solution of epinephrine hydrochloride in water. When administered by intravenous route the 1:1,000 solution should be diluted to 1:10,000 with saline; by endotracheal route the 1:1,000 solution is diluted with 3 to 5 mL of saline.

Norepinephrine

Norepinephrine is the neurotransmitter of sympathetic postganglionic fibers and of certain tracts in the central nervous system and constitutes 1/10 to 1/5 of the catecholamines in the adrenal medulla. It has β_1- and α-adrenergic effects, but in contrast to epinephrine and isoproterenol, norepinephrine does not stimulate β_2 receptors.

Intravenous infusion of norepinephrine causes an increase in peripheral resistance and a rise in systolic and diastolic blood pressure, with no change (or a decrease) in cardiac output; therefore, its use is limited to the management of hypotension and was demonstrated to be efficacious in extreme situations such as refractory septic shock (92). It has no indication in situations that require increased myocardial contraction force. In addition, norepinephrine may induce arrhythmias, tissue ischemia secondary to extreme vasoconstriction, and skin necrosis if cutaneous infiltration occurs. The mechanisms and extent of absorption, metabolism, and excretion are similar to those of epinephrine. It is administered by intravenous infusion at an initial dose of 0.1 μg per kg per minute and increased until the desired effect is obtained or up to 1 μg per kg per minute.

Isoproterenol

Isoproterenol (isoprenaline) acts on β_1- and β_2-adrenergic receptors, with minimal effect on α receptors. It is used in patients with depressed contractility and low cardiac output. It may reduce blood pressure, especially in patients with hypovolemia, but a reduction in systemic vascular resistance may be beneficial in some patients with elevated systemic resistance and low cardiac output. Isoproterenol may favorably reduce PVR in patients with pulmonary hypertension. Intravenous infusion of isoproterenol causes positive inotropic and chronotropic effects, decreased peripheral resistance and diastolic pressure, and increased renal blood flow. The resulting greater cardiac output may raise systolic pressure. Bradycardia due to AV block or sinus node dysfunction may be managed temporarily by infusing isoproterenol until more definitive therapy is available. Isoproterenol is rapidly absorbed when administered as aerosol, and it is metabolized primarily by COMT. Although less pronounced, its side effects are similar to those of epinephrine.

Dopamine

This sympathomimetic amine is a metabolic precursor of norepinephrine and epinephrine and acts as a central neurotransmitter. It acts on dopamine receptors of the brain and vascular beds in the kidney, brain, and coronaries. It has a positive inotropic effect on the myocardium resulting from direct stimulation of β_1-adrenergic receptors and also from the effect of norepinephrine released by cardiac sympathetic nerve terminals. It has a less marked chronotropic effect than isoproterenol. At low therapeutic doses (2 to 5 μg per kg per minute), it has a predominant β_1-adrenergic action and the increase in cardiac output parallels the increase in heart rate; at higher doses, dopamine has increasing α-adrenergic action. In addition, at low doses it causes renal vasodilation and promotes diuresis by stimulating renal D_1- and D_2-dopaminergic receptors and increases systolic pressure with little or no effect on diastolic pressure. Because it increases pulmonary artery pressure, it should be used with caution if at all, in patients with elevated PVR. At high doses (>10 μg per kg per minute), it stimulates arteriolar α-adrenergic receptors, causing vasoconstriction (including renal vasoconstriction) and hypertension.

In contrast to the response to isoproterenol, which is equal at all ages, the inotropic response to dopamine in the young animal increases with advancing age (89); this explains the greater dopamine requirements of young infants to obtain a therapeutic effect. This may be due to decreased levels of releasable norepinephrine of the immature myocardium and/or greater dopamine clearance in infancy as compared to later in childhood (93).

Dopamine does not cross the blood–brain barrier; it is metabolized by monoaminooxidase and COMT and therefore is effective only when given parenterally. No adverse effects have been recorded in infants, children, and adolescents with a dose of 0.3 to 25 μg per kg per minute (89). However, excessive dosing can cause side effects that represent enhanced sympathomimetic activity. Extravasations may cause ischemic necrosis. Phentolamine may be used when gangrene of the fingers or toes is feared following prolonged administration of the drug.

Dobutamine

Dobutamine is a synthetic β-sympathomimetic amine that has a potent inotropic action. It has little effect on heart rate in adults but significant chronotropic effects in young children. It is a mixture of L and D isomers, and its pharmacologic effects are explained by their different action on α_1- (L isomer) and β_1- and β_2-adrenergic (D isomer) receptors. It does not stimulate renal dopamine receptors and has no effect on renal vasculature; low-dose dopamine may be added to the dobutamine infusion if increased renal cortical flow is desired. High doses of dobutamine may cause elevation of systemic arterial pressure. Increasing plasma concentrations correlate with improvement in cardiac function in adults with low output failure (93). The combination of dobutamine with dopamine improves cardiac performance at lower doses of each drug, preserving the renal vasodilatory effect of dopamine and reducing the potential for toxic reaction. Wide variability in drug clearance and in hemodynamic response requires individual titration of dobutamine therapy. It is effective even in preterm infants with low systemic blood flow (94).

Dobutamine plasma half-life is about 2 minutes, and its clearance in children is around 100 mL per kg per minute (95).

Dobutamine stress testing was shown useful in cardiac magnetic resonance after Fontan operation (96) and in echocardiography in pediatric heart transplant patients (97).

NEWER INOTROPIC AGENTS

Some patients in cardiac failure remain symptomatic despite conventional therapy, including diuretics, angiotensive converting-enzyme inhibitors, and digoxin. Newer cardiotonics may be used in these patients which not only increase the contractility of the myocardium but also have vasodilating properties and the potential of a greater therapeutic index as compared with digoxin. Their inotropic effect is obtained by a mechanism different than inhibition of Na^+, K^+-ATPase, or β-adrenergic receptor stimulation (98,99). Data are available on these agents in the developing organism (5,100–103).

PHOSPHODIESTERASE INHIBITORS

Inamrinone and Milrinone

Inamrinone (or amrinone) and milrinone are potent bipyridine derivatives that selectively inhibit cyclic AMP-specific cardiac phosphodiesterase and result in a positive inotropic effect, additive to that of digitalis. Infusion of inamrinone results in an increase in cardiac output with reduction in filling pressures and systemic vascular resistance. Heart rate is affected minimally by inamrinone at conventional doses. Inamrinone reduces pulmonary artery pressure without producing systemic hypotension in infants and children with intracardiac left-to-right shunt. Inamrinone may be effective in postoperative low-output states, and in this setting it has had the broadest application.

Both agents are well absorbed following oral administration, rapidly distributed in the body, and excreted in the urine. Inamrinone undergoes biotransformation in the liver to an N-acetyl derivative and other metabolites. The plasma elimination half-lives of inamrinone and milrinone in adults are around 4 and 1.5 hours, respectively. Plasma half-life of milrinone is about 3 hours in infants and 2 hours in older children (100). Neonates have a longer half-life and slower clearance of inamrinone than infants (101,102). The body clearance of both drugs is reduced in cardiac failure.

Inamrinone is metabolized by *N*-acetyltransferase, and its clearance is greater in fast acetylators (103). Clearance of milrinone is a function of age; its V_d was found to be 482 mL per kg in children after cardiac surgery (104).

Dosing regimens of milrinone have been designed for neonates (102,105). High dose of milrinone after pediatric congenital heart surgery reduces the risk for low cardiac output syndrome in infants and children (106) probably by a direct myocardial effect (107). Milrinone has been successfully administered in children with enterovirus-induced pulmonary edema (108) and in newborns with persistent pulmonary hypertension (109) and combined with nitric oxide, stabilizes pulmonary hemodynamics after Fontan operation (110).

Inamrinone acts rapidly following intravenous administration, whereas after oral dosing its effect peaks within 3 hours and lasts for 4 to 6 hours. The inotropic action of inamrinone is age dependent (5,111). Inamrinone and milrinone have direct vasodilator effects in newborn animals (112). Inamrinone has been shown to be useful in refractory septic shock (113). These bipyridines are efficacious in acute or decompensated cardiac failure, but their long-term use has resulted in serious side effects and increased morbidity in adults (114). Toxicity is related to dose and route of administration and includes gastrointestinal intolerance, hepatotoxicity, fever, and thrombocytopenia. Milrinone is better tolerated than inamrinone.

Enoximone

Enoximone is an imidazole derivative available in intravenous and oral forms; it has a wide margin of safety. In addition to its positive inotropic effect it causes vasodilation. Its terminal plasma half-life is 6 hours in the adult; it is excreted in the urine as a sulfoxide metabolite (115). No relationship has been established between the plasma concentration of the parent drug or its sulfoxide metabolite and the pharmacologic effect.

Enoximone may restore myocardial contractility in volume and catecholamine refractory septic shock (116). Adverse effects (nausea, diarrhea, headache, abnormal liver function tests) occur in as many as one-fourth of the patients (117).

PRELOAD- AND AFTERLOAD-REDUCING DRUGS

Drugs that modify the workload of the heart in children are standard therapy in patients with heart failure (7,118). The aim of preload-reducing therapy is to decrease the elevated pressure and congestion in the venous bed (systemic or pulmonary), the ventricular filling, and the ventricular dilation of the patient in heart failure. Afterload-reducing agents are arteriolar vasodilators that tend to lower the elevated resistance to left ventricular ejection (afterload) and to improve stroke volume. The increased systemic vascular resistance in heart failure is caused by compensatory homeostatic mechanisms that aim to maintain systemic arterial pressure (i.e., elevated sympathetic tone and circulating catecholamines) and stimulation of the renin–angiotensin system. Systemic vasodilators are particularly useful in severe mitral or aortic regurgitation, systemic hypertension, cardiomyopathy, myocardial ischemia, and in postoperative cardiac surgical patients. Because volume or pressure loading may decrease myocardial contractility, systemic vasodilators used in severe cardiac failure are usually administered in combination with inotropic drugs.

Preload- and afterload-reducing drugs cause variable regional vasodilation. Direct-acting agents such as hydralazine, nitroprusside, and nitrates cause rather uniform arteriolar and/or venous vasodilation. On the other hand, the effect of α-adrenergic blocking agents and ACE inhibitors is limited to specific beds. Table 42.3 summarizes the main systemic vasodilators used in the treatment of cardiac failure in infants and children and their recommended doses. This simplified classification reflects their main site of action; however, the physiologic response to vasodilation is often more complex in the patient with heart failure.

Nitrovasodilators

The organic nitrates directly relax vascular smooth muscle and, consequently, dilate peripheral arteries and veins. Both preload and afterload are reduced; thereby reducing left ventricular filling pressures and increasing cardiac output. Relaxation is mediated by nitric oxide, which activates guanylate cyclase, resulting in increased formation of cyclic guanosine 3,5-monophosphate (cGMP) in vascular smooth muscle cells. Activation of cAMP-dependent protein kinase affects the phosphorylation state of key regulatory proteins and results in vasodilation.

Nitroglycerin

The mechanism of action of nitroglycerin is dilation of the venous capacitance vessels, with lesser effects on arterioles. Thus, right and left atrial pressures are reduced. Pulmonary and systemic arterial pressures may also fall and reflex tachycardia may occur. Nitroglycerin is not as effective as nitroprusside in lowering blood pressure in healthy children undergoing major surgery (119). In adult patients with myocardial ischemia, nitroglycerin ameliorates ischemia, presumably because of improvement in the ratio of myocardial oxygen supply and demand (120).

Nitroglycerin is of value in children with low cardiac output syndrome after cardiac surgery (121). Nitroglycerin has been used as a pulmonary vasodilator in children with variable success, depending on the cause and duration of pulmonary hypertension (122–124). Data suggest that nitroglycerin at higher doses may be useful for some cases of reactive pulmonary hypertension, but fixed pulmonary vascular disease, sepsis, and chronic lung disease do not respond. Sublingual nitroglycerin may provoke vasovagal syncope under controlled laboratory settings as head-up tilt-table test in children and adolescents with unexplained syncope (125).

TABLE 42.3 Dosing of Preload- and Afterload-Reducing Drugs

Drug	*Mechanism of Action*	*Route and Dosage*
Venous Muscle Relaxant		
Nitroglycerin	Direct vasodilation (increase in cyclic GMP)	i.v., titrate: 0.5–20 μg/kg/min (maximum 20 μg/kg/min)
Arteriolar Vasodilators		
Hydralazine	Direct vasodilation	i.v., 1.5 μg/kg/min or 0.1–0.5 mg/kg q6 hr
Nifedipine	Calcium channel blocker	p.o., 0.25–1 mg/kg/dose q6–8 hr (maximum 200 mg/d)
		p.o. or sublingual, 0.1–0.5 mg/kg/dose q6–8 hr (caution in neonates)
Mixed Vasodilators		
Nitroprusside	Direct vasodilation (increase in cyclic GMP)	i.v., titrate: 0.5–8 μg/kg/min
Phentolamine	Competitive α_1- and α_2-adrenergic blocker	i.v., 0.05–1 mg/kg/dose (maximum 5 mg)
Prazosin	Competitive α_1-adrenergic blocker	p.o. first dose 5 μg/kg; increase as needed up to 100 μg/kg/d (q6 hr)
Captopril	Angiotensin-converting-enzyme inhibitor	p.o., neonates: 0.1–0.4 mg/kg/dose (q6–24 hr) Infants: 0.5–6 mg/kg/d (q6–24 hr) Older children: 12 mg/dose (q12–24 hr)
Enalapril	Angiotensin-converting-enzyme inhibitor	p.o., infants and children: 0.1–0.5 mg/kg/d (q.d., b.i.d.) Adolescents and adults: 2.5–5 mg/d (q.d.), titrate to maximum 40 mg/d

GMP; Guanosine-3,5-monophosphate; iv., intravenous; p.o., oral; q, every; q.d., daily; b.i.d., twice daily.

Nitroprusside

Nitroprusside is a vasodilator that acts directly on vascular smooth muscle and leads to veno- and arteriolar dilation; it is more potent in reducing afterload than is nitroglycerine. Its mechanism of action is through release of nitric oxide, which then reacts with a variety of thiols to produce unstable S-nitrosothiols, potent activators of guanylate cyclase. The rise in intracellular cAMP activates cAMP-dependent protein kinases, leading to smooth muscle relaxation and vasodilation (126).

Nitroprusside decreases central venous, pulmonary capillary wedge, and left ventricular end-diastolic and systemic arterial pressures. It reduces pulmonary congestion and dyspnea and may increase cardiac output. Sodium nitroprusside increases the forward stroke volume in mitral and aortic regurgitation.

Progressive increases in the cardiac index in children with hypertensive crisis receiving nitroprusside may simulate nitroprusside tachyphylaxis, and higher doses are required to achieve equivalent blood pressure control (127). Thus, invasive hemodynamic monitoring is required during nitroprusside infusion for hypertensive crisis.

The results of nitroprusside administration in congestive heart failure vary, depending on the cause of heart failure: it may increase Qp/Qs and hemodynamic deterioration in children with large left-to-right shunts and congestive heart failure (128) and may cause improvement in patients with dilated cardiomyopathy (129).

The major side effects of nitroprusside are predictable from its hemodynamic and metabolic properties. Systemic hypotension is a major risk following a sudden bolus of nitroprusside. Patients should have intravenous access established so that intravascular volume can be expanded rapidly. If necessary, children can be placed in the Trendelenburg position, which shifts blood volume to the central circulation and restores adequate blood pressure. Invasive arterial pressure monitoring allows immediate detection of sudden hypotension.

Cyanide and, to a lesser extent, thiocyanate toxicity are the most feared metabolic complications. Cyanide accumulation should be suspected when tachyphylaxis, increased mixed venous O_2 saturation, or metabolic acidosis is encountered during nitroprusside administration. High doses can induce carboxyhemoglobinemia, probably by inducing hemeoxygenase (130). In adults, 12.5 mg of hydroxocobalamin administered more than 30 minutes has prevented accumulation of cyanide and acidosis. Initial treatment of cyanide toxicity is by breaking amyl nitrite pearls onto gauze and having the vapor be inhaled.

Nitric Oxide

Nitric oxide is tonically produced by vascular endothelium by the conversion of arginine into citrulline. This causes relaxation of vascular smooth muscle and occurs in all vascular beds. Nitric oxide is a radical species (NO) and has a very short half-life. Nitric oxide is inactivated by binding to hemoglobin with a strong affinity (131,132). Inhaled nitric oxide is a potent and selective pulmonary vasodilator in pediatric patients with pulmonary arterial hypertension resulting from congenital heart disease (133–137). The nitric oxide precursor citrulline has been suggested as a potential therapy for postoperative pulmonary hypertension in children undergoing congenital heart surgery (138).

INHIBITION OF THE RENIN–ANGIOTENSIN SYSTEM

Angiotensin II plays an important role in the pathophysiology of heart failure and in the pathologic remodeling of the myocardium. It is a potent vasoconstrictor; it also promotes sodium and water retention by its effects on renal hemodynamics and on aldosterone release. In addition, it contributes to vascular hyperplasia and to myocardial hypertrophy, stimulates myocyte death, is arrhythmogenic, and potentiates catecholamine release. Angiotensin II is formed by cleavage of angiotensin I by the ACE and also by non–ACE-dependent pathways.

ACE inhibitors block angiotensin II and aldosterone formation, potentiate the effects of diuretics, and diminish sympathetic activity. They cause both arterial and venous dilation and consequently increase cardiac output and decrease right and left filling pressures and end-diastolic volumes.

The renin–angiotensin system may be inhibited also through inhibition of angiotensin AT_1 receptors.

Captopril

Captopril was the first clinically available drug in the class of ACE inhibitors. Captopril lowers systemic vascular resistance and increases venous capacitance. Blood pressure does not change significantly if cardiac output can increase to compensate for the fall in systemic vascular resistance.

Captopril is rapidly and extensively absorbed from the gastrointestinal tract. Its absorption is decreased by food; 40% to 50% is eliminated unchanged by renal excretion and the remainder by hepatic metabolism. The half-life is less than 3 hours and increases in cases of renal impairment (139).

The recommended dosing of captopril depends on age. For newborns, the usual initial dosing is 0.5 mg per kg twice or thrice daily. It should be adjusted as needed and tolerated while monitoring the blood pressure response over the 2 hours after dosing. If the blood pressure falls by more than 10%, the dose should be temporarily reduced. If no decrease in blood pressure is noted, the dose can be increased. Older infants and children generally require 3 to 4 mg per kg per day. However, in patients who are sodium and water depleted, the initial dose should be reduced.

Captopril has been used successfully in patients with congestive heart failure due to dilated cardiomyopathy and large left-to-right shunts, in patients with mitral and aortic regurgitation, and in systemic hypertension, conditions which are characterized by a hypereninemic state (140–145). There are few significant complications from captopril. Hypotension is the major hemodynamic complication; it is more common at high doses and in young infants. Renal insufficiency occurs rarely (146).

Enalapril

Enalapril is a prodrug that is hydrolyzed by a serum esterase to the active compound, enalaprilat. Approximately 60% of enalapril is absorbed from the gastrointestinal tract; absorption is unaffected by the presence of food. It is mostly eliminated by renal excretion and partly fecal elimination. Its half-life is 11 hours and is increased in renal failure.

The initial oral dosage for infants and children is 0.1 mg per kg per day. The dosage may be adjusted as needed and tolerated, up to a maximum of 0.5 mg per kg per day. Enalapril is effective in children and infants with hypertension (147), volume-overloaded left ventricle, left-to-right shunt, and valvular regurgitation (148,149). It prevents cardiac function deterioration in left ventricular end-systolic wall stress in long-term survivors of pediatric cancer (150).

NEWER TRENDS IN THE TREATMENT OF CONGESTIVE HEART FAILURE

Spironolactone

Traditionally, the role of aldosterone in heart failure was thought to be a result of its effects on epithelial cells, where it induces sodium reabsorption and potassium excretion with subsequent hemodynamic effects from intravascular volume expansion. On this basis, spironolactone, a nonselective aldosterone antagonist, has been used for the treatment of congestive heart failure to block aldosterone-mediated effects in epithelial cells. The Randomized Aldactone Evaluation Study (RALES), in which a low spironolactone dose was added to existing therapy in adult patients with heart failure, showed a significant reduction in morbidity and mortality (151). Those results suggest that saliuresis is not required for its beneficial effect and that the role of aldosterone in the pathophysiology of cardiovascular disease is more complex. Classical effects of aldosterone are mediated via its nuclear receptor. Novel nonepithelial effects of aldosterone are mediated via a second-messenger system, which involves activation of the sodium/hydrogen antiporter (152). These effects of aldosterone have been demonstrated in the kidney, vascular smooth muscle cell, and leucocytes, and in the regulation of rapid corticotropin suppression. Experimental evidence demonstrates that cardiovascular damage induced by aldosterone can be prevented by administration of a selective mineralocorticoid receptor antagonist (153).

β-Blockers

In the past the use of β-blockers was considered contraindicated in patients with heart failure due to their negative inotropic effect. However, increase in left ventricular ejection fraction and improvement in symptoms have been demonstrated in adults with heart failure. The improved ventricular fraction is attributed to prevention of the β-adrenergic receptor-mediated adverse effects of norepinephrine on the myocardium. The experience with the use of β-blocker agents in children with heart failure has been considered similar to the much more extensive reported evidence in adults (154). Specifically, carvedilol was suggested to have a role in the treatment of pediatric patients with congestive heart failure not responding to standard therapy. It has been shown that infants and children with heart failure with dilated cardiomyopathy and with congenital heart disease who did not respond to standard therapy, and treated with carvedilol, show improvement in clinical parameters and ejection fraction (155,156). However, preliminary results of another randomized placebo controlled trial suggested that carvedilol lacks clinical value in children and adolescents with symptomatic systolic heart failure (157).

ANTIARRHYTHMIC AGENTS

Several drugs are currently available for the treatment of dysrhythmias in pediatric patients. None of them is universally effective. Most produce frequent or severe side effects, and extensive pediatric use has been limited to only a few. Insufficient pharmacokinetic data are available concerning both "classical" and "newer" antiarrhythmic agents in infants and children, and dosage is derived from clinical experience. As many arrhythmias are rare or occur as emergencies, the use of antiarrhythmic agents in children is not based on classical randomized, controlled trials. Final recommendations of rational dosages should await reports on the relationship of pharmacokinetic processes to their therapeutic and toxic effects. Currently, the safety and efficacy of radio frequency ablation procedures make complex drug therapy or use of agents with significant potential side effects unnecessary. Short-term use of antiarrhythmic drugs is now considered while awaiting ablation (158,159).

Classification of antiarrhythmic agents is complex; they exert multiple actions that vary in different tissues and generate active metabolites that produce different effects than the parent drug. The Vaughan Williams antiarrhythmic drug classification scheme is the most widely recognized mean of grouping drugs with somewhat similar antiarrhythmic effects (160). A system that classifies antiarrhythmic actions rather than drugs has been proposed (Table 42.4) (161). Another classification based on the desired target mechanism underlying a tachyarrhythmia was proposed by the Task Force of the European Society of Cardiology: channel-active antiarrhythmic agents, receptor–mediated antiarrhythmic agents, and pump-active antiarrhythmic agents (162).

The therapeutic indications and dosages of antiarrhythmic agents are summarized in Tables 42.5 and 42.6. Drug interactions, both pharmacokinetic and pharmacodynamic, are common in combination therapy for cardiac antiarrhythmias and between antiarrhythmic agents and other drugs (Table 42.7). Most published pediatric experience exists with digoxin, propranolol, propafenone, flecainide, amiodarone, sotalol, and adenosine. Some of them have unique pharmacokinetics. Propranolol, amiodarone, and verapamil have poor bioavailability and are highly protein bound. Amiodarone has a very large volume of distribution (66 L per kg) and esmolol a very small one (0.13 L per kg). Some agents have extreme plasma elimination half-lives: amiodarone (terminal half-life of about 30 days), esmolol (6 minutes), and adenosine ($<$10 seconds). Because of individual differences in the rate of biotransformation, the plasma $t_{1/2}$ of propafenone may vary fourfolds (4 to 16 hours). Plasma elimination half-life of propranolol in infants is shorter than in children (3 to 4 hours vs. 6 hours)

TABLE 42.4 Classification of Antiarrhythmic Agents by Their Mechanism of Action

Class	*Mechanism of Action*	*Drugs*	*Effect on ECG*
I	Fast sodium channel blockade; depress phase 0		
IA	Prolongs repolarization and refractory period	Quinidine Procainamide Disopyramide	Prolong QRS and QTc
IB	Shortens repolarization	Lidocaine Tocainide Mexiletine Phenytoin	Minimal effect on PR, QRS, and QTc
IC	Slows conduction; little effect on repolarization	Encainide Flecainide Lorcainide Propafenone	Prolong PR, QRS, and QTc
Unclassified	Combined effects of IA, IB, and/or IC	Ethmozine	May prolong PR and QRS
II	β-Adrenergic blockage	Propranolol Timolol Metoprolol	Prolongs PR
III	Prolongs repolarization and refractory period	Amiodarone Bretylium	Prolong PR and QTc
IV	Slow calcium channel blockade	Verapamil Diltiazem Nifedipine	Prolongs PR

QTc, QT interval corrected for heart rate.

whereas the reverse is the case with flecainide (27 hours in infants and 8 to 12 hours in children) (163–165). Maternal treatment with digoxin, propranolol, verapamil, quinidine, procainamide, and flecainide is considered compatible with breast-feeding, whereas amiodarone is not recommended in nursing mothers (166).

β-BLOCKING AGENTS

As a class, β-blockers exert their electrophysiologic effect by competitive inhibition of endogenous catecholamines at β-adrenergic receptors. This inhibits pacemaker potentials and decreases phase 4 spontaneous depolarization. The

TABLE 42.5 Therapeutic Indications of Antiarrhythmic Drugs

Drug	*Therapeutic Indications*	*Comments*
Quinidine	PVD, VT	Contraindicated in long-QT syndrome
Procainamide	PVD, VT	Contraindicated in myasthenia gravis and complete heart block
Disopyramide	PVD, VT (non–life-threatening)	
Lidocaine	VT	
Phenytoin	Digoxin-induced tachyarrhythmias	Infuse slowly
Mexiletine	VA in CHD	May replace phenytoin in patients with phenytoin side effects
Encainide	PJRT, SVT refractory to digoxin, propranolol, verapamil	Greater efficacy when combined with verapamil or propranolol
Flecainide	Refractory to digoxin, propranolol, verapamil	
Propafenone	Life-threatening postoperative JET	Use colloid during loading to maintain BP
Ethmozine	AET originating in right atrium	
Propranolol	SVA, VA, digitalis-induced arrhythmias	Contraindicated in asthma and heart block
Amiodarone	Refractory and life-threatening arrhythmias in CHD, myocarditis, cardiomyopathies	Screen thyroid function, monitor HR in sick sinus syndrome, use with caution with other antiarrhythmics. Decrease digoxin dose to ½ (kinetic and dynamic interaction)
Verapamil	Reentrant SVT	Contraindicated in severe low cardiac output, intracardiac right-to-left shunt, patients receiving β-blockers. Use with extreme caution in infants

AET, atrial ectopic tachycardia; BP, blood pressure; CHD, congenital heart disease; HR, heart rate; JET, junctional ectopic tachycardia; PAF, paroxysmal atrial flutter/fibrillation; PJRT, permanent junction reciprocating tachycardia (atypical atrioventricular node reentry); PVD, premature ventricular depolarization; SVT, supraventricular tachycardia; SVA, supraventricular arrhythmia; VA, ventricular arrhythmia; VT, ventricular tachycardia.

TABLE 42.6 Doses of Antiarrhythmic Agents

Drug	*Route*	*Dosage*
Procainamide	i.v.	Initial: 3–6 mg/kg over 5 min; may repeat q5–10 min to maximum 15 mg/kg/total loading dose (maximum dose 500 mg)
		Maintenance: 0.02–0.08 mg/kg/min; (maximum 2 g/d)
	p.o.	15–50 mg/kg/d (q3–6 hr) (max 4 g/d)
Disopyramide	p.o.	<1 yr: 10–30 mg/kg/d (q6 hr)
		1–4 yr: 10–20 mg/kg/d (q6 hr)
		4–12 yr: 10–15 mg/kg/d (q6 hr)
		12–18 yr: 6–15 mg/kg/d (q6 hr)
Lidocaine	i.v.	Initial: 1–3 mg/kg
		Maintenance: 0.01–0.05 mg/kg/min
Phenytoin	i.v.	1.25 mg/kg over 5 min; may repeat to total dose 15 mg/kg
	p.o.	5–10 mg/kg/d (q8–12 hr)
Mexiletine		1.5–5 mg/kg/d (q8 hr)
Flecainide	p.o.	3–6 mg/kg/d (q8–12 hr); increase if necessary to maximum 20 mg/kg
Propafenone	i.v.	Loading: boluses of 0.2 mg/kg q 10 min until ventricular rate <150/min or maximum 2 mg/kg
		Maintenance: 4–10 μg/kg/min
Moricizine	p.o.	200 mg/m^2/d (q8 hr); increase q2–3 d to maximum 600 mg/m^2/d
Propranolol	i.v.	0.01–0.1 mg/kg over 10 min (may repeat q6–8 hr; maximum 1 mg in infants, 3 mg in children)
	p.o.	0.5–1 mg/kg/d (q6–8 hr); increase to 2–5 mg/kg/d
Amiodarone	i.v.	5–7 mg/kg over 30 min, followed by 7–10 μg/kg/min
	p.o.	Loading: 10–15 mg/kg/d (q12 hr) for 7–10 d
		Maintenance: 2–5 mg/kg/d for 1–2 mo; then decrease or increase according to response
Verapamil	i.v.	Children:
	p.o.	0.1 mg/kg over 30 s; may repeat after 15-min interval
		4–8 mg/kg/d (q6–8 hr)
Sotalol	p.o.	100 mg/m^2/d (q8–12 hr). May increase to 200 mg/m^2/d
Adenosine	i.v.	Initial: 100–150 μg/kg (rapid bolus); if not effective, increase dose q 2 min by 50 μg/kg to maximum dose 250 μg/kg

i.v., intravenous; p.o., oral; q, every.

TABLE 42.7 Pharmacokinetic Interactions with Antiarrhythmic Agents

Antiarrhythmic Agent	*Interacting Drug*	*Resultant Interaction*
Quinidine	Cimetidine	Inhibition of quinidine metabolism
	Phenytoin	Induction of quinidine and reduced serum quinidine concentrations
	Phenobarbital	Increased prothrombin time
	Warfarin	Digoxin toxicity
	Digoxin	Inhibits specific liver cytochrome P-450
	Debrisoquine	Postural hypotension
	Nitroglycerin	Increased serum quinidine
	Amiodarone	
Disopyramide	Phenytoin	Induction of disopyramide metabolism
	Phenobarbital	
Mexiletine	Phenobarbital	Increased clearance of mexiletine
	Phenytoin	
	Rifampin	
Mexiletine	Cimetidine	Slows mexiletine absorption
Encainide	Cimetidine	Increased serum concentration of encainide and metabolites
Amiodarone	Various drugs	Amiodarone blocks cytochrome P-450 metabolites
Amiodarone	Warfarin	Potentiation of warfarin effect
Amiodarone	Procainamide	Increased serum procainamide
Amiodarone	Flecainide	Increased serum flecainide
Lidocaine	Beta blockers	Increased serum lidocaine
	Cimetidine	

β-blockers counteract the catecholamine effects of increased membrane excitability, acceleration of phase 0 velocity, and increased delayed after-depolarizations (167).

Propranolol

Propranolol is the most commonly used β-blocking agent. It is a nonselective β_1- and β_2-adrenergic blocking agent used in diseases of the cardiovascular system such as hypertension, tetralogy of Fallot, hypertrophic obstructive cardiomyopathy, and arrhythmias, as well as neonatal thyrotoxicosis and other conditions. It exerts negative inotropic and chronotropic effects on the heart that result in decreased cardiac output.

The effective refractory period of the AV node is increased by propranolol, and thus this agent slows the ventricular response to rapid atrial arrhythmias and abolishes supraventricular arrhythmias which require reentry in the AV node (168). This electrophysiologic effect explains most of its antiarrhythmic actions. At high concentrations, (rarely needed for antiarrhythmia control) it has nonspecific "quinidine-like" actions, such as a decrease in membrane responsiveness of Purkinje cells (169). Important noncardiac effects of propranolol include decreased blood glucose concentration and plasma renin activity and bronchoconstriction.

Propranolol has complex pharmacokinetics (169). It is effectively absorbed in the intestine; however, the bioavailability is low due to first-pass effect (170). Its elimination decreases when hepatic blood flow decreases (such as in low cardiac output). For those reasons the use of propranolol based on unit of body weight or surface area is only an approximation for initial treatment.

Following maternal dosage, the infant receives propranolol by placental transfer and by breast milk (171,172). The use of propranolol in pregnancy has been associated with several fetal, obstetric, and neonatal complications: decreased placental size and intrauterine growth retardation, fetal depression at birth, and postnatal hypoglycemia, bradycardia, and hyperbilirubinemia (172). The increased muscular tone of the uterus and decreased uterine flow induced by propranolol and/or effects of this drug on maternal heart rate or blood pressure could explain the decreased placental size and retardation of fetal growth.

As compared to propranolol other β-adrenergic blocking agents such as atenolol and acebutolol appear to cross more effectively into breast milk, probably because of substantially lower protein binding, and cases of neonatal toxicity with these agents have been described.

The use of propranolol in infants and children with tetralogy of Fallot and with hypertrophic obstructive cardiomyopathy results in clinical improvement (173,174); treatment failures correlate with low doses (and low serum concentrations) (173). A dose of 2 to 6 mg per kg per day is recommended for the management of hypoxemic spells in infants with tetralogy of Fallot (173). Although it is not a drug of choice today, much higher doses were recommended in the long-term management of supraventricular tachycardia and hypertension in children; those doses (up to 16 mg per kg) resulted in plasma concentrations in the range of 100 to 700 ng per mL with no reported side effects. However, caution should be exercised with the use of high doses; because of its β-adrenergic blocking properties, propranolol may decrease cardiac contractility and produce AV conduction disturbances, bradycardia, hypo- or hyperglycemia, gastrointestinal alterations, and bronchospasm. Coadministration of intravenous propranolol with calcium channel blockers is contraindicated because of the significant synergistic negative effects on contractility.

In patients scheduled for cardiac surgery it has been recommended that propranolol therapy be discontinued several days prior to the operative procedures (175).

Atenolol

Atenolol is a commonly used long-acting selective β_1-blocker (176,177). The drug is hydrophilic and does not cross the blood–brain barrier. Atenolol reaches peak concentration 2 to 3 hours after an oral dose. It can be given once or twice a day with a half-life of up to 9 to 10 hours. Since atenolol does not cross the blood–brain barrier, the side effect profile is considerably reduced compared with propranolol. Although atenolol is a selective β_1-agent, the risk of bronchospasm is not eliminated completely.

Nadolol

Nadolol is a nonselective β-adrenergic blocking agent. Peak plasma concentration occurs 3 to 4 hours after administration; the elimination time is 20 to 24 hours and thus, it can be given in one daily dose. It is used in pediatric patients for both supraventricular tachycardias and ventricular arrhythmias (178).

Esmolol

Esmolol is a short-acting intravenous cardioselective β-blocking agent. It has fast onset of action and a short half-life, allowing for rapid resolution of effect following discontinuation. Rapid clearance by erythrocyte esterases results in an average half-life of 9 minutes in adults and 2 to 4 minutes in younger patients. Effects include a decrease in heart rate, blood pressure, and cardiac index, with recovery of cardiac function within 10 to 15 minutes following discontinuation (179). Noncardiac adverse effects are minimal.

CALCIUM CHANNEL BLOCKERS

These drugs are a heterogeneous group of highly lipid-soluble compounds that inhibit the entry of calcium ions into the cell or their mobilization from intracellular stores. Their pharmacologic effects are most prominent and have been best characterized in the cardiovascular system, but they also affect other tissues.

Verapamil

Verapamil has more potent cardiac effects than nifedipine at doses sufficient to produce vasodilation. It was originally used as an antianginal drug; later it was found useful in the management of cardiac arrhythmias (180,181) and of hypertrophic cardiomyopathy in adults and children (182). Verapamil prolongs AV junctional conduction time (antero- and retrograde) and the refractory period of the

AV node and depresses sinus node automaticity. It also causes direct negative chronotropic and inotropic effects, resulting in worsening of the ventricular function in patients with congestive heart failure. The potentially more advantageous diltiazem has similar electrophysiologic effects as verapamil and minimal negative inotropic effects; however, experience with this agent in cardiac arrhythmias in children is limited.

Verapamil improves left ventricular diastolic relaxation and filling and symptomatology in adults and children with hypertrophic cardiomyopathy (182); it is unclear, however, whether the long-term prognosis of this condition is also improved.

Verapamil is well absorbed following oral administration but only about 20% reaches the systemic circulation due to a marked first-pass effect. It is highly bound to plasma protein. It undergoes N-demethylation to the biologically active norverapamil. Its bioavailability increases and the degree of its biotransformation decreases during chronic therapy, which results in prolongation of its plasma half-life and in higher plasma concentration (183). Pharmacokinetic data for verapamil are similar in adults and infants (184), but older children have a longer plasma half-life and a smaller body clearance as compared with adults (185). Serious side effects may occur in infants after even a single standard intravenous dose; therefore, it should be used with great caution in this age group (186).

In children with supraventricular tachycardia verapamil is used mainly intravenously. Adverse effects of verapamil are dose related and an extension of its pharmacology.

Intravenous calcium chloride (10 mg per kg) followed by normal saline (10 mL per kg, rapidly) and/or sympathomimetic amines and atropine (0.01 mg per kg) are recommended if hypotension, sinus bradycardia, and/or advanced AV block occurs as a result of verapamil therapy (186). The use of verapamil with β-adrenergic blockers is contraindicated; both agents prolong the refractory period of the AV node, and combination therapy may result in hypotension, bradycardia, asystole, and death. Coadministration of verapamil and disopyramide may also be lethal (187). Simultaneous administration of verapamil (but not nifedipine or diltiazem) with digoxin increases serum digoxin concentrations; this seems to be due to inhibition of the renal tubular secretion of digoxin (188). Administration of verapamil to patients on warfarin therapy may cause prolongation of prothrombin time, perhaps as a result of warfarin displacement from protein-binding sites (187).

Amiodarone

Amiodarone is a highly effective agent used in a variety of severely symptomatic and uncontrolled life-threatening arrhythmias. It is a potent agent for control of a variety of tachyarrhythmias (189,190). Chemically, it is an iodinated benzofuran with a structure similar to thyroxine. It prolongs the action potential of all cardiac cell types and lengthens AV nodal conduction. In addition, it has α- and β-blocker effects (191).

Amiodarone has unique and complex pharmacokinetic properties (192) that have not been well characterized in children. Its absorption following oral administration is slow and erratic, its bioavailability is low, and its onset of action is delayed for days (4 to 10) in children and several weeks in adults. It is very highly bound to plasma proteins (99.9%). It accumulates in tissues, is metabolized by the liver, eliminated in bile, and undergoes enterohepatic circulation). Its concentration in myocardium is about 50 times greater than in plasma. Its initial $t_{1/2}$ is 3 to 10 days and the terminal $t_{1/2}$ is 26 to 107 days. Because of its long terminal life, its effects may persist for a considerable period after discontinuation of the drug. A major metabolite, desethylamiodarone, accumulates and reaches plasma concentration similar to the parent drug in adults during long-term oral treatment; its antiarrhythmic potency is unclear. At effective doses, lower serum concentrations of amiodarone and desethylamiodarone are reached in children than in adults; at similar plasma concentrations of amiodarone, lower concentrations of desethylamiodarone are reached in infants than in children (193). Serum concentrations of amiodarone and desethylamiodarone do not distinguish between responders and nonresponders. On the other hand, severe toxicity seems to correlate with amiodarone serum concentrations greater than 2.5 μg per mL and desethylamiodarone greater than 3.0 μg per mL (194). Transplacental passage of amiodarone and desethylamiodarone has been estimated as 10% and 25%, respectively. Maternal milk contains higher concentrations of amiodarone and desethylamiodarone than plasma; in one study, daily ingestion by a breast-fed infant was estimated as 1.5 and 0.5 mg per kg body weight, respectively, with no untoward effects (192).

Amiodarone is used for a variety of resistant tachyarrhythmias. An oral loading protocol, using 10 to 15 mg per kg per day, is often used for 5 to 10 days. This dose is usually split in a twice-daily schedule to avoid gastrointestinal side effects. Some centers advocate loading for 3 to 5 days, using up to 50 mg per kg per day.

Intravenous dosing of amiodarone has a rapid action, and the effect after the first dose persists for 1 to 6 hours. Intravenous amiodarone is recommended in young patients by administering 5 mg per kg bolus divided into five 1 mg per kg aliquots, each given over 5 minutes or as two 2.5 mg per kg boluses (195,196). The reported average successful load is 6 mg per kg. Amiodarone is also given as infusions, mostly in patients with ventricular tachyarrhythmias, at 10 to 15 mg per kg per day. During chronic therapy it is given orally once a day, after a loading intravenous or oral dose. As compared to low and medium dosing regimens, higher doses showed better overall efficacy; however, adverse events were common and appeared to be dose related (197).

Most adverse effects are reversible and include rash, photosensitivity, blue or green skin discoloration, hepatitis, peripheral neuropathy, keratopathy, thyroid dysfunction, and behavioral changes (195,196). Those toxicities are less frequent in children than in adults. Pulmonary toxicity may be lethal in adults; it has not been reported in children. Hypotension may follow intravenous administration. Proarrhythmia events, which are rare, include AV block, sinus node dysfunction, torsades de pointes, and rapid ventricular response during atrial flutter if there is an accessory connection (198,199). Amiodarone increases warfarin effect, digoxin and phenytoin concentrations, and class I antiarrhythmic toxicity.

OTHER ANTIARRHYTHMIC DRUGS USED FREQUENTLY IN PEDIATRIC PATIENTS

Sotalol

Sotalol is often substituted for amiodarone to avoid the amiodarone side effect profile. Sotalol hydrochloride is a racemic mixture of D- and L-isomers. Both isomers have class III effects. In addition, the L-isomer has nonselective β-blocking activity without intrinsic sympathomimetic or anesthetic properties. Complex electrophysiologic effects include reduction in delayed rectifier and inward rectifier potassium currents, prolonging action potential, and concomitantly refractoriness of all cardiac tissue and accessory pathways. Sotalol is a nonselective β-blocker with class III effects. The β-blocking effects slow the AV nodal conduction and the sinus rate. The ECG effects manifest as prolongation of the QT interval. The prolonged action potential may increase calcium conduction and therefore contractility. This effect helps balance the negative inotropic effect of β-blockade and facilitates use in patients with impaired ventricular function (200). Sotalol is used in a wide range of arrhythmias, including atrial flutter and atrial fibrillation (200,201). Pediatric applications include supraventricular tachycardia, atrial flutter, ectopic atrial tachycardia, and junctional ectopic tachycardia (202–204). Sotalol is partially or completely effective for refractory tachyarrhythmias in patients with congenital heart disease, and nonpharmacological interventions improve its efficacy (205).

Sotalol has excellent enteric absorption and peak concentrations are present after 2 hours. The elimination half-life in adults ranges from 7 to 12 hours. It is minimally metabolized, there are no active metabolites, and levels are not clinically helpful. The drug is excreted in the urine. Sotalol crosses the placenta and is excreted in breast milk.

The starting dose is 100 mg per m^2 per day. The drug is given on a three-times or twice-daily schedule, often based on the response of incessant supraventricular tachycardias. The dose can be increased to 200 mg per m^2 per day. Sotalol has the side effect profile of β-blockers with mild negative inotropic effects. Unlike other β-blockers, sotalol prolongs the QT interval because of class III effects. The most serious adverse side effect is torsades de pointes, with an incidence approximating that of quinidine-induced torsades. Use should be avoided in patients with hypokalemia or hypomagnesemia.

Flecainide

Flecainide is the most commonly used class IC drug in pediatrics. It is a powerful sodium channel blocker that markedly depresses phase 0 and slows conduction. Like other IC agents it has slow onset and offset kinetics. It shortens the effective refractory period in Purkinje fibers but lengthens them in atrial and ventricular myocardium. The slowing of conduction and slow kinetics prolong both the PR interval and QRS in sinus rhythm. Flecainide slows conduction and increases the effective refractory period of accessory pathways and the fast retrograde limb in AV nodal reentry tachycardia. There is little effect on the sinus node except exacerbation of bradycardia in patients with sinus node dysfunction. Flecainide is associated with proarrhythmia (206). It is primarily used in the treatment of paroxysmal and incessant forms of supraventricular and ventricular tachycardia in children (207–209). Flecainide has been used in combination with amiodarone for refractory tachyarrhythmias in infants (210).

After an oral dose, flecainide reaches its peak concentration in 1 to 2 hours. Milk products block flecainide absorption, and, when patients are put on clear liquid diets, levels can rise substantially (211). Doses should be reduced by 25% to 30% in this setting. Flecainide is metabolized in the liver and about 40% is excreted unchanged in the urine. There are two metabolites with weak membrane effects. The elimination half-life varies with age: it may be as long as 27 hours in newborns in the first day, 11 hours in patients younger than 4 to 6 months, 8 hours in children aged 6 to 10 years, and 12 hours in adolescents (212). Flecainide crosses the placenta readily and reaches a concentration in the fetus of approximately 70% that of maternal levels (213).

Adverse effects include dizziness, headache, fatigue, tremor, blurry vision, nausea, vomiting, and anorexia. Severe proarrhythmia, affecting 1% to 3% of patients, occurs primarily in patients with abnormal hearts such as during the treatment of atrial flutter following congenital heart surgery (206).

Propafenone

Propafenone is a sodium channel blocker structurally similar to β-receptor antagonists resulting in β-blocking activity. It reduces phase 0 upstroke velocity and slows impulse conduction. It prolongs the effective refractory period of atrial and ventricular myocardium. It also prolongs the effective refractory period and blocks the antegrade and retrograde conduction of accessory pathways (214). ECG effects include prolongation of the PR interval and QRS. Propafenone has additional calcium channel antagonism that suppresses some forms of automaticity and produces a negative inotropic effect (214). In children it is effective in the treatment of supraventricular and ventricular tachycardias (215). An important reported efficacy is in incessant forms of supraventricular tachycardia such as ectopic atrial and junctional ectopic tachycardias (216).

Propafenone reaches peak concentration 2 to 3 hours after an oral dose. It is rapidly and completely absorbed but demonstrates variable first-pass hepatic clearance and only 3% to 40% reaches the systemic circulation. An increase in dose causes a disproportionate increase in plasma concentrations. Most patients rapidly metabolize it to active metabolites via the hepatic cytochrome P-450 system to 5-OH propafenone and have a half-life of 3 to 12 hours. Some patients (6% to 10%) have genetically determined slow metabolic clearance with prolonged half-life (10 to 32 hours) and high serum levels at normal doses (215), whereas extensive metabolizers (97% of patients studied) have a half-life of about 5 hours.

Like flecainide, propafenone should he used with caution, if at all, in patients with a structurally abnormal heart. A higher risk of arrest and sudden death was reported in this subpopulation (217). Other side effects with oral therapy are also like those of flecainide: blurry vision, paresthesias, and nausea.

Adenosine

Adenosine, an endogenous purine nucleoside found in multiple tissues, is an important modulator of cardiac electrophysiologic function. It exerts its primary action via a specific adenosine receptor, A_1, which is linked to potassium channels via the G protein system. The direct actions of adenosine primarily affect sinus and AV nodal tissue and atrial myocardium; it has no influence on ventricular myocardium. Indirect actions arise from antagonism of catecholamine-induced adenylate cyclase, resulting in decreased cyclic adenosine monophosphate, inward calcium, and sinus node pacemaker currents (218,219).

Electrophysiologic effects of adenosine include decreased rate of spontaneous sinus node firing, slowing or block of AV nodal conduction, and shortening of atrial action potential. During atrial or ventricular pacing adenosine can produce high degrees of AV nodal block, unmasking antegrade or retrograde conduction in accessory pathways.

Adenosine has altered the emergency therapy of supraventricular tachycardia and replaced the use of verapamil in children, including premature neonates (220–222).

Adenosine is rapidly metabolized by erythrocytes and endothelial tissue, resulting in a half-life of 1 to 5 seconds. The drug is given as a rapid intravenous bolus at initial doses of 100 to 150 μg per kg, followed by saline flush. Its effects are seen in 7 to 20 seconds. It is therefore a powerful therapeutic and diagnostic agent. Effects are pronounced when the drug is given centrally as opposed to peripherally.

The dose may be doubled, up to a maximum of 300 μg per kg (the maximal adult dose is 6 to 12 mg) (223). Methylxanthines are adenosine receptor antagonists; so higher doses are required by patients taking theophylline (224).

Adenosine may cause transient hypotension, facial flushing, and mild bronchospasm (225). Ventricular ectopy is not unusual and may be the mechanism of termination of some reciprocating tachycardias rather than adenosine-induced AV block. Occasionally, atrial fibrillation results from adenosine administration. Dipyridamole and diazepam can inhibit its cellular uptake and potentiate its effect.

REFERENCES

1. Greenberg B. Treatment of heart failure: state of the art and prospectives. *J Cardiovasc Pharmacol* 2001;38 (Suppl 2):S59–S63.
2. White RD, Lietman PS. A reappraisal of digitalis for infants with left-to-right shunts and "heart failure." *J Pediatr* 1978;92:867–870.
3. Driscoll DJ, Gillete PC, Ezrailson EG, et al. Inotropic response of the neonatal canine myocardium to dopamine. *Pediatr Res* 1978;12: 42–45.
4. Friedman WF, George BL. New concepts and drugs in the treatment of congestive heart failure. *Pediatr Clin North Am* 1984;31: 1197–1227.
5. Binab O, Legato MJ, Danilo P Jr, et al. Developmental changes in the cardiac effects of amrinone in the dog. *Circ Res* 1983;52: 747–752.
6. Perkin RM, Levin DL, Webb R, et al. Dobutamine: a hemodynamic evaluation in children with shock. *J Pediatr* 1982;100: 977–983.
7. Friedman WF, George BL. Treatment of congestive heart failure by altering loading conditions of the heart. *J Pediatr* 1985;106:697–706.
8. Rudolph AM. Developmental considerations in neonatal failure. *Hasp Pract (Off Ed)* 1985;20:53–70.
9. Sheldon CA, Friedman WF, Sybers HD. Scanning electron microscopy of fetal and neonatal lamb cardiac cells. *J Mol Cell Cardiol* 1976;8:853–862.
10. McPherson PA, Kramer MF, Covell JW, et al. A comparison of the active stiffness of fetal and adult cardiac muscle. *Pediatr Res* 1976; 10:660–664.
11. Romero TE, Friedman WF. Limited left ventricular response to volume overload in the neonatal period: a comparative study with the adult animal. *Pediatr Res* 1979;13:910–915.
12. Geis WP, Tatooles CJ, Priola DV, et al. Factors influencing neurohormonal control of the heart in the newborn. *Am J Physiol* 1975;228:1685–1689.
13. Pappano AJ. Ontogenic development of autonomic neuroeffector transmission and transmitter reactivity in embryonic and fetal hearts. *Pharmacol Rev* 1977;29:3–33.
14. Klopfenstein HS, Rudolph AM. Postnatal changes in the circulation and responses to volume loading in sheep. *Circ Res* 1978;42: 839–845.
15. Goldberg BP, Baskin SI, Roberts J. Effects of aging on ionic movements of atrial muscle. *Fed Proc* 1974;34:188–190.
16. Battaglia FC, Meschia G. Principal substrates of fetal metabolism. *Physiol Rev* 1978;58:449–527.
17. Uretzky BF, Young JB, Shabidi FE, et al. Randomized trial assessing the effect of digoxin withdrawal in patients with mild to moderate chronic congestive heart failure: results of the PROVED trial. *J Am Coll Cardiol* 1993;22:955–962.
18. Evered DC. The binding of digoxin by the serum proteins. *Eur J Pharmacol* 1972;18:236–244.
19. Fricke U, Hullbom U, Klaus W. Inotropic action, myocardial uptake and subcellular distribution of ouabain, digoxin and digitoxin in isolated rat hearts. *Naunyn Schmiedebergs Arch Pharmacol* 1975;288:195–214.
20. Gardner JD, Kilno DR, Swartz TI, et al. Effects of digoxin-specific antibodies on accumulation and binding of digoxin by human erythrocytes. *J Clin Invest* 1973;52:1820–1833.
21. Godfraind T, Lesne M. The uptake of cardiac glycosides in relation to their actions in isolated cardiac muscle. *Br J Pharmacol* 1972; 46:488–497.
22. Kim ND, Bailey LE, Drese FE. Correlation of the subcellular distribution of digoxin with the positive inotropic effect. *J Pharmacol Exp Ther* 1972;18:377–385.
23. Okarma TB, Tramell P, Kalman SM. The surface interaction between digoxin and cultured heart cells. *J Pharmacol Exp Ther* 1972;183:559–576.
24. Lee KS, Klaus W. The subcellular basis for the mechanism of inotropic action of cardiac glycosides. *Pharmacol Rev* 1971;23: 193–261.
25. Akera T. Membrane adenosinetriphosphatase: a digitalis receptor? *Science* 1977;198:569–574.
26. Okita GT. Dissociation of Na^+, K^+-ATPase inhibition from digitalis inotropy. *Fed Proc* 1977;36:2225–2230.
27. Schwartz A, Adams RJ. Studies on the digitalis receptor. *Circ Res* 1980;46:154–160.
28. Ferguson DW, Berg WI, Sanders IC, et al. Sympathoinhibitory responses to digitalis glycosides in heart failure patients: direct evidence from sympathetic neural recording. *Circulation* 1989; 80:65–77.
29. Krun H, Bigger IT, Goldsmith RL, et al. Effect of long-term digoxin therapy on autonomic function in patients with chronic heart failure. *J Am Coll Cardiol* 1995;25:289–294.
30. Eichhorn EJ, Gheorghiade M. Digoxin: new perspective on an old drug. *N Engl J Med* 2002;347:1394–1395.
31. Sabati M, Borga O, Hultvist-Bengtsson U. The role of P-glycoprotein in intestinal regional absorption of digoxin in rats. *Eur J Pharm Sci* 2001;14:21–27.
32. Kopke JA, Gerloff T, Mai I, et al. Modulation of steady state kinetics of digoxin by haplotypes of P-glycoprotein MDRI gene. *Clin Pharmacol Ther* 2002;72:584–594.
33. Nakamura T, Kakumoto M, Yamashita K, et al. Factors influencing the prediction of steady state concentration of digoxin. *Biol Pharm Bull* 2001;24:403–408.

34. Vestuyfi C, Strabach S, El-Morabet, et al. Dipyridamole enhances digoxin bioavailability via P glycoprotein inhibition. *Clin Pharmacol Ther* 2003;73:51–60.
35. Morselli PL, Assael BM, Gomeni R, et al. Digoxin pharmacokinetics during human development. In: Morselli PL, Garrattini S, Sereni F, eds. *Basic and therapeutic aspects of perinatal pharmacology.* New York, NY: Raven Press, 1975:377–392.
36. Andersson KE, Bertler A, Wettrell G. Post-mortem distribution and tissue concentration of digoxin in infants and adults. *Acta Paediatr Scand* 1975;64:497–504.
37. Gorodischer R, Jusko WI, Yaffe SJ. Tissue and erythrocyte distribution of digoxin in infants. *Clin Pharmacol Ther* 1976;19:256–263.
38. Kim PW, Krasula RW, Soyka LF, et al. Post-mortem tissue digoxin concentration in infants and children. *Circulation* 1975;52: 1128–1131.
39. Kerjalainen J, Ojala K, Reissel P. Tissue concentrations of digoxin in an autopsy material. *Acta Pharmacol Toxicol (Copenh)* 1974;34:385–390.
40. Hartel G, Kyllonen K, Merikallio E, et al. Human serum and myocardium digoxin. *Clin Pharmacol Ther* 1976;19:153–157.
41. Koren G, Farine D, Grundmann H, et al. Endogenous digoxin-like substances in uneventful and high-risk pregnancies. *Dev Pharmacol Ther* 1988;11:82–87.
42. Gault MH, Vasedv SC, Longerich LL, et al. Plasma digitalis-like factor(s) increase with salt loading. *N Engl J Med* 1984;309:1459.
43. Martinka E, Ocenasova A, Kamenistiakova L, et al. Endogenous digoxin-like immunoactivity in subjects with diabetes mellitus and hypertension. *Am J Hypertens* 1998;11:667–677.
44. Devynck MA, Pemollet MG, Rosenfeld JB, et al. Measurements of digitalis-like compound in plasma: application in studies of essential hypertension. *Br Med J* 1983;287:631–634.
45. Dasgupta A. Endogenous and exogenous digoxin-like immunoreactive substances: impact on therapeutic drug monitoring of digoxin. *Am J Clin Pathol* 2002;118:132–140.
46. Koren G, Fame D, Marlsky D, et al. Significance of the endogenous digoxin-like substances in infants and mothers. *Clin Pharmacol Ther* 1984;36:759–764.
47. Tzuo MC, Reuning RH, Sams RA. Quantification of interference in digoxin immunoassay in renal, hepatic, and diabetic disease. *Clin Pharmacol Ther* 1997;61:429–441.
48. Crossy MJ, Dasgupta A. Effect of digoxin-like immunoreactive substances and digoxin FAB antibodies on the new digoxin microparticle enzyme immunoassay. *Ther Drug Monit* 1997;19:185–190.
49. Chicella M, Branim B, Lee KR, et al. Comparison of microparticle enzyme and fluorescence polarization immunoassay in pediatric patients not receiving digoxin. *Ther Drug Monit* 1998;20:347–351.
50. Doherty JE, Flanagan WI, Dalrymple GV, et al. Tritiated digoxin. Excretion and turnover times in normal donors before and after nephrectomy and the recipient of the kidney after transplantation. *Am J Cardiol* 1972;29:470–474.
51. Halkin H, Scheiner LB, Perk CC, et al. Determinants of the renal clearance of digoxin. *Clin Pharmacol Ther* 1975;17:385–394.
52. Jusko WJ, Szefler SJ, Goldgarb AL. Pharmacokinetic design of digoxin dosage regimen in relation to renal function. *J Clin Pharmacol* 1974;14:525–535.
53. Gorodischer R, Jusko WI, Yaffe SJ. Renal clearance of digoxin in young infants. *Res Commun Chem Pathol Pharmacol* 1977;16: 363–374.
54. Halkin H, Radomsky M, Millman P, et al. Steady state serum concentration and renal clearance of digoxin in neonates, infants and children. *Eur J Clin Pharmacol* 1978;13:113–117.
55. Pinto N, Halachmi N, Verjee Z, et al. Ontogeny of renal P-glycoprotein expression in mice: correlation with digoxin clearance. *Pediatr Res* 2005;58:1284–1289.
56. Koup JR, Jusko WI, Elwood CM, et al. Digoxin pharmacokinetics: role of renal failure in dosage regime design. *Clin Pharmacol Ther* 1975;18:19.
57. Brown DD, Donnois JC, Abraham GN, et al. Effect of furosemide on the renal excretion of digoxin. *Clin Pharmacol Ther* 1976;20: 395–400.
58. Roden DM. Antiarrhythmic drugs. In: Brunton LL, Lazo JS, Parker KL, eds. *Goodman & Gilman's the pharmacological basis of therapeutics*, 11th ed. New York, NY: McGraw-Hill, 2006:899–932.
59. Wettrell G, Andersson KE. Clinical pharmacokinetics of digoxin in infants. *Clin Pharmacokinet* 1977;2:17–31.
60. Warburton D, Bell EF, Oh W. Pharmacokinetics and echocardiographic effects of digoxin in low birth weight infants with left-to-right shunting due to patent ductus arteriosus. *Dev Pharmacol Ther* 1980;1:189–200.
61. Lundell BPW, Boreus LO. Digoxin therapy and left ventricular performance in premature infants with patent ductus arteriosus. *Acta Pediatr Scand* 1983;72:339–344.
62. Sandor GO, Bloom KR, Izukawa T, et al. Noninvasive assessment of left ventricular function related to serum digoxin levels in neonates. *Pediatrics* 1980;65:541–546.
63. Berman W Jr, Yabek SM, Dillan T, et al. Effects of digoxin in infants with a congested circulatory state due to a ventricular septal defect. *N Engl J Med* 1983;308:363–366.
64. Sahn DJ, Vaucher Y, Williams DE, et al. Echocardiographic detection of large left to right shunts and cardiomyopathies in infants and children. *Am J Cardiol* 1976;73:73–76.
65. Pinsky WW, Jacobsen JR, Gillette PC, et al. Dosage of digoxin in premature infants. *J Pediatr* 1979;96:639–643.
66. Kimball TR, Dniels SR, Meyer RA, et al. Effect of digoxin on contractility and symptoms in infants with a large ventricular septal defect. *Am J Cardiol* 1991;68:1377–1382.
67. Packer M, Gheorghiade M, Young JB, et al. Withdrawal of digoxin from patients with chronic heart failure treated with angiotensin-converting enzyme inhibitors. RADIANCE study. *N Engl J Med* 1993;329:1–7.
68. Patel D, Cuneo B, Viesca R, et al. Digoxin for the treatment of fetal congestive heart failure with sinus rhythm assessed by cardiovascular profile score. *J Matern Fetal Neonatal Med* 2008;21: 477–482.
69. Hallberg P, Michaelsson K, Mellhus H. Digoxin therapy for the treatment of heart failure. *N Engl J Med* 2003;348:661–663.
70. Koren G. Interaction between digoxin and commonly coadministered drugs in children. *Pediatrics* 1985;75:1032–1037.
71. Ratnapalan S, Griffiths K, Costei AM, et al. Digoxin-carvedilol interactions in children. *J Pediatr* 2003;142:572–574.
72. Koren G, Zarfin Y, Perlman M, et al. Effects of indomethacin on digoxin pharmacokinetics in preterm infants. *Pediatr Pharmacol (New York)* 1984;4:25–30.
73. Strauss MH, Dorian P, Cardella C, et al. Digoxin cyclosporine interaction: a new phenomenon. *Clin Invest Med* 1986;9:A16.
74. Halkin H, Radomsky M, Blieden L, et al. Steady state serum digoxin concentration in relation to digitalis toxicity in neonates and infants. *Pediatrics* 1978;61:184.
75. Koren G, Parker R. Interpretation of excessive serum concentrations of digoxin in children. *Am J Cardiol* 1985;55:1210–1214.
76. Shapin W, Narahara K, Taubert K. Relationship of plasma digitoxin and digoxin to cardiac response following intravenous digitalization in man. *Circulation* 1970;42:1065–1072.
77. Steiness E, Waldorf S, Hansen P, et al. Reduction of digoxin-induced inotropism during quinidine administration. *Clin Pharmacol Ther* 1980;27:791–795.
78. Ingelfinger JA, Goldman P. The serum digitalis concentration. Does it diagnose digitalis toxicity? *N Engl J Med* 1976;294:867.
79. Belz OO, Aust PE, Munkes R. Digoxin plasma concentrations and nifedipine. *Lancet* 1981;1:844–845.
80. Shapiro W. Correlative studies of serum digoxin levels and the arrhythmias of digitalis intoxication. *Am J Cardiol* 1978;41:852–859.
81. Tsien RW. Cyclic AMP and contractile activity in the heart. *Adv Cyclic Nucleotide Res* 1977;8:363.
82. Hyman AL, Lippton HL, Kadowitz PI. Autonomic regulation of the pulmonary circulation. *J Cardiovasc Pharmacol* 1985;7(Suppl 3): s80–s95.
83. Barrington K, Chan W. The circulatory of epinephrine on infusion in the anesthetized piglet. *Pediatr Res* 1993;33:190–194.
84. Cutaia M, Porcelli RI. Pulmonary vascular reactivity after repetitive exposure to selected biologic amines. *J Appl Physiol* 1983;55: 1868–1876.
85. Meadow WL, Rudinsky BF, Strates E. Selective elevation of systemic blood pressure by epinephrine during sepsis-induced pulmonary hypertension in piglets. *Pediatr Rev* 1986;20:872.
86. Porcelli RI, Cutaia MV. Pulmonary vascular reactivity to biogenic amines during acute hypoxia. *Am J Physiol* 1988;255:H329–H334.
87. Lock IE, Olley PM, Coceani F. Enhanced β-adrenergic receptor responsiveness in hypoxic neonatal pulmonary circulation. *Am J Physiol* 1981;240:H697–H703.

88. Fisher DG, Schwartz PH, Davis AL. Pharmacokinetics of exogenous epinephrine in critically ill children. *Crit Care Med* 1993;21: 111–117.
89. Driscoll DJ, Gillette PC, McNamara DG. The use of dopamine in children. *J Pediatr* 1978;92:309–314.
90. Steinberg C, Notterdam DA. Pharmacokinetics of cardiovascular drugs in children. *Clin Pharmacokinet* 1994;27:345–347.
91. Kao B, Stewart de Ramirez SA, Belfort MB, et al. Inhaled epinephrine for the treatment of transient tachypnea of the newborn. *J Perinatol* 2008;28:205–210.
92. Tourneux P, Rakza T, Abazine A, et al. Noradrenaline for management of septic shock refractory to fluid loading and dopamine or dobutamine in full-term newborn infants. *Acta Paediatr* 2008;97: 177–180.
93. Leier CV, Unverferth DV. Dobutamine. *Ann Intern Med* 1983; 99:490–496.
94. Osborn D, Evans N, Kluckow M. Randomized trial of dobutamine versus dopamine in preterm infants with low systemic blood flow. *J Pediatr* 2002;140:183–191.
95. Habib DM, Padburg IF, Anas NG, et al. Dobutamine pharmacokinetics and pharmacodynamics in pediatric intensive care patients. *Crit Care Med* 1992;20:601–608.
96. Robbers-Visser D, Jan Ten Harkel D, Kapusta L, et al. Usefulness of cardiac magnetic resonance imaging combined with low-dose dobutamine stress to detect an abnormal ventricular stress response in children and young adults after Fontan operation at young age. *Am J Cardiol* 2008;101:1657–1662.
97. Dipchand AI, Bharat W, Manlhiot C, et al. A prospective study of dobutamine stress echocardiography for the assessment of cardiac allograft vasculopathy in pediatric heart transplant recipients. *Pediatr Transplant* 2008;12:570–576.
98. Colucci WS, Wright RF, Braunwald E. New positive inotropic agents in the treatment of congestive heart failure. *N Engl J Med* 1986;14:290–299, 349–358.
99. Rocci ML, Wilson H. The pharmacokinetics and pharmacodynamics of newer inotropic agents. *Clin Pharmacokinet* 1977;13: 91–109.
100. Ramamoorthy C, Anderson GD, Williams GD, et al. Pharmacokinetics and side effects of milrinone in infants and children after open heart surgery. *Anesth Analg* 1998;86:283–289.
101. Allen-Webb EM, Ross MP, Pappas JB, et al. Age-related amrinone pharmacokinetics in a pediatric population. *Crit Care Med* 1994; 22:1016–1024.
102. Paradisis M, Jiang X, McLachlan AJ, et al. Population pharmacokinetics and dosing regimen design of milrinone in preterm infants. *Arch Dis Child Fetal Neonatal Ed* 2007;92:F204–F209.
103. Hamilton RA, Kawalsky SF, Wright EM, et al. Effect of acetylator phenotype on amrinone pharmacokinetics. *Clin Pharmacol Ther* 1986;40:615–619.
104. Bailey JM, Hoffman TM, Wessel DL, et al. A population pharmacokinetic analysis of milrinone in pediatric patients after cardiac surgery. *J Pharmacokinet Pharmacodyn* 2004;31:43–59.
105. Zuppa A, Nicolson SC, Adamson PC, et al. Population pharmacokinetics of milrinone in neonates with hypoplastic left heart syndrome undergoing stage I reconstruction. *Anesth Analg* 2006; 102:1062–1069.
106. Hoffman TM, Wernovsky G, Atz AM, et al. Efficacy and safety of milrinone in preventing low cardiac output syndrome in infants and children after corrective surgery for congenital heart disease. *Circulation* 2003;107:996–1002.
107. Duggal B, Pratap U, Slavik Z, et al. Milrinone and low cardiac output following cardiac surgery in infants: is there a direct myocardial effect? *Pediatr Cardiol* 2005;26:642–645.
108. Wang SM, Lei HY, Huang MC, et al. Therapeutic efficacy of milrinone in the management of enterovirus 71-induced pulmonary edema. *Pediatr Pulmonol* 2005;39:219–223.
109. McNamara PJ, Laique F, Muang-In S, et al. Milrinone improves oxygenation in neonates with severe persistent pulmonary hypertension of the newborn. *J Crit Care* 2006;21:217–222.
110. Cai J, Su Z, Shi Z, et al. Nitric oxide and milrinone: combined effect on pulmonary circulation after Fontan procedure: a prospective, randomized study. *Ann Thorac Surg* 2008;86:882–888.
111. Binah O, Rosen MR. Developmental changes in the interactions of amrinone and ouabain in canine ventricular muscle. *Dev Pharmacol Ther* 1983;6:333–346.
112. Coo JY, Olley PM, Vella G, et al. Bipyridine derivatives lower arteriolar resistance and improve left ventricular function in newborn lambs. *Pediatr Res* 1987;22:422–428.
113. Irazuzta JE, Pretzlaff RK, Rowin ME. Amrinone in pediatric refractory septic shock: an open-label pharmacodynamic study. *Pediatr Crit Care Med* 2001;2:24–28.
114. Stevenson LW. Inotropic therapy for heart failure. *N Engl J Med* 1998;339:1848–1850.
115. Okerholm RO, Chan KY, Lang IF, et al. Biotransformation and pharmacokinetic overview of enoximone and its sulfoxide metabolite. *Am J Cardiol* 1987;60:21C–26C.
116. Ringe HI, Varnholt V, Gaetdicke G. Cardiac rescue with enoximone in volume and catecholamine refractory septic shock. *Pediatr Crit Care Med* 2003;4:471–475.
117. Jessup M, Ulrich S, Samaha J, et al. Effects of low dose enoximone for chronic congestive heart failure. *Am J Cardiol* 1987;60: 80C–84C.
118. Cohn IN, Franciosa JA. Vasodilator therapy in cardiac failure. *N Engl J Med* 1977;297:27–31, 254–258.
119. Yaster M, Simmons RS, Tolo VT, et al. A comparison of nitroglycerine and nitroprusside for inducing hypotension in children: a double-blind study. *Anesthesiology* 1986;65:175–179.
120. Chiarello M, Gold HK, Leinbach RC, et al. Comparison between the effects of nitroprusside and nitroglycerine on ischemic injury during acute myocardial infarction. *Circulation* 1976;54:766–773.
121. Benson LN, Bohn D, Edmonds IF, et al. Nitroglycerin therapy in children with low cardiac index after heart surgery. *Cardiovasc Med* 1979;4:207–215.
122. Damen S, Hitchcock F. Reactive pulmonary hypertension after a switch operation. Successful treatment with glyceryl trinitrate. *Br Heart J* 1985;153:223–225.
123. Ilbawi MN, Idriss FS, DeLeon SY, et al. Hemodynamic effects of intravenous nitroglycerin in pediatric patients after heart surgery. *Circulation* 1985;72:(pt 2):101–107.
124. Rudinsky BF, Komar U, Strates E, et al. Neither nitroglycerin nor nitroprusside selectively reduces sepsis-induced pulmonary hypertension in piglets. *Crit Care Med* 1987;15:1127–1130.
125. Dindar A, Cetin B, Ertuğrul T, et al. Sublingual isosorbide dinitrate-stimulated tilt test for diagnosis of vasovagal syncope in children and adolescents. *Pediatr Cardiol* 2003;24:270–273.
126. Ignarro L, Lippton H, Edwards SC, et al. Mechanism of vascular smooth muscle relaxation by organic nitrates, nitrites, nitroprusside and nitric oxide: evidence for the involvement of S-nitrosothiols as active intermediates. *J Pharmacol Exp Ther* 1981;218:739–749.
127. Rouby T, Gory O, Bourrelli B, et al. Resistance to sodium nitroprusside in hypertensive patients. *Crit Care Med* 1982;10:301–304.
128. Beekman RH, Rocchini AP, Rosenthal A. Hemodynamic effects of nitroprusside in infants with a large ventricular septal defect. *Circulation* 1981;64:553–558.
129. Dillon TR, Janos OO, Meyer RA, et al. Vasodilator therapy for congestive heart failure. *J Pediatr* 1980;96:623–629.
130. López-Herce J, Borrego R, Bustinza A, et al. Elevated carboxyhemoglobin associated with sodium nitroprusside treatment. *Intensive Care Med* 2005;31:1235–1238.
131. Million O, Ziltner F, Baumann R. Oxygen pressure-dependent control of carbonic anhydrase synthesis in chick embryonic erythrocytes. *Am J Physiol* 1991;261:Rl188–Rl196.
132. Hermon NM, Brda G, Goleji J, et al. Methemoglobin formation in children with congenital heart disease treated with inhaled nitric oxide after cardiac surgery. *Intensive Care Med* 2003;29:447–452.
133. Lee ML, Chiu IS. Inhaled nitric oxide for persistent pulmonary hypertension in a neonate with pulmonary atresia and intact ventricular septum after radiofrequency valvulotomy, balloon valvuloplasty and Blalock-Taussig shunt. *Int J Cardiol* 2003;87:273–277.
134. Riddle EM, Feltes TF, Rosen K, et al. Association of nitric oxide dose and methemoglobin levels in patients with congenital heart disease and pulmonary hypertension. *Am J Cardiol* 2002;90:442–444.
135. Komai H, Naito Y, Kimura H. PMTD: nitric oxide synthase expression in lungs of pulmonary hypertensive patients with heart disease. *Cardiovasc Pathol* 2001;10:29–32.
136. Ryan A, Tobias JD. A 5-year survey of nitric oxide use in a pediatric intensive care unit. *Am J Ther* 2007;14:253–258.
137. Roofthooft MT, Bergman KA, Waterbolk TW, et al. Persistent pulmonary hypertension of the newborn with transposition of the great arteries *Ann Thorac Surg* 2007;83:1446–1450.

138. Barr FE, Tirona MB, Rice G, et al. Pharmacokinetics and safety of intravenously administered citrulline in children undergoing congenital heart surgery: potential therapy for postoperative pulmonary hypertension. *J Thorac Cardiovasc Surg* 2007;134:319–326.
139. Levy M, Koren G, Klein J, et al. Captopril pharmacokinetics, blood pressure response and plasma renin activity in normotensive children with renal scarring. *Dev Pharmacol Ther* 1991;16: 185–193.
140. Lewis AB, Chabot M. The effect of treatment with angiotensin-converting enzyme inhibitors on survival of pediatric patients with dilated cardiomyopathy. *Pediatr Cardiol* 1993;14:9–12.
141. Webster MW, Neutze JM, Calder AL. Acute hemodynamic effects of converting enzyme inhibition in children with intracardiac shunts. *Pediatr Cardiol* 1992;13:129.
142. Alehan D, Ozkutlu S. Beneficial effects of 1-year captopril therapy with chronic aortic regurgitation who have no symptoms. *Am Heart J* 1998;135:598–603.
143. Sinaiko AR, Mirkin BL, Hedrick DA, et al. Antihypertensive effect of and elimination time kinetics of captopril in hypertensive children with renal disease. *J Pediatr* 1983;103:799–805.
144. Mori Y, Nakazawa M, Tomimatsu H, et al. Long-term effect of angiotensin-converting enzyme in volume overloaded heart during growth: a controlled pilot study. *J Am Coll Cardiol* 2000;36:270–275.
145. Momma K. ACE inhibitors in pediatric patients with heart failure. *Paediatr Drugs* 2006;8:55–69.
146. Shaw NJ, Wilson N, Dickinson DF. Captopril in heart failure secondary to left to right shunts. *Arch Dis Child* 1988;63:360–363.
147. Wells T, Frame V, Soffer B, et al. A double-blind, placebo controlled, dose response of the effectiveness and safety of enalapril for children with hypertension. *J Clin Pharmacol* 2002;42:870–880.
148. Calabro R, Pisacane C, Pacileo G, et al. Hemodynamic effects of a single oral dose of enalapril among children with asymptomatic chronic mitral regurgitation. *Am Heart J* 1999;138:955–961.
149. Nakamura H, Ishii M, Sugimura T, et al. The kinetic profile of enalapril and enalaprilat and their possible developmental changes in pediatric patients with congestive heart failure. *Clin Pharmacol Ther* 1994;56:160–168.
150. Silber JH, Cnaan A, Clark BJ, et al. Enalapril to prevent cardiac function decline in long-term survivors of pediatric cancer exposed to anthracyclines *J Clin Oncol* 2004;22:820–828.
151. Pitt B, Zannad F, Remme WJ, et al. The effect of spironolactone on morbidity and mortality in patients with severe heart failure. *N Engl J Med* 1999;341:709–717.
152. Horisberger JD, Rossier BC. Aldosterone regulation of gene transcription leading to control of ion transport. *Hypertension* 1992;19:221–227.
153. Rocha R, Williams GH. Rational for the use of aldosterone antagonists in congestive heart failure. *Drugs* 2002;62:723–731.
154. Bruns LA, Canter CE. Should β-blockers be used for the treatment of pediatric patients with chronic heart failure? *Pediatr Drugs* 2002;4:771–778.
155. Laer S, Mir TS, Behn F, et al. Carvedilol therapy in pediatric patients with congestive heart failure: a study investigating clinical and pharmacokinetic parameters. *Am Heart J* 2002;143:916–922.
156. Bajcetic M, Kokic AN, Djukic M, et al. Effects of carvedilol on left ventricular function and oxidative stress in infants and children with idiopathic dilated cardiomyopathy: a 12-month, two-center, open-label study. *Clin Ther* 2008;30:702–714.
157. Shaddy RE, Boucek MM, Hsu DT, et al. Carvedilol for children and adolescents with heart failure: a randomized controlled trial. *JAMA* 2007;298:1171–1179.
158. Kugler ID, Danford DA, Dial BJ, et al. Radiofrequency catheter ablation for tachyarrhythmias in children and adolescents. The Pediatric Electrophysiology Society. *N Engl J Med* 1994;330: 1481–1487.
159. Perry JC, Iverson P, Kugler JD. Radiofrequency catheter ablation of tachyarrhythmias in young patients with structurally abnormal hearts. *Pacing Clin Electrophysiol* 1996;19:579.
160. Vaughan Williams EM. Classification of antiarrhythmic drugs. In: Sandoe E, Flensted-Jenscti E, Olsen KH, eds. *Cardiac arrhythmias.* Sodertalje, Sweden: Astra, 1970:149–472.
161. Harrison DC. Antiarrhythmic drug classification: new science and practical applications. *Am J Cardiol* 1985;50:185–187.
162. Task Force of the Working Group or Arrhythmias of the European Society of cardiology. The Sicilian Gambit. A new approach to the classification of antiarrhythmic drugs based on their actions on arrhythmogenic mechanisms. *Circulation* 1991;84:183.
163. Bink-Boelkens MT. Pharmacologic management of arrhythmias. *Pediatr Cardiol* 2000;21:508–515.
164. Dubin A. Antiarrhythmic drug therapy in neonates. *Prog Pediatr Cardiol* 2000;11:55–63.
165. Woosley RL, Funck-Brentano C. Overview of the clinical pharmacology of antiarrhythmic drugs. *Am J Cardiol* 1988;61:61A–69A.
166. Taddio A, Ito S. Drugs and breast feeding. In: Koren G, ed. *Maternal–fetal toxicity*, 3rd ed. New York, NY: Marcel Dekker, Inc., 2001:177–232.
167. Frishman WH, Cavusoglu E. β-Adrenergic blockers and their role in the therapy of arrhythmias. In: Podrid PJ, Kowey PR, eds. *Cardiac arrhythmia: mechanisms, diagnosis, and management.* Baltimore, MD: Williams & Wilkins, 1995:421–434.
168. Wu D, Denes P, Dhingra R, et al. The effects of propranolol in induction of AV nodal resistant paroxsysmal tachycardia. *Circulation* 1974;50:665–677.
169. Nies AS, Shand DG. Clinical pharmacology of propranolol. *Circulation* 1975;52:6–15.
170. Nies AS, Shand DG, Wilkinson GR. Metered hepatic blood flow and drug disposition. *Clin Pharmacokinet* 1976;1:135–155.
171. Langer A, Hung GT, McA'Nulty JA, et al. Adrenergic blockade: a new approach to hyperthyroidism during pregnancy. *Obstet Gynecol* 1974;144:181.
172. Habib A, McCarthy JS. Effects on the neonate of propranolol administered during pregnancy. *J Pediatr* 1977;91:808.
173. Garson A Jr, Gillette PC, McNamara DG. Propranolol: the preferred palliation for tetralogy of Fallot. *Am J Cardiol* 1981;47: 1098–1104.
174. Shand DG, Sell CG, Oates JA. Hypertrophic obstructive cardiomyopathy in an infant. Propranolol therapy for three years. *N Engl J Med* 1971;285:843.
175. Viljoen JF, Estafanous FG, Kellner GA. Propranolol and cardiac surgery. *J Thorac Cardiovasc Surg* 1972;64:826.
176. Trippel DI, Gillette PC. Atenolol in children with ventricular arrhythmias. *Am Heart J* 1990;119:1312–1316.
177. Trippel DL, Gillette PC. Atenolol in children with supraventricular tachycardia. *Am J Cardiol* 1989;64:233–236.
178. Mehta AV, Chidainbaram B. Efficacy and safety of intravenous and oral nadolol for supraventricular tachycardia in children. *J Am Coll Cardiol* 1992;19:630–635.
179. Cueno BF, Zales VR, Blahunka PC, et al. Pharmacodynamics and pharmacokinetics of esmolol, a short-acting 3-blocking agent, in children. *Pediatr Cardiol* 1994;15:296–301.
180. Shahar E, Barzilay Z, Frand M. Verapamil in the treatment of paroxysmal supraventricular tachycardia in infants and children. *J Pediatr* 1981;98:323–326.
181. Porter CJ, Gilette PC, Garson A, et al. Effects of verapamil on supraventricular tachycardia in children. *Am J Cardiol* 1981;48:487.
182. Shaffer EM, Rocchini AP, Spicer RL, et al. Effects of verapamil on left ventricular diastolic filling in children with hypertrophic cardiomyopathy. *Am J Cardiol* 1988;61:413–417.
183. Hamman SR, Blouin RA, McAllister RG Jr. Clinical pharmacokinetics of verapamil. *Clin Pharmacokinet* 1984;9:26–41.
184. De Vonderweid U, Benettoni A, Piovan D, et al. Use of oral verapamil in long-term treatment of neonatal paroxysmal supraventricular tachycardia. A pharmacokinetic study. *Int J Cardiol* 1984; 5:581.
185. Wagner JG, Rocchini AP, Vasiliades J. Prediction of steady-state verapamil plasma concentrations in children and adults. *Clin Pharmacol Ther* 1982;32:172–181.
186. Epstein ML, Kiel EA, Victorica BE. Cardiac decompensation following verapamil therapy in infants with supraventricular tachycardia. *Pediatrics* 1985;75:737–740.
187. Porter CJ, Garson A, Gilette PC. Verapamil: an effective calcium blocking agent for pediatric patients. *Pediatrics* 1983;71:748–755.
188. Koren G, Soldin S, MacLeod SM. Digoxin–verapamil interaction: in vitro studies in rat tissue. *J Cardiovasc Pharmacol* 1983;5:443.
189. Garson A Jr, Gillette PC, Mcvey P, et al. Amiodarone treatment of critical arrhythmias in children and young adults. *J Am Coll Cardiol* 1984;4:749–755.
190. Coumel P, Fidelle J. Amiodarone in the treatment of cardiac arrhythmias in children: one hundred thirty-five cases. *Am Heart J* 1980;100:1063–1069.

191. Singh BN. Amiodarone: historical development and pharmacologic profile. *Am Heart J* 1983;106:788–797.
192. Bucknall CA, Keeton BR, Curry PVI, et al. Intravenous and oral amiodarone for arrhythmias in children. *Br Heart J* 1986;56: 278–284.
193. Kannan R, Yabek SM, Garson A, et al. Amiodarone efficacy in a young population: relationship to serum amiodarone and desethylamiodarone levels. *Am Heart J* 1987;114:283–287.
194. Latini T, Tognoni G, Kates RE. Clinical pharmacokinetics of amiodarone. *Clin Pharmacokinet* 1984;9:136.
195. Perry JC, Knilans TK, Marlow D, et al. Intravenous amiodarone for life-threatening tachyarrhythmias in children and young adults. *J Am Coll Cardiol* 1993;22:95–98.
196. Figa FH, Gow RM, Hamilton RM, et al. Clinical efficacy and safety of intravenous amiodarone in infants and children. *Am J Cardiol* 1993;74:573–577.
197. Saul JP, Scott WA, Brown S, et al. Intravenous amiodarone for incessant tachyarrhythmias in children: a randomized, double-blind, antiarrhythmic drug trial. *Circulation* 2005;112:3470–3477.
198. Guccione P, Paul T, Garson A Jr. Long-term follow-up of amiodarone therapy in the young: continued efficacy, unimpaired growth, moderate side effects. *J Am Coll Cardiol* 1990;15: 1118–1124.
199. Paul T, Guccione P. New antiarrhythmic drugs in pediatric use: amiodarone. *Pediatr Cardiol* 1994;15:132–138.
200. Singh BN. Antiarrhythmic actions of DL-sotalol in ventricular and supraventricular arrhythmias. *J Cardiovasc Pharmacol* 1992;20: S75–S90.
201. EP Walsh, JP Saul, Triedman JK, eds. *Cardiac arrhythmias in children and adults with congenital heart disease.* Philadelphia, PA: Lippincott Williams & Wilkins, 2001.
202. Zanetti LAF. Sotalol: a new class III antiarrhythmic agent. *Clin Pharm* 1993;12:883–891.
203. Macagnes P, Tipple M, Fournier A. Effectiveness of oral sotalol for treatment of pediatric arrhythmias. *Am J Cardiol* 1992;69: 751–775.
204. Tipple M, Sandor C. Efficacy and safety of oral sotalol in early infancy. *Pacing Clin Electrophysiol* 1991;14:2062–2206.
205. Miyazaki A, Ohuchi H, Kurosaki KI, et al. Efficacy and safety of sotalol for refractory tachyarrhythmias in congenital heart disease. *Circ J* 2008;72:1998–2003.
206. The Cardiac Arrhythmia Suppression Trial (CAST). Investigators: preliminary report: effect of encainide and flecainide on mortality in a randomized trial of arrhythmia suppression after myocardial infarction. *N Engl J Med* 1989;321:406.
207. Perry JC, Garson A Jr. Flecainide acetate for treatment of tachyarrhythmias in children: review of world literature on efficacy, safety, and dosing. *Am Heart J* 1992;124:1614–1621.
208. Fish FA, Gillette PC, Benson DW Jr, et al. Proarrhythmia, cardiac arrest and death in young patients receiving encainide and flecainide. *J Am Coll Cardiol* 1991;18:356–365.
209. Perry JC, McQuinn RL, Smith RT Jr, et al. Flecainide acetate for resistant arrhythmias in the young: efficacy and pharmacokinetics. *J Am Coll Cardiol* 1989;14:185–191.
210. Fenrich AL Jr, Perry JC, Friedman RA. Flecainide and amiodarone: combined therapy for refractory tachyarrhythmias in infancy. *J Am Coll Cardiol* 1995;25:1195–1198.
211. Russell GAB, Martin RP. Flecainide toxicity. *Arch Dis Child* 1989;64:860–862.
212. Perly JC, McQuinn RL, Smith RT Jr, et al. Flecainide acetate for resistant arrhythmias in the young: efficacy and pharmacokinetics. *J Am Coll Cardiol* 1989;14:185–191.
213. Perry JC, Ayres NA, Carpenter RJ Jr. Fetal supraventricular tachycardia treated with flecainide acetate. *J Pediatr* 1991;118:303–305.
214. Paul T, Janousek J. New antiarrhythmic drugs in pediatric use: propafenone. *Pediatr Cardiol* 1994;15:190–197.
215. Janousek J, Paul T, Reimer A, et al. Usefulness of propafenone for supraventricular arrhythmias in infants and children. *Am J Cardiol* 1993;72:294–300.
216. Beaufort CCM, Bink-Boelkens MTE. Oral propafenone as treatment for incessant supraventricular and ventricular tachycardia in children. *Am J Cardiol* 1993;72:1213–1214.
217. Tili J, Herxheimer A. Death of a child with supraventricular tachycardia. *Lancet* 1992;339:1597–1598.
218. Lerman RB, Belardinelli L. Cardiac electrophysiology of adenosine: basic and clinical concepts. *Circulation* 1991;83:1499–1509.
219. Engeistein ED, Lippman N, Stein KM, et al. Mechanism-specific effects of adenosine on atrial tachycardia. *Circulation* 1994;89: 2645–2654.
220. Rossi AF, Steinberg LG, Ripel G, et al. Use of adenosine in the management of perioperative arrhythmias in the pediatric cardiac intensive care unit. *Crit Care Med* 1992;20:1107–1111.
221. Eubanks AP, Artman M. Administration of adenosine to a newborn of 26 weeks' gestation. *Pediatr Cardiol* 1994;15:157–158.
222. Fletcher S, Fyfe DA, Gillette PC, et al. The utility of adenosine to terminate supraventricular tachycardia in a premature hydropic infant. *Am Heart J* 1991;121:1818–1819.
223. Overholt ED, Rheuban KS, Gutgesell HP, et al. Usefulness of adenosine for arrhythmias in infants and children. *Am J Cardiol* 1988;61:336–340.
224. Berul CI. Higher adenosine dosage required for supraventricular tachycardia in infants treated with theophylline. *Clin Pediatr (Phila)* 1993;32:167–168.
225. Tili J, Shinebourne EA, Rigby ML, et al. Efficacy and safety of adenosine in the treatment of supraventricular tachycardia in infants and children. *Br Heart J* 1989;62:204–211.

CHAPTER

43

Jean-Pierre Guignard

Diuretics

INTRODUCTION

Diuretics promote the excretion of water and electrolytes. They are primarily used in states of inappropriate salt and water retention. Such states can be secondary to renal diseases (nephrotic syndrome, glomerulonephritis, chronic renal failure), congestive heart failure (CHF), and liver disease (cirrhosis). Diuretics are also used in a variety of clinical situations in which an increase in sodium excretion is not the primary goal of treatment. Such conditions include acute renal failure (ARF), electrolyte disturbances (hypo- or hyperkalemia, hypercalcemia, hypercalciuria) and nephrogenic diabetes insipidus. Effective therapeutic goals when using diuretics require thorough knowledge of the renal regulation of water and electrolytes.

RENAL FUNCTION

Urine formation starts by the ultrafiltration of plasma through the glomerular capillary wall. The rate of glomerular filtration (GFR) is determined by the net filtration pressure across the glomerular capillaries and the glomerular ultrafiltration coefficient (K_f), which is the product of the surface area and the permeability of the glomerular capillaries:

$$\text{GFR} = K_f \times \text{net filtration pressure}$$

Changes in systemic arterial pressure, in intrarenal arteriolar resistance, and in the plasma oncotic pressure modulate GFR (1). Both renal perfusion and GFR are controlled by hormones and autacoids such as angiotensin II, the prostaglandins, endothelin, bradykinin, and nitric oxide, and by the sympathetic nervous system. The filtration process does not produce significant changes in the concentration of small solutes. Modifications of the filtrate occur by the reabsorption and secretion of solutes across the renal tubular cells and by the reabsorption of water.

TRANSPORT OF SOLUTES

Reabsorption of solutes is achieved by active or passive transport across the tubular cell membranes, using a transcellular or a paracellular route. Primary active transport requires a source of metabolic energy, provided by adenosine triphosphate (ATP) hydrolysis. The most important active process in the nephron is the Na^+, K^+-ATPase located on the basolateral side of the tubular cells. Other primary active transport mechanisms include various ATPases: Ca^{2+}-ATPase, H^+-ATPase, and a H^+, K^+-ATPase. Secondary active transport of solutes along (**symport**) or against (**antiport**) the Na^+ gradient created by its primary active transport occurs via specific protein carrier molecules (**transporters**). Some proteins in the cell membranes, termed **uniporters**, transport only a single substance down the concentration gradient. Such is the case for glucose moving across the basolateral membrane of proximal tubular cells. Finally, cell membranes contain channels allowing the rapid passage of specific ions (Na^+, K^+, Cl^-) across cellular membranes (2). Transport via channels or uniporters is sometimes referred to as *facilitated diffusion*.

Water flows passively down the osmotic gradient created by the active transport of solutes. The water reabsorbed along the nephron carries solutes, a process termed *solvent drag*. Macromolecules are transported by *endocytosis*, a process also using the energy provided by the ATPases.

REABSORPTION OF SODIUM

The renal tubule can reabsorb up to 99% of the filtered load of sodium. Two-thirds are reabsorbed in the proximal tubule, 25% in the ascending limb of loop of Henle, and 10% in the distal tubule and collecting duct. The driving force for Na^+ reabsorption is the Na^+, K^+-ATPase in the basolateral membrane of the tubular cell. The gradient created by the active pumping of Na^+ out of the cell allows the passive entry of Na^+ at the luminal membrane, along its electrochemical gradient. The basolateral pump also provides energy for the secondary antiport or symport transport of such solutes as Cl^-, HCO_3^-, Ca^{2+}, phosphate, glucose, urea, and amino acids (1).

In the early proximal tubule the reabsorption of Na^+ is coupled to that of HCO_3^- and a number of organic molecules. Many of these solutes are almost completely removed from the tubular fluid in the first part of the proximal tubule. In the second half of the proximal tubule, Na^+ is reabsorbed with Cl^-.

The thick ascending limb of loop of Henle reabsorbs approximately 25% of the filtered load of Na^+. It is impermeable to water. The movement of Na^+ across the luminal membrane is mediated by the Na^+, 2 Cl^-, K^+ symporter. The Na^+ that is reabsorbed is deposited in the medullary interstitium, where it is trapped by the countercurrent multiplier mechanism, together with urea. The integrity of the Na^+, K^+-ATPase and of the Na^+, 2 Cl^-, K^+ cotransport is necessary for the generation of a hypertonic medulla required to concentrate the urine.

The early distal tubule forms part of the juxtaglomerular apparatus that provides the feedback control of single nephron GFR. In this part of the nephron, which is also impermeable to water, the continuous avid reabsorption of Na^+ results in the dilution of urine. This segment is thus referred to as the *diluting segment.*

The late distal tubule and collecting duct are composed of two distinct cell types, the principal cells and the intercalated cells. The principal cells reabsorb Na^+ and water and secrete K^+, a process controlled by aldosterone. The intercalated cells reabsorb K^+ and secrete H^+ in the tubular lumen. These cells play an important role in regulating acid–base balance. In the distal tubule and collecting duct, part of sodium enters the luminal membrane via an epithelial Na^+ channel ($E_{NA}C$).

The medullary collecting duct reabsorbs ~3% of the filtered load of Na^+. Active H^+ secretion against steep concentration gradients occurs in this segment, which is essential for the excretion of fixed acids. The permeability of the collecting duct cells to water is under the influence of arginine vasopressin (AVP), also known as the antidiuretic hormone (ADH) (1).

TRANSPORT OF WATER

The proximal tubule is highly permeable to water, much of which passes through the cells via aquaporin-1 water channels present in both the apical and the basolateral cell membranes (3). While the descending limb of loop of the Henle is highly permeable to water, the thin and thick ascending segments of the loop are almost totally impermeable. The permeability of the collecting duct to water is under the control of AVP. This hormone increases the permeability of the cortical tubular cells by incorporating aquaporin-2 water channels in the apical membrane (3). In the presence of AVP, the permeability of this segment to water is thus increased, allowing the diffusion of free water out of the tubular lumen into the highly hypertonic interstitium (1).

TRANSPORT OF OTHER CATIONS AND ANIONS (K^+, Ca^{2+}, Pi)

POTASSIUM

The kidneys play a major role in maintaining K^+ balance. Two-thirds of the filtered K^+ are reabsorbed in the proximal tubule and 20% in the ascending limb of loop of Henle. The regulation of K^+ excretion occurs via the secretion of K^+ in the distal tubule and collecting duct. When the dietary intake of K^+ is too large, K^+ excretion can exceed the K^+ filtered load. Three major factors control the rate of distal K^+ secretion: (a) the activity of the Na^+, K^+-ATPase; (b) the electrochemical gradient for K^+ across the apical membrane; and (c) the permeability of the apical membrane to K^+. The excretion of K^+ is regulated by the plasma K^+ concentration, the acid–base balance, aldosterone, and AVP.

CALCIUM

Seventy percent of the filtered Ca^{2+} is reabsorbed in the proximal tubule, 20% in the thick ascending limb of loop of Henle, 9% in the distal tubule, and 1% in the collecting duct. In the proximal tubule, Ca^{2+} enters the apical membrane by diffusing through a paracellular route or Ca^{2+} channels, down the electrochemical gradient created by the primary and secondary active transport of Ca^{2+} out of the basolateral membrane (Ca^{2+}-ATPase; Na^+-Ca^{2+} antiport). Reabsorption of Ca^{2+} in the ascending limb is largely passive down the electrochemical gradient created by the active reabsorption of Na^+. The reabsorption of Na^+ and Ca^{2+} changes in parallel in both the proximal and the thick ascending limb of loop of Henle. This accounts for the occurrence of parallel changes in Ca^{2+} and Na^+ excretion. In the distal tubule the reabsorption of Ca^{2+} is entirely active and independent from that of Na^+. The renal excretion of Ca^{2+} is regulated by parathyroid hormone, calcitriol, and calcitonin (1).

PHOSPHATE

The proximal tubule reabsorbs 80% of the filtered load of Pi and the distal tubule 10%. The remaining 10% is excreted in the urine. Pi enters the apical membrane by a $2Na^+$–Pi symporter and exits the cell across the basolateral membrane by a Pi–anion antiporter. The excretion of Pi is mainly regulated by parathyroid hormone. Extracellular fluid (ECF) volume expansion decreases the reabsorption of Pi. Other factors depressing the reabsorption of Pi include metabolic acidosis and the glucocorticoids (1).

SECRETION OF ORGANIC CATIONS AND ANIONS

The proximal tubule reabsorbs solutes and water and also secretes various organic cations and anions, many of which are end products of metabolism. The transport mechanisms for both organic cations and anions are nonspecific, so that several cations and several anions can compete for the cationic or the anionic secretory pathways. In addition to endogenous organic cations and anions, various exogenous drugs are also eliminated by secretion. Such is the case for the anionic diuretics (acetazolamide, thiazides, furosemide, bumetanide) or cationic diuretics (amiloride) (1).

REGULATION OF Na^+ AND WATER TRANSPORT

In addition to the glomerular tubular balance that via Starling forces adapts the reabsorption of Na^+ to its filtered load, Na^+ transport is regulated by various hormones and paracrine factors. Angiotensin II, aldosterone, the atrial natriuretic peptide (ANP), the prostaglandins, the catecholamines, and dopamine play major roles (1).

ANGIOTENSIN II

Angiotensin II stimulates proximal Na^+ and water reabsorption by increasing the apical Na^+/H^+ exchange. It is an important secretagogue for aldosterone. By acting on the zona glomerulosa of the adrenal cortex to release aldosterone, it indirectly favors distal Na^+ reabsorption. Angiotensin II release is activated by a decrease in extracellular fluid volume and renal perfusion.

ALDOSTERONE

Aldosterone stimulates the distal reabsorption of Na^+ by increasing the permeability of the collecting tubule luminal membrane to Na^+. Aldosterone also favors the secretion of K^+ and H^+ and increases the reabsorption of Cl^-. Aldosterone stimulates the Na^+, K^+-ATPase and the production of ATP. The secretion of aldosterone by the adrenal cortex is stimulated by angiotensin II, hyperkalemia, and severe hyponatremia.

ATRIAL NATRIURETIC PEPTIDE

The heart produces two natriuretic peptides: the ANP stored in the atrial myocytes and the brain natriuretic peptide (BNP) stored in the ventricular myocytes. Both peptides are released when the heart dilates. The kidneys produce a related natriuretic peptide termed urodilatin. In general, the natriuretic peptides antagonize the actions of the renin–angiotensin–aldosterone system. The 28-amino acids peptide is released when atrial stretch receptors sense an increase in the effective circulating volume. ANP stimulates the excretion of Na^+ by (a) increasing GFR via vasodilatation of the afferent arterioles; (b) inhibiting renin release and the secretion of aldosterone; (c) inhibiting the Na^+, K^+-ATPase in the inner medullary collecting duct, and (d) closing the epithelial Na^+ channels.

PROSTAGLANDINS

The prostaglandins, synthesized by the cyclooxygenases in the renal cortex, the medullary interstitium, and the collecting duct epithelial cells, increase Na^+ excretion. They do it by increasing GFR and by inhibiting Na^+ reabsorption in the collecting duct.

NOREPINEPHRINE AND EPINEPHRINE

Norepinephrine and epinephrine released from sympathetic nerves and the adrenal medulla, respectively, stimulate Na^+ reabsorption in the proximal tubule, the thick ascending limb of the loop of Henle, the distal tubule, and the collecting duct.

DOPAMINE

Dopamine, synthesized by proximal tubular cells and dopaminergic nerves, increases the excretion of Na^+ by inhibiting Na^+ proximal reabsorption.

ANTIDIURETIC HORMONE (ARGININE VASOPRESSIN)

Water following Na^+ passively, its reabsorption is increased by all the factors that stimulate Na^+ reabsorption. The hormone that really regulates water balance is AVP, a nonapeptide with a molecular weight of 1,099 daltons.

Three types of receptors mediate the actions of AVP. V_{1A} receptors are located on vascular smooth muscle and mediate vasoconstriction. V_{1B} receptors are present in the anterior pituitary gland and mediate the release of adrenocorticotropic hormone. The V_2 receptors are located in the renal distal tubule and collecting duct. AVP binding to the V_2 receptors leads to activation of an adenylyl cyclase with subsequent rise in intracellular cyclic AMP. This second messenger mediates the translocation of intracellular vesicles containing the water channel aquaporin-2 into the apical plasma membrane (3) and increases the transcription of aquaporin 2 (AQP-2). AVP-regulated AQP-2 shuttling is the primary determinant for water permeability of the collecting duct and, consequently, for the antidiuresis. In addition, AVP stimulates Na^+–K^+–$2Cl^-$ cotransport in the ascending limb of loop of Henle via V_2 receptors.

The release of AVP is rapid, its plasma half-life is short (10 to 15 minutes), thus allowing a fine regulation of the plasma osmolality. Small changes in P_{osm} ($\pm$3 mOsm per kg H_2O) activate or inhibit AVP release. Osmoreceptors, located in the supraoptic nucleus of the hypothalamus, regulate the release of AVP. Volo- and baroreceptors also affect AVP release. Because of the greater sensitivity of the osmoreceptors, their influence predominates when changes in osmolality and plasma volume are moderate. When large changes in plasma volume occur, however, the influence of the volo- and baroreceptors predominates over that of the osmoreceptors, leading to "inappropriate" secretion of AVP, with consequent water retention and hemodilution. Nonosmotic stimulation or inhibition of AVP release occurs as a consequence of drugs (nicotine, morphine, barbiturates), pain, and respiratory or cerebral distress (1).

BODY FLUID HOMEOSTASIS

The kidney is responsible for maintaining the ECF fluid volume and osmolality constant in spite of large changes in salt and water intake.

BODY FLUID VOLUME

NaCl, the major osmotically active solute in ECF, determines its volume. The balance between the intake and the renal excretion of Na^+ thus regulates ECF volume, and as a consequence cardiac output and blood pressure. Long-term changes in Na^+ excretion are regulated by aldosterone. More rapid changes in Na^+ excretion are achieved by changes in GFR and/or by various intrarenal hormones that regulate Na^+ reabsorption.

ECF volume is closely related to plasma volume. Alterations in plasma volume are sensed both on the venous and on the arterial side of the circulation. Arterial sensors perceive the adequacy of blood flow in the arterial circuit, a parameter coined as *effective circulating volume.* This volume is also sensed by baroreceptors located in the juxtaglomerular apparatus of the kidney. A decrease in renal perfusion pressure activates the renin–angiotensin–aldosterone system. Changes in the effective circulating volume activate other intrarenal hormones that modulate Na^+ reabsorption either directly by an action on tubular transport or indirectly by changes in GFR (1).

BODY FLUID OSMOLALITY

The plasma osmolality is maintained within narrow limits. A 2% to 3% increase in P_{osm} stimulates the osmoreceptors with the consequent release of AVP, leading to the reabsorption of free water in the collecting duct. Urine flow rate decreases and the osmolality of the urine increases. The opposite happens when P_{osm} decreases by 2% to 3%. The concentration of urine can vary from 40 to 1,400 mOsm per kg H_2O, depending on whether AVP is completely absent or maximally stimulated. Concentration of the urine requires the presence of a hypertonic medullary interstitium. Impaired NaCl transport in the thick ascending limb of loop of Henle or defective countercurrent multiplier mechanisms results in a decrease in maximal urine osmolality (1).

DEVELOPMENTAL ASPECTS OF RENAL FUNCTION AND BODY FLUID HOMEOSTASIS

In the human fetus, urine formation starts around the 10th to 12th week of gestation. The urine is normally hypotonic, indicating that the kidney actively reabsorbs electrolytes and solutes from the glomerular ultrafiltrate. The fetal kidney responds to diuretics administered to the mother by increasing its urine flow rate. The full complement of nephrons is achieved around the 35th week of gestation. GFR and renal plasma flow increase progressively throughout gestation but remain relatively low. GFR at birth is equal to 20 mL per minute per 1.73 m^2 in term infants and doubles in the first 2 weeks of life. It reaches mature levels of 100 mL per minute per 1.73 m^2 by the 6th to 12th month of postnatal age. GFR is lower at birth in premature neonates and develops at a somewhat lower velocity (4,5).

The reabsorption of filtered solute also undergoes maturational changes. Proximal Na^+ reabsorption increases in parallel with an increase in the activity of the Na^+, K^+-ATPase and in the number of the glucose- and bicarbonate-Na^+ cotransporters. Reabsorption in the loop of Henle also increases along with the activity of the Na^+, K^+-ATPase in this segment. Resistance of the distal tubule to aldosterone has been claimed to be partly responsible for Na^+ wasting in the first weeks of premature infants (6).

In early postnatal life, several transporters and enzymes involved in the reabsorption of bicarbonate are weakly expressed, resulting in a relatively low HCO_3^- excretion threshold. The overall reabsorption of various electrolytes and solutes also undergoes maturational changes linked to the maturation of the transporters, symporters, and antiporters.

The distribution of water in the various compartments of the body varies with age. The ECF volume decreases from 60% body weight at 28 weeks of gestation to 42% at term and 20% at 3 months of age. These changes reflect the excretion of excessive ECF and a gradual increase in the amount of fat tissues. Although the volume of body fluid varies during growth, the tonicity of ECF is kept constant by the kidney, which excretes or retains appropriate amounts of water (7).

The newborn, premature or at term, is able to decrease urine osmolality to values as low as 40 mOsm per kg H_2O. Free-water excretion depends on the distal reabsorption of Na^+ and hence on the amount of Na^+ delivered to the distal tubule. Because of the low GFR present in the newborn infant, the ability to excrete large amounts of free water is limited (7).

The concentrating ability is limited in newborn infants, the more so in the preterm neonates. The relative ineffectiveness of the concentrating mechanism in the neonate has been ascribed to (a) a low corticomedullary concentration gradient; (b) shortness of the loops of Henle; (c) decreased formation of cAMP in response to ADH; and (d) interference of the elevated levels of prostaglandins with the vasopressin-stimulated cAMP synthesis.

In spite of elevated aldosterone levels, premature neonates frequently have difficulties in maintaining a positive Na^+ balance on a Na^+ intake of 1 to 2 mmol per kg per day on the 2nd to 4th week of life. Deficient proximal NaCl reabsorption and relative resistance to aldosterone have been claimed to be responsible for Na^+ wasting. Both the renin–angiotensin system and the osmo- voloreceptors control system of ADH are efficient in the early newborn period. Hyponatremia is frequently seen, however, as the consequence of inappropriate secretion of ADH secondary to respiratory or cerebral distress (7,8).

CLINICAL USE OF DIURETICS

Diuretics are used in sodium-retaining states with or without the formation of edema, in situations of arterial hypertension or electrolyte imbalances, in oliguric renal failure, and in nephrogenic diabetes insipidus (9–12). Diuretics can be used to test the integrity of distal tubular function.

EDEMATOUS STATES

Salt and water retention with edema formation can occur as a primary event or as a consequence of reduced effective circulating volume with secondary hyperaldosteronism. The use of diuretics can be lifesaving when Na retention is associated with an expansion of the ECF volume. It may on the contrary further compromise the situation when sodium retention occurs in response to homeostatic mechanisms mobilized to defend the circulating volume. The use of diuretics therefore requires careful monitoring of the patient's hemodynamic states and an understanding of his or her underlying condition (6,13).

Congestive Heart Failure

CHF is associated with an increase in pressure in the venous circulation. The increased capillary pressure favors the movement of fluid into the interstitium, resulting in the formation of edema. Failure of the heart to provide normal tissue perfusion is sensed as a decrease in effective circulating volume by the kidney, which is stimulated to retain NaCl and water. The presence of edema thus represents a side effect of the compensatory renal response to defend the effective circulating volume. The treatment of this condition consists in restoring normal cardiac output. By mobilizing the edematous fluid, diuretics improve the symptoms of CHF. The pulmonary edema secondary to left-sided heart failure requires the urgent use of diuretics to reduce the life-threatening pulmonary congestion (11).

Nephrotic Syndrome

The nephrotic syndrome is characterized by an increase in the permeability of the glomerular barrier to proteins, heavy proteinuria, hypoproteinemia, and the formation of edema. Two pathogenic mechanisms have been proposed to explain the formation of edema. In the *underfill hypothesis,* decreased plasma oncotic pressure results in decreased effective circulating volume with consequent secondary hyperaldosteronism and hypervasopressinism, leading to progressive salt and water retention. In this situation, usually seen at the onset of the minimal changes in nephrotic syndrome, the hypovolemia is manifested by clinical signs such as tachycardia, abdominal pain, and poorly perfused limbs. Elevated hematocrit and very low urinary sodium (<10 mmol per L) confirm the state of hypovolemia. Diuretics should only be used with great caution in this condition and only after correction of the hypovolemia by albumin infusion.

In the *overfill theory* (14), the edema is caused by the primary retention of Na^+ and water, with increased plasma volume, increased hydrostatic capillary pressure, and leak of fluid into the interstitium. The pathogenesis of saline retention in the overfill hypothesis is not yet clear. Decrease in the activity of the ANP has been claimed to be responsible for the increased Na^+ retention. These patients benefit from diuretic administration.

The *underfill* and the *overfill* theories are not necessarily exclusive. The predominance of a mechanism may depend on the stage and nature of the nephrotic syndrome, the rate of development of proteinuria, and the plasma oncotic pressure (14,15).

Liver Diseases

The occurrence of edema in patients with liver disease is secondary to decreased albumin synthesis, decreased oncotic pressure, and decreased effective circulating volume. The kidney responds by increasing salt and water retention. As ascitis develops, there is a rise in intra-abdominal pressure, a phenomenon that impairs venous drainage from the lower limbs. Although diuretic therapy for ascitis fails to improve survival in children, it benefits quality of life and limits complications such as bacterial peritonitis (16). Defective liver function also results in impaired inactivation of salt- and water-retaining hormones, such as aldosterone or vasopressin.

ARTERIAL HYPERTENSION

Arterial hypertension may be secondary to salt retention and expansion of the ECF volume. Na^+ retention may be directly related to excessive synthesis of aldosterone in primary hyperaldosteronism. In the renal vascular form of hypertension, increased formation of angiotensin II elevates the blood pressure by inducing vasoconstriction and by stimulating sodium reabsorption. In essential hypertension, the retention of Na^+ is not obvious. It has been recently hypothesized that impaired extrusion of Na^+ out of the cells, secondary to defective Na^+/Ca^{2+} counter transport could lead to an increase in intracellular Ca^{2+} with consequent increased vascular contractility (17). By leading to ECF volume contraction, diuretics decrease the blood pressure. They are often used as first-line drugs in the treatment of arterial hypertension (18,19). In adults, low-dose diuretics (hydrochlorothiazide 12.5 mg; torasemide 2.5 mg) constitute effective one-daily monopharmacotherapies for mild-to-moderate uncomplicated essential hypertension (17).

ELECTROLYTES IMBALANCE

Diuretics can be used in various situations associated with dyselectrolytemia. They can increase K^+ excretion in hyperkalemic states (loop diuretics, thiazides), increase calcium excretion in hypercalcemia (loop diuretics), or decrease the rate of calcium excretion in hypercalciuric states (thiazides). Increased HCO_3^- excretion can be achieved by the acetazolamide, whereas increased H^+ excretion can be stimulated by loop diuretics.

NEPHROGENIC DIABETES INSIPIDUS

This condition is characterized by the resistance of the collecting duct to the action of ADH. It can be due either to a X-linked congenital defect in the V2 receptors or to an autosomal recessive mutation in the aquaporin-2 molecule. The patient with diabetes insipidus excretes large amounts of dilute urine. The thiazides can reduce the extracellular space volume by impairing sodium distal reabsorption and increasing NaCl excretion. This decrease in ECF volume stimulates proximal salt and water retention, thus eventually leading to reduced urine flow rate. Prolonged treatment with hydrochlorothiazide–amiloride appears to be more effective and better tolerated than with just hydrochlorothiazide. Such treatment is as efficacious as the association hydrochlorothiazide–indomethacin, with fewer severe side effects (20).

ACUTE RENAL FAILURE

Because they have been shown to variably increase total renal blood flow, loop diuretics are often administered to patients with oliguric renal insufficiency, in the hope of

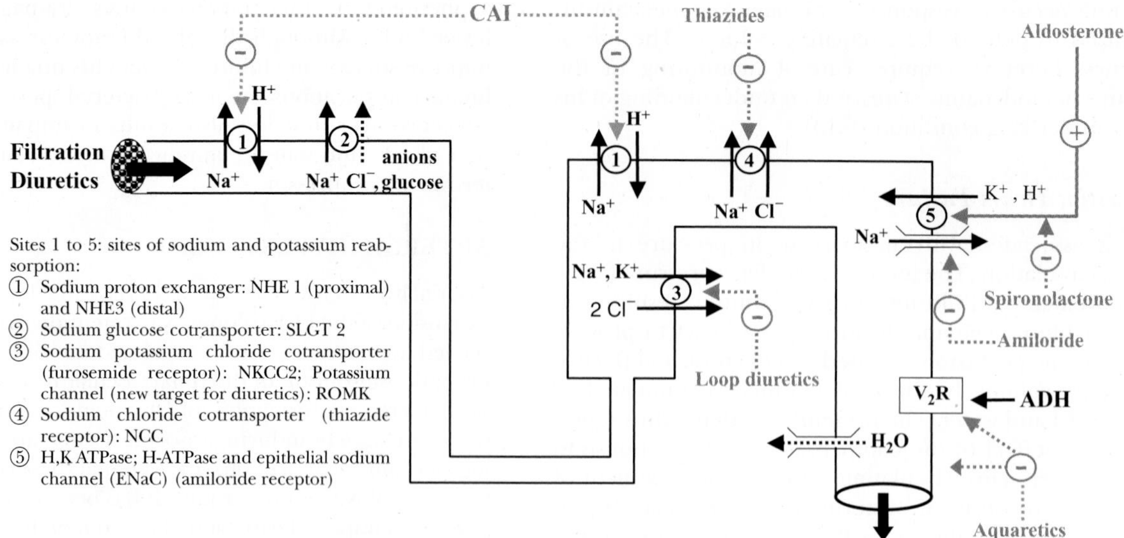

Figure 43.1. Sodium reabsorption along the nephron and sites of action of diuretic agents. ADH, Antidiuretic hormone; CAI, carbonic anhydrase inhibitors.

promoting diuresis and improving GFR and renal perfusion (31). Although diuretic administration may convert oliguric ARF to nonoliguric ARF, there is no evidence that this treatment can ameliorate renal function or improve the outcome of patients with ARF (21).

DIFFERENTIAL DIAGNOSIS OF CONGENITAL TUBULOPATHIES

Diuretics such as acetazolamide, furosemide, or hydrochlorothiazide can be used to test distal tubular acidification or distal sodium reabsorption defects.

CLASSIFICATION OF DIURETICS

Diuretics can be classified according to their site and mode of action (Fig. 43.1, Table 43.1). They all increase sodium and water excretion and variably modify electrolyte excretion (Table 43.2). *Filtration diuretics* increase salt and water excretion by primarily increasing GFR. *Osmotic diuretics* depress salt and electrolyte reabsorption in the proximal tubule and in loop of Henle. *Inhibitors of carbonic anhydrase* act primarily on the proximal tubule. The most commonly used diuretics inhibit Na^+ reabsorption either in the ascending limb of loop of Henle (*loop diuretics*), in the distal convoluted tubule (*thiazide and thiazide-like diuretics*), or in the late distal tubule and collecting duct (*K^+-sparing* diuretics) (12,10). New diuretics are being developed with different modes of action (*natriuretic peptides, adenosine antagonists, vasopressin antagonists*). All diuretics share adverse effects, which are actually extension of their primary effects on electrolyte excretion (Table 43.3), as well as nonelectrolyte adverse effects (Table 43.4).

FILTRATION DIURETICS

Agents that increase diuresis by increasing GFR are sometimes called *filtration diuretics.* These agents include the glucocorticoids and theophylline, as well as inotropic agents such as isoproterenol, dopamine and dobutamine. By increasing GFR, these drugs only moderately increase Na^+ excretion. Part of the natriuresis achieved by filtration diuretics reflects inhibition of tubular Na^+ reabsorption rather than an increase in the Na^+ filtered load only.

TABLE 43.1 Clinical Use of Diuretics

Osmotic diuretics
Oliguric acute renal failure
Cerebral edema
Elevated intrarenal pressure
Carbonic anhydrase inhibitors
Acute mountain sickness
Glaucoma
Epilepsy
Production of alkaline diuresis
Assessment of distal urinary acidification
Loop diuretics
Edematous states
Hypercalcemia
Hyperkalemia
Respiratory disorders in neonates
Oliguric states and prerenal failure
Nephrotic syndrome
Severe hyponatremia
Assessment of distal urinary acidification
Thiazides
Edematous states
Arterial hypertension
Hypercalciuria
Bronchopulmonary dysplasia
Nephrogenic diabetes insipidus
Diagnosis of renal tubular hypokalemic disorders
Potassium-sparing diuretics
Adjunctive therapy with loop or thiazide diuretics
Prevention of hypokalemia
Aquaretics
Promotion of free-water excretion
Hyponatremic states, congestive heart failure

TABLE 43.2 Acute Effects of Diuretics on Electrolyte Excretion[a]

	Na^+	K^+	Ca^{2+}	Mg^{2+}	H^+	Cl^-	HCO_3^-	$H2PO_4^-$	*Uric Acid: Acute*	*Uric Acid: Chronic*
Osmotic diuretics	↑↑	↑	↑	↑↑	?	↑	↑	↑	↑	?
Carbonic anhydrase inhibitors	↑	↑↑	=	~	↓	(↑)	↑↑	↑↑	?	↓
Loop diuretics	↑↑	↑↑	↑↑	↑↑	↑	↑↑	↑	↑	↑	↓
Thiazide diuretics	↑	↑↑	~	V↑	↑	↑	↑	↑	↑	↓
K^+-sparing diuretics	↑	↓	↓	↓	↓	↑	(↑)	=	?	↓

↑↑, marked increase; ↑, moderate increase; (↑), slight increase; ↓, decrease; = , no change; ~, variable effects; V(↑), variable increase; ?, insufficient data.

[a]In the absence of significant volume depletion, which would trigger complex adjustments.

Adapted from Jackson EK. Diuretics. In: Goodman and Gilman's. The Pharmacological basis of Therapeutics (Harman JG, Limbird LE, eds). McGraw-Hill Med. Publ. Div., 10th ed. 2001, p. 764, with permission.

DOPAMINERGIC AGENTS

Dopamine, a naturally occurring catecholamine, acts on the specific dopaminergic receptors DA_1 and DA_2, and also activates the α- and the β-adrenoreceptors. Dopamine may improve renal function by (a) increasing cardiac output through stimulation of the β-adrenergic receptors, (b) increasing blood pressure by inotropic and vasoactive mechanisms, (c) increasing renal perfusion via stimulation of the dopamine receptors in the renal vessels, and (d) directly inhibiting sodium reabsorption (22). The beneficial effects of low-dose dopamine in oliguric states are variable and, when present, modest. Because of a great overlap in the response to dopamine and significant individual variation, no dose is clearly only a beneficial renal dose (23). Even at low doses, dopamine may increase cardiac contractility and systemic vascular resistance and produce tachycardia, arrhythmia, tissue necrosis, and digital gangrene (24). Dopamine also blunts hypoxic ventilatory drive and may increase pulmonary shunt fraction in critically ill patients. Until efficacy and safety are demonstrated in control prospective studies, the use of dopamine as a renal protective agent remains questionable (25). The price of the modest improvement in urine output and sodium excretion with dopamine may be too high.

The same conclusion applies to dopexamine, a dopaminergic agent devoid of action on the α-receptors (26), and probably also to dobutamide, a dopaminergic agent that stimulates the β_1-adrenoreceptors, with little effect on the β_2- and the α-receptors (27).

OSMOTIC DIURETICS

CHEMISTRY

Osmotic diuretics are agents that inhibit the reabsorption of solute and water by altering osmotic driving forces along the nephron. Osmotic diuretics include mannitol, glycerin, isosorbide, and urea. Mannitol, a hexahydric alcohol related to mannose, with a molecular weight of 182 daltons, is most commonly used (28).

MECHANISMS AND SITES OF ACTION

Freely filtered and (mostly) not reabsorbed, osmotic diuretics increase the tubular fluid osmolality, thus impairing the diffusion of water out of the tubular lumen, as well as that of NaCl by a solvent drag effect. The osmotic diuretics act in the proximal tubule and in the loop of

TABLE 43.3 Electrolytes Disturbances Induced by Diuretics

	Osmotic	*Carbon Anhydrase Inhibitors*	*Loop*	*Thiazides*	*K^+-Sparing*
Hypovolemia	+++	–	+++	+	+
Hyponatremia	++	–	++	+++	–
Hypokalemia	++	+	+++	++	–
Hyperkalemia	–	–	–	–	++
Hypercalciuria	+	–	++	–	–
Hypercalcemia	–	–	–	+	–
Hypomagnesemia	+	–	+	+	–
Hypophosphatemia	+	–	+	+	–
Hyperuricemia	–	–	++	++	–
Metabolic acidosis	+	++	–	–	+
Metabolic alkalosis	+	–	++	++	–

Adapted from Sherbotie JR, Kaplan B. Diuretics. In: Pediatr Pharmacol (Aranda J, Yaffé S, eds), chapter 46, Philadelphia, WB Saunders Co, 1992:524–534, with permission.

TABLE 43.4 Nonelectrolytic Side Effects of Diuretics

Osmotic diuretics		Congestive heart failure and pulmonary edema; nausea, vomiting
Carbonic anhydrase inhibitors		Drowsiness, fatigue, central nervous system depression, paresthesia, calculus formation
Loop diuretics		Ototoxicity (usually reversible), nephrocalcinosis in neonates, patent ductus arteriosus in neonates, hyperuricemia, hyperglycemia, hyperlipidemia, hypersensitivity
Thiazides		Hyperglycemia, insulin resistance, hyperlipidemia, hypersensitivity (fever, rash, purpura, anaphylaxis, interstitial nephritis), hyperuricemia
K^+-sparing	Amiloride	Diarrhea, headache
	Triamterene	Glucose intolerance, interstitial nephritis, blood dyscrasias
	Spironolactone	Gynecomastia, hirsutism, peptic ulcers, ataxia, headache

Henle. By attracting water from the intracellular compartment, osmotic diuretics increase ECF volume and renal blood flow. Increased medullary blood flow washes out the hypertonic medulla, thus impairing the concentrating mechanism. By inhibiting NaCl reabsorption out of the water-impermeable thick ascending limb, osmotic diuretics also impair the dilution of urine. Osmotic diuretics increase nonspecifically the excretion of all electrolytes. The natriuresis induced by osmotic diuretics is only about 10% of the filtered load.

PHARMACOKINETIC PROPERTIES

While isosorbide and glycerin can be given orally, mannitol and urea must be administered intravenously. Glycerin is mostly metabolized. Mannitol, urea, and isosorbide are excreted in the urine. The half-life of mannitol is 0.25 to 1.5 hours; it is prolonged in patients with renal failure.

EFFICACY AND THERAPEUTIC USES

Osmotic diuretics increase the excretion of Na^+, K^+, Cl^-, Mg^{2+}, Ca^{2+}, Cl^-, and HCO_3^-. They improve renal perfusion without significantly affecting GFR. Mannitol is used to increase urine flow rate in patients with prerenal failure, to promote the excretion of toxic substances by forced diuresis, and to reduce elevated intracranial and intraocular pressures.
Drug dosage: **see Table 43.5**

Specific Indications

Oliguric Prerenal Failure
Mannitol is infused in oliguric euvolemic patients at a dose of 2 to 5 mL per kg of body weight of 20% mannitol, intravenously over 5 minutes. The diuretic response appears within 1 to 3 hours. While mannitol may promote diuresis, it does not significantly protect GFR (21). In patients receiving radiocontrast agents, mannitol does not appear better than simple hydration with 0.45% NaCl (29). Mannitol is also sometimes used to prevent the occurrence of ARF in patients undergoing cardiac surgery (30). In low–birth-weight infants, mannitol increases the risk of intraventricular (cerebral) hemorrhage; its use should therefore be avoided (31).

Dialysis Disequilibrium
Mannitol can be used to prevent the occurrence of the dialysis disequilibrium syndrome. By compensating the decrease in plasma osmolality induced by dialytic removal of solutes during the dialysis session, mannitol prevents the occurrence of cerebral edema. Mannitol is infused in the second half of the dialysis session at a dose of 2 to 5 mL per kg of 20% mannitol.

Intracranial and Ocular Pressure
Osmotic diuretics are used to reduce cerebral edema and to decrease intraocular pressure in glaucoma, as well as preoperatively in patients requiring ocular surgery.

ADVERSE EFFECTS—INTERACTIONS

Circulatory overload and CHF can occur as a consequence of inadequate expansion of extracellular fluid volume. Fluid and electrolyte imbalance can occur after overuse of mannitol. Extravasation can lead to tissue necrosis.

INHIBITORS OF CARBONIC ANHYDRASE

CHEMISTRY

Acetazolamide, a sulfonamide derivative, is the main inhibitor of carbonic anhydrase used in humans.

MECHANISMS AND SITES OF ACTION

Inhibition of carbonic anhydrase, present in all tubular cells and in the brush border of proximal tubular cells, results in depressed cellular formation and subsequent secretion of H^+. As a consequence, the HCO_3^- ions that are normally reabsorbed by combining with H^+ in the tubular lumen are excreted in the urine. Decreased H^+

TABLE 43.5 Dosages of Common Diuretics

Drug	Route/Interval (q hr)	Dosage (mg/kg/day)	Half-Life $t_{1/2}$ (hr)	Comments
Mannitol	i.v., 2–4	200–500	0.3–2	Risk of expansion of ECV
Acetazolamide	p.o., 6–8	5	6–9	Not effective at GFR <20[a]; self-limited action as plasma HCO_3^- falls
Furosemide	p.o., 12–24	1–2	~1.5	Effective at GFR <10[a]
	i.v., 12–24	0.5–1.5	~1.5	Doses may be increased up to 5 mg/kg in CRF
	c.i.v.i.	100–200 μg/kg/hr		Hypokalemia; Mg, Ca depletion; ototoxicity; metabolic alkalosis
Torasemide	p.o.	0.5–1	~3.5	Longer $t_{1/2}$ and larger duration than furosemide; effective at GFR <10[a]; idem furosemide
Ethacrynic acid	p.o., 12–24	1–2	~1	Effective at GFR <10[a]; idem furosemide
Bumetanide	p.o., 12–24	0.01–0.10	~1	Effective at GFR <10[a]; idem furosemide
	i.v., 12–24	0.01–0.05		
	c.i.v.i.	5–10 μg/kg/hr	~1	
Hydrochlorothiazide	p.o. 12–24	1–3	~2.5	Not effective at GFR <20[a]; hypokalemia, metabolic alkalosis
Chlorthalidone	p.o., 24–48	0.5–2.0	45	Not effective at GFR <20[a]; hypokalemia, metabolic alkalosis
Metolazone	p.o. 12–24	0.2–0.4	8–10	Effective at GFR <20[a]; hypokalemia
Spironolactone	p.o. 6–12	1–3	~1.6	Delayed effect. Avoid in CRF or K supplementation hyperkalemia, acidosis
Canreonate-K	i.v. 24	4–10	~16	Single i.v. dose; hyperkalemia, acidosis
Triamterene	p.o. 12–24	2–4	~4.2	Avoid in CRF or K supplementation hyperkalemia, acidosis
Amiloride	p.o. 24	0.5	~21	Avoid in CRF or K supplementation hyperkalemia, acidosis

civi, constant i.v. infusion; CRF, chronic renal failure; ECV, extracellular volume; i.v., intravenous; p.o., oral; q, every.
[a]GFR, glomerular filtration rate (mL/min/1.73 m^2).

secretion is associated with decreased Na^+ reabsorption. In the distal tubule, K^+ secretion is enhanced because of the increased delivery of Na^+ to the late distal tubule and because of reduced H^+ available for secretion in exchange with Na^+ (1). Carbonic anhydrase inhibitors are weak diuretics, at best producing the excretion of 5% of the Na^+ and water filtered load. The action of carbonic anhydrase inhibitors is self-limiting. The excretion of HCO_3^- decreases in parallel with the development of metabolic acidosis in response to carbonic anhydrase inhibition.

PHARMACOKINETIC PROPERTIES

Acetazolamide is readily absorbed; it has a 100% oral availability and a half-life of 6 to 9 hours. It is eliminated in the urine. Acetazolamide crosses the placental barrier and is secreted in breast milk.

EFFICACY AND THERAPEUTIC USES

Acetazolamide increases the urinary excretion of bicarbonate, sodium, and potassium, promoting alkaline diuresis. The mild metabolic acidosis induced by the continuous administration of acetazolamide limits the diuretic effects of the agent. Acetazolamide is consequently not used presently for its natriuretic effect. It may be useful to alkalinize the urine when necessary, as for instance, when chemotherapy is given. Acetazolamide has useful specific indications related to its ability to inhibit the carbonic anhydrase in different systems. Such indications are mountain sickness, glaucoma, and specific respiratory disorders. Acetazolamide can be a beneficial adjunctive agent in the pharmacotherapy of refractory epilepsy (32).

SPECIFIC INDICATIONS

Assessment of Distal Tubular Acidification

Acetazolamide can also be used to assess reliably the distal acidification ability by measuring the urine minus blood PCO_2 in alkaline urine (33).
Drug dosage: **see Table 43.5**

ADVERSE EFFECTS—INTERACTIONS

The occurrence of metabolic acidosis is common if the urinary losses of HCO_3^- are not substituted. Paresthesias, drowsiness, rash, and fever are not uncommon. Formation of renal calculi, rare blood dyscrasias, and hepatic failure are occasionally seen.

LOOP DIURETICS: INHIBITION OF Na^+, K^+, $2Cl^-$ SYMPORT

CHEMISTRY

Loop diuretics form a group of diuretics with diverse chemical structures (9,34). Furosemide and bumetanide are sulfonamide derivatives, torasemide is a sulfonylurea, and ethacrynic acid is a phenoxyacetic acid derivative.

MECHANISMS AND SITES OF ACTION

Loop diuretics block the Na^+, K^+, $2Cl^-$ symporter in the thick ascending limb of loop of Henle, where 25% of NaCl filtered load are reabsorbed. They are consequently highly efficacious, as only a small proportion of the filtered load of sodium that escapes reabsorption in the loop can be reabsorbed downstream. Loop diuretics act from within the tubular lumen where they are secreted via the organic acid pump. The effect of loop diuretics is more closely related to their urinary excretion rate than to their plasma concentration. By inhibiting NaCl reabsorption in loop of Henle, loop diuretics abolish the lumen positive voltage and thus the driving force for Ca^{2+} and Mg^{2+} reabsorption. They consequently increase Ca^{2+} and Mg^{2+} excretion. Loop diuretics significantly increase K^+ excretion. Inhibition of NaCl transport upstream of the distal tubule results in increased Na^+ delivery to the late portion of the distal tubule and cortical collecting duct. This part of the nephron responds by increasing K^+ and H^+ secretion. This secretion is also stimulated by the state of secondary hyperaldosteronism usually present as a consequence of diuretic-induced decrease in ECF volume. By inhibiting NaCl reabsorption in the water-impermeable thick ascending limb of loop of Henle, loop diuretics interfere both with the diluting and the concentrating mechanism. Loop diuretics do not inhibit $HCO3^-$ reabsorption.

PHARMACOKINETIC PROPERTIES

Furosemide is rapidly absorbed from the gastrointestinal tract, with a bioavailability close to 60% to 70%. It is 99% bound to plasma albumin. Furosemide and ethacrynic acid displace bilirubin from albumin-binding sites (10). Furosemide is mainly excreted unchanged in the urine. The diuretic response to loop diuretics appears within a few minutes after intravenous administration and within 30 to 60 minutes after oral administration. The effect does not last more than 2 hours after intravenous injection and 6 hours after oral administration. Nonrenal clearance is increased in patients with chronic renal failure. The half-life is prolonged in patients with renal and liver insufficiency and in premature and term neonates in whom half-lives as long as 45 hours have been observed. Although the pharmacology of furosemide has been well studied in children (35) and neonates (36), that of other loop diuretics is not as well defined. The pharmacokinetics and pharmacodynamics of bumetanide have been studied in critically ill children (37) and critically ill infants (38). Diuretic efficiency of bumetanide was maximal at doses of 0.005 to 0.010 mg per kg (39). The efficacy of torasemide has been assessed in immature animals (40), and its efficacy and safety in children with heart failure. A significant improvement in heart failure was observed, along with a potassium-sparing effect that was subscribed to the antialdosterone properties of this agent (41). Loop diuretics cross the placental barrier and are secreted in breast milk.

EFFICACY AND THERAPEUTIC USES

Loop diuretics are the most potent natriuretic agents, also markedly increasing Cl^-, K^+, Ca^{2+}, and Mg^{2+} excretion (9). They have steep dose-response curves. They remain active in patients with advanced renal failure. Loop diuretics are the most frequently used diuretics in children, infants, and neonates. Specific indications include oliguric states associated with prerenal failure, various respiratory disorders such as respiratory distress syndrome (RDS), bronchopulmonary dysplasia and asthma, indomethacin-associated oliguria, and hypercalcemic states. Loop diuretics can decrease blood pressure in hypertensive children, but their short duration of action makes them less suitable than the thiazides in this indication.

Continuous Intravenous Infusion of Loop Diuretics

Clinical trials in infants indicate that continuous infusion therapy can produce more efficient and better-controlled diuresis with less fluid shifts and greater hemodynamic stability (42). Administration of a small loading dose of the diuretic before starting the continuous infusion accelerates the diuretic response (34). Alternatively, starting with a relatively high continuous infusion dose (0.2 mg per kg per hour) of furosemide may be optimal (43). In hemodynamically stable postoperative cardiac patients, intermittent furosemide has been claimed to be more efficacious than continuous infusion of furosemide (44).

Indications

Edematous States

CHF is the most common indication to the use of loop diuretics in neonates and infants. In infants with severe CHF, the diuretic effect of furosemide is inversely related to serum aldosterone levels. The concomitant administration of a K^+-sparing diuretic improves the response to loop diuretics (45). Furosemide increases the peripheral venous capacitance and can thus be useful independently from its diuretic effect. In adults, torasemide has been shown to be at least as effective as furosemide in reducing salt and water retention (46), to have a longer duration of action, and to reduce overall treatment costs of CHF in comparison with furosemide (47).

Nephrotic Syndrome

In hypovolemic patients with massive nephrotic edema, intravenous furosemide can be used to promote sodium and water excretion. In hypovolemic patients, furosemide (1 to 2 mg per kg) should be given only after the expansion of the extracellular space with intravenous albumin (5 mL per kg of 20% albumin in 60 minutes). This regimen usually results in a loss of 1% to 2% of body weight. The dose can be repeated. The effect is transient but may be useful in patients with severe ascitis and/or pulmonary edema. The therapy may be associated with potentially serious complications such as CHF or respiratory distress (48). Coadministration of intravenous furosemide and mannitol (5 mL per kg of a 20% solution) could be a safe, inexpensive, and effective alternative to the classic furosemide–albumin regimen (49). In hypervolemic patients, the use of furosemide alone appears safe and effective (50).

Specific Indications

Oliguric States

Furosemide is frequently used in oliguric states secondary to prerenal or renal failure, in the hope of promoting diuresis and improving renal function. Although furosemide may increase urine output and facilitate the clinical management of the patient, it is unlikely to improve GFR. By inducing diuresis and possibly hypovolemia, loop diuretics carry the risk of further stressing the oliguric kidney. There is as yet no clinical (21) or experimental (51) evidence that loop diuretics can prevent ARF or improve the outcome of patients with ARF.

Respiratory Distress Syndrome

Furosemide administration has produced conflicting results in preterm neonates with RDS (10). While furosemide usually acutely induces diuresis, and a transient improvement in pulmonary function, a recent critical review of the literature (52) failed to support the routine administration of furosemide (or any diuretic) in preterm infants with RDS and concluded that elective administration of diuretics should be weighed against the risk of inducing cardiovascular complications.

Preterm Infants with or Developing Chronic Lung Disease

Loop diuretics have been given to preterm infants with chronic lung disease (CLD) in the hope of decreasing the need for oxygen or ventilatory support. A critical review of the available data of the literature concluded that in preterm infants younger than 3 weeks developing CLD, furosemide had either inconstant effects or no detectable effects (53). In infants older than 3 weeks with CLD, the acute intravenous administration of furosemide (1 mg per kg) improved lung compliance and airway resistance for 1 hour. Chronic administration of furosemide improved both oxygenation and lung compliance. However, the reviewers concluded that routine or sustained use of loop diuretics in infants with or developing CLD could not be recommended until randomized trials assessing their effects on survival, duration of ventilatory support and oxygen administration, potential complications, and long-term outcome are available (53). A similar conclusion was drawn from studies on the effect of aerosolized furosemide in preterm infants with CLD. Although not enough information was available in premies younger than 3 weeks, data in preterm infants older than 3 weeks with CLD showed that a single dose of aerosolized furosemide improved pulmonary mechanisms. But in view of the lack of data from randomized trials concerning the effects on important clinical outcomes, routine or sustained use of aerosolized loop diuretics in infants with or developing CLD cannot be recommended (54).

Posthemorrhagic Ventricular Dilatation

A critical review of randomized trials in newborn infants with posthemorrhagic ventricular dilatation (55) concluded that acetazolamide and furosemide therapy is neither effective nor safe in treating preterm infants with posthemorrhagic ventricular dilatation. The largest trial in 177 infants showed that acetazolamide and furosemide treatment resulted in a borderline increase in the risk for motor impairment at 1 year and in an increased risk for nephrocalcinosis, without decreasing the risk for disability, chronic motor impairment, or death (55).

Indomethacin-induced Oliguria

Oliguria occurs frequently after administration of indomethacin to close a patent ductus arteriosus (PDA). Inhibition of prostaglandin synthesis by indomethacin is responsible for the oliguria. Because furosemide increases prostaglandin production, it could potentially help prevent indomethacin-related toxicity and also decrease ductal response to indomethacin. Available studies indicate that furosemide increased urine output in all patients, leading to a 5% weight loss during a three-dose course. It increases creatinine clearance only in patients with initial blood urea nitrogen/creatinine ratio of less than 20 mg per mg. A critical review concluded that there was as yet not enough evidence to support the administration of furosemide to preterm infants treated with indomethacin for PDA (56). Also noteworthy is the conclusion that there is as yet not enough evidence from randomized trials to show that there is any value in giving dopamine to prevent renal dysfunction in indomethacin-treated preterm infants (57).

Hypercalcemic States

Loop diuretics can promote calcium excretion and decrease hypercalcemia. Isotonic saline must be infused concomitantly to prevent volume depletion.

Severe Hyponatremia

Severe hyponatremia can be treated by loop diuretics and the concomitant isovolumetric infusion of hypertonic saline.

Intratracheal Furosemide

Direct intratracheal administration of furosemide has been claimed to produce beneficial effects in children with asthma, in infants with bronchopulmonary dysplasia, and in toddlers with compromised lung mechanics after cardiac surgery. In the latter study, a systemic effect was observed within 15 minutes after intratracheal instillation of the agent (58).

Assessment of Distal Renal Acidification

The simultaneous administration of furosemide and fludrocortisone has been shown to be an easy, effective, and well-tolerated alternative to standard ammonium chloride loading to assess urinary acidification and confirm the diagnosis of distal renal tubular acidosis (59).

Drug dosage: **see Table 43.5**

ADVERSE EFFECTS—INTERACTIONS

Because of their efficacy, common adverse effects including volume depletion, postural hypotension, dizziness and syncope, hyponatremia, and hypokalemia are commonly observed. These effects are dose dependent and often occur after overzealous use of large doses of diuretics or chronic administration.

Hypochloremic Metabolic Alkalosis

This condition occurs frequently as a consequence of direct stimulation by loop diuretics of H^+ secretion in the collecting tubule.

Hypercalciuria

Elevated Ca^{2+} urinary losses in response to loop diuretics are associated with a significant risk of *nephrocalcinosis* in premature infants (60), of secondary hyperparathyroidism, of bone resorption, and of rickets. When prolonged, hypercalciuria may lead to renal impairment (61). Although thiazide diuretics decrease calcium and oxalate excretion, adding thiazides to loop diuretics did not appear beneficial (62).

Patent Ductus Arteriosus

The suggestion that by stimulating prostaglandin synthesis furosemide could promote PDA has not been confirmed. The beneficial renal effect of combining furosemide and indomethacin is still controversial (34).

Ototoxicity

The use of furosemide has been identified as an independent risk factor for sensorineural hearing loss in preterm infants (63). Hearing loss may be transient or permanent. It is usually associated with elevated blood concentrations of loop diuretics. The coadministration of loop diuretics and aminoglycosides increases the risk of ototoxicity. By avoiding elevated peak concentrations of furosemide, the continuous infusion decreases the risk of ototoxicity (34).

Chronic Use

Increased distal delivery of Na^+ as a consequence of loop diuretic administration leads to hypertrophy of distal nephrons with consequent hyperreabsorption of Na^+.

Miscellaneous

Pancreatitis, jaundice, deterioration of glucose tolerance, thrombocytopenia, and serious skin disorders occur occasionally. The majority of adverse effects occur with the use of high doses.

Interactions

Drug interactions may occur with the coadministration of nephrotoxic antibiotics, nonsteroidal anti-inflammatory drugs, anticoagulants, and cisplatin.

DISTAL CONVOLUTED TUBULE: INHIBITORS OF Na^+, Cl^- SYMPORT

CHEMISTRY

The benzothiadiazide derivatives are sulfonamides. They are weak diuretics that inhibit the reabsorption of NaCl at the diluting site in the early distal tubule. The main thiazides include chlorothiazide and hydrochlorothiazide. Thiazide-like agents such as chlorthalidone and metolazone belong to this group.

MECHANISMS AND SITES OF ACTION

The thiazides are organic anions that gain access to the tubular lumen by filtration and by secretion in the proximal tubule. They decrease NaCl reabsorption in the distal convoluted tubule by inhibiting the Na^+–Cl^- apical symporter. This symporter, sometimes called ENCC1 or TSC, is predominantly expressed in the epithelial cells of the distal convoluted tubule. Its expression is upregulated by aldosterone (1). To reach their site of action on the luminal side of the tubular cells, the thiazides must be secreted by the anionic organic acid pathway in the proximal tubule. Approximately 4% to 5% of the Na^+ filtered load is being reabsorbed in the distal collecting duct, and inhibition of Na^+ reabsorption at this site can only modestly increase NaCl excretion. Some of the thiazides also slightly increase the excretion of HCO_3^- by weakly inhibiting the carbonic anhydrase. By increasing Na^+ delivery to the late distal tubule, the thiazides lead to increased reabsorption of Na^+ in the late distal tubule, in exchange for K^+ and H^+, which are lost in the urine. By inhibiting NaCl reabsorption in the early distal tubule, the thiazides blunt the ability to dilute the urine. They do not interfere with the concentrating mechanism. The thiazides stimulate Ca^{2+} reabsorption in the distal tubule, probably by opening the apical membrane Ca^{2+} channels. The thiazides (but not metolazone) are ineffective at GFRs below 30 mL per minute per 1.73 m^2.

PHARMACOKINETIC PROPERTIES

The thiazides are fairly rapidly absorbed after oral administration. They variably bind to plasma proteins. They are eliminated unchanged, exclusively (chlorothiazide, hydrochlorothiazide, chlortalidone) or in great part (~80%) (metolazone) in the urine. Administration of thiazides initiates diuresis in 2 hours, an effect that lasts for 12 hours. The response to metolazone is somewhat more rapid (1 hour) and lasts longer (12 to 24 hours). The thiazides cross the placental barrier and are secreted in breast milk.

EFFICACY AND THERAPEUTIC USES

Thiazide diuretics moderately increase the excretion of Na^+, Cl^-, and water. All thiazides (chlorothiazide, hydrochlorothiazide) and thiazide-like diuretics have overall similar effects when used in maximal doses. When administered chronically, they decrease the excretion of Ca^{2+}, as well as that of uric acid, probably as a consequence of increased proximal reabsorption due to volume depletion. The excretion of Mg^{2+} is somewhat increased, as is the excretion of K^+ and fixed acids. Increased Na^+ delivery to the late distal tubule and collecting duct is responsible for the increased excretion of K^+ and fixed acids. Because of the risk of inducing hypokalemia, prophylactic coadministration of K^+-sparing diuretics may be indicated to prevent the occurrence of severe hypokalemia.

Alternatively, potassium supplementation may be useful in patients at risk. Magnesium supplementation may also be necessary. The thiazides, but not metolazone, increase the excretion of HCO_3^-. In the absence of significant volume depletion, the thiazides do not normally influence renal hemodynamics and GFR. In contrast with the thiazides and chlortalidone, metolazone remains effective at GFRs below 30 mL per minute per 1.73 m^2.

Indications

The main indications for the administration of thiazide diuretics include edematous states, hypertension, and a few specific indications.

Specific Indications

Hypercalciuria

The thiazides decrease calcium excretion and this effect may be useful in states of idiopathic hypercalciuria, as well as to prevent calcium losses in patients receiving glucocorticoids (64). They have been associated with loop diuretics to decrease the risk of hypercalciuria and nephrocalcinosis in very low–birth-weight infants undergoing loop diuretic therapy, with disappointing results (8). The thiazides have been used to prevent renal stone formation in susceptible patients. The use of thiazides has been associated with a rise in total serum cholesterol and in the low-density lipoprotein/low-density lipoprotein ratio, indicating that the risks and benefits of the thiazide therapy should be considered before starting treatment (65). In children with X-linked hypophosphatemia on renal phosphate and vitamin D therapy, hydrochlorothiazide decreased the urinary excretion of calcium but did not reverse the nephrocalcinosis (66).

Proximal Tubular Renal Acidosis

The thiazides have been used to raise the plasma bicarbonate concentration in proximal renal tubular acidosis. This effect is the consequence of volume contraction induced by the thiazides, a chronic condition that is deleterious for growth.

Nephrogenic Diabetes Insipidus

The thiazides have been successfully used in children with nephrogenic diabetes insipidus. By inducing volume contraction, they enhance the proximal tubular reabsorption of water and electrolytes, thus significantly decreasing urine output. While usefully decreasing urine output, volume contraction may inhibit growth in young children with nephrogenic diabetes insipidus. The concomitant use of hydrochlorothiazide and amiloride obviates the need for the K^+ supplementation and has been shown as useful as the standard treatment with hydrochlorothiazide and indomethacin (20,67) in reducing urine output.

Chronic Lung Disease

Thiazide and thiazide-like diuretics have been used in the hope of improving pulmonary mechanisms and clinical outcome in preterm infants with CLD. A critical analysis of available well-planned studies led to the conclusion that in preterm infants older than 8 weeks with CLD, a 4-week treatment with thiazides and spironolactone reduced the need for furosemide, improved lung compliance, decreased the risk of death, and tended to decrease the risk for lack of extubation after 8 weeks in intubated infants who did not have access to corticosteroids, bronchodilators, or aminophylline. There was little evidence to support any benefit on the need for ventilatory support, length of hospital stay, or long-term outcome in infants receiving current therapy. There was also no evidence to support the hypothesis that adding spironolactone to thiazides or metolazone to furosemide improved the outcome of preterm infants (68). The addition of K^+-sparing diuretics to thiazide did, however, decrease the risk of hypokalemia.

DIAGNOSIS OF RENAL TUBULAR HYPOKALEMIC DISORDERS

Assessment of the maximal diuretic response induced by the administration of hydrochlorothiazide (1 mg per kg, orally) allows to differentiate Gielmann's from Bartter's syndrome, the former presenting with a blunted response to the diuretic agent (69).

Drug dosage: **see Table 43.5**

ADVERSE EFFECTS—INTERACTIONS

Thiazides may adversely affect water balance and induce electrolyte imbalances (Table 43.3). Other side effects include gastrointestinal disturbances, hypersensitivity reactions, cholestatic jaundice, pancreatitis, thrombocytopenia, and hyperglycemia in diabetic and susceptible patients, and hyperlipidemia. Precipitation of hepatic encephalopathy has been observed in patients with hepatic cirrhosis. The thiazides displace bilirubin from albumin and should be cautiously administered to patients with jaundice.

LATE DISTAL AND CORTICAL COLLECTING DUCT: K^+-SPARING DRUGS

CHEMISTRY

Two types of diuretics form the group of K^+-sparing diuretics: (a) the inhibitors of a renal epithelial Na^+ channels and (b) the antagonists of mineralocorticoid receptors. The overall effects of these two groups of diuretics differ only in their mode of action.

MECHANISMS AND SITES OF ACTION

The antagonists of the action of aldosterone on the principal cells of the collecting duct increase Na^+ excretion and decrease K^+ and H^+ secretion. Spironolactone, the main agent in this group, competitively inhibits the binding of aldosterone to the mineralocorticoid receptor, thus decreasing the synthesis of aldosterone-induced proteins. The aldosterone antagonists have greater effects in situations of hyperaldosteronism. They do not modify the renal hemodynamics. Highly selective antagonists of the mineralocorticoid receptor are currently under investigation (70).

The epithelial Na^+ channel blockers amiloride and triamterene block the entry of Na^+ into the cell through the

Na^+-selective channels ($E_{NA}C$) in the apical membrane. Because of changes in electrical profile across the apical membrane, the diffusion of both H^+ and K^+ from cells into tubular fluid decreases. Activation of the renin–angiotensin–aldosterone system by the diuretics also impairs the excretion of K^+, H^+, Ca^{2+}, and Mg^{2+}. $E_{NA}C$ blockers do not affect renal hemodynamics.

PHARMACOKINETIC PROPERTIES

Spironolactone is rapidly absorbed from the gastrointestinal tract, with a bioavailability close to 90%. It is 90% bound to plasma proteins and is excreted mainly in the urine and to a lesser extent in the feces. Spironolactone has a slow onset of action, requiring 2 to 3 days for maximum effect.

Cancreonate–potassium has similar actions to those of spironolactone. It is available for intravenous administration.

Amiloride is incompletely absorbed from the gastrointestinal tract with a bioavailability of only 50%. It is not bound to plasma proteins and is excreted unchanged in the urine. Its half-life is 6 to 9 hours. It is prolonged in patients with hepatic or renal failure.

Triamterene is unreliably absorbed. It is metabolized by hepatic conjugation. One-fifth of the dose is excreted unchanged in the urine. Its half-life is 1 to 3 hours.

All K^+-sparing diuretics cross the placental barrier and are secreted in breast milk.

EFFICACY AND THERAPEUTIC USES

K^+-sparing diuretics are also often used in association with thiazide diuretics in the management of preterm infants with CLD. Although they certainly decrease the risk of hypokalemia and facilitate the clinical management of the infants, there is as yet no definite proof that their association to thiazide improves the long-term outcome of preterm infants with CLD.

The overall effects on electrolyte excretion are similar for spironolactone, amiloride, and triamterene. They are weak natriuretic agents that reduce the excretion of potassium and hydrogen ions. K^+-sparing diuretics are mainly used in Na^+-retaining states in association with loop or thiazide diuretics. They enhance the natriuretic effect while at the same time limiting K^+ losses. Refractory edema secondary to CHF, cirrhosis of the liver, and the nephrotic syndrome represent the most common indications for the use of K-sparing diuretics. In these conditions associated with secondary hyperaldosteronism, spironolactone is the first-choice agent provided renal function is not impaired (71). Because they induce K^+ retention, K^+-sparing diuretics should not be used in patients with impaired renal function or in those receiving K^+ supplementation. They should also be avoided in patients prone to develop metabolic acidosis. The respiratory function and sputum excretion of patients with cystic fibrosis have been improved by the inhalation of 10^{-3} M amiloride, possibly by the blocking effect of $E_{NA}C$ in pulmonary tissue (72). A multicenter randomized double-blind placebo-controlled trial has not confirmed the beneficial effect of aerosolized amiloride (73). Amiloride has been successfully used in association with hydrochlorothiazide in patients with nephrogenic diabetes insipidus, obviating the need for using indomethacin (20).

***Drug dosage:* see Table 43.5.**

ADVERSE EFFECTS—INTERACTIONS

The main adverse effect of K^+-sparing diuretics is to increase the K^+ plasma concentration to harmful levels. Close monitoring of K^+ concentration is thus mandatory. Gastrointestinal disturbances, dizziness, photosensitivity, and blood dyscrasias have been reported after the use of triamterene.

Significant adverse effects have been observed with spironolactone: gynecomastia, hirsutism, impotence, and menstrual irregularities can occur. Gynecomastia in males is related to both the dose and duration of treatment. Breast enlargement and tenderness occur in women. The pathogenesis of the adverse effects of spironolactone on the endocrine system is probably related to an antiadrenergic action and to reduced 17 hydroxylase activity.

Interactions

K^+-sparing diuretics should not be used in patients receiving angiotensin-converting enzyme inhibitors, as the association can worsen the risk of hyperkalemia.

The half-life of amiloride is prolonged in patients with hepatic or renal failure.

NEW DEVELOPMENT IN DIURETIC THERAPY

Three categories of diuretics are under development:

1. The natriuretic peptides
2. The adenosine A_1 receptor antagonists
3. The AVP antagonists

Natriuretic Peptides

The ANP and the B-type natriuretic peptide (BNP) are two peptides with natriuretic and diuretic properties (74). Both are released by cardiac cells in the atria in response to increased blood volume. ANP (28 amino acids) and BNP (32 amino acids) act via the natriuretic peptide receptor A (NPR-A). In addition to increasing the excretion of Na^+, both peptides inhibit the sympathetic system and the renin–angiotensin–aldosterone system. They also relax vascular smooth muscle. The ANP and BNP are degraded by the metalloproteinase neutral endopeptidase 24.11 (NEP). Urodilatin is a noncirculating natriuretic peptide (32 amino acids) secreted by distal tubular cells and is not degraded by the NEP located in the proximal tubular cells (75).

ANP favors filtration by relaxing the afferent artery and the mesangial cells (76). The NPs inhibit Na^+ proximal reabsorption and decrease distal Na^+ reabsorption indirectly by blunting angiotensin II and aldosterone synthesis and directly by inhibiting the thiazide-sensitive Na^+ channel. ANP increases diuresis by inhibiting the action of AVP on water permeability.

Therapy

Enhancing the activity of the NPs could help patients presenting with inappropriate salt and water retention (77).

This can be achieved by (a) administration of exogenous ANP and BNP, (b) using nonpeptide antagonists of the NP-A-receptor, and (c) using NEP 24.11 inhibitors. Studies with BNP (77) have produced promising results in situations of heart failure. Recent clinical trials have, however, cast doubt on the safety and effectiveness of the ANP and BNP analogues (78).

The use of NEP 24.11 also appears promising, resulting in significant natriuresis and diuresis. Because NEP also inhibits the degradation of angiotensin II, angiotensin-converting enzyme (ACE) inhibitors should be associated with NEP 24.11 inhibitors in order to prevent vasoconstriction that may be secondary to stimulation of the renin–angiotensin–aldosterone system in response to loss of Na^+ and water. Drugs like omapatrilat, which inhibit both the ACE and the NEP, are being successfully investigated in adults presenting with chronic heart failure (79). Pediatric studies are not available.

Adenosine A_1 Receptor Antagonists

Adenosine is produced in the kidney. In physiologic conditions, it participates in the regulation of GFR, renin secretion, and sodium reabsorption (80). Adenosine acts on four types of receptors, the A_1, A_{2A}, A_{2B}, and A_3 (81). The A_1 receptors are widely distributed in the kidney and found in the renal vasculature, glomeruli, juxtaglomerular apparatus, cortical tubules, ascending limbs of loops of Henle, and collecting duct cells (82). Stimulation of the A_1 receptors inhibits adenylate cyclase and activates K^+ channels. A_1 receptors participate in the tubuloglomerular feedback mechanism by vasoconstricting the afferent arteriole. Intact adenosine A_1 receptors are required for the diuretic and natriuretic action of theophylline and caffeine (83,84). The A_2 receptors activate adenylate cyclase and vasodilate the efferent arteriole (81).

Theophylline is a nonselective antagonist of adenosine receptors (85). When used in low doses (0.5 mg per kg) in newborn rabbits, theophylline increased Na^+ and water excretion (86). This natriuretic response, which occurs without change in GFR, could be mediated by blockade of the A_1 receptors. When used in oliguric acute hypoxemic vasomotor nephropathy in newborn animals, theophylline protects renal function and increases urine output (86). The same benefit has been observed in randomized clinical studies with the prophylactic use of theophylline in term neonates with perinatal asphyxia (87–90) and with the curative use of theophylline in preterm neonates with RDS (91) and in critically ill children (92). In all studies, the renal benefit of theophylline was observed without apparent adverse effects on the central nervous system. Further large clinical trials should confirm the usefulness of low-dose theophylline as a diuretic and renal protective agent.

Arginine Vasopressin Antagonists

AVP, the ADH, acts on three types of receptors: (a) the V_{1A} receptors mediating vasoconstriction, (b) the V_{1B} mediating the release of adrenocorticotropic hormone, and (c) the V_2 receptors mediating free-water reabsorption in the collecting duct. AVP also stimulates Na^+–K^+–$2Cl^-$ cotransport in the ascending limb of loop of Henle via V_2 receptors.

Orally active nonpeptide-selective V_2 antagonists have been developed (93,94). They include the following agents: lixivaptan, tolvaptan, and satavaptan. Experimental and adult human studies demonstrate that these agents increase the excretion of free water and decrease the urine osmolality in a dose-dependent manner. They may thus prove useful in treating hyponatremic states (74,94).

Blockade of V_2 receptors results in increased levels of AVP. This can lead to stimulation of the V_1 receptors and result in vasoconstriction. Combined V_{1A} and V_2 receptors blockade may prevent this adverse hemodynamic response. The use of the V_{1A} + V_2 receptor antagonist conivaptan in adult patients with chronic heart failure resulted in improved diuresis, pulmonary capillary wedge pressure, cardiac index, systemic and pulmonary resistance, blood pressure, and heart rate remaining unchanged (95). These promising results in patients with heart failure were not confirmed by subsequent studies (96), leading to the conclusion that conivaptan could not be recommended for patients with CHF, unless the benefit of correcting the associated hyponatremia outweighs the potential risk of adverse effects.

Based on currently available adult studies, oral or intravenous conivaptan, a dual V_{1A} + V_2 receptor antagonist, appears to be effective in inducing aquaresis to correct hyponatremia with short-term use in both hypovolemic and hypervolemic patients (96). One of the most concerning issues with the use of any V_2 receptor antagonist in the treatment of hyponatremia is the rate of correction of serum sodium concentration. The occurrence of hypokalemia in up to 22% of patients is also of considerable concern. This hypokalemia could be due to renal potassium wasting secondary to increased diuresis with consequent facilitated potassium secretion.

Worth mentioning is the observation that AVP is a powerful modulator of cystogenesis. AVP V_2 receptor antagonists indeed inhibit the formation and growth of renal cysts in animal models of cystic kidney disease, presumably by down-regulating cAMP signaling, cell proliferation, and chloride-driven fluid secretion. Clinical studies in patients with autosomal polycystic kidney disease (PKD) are presently being performed. Preliminary results of phase 2 and phases 2 to 3 clinical trials suggest that the antagonist tolvaptan is safe and well tolerated in autosomal dominant PKD (97). These results provide further support for clinical trials of V_2 receptor antagonists in PKD.

The use of V_2 or V_{1A} + V_2 receptor antagonists has not been validated in neonates, infants, or children.

REFERENCES

1. Giebisch G, Windhager E. The urinary system. Part VI. In: Boron WF, Boulpaep EL, eds. *Medical Physiology*. Philadelphia, PA: Saunders, 2003:735–876.
2. Garty H, Palmer LG. Epithelial sodium channels: function, structure, and regulation. *Physiol Rev* 1997;77:359–396.
3. Yamamoto T, Sasaki S. Aquaporins in the kidney: emerging new aspects. *Kidney Int* 1998;54:1041–1051.
4. Guignard JP. Renal function in the newborn infant. *Pediatr Clin North Am* 1982;29:777–790.
5. Guignard JP, John EG. Renal function in the tiny, premature infant. *Clin Perinatol* 1986;13:377–401.
6. Guignard JP, Gouyon JB. Body fluid homeostasis in the newborn infant with congestive heart failure: effects of diuretics. *Clin Perinatol* 1988;15:447–466.

7. Guignard JP. Renal morphogenesis and development of renal function. In: Taeusch HW, Ballard RA, Gleason CA, eds. *Avery's diseases of the newborn*, 8th ed. Philadelphia, PA: WB Saunders Co, 2005:1257–1266.
8. Guignard JP. Postnatal development of glomerular filtration rate in neonates. In: Polin RA, Fox WW, Abman SH, eds. *Fetal and neonatal medicine*, 3rd ed, vol 2. Orlando: WB Saunders Co, 2004:1256–1266.
9. Brater DC. Diuretic therapy. *N Engl J Med* 1998;339:387–395.
10. Chemtob S, Kaplan BS, Sherbotie JR, et al. Pharmacology of diuretics in the newborn. *Pediatr Clin North Am* 1989;36:1231–1250.
11. Lowrie L. Diuretic therapy of heart failure in infants and children. *Prog Pediatr Cardiol* 2000;12:45–55.
12. Wells TG. The pharmacology and therapeutics of diuretics in the pediatric patient. *Pediatr Clin North Am* 1990;37:463–504.
13. Morrison RT. Edema and principles of diuretic use. *Med Clin North Am* 1997;81:689–704.
14. Schrier RW, Fassett RG. A critique of the overfill hypothesis of sodium and water retention in the nephrotic syndrome. *Kidney Int* 1998;53:1111–1117.
15. Vande Walle JG, Donckerwolcke RA. Pathogenesis of edema formation in the nephrotic syndrome. *Pediatr Nephrol* 2001;16:283–293.
16. Sabri M, Saps M, Peters JM. Pathophysiology and management of pediatric ascites. *Curr Gastroenterol Rep* 2003;5:240–246.
17. Reyes AJ. Diuretics in the therapy of hypertension. *J Hum Hypertens* 2002;16(Suppl 1):S78–S83.
18. Dupont AG. The place of diuretics in the treatment of hypertension: a historical review of classical experience over 30 years. *Cardiovasc Drugs Ther* 1993;7(Suppl 1):55–62.
19. Freis ED. The efficacy and safety of diuretics in treating hypertension. *Ann Intern Med* 1995;122:223–226.
20. Kirchlechner V, Koller DY, Seidl R, et al. Treatment of nephrogenic diabetes insipidus with hydrochlorothiazide and amiloride. *Arch Dis Child* 1999;80:548–552.
21. Kellum JA. Use of diuretics in the acute care setting *Kidney Int Suppl* 1998;66:S67–S70.
22. Seri I. Cardiovascular, renal, and endocrine actions of dopamine in neonates and children. *J Pediatr* 1995;126:333–344.
23. Dasta JF, Kirby MG. Pharmacology and therapeutic use of low-dose dopamine. *Pharmacotherapy* 1986;6:304–310.
24. Baldwin L, Henderson A, Hickman P. Effect of postoperative low-dose dopamine on renal function after elective major vascular surgery. *Ann Intern Med* 1994;120:744–747.
25. Gambaro G, Bertaglia G, Puma G, et al. Diuretics and dopamine for the prevention and treatment of acute renal failure: a critical reappraisal. *J Nephrol* 2002;15:213–219.
26. Jaton T, Thonney M, Guignard JP. Failure of dopexamine to protect the hypoxemic newborn rabbit kidney. *Dev Pharmacol Ther* 1991;17:161–166.
27. Driscoll DJ, Gillette PC, Lewis RM, et al. Comparative hemodynamic effects of isoproterenol, dopamine, and dobutamine in the newborn dog. *Pediatr Res* 1979;13:1006–1009.
28. Better OS, Rubinstein I, Winaver JM, et al. Mannitol therapy revisited (1940–1997). *Kidney Int* 1997;52:886–894.
29. Solomon R, Werner C, Mann D, et al. Effects of saline, mannitol, and furosemide to prevent acute decreases in renal function induced by radiocontrast agents. *N Engl J Med* 1994;331: 1416–1420.
30. Rigden SP, Dillon MJ, Kind PR, et al. The beneficial effect of mannitol on post-operative renal function in children undergoing cardiopulmonary bypass surgery. *Clin Nephrol* 1984;21:148–151.
31. Gouyon JB, Guignard JP. Drugs and acute renal insufficiency in the neonate. *Biol Neonate* 1986;50:177–181.
32. Reiss WG, Oles KS. Acetazolamide in the treatment of seizures. *Ann Pharmacother* 1996;30:514–519.
33. Alon U, Hellerstein S, Warady BA. Oral acetazolamide in the assessment of (urine-blood) PCO_2. *Pediatr Nephrol* 1991;5:307–311.
34. Eades SK, Christensen ML. The clinical pharmacology of loop diuretics in the pediatric patient. *Pediatr Nephrol* 1998;12:603–616.
35. Prandota J. Clinical pharmacology of furosemide in children: a supplement. *Am J Ther* 2001;8:275–289.
36. Mirochnick MH, Miceli JJ, Kramer PA, et al. Furosemide pharmacokinetics in very low birth weight infants. *J Pediatr* 1988;112:653–657.
37. Marshall JD, Wells TG, Letzig L, et al. Pharmacokinetics and pharmacodynamics of bumetanide in critically ill pediatric patients. *J Clin Pharmacol* 1998;38:994–1002.
38. Sullivan JE, Witte MK, Yamashita TS, et al. Pharmacokinetics of bumetanide in critically ill infants. *Clin Pharmacol Ther* 1996;60: 405–413.
39. Sullivan JE, Witte MK, Yamashita TS, et al. Dose-ranging evaluation of bumetanide pharmacodynamics in critically ill infants. *Clin Pharmacol Ther* 1996;60:424–434.
40. Dubourg L, Mosig D, Drukker A, et al. Torasemide is an effective diuretic in the newborn rabbit. *Pediatr Nephrol* 2000;14:476–479.
41. Senzaki H, Kamiyama M, Masutani S, et al. Efficacy and safety of torasemide in children with heart failure. *Arch Dis Child* 2008;93: 768–771.
42. Luciani GB, Nichani S, Chang AC, et al. Continuous versus intermittent furosemide infusion in critically ill infants after open heart operations. *Ann Thorac Surg* 1997;64:1133–1139.
43. van der Vorst MM, Ruys-Dudok van Heel I, Kist-van Holthe JE, et al. Continuous intravenous furosemide in haemodynamically unstable children after cardiac surgery. *Intensive Care Med* 2001;27:711–715.
44. Klinge JM, Scharf J, Hofbeck M, et al. Intermittent administration of furosemide versus continuous infusion in the postoperative management of children following open heart surgery. *Intensive Care Med* 1997;23:693–697.
45. Baylen BG, Johnson G, Tsang R, et al. The occurrence of hyperaldosteronism in infants with congestive heart failure. *Am J Cardiol* 1980;45:305–310.
46. Knauf H, Mutschler E. Clinical pharmacokinetics and pharmacodynamics of torasemide. *Clin Pharmacokinet* 1998;34:1–24.
47. Young M, Plosker GL. Torasemide: a pharmacoeconomic review of its use in chronic heart failure. *Pharmacoeconomics* 2001;19:679–703.
48. Haws RM, Baum M. Efficacy of albumin and diuretic therapy in children with nephrotic syndrome. *Pediatrics* 1993;91:1142–1146.
49. Lewis MA, Awan A. Mannitol and frusemide in the treatment of diuretic oedema in nephrotic syndrome. *Arch Dis Child* 1999;80: 184–185.
50. Kapur G, Valentini RP, Imam, et al. Treatment of severe edema in children with nephrotic syndrome with diuretics alone—a prospective study. *Clin J Am Soc Nephrol* 2009;4:907–913.
51. Dubourg L, Drukker A, Guignard J-P. Failure of the loop diuretic torasemide to improve renal function of hypoxemic vasomotor nephropathy in the newborn rabbit. *Pediatr Res* 2000;47: 504–508.
52. Brion LP, Soll RF. Diuretics for respiratory distress syndrome in preterm infants. *Cochrane Database Syt Rev* 2008;(1):CD001454.
53. Brion LP, Primhak RA. Intravenous or enteral loop diuretics for preterm infants with (or developing) chronic lung disease: *Cochrane Database Syst Rev* 2002;(1):CD001453.
54. Brion LP, Primhak RA, Yong W. Aerosolized diuretics for preterm infants with (or developing) chronic lung disease. *Cochrane Database Syst Rev* 2006;(3):CD001694.
55. Whitelaw A, Kennedy CR, Brion LP. Diuretic therapy for newborn infants with posthemorrhagic ventricular dilatation. *Cochrane Database Syst Rev* 2001;(2):CD 002270).
56. Brion LP, Campbell DE. Furosemide for symptomatic patent ductus arteriosus in indomethacin-treated infants. *Cochrane Database Syst Rev* 2001;(3):CD 001148.
57. Barrington K, Brion LP. Dopamine versus no treatment to prevent renal dysfunction in indomethacin-treated preterm newborn infants. *Cochrane Database Syst Rev* 2002;(3):CD 003213.
58. Aufricht C, Votava F, Marx M, et al. Intratracheal furosemide in infants after cardiac surgery: its effects on lung mechanics and urinary output, and its levels in plasma and tracheal aspirate. *Intensive Care Med* 1997;23:992–997.
59. Walsh SB, Shirley DG, Wrong OM, et al. Urinary acidification assessed by simultaneous furosemide and fludrocortisone treatment: an alternative to ammonium chloride. *Kidney Int* 2007;71: 1310–1316.
60. Gimpel C, Krause A, Franck P, et al. Exposure to furosemide as the strongest risk factor for nephrocalcinosis in preterm infants [published online ahead of print May 14, 2009]. *Pediatr Int* 2010; 52:51–56.
61. Downing GJ, Egelhoff JC, Daily DK, et al. Kidney function in very low birth weight infants with furosemide-related renal calcifications at ages 1 to 2 years. *J Pediatr* 1992;120:599–604.
62. Campfield T, Braden G, Flynn-Valone P, et al. Effect of diuretics on urinary oxalate, calcium, and sodium excretion in very low birth weight infants. *Pediatrics* 1997;99:814–818.

63. Borradori C, Fawer CL, Buclin T, et al. Risk factors of sensorineural hearing loss in preterm infants. *Biol Neonate* 1997;71:1–10.
64. Lukert BP, Raisz LG. Glucocorticoid-induced osteoporosis: pathogenesis and management. *Ann Intern Med* 1990;112:352–364.
65. Reusz GS, Dobos M, Tulassay T. Hydrochlorothiazide treatment of children with hypercalciuria: effects and side effects. *Pediatr Nephrol* 1993;7:699–702.
66. Seikaly MG, Baum M. Thiazide diuretics arrest the progression of nephrocalcinosis in children with X-linked hypophosphatemia. *Pediatrics* 2001;108:E6.
67. Knoers N, Monnens LA. Amiloride-hydrochlorothiazide versus indomethacin-hydrochlorothiazide in the treatment of nephrogenic diabetes insipidus. *J Pediatr* 1990;117:499–502.
68. Brion LP, Primhak RA, Ambrosio-Perez I. Diuretics acting on the distal renal tubule for preterm infants with (or developing) chronic lung disease. *Cochrane Database Syst Rev* 2002;(1):CD 001817.
69. Colussi G, Bettinelli A, Tedeschi S, et al. A thiazide test for the diagnosis of renal tubular hypokalemic disorders. *Clin J Am Soc Nephrol* 2007;2:454–460.
70. Delyani JA. Mineralocorticoid receptor antagonists: the evolution of utility and pharmacology. *Kidney Int* 2000;57:1408–1411.
71. Buck ML. Clinical experience with spironolactone in pediatrics. *Ann Pharmacother* 2005;39:823–828.
72. Hofmann T, Senier I, Bittner P, et al. Aerosolized amiloride: dose effect on nasal bioelectric properties, pharmacokinetics, and effect on sputum expectoration in patients with cystic fibrosis. *J Aerosol Med* 1997;10:147–158.
73. Pons G, Marchand MC, d'Athis P, et al. French multicenter randomized double-blind placebo-controlled trial on nebulized amiloride in cystic fibrosis patients. The amiloride-AFLM Collaborative Study Group. *Pediatr Pulmonol* 2000;30:25–31.
74. Costello-Boerrigter LC, Boerrigter G, Burnett JC Jr. Revisiting salt and water retention: new diuretics, aquaretics, and natriuretics. *Med Clin North Am* 2003;87:475–491.
75. Forssmann W, Meyer M, Forssmann K. The renal urodilatin system: clinical implications. *Cardiovasc Res* 2001;51:450–462.
76. Semmekrot B, Guignard J-P. Atrial natriuretic peptide during early human development. *Biol Neonate* 1991;60:341–349.
77. Colucci WS, Elkayam U, Horton DP, et al. Intravenous nesiritide, a natriuretic peptide, in the treatment of decompensated congestive heat failure. Nesiritide Study Group. *N Engl J Med* 2000;343: 246–253.
78. Potter LR, Yoder AR, Flora DR, et al. Natriuretic peptides: their structures, receptors, physiologic functions and therapeutic applications. *Handb Exp Pharmacol* 2009;191:341–366.
79. Chen HH, Lainchbury JG, Burnett JC Jr. Natriuretic peptide receptors and neutral endopeptidase in mediating the renal actions of a new therapeutic synthetic natriuretic peptide dendroaspis natriuretic peptide. *J Am Coll Cardiol* 2002;40:1186–1191.
80. Di Sole F. Adenosine and renal tubular function. *Curr Opin Nephrol Hypertens* 2008;17:399–407.
81. Fredholm BB, Arslan G, Halldner, et al. Structure and function of adenosine receptors and their genes. *Naunyn Schmiedebergs Arch Pharmacol* 2000;362:364–374.
82. Welch WJ. Adenosine type 1 receptor antagonists in fluid retaining disorders. *Expert Opin Investig Drugs* 2002;11:1553–1562.
83. Wilcox CS, Welch WJ, Schreiner GF, et al. Natriuretic and diuretics actions of a highly selective adenosine A_1 receptor antagonist. *J Am Soc Nephrol* 1999;10:714–720.
84. Rieg T, Steigele H, Schnermann J, et al. Requirement of intact adenosine A1 receptors for the diuretic and natriuretic action of the methylxanthines theophylline and caffeine. *J Pharmacol Exp Ther* 2005;313:403–409.
85. Biaggioni I, Paul S, Puckett A, et al. Caffeine and theophylline as adenosine receptor antagonists in humans. *J Pharmacol Exp Ther* 1991;258:588–593.
86. Gouyon JB, Guignard JP. Theophylline prevents the hypoxemia-induced renal hemodynamic changes in rabbits. *Kidney Int* 1988;33: 1078–1083.
87. Huet F, Semama D, Grimaldi M, et al. Effects of theophylline on renal insufficiency in neonates with respiratory distress syndrome. *Intensive Care Med* 1995;21:511–514.
88. Jenik AG, Ceriani Cernadas JM, Gorenstein A, et al. A randomized, double-blind, placebo-controlled trial of the effects of prophylactic theophylline on renal function in term neonates with perinatal asphyxia. *Pediatrics* 2000;105(4):E45.
89. Bakr AF. Prophylactic theophylline to prevent renal dysfunction in newborns exposed to perinatal asphyxia—a study in a developing country. *Pediatr Nephrol* 2005;20:1249–1252.
90. Bhat MA, Shah ZA, Makhdoomi MA, et al. Theophylline for renal function in term neonates with perinatal asphyxia: a randomized, placebo-controlled trial. *J Pediatr* 2006;149:180–184.
91. Cattarelli D, Spandrio M, Gasparoni A, et al. A randomised, double blind, placebo controlled trial of the effect of theophylline in prevention of vasomotor nephropathy in very preterm neonates with respirators distress syndrome. *Arch Dis Child Fetal Neonatal Ed* 2006;91:F80–F84.
92. Bell M, Jackson E, Mi Z, et al. Low-dose theophylline increases urine output in diuretic-dependent critically ill children. *Intensive Care Med* 1998;24:1009–1110.
93. Costello-Boerrigter LC, Boerrigter G, Burnett JC. Pharmacology of vasopressin antagonists. *Heart Fail Rev* 2009;14:75–82.
94. Kumar S, Berl T. Vasopressin antagonists in the treatment of water-retaining disorders. *Semin Nephrol* 2008;28:279–288.
95. Udelson JE, Smith WB, Hendrix GH, et al. Acute hemodynamic effects of conivaptan, a dual V(1 A) and V(2) vasopressin receptor antagonist, in patients with advanced heart failure. *Circulation* 2001;104:2417–2423.
96. Hline SS, Pham PT, Pham PT, et al. Conivaptan: a step forward in the treatment of hyponatremia? *Ther Clin Risk Manag* 2008;4:315–326.
97. Torres VE. Vasopressin antagonists in polycystic kidney disease. *Semin Nephrol* 2008;28:306–317.

CHAPTER

44

Stacey L. Berg
Lisa R. Bomgaars
David G. Poplack

Clinical Pharmacology of Antineoplastic Drugs

Challenges inherent in administering antineoplastic therapy safely to children are numerous. Among the most critical issues are the toxicity of antineoplastic drugs and the developmental heterogeneity of the pediatric population. Antineoplastic agents have the lowest therapeutic index of any drugs in clinical use. Because cancer is life-threatening, clinicians and patients are willing to tolerate toxicity from anticancer agents that would be intolerable for any other class of drugs. Furthermore, these agents are virtually always used in combination, even when the interactions among the agents selected are poorly understood. Children of any age, from newborn to adolescent, may require therapy, yet the impact of developmental factors on the pharmacology of antineoplastic drugs is seldom known. In particular, neonates and young infants, who are most likely to differ physiologically from older children and adults, represent such a small number of pediatric cancer cases that there is relatively little opportunity to study the clinical pharmacology of drugs in this population, even though it may be most vulnerable to ignorance.

In this chapter, we apply general principles of pharmacology to an overview of the antineoplastic drugs commonly used to treat childhood cancer. The approach to understanding drugs by studying their absorption, distribution, metabolism, and elimination can be applied to the antineoplastic agents. However, because these agents do not comprise one homogeneous class, it is helpful also to consider mechanism of action as a general characteristic that must be understood about each drug before the pharmacology of the agent can be fully appreciated. In this chapter, we illustrate the way that each basic principle may be applied to antineoplastic agents using specific drugs as examples, then discuss the way that understanding individual drugs can be used to design the combination chemotherapy regimens that are the cornerstone of anticancer treatment for children. Finally, we review special considerations in the pharmacology of antineoplastic drugs in infants and younger children.

MECHANISMS OF ACTION

Understanding drug mechanism of action is useful in making rational decisions about the dose and administration schedule for individual drugs as well as about logical ways to combine drugs into multiagent regimens. For example, antimetabolites are considered cell cycle phase specific because they produce cytotoxicity during S phase, when they can be incorporated as fraudulent substrates into replicating DNA. Thus, these agents are often administered by prolonged infusion or in multiple daily doses to increase the likelihood that drug will be present when cells are passing through S phase. Similarly, logical combinations of agents may be based on nonoverlapping mechanisms of resistance or nonoverlapping toxicities, but they may also take advantage of mechanism of action by inhibiting the same intracellular process at different points in its pathway or by taking advantage of lesions induced by one drug to potentiate the activity of another (as discussed later) (1). Some commonly used anticancer drugs and their mechanisms of action are listed in Table 44.1.

Many anticancer drugs work by interfering at some stage with the synthesis or function of DNA and RNA in tumor cells. These disruptions usually induce apoptosis as the final common pathway of cell death and are not tumor specific (2–5). In the past, potential anticancer drugs were usually identified in general screens for cytotoxicity, such as the National Cancer Institute panel of tumor cell lines (6,7). More recently, however, advances in understanding tumor biology, especially at the molecular level, have led to the rational development of agents that act more specifically on abnormal molecules or pathways within tumor cells. These targeted agents may theoretically be both more active against tumors and less toxic to normal tissues. The enthusiasm generated by this approach makes it likely that the proportion of molecularly targeted new drugs will increase and that there will be less emphasis on the development of nonspecific cytotoxic agents in the future (8,9). However, the ability to apply these new targeted agents properly will depend on detailed understanding of the

TABLE 44.1 Mechanism of Action of Commonly Used Anticancer Drugs

Drug Class	*Examples*	*Mechanism of Action*
Alkylating agents	Cyclophosphamide	Forms DNA cross-links
	Ifosfamide	
	Cisplatin	
	Carboplatin	
	Temozolomide	
Anthracyclines	Daunomycin	Intercalates into DNA; inhibits topoisomerase II
	Doxorubicin	
	Idarubicin	
Epipodophyllotoxins	Etoposide (VP-16)	
	Teniposide (VM-26)	Inhibits topoisomerase II
Antimetabolites	Methotrexate	
	Cytarabine	Inhibits dehydrofolate reductase
	6-Mercaptopurine	Forms fraudulent substrates
Vinca alkaloids	Vincristine	Inhibits microtubule assembly
Taxanes	Paclitaxel	Stabilizes microtubules
	Docetaxel	
Camptothecin analogues	Topotecan	Inhibits topoisomerase I
	Irinotecan	
Molecularly targeted agents	Imatinib mesylate (Gleevec)	Inhibits bcr–abl tyrosine kinase, c-Kit, and PDGF-R pathways
	Bevacizumab (Avastin)	Inhibits VEGF
	Erlotinib (Tarceva)	Inhibits EGRF

EGRF, epidermal growth factor receptor; PDGF-R, platelet-derived growth factor receptor; VEGF, vascular endothelial growth factor.

drug's targeted pathway in the pathogenesis of pediatric malignancies (10).

Many conventional anticancer agents exert their cytotoxicity by producing inter- and intrastrand cross-links or strand breaks in DNA. Alkylating agents such as nitrogen mustard, cyclophosphamide, ifosfamide, melphalan, and dacarbazine form covalent bonds with intracellular molecules, including DNA as the primary target. The bifunctional alkylating agents, which include nitrogen mustard, the oxazaphosphorines cyclophosphamide and ifosfamide, and melphalan, have two reactive groups that can form intra- and interstrand cross-links that inactivate DNA (11). Although cisplatin and carboplatin are not classical alkylating agents, they also undergo similar chemical reactions to form covalent bonds and cross-links like those formed by alkylating agents (12).

The anthracycline antitumor antibiotics doxorubicin, daunomycin, and idarubicin and the related compound actinomycin D have planar multiring structures that can intercalate into the double helix of DNA, interfering with its replication and transcription. The cytotoxicity of the anthracyclines results from DNA strand breaks that are mediated by the enzyme topoisomerase-II; the exact mechanism of action is not fully explicated (13). The anthracyclines also undergo enzymatic reduction to form free radicals that undergo further reactions to produce to hydrogen peroxide and hydroxyl radicals. It is not known whether these highly reactive compounds contribute to the antitumor effect of the anthracyclines, but they may contribute in part to their well-known cardiac toxicity (13–15). The principal metabolites of the anthracyclines are the corresponding alcohols, doxorubicinol, daunomycinol, and idarubicinol, formed by the action of aldoketoreductase (see below).

The epipodophyllotoxins etoposide (VP-16) and teniposide (VM-26) also interact with topoisomerase II to produce DNA strand breaks, but they do not intercalate into DNA. Topoisomerase-II is normally responsible for opening and rejoining DNA during replication, but in the presence of an epipodophyllotoxin, the strand-closing reaction is blocked (16,17).

The antimetabolites, structural analogues of normal intracellular molecules, act as fraudulent substrate enzymes in critical biochemical pathways. Antimetabolites are among the oldest anticancer agents in clinical use, and they can be viewed as rationally synthesized agents because they are specifically designed to take advantage of well-characterized biochemical pathways, although the pathways are not specific to tumor cells. Antimetabolites exert their cytotoxicity by inhibiting enzymatically catalyzed steps in the synthesis of nucleic acids or by being incorporated into DNA or RNA, resulting in defective products. The antimetabolites most commonly used in children include cytarabine (ara-C), 6-mercaptopurine (MP), thioguanine (TG), and methotrexate. Newer antimetabolites include nelarabine (Ara-G) (18–20) gemcitabine (21–23), capecitabine (24,25), and clofarabine (26). While the role of gemcitabine and capecitabine in pediatric cancer treatment is not yet established, nelarabine is active in pediatric patients with refractory T-cell malignancies (27) and approved for use in that setting, and clofarabine is active and approved for use in patients with relapsed or refractory acute lymphoblastic leukemia (28). The role of these agents in frontline therapy combinations has not yet been defined. Many antimetabolites act as prodrugs that require metabolic activation; this feature will be discussed in detail in the section on biotransformation.

Tubulin, a structural protein that polymerizes to form microtubules, which are critical for successful completion of mitosis, is the intracellular target for several classes of anticancer agents. The *Vinca* alkaloids vincristine and vinblastine bind to tubulin, thus blocking microtubule assembly, preventing the formation of the mitotic spindle, and inhibiting mitosis (16). In contrast, the taxanes paclitaxel and its semisynthetic analogue docetaxel also interact with microtubules, but these agents block mitosis by stabilizing microtubules, preventing their normal disassembly (29–31). Although taxanes have well-defined roles in the treatment of adult cancers, they appear to have limited utility in pediatric tumors and are not widely used.

The bacterial enzyme L-asparaginase has a mechanism of action unique among anticancer agents. This drug, first identified in the 1950s in guinea pig serum (32), depletes the circulating pool of the amino acid L-asparagine, which is nonessential in mammals. Lymphoblasts, however, lack the enzyme that converts aspartic acid to asparagine and therefore are dependent on the presence of L-asparagine to maintain protein synthesis (33). L-asparaginase therapy is an important component of lymphoblastic leukemia treatment. L-asparaginase is commonly administered as either the "native" *E. coli*-produced product which requires frequent (three times a week) administration or a pegylated product with a longer half-life (34,35).

The camptothecin analogues topotecan and irinotecan are agents that exert their antitumor effect by inhibiting topoisomerase-I, a nuclear enzyme involved in DNA uncoiling during replication (36). Treatment with camptothecins leads to formation of DNA–topoisomerase-I adducts and single-strand DNA breaks (36).

Many new molecular-targeted agents are in development, although for the most part their efficacy in pediatric anticancer therapy is not yet determined. One agent that clearly does have a role is the tyrosine kinase inhibitor imatinib mesylate (Gleevec). This agent inhibits the bcr–abl tyrosine kinase that results from the Philadelphia (9,22) chromosome translocation in chronic myelogenous leukemia (37,38). It also inhibits platelet-derived growth factor receptor (PDGF-R), stem cell factor receptor, and c-*kit*-mediated signaling (39–41). Imatinib mesylate is active in most patients with chronic myelogenous leukemia as well as in some patients with Philadelphia chromosome–positive acute lymphocytic leukemia (ALL) (38,42–49). A number of other molecularly targeted agents also have been approved for use in adult malignancies. A particularly compelling target is the vascular endothelial growth factor pathway (50); bevacizumab (Avastin) is the prototype in this class and is used in combination with chemotherapy in adult lung and colon cancer (51,52). Bevacizumab is actively being studied in a range of childhood cancers. Erlotinib (Tarceva) targets the epidermal growth factor receptor tyrosine kinase (53) and is also being studied in children.

PHARMACOKINETICS

Pharmacokinetics is the study of drug absorption, distribution, metabolism, and excretion. Understanding these processes may help determine the proper dose, schedule, and route of administration for anticancer agents. In addition, modeling the pharmacokinetic behavior of a drug may yield important insights into relationships among things like dose and toxicity and response. In children, this understanding is particularly important because developmental physiologic differences between children and adults, such as degree of drug absorption, plasma protein or tissue binding, distribution of drug in the various tissues of the body, and excretory organ function, may mean that the appropriate dose and schedule of administration of a given drug might be quite different in children from adults. In addition, understanding drug elimination pathways can be helpful when recommending dose adjustments for patients with hepatic or renal dysfunction (54).

Among the most important pharmacokinetic concepts is systemic drug exposure, quantified by determining the area under the plasma concentration–time curve, or AUC. Measuring systemic drug exposure can be labor intensive and often involves collaborative research efforts. For drugs administered by prolonged continuous infusion, determination of the steady-state plasma drug concentration is adequate. However, for drugs administered intermittently, determination of the AUC generally requires sampling at multiple points over a prolonged period. However, detailed pharmacokinetic modeling may permit development of a limited sampling strategy in which the AUC can be predicted from a small number of pharmacokinetic samples after drug distribution is thoroughly described in a relatively small initial group of patients (55–57). In addition, parameters other than AUC should also be evaluated for clinical correlations. For example, methotrexate toxicity depends more on the time that drug concentrations stay above certain levels than on the AUC (as discussed later).

ABSORPTION

Absorption refers to the movement of an agent from a peripheral site into the systemic circulation. Because oral administration is the most important nonintravenous route of anticancer drug administration, it is important to consider limitations produced by the gastrointestinal tract. After oral administration, drugs may be degraded by acids in the stomach, adsorbed by food or other medications, metabolized by enzymes in gut luminal cells, extracted by the liver in first-pass metabolism before a systemic effect can be produced, or simply not absorbed because of physicochemical characteristics of the drug molecule. The rate and extent of drug absorption after oral compared with intravenous administration is referred to as bioavailability. Before a drug can be incorporated into anticancer treatment regimen, its bioavailability must be understood. The most reliable way to study bioavailability is to compare plasma AUCs after oral and intravenous administration in the same patient; bioavailability is usually expressed as the fraction of the AUC after intravenous administration produced by oral administration.

The two agents most commonly administered by mouth in childhood anticancer therapy are methotrexate and mercaptopurine (MP), which are used in nearly all maintenance regimens for ALL. Both these agents exhibit considerable variation in bioavailability (58–63). Concomitant food administration diminishes the absorption of both agents (64,65). There may also be diurnal variation in the absorption or elimination of these drugs, as suggested by the observation that children who take oral methotrexate and MP in the evening appear to have lower risk of relapse than those who take them in the morning (66–69).

Bioavailability of methotrexate at low doses (7.5 to 40 mg per m^2) is quite variable. In one study, absorption ranged from 23% to 95% (58). Furthermore, methotrexate absorption appears to be saturable, with a plateau in AUC observed at doses of 30 mg per m^2 (58,70,71). Therefore, the relationship between dose and AUC is not linear for oral methotrexate. To overcome these limitations, intramuscular administration is sometimes used instead of oral administration of methotrexate. In one study of children with ALL, intramuscular injection of methotrexate resulted in approximately twice the bioavailability of oral administration, and at doses exceeding 40 mg per m^2 intramuscular absorption did not show the same nonlinearity as oral administration (71).

Oral administration of MP also results in variable systemic exposure. MP undergoes extensive first-pass metabolism in the liver and gut mucosa by the enzyme xanthine oxidase (63,72). In addition, there is considerable interpatient variability of plasma MP concentrations even when the dose is administered under fasting conditions (61–63). Intrapatient variability has also been observed with repeated monitoring of individual patients (73).

Other agents may have more predictable bioavailability after oral administration. The absorption of prednisone and dexamethasone is greater than 80% (74,75), although variability in the absorption of prednisone has been reported in children (76). Oral busulfan is rapidly absorbed, with a bioavailability of 70% in children (77,78). Interestingly, there appears to be circadian variation in busulfan plasma concentrations, with the highest troughs occurring in the early morning (79).

DISTRIBUTION

Distribution of a drug refers to its transfer among various tissues, blood, tumor, and any other compartments. Although it is possible to measure drug concentrations in different tissues under laboratory conditions, it is not feasible to do so in most clinical settings. Drug concentrations in various compartments can be estimated using pharmacokinetic modeling techniques, but the compartments referred to in models do not usually correlate directly with physiologic compartments. However, the use of pharmacokinetic models, in addition to preclinical studies, permits some conclusions to be drawn about the distribution of most anticancer agents. For example, the pharmacokinetic behavior of both the anthracyclines and the *Vinca* alkaloids is consistent with extensive tissue binding. Disappearance of these drugs from plasma drug during the distributive phase is extremely rapid, with a distribution half-life of less than 10 minutes. These agents also exhibit volumes of distribution that are much larger than the circulatory volume (several hundred L per m^2) as well as a prolonged terminal half-lives (80,81). In addition, tissue levels of anthracyclines, which bind extensively to DNA, are 10- to 500-fold higher than plasma concentrations of the drugs (13).

Methotrexate distributes widely in total body water (82). This is important in relationship to drug toxicity because methotrexate distributes freely into extravascular fluid collections such as pleural effusions or ascites. These fluid collections can contain substantial amounts of methotrexate after high-dose administration and can act as depots that release drug slowly back to other issues, resulting in prolonged systemic drug exposure and increased toxicity (83). Thus, methotrexate should be administered with caution to patients with ascites or pleural effusions, and consideration should be given to draining such fluid collections prior to methotrexate therapy.

Distribution of drugs into the central nervous system (CNS) represents a special challenge in anticancer therapy. Both primary and metastatic CNS tumors are very common in children, and drugs must cross the blood–brain barrier (BBB) to gain access to these tumors. In many tumors the BBB is at least partially disrupted by the tumor itself (84). In other cases, the BBB is relatively intact. Drugs that are poorly soluble in lipids, undergo significant ionization in plasma, or are highly protein bound are unlikely to penetrate extensively across the BBB (85–87). Because it is very difficult to measure drug penetration into tumor or brain tissue, the concentration of drug in the cerebrospinal fluid (CSF) is often used as a surrogate marker for CNS penetration. CNS drug penetration is most accurately described expressed as the ratio of drug AUC in CSF to drug AUC in plasma. The majority of anticancer drugs in clinical use do not cross the intact BBB to any significant extent (Table 44.2). CSF:plasma ratios for the *Vinca* alkaloids, anthracyclines, and epipodophyllotoxins

TABLE 44.2 Central Nervous System Penetration of Common Anticancer Agents

Drug	*Cerebrospinal Fluid: Plasma Ratio (%)*
Alkylating agents	
Cyclophosphamide	50/15[a]
Ifosfamide	30/15[a]
Platinum analogues	
Cisplatin	<10
Carboplatin	<5
Antimetabolites	
Methotrexate	3
Cytarabine	15
Antitumor antibiotics	
Anthracyclines	ND[b]
Dactinomycin	ND[b]
Plant alkaloids	
Vinca alkaloids	5
Epipodophyllotoxins	<5
Topoisomerase-I inhibitors	
Topotecan	30
Irinotecan	14
Miscellaneous	
Prednisolone	<10
Dexamethasone	15

[a]Includes parent compound/active metabolite.
[b]Drug not detectable in cerebrospinal fluid.
From Berg S, Balis F, Poplack D. Cancer chemotherapy. In: Nathan D, Orkin S, eds. *Hematology of infancy and childhood*, 5th ed. Oxford: Elsevier, 1998:1201–1232, with permission.

are less than 10%. A few agents, such as thiotepa and the nitrosoureas, penetrate well. Several useful agents, such as cytarabine and methotrexate, do not penetrate well but can be administered in such high systemic doses that even though the CSF:plasma ratio is low, the CSF concentration is still cytotoxic (88–94). However, such high-dose systemic approaches produce significant systemic toxicity. The most common approach to overcome this problem is the direct intrathecal administration of anticancer agents. Methotrexate and cytarabine remain the mainstay of intrathecal therapy, although other agents, such as thiotepa (95), DepoCyt (liposomally encapsulated cytarabine) (96–99), topotecan (100), gemcitabine (101,102), and busulfan (103) have also been studied.

BIOTRANSFORMATION

Biotransformation, or metabolism, of anticancer drugs can result in production of active agents or inactivation of the agents. Some commonly administered anticancer agents are really prodrugs that require metabolic transformation before they have antitumor activity (Table 44.3). Other drugs are active in the form administered but undergo metabolism to additional active species that may contribute importantly to activity or toxicity. For these agents, all active moieties must be considered in evaluating the relationship between pharmacokinetic parameters like AUC or half-life and pharmacodynamic parameters like response or toxicity. Drug activation most commonly occurs in the liver, where the bulk of drug metabolism takes place. Some drugs, especially antimetabolites, may be activated in their target tissues as they are incorporated into DNA, RNA, or other macromolecules. A few drugs, such as alkylating agents, undergo spontaneous chemical decomposition in solution to cytotoxic reactive intermediates. Interpatient variability in metabolic activation may be an important part of interpatient variability in drug activity or especially toxicity at a given dose. Saturation of drug-metabolizing enzymes at high dose levels may lead to nonlinear dose-response curves. Interaction or competition with other drugs for a metabolic pathway, or even a drug's induction of its own metabolic pathways, could also result in unexpected alterations in exposure to active species. In designing plans for regional therapy, such as intrathecal or intra-arterial drug administration, it is important to remember that agents requiring activation at a distant site will not be useful.

TABLE 44.3 Agents That Function as Prodrugs or Have Active Metabolite Species

Class of Drug	*Prodrug*	*Active Species*
Antimetabolites	Cytarabine	Arabinosylcytidine triphosphate
	Methotrexate	Methotrexate; methotrexate polyglutamates
	Mercaptopurine Thioguanine	Thioguanine nucleotides
Alkylating agents	Cyclophosphamide Ifosfamide	4-Hydroxymetabolites
Anthracyclines	Idarubicin	Idarubicin; idarubicinol
Topoisomerase inhibitors	Irinotecan	SN-38

As mentioned, most antimetabolites are activated at their target sties. For example, after entering cells, cytarabine is converted to the active nucleotide arabinosylcytosine triphosphate (Ara-CTP) in three phosphorylation steps catalyzed by deoxycytidine kinase, deoxycytidylate kinase, and nucleoside diphosphate kinase (104,105). Ara-CTP then acts as a fraudulent substrate for DNA replicative and repair enzymes. The pharmacokinetic parameters of the active intracellular metabolites are more predictive of response than plasma levels of the parent drug. For example, studies have shown little correlation between the pharmacokinetic parameters of cytarabine in plasma and leukemic cell concentrations of Ara-CTP. Ara-CTP retention in blasts correlates with response better than plasma drug concentrations (106–108). Furthermore, decreased deoxycytidine kinase activity, resulting in decreased accumulation of Ara-CTP, is a primary mechanism of Ara-C resistance (109–112).

The antimetabolite methotrexate is not strictly a prodrug, since its parent form strongly inhibits dihydrofolate reductase and blocks the conversion of naturally occurring folates to their active, chemically reduced form. This in turn results in depletion of purines and thymidylate and eventually to inhibition of DNA synthesis (113,114). However, intracellular polyglutamation of methotrexate enhances the drug's inhibitory effect on several critical synthetic enzymes in both the purine and the pyrimidine synthetic pathways, as well as increasing its intracellular retention. The enzyme responsible for polyglutamation of folates and methotrexate, folylpolyglutamate synthetase, is expressed in higher amounts in the leukemic blasts from children with ALL than in those from children with acute nonlymphoblastic leukemia. In addition, higher folylpolyglutamate synthetase activity in B-cell leukemic blasts compared with T-cell blasts may also partially explain the better response to methotrexate-based maintenance therapy in B-lineage leukemias, as these cells accumulate methotrexate polyglutamates to a significantly greater extent (115,116).

The oxazaphosphorines cyclophosphamide and ifosfamide are prodrugs that require hepatic activation. Hydroxylation of the 4-carbon position on the ring yields the primary 4-hydroxyl metabolites, which are in spontaneous equilibrium with the open-ring aldehydes. The 4-hydroxyl metabolites are cytotoxic in vitro and are believed to be the transport forms of the active alkylating species phosphoramide mustard and ifosfamide mustard, which are formed by spontaneous elimination of acrolein from the open-ring aldehydes (11,117,118). After administration of the same dose, activated cyclophosphamide metabolites are present at about three times the concentration of activated ifosfamide metabolites (119). In addition, the activation of ifosfamide is saturable near the maximum tolerated dose (117), whereas saturable elimination of cyclophosphamide becomes apparent only at very high doses (4 to 6 g per m^2) used in bone marrow transplant regimens (120).

The primary metabolites of the anthracyclines are the corresponding alcohols doxorubicinol, daunomycinol, and idarubicinol. The AUCs of daunomycinol and idarubicinol exceed those of the parent drug after intravenous administration, whereas the AUC of doxorubicin exceeds that of doxorubicinol (13,121–124). Doxorubicinol and daunomycinol are less cytotoxic than the parent drugs, but idarubicinol is equitoxic to idarubicin in vitro and may contribute importantly to overall drug activity (125,126). Some data suggest that anthracycline-induced cardiac toxicity may be mediated by the alcohol metabolites and not by parent drug (127–130).

The epipodophyllotoxins are also extensively metabolized. Some of the metabolites retain anticancer activity, whereas others appear to be less active than the parent drug. The relative importance of the metabolites is not well understood (131–133).

ELIMINATION

The role of biotransformation in the elimination of drugs from the body is even more important than its role in drug activation. Metabolism, along with renal or biliary excretion, is the primary pathway for drug clearance. Clearance determines the systemic exposure to a drug. Because drug exposure is often related to toxicity, delayed elimination can lead to increased toxicity. Therefore, understanding the route of elimination is important in understanding potential toxicities in patients with organ dysfunction, especially renal or hepatic dysfunction.

Because hepatic or renal clearance plays an important role in the elimination of most drugs, it would appear to make sense to reduce the dose administered in patients with evidence of hepatic and renal dysfunction (54). Unfortunately, there are no tests of hepatic and renal functions that are clearly predictive of delayed drug elimination, and for most recommended dose modifications, there are less pharmacokinetic or clinical data available to validate the recommendations. For most agents, therapeutic monitoring, or measurement of plasma drug concentrations to predict toxicity or guide further dosing, is not available. Complicating the problem is the concern that empiric dose modifications, while avoiding toxicity, might compromise anticancer effect in patients with mild to moderate organ dysfunction (134). For young children, in whom developmental changes in organ function are overlaid on drug- or disease-related organ dysfunction, the dilemma of dose modification is even more acute. Rational guidelines for dose modification or therapeutic monitoring will be developed only through systematic study of anticancer drug pharmacokinetics in children with varying degrees of organ dysfunction.

The only anticancer drug for which therapeutic monitoring is standard is methotrexate. One reason for this is that, in contrast to most other anticancer drugs, methotrexate toxicity is related to the length of time that drug concentration exceeds a specific threshold concentration rather than to the drug AUC. This greatly simplifies monitoring because it is easier to measure a drug's concentration at a particular moment than to predict a drug's AUC in real time. Furthermore, even though it is obviously not possible to reduce the methotrexate dose retrospectively in the face of toxic levels, this is the one agent for which a reliable antidote exists that can lessen toxicity. As discussed previously, methotrexate works by inhibiting dihydrofolate reductase, resulting in depletion of reduced folate pools. Leucovorin (folinic acid) provides an exogenous source of reduced folates and effectively rescues cells from methotrexate toxicity (82,135–137).

Seventy percent to 90% of a methotrexate dose is renally excreted through glomerular filtration and tubular secretion and reabsorption (83,138,139). Methotrexate clearance is delayed in patients with significant renal dysfunction, which can result in significant toxicity even after a relatively low dose of the drug. Adequate renal function should be confirmed prior to administration of high-dose methotrexate therapy. Serum methotrexate concentration and renal function should be monitored during and after the dose. Patients with delayed methotrexate clearance should receive leucovorin until the plasma methotrexate concentration falls below 0.1 μmol per L (10^{-7} M). In addition, the leucovorin dose may have to be adjusted according to the serum concentration of methotrexate (140). In patients with significant renal dysfunction after methotrexate or with the life-threatening emergency of intrathecal methotrexate overdose, the administration of glucarpidase (formerly carboxypeptidase G2), an enzyme that cleaves methotrexate to inactive metabolites, can reduce methotrexate concentrations rapidly and appears to ameliorate toxicity significantly (141,142).

Aside from methotrexate, most antimetabolites are metabolized by the same degradative pathways as their endogenous counterparts. Cytarabine is rapidly deaminated to uridine arabinoside (ara-U), which is not cytotoxic, by the ubiquitous enzyme cytidine deaminase. Similarly, MP and fluorouracil are catabolized through purine and pyrimidine degradative pathways to inactive metabolites. MP is also inactivated through S-methylation, which is catalyzed by thiopurine methyltransferase (TPMT). TPMT activity is inversely related to the amount of active thioguanine nucleotides formed from MP and TG (143). A common polymorphism in the TPMT gene results in a trimodal distribution of enzyme activity (143). One in 300 patients has very low TPMT activity and is extremely sensitive to thiopurines, and erythrocyte thioguanine nucleotide levels in these TPMT-deficient patients are markedly elevated (144,145). Even a short course of therapy can result in profound myelosuppression in TPMT deficiency, and there is debate about whether determination of TPMT genotype should be routine when thiopurine administration is planned (146–148).

The primary mechanism of clearance for chemically reactive agents like nitrogen mustard is spontaneous chemical decomposition to inactive intermediates. This mechanism does not depend on normal hepatic or renal function, and therefore dose modification for these agents is not usually predicated on organ dysfunction. Similarly, cisplatin, in its active, unbound form, is "eliminated" by aquation followed by formation of covalent bonds to plasma or tissue proteins. Once bound to proteins, the drug is inactive. Approximately 25% of the dose is eliminated through renal excretion (149–151). However, even in patients with no renal function, full-dose cisplatin is tolerated (152), and the terminal half-life is not prolonged (153), presumably because the active platinum species bind rapidly with plasma and tissue proteins, leading to inactivation. Nonetheless, cisplatin dosing is routinely modified in patients with renal dysfunction because cisplatin is nephrotoxic and renal function could be further impaired.

Carboplatin is less chemically reactive than cisplatin, and renal excretion rather than tissue binding is the primary route of carboplatin elimination (154). Plasma carboplatin exposure is linearly related to glomerular filtration rate. Formulas have been developed to adjust the carboplatin dose based on the glomerular filtration rate to achieve either a target AUC (155–158) or a desired level of thrombocytopenia (159).

The anthracyclines are eliminated primarily by hepatic biotransformation and biliary excretion. In addition, enzymatic reduction of the anthraquinone ring produces free radical forms that then spontaneously eliminate the sugar moiety, giving rise to inactive deoxyaglycone metabolites (13). Delayed clearance of doxorubicin with increased toxicity was reported in early studies in both adults and children with hepatic dysfunction (160,161). However, other studies have shown no significant difference in plasma pharmacokinetics or toxicity in patients with mild hepatic dysfunction compared with patients with normal hepatic function (134). In a study in patients with acute nonlymphocytic leukemia incorporating decreased doses of doxorubicin in patients with abnormal liver function tests, dose modification was associated with lower plasma drug levels, less toxicity, and a diminished duration of response and survival (162). The usual recommendation is to reduce the doxorubicin dose in patients with direct bilirubin elevations, although some patients with hyperbilirubinemia may not require dose modification (163–167). The anthracyclines can also be conjugated with a sulfate or glucuronide group as a further detoxification step. Decreased clearance of doxorubicinol, an active metabolite of doxorubicin, has been reported in children with more than 30% body fat (168). Additional study of the effects of body composition on anthracycline pharmacokinetics is needed to fully elucidate the effect on clinical outcomes.

The oxazaphosphorines, which, as noted, require oxidation by hepatic microsomal enzymes at the 4-position for activation, are also inactivated by further oxidation at the same site. This reaction is catalyzed by aldehyde dehydrogenase. Enzymatic cleavage of the chloroethyl side chain of these compounds yields the potentially toxic byproduct chloracetaldehyde. This pathway is more important for ifosfamide than cyclophosphamide metabolism, and chloracetaldehyde has been implicated in toxicities that are more common with ifosfamide, including its neurotoxic and nephrotoxic effects (117,169).

The epipodophyllotoxin analogues etoposide and teniposide are both extensively metabolized, but the renal elimination of these two drugs differs. Renal excretion accounts for 30% to 40% of the total systemic clearance of etoposide (170,171), but only 10% of teniposide clearance (172,173). The greater protein binding of teniposide probably explains this difference, as only unbound drug is renally excreted. In one study, a statistically significant correlation between etoposide clearance and creatinine clearance was reported, whereas abnormal liver function did not appear to affect clearance (174). These studies have led to the recommendation that etoposide dose should be reduced in patients with renal dysfunction, but dose modification may not be necessary in those with abnormal liver function tests.

The metabolism of the *Vinca* alkaloids is poorly understood despite the common use of these agents, especially in childhood cancer. Part of the reason is that assays for measuring parent drug or metabolites have been difficult to develop. Recent data suggest that the CYP3A4 and CYP3A5 pathways have a role in the metabolism of these agents (175,176).

Variability among individuals produced by genetic polymorphisms of drug-metabolizing enzymes is increasingly being recognized as a major factor in anticancer drug therapy. This field is developing very quickly, and many single-nucleotide polymorphisms in enzymes affecting drug metabolism and chemosensitivity have been identified, such as the cytochrome P-450 system, pathways responsible for conjugation reactions, including acetylation, sulfation, glucuronidation, and methylation, and DNA repair pathways (177–184). For example, TPMT, discussed previously, is probably the best-studied genetic polymorphism affecting anticancer drug metabolism. Appreciation of the effect of TPMT polymorphisms and treatment toxicity led to inclusion of this information in the drug label in 2004 (185). Similarly, fluorouracil is also metabolized by a gene with well-described polymorphism, dihydropyrimidine dehydrogenase. Patients with dihydropyrimidine dehydrogenase deficiency are at risk for severe fluorouracil toxicity (186). Patients with polymorphisms in the UGT1A1 promoter have reduced glucuronidation of the active irinotecan metabolite SN-38 and are at increased risk for neutropenia (187). Evaluation of the pharmacogenetics and pharmacogenomics of anticancer agents is an active area of research and is likely to have a major impact on individualization of anticancer drug dosing in the future (188–191).

COMBINATION CHEMOTHERAPY

Anticancer agents are almost always used in combinations, not administered singly. Both clinical experience and experimental models support this approach. For example, in the early days of chemotherapy for children with ALL, single-agent therapy produced disease remission in many cases, but these remissions were brief. When drugs were combined, however, both the number of patients entering remission and the duration of the remissions improved (192,193). These observations are consistent with the Goldie–Coldman, or somatic mutation, model of drug resistance (194,195). Goldie and Coldman proposed that resistance to a particular drug arises from a spontaneous, random genetic mutation in a single cell within a tumor. Once such a mutation occurs, the tumor can no longer be cured by that drug because eventually the progeny of the original resistant cell will dominate the population and the entire tumor will be effectively resistant. The probability of such a mutation's occurring depends on the intrinsic genetic instability of the tumor. The chance of a tumor's acquiring resistance to multiple drugs in a combination, however, is orders of magnitude lower, because the probability of multiple mutations all taking place in a single cell is the product of the probabilities of all the single mutations. Thus, even if a cell or subpopulation is resistant to one agent in the combination, other agents should still be effective.

The Goldie–Coldman hypothesis does not take into account the phenomenon of multidrug resistance (MDR). MDR refers to the situation in which a single genetic

TABLE 44.4 Some Common Combination Chemotherapy Regimens

Nickname	*Components*
VAC	Vincristine Dactinomycin Cyclophosphamide
VAdriaC	Vincristine Adriamycin Cyclophosphamide
VP/Ifos	Ifosfamide Etoposide
MOPP	Nitrogen mustard Vincristine (Oncovin) Prednisone Procarbazine
CHOP	Cyclophosphamide Adriamycin Vincristine Prednisone
ICE	Ifosfamide Carboplatin Etoposide

mutation, such as amplification of the *mdr1* gene, confers resistance to a broad range of antineoplastic agents, including drugs to which the tumor has never been exposed (196–204). Clearly in this setting the odds of a tumor's being resistant to all the agents in a combination could be much higher than if the tumor had to acquire resistance to each drug separately.

Despite this theoretical underpinning, the development of combination chemotherapy regimens remains empiric in most cases. In general, drugs selected for combinations are all known to show single-agent activity against the tumor type for which the combination is designed. Consistent with the Goldie–Coldman model, drugs are also selected for "non–cross-resistance," meaning that the known mechanisms by which tumors acquire resistance to the drugs are different for the different agents being combined. In addition, the mechanisms of antitumor action of the drugs should differ. Ideally, agents would be synergistically active, but since synergy is difficult to identify even with complex preclinical modeling, the mechanisms of action should at least not be obviously antagonistic. In a few instances, known drug interactions can be advantageous in combination therapy. For example, although the folate analogue leucovorin has no independent antitumor activity, it increases the cytotoxic effect of fluorouracil by enhancing the binding of fluorouracil to its target, thymidylate synthase (40,205). Finally, the agents selected for a combination should have nonoverlapping toxicities whenever possible to permit the administration of all the agents at their maximum tolerated doses. Some of the commonly used drug combinations are listed in Table 44.4 (206–213). Clearly, a thorough knowledge of the clinical pharmacology of individual anticancer drugs is required in the design of optimal combination regimens.

SPECIAL CONSIDERATIONS IN INFANTS AND YOUNGER CHILDREN

Critical developmental changes in body composition, renal and hepatic function, and other determinants of drug disposition are discussed in other chapters of this book. Antineoplastic agents are affected by these changes just as other classes of drugs are. Because the therapeutic index of chemotherapy drugs is so low, understanding developmental issues is particularly critical for pediatric oncologists. Unfortunately, data directly related to the effects of these issues on anticancer drug pharmacokinetics and pharmacodynamics are scanty. Most drugs have been insufficiently studied, especially in infants, to provide conclusive recommendations about age-specific dosing regimens or other modifications.

Even the apparently obvious rationale of proportioning a drug's dose to the patient's size has come into question recently. Anticancer drug doses for children and adults are usually based on body surface area (BSA). The argument for this has been that (a) "It is natural to proportion dosage

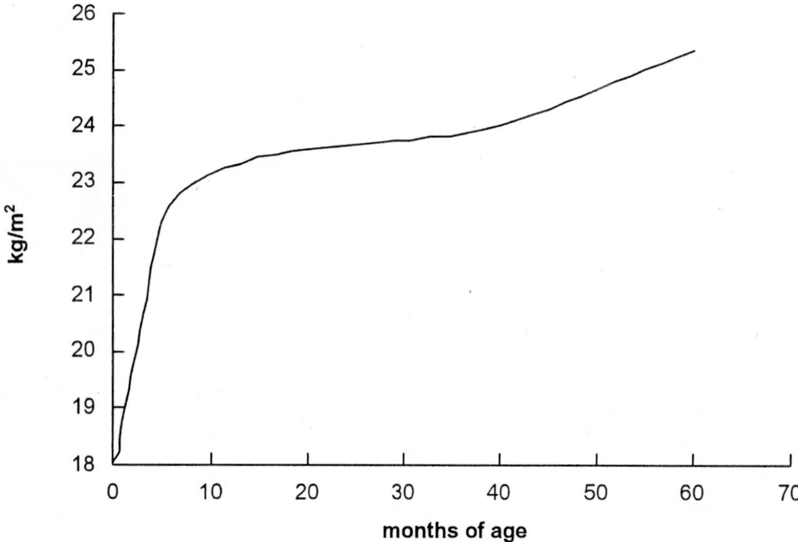

Figure 44.1. Ratio of body weight to body surface area from birth to 70 months of age.

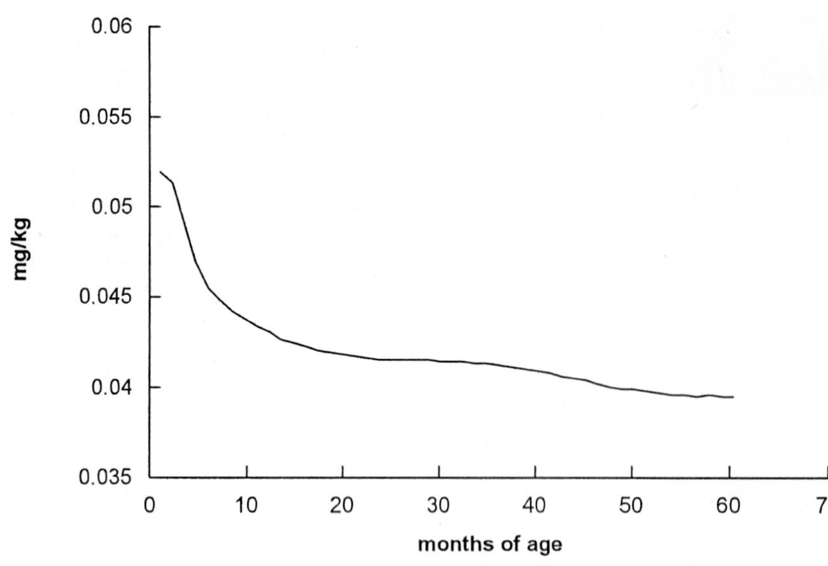

Figure 44.2. Change in dose of drug per kilogram of body weight after administration of a fixed dose per square meter of body surface area from birth to 70 months of age.

according to size of patient" (214) and (b) BSA is a better predictor than weight of excretory organ function (215). However, it is common for anticancer drug AUC to vary as much as 10-fold among children even if the same dose is administered (164). Furthermore, there is controversy in adult oncology over whether BSA-based dosing actually offers any advantage over simply choosing a fixed dose for use in all adults (216,217). Opponents of BSA-based dosing point out that calculation of BSA using formulas that incorporate height and weight is intrinsically inaccurate (218). In addition, for many anticancer drugs there is a poor correlation between dose (normalized to BSA) and pharmacokinetic parameters or toxicity (219–222). In drugs that exhibit large interpatient variability, pharmacodynamic end points may correlate reasonably well with AUC, but AUC may not correlate with dose. For this reason, some authors have advocated administering anticancer drugs to produce targeted AUCs, rather than using specific doses, as a more rational strategy for optimizing chemotherapy (223–229).

Further confounding this issue is the fact that the ratio of weight to BSA is not constant in young children but varies from approximately 18 kg per m^2 at 1 month of age to nearly 40 kg per m^2 by adulthood (Fig. 44.1) (230). Conversely, if a uniform BSA-based dose is given to all children, infants receive a much higher weight-based dose (Fig. 44.2) (230). Based on observations of increased toxicity in infants younger than 1 year receiving actinomycin D or vincristine doses based on BSA, many protocols utilize weight-based dosing for infants and young children in contrast to BSA-based dosing for older children (231–233). It is worth noting that this topic is so unsettled that it was the major focus of conversation at a conference sponsored by the National Cancer Institute as recently as 2003 (234). Nonetheless, for children, in whom the variation in body size is much greater than that among adults, some variation in size-based dosing remains appropriate (218).

In contrast to the controversy surrounding the right way to dose systemically administered anticancer agents, there is relative clarity over dosing intrathecal chemotherapy, where only age is considered. The CSF volume approaches adult size by about 3 years of age, whereas BSA obviously does not do so until the late teenage years. Bleyer (235) demonstrated that there was a direct correlation between patient age and CSF methotrexate concentration when intrathecal methotrexate was dosed on the basis of BSA. Older patients were more likely to have neurotoxicity, whereas younger patients were more likely to have ineffective therapy when a BSA-based dose of 12 mg per m^2 was given (235). In contrast, when methotrexate was given at a constant 12-mg dose to all patients older than 3 years regardless of size, methotrexate levels were significantly less variable and meningeal relapse became less frequent in younger children (235,236). In contrast to BSA-based calculations for doses of systemically administered drugs, the dose for intrathecal methotrexate is based on patient age, with a constant dose administered to all patients older than 3 years (Table 44.5).

CONCLUSIONS

Anticancer drug therapy in children is remarkably effective: The cure rate for all children with cancer now approaches 80% (237). Nonetheless, therapy for some tumors, such as brain tumors, lags behind, and for all cancer treatment in

TABLE 44.5 Age-Based Dosing for Intrathecal Methotrexate

Patient Age (yr)	*Methotrexate Dose (mg)*
<1	6
1	8
2	10
≥3	12

From Bleyer WA. Clinical pharmacology of intrathecal methotrexate. II. An improved dosage regimen derived from age-related pharmacokinetics. *Cancer Treat Rep* 1977;61:1419–1425, with permission.

children, both acute and long-term morbidity of therapy remains a difficult problem. Further improvements will come about only through pharmacologically guided preclinical research and clinical trials.

REFERENCES

1. Wittes RE, Goldin A. Unresolved issues in combination chemotherapy. *Cancer Treat Rep* 1986;70:105–125.
2. Fisher DE. Apoptosis in cancer therapy: crossing the threshold. *Cell* 1994;78:539–542.
3. Kerr JF, Winterford CM, Harmon BV. Apoptosis. Its significance in cancer and cancer therapy. *Cancer* 1994;73:2013–2026.
4. Kohn KW, Jackman J, O'Connor PM. Cell cycle control and cancer chemotherapy. *J Cell Biochem* 1994;54:440–452.
5. Sachs L, Lotem J. Control of programmed cell death in normal and leukemic cells: new implications for therapy. *Blood* 1993;82: 15–21.
6. Cragg GM. Natural product drug discovery and development: the United States National Cancer Institute role. *P R Health Sci J* 2002;21:97–111.
7. Cragg GM, Newman DJ. Discovery and development of antineoplastic agents from natural sources. *Cancer Invest* 1999;17:153–163.
8. Druker BJ. STI571 (Gleevec) as a paradigm for cancer therapy. *Trends Mol Med* 2002;8:S14–S18.
9. Parr AL, Myers TG, Holbeck SL, et al. Thymidylate synthase as a molecular target for drug discovery using the National Cancer Institute's Anticancer Drug Screen. *Anticancer Drugs* 2001;12: 569–574.
10. Balis FM, Fox E, Widemann BC, et al. Clinical drug development for childhood cancers. *Clin Pharmacol Ther* 2009;85:127–129.
11. Colvin M, Chabner BA. Alkylating agents. In: Chabner BA, ed. *Cancer chemotherapy principles and practice.* Philadelphia, PA: Lippincott, 1990:276–313.
12. Reed E, Kohn KW. Platinum analogues. In: Chabner BA, ed. *Cancer chemotherapy principles and practice.* Philadelphia, PA: Lippincott, 1990:465–490.
13. Myers CE, Chabner BA. Anthracyclines. In: Chabner BA, ed. *Cancer chemotherapy principles and practice.* Philadelphia, PA: Lippincott, 1990:356–381.
14. Bachur NR, Gordon SL, Gee MV. A general mechanism for microsomal activation of quinone anticancer agents to free radicals. *Cancer Res* 1978;38:1745–1750.
15. Gianni L, Herman EH, Lipshultz SE, et al. Anthracycline cardiotoxicity: from bench to bedside. *J Clin Oncol* 2008;26: 3777–3784.
16. Bender RA, Hamel E, Hande KR. Plant alkaloids. In: Chabner BA, ed. *Cancer chemotherapy principles and practice.* Philadelphia, PA: Lippincott, 1990:253–275.
17. van Maanen JM, Retel J, de Vries J, et al. Mechanism of action of antitumor drug etoposide: a review. *J Natl Cancer Inst* 1988;80: 1526–1533.
18. Kisor DF, Plunkett W, Kurtzberg J, et al. Pharmacokinetics of nelarabine and 9-beta-D-arabinofuranosyl guanine in pediatric and adult patients during a phase I study of nelarabine for the treatment of refractory hematologic malignancies. *J Clin Oncol* 2000;18:995–1003.
19. Kurtzberg J, Ernst TJ, Keating MJ, et al. Phase I study of 506U78 administered on a consecutive 5-day schedule in children and adults with refractory hematologic malignancies. *J Clin Oncol* 2005;23:3396–3403.
20. Lambe CU, Averett DR, Paff MT, et al. 2-Amino-6-methoxypurine arabinoside: an agent for T-cell malignancies. *Cancer Res* 1995;55: 3352–3356.
21. Abbruzzese JL. Phase I studies with the novel nucleoside analog gemcitabine. *Semin Oncol* 1996;23:25–31.
22. Plunkett W, Huang P, Searcy CE, et al. Gemcitabine: preclinical pharmacology and mechanisms of action. *Semin Oncol* 1996;23:3–15.
23. Plunkett W, Huang P, Xu YZ, et al. Gemcitabine: metabolism, mechanisms of action, and self-potentiation. *Semin Oncol* 1995;22:3–10.
24. Budman DR. Capecitabine. *Invest New Drugs* 2000;18:355–363.
25. Schilsky RL. Pharmacology and clinical status of capecitabine. *Oncology (Williston Park)* 2000;14:1297–1306; discussion 1309–1311.
26. Bonate PL, Arthaud L, Cantrell WR, et al. Discovery and development of clofarabine: a nucleoside analogue for treating cancer. *Nat Rev Drug Discov* 2006;5:855–863.
27. Berg SL, Blaney SM, Devidas M, et al. Phase II study of nelarabine (compound 506U78) in children and young adults with refractory T-cell malignancies: a report from the Children's Oncology Group. *J Clin Oncol* 2005;23:3376–3382.
28. Jeha S, Gaynon PS, Razzouk BI, et al. Phase II study of clofarabine in pediatric patients with refractory or relapsed acute lymphoblastic leukemia. *J Clin Oncol* 2006;24:1917–1923.
29. Ringel I, Horwitz SB. Studies with RP 56976 (taxotere): a semisynthetic analogue of taxol. *J Natl Cancer Inst* 1991;83:288–291.
30. Schiff PB, Fant J, Horwitz SB. Promotion of microtubule assembly in vitro by taxol. *Nature* 1979;277:665–667.
31. Schiff PB, Horwitz SB. Taxol stabilizes microtubules in mouse fibroblast cells. *Proc Natl Acad Sci U S A* 1980;77:1561–1565.
32. Broome J. Evidence that the L-asparaginase activity of guinea pig serum is responsible for its antilymphoma effects. *Nature* 1961; 191:1114–1115.
33. Holcenberg JS. Enzymes as drugs. *Annu Rev Pharmacol Toxicol* 1977;17:97–116.
34. Avramis VI, Sencer S, Periclou AP, et al. A randomized comparison of native *Escherichia coli* asparaginase and polyethylene glycol conjugated asparaginase for treatment of children with newly diagnosed standard-risk acute lymphoblastic leukemia: a Children's Cancer Group study. *Blood* 2002;99:1986–1994.
35. Silverman LB, Gelber RD, Dalton VK, et al. Improved outcome for children with acute lymphoblastic leukemia: results of Dana-Farber Consortium Protocol 91-01. *Blood* 2001;97:1211–1218.
36. Slichenmyer WJ, Rowinsky EK, Donehower RC, et al. The current status of camptothecin analogues as antitumor agents. *J Natl Cancer Inst* 1993;85:271–291.
37. Deininger MW, Goldman JM, Lydon N, et al. The tyrosine kinase inhibitor CGP57148B selectively inhibits the growth of BCR-ABL-positive cells. *Blood* 1997;90:3691–3698.
38. Druker BJ, Tamura S, Buchdunger E, et al. Effects of a selective inhibitor of the Abl tyrosine kinase on the growth of Bcr-Abl positive cells. *Nat Med* 1996;2:561–566.
39. Buchdunger E, Cioffi CL, Law N, et al. Abl protein–tyrosine kinase inhibitor STI571 inhibits in vitro signal transduction mediated by c-kit and platelet-derived growth factor receptors. *J Pharmacol Exp Ther* 2000;295:139–145.
40. Carroll M, Ohno-Jones S, Tamura S, et al. CGP 57148, a tyrosine kinase inhibitor, inhibits the growth of cells expressing BCR-ABL, TEL-ABL, and TEL-PDGFR fusion proteins. *Blood* 1997;90: 4947–4952.
41. Heinrich MC, Griffith DJ, Druker BJ, et al. Inhibition of c-kit receptor tyrosine kinase activity by STI 571, a selective tyrosine kinase inhibitor. *Blood* 2000;96:925–932.
42. Champagne MA, Capdeville R, Krailo M, et al. Imatinib mesylate (STI571) for treatment of children with Philadelphia chromosome-positive leukemia: results from a Children's Oncology Group phase 1 study. *Blood* 2004;104:2655–2660.
43. Druker BJ, Talpaz M, Resta DJ, et al. Efficacy and safety of a specific inhibitor of the BCR-ABL tyrosine kinase in chronic myeloid leukemia. *N Engl J Med* 2001;344:1031–1037.
44. Johnson JR, Bross P, Cohen M, et al. Approval summary: imatinib mesylate capsules for treatment of adult patients with newly diagnosed Philadelphia chromosome-positive chronic myelogenous leukemia in chronic phase. *Clin Cancer Res* 2003;9: 1972–1979.
45. Kantarjian HM, Cortes JE, O'Brien S, et al. Imatinib mesylate therapy in newly diagnosed patients with Philadelphia chromosome-positive chronic myelogenous leukemia: high incidence of early complete and major cytogenetic responses. *Blood* 2003;101:97–100.
46. Kantarjian HM, O'Brien S, Cortes JE, et al. Treatment of Philadelphia chromosome-positive, accelerated-phase chronic myelogenous leukemia with imatinib mesylate. *Clin Cancer Res* 2002;8:2167–2176.
47. Kantarjian HM, Talpaz M. Imatinib mesylate: clinical results in Philadelphia chromosome-positive leukemias. *Semin Oncol* 2001; 28:9–18.
48. Kantarjian HM, Talpaz M, O'Brien S, et al. Imatinib mesylate for Philadelphia chromosome-positive, chronic-phase myeloid leukemia

after failure of interferon-alpha: follow-up results. *Clin Cancer Res* 2002;8:2177–2187.
49. Kolb EA, Pan Q, Ladanyi M, et al. Imatinib mesylate in Philadelphia chromosome-positive leukemia of childhood. *Cancer* 2003;98: 2643–2650.
50. Ferrara N. Vascular endothelial growth factor as a target for anticancer therapy. *Oncologist* 2004;9(Suppl 1):2–10.
51. Cohen MH, Gootenberg J, Keegan P, et al. FDA drug approval summary: bevacizumab (Avastin) plus Carboplatin and Paclitaxel as first-line treatment of advanced/metastatic recurrent nonsquamous non-small cell lung cancer. *Oncologist* 2007;12:713–718.
52. Cohen MH, Gootenberg J, Keegan P, et al. FDA drug approval summary: bevacizumab plus FOLFOX4 as second-line treatment of colorectal cancer. *Oncologist* 2007;12:356–361.
53. Cohen MH, Johnson JR, Chen YF, et al. FDA drug approval summary: erlotinib (Tarceva) tablets. *Oncologist* 2005;10:461–466.
54. Powis G. Effects of disease states on pharmacokinetics of anticancer drugs. In: Ames MM, Powis G, Kovach JS, eds. *Pharmacokinetics of anticancer agents in humans.* Amsterdam: Elsevier, 1983:365–397.
55. Bomgaars LR, Bernstein M, Krailo M, et al. Phase II trial of irinotecan in children with refractory solid tumors: a Children's Oncology Group Study. *J Clin Oncol* 2007;25:4622–4627.
56. Egorin MJ, Forrest A, Belani CP, et al. A limited sampling strategy for cyclophosphamide pharmacokinetics. *Cancer Res* 1989;49: 3129–3133.
57. Ratain MJ, Vogelzang NJ. Limited sampling model for vinblastine pharmacokinetics. *Cancer Treat Rep* 1987;71:935–939.
58. Balis FM, Savitch JL, Bleyer WA. Pharmacokinetics of oral methotrexate in children. *Cancer Res* 1983;43:2342–2345.
59. Kearney PJ, Light PA, Preece A, et al. Unpredictable serum levels after oral methotrexate in children with acute lymphoblastic leukaemia. *Cancer Chemother Pharmacol* 1979;3:117–120.
60. Koren G, Solh H, Klein J, et al. Disposition of oral methotrexate in children with acute lymphoblastic leukemia and its relation to 6-mercaptopurine pharmacokinetics. *Med Pediatr Oncol* 1989;17: 450–454.
61. Lennard L, Keen D, Lilleyman JS. Oral 6-mercaptopurine in childhood leukemia: parent drug pharmacokinetics and active metabolite concentrations. *Clin Pharmacol Ther* 1986;40:287–292.
62. Sulh H, Koren G, Whalen C, et al. Pharmacokinetic determinants of 6-mercaptopurine myelotoxicity and therapeutic failure in children with acute lymphoblastic leukemia. *Clin Pharmacol Ther* 1986;40:604–609.
63. Zimm S, Collins JM, Riccardi R, et al. Variable bioavailability of oral mercaptopurine. Is maintenance chemotherapy in acute lymphoblastic leukemia being optimally delivered? *N Engl J Med* 1983;308:1005–1009.
64. Pinkerton CR, Welshman SG, Glasgow JF, et al. Can food influence the absorption of methotrexate in children with acute lymphoblastic leukaemia? *Lancet* 1980;2:944–946.
65. Riccardi R, Balis FM, Ferrara P, et al. Influence of food intake on bioavailability of oral 6-mercaptopurine in children with acute lymphoblastic leukemia. *Pediatr Hematol Oncol* 1986;3:319–324.
66. Balis FM, Jeffries SL, Lange B, et al. Chronopharmacokinetics of oral methotrexate and 6-mercaptopurine: is there diurnal variation in the disposition of antileukemic therapy? *Am J Pediatr Hematol Oncol* 1989;11:324–326.
67. Koren G, Ferrazzini G, Sohl H, et al. Chronopharmacology of methotrexate pharmacokinetics in childhood leukemia. *Chronobiol Int* 1992;9:434–438.
68. Koren G, Langevin AM, Olivieri N, et al. Diurnal variation in the pharmacokinetics and myelotoxicity of mercaptopurine in children with acute lymphocytic leukemia. *Am J Dis Child* 1990;144: 1135–1137.
69. Rivard GE, Infante-Rivard C, Hoyoux C, et al. Maintenance chemotherapy for childhood acute lymphoblastic leukaemia: better in the evening. *Lancet* 1985;2:1264–1266.
70. Balis FM, Mirro J Jr, Reaman GH, et al. Pharmacokinetics of subcutaneous methotrexate. *J Clin Oncol* 1988;6:1882–1886.
71. Teresi ME, Crom WR, Choi KE, et al. Methotrexate bioavailability after oral and intramuscular administration in children. *J Pediatr* 1987;110:788–792.
72. Zimm S, Collins JM, O'Neill D, et al. Inhibition of first-pass metabolism in cancer chemotherapy: interaction of 6-mercaptopurine and allopurinol. *Clin Pharmacol Ther* 1983;34:810–817.
73. Balis F, Holcenberg J, et al. CCG 105PH: population pharmacokinetics of oral methotrexate and mercaptopurine in children with acute lymphoblastic leukemia. *Proc Am Soc Clin Oncol* 1993; 12:318.
74. Duggan DE, Yeh KC, Matalia N, et al. Bioavailability of oral dexamethasone. *Clin Pharmacol Ther* 1975;18:205–209.
75. Pickup ME. Clinical pharmacokinetics of prednisone and prednisolone. *Clin Pharmacokinet* 1979;4:111–128.
76. Green OC, Winter RJ, Kawahara FS, et al. Plasma levels, half-life values, and correlation with physiologic assays for growth and immunity. *J Pediatr* 1978;93:299–303.
77. Hassan M, Ljungman P, Bolme P, et al. Busulfan bioavailability. *Blood* 1994;84:2144–2150.
78. Regazzi MB, Locatelli F, Buggia I, et al. Disposition of high-dose busulfan in pediatric patients undergoing bone marrow transplantation. *Clin Pharmacol Ther* 1993;54:45–52.
79. Vassal G, Challine D, Koscielny S, et al. Chronopharmacology of high-dose busulfan in children. *Cancer Res* 1993;53:1534–1537.
80. Groninger E, Meeuwsen-de Boar T, Koopmans P, et al. Pharmacokinetics of vincristine monotherapy in childhood acute lymphoblastic leukemia. *Pediatr Res* 2002;52:113–118.
81. Robert J. Anthracyclines. In: Grochow L, Ames M, eds. *A clinician's guide to chemotherapy pharmacokinetics and pharmacodynamics.* Baltimore, MD: Williams & Wilkins, 1998:93–173.
82. Pratt CB, Roberts D, Shanks EC, et al. Clinical trials and pharmacokinetics of intermittent high-dose methotrexate-"leucovorin rescue" for children with malignant tumors. *Cancer Res* 1974;34: 3326–3331.
83. Allegra CJ. Antifolates. In: Chabner BA, ed. *Cancer chemotherapy principles and practice.* Philadelphia, PA: Lippincott, 1990:110–153.
84. Strother D, Pollack I, Fisher P, et al. Tumors of the central nervous system. In: Pizzo PA, Poplack DG, eds. *Principles and practice of pediatric oncology.* Philadelphia, PA: Lippincott Williams & Wilkins, 2002:751–824.
85. Koch-Weser J, Sellers EM. Binding of drugs to serum albumin (first of two parts). *N Engl J Med* 1976;294:311–316.
86. Mellett LB. Physicochemical considerations and pharmacokinetic behavior in delivery of drugs to the central nervous system. *Cancer Treat Rep* 1977;61:527–531.
87. Poplack D, Bleyer W, Horowitz M. Pharmacology of antineoplastic agents in cerebrospinal fluid. In: Wood J, ed. *Neurobiology of cerebrospinal fluid.* New York, NY: Plenum Press, 1980:561–578.
88. Balis FM, Savitch JL, Bleyer WA, et al. Remission induction of meningeal leukemia with high-dose intravenous methotrexate. *J Clin Oncol* 1985;3:485–489.
89. Donehower RC, Karp JE, Burke PJ. Pharmacology and toxicity of high-dose cytarabine by 72-hour continuous infusion. *Cancer Treat Rep* 1986;70:1059–1065.
90. Evans WE, Hutson PR, Stewart CF, et al. Methotrexate cerebrospinal fluid and serum concentrations after intermediate-dose methotrexate infusion. *Clin Pharmacol Ther* 1983;33:301–307.
91. Frick J, Ritch PS, Hansen RM, et al. Successful treatment of meningeal leukemia using systemic high-dose cytosine arabinoside. *J Clin Oncol* 1984;2:365–368.
92. Frick JC, Hansen RM, Anderson T, et al. Successful high-dose intravenous cytarabine treatment of parenchymal brain involvement from malignant lymphoma. *Arch Intern Med* 1986;146:791–792.
93. Morra E, Lazzarino M, Brusamolino E, et al. The role of systemic high-dose cytarabine in the treatment of central nervous system leukemia. Clinical results in 46 patients. *Cancer* 1993;72:439–445.
94. Shapiro WR, Young DF, Mehta BM. Methotrexate: distribution in cerebrospinal fluid after intravenous, ventricular and lumbar injections. *N Engl J Med* 1975;293:161–166.
95. Grossman SA, Finkelstein DM, Ruckdeschel JC, et al. Randomized prospective comparison of intraventricular methotrexate and thiotepa in patients with previously untreated neoplastic meningitis. Eastern Cooperative Oncology Group. *J Clin Oncol* 1993;11: 561–569.
96. Bomgaars L, Geyer JR, Franklin J, et al. Phase I trial of intrathecal liposomal cytarabine in children with neoplastic meningitis. *J Clin Oncol* 2004;22:3916–3921.
97. Glantz MJ, Jaeckle KA, Chamberlain MC, et al. A randomized controlled trial comparing intrathecal sustained-release cytarabine (DepoCyt) to intrathecal methotrexate in patients with neoplastic meningitis from solid tumors. *Clin Cancer Res* 1999;5:3394–3402.

98. Glantz MJ, LaFollette S, Jaeckle KA, et al. Randomized trial of a slow-release versus a standard formulation of cytarabine for the intrathecal treatment of lymphomatous meningitis. *J Clin Oncol* 1999;17:3110–3116.
99. Jaeckle KA, Phuphanich S, Bent MJ, et al. Intrathecal treatment of neoplastic meningitis due to breast cancer with a slow-release formulation of cytarabine. *Br J Cancer* 2001;84:157–163.
100. Blaney SM, Heideman R, Berg S, et al. Phase I clinical trial of intrathecal topotecan in patients with neoplastic meningitis. *J Clin Oncol* 2003;21:143–147.
101. Bernardi RJ, Bomgaars L, Fox E, et al. Phase I clinical trial of intrathecal gemcitabine in patients with neoplastic meningitis. *Cancer Chemother Pharmacol* 2008;62:355–361.
102. Chen YM, Chen MC, Tsai CM, et al. Intrathecal gemcitabine chemotherapy for non-small cell lung cancer patients with meningeal carcinomatosis—a case report. *Lung Cancer* 2003;40: 99–101.
103. Gururangan S, Petros WP, Poussaint TY, et al. Phase I trial of intrathecal spartaject busulfan in children with neoplastic meningitis: a Pediatric Brain Tumor Consortium Study (PBTC-004). *Clin Cancer Res* 2006;12:1540–1546.
104. Chabner BA. Cytidine analogues. In: Chabner BA, Collins JM, eds. *Cancer chemotherapy principles and practice.* Philadelphia, PA: Lippincott, 1990:154–179.
105. Kufe DW, Spriggs DR. Biochemical and cellular pharmacology of cytosine arabinoside. *Semin Oncol* 1985;12:34–48.
106. Estey E, Plunkett W, Dixon D, et al. Variables predicting response to high dose cytosine arabinoside therapy in patients with refractory acute leukemia. *Leukemia* 1987;1:580–583.
107. Liliemark JO, Plunkett W, Dixon DO. Relationship of 1-beta-D-arabinofuranosylcytosine in plasma to 1-beta-D-arabinofuranosylcytosine 5′-triphosphate levels in leukemic cells during treatment with high-dose 1-beta-D-arabinofuranosylcytosine. *Cancer Res* 1985;45:5952–5957.
108. Plunkett W, Iacoboni S, Estey E, et al. Pharmacologically directed ara-C therapy for refractory leukemia. *Semin Oncol* 1985; 12:20–30.
109. Bergman AM, Pinedo HM, Peters GJ. Determinants of resistance to 2′,2′-difluorodeoxycytidine (gemcitabine). *Drug Resist Updat* 2002;5:19–33.
110. Hagenbeek A, Martens AC, Colly LP. In vivo development of cytosine arabinoside resistance in the BN acute myelocytic leukemia. *Semin Oncol* 1987;14:202–206.
111. Kees UR, Ford J, Dawson VM, et al. Development of resistance to 1-beta-D-arabinofuranosylcytosine after high-dose treatment in childhood lymphoblastic leukemia: analysis of resistance mechanism in established cell lines. *Cancer Res* 1989;49:3015–3019.
112. Stam RW, den Boer ML, Meijerink JP, et al. Differential mRNA expression of Ara-C-metabolizing enzymes explains Ara-C sensitivity in MLL gene-rearranged infant acute lymphoblastic leukemia. *Blood* 2003;101:1270–1276.
113. Chu E, Allegra C. Antifolates. In: Chabner B, Longo D, eds. *Cancer chemotherapy and biotherapy principles and practice.* Philadelphia, PA: Lippincott–Raven, 1996:109–148.
114. Goldman ID, Matherly LH. The cellular pharmacology of methotrexate. *Pharmacol Ther* 1985;28:77–102.
115. Barredo JC, Synold TW, Laver J, et al. Differences in constitutive and post-methotrexate folylpolyglutamate synthetase activity in B-lineage and T-lineage leukemia. *Blood* 1994;84:564–569.
116. Galpin AJ, Schuetz JD, Masson E, et al. Differences in folylpolyglutamate synthetase and dihydrofolate reductase expression in human B-lineage versus T-lineage leukemic lymphoblasts: mechanisms for lineage differences in methotrexate polyglutamylation and cytotoxicity. *Mol Pharmacol* 1997;52:155–163.
117. Brade WP, Herdrich K, Varini M. Ifosfamide–pharmacology, safety and therapeutic potential. *Cancer Treat Rev* 1985;12:1–47.
118. Grochow LB, Colvin M. Clinical pharmacokinetics of cyclophosphamide. *Clin Pharmacokinet* 1979;4:380–394.
119. Wagner T, Heydrich D, Jork T, et al. Comparative study on human pharmacokinetics of activated ifosfamide and cyclophosphamide by a modified fluorometric test. *J Cancer Res Clin Oncol* 1981;100:95–104.
120. Chen TL, Passos-Coelho JL, Noe DA, et al. Nonlinear pharmacokinetics of cyclophosphamide in patients with metastatic breast cancer receiving high-dose chemotherapy followed by autologous bone marrow transplantation. *Cancer Res* 1995;55: 810–816.
121. Gil P, Favre R, Durand A, et al. Time dependency of adriamycin and adriamycinol kinetics. *Cancer Chemother Pharmacol* 1983;10: 120–124.
122. Greene RF, Collins JM, Jenkins JF, et al. Plasma pharmacokinetics of adriamycin and adriamycinol: implications for the design of in vitro experiments and treatment protocols. *Cancer Res* 1983;43:3417–3421.
123. Huffman DH, Bachur NR. Daunorubicin metabolism in acute myelocytic leukemia. *Blood* 1972;39:637–643.
124. Reid JM, Pendergrass TW, Krailo MD, et al. Plasma pharmacokinetics and cerebrospinal fluid concentrations of idarubicin and idarubicinol in pediatric leukemia patients: a Childrens Cancer Study Group report. *Cancer Res* 1990;50:6525–6528.
125. Kuffel MJ, Ames MM. Comparative resistance of idarubicin, doxorubicin and their C-13 alcohol metabolites in human MDR1 transfected NIH-3T3 Cells. *Cancer Chemother Pharmacol* 1995;36: 223–226.
126. Reid J, Kuffel MJ, et al. Cytotoxic concentrations of idarubicinol, the alcohol metabolite of idarubicin, are present in CSF following administration of idarubicin to children with relapsed leukemia. *Proc Am Assoc Cancer Res* 1989;30:250.
127. Cusack BJ, Young SP, Driskell J, et al. Doxorubicin and doxorubicinol pharmacokinetics and tissue concentrations following bolus injection and continuous infusion of doxorubicin in the rabbit. *Cancer Chemother Pharmacol* 1993;32:53–58.
128. de Jong J, Schoofs PR, Snabilie AM, et al. The role of biotransformation in anthracycline-induced cardiotoxicity in mice. *J Pharmacol Exp Ther* 1993;266:1312–1320.
129. Olson RD, Mushlin PS, Brenner DE, et al. Doxorubicin cardiotoxicity may be caused by its metabolite, doxorubicinol. *Proc Natl Acad Sci U S A* 1988;85:3585–3589.
130. Stewart DJ, Grewaal D, Green RM, et al. Concentrations of doxorubicin and its metabolites in human autopsy heart and other tissues. *Anticancer Res* 1993;13:1945–1952.
131. Gantchev TG, Hunting DJ. The ortho-quinone metabolite of the anticancer drug etoposide (VP-16) is a potent inhibitor of the topoisomerase II/DNA cleavable complex. *Mol Pharmacol* 1998; 53:422–428.
132. Lovett BD, Strumberg D, Blair IA, et al. Etoposide metabolites enhance DNA topoisomerase II cleavage near leukemia-associated MLL translocation breakpoints. *Biochemistry* 2001;40:1159–1170.
133. Pommier Y, Fesen M, Goldwasser F. Topoisomerase II inhibitors: the epipodophyllotoxins, m-AMSA, and the ellipticine derivatives. In: Chabner B, Longo D, eds. *Cancer chemotherapy and biotherapy principles and practice.* Philadelphia, PA: Lippincott–Raven, 1996:435–461.
134. Sulkes A, Collins JM. Reappraisal of some dosage adjustment guidelines. *Cancer Treat Rep* 1987;71:229–233.
135. Frei E III, Jaffe N, Tattersall MH, et al. New approaches to cancer chemotherapy with methotrexate. *N Engl J Med* 1975;292:846–851.
136. Hitchings GH, Burchall JJ. Inhibition of folate biosynthesis and function as a basis for chemotherapy. *Adv Enzymol Relat Areas Mol Biol* 1965;27:417–468.
137. Stoller RG, Hande KR, Jacobs SA, et al. Use of plasma pharmacokinetics to predict and prevent methotrexate toxicity. *N Engl J Med* 1977;297:630–634.
138. Huffman DH, Wan SH, Azarnoff DL, et al. Pharmacokinetics of methotrexate. *Clin Pharmacol Ther* 1973;14:572–579.
139. Liegler DG, Henderson ES, Hahn MA, et al. The effect of organic acids on renal clearance of methotrexate in man. *Clin Pharmacol Ther* 1969;10:849–857.
140. Bleyer WA. Antineoplastic agents. In: Yaffe SJ, ed. *Pediatric pharmacology: therapeutic principles in practice.* New York, NY: Grune & Stratton, 1980:349–377.
141. Widemann BC, Balis FM, Murphy RF, et al. Carboxypeptidase-G2, thymidine, and leucovorin rescue in cancer patients with methotrexate-induced renal dysfunction. *J Clin Oncol* 1997;15: 2125–2134.
142. Widemann BC, Balis FM, Shalabi A, et al. Treatment of accidental intrathecal methotrexate overdose with intrathecal carboxypeptidase G2. *J Natl Cancer Inst* 2004;96:1557–1559.
143. Lennard L, Lilleyman JS, Van Loon J, et al. Genetic variation in response to 6-mercaptopurine for childhood acute lymphoblastic leukaemia. *Lancet* 1990;336:225–229.

144. Evans WE, Horner M, Chu YQ, et al. Altered mercaptopurine metabolism, toxic effects, and dosage requirement in a thiopurine methyltransferase-deficient child with acute lymphocytic leukemia. *J Pediatr* 1991;119:985–989.
145. Lennard L, Van Loon JA, Weinshilboum RM. Pharmacogenetics of acute azathioprine toxicity: relationship to thiopurine methyltransferase genetic polymorphism. *Clin Pharmacol Ther* 1989;46: 149–154.
146. Marra CA, Esdaile JM, Anis AH. Practical pharmacogenetics: the cost effectiveness of screening for thiopurine s-methyltransferase polymorphisms in patients with rheumatological conditions treated with azathioprine. *J Rheumatol* 2002;29:2507–2512.
147. McLeod HL, Coulthard S, Thomas AE, et al. Analysis of thiopurine methyltransferase variant alleles in childhood acute lymphoblastic leukaemia. *Br J Haematol* 1999;105:696–700.
148. McLeod HL, Krynetski EY, Relling MV, et al. Genetic polymorphism of thiopurine methyltransferase and its clinical relevance for childhood acute lymphoblastic leukemia. *Leukemia* 2000;14: 567–572.
149. Jacobs C, Kalman SM, Tretton M, et al. Renal handling of cis-diamminedichloroplatinum(II). *Cancer Treat Rep* 1980;64:1223–1226.
150. Reece PA, Stafford I, Davy M, et al. Disposition of unchanged cisplatin in patients with ovarian cancer. *Clin Pharmacol Ther* 1987;42: 320–325.
151. Vermorken JB, van der Vijgh WJ, Klein I, et al. Pharmacokinetics of free and total platinum species after rapid and prolonged infusions of cisplatin. *Clin Pharmacol Ther* 1986;39:136–144.
152. Gouyette A, Lemoine R, Adhemar JP, et al. Kinetics of cisplatin in an anuric patient undergoing hemofiltration dialysis. *Cancer Treat Rep* 1981;65:665–668.
153. Belt RJ, Himmelstein KJ, Patton TF, et al. Pharmacokinetics of non-protein-bound platinum species following administration of cis-dichlorodiammineplatinum(II). *Cancer Treat Rep* 1979;63: 1515–1521.
154. van der Vijgh WJ. Clinical pharmacokinetics of carboplatin. *Clin Pharmacokinet* 1991;21:242–261.
155. Bin P, Boddy AV, English MW, et al. The comparative pharmacokinetics and pharmacodynamics of cisplatin and carboplatin in paediatric patients: a review. *Anticancer Res* 1994;14:2279–2283.
156. Calvert AH. Dose optimisation of carboplatin in adults. *Anticancer Res* 1994;14:2273–2278.
157. Marina NM, Rodman J, Shema SJ, et al. Phase I study of escalating targeted doses of carboplatin combined with ifosfamide and etoposide in children with relapsed solid tumors. *J Clin Oncol* 1993;11:554–560.
158. Newell DR, Pearson AD, Balmanno K, et al. Carboplatin pharmacokinetics in children: the development of a pediatric dosing formula. The United Kingdom Children's Cancer Study Group. *J Clin Oncol* 1993;11:2314–2323.
159. Egorin MJ, Van Echo DA, Tipping SJ, et al. Pharmacokinetics and dosage reduction of cis-diammine(1,1-cyclobutanedicarboxylato)platinum in patients with impaired renal function. *Cancer Res* 1984;44:5432–5438.
160. Benjamin RS, Wiernik PH, Bachur NR. Adriamycin chemotherapy—efficacy, safety, and pharmacologic basis of an intermittent single high-dosage schedule. *Cancer* 1974;33:19–27.
161. Evans WE, Crom WR, Sinkule JA, et al. Pharmacokinetics of anticancer drugs in children. *Drug Metab Rev* 1983;14:847–886.
162. Brenner DE, Wiernik PH, Wesley M, et al. Acute doxorubicin toxicity. Relationship to pretreatment liver function, response, and pharmacokinetics in patients with acute nonlymphocytic leukemia. *Cancer* 1984;53:1042–1048.
163. Chang PC, Brenner DE, Riggs CE, et al. Adriamycin toxicity: preliminary guidelines for dosage reduction. *Clin Res* 1979;27:382A.
164. Crom WR, Glynn-Barnhart AM, Rodman JH, et al. Pharmacokinetics of anticancer drugs in children. *Clin Pharmacokinet* 1987; 12:168–213.
165. Cupp MJ, Higa GM. Doxorubicin dosage guidelines in a patient with hyperbilirubinemia of Gilbert's syndrome. *Ann Pharmacother* 1998;32:1026–1029.
166. Gurevich I, Akerley W. Treatment of the jaundiced patient with breast carcinoma: case report and alternate therapeutic strategies. *Cancer* 2001;91:660–663.
167. Kaye SB, Cummings J, Kerr DJ. How much does liver disease affect the pharmacokinetics of adriamycin? *Eur J Cancer Clin Oncol* 1985;21:893–895.
168. Thompson PA, Rosner GL, Matthay KK, et al. Impact of body composition on pharmacokinetics of doxorubicin in children: a Glaser Pediatric Research Network study. *Cancer Chemother Pharmacol* 2008;64:243–251.
169. Pratt CB, Green AA, Horowitz ME, et al. Central nervous system toxicity following the treatment of pediatric patients with ifosfamide/mesna. *J Clin Oncol* 1986;4:1253–1261.
170. Allen LM, Creaven PJ. Comparison of the human pharmacokinetics of VM-26 and VP-16, two antineoplastic epipodophyllotoxin glucopyranoside derivatives. *Eur J Cancer* 1975;11:697–707.
171. Hande KR, Wedlund PJ, Noone RM, et al. Pharmacokinetics of high-dose etoposide (VP-16-213) administered to cancer patients. *Cancer Res* 1984;44:379–382.
172. D'Incalci M, Rossi C, Sessa C, et al. Pharmacokinetics of teniposide in patients with ovarian cancer. *Cancer Treat Rep* 1985;69:73–77.
173. Holthuis JJ, de Vries LG, Postmus PE, et al. Pharmacokinetics of high-dose teniposide. *Cancer Treat Rep* 1987;71:599–603.
174. D'Incalci M, Rossi C, Zucchetti M, et al. Pharmacokinetics of etoposide in patients with abnormal renal and hepatic function. *Cancer Res* 1986;46:2566–2571.
175. Dennison JB, Jones DR, Renbarger JL, et al. Effect of CYP3A5 expression on vincristine metabolism with human liver microsomes. *J Pharmacol Exp Ther* 2007;321:553–563.
176. Dennison JB, Kulanthaivel P, Barbuch RJ, et al. Selective metabolism of vincristine in vitro by CYP3A5. *Drug Metab Dispos* 2006; 34:1317–1327.
177. Carlini EJ, Raftogianis RB, Wood TC, et al. Sulfation pharmacogenetics: SULT1A1 and SULT1A2 allele frequencies in Caucasian, Chinese and African-American subjects. *Pharmacogenetics* 2001;11: 57–68.
178. Iyer L, King CD, Whitington PF, et al. Genetic predisposition to the metabolism of irinotecan (CPT-11). Role of uridine diphosphate glucuronosyltransferase isoform 1A1 in the glucuronidation of its active metabolite (SN-38) in human liver microsomes. *J Clin Invest* 1998;101:847–854.
179. Iyer L, Whitington P, Roy S, et al. Genetic basis for the glucuronidation of SN-38: role of UGT*1 isoform. *Clin Pharmacol Ther* 1997;61:164.
180. Kuehl P, Zhang J, Lin Y, et al. Sequence diversity in CYP3 A promoters and characterization of the genetic basis of polymorphic CYP3A5 expression. *Nat Genet* 2001;27:383–391.
181. Raftogianis RB, Wood TC, Otterness DM, et al. Phenol sulfotransferase pharmacogenetics in humans: association of common SULT1A1 alleles with TS PST phenotype. *Biochem Biophys Res Commun* 1997;239:298–304.
182. Ratain MJ, Mick R, Berezin F, et al. Paradoxical relationship between acetylator phenotype and amonafide toxicity. *Clin Pharmacol Ther* 1991;50:573–579.
183. Reid J, Buckner J, Schaaf L, et al. Anticonvulsants alter the pharmacokinetics of irinotecan (CPT-11) in patients with recurrent glioma. *Proc Am Soc Clin Onocl* 2000;19:A160.
184. Weinshilboum RM, Otterness DM, Szumlanski CL. Methylation pharmacogenetics: catechol O-methyltransferase, thiopurine methyltransferase, and histamine N-methyltransferase. *Annu Rev Pharmacol Toxicol* 1999;39:19–52.
185. Robert J, Rigal-Huguet F, Hurteloup P. Comparative pharmacokinetic study of idarubicin and daunorubicin in leukemia patients. *Hematol Oncol* 1992;10:111–116.
186. Diasio RB, Beavers TL, Carpenter JT. Familial deficiency of dihydropyrimidine dehydrogenase. Biochemical basis for familial pyrimidinemia and severe 5-fluorouracil-induced toxicity. *J Clin Invest* 1988;81:47–51.
187. Innocenti F, Undevia SD, Iyer L, et al. Genetic variants in the UDP-glucuronosyltransferase 1A1 gene predict the risk of severe neutropenia of irinotecan. *J Clin Oncol* 2004;22:1382–1388.
188. Huang RS, Ratain MJ. Pharmacogenetics and pharmacogenomics of anticancer agents. *CA Cancer J Clin* 2009;59:42–55.
189. Nagasubramanian R, Innocenti F, Ratain MJ. Pharmacogenetics in cancer treatment. *Annu Rev Med* 2003;54:437–452.
190. Relling MV, Dervieux T. Pharmacogenetics and cancer therapy. *Nat Rev Cancer* 2001;1:99–108.
191. Watters JW, McLeod HL. Cancer pharmacogenomics: current and future applications. *Biochim Biophys Acta* 2003;1603:99–111.
192. Henderson EH, Samaha RJ. Evidence that drugs in multiple combinations have materially advanced the treatment of human malignancies. *Cancer Res* 1969;29:2272–2280.

193. Poplack DG. Acute lymphoblastic leukemia and less frequently occurring leukemias in the young. In: Levine A, ed. *Cancer in the young.* New York, NY: Masson, 1982:405–460.
194. Goldie JH, Coldman AJ. The genetic origin of drug resistance in neoplasms: implications for systemic therapy. *Cancer Res* 1984;44: 3643–3653.
195. Goldie JH, Coldman AJ. Application of theoretical models to chemotherapy protocol design. *Cancer Treat Rep* 1986;70:127–131.
196. Fojo AT, Ueda K, Slamon DJ, et al. Expression of a multidrug-resistance gene in human tumors and tissues. *Proc Natl Acad Sci U S A* 1987;84:265–269.
197. List AF. Non-P-glycoprotein drug export mechanisms of multidrug resistance. *Semin Hematol* 1997;34:20–24.
198. Michieli M, Damiani D, Ermacora A, et al. P-glycoprotein (PGP), lung resistance-related protein (LRP) and multidrug resistance-associated protein (MRP) expression in acute promyelocytic leukaemia. *Br J Haematol* 2000;108:703–709.
199. Moscow JA, Schneider E, Ivy SP, et al. Multidrug resistance. *Cancer Chemother Biol Response Modif* 1997;17:139–177.
200. Pastan I, Gottesman M. Multiple-drug resistance in human cancer. *N Engl J Med* 1987;316:1388–1393.
201. Roninson IB, Abelson HT, Housman DE, et al. Amplification of specific DNA sequences correlates with multi-drug resistance in Chinese hamster cells. *Nature* 1984;309:626–628.
202. Roninson IB, Chin JE, Choi KG, et al. Isolation of human mdr DNA sequences amplified in multidrug-resistant KB carcinoma cells. *Proc Natl Acad Sci U S A* 1986;83:4538–4542.
203. Scotto KW, Biedler JL, Melera PW. Amplification and expression of genes associated with multidrug resistance in mammalian cells. *Science* 1986;232:751–755.
204. Shen DW, Fojo A, Chin JE, et al. Human multidrug-resistant cell lines: increased mdr1 expression can precede gene amplification. *Science* 1986;232:643–645.
205. Grem JL. Fluorinated pyrimidines. In: Chabner BA, Collins JM, eds. *Cancer chemotherapy principles and practice.* Philadelphia, PA: Lippincott, 1990:180–224.
206. Burgert EO. Ewing's sarcoma. *Curr Concepts Oncol* 1986;8:11–17.
207. Dahl GV, Rivera GK, Look AT, et al. Teniposide plus cytarabine improves outcome in childhood acute lymphoblastic leukemia presenting with a leukocyte count greater than or equal to 100 × 10(9)/L. *J Clin Oncol* 1987;5:1015–1021.
208. Geyer JR, Pendergrass TW, Milstein JM, et al. Eight drugs in one day chemotherapy in children with brain tumors: a critical toxicity appraisal. *J Clin Oncol* 1988;6:996–1000.
209. Hays DM. Rhabdomyosarcoma: management in children and young adult. *Curr Concepts Oncol* 1986;8:3–10.
210. Magrath IT, Janus C, Edwards BK, et al. An effective therapy for both undifferentiated (including Burkitt's) lymphomas and lymphoblastic lymphomas in children and young adults. *Blood* 1984; 63:1102–1111.
211. Maurer HM, Beltangady M, Gehan EA, et al. The Intergroup Rhabdomyosarcoma Study-I. A final report. *Cancer* 1988;61: 209–220.
212. Miser JS, Kinsella TJ, Triche TJ, et al. Ifosfamide with mesna uroprotection and etoposide: an effective regimen in the treatment of recurrent sarcomas and other tumors of children and young adults. *J Clin Oncol* 1987;5:1191–1198.
213. Reaman GH, Ladisch S, Echelberger C, et al. Improved treatment results in the management of single and multiple relapses of acute lymphoblastic leukemia. *Cancer* 1980;45:3090–3094.
214. Dawson W. Relations between age and weight and doses of drugs. *Ann Intern Med* 1940;13:1594–1615.
215. Pinkel D. The use of body surface area as a criterion of drug dosage in cancer chemotherapy. *Cancer Res* 1958;18:853–856.
216. Hempel G, Boos J. Flat-fixed dosing versus body surface area based dosing of anticancer drugs: there is a difference. *Oncologist* 2007;12:924–926.
217. Mathijssen RH, de Jong FA, Loos WJ, et al. Flat-fixed dosing versus body surface area based dosing of anticancer drugs in adults: does it make a difference? *Oncologist* 2007;12:913–923.
218. Gurney H. Dose calculation of anticancer drugs: a review of the current practice and introduction of an alternative. *J Clin Oncol* 1996;14:2590–2611.
219. Baker SD, Verweij J, Rowinsky EK, et al. Role of body surface area in dosing of investigational anticancer agents in adults, 1991–2001. *J Natl Cancer Inst* 2002;94:1883–1888.
220. Grochow LB, Baraldi C, Noe D. Is dose normalization to weight or body surface area useful in adults? *J Natl Cancer Inst* 1990;82: 323–325.
221. Gurney HP, Ackland S, Gebski V, et al. Factors affecting epirubicin pharmacokinetics and toxicity: evidence against using body-surface area for dose calculation. *J Clin Oncol* 1998;16: 2299–2304.
222. Ratain MJ. Body-surface area as a basis for dosing of anticancer agents: science, myth, or habit? *J Clin Oncol* 1998;16:2297–2298.
223. Evans WE, Relling MV. Clinical pharmacokinetics–pharmacodynamics of anticancer drugs. *Clin Pharmacokinet* 1989;16:327–336.
224. Evans WE, Rodman JH, Relling MV, et al. Concept of maximum tolerated systemic exposure and its application to phase I–II studies of anticancer drugs. *Med Pediatr Oncol* 1991;19:153–159.
225. Graham MA, Workman P. The impact of pharmacokinetically guided dose escalation strategies in phase I clinical trials: critical evaluation and recommendations for future studies. *Ann Oncol* 1992;3:339–347.
226. Lowis SP, Price L, Pearson AD, et al. A study of the feasibility and accuracy of pharmacokinetically guided etoposide dosing in children. *Br J Cancer* 1998;77:2318–2323.
227. Rodman JH, Abromowitch M, Sinkule JA, et al. Clinical pharmacodynamics of continuous infusion teniposide: systemic exposure as a determinant of response in a phase I trial. *J Clin Oncol* 1987;5: 1007–1014.
228. van den Bongard HJ, Mathot RA, Beijnen JH, et al. Pharmacokinetically guided administration of chemotherapeutic agents. *Clin Pharmacokinet* 2000;39:345–367.
229. Woo MH, Relling MV, Sonnichsen DS, et al. Phase I targeted systemic exposure study of paclitaxel in children with refractory acute leukemias. *Clin Cancer Res* 1999;5:543–549.
230. McLeod HL, Relling MV, Crom WR, et al. Disposition of antineoplastic agents in the very young child. *Br J Cancer Suppl* 1992; 18:S23–S29.
231. Green DM, Finklestein JZ, Norkool P, et al. Severe hepatic toxicity after treatment with single-dose dactinomycin and vincristine. A report of the National Wilms' Tumor Study. *Cancer* 1988;62: 270–273.
232. Green DM, Norkool P, Breslow NE, et al. Severe hepatic toxicity after treatment with vincristine and dactinomycin using single-dose or divided-dose schedules: a report from the National Wilms' Tumor Study. *J Clin Oncol* 1990;8:1525–1530.
233. Woods WG, O'Leary M, Nesbit ME. Life-threatening neuropathy and hepatotoxicity in infants during induction therapy for acute lymphoblastic leukemia. *J Pediatr* 1981;98:642–645.
234. *Cancer pharmacology in infants and young children.* Arlington, VA: Children's Oncology Group, National Cancer Institute, Cancer Therapy Evaluation Program, 2003.
235. Bleyer AW. Clinical pharmacology of intrathecal methotrexate. II. An improved dosage regimen derived from age-related pharmacokinetics. *Cancer Treat Rep* 1977;61:1419–1425.
236. Bleyer WA, Coccia PF, Sather HN, et al. Reduction in central nervous system leukemia with a pharmacokinetically derived intrathecal methotrexate dosage regimen. *J Clin Oncol* 1983;1: 317–325.
237. Linabery AM, Ross JA. Childhood and adolescent cancer survival in the US by race and ethnicity for the diagnostic period 1975–1999. *Cancer* 2008;113:2575–2596.

CHAPTER

45

Amrish Jain
Rudolph P. Valentini
Tej K. Mattoo
Scott A. Gruber

Immunosuppressive and Immunomodulatory Drugs

INTRODUCTION

Organ transplantation has been performed successfully in infants, children, and adolescents for over four decades and is the standard of care for end-stage organ disease. In many centers across the world, increasing numbers of kidney, heart, liver, and other solid-organ transplants are being performed. The goal of organ transplantation has been to achieve long-term graft outcome. This has been possible as a result of major advances in understanding of immunobiology and use of novel immunosuppressive and immunomodulatory drug regimens. To understand the basis of immunosuppressive protocols and rationalize current transplantation practices, a brief history of transplant immunosuppression is provided.

HISTORICAL OVERVIEW

Major advances in immunosuppressive therapy can be related to a surge in the interest in organ transplantation after World War II. Alexis Carrel made the early observation that allografts were quickly destroyed, whereas autotransplants maintained long-term graft function. He surmised that allograft loss was due to biologic phenomena rather than technical problems (1). Modern transplant immunology developed in the 1940s with Gibson and Medawar's work established an immune basis for graft rejection and the need for immunosuppressive therapy (2). Initial efforts at immunosuppression with total body irradiation yielded very poor results. In 1954, the first successful live-donor kidney transplant was performed between identical twins by Murray et al. (3).

The era of drug therapy for immunosuppression was launched after Schwartz and Dameshek (4) demonstrated drug-assisted deletional tolerance using 6-mercaptopurine in 1959. Its analogue, azathioprine (AZA), in combination with corticosteroids, formed the mainstay of early immunosuppressive protocols in the 1960s. The addition of polyclonal antibodies in the 1970s marked the introduction of biologic agents (5). Much of the current success of organ transplantation can be attributed to discovery of the potent immunosuppressive agent cyclosporin A (CsA) by Borel in 1972 (6,7). The widespread clinical use of CsA in the early 1980s increased 1-year renal graft survival from about 50% to more than 80%. OKT3, the first monoclonal antibody (MAb) to be used in clinical transplantation, gained widespread acceptance despite its side effects in the mid 1980s as an adjunct to CsA, AZA, and prednisone (PRED). In the 1990s, the immunosuppressive armamentarium expanded rapidly with addition of mycophenolate mofetil (MMF), tacrolimus (TAC), and murine as well as humanized interleukin-2 receptor (IL-2R) MAbs. In 1999, sirolimus (SRL) was introduced and in the 21st century, it became a rescue agent in patients with calcineurin inhibitor-induced nephrotoxicity. Table 45.1 summarizes the major historical landmarks in transplant immunosuppression over the past several decades.

Advances in the pharmacology of these drugs, along with widespread use of therapeutic drug monitoring (TDM), has resulted in increased antirejection efficacy and reduced toxicity while ensuring high graft survival rates and overall improvements in the quality of life for transplant recipients. The current decade has focused on adding novel biologic agents to the armamentarium to achieve improved long-term graft survival. On the other hand, the concept of tolerance or near tolerance is fast emerging. Now, the goal of transplantation is to achieve a state where the graft continues to function well with minimal immunosuppression and avoid posttransplant infections, malignancies, and increased cardiovascular risk. Thus, achieving a balance between over- and under-immunosuppression has become the goal of organ transplantation.

Pediatric solid-organ transplants constituted only 7.0% of the 27,963 transplants performed in the United States in 2008 (8). The recent USRDS data documents a fourfold increase in the transplant prevalence rate in pediatric renal transplant recipients since 1980 (9). Hence, more data are now becoming available on the pharmacology of immunosuppressants in children. However, for newer therapies, few studies exist and only limited data are available in the pediatric population. Although many drugs

TABLE 45.1 Landmarks in Each Decade in the History of Transplant Immunosuppression

Year in Transplant History	*Milestone in Transplant Immunosuppression*
1950s	Successful live donor kidney transplant between identical twins
1960s	Introduction of azathioprine and use in combination with corticosteroids
1970s	Availability of antithymocyte globulin (ATG) and antilymphocyte globulin (ALG)
1980s	Cyclosporine introduction
1985	Use of OKT3, first monoclonal antibody
1990s	Tacrolimus, mycophenolate mofetil, daclizumab and basiliximab availability
1999	Sirolimus
2000s	Steroid and calcineurin-inhibitor avoidance/sparing protocols

TABLE 45.2 Immunosuppressive Agents Categorized According to Mechanism of Action

Mechanism of Action	*Drugs*
Polyclonal antibodies	Antithymocyte globulin Thymoglobulin (rabbit) ATGAM (equine)
Monoclonal antibodies	Anti-CD3 antibody: OKT3 (murine) Anti-CD52 antibody: Alemtuzumab (human) Anti-CD20 antibody: Rituximab Anti-CD25 antibody: Daclizumab (human) Basiliximab (chimeric)
Calcineurin inhibitors	Cyclosporine Tacrolimus
Target of rapamycin inhibitors	Sirolimus Everolimus
Antimetabolites	Azathioprine
Purine synthesis inhibitors	Mycophenolate mofetil
Others	Corticosteroids Intravenous immunoglobulin

have immunosuppressive properties, this chapter will focus on those agents primarily used as immunosuppressants for organ transplantation in children. A detailed discussion of the pharmacology of other drugs that may also have immunosuppressive and immunomodulatory properties, such as chemotherapeutic agents and biologicals, can be found in other sections of this book.

CLASSIFICATION

The immunosuppressive and immunomodulatory drugs can be pharmacologically categorized on the basis of their mechanism of action. The three-signal model of T-cell activity and proliferation is helpful in understanding the molecular mechanisms and site of action of various immunosuppressive drugs (10). Signal 1 features antigen-presenting cells (APCs; macrophages and dendritic cells) presenting the foreign antigen to the T lymphocyte, activating the T-cell receptor (TCR), which further relays the signal through the transduction apparatus known as the CD3 complex. Signal 2 is a nonantigen-specific costimulatory signal which occurs as a result of binding of the B7 molecule on the APC to CD28 on the T cell. Both signal 1 and signal 2 activate signal transduction pathways: the calcium–calcineurin pathway, mitogen-activated protein (MAP) pathway, and the nuclear factor-κB (NF-κB) pathway. This in turn leads to increased expression of interleukin-2 (IL-2), which through its receptor (IL-2R) activates the cell cycle (signal 3). Signal 3 activation requires the enzyme target of rapamycin for translation of mRNA and cell proliferation. Thus, various drugs act on different cellular signals and achieve immunosuppression by a number of mechanisms: depleting lymphocytes, diverting lymphocyte traffic, or blocking lymphocyte response pathways. Table 45.2 lists the immunosuppressive drugs and their mechanism of action. Figures 45.1 and 45.2 depict a schematic representation of the three-signal model along with the site of action of common immunosuppressive drugs.

Immunosuppressive agents are also classified on the basis of the phase of transplantation for which they are used (Table 45.3). Different immunosuppressive drugs are used for induction versus maintenance of immunosuppression, while others may be used for the treatment and reversal of graft rejection. The commonly used agents in immunosuppressive protocols are discussed in greater detail in the following section.

CALCINEURIN INHIBITORS

INTRODUCTION

The two drugs in the class of calcineurin inhibitors (CIs), CsA and TAC, form the backbone of current immunosuppressive protocols (Table 45.2). They share a common

TABLE 45.3 Immunosuppressive Agents Categorized According to Phase of Immunosuppression

Phase of Immunosuppression	*Drugs*
Induction phase	Daclizumab Basiliximab Thymoglobulin OKT3 Corticosteroids
Maintenance phase	Cyclosporine Tacrolimus Mycophenolate mofetil, azathioprine Sirolimus Corticosteroids
Treatment of rejection	Corticosteroids Thymoglobulin Intravenous immunoglobulin Rituximab

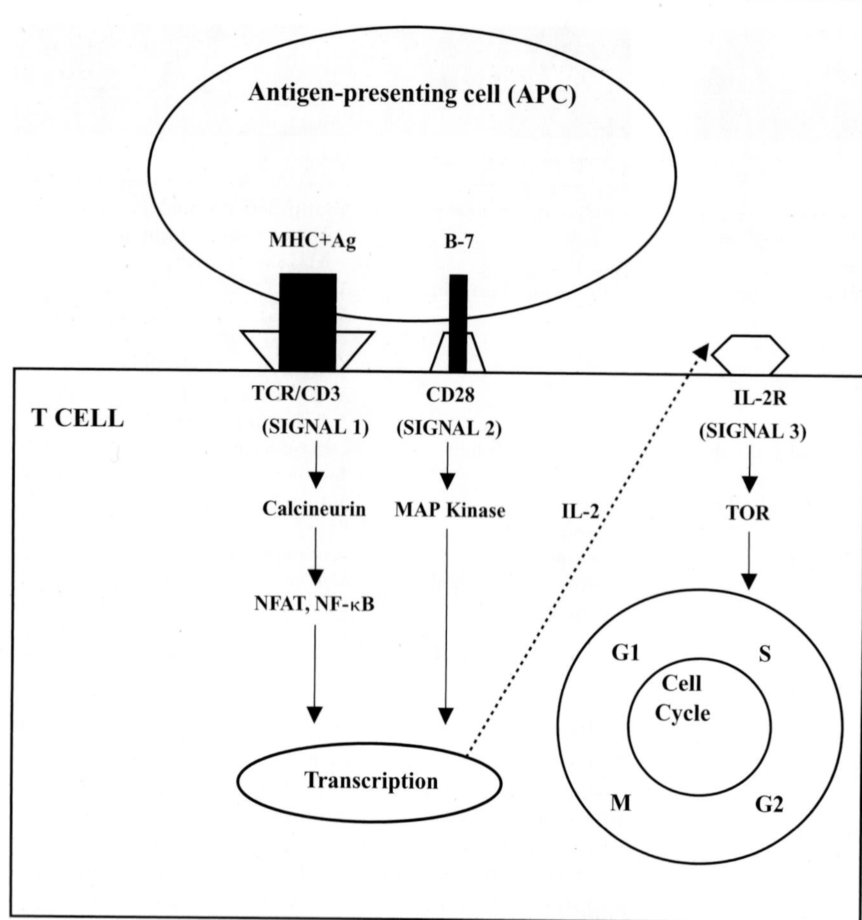

Figure 45.1. The three-signal model in T-cell activation of immunosuppressive agents. APC, antigen-presenting cell; IL-2R, interleukin-2 receptor; MAP kinase, mitogen-activated protein kinase; MHC, major histocompatibility complex; NFAT, nuclear factor of activated T cell; NF-κB, nuclear factor-κB; TCR, T-cell receptor; TOR, target of rapamycin.

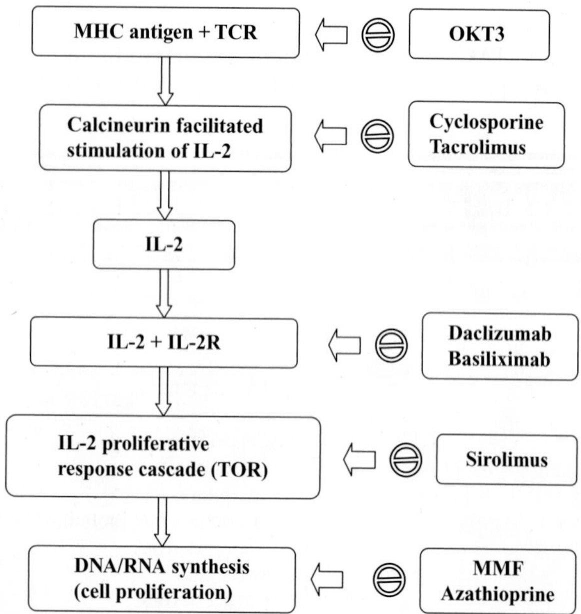

Figure 45.2. Site of action of common immunosuppressive agents. MHC, major histocompatibility complex; MMF, mycophenolate mofetil; TCR, T-cell receptor; TOR, target of rapamycin.

mechanism of action, although they differ markedly in their biochemical structure and properties. CsA revolutionized immunosuppressive therapy for solid-organ transplantation after the Food and Drug Administration (FDA) approved it in 1983. Before the introduction of CsA, there was a failure rate of 50% of renal grafts by 1 year as compared with 80% 1-year graft survival following its incorporation into most immunosuppressive protocols (11). TAC, which came into use in the 1990s, is 10 to 100 times more potent on a molar basis, and has increased antirejection efficacy and a slightly different side-effect profile when compared with CsA (12). TAC was used initially in liver transplantation and subsequently in renal transplantation. Currently, the vast majority of the renal, liver, and pancreas transplants, and virtually all small bowel transplants, are being performed using TAC-based protocols.

CHEMISTRY

CsA is a nonpolar, hydrophobic, small cyclic polypeptide antibiotic produced by the fungi *Beauveria nivea* (formerly

Tolypocladium inflatum Gams or *Trichoderma polysporum*) and *Cylindrocarpon lucidum* Booth. It has a molecular weight of 1,203 with 11 amino acids. Amino acids at the 1, 2, 3, and 11 positions form the active site, and its cyclic structure is critical for immunosuppression. TAC is a macrolide antibiotic with limited antimicrobial activity that is derived from the fungus *Streptomyces tsukubaensis*, originally isolated from a soil sample taken from the base of Mount Tsukuba in Japan.

MECHANISM OF ACTION AND PHARMACOLOGIC EFFECTS

T cells are stimulated by binding of an antigen to the TCR–CD3 complex (signal 1; Fig. 45.1). This leads to intracellular release of Ca^{2+}, and causes Ca^{2+}/calmodulin-dependent activation of calcineurin, a serine/threonine phosphatase. The phosphatase activity of calcineurin is crucial to the dephosphorylation of a nuclear regulatory protein known as the nuclear factor of activated T cells, which allows it to translocate into the nucleus and activate, directly or indirectly, transcription of genes encoding critical cytokines important in initiating the immune response, including IL-2, IL-4, interferon-γ (IFN-γ), and tumor necrosis factor α (TNF-α) (13,14).

Despite differences in molecular structure, both CsA and TAC bind to ubiquitous cytosolic proteins called "immunophilins." CsA binds to cyclophilin, and TAC, previously known as FK506, binds to the FK-binding protein FKBP12. These drug–immunophilin complexes bind to a calcineurin–calmodulin–calcium complex resulting in noncompetitive inhibition of calcineurin's phosphatase activity, thereby blocking the immune response. IL-2 is the most important T-cell growth factor and acts in an autocrine as well as paracrine fashion (13,14). Thus, as a result of calcineurin inhibition, there is marked decrease in IL-2 production and downstream lymphocyte proliferation. Since T cells contain relatively low levels of calcineurin, CIs are potent and selective inhibitors of T-cell activation. At therapeutic drug levels, calcineurin activity is reduced by about 50% (15). Although TAC is 10- to 100-fold more active than CsA on a molecular level, TAC does not inhibit secondary proliferation of activated T cells in response to IL-2 (12,16). It also does not appear to modify mononuclear phagocyte or natural killer cell function (16).

Other well-described effects of CsA include increased transforming growth factor β (TGF-β) production, sympathetic activation, vasoconstriction, increased plasma endothelin-1 levels, and upregulation of angiotensin-II receptors on vascular smooth muscle. These actions may explain some of the side effects of the drug, such as hypertension. Enhancement of TGF-β expression may contribute not only to immunosuppressive activity but also to renal interstitial fibrosis (17) and development of posttransplant neoplasias.

PHARMACOKINETICS

The pharmacokinetics of both CsA and TAC are characterized by high inter- and intraindividual variability and a narrow therapeutic index. Thus, close TDM is essential to identify under-immunosuppression resulting in graft failure as well as over-immunosuppression leading to toxicity, infections, and/or malignancy.

Absorption

CsA is primarily absorbed from the upper small intestine, with no apparent absorption from the colon (18). The original oil-based formulation of CsA (Sandimmune; Sandoz, Basel, Switzerland) was approved by the FDA in 1983 and was characterized by wide inter- and intrapatient variation in its bioavailability, especially in young children. The absorption of oral Sandimmune is highly bile dependent, and thus absorption is unpredictable in patients with liver transplant, cholestasis, biliary disorder, diarrhea, and malabsorption. A microemulsion formulation (Neoral; Novartis, Basel, Switzerland) was approved in 1995 because of its better absorption profile, since it is less dependent on bile, food, or other factors for its dispersion. Food tends to increase the absorption of CsA and its bioavailability also increases with time posttransplant, possibly because of improved absorption from nonuremic gut in the posttransplant period. Bowel length, interaction with other drugs, presystemic metabolism in the gut wall, and type of transplant are all contributing factors to the variation of bioavailability patterns in pediatric transplant patients.

Bioavailability of oral preparations averages 30% to 45%; hence, a 1:3 ratio is used to convert intravenous to oral dosing. Time to peak blood concentration (T_{max}) ranges between 1 and 4 hours depending on the formulation, patient age, transplant type, and time after transplant. In general, Neoral shows a faster peak and greater area under the curve (AUC) when compared with Sandimmune. In children with a renal transplant, a 70% increase in AUC and 92% increase in peak cyclosporine level (C_{max}) were observed following 1:1 conversion from Sandimmune to Neoral (19). Similar patterns have also been observed in pediatric liver transplant recipients (20).

Distribution

CsA is widely distributed to tissues outside the intravascular space. In the blood, up to 50% of the drug is in erythrocytes, about 40% is in plasma, and the rest is in other cells (21). Plasma CsA is 90% protein bound, mostly to low-density lipoproteins (21). The binding of low-density lipoprotein receptor with CsA is implicated as a cause of hyperlipidemia in transplant patients. On the other hand, lipoprotein binding is important for transfer of CsA across plasma membranes, and toxic effects may be reduced by lowering cholesterol levels. The volume of distribution (V_d) of CsA is 3 to 5 L per kg (21) and does not appear to differ between pediatric and adult transplant recipients. However, systemic clearance is comparatively higher in the pediatric population, with the highest clearance being in infants (22). The half-life of parent drug is approximately 8 hours.

Metabolism

CsA is extensively metabolized by the cytochrome P450 3A4 (CYP3A4) system in the liver, and to some extent in the gastrointestinal tract and kidneys. The intestinal CYP3A4 and P-glycoprotein, a drug efflux pump on the luminal surface of the intestinal epithelium, are responsible for first-pass metabolism (23,24). Marked interindividual and ethnic differences in activity of these enzyme systems, due to genetic polymorphisms, account for reduced and variable oral absorption (25).

The liver is the primary site of drug metabolism, but gastrointestinal metabolism may contribute up to half of CsA metabolism. CsA may be metabolized to more than 25 compounds, although most of the immunosuppressive activity and toxicity is attributable to the parent drug. Some CsA metabolites may have nephrotoxic and immunosuppressive potential, and one of the metabolites, M17, exhibits plasma levels similar to the parent compound. Excretion is primarily via the biliary route, and only about 6% of the dose is excreted in the urine (21). In cases of renal dysfunction, the dose does not require modification. Also, CsA is not dialyzable and can be given during dialysis without dose modification. CsA crosses the placenta and is distributed in mother's milk, but it does not cross the blood–brain barrier.

Dosing

The usual initial oral dose of CsA is 8 to 12 mg per kg per day, given in two to three divided doses during the induction phase, with target trough levels of 150 to 300 ng per mL. Higher doses are needed in the immediate posttransplant period to maintain higher blood levels (see later discussion) in the face of decreased absorption, which improves with time. Some authors recommend 300 mg per m^2 daily dose in children, with whole-blood concentrations within the range of 150 to 250 ng per mL for the first 6 weeks and 100 to 200 ng per mL thereafter (26). In general, pediatric patients require higher doses of CsA per kilogram of body weight to achieve target whole-blood concentrations of drug equivalent to that used in the adults. Younger patients (<8 years of age) may be managed more effectively with a thrice-daily administration schedule rather than the conventional twice-daily dosing used in the older pediatric and adult transplant populations (22). The comparatively higher doses and more frequent administration schedule used in pediatric transplant recipients are a consequence of age-related differences in bioavailability and increased metabolic clearance of the drug in younger patients (22). Several generic formulations of CsA are now available that have been deemed bioequivalent to Neoral by the FDA. However, bioavailability may vary, and more frequent TDM is recommended when switching between different formulations.

TAC shares many pharmacokinetic features with CsA but has its own unique characteristics as well. TAC is rapidly absorbed from the small intestine, when administered orally. Peak levels are reached within 1 to 2 hours, unlike CsA which may take 1 to 4 hours (27). Unlike Sandimmune, its absorption is bile independent, thus making it the preferred agent in liver transplant patients. In spite of its relative effectiveness and consistency of absorption, the drug has poor oral bioavailability (25% on average). TAC has wide inter- and intrapatient variability (6,28,29) due to extensive first-pass metabolism in the gastrointestinal tract and liver similar to that of CsA (30). Intravenous-to-oral conversion is therefore estimated by a 1:4 or 1:5 dose ratio. Pharmacokinetic profiling demonstrates both prolonged T_{max} and low C_{max} values following oral administration, indicating slow and poor absorption (31). The concomitant presence of food decreases both C_{max} and AUC. Gastric emptying of solids is faster in patients receiving TAC as compared with CsA, an effect that may be beneficial for patients with gastric motility disorders. Also, of interest is the role of transporter proteins, P-glycoprotein in the gut wall, which results in up to 50% of drug being excreted back into the lumen (32). This explains why drug concentrations tend to be higher during episodes of diarrhea, as the injured gut wall loses transporter capacity.

In the blood, TAC is highly bound to erythrocytes, partly accounting for its extensive V_d. Indeed, V_d ranges from 2.6 to 2.76 L per kg in pediatric liver transplant patients based on whole-blood levels (29,30,33). Seventy-two percent to 98% of plasma TAC is bound to plasma proteins (30). This is unlike CsA, which is more bound to lipoproteins, and hence TAC causes less hyperlipidemia than CsA. TAC is primarily metabolized via demethylation and hydroxylation by the hepatic CYP3A4 enzyme system into 10 or more metabolites. Although some metabolites may have biological activity, most of the immunosuppressive activity and toxicity is due to parent drug. The half-life of TAC is 8 hours, similar to that of CsA. Clearance is mainly via biliary excretion, whereas urinary excretion is negligible and no dose change is required in patients with renal dysfunction.

TAC is usually administered orally at 0.1 to 0.3 mg per kg per day in two divided doses. Most pharmacokinetic studies in children show that the dose required to maintain target blood concentrations is two to three times higher per kilogram of body weight than that in adults (31,34,35). This is related to the larger V_d and higher blood clearance of drug in the pediatric population, which are about twice that observed in adults, unlike CsA (30,31,33,36). Pediatric renal transplant recipients may have lower C_{max} and AUC values than liver transplant patients, consistent with decreased hepatic clearance in the latter group (34). Hepatitis C virus-positive patients may also require lower drug doses based on decreased liver metabolism (37,38). In general, patients with liver disease and older patients require longer dose intervals as compared with pediatric patients. Patients of African American ethnicity may also require larger doses of TAC at shorter intervals.

THERAPEUTIC DRUG MONITORING

The measurement of CsA and TAC levels is a routine practice in the management of all transplant patients because of the wide variability in pharmacokinetics and strong correlation between level of drug and the incidence of graft rejection and toxicity (39,40). However, controversy prevails regarding the optimal strategy for monitoring drug concentrations. Interpretation of drug concentration depends on sample matrix, assay methodology, type of organ transplant, and time posttransplantation.

CsA concentrations can be measured in whole blood or plasma. Whole-blood measurement is now preferred due to the wide distribution of the drug in red blood cells and the temperature dependence of plasma levels. Clinicians need to emphasize the assay used to detect these levels, since different methods are available. High-performance liquid chromatography (HPLC) is the reference standard for parent drug measurement but is not suitable for routine clinical use. The commonly used immunoassays for whole-blood sample measurement of CsA are the fluorescence polarization immunoassay and the enzyme-multiplied immunoassay technique. The commonly used assays cross-react with CsA metabolites to different degrees, and therefore target blood levels are specific to the assay technique utilized (6,41). Clinical outcomes correlate best with AUC, which provides the best estimate of total drug exposure in an individual. Because AUC estimation requires multiple blood draws at specific times, surrogates for drug exposure are utilized. Trough level (C0) is easier to obtain and is not greatly affected by small inaccuracies in the time of blood collection, and therefore is most commonly used. However, trough levels correlate poorly with AUC or with calcineurin phosphatase activity in renal transplant patients (39,40). Similar relationships have also been noted in pediatric liver transplant patients.

Neoral has a more consistent initial absorption profile than does Sandimmune. With the microemulsion formulation, CsA levels at 2 hours postdose (C2) have been found to correlate better with total drug exposure and immunosuppressive efficacy than C0 levels (42). A C2 blood sample also has a higher proportion of parent drug when compared with a C0 sample; this results in better agreement in C2 levels measured by different assay methodologies than occurs with C0 concentrations, which have a greater proportion of metabolites. However, error margins are greater for C2 levels if the sample is not collected within a narrow (±15 minute) time window. Overall, C2 monitoring has not been universally adopted but is rapidly gaining ground (43–45). Many pediatric centers now advocate measurement of C2 levels when monitoring CsA therapy in children (46–48).

Similar to CsA, TAC is a drug with a narrow therapeutic index. Because of variable bioavailability and clearance, TDM is mandatory for optimizing clinical outcome. Whole blood is preferred to plasma, as the preferred means for measurement of TAC levels because at least 75% to 80% of drug is bound to erythrocytes. The Abbott microparticle immunoassay methodology is widely used because of its ease and simplicity; however, the DiaSorin enzyme-linked immunosorbent assay provides less metabolite cross-reactivity. Unlike CsA, the 12-hour trough level of TAC correlates well with AUC and clinical outcomes and is the accepted standard for monitoring TAC therapy. Guidelines provided for target levels in adults (10 to 15 ng per mL in the first 3 to 6 months posttransplant) seem applicable to the pediatric age group, but more clinical outcome data are needed (6,49,50). Currently, target TAC trough whole-blood level guidelines followed at the Children's Hospital of Michigan (CHM) pediatric renal transplant program are shown in Table 45.4.

TABLE 45.4 Target Ranges for Tacrolimus Whole-Blood Trough Levels in Pediatric Renal Transplant Patients at Children's Hospital of Michigan

Months After Transplantation	*Fluorescence Polarization Immunoassay (ng/mL)*
0–3	10–12
4–6	8–10
7–9	6–8
10–12	4–6
>12	4–6

ADVERSE EFFECTS

CsA and TAC have similarities as well as differences in their toxicity profiles. Renal, metabolic, hematologic, neurologic, gastrointestinal, cosmetic, and other side effects are summarized in Table 45.5.

Renal Toxicity

The most common dose-limiting side effect of CIs is nephrotoxicity. CI-induced acute renal toxicity is due to a decrease in renal blood flow and glomerular filtration rate (GFR) produced by a dose-dependent, reversible vasoconstriction affecting primarily afferent arterioles, resulting in a picture of "prerenal dysfunction" with intact tubular function. Vasoconstriction is the combined effect of increased thromboxane and endothelin production, increased sympathetic activity and nitric oxide synthase inhibition with a decrease in nitric oxide, a preglomerular arteriolar relaxant. This renal vasoconstriction may manifest clinically as a delay in recovery of early graft function in kidney transplant patients, a rise in serum creatinine, or worsening hypertension. Renal vasoconstriction is more prominent with CsA than with TAC, also accounting for increasing sodium retention and hypertension. Acute microvascular disease can be caused by either of the CIs and has been

TABLE 45.5 Adverse Effects of Calcineurin Inhibitors

Organ System	*Toxicity*
Renal	Acute vasoconstriction—prerenal dysfunction Chronic interstitial fibrosis Thrombotic microangiopathy—hemolytic uremic syndrome-like picture Salt and water retention, hyperkalemia, hypomagnesemia
Gastrointestinal	Anorexia, nausea, vomiting, abdominal discomfort, diarrhea
Hepatobiliary	Elevated transaminases, cholelithiasis
Neurologic	Tremors, seizures, headache, insomnia, encephalopathy
Metabolic/endocrine	Diabetes mellitus, hyperlipidemia, hyperuricemia
Cosmetic	Gingival hyperplasia, hirsutism, hypertrichosis, alopecia, gynecomastia
Cardiovascular	Hypertension

shown to produce thrombotic microangiopathy, resulting in a hemolytic uremic syndrome (HUS)-like picture due to a direct toxic effect on vascular endothelial cells inhibiting prostacyclin production.

Chronic toxicity from CIs can lead to characteristic afferent arteriolar hyalinosis and patchy or striped interstitial fibrosis on renal biopsy. These lesions appear to be a result of long-standing renal vasoconstriction along with ischemia. The resulting chronic renal ischemia increases the accumulation of extracellular matrix proteins in the interstitium. Interstitial fibrosis is felt to be the result of a CI-stimulated increase in TGF-β production. Thus, resulting in chronic allograft nephropathy and ultimately leading to poor graft survival.

Fluid and Electrolyte Abnormalities

CsA is a more potent renal vasoconstrictor and as a result causes more sodium retention, edema, and hypertension when compared with TAC. Other side effects include hyperkalemia and mild hyperchloremic acidosis (a picture of type-IV renal tubular acidosis). Concomitant administration of a β-blocker, angiotensin-converting-enzyme (ACE) inhibitor, and/or angiotensin-receptor blocker may further exaggerate hyperkalemia. Hypomagnesemia is more common with TAC than with CsA. Hyperuricemia is also a common abnormality, although gouty attacks are more common with CsA than with TAC.

Glucose Metabolism Disorders

Posttransplant diabetes mellitus (PTDM) is a serious adverse effect of CsA and TAC therapy. A meta-analysis demonstrated a significantly higher incidence of PTDM among TAC-treated adult renal transplant recipients when compared with CsA recipients (51). Interestingly, a prospective randomized trial in children showed no differences in the PTDM rate (52). The proposed mechanism of CI-induced PTDM includes a direct toxic effect on β islet cells and an increase in peripheral insulin resistance.

Dyslipidemia

CsA has an adverse effect on lipid profile leading to hypercholesterolemia and hypertriglyceridemia. The binding of low-density lipoprotein receptor with CsA is implicated as a cause of hyperlipidemia in transplant patients and may also be related to abnormal low-density lipoprotein feedback to the liver. The effect may be less marked with TAC, and switching from CsA to TAC may improve the lipid profile.

Malignancies

Patients receiving immunosuppressants are at increased risk for development of infections, posttransplant lymphoproliferative disorder (PTLD), and other viral-associated malignancies. This risk is related to the overall intensity of immunosuppression rather than to specific individual agents. Although large studies focusing on the toxicity of these drugs in the pediatric population are not available, their adverse reaction profile in children appears to be similar to that in the adult population. However, the incidence of PTLD is higher in pediatric allograft recipients because these patients tend to be more heavily immunosuppressed (receive antilymphocyte antibody for induction and/or treatment of acute rejection) and are more likely to be Epstein–Barr virus (EBV) seronegative and receive EBV-seropositive donor organs. Although PTLD was initially shown to be more common with TAC, a randomized controlled trial in the pediatric population did not report increased malignancy with TAC when compared with CsA (52).

Neurotoxicity

Coarse tremors, headaches, and insomnia are dose related and more common with TAC. Seizures and leukoencephalopathy have also been reported.

Hematologic Toxicity

Hemolytic anemia with thrombocytopenia may occur as a part of HUS in transplant patients. We reported a pediatric case of autoimmune hemolytic anemia requiring multiple transfusions, which improved after withdrawal of CI and substitution with SRL (53).

Cosmetic

Gingival hyperplasia and hypertrichosis are more common with CsA than with TAC. CsA may also cause gynecomastia in men and breast enlargement in women. TAC may produce hair loss and alopecia.

To summarize, although there are similarities in their side-effect profiles, CsA has a greater tendency to produce gingival hyperplasia, hirsutism, hyperlipidemia, and hypertension. TAC is more likely to cause PTDM and neurotoxicity. In a randomized trial of TAC versus CsA microemulsion in pediatric renal transplant recipients, 95% to 100% of patients experienced at least one adverse event (52), most commonly hypertension, hypomagnesemia, and urinary tract infections. Hypomagnesemia and diarrhea were more common with TAC use, whereas hypertrichosis, flu syndrome, and gingival hyperplasia were more frequently seen with CsA. In this study, no differences were noted in the incidence of posttransplant infections, diabetes mellitus, or lymphoproliferative disorders.

DRUG INTERACTIONS

Because of the prime importance of the intestinal P-glycoprotein and CYP3A4 systems in absorption and metabolism of CIs, a large number of drugs that affect these systems can cause significant interactions (24,54), as shown in Table 45.6. Additive toxicity may also occur with other drugs, such as hyperkalemia with ACE inhibitors; nephrotoxicity with aminoglycosides, amphotericin B, and nonsteroidal anti-inflammatory drugs; and myopathy and rhabdomyolysis with lipid-lowering agents.

THERAPEUTIC EFFICACY AND PHARMACOECONOMICS

The clinician has to balance efficacy and toxicity when choosing a CI for transplant patients. A recently analyzed

TABLE 45.6 Drug Interactions with Calcineurin Inhibitors by Commonly Used Agents Affecting Cytochrome P450 3A4 (CYP3A4) and P-glycoprotein

CYP3A Inducer (↓ Drug Level)	*CYP3A Inhibitor (↑Drug Level)*	*P-glycoprotein Inducer (↓ Drug Level)*	*P-glycoprotein Inhibitor (↑Drug Level)*
Anticonvulsants	Antifungals	Anticonvulsants	Antifungals
Phenobarbital	Ketoconazole	Phenobarbital	Ketoconazole
Phenytoin	Itraconazole	Phenytoin	
Carbamazepine	Fluconazole	Carbamazepine	
	Voriconazole		
Antitubercular	Macrolide antibiotics	Antitubercular	Calcium channel blockers
Rifampin	Erythromycin	Rifampin	Verapamil
Rifabutin	Clarithromycin	Rifabutin	Diltiazem
Isoniazid			Nicardipine
Antiarrhythmics	Calcium channel blockers	Miscellaneous	Miscellaneous
Amiodarone	Verapamil	St John's wort	Protease inhibitors
Quinidine	Diltiazem		Wild cherry
	Nicardipine		
	Amlodipine		
Miscellaneous	Miscellaneous		
St John's wort	Glucocorticoids		
Carvedilol	Grapefruit juice		
	Protease inhibitors		
	NSAIDs		
	Metronidazole		
	Cimetidine		

meta-analysis of 30 randomized controlled trials in adult renal transplant patients (55) showed TAC to be more effective than the microemulsion formulation of cyclosporine in preventing rejection episodes. However, a higher rate of diabetes and PTLD was reported in the TAC study group. In the pediatric population, there is a paucity of studies comparing the two CI drugs. A randomized controlled trial in pediatric renal transplants demonstrated that at 4 years, patient survival was similar but graft survival significantly favored TAC. In children, both PTDM and PTLD were reported to be similar in the TAC and CsA study groups (56). Also, the medication costs were not significantly different over the 4-year posttransplant period (16). Because graft survival is better with TAC, it has a pharmacoeconomic advantage over CsA as also shown in adult trials.

MYCOPHENOLATE MOFETIL

The prodrug mycophenolate mofetil (MMF) is a 2-morpholinoethyl ester of mycophenolic acid (MPA), the active immunosuppressive metabolite. MPA was initially isolated as a fermentation product of the fungus *Penicillium* in 1898, but its immunosuppressive properties were not fully recognized until the 1970s. Approved by the FDA in 1995, it is primarily used as an adjunctive agent in combination with CIs and steroids as maintenance therapy for prevention of acute transplant rejection. It has almost completely replaced AZA in this role.

MECHANISM OF ACTION

MPA acts by blocking de novo purine synthesis in lymphocytes. Purines can be generated by de novo synthesis or by recycling (salvage pathway), and lymphocytes preferentially use the former. MPA is a selective and noncompetitive inhibitor of inosine monophosphate dehydrogenase 2 (IMPDH2), the rate-limiting enzyme in the de novo purine biosynthetic pathway for converting inosine monophosphate to guanosine monophosphate (GMP). Depletion of GMP by MPA has a relatively selective antiproliferative effect on lymphocytes. In vitro, MMF blocks the proliferation of T and B cells, and inhibits clonal expansion. This results in inhibition of antibody production, generation of cytotoxic T cells, and development of delayed-type hypersensitivity. Because of greater dependence of lymphocytes on de novo synthesis of purines as compared to the "salvage" pathway, MPA is a more selective inhibitor of T- and B-cell proliferation than AZA (9). MPA may also be beneficial in patients with chronic rejection by delaying and preventing proliferative arteriolopathy.

PHARMACOKINETICS

The pharmacokinetics of MMF appear to be similar in both the pediatric and adult transplant population. However, pharmacokinetic data in children are less available, with the focus mainly on renal transplant recipients (6,57–63).

MMF is rapidly and completely absorbed after oral administration with the mofetil moiety helping to improve oral bioavailability. It undergoes immediate hydrolysis by esterases into the active compound, MPA (6). Peak concentrations are noted within 1 to 2 hours postdose, and absorption may be faster in pediatric liver transplant patients than in adults (58,63). The presence of food prolongs T_{max} and decreases C_{max} by 40%. MPA undergoes significant enterohepatic recirculation (6). It is highly bound to serum albumin, but the free drug is pharmacologically active (6). MPA is primarily metabolized in the liver by β-glucuronidase to MPA glucuronide (MPAG), an inactive metabolite that may undergo enterohepatic recirculation. The excretion of MPAG in the gut may account for a second peak at 5 to 6 hours and may contribute to gastrointestinal side effects. MPAG is finally excreted in the urine. The half-life of the drug is 17 hours.

MMF is available as capsules, tablets, oral suspension, and intravenous solution. An enteric-coated form of MPA (myfortic) is also available. MMF is given in a dose of 600 mg per m^2 twice daily up to a maximum of 1 to 1.5 g per dose. At the CHM renal transplant program, we reduce the dose of MMF to 400 mg per m^2 twice daily once TAC is introduced to the regimen and approaching therapeutic levels. No dose adjustment is necessary in patients with hepatic impairment; however, in the presence of renal insufficiency (GFR $<$ 25 mL per minute), dose reduction may be necessary to prevent drug-induced toxicity due to increased MPAG and free MPA levels (64). Neither MMF nor MPA is dialyzable.

THERAPEUTIC DRUG MONITORING

MMF pharmacokinetic profiling demonstrates higher intraindividual variability in the immediate posttransplant period, which decreases over time while interindividual variability persists (65). Overall, AUC and C_{max} increase with time after transplantation (6,65). In pediatric renal transplant patients, MPA AUC was found to inversely correlate with the development of acute rejection, whereas the free MPA level was a better predictor of adverse effects (60). A literature review noted that TDM monitoring has limitations and has revealed conflicting results. A predose trough level appears less reliable as a predictor of risk of rejection (66). Although evidence is limited, a total MPA AUC value between 30 and 60 μg per mL by HPLC has been suggested for at least the first 6 months postrenal or heart transplantation when used in combination with steroids and CsA (67). The steady-state trough MPA concentration is to be maintained between 1 and 3.5 μg per mL for a favorable clinical outcome. A recent study in adult renal transplants demonstrated that creatinine clearance significantly correlated with 12-hour trough MPA level, suggesting its usefulness (68). Such findings in several other studies indicate that routine or selective pharmacokinetic or pharmacodynamic TDM of MMF may be advisable, but the ideal strategy, based on either trough MPA levels or IMPDH activity, remains debatable. Most studies have found AUC to be the most useful predictor, but this is not practical due to the multiple blood draws required (69).

ADVERSE EFFECTS

MMF commonly produces gastrointestinal side effects, including diarrhea (most prominent), abdominal pain, nausea, vomiting, and enterocolitis. Diarrhea can be seen in up to one-third of patients. Esophagitis and gastritis may also occur and, rarely, gastrointestinal bleeding or perforation may ensue. The gastrointestinal side effects may be improved after reduction in dosage or splitting among three or four doses. The gastrointestinal side effects of the enteric-coated formulation have not been found to be significantly different from those of MMF. In spite of its more selective action on lymphocytes, MMF can produce severe leukopenia, anemia, and thrombocytopenia as a result of bone marrow suppression. MMF dosing should be discontinued or reduced if the absolute neutrophil count is less than 1,300 per mm^3. An increased incidence of herpes simplex, varicella zoster, and cytomegalovirus (CMV) infections has been noted with MMF use when compared with AZA. MMF does not have any nephro-, neuro-, or hepatotoxicity. Finally, MMF should be avoided in conditions of hereditary hypoxanthine–guanine phosphoribosyltransferase deficiency, such as the Lesch–Nyhan and Kelley–Seegmiller syndromes.

DRUG INTERACTIONS

Concurrent administration of antacids, cholestyramine, or iron should be avoided with MMF because they decrease its bioavailability. Bile sequestrants reduce MPA AUC by interfering with enterohepatic circulation. MPA levels decrease from baseline requiring an increase in MMF dose by almost 50% when used in combination with CsA as a result of a decrease in enterohepatic circulation. This is in contrast to MMF usage with TAC or SRL, where no effect is seen, and therefore no MMF dose adjustment is needed (70). Glucocorticoids have been shown to reduce MMF bioavailability in adult renal transplant recipients by inducing glucuronyl transferase expression and thereby increasing MPA metabolism (71), but the clinical significance of this effect is not clear. MMF and AZA should not be given at the same time, as hematologic toxicity may be additive.

THERAPEUTIC EFFICACY

MMF is indicated for prophylaxis of allogeneic kidney, heart, and liver transplant rejection along with CIs and steroids. MMF has been associated with improved graft survival and improved renal function in combination with steroids and CI. It has been used to support immunosuppression while withdrawing CIs in patients with chronic CI toxicity. There have been studies with CI avoidance and using SRL and/or MMF instead. Also, use of MMF with reduction of CI has a favorable effect on blood pressure (72). Its use in primary glomerulopathy, lupus nephritis, rheumatoid arthritis, graft versus host disease after bone marrow transplantation, and atopic dermatitis has been gaining popularity based on clinical trials, though it is not yet FDA approved for these indications.

AZATHIOPRINE

A prodrug for 6-mecaptopurine (6-MP), AZA was responsible for the initial success of renal transplantation when used in combination with corticosteroids for immunosuppression. After the introduction of CsA, it formed the second component of "standard" triple-drug therapy (CsA, AZA, PRED). Currently, however, its use has virtually been completely replaced by MMF because of the latter's higher lymphocyte selectivity and greater antirejection efficacy.

MECHANISM OF ACTION

AZA suppresses the proliferation of B and T cells and decreases the number of monocytes circulating in the blood by arresting the cell cycle of promyelocytes in the bone marrow. Thus, AZA is an S-phase-specific agent that inhibits DNA synthesis by interfering with purine biosynthesis. This antiproliferative effect is a result of its metabolites, which include 6-mercaptopurine, 6-thiouric acid, 6-methylmercaptopurine, and 6-thioguanine. They also block the de novo pathway by formation of thioinosinic acid, accounting for the specificity of action on lymphocytes.

PHARMACOKINETICS

There are few pharmacokinetic studies in the pediatric population (6). Data from studies in adults demonstrate that AZA is rapidly absorbed after oral administration and is converted to 6-MP. When administered orally, about 50% of the dose is absorbed. Hence, intravenous to oral dose equivalence is 1:2. AZA is primarily metabolized by the liver to 6-MP, and further converted to the active metabolite thioinosinic acid by hypoxanthine–guanine phosphoribosyltransferase and subsequently, the metabolites are excreted by the kidney. About 1% of Caucasians are homozygous for an abnormal allele causing deficiency of thiopurine methyltransferase (TPMT), a key enzyme in AZA metabolism. These individuals are at high risk for developing drug-induced toxicity and can be potentially identified by TPMT genotyping (73). The drug is not significantly dialyzed and dose reduction may be needed with renal failure.

Dosing

AZA is administered orally at 2 to 3 mg per kg per day when used as a primary immunosuppressant. However, it is most commonly used in combination with CIs at a dose of 1 to 2 mg per kg per day. Allopurinol will increase the levels of the metabolite thioinosinic acid, and AZA dose may have to be reduced by two-third in patients requiring coadministration. TDM is not performed in patients on AZA, since therapeutic activity and toxicity is related to tissue levels and is independent of blood levels.

Side Effects

Its major toxicity is myelosuppression, predominantly leukopenia. It may also lead to anemia and thrombocytopenia and red cell aplasia in occasional cases. The hematologic side effects are dose related and may occur late in therapy. They are usually reversible on discontinuation or on dose reduction. Other adverse effects include gastrointestinal disturbances, hepatitis (reversible elevation in transaminases and bilirubin levels), and rarely pancreatitis. AZA also increases susceptibility to infections and is also associated with skin cancer development.

THERAPEUTIC EFFICACY

AZA is still infrequently used as an adjunctive agent in immunosuppressive protocols to prevent allograft rejection. It is also used in other disorders such as rheumatoid arthritis.

SIROLIMUS (RAPAMYCIN)

Sirolimus (SRL) is a lactone macrolide antibiotic derived from the fungus *Streptomyces hygroscopicus*, originally isolated from a soil sample taken from Easter Island (Rapa Nui, hence the name rapamycin) in 1975. Although it was being investigated as an antifungal and antitumor agent, its lymphopenic properties became apparent, which led to its use as an immunosuppressant (74). The FDA approved it in 1999 for clinical use in preventing renal allograft rejection. It is 100 times more potent than CsA in vitro, and because of different mechanisms of action, it works synergistically with CIs.

MECHANISM OF ACTION

SRL is similar to TAC in its molecular structure and also binds to the cytosolic protein FKBP12 (74). However, TAC acts as a CI, and SRL acts on signal 3. Thus, both act on different sites in the signal transduction pathway in spite of competition for the same cellular receptor, resulting in immunosuppressive synergism in vivo (14,74,75). SRL primarily inhibits T-cell proliferation in response to various stimuli, such as cytokines, alloantigens, and mitogens. The SRL–FKBP complex binds to the mammalian target of rapamycin protein, a key regulatory kinase, which blocks the activation of the 70-kDa S6 protein kinases necessary for cellular proliferation. The final result is an inhibition of DNA and protein synthesis and eventual arrest of cell-cycle progression in the mid to late G1 phase (14,74,75). Unlike CsA or TAC, SRL blocks IL-2-mediated signal transduction and cell proliferation and blocks lymphocyte response to IL-4, IL-7, and other cytokines. SRL also inhibits antigen- and cytokine-mediated B-cell proliferation independent of its effect on T helper cells. Finally, cytokine-dependent differentiation of B cells into antibody-producing cells is blocked, resulting in decreased immunoglobulin synthesis (75).

PHARMACOKINETICS

Similar to CIs, SRL also has poor bioavailability, demonstrates wide intra- and interpatient variability, has the potential for drug interactions by virtue of metabolism by CYP3A4, has its own side-effect profile, and requires TDM (76–78) (Table 45.7). SRL is absorbed from the gastrointestinal tract, absorption being delayed by a fatty meal. The peak concentration is reached in 1 to 2 hours with excellent penetration in most tissues. Its long half-life (average 62 hours) requires a loading dose but permits convenient once-daily dosing. SRL is a substrate for both CYP3A4 and P-glycoprotein. It is extensively metabolized in the liver by *O*-methylation and/or hydroxylation, and the parent drug accounts for more than 90% of its immunosuppressive activity. The drug is primarily excreted by the biliary system and renal excretion is minimal. Hence, dose adjustment is required in patients with liver dysfunction and not in patients with kidney dysfunction.

Very little information is available regarding the pharmacokinetic profile of SRL in the pediatric population. Children 4 to 10 years of age with renal transplants may have increased mean time to maximum concentration,

TABLE 45.7 Summary of Sirolimus Pharmacokinetic Parameters in Adults

Bioavailability (%)	14 (6)
Absorption	Delayed by high-fat meal (79)
T_{max} (hr)	1 (0.33–5) (6)
Blood distribution	Red blood cells 95%, plasma 3% (80), no temperature or concentration dependence
$t_{1/2}$ (hr)	35–95 (6,81)
Clearance (mL/hr/kg)	87–416 (6,81)
Metabolism	Liver and intestines, substrate for P-glycoprotein and cytochrome P450 3A (6,80,81); 56% metabolites in trough whole-blood levels (80)
Excretion	Feces

increased weight-normalized apparent oral-dose clearance, and a shorter half-life, indicating that higher doses corrected for body surface area and weight may be required to maintain similar drug concentrations (76).

TDM and Dosing

SRL is available as 1-, 2-, or 5-mg tablets or an oral solution. Whole-blood trough levels correlate well with AUC and are considered adequate for TDM, and a target range of 5 to 15 ng per mL has been recommended in adults (82,83). Since SRL has a long half-life, once dose adjustments have been made, levels should be checked 5 to 7 days later. Also, once steady state is reached, frequent monitoring of levels may not be required.

Drug Interaction

In adult kidney transplant recipients, SRL C_{max}, and AUC are markedly increased if CsA microemulsion and SRL are administered at the same time when compared with administration 4 hours apart (84). However, this effect was not seen in a small number of pediatric patients (76). It has been recommended that there be at least a 4-hour difference in the timing of full-dose CsA and SRL administration because both share the same metabolic pathway. In contrast, it has been suggested that when using low doses of either CsA or TAC, spacing of drug delivery is not important as long as TDM is used (42,85). Overall, simultaneous use of CsA and SRL may increase toxicity of CsA and may have a similar effect with regard to TAC combination. SRL levels may also be increased with use of CsA. Other drug interactions, similar to those with CsA and TAC, can occur with antifungals, anticonvulsants, and other drugs inhibiting or inducing CYP3A4 and the P-glycoprotein system.

ADVERSE EFFECTS

Common adverse effects include hypercholesterolemia, hypertriglyceridemia, myelosuppression (with thrombocytopenia being most prominent), increased incidence of lymphoceles, oral ulcers, and delayed wound healing (86). Nephrotoxicity occurs often as a result of SRL increasing

TABLE 45.8 Common Adverse Effects of Sirolimus

Organ System	*Toxicity*
Renal	Prolonged delayed graft function
	Proteinuria
	Hypokalemia
	Hypophosphatemia
Metabolic	Hypertriglyceridemia
	Hypercholesterolemia
Hematologic	Bone marrow suppression
	Anemia, leucopenia, thrombocytopenia
	Thrombotic microangiopathy
Gastrointestinal	Diarrhea
	Mouth ulcers
Pulmonary	Pneumonitis
Cosmetic	Impaired wound healing
Others	Lymphocele
	Reflex sympathetic dystrophy

CI toxicity. SRL is known to prolong delayed graft function and also causes proteinuria. Again, data in the pediatric age group are very limited (76). Table 45.8 summarizes the common side effects of SRL.

THERAPEUTIC USE

SRL is increasingly being used in pediatric transplant patients, and its role is still evolving. SRL has been shown to decrease the occurrence and severity of acute allograft rejection in combination with either CsA or TAC. Along these lines, it may assist in reducing CI dose and toxicity (87) and in permitting withdrawal of steroids from the immunosuppressive regimen. Use of SRL has potential for the prevention and/or treatment of chronic rejection (88,89) and in the development of CI-free protocols (90). Accordingly, SRL has helped in the design of CI withdrawal, CI avoidance, and corticosteroid-sparing regimens. A single-center experience with combination SRL/TAC/PRED maintenance therapy along with basiliximab induction in pediatric renal transplant recipients yielded a 100% 1-year graft and patient survival (91). Another single-center report demonstrated rejection-free graft survival in pediatric renal allograft recipients with a SRL/TAC/PRED regimen (91). A combined study in the adult and pediatric renal transplant population demonstrated the efficacy of steroid-free maintenance immunosuppression with an SRL-based regimen (92). A study involving 66 pediatric renal transplant patients reported a low rejection rate of 11% at 6 months with use of SRL/CI/PRED. However, 20% of the study population also reported significant adverse effects including pneumonitis and wound dehiscence (93). In pediatric heart and lung transplants, successful conversion to SRL in the late posttransplant period was reported without significant adverse effects (94,95). Interestingly, adult studies have also reported a low incidence of malignancies in patients receiving SRL-based regimens. Pooled data from five multicenter adult trials reported that SRL-based immunosuppression was associated with a reduced 2-year malignancy rate (96). In one of the studies, we reported a reduced incidence of CMV infection with a regimen using SRL versus TAC (97). The antiviral and antineoplastic effects of SRL are novel when compared with CIs and need further study in the pediatric population.

ANTILYMPHOCYTE ANTIBODIES

Polyclonal antibodies (antilymphocyte globulins) were among the earliest immunosuppressants used in organ transplantation in the 1960s along with AZA and PRED. Since then, the availability of MAbs, such as OKT3 and anti-IL-2 receptor antibodies, has expanded the spectrum of biologic agents in transplantation. Although mainly used for induction therapy to reduce the incidence of graft rejection in the early posttransplant period or to treat severe or steroid-resistant acute rejection episodes, these agents are also finding wider application in delaying CI introduction or in permitting steroid avoidance or withdrawal.

POLYCLONAL ANTIBODIES: ATGAM AND THYMOGLOBULIN

Two antithymocyte globulin preparations are commercially available in the United States, ATGAM and Thymoglobulin, prepared by immunizing horses or rabbits, respectively, with human thymic lymphocytes followed by harvesting the immunoglobulin G (IgG) fraction of immune sera. These preparations contain several antibodies that react with many different clones of cells and with a variety of molecules on lymphocytes.

Mechanism of Action

Their immunosuppressive effect is primarily due to lymphocyte depletion resulting from opsonization leading to complement-mediated lysis or mononuclear phagocytosis and induction of Fas-mediated apoptosis (98). However, nondepletive actions such as partial T-cell activation due to binding of multiple cell surface receptors inducing anergy may also be important (99).

Dosing

In pediatric renal transplant patients, 5 days of Thymoglobulin therapy was found to produce equal or greater immunosuppression than 10 days of ATGAM treatment (100). ATGAM at 15 mg per kg per day for 10 days and Thymoglobulin at 2 mg per kg per day for 5 days produced a rapid reduction in CD3, CD4, and CD8 lymphocytes to 2% to 15% of baseline within 24 hours. By day 10, the numbers increased to 14% to 34% with Thymoglobulin and 52% to 56% with ATGAM (100). In general, Thymoglobulin is considered the more potent preparation, may have beneficial effects in reducing the incidence of delayed graft function, and is more widely used.

Thymoglobulin is usually administered in a dose of 1.5 mg per kg per day for a 4- to 7-day period. The first dose is administered intraoperatively, when Thymoglobulin is used as an induction agent. It is infused over a 4- to 8-hour period via a central venous catheter. In rare circumstances, it may be infused through a peripheral vein by adding hydrocortisone and heparin to the infusion and increasing the volume to prevent thrombophlebitis. A skin test is recommended prior to ATGAM administration to prevent anaphylaxis. Premedication with steroids, antihistamine, and acetaminophen is used in most centers, especially for the first two doses before ATGAM administration. Dose adjustment according to absolute CD3 (<10 to 20) or absolute lymphocyte (<250) count is performed in some centers.

Side Effects

Chills, fever, and arthralgia are the most common side effects; anaphylaxis has occurred in rare instances. This "cytokine release syndrome" is less common with Thymoglobulin. Because of polyspecificity, these agents not infrequently produce leukopenia and thrombocytopenia, necessitating dose reduction or occasionally temporary cessation. They also tend to cause increasing susceptibility to viral infections especially CMV, as a result of prolonged depletion of lymphocytes. A summary of their side effects is shown in Table 45.9.

TABLE 45.9 Comparison of Side Effects of Polyclonal and Monoclonal Antibodies (109)

Side Effects	*Thymoglobulin*	*Basiliximab*	*Daclizumab*
Fever, chills, arthralgia	++	+	+
Cytokine-release syndrome	+	–	–
Anaphylaxis	+	Rare	Rare
Antibody formation	++	Rare	Rare
Hematologic		None	None
Lymphopenia	++		
Neutropenia	++		
Thrombocytopenia	+		
Anemia	+		
Infections	++	+	+
Hypotension	+	–	–
Hypertension	–	+	+
Hyperglycemia	–	+	+
Hirsutism	–	+	+
Pruritus	–	–	+

Therapeutic Efficacy

Thymoglobulin is used as an induction agent in high-risk patients who have high panel-reactive antibody and are a repeat transplant. Thymoglobulin is also used to treat steroid-resistant rejection and acute humoral rejection.

MONOCLONAL ANTIBODIES: OKT3, BASILIXIMAB, AND DACLIZUMAB

Mouse Monoclonal Anti-CD3 Antibody: OKT3

OKT3 was the first MAb to be available for organ transplant immunosuppression in 1987. It is a murine antibody produced by hybridizing mouse B cells with a myeloma cell line. After the initial dose, T cells are rapidly depleted from the circulation, and when they reappear in a few days, the modulated cells have a very low density of CD3/TCR and are therefore ineffective (101). OKT3 is highly effective in reversing acute rejection when used as primary therapy or for steroid-resistant cases (102–105). It is also effective as induction therapy for prevention of acute rejection. The usual daily dose is 0.1 mg per kg up to a maximum of 5 mg given intravenously daily for 7 to 14 days. Development of neutralizing (human-antimouse) antibodies may render OKT3 ineffective when used again after the initial course, and therapeutic monitoring with CD3 cell counts is recommended (101). A common adverse effect is the cytokine release syndrome, which is an influenza-like syndrome that results from release of IL-2, IFN-γ, TNF-α, and other cytokines following administration of the first dose of OKT3. Other toxicities/adverse effects that may follow include pulmonary edema, nephrotoxicity, headaches, aseptic meningitis, and encephalopathy. Excessive immunosuppression, with an increased incidence of viral (CMV) infections and PTLD, is a concern following administration of OKT3 as with the polyclonal antibodies. OKT3 is rarely used now due to the introduction of other antibody preparations with less toxicity and equal or greater efficacy.

MONOCLONAL ANTI-CD25 ANTIBODY: BASILIXIMAB AND DACLIZUMAB

The use of polyclonal antibodies for induction has decreased in the last decade and is being replaced by monoclonal antibodies. The 2008 North American Pediatric Renal Trials and Collaborative Studies (NAPRTCS) report suggests that use of polyclonal antibodies versus monoclonal antibodies was 28% versus 22% in 1996 as compared with 14% versus 40% in 2008, respectively (106). The two commonly used monoclonal antibodies are basiliximab (24%) and daclizumab (9.5%) (107).

Mechanism of Action

The anti-IL-2R antibodies basiliximab and daclizumab exert their immunosuppressive effect by binding to the α chain of the IL-2R (anti-CD25). The α chain of IL-2R is expressed on activated T lymphocytes and binding with IL-2 triggers the activated T cell to undergo rapid proliferation. Thus, blockade of CD25 prevents IL-2-induced T-cell activation and causes only minimal depletion of T cells. Basiliximab is a chimeric antibody which has murine heavy- and light-chain variable regions grafted onto human immunoglobulin constant domains. Daclizumab is a humanized Mab, which has murine hypervariable regions molecularly engineered into a human IgG backbone (108).

TABLE 45.10 Pharmacokinetics of Basiliximab and Daclizumab in Children (109)

Pharmacokinetic Parameter	*Basiliximab*	*Daclizumab*
Dose	10–20 mg	1–2 mg/kg
Total doses	2	2–5
Dose interval	Day 0 and 4	Day 0 and every 2 weeks
Trough level (μg/mL)	0.2	5
Volume of distribution (L)	5	3.4
Half-life (d)	10	13
Clearance (mL/hr)	17	10
Efficacy (d)	37	90

Pharmacokinetics

Both basiliximab and daclizumab saturate the IL-2R in vivo at serum concentrations of more than 0.2 and 1.0 mg per L, respectively. In adults, basiliximab is usually given in a 20-mg dose on days 0 and 4 postoperatively, and possesses a serum half-life of 7 days while maintaining receptor saturation for 30 to 45 days. Daclizumab is dosed at 1 mg per kg every other week for five doses. It has a half-life of 20 days, and saturates receptors for 90 to 120 days (108). A comparison of pharmacokinetics of the two drugs is shown in Table 45.10 (109,110). Dual-dose regimens with higher individual doses are being evaluated for daclizumab and could prove to be equally or more efficacious. We reported the use of two-dose daclizumab for the first time in pediatric renal transplantation with an acceptable incidence of acute rejection episodes (11.5%) without an increase in adverse events (111). In liver transplant patients, basiliximab has been found to have a shorter half-life of about 4 days and IL-2R blockade lasting 13 to 41 days because of loss of antibody in ascitic fluid and perioperative blood loss. However, satisfactory immunosuppression was achieved despite altered pharmacokinetics. Similar pharmacokinetic changes were also noted for daclizumab in adult liver transplant recipients (112). Thus, modified MAbs have a prolonged serum half-life and high affinity for human epitopes, can be given preoperatively, are easy to infuse in a peripheral vein even in an outpatient setting, have low immunogenicity, and can be reused without the development of human-antimouse antibodies (113).

Therapeutic Efficacy

In randomized, placebo-controlled phase III trials in adult deceased-donor renal transplant patients, induction therapy with either antibody resulted in lower rates of acute rejection in the first 6 months and a delay in the onset of the first rejection episode. In some studies, a reduced need for antilymphocyte therapy in treating steroid-resistant acute rejection and lower serum creatinine levels were also noted. In 24 children undergoing primary renal transplantation receiving daclizumab, TAC, and MMF, no acute rejection episodes were noted in the first 6 months (114). Basiliximab has been used in pediatric renal transplant patients at the adult dose if weight is more than 35 kg and at half-dose (10 mg) if weight is less than 35 kg. IL-2R blockade lasted for up to 6 weeks, and acute rejection developed in 21% of patients (115). Two other studies in pediatric renal allograft recipients found these doses to be efficacious (116,117). An extended course of daclizumab induction therapy in combination with TAC and MMF in 10 children undergoing renal transplantation allowed for steroid-free immunosuppression, with 100% patient and graft survival over a mean follow-up period of 9 months (118).

Side Effects

The safety profile of anti-IL-2R antibodies makes them an attractive choice for induction therapy (6,112,119). They do not result in cytokine release syndrome, thrombocytopenia, or anti-idiotype antibody development, and their use per se has not been associated with an increased incidence of CMV infection and PTLD. However, long-term studies, especially in children, are lacking. A comparison of the side effects of polyclonal versus monoclonal antibodies is shown in Table 45.9.

GLUCOCORTICOIDS

Although there is much interest in developing and testing steroid-sparing, steroid-withdrawal, and steroid-avoidance immunosuppressive protocols in solid-organ transplantation (120,121), glucocorticoids continue to be involved in all phases of posttransplant management, including induction and maintenance therapy for prevention of allograft rejection and first-line treatment of acute rejection episodes.

MECHANISM OF ACTION

Steroids have an effect on almost all components of the immune and inflammatory response, which contributes to their global immunosuppressive effect. Steroids complex with cytoplasmic glucocorticoid receptors, which translocate into the nucleus and bind to glucocorticoid response elements in the promoter region of critical cytokine genes, thus inhibiting their transcription (122,123). Steroids also reduce transcription of NF-κB-dependent cytokines by inducing transcription of the IκBα gene. IκBα protein then binds to NF-κB and prevents its translocation into the nucleus (14,124,125). The reduced production of immunoregulatory and proinflammatory cytokines, such as TNF-α, IL-1, IL-2, IL-6, IL-8, and IFN-γ, inhibits T-cell proliferation, prevents upregulation of adhesion molecules, and reduces the intensity of the inflammatory response. Glucocorticoids also increase production of Th2 cytokines such as IL-4, IL-10, and IL-13, which have anti-inflammatory and antiproliferative effect (123,126).

PHARMACOKINETICS

Glucocorticoids are primarily metabolized in the liver by cytochrome P450 microsomal enzymes. The hydroxyl derivatives are then conjugated with glucuronic acid, forming water-soluble compounds that are excreted by the kidneys. Because no TDM system is available for glucocorticoids, it is important to keep in mind possible pharmacokinetic interactions with other inducers or inhibitors of the cytochrome P450 system or with drugs metabolized by the same microsomal enzymes.

Dosing

The commonly used formulations are intravenous methylprednisolone and oral PRED. For pediatric renal transplantation at the CHM, methylprednisolone is given at a dose of 10 mg per kg intraoperatively, 2 mg per kg in two divided doses on day 1, and then tapered to oral PRED 0.6 mg per kg per day by day 7 and 0.15 mg per kg per day by 6 months. When used for acute rejection episodes, methylprednisolone 10 mg per kg is given for 3 to 5 days, followed by a tapering schedule of oral PRED.

Side Effects

Glucocorticoid-induced side effects include cushingoid habitus, hypertension, hyperlipidemia, osteopenia, growth retardation, aseptic necrosis of the femoral head, cataracts, hyperglycemia, psychopathologic effects, impaired wound healing, and acne.

THERAPEUTIC USE

Steroids are used in the induction and maintenance phases of immunosuppression and are also the first line of treatment for acute rejection. Side effects remain a significant concern for transplant recipients, even though lower doses are being used now due to availability of other powerful immunosuppressants (127,128). Along these lines, the number of patients receiving alternate-day steroids at 6 years posttransplant is about 31% (127), and median daily PRED dose has also decreased over the first 2 years following transplantation. Better growth has been demonstrated in children receiving alternate-day steroid therapy without a significant change in serum creatinine. Thus, various strategies are being developed to minimize the side effects: reduction of total daily dose, use of alternate-day dosing regimens, and steroid withdrawal in the posttransplant period or complete steroid avoidance (129–133).

CURRENT DESIGN OF IMMUNOSUPPRESSIVE PROTOCOLS

The incidence of acute rejection is highest in the early posttransplant period, with the majority of acute rejection episodes occurring in the first 3 months. Acute rejection is perhaps the single most important risk factor for subsequent development of chronic allograft nephropathy and graft loss in renal transplant recipients. This concept is incorporated in the typical design of immunosuppressive regimens, which call for intensified immunosuppression within the first week(s) posttransplant, called the induction phase, followed by a long-term maintenance phase.

INDUCTION PHASE

Although the goal of induction immunosuppression is to prevent acute rejection, several other factors affecting graft and renal function (in extrarenal transplants) have to be considered when choosing an induction regimen. High-dose, rapidly tapering steroids and MMF are part of almost all induction regimens. The choice of CI and/or antilymphocyte antibody used for induction varies depending on the organ transplanted, individualized donor and recipient risk factors for acute rejection and delayed graft function, and a center's preferences. The use of antibody induction is more widespread in the United States than in Europe. The nephrotoxicity of CIs and the better safety profile of newer antibody preparations have been the major factor favoring a trend toward antibody-based induction therapy. NAPRTCS data indicate that antibody induction was used in 54% of pediatric renal transplants (anti-IL-2R antibodies 34%, polyclonal antibodies 14%, others 6%, OKT3 0%) in 2007 (106). IL-2R MAbs are not considered as potent as polyclonal antibodies because only the IL-2Rα chain is blocked, and they are most often used concomitantly with CIs in induction therapy. Therefore, in patients who have received prior transplants or who have increased panel-reactive antibody and are at increased risk for rejection, or in deceased-donor recipients at high risk for delayed graft function where delayed introduction of CIs is desired, polyclonal antibodies are often preferred. In living-donor transplants, anti-IL-2R MAb with early CI use may be the preferred approach. However, comparable rates of acute rejection have been observed with either strategy in a randomized trial (134). Polyclonal antibody is given for the initial 4 to 7 days in the setting of delayed graft function, and CIs are usually withheld or started at low doses until the serum creatinine falls below 3 mg per dL (sequential therapy). Advantages of antibody induction include a reduced incidence and delayed onset of the first acute rejection episode (113–115,119,135–137), avoidance of CI nephrotoxicity in a newly implanted graft, and improved long-term function of deceased-donor transplants. A novel strategy utilizing extended induction with daclizumab until 6 months after transplant has been reported in children with the aim to reduce steroid use (138).

MAINTENANCE PHASE

CsA/AZA/PRED was the classic triple-therapy combination used in virtually all renal allograft recipients in the early 1990s, but TAC and MMF have gained substantial ground on CsA and AZA, respectively. NAPRTCS data in pediatric renal transplant recipients demonstrate that at 1 year posttransplant, 88% of patients were on CsA/AZA/PRED in 1992, compared with only 11% in 2007. Use of AZA decreased from 90% in 1987 to 15% to 20% in 2000 and to 3.5% in 2007 (106). When MMF was used in place of AZA, significant decreases in rejection rates were noted (139,140). The utilization of various drugs and regimens in NAPRTCS data at 30 days postrenal transplant is shown in Table 45.11. In the 2008 report, 26.5% of patients received CsA/MMF/PRED and 29% received TAC/MMF/PRED as their long-term maintenance regimen. The incidence of acute rejection both at 6 and 12 months as well as the incidence of steroid-resistant rejection was lower in the TAC versus CsA group (26,52). The TAC group also had a significantly higher GFR at 1 year posttransplant (26). Along these lines, triple therapy consisting of a CI, MMF, and PRED is the most commonly employed immunosuppressive strategy for maintaining long-term graft function and avoiding rejection over the lifetime of an allograft. Since its introduction a few years ago, SRL has been used as a secondary agent in combination with CIs and PRED in place of MMF or as a primary agent together with MMF and PRED (in a "CI-free" regimen) as maintenance immunosuppression.

TABLE 45.11 Utilization of Various Drug Regimens at 30 Days Postpediatric Renal Transplantation: 2008 NAPRTCS Annual Report (106)

Maintenance Drug Regimen	*Utilization (%)*
PRED/TAC/MMF	29.0
PRED/CsA/MMF	26.5
PRED/CsA/AZA	14.9
PRED/CsA	8.6
PRED/TAC	7.7
TAC/MMF	3.3
PRED/TAC/AZA	2.1
Other combinations	8.0

AZA, azathioprine; CsA, cyclosporin A; MMF, mycophenolate mofetil; PRED, prednisone; TAC, tacrolimus.

Thus, increasing utilization of potent induction and maintenance immunosuppressive medications has improved long-term graft survival and also helped in achieving the short-term goal of reduced rejection rates. On the other hand, we have seen an increase in infections and PTLD and hence immunosuppression minimization is being studied. The approach is targeted to either avoid or withdraw corticosteroids or CIs early on and normalize growth curves with minimal drug nephrotoxicity.

ACKNOWLEDGMENTS

We are thankful to Dr. Neena R. Gupta and Dr. Darla K. Granger for their contribution to the initial version of this chapter.

REFERENCES

1. Papalois VE, Najarian JS. Pediatric kidney transplantation: historic hallmarks and a personal perspective. *Pediatr Transplant* 2001; 5:239–245.
2. Gibson T, Medawar PB. The behavior of skin homografts in man. *J Anat* 1943;77:299–310.
3. Murray JE, Merrill JP, Harrison JH. Kidney Transplantation between seven pairs of identical twins. *Ann Surg* 1958;148: 343–359.

4. Schwartz R, Dameshek W. Drug-induced immunological tolerance. *Nature* 1959;183:1682–1683.
5. Starzl TE, Marchioro TL, Porter KA, et al. The use of heterologous antilymphoid agents in canine renal and liver homotransplantation and in human renal homotransplantation. *Surg Gynecol Obstet* 1967;124:301–308.
6. del Mar Fernández De Gatta M, Santos-Buelga D, Dominguez-Gil A, et al. Immunosuppressive therapy for paediatric transplant patients: pharmacokinetic considerations. *Clin Pharmacokinet* 2002; 41:115–135.
7. Borel JF, Feurer C, Gubler HU, et al. Biological effects of cyclosporin A: a new antilymphocytic agent. *Agents Actions* 1976; 6:468–475.
8. Organ Procurement and Transplant Network. http://optn.transplant.hrsa.gov/latestData/viewDataReports.asp. Accessed September 1, 2009.
9. United States Renal Data System. http://www.usrds.org/2008. Accessed September 1, 2009.
10. Pietra BA. Transplantation immunology 2003: simplified approach. *Pediatr Clin N Am 2003*;50:1233–1259.
11. Kari JA, Trompeter RS. What is the calcineurin inhibitor of choice for pediatric renal transplantation? *Pediatr Transplant* 2004; 8:437–444.
12. Scott LJ, McKeage K, Keam SJ, et al. Tacrolimus: a further update of its use in the management of organ transplantation. *Drugs* 2003;63:1247–1297.
13. Hutchinson IV, Bagnall W, Bryce P, et al. Differences in the mode of action of cyclosporine and FK 506. *Transplant Proc* 1998; 30:959–960.
14. Suthanthiran M, Strom TB. Immunoregulatory drugs: mechanistic basis for use in organ transplantation. *Pediatr Nephrol* 1997;11: 651–657.
15. Batiuk TD, Pazderka F, Halloran PF. Calcineurin activity is only partially inhibited in leukocytes of cyclosporine-treated patients. *Transplantation* 1995;59:1400–1404.
16. Filler G. Calcineurin inhibitors in pediatric renal transplant recipients. *Pediatr Drugs* 2007;9:165–174.
17. Khanna AK, Cairns VR, Becker CG, et al. TGF-beta: a link between immunosuppression, nephrotoxicity, and CsA. *Transplant Proc* 1998;30:944–945.
18. Drewe J, Beglinger C, Kissel T. The absorption site of cyclosporin in the human gastrointestinal tract. *Br J Clin Pharmacol* 1992;33: 39–43.
19. Kelles A, Herman J, Tjandra-Maga TB, et al. Sandimmune to Neoral conversion and value of abbreviated AUC monitoring in stable pediatric kidney transplant recipients. *Pediatr Transplant* 1999;3:282–287.
20. Dunn S, Cooney G, Sommerauer J, et al. Pharmacokinetics of an oral solution of the microemulsion formulation of cyclosporine in maintenance pediatric liver transplant recipients. *Transplantation* 1997;63:1762–1767.
21. Dunn CJ, Wagstaff AJ, Perry CM, et al. Cyclosporin: an updated review of the pharmacokinetic properties, clinical efficacy and tolerability of a microemulsion-based formulation (Neoral) in organ transplantation. *Drugs* 2001;61:1957–2016.
22. Cooney GF, Habucky K, Hoppu K. Cyclosporin pharmacokinetics in paediatric transplant recipients. *Clin Pharmacokinet* 1997; 32:481–495.
23. Roberts MS, Magnusson BM, Burczynski FJ, et al. Enterohepatic circulation: physiological, pharmacokinetic and clinical implications. *Clin Pharmacokinet* 2002;41:751–790.
24. van Gelder T. Drug interactions with tacrolimus. *Drug Saf* 2002;25:707–712.
25. Macphee IA, Fredericks S, Tai T, et al. Tacrolimus pharmacogenetics: polymorphisms associated with expression of cytochrome p4503A5 and P-glycoprotein correlate with dose requirement. *Transplantation* 2002;74:1486–1489.
26. Filler G, Trompeter R, Webb NJ, et al. One year glomerular filtration rate predicts graft survival in pediatric renal recipients: a randomized trial of tacrolimus vs cyclosporine microemulsion. *Transplant Proc* 2002;34:1935–1938.
27. Montini G, Ujka F, Varagnolo C, et al. The pharmacokinetics and immunosuppressive response of tacrolimus in pediatric renal transplant recipients. *Pediatr Nephrol* 2006;21:719–724.
28. Venkataramanan R, Swaminathan A, Prasad T, et al. Clinical pharmacokinetics of tacrolimus. *Clin Pharmacokinet* 1995;29:404–430.
29. Yasuhara M, Hashida T, Toraguchi M, et al. Pharmacokinetics and pharmacodynamics of FK 506 in pediatric patients receiving living-related donor liver transplantations. *Transplant Proc* 1995;27: 1108–1110.
30. Wallemacq PE, Verbeeck RK. Comparative clinical pharmacokinetics of tacrolimus in paediatric and adult patients. *Clin Pharmacokinet* 2001;40:283–295.
31. Shishido S, Asanuma H, Tajima E, et al. Pharmacokinetics of tacrolimus in pediatric renal transplant recipients. *Transplant Proc* 2001;33:1066–1068.
32. Christians U, Strom T, Zhang YL, et al. Active drug transport of immunosuppressants: new insights for pharmacokinetics and pharmacodynamics. *Ther Drug Monit* 2006;28:39–44.
33. Wallemacq PE, Furlan V, Moller A, et al. Pharmacokinetics of tacrolimus (FK506) in paediatric liver transplant recipients. *Eur J Drug Metab Pharmacokinet* 1998;23:367–370.
34. Filler G, Grygas R, Mai I, et al. Pharmacokinetics of tacrolimus (FK 506) in children and adolescents with renal transplants. *Nephrol Dial Transplant* 1997;12:1668–1671.
35. McDiarmid SV, Colonna JO, Shaked A, et al. Differences in oral FK506 dose requirements between adult and pediatric liver transplant patients. *Transplantation* 1993;55:1328–1332.
36. Mehta P, Beltz S, Kedar A, et al. Increased clearance of tacrolimus in children: need for higher doses and earlier initiation prior to bone marrow transplantation. *Bone Marrow Transplant* 1999;24: 1323–1327.
37. Manzanares C, Moreno M, Castellanos F, et al. Influence of hepatitis C virus infection on FK 506 blood levels in renal transplant patients. *Transplant Proc* 1998;30:1264–1265.
38. Moreno M, Manzanares C, Castellano F, et al. Monitoring of tacrolimus as rescue therapy in pediatric liver transplantation. *Ther Drug Monit* 1998;20:376–379.
39. Lindholm A, Kahan BD. Influence of cyclosporine pharmacokinetics, trough concentrations, and AUC monitoring on outcome after kidney transplantation. *Clin Pharmacol Ther* 1993;54: 205–218.
40. Mahalati K, Belitsky P, Sketris I, et al. Neoral monitoring by simplified sparse sampling area under the concentration–time curve: its relationship to acute rejection and cyclosporine nephrotoxicity early after kidney transplantation. *Transplantation* 1999;68: 55–62.
41. Shaw LM, Holt DW, Keown P, et al. Current opinions on therapeutic drug monitoring of immunosuppressive drugs. *Clin Ther* 1999;21:1632–1652.
42. Kahan BD, Keown P, Levy GA, et al. Therapeutic drug monitoring of immunosuppressant drugs in clinical practice. *Clin Ther* 2002;24:330–350.
43. Cole E, Midtvedt K, Johnston A, et al. Recommendations for the implementation of Neoral C_2 monitoring in clinical practice. *Transplantation* 2002;73:S19–S22.
44. Levy G, Thervet E, Lake J, et al. Patient management by Neoral C_2 monitoring: an international consensus statement. *Transplantation* 2002;73:S12–S18.
45. Nashan B, Cole E, Levy G, et al. Clinical validation studies of Neoral C_2 monitoring: a review. *Transplantation* 2002;73:S3–S11.
46. Dello Strologo L, Pontesilli C, Rizzoni G, et al. C2 monitoring: a reliable tool in pediatric renal transplant recipients. *Transplantation* 2003;76:444–445.
47. Ferraresso M, Ghoi L, Zacchello G, et al. Pharmacokinetic of cyclosporine microemulsion in pediatric kidney recipients receiving a quadruple immunosuppressive regimen: the value of C2 blood levels. *Transplantation* 2005;79:1164–1168.
48. Pape L, Ehrich JH, Offner G. Advantages of cyclosporine A using 2-h levels in pediatric kidney transplantation. *Pediatr Nephrol* 2004; 19:1035–1038.
49. Jusko WJ, Thomson AW, Fung J, et al. Consensus document: therapeutic monitoring of tacrolimus (FK-506). *Ther Drug Monit* 1995;17:606–614.
50. Shapiro R. Tacrolimus in pediatric renal transplantation: a review. *Pediatr Transplant* 1998;2:270–276.
51. Webster A, Woodroffe RC, Taylor RS, et al. Tacrolimus versus cyclosporine as primary immunosuppression for kidney transplant recipients. *Cochrane Database Syst Rev* 2005;4:CD003961.
52. Trompeter R, Filler G, Webb NJ, et al. Randomized trial of tacrolimus versus cyclosporin microemulsion in renal transplantation. *Pediatr Nephrol* 2002;17:141–149.

53. Valentini RP, Imam A, Warrier I, et al. Sirolimus rescue for tacrolimus-associated post-transplant autoimmune hemolytic anemia. *Pediatr Transplant* 2006;10:358–361.
54. Campana C, Regazzi MB, Buggia I, et al. Clinically significant drug interactions with cyclosporin. An update. *Clin Pharmacokinet* 1996;30:141–179.
55. Webster A, Woodroffe RC, Taylor RS, et al. Tacrolimus versus cyclosporine as primary immunosuppression for kidney transplant recipients: meta analysis and meta-regression of randomized trial data. *BMJ* 2005;331:810–822.
56. Filler G, Webb NJ, Milford DV, et al. Four-year data after pediatric renal transplantation: a randomized trial of Tacrolimus vs cyclosporine microemulsion. *Pediatr Transplant* 2005;9: 498–503.
57. Aigrain EJ, Shaghaghi EK, Baudouin V, et al. Pharmacokinetics of mycophenolate mofetil in eight pediatric renal transplant patients. *Transplant Proc* 2000;32:388–390.
58. Jacqz-Aigrain E, Khan SE, Baudouin V, et al. Pharmacokinetics and tolerance of mycophenolate mofetil in renal transplant children. *Pediatr Nephrol* 2000;14:95–99.
59. Weber LT, Shipkova M, Armstrong VW, et al. Comparison of the Emit immunoassay with HPLC for therapeutic drug monitoring of mycophenolic acid in pediatric renal-transplant recipients on mycophenolate mofetil therapy. *Clin Chem* 2002;48: 517–525.
60. Weber LT, Shipkova M, Armstrong VW, et al. The pharmacokinetic–pharmacodynamic relationship for total and free mycophenolic acid in pediatric renal transplant recipients: a report of the German study group on mycophenolate mofetil therapy. *J Am Soc Nephrol* 2002;13:759–768.
61. Weber LT, Schutz E, Lamersdorf T, et al. Therapeutic drug monitoring of total and free mycophenolic acid (MPA) and limited sampling strategy for determination of MPA-AUC in paediatric renal transplant recipients. The German Study Group on Mycophenolate Mofetil (MMF) Therapy. *Nephrol Dial Transplant* 1999;14(Suppl 4):34–35.
62. Weber LT, Schutz E, Lamersdorf T, et al. Pharmacokinetics of mycophenolic acid (MPA) and free MPA in paediatric renal transplant recipients—a multicentre study. The German Study Group on Mycophenolate Mofetil (MMF) Therapy. *Nephrol Dial Transplant* 1999;14(Suppl 4):33–34.
63. Brown NW, Aw MM, Mieli-Vergani G, et al. Mycophenolic acid and mycophenolic acid glucuronide pharmacokinetics in pediatric liver transplant recipients: effect of cyclosporine and tacrolimus comedication. *Ther Drug Monit* 2002;24:598–606.
64. Kaplan B, Gruber SA, Nallamathou R, et al. Decreased protein binding of mycophenolic acid associated with leukopenia in a pancreas transplant recipient with renal failure. *Transplantation* 1998;65:1127–1129.
65. Weber LT, Lamersdorf T, Shipkova M, et al. Area under the plasma concentration–time curve for total, but not for free, mycophenolic acid increases in the stable phase after renal transplantation: a longitudinal study in pediatric patients. German Study Group on Mycophenolate Mofetil Therapy in Pediatric Renal Transplant Recipients. *Ther Drug Monit* 1999;21: 498–506.
66. Arns W, Cibrik DM, Walker RG, et al. Therapeutic drug monitoring of mycophenolic acid in solid organ transplant patients treated with mycophenolate mofetil: review of the literature. *Transplantation.* 2006;82:1004–1012.
67. Shaw LM, Holt DW, Oellerich M, et al. Current issues in therapeutic drug monitoring of mycophenolic acid: report of a roundtable discussion. *Ther Drug Monit* 2001;23:305.
68. Sánchez Fructuoso AI, de la Higuera MA, Garcia-Ledesma P, et al. Graft outcome and mycophenolic acid trough level monitoring in kidney transplantation. *Transplant Proc* 2009;41: 2102–2103.
69. Mourad M, Wallemacq P, Konig J, et al. Therapeutic monitoring of mycophenolate mofetil in organ transplant recipients: is it necessary?. *Clin Pharmacokinet* 2002;41:319–327.
70. Filler G, Zimmering M, Mai I. Pharmacokinetics of mycophenolate mofetil are influenced by concomitant immunosuppression. *Pediatr Nephrol* 2000;14:100–104.
71. Cattaneo D, Perico N, Gaspari F, et al. Glucocorticoids interfere with mycophenolate mofetil bioavailability in kidney transplantation. *Kidney Int* 2002;62:1060–1067.
72. Zimmerhackl LB, Wiesmayr S, Kirste G, et al. Mycophenolate mofetil (Cellcept) in pediatric renal transplantation. *Transplant Proc* 2006;38:2038–2040.
73. Yagil Y, Yagil C. Insights into pharmacogenomics and its impact upon immunosuppressive therapy. *Transpl Immunol* 2002;9: 203–209.
74. Abraham RT, Wiederrecht GJ. Immunopharmacology of rapamycin. *Annu Rev Immunol* 1996;14:483–510.
75. Sehgal SN, Rapamune (RAPA, rapamycin, sirolimus): mechanism of action; immunosuppressive effect results from blockade of signal transduction and inhibition of cell cycle progression. *Clin Biochem* 1998;31:335–340.
76. Ettenger RB, Grimm EM. Safety and efficacy of TOR inhibitors in pediatric renal transplant recipients. *Am J Kidney Dis* 2001;38: S22–S28.
77. Gallant-Haidner HL, Trepanier DJ, Freitag DG, et al. Pharmacokinetics and metabolism of sirolimus. *Ther Drug Monit* 2000;22:31–35.
78. Mahalati K, Kahan BD. Clinical pharmacokinetics of sirolimus. *Clin Pharmacokinet* 2001;40:573–585.
79. Zimmerman JJ, Ferron GM, Lim HK, et al. The effect of a high-fat meal on the oral bioavailability of the immunosuppressant sirolimus (rapamycin). *J Clin Pharmacol* 1999;39:1155–1161.
80. Trepanier DJ, Gallant H, Legatt DF, et al. Rapamycin: distribution, pharmacokinetics and therapeutic range investigations: an update. *Clin Biochem* 1998;31:345–351.
81. Ingle GR, Sievers TM, Holt CD. Sirolimus: continuing the evolution of transplant immunosuppression. *Ann Pharmacother* 2000;34: 1044–1055.
82. Meier-Kriesche HU, Kaplan B. Toxicity and efficacy of sirolimus: relationship to whole-blood concentrations. *Clin Ther* 2000; 22(Suppl B):B93–B100.
83. Kahan BD, Napoli KL, Kelly PA, et al. Therapeutic drug monitoring of sirolimus: correlations with efficacy and toxicity. *Clin Transplant* 2000;14:97–109.
84. Kaplan B, Meier-Kriesche HU, Napoli KL, et al. The effects of relative timing of sirolimus and cyclosporine microemulsion formulation coadministration on the pharmacokinetics of each agent. *Clin Pharmacol Ther* 1998;63:48–53.
85. McAlister VC, Mahalati K, Peltekian KM, et al. A clinical pharmacokinetic study of tacrolimus and sirolimus combination immunosuppression comparing simultaneous to separated administration. *Ther Drug Monit* 2002;24:346–350.
86. Kahan BD. The limitations of calcineurin and mTOR inhibitors: new directions for immunosuppressive strategies. *Transplant Proc* 2002;34:130–133.
87. Kahan BD, Julian BA, Pescovitz MD, et al. Sirolimus reduces the incidence of acute rejection episodes despite lower cyclosporine doses in Caucasian recipients of mismatched primary renal allografts: a phase II trial. Rapamune Study Group. *Transplantation* 1999;68:1526–1532.
88. Kahan BD. The potential role of rapamycin in pediatric transplantation as observed from adult studies. *Pediatr Transplant* 1999; 3:175–180.
89. Kahan BD. Sirolimus and FTY720: new approaches to transplant immunosuppression. *Transplant Proc* 2002;34:2520–2522.
90. Pescovitz MD, Govani M. Sirolimus and mycophenolate mofetil for calcineurin-free immunosuppression in renal transplant recipients. *Am J Kidney Dis* 2001;38:S16–S21.
91. El Sabrout R, Weiss R, Butt F, et al. Rejection-free protocol using sirolimus–tacrolimus combination for pediatric renal transplant recipients. *Transplant Proc* 2002;34:1942–1943.
92. Mital D, Podlasek W, Jensik SC. Sirolimus-based steroid-free maintenance immunosuppression. *Transplant Proc* 2002;34:1709–1710.
93. Hymes LC, Warshaw BL. Sirolimus in pediatric patients: results in the first 6 months post-renal transplant. *Pediatr Transplant* 2005; 9:520–522.
94. Sindhi R, Seward J, Mazariegos G, et al. Replacing calcineurin inhibitors with m TOR inhibitors in children. *Pediatr Transplant* 2005;9:391–397.
95. Lobach NE, Pollock-Barziv SM, West LJ, et al. Sirolimus immunosuppression in pediatric heart transplant recipients: a single center experience. *J Heart Lung Transplant* 2005;24:184–189.
96. Mathew T, Kreis H, Friend P. Two-year incidence of malignancy in sirolimus-treated renal transplant recipients; results from five multicenter studies. *Clin Transplant* 2004;18:446–449.

97. Gruber SA, Garnick J, Morawski K, et al. Cytomegalovirus prophylaxis with valganciclovir in African-American renal allograft recipients based on donor/recipient serostatus. *Clin Transplant* 2005;18:273–278.
98. Brennan DC. Polyclonal antibodies in immunosuppression. *Transplant Proc* 2001;33:1002–1004.
99. Merion RM, Howell T, Bromberg JS. Partial T-cell activation and anergy induction by polyclonal antithymocyte globulin. *Transplantation* 1998;65:1481–1489.
100. Brophy PD, Thomas SE, McBryde KD, et al. Comparison of polyclonal induction agents in pediatric renal transplantation. *Pediatr Transplant* 2001;5:174–178.
101. Alkhunaizi A, Norman D. Induction immunosuppressive therapy. In: Owen W, Pereira BJG, Sayegh MH, eds. *Dialysis and transplantation: a companion to Brenner and Rector's The Kidney*. Philadelphia, PA: WB Saunders, 2000:546–560.
102. Ortho Multicenter Transplant Study Group. A randomized clinical trial of OKT3 monoclonal antibody for acute rejection of cadaveric renal transplants. *N Engl J Med* 1985;313:337–342.
103. Kamath S, Dean D, Peddi VR, et al. Primary therapy with OKT3 for biopsy-proven acute renal allograft rejection. *Transplant Proc* 1998;30:1178–1180.
104. Norman DJ, Leone MR. The role of OKT3 in clinical transplantation. *Pediatr Nephrol* 1991;5:130–136.
105. Leone MR, Barry JM, Alexander SR, et al. Monoclonal antibody OKT3 therapy in pediatric kidney transplant recipients. *J Pediatr* 1990;116:S86–S91.
106. Harmon W, Fine R, Alexander S, et al. NAPRTCS 2008 Annual Report, 2008. https://web.emmes.com/study/ped/annlrept2008.pdf.
107. Pescovitz MD. Use of antibody induction in pediatric renal transplantation. *Curr Opin Organ Transplant* 2008;13:495–499.
108. Cibrik DM, Kaplan B, Meier-Kriesche HU. Role of anti-interleukin-2 receptor antibodies in kidney transplantation. *BioDrugs* 2001;15:655–666.
109. Filippo SD. Anti-IL-2 receptor antibody vs. polyclonal anti-lymphocyte antibody as induction therapy in pediatric transplantation. *Pediatr Transplant* 2005;9:373–380.
110. Pescovitz MD, Knechtle S, Alexander SR, et al. Safety and pharmacokinetics of daclizumab in pediatric renal transplant recipients. *Pediatr Transplant* 2008;12:447–455.
111. Jain A, Valentini RP, Gruber SA, et al. Two-dose daclizumab induction in pediatric renal transplantation. *Pediatr Transplant* 2009;13:490–494.
112. Kelly DA. The use of anti-interleukin-2 receptor antibodies in pediatric liver transplantation. *Pediatr Transplant* 2001;5:386–389.
113. Vincenti F. The role of newer monoclonal antibodies in renal transplantation. *Transplant Proc* 2001;33:1000–1001.
114. Ciancio G, Burke GW, Suzart K, et al. Effect of daclizumab, tacrolimus, and mycophenolate mofetil in pediatric first renal transplant recipients. *Transplant Proc* 2002;34:1944–1945.
115. Vester U, Kranz B, Testa G, et al. Efficacy and tolerability of interleukin-2 receptor blockade with basiliximab in pediatric renal transplant recipients. *Pediatr Transplant* 2001;5:297–301.
116. Kovarik JM, Offner G, Broyer M, et al. A rational dosing algorithm for basiliximab (Simulect) in pediatric renal transplantation based on pharmacokinetic–dynamic evaluations. *Transplantation* 2002;74:966–971.
117. Offner G, Broyer M, Niaudet P, et al. A multicenter, open-label, pharmacokinetic/pharmacodynamic safety, and tolerability study of basiliximab (Simulect) in pediatric *de novo* renal transplant recipients. *Transplantation* 2002;74:961–966.
118. Sarwal MM, Yorgin PD, Alexander S, et al. Promising early outcomes with a novel, complete steroid avoidance immunosuppression protocol in pediatric renal transplantation. *Transplantation* 2001;72:13–21.
119. Ettenger RB. Antibody therapy as an induction regimen in pediatric renal transplantation. *Transplant Proc* 1999;31:2677–2678.
120. Ponticelli C, Tarantino A, Montagnino G. Steroid withdrawal in renal transplant recipients. *Transplant Proc* 2001;33:987–988.
121. Ponticelli C. Steroid-free immunosuppression. *Transplant Proc* 2001;33:3259–3260.
122. Almawi WY, Hess DA, Rieder MJ. Multiplicity of glucocorticoid action in inhibiting allograft rejection. *Cell Transplant* 1998;7:511–523.
123. Almawi WY, Abou Jaoude MM, Li XC. Transcriptional and post-transcriptional mechanisms of glucocorticoid antiproliferative effects. *Hematol Oncol* 2002;20:17–32.
124. Almawi WY, Melemedjian OK. Negative regulation of nuclear factor-kappaB activation and function by glucocorticoids. *J Mol Endocrinol* 2002;28:69–78.
125. Tsoulfas G, Geller DA. NF-kappaB in transplantation: friend or foe? *Transpl Infect Dis* 2001;3:212–219.
126. Almawi WY, Melemedjian OK, Rieder MJ. An alternate mechanism of glucocorticoid anti-proliferative effect: promotion of a Th2 cytokine-secreting profile. *Clin Transplant* 1999;13:365–374.
127. Ettenger R. The practical problems of prednisone in pediatric renal transplantation. *Transplant Proc* 2001;33:989–991.
128. Ponticelli C, Tarantino A, Montagnino G, et al. Use of steroids in renal transplantation. *Transplant Proc* 1999;31:2210–2211.
129. Delucchi A, Valenzuela M, Ferrario M, et al. Early steroid withdrawal in pediatric renal transplant on newer immunosuppressive drugs. *Pediatr Transplant* 2007;11:743–748.
130. Jensen S, Jackson J, Riley L, et al. Tacrolimus-based immunosuppression with steroid withdrawal in pediatric kidney transplantation—4-year experience at a moderate volume center. *Pediatr Transplant* 2003;7:119–124.
131. Oberholzer J, John E, Lumpaopong A, et al. Early discontinuation of steroids is safe and effective in pediatric transplant recipients. *Pediatr Transplant* 2005;9:456–463.
132. Vidhun J, Sarwal M. Corticosteroid avoidance in pediatric renal transplantation. *Pediatr Nephrol* 2005;20:418–426.
133. Silverstein DM, Aviles DH, Le Blanc PM, et al. Results of one-year follow-up steroid-free immunosuppression in pediatric renal transplant patients. *Pediatr Transplant* 2005;9:1–9.
134. Sollinger H, Kaplan B, Pescovitz MD, et al. Basiliximab versus antithymocyte globulin for prevention of acute renal allograft rejection. *Transplantation* 2001;72:1915–1919.
135. Loertscher R. The utility of monoclonal antibody therapy in renal transplantation. *Transplant Proc* 2002;34:797–800.
136. Vincenti F. Interleukin-2 receptor monoclonal antibodies in renal transplantation: current use and emerging regimens. *Transplant Proc* 2001;33:3169–3171.
137. Warady BA, Hebert D, Sullivan EK, et al. Renal transplantation, chronic dialysis, and chronic renal insufficiency in children and adolescents. The 1995 Annual Report of the North American Pediatric Renal Transplant Cooperative Study. *Pediatr Nephrol* 1997;11:49–64.
138. Sarwal MM, Vidhun JR, Alexander SR, et al. Continued superior outcomes with modification and lengthened follow-up of a steroid avoidance pilot with extended daclizumab induction in pediatric renal transplantation. *Transplantation* 2003;76:1331–1339.
139. Virji M, Carter JE, Lirenman DS. Single-center experience with mycophenolate mofetil in pediatric renal transplant recipients. *Pediatr Transplant* 2001;5:293–296.
140. Jungraithmayr T, Staskewitz A, Kirste G, et al. Pediatric renal transplantation with mycophenolate mofetil-based immunosuppression without induction: results after three years. *Transplantation* 2003;75:454–461.

CHAPTER

46

Sinno H. P. Simons
Brian J. Anderson
Dick Tibboel

Analgesic Agents

INTRODUCTION

It was generally believed that neonates were unable to experience pain (1). The importance of antinociceptive therapy in children, infants, and newborns has been increasingly acknowledged over the past two decades, leading to a burst of research and increased use of analgesic agents in this population. Research has concentrated on the development of pain assessment instruments and clinical trials investigating the effectiveness and safety of analgesics in infants. Many instruments containing behavioral and physiologic items have proved to be useful and reliable measures of postoperative and procedural pain in different age groups and to a lesser extent for individuals with mental handicaps. Knowledge about analgesic effects has been enlarged using pain assessment tools in randomized trials comparing different dose regimen and different agents (2). These trials have gained more insight into the specific pharmacokinetics (PK) and pharmacodynamics (PD) of analgesics in infants (3,4). PK and PD knowledge has increased over the past few years, but more research is necessary (5).

Pediatric pharmacokinetics is altered with age through the maturation of enzyme systems and physiologic processes responsible for absorption and elimination (6–8). Changing body composition alters disposition. Pharmacodynamic changes with age are poorly documented, although out of infancy they are commonly similar to adults (9). Purported pharmacodynamic differences between children and adults for drugs such as morphine, for example, disappear once PK differences are accounted for (10,11).

Analgesics in pediatric patients can be broadly divided into opioids and nonopioids.

OPIOIDS

Opioid analgesics include naturally occurring agents (opium alkaloids) and synthetic opioid agonists that elicit morphine-like activity. The analgesic effects of opioids occur by activation of μ-, κ-, and/or δ-receptors in the central nervous system (CNS) (12). Each class of receptors is divided into subtypes that have different clinical effects. Analgesia is obtained by spinal or supraspinal activation of opioid receptors, leading to decreased neurotransmitter release from nociceptive neurons, inhibiting the ascending neuronal pain pathways and altering perception and response to pain (13). Opioid receptors also exist outside the CNS in the dorsal root ganglia and on peripheral terminals of primary afferent neurons (14).

The World Health Organization (WHO) Analgesic Ladder is a generally accepted guideline for the supply of analgesics; it was originally developed for the treatment of cancer pain. Mild pain should be treated with nonopioid analgesics [acetaminophen or nonsteroidal anti-inflammatory drugs (NSAIDs)], moderate pain should be treated with "weaker" opioids or combination products, and severe pain should be treated with stronger opioids (World Health Organization; Cancer Pain Relief; Albany NY: WHO Publications Center, 1986) (15). Opioids in children, infants, and newborns are reserved for moderate-to-severe types of pain, such as postoperative pain, sickle cell disease, and palliative care (16), or as an additive to acetaminophen or NSAIDs if pain is moderate. Furthermore, opioids may be used in the intensive care unit for pain or stress related to artificial ventilation, surgical procedures [chest tube placement, vessel canulation for extracorporeal membrane oxygenation (ECMO)], or painful conditions such as necrotizing enterocolitis. The most frequently used opioids are fentanyl and morphine, but codeine, oxycodone, methadone, hydromorphone, and meperidine are used in children, as well as fentanyl derivatives such as alfentanil and sufentanil. Recommended starting doses are shown in Table 46.1. All doses should, however, be adjusted to clinical circumstances and titrated to the individual patients' needs. Doses aim to achieve a target concentration, but the correlations between the analgesic plasma concentrations and validated pain scores are weak (17,18).

Opioids produce adverse effects that may be minimized by appropriate drug selection and dosing. Respiratory depression, hypotension, glottic and chest wall rigidity, constipation, urinary retention, seizures, sedation, and bradycardia are well described. Continuous monitoring and frequent assessment of vital signs should be performed during opioid administration. Naloxone is a competitive opioid receptor agonist that reverses many of these side effects in appropriate dosage. Naloxone also antagonizes endorphin effects, and some morphine side effects can be

TABLE 46.1 Opioid Analgesics: Recommended Starting Doses in Neonates and Children[a]

Drug	*Equianalgesic Doses (mg)*		*Usual Starting Intravenous Or Subcutaneous Doses and Intervals*		Parenteral: Oral Dose Ratio	*Usual Starting Oral Doses and Intervals*	
	Parenteral	*Oral*	*Child <50 kg*	*Child ≥50 kg*		*Child <50 kg*	*Child ≥50 kg*
Codeine	120	200	NR	NR	1:2	0.5–1.0 mg/kg every 3–4 hr	30–60 mg every 3–4 hr
Morphine	10	30 (long term) 60 (single dose)	Bolus: 0.1 mg/kg every 2–4 hr Infusion: 0.03 mg/kg/hr	Bolus: 5–8 mg every 2–4 hr Infusion: 1.5 mg/hr	1:3 (long term) 1:6 (single dose)	Immediate release: 0.3 mg/kg every 3–4 hr Sustained release: 20–35 kg: 10–15 mg every 8–12 hr 35–50 kg: 15–30 mg every 8–12 hr	Immediate release: 15–20 mg every 3–4 hr Sustained release: 30–45 mg every 8–12 hr
Oxycodone	NA	15–20	NA	NA	NA	0.1–0.2 mg/kg every 3–4 hr	5–10 mg every 3–4 hr
Methadone[b]	10	10–20	0.1 mg/kg every 4–8 hr	5–8 mg every 4–8 hr	1:2	0.1–0.2 mg/kg every 4–8 hr	5–10 mg every 4–8 hr
Fentanyl	100 μg (0.1 mg)	NA	Bolus: 0.5–1.0 μg/kg every 1–2 hr Infusion: 0.5–2.0 μg/kg/hr	Bolus: 25–50 μg every 1–2 hr Infusion: 25–100 μg/hr	NA	NA	NA
Hydromorphone	1.5–2	6–8	Bolus: 0.02 mg every 2–4 hr Infusion: 0.006 mg/kg/hr	Bolus: 1 mg every 2–4 hr Infusion: 0.3 mg/hr	1:4	0.04–0.08 mg/kg every 3–4 hr	2–4 mg every 3–4 hr
Meperidine (pethidine)[c]	75–100	300	Bolus: 0.8–1.0 mg/kg every 2–3 hr	Bolus: 50–75 mg every 2–3 hr	1:4	2–3 mg/kg every 3–4 hr	100–150 mg every 3–4 hr

NA, not applicable; NR, not recommended.

[a]Doses are for patients older than 6 months. In infants younger than 6 months, initial per-kilogram doses should begin at roughly 25% of the per-kilogram doses recommended here. Higher doses are often required for patients receiving mechanical ventilation. All doses are approximate and should be adjusted according to clinical circumstances. Recommendations are adapted from previous summary tables, including those of a consensus statement from the World Health Organization and the International Association for the Study of Pain (348).

[b]Methadone requires additional vigilance because it can accumulate and produce delayed sedation. If sedation occurs, doses should be withheld until sedation resolves. Thereafter, doses should be substantially reduced, or the interval between doses should be extended to 8 to 12 hr, or both.

[c]The use of meperidine should generally be avoided if other opioids are available, especially with long-term use, because its metabolite can cause seizures.

From Berde CB, Sethna NF, Analgesics for the treatment of pain in children. *N Engl J Med* 2002; 347(14):1094–1103, with permission.

TABLE 46.2 Onset, Peak, and Duration of Effects as well as Lipid Solubility of Opioids

	Morphine	*Meperidine*	*Fentanyl*	*Sufentanil*	*Alfentanil*	*Remifentanil*
Peak effect (min)	45–90	20	3–4	5–6	1–2	1
Duration	4–5 hr	2–4 hr	30 min	30 min	15 min	5–10 min
Oil/H_2O	1.4	39	860	1.8	13.4	17.9

Adapted from The World Wide Anaesthetist. http://www.anaesthetist.com, with permission.

managed alternatively (e.g., neuromuscular blocking drugs for fentanyl muscle rigidity).

MORPHINE

Mechanism of Action/Metabolism

The most common opioid used for pediatric pain is morphine. Morphine is a member of the morphinan-framed alkaloids. The drug is soluble in water, but lipid solubility is poor compared with that of other opioids (Table 46.2). Although morphine may also act on κ-opioid receptor subtypes (19), the analgesic effect of morphine is mainly caused by an activation of μ-receptors, as confirmed by a lack of analgesic effect of morphine in murine studies using μ-receptor knockout mice (20–22). Alterations of the morphine molecular structure change the pharmacologic activity and may have important clinical consequences (Fig. 46.1). The most important positions on the morphine molecule, next to the nitrogen atom (probably responsible for the analgesic activity, as modifications reduce penetration into the CNS), are the phenolic hydroxyl at position 3 and the alcoholic hydroxyl at position 6. Morphine is mainly metabolized by the enzyme UDP-glucuronosyl transferase 2B7 (UGT2B7) into morphine-3-glucuronide (M3G) and morphine-6-glucuronide (M6G) (23). Contributions to both

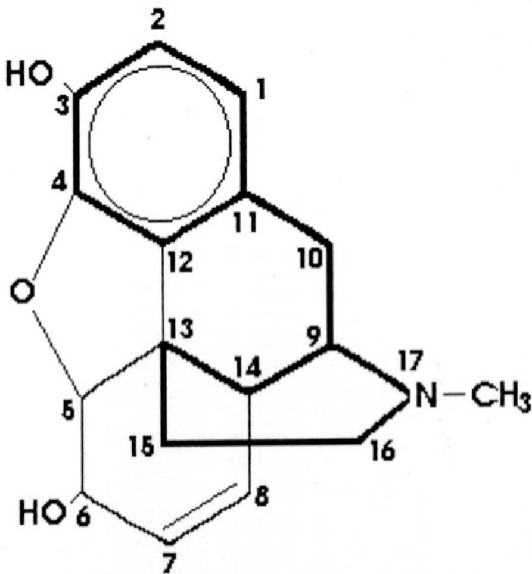

Figure 46.1. The morphine molecule. The structure of morphine and all opium derivatives is characterized by the piperidine ring, which is indicated with bold lines. (From *Goodman and Gilman's The pharmacological basis of therapeutics.* New York: Pergamon Press, 1990:485–531, with permission.)

the desired effect (analgesia) and the undesired effects (nausea, respiratory depression) of M6G are the subject of clinical controversy (24–26,27–29,30). M3G has been suggested to antagonize the antinociceptive and respiratory depressive effects of morphine and M6G (31,32), and contributes to the development of tolerance. The enzyme responsible for morphine glucuronidation, UGT2B7 (6), is mainly found in the liver, but also exists in the intestines and kidneys (33). Sulfation is a minor pathway (34,35). The metabolites are cleared by the kidneys and partly by biliary excretion. Some recirculation of morphine occurs due to β-glucuronidase activity in the gut (36). Impaired renal function leads to accumulation of M3G and M6G (37).

Morphine may be administered by different routes. Administration in premature newborns is limited to the intravenous route. The painful administration of intramuscular morphine injections is frowned upon. Subcutaneous intermittent boluses through an indwelling catheter offer an alternative route (38). The large variability observed after rectal administration is a major disadvantage of this route, although clinically frequently used (39). Oral morphine, either as elixir or slow-release formulations, offers a good alternative despite a high first-pass effect. Epidural or intrathecal administration may cause delayed respiratory depression due to slow rostral migration within the cerebrospinal fluid (CSF) (40). Patient-controlled analgesia (PCA) is possible in some children aged as young as 6 years, and nurse-controlled analgesia can be used effectively in younger children (41).

Pharmacodynamics

There is a delay between analgesic effect and plasma concentration. The effect compartment equilibration half-time (T_{eq}) for morphine is approximately 17 minutes in adults (42), but is anticipated to be shorted with decreasing age. A concentration–response relationship for morphine analgesia in children has not been described, although adverse effect relationships for both vomiting (43) and respiratory depression are reported (44). The effectiveness of intravenous morphine in infants using validated pain assessment tools has been studied in different age groups. After major surgery, continuous morphine doses of 10 to 40 μg per kg have been shown to be effective in alleviating pain in infants and children 0 to 14 years of age (45). No difference in analgesic effect was found between continuous and intermittent dosing. Randomized controlled trials showed different pharmacodynamic effects of intravenous morphine in premature neonates requiring artificial ventilation with continuous doses of 10 to 30 μg per kg (46,47). Morphine did not reduce pain responses during endotracheal suctioning (48). Chay et al. reported mean morphine concentrations required to produce adequate sedation in 50% of neonates to be 125 ng per mL (49), but analgesic target plasma concentrations for postoperative morphine analgesia are generally believed to be around 15 to 20 ng per mL (50,51). The large PK and PD variability means that morphine is often titrated to effect using small incremental doses (0.02 mg per kg) in children suffering postoperative pain (52). As morphine should not be routinely prescribed for ventilated newborns, it should be used only in those newborns who have increased pain scores and doses again should be titrated to the individual needs of each neonate (46,47).

Pharmacokinetics

Morphine clearance matures with postconceptual age (6,50) and reaches adult rates at 6 to 12 months (Table 46.3). Fetuses have been shown to be capable of metabolizing morphine from 15 weeks of gestation (53,54). In premature newborns, morphine clearance increases with gestation and postnatal age (48). Morphine plasma concentrations show large between individual variability (55). Clinical circumstances, such as type of surgery, concurrent illness, and infants requiring ECMO (56), also have reduced morphine clearance. Protein binding of morphine is low, from 20% in premature neonates (57) to 35% in adults (58), and has no impact on disposition changes with age (59).

Respiratory depression may occur at concentrations of 20 ng per mL (51). Respiratory depression, as measured by carbon dioxide response curves or by arterial oxygen tension, is similar in children aged 2 to 570 days at the same morphine concentration (44). Furthermore, intrathecal dosing causes similar respiratory depression at similar CSF concentrations in children aged 4 months to 15 years (60). Hypotension, bradycardia, and flushing are part of the histamine response to morphine and are associated with a rapid intravenous bolus administration. Morphine in preterm newborns has only small effects on blood pressure, but the effect might be more significant in extreme premature infants and dependant of the morphine doses (61,62). The incidence of vomiting in children after tonsillectomy is related to morphine dose. Doses above 0.1 mg per kg were associated with a more than 50% incidence of vomiting (43).

TABLE 46.3 Age-Related Clearances of Morphine and Fentanyl Standardized to a 70-kg Person

	CL (Allometric ¾ Power Model) (L Per hr Per 70 kg)		
	Morphine		*Fentanyl*
Neonate (<1 wk)	13.1 (8.7)	Neonate (<1 mo)	31.5 (5.2)
Neonate (1 wk–2 mo)	18.4 (7.9)		
Infant (2–6 mo)	48.8 (15.6)	Infant (1–6 mo)	41.1 (3.2)
Infant (6 mo–2.5 yr)	51 (13–68)	Child (1–5 yr)	34.1 (12.3)
Adult	63 (4)	Adult	43.0 (7.3)

Adapted from Anderson BJ, Meakin GH. Scaling for size: some implications for paediatric anaesthesia dosing. *Paediatr Anaesth* 2002;12:205–219, with permission.

CODEINE

Codeine, or methylmorphine, is a morphine-like opioid with 1/10 the potency of morphine. It is mainly metabolized by glucuronidation, but minor pathways are *N*-demethylation to norcodeine and *O*-demethylation to morphine. Around 10% of codeine is metabolized to morphine. As codeine's affinity for opioid receptors is very low, the analgesic effect of codeine is mainly due to its metabolite, morphine (63). The cytochrome P450 (CYP) enzyme CYP2D6 catalyzes the metabolism of codeine to morphine. A genetic polymorphism of this enzyme causes distinct phenotypes responsible for the presence of ultrarapid extensive, extensive, and slow codeine metabolizers in the population (64,65). Between 7% and 10% of the population are believed to be slow metabolizers of codeine (65–67), but this percentage has been reported to be much higher (65,66). Although codeine has been shown to cause no analgesic effect in the poor metabolizers, side effects persist (67). High incidences of adverse effects might be expected in patients who have an ultrarapid extensive metabolism. These patients achieve higher morphine concentrations. Codeine metabolites and 10% of unmetabolized codeine are excreted in the urine. The plasma half-life of codeine is 3 to 4 hours.

Codeine can be given by intramuscular, oral, and rectal routes. Intravenous codeine is not recommended because of hypotensive effects (68). Rectal codeine achieves lower concentrations than intramuscular codeine because of incomplete, slower, more variable absorption (69). In children, it is generally given in doses of 1 to 3 mg per kg per day. Codeine is often used in combination with acetaminophen or NSAIDs. The addition of codeine to acetaminophen has been shown to improve postoperative pain relief in infants (70). The analgesic effect of acetaminophen (10 to 15 mg per kg) and codeine (1 to 1.5 mg per kg) was comparable to that of ibuprofen (5 to 10 mg per kg) in children after tonsillectomy (71).

Peak plasma concentration (C_{max}) occurs after 1 hour (T_{max}) after oral administration. The plasma half-life is 3 to 3.5 hours. The C_{max} is reached 30 minutes after intramuscular injection (63). The pharmacokinetics of codeine is poorly described in children despite use over decades. A volume of distribution (V) of 3.6 L per kg and a clearance (CL) of 0.85 L per hour have been described in adults, but there are few data detailing pediatric pharmacokinetic developmental changes. The neonatal half-life is longer due to immature clearance (e.g., 4.5 hours), while that of an infant is shorter (e.g., 2.6 hours) (72). Administration (especially of codeine preparations with an antihistamine and a decongestant) in the neonate may cause intoxication (73). Recently, a newborn died from morphine poisoning when his mother used codeine while breastfeeding. The mother, an ultrarapid metabolizer, produced much more morphine when taking codeine than most people do (74,75). Codeine has been used in infants and neonates after major surgery as an adjunct to acetaminophen or NSAIDs (optimal oral codeine dosage 1 to 1.5 mg per kg every 4 to 6 hours, oral acetaminophen 20 mg per kg every 6 hours in infants older than 3 months) (76).

The adverse effects of codeine are broadly similar to those of other opioids. Adverse effects at low doses appear to be directly related to morphine plasma concentrations, but are caused by codeine at higher doses (77). There is a broad belief that codeine causes fewer side effects, such as sedation and respiratory depression, compared with other opioids, but there is little evidence for this.

The analgesic effect of codeine is dependent on its conversion to morphine. Consequently, other medications competing for the CYP2D6 enzyme (e.g., quinidine) may decrease the analgesic effect of codeine.

OXYCODONE

Oxycodone is a semisynthetic analgesic that is available as an immediate-release product (oral solution and capsule) as well as a controlled-release tablet for 12-hourly administration. Immediate-release and controlled-release preparations of oxycodone have similar efficacy and comparable side-effect profiles in adults (78). The relative bioavailability of intranasal, oral, and rectal formulations was approximately 50% that of intravenous in adults. The buccal and sublingual absorption of oxycodone is similar in young children (79). Intramuscular administration provides relatively constant drug absorption, while buccal and gastric administration is associated with large interindividual variation in the rate of absorption (80). Mean values of drug clearance and volume of distribution (V_{ss}) were 15.2 (SD 4.2) mL per minute per kg and 2.1 (SD 0.8) L per kg in children after ophthalmic surgery (81).

Oxycodone is very expensive, and drugs such as controlled-release morphine and methadone offer cheaper alternatives (78). Controlled-release oxycodone may be appropriate if the patient cannot tolerate other controlled-release or long-acting opioid analgesics. Olkkola et al. showed that oxycodone (0.1 mg per kg) in children after ophthalmic surgery caused greater ventilatory depression compared with other opioids (81).

METHADONE

Methadone is a synthetic opioid with an analgesic potency similar to that of morphine but with a more rapid distribution and a slower elimination. Methadone is used as a maintenance drug in opioid-addicted adults to prevent withdrawal. Methadone might have beneficial effects because it is a long-acting synthetic opioid with a very high bioavailability by the enteral route. Although only few data on the efficacy and safety of methadone are available, methadone is widely used for the treatment of opioid withdrawal in neonates and children (82,83). Intravenous methadone has been shown to be an effective analgesic for postoperative pain relief (84), and oral administration has been recommended as the first-line opioid for severe and persistent pain in children (85). It also seems to be a safe enteral alternative for intravenous opioids in palliative pediatric oncological patients (86). Although a predominant role for methadone in the management of prolonged pain in neonates has been suggested, use needs to be evaluated in a clinical research setting (87). The few data on methadone pharmacokinetics show a slow elimination half-life with large interindividual variability (3.8 to 62 hours) (87). Methadone's lipid solubility is greater than that of morphine (88). The increased lipid solubility and longer duration of effect give this drug potential for single-shot epidural use.

HYDROMORPHONE

Hydromorphone is a semisynthetic congener of morphine with a potency of around 5 to 7.5 times that of morphine (89). Hydromorphone is metabolized to hydromorphone-3-glucuronide and also, to a lesser extent, to dihydroisomorphine and dihydromorphine (90). The intravenous:oral dose ratio is 1:5, as there is high first-pass metabolism (91). A clearance of 51.7 mL per minute per kg (range, 28.6 to 98.2) is reported in children (92).

Hydromorphone is used for chronic cancer pain and for postoperative analgesia. The side-effect profile is comparable to that of other strong opioids, and hydromorphone does not convincingly demonstrate clinical superiority in adults over other strong opioid analgesics (93). Goodarzi showed that epidural hydromorphone caused fewer side effects than morphine and fentanyl in children undergoing orthopedic procedures (94). PCA with hydromorphone seems to result in similar analgesia and side effects compared to morphine in children for the management of mucositis pain after bone marrow transplantation (89). Plasma concentrations of around 4.7 ng per mL (range 1.9 to 8.9 ng per mL) relieve mucositis in children given PCA devices. Time to peak concentration is 4 to 6 hours and clearance is 51.7 mL per minute per kg in children (89,92).

MEPERIDINE (PETHIDINE)

Meperidine is a weak opioid, primarily μ-receptor, agonist that has a potency of 1/10 that of morphine. The analgesic effects are detectable within 5 minutes of intravenous administration and peak effect is reached within 10 minutes (36,95). In adults, meperidine is metabolized to meperidinic acid and normeperidine. Meperidine clearance in infants and children is approximately 10 mL per minute per kg (96,97). Elimination in neonates is greatly reduced, and elimination half-time in neonates, who have received pethidine by placental transfer, may be two to seven times longer than that in adults (98).

Meperidine was initially synthesized as an anticholinergic agent but was soon discovered to have analgesic properties. Although meperidine's anticholinergic effects were demonstrated in vivo, the anticholinergic effects on the biliary and renal tracts have not been demonstrated in vivo. Studies have clearly demonstrated that meperidine is no more efficacious in treating biliary or renal tract spasm than comparative μ-opioids. Meperidine was portrayed in practice and teaching as having unique clinical advantages (99). Because morphine results in better analgesia with fewer side effects, there are no particular advantages of meperidine as an analgesic (100). Accumulation of the metabolite normeperidine results in seizures and dysphoria (3).

Intramuscular administration of meperidine was frequently used in pediatric patients, but this route of administration is used uncommonly now because it is painful. Meperidine's local anesthetic properties have been found useful for epidural techniques (101).

FENTANYL

Fentanyl is a synthetic opioid that acts as a "morphine-like agonist." Its potency is about 50- to 100-fold that of morphine, with a large postulated effect on the μ-receptor. A plasma concentration of 15 to 30 ng per mL is required to provide total intravenous anesthesia (102,103). Fentanyl has a wide margin of safety and beneficial effects on hemodynamic stability (104,105) and has a rapid onset (T_{eq} = 6.6 minutes) and a short duration of action. This is probably due to the relative increased lipid solubility and molecular conformation, enabling efficient penetration of the blood–brain barrier. Fentanyl may be the preferred analgesic agent for critically ill patients with hemodynamic instability, patients with symptoms related to histamine release during morphine infusion, or patients with morphine tolerance. Because of its rapid onset of action and short duration of effect, fentanyl efficiently alleviates procedural pain (106). It has been used in neonates on artificial ventilation (107) with bronchopulmonary dysplasia, pulmonary hypertension, and/or diaphragmatic hernia. One study showed a need to escalate dose during ECMO, indicating a rapid development of tolerance (108). Overall, the use of synthetic opioids shows a more rapid tolerance (3 to 5 days) than that of morphine (2 weeks) and heroin (weeks) (87,109).

Fentanyl metabolism is related to the activity of the hepatic cytochrome P450 system (CYP3A4) and is metabolized by oxidative *N*-dealkylation into norfentanyl and hydroxylized (110,111). All metabolites are inactive, and a small amount of fentanyl is renally eliminated unmetabolized (112).

Fentanyl has been shown to effectively prevent preterm neonates from surgical stress responses and to improve postoperative outcome (113). Single fentanyl doses (3 μg per kg) and infusion (1.1 μg per kg per hour) reduced physiologic and behavioral measures of pain and stress during mechanical ventilation in preterm neonates (114,115) as effectively as morphine (107). International recommended starting doses are, however, smaller, as is shown in Table 46.1. In older infants and children, fentanyl has been shown to be effective for the management of peri- and postoperative pain (116) and for the management of procedural pain. Fentanyl clearance may be impaired due to decreased hepatic blood flow (e.g., from increased intra-abdominal pressure) (117) in neonates after major abdominal surgery (e.g., omphalocele). Fentanyl also has a propensity for muscular rigidity (118). Transdermal fentanyl can be used for severe cancer-related pain (119) or in palliative pediatric care (16). Fentanyl plasma concentrations are not measurable until 2 hours after application, and there is an 8 to 16 hours latency until full clinical fentanyl effects are observed. Following removal, serum fentanyl concentrations decline gradually and fall to 50% in approximately 16 hours. This prolonged apparent elimination half-life occurs because fentanyl continues to be absorbed from the skin, where a fentanyl depot concentrates (120). The systemic availability of fentanyl by this route is approximately 30% of that found using the intravenous route (121). Oral transmucosal fentanyl provides consistent analgesia for brief painful procedures (122). Transdermal and transmucosal fentanyl have not been studied in newborns.

Because fentanyl has very high lipid solubility, it is widely distributed in tissues. Its short duration of effect is due to redistribution to deep, lipid-rich compartments. Accumulation of fentanyl in lipid-rich tissues may redistribute slowly after discontinuation of therapy, resulting in prolonged periods of sedation and respiratory depression after an extended period of use (123). The context-sensitive half-time after an infusion of 1 hour is approximately 20 minutes, but it is 270 minutes after an 8-hour infusion (124).

The clearance of fentanyl appears to be somewhat immature at birth but increases dramatically after birth. Fentanyl clearance is 70% to 80% of adult values in term neonates (Table 46.3) and, standardized to a 70-kg person, appears to reach adult levels within the first 2 weeks of life (123,125). The volume of distribution of fentanyl at steady state is around 5.9 L per kg in term-born neonates and decreases with age to 4.5 L per kg during infancy, 3.1 L per kg during childhood, and 1.6 L per kg in adults (126). Initial plasma concentrations in pediatric patients are lower than in adults due to larger distribution volumes.

The intraoperative use of 3 μg per kg fentanyl in infants did not result in respiratory depression or hypoxemia in a placebo-controlled trial (116). Only 3 of 2,000 nonintubated infants and children experienced short apneic episodes after a low dose of fentanyl for the repair of facial lacerations (127). Fentanyl has similar respiratory depression in infants and adults when plasma concentrations are similar (128).

Fentanyl, alfentanil, and sufentanil are metabolized by CYP3A4, and other drugs that also use this enzyme (e.g., cyclosporine, erythromycin) may decrease clearance, leading to increased fentanyl plasma concentrations (129,130). Acetaminophen has been shown to interact with fentanyl metabolism in vitro (131), although the clinical importance of this interaction is probably unimportant.

Research investigating DNA polymorphisms has shown genetic variability of CYP3A4 with slow and rapid metabolizers. One explanation for between individual variability in clearance across a patient population appears to be the efficiency of drug metabolism arising from differences in enzyme expression levels and/or from the presence of allelic variants of the enzyme with compromised catalytic ability.

ALFENTANIL

Alfentanil is a synthetic opioid that is chemically a derivate of fentanyl. It has a rapid onset (T_{eq} = 0.9 minute), a brief duration of action, and one-fourth the potency of fentanyl. Alfentanil has lower lipid solubility and causes less histamine release (18) than fentanyl. It is used as a procedural analgesic for pediatric patients because the onset of analgesia is rapid (132). Sufficient analgesia during endotracheal intubation and suctioning has been found using 10 to

20 μg per kg alfentanil in preterm neonates (132–134). A target plasma concentration of 400 ng per mL is used in anesthesia. Metabolism is comparable to that in adults, that is, phase 1 via oxidative *N*-dealkylation by CYP3A4 (99) and *O*-dealkylation, and then phase 2 conjugation to renally excreted end products (135). Alfentanil plasma protein binding increases from 65% in preterm neonates and 79% in term infants to around 90% in adults (136,137). The volume of distribution is smaller in infants than in adults (138). Clearances of alfentanil, standardized to a 70-kg person, are similar at different ages (250 to 500 mL per minute per 70 kg) except for the neonatal age group, in which clearances are decreased (20 to 60 mL per minute per 70 kg). Consequently, elimination half-life in children (40 to 68 minutes) is higher in the neonatal period. In premature neonates, the half-life is as long as 6 to 9 hours (139,140). Children with chronic renal failure or chronic hepatic disease do not show impaired clearance of alfentanil (141). Alfentanil cannot be used without neuromuscular blocking drugs in newborns because of a very high incidence of rigidity (132,142).

SUFENTANIL

Sufentanil is a most potent opioid analgesic, and is 5 to 10 times more potent than fentanyl, with a T_{eq} of 6.2 minutes. A concentration of 5 to 10 ng per mL is required for total intravenous anesthesia, 0.2 to 0.4 ng per mL for analgesia.

Elimination of sufentanil has been suggested by *O*-demethylation and *N*-dealkylation in animal studies. Like fentanyl and alfentanil, the P450 CYP3A4 enzyme is responsible for the *N*-dealkylation (110). The amount of free sufentanil decreases with age (neonates 19%; infants 11%; children/adults 8%) and is strongly correlated with the α-1-acid glycoprotein plasma concentration (136). The lower concentration of α-1-acid glycoprotein in newborns and infants contributes to the increased free fraction of sufentanil in these age groups. Although sufentanil, fentanyl, alfentanil, and remifentanil have high protein binding (>70%) and have high hepatic (or nonhepatic for remifentanil) extraction ratios, protein binding changes are probably clinically unimportant (59) because dose is titrated to effect, and clearance variability has greater impact.

REMIFENTANIL

Remifentanil resembles fentanyl, sufentanil, and alfentanil in chemical structure. It is a selective μ-receptor agonist with a higher potency than alfentanil. Because the inhibitory neurotransmitter glycine is used as a carrier for remifentanil, it should not be used for spinal or epidural applications (143), and because of its short duration of action, it is usually given as an infusion (T_{eq} = 1.16 minutes) (144,145). A concentration of 2 to 4 ng per mL supplements anesthesia for major surgery. Analgesic concentrations are 0.2 to 0.4 ng per mL.

Remifentanil is metabolized to carbonic acid. The metabolism is independent of liver and renal function. Remifentanil reacts with nonspecific esterase in tissue and erythrocytes (146,147). Carbonic acid is excreted through the kidneys. Clearances decreases with age, with rates of 90 mL per kg per minute in infants younger than 2 years, 60 mL per kg per minute between 2 and 12 years of age, and 40 mL per kg per minute in adults (148–150). Volume of distribution in children is smaller (200 to 300 mL per kg) than in adults (400 mL per kg), and might by increased in young infants (450 mL per kg). Elimination half-life seems to be constant, around 3 to 6 minutes (40,151).

Administration of 1 μg per kg intravenously followed by 0.1 to 1.0 μg per kg per minute results in sufficient analgesia during surgery in children (152–155). Because of its short duration, remifentanil seems to be ideally suited for pediatric neurosurgical patients who may require neurologic assessment at completion of surgery (156). Its use is accompanied by a high incidence of life-threatening respiratory depression at subtherapeutic concentrations (157). As a result of a rapid development of μ-receptor tolerance with remifentanil use, higher subsequent opioid doses are required.

Intravenous remifentanil doses of 0.25 μg per kg per minute appear to be safe and effective in neonates (158,159), but data concerning the use of remifentanil in this group are few.

NONOPIOIDS

ACETAMINOPHEN

Mechanism of Action

Acetaminophen (paracetamol) has been used in clinical practice for more than 100 years and is the most commonly prescribed pediatric medicine. Acetanilid, the parent compound of acetaminophen, was introduced in 1886. Toxicity-related problems with acetanilid led to the introduction of acetaminophen (*N*-acetyl-*p*-amino-phenol) by von Mering in 1893. The popularity of acetaminophen over the nonsteroidal anti-inflammatory agents ascended after the reported association between Reye syndrome and aspirin in the 1980s (160). Acetaminophen is widely used in the management of pain and fever but is lacking anti-inflammatory effects.

Acetaminophen has a central analgesic effect that is mediated through activation of descending serotonergic pathways. Debate exists about its primary site of action, which may be inhibition of prostaglandin synthesis or through an active metabolite influencing cannabinoid receptors. Prostaglandin H_2 synthetase (PGHS) is the enzyme responsible for metabolism of arachidonic acid to the unstable prostaglandin H_2. The two major forms of this enzyme are the constitutive PGHS-1 and the inducible PGHS-2. PGHS comprises two sites: a cyclooxygenase (COX) site and a peroxidise (POX) site. The conversion of arachidonic acid to prostaglandin G2 (PGG_2) is dependent on a tyrosine-385 radical at the COX site. Formation of a ferryl protoporphyrin IX radical cation from the reducing agent Fe^{3+} at the POX site is essential for conversion of tyrosine-385 to its radical form. Acetaminophen acts as a reducing cosubstrate on the POX site and lessens availability of the ferryl protoporphyrin IX radical cation. This effect can be reduced by the presence of hydroperoxide-generating lipoxygenase enzymes within the cell (peroxide tone) or by swamping the POX site with substrate such as PGG_2. Peroxide tone and swamping explain acetaminophen's lack of peripheral analgesic effect, platelet effect, and anti-inflammatory effects. Alternatively, acetaminophen effects may be mediated by an active metabolite (*p*-aminophenol). *P*-aminophenol is conjugated with arachidonic acid by fatty acid amide hydrolase to form AM404. AM404 exerts effect through cannabinoid receptors (161).

Pharmacodynamics

Antipyresis

Brown et al. (162) reported a linked-population PK–PD model for antipyresis using mixed-effect models. The acetaminophen PK parameters were similar to those reported by others (163,164). The link component yielded a K_{eo} (ln $2/T_{eq}$) of 0.58 (SE 0.06) per hour (T_{eq} 71, SE 7 minutes); the sigmoid E_{max} component yielded an EC_{50} of 4.63 g per L and a Hill coefficient N of 3.98 (SE 0.42). The predicted maximum effect response was 1.38°C, but this was possibly constrained by the temperature enrollment criteria and a failure to explore higher doses. These authors noted two major additional factors that influence interpretation of the relationship between plasma concentration and fever reduction: the cyclical nature of fever and the initial temperature at when acetaminophen was given.

Analgesia

Korpela et al. (165) studied day-stay surgical children randomized to receive a single dose of 0, 20, 40, or 60 mg per kg of rectal acetaminophen. In the postanesthesia care unit, pain scores were significantly lower in the 40 and 60 mg per kg groups compared with placebo and 20 mg per kg groups. Acetaminophen resulted in a dose-related reduction in the number of children who required postoperative rescue opioid, with significance reached with 40 or 60 mg per kg doses. Calculated dose of acetaminophen at which 50% of the children did not require a rescue opioid was 35 mg per kg. However, neither the antipyretic nor the analgesic effect of acetaminophen is directly related to plasma concentration. Time delays of approximately 1 hour between peak concentration and peak effect are reported (166,167). The time delay is similar to that described for acetaminophen CSF kinetics (168).

Pain fluctuations, pain type, and placebo effects complicate interpretation of clinical studies (169). Anderson et al. (164) reported pharmacodynamic population parameter estimates [population variability coefficient of variation (CV)] in children after tonsillectomy. An E_{max} model in which the greatest possible pain relief (visual analogue scale 0 to 10) equates to an E_{max} of 10 were $E_{max} = 5.17$ (64%) and $EC_{50} = 9.98$ (107%) mg per L. The equilibration half-time (T_{eq}) of the analgesic effect compartment was 53 (217%) minutes. A target effect compartment concentration of 10 mg per L is associated with a pain reduction of 2.6/10. Effect site concentrations associated with analgesia for the pains experienced as a neonate are unknown.

The use of an intravenous acetaminophen formulation allows greater dosing accuracy, less pharmacokinetic variability attributable to absorption, and more rapid speed of effect onset (169). A new intravenous acetaminophen preparation, with mannitol, cysteine, and sodium phosphate as carriers, has circumvented problems of injection site pain associated with the earlier prodrug (propacetamol). Infusions over 15 minute of intravenous acetaminophen 15 mg per kg following inguinal hernia repair in children resulted in a steep reduction in pain relief between 15 and 30 minute (170), consistent with a delay achieving effect site concentrations in the brain. Intravenous acetaminophen has been successfully used for neonatal analgesia (171) and two European centers have published dosing guidelines in neonates (172,173). These regimens attempt to achieve a steady-state target concentration of 10 mg per L.

Pharmacokinetics

Oral Absorption

Bioavailability. Acetaminophen has low first-pass metabolism, and the hepatic extraction ratio is 0.11 to 0.37 in adults (174). The relative bioavailability of rectal compared with oral acetaminophen formulations ($F_{rectal/oral}$) has been reported as 0.52 (range 0.24 to 0.98) (175) and even as low as 0.3 (176). The relative bioavailability is higher in neonates, where it is possible suppository insertion height may result in a different rectal venous drainage pattern. Hopkins et al. (177) noted that the area under the curve (AUC) in neonates after suppository administration was significantly greater than in infants and in older children. Van der Marel et al. (178) noted a similar finding in children aged 10.3 (SD 2.3) months after craniofacial surgery. The mean AUC was 171.2 mg per hour per L after rectal suppository compared with 111.9 mg per hour per L after elixir, although some of this difference was attributable to vomiting after oral elixir. The relative bioavailability of rectal formulations appears to be age related. The bioavailability of the capsule suppository relative to elixir decreased with age from 0.92 (22%) at 28 weeks postconception to 0.86 at 2 years of age; the triglyceride base decreased from 0.86 (35%) at 28 weeks postconception to 0.5 at 2 years of age (Fig. 46.2). The relative bioavailability of a rectal solution was 0.66 (179).

Rate of absorption. Acetaminophen has a pK_a of 9.5, and in the alkaline medium of the duodenum, acetaminophen is nonionized. Consequently, absorption of the nonionized

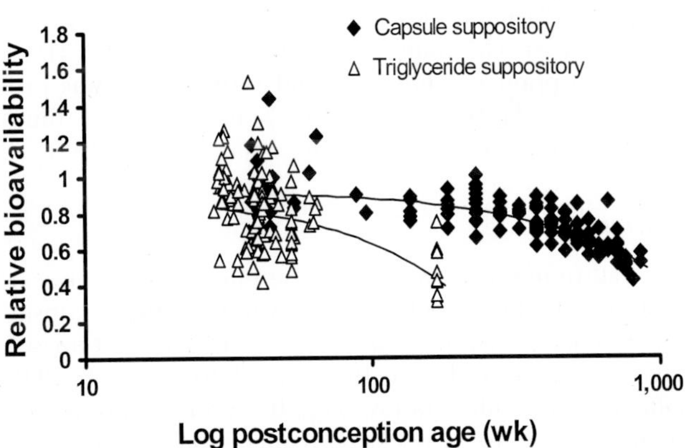

Figure 46.2. Changes in relative bioavailability of triglyceride-based and capsule suppository formulations with age. (From Anderson BJ, van Lingen RA, Hansen TG, et al. Acetaminophen developmental pharmacokinetics in premature neonates and infants: a pooled population analysis. *Anaesthesiology* 2002;96: 1336–1345, with permission.)

form from the duodenum to the systemic circulation is rapid ($T_{1/2,abs}$ = 6.8, SD 0.9 minute in adult volunteers) (180). A pharmacokinetic model using a first-order input model with a lag time has been used to describe absorption. Brown et al. (181) reported rapid absorption ($T_{1/2,abs}$ = 2.7, SE 1.2 minutes, T_{lag} = 4.2, SE 0.4 minute) parameters in febrile children given elixir orally. Similar absorption half-lives have been estimated in children given acetaminophen as an elixir before tonsillectomy ($T_{1/2,abs}$ = 4.5 minutes, CV = 63%, T_{lag} = 0) (181). These children had undergone fasting for at least 6 hours prior to surgery, and gastric transit times were rapid. Absorption in children younger than 3 months was delayed by a factor of 3.68 (182). Acetaminophen absorption depends on gastric emptying, and gastric emptying is slow and erratic in the neonate (183). Normal adult rates may not be reached until 6 to 8 months (184). Gastric pH is near neutral in neonates. This increases the unionized form available for absorption for acetaminophen (185). The stomach, however, is a poor route of entry to the circulation. The increased surface area, blood flow, and permeability of the small intestine favor the intestinal route. Oral absorption was considerably delayed in premature neonates in the first few days of life (186).

Rectal Absorption

Rectal acetaminophen is widely used in children presenting for surgical procedures because of gastrointestinal dysfunction or preoperative fasting guidelines that disallow food or fluids up to 6 hours before surgery. It is also preferable in children with nausea and vomiting. Some cultures have a greater preference for this route over oral administration (e.g., France vs. England (187). Absorption through the rectal route is slow and erratic (188,189). Data in preterm neonates are scarce (190).

Birmingham et al. (191) reported a first-order input model with a zero-order dissolution time to describe absorption characteristics of a triglyceride-base suppository in children. Others have reported a first-order absorption model with lag time. Regardless of the model, absorption is slow, with large variability (192). For example, absorption parameters for the triglyceride base and capsule suppository were $T_{1/2,abs}$ = 1.34 hours (CV = 90%), T_{lag} = 0.14 hour (31%) and $T_{1/2,abs}$ = 0.65 hour (63%), T_{lag} = 0.54 hour (31%). The absorption half-life for rectal formulations was prolonged in infants younger than 3 months (1.51 times greater) compared with values in older children (168).

Clearance

Several studies have shown that the rate constant for acetaminophen glucuronide formation in neonates is considerably smaller than in adults, but the rate constant for sulfate formation is larger than in adults (190,193,194). Glucuronide/sulfate ratios range from 0.12 in premature neonates of 28 to 32 weeks postconception age to 0.28 in those at 32 to 36 weeks postconception to 0.34 in term neonates 0 to 2 days old. Ratios of 0.75 in children aged 1 to 9 years, 1.61 in those aged 12 years, and 1.8 in adults were reported. Approximately 4% of acetaminophen is excreted in urine unmetabolized and the amount is dependent on urine flow (195).

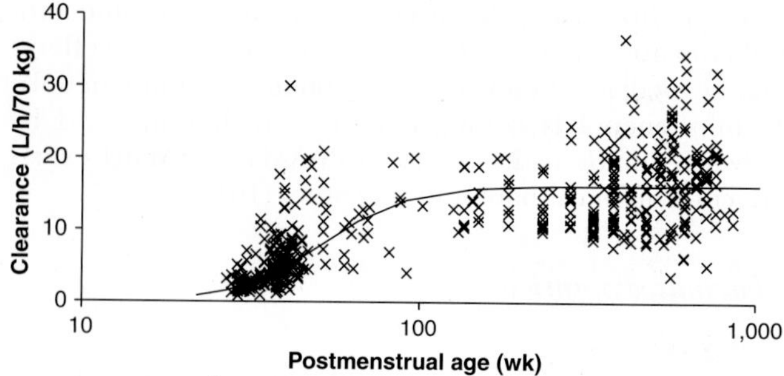

Figure 46.3. Clearance changes with age. Individual predicted clearances, standardized to a 70-kg person, from the NONMEM program's post hoc step are plotted against age. The thin line demonstrates the predicted nonlinear relationship between clearance and age. (From Anderson BJ, Allegaert K. Intravenous neonatal acetaminophen dosing; the magic of ten days. *Pediatr Anesth* 2009;19:289–295, with permission.)

Population parameter estimates (between subject variability, %) were central volume (V_2/F_{oral}) 24.0 (54.7%), peripheral volume of distribution (V_3/F_{oral}) 30.4 (31.7%), clearance (CL/F_{oral}) 16.3 (40.4%), and intercompartment clearance (Q/F_{oral}) 54.7 (116%). Clearance increased from 27 weeks PCA (1.87 L per hour per 70 kg) to reach 84% of the mature value by 1 year of age (standardized to a 70-kg person using allometric "¼ power" models) (196). Figure 46.3 shows age-related clearance estimates. Between occasion variability for clearance (CL/F_{oral}) was 18.5%.

Volume of Distribution

The population distribution volumes are similar to those reported in adults (56 to 70 L) (197). The volume of distribution for acetaminophen in mammals (197), including humans, is 49 to 70 L per 70 kg, as we would expect from the allometric size model with a power function of 1. Peripheral volume of distribution decreased from 27 weeks PCA (45.01 per 70 kg) to reach 110% of its mature value by 6 months of age (Fig. 46.4). Central volume of distribution and intercompartment clearance did not change with age. Between occasion variability for the peripheral volume of distribution (V_3/F_{oral}) was 19.3% (196).

Fetal body composition and water distribution alter considerably during the third trimester, and over the first few months of life probably reflects neonatal body composition and the rapid changes in body water distribution in early life because acetaminophen has a low molecular weight and reasonable lipid solubility (198) and acetaminophen crosses cell membranes easily, distributing throughout all tissues and fluids (199). The tissue:plasma concentration ratios are close to unity at equilibrium (199).

Disease States

The effects of altered physiology such as fever (200), anesthesia (201), or mildly impaired hepatic dysfunction (202,203) on pharmacokinetic parameters have received little attention, but appear to have minimal impact in children.

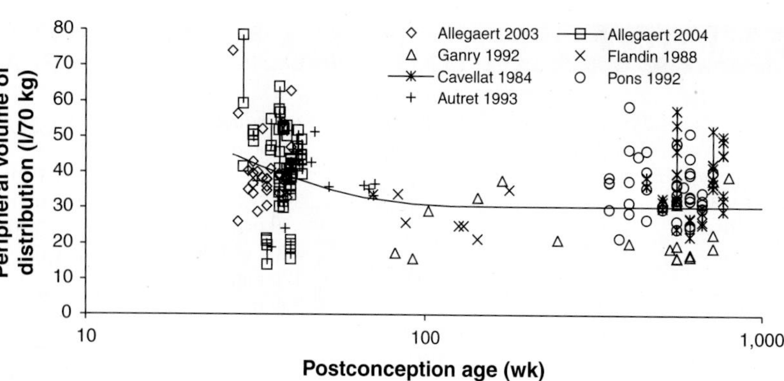

Figure 46.4. Peripheral volume of distribution changes with age. Individual predicted volumes, standardized to a 70-kg person, against age. The solid line demonstrates the nonlinear relationship between volume of distribution and age. Those children given multiple doses have volume of distribution estimates linked by a fine line to demonstrate between occasion variability. (From Anderson BJ, Pons G, Autret-Leca E, et al. Paediatric intravenous acetaminophen (propacetamol) pharmacokinetics; a population analysis. *Pediatr Anesth* 2005;15:282–292, with permission.)

Toxicity

Chronic Use of Acetaminophen

Acetaminophen overdose results in increased production of highly reactive electrophilic arylating metabolites by the hepatic cytochrome P450-dependent mixed-function oxidase enzyme system (204). The toxic metabolite of acetaminophen, *N*-acetyl-*p*-benzoquinone imine (NAPQI), is formed by the CYP2E1, 1A2, and 3A4 (205). This metabolite binds to intracellular hepatic macromolecules to produce cell necrosis and damage. Acetaminophen concentrations may rise in pediatric patients with low clearance after regular doses of 15 mg per kg every 4 hours (206). There is evidence of glutathione depletion in adult volunteers given doses of 0.5 and 3 g acetaminophen separated by 4 to 10 days (207). Penna and Buchanan (208) reported 7 deaths and 11 cases of hepatotoxicity associated with acetaminophen in children. Mortality due to hepatotoxicity was associated with doses greater than 300 mg per day per kg for 1 to 6 days. Survival was usually seen in those children suffering hepatotoxicity due to acetaminophen greater than 150 mg per day per kg for 2 to 8 days. Subsequent guidelines (209,210) recommend that doses should not exceed 90 mg per day per kg.

Significant hepatic and renal disease, malnutrition, and dehydration increase the propensity for toxicity. Medications that induce the hepatic CYP2E1, 1A2, and 3A4 systems (e.g., phenobarbitone, phenytoin, and rifampicin) may also increase the risk of hepatotoxicity. The coingestion of therapeutic drugs, foodstuffs, or other xenobiotics has potential to induce these enzymes (211). The influence of disease on acetaminophen toxicity is unknown. It has been speculated that ingestion of acetaminophen increases the potential for liver injury by another cause, such as a viral agent (212). Hepatotoxicity causing death or requiring liver transplantation has been reported with doses above 75 mg per kg per day in children and 90 mg per kg per day in infants (211,213–215). It is possible that even these regimens may cause hepatotoxicity if used for longer than 2 to 3 days (211). These reports (211,213–215) and others from Australia (216,217) and Scotland (218) are concerning. Kozer et al. (219) demonstrated that ill children receiving repeated large doses of acetaminophen (>90 mg per kg per day) may show abnormalities in liver function. It is unknown whether there is a difference in the propensity to toxicity between children given acetaminophen for fever and those given acetaminophen for postoperative analgesia.

Hepatic enzyme profiles have been used as a surrogate assessment in two neonatal studies (220,221). Neither group of authors noted hepatic changes during the treatment periods that extended over a median of 4 days, but the value of hepatic changes is debated (222). It is currently impossible to predict which individuals have an enhanced susceptibility to cellular injury from acetaminophen. One area of future investigation is the role of single nuclear polymorphisms in NAPQI production.

Single Dose of Acetaminophen

The plasma concentration associated with toxicity after a single dose of acetaminophen in children is extrapolated from adult data. The Rumack and Matthew (223) acetaminophen toxicity nomogram is widely used to guide management of acetaminophen overdose in adults and children. This nomogram was derived from a study by Prescott et al. (224) of 30 adult patients who ingested an overdose of acetaminophen. In poisoned patients with similar initial concentrations, the half-life in those without liver damage was 2.9 (SE 0.3) hours and in those with liver damage was 7.6 (SE 0.8) hours. Acetaminophen concentrations of more than 300 mg per L at 4 hours were always associated with severe hepatic lesions, but none were observed in patients with concentrations less than 150 mg per L. The half-life was less than 4 hours in all patients without liver damage.

Clearance is a nonlinear function of weight, whereas volume is a linear function of weight. Dose is usually expressed as a linear function of weight. The 4-hour concentration in children is determined by clearance, not volume, because absorption is rapid after oral elixir. As a consequence, younger children (1 to 5 years) require larger doses than older children and adults to achieve similar concentrations at 4 hours (225,226). This has been demonstrated in animals. Young rats have a higher median lethal dose than older rats (227). More drug is required to produce a hepatotoxic reaction (227). Children (1 to 5 years) with reported accidental ingestion of more than 250 mg per kg (compare to 150 mg per kg in adults) can have serum concentration measured at 2 hours after ingestion rather than the 4-hour time point recommended in adults.

Children younger than 6 years are thought to be less susceptible to toxicity than older children and adults (223). Less than 5% of children younger than 6 years with acetaminophen concentrations above the Rumack–Matthew treatment line will develop transient hepatic abnormalities (228). This may, in part, be attributable to the shorter

TABLE 46.4 Suggested Acetaminophen Dosing[a,b]

Age	*Typical Body Weight (kg)*	*Acetaminophen Clearance (L/hr/kg)*	*Acetaminophen Dose (oral)*
Neonate	3.3	0.21	50 mg, 8 hr
3 mo	6	0.25	90 mg, 6 hr
6 mo	7.5	0.27	120 mg, 6 hr
1 yr	10	0.29	120 mg, 4 hr
5 yr	18	0.25	250 mg, 4 hr
8 yr	24	0.24	300 mg, 4 hr
12 yr	38	0.21	375 mg, 4 hr
16 yr	50	0.3	500 mg, 4 hr
Adult	70	0.3	1000 mg, 6 hr

[a]The maintenance dose of acetaminophen for a patient is calculated as follows: *acetaminophen maintenance dose = acetaminophen clearance × target concentration.* Individual clearance values can be predicted from weight and age (182,186). Most of the age-related changes in clearance are complete by 1 year of age. There are also size-related changes in clearance so that the value per kg continues to decrease as weight increases in children (179,343). Clearance in adults is reported as higher than in children. The doses have been calculated to maintain a target serum acetaminophen concentration of 10 mg/L. Doses in adults are limited by concerns about hepatotoxicity.

[b]For patients more than 20% overweight, use ideal body weight. Children prefer elixir to capsules or tablets. It is important to note that elixir formulation is available in different formulation strengths when prescribing the dose by volume. Proprietary cough and cold medications containing acetaminophen are also available. Concurrent use of such medications can result in inadvertent acetaminophen toxicity. The relative bioavailability of rectal formulations is reduced out of the neonatal period and dose can be increased by 30%. Dose is reduced in premature neonates (e.g., 24 and 45 mg/kg/d at 30 and 34 wk postconception, respectively) (186).

half-life seen in children. In addition, young rats have been reported to have an increase rate of glutathione synthesis compared with older rats, as well as a capacity to increase glutathione levels after depletion (229). Glutathione may then provide increased detoxification.

Neonates can produce hepatotoxic metabolites (e.g., NAPQI), but there are suggestions of a lower activity of cytochrome P450 in neonates. This may explain the low occurrence of acetaminophen-induced hepatotoxicity seen in neonates (193,230), despite reports of high serum concentrations in newborn neonates (193,230). Placental transfer from the mother achieved these concentrations.

Adults may be more susceptible to hepatic damage due to acetaminophen's complex interaction with alcohol (207). Alcohol induces the enzyme system and is a substrate for CYP2E1. If, after enzyme induction by alcohol, acetaminophen is ingested without alcohol, then increased formation of NAPQI occurs (207). Lower amounts of P450 cytochrome oxidase system metabolites have been reported in children (231). Underreporting of dosing during parasuicide attempts (232) and absorption variability due to other drugs (e.g., dextropropoxyphene (233) or acetaminophen formulation also contribute to the increased toxicity seen in adults. Suggested acetaminophen dosing for different age groups is shown in Table 46.4.

NONSTEROIDAL ANTI-INFLAMMATORY DRUGS

MECHANISM OF ACTION

The nonsteroidal anti-inflammatory drugs (NSAIDs) are a heterogeneous group of compounds that share common antipyretic, analgesic, and anti-inflammatory effects (Table 46.5). Their major action is through inhibition of prostaglandin synthesis. NSAIDs act by reducing prostaglandin biosynthesis through inhibition of PGHS. The two major forms of this enzyme are the constitutive PGHS-1 and the inducible PGHS-2 (COX-1 and COX-2). This enzyme converts arachidonic acid to cyclic endoperoxides. Most NSAIDs block the function of both isozymes to varying degrees (234). The prostanoids produced by COX-1 isozyme protect the gastric mucosa, regulate renal blood flow, and induce platelet aggregation. NSAID-induced gastrointestinal toxicity, for example, is generally believed to occur through blockade of COX-1 activity, whereas the anti-inflammatory effects of NSAIDs are thought to occur primarily through inhibition of the inducible isoform, COX-2. Some of the NSAIDs may also inhibit the lipoxygenase pathway by an action on hydroperoxy fatty acid peroxidase.

PHARMACODYNAMICS

The NSAIDs are commonly used in children for antipyresis and analgesia. The anti-inflammatory properties of the NSAIDs have, in addition, been used in such diverse disorders as juvenile idiopathic arthritis, renal and biliary colic, dysmenorrhea, Kawasaki disease, and cystic fibrosis (235–238). The NSAIDs indomethacin and ibuprofen are also used to treat delayed closure of patent ductus arteriosus in premature infants (239). Acetaminophen and NSAIDs are often given together for the management of pain or fever. Despite the widespread use of this combination, debate exists about benefits (240–242). It is unknown whether

TABLE 46.5 Classification of Nonsteroidal Anti-Inflammatory Drugs According to their Chemical Structure

Akanones	**Anthranilic acids**	**Arylpropionic acids**
Nabumetone	Mefenamic acid	Fenoprofen
Diarylheterocyclics	Meclofenamic acid	Ibuprofen
Celecoxib	Tolfenamic acid	Flurbiprofen
Rofecoxib	**Heteroaryl acetic acids**	Ketoprofen
Enolic acids	Diclofenac	Naproxen
Meloxicam	Ketorolac	Tiaprofenic acid
Phenylbutazone	Tolmetin	**Indole and indene**
Piroxicam	**Salicylic acid derivatives**	**acetic acids**
Tenoxicam	Aspirin	Etodolac
Others	Sodium salicylate	Indomethacin
Nimesulide		Sulindac

From Litalien C, Jacqz-Aigrain E. Risks and benefits of nonsteroidal anti-inflammatory drugs in children: a comparison with paracetamol. *Paediatr Drugs* 2001;3:817–858, with permission.

there is synergy or additivity of effect when the two drugs are used together.

Analgesia

There are no linked PK–PD studies investigating NSAID analgesia in children. Pain relief attributable to NSAIDs has been compared to pain relief from other analgesics or analgesic modalities (e.g., caudal blockade, acetaminophen, and morphine) (243,244,245). Morphine is accepted as a standard analgesic in children (see earlier) and is often used for comparative studies with other analgesic medications. Studies comparing ketorolac (0.75 to 1 mg per kg) with morphine (0.1 mg per kg) for analgesia after pediatric tonsillectomy (246), strabismus surgery (247), or general surgery have demonstrated similar degrees of analgesia with reduced emesis with some increased bleeding in children given ketorolac. Diclofenac and ketorolac are both reported to reduce morphine use by up to 40% in children after a surgical insult (248–250).

A large number of studies have been done comparing acetaminophen to an NSAID for either analgesia or antipyresis in children. Most show either a similar effect or a slightly superior effect with an NSAID (240,251–262). At therapeutically equivalent doses, NSAIDs appear to be equally efficacious (263). Maunuksela and Olkkola (264) suggested that 1 mg per kg of rectal diclofenac = 10 mg per kg of oral ibuprofen = 40 mg per kg of rectal acetaminophen = 5 mg per kg of intravenous ketoprofen = 0.5 mg per kg of intravenous ketorolac.

These data confirm that NSAIDs in children are effective analgesic drugs, improving the quality of analgesia, but they do not quantify the effect. It is not possible to develop an understanding of the dose–effect relationship from these data. Nor is it possible to determine whether equipotent doses are being compared.

Relative efficacy may be determined indirectly from comparisons of each analgesic with placebo. By using a measure of at least 50% pain relief as a common descriptor of analgesic effectiveness, it is possible to produce a rank order of analgesic effectiveness (265). Collins et al. used this principle to determine the number-needed-to-treat (NNT) descriptor of effectiveness in adults (265). A single dose of ibuprofen 400 mg had an NNT of 2.7 for at least 50% pain relief compared with placebo (265). This means that one of every three patients with pain of moderate to severe intensity will experience at least 50% pain relief with ibuprofen, which they would not have had with placebo. The equivalent NNTs for ibuprofen 200 and 600 mg were 3.3 and 2.4, respectively, and those for diclofenac 25, 50, and 100 mg were 2.6, 2.3, and 1.8, respectively (Table 46.6). NSAID concentration–response relationships are rare in children. An aspirin therapeutic articular concentration of 150 to 300 mg per L has been suggested in adults for rheumatoid arthritis (266). Adult patients suffering rheumatoid arthritis with naproxen trough concentrations below 18 mg per L had no clinical response, whereas 76% of those with concentrations above 50 mg per L responded (267). The clinical effectiveness and free synovial concentrations of naproxen are also correlated (268,269). NSAID concentration–response relationships have been described for adults (17,270,271). Mandema and Stanski (271) studied patients (n = 522) given a single oral or intramuscular administration of placebo or a single intramuscular dose of 10, 30, 60, or 90 mg ketorolac for postoperative pain relief after orthopedic surgery. Mixed effects models were used. In this period, 288 patients received additional medication because of insufficient pain relief. Pain relief was found to be a function of drug concentration (E_{max} model), time (waxing and waning of placebo effect), and an individual random effect. The E_{max}, EC_{50}, and T_{eq} were 8.5/10, 0.37 mg per L, and 24 minutes, respectively.

TABLE 46.6 Number Needed to Treat (NNT) for Ibuprofen and Diclofenac in Adults

Ibuprofen (mg)	*NNT (95% CI)*	*Diclofenac (mg)*	*NNT (95% CI)*
50	3.6 (2.5–6.1)	25	2.6 (1.9–4.5)
100	5.6 (3.8–9.9)	50	2.3 (2.1–2.7)
200	3.3 (2.8–4)	100	1.8 (1.5–2.1)
400	2.7 (2.5–3)		
600	2.4 (1.9–3.3)		
800	1.6 (1.3–2.2)		

CI, confidence interval.
Adapted from Collins SL, Moore RA, McQuay HJ, et al. Single dose ibuprofen and diclofenac for postoperative pain. *Cochrane Database Syst Rev* 2002;(3), with permission.

Interpretation of PK–PD relationships is also complicated by active metabolites. Diclofenac's 4′-hydroxyl metabolite has 30% of the anti-inflammatory and antipyretic activity of the parent compound. Approximately 20% of the parent drug is processed (CYP2C9) to this metabolite. Despite the impact of this metabolite, there are reasonable data to support the contention that diclofenac 50 mg is as effective as diclofenac 100 mg in adults (272). Little or no information on developmental differences in arachidonic acid release, prostaglandin formation, or COX-2 expression is available for the pediatric population. It has been assumed that attaining similar adult exposure to 50 mg in children should give similar effectiveness. This argument has been used to support a single dose of diclofenac 1 mg per kg in children 1 to 12 years as equivalent to 50 mg in adults (273).

Antipyresis

Ibuprofen is the most common NSAID antipyretic studied (162,163,274,275). Brown et al. (162) reported a linked-population PK–PD model for antipyresis using mixed-effects models. The link component yielded a K_{eo} of 0.70 (SE 0.11) and 0.57 (SE 0.11) per hour for ibuprofen 5 and 10 mg per kg, respectively; the sigmoid E_{max} component yielded EC_{50} and Hill coefficient (N) values of 11.33 (SE 1.35) and 3.97 (SE 0.58) mg per L for ibuprofen 5 mg per kg, respectively, and 12.83 (SE 1.89) and 4.27 (SE 0.63) mg per L for ibuprofen 10 mg per kg. Similar results were reported by Troconiz et al. (274).

The interpretation of the concentration–response relationship is confounded by the disease process, initial temperature, dosing regimens, and fever fluctuation, ensuring that direct comparison between acetaminophen and ibuprofen is difficult. A large number of studies have suggested that the clinical effectiveness of these two drugs is similar. No clinical trials have been conducted that demonstrate superior effect when both drugs are used compared with one alone.

Patent Ductus Arteriosus Closure

Both indomethacin and ibuprofen are used to expedite patent ductus arteriosus closure in premature neonates by inhibiting prostaglandin synthesis, namely, PGE_2 (239,276,277). Shaffer et al. (277) examined factors affecting PDA closure after indomethacin treatment in poor responders, neonates weighing less than 100 g and/or 10 days of postnatal age or older. Closure appears dependent on a critical predose serum concentration of 1.9 mg per L in neonates younger than 10 days and 1.4 mg per L in neonates 10 days of age or older. Dose and duration of treatment were increased in the older group, assumably due to increased clearance.

Cystic Fibrosis

High-dose ibuprofen therapy has been demonstrated to slow down deterioration in pulmonary function in children with cystic fibrosis with mild lung disease. Therapeutic drug monitoring has been recommended to maintain peak concentrations within the range of 50 to 100 mg per L to ensure efficacy (278).

PHARMACOKINETICS

The pharmacokinetics of NSAIDs has been reviewed by Litalien and Jacqz-Aigrain (279). Pharmacokinetic age-related changes and covariate effects are poorly documented for many of the NSAIDs. There is a paucity of data in infants younger than 6 months (Table 46.7).

NSAID formulations may be administered orally, topically, intraocularly, intra-articularly, intravenously, intramuscularly, and rectally. NSAIDs are rapidly absorbed in the gastrointestinal tract after oral administration. Time to maximal concentration is generally 1 to 2 hours, but depends on formulation and concomitant food intake. Troconiz et al. (274) reported a $T_{1/2,abs}$ of 0.85 hour for ibuprofen suspension in febrile children. Absorption due to the dissolution time of diclofenac tablets is slower than that associated with effervescent or liquid formulations (280,281). An absorption lag time of 1 hour has been reported in children given enteric-coated diclofenac tablets (262). The relative bioavailability of oral preparations approaches 1 compared to intravenous administration. The rate and extent of rectal administration of NSAIDs such as ibuprofen, diclofenac, flurbiprofen, indomethacin, and nimesulide is less than those by oral routes (188). The relative bioavailability of suppository compared to oral flurbiprofen was 99.8% in children 6 to 12 years old (282).

NSAID PK is usually described using a one-compartment, first-order elimination model. The apparent volume of distribution (V/F) is small in adults (<0.2 L per kg, suggesting minimal tissue binding) but is larger in children; for example, ketorolac V/F in children 4 to 8 years old is twice that of adults (283,284). Premature neonates (22 to 31 weeks' gestational age) given intravenous ibuprofen had a V/F of 0.62 (SD 0.04) L per kg (285). Van Overmeire et al. (276) reported a dramatic reduction in ibuprofen central volume (V_c/F) following closure of the PDA in premature neonates (0.244 vs. 0.171 L per kg). The NSAIDs, as a group, are weakly acidic, lipophilic, and highly protein bound. The bound fraction in children (e.g., etodolac, 93.9% vs. 95.5%) (286) and premature neonates (e.g., ibuprofen, 94.9% vs. 98.7%) (285) is slightly lower than in adults. Binding of NSAIDs to plasma proteins is a saturable process. The impact of this reduced protein binding is probably minimal with routine dosing because NSAIDs cleared by the liver have a low hepatic extraction ratio (59). In addition, they have a long equilibration time between plasma and effect compartments (59). Substantial intra-articular tissue concentrations of NSAIDs are attained after systemic administration, and elimination half-times are longer in synovial fluid than in plasma, contributing to their effectiveness in arthritis (287,288).

NSAIDs undergo extensive phase I and phase II enzyme biotransformation in the liver, with subsequent excretion into urine or bile. Enterohepatic recirculation occurs when a significant amount of an NSAID or its conjugated metabolites are excreted into the bile and then reabsorbed in the distal intestine. NSAID elimination is not dependent on hepatic blood flow. Hepatic NSAID elimination is dependent on the free fraction of NSAID within the plasma and the intrinsic enzyme activities of the liver. Renal elimination is not an important elimination pathway for NSAIDs, except for azapropazone. Pharmacokinetic parameter estimate variability is large, partly attributable to covariate effects of age, size, and pharmacogenomics. Ibuprofen, for example, is metabolized by the CYP2C9 and CYP2C8 subfamily (129,289). It is known that considerable variation exists in the expression of CYP2 C activities among individuals, and functional polymorphism of the gene coding for CYP2C9 has been described. It has been demonstrated in human liver microsomes that intrinsic ibuprofen clearance was much higher for the CYP2C9 (Arg 144) variant than for the CYP2C9 (Cys 144) variant (290). From the literature on phenytoin metabolism, it seems that CYP2C9 activity is low immediately after birth, subsequently increasing progressively to peak activity at a young age (130).

There is relatively little transfer from maternal to fetal blood. Excretion of NSAIDs into breast milk of lactating mothers is low. Infant exposure to ketorolac via breast milk is estimated to be 0.4% of maternal exposure (291).

NSAID elimination is all too frequently described only in terms of half-life, which is therefore confounded by volume of distribution. The plasma half-lives of NSAIDs in adults range from 0.25 to greater than 70 hours, indicating wide differences in clearance rates. Elimination half-lives are longer in neonates than in children. An elimination half-life of 30.5 ± 4.2 hours was reported in premature infants receiving ibuprofen within the first 12 hours of life (285), in contrast with 1.6 ± 0.7 hours in infants and children aged 3 months to 10 years (163). Clearance increases from birth, but is confounded by age and weight (292). Ibuprofen clearance increases from 2.06 mL per hour per kg at 22 to 31 weeks PCA (285), 9.49 mL per hour per kg

TABLE 46.7 Pharmacokinetic Parameter Estimates[a]

Age	*No.*	*Formulation*	*CL/F (mL/hr/kg)*	*V/F (L/kg)*	$T_{1/2}$ *(hr)*	*Ref.*
Salicylic acid						
0.3–4 yr	6	Suspension	ND	0.3 (0.1)	4 (2.1)	337
0.8–1.8 yr	5	Suspension	ND	0.3 (0.06)	5.6 (6.4)	337
5.5 (0.8) yr	10	Tablet	22.1 (1.8)	0.113 (0.005)	3.24	194
Diclofenac						
4.3–6.8 yr	10	i.v.	462 (90)	0.9 (0.25)	1.3 (0.3)	283
5–15 yr	11	Tablet	754 (207)	0.71 (0.23)	0.65 (0.14)	253
Etodolac						
8.1–14.8 yr	11	Tablet	53.3 (13.3)	0.49 (0.12)	6.5 (1.4)	275
Fenclofenac						
3–17 yr	17	Tablet	. . .	. . .	25.4	338
Flurbiprofen						
6–8 yr	4	Suspension/	26 (25–27)	0.15	2.71 (2.21–3.45)	271
		suppository	25 (22–30)	0.17	3.22 (2.88–3.75)	
12 yr	4	Suspension/	33 (24–48)	0.14	3.07 (2.76–3.48)	271
		suppository	43 (27–69)	0.19	3.15 (2.81–3.85)	
Ibuprofen						
22–31 wk	21 d	i.v.	2.06 (0.33)	0.062 (0.004)	30.5	274
28.6 (1.9) wk	13 d	i.v.	9.49 (6.82)	0.357 (0.121)	43.1 (26.1)	265
0.5–1.5 yr	11	Suspension	110 (40)	0.20 (0.09)	1.6 (0.4)	339
11 mo–11 yr	18	Suspension	57.6	0.164	1.97	154
3 mo–12 yr	28	Suspension	80 (SE 10)	0.16 (SE 0.02)	1.44 (SE 0.15)	153
3 mo–12 yr	39	Suspension	110 (SE 10)	0.22 (SE 0.02)	1.37 (SE 0.09)	153
5.2 (1.7) yr	22	Suspension	140 (32)	0.27 (0.11)	1.4 (0.5)	231
5.2 (2.5) yr	4	Tablet	114 (26)	0.26 (0.1)	1.6 (0.4)	231
4–16 yr	103[b]	Suspension/	71 (CV 24%)	V_c 0.06,	. . .	263
		granules	(4.05 L/hr/70 kg)	V_p 0.1 (CV 65%)		
Celecoxib						
11.3 (3.9)	11[c]	Tablet	1,400 (1,000)	7.9 (7.8)	3.7 (1.1)	287
Indomethacin						
28.8 (2.5) wk[d]	83[e]	i.v.	2.63 × wt (kg) + 0.244 PNA (d) mL/hr (CV 77%)	0.28 × wt (kg) + 0.0041 PNA (d) L (CV 28%)		282
5.7 (4.7) d[f]						
1.2–4.6 yr	14	i.v.	192 (102)	0.74 (0.75)	6.1 (4.9)	340
Ketoprofen						
7 mo–16 yr	18	i.v.	90 (60–130)	0.16 (0.12–0.21)	1.3 (0.8–1.7)	341
Ketorolac						
1–16 yr	36	i.v.	34.2 (10.2)	0.113 (0.033)	. . .	186
4–8 yr	10	i.v.	42 (30–58)	0.26 (0.19–0.44)	6.1 (3.5–10)	272
3–18 yr	50	i.v.	66 (30)	0.35 (0.2)	4.1 (2.3)	285
3.3–8 yr	7	i.v.	80 (50)	0.26 (0.17)	2.26 (1.35)	284
2.6–7.3 yr	7	i.v.	70 (30)	0.21 (0.08)	2.09 (0.57)	284
Naproxen						
8.1–14.1 yr	12	Tablet	9.2 (2.6)	0.11 (0.02)	8.1 (2.1)	342
10.4–14.1 yr	10	Suspension	9 (2.4)	0.13 (0.03)	9.6 (3.2)	342
Nimesulide						
7–9 yr	16	Granules	138.6	0.41	2.4	286
Piroxicam						
6.7–15.9 yr	10	Tablet	3.4 (1.1)	0.16 (0.05)	32.6 (6.5)	186
Tiaprofenic acid						
3.5–10.6 yr	12	Suspension	94 (40–275)	0.32 (0.08–0.91)	2.4 (1.4–5.8)	59
0.5–3 yr	10	Suspension	90 (10)	0.23 (0.06)	1.82 (0.48)	343
Tolfenamic acid						
2–14 yr	6	Suspension	230 (25)	. . .	2.82 (0.21)	344

[a]Variability is given in parentheses as SD, range, or SE. CL/*F*, apparent drug plasma clearance; i.v., intravenous; $T_{1/2}$, elimination half-life; *V/F*, apparent volume of distribution; V_c, initial volume of distribution; V_p, apparent volume of distribution of peripheral compartment, ND, not determined, CV, coefficient of variation; PNA, postnatal age.
[b]Data reported using allometric model. Estimate presented for a 30-kg individual.
[c]Oncology children having cytotoxic chemotherapy.
[d]Age is gestational age (wk).
[e]Covariates age and weight included in parameter estimates.
[f]Age is postnatal age (d).
Modified from Litalien C, Jacqz-Aigrain E. Risks and benefits of nonsteroidal anti-inflammatory drugs in children: a comparison with paracetamol. *Paediatr Drugs* 2001:3;817–858.

TABLE 46.8 Ketorolac Age-Related Pharmacokinetic Changes[a]

Age (yr)	Weight (kg)	V_{ss} (SD) (L/kg)	CL (SD) (L/min/kg)	CL_{std} (SD) (L/min/ 70 kg)
1–3	12	0.111 (0.025)	0.6 (0.2)	27.0 (9.0)
4–7	20	0.128 (0.047)	0.61 (0.22)	31.2 (11.3)
8–12	30	0.099 (0.014)	0.54 (0.15)	30.6 (8.5)
12–16	50	0.116 (0.040)	0.51 (0.12)	32.8 (7.7)
Adult (281)	70	0.11	0.3–0.55	21–38.5

[a] V_{ss}, volume of distribution at steady state; CL_{std}, total body clearance standardized to a 70-kg person using an allometric ¾ power model; $n = 36$. Weight is estimated. Data are from Dsida RM, Wheeler M, Birmingham PK, et al. Age-stratified pharmacokinetics of ketorolac tromethamine in pediatric surgical patients. *Anesth Analg* 2002;94:266–270.

at 28 weeks PCA (276), to 140 mL per hour per kg at 5 years (238). Similar maturation is now reported for indomethacin (293,294). Clearance (L per hour per kg) is generally increased in childhood both for the established NSAIDs (225,283,294–298) and for the newer COX-2 inhibitors (299), as we might expect when size is unaccounted for. Age-related ketorolac pharmacokinetic parameter estimates after 0.5 mg per kg intravenously are shown in Table 46.8. Elimination clearance, corrected for size using an allometric ¾ power model, is similar to adult estimates from 1 year of age.

NSAIDs exhibit stereoselectivity. Ibuprofen stereoselectivity has been reported in premature neonates (<28 weeks' gestation). R- and S-ibuprofen half-lives were about 10 hours and 25.5 hours, respectively. The mean clearance of R-ibuprofen (12.7 mL per hour) was about 2.5-fold higher than for S-ibuprofen (5.0 mL per hour) (300). The lower clearance and longer half-life of S-ibuprofen suggests that pharmacokinetic predictions based on racemic assays may underestimate the duration of pharmacologic effect. Single isomer NSAIDs are appearing for the treatment of acute pain and may have fewer adverse effects than traditional NSAIDs (301,302).

Reports of the use of COX-2 selective inhibitors in children are appearing in the literature (303,304), but their future use is uncertain following reports of atherothrombosis in adults (305). Future benefits may be derived from nitric oxide releasing NSAIDs that have increased potency and reduced side effects (306).

DRUG INTERACTIONS

NSAIDs undergo drug interactions through protein-binding displacement, altered clearance, and competition for active renal tubular secretion with other organic acids. High protein binding among the NSAIDs has been used to explain drug interactions with oral anticoagulant agents, oral hypoglycemics, sulfonamides, bilirubin, and other protein-bound drugs. An influential paper by Aggeler et al. (307) showed that warfarin administered with phenylbutazone increased plasma warfarin concentrations and prothrombin time in normal volunteers. Phenylbutazone displaces warfarin from its albumin-binding sites in vitro, and this observation cannot be extrapolated to an in vivo effect. The observed effect is due to changes in drug metabolic clearance and not from changes in protein binding (59).

The NSAIDs can reduce the antihypertensive effect of angiotensin-converting enzyme inhibitors and β-blockers with possible loss of blood pressure control and can attenuate the natriuretic effect of thiazide diuretics and frusemide. Concurrent administration of probenecid decreases NSAID renal clearance. Lithium and methotrexate concentrations may be increased due to decreased renal clearance. Significant drug interactions have also been demonstrated for aspirin (acetylsalicylic acid), digoxin, cyclosporine, cholestyramine, and colestipol (288).

RENAL FAILURE

Renally excreted NSAIDs such as azapropazone may accumulate in renal failure. Ketoprofen and naproxen are metabolized via the acylglucuronidation pathway, and also may accumulate in renal failure. Renal impairment is a risk factor for NSAID-induced renal toxicity (263).

HEPATIC DISEASE

Hypoalbuminemia will alter the V/F of an NSAID. NSAIDs that are mainly eliminated by hepatic oxidative metabolism may require dose reduction, or should be avoided in the presence of significant liver disease (ibuprofen, piroxicam, tenoxicam, diclofenac, flurbiprofen, nabumetone, sulindac) (263).

SAFETY ISSUES

The most common adverse events in NSAID recipients are nausea, dizziness, and headache. NSAIDs have potential to cause gastrointestinal irritation, blood clotting disorders, renal impairment, neutrophil dysfunction, and bronchoconstriction (308,309), effects postulated to be related to COX-1/COX-2 ratios (Table 46.9), although this concept may be an oversimplification (310,311). For example, the COX-2 inhibitors rofecoxib and celecoxib produce qualitative changes in urinary prostaglandin excretion, glomerular filtration rate, sodium retention, and their consequences similar to nonselective NSAIDs. COX-2 is constitutively expressed in renal tissues of all species. It seems unlikely that these COX-2 inhibitors will offer renal safety benefits over nonselective NSAID therapies. It is reasonable to assume

TABLE 46.9 Relative Cyclooxygenase-1/ Cyclooxygenase-2 (COX-1/COX-2) Specificity Ratios

COX-2/COX-1 > 1	COX-2/COX-1 ≈ 1	COX-2/COX-1 < 1
Aspirin	Diclofenac	Celecoxib
Ibuprofen	Naproxen	Meloxicam
Indomethacin		Nimesulide
Tolfenamic acid		Rofecoxib

From Litalien C, Jacqz-Aigrain E. Risks and benefits of nonsteroidal anti-inflammatory drugs in children: a comparison with paracetamol. *Paediatr Drugs* 2001;3:817–858.

that all NSAIDs, including COX-2-selective inhibitors, share a similar risk for adverse renal effects (312).

Renal Effects

The effect of short-term treatment with NSAIDs on healthy kidneys is negligible. Ibuprofen reduced the glomerular filtration rate by 20% in premature neonates, affecting aminoglycoside clearance, and this effect appears independent of gestational age (313,314). Large studies involving ibuprofen (315,316,317) and ketorolac (318,319) have shown little risk. Similar data are reported in children suffering juvenile rheumatoid arthritis (JIA) given NSAIDs as long-term treatment (319,320). However, renal compromise is described in children compromised by dehydration, hypovolemia, hypotension, or preexisting renal disease (284,321–325). NSAIDs may also potentiate the toxicity of other drugs such as aminoglycosides and cyclosporin (326,327).

Gastrointestinal Effects

Adverse gastrointestinal effects are significant in adults, particularly in those with peptic ulcer disease, caused by *Helicobacter pylori*, or *with* advanced age (328–330). The risk of acute gastrointestinal bleeding in children given short-term ibuprofen was estimated to be 7.2 in 100,000 (95% CI, 2 to 18 in 100,000) (315,317) and was not different from those children given acetaminophen. Similar data are reported in children given ketorolac for acute pain (284). The incidence of clinically significant gastropathy is comparable in adults and children given NSAIDs for JIA (331,332), but gastroduodenal injury may be very much higher (75%) depending on assessment criteria (e.g., abdominal pain, anemia, and endoscopy) (333).

Bleeding Propensity

The commonly used NSAIDs such as ketorolac, diclofenac, ibuprofen, and ketoprofen have reversible antiplatelet effects, which are attributable to the inhibition of thromboxane synthesis. This side effect is of concern during the perioperative period (334,335). Bleeding time is usually slightly increased, but it remains within normal limits in children with normal coagulation systems. Ketorolac can be used to treat pain after congenital heart surgery without an increased risk of bleeding complications (336). Neonates given prophylactic ibuprofen to induce patent ductus arteriosus closure did not have an increased frequency of intraventricular hemorrhage (337). A Cochrane review has established that even after tonsillectomy, NSAIDs did not cause any increase in bleeding that required a return to theater in children (338). There was significantly less nausea and vomiting with NSAIDs compared with alternative analgesics, suggesting that their benefits outweigh their negative aspects.

Studies involving the use of ketorolac analgesia for tonsillectomy have reported increased bleeding in children, attributable to the dose used and whether it is given preoperatively or postoperatively (339). The risk associated with the drug was larger and clinically important when ketorolac was used in higher doses, in older subjects, and for more than 5 days.

Asthma

Aspirin or NSAID exacerbated respiratory disease (ERD) is more a disorder of adults, but exacerbations in children and teenagers have been reported. These cases are countered by reports of beneficial reduction of asthma symptoms where ibuprofen was administered for antipyresis (340). Palmer concluded that benefit is likely seen in younger children with mild episodic asthma and that aspirin-ERD is a concern in one in three teenagers with severe asthma and coexistent nasal disease. COX-2 inhibitors are reported as safe in NSAID-ERD (341).

REFERENCES

1. Anand KJS, Hickey PR. Pain and its effects in the human neonate and fetus. *N Engl J Med* 1987;317(21):1321–1329.
2. Hummel P, van Dijk M. Pain assessment: current status and challenges. *Semin Fetal Neonatal Med* 2006;11(4):237–245.
3. Berde CB, Sethna N. Analgesics for the treatment of pain in children. *N Engl J Med* 2002;347(14):1094–1103.
4. Bellu R, de Waal KA, Zanini R. Opioids for neonates receiving mechanical ventilation. *Cochrane Database Syst Rev* 2008(1): CD004212.
5. Anderson BJ, Palmer GM. Recent developments in the pharmacological management of pain in children. *Curr Opin Anaesthesiol* 2006;19(3):285–292.
6. Faura CC, Collins SL, Moore RA, et al. Systematic review of factors affecting the ratios of morphine and its major metabolites. *Pain* 1998;74(1):43–53.
7. de Wildt SN, Kearns GL, Leeder JS, et al. Glucuronidation in humans. Pharmacogenetic and developmental aspects. *Clin Pharmacokinet* 1999;36(6):439–452.
8. de Wildt SN, Kearns GL, Leeder JS, et al. Cytochrome P450 3 A: ontogeny and drug disposition. *Clin Pharmacokinet* 1999;37(6): 485–505.
9. Stephenson T. How children's responses to drugs differ from adults. *Br J Clin Pharmacol* 2005;59(6):670–673.
10. Anderson BJ, Allegaert K, Holford NH. Population clinical pharmacology of children: general principles. *Eur J Pediatr* 2006; 165(11):741–746.
11. Anderson BJ, Allegaert K, Holford NH. Population clinical pharmacology of children: modelling covariate effects. *Eur J Pediatr* 2006;165(12):819–829.
12. Inturrisi CE. Clinical pharmacology of opioids for pain. *Clin J Pain* 2002;18(Suppl 4):S3–S13.
13. Suresh S, Anand KJS. Opioid tolerance in neonates: mechanisms, diagnosis, assessment, and management. *Semin Perinatol* 1998; 22(5):425–433.
14. Stein C, Machelska H, Binder W, et al. Peripheral opioid analgesia. *Curr Opin Pharmacol* 2001;1(1):62–65.
15. McGrath PA. Development of the World Health Organization Guidelines on Cancer Pain Relief and Palliative Care in Children. *J Pain Symptom Manage* 1996;12(2):87–92.
16. Zernikow B, Michel E, Craig F, et al. Pediatric palliative care: use of opioids for the management of pain. *Paediatr Drugs* 2009;11(2): 129–151.
17. Suri A, Estes KS, Geisslinger G, et al. Pharmacokinetic–pharmacodynamic relationships for analgesics. *Int J Clin Pharmacol Ther* 1997;35(8):307–323.
18. Olkkola KT, Hamunen K. Pharmacokinetics and pharmacodynamics of analgesic drugs. In: Anand KJ, Stevens B, McGrath P, eds. *Pain in neonates*, 2nd revised and enlarged edition. Amsterdam, Netherlands: Elsevier, 2000:135–158.
19. Rahman W, Dashwood MR, Fitzgerald M, et al. Postnatal development of multiple opioid receptors in the spinal cord and development of spinal morphine analgesia. *Brain Res Dev Brain Res* 1998;108(1–2):239–254.
20. Loh HH, Liu HC, Cavalli A, et al. mu Opioid receptor knockout in mice: effects on ligand-induced analgesia and morphine lethality. *Brain Res Mol Brain Res* 1998;54(2):321–326.

21. Matthes HW, Maldonado R, Simonin F, et al. Loss of morphine-induced analgesia, reward effect and withdrawal symptoms in mice lacking the mu-opioid-receptor gene. *Nature* 1996;383(6603):819–823.
22. Sora I, Takahashi N, Funada M, et al. Opiate receptor knockout mice define mu receptor roles in endogenous nociceptive responses and morphine-induced analgesia. *Proc Natl Acad Sci U S A* 1997;94(4):1544–1549.
23. Coffman BL, Rios GR, King CD, et al. Human UGT2B7 catalyzes morphine glucuronidation. *Drug Metab Dispos* 1997;25(1):1–4.
24. Wittwer E, Kern SE. Role of morphine's metabolites in analgesia: concepts and controversies. *AAPS J* 2006;8(2):E348–E352.
25. Romberg R, Olofsen E, Sarton E, et al. Pharmacokinetic–pharmacodynamic modeling of morphine-6-glucuronide-induced analgesia in healthy volunteers: absence of sex differences. *Anesthesiology* 2004;100(1):120–133.
26. van Dorp EL, Romberg R, Sarton E, et al. Morphine-6-glucuronide: morphine's successor for postoperative pain relief? *Anesth Analg* 2006;102(6):1789–1797.
27. Osborne PB, Chieng B, Christie MJ. Morphine-6 beta-glucuronide has a higher efficacy than morphine as a mu-opioid receptor agonist in the rat locus coeruleus. *Br J Pharmacol* 2000;131(7):1422–1428.
28. Murthy BR, Pollack GM, Brouwer KL. Contribution of morphine-6-glucuronide to antinociception following intravenous administration of morphine to healthy volunteers. *J Clin Pharmacol* 2002;42(5):569–576.
29. Osborne R, Thompson P, Joel S, et al. The analgesic activity of morphine-6-glucuronide. *Br J Clin Pharmacol* 1992;34(2):130–138.
30. Thompson PI, Joel SP, John L, et al. Respiratory depression following morphine and morphine-6-glucuronide in normal subjects. *Br J Clin Pharmacol* 1995;40(2):145–152.
31. Gong QL, Hedner J, Bjorkman R, et al. Morphine-3-glucuronide may functionally antagonize morphine-6-glucuronide induced antinociception and ventilatory depression in the rat. *Pain* 1992; 48(2):249–255.
32. Smith MT, Watt JA, Cramond T. Morphine-3-glucuronide—a potent antagonist of morphine analgesia. *Life Sci* 1990;47(6):579–585.
33. Fisher MB, Vandenbranden M, Findlay K, et al. Tissue distribution and interindividual variation in human UDP-glucuronosyltransferase activity: relationship between UGT1A1 promoter genotype and variability in a liver bank. *Pharmacogenetics* 2000; 10(8):727–739.
34. Choonara I, Ekbom Y, Lindstrom B, et al. Morphine sulphation in children. *Br J Clin Pharmacol* 1990;30(6):897–900.
35. McRorie TI, Lynn AM, Nespeca MK, et al. The maturation of morphine clearance and metabolism. *Am J Dis Child* 1992;146(8):972–976.
36. Koren G, Maurice L. Pediatric uses of opioids. *Pediatr Clin North Am* 1989;36(5):1141–1156.
37. Choonara IA, McKay P, Hain R, et al. Morphine metabolism in children. *Br J Clin Pharmacol* 1989;28(5):599–604.
38. Lamacraft G, Cooper MG, Cavalletto BP. Subcutaneous cannulae for morphine boluses in children: assessment of a technique. *J Pain Symptom Manage* 1997;13(1):43–49.
39. Lundeberg S, Beck O, Olsson GL, et al. Rectal administration of morphine in children. Pharmacokinetic evaluation after a single-dose. *Acta Anaesthesiol Scand* 1996;40(4):445–451.
40. Reich A, Beland B, van Aken H. Intravenous narcotics and analgesic agents. In: Bissonnette B, Dalens BJ, eds. *Pediatric anesthesia*. New York: McGraw-Hill, 259–277.
41. Schiessl C, Gravou C, Zernikow B, et al. Use of patient-controlled analgesia for pain control in dying children. *Support Care Cancer* 2008;16(5):531–536.
42. Inturrisi CE, Colburn WA. Application of pharmacokinetic–pharmacodynamic modeling to analgesia. In: Foley KM, Inturrisi CE, eds. *Advances in pain research and therapy opioid analgesics in the management of clinical pain*. New York: Raven Press, 1986:441–452.
43. Anderson BJ, Ralph CJ, Stewart AW, et al. The dose-effect relationship for morphine and vomiting after day-stay tonsillectomy in children. *Anaesth Intensive Care* 2000;28(2):155–160.
44. Lynn AM, Nespeca MK, Opheim KE, et al. Respiratory effects of intravenous morphine infusions in neonates, infants, and children after cardiac surgery. *Anesth Analg* 1993;77(4):695–701.
45. van Dijk M, Bouwmeester NJ, Duivenvoorden HJ, et al. Efficacy of continuous versus intermittent morphine administration after major surgery in 0–3-year-old infants; a double-blind randomized controlled trial. *Pain* 2002;98(3):305–313.
46. Simons SHP, van Dijk M, van Lingen RA, et al. Routine morphine infusion in preterm neonates who received ventilatory support: a randomized controlled trial. *JAMA* 2003;290:2419–2427.
47. Anand KJ, Hall RW, Desai N, et al. Effects of morphine analgesia in ventilated preterm neonates: primary outcomes from the NEOPAIN randomised trial. *Lancet* 2004;363(9422):1673–1682.
48. Anand KJ, Anderson BJ, Holford NH, et al. Morphine pharmacokinetics and pharmacodynamics in preterm and term neonates: secondary results from the NEOPAIN trial. *Br J Anaesth* 2008; 101(5):680–689.
49. Chay PC, Duffy BJ, Walker JS. Pharmacokinetic–pharmacodynamic relationships of morphine in neonates. *Clin Pharmacol Ther* 1992; 51(3):334–342.
50. Kart T, Christrup LL, Rasmussen M. Recommended use of morphine in neonates, infants and children based on a literature review: Part 2—Clinical use. *Paediatr Anaesth* 1997;7(2):93–101.
51. Lynn A, Nespeca MK, Bratton SL, et al. Clearance of morphine in postoperative infants during intravenous infusion: the influence of age and surgery. *Anesth Analg* 1998;86(5):958–963.
52. Anderson BJ, Persson M, Anderson M. Rationalising intravenous morphine prescriptions in children. *Acute Pain* 1999;2:59–67.
53. Pacifici GM, Sawe J, Kager L, et al. Morphine glucuronidation in human fetal and adult liver. *Eur J Clin Pharmacol* 1982;22(6):553–558.
54. Pacifici GM, Franchi M, Giuliani L, et al. Development of the glucuronyltransferase and sulphotransferase towards 2-naphthol in human fetus. *Dev Pharmacol Ther* 1989;14(2):108–114.
55. Knibbe CA, Krekels EH, van den Anker JN, et al. Morphine glucuronidation in preterm neonates, infants and children younger than 3 years. *Clin Pharmacokinet* 2009;48(6):371–385.
56. Peters JW, Anderson BJ, Simons SH, et al. Morphine pharmacokinetics during venoarterial extracorporeal membrane oxygenation in neonates. *Intensive Care Med* 2005;31(2):257–263.
57. Bhat R, Chari G, Gulati A, et al. Pharmacokinetics of a single dose of morphine in preterm infants during the first week of life. *J Pediatr* 1990;117(3):477–481.
58. Olsen GD. Morphine binding to human plasma proteins. *Clin Pharmacol Ther* 1975;17(1):31–35.
59. Benet LZ, Hoener BA. Changes in plasma protein binding have little clinical relevance. *Clin Pharmacol Ther* 2002;71(3):115–121.
60. Nichols DJ, Yaster M, Lynn AM, et al. Disposition and respiratory effects of intrathecal morphine in children. *Anesthesiology* 1993;79:733–738.
61. Hall RW, Kronsberg SS, Barton BA, et al. Morphine, hypotension, and adverse outcomes among preterm neonates: who's to blame? Secondary results from the NEOPAIN trial. *Pediatrics* 2005;115(5):1351–1359.
62. Simons SH, Roofthooft DW, van Dijk M, et al. Morphine in ventilated neonates: its effects on arterial blood pressure. *Arch Dis Child Fetal Neonatal Ed* 2006;91(1):F46–F51.
63. William DG, Hatch DJ, Howard RF. Codeine phosphate in paediatric medicine. *Br J Anaesth* 2001;86(3):413–421.
64. Chen ZR, Somogyi AA, Bochner F. Polymorphic *O*-demethylation of codeine. *Lancet* 1988;2(8616):914–915.
65. Sindrup SH, Brosen K. The pharmacogenetics of codeine hypoalgesia. *Pharmacogenetics* 1995;5(6):335–346.
66. Williams DG, Patel A, Howard RF. Pharmacogenetics of codeine metabolism in an urban population of children and its implications for analgesic reliability. *Br J Anaesth* 2002;89(6):839–845.
67. Eckhardt K, Li S, Ammon S, et al. Same incidence of adverse drug events after codeine administration irrespective of the genetically determined differences in morphine formation. *Pain* 1998; 76(1–2):27–33.
68. Parke TJ, Nandi PR, Bird KJ, et al. Profound hypotension following intravenous codeine phosphate. Three case reports and some recommendations. *Anaesthesia* 1992;47(10):852–854.
69. McEwan A, Sigston PE, Andrews KA, et al. A comparison of rectal and intramuscular codeine phosphate in children following neurosurgery. *Paediatr Anaesth* 2000;10(2):189–193.
70. Tobias JD, Lowe S, Hersey S, et al. Analgesia after bilateral myringotomy and placement of pressure equalization tubes in

children: acetaminophen versus acetaminophen with codeine. *Anesth Analg* 1995;81(3):496–500.
71. St Charles CS, Matt BH, Hamilton MM, et al. A comparison of ibuprofen versus acetaminophen with codeine in the young tonsillectomy patient. *Otolaryngol Head Neck Surg* 1997;117(1):76–82.
72. Quiding H, Olsson GL, Boreus LO, et al. Infants and young children metabolise codeine to morphine. A study after single and repeated rectal administration. *Br J Clin Pharmacol* 1992;33(1):45–49.
73. Magnani B, Evans R. Codeine intoxication in the neonate. *Pediatrics* 1999;104(6):e75.
74. Ciszkowski C, Madadi P, Phillips MS, et al. Codeine, ultrarapid-metabolism genotype, and postoperative death. *N Engl J Med* 2009;361(8):827–828.
75. Madadi P, Shirazi F, Walter FG, et al. Establishing causality of CNS depression in breastfed infants following maternal codeine use. *Paediatr Drugs* 2008;10(6):399–404.
76. Cunliffe M. Codeine phosphate in children: time for re-evaluation? *Br J Anaesth* 2001;86(3):329–331.
77. Poulsen L, Brosen K, Arendt-Nielsen L, et al. Codeine and morphine in extensive and poor metabolizers of sparteine: pharmacokinetics, analgesic effect and side effects. *Eur J Clin Pharmacol* 1996;51(3–4):289–295.
78. Rischitelli DG, Karbowicz SH. Safety and efficacy of controlled-release oxycodone: a systematic literature review. *Pharmacotherapy* 2002;22(7):898–904.
79. Kokki H, Rasanen I, Lasalmi M, et al. Comparison of oxycodone pharmacokinetics after buccal and sublingual administration in children. *Clin Pharmacokinet* 2006;45(7):745–754.
80. Kokki H, Rasanen I, Reinikainen M, et al. Pharmacokinetics of oxycodone after intravenous, buccal, intramuscular and gastric administration in children. *Clin Pharmacokinet* 2004;43(9):613–622.
81. Olkkola KT, Hamunen K, Seppala T, et al. Pharmacokinetics and ventilatory effects of intravenous oxycodone in postoperative children. *Br J Clin Pharmacol* 1994;38(1):71–76.
82. Suresh S, Anand KJS. Opioid tolerance in neonates: a state of the art review. *Paediatr Anaesth* 2001;11:511–521.
83. Tobias JD. Tolerance, withdrawal, and physical dependency after long-term sedation and analgesia of children in the pediatric intensive care unit. *Crit Care Med* 2000;28(6):2122–2132.
84. Berde CB, Beyer JE, Bournaki MC, et al. Comparison of morphine and methadone for prevention of postoperative pain in 3- to 7-year-old children. *J Pediatr* 1991;119(1, pt 1):136–141.
85. Shir Y, Shenkman Z, Shavelson V, et al. Oral methadone for the treatment of severe pain in hospitalized children: a report of five cases. *Clin J Pain* 1998;14(4):350–353.
86. Davies D, DeVlaming D, Haines C. Methadone analgesia for children with advanced cancer. *Pediatr Blood Cancer* 2008;51(3):393–397.
87. Chana SK, Anand KJS. Can we use methadone for analgesia in neonates? *Arch Dis Child Fetal Neonatal Ed* 2001;85(2):F79–F81.
88. Berkowitz BA. The relationship of pharmacokinetics to pharmacological activity: morphine, methadone and naloxone. *Clin Pharmacokinet* 1976;1(3):219–230.
89. Collins JJ, Geake J, Grier HE, et al. Patient-controlled analgesia for mucositis pain in children: a three-period crossover study comparing morphine and hydromorphone. *J Pediatr* 1996;129(5):722–728.
90. Hagen N, Thirlwell MP, Dhaliwal HS, et al. Steady-state pharmacokinetics of hydromorphone and hydromorphone-3-glucuronide in cancer patients after immediate and controlled-release hydromorphone. *J Clin Pharmacol* 1995;35(1):37–44.
91. Volles DF, McGory R. Perspectives in pain management: pharmacokinetic considerations. *Critical Care Clinics* 1999;15(1):55–75.
92. Babul N, Darke AC, Hain R. Hydromorphone and metabolite pharmacokinetics in children. *J Pain Symptom Manage* 1995;10(5):335–337.
93. Quigley C. A systematic review of hydromorphone in acute and chronic pain. *J Pain Symptom Manage* 2003;25(2):169–178.
94. Goodarzi M. Comparison of epidural morphine, hydromorphone and fentanyl for postoperative pain control in children undergoing orthopaedic surgery. *Paediatr Anaesth* 1999;9(5):419–422.
95. Jaffe JH, Martine WR. Opioid analgesics and antagonists. In: Goodman Gilman A, Rall TW, Nies AS, Taylor P, eds. *The pharmacological basis of therapeutics.* New York: Pergamon Press, 1990:485–531.
96. Hamunen K, Maunuksela EL, Seppala T, et al. Pharmacokinetics of i.v. and rectal pethidine in children undergoing ophthalmic surgery. *Br J Anaesth* 1993;71(6):823–826.
97. Pokela ML, Olkkola KT, Koivisto M, et al. Pharmacokinetics and pharmacodynamics of intravenous meperidine in neonates and infants. *Clin Pharmacol Ther* 1992;52(4):342–349.
98. Caldwell J, Wakile LA, Notarianni LJ, et al. Maternal and neonatal disposition of pethidine in childbirth—a study using quantitative gas chromatography-mass spectrometry. *Life Sci* 1978;22(7):589–596.
99. Latta KS, Ginsberg B, Barkin RL. Meperidine: a critical review. *Am J Ther* 2002;9(1):53–68.
100. Vetter TR. Pediatric patient-controlled analgesia with morphine versus meperidine. *J Pain Symptom Manage* 1992;7(4):204–208.
101. Ngan Kee WD. Intrathecal pethidine: pharmacology and clinical applications. *Anaesth Intensive Care* 1998;26(2):137–146.
102. Scott JC, Stanski DR. Decreased fentanyl and alfentanil dose requirements with age. A simultaneous pharmacokinetic and pharmacodynamic evaluation. *J Pharmacol Exp Ther* 1987;240(1):159–166.
103. Wynands JE, Townsend GE, Wong P, et al. Blood pressure response and plasma fentanyl concentrations during high- and very high-dose fentanyl anesthesia for coronary artery surgery. *Anesth Analg* 1983;62(7):661–665.
104. Yaster M, Koehler RC, Traystman RJ. Effects of fentanyl on peripheral and cerebral hemodynamics in neonatal lambs. *Anesthesiology* 1987;66(4):524–530.
105. Hickey PR, Hansen DD, Wessel DL, et al. Blunting of stress responses in the pulmonary circulation of infants by fentanyl. *Anesth Analg* 1985;64(12):1137–1142.
106. Barrington KJ, Byrne PJ. Premedication for neonatal intubation. *Am J Perinatol* 1998;15(4):213–216.
107. Saarenmaa E, Huttunen P, Leppaluoto J, et al. Advantages of fentanyl over morphine in analgesia for ventilated newborn infants after birth: a randomized trial. *J Pediatr* 1999;134(2):144–150.
108. Arnold JH, Truog RD, Scavone JM, et al. Changes in the pharmacodynamic response to fentanyl in neonates during continuous infusion. *J Pediatr* 1991;119(4):639–643.
109. Franck LS, Vilardi J, Durand D, et al. Opioid withdrawal in neonates after continuous infusions of morphine or fentanyl during extracorporeal membrane oxygenation. *Am J Crit Care* 1998;7(5):364–369.
110. Tateishi T, Krivoruk Y, Ueng YF, et al. Identification of human liver cytochrome P-450 3A4 as the enzyme responsible for fentanyl and sufentanil *N*-dealkylation. *Anesth Analg* 1996;82(1):167–172.
111. Labroo RB, Paine MF, Thummel KE, et al. Fentanyl metabolism by human hepatic and intestinal cytochrome P450 3A4: implications for interindividual variability in disposition, efficacy, and drug interactions. *Drug Metab Dispos* 1997;25(9):1072–1080.
112. Jacqz-Aigrain E, Burtin P. Clinical pharmacokinetics of sedatives in neonates. *Clin Pharmacokinet* 1996;31(6):423–443.
113. Anand KJS, Sippell WG, Aynsley-Green A. Randomised trial of fentanyl anaesthesia in preterm babies undergoing surgery: effects on the stress response. *Lancet* 1987;1(8524):62–66.
114. Guinsburg R, Kopelman BI, Anand KJS, et al. Physiological, hormonal, and behavioral responses to a single fentanyl dose in intubated and ventilated preterm neonates. *J Pediatr* 1998;132(6):954–959.
115. Lago P, Benini F, Agosto C, et al. Randomised controlled trial of low dose fentanyl infusion in preterm infants with hyaline membrane disease. *Arch Dis Child Fetal Neonatal Ed* 1998;79(3):F194–F197.
116. Barrier G, Attia J, Mayer MN, et al. Measurement of post-operative pain and narcotic administration in infants using a new clinical scoring system. *Intensive Care Med* 1989;15(Suppl 1):S37–S39.
117. Gauntlett IS, Fisher DM, Hertzka RE, et al. Pharmacokinetics of fentanyl in neonatal humans and lambs: effects of age. *Anesthesiology* 1988;69(5):683–687.
118. Taddio A. Opioid analgesia for infants in the neonatal intensive care unit. *Clin Perinatol* 2002;29(3):493–509.
119. Collins JJ, Dunkel IJ, Gupta SK, et al. Transdermal fentanyl in children with cancer pain: feasibility, tolerability, and pharmacokinetic correlates. *J Pediatr* 1999;134(3):319–323.
120. Grond S, Radbruch L, Lehmann KA. Clinical pharmacokinetics of transdermal opioids: focus on transdermal fentanyl. *Clin Pharmacokinet* 2000;38(1):59–89.

121. Sebel PS, Barrett CW, Kirk CJ, et al. Transdermal absorption of fentanyl and sufentanil in man. *Eur J Clin Pharmacol* 1987;32(5):529–531.
122. Schechter NL, Weisman SJ, Rosenblum M, et al. The use of oral transmucosal fentanyl citrate for painful procedures in children. *Pediatrics* 1995;95(3):335–339.
123. Koehntop DE, Rodman JH, Brundage DM, et al. Pharmacokinetics of fentanyl in neonates. *Anesth Analg* 1986;65(3):227–232.
124. Hughes MA, Glass PS, Jacobs JR. Context-sensitive half-time in multicompartment pharmacokinetic models for intravenous anesthetic drugs. *Anesthesiology* 1992;76(3):334–341.
125. van Lingen R, Simons S, Anderson B, et al. The effects of analgesia in the vulnerable infant during transition from the intrauterine to the extrauterine environment. *Clin Perinatol* 2002;29(3):511–534.
126. Johnson KL, Erickson JP, Holley FO, et al. Fentanyl pharmacokinetics in the paediatric population. *Anesthesiology* 1984;61:A441.
127. Billmire DA, Neale HW, Gregory RO. Use of i.v. fentanyl in the outpatient treatment of pediatric facial trauma. *J Trauma* 1985;25(11):1079–1080.
128. Hertzka RE, Gauntlett IS, Fisher DM, et al. Fentanyl-induced ventilatory depression: effects of age. *Anesthesiology* 1989;70(2):213–218.
129. Touw DJ. Clinical implications of genetic polymorphisms and drug interactions mediated by cytochrome P-450 enzymes. *Drug Metabol Drug Interact* 1997;14(2):55–82.
130. Tanaka E. Clinically important pharmacokinetic drug–drug interactions: role of cytochrome P450 enzymes. *J Clin Pharm Ther* 1998;23(6):403–416.
131. Feierman DE. The effect of paracetamol (acetaminophen) on fentanyl metabolism in vitro. *Acta Anaesthesiol Scand* 2000;44(5):560–563.
132. Saarenmaa E, Huttunen P, Leppaluoto J, et al. Alfentanil as procedural pain relief in newborn infants. *Arch Dis Child Fetal Neonatal Ed* 1996;75(2):F103–F107.
133. Pokela ML. Effect of opioid-induced analgesia on beta-endorphin, cortisol and glucose responses in neonates with cardiorespiratory problems. *Biol Neonate* 1993;64(6):360–367.
134. Pokela ML, Koivisto M. Physiological changes, plasma beta-endorphin and cortisol responses to tracheal intubation in neonates. *Acta Paediatr* 1994;83(2):151–156.
135. Davis PJ, Cook DR. Clinical pharmacokinetics of the newer intravenous anaesthetic agents. *Clin Pharmacokinet* 1986;11(1):18–35.
136. Meuldermans W, Woestenborghs R, Noorduin H, et al. Protein binding of the analgesics alfentanil and sufentanil in maternal and neonatal plasma. *Eur J Clin Pharmacol* 1986;30(2):217–219.
137. Wilson AS, Stiller RL, Davis PJ, et al. Fentanyl and alfentanil plasma protein binding in preterm and term neonates. *Anesth Analg* 1997;84(2):315–318.
138. Meistelman C, Saint-Maurice C, Lepaul M, et al. A comparison of alfentanil pharmacokinetics in children and adults. *Anesthesiology* 1987;66(1):13–16.
139. Marlow N, Weindling AM, Van Peer A, et al. Alfentanil pharmacokinetics in preterm infants. *Arch Dis Child* 1990;65(4, Special No.):349–351.
140. Killian A, Davis PJ, Stiller RL, et al. Influence of gestational age on pharmacokinetics of alfentanil in neonates. *Dev Pharmacol Ther* 1990;15(2):82–85.
141. Davis PJ, Killian A, Stiller RL, et al. Pharmacokinetics of alfentanil in newborn premature infants and older children. *Dev Pharmacol Ther* 1989;13(1):21–27.
142. Pokela ML, Ryhanen PT, Koivisto ME, et al. Alfentanil-induced rigidity in newborn infants. *Anesth Analg* 1992;75(2):252–257.
143. Thompson JP, Rowbotham DJ. Remifentanil—an opioid for the 21st century. *Br J Anaesth* 1996;76(3):341–343.
144. Patel SS, Spencer CM. Remifentanil. *Drugs* 1996;52(3):417–427; discussion 28.
145. Duthie DJ. Remifentanil and tramadol. *Br J Anaesth* 1998;81(1):51–57.
146. Egan TD. Remifentanil pharmacokinetics and pharmacodynamics. A preliminary appraisal. *Clin Pharmacokinet* 1995;29(2):80–94.
147. Dershwitz M, Hoke JF, Rosow CE, et al. Pharmacokinetics and pharmacodynamics of remifentanil in volunteer subjects with severe liver disease. *Anesthesiology* 1996;84(4):812–820.
148. Rigby-Jones AE, Priston MJ, Sneyd JR, et al. Remifentanil-midazolam sedation for paediatric patients receiving mechanical ventilation after cardiac surgery. *Br J Anaesth* 2007;99(2):252–261.
149. Rigby-Jones AE, Priston MJ, Thorne GC, et al. Population pharmacokinetics of remifentanil in critically ill post cardiac neonates, infants and children. *Br J Anaesth* 2005;95:578P–579P.
150. Davis PJ, Wilson AS, Siewers RD, et al. The effects of cardiopulmonary bypass on remifentanil kinetics in children undergoing atrial septal defect repair. *Anesth Analg* 1999;89(4):904–908.
151. Ross AK, Davis PJ, Dear Gd GL, et al. Pharmacokinetics of remifentanil in anesthetized pediatric patients undergoing elective surgery or diagnostic procedures. *Anesth Analg* 2001;93(6):1393–1401, table of contents.
152. Marsh DF, Hodkinson B. Remifentanil in paediatric anaesthetic practice. *Anaesthesia* 2009;64(3):301–308.
153. Davis PJ, Lerman J, Suresh S, et al. A randomized multicenter study of remifentanil compared with alfentanil, isoflurane, or propofol in anesthetized pediatric patients undergoing elective strabismus surgery. *Anesth Analg* 1997;84(5):982–989.
154. Prys-Roberts C, Lerman J, Murat I, et al. Comparison of remifentanil versus regional anaesthesia in children anaesthetised with isoflurane/nitrous oxide. International Remifentanil Paediatric Anaesthesia Study group. *Anaesthesia* 2000;55(9):870–876.
155. Donmez A, Kizilkan A, Berksun H, et al. One center's experience with remifentanil infusions for pediatric cardiac catheterization. *J Cardiothorac Vasc Anesth* 2001;15(6):736–739.
156. German JW, Aneja R, Heard C, et al. Continuous remifentanil for pediatric neurosurgery patients. *Pediatr Neurosurg* 2000;33(5):227–229.
157. Litman RS. Conscious sedation with remifentanil during painful medical procedures. *J Pain Symptom Manage* 2000;19(6):468–471.
158. Chiaretti A, Pietrini D, Piastra M, et al. Safety and efficacy of remifentanil in craniosynostosis repair in children less than 1 year old. *Pediatr Neurosurg* 2000;33(2):83–88.
159. Davis PJ, Galinkin J, McGowan FX, et al. A randomized multicenter study of remifentanil compared with halothane in neonates and infants undergoing pyloromyotomy. I. Emergence and recovery profiles. *Anesth Analg* 2001;93(6):1380–1386, table of contents.
160. Commitee on Infectious Disease AAoP. Aspirin and Reye syndrome. *Pediatrics* 1982;69(6):810–812.
161. Anderson BJ. Paracetamol (acetaminophen): mechanisms of action. *Paediatr Anaesth* 2008;18(10):915–921.
162. Brown RD, Kearns GL, Wilson JT. Integrated pharmacokinetic–pharmacodynamic model for acetaminophen, ibuprofen, and placebo antipyresis in children. *J Pharmacokinet Biopharm* 1998;26(5):559–579.
163. Kelley MT, Walson PD, Edge JH, et al. Pharmacokinetics and pharmacodynamics of ibuprofen isomers and acetaminophen in febrile children. *Clin Pharmacol Ther* 1992;52(2):181–189.
164. Anderson BJ, Woollard GA, Holford NHG. Acetaminophen analgesia in children: placebo effect and pain resolution after tonsillectomy. *Eur J Clin Pharmacol* 2001;57:559–569.
165. Korpela R, Korvenoja P, Meretoja OA. Morphine-sparing effect of acetaminophen in pediatric day-case surgery. *Anesthesiology* 1999;91:442–447.
166. Arendt Nielsen L, Nielsen JC, Bjerring P. Double-blind, placebo controlled comparison of paracetamol and paracetamol plus codeine—a quantitative evaluation by laser induced pain. *Eur J Clin Pharmacol* 1991;40(3):241–247.
167. Nielsen JC, Bjerring P, Arendt Nielsen L, et al. Analgesic efficacy of immediate and sustained release paracetamol and plasma concentration of paracetamol. Double blind, placebo-controlled evaluation using painful laser stimulation. *Eur J Clin Pharmacol* 1992;42(3):261–264.
168. Anderson BJ, Holford NHG, Woollard GA, et al. Paracetamol plasma and cerebrospinal fluid pharmacokinetics in children. *Br J Clin Pharmacol* 1998;46(3):237–243.
169. Anderson BJ, Gibb IA. Paracetamol (acetaminophen) pharmacodynamics; interpreting the plasma concentration. *Arch Dis Child* 2008;93(3):241–247.
170. Murat I, Baujard C, Foussat C, et al. Tolerance and analgesic efficacy of a new i.v. paracetamol solution in children after inguinal hernia repair. *Paediatr Anaesth* 2005;15(8):663–670.
171. Agrawal S, Fitzsimons JJ, Horn V, et al. Intravenous paracetamol for postoperative analgesia in a 4-day-old term neonate. *Paediatr Anaesth* 2007;17(1):70–71.
172. Allegaert K, Murat I, Anderson BJ. Not all intravenous paracetamol formulations are created equal. *Paediatr Anaesth* 2007;17(8):811–812.

173. Bartocci M, Lundeberg S. Intravenous paracetamol: the "Stockholm protocol" for postoperative analgesia of term and preterm neonates. *Paediatr Anaesth* 2007;17(11):1120–1121.
174. Rawlins MD, Henderson BD, Hijab AR. Pharmacokinetics of paracetamol (acetaminophen) after intravenous and oral administration. *Eur J Clin Pharmacol* 1977;11:283–286.
175. Montgomery CJ, McCormack JP, Reichert CC, et al. Plasma concentrations after high-dose (45 mg.kg-1) rectal acetaminophen in children. *Can J Anaesth* 1995;42(11):982–986.
176. Dange SV, Shah KU, Deshpande AS, et al. Bioavailability of acetaminophen after rectal administration. *Indian Pediatr* 1987;24(4): 331–332.
177. Hopkins CS, Underhill S, Booker PD. Pharmacokinetics of paracetamol after cardiac surgery. *Arch Dis Child* 1990;65(9): 971–976.
178. van der Marel CD, van Lingen RA, Pluim MA, et al. Analgesic efficacy of rectal versus oral acetaminophen in children after major craniofacial surgery. *Clin Pharmacol Ther* 2001;70(1):82–90.
179. Anderson BJ, Meakin GH. Scaling for size: some implications for paediatric anaesthesia dosing. *Paediatr Anaesth* 2002;12(3): 205–219.
180. Clements JA, Heading RC, Nimmo WS, et al. Kinetics of acetaminophen absorption and gastric emptying in man. *Clin Pharmacol Ther* 1978;24(4):420–431.
181. Brown RD, Wilson JT, Kearns GL, et al. Single-dose pharmacokinetics of ibuprofen and acetaminophen in febrile children. *J Clin Pharmacol* 1992;32(3):231–241.
182. Anderson BJ, Woollard GA, Holford NH. A model for size and age changes in the pharmacokinetics of paracetamol in neonates, infants and children. *Br J Clin Pharmacol* 2000;50(2):125–134.
183. Gupta M, Brans Y. Gastric retention in neonates. *Pediatrics* 1978;62:26–29.
184. Grand RJ, Watkins JB, Torti FM. Development of the human intestinal tract: a review. *Gastroenterology* 1976;70:790–810.
185. Forrest JA, Clements JA, Prescott LF. Clinical pharmacokinetics of paracetamol. *Clin Pharmacokinet* 1982;7(2):93–107.
186. Anderson BJ, van Lingen RA, Hansen TG, et al. Acetaminophen developmental pharmacokinetics in premature neonates and infants: a pooled population analysis. *Anesthesiology* 2002;96(6): 1336–1345.
187. Seth N, Llewellyn NE, Howard RF. Parental opinions regarding the route of administration of analgesic medication in children. *Paediatr Anaesth* 2000;10(5):537–544.
188. van Hoogdalem E, de Boer AG, Breimer DD. Pharmacokinetics of rectal drug administration, Part I. General considerations and clinical applications of centrally acting drugs. *Clin Pharmacokinet* 1991;21(1):11–26.
189. van Hoogdalem EJ, de Boer AG, Breimer DD. Pharmacokinetics of rectal drug administration, Part II. Clinical applications of peripherally acting drugs, and conclusions. *Clin Pharmacokinet* 1991;21(2):110–128.
190. van Lingen RA, Deinum JT, Quak JM, et al. Pharmacokinetics and metabolism of rectally administered paracetamol in preterm neonates. *Arch Dis Child Fetal Neonatal Ed* 1999;80(1):F59–F63.
191. Birmingham PK, Tobin MJ, Henthorn TK, et al. Twenty-four-hour pharmacokinetics of rectal acetaminophen in children: an old drug with new recommendations. *Anesthesiology* 1997;87(2): 244–252.
192. Gaudreault P, Guay J, Nicol O, et al. Pharmacokinetics and clinical efficacy of intrarectal solution of acetaminophen. *Can J Anaesth* 1988;35:149–152.
193. Levy G, Garrettson LK, Soda DM. Evidence of placenta transfer of acetaminophen. *Pediatrics* 1975;55:895.
194. Miller RP, Roberts RJ, Fischer LJ. Acetaminophen elimination kinetics in neonates, children, and adults. *Clin Pharmacol Ther* 1976;19(3):284–294.
195. Miners JO, Osborne NJ, Tonkin AL, et al. Perturbation of paracetamol urinary metabolic ratios by urine flow rate. *Br J Clin Pharmacol* 1992;34(4):359–362.
196. Anderson BJ, Pons G, Autret-Leca E, et al. Pediatric intravenous paracetamol (propacetamol) pharmacokinetics: a population analysis. *Paediatr Anaesth* 2005;15(4):282–292.
197. Prescott LF. Paracetamol (acetaminophen). *A critical bibliographic review*, 1st ed. London: Taylor and Francis Publishers, 1996.
198. van Bree JB, de Boer AG, Danhof M, et al. Characterization of an "in vitro" blood-brain barrier: effects of molecular size and lipophilicity on cerebrovascular endothelial transport rates of drugs. *J Pharmacol Exp Ther* 1988;247(3):1233–1239.
199. Alam SN, Roberts RJ, Fischer LJ. Age-related differences in salicylamide and acetaminophen conjugation in man. *J Pediatr* 1977; 90(1):130–135.
200. Wilson JT, Brown RD, Bocchini JA Jr, et al. Efficacy, disposition and pharmacodynamics of aspirin, acetaminophen and choline salicylate in young febrile children. *Ther Drug Monit* 1982;4(2): 147–180.
201. Reilly CS, Nimmo WS. Drug absorption after general anaesthesia for minor surgery. *Anaesthesia* 1984;39(9):859–861.
202. al Obaidy SS, Li Wan Po A, McKiernan PJ, et al. Assay of paracetamol and its metabolites in urine, plasma and saliva of children with chronic liver disease. *J Pharm Biomed Anal* 1995;13(8): 1033–1039.
203. al Obaidy SS, McKiernan PJ, Li Wan Po A, et al. Metabolism of paracetamol in children with chronic liver disease. *Eur J Clin Pharmacol* 1996;50(1–2):69–76.
204. Miner DJ, Kissinger PT. Evidence for the involvement of *N*-acetyl-*p*-quinoneimine in acetaminophen poisoning. *Annu Rev Pharmacol Toxicol* 1983;12:251.
205. Slattery JT, Nelson SD, Thummel KE. The complex interaction between ethanol and acetaminophen. *Clin Pharmacol Ther* 1996; 60(3):241–246.
206. Nahata MC, Powell DA, Durrell DE, et al. Acetaminophen accumulation in pediatric patients after repeated therapeutic doses. *Eur J Clin Pharmacol* 1984;27(1):57–59.
207. Slattery JT, Wilson JM, Kalhorn TF, et al. Dose-dependent pharmacokinetics of acetaminophen: evidence of glutathione depletion in humans. *Clin Pharmacol Ther* 1987;41:413–418.
208. Penna A, Buchanan N. Paracetamol poisoning in children and hepatotoxicity. *Br J Clin Pharmacol* 1991;32(2):143–149.
209. Temple AR. Pediatric dosing of acetaminophen. *Pediatr Pharmacol (New York)* 1983;3(3–4):321–327.
210. Shann F. Paracetamol: when, why and how much. *J Paediatr Child Health* 1993;29(2):84–85.
211. Kearns GL, Leeder JS, Wasserman GS. Acetaminophen overdose with therapeutic intent. *J Pediatr* 1998;132(1):5–8.
212. Alonso EM, Sokol RJ, Hart J, et al. Fulminant hepatitis associated with centrilobular necrosis in young children. *J Pediatr* 1995; 127:888–894.
213. Heubi JE, Barbacci MB, Zimmerman HJ. Therapeutic misadventures with acetaminophen: hepatoxicity after multiple doses in children. *J Pediatr* 1998;132(1):22–27.
214. Heubi JE, Bien JP. Acetaminophen use in children: more is not better. *J Pediatr* 1997;130:175–177.
215. Rivera Penera T, Gugig R, Davis J, et al. Outcome of acetaminophen overdose in pediatric patients and factors contributing to hepatotoxicity. *J Pediatr* 1997;130(2):300–304.
216. Hynson JL, South M. Childhood hepatotoxicity with paracetamol doses less than 150 mg/kg per day. *Med J Aust* 1999;171:497.
217. Miles FK, Kamath R, Dorney SFA, et al. Accidental paracetamol overdosing and fulminant hepatic failure in children. *Med J Aust* 1999;171:472–475.
218. Morton NS, Arana A. Paracetamol-induced fulminant hepatic failure in a child after 5 days of therapeutic doses. *Paediatr Anaesth* 1999;9:463–465.
219. Kozer E, Barr J, Bulkowstein M, et al. A prospective study of multiple supratherapeutic acetaminophen doses in febrile children. *Vet Hum Toxicol* 2002;44(2):106–109.
220. Palmer GM, Atkins M, Anderson BJ, et al. I.V. acetaminophen pharmacokinetics in neonates after multiple doses. *Br J Anaesth* 2008;101(4):523–530.
221. Allegaert K, Rayyan M, De Rijdt T, et al. Hepatic tolerance of repeated intravenous paracetamol administration in neonates. *Paediatr Anaesth* 2008;18(5):388–392.
222. Anderson BJ, Allegaert K. Intravenous neonatal paracetamol dosing: the magic of 10 days. *Paediatr Anaesth* 2009;19(4):289–295.
223. Rumack BH, Matthew H. Acetaminophen poisoning and toxicity. *Pediatrics* 1975;55:871–876.
224. Prescott LF, Wright N, Roscoe P, et al. Plasma paracetamol half-life and hepatic necrosis in patients with paracetamol overdose. *Lancet* 1971;1:519–522.
225. Anderson BJ, Holford NHG, Armishaw JC, et al. Predicting concentrations in children presenting with acetaminophen overdose. *J Pediatrics* 1999;135(3):290–295.

226. Mohler CR, Nordt SP, Williams SR, et al. Prospective evaluation of mild to moderate pediatric acetaminophen exposures. *Ann Emerg Med* 2000;35:239–244.
227. Mancini RE, Sonawane BR, Yaffe SJ. Developmental susceptibility to acetaminophen toxicity. *Res Commun Chem Pathol Pharmacol* 1980;27(3):603–606.
228. Rumack BH. Acetaminophen overdose in children and adolescents. *Pediatr Clin North Am* 1986;33(3):691–701.
229. Lauterburg BH, Vaishnav Y, Stillwell WG, et al. The effects of age and glutathione depletion on hepatic glutathione turnover in vivo determined by acetaminophen probe analysis. *J Pharmacol Exp Ther* 1980;213(1):54–58.
230. Roberts I, Robinson MJ, Mughal MZ, et al. Paracetamol metabolites in the neonate following maternal overdose. *Br J Clin Pharmacol* 1984;18(2):201–206.
231. Peterson RG, Rumack BH. Pharmacokinetics of acetaminophen in children. *Pediatrics* 1978;62:877.
232. Canalese J, Gimson AE, Davis M, et al. Factors contributing to mortality in paracetamol-induced hepatic failure. *Br Med J Clin Res Ed* 1981;282(6259):199–201.
233. Tighe TV, Walter FG. Delayed toxic acetaminophen level after initial four hour nontoxic level. *J Toxicol Clin Toxicol* 1994;32(4):431–434.
234. Mitchell JA, Akarasereenont P, Thiemermann C, et al. Selectivity of nonsteroidal antiinflammatory drugs as inhibitors of constitutive and inducible cyclooxygenase. *Proc Natl Acad Sci U S A* 1993;90(24):11693–11697.
235. Oermann CM, Sockrider MM, Konstan MW. The use of anti-inflammatory medications in cystic fibrosis: trends and physician attitudes. *Chest* 1999;115(4):1053–1058.
236. Konstan MW, Byard PJ, Hoppel CL, et al. Effect of high-dose ibuprofen in patients with cystic fibrosis. *N Engl J Med* 1995; 332(13):848–854.
237. Konstan MW, Hoppel CL, Chai BL, et al. Ibuprofen in children with cystic fibrosis: pharmacokinetics and adverse effects. *J Pediatr* 1991;118(6):956–964.
238. Scott CS, Retsch-Bogart GZ, Kustra RP, et al. The pharmacokinetics of ibuprofen suspension, chewable tablets, and tablets in children with cystic fibrosis. *J Pediatr* 1999;134(1):58–63.
239. Van Overmeire B, Smets K, Lecoutere D, et al. A comparison of ibuprofen and indomethacin for closure of patent ductus arteriosus. *N Engl J Med* 2000;343(10):674–681.
240. Pickering AE, Bridge HS, Nolan J, et al. Double-blind, placebo-controlled analgesic study of ibuprofen or rofecoxib in combination with paracetamol for tonsillectomy in children. *Br J Anaesth* 2002;88(1):72–77.
241. Viitanen H, Tuominen N, Vaaraniemi H, et al. Analgesic efficacy of rectal acetaminophen and ibuprofen alone or in combination for paediatric day-case adenoidectomy. *Br J Anaesth* 2003; 91(3):363–367.
242. Gazal G, Mackie IC. A comparison of paracetamol, ibuprofen or their combination for pain relief following extractions in children under general anaesthesia: a randomized controlled trial. *Int J Paediatr Dent* 2007;17(3):169–177.
243. Splinter WM, Reid CW, Roberts DJ, et al. Reducing pain after inguinal hernia repair in children: caudal anesthesia versus ketorolac tromethamine. *Anesthesiology* 1997;87(3):542–546.
244. Ryhanen P, Adamski J, Puhakka K, et al. Postoperative pain relief in children. A comparison between caudal bupivacaine and intramuscular diclofenac sodium. *Anaesthesia* 1994;49(1):57–61.
245. Moores MA, Wandless JG, Fell D. Paediatric postoperative analgesia. A comparison of rectal diclofenac with caudal bupivacaine after inguinal herniotomy. *Anaesthesia* 1990;45(2):156–158.
246. Gunter JB, Varughese AM, Harrington JF, et al. Recovery and complications after tonsillectomy in children: a comparison of ketorolac and morphine. *Anesth Analg* 1995;81(6):1136–1141.
247. Munro HM, Riegger LQ, Reynolds PI, et al. Comparison of the analgesic and emetic properties of ketorolac and morphine for paediatric outpatient strabismus surgery. *Br J Anaesth* 1994;72(6): 624–628.
248. Morton NS, O'Brien K. Analgesic efficacy of paracetamol and diclofenac in children receiving PCA morphine. *Br J Anaesth* 1999;82(5):715–717.
249. Vetter TR, Heiner EJ. Intravenous ketorolac as an adjuvant to pediatric patient-controlled analgesia with morphine. *J Clin Anesth* 1994;6(2):110–113.
250. Oztekin S, Hepaguslar H, Kar AA, et al. Preemptive diclofenac reduces morphine use after remifentanil-based anaesthesia for tonsillectomy. *Paediatr Anaesth* 2002;12(8):694–699.
251. Watcha MF, Ramirez Ruiz M, White PF, et al. Perioperative effects of oral ketorolac and acetaminophen in children undergoing bilateral myringotomy. *Can J Anaesth* 1992;39(7):649–654.
252. Baer GA, Rorarius MG, Kolehmainen S, et al. The effect of paracetamol or diclofenac administered before operation on postoperative pain and behaviour after adenoidectomy in small children. *Anaesthesia* 1992;47(12):1078–1080.
253. Bennie RE, Boehringer LA, McMahon S, et al. Postoperative analgesia with preoperative oral ibuprofen or acetaminophen in children undergoing myringotomy. *Paediatr Anaesth* 1997;7(5): 399–403.
254. Bertin L, Pons G, d'Athis P, et al. A randomized, double-blind, multicentre controlled trial of ibuprofen versus acetaminophen and placebo for symptoms of acute otitis media in children. *Fundam Clin Pharmacol* 1996;10(4):387–392.
255. Figueras Nadal C, Garcia de Miguel MJ, Gomez Campdera A, et al. Effectiveness and tolerability of ibuprofen-arginine versus paracetamol in children with fever of likely infectious origin. *Acta Paediatr* 2002;91(4):383–390.
256. Purssell E. Treating fever in children: paracetamol or ibuprofen? *Br J Community Nurs* 2002;7(6):316–320.
257. Tawalbeh MI, Nawasreh OO, Husban AM. Comparative study of diclofenac sodium and paracetamol for treatment of pain after adenotonsillectomy in children. *Saudi Med J* 2001;22(2): 121–123.
258. Van Esch A, Van Steensel Moll HA, Steyerberg EW, et al. Antipyretic efficacy of ibuprofen and acetaminophen in children with febrile seizures. *Arch Pediatr Adolesc Med* 1995;149(6): 632–637.
259. Walson PD, Galletta G, Braden NJ, et al. Ibuprofen, acetaminophen, and placebo treatment of febrile children. *Clin Pharmacol Ther* 1989;46(1):9–17.
260. Goyal PK, Chandra J, Unnikrishnan G, et al. Double blind randomized comparative evaluation of nimesulide and paracetamol as antipyretics. *Indian Pediatr* 1998;35(6):519–522.
261. Johnson GH, Van Wagoner JD, Brown J, et al. Bromfenac sodium, acetaminophen/oxycodone, ibuprofen, and placebo for relief of postoperative pain. *Clin Ther* 1997;19(3):507–519.
262. Romsing J, Ostergaard D, Senderovitz T, et al. Pharmacokinetics of oral diclofenac and acetaminophen in children after surgery. *Paediatr Anaesth* 2001;11(2):205–213.
263. Davies NM, Skjodt NM. Choosing the right nonsteroidal anti-inflammatory drug for the right patient: a pharmacokinetic approach. *Clin Pharmacokinet* 2000;38(5):377–392.
264. Maunuksela E-L, Olkkola KT. Nonsteroidal anti-inflammatory drugs in pediatric pain management. In: Schechter NL, Berde CB, Yaster M, eds. *Pain in infants, children, and adolescents*, 2nd ed. Philadelphia, PA: Lippincott Williams & Wilkins, 2003:171–180.
265. Collins SL, Moore RA, McQuay HJ, et al. Single dose oral ibuprofen and diclofenac for postoperative pain. *Cochrane Database Syst Rev* 2009;8(3):CD001548.
266. Needs CJ, Brooks PM. Clinical pharmacokinetics of the salicylates. *Clin Pharmacokinet* 1985;10(2):164–177.
267. Day RO, Furst DE, Dromgoole SH, et al. Relationship of serum naproxen concentration to efficacy in rheumatoid arthritis. *Clin Pharmacol Ther* 1982;31(6):733–740.
268. Day RO, Francis H, Vial J, et al. Naproxen concentrations in plasma and synovial fluid and effects on prostanoid concentrations. *J Rheumatol* 1995;22(12):2295–2303.
269. Bertin P, Lapicque F, Payan E, et al. Sodium naproxen: concentration and effect on inflammatory response mediators in human rheumatoid synovial fluid. *Eur J Clin Pharmacol* 1994;46(1):3–7.
270. Boni JP, Korth-Bradley JM, Martin P, et al. Pharmacokinetics of etodolac in patients with stable juvenile rheumatoid arthritis. *Clin Ther* 1999;21(10):1715–1724.
271. Mandema JW, Stanski DR. Population pharmacodynamic model for ketorolac analgesia. *Clin Pharmacol Ther* 1996;60(6):619–635.
272. McQuay HJ, Moore RA. Postoperative analgesia and vomiting, with special reference to day-case surgery: a systematic review. *Health Technol Assess* 1998;2(12):1–236.
273. Standing JF, Howard RF, Johnson A, et al. Population pharmacokinetics of oral diclofenac for acute pain in children. *Br J Clin Pharmacol* 2008;66(6):846–853.

274. Troconiz IF, Armenteros S, Planelles MV, et al. Pharmacokinetic–pharmacodynamic modelling of the antipyretic effect of two oral formulations of ibuprofen. *Clin Pharmacokinet* 2000;38(6):505–518.
275. Kauffman RE, Nelson MV. Effect of age on ibuprofen pharmacokinetics and antipyretic response. *J Pediatr* 1992;121(6):969–973.
276. Van Overmeire B, Touw D, Schepens PJ, et al. Ibuprofen pharmacokinetics in preterm infants with patent ductus arteriosus. *Clin Pharmacol Ther* 2001;70(4):336–343.
277. Shaffer CL, Gal P, Ransom JL, et al. Effect of age and birth weight on indomethacin pharmacodynamics in neonates treated for patent ductus arteriosus. *Crit Care Med* 2002;30(2):343–348.
278. Beringer P, Aminimanizani A, Synold T, et al. Development of population pharmacokinetic models and optimal sampling times for ibuprofen tablet and suspension formulations in children with cystic fibrosis. *Ther Drug Monit* 2002;24(2):315–321.
279. Litalien C, Jacqz-Aigrain E. Risks and benefits of nonsteroidal anti-inflammatory drugs in children: a comparison with paracetamol. *Paediatr Drugs* 2001;3(11):817–858.
280. Silva LC, Simoes IG, Lerner FE, et al. Comparative bioavailability of two different diclofenac formulations in healthy volunteers. *Arzneimittelforschung* 1999;49(11):920–924.
281. Lötsch J, Kettenmann B, Renner B, et al. Population pharmacokinetics of fast release oral diclofenac in healthy volunteers: relation to pharmacodynamics in an experimental pain model. *Pharm Res* 2000;17(1):77–84.
282. Scaroni C, Mazzoni PL, D'Amico E, et al. Pharmacokinetics of oral and rectal flurbiprofen in children. *Eur J Clin Pharmacol* 1984;27(3):367–369.
283. Olkkola KT, Maunuksela EL. The pharmacokinetics of postoperative intravenous ketorolac tromethamine in children. *Br J Clin Pharmacol* 1991;31(2):182–184.
284. Forrest JB, Heitlinger EL, Revell S. Ketorolac for postoperative pain management in children. *Drug Saf* 1997;16(5):309–329.
285. Aranda JV, Varvarigou A, Beharry K, et al. Pharmacokinetics and protein binding of intravenous ibuprofen in the premature newborn infant. *Acta Paediatr* 1997;86(3):289–293.
286. Boni J, Korth-Bradley J, McGoldrick K, et al. Pharmacokinetic and pharmacodynamic action of etodolac in patients after oral surgery. *J Clin Pharmacol* 1999;39(7):729–737.
287. Rolf C, Engstrom B, Beauchard C, et al. Intra-articular absorption and distribution of ketoprofen after topical plaster application and oral intake in 100 patients undergoing knee arthroscopy. *Rheumatology (Oxford)* 1999;38(6):564–567.
288. Davies NM, Anderson KE. Clinical pharmacokinetics of diclofenac. Therapeutic insights and pitfalls. *Clin Pharmacokinet* 1997;33(3):184–213.
289. Gal P, Ransom JL, Schall S, et al. Indomethacin for patent ductus arteriosus closure. Application of serum concentrations and pharmacodynamics to improve response. *J Perinatol* 1990;10(1):20–26.
290. Hamman MA, Thompson GA, Hall SD. Regioselective and stereoselective metabolism of ibuprofen by human cytochrome P450 2C. *Biochem Pharmacol* 1997;54(1):33–41.
291. Brocks DR, Jamali F. Clinical pharmacokinetics of ketorolac tromethamine. *Clin Pharmacokinet* 1992;23(6):415–427.
292. Wiest DB, Pinson JB, Gal PS, et al. Population pharmacokinetics of intravenous indomethacin in neonates with symptomatic patent ductus arteriosus. *Clin Pharmacol Ther* 1991;49(5):550–557.
293. Smyth JM, Collier PS, Darwish M, et al. Intravenous indometacin in preterm infants with symptomatic patent ductus arteriosus. A population pharmacokinetic study. *Br J Clin Pharmacol* 2004;58(3):249–258.
294. Korpela R, Olkkola KT. Pharmacokinetics of intravenous diclofenac sodium in children. *Eur J Clin Pharmacol* 1990;38(3):293–295.
295. Gonzalez-Martin G, Maggio L, Gonzalez-Sotomayor J, et al. Pharmacokinetics of ketorolac in children after abdominal surgery. *Int J Clin Pharmacol Ther* 1997;35(4):160–163.
296. Kauffman RE, Lieh-Lai MW, Uy HG, et al. Enantiomer-selective pharmacokinetics and metabolism of ketorolac in children. *Clin Pharmacol Ther* 1999;65(4):382–388.
297. Ugazio AG, Guarnaccia S, Berardi M, et al. Clinical and pharmacokinetic study of nimesulide in children. *Drugs* 1993;46(Suppl 1):215–218.
298. Bertin L, Rey E, Pons G, et al. Pharmacokinetics of tiaprofenic acid in children after a single oral dose. *Eur J Clin Pharmacol* 1991;41(3):251–253.
299. Stempak D, Gammon J, Klein J, et al. Single-dose and steady-state pharmacokinetics of celecoxib in children. *Clin Pharmacol Ther* 2002;72(5):490–497.
300. Gregoire N, Gualano V, Geneteau A, et al. Population pharmacokinetics of ibuprofen enantiomers in very premature neonates. *J Clin Pharmacol* 2004;44(10):1114–1124.
301. Jackson ID, Heidemann BH, Wilson J, et al. Double-blind, randomized, placebo-controlled trial comparing rofecoxib with dexketoprofen trometamol in surgical dentistry. *Br J Anaesth* 2004;92(5):675–680.
302. Gaitan G, Herrero JF. Subanalgesic doses of dexketoprofen and HCT-2037 (nitrodexketoprofen) enhance fentanyl antinociception in monoarthritic rats. *Pharmacol Biochem Behav* 2005;80(2):327–332.
303. Sheeran PW, Rose JB, Fazi LM, et al. Rofecoxib administration to paediatric patients undergoing adenotonsillectomy. *Paediatr Anaesth* 2004;14(7):579–583.
304. Joshi W, Connelly NR, Reuben SS, et al. An evaluation of the safety and efficacy of administering rofecoxib for postoperative pain management. *Anesth Analg* 2003;97(1):35–38.
305. Krotz F, Schiele TM, Klauss V, et al. Selective COX-2 inhibitors and risk of myocardial infarction. *J Vasc Res* 2005;42(4):312–324.
306. Levin RI. Theriac found? Nitric oxide-aspirin and the search for the universal cure. *J Am Coll Cardiol* 2004;44(3):642–643.
307. Aggeler PM, O'Reilly RA, Leong L, et al. Potentiation of anticoagulant effect of warfarin by phenylbutazone. *N Engl J Med* 1967;276(9):496–501.
308. Kam PC, See AU. Cyclo-oxygenase isoenzymes: physiological and pharmacological role. *Anaesthesia* 2000;55(5):442–449.
309. Simon AM, Manigrasso MB, O'Connor JP. Cyclo-oxygenase 2 function is essential for bone fracture healing. *J Bone Miner Res* 2002;17(6):963–976.
310. Lipsky PE, Brooks P, Crofford LJ, et al. Unresolved issues in the role of cyclooxygenase-2 in normal physiologic processes and disease. *Arch Intern Med* 2000;160(7):913–920.
311. McCrory CR, Lindahl SG. Cyclooxygenase inhibition for postoperative analgesia. *Anesth Analg* 2002;95(1):169–176.
312. Brater DC, Harris C, Redfern JS, et al. Renal effects of COX-2-selective inhibitors. *Am J Nephrol* 2001;21(1):1–15.
313. Allegaert K, Cossey V, Langhendries JP, et al. Effects of co-administration of ibuprofen-lysine on the pharmacokinetics of amikacin in preterm infants during the first days of life. *Biol Neonate* 2004;86(3):207–211.
314. Allegaert K, Anderson BJ, Cossey V, et al. Limited predictability of amikacin clearance in extreme premature neonates at birth. *Br J Clin Pharmacol* 2005;61:39–48.
315. Lesko SM, Mitchell AA. An assessment of the safety of pediatric ibuprofen. A practitioner-based randomized clinical trial. *JAMA* 1995;273(12):929–933.
316. Lesko SM, Mitchell AA. Renal function after short-term ibuprofen use in infants and children. *Pediatrics* 1997;100(6):954–957.
317. Lesko SM, Mitchell AA. The safety of acetaminophen and ibuprofen among children younger than two years old. *Pediatrics* 1999;104(4):e39.
318. Houck CS, Wilder RT, McDermott JS, et al. Safety of intravenous ketorolac therapy in children and cost savings with a unit dosing system. *J Pediatr* 1996;129(2):292–296.
319. Flato B, Vinje O, Forre O. Toxicity of antirheumatic and anti-inflammatory drugs in children. *Clin Rheumatol* 1998;17(6):505–510.
320. Szer IS, Goldenstein-Schainberg C, Kurtin PS. Paucity of renal complications associated with nonsteroidal antiinflammatory drugs in children with chronic arthritis. *J Pediatr* 1991;119(5):815–817.
321. van Biljon G. Reversible renal failure associated with ibuprofen in a child. A case report. *S Afr Med J* 1989;76(1):34–35.
322. Moghal NE, Hulton SA, Milford DV. Care in the use of ibuprofen as an antipyretic in children. *Clin Nephrol* 1998;49(5):293–295.
323. Primack WA, Rahman SM, Pullman J. Acute renal failure associated with amoxicillin and ibuprofen in an 11-year-old boy. *Pediatr Nephrol* 1997;11(1):125–126.
324. Buck ML, Norwood VF. Ketorolac-induced acute renal failure in a previously healthy adolescent. *Pediatrics* 1996;98(2, pt 1):294–296.

325. Ray PE, Rigolizzo D, Wara DR, et al. Naproxen nephrotoxicity in a 2-year-old child. *Am J Dis Child* 1988;142(5):524–525.
326. Sheiner LB. A new approach to the analysis of analgesic drug trials, illustrated with bromfenac data. *Clin Pharmacol Ther* 1994; 56(3):309–322.
327. Kovesi TA, Swartz R, MacDonald N. Transient renal failure due to simultaneous ibuprofen and aminoglycoside therapy in children with cystic fibrosis. *N Engl J Med* 1998;338(1):65–66.
328. Feldman M, McMahon AT. Do cyclooxygenase-2 inhibitors provide benefits similar to those of traditional nonsteroidal anti-inflammatory drugs, with less gastrointestinal toxicity? *Ann Intern Med* 2000;132(2):134–143.
329. Silverstein FE, Faich G, Goldstein JL, et al. Gastrointestinal toxicity with celecoxib vs nonsteroidal anti-inflammatory drugs for osteoarthritis and rheumatoid arthritis: the CLASS study: a randomized controlled trial. Celecoxib Long-term Arthritis Safety Study. *JAMA* 2000;284(10):1247–1255.
330. Bombardier C, Laine L, Reicin A, et al. Comparison of upper gastrointestinal toxicity of rofecoxib and naproxen in patients with rheumatoid arthritis. VIGOR Study Group. *N Engl J Med* 2000;343(21):1520–1528.
331. Keenan GF, Giannini EH, Athreya BH. Clinically significant gastropathy associated with nonsteroidal antiinflammatory drug use in children with juvenile rheumatoid arthritis. *J Rheumatol* 1995; 22(6):1149–1151.
332. Dowd JE, Cimaz R, Fink CW. Nonsteroidal antiinflammatory drug-induced gastroduodenal injury in children. *Arthritis Rheum* 1995; 38(9):1225–1231.
333. Mulberg AE, Linz C, Bern E, et al. Identification of nonsteroidal antiinflammatory drug-induced gastroduodenal injury in children with juvenile rheumatoid arthritis. *J Pediatr* 1993;122(4):647–649.
334. Souter AJ, Fredman B, White PF. Controversies in the perioperative use of nonsteroidal antiinflammatory drugs. *Anesth Analg* 1994;79(6):1178–1190.
335. Rusy LM, Houck CS, Sullivan LJ, et al. A double-blind evaluation of ketorolac tromethamine versus acetaminophen in pediatric tonsillectomy: analgesia and bleeding. *Anesth Analg* 1995;80(2):226–229.
336. Gupta A, Daggett C, Drant S, et al. Prospective randomized trial of ketorolac after congenital heart surgery. *J Cardiothorac Vasc Anesth* 2004;18(4):454–457.
337. Ment LR, Vohr BR, Makuch RW, et al. Prevention of intraventricular hemorrhage by indomethacin in male preterm infants. *J Pediatr* 2004;145(6):832–834.
338. Cardwell M, Siviter G, Smith A. Non-steroidal anti-inflammatory drugs and perioperative bleeding in paediatric tonsillectomy. *Cochrane Database Syst Rev* 2005;(2):CD003591.
339. Strom BL, Berlin JA, Kinman JL, et al. Parenteral ketorolac and risk of gastrointestinal and operative site bleeding. A postmarketing surveillance study. *JAMA* 1996;275(5):376–382.
340. Lesko SM. The safety of ibuprofen suspension in children. *Int J Clin Pract Suppl* 2003;(135):50–53.
341. Palmer GM. A teenager with severe asthma exacerbation following ibuprofen. *Anaesth Intensive Care* 2005;33(2):261–265.
342. Anderson BJ, McKee AD, Holford NH. Size, myths and the clinical pharmacokinetics of analgesia in paediatric patients. *Clin Pharmacokinet* 1997;33(5):313–327.
343. Pariente-Khayat A, Dubois MC, Vauzelle-Kervroedan F, et al. Pharmacokinetics of tiaprofenic acid in infants after a single oral dose. *Int J Clin Pharmacol Ther* 1996;34:342–344.
344. Niopas I, Georgarakis M, Sidi-Frangandrea V, et al. Pharmacokinetics of tolfenamic acid in pediatric patients after single oral dose. *Eur J Drug Metab Pharmacokinet* 1995;20:293–296.

Santhanam Suresh
Charles J. Coté

CHAPTER

47

Local Anesthetic Solutions for Regional Anesthesia in Infants, Children, and Adolescents

The use of local anesthetics has increased in the pediatric population because of the rising interest in the use of regional anesthetic techniques by a variety of specialists as a means for providing analgesia (1). To improve both safety and effectiveness the practitioner should have a clear understanding of the pharmacology of local anesthetic solutions. In this chapter, we will review basic mechanisms or local anesthetics, methods to reduce potential toxicity, and new directions for resuscitation should a local anesthetic overdose or unintended intravenous injection occur.

MECHANISM OF ACTION OF LOCAL ANESTHETICS

Sodium channels are necessary for the propagation and generation of nerve impulses. Local anesthetics reversibly bind to Na^+ channels of the nerve thereby inhibiting the propagation of nerve impulses. Although individual sensory axons and other parts of the nervous system have different types of Na^+ channels, the general action of the local anesthetics on these channels is the same (2). The drugs bind to their target sites on the channels in bare nerve membranes rapidly, in about 1 to 10 seconds at the 50% inhibitory drug concentration (IC_{50}) and dissociate in about the same time. The IC_{50} concentrations are much lower than the clinically injected concentrations, for example, IC_{50} for channel inhibition by lidocaine is 0.2 mmol per L, but a successful block requires an injection of a 1% solution, almost 40 mmol per L. This is due to the fact that less than one molecule in 20 of the injected dose of 1% lidocaine is found within the nerve during blockade (3). The major reasons for this inefficient delivery system are (a) the protonated drug has a pH of 5 to 6 and thus poorly penetrates the perineural area and (b) the extraneural and intraneural vasculature rapidly removes the local anesthetic from the area around the nerve (4). Sodium channels can be inhibited in two ways: (a) by a conformational mechanism (where the activation gating is suppressed; mainly neutral anesthetics) or (b) by an occlusion mechanism (where the pore is blocked; mainly charged local anesthetics). Most tertiary amine local anesthetics are in dynamic equilibrium between charged and neutral forms; hence, they inhibit Na^+ channels through both mechanisms. Two major methods to increase the delivery of local anesthetics to their effect site are (a) to neutralize (alkalinize) the injectate thereby increasing the fraction of uncharged drug molecules to promote perineural penetration and (b) to add a vasoconstrictor such as epinephrine to decrease the rate of vascular removal.

Alkalinization of local anesthetics is often advocated as a means for improving drug delivery to the nerve tissue; however, if the pH exceeds 7, the solution becomes less soluble hence leading to precipitation (5). Therefore, it is crucial not to overneutralize the local anesthetic solution; adding bicarbonate should occur just prior to injection so as to avoid precipitation. This may particularly be a problem with bupivacaine and ropivacaine where a small amount of bicarbonate (0.1 mEq Na HCO_3 per 10 mL) may cause precipitation within a matter of minutes (5,6). Conversely, this explains the diminished effectiveness when injecting local anesthetic into areas of infection where tissue acidity causes the local anesthetics to be in a more protonized state and therefore less able to cross biologic membranes. Vasoconstrictors are effective in prolonging a block only for local anesthetics that do not have intrinsic vasoconstrictive properties (e.g., bupivacaine but not ropivacaine) and those that are hydrolyzed by local esterases (e.g., chloroprocaine).

Another very important factor is that hydrophobic local anesthetics more rapidly cross the fat layer of biologic membranes. Thus, the more fat-soluble agents cross into neural tissue more readily (e.g., bupivacaine) than those that are more hydrophilic (e.g., procaine). Another method to speed the onset, prolong the duration of local anesthetic action, and increase the intensity of the block is

TABLE 47.1 Relative Potency of Local Anesthetics

	Short Duration	*Medium Duration*		*Long Duration*		
	2-Chloroprocaine	*Lidocaine*	*Mepivacaine*	*Bupivacaine*	*Ropivacaine*	*Tetracaine*
Peripheral nerve	NA	1.0	2.6	3.6	3.6	NA
Spinal	NA	1.0	1.0	9.6	NA	6.3
Epidural	2.0	1.0	1.0	4.0	4.0	NA

NA, Data not available.
From Hassan HG, Renck H, Akerman B, et al. On the relative potency of amino-amide local anaesthetics in vivo. *Acta Anaesthesiol Scand* 1994;38:505–509.

to increase the concentration of the drug (e.g., 2% vs. 0.5% lidocaine) (bearing in mind the safe dosing limits, see below). Conversely, if the intended effect of the local anesthetic injection is primarily to produce analgesia (e.g., pure sensory blockade vs. sensory plus motor blockade) a more dilute concentration of local anesthetic solution generally will preferentially block sensory fibers while sparing motor fibers, for example, for postoperative caudal/epidural analgesia or for continuous catheter peripheral nerve blockade. The relative potency of local anesthetics for a variety of clinical applications varies considerably (Table 47.1).

TACHYPHYLAXIS

This is a clinical phenomenon whereby repeated injections of the same dose of local anesthetic solution lead to decreasing pharmacodynamic effects. An interesting clinical phenomenon to tachyphylaxis is the dependence on dosing intervals. If the dosing intervals are short enough that no pain is perceived, tachyphylaxis does not occur. Conversely, if the patient's pain has recurred prior to redosing, tachyphylaxis may be observed. This is thought to be due to a central sensitization (so called "wind-up") phenomenon (7).

TOXICITY OF LOCAL ANESTHETICS SOLUTIONS

Toxicity of local anesthetic solutions includes central nervous system (CNS), cardiac toxicity, allergic reactions, and local tissue toxicity (Table 47.2). In general, CNS toxicity manifests as circumoral tingling followed by lightheadedness, dizziness, tinnitus, garrulousness, slurred speech, visual disturbances, and seizures. Cardiac toxicity may manifest initially as hypertension and tachycardia (due to intravascular injection of epinephrine within the local anesthetic solution) followed by vasodilation, hypotension, cardiac arrhythmias, and severe cardiac dysfunction leading to cardiac arrest. Since children usually receive high-dose local anesthetics while under anesthesia the vast majority of symptoms are masked. Electrocardiographic monitoring can be particularly helpful, since doubling or tripling of the amplitude of the T wave and ST-segment elevation often indicate intravascular injection of epinephrine, particularly with bupivacaine (Fig. 47.1) (8). The CNS manifestations of local anesthetic overdose or intravascular injection are readily offset with intravenous benzodiazepines but such administration will not block the cardiac depression. Cardiac depression, particularly with the amides, is very difficult to reverse. During the past several years the successful use of intralipid for the management of local anesthetic toxicity has been reported. The original discovery was based on the observation that an adult with carnitine deficiency seemed to be very sensitive to cardiac arrhythmias induced by bupivacaine (9). Since carnitine is essential for fatty acid mitochondrial transport to the heart the authors postulated that bupivacaine may cause further impairment of fatty acid transport (9). Instead, the authors found the opposite of their postulation. Their laboratory dose escalation experiment with Sprague-Dawley rats that were pretreated or received 10%, 20%, or 30% intralipid compared with saline found a shift in the dose response to bupivacaine-induced cardiac arrest: approximately 18 mg per kg for saline, approximately 28 mg per kg for 10% intralipid, approximately 50% for 20% intralipid, and approximately

TABLE 47.2 Toxicity of Local Anesthetics

Systemic toxicity
(1) Central nervous system
  a. Lightheadedness and dizziness
  b. Visual and auditory disturbances
  c. Muscle twitching and tremors
  d. Generalized convulsions
(2) Cardiovascular toxicity
  a. Direct cardiac effects
    i. Depresses rapid phase of depolarization of Purkinje fibers leading to cardiac dysrhythmias
    ii. Depresses spontaneous pacemaker activity in the sinus node
    iii. Negative inotropic effect on the heart
    iv. Depresses myocardial contractility by affecting calcium influx and triggered release
  b. Direct peripheral vascular effects
    i. Biphasic effect; low concentrations cause vasoconstriction while high concentrations cause vasodilation
    ii. Animal studies have shown increase in pulmonary vascular resistance
    iii. Acidosis and hypoxia markedly increase the toxicity of local anesthetic solutions.
  c. Ventricular arrhythmias
    i. Ventricular fibrillation
    ii. Reentrant arrhythmias similar to torsades de pointes (140).

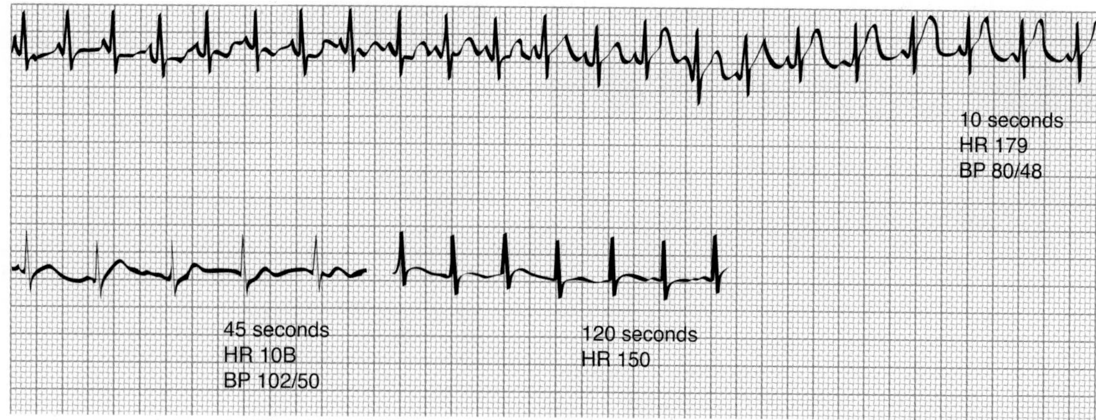

Figure 47.1. Electrocardiographic changes associated with the intravenous injection of bupivacaine and epinephrine 1:200,000. Note the marked increase in the height of the T wave (8). (Reproduced from Freid EB, Bailey AG, Valley RD. Electrocardiographic and hemodynamic changes associated with unintentional intravascular injection of bupivacaine with epinephrine in children. *Anesthesiology* 1993;79:394–398, with permission.)

82% for 30% intralipid (10). The authors subsequently demonstrated accelerated removal of bupivacaine and recovery from bupivacaine-induced cardiac toxicity in an isolated rat heart model (11). Thus, it appears that intralipid is protective of bupivacaine-induced cardiac toxicity. The authors then performed a large animal study and found that 4-mL per kg of 20% intralipid substantially improved survival from bupivacaine-induced cardiac arrest (12). The premise that lipids can act as a sink to counteract the cardiovascular effects of amide anesthetic solutions has been shown to be very effective in animal experiments (13). Since the publication of these animal experiments a number of case reports of the use of lipid for management of local anesthetic toxicity seem to substantiate the efficacy of this treatment (14–17). Further investigations suggest that long-chain triglyceride infusions may be more efficacious than medium-chain triglyceride infusions and that recurrence of cardiac toxicity may occur after initial rescue (18,19). One pediatric patient was rescued with 3 mL per kg of 20% intralipid followed by an infusion of 0.25 mL per kg per minute until resuscitation (20). An expanded description of the literature and the evolvement of this therapy can be found on www.lipidrescue.org maintained by the University of Illinois in Chicago. These multiple case reports of successful management of toxicity using intralipid are very encouraging but much further research is needed in terms of determining the most effective dose, concentration, and duration of intralipid infusions (21–24). Our recommendation is to have intralipid available in any location where a long-acting amide local anesthetic solution is being utilized. The intralipid solution (20% emulsion) should be administered as soon as the local anesthetic toxicity is suspected. A continuous infusion of lipid emulsion is recommended for about 1 hour following exposure to local anesthetic toxicity. Note that this is a guideline based upon individual clinical reports in adults and children and that the most important issue always remains excellent chest compressions to maintain perfusion and pulmonary ventilation to ensure oxygenation while instituting the administration of the intralipid (25). The use of antiarrhythmics such as amiodarone and inotropics to support cardiac function is essential; intralipid should be viewed as an important supplement to the resuscitation (19). Probably the most important safety factor is to always double check the proposed dose (Table 47.3) and the concentration (Table 47.4) of the local anesthetic to be used so as to remain within recommended limits, combine the local anesthetic with low-dose epinephrine where appropriate (Table 47.5) so as to slow the absorption and to have a marker of vascular injection (electrocardiographic changes), and administer the block in graded

TABLE 47.3 Maximum Recommended Doses and Duration of Action of Commonly Used Local Anesthetics

Local Anesthetic	*Maximum Dose (mg/kg)*[a]	*Duration of Action (min)*[b]
Procaine	10	60–90
2-Chloroprocaine	20	30–60
Tetracaine	1.5	180–600
Lidocaine	7	90–200
Mepivacaine	7	120–240
Bupivacaine	2.5	180–600
Ropivacaine	3	120–240

[a]These are maximum doses of local anesthetics. Doses of amides should be decreased by 30% in infants younger than 6 months. When lidocaine is being administered intravascularly (e.g., during intravenous regional anesthesia), the dose should be decreased to 3–5 mg/kg; there is no need to administer long-acting local anesthetic agents for intravenous regional anesthesia, and such a practice is potentially dangerous.
[b]Duration of action is dependent on concentration, total dose, site of administration, and the patient's age.
Reproduced from Polaner DM, Suresh S, Coté CJ. Regional anesthesia. In: Coté CJ, Lerman J, Todres ID, eds. *A practice of anesthesia for infants and children*, 4th ed. Philadelphia, PA: Saunders Elsevier, 2009:871, with permission.

TABLE 47.4 Local Anesthetic Concentration and Its Conversion to Milligrams Per Milliliter

Concentration (%)	*mg/mL*
3.0	30
2.5	25
2.0	20
1.0	10
0.5	5
0.25	2.5
0.125	1.25

Reproduced from Polaner DM, Suresh S, Coté CJ. Regional anesthesia. In: Coté CJ, Lerman J, Todres ID, eds. *A Practice of anesthesia for infants and children*, 4th ed. Philadelphia, PA: Saunders Elsevier, 2009:872, with permission.

doses with multiple aspirations so as to reduce unintended intravascular administration.

CLASSES OF LOCAL ANESTHETIC SOLUTIONS

Local anesthetics are represented by two main classes of drugs, the amino-amides (amides) and the amino-esters (esters) (Table 47.6). The main differences between the two classes are that the amides undergo enzymatic degradation by the liver whereas the esters are hydrolyzed by plasma cholinesterases (26); these differences play an important role in the metabolism and safe use of local anesthetics particularly in the neonate and infant.

AMIDES

The local anesthetics belonging to this class include lidocaine, bupivacaine, ropivacaine, and levobupivacaine; however, levobupivacaine is not available for commercial use in North America. These are the most commonly used local anesthetics in infants and children. Although the selection of these agents is related to the time of onset and the desired duration of the local anesthetic effect, careful attention must be paid to the potential toxic effects. For example, the ability of the neonate's liver to biotransform and to oxidize and reduce the local anesthetics is vastly diminished compared with that of the adult (27). At approximately 3 to 6 months of age, the ability to conjugate drugs achieves adult levels (28,29). Another consideration is that older children will absorb local anesthetics more rapidly than do adults and therefore achieve higher blood levels of local anesthetic; for example, higher blood levels have been found in children undergoing intercostal nerve blocks than in adults (30). After caudal administration of local anesthetic solution, peak plasma concentrations are obtained in children and adults in about 30 minutes (31). The steady-state volume of distribution (V_{dss}) for amides is increased in children compared with adults although clearance (Cl) is similar (31,32). Since the elimination half-life ($t_{1/2}$) is related to the volume of distribution and clearance as follows $t_{1/2} = (0.693 \times V_{dss})/Cl$, the larger steady-state volume of distribution results in prolongation of the elimination half-life. This may not play an important role in single-dose injections but may play a vital role in continuous infusions or repeated injections. The risk with repeated doses has been demonstrated to be greater in infants and children than in adults (33,34).

TABLE 47.5 Epinephrine Dilution and Conversion to Micrograms Per Milliliter

Epinephrine Dilution	*μg/mL*
1:100,000	10
1:200,000	5
1:400,000	2.5
1:800,000	1.25

Reproduced from Polaner DM, Suresh S, Coté CJ. Regional anesthesia. In: Coté CJ, Lerman J, Todres ID, eds. *A practice of anesthesia for infants and children*, 4th ed. Philadelphia, PA: Saunders Elsevier, 2009:871, with permission.

TABLE 47.6 Commonly Used Local Anesthetics

Esters	*Amides*
Procaine	Lidocaine
Tetracaine	Mepivacaine
2-Chloroprocaine	Bupivacaine
	Ropivacaine
	Etidocaine

Reproduced from Polaner DM, Suresh S, Coté CJ. Regional anesthesia. In: Coté CJ, Lerman J, Todres ID, eds. *A practice of anesthesia for infants and children*, 4th ed. Philadelphia, PA: Saunders Elsevier, 2009:868, with permission.

The systemic absorption of local anesthetics is very dependent upon the site of injection. A common rule of thumb is to remember the nemonic **ICE-Blocks** (***I***ntercostal > ***C***audal > ***E***pidural > peripheral nerve ***B***locks) in order of increased risk for toxicity (30). This relationship is very important to bear in mind since the same dose of local anesthetic when administered as a peripheral nerve block may be toxic when used for intercostal nerve blocks.

BUPIVACAINE

This is the most commonly used local anesthetic solution in infants and children in North America. The pharmacokinetics as well as the pharmacodynamics has been well studied in infants and children (31,32,35–38). The average duration of analgesia is about 5 to 6 hours after a single bolus injection (39,40). The concentration of the local anesthetic used depends on the site, the desired density of blockade, postoperative "street readiness," and the potential for toxicity. The concomitant use of other local anesthetic solutions including infiltration anesthesia has to be taken into consideration before a total dose (mg per kg) of local anesthetic solution is taken into consideration.

Pharmacology

Bupivacaine is bound to α-1-acid glycoprotein. It is a racemic mixture of the levo and dextro-enantiomers. Although the levo-enantiomer is the active form that provides the clinical effect of the local anesthetic solution, the dextro-enantiomer causes the adverse effects related to local anesthesia including cardiac and CNS toxicity. The cytochrome involved with metabolism of bupivacaine is CYP3A4, which may be immature in neonates and infants younger than 6 months, thus accounting in part for the delayed clearance compared with that in older children and the need to reduce total drug exposure, particularly if administered by a continuous infusion (see below) (41,42).

Toxicity

The major adverse effect of bupivacaine is toxicity related to the cardiovascular system and the CNS. Local anesthetics have the ability to cross the blood–brain barrier and cause alterations in CNS functions. As the systemic concentration of the local anesthetic increases, the risk of complications from toxicity increases exponentially (43). In pediatric patients, the incidence of cardiac toxicity occurs sooner than neurotoxicity. This may be partly due to the fact that children may be anesthetized thereby masking the CNS manifestations of toxicity until significant cardiac toxicity is observed (44,45). This may also be affected by the concomitant use of volatile agents (46).

Application and Dosing

Bupivacaine can be used for most peripheral nerve blocks as well as for epidural and caudal infusions in infants and children. The maximum dosage suggested for bolus injections in the caudal space or epidural space for older children is 4 mg per kg and for neonates and infants is 2 mg per kg. Dosage recommendations for continuous infusions are 0.4 mg per kg per hour in older children and 0.2 mg per kg per hour in neonates and infants (47). An example of a continuous infusion in a 10-kg infant will be 0.2 mg per kg per hour; this will be equivalent to 2 mL per hour of a 0.1% solution of bupivacaine (1 mg per mL of bupivacaine). The concentration of the solution used for peripheral nerve blocks is usually 0.25% or 0.5% bearing in mind the ceiling limit for maximum dosage.

ROPIVACAINE

This is a newer amide local anesthetic. It is a levo-enantiomer with less cardiovascular and CNS side effects compared with bupivacaine. The lethal dose in rats is higher than that of bupivacaine. (LD_{50}) (48,49). Ropivacaine seems to have less motor blockade when compared with bupivacaine especially when a concentration of 0.375% or greater is used. This may offer some advantages in an outpatient setting (50). Several pediatric trials have demonstrated a longer duration of action of ropivacaine when compared with mepivacaine for peripheral nerve blocks (51).

Pharmacology

Just as with bupivacaine, ropivacaine is 95% protein bound to α-1-acid glycoprotein (41). With both drugs the lower α-1-acid glycoprotein concentration in neonates makes them more susceptible to toxicity. A number of studies have examined the absorption of ropivacaine in children (52–58). Absorption seems to be a bit slower than a similar dose of bupivacaine, perhaps in part related to its intrinsic vasoconstrictive properties and to reduced metabolism (58). The cytochrome involved with metabolism of ropivacaine (CYP1A2) is also immature in neonates and infants, thus necessitating a reduced dose just as with bupivacaine (41). A caudal block with ropivacaine 2 mg per kg in children aged 1 to 8 years resulted in plasma concentrations of ropivacaine well below toxic levels in adults (56). This dose was also noted to produce less motor block but provide adequate analgesia. The mean C_{max} of total ropivacaine at 2 mg per kg was 0.47 mg per L. A threshold of CNS toxicity was noted at a plasma concentration of 0.6 mg per L. Body-weight-adjusted clearance (Cl) was the same as in adults (5 mL per minute per kg). Ropivacaine clearance depends on the unbound fraction of ropivacaine rather than the liver blood flow.

Toxicity

Although an improved safety profile of ropivacaine compared with bupivacaine has been demonstrated in animal experiments (49), there have been reports of CNS toxicity with the use of epidural ropivacaine (59,60). Hence, it is important that an overdose of ropivacaine is avoided in infants and children. One study found stable unbound plasma concentration in children aged 1 to 9 years following infusions of 24 to 72 hours at a rate of 0.4 mg per kg (61). Another study in children 12 to 25 kg demonstrated that single-shot caudal administration of 1 to 3 mg per kg results in unbound ropivacaine concentrations well below the toxic level reported in adults (62). Our recommended dose is bolus dose of 2 mg per kg and an infusion rate of 0.2 mg per kg per hour.

LEVOBUPIVACAINE

This is a newer levo-enantiomer that also has fewer adverse cardiovascular effects and less motor blockade than bupivacaine (63–67).

Pharmacology

A population-based pharmacokinetic study in infants younger than 3 months found markedly reduced clearance (approximately half that of adults) which the authors ascribed to immaturity of CYP3A4 and CYP1A2 (68). Thus, a lower dose would be indicated in this population. Pharmacokinetic studies in older children demonstrate a similar profile as bupivacaine (68,69). Several pediatric trials have demonstrated its efficacy for a variety of blocks (66,70–75). Since this drug is not available in the United States, levobupivacaine is not used abundantly in general pediatric anesthesiology practice.

Toxicity

Levobupivacaine appears to have a better safety profile than bupivacaine (76). Levobupivacaine, in the animal model, has been shown to have (a) less cardiotoxicity than bupivacaine, (b) less myocardial depression than bupivacaine, and (c) it is less likely to cause fatal dysrhythmias than bupivacaine (77).

LIDOCAINE

Lidocaine is perhaps the most commonly used short-acting but rapid onset amide local anesthetic. In the operating room it is used as a topical anesthetic for airway manipulations, for facilitating insertion of intravenous catheters, intravenously as a means to reduce the pain of intravenous drug administration (e.g., propofol), and often combined with bupivacaine (equal volumes of 1% lidocaine with epinephrine 1:200,000 and 0.5% bupivacaine with epinephrine 1:200,000) for a more rapid onset of analgesia for local infiltration of surgical incisions at the end of the case. It is important to understand that lidocaine is rapidly and nearly completely absorbed from mucosal membranes so that appropriate total dose calculation is important (78,79). Likewise, in the emergency room this is the most frequent local anesthetic used for skin infiltration as well as in the cardiac catheterization laboratory and radiology suites. Dilute lidocaine (0.25% to 0.5%) has also been used for intravenous regional anesthesia for forearm fracture reduction (80–82). Note that lidocaine (maximum dose of 5 mg per kg or 1 mL per kg) is the only local anesthetic with a sufficient safely profile for this technique. Deaths have occurred when bupivacaine was used for intravenous regional anesthesia (83,84). Small doses of lidocaine (5 mL of a 2% solution) have been used to provide topical analgesia to children with oral mucositis with only minor systemic absorption (85). Regardless of the site of injection, the total dose must be calculated as systemic toxicity and significant absorption may occur (86–88).

Pharmacokinetics

Study of intravenous lidocaine in children under general anesthesia revealed that the distribution half-life (3.2 minutes), elimination half-life (58 minutes), volume of distribution (1.1. L per kg), and total plasma clearance (11 mL per minute per kg) were similar in adults and in children 6 months or older (89). Similar pharmacokinetic parameters were found following epidural administration (90).

Toxicity

As with all local anesthetics, toxicity is generally manifest as CNS excitation (seizures) and secondarily with cardiac manifestations (hypotension, cardiac arrest). Fortunately, the cardiac toxicity is far less than with the other amide local anesthetics, thereby making successful resuscitation more likely (91–93).

ESTERS

Ester local anesthetics are metabolized by plasma cholinesterases. As a result, in populations with lower pseudocholinesterases (26,94), there is an increase in the duration of local anesthetic activity particularly in infants and neonates. Overall, however, because there is no metabolism by liver or kidney, the safety profile is improved compared with amide local anesthetics offering improved safety when used as a continuous infusion over 24 to 72 hours in neonates and infants (95,96). Chloroprocaine is the only drug in this class that is commonly used in children.

Toxicity

Toxicity is based on the absence of pseudocholinesterase in the neonate.

Dosing

After a bolus dose of 1 mL per kg, a continuous infusion of chloroprocaine at 0.3 mL per kg of a 3% 2-chloroprocaine is recommended to achieve a level of T4 to T2 (96). This will be effective in producing complete surgical anesthesia for neonates undergoing hernia repair. Although the drug is not commonly used in pediatric practice, the advantage of its use is the capacity to provide complete motor block that is not prolonged.

TOPICAL ANESTHESIA

Several local topical anesthetic preparations are now commonly used to reduce procedural pain in neonates, infants, and children (97–104). The most common local anesthetic preparations for topical use include lidocaine, amethocaine, tetracaine, benzocaine, and prilocaine. When applied to skin they produce effective but relatively short duration of analgesia. It is essential to avoid application to mucus membranes, to prevent ingestion, and to remain within the recommended limits so as to avoid toxicity or death (105–109). One of the first commercially available topical anesthetic formulations was EMLA cream (Eutectic Mixture of Local Anesthetic) which is a mixture of lidocaine 2.5% and prilocaine 2.5%. This is used extensively for topical anesthesia in neonates particularly for circumcision as well for venipunctures (110–115). The preparation has to be applied under an occlusive bandage for 45 to 60 minutes to obtain effective cutaneous analgesia. Although the incidence of methemoglobinemia from prilocaine is not very common in neonates, caution should be exercised when applying large doses of EMLA (105–107,116). Although EMLA can provide good analgesia it may not provide similar analgesia to a dorsal nerve block with local anesthetic solution (115). A newer topical anesthetic solution that offers a faster rate of onset is a 4% or 5% liposomal lidocaine solution (LMX-4 formerly ELA-max 4, ELA-max 5). With this topical cream there is no need for an occlusive dressing and it has the same efficacy as EMLA but with a more rapid onset (30 minutes vs. 60 minutes) (117–120). Liposome-encapsulated lidocaine and tetracaine have been shown to remain in the epidermis after topical application affording a fast and lasting local anesthetic effect (121,122). Amethocaine 4% (Ametop) (tetracaine) is another recent addition to the topical analgesic local anesthetics also with a slightly fast onset than EMLA (123). In one study it has been shown to have similar efficacy to EMLA (124). A Cochrane review concluded that amethocaine was superior to EMLA for venipuncture whereas another described a more rapid onset (102). A newer needleless, jet-infused local anesthetic administration system called the J-tip (125) offers the ability to provide adequate analgesia without needle insertion with immediate onset of analgesia to a very limited area that one study demonstrated to be superior to a 30-minute application of LMX-4 or a 60-minute application of EMLA (126,127). Other methods for local enhancement of onset are being investigated; these include the use of local heating with ultrasound (128,129), iontophoresis (130–132), and lidocaine transdermal patches (133). Topical anesthesia through cut skin may be provided by a mixture of tetracaine, epinephrine, and cocaine (known as TAC). TAC is used in pediatric emergency departments for suturing lacerations (134,135) TAC is provided as tetracaine 0.5%, epinephrine 1:2,000, and cocaine 10% to 11.8%. A more dilute solution of cocaine may be able to provide similar topical anesthesia without the risk of complications. The maximum dose is 0.05 mL per kg in children. TAC is ineffective when applied to intact skin and has to be applied to abraded skin or lacerated skin. There are reports of toxicity associated with topical absorption of TAC (136–138). Because of the potential for abuse, a newer tetracaine–phenylephrine solution has been shown to be as effective as TAC.

TUMESCENTS

Subcutaneous infiltration of local anesthetic solution is commonly used by plastic surgeons particularly for liposuction surgery. Total doses of lidocaine up to 35 to 40 mg per kg have been shown to be safe while used as a tumescent. Additional use of local anesthetics including infiltration anesthesia should be carefully evaluated and it should be noted that peak plasma levels occurred at 6 to 12 hours postoperatively suggesting that delayed onset of toxicity is possible (139).

REFERENCES

1. Suresh S, Wheeler M. Practical pediatric regional anesthesia. *Anesthesiol Clin North America* 2002;20:83–113.
2. Butterworth JF, Strichartz GR. Molecular mechanisms of local anesthesia: a review. *Anesthesiology* 1990;72:711–734.
3. Strichartz GR, Berde CB. Local anesthetics. In: Miller RD, ed. *Anesthesia*, 6th ed. New York, NY: Churchill Livingstone, 2005: 573–603.
4. Strichartz GR. Local anesthetic pharmacology. In: Benzon HT, Raja S, Borsook D, Molloy RE, Strichartz GR, eds. *Essentials of pain medicine and regional anesthesia*, 1st ed. New York, NY: Churchill Livingstone, 1999:340–351.
5. Fulling PD, Peterfreund RA. Alkalinization and precipitation characteristics of 0.2% ropivacaine. *Reg Anesth Pain Med* 2000;25: 518–521.
6. Peterfreund RA, Datta S, Ostheimer GW. pH adjustment of local anesthetic solutions with sodium bicarbonate: laboratory evaluation of alkalinization and precipitation. *Reg Anesth* 1989;14:265–270.
7. Woolf CJ. Central sensitization: uncovering the relation between pain and plasticity. *Anesthesiology* 2007;106:864–867.
8. Freid EB, Bailey AG, Valley RD. Electrocardiographic and hemodynamic changes associated with unintentional intravascular injection of bupivacaine with epinephrine in infants. *Anesthesiology* 1993; 79:394–398.
9. Weinberg GL, Laurito CE, Geldner P, et al. Malignant ventricular dysrhythmias in a patient with isovaleric acidemia receiving general and local anesthesia for suction lipectomy. *J Clin Anesth* 1997;9:668–670.
10. Weinberg GL, VadeBoncouer T, Ramaraju GA, et al. Pretreatment or resuscitation with a lipid infusion shifts the dose-response to bupivacaine-induced asystole in rats. *Anesthesiology* 1998;88: 1071–1075.
11. Weinberg GL, Ripper R, Murphy P, et al. Lipid infusion accelerates removal of bupivacaine and recovery from bupivacaine toxicity in the isolated rat heart. *Reg Anesth Pain Med* 2006;31:296–303.
12. Weinberg G, Ripper R, Feinstein DL, et al. Lipid emulsion infusion rescues dogs from bupivacaine-induced cardiac toxicity. *Reg Anesth Pain Med* 2003;28:198–202.
13. Weinberg G. Lipid rescue resuscitation from local anaesthetic cardiac toxicity. *Toxicol Rev* 2006;25:139–145.
14. Spence AG. Lipid reversal of central nervous system symptoms of bupivacaine toxicity. *Anesthesiology* 2007;107:516–517.
15. Whiteside J. Reversal of local anaesthetic induced CNS toxicity with lipid emulsion. *Anaesthesia* 2008;63:203–204.
16. Mathieu S, Cranshaw J. Treatment of severe local anaesthetic toxicity. *Anaesthesia* 2008;63:202–203.
17. McCutchen T, Gerancher JC. Early intralipid therapy may have prevented bupivacaine-associated cardiac arrest. *Reg Anesth Pain Med* 2008;33:178–180.
18. Mazoit JX, Le GR, Beloeil H, et al. Binding of long-lasting local anesthetics to lipid emulsions. *Anesthesiology* 2009;110:380–386.
19. Marwick PC, Levin AI, Coetzee AR. Recurrence of cardiotoxicity after lipid rescue from bupivacaine-induced cardiac arrest. *Anesth Analg* 2009;108:1344–1346.
20. Ludot H, Tharin JY, Belouadah M, et al. Successful resuscitation after ropivacaine and lidocaine-induced ventricular arrhythmia following posterior lumbar plexus block in a child. *Anesth Analg* 2008;106:1572–1574.
21. Brull SJ. Lipid emulsion for the treatment of local anesthetic toxicity: patient safety implications. *Anesth Analg* 2008;106: 1337–1339.
22. Picard J, Ward SC, Zumpe R, et al. Guidelines and the adoption of "lipid rescue" therapy for local anaesthetic toxicity. *Anaesthesia* 2009;64:122–125.
23. Weinberg GL. Limits to lipid in the literature and lab: what we know, what we don't know. *Anesth Analg* 2009;108:1062–1064.
24. Groban L, Butterworth J. Lipid reversal of bupivacaine toxicity: has the silver bullet been identified? *Reg Anesth Pain Med* 2003; 28:167–169.
25. Moore DC. Lipid rescue from bupivacaine cardiac arrest: a result of failure to ventilate and maintain cardiac perfusion? *Anesthesiology* 2007;106:636–637.
26. Raj PP, Ohlweiler D, Hitt BA, et al. Kinetics of local anesthetic esters and the effects of adjuvant drugs on 2-chloroprocaine hydrolysis. *Anesthesiology* 1980;53:307–314.
27. Besunder JB, Reed MD, Blumer JL. Principles of drug biodisposition in the neonate. A critical evaluation of the pharmacokinetic–pharmacodynamic interface (part II). *Clin Pharmacokinet* 1988;14: 261–286.
28. Rane A, Sjoqvist F. Drug metabolism in the human fetus and newborn infant. *Pediatr Clin North Am* 1972;19:37–49.
29. Levy G. Pharmacokinetics of fetal and neonatal exposure to drugs. *Obstet Gynecol* 1981;58(Suppl):9S–16S.
30. Rothstein P, Arthur GR, Feldman HS, et al. Bupivacaine for intercostal nerve blocks in children: blood concentrations and pharmacokinetics. *Anesth Analg* 1986;65:625–632.
31. Ecoffey C, Desparmet J, Maury M, et al. Bupivacaine in children: pharmacokinetics following caudal anesthesia. *Anesthesiology* 1985; 63:447–448.
32. Murat I, Montay G, Delleur MM, et al. Bupivacaine pharmacokinetics during epidural anaesthesia in children. *Eur J Anaesthesiol* 1988;5:113–120.
33. Berde C. Epidural analgesia in children. *Can J Anaesth* 1994;41: 555–560.
34. Luz G, Wieser C, Innerhofer P, et al. Free and total bupivacaine plasma concentrations after continuous epidural anaesthesia in infants and children. *Paediatr Anaesth* 1998;8:473–478.
35. Frawley G, Ragg P, Hack H. Plasma concentrations of bupivacaine after combined spinal epidural anaesthesia in infants and neonates. *Paediatr Anaesth* 2000;10:619–625.
36. Larsson BA, Lonnqvist PA, Olsson GL. Plasma concentrations of bupivacaine in neonates after continuous epidural infusion. *Anesth Analg* 1997;84:501–505.

37. Mazoit JX, Denson DD, Samii K. Pharmacokinetics of bupivacaine following caudal anesthesia in infants. *Anesthesiology* 1988;68: 387–391.
38. Meunier JF, Goujard E, Dubousset AM, et al. Pharmacokinetics of bupivacaine after continuous epidural infusion in infants with and without biliary atresia. *Anesthesiology* 2001;95:87–95.
39. Payne KA, Hendrix MR, Wade WJ. Caudal bupivacaine for postoperative analgesia in pediatric lower limb surgery. *J Pediatr Surg* 1993;28:155–157.
40. Fisher QA, McComiskey CM, Hill JL, et al. Postoperative voiding interval and duration of analgesia following peripheral or caudal nerve blocks in children. *Anesth Analg* 1993;75:173–177.
41. Mazoit JX, Dalens BJ. Pharmacokinetics of local anaesthetics in infants and children. *Clin Pharmacokinet* 2004;43:17–32.
42. Weston PJ, Bourchier D. The pharmacokinetics of bupivacaine following interpleural nerve block in infants of very low birthweight. *Paediatr Anaesth* 1995;5:219–222.
43. Berde CB. Toxicity of local anesthetics in infants and children. *J Pediatr* 1993;122:S14–S20.
44. Groban L, Deal DD, Vernon JC, et al. Cardiac resuscitation after incremental overdosage with lidocaine, bupivacaine, levobupivacaine, and ropivacaine in anesthetized dogs. *Anesth Analg* 2001;92: 37–43.
45. Chang DH, Ladd LA, Copeland S, et al. Direct cardiac effects of intracoronary bupivacaine, levobupivacaine and ropivacaine in the sheep. *Br J Pharmacol* 2001;132:649–658.
46. Badgwell JM, Heavner JE, Kytta J. Bupivacaine toxicity in young pigs is age-dependent and is affected by volatile anesthetics. *Anesthesiology* 1990;73:297–303.
47. Berde CB. Convulsions associated with pediatric regional anesthesia. *Anesth Analg* 1992;75:164–166.
48. Kohane DS, Sankar WN, Shubina M, et al. Sciatic nerve blockade in infant, adolescent, and adult rats: a comparison of ropivacaine with bupivacaine. *Anesthesiology* 1998;89:1199–1208.
49. Dony P, Dewinde V, Vanderick B, et al. The comparative toxicity of ropivacaine and bupivacaine at equipotent doses in rats. *Anesth Analg* 2000;91:1489–1492.
50. Da Conceicao MJ, Coelho L. Caudal anaesthesia with 0.375% ropivacaine or 0.375% bupivacaine in paediatric patients. *Br J Anaesth* 1998;80:507–508.
51. Fernandez-Guisasola J, Andueza A, Burgos E, et al. A comparison of 0.5% ropivacaine and 1% mepivacaine for sciatic nerve block in the popliteal fossa. *Acta Anaesthesiol Scand* 2001;45:967–970.
52. Koinig H, Krenn CG, Glaser C, et al. The dose-response of caudal ropivacaine in children. *Anesthesiology* 1999;90:1339–1344.
53. Habre W, Bergesio R, Johnson C, et al. Pharmacokinetics of ropivacaine following caudal analgesia in children. *Paediatr Anaesth* 2000;10:143–147.
54. Wulf H, Peters C, Behnke H. The pharmacokinetics of caudal ropivacaine 0.2% in children. A study of infants aged less than 1 year and toddlers aged 1–5 years undergoing inguinal hernia repair. *Anaesthesia* 2000;55:757–760.
55. Hansen TG, Ilett KF, Reid C, et al. Caudal ropivacaine in infants: population pharmacokinetics and plasma concentrations. *Anesthesiology* 2001;94:579–584.
56. Lonnqvist PA, Westrin P, Larsson BA, et al. Ropivacaine pharmacokinetics after caudal block in 1–8 year old children. *Br J Anaesth* 2000;85:506–511.
57. McCann ME, Sethna NF, Mazoit JX, et al. The pharmacokinetics of epidural ropivacaine in infants and young children. *Anesth Analg* 2001;93:893–897.
58. Bosenberg AT, Thomas J, Cronje L, et al. Pharmacokinetics and efficacy of ropivacaine for continuous epidural infusion in neonates and infants. *Paediatr Anaesth* 2005;15:739–749.
59. Abouleish EI, Elias M, Nelson C. Ropivacaine-induced seizure after extradural anaesthesia. *Br J Anaesth* 1998;80:843–844.
60. Eledjam JJ, Gros T, Viel E, et al. Ropivacaine overdose and systemic toxicity. *Anaesth Intensive Care* 2000;28:705–707.
61. Berde CB, Yaster M, Meretoja O, et al. Stable plasma concentrations of unbound ropivacaine during postoperative epidural infusion for 24–72 hours in children. *Eur J Anaesthesiol* 2008;25: 410–417.
62. Bosenberg AT, Thomas J, Lopez T, et al. Plasma concentrations of ropivacaine following a single-shot caudal block of 1, 2 or 3 mg/kg in children. *Acta Anaesthesiol Scand* 2001;45:1276–1280.
63. McLeod GA, Burke D. Levobupivacaine. *Anaesthesia* 2001;56: 331–341.
64. Foster RH, Markham A. Levobupivacaine: a review of its pharmacology and use as a local anaesthetic. *Drugs* 2000;59:551–579.
65. Ivani G, Borghi B, van Oven H. Levobupivacaine. *Minerva Anestesiol* 2001;67:20–23.
66. Ivani G, De Negri P, Lonnqvist PA, et al. A comparison of three different concentrations of levobupivacaine for caudal block in children. *Anesth Analg* 2003;97:368–371.
67. Locatelli B, Ingelmo P, Sonzogni V, et al. Randomized, double-blind, phase III, controlled trial comparing levobupivacaine 0.25%, ropivacaine 0.25% and bupivacaine 0.25% by the caudal route in children. *Br J Anaesth* 2005;94:366–371.
68. Chalkiadis GA, Eyres RL, Cranswick N, et al. Pharmacokinetics of levobupivacaine 0.25% following caudal administration in children under 2 years of age. *Br J Anaesth* 2004;92:218–222.
69. Cortinez LI, Fuentes R, Solari S, et al. Pharmacokinetics of levobupivacaine (2.5 mg/kg) after caudal administration in children younger than 3 years. *Anesth Analg* 2008;107:1182–1184.
70. Gunter JB, Gregg T, Varughese AM, et al. Levobupivacaine for ilioinguinal/iliohypogastric nerve block in children. *Anesth Analg* 1999;89:647–649.
71. Lerman J, Nolan J, Eyres R, et al. Efficacy, safety, and pharmacokinetics of levobupivacaine with and without fentanyl after continuous epidural infusion in children: a multicenter trial. *Anesthesiology* 2003;99:1166–1174.
72. Astuto M, Disma N, Arena C. Levobupivacaine 0.25% compared with ropivacaine 0.25% by the caudal route in children. *Eur J Anaesthesiol* 2003;20:826–830.
73. Ala-Kokko TI, Raiha E, Karinen J, et al. Pharmacokinetics of 0.5% levobupivacaine following ilioinguinal–iliohypogastric nerve blockade in children. *Acta Anaesthesiol Scand* 2005;49: 397–400.
74. Frawley GP, Downie S, Huang GH. Levobupivacaine caudal anesthesia in children: a randomized double-blind comparison with bupivacaine. *Paediatr Anaesth* 2006;16:754–760.
75. Yao YS, Qian B, Chen BZ, et al. The optimum concentration of levobupivacaine for intra-operative caudal analgesia in children undergoing inguinal hernia repair at equal volumes of injectate. *Anaesthesia* 2009;64:23–26.
76. Giaufre E, Dalens B, Gombert A. Epidemiology and morbidity of regional anesthesia in children: a one-year prospective survey of the French-Language Society of Pediatric Anesthesiologists. *Anesth Analg* 1996;83:904–912.
77. Huang YF, Pryor ME, Mather LE, et al. Cardiovascular and central nervous system effects of intravenous levobupivacaine and bupivacaine in sheep. *Anesth Analg* 1998;86:797–804.
78. Amitai Y, Zylber-Katz E, Avital A, et al. Serum lidocaine concentrations in children during bronchoscopy with topical anesthesia. *Chest* 1990;98:1370–1373.
79. Eyres RL, Bishop W, Oppenheim RC, et al. Plasma lignocaine concentrations following topical laryngeal application. *Anaesth Intensive Care* 1983;11:23–26.
80. Werk LN, Lewis M, Armatti-Wiltrout S, et al. Comparing the effectiveness of modified forearm and conventional minidose intravenous regional anesthesia for reduction of distal forearm fractures in children. *J Pediatr Orthop* 2008;28:410–416.
81. Bratt HD, Eyres RL, Cole WG. Randomized double-blind trial of low- and moderate-dose lidocaine regional anesthesia for forearm fractures in childhood. *J Pediatr Orthop* 1996;16:660–663.
82. Colizza WA, Said E. Intravenous regional anesthesia in the treatment of forearm and wrist fractures and dislocations in children. *Can J Surg* 1993;36:225–228.
83. Heath ML. Deaths after intravenous regional anaesthesia. *Br Med J (Clin Res Ed)* 1982;285:913–914.
84. Moore DC. Bupivacaine toxicity and Bier block: the drug, the technique, or the anesthetist. *Anesthesiology* 1984;61:782.
85. Elad S, Cohen G, Zylber-Katz E, et al. Systemic absorption of lidocaine after topical application for the treatment of oral mucositis in bone marrow transplantation patients. *J Oral Pathol Med* 1999; 28:170–172.
86. Cassidy SC, Jones PR, Cox S, et al. Serum lidocaine concentrations after subcutaneous administration in patients undergoing cardiac catheterization in a pediatric institution. *J Pediatr* 1996;129: 464–466.

87. Ryan CA, Robertson M, Coe JY. Seizures due to lidocaine toxicity in a child during cardiac catheterization. *Pediatr Cardiol* 1993; 14:116–118.
88. Gunter JB. Benefit and risks of local anesthetics in infants and children. *Paediatr Drugs* 2002;4:649–672.
89. Finholt DA, Stirt JA, DiFazio CA, et al. Lidocaine pharmacokinetics in children during general anesthesia. *Anesth Analg* 1986; 65:279–282.
90. Ecoffey C, Desparmet J, Berdeaux A, et al. Pharmacokinetics of lignocaine in children following caudal anaesthesia. *Br J Anaesth* 1984;56:1399–1402.
91. Mather LE, Copeland SE, Ladd LA. Acute toxicity of local anesthetics: underlying pharmacokinetic and pharmacodynamic concepts. *Reg Anesth Pain Med* 2005;30:553–566.
92. Casati A, Putzu M. Bupivacaine, levobupivacaine and ropivacaine: are they clinically different? *Best Pract Res Clin Anaesthesiol* 2005;19:247–268.
93. Groban L. Central nervous system and cardiac effects from long-acting amide local anesthetic toxicity in the intact animal model. *Reg Anesth Pain Med* 2003;28:3–11.
94. Kuhnert BR, Philipson EH, Pimental R, et al. A prolonged chloroprocaine epidural block in a postpartum patient with abnormal pseudocholinesterase. *Anesthesiology* 1982;56:477–478.
95. Tobias JD, Rasmussen GE, Holcomb GW, et al. Continuous caudal anaesthesia with chloroprocaine as an adjunct to general anaesthesia in neonates. *Can J Anaesth* 1996;43:69–72.
96. Henderson K, Sethna NF, Berde CB. Continuous caudal anesthesia for inguinal hernia repair in former preterm infants. *J Clin Anesth* 1993;5:129–133.
97. Cregin R, Rappaport AS, Montagnino G, et al. Improving pain management for pediatric patients undergoing nonurgent painful procedures. *Am J Health Syst Pharm* 2008;65:723–727.
98. Khan AN, Sachdeva S. Current trends in the management of common painful conditions of preschool children in United States pediatric emergency departments. *Clin Pediatr (Phila)* 2007; 46:626–631.
99. Lemyre B, Hogan DL, Gaboury I, et al. How effective is tetracaine 4% gel, before a venipuncture, in reducing procedural pain in infants: a randomized double-blind placebo controlled trial. *BMC Pediatr* 2007;7:7.
100. Eidelman A, Weiss JM, Lau J, et al. Topical anesthetics for dermal instrumentation: a systematic review of randomized, controlled trials. *Ann Emerg Med* 2005;46:343–351.
101. Anand KJ, Johnston CC, Oberlander TF, et al. Analgesia and local anesthesia during invasive procedures in the neonate. *Clin Ther* 2005;27:844–876.
102. O'Brien L, Taddio A, Lyszkiewicz DA, et al. A critical review of the topical local anesthetic amethocaine (Ametop) for pediatric pain. *Paediatr Drugs* 2005;7:41–54.
103. Priestley S, Kelly AM, Chow L, et al. Application of topical local anesthetic at triage reduces treatment time for children with lacerations: a randomized controlled trial. *Ann Emerg Med* 2003; 42:34–40.
104. Houck CS, Sethna NF. Transdermal analgesia with local anesthetics in children: review, update and future directions. *Expert Rev Neurother* 2005;5:625–634.
105. American Academy of Pediatrics. Committee on Drugs. Alternate routes of drug administration—advantages and disadvantages. *Pediatrics* 1997;100:143–152.
106. Curtis LA, Dolan TS, Seibert HE. Are one or two dangerous? Lidocaine and topical anesthetic exposures in children. *J Emerg Med* 2008;37(1):32–39.
107. Raso SM, Fernandez JB, Beobide EA, et al. Methemoglobinemia and CNS toxicity after topical application of EMLA to a 4-year-old girl with molluscum contagiosum. *Pediatr Dermatol* 2006;23: 592–593.
108. Hua YM, Hung CH, Yuh YS. Acute intoxication of lidocaine and chlorpheniramine: report of one case. *Acta Paediatr Taiwan* 2005; 46:385–387.
109. Dahshan A, Donovan GK. Severe methemoglobinemia complicating topical benzocaine use during endoscopy in a toddler: a case report and review of the literature. *Pediatrics* 2006;117: e806–e809.
110. Corbett JV. EMLA cream for local anesthesia. *MCN Am J Matern Child Nurs* 1995;20:178.
111. Chang PC, Goresky GV, O'Connor G, et al. A multicentre randomized study of single-unit dose package of EMLA patch vs EMLA 5% cream for venepuncture in children. *Can J Anaesth* 1994;41:59–63.
112. Gourrier E, Karoubi P, el HA, et al. Use of EMLA cream in a department of neonatology. *Pain* 1996;68:431–434.
113. Stevens B, Johnston C, Taddio A, et al. Management of pain from heel lance with lidocaine-prilocaine (EMLA) cream: is it safe and efficacious in preterm infants? *J Dev Behav Pediatr* 1999;20:216–221.
114. Taddio A, Ohlsson K, Ohlsson A. Lidocaine–prilocaine cream for analgesia during circumcision in newborn boys. *Cochrane Database Syst Rev* 2000;(2):CD000496.
115. Lander J, Brady-Fryer B, Metcalfe JB, et al. Comparison of ring block, dorsal penile nerve block, and topical anesthesia for neonatal circumcision: a randomized controlled trial. *JAMA* 1997;278:2157–2162.
116. Brisman M, Ljung BM, Otterbom I, et al. Methaemoglobin formation after the use of EMLA cream in term neonates. *Acta Paediatr* 1998;87:1191–1194.
117. Eichenfield LF, Funk A, Fallon-Friedlander S, et al. A clinical study to evaluate the efficacy of ELA-Max (4% liposomal lidocaine) as compared with eutectic mixture of local anesthetics cream for pain reduction of venipuncture in children. *Pediatrics* 2002;109:1093–1099.
118. Koh JL, Harrison D, Myers R, et al. A randomized, double-blind comparison study of EMLA and ELA-Max for topical anesthesia in children undergoing intravenous insertion. *Paediatr Anaesth* 2004;14:977–982.
119. Smith DP, Gjellum M. The efficacy of LMX versus EMLA for pain relief in boys undergoing office meatotomy. *J Urol* 2004;172: 1760–1761.
120. Kleiber C, Sorenson M, Whiteside K, et al. Topical anesthetics for intravenous insertion in children: a randomized equivalency study. *Pediatrics* 2002;110:758–761.
121. Fisher R, Hung O, Mezei M, et al. Topical anaesthesia of intact skin: liposome-encapsulated tetracaine vs EMLA. *Br J Anaesth* 1998; 81:972–973.
122. Gesztes A, Mezei M. Topical anesthesia of the skin by liposome-encapsulated tetracaine. *Anesth Analg* 1988;67:1079–1081.
123. O'Brien L, Taddio A, Ipp M, et al. Topical 4% amethocaine gel reduces the pain of subcutaneous measles–mumps–rubella vaccination. *Pediatrics* 2004;114:e720–e724.
124. Arendts G, Stevens M, Fry M. Topical anaesthesia and intravenous cannulation success in paediatric patients: a randomized double-blind trial. *Br J Anaesth* 2008;100:521–524.
125. Cooper JA, Bromley LM, Baranowski AP, et al. Evaluation of a needle-free injection system for local anaesthesia prior to venous cannulation. *Anaesthesia* 2000;55:247–250.
126. Spanos S, Booth R, Koenig H, et al. Jet injection of 1% buffered lidocaine versus topical ELA-Max for anesthesia before peripheral intravenous catheterization in children: a randomized controlled trial. *Pediatr Emerg Care* 2008;24:511–515.
127. Jimenez N, Bradford H, Seidel KD, et al. A comparison of a needle-free injection system for local anesthesia versus EMLA for intravenous catheter insertion in the pediatric patient. *Anesth Analg* 2006;102:411–414.
128. Zempsky WT, Anand KJ, Sullivan KM, et al. Lidocaine iontophoresis for topical anesthesia before intravenous line placement in children. *J Pediatr* 1998;132:1061–1063.
129. Spierings EL, Brevard JA, Katz NP. Two-minute skin anesthesia through ultrasound pretreatment and iontophoretic delivery of a topical anesthetic: a feasibility study. *Pain Med* 2008;9:55–59.
130. Zempsky WT, Robbins B, McKay K. Reduction of topical anesthetic onset time using ultrasound: a randomized controlled trial prior to venipuncture in young children. *Pain Med* 2008;9: 795–802.
131. Miller KA, Balakrishnan G, Eichbauer G, et al. 1% lidocaine injection, EMLA cream, or "numby stuff" for topical analgesia associated with peripheral intravenous cannulation. *AANA J* 2001;69:185–187.
132. Squire SJ, Kirchhoff KT, Hissong K. Comparing two methods of topical anesthesia used before intravenous cannulation in pediatric patients. *J Pediatr Health Care* 2000;14:68–72.
133. Leopold A, Wilson S, Weaver JS, et al. Pharmacokinetics of lidocaine delivered from a transmucosal patch in children. *Anesth Prog* 2002;49:82–87.

134. Blackburn PA, Butler KH, Hughes MJ, et al. Comparison of tetracaine–adrenaline–cocaine (TAC) with topical lidocaine–epinephrine (TLE): efficacy and cost [see comments]. *Am J Emerg Med* 1995;13:315–317.
135. Kuhn M, Rossi SO, Plummer JL, et al. Topical anaesthesia for minor lacerations: MAC versus TAC. *Med J Aust* 1996;164: 277–280.
136. Bonadio WA. Safe and effective method for application of tetracaine, adrenaline, and cocaine to oral lacerations. *Ann Emerg Med* 1996;28:396–398.
137. Bonadio WA, Wagner V. TAC (tetracaine, adrenaline, cocaine) for the repair of minor dermal lacerations. *Pediatr Emerg Care* 1988; 4:82.
138. Bonadio WA. TAC: a review. *Pediatr Emerg Care* 1989;5:128–130.
139. Samdal F, Amland PF, Bugge JF. Plasma lidocaine levels during suction-assisted lipectomy using large doses of dilute lidocaine with epinephrine. *Plast Reconstr Surg* 1994;93:1217–1223.
140. Kasten GW. Amide local anesthetic alterations of effective refractory period temporal dispersion: relationship to ventricular arrhythmias. *Anesthesiology* 1986;65:61–66.

CHAPTER

48

Sylvain Chemtob
Véronique G. Dorval

Nonsteroidal Anti-Inflammatory Drugs

Inflammation is among the most important tissue responses to injury; it is observed in all acquired disorders as well as genetic conditions modified by environmental exposures. The outcome of the inflammatory response may be beneficial as is the case in limiting invading organisms. On the other hand, the outcome may be deleterious if chronic inflammation ensues, as seen with chronic rheumatic disorders, which lead to pain and destruction of bone and cartilage resulting in potentially severe disability. Inflammation involves a complex sequence paradigm implicating responses of a number of cell types, such that upon early activation of endothelium, leukocytes and monocytes are chemoattracted to the site to contain the injury. The elimination of triggering noxious stimulus is associated with sacrifice of certain cells. Repair involves repopulation of some cells associated with revascularization.

There are numerous mediators of inflammation and their properties are intertwined with one another. For instance, effects of chemokines, interleukins, leukotrienes, and histamine are interlinked in lung inflammation associated with asthma; while in degenerative arthritis interleukins (especially IL-1 and IL-18) interact with prostanoids. Growth factors such as platelet-derived growth factor and vascular endothelial growth factor participate in these processes, especially during the repair phases. In this chapter, we shall focus on lipid mediators modulated by nonsteroidal anti-inflammatory drugs (NSAIDs); we will also cover some pharmacology of acetaminophen which, although not classically an NSAID, may exert its effects (at least in part) via cyclooxygenases (COXs). A review of prostanoid biochemistry and pharmacology will be presented relevant to the mode of action of NSAIDs. Applications of NSAIDs particularly in pyrosis, arthritic conditions, and in indications applicable to the neonate, notably patent ductus arteriosus (PDA) and intraventricular cerebral hemorrhage, will be covered. Detailed descriptions of other agents indicated in pyresis, pain, asthma, some of which also act via prostanoids, will be covered elsewhere in this book.

SYNTHESIS OF PROSTANOIDS

Prostanoids are important autacoids which exert diverse physiological and pathophysiological effects in various systems. These involve modulation of neuronal activity, pyrexia and sleep induction, alterations in platelet aggregation, relaxation and contraction of smooth muscle, regulation of ion and water transport in kidneys as well as of gastrointestinal motility and secretion. There are five physiologically major prostanoids that are well characterized, prostaglandin E_2 (PGE_2), $PGF_{2\alpha}$, PGD_2, PGI_2, and thromboxane A_2 (TXA_2); other prostanoid-like compounds, such as isoprostanes, also exert biological effects through receptor sites that are not yet clearly identified (1–3), and these will not be covered in this review.

Prostanoids derive from arachidonic acid released from phospholipids. Cyclooxygenase (COX) is the enzyme responsible for the committed step in the conversion of arachidonic acid to prostanoids (Fig. 48.1). There are two separate genes encoding COX proteins, COX-1 and COX-2; a splice variant of COX-1, termed COX-3, has also been unidentified (4). COX-1 is mostly constitutive, and COX-2 is highly and readily expressed during inflammation. However, COX-1 also contributes significantly to prostaglandin generation in inflamed tissue (5,6). Along the same lines, COX-2 is normally expressed in a number of tissues independent of inflammatory stimuli, especially during development. For instance, COX-2 is highly expressed in kidneys, and disruption of its gene (in mice) leads to fatal renal failure (7,8); adverse renal effects have also been observed with COX-2 inhibitors (9). COX-2 is also normally expressed in perinatal brain (10).

Both COX-1 and COX-2 catalyze the same reactions by converting arachidonic acid into PGH_2. PGH_2 is then converted into specific prostanoids by individual enzymes. PGE_2 formation is catalyzed by at least one cytosolic and two microsomal isoforms (11–13); PGD_2 by three PGD_2 synthases of which the principal one is lipocalin PGD_2 synthase; and $PGF_{2\alpha}$, PGI_2, and TXA_2 by specific individual

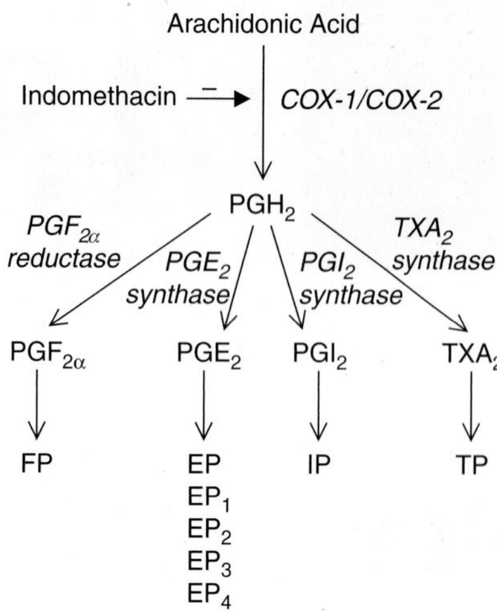

Figure 48.1. Arachidonic acid metabolism via the cyclooxygenase pathway. Nonsteroidal anti-inflammatory drugs (NSAIDs), such as indomethacin, inhibit cyclooxygenase (COX) conversion of arachidonic acid into prostaglandin H_2 (PGH_2).

enzymes; synthases for the latter two exhibit cytochrome P450 properties, and belong to corresponding CYP8 and CYP5 subfamilies, respectively.

COX-3 [and partial COX-1 proteins (a and b)] is derived from the COX-1 gene. COX-3 retains intron 1 of the COX-1 gene, while partial COX-1 protein does not contain a core central sequence of COX-1 (amino acids 119 to 337) (4). These proteins are capable of catalyzing prostaglandin formation and seem to be expressed in brain and heart. Bioactivity of COX-3 revealed that it is inhibited by acetaminophen and phenacetin (acetaminophen prodrug) at IC_{50} of 100 to 500 μM. However, all NSAIDs tested were found to be inhibitors of COX-3 with even greater potency than acetaminophen and phenacetin, especially for diclofenac which had an IC_{50} of 8 nM compared with 35 to 40 nM for COX-1 and COX-2; more recent studies reveal interesting observations pointing to actions of acetaminophen primarily through COX-2 including in humans (14,15). Thus, although COX-3 may be a target for acetaminophen, its relevance regarding acetaminophen effects in the clinical setting is questionable.

PROSTANOID RECEPTORS

Prostanoids exert their effects through respective receptors. On the basis of pharmacological characterization, which was confirmed biochemically, distinct receptors have been identified for prostanoids. A classification for prostanoid receptors was proposed and adopted such that for PGD_2, PGE_2, $PGF_{2\alpha}$, PGI_2, and TXA_2, they are classified, respectively, as DP, EP, FP, IP, and TP; EP receptors are further divided into EP_1, EP_2, EP_3, and EP_4 (16,17). The eight known types of prostanoid receptors are each encoded by an individual gene. The cloning of the prostanoid receptors identified another degree of heterogeneity secondary to mRNA splicing. Splice variants have been identified for the EP_1, EP_3, FP, and TP receptor homologues of various species. There are currently nine known subtypes of the human EP_3 receptor: $EP_{3\text{-}1a}$, $EP_{3\text{-}1b}$, $EP_{3\text{-}II}$, $EP_{3\text{-}III}$, $EP_{3\text{-}IV}$, $EP_{3\text{-}V}$, $EP_{3\text{-}VI}$, $EP_{3\text{-}e}$, and $EP_{3\text{-}f}$ (18–20); subtypes of the EP_3 receptors are distinguished by variances in the tail of the carboxy-terminal portion. Human subtypes also exist for the TP receptor (21), specifically TP_α and TP_β, which as for EP_3 subtypes vary by the tail of their carboxy-terminal end. Although splice variants have been identified for the rat EP_1 (22) and the ovine FP (23) receptors, which also differ by their carboxyl-terminal portions, human homologues to EP_1 and FP subtypes have not been detected.

Sequence homology is mainly based on signaling pathway than on preferential ligand (24–26). The effects of prostanoid receptors on smooth muscle reflect this relationship. Thus, EP_2, EP_4, DP, and IP induce smooth muscle relaxation and are more closely related to each other than to the other prostanoid receptors. Similarly, EP_1, FP, and TP receptors cause smooth muscle contraction and form another group based on sequence homology.

Prostanoid receptors are rhodopsin-type containing seven transmembrane domains, an extracellular amino- and intracellular carboxy-terminus, and belong to the superfamily of G protein-coupled receptors. There are 28 amino acid residues conserved within all prostanoid receptor sequences, and 8 of these are shared with other G protein-coupled receptors. These conserved regions are thought to play fundamental roles in the structure of the prostanoid binding domains. These residues are believed to be particularly important in receptor structure and/or function. For instance, an arginine in the seventh transmembrane domain conserved between all prostanoid receptors was proposed to be the binding site for the carboxyl moiety of the prostanoids (27,28); the conserved motif in the second extracellular loop may also function in this regard (27). In addition, glycosylation is required for ligand binding of certain prostanoid receptors (29).

Three clusters of related receptors have been defined based on their signaling: (i) DP, IP, EP_2, and EP_4; (ii) EP_1, FP, and TP; and (iii) EP_3. Prostanoid receptors in group (i) are linked to heterotrimeric G proteins that are composed of a G_α subunit that generally stimulates adenylate cyclase (designated $G_{\alpha s}$) to produce cyclic AMP. Accordingly, its dominant effect on smooth muscle is relaxation. Prostanoid receptors in group (ii) couple mostly to increases in intracellular free Ca^{2+} through the activation by $G_{\alpha q}$ of phospholipase C, with subsequent inositol phosphate liberation. In smooth muscle, stimulation of this group of receptors leads to contraction. Group (iii), which constitutes the EP_3 subtypes of the prostanoid receptor family, employs as its primary effector pathway inhibition of adenylate cyclase through the $G_{\alpha i}$ family (30). However, because of the variant molecular nature of EP_3, the latter can couple to a variety of G proteins.

The effects of PGE_2 and PGD_2 in inflammation are well established (31). PGE_2 through its EP_3 receptor is also significantly implicated in pyrexia (32), whereas PGD_2 via its DP receptor seems to contribute to allergen-evoked bronchoconstriction (33); moreover, the PGD_2 metabolite 15-deoxy-Δ-PGJ_2 (12,14) is a potent immune modulator.

NONSTEROIDAL ANTI-INFLAMMATORY DRUGS

NSAIDs are a heterogeneous group of agents, which inhibit COX activity (Fig. 48.1). NSAIDs can be classified

TABLE 48.1 Classification of Nonsteroidal Anti-Inflammatory Drugs

Basic Chemical Structure	*Specific Drugs*
Salicylic acid derivatives	Aspirin
	Sodium salicylate
Arylpropionic acids	Fenoprofen
	Flurbiprofen
	Ibuprofen
	Naproxen
	Ketoprofen
Heteroaryl acetic acids	Diclofenac
	Ketorolac
	Tolmetin
Indole and indene acetic acids	Etodolac
	Indomethacin
	Sulindac
Anthranilic acids (fenamates)	Mefenamic acid
	Meclofenamic acid
	Tolfenamic acid
Enolic acids	Meloxicam
	Piroxicam
	Phenylbutazone
	Tenoxicam
Alkanones	Nabumetone
Diarylheterocyclics (coxibs)	Celecoxib
	Rofecoxib
	Valdecoxib
Others	Nimesulide

based on chemical structure (Table 48.1). More recently, specific COX-2 inhibitors have been developed, and older NSAIDs found to exhibit COX-2-preferential properties; the latter has been the case for nimesulide, meloxicam, and etodolac (34).

NSAIDs exert antipyretic, anti-inflammatory, and antinociceptive effects. Despite the pleiotropic nature of prostaglandins in various physiological and pathological processes, the effects of NSAIDs cannot be solely attributed to inhibition of COX. Indeed, COX inhibitors exert a number of COX-independent actions. For instance, doses of aspirin needed to treat chronic inflammatory conditions are much higher than those required to inhibit prostaglandin synthesis. A number of cellular mechanisms affected by NSAIDs, such as angiogenesis, apoptosis, and cell cycle progression, have been observed at NSAID concentrations 100- to 1,000-fold greater than those needed to inhibit prostaglandin formation. In this process, a number of targets other than COX have been identified for NSAIDs, including nuclear factor κB (NF-κB), mitogen-activated protein kinase (Erk2), ribosomal S6 kinase 2, signal transducer and activator of transcription-1 (STAT1), peroxisome proliferator-activated receptor γ (PPARγ), and Akt protein kinase (35–38). However, the effects of NSAIDs on these various targets differ between NSAIDs (39). Moreover, although effects on COX are relatively restricted to the S-stereoisomers, R-stereoisomers act on some of the targets mentioned above.

Nonetheless, a major mechanism of action of NSAIDs is through inhibition of prostaglandin biosynthesis. This is consistent with proinflammatory of certain prostaglandins (34), the fever-inducing actions of PGE_2 via its EP_3 receptors, and nociceptive actions of PGI_2. The mechanism of action of acetaminophen is still debatable. Although attempts to explain its main mechanism of action in vivo through the inhibition of COX-3 have lately mostly been rejected (40,41), recent studies point to significant COX-2 inhibition (14) particularly in the physiological setting when arachinodic acid levels and peroxide tone are relatively low (42,43). Although, its primary site of action appears to be inhibition of PG synthesis, nociceptive modulation by acetaminophen may also arise from activation of descending serotonergic pathways (44,45). Elucidating these mechanisms at the molecular level is currently ongoing.

PHARMACOKINETIC PROPERTIES OF NSAIDs

A detailed review on pharmacokinetics of NSAIDs in children is reported (46). Pharmacokinetics in children is notable by interindividual differences. In general, NSAIDs are rapidly absorbed from the intestine to reach maximal plasma concentrations within 1 to 2 hours. They tend to distribute in a small volume of distribution and are highly bound to plasma proteins; but in children, the apparent volume of distribution is greater than that in adults as shown for diclofenac, ibuprofen, ketorolac, and nimesulide for reasons that are not yet clear. Assuming, a comparable concentration–efficacy relationship, children may require higher loading doses. NSAIDs are metabolized via phase I and II biotransformations. Conjugation occurs mostly with glucuronic acid and sulfate producing mostly inactive compounds. Approximately 60% to 70% of metabolized agents are excreted in urine and the rest in feces.

Aspirin is rapidly absorbed enterally with a t_{max} of 2 hours. It is readily deacetylated by intestinal, hepatic, and blood esterases. Aspirin is metabolized by liver enzymes mostly into salicyluric acid, salicyl phenolic glucuronide, and salicyl acyl glucuronide and altogether account for 90% of metabolites which are inactive and eliminated by the kidneys; because of the ionized form of this acid, its renal elimination is favored in alkaline urine. Interestingly, aspirin metabolism is relatively rapidly saturated, such that its kinetics proceeds from first to zero order; accordingly, the half-life of aspirin changes as a function of dose.

Acetaminophen is very commonly used in the pediatric population. Orally administered acetaminophen is rapidly (t_{max} = 1 hour) and nearly fully absorbed (>90%). In contrast, rectally administered acetaminophen is variable with mean bioavailability of 47% in children. Contrary to most NSAIDs, this drug has low protein binding. Its elimination occurs by conjugation to glucuronide and sulfates, the latter being the dominant form in children up to 9 years of age. A small amount of acetaminophen is oxidized by CYP enzymes. This latter pathway generates electrophilic compounds which require glutathione for detoxification; in overdose, this pathway is overutilized resulting in glutathione depletion and hepatic toxicity.

Specific COX-2 inhibitors have been approved by the Food and Drug Administration (United States) for a number of inflammatory and nociceptive indications; however, increased cardiovascular morbidity (and mortality) with a number of recently developed COX-2 inhibitors has resulted in limiting their applications particularly in adult patients (47,48). Selective COX-2 inhibitors, such as celecoxib, rofecoxib, valdecoxib, as well as meloxicam (semi-selective COX-2 inhibitor), are readily absorbed enterally within 2 to 3 hours for the coxibs and 5 to 6 hours for meloxicam. Celecoxib, valdecoxib, and meloxicam are mainly metabolized by CYP2C9 and to some extent by CYP3A4 (49) and exhibit in the adult a $t_{1/2}$ of 11 and 20 hours, respectively. In children, celecoxib is also well absorbed orally but is cleared much faster with a $t_{1/2}$ of approximately 4 hours (50). Rofecoxib is metabolized by CYP1A2 and cytosolic liver enzymes (51) and has a $t_{1/2}$ of 17 hours; its disposition in children is reported to be similar to that in adults (52).

ANTIPYRETIC EFFICACY OF NSAIDs AND ACETAMINOPHEN

Fever represents the major indication of NSAIDs and acetaminophen in children. Of the NSAIDs, ibuprofen, approved in the United States for this indication, is by far the most commonly utilized in developed countries; aspirin, which has been mostly abandoned because of the risk of Reye syndrome, is still used in underdeveloped parts of the world. Doses of 10 mg per kg ibuprofen and 15 mg per kg acetaminophen have been found to exert similar antipyretic efficacy (53). Higher doses of ibuprofen (specifically 10 compared to 5 mg per kg) were more effective in lowering higher core temperatures (54).

NSAIDs IN JUVENILE RHEUMATOID ARTHRITIS AND OTHER INFLAMMATORY CONDITIONS OF CHILDHOOD

A number of randomized trials have evaluated the efficacy of NSAIDs in juvenile rheumatoid arthritis [for review, see reference no. (46)]. Overall diverse NSAIDs have been found to be equivalently effective, consistent with observations in the adult. Response is also dependent upon duration of therapy and increases with the latter to achieve approximately 80% efficacy after 8 weeks of treatment. Prolonged treatment with NSAIDs as needed for juvenile rheumatoid arthritis seems to augment the risk of gastroduodenal injury to a prevalence of 50% or more (19). On the other hand, significant renal complications are uncommon (55). Pseudoporphyria is an infrequent complication of NSAIDs, essentially limited to naproxen; the condition resolves upon drug discontinuation. Selective COX-2 inhibitors seem to be as effective as nonselective COX inhibitors, but exert fewer gastrointestinal complications (56,57). Although acetaminophen acts principally via COX-2 (14,15), its anti-inflammatory properties are limited as is its efficacy in severe rheumatoid arthritis (1,24,58).

Aspirin is commonly utilized in Kawasaki disease, but its efficacy remains controversial; however, aspirin combined with intravenous immunoglobulins is effective in this condition (59), but in acute Kawasaki it may cause thromboembolism (60). Similarly, the benefits of ibuprofen on lung function in cystic fibrosis have been confirmed in randomized trials (61,62).

ADVERSE EFFECTS SECONDARY TO NSAIDs AND ACETAMINOPHEN

Adverse effects of NSAIDs in children are similar in nature to those described in adults. Ibuprofen seems to exert a 7.2/100,000 risk of gastrointestinal bleeding (63). Mild reversible renal impairment is also observed in 8% to 10% of patients (64); dehydration doubles the risk. Other potential adverse effects of ibuprofen include aseptic meningitis and increased susceptibility of enhanced infections associated with group A β-hemolytic streptococci in children with varicella.

TABLE 48.2 Contraindications for Use of Nonsteroidal Anti-Inflammatory Drugs (NSAIDs)

Allergy to NSAIDs
Nasal polyps
Angioedema or bronchospastic reactivity to NSAIDs
Hypovolemia and dehydration (enhances risk for renal failure)
Peptic ulcer disease
Renal insufficiency
Hepatic insufficiency
Bleeding disorders
Viral illness (only for aspirin: risk of Reye syndrome)

Acetaminophen is relatively safe. High doses are associated with hepatotoxicity. Limitation of acetaminophen doses to less than 60 mg per kg per day virtually abolishes the risk of hepatotoxicity, unless used with other hepatotoxic agents (65).

Overall, NSAIDs have a good tolerance record. Nonetheless, in certain cases, they should be contraindicated (Table 48.2). In light of the cardiovascular effects recently associated with long-term COX-2 inhibitors use in adult, the dosing, tolerance, and safety of selective COX-2 inhibitors in children may need to be revisited.

NSAIDs FOR PATENT DUCTUS ARTERIOSUS OF THE NEWBORN

Patent ductus arteriosus (PDA) is a common complication of the preterm infant. Its incidence is inversely related to gestational age. A patent DA is essential for fetal well-being because it allows 90% of the right ventricular output to bypass the high-resistance pulmonary vascular bed in utero. Prostaglandins play a major role in maintaining ductal patency during fetal life (66). Of the prostaglandins, PGE_2 is the most important ductus arteriosus (DA) relaxant. Accordingly, inhibition in prostaglandin formation favors ductal constriction. Two COX inhibitors, indomethacin and, more recently, ibuprofen (2006), have been approved for the treatment of ductal patency in North America.

Indomethacin

Indomethacin is successful in closing 70% to 90% of patent DA in preterm infants (67). However, the response is variable due to physiological constraints of the more immature DA (68) and differing volume of distribution (69). Accordingly, optimal therapeutic dosing is difficult to establish; acceptable doses range from 0.1 to 0.25 mg per kg administered every 12 to 24 hours.

Numerous randomized trials have been performed to date to evaluate the efficacy of indomethacin in DA closure. A review of the prophylactic (first 24-hour postnatal), presymptomatic (mostly within 72 hours of age), and symptomatic (usually 8 to 10 days of age) trials has recently been published (70). Interestingly, the rate of success in DA closure is irrespective of the age of onset within ages studied. Despite its efficacy in the majority of preterm infants, response to indomethacin seems to be diminished in children of lowest gestational age. In these cases, it has been observed that PGE_2 production resurges within 5 days of indomethacin treatment (~36 hour) (71,72). To circumvent this problem, prolonged treatments (5 to 7 days) with indomethacin were found to minimize ductal reopening (73–75). Evaluation of longer term morbidities revealed that overall the duration of oxygen therapy, hospital stay, the rate of bronchopulmonary dysplasia, and of death were unaffected by indomethacin treatment. Similarly, the rate of necrotizing enterocolitis and of retinopathy of prematurity was not significantly altered with the surprising exception of the collaborative trial (67).

The large trial of indomethacin prophylaxis in preterms (named by the acronym TIPP trial) revealed similar conclusions. Prophylactic indomethacin reduces the rate of PDA in preterm infants, but the rate of bronchopulmonary dysplasia does not seem to be diminished (76,77); this may partly be explained by harmful side effects of indomethacin on oxygenation and edema formation (77). On the other hand, the prophylactic administration of indomethacin during the first week of life significantly reduced the risk of serious pulmonary hemorrhage (78). Prophylactic indomethacin also reduced the rate of severe (grade 4) intraventricular hemorrhage as confirmed in the multicenter studies (76,79), but this did not lead to improved neurodevelopmental outcome (76,80,81), which may be due to direct cerebral hemodynamic compromising effects of indomethacin (82,83); accordingly, the cost-effectiveness of prophylactic indomethacin cannot so far be upheld (84). With this in mind along with the associated rapid decrease in renal (32,82) as well as mesenteric blood flow (82,85) in response to indomethacin bolus injections, continuous slow-rate infusion of indomethacin has been suggested. Using a 36-hour infusion of indomethacin, ductal closure rate was found to be similar to that after bolus injection without the cerebral, renal, and mesenteric hemodynamic compromise seen with the latter (73,82,86).

Ibuprofen

Other strategies to avoid major organ hemodynamic curtailment associated with indomethacin have been proposed in the last few years through the use of alternative NSAIDs. In this regard, ibuprofen has been evaluated since it was found to cause markedly lesser decrease in cerebral, renal, and mesenteric blood flow of the neonate (87–89).

Six randomized trials of symptomatic patent DA compared intravenous ibuprofen to indomethacin (Table 48.3). A recently published large multicenter double-blind randomized trial compared intravenous ibuprofen to placebo on ductal closure and confirmed efficacy and safety of ibuprofen in extremely low-birth-weight infants (90). Overall, the efficacy of ibuprofen was found to be comparable to that of indomethacin. Oliguria was the only variable found to be decreased in ibuprofen-treated infants. Otherwise there was no statistically significant difference between the drugs with regard to mortality, surgical ligation, duration of ventilator support, intraventricular hemorrhage, periventricular leukomalacia, necrotizing enterocolitis, retinopathy of prematurity, sepsis, time to full feeds, gastrointestinal bleed, and duration of hospital stay (22); yet, a tendency toward decreased periventricular leukomalacia was observed in the large US multicenter trial (90).

The relative unavailability of IV ibuprofen in many developing countries has fuelled the assessment of safety and efficacy of oral ibuprofen in the treatment or prophylaxis of PDA. Seven small studies (Table 48.4) to date have reported successful ductal closure with oral ibuprofen. Dosing employed in these studies was directly extrapolated from the intravenous trials. Pharmacokinetic studies revealed lower plasma ibuprofen concentration following oral compared with intravenous administration (91,92). To explain why efficacy and side effect profiles appear to be similar for the two routes of administration, it has been proposed that a more gradual rise in ibuprofen plasma levels and longer half-life from the oral administration could potentially lead to a more sustained inhibition of prostaglandin synthesis despite the lower plasma levels (29,91,93). Although none of the studies on oral ibuprofen reported gastrointestinal adverse events, the safety of the osmolarity of oral ibuprofen formulations and its potential impact on the preterm gut has been raised as a concern (10). Additional adequately powered studies are needed to confirm equivalent efficacy between intravenous and oral routes of administration of ibuprofen in the treatment of PDA.

The trials of prophylactic ibuprofen in preterm infants published to date reveal that prophylactic ibuprofen significantly augmented the rate of DA closure. Other than a slight increase in serum creatinine levels, no other differences in various parameters evaluated were found; notably, there was no statistical difference in mortality, surgical ligation, chronic lung disease, intraventricular hemorrhage, necrotizing enterocolitis, time to full feeds, gastrointestinal bleed, and duration of hospital stay (94). One trial reported pulmonary hypertension in three children treated with prophylactic ibuprofen (95); however, there was no echocardiography performed prior to ibuprofen administration, questioning whether this is a valid side effect. Unlike indomethacin prophylaxis, the prophylactic treatment with ibuprofen has not been shown to reduce the risk of intraventricular hemorrhage in preterm infants (96–98); however, it is important to emphasize that despite the reduction in intraventricular hemorrhage using prophylactic indomethacin, neurodevelopmental outcome is unaffected (76,80,81). Pharmacokinetic data reveal greater plasma clearance of ibuprofen relative to indomethacin and comparable half-lives and protein binding (Table 48.5) (99–102). Ibuprofen peak concentrations seem to be higher in the first postnatal day compared with the third day; a contracted volume of distribution and higher clearance of ibuprofen with increasing postnatal age seem to be responsible for the differences, requiring higher dosing of ibuprofen to reach effective concentrations (103).

Hence, ibuprofen and indomethacin are equivalently effective in closing patent DA. Apart from a diminished rate of oliguria with ibuprofen, adverse effects studied so far are comparable for the two drugs. Studies have shown

TABLE 48.3 Intravenous Ibuprofen and Ibuprofen–Indomethacin Comparative Randomized Trials for Closure of Patent Ductus Arteriosus

Authors (Reference)	*n*	*Gestational Age (wk)*	*Age at Onset of Treatment (d)*	*Ibuprofen Dose (mg/kg i.v.)*[a]	*Indomethacin Dose (mg/kg i.v.)*[b]	*Ductus Arteriosus Closure Rate (%)*		*Undesired Effects*	
						Indomethacin	*Ibuprofen*	*Indomethacin*	*Ibuprofen*
Van Overmeire (125)	40	<33	2–3	10/5/5	0.2 × 3	75	80	Oliguria (80%) ↑ creatinine	Oliguria (5%)
Pezzati (89)	17	<33	2	10/5/5	0.2/0.1/0.1	100	100	Oliguria (80%) ↑ creatinine ↓ CBFV[c]	
Patel (88)	33	<35	3–21	10/5/5	0.2–0.25 × 3	93	78	↓ CBFV	
Lago (126)	175	≤34	2–3	10/5/5	0.2 × 3	82	86	Oliguria (15%) ↑ creatinine	Oliguria (1%)
Van Overmeire (127)	148	≤34	2–4	10/5/5	0.2 × 3	66	70	Oliguria (19%) ↑ creatinine	Oliguria (7%)
Su (128)	63	<32	2–7	10/5/5	0.2 × 3	81	84	Oliguria: > post ibuprofen ↑ creatinine	
Varvarigou[d] (129)	23[e]	<31	≤3 hr	10/5/5	. . .		100		
Dani (96)	40	<34	3	10/5/5	. . .		90		
	40[d]	<34	1	10/5/5	. . .		92		
De Carolis[d] (130)	46	<31	~2 hr	10/5/5	. . .		87		

[a]Sequential daily doses.
[b]Every 12-hr dosing.
[c]CBFV refers to cerebral blood flow velocity.
[d]Prophylactic treatments with ibuprofen; other studies are symptomatic treatments.
[e]Eleven additional babies treated with only one dose ibuprofen (10 mg/kg) had closure rate comparable to saline-treated group ($n = 11$).

TABLE 48.4 Oral Ibuprofen Randomized and Nonrandomized Trials for Closure of Patent Ductus Arteriosus

Authors (Reference)	n	Gestational Age (wk)	Age at Onset of Treatment (d)	Ibuprofen Dose (mg/kg p.o.)[a]	Control	Ductus Arteriosus Closure Rate (%)		Undesired Effects	
						Control[b]	Oral Ibuprofen	Control	Ibuprofen
Randomized									
Supapannachart (131)	18	<34	<10	10/10/10	i.v. Indo[c] 0.2 × 3	89	78	Oliguria	
Chotigeat (132)	30	<35	<10	10/5/5	i.v. Indo[c] 0.2 × 3	67	47	NEC[d]: 67%	NEC: 40%
Aly et al. (133)	21	<35	2–7	10/5/5	i.v. Indo[c] 0.2 × 3	78	83	2 severe lung hemorrage	
Cherif (134)	64	<32	3	10/5/5[e]	3 i.v. Ibu[a] 10/5/5	70	70.3	Increased creatinine	
Nonrandomized									
Hariprasad (135)	13	35–28	3–5	10/5/5[c]	. . .		84.6		
Heyman (136)	22	<32	2	10/5/5[f]	. . .		95.5	31.2% adverse events	9.3% adverse events
Cherif (137)	40	26–31.5	2–4	10/5/5g	. . .		95		

[a]Sequential daily doses.
[b]Control groups: indo = i.v. indomethacin, ibu = i.v. ibuprofen.
[c]Every 12-hr dosing.
[d]NEC refers to necrotizing enterocolitis.
[e]DA closed after one or two doses in 19 subject in oral ibuprofen group, 20 subjects in the intravenous group.
[f]DA closed, respectively, in 14, 6, and 2 subjects after one, two, and three doses.
[g]DA closed, respectively, in 24, 10, and 6 subjects after one, two, and three doses.

TABLE 48.5 Pharmacokinetics of Ibuprofen and Indomethacin in Preterm Infants

Parameters	*Ibuprofen*	*Indomethacin*
C_{max} (μg/mL)	28.4–180.6[a]	0.027–0.31
Cl (mL/kg/hr)	2.1–8.3[a]	4.6–20.1
$t_{1/2}$ (hr)	40–58.4	30–90
Protein binding (%)	95	98

[a]Higher C_{max} and lower Cl on first postnatal day.

that ibuprofen can exert a displacement of protein-bound bilirubin (104). Nonetheless, the high plasma concentration of ibuprofen required for this displacement to occur is not reached when conventional doses of ibuprofen are administered in the treatment of PDA (105). One retrospective cohort study reported higher peak serum bilirubin concentration in infants treated with ibuprofen compared with indomethacin; however, there were no differences as to the duration of phototherapy or the neurodevelopmental outcomes at 2 years in the two groups (39). Additional long-term neurodevelopmental outcomes are needed for more in-depth evaluation of ibuprofen.

COX-1, COX-2, and PGE_2 Receptors in the DA

COX-2 inhibitors have been introduced with the claim that they cause fewer adverse effects. So far, few human studies using COX-2 inhibitors have examined their effects on ductal patency and these have not been direct administrations to newborns. Animal experiments have revealed in some species expression of COX-2 in the fetal DA (106,107), which appears to increase with advancing gestation and contributes to most of the local PGE_2 generation (108). However, selective inhibition of COX-2 (including celecoxib) increases ductal tone to a lesser extent than COX-1 or nonselective COX inhibitors (106,108). Interestingly, COX-2 deficiency in the DA may interfere with DA closure (109,110), suggesting that COX-2 may be required for DA closure. Consistent with these observations, a randomized trial for women at risk of preterm delivery revealed that maternal administration of the selective COX-2 inhibitor celecoxib did not cause fetal ductal closure (50), whereas the semiselective COX-2 inhibitor nimesulide may not be as safe to the fetus as it caused ductal contraction comparable to that seen with indomethacin (111). More importantly, even if selective COX-2 inhibitors do not close DA in the fetus and may be ineffective in the preterm neonate, adverse renal effects are a serious concern (112) and possibly particularly to the neonate (113). Hence, along with the current relative moratorium on COX-2 inhibitors because of potential serious adverse effects, benefits of COX-2 inhibitors cannot be justified.

Microsomal PGE synthase is the principal generator of PGE_2 in the DA (114). Genetic deletion and pharmacological-induced diminished expression of microsomal PGE synthase (115) is associated with increased DA tone; this suggests that microsomal PGE synthase may be a potential target for DA closure.

The fetal DA expresses EP_2, EP_3, and EP_4 receptors of PGE_2 (116–118). Interestingly, stimulation of all three receptors evokes DA relaxation (117). Ontogenic changes in PGE_2 receptor profile in the DA are still debated. The relative role of each of the PGE_2 receptor in physiologic DA relaxation remains to be determined. EP_4 is presumably an important target (6), but its specific function is controversial. On one hand, stimulation of EP_4 opens the DA (119,120) and antagonism of EP_4 closes it (121,122). On the other hand, genetic disruption of EP_4 is associated with patent DA (123) while chronic stimulation of EP_4 promotes hyaluronan-mediated neointimal formation of the DA (124). Hence, as suggested above for COX-2 (109,110), it may be conceivable that EP_4 participates in triggering the ultimate closure of the DA.

In certain congenital heart malformations (e.g., transposition of great vessels, tetralogy of Fallot, coarctation of aorta), patency of DA after delivery is essential for adequate systemic circulation, which is DA dependent. At present, this is clinically achieved by administration of PGE_1. More selective EP stimulation may offer advantages. EP_2 is present in the DA of the term newborn and its stimulation maintains DA patency in newborn animals (108); this has yet to be confirmed in humans.

ACKNOWLEDGMENTS

The authors thank the following agencies that contributed to personal works presented: Canadian Institutes of Health Research (CIHR), Fonds de la Recherche en Santé du Québec, and Heart & Stroke Foundation of Québec. S. Chemtob is recipient of a Canada Research Chair.

REFERENCES

1. Ring EF, Collins AJ, Bacon PA, et al. Quantitation of thermography in arthritis using multi-isothermal analysis. II. Effects of nonsteroidal anti-inflammatory therapy on the thermographic index. *Ann Rheum Dis* 1974;33:353–356.
2. Roberts LJ II, Brame CJ, Chen Y, et al. Novel eicosanoids. Isoprostanes and related compounds. *Methods Mol Biol* 1999; 120:257–285.
3. Roberts LJ II, Morrow JD. The generation and actions of isoprostanes. *Biochim Biophys Acta* 1997;1345:121–135.
4. Chandrasekharan NV, Dai H, Roos KL, et al. COX-3, a cyclooxygenase-1 variant inhibited by acetaminophen and other analgesic/antipyretic drugs: cloning, structure, and expression. *Proc Natl Acad Sci U S A* 2002;99:13926–13931.
5. Gretzer B, Ehrlich K, Maricic N, et al. Selective cyclo-oxygenase-2 inhibitors and their influence on the protective effect of a mild irritant in the rat stomach. *Br J Pharmacol* 1998;123:927–935.
6. Siegle I, Klein T, Backman JT, et al. Expression of cyclooxygenase 1 and cyclooxygenase 2 in human synovial tissue: differential elevation of cyclooxygenase 2 in inflammatory joint diseases. *Arthritis Rheum* 1998;41:122–129.
7. Dinchuk JE, Car BD, Focht RJ, et al. Renal abnormalities and an altered inflammatory response in mice lacking cyclooxygenase II. *Nature* 1995;378:406–409.
8. Morham SG, Langenbach R, Loftin CD, et al. Prostaglandin synthase 2 gene disruption causes severe renal pathology in the mouse. *Cell* 1995;83:473–482.
9. Gambaro G, Perazella MA. Adverse renal effects of anti-inflammatory agents: evaluation of selective and nonselective cyclooxygenase inhibitors. *J Intern Med* 2003;253:643–652.

10. Pereira-da-Silva L, Pita A, Virella D, et al. Orals ibuprofen for patent ductus arteriosus closure in preterm infants: does high osmolality matter? *Am J Perinatol* 2008;43:71–74.
11. Ogorochi T, Ujihara M, Narumiya S. Purification and properties of prostaglandin H-E isomerase from the cytosol of human brain: identification as anionic forms of glutathione S-transferase. *J Neurochem* 1987;48:900–909.
12. Tanikawa N, Ohmiya Y, Ohkubo H, et al. Identification and characterization of a novel type of membrane-associated prostaglandin E synthase. *Biochem Biophys Res Commun* 2002;291:884–889.
13. Watanabe K, Kurihara K, Tokunaga Y, et al. Two types of microsomal prostaglandin E synthase: glutathione-dependent and -independent prostaglandin E synthases. *Biochem Biophys Res Commun* 1997;235: 148–152.
14. Hinz B, Cheremina O, Brune K. Acetaminophen (paracetamol) is a selective cyclooxygenase-2 inhibitor in man. *FASEB J* 2008;22: 383–390.
15. Kis B, Snipes JA, Simandle SA, et al. Acetaminophen-sensitive prostaglandin production in rat cerebral endothelial cells. *Am J Physiol* 2005;288:R897–R902.
16. Coleman RA, Kennedy I, Sheldrick RLG. New evidence with selective agonists and antagonists for the subclassification of PGE2-sensitive (EP) receptors. Adv Prostaglandin Thromboxane Leukot Res 1987;17A:467–470.
17. Coleman RA, Smith WL, Narumiya S. International union of pharmacology classification of prostanoid receptors: properties, distribution, and structure of the receptors and their subtypes. *Pharmacol Rev* 1994;46:205–229.
18. Adam M, Boie Y, Rushmore TH, et al. Cloning and expression of three isoforms of the human EP3 prostanoid receptor. *FEBS Lett* 1994;338:170–174.
19. Kotani M, Tanaka I, Ogawa Y, et al. Structural organization of the human prostaglandin EP3 receptor subtype gene (PTGER3). *Genomics* 1997;40:425–434.
20. Regan JW, Bailey TJ, Donello JE, et al. Molecular cloning and expression of human EP3 receptors: evidence of three variants with differing carboxyl termini. *Br J Pharmacol* 1994;112:377–385.
21. Raychowdhury MK, Yukawa M, Collins LJ, et al. Alternative splicing produces a divergent cytoplasmic tail in the human endothelial thromboxane A_2 receptor. *J Biol Chem* 1994;269:19256–19261.
22. Ohlsson A, Walia R, Shah S. Ibuprofen for the treatment of a patent ductus arteriosus in preterm and/or low birth weight infants. *Cochrane Database Syst Rev* 2003;2:CD003481.
23. Pierce KL, Bailey TJ, Hoyer PB, et al. Cloning of a carboxyl-terminal isoform of the prostanoid FP receptor. *J Biol Chem* 1997;272: 883–887.
24. Boardman PL, Hart FD. Clinical measurement of the anti-inflammatory effects of salicylates in rheumatoid arthritis. *BMJ* 1967;74:264–278.
25. Regan JW, Bailey TJ, Pepperl DJ, et al. Cloning of a novel human prostaglandin receptor with characteristics of the pharmacologically defined EP2 subtype. *Mol Pharmacol* 1994;46:213–220.
26. Toh H, Ichikawa A, Narumiya S. Molecular evolution of receptors for eicosanoids. *FEBS Lett* 1995;361:17–21.
27. Audoly L, Breyer RM. The second extracellular loop of the prostaglandin EP3 receptor is an essential determinant of ligand selectivity. *J Biol Chem* 1997;272:13475–13478.
28. Huang C, Tai HH. Expression and site-directed mutagenesis of mouse prostaglandin E2 receptor EP3 subtype in insect cells. *Biochem J* 1995;307:493–498.
29. Chiang N, Tai HH. The role of *N*-glycosylation of human thromboxane A_2 receptor in ligand binding. *Arch Biochem Biophys* 1998; 352:207–213.
30. Negishi M, Ito S, Yokohama H, et al. Functional reconstitution of prostaglandin E receptor from bovine adrenal medulla with guanine nucleotide binding proteins. *J Biol Chem* 1988;263: 6893–6900.
31. Harris SG, Padilla J, Koumas L, et al. Prostaglandins as modulators of immunity. *Trends Immunol* 2002;23:144–150.
32. van Bel F, Guit GL, Schipper J, et al. Indomethacin-induced changes in renal blood flow velocity waveform in premature infants investigated with color Doppler imaging. *J Pediatr* 1991;118: 621–626.
33. Matsuoka T, Hirata M, Tanaka H, et al. Prostaglandin D2 as a mediator of allergic asthma. *Science* 2000;287:2013–2017.
34. Riendeau D, Percival MD, Boyce S, et al. Biochemical and pharmacological profile of a tetrasubstituted furanone as a highly selective COX-2 inhibitor. *Br J Pharmacol* 1997;121:105–117.
35. Hsu AL, Ching TT, Wang DS, et al. The cyclooxygenase-2 inhibitor celecoxib induces apoptosis by blocking Akt activation in human prostate cancer cells independently of Bcl-2. *J Biol Chem* 2000;275:11397–11403.
36. Jones MK, Wang H, Peskar BM, et al. Inhibition of angiogenesis by nonsteroidal anti-inflammatory drugs: insight into mechanisms and implications for cancer growth and ulcer healing. *Nat Med* 1999;5:1418–1423.
37. Kopp E, Ghosh S. Inhibition of NF-kappa B by sodium salicylate and aspirin. *Science* 1994;265:956–959.
38. Lehmann JM, Lenhard JM, Oliver BB, et al. Peroxisome proliferator-activated receptors alpha and gamma are activated by indomethacin and other non-steroidal anti-inflammatory drugs. *J Biol Chem* 1997;272:3406–3410.
39. Rheinlaender C, Helfenstein D, Walch E, et al. Total serum bilirubin levels during cyclooxygenase inhibitor treatment for patent ductus arteriosus in preterm infants. *Acta Paediatr* 2009; 98:36–42.
40. Kis B, Snipes JA, Busija DW. Acetaminophen and the cyclooxygenase-3 puzzle: sorting out facts, fictions, and uncertainties. *J Pharmacol Exp Ther* 2005;315:1–7.
41. Li S, Dou W, Tang Y, Goorha S, et al. Acetaminophen: antipyretic of hypothermic in mice? In either case, PGHS-1b (COX-3) is irrelevant. *Prostaglandins Other Lipid Mediat* 2008;85:89–99.
42. Boutaud O, Aronoff DM, Richardson JH, et al. Determinants of the cellular specificity of acetaminophen as an inhibitor of prostaglandin H_2 synthase. *Proc Natl Acad Sci U S A* 2002;99: 7130–7135.
43. Graham GG, Scott KF. Mechanism of action of paracetamol. *Am J Ther* 2005;12(1):46–55.
44. Pickering G, Esteves V, Loriot MA, et al. Acetaminophen reinforces descending inhibitory pain pathways. *Clin Pharmacol Ther* 2008;84:47–51.
45. Pickering G, Loriot MA, Libert F, et al. Analgesic effects of acetaminophen in humans: first evidence of a central serotonergic mechanism. *Clin Pharmacol Ther* 2006;79:371–378.
46. Litalien C, Jacqz-Aigrain E. Risks and benefits of nonsteroidal anti-inflammatory drugs in children: a comparison with paracetamol. *Paediatr Drugs* 2001;3:817–858.
47. Fosbøl EL, Gislason GH, Jacobsen S, et al. Risk of myocardial infarction and death associated with the use of nonsteroidal anti-inflammatory drugs (NSAIDs) among healthy individuals: a nationwide cohort study. *Clin Pharmacol Ther* 2009;85:190–197.
48. McGettigan P, Henry D. Cardiovascular risk and inhibition of cyclooxygenase: a systematic review of the observational studies of selective and nonselective inhibitors of cyclooxygenase 2. *JAMA* 2006;296:1633–1644.
49. Rodrigues AD. Impact of CYP2C9 genotype on pharmacokinetics: are all cyclooxygenase inhibitors the same? *Drug Metab Dispos* 2005;33:1567–1575.
50. Stika CS, Gross GA, Leguizamon G, et al. A prospective randomized safety trial of celecoxib for treatment of preterm labor. *Am J Obstet Gynecol* 2002;187:653–660.
51. Karjalainen MJ, Neuvonen PJ, Backman JT. Rofecoxib is a potent, metabolism-dependent inhibitor of CYP1A2: implications for in vitro prediction of drug interactions. *Drug Metab Dispos* 2006;34: 2091–2096.
52. Prescilla RP, Frattarelli DA, Haritos D, et al. Pharmacokinetics of rofecoxib in children with sickle cell hemoglobinopathy. *J Pediatr Hematol Oncol* 2004;26:661–664.
53. Walson PD, Galletta G, Chomilo F, et al. Comparison of multidose ibuprofen and acetaminophen therapy in febrile children. *Am J Dis Child* 1992;146:626–632.
54. Walson PD, Galletta G, Braden NJ, et al. Ibuprofen, acetaminophen, and placebo treatment of febrile children. *Clin Pharmacol Ther* 1989;46:9–17.
55. Allen RC, Petty RE, Lirenman DS, et al. Renal papillary necrosis in children with chronic arthritis. *Am J Dis Child* 1986;140: 20–22.
56. Foeldvari I, Szer IS, Zemel LS, et al. A prospective study comparing celecoxib with naproxen in children with juvenile rheumatoid arthritis. *J Rheumatol* 2009;36:174–182.

57. Reiff A, Lovell DJ, Adelsberg JV, et al. Evaluation of the comparative efficacy and tolerability of rofecoxib and naproxen in children and adolescents with juvenile rheumatoid arthritis: a 12-week randomized controlled clinical trial with a 52-week open-label extension. *J Rheumatol* 2006;33:985–995.
58. Seppala E, Missila M, Isomaki H, et al. Comparison of the effects of different anti-inflammatory drugs on synovial fluid prostanoid concentration in patients with rheumatoid arthritis. *Clin Rheumatol* 1985;4:315–320.
59. De Rosa G, Pardeo M, Rigante D. Current recommendations for the pharmacologic therapy in Kawasaki syndrome and management of its cardiovascular complications. *Eur Rev Med Pharmacol Sci* 2007;11:301–308.
60. Baba R. Effect of immunoglobulin therapy on blood viscosity and potential concerns of thromboembolism, especially in patients with acute Kawasaki disease. *Recent Pat Cardiovasc Drug Discov* 2008; 3:141–144.
61. Konstan MW, Byard PJ, Hoppel CL, et al. Effect of high-dose ibuprofen in patients with cystic fibrosis. *N Engl J Med* 1995;332: 848–854.
62. Lands LC, Stanojevic S. Oral non-steroidal anti-inflammatory drug therapy for cystic fibrosis. *Cochrane Database Syst Rev* 2007;4: CD001505.
63. Lesko SM, Mitchell AA. An assessment of the safety of pediatric ibuprofen. A practitioner-based randomized clinical trial. *JAMA* 1995;273:929–933.
64. Lesko SM, Mitchell AA. Renal function after short-term ibuprofen use in infants and children. *Pediatrics* 1997;100:954–957.
65. Heubi JE, Barbacci MB, Zimmerman HJ. Therapeutic misadventures with acetaminophen: hepatoxicity after multiple doses in children. *J Pediatr* 1998;132:22–27.
66. Coceani F, Oley PM. The response of the ductus arteriosus to prostaglandins. *Can J Physiol Pharmacol* 1973;51:220–225.
67. Gersony WM, Peckham GJ, Ellison RC, et al. Effects of indomethacin in premature infants with patent ductus arteriosus: results of a national collaborative study. *J Pediatr* 1983;102:895–906.
68. Clyman RI, Chen YQ, Chemtob S, et al. In utero remodeling of the fetal lamb ductus arteriosus: the role of antenatal indomethacin and avascular zone thickness on vasa vasorum proliferation, neointima formation, and cell death. *Circulation* 2001;103: 1806–1812.
69. Gal P, Ransom JL, Weaver RL, et al. Indomethacin pharmacokinetics in neonates: the value of volume of distribution as a marker of permanent patent ductus arteriosus closure. *Ther Drug Monit* 1991;13:42–45.
70. Benitz WE. Treatment of persistent patent ductus arteriosus in preterm infants: time to accept the null hypothesis? *J Perinatol* 2010;30:241–252.
71. Clyman RI, Campbell D, Heymann MA, et al. Persistent responsiveness of the neonatal ductus arteriosus in immature lambs: a possible cause for reopening of patent ductus arteriosus after indomethacin-induced closure. *Circulation* 1985;71:141–145.
72. Seyberth HW, Muller H, Wille L, et al. Recovery of prostaglandin production associated with reopening of the ductus arteriosus after indomethacin treatment in preterm infants with respiratory distress syndrome. *Pediatr Pharmacol (New York)* 1982;2:127–141.
73. Hammerman C, Aramburo MJ. Prolonged indomethacin therapy for the prevention of recurrences of patent ductus arteriosus. *J Pediatr* 1990;117:771–776.
74. Leonhardt A, Isken V, Kuhl PG, et al. Prolonged indomethacin treatment in preterm infants with symptomatic patent ductus arteriosus: efficacy, drug level monitoring, and patient selection. *Eur J Pediatr* 1987;146:140–144.
75. Rhodes PG, Ferguson MG, Reddy NS, et al. Effects of prolonged versus acute indomethacin therapy in very low birth-weight infants with patent ductus arteriosus. *Eur J Pediatr* 1988;147:481–484.
76. Schmidt B, Davis P, Moddemann D, et al. Long-term effects of indomethacin prophylaxis in extremely-low-birth-weight infants. *N Engl J Med* 2001;344:1966–1972.
77. Schmidt B, Robert RS, Fanaroff A, et al. Indomethacin prophylaxis, patent ductus arteriosus, and the risk of bronchopulmonary dysplasia: further analyses from the Trial of Indomethacin Prophylaxis in Preterms (TIPP). *J Pediatr* 2006;148:730–734.
78. Alfaleh K, Smyth JA, Roberts RS, et al. Prevention and 18-month outcomes of serious pulmonary hemorrhage in extremely low birth weight infants: results from the trial of indomethacin prophylaxis in preterms. *Pediatrics* 2008;121:e233–e238.
79. Ment LR, Oh W, Ehrenkranz RA, et al. Low-dose indomethacin and prevention of intraventricular hemorrhage: a multicenter randomized trial. *Pediatrics* 1994;93:543–550.
80. Ment LR, Vohr B, Allan W, et al. Outcome of children in the indomethacin intraventricular hemorrhage prevention trial. *Pediatrics* 2000;105:485–491.
81. Vohr BR, Allan WC, Westerveld M, et al. School-age outcomes of very low birth weight infants in the indomethacin intraventricular hemorrhage prevention trial. *Pediatrics* 2003;111:340–346.
82. Christmann V, Liem KD, Semmekrot BA, et al. Changes in cerebral, renal and mesenteric blood flow velocity during continuous and bolus infusion of indomethacin. *Acta Paediatr* 2002;91:440–446.
83. Ohlsson A, Bottu J, Govan J, et al. Effect of indomethacin on cerebral blood flow velocities in very low birth weight neonates with a patent ductus arteriosus. *Dev Pharmacol Ther* 1993;20:100–106.
84. Zupancic JA, Richardson DK, O'Brien BJ, et al. Retrospective economic evaluation of a controlled trial of indomethacin prophylaxis for patent ductus arteriosus in premature infants. *Early Hum Dev* 2006;82:97–103.
85. Van Bel F, Van Zoeren D, Schipper J, et al. Effect of indomethacin on superior mesenteric artery blood flow velocity in preterm infants. *J Pediatr* 1990;116:965–970.
86. Hammerman C, Shchors I, Jacobson S, et al. Ibuprofen versus continuous indomethacin in premature neonates with patent ductus arteriosus: is the difference in the mode of administration? *Pediatr Res* 2008;64:291–297.
87. Mosca F, Bray M, Lattanzio M, et al. Comparative evaluation of the effects of indomethacin and ibuprofen on cerebral perfusion and oxygenation in preterm infants with patent ductus arteriosus. *J Pediatr* 1997;131:549–554.
88. Patel J, Roberts I, Azzopardi D, et al. Randomized double-blind controlled trial comparing the effects of ibuprofen with indomethacin on cerebral hemodynamics in preterm infants with patent ductus arteriosus. *Pediatr Res* 2000;47:36–42.
89. Pezzati M, Vangi V, Biagiotti R, et al. Effects of indomethacin and ibuprofen on mesenteric and renal blood flow in preterm infants with patent ductus arteriosus. *J Pediatr* 1999;135:733–738.
90. Aranda JV, Clyman R, Cox B, et al. A randomized, double-blind, placebo controlled trial on intravenous ibuprofen L-lysin for the early closure of non symptomatic patent ductus arteriosus within 72 hours of birth in extremely low-birth-weight infants. *Am J Perinatol* 2009;26:235–245.
91. Sangtawesin C, Sangtewesin V, Raksasinborisut C, et al. Oral ibuprofen prophylaxis for symptomatic patent ductus arteriosus of prematurity. *J Med Assoc Thai* 2006;89:314–321.
92. Sharma PK, Garg SK, Norang, A. Pharmacokinetics of oral ibuprofen in premature infants. *J Clin Pharmacol* 2003;43:968–973.
93. Sangtawesin C, Sangtewesin V, Lertsutthiwong W, et al. Prophylaxis of symptomatic patent ductus arteriosus with ibuprofen in very low birth weight infants. *J Med Assoc Thai* 2008;91:S28–S34.
94. Shah SS, Ohlsson A. Ibuprofen for the prevention of patent ductus arteriosus in preterm and/or low birth weight infants. *Cochrane Database Syst Rev* 2003;2:CD004213.
95. Gournay V, Savagner C, Thiriez G, et al. Pulmonary hypertension after ibuprofen prophylaxis in very preterm infants. *Lancet* 2002; 359:1486–1488.
96. Dani C, Bertini G, Pezzati M, et al. Prophylactic ibuprofen for the prevention of intraventricular hemorrhage among preterm infants: a multicenter, randomized study. *Pediatrics* 2005;115:1529–1535.
97. Shah SS, Ohlsson A. Ibuprofen for the prevention of patent ductus arteriosus in preterm and/or low birth weight infants. *Cochrane Database Syst Rev* 2006;1:CD004213.
98. Van Overmeire B, Allegaert K, Casaer A, et al. Prophylactic ibuprofen in premature infants: a multicentre, randomised, double-blind, placebo-controlled trial. *Lancet* 2004;364:1945–1949.
99. Aranda JV, Varvarigou A, Beharry K, et al. Pharmacokinetics and protein binding of intravenous ibuprofen in the premature newborn infant. *Acta Paediatr* 1997;86:289–293.
100. Bhat R, Vidyasagar D, Vadapalli M, et al. Disposition of indomethacin in preterm infants. *J Pediatr* 1979;95:313–316.
101. Bianchetti G, Monin P, Marchal F, et al. Pharmacokinetics of indomethacin in the premature infant. *Dev Pharmacol Ther* 1980;1: 111–124.

102. Van Overmeire B, Touw D, Schepens PJ, et al. Ibuprofen pharmacokinetics in preterm infants with patent ductus arteriosus. *Clin Pharmacol Ther* 2001;70:336–343.
103. Hirt D, Van Overmeire B, Treluyer JM, et al. An optimized ibuprofen dosing scheme for preterm neonates with patent ductus arteriosus, based on a population pharmacokinetic and pharmacodynamic study. *Br J Clin Pharmacol* 2008;65:629–636.
104. Cooper-Peel C, Brodersen R, Robertson A. Does ibuprofen affect bilirubin-albumin binding in newborn infant serum? *Pharmacol Toxicol* 1996;79:297–299.
105. Ambat MT, Ostrea EM Jr, Aranda JV. Effects of ibuprofen L-lysinate on bilirubin binding to albumin as measured by saturation index and horseradish peroxidase assays. *J Perinatol* 2008;28:287–290.
106. Clyman RI, Hardy P, Waleh N, et al. Cyclooxygenase-2 plays a significant role in regulating the tone of the fetal lamb ductus arteriosus. *Am J Physiol* 1999;276:R913–R921.
107. Coceani F, Ackerley C, Seidlitz E, et al. Function of cyclo-oxygenase-1 and cyclo-oxygenase-2 in the ductus arteriosus from foetal lamb: differential development and change by oxygen and endotoxin. *Br J Pharmacol* 2001;132:241–251.
108. Guerguerian AM, Hardy P, Bhattacharya M, et al. Expression of cyclooxygenases in ductus arteriosus of fetal and newborn pigs. *Am J Obstet Gynecol* 1998;179:1618–1626.
109. Loftin CD, Trivedi DB, Tiano HF, et al. Failure of ductus arteriosus closure and remodeling in neonatal mice deficient in cyclooxygenase-1 and cyclooxygenase-2. *Proc Natl Acad Sci U S A* 2001;98: 1059–1064.
110. Trivedi DB, Sugimoto Y, Loftin CD. Attenuated cyclooxygenase-2 expression contributes to patent ductus arteriosus in preterm mice. *Pediatr Res* 2006;60:669–674.
111. Sawdy RJ, Lye S, Fisk NM, et al. A double-blind randomized study of fetal side effects during and after the short-term maternal administration of indomethacin, sulindac, and nimesulide for the treatment of preterm labor. *Am J Obstet Gynecol* 2003;188:1046–1051.
112. Giovanni G, Giovanni P. Do non-steroidal anti-inflammatory drugs and COX-2 selective inhibitors have different renal effects? *J Nephrol* 2002;15:480–488.
113. Peruzzi L, Gianoglio B, Porcellini G, et al. Neonatal chronic kidney failure associated with cyclo-oxygenase-2 inhibitors administered during pregnancy. *Minerva Urol Nefrol* 2001;53: 113–116.
114. Bouayad A, Fouron JC, Hou X, et al. Developmental regulation of prostaglandin E_2 synthase in porcine ductus arteriosus. *Am J Physiol* 2004;286:R903–R909.
115. Baragatti B, Sodini D, Uematsu S, et al. Role of microsomal prostaglandin E synthase-1 (mPGES1)-derived PGE2 in patency of the ductus arteriosus in the mouse. *Pediatr Res* 2008;64: 523–527.
116. Bhattacharya M, Asselin P, Hardy P, et al. Developmental changes in prostaglandin E(2) receptor subtypes in porcine ductus arteriosus. Possible contribution in altered responsiveness to prostaglandin E(2). *Circulation* 1999;100:1751–1756.
117. Bouayad A, Kajino H, Waleh N, et al. Characterization of PGE2 receptors in fetal and newborn lamb ductus arteriosus. *Am J Physiol* 2001;280:H2342–H2349.
118. Stempak D, Gammon J, Klein J, et al. Single-dose and steady-state pharmacokinetics of celecoxib in children. *Clin Pharmacol Ther* 2002;72:490–497.
119. Kajino H, Taniguchi T, Fujieda K, et al. An EP4 receptor agonist prevents indomethacin-induced closure of rat ductus arteriosus in vivo. *Pediatr Res* 2004;56:586–590.
120. Momma K, Toyoshima K, Takeuchi D, et al. In vivo reopening of the neonatal ductus arteriosus by a prostanoid EP4-receptor agonist in the rat. *Prostaglandins Other Lipid Mediat* 2005;78: 117–128.
121. Momma K, Toyoshima K, Takeuchi D, et al. In vivo constriction of the fetal and neonatal ductus arteriosus by a prostanoid EP4-receptor antagonist in rats. *Pediatr Res* 2005;58:971–975.
122. Wright DH, Abran D, Bhattacharya M, et al. Prostanoid receptors: ontogeny and implications in vascular physiology. *Am J Physiol* 2001;281:R1343–R1360.
123. Nguyen M, Camenisch T, Snouwaert JN, et al. The prostaglandin receptor EP4 triggers remodelling of the cardiovascular system at birth. *Nature* 1997;390:78–81.
124. Yokoyama U, Minamisawa S, Quan H, et al. Chronic activation of the prostaglandin receptor EP4 promotes hyaluronan-mediated neointimal formation in the ductus arteriosus. *J Clin Invest* 2006;116:3026–3034.
125. Van Overmeire B, Follens I, Hartmann S, et al. Treatment of patent ductus arteriosus with ibuprofen. *Arch Dis Child Fetal Neonatal Ed* 1997;76:F179–F184.
126. Lago P, Bettiol T, Salvadori S, et al. Safety and efficacy of ibuprofen versus indomethacin in preterm infants treated for patent ductus arteriosus: a randomised controlled trial. *Eur J Pediatr* 2002;161:202–207.
127. Van Overmeire B, Smets K, Lecoutere D, et al. A comparison of ibuprofen and indomethacin for closure of patent ductus arteriosus. *N Engl J Med* 2000;343:674–681.
128. Su PH, Chen JY, Su CM, et al. Comparison of ibuprofen and indomethacin therapy for the patent ductus arteriosus in preterm infants. *Pediatr Int* 2003;45:665–670.
129. Varvarigou A, Bardin CL, Beharry K, et al. Early ibuprofen administration to prevent patent ductus arteriosus in premature newborn infants. *JAMA* 1996;275:539–544.
130. De Carolis MP, Romagnoli C, Polimeni V, et al. Prophylactic ibuprofen therapy of patent ductus arteriosus in preterm infants. *Eur J Pediatr* 2000;159:364–368.
131. Supapannachart S, Limrungsikul A, Khowsathit P. Oral ibuprofen and indomethacin for treatment of patent ductus arteriosus in premature infants: a randomized trial at Ramathibodi Hospital. *J Med Assoc Thai* 2002;85:S1252–1258.
132. Chotigeat U, Jirapap K, Layangkool T. A Comparison of oral ibuprofen and intravenous indomethacin for the closure of patent ductus arteriosus in preterm infants. *J Med Assoc Thai* 2003;86:S563–569.
133. Aly H, Lofty W, Badrawi N, Ghawa M, Abdel-Meguid IE, Hammad TA. Oral ibuprofen and the PDA in premature infants: a randomized pilot study. *Am J Perinatol* 2007;24:267–270.
134. Cherif A, Khrouf N, Jabnoun S, et al. Randomized pilot study comparing oral ibuprofen with intravenous ibuprofen in very low birth weight infants with patent ductus arteriosus. *Pediatrics* 2008;122:e1256–261.
135. Hariprasad P, Sundarrajan V, Srimathy G, et al. Oral ibuprofen for closure of hemodynamically significant PDA in premature neonates. *Indian Pediatr* 2002;39:99–100.
136. Heyman E, Morag I, Batash D, Keidar R, Baram S, Berkovitch M. Closure of patent ductus arteriosus with oral ibuprofen suspension in premature newborns; a pilot study. *Pediatrics.* 2003;112: 354–358.
137. Cheriff A, Janoun S, Krouf N. Oral ibuprofen in the early curative closure of patent ductus arteriosus in very premature infants. *Am J Perinatol* 2007;24:3339–346.

CHAPTER

49

Thomas G. Wells
Mohammad Ilyas
Russell W. Chesney
Deborah P. Jones

Antihypertensive Agents

Until 1997, few antihypertensive agents were studied systematically in children, and very few were labeled for use in patients younger than 18 years (1). As new drugs were introduced into the market, pediatricians had to choose between the use of promising new agents without the benefit of controlled studies in a pediatric population and continued use of older but familiar agents. The First and Second Task Force Reports on Blood Pressure Control in Children offered treatment schemes based on strategies that were used in adults at the time (2,3). These schemes tacitly recognized the need to use drugs that were not labeled for use in children. Off-label use, with all of its implied risks, was often the only viable option available to physicians who treated children with hypertension (1). Newer drugs promised not only new approaches to the treatment of hypertension but also, in many cases, fewer adverse effects.

Recognizing the need to address this inequity, several federal initiatives designed to include children in the drug development process were proposed. In 1994, the Food and Drug Administration (FDA) promulgated the Pediatric Rule, which was expanded in 1998 and required manufacturers to perform limited studies in children if a new drug offered any potential health benefits in the pediatric population (4,5). With the passage of the FDA Modernization Act (FDAMA) in 1997 and later the Best Pharmaceuticals for Children Act (BPCA) in 2002, pharmaceutical firms were granted meaningful incentives in exchange for conducting appropriate pediatric studies (6,7).

The enabling legislation and regulatory requirements led to a dramatic increase in the number of pediatric trials. As a result, the number of anti-hypertensive medications with pediatric labeling has increased (8,9) (Table 49.1). In addition, several extemporaneously compounded liquid solutions were developed and tested for short-term stability and bioequivalence (10–12). Because very few drugs used to treat hypertension in children are manufactured as commercially available solutions or suspensions, these extemporaneous formulations represented a significant advance in treating younger children who are unable to swallow tablets or capsules.

HYPERTENSION IN CHILDREN

As many as 10% to 13% of children will have elevated blood pressure (BP) on a single measurement (13,14), but persistent hypertension is observed in only 1% to 2.5% of the pediatric population (15–18). More recent data estimates that the prevalence of pre-hypertension is nearly 10% and established hypertension 4%, with greater burden on minority children (19). Despite the availability of widely accepted normative BP data (20), the accurate diagnosis of persistent hypertension can be difficult. Errors in cuff selection and technique are still common despite publication of accepted methods for performing casual BP measurement in children (18). Labile BP and the "white coat" effect complicate the diagnosis in children with high normal BP or borderline to moderate hypertension (21,22). The use of ambulatory blood pressure monitoring (ABPM) in these children has helped to separate those who require evaluation and treatment from those who need only longitudinal observation (20,23,24). Accurate diagnosis is extremely important because failure to diagnose and adequately control clinically significant hypertension may result in the development of target organ damage (25–30). Conversely, improper diagnosis and subsequent treatment of normotensive children may risk unnecessary exposure to adverse events.

Selection of appropriate therapy often depends on the suspected cause of hypertension. Secondary causes of hypertension, particularly renal and renovascular diseases, are commonly observed among preadolescent children (Table 49.2) (20,31,32). During adolescence, secondary causes of hypertension continue to occur, but the prevalence of primary hypertension increases dramatically (20,33). It is likely that obesity, insulin resistance, and genetically determined factors contribute to the development of hypertension in some adolescents (34–37). Both primary and secondary hypertension in children and adolescents may result in significant target organ damage (25–30). It is particularly important that these children receive adequate antihypertensive therapy. The working group has recommended that pharmacologic treatment be initiated in individuals with symptomatic hypertension,

TABLE 49.1 Antihypertensive Medications with Pediatric Labeling (8)

Amlodipine[a]	Furosemide
Benazepril[a]	Hydralazine
Candesartan[a]	Irbesartan[a]
Captopril	Lisinopril[a]
Chlorothiazide	Losartan[a]
Diazoxide	Metoprolol[a]
Enalapril[a]	Minoxidil
Eplerenone[a]	Propranolol
Fenoldopam[a]	Spironolactone
Fosinopril[a]	Valsartan[a]

[a]Denotes post-Food and Drug Administration Modernization Act.

secondary hypertension, evidence of target organ damage (left ventricular hypertrophy), diabetes (type 1 and 2), and persistent hypertension after attempted life-style change (20). Unfortunately, these recommendations lack the support of clinical trials.

Dietary modifications, weight reduction, and aerobic exercise are useful interventions in almost all children with hypertension (20). These nonpharmacologic therapies are often employed initially as the sole treatment in children with prehypertension (90th to 95th percentile) and stage I (95th to 99th percentile) primary hypertension who do not exhibit target organ damage and have few, if any, additional cardiovascular risk factors (38). It is important to note that nonpharmacologic therapies often augment the effectiveness of selected antihypertensive agents in both primary and secondary hypertension in children [e.g., sodium chloride restriction and angiotensin-converting enzyme (ACE) inhibitor therapy].

TABLE 49.3 Individualization of Antihypertensive Therapy in Children: Factors to Consider

Diagnosis: primary versus secondary cause for hypertension
Severity of hypertension
Patient compliance issues
- School and activity schedules
- Supportive parent(s)/guardian(s)
- Self-motivation
- Dosing interval
- Cost

Patient demographics
- Race
- Gender
- Age

Concurrent diseases or medical conditions
Concurrent nonpharmacologic therapies
Concomitant drug therapy
Available formulations
Athletic participation

In children, as in adults, many physicians have abandoned the traditional stepped-care approach to therapy. Individualized selection of therapeutic agents in children depends on many factors (Table 49.3).

CLASSIFICATION OF ANTIHYPERTENSIVE AGENTS

A scheme for classifying antihypertensive agents is presented in Table 49.4. Diuretics, although quite useful in the treatment of hypertension in children, are considered elsewhere (Chapter 43). Angiotensin-II-receptor antagonists (ARBs),

TABLE 49.2 Causes of Hypertension in Children (3,30–43)

Neonates (0–1 mo)	*Infants/Toddlers (1–24 mo)*	*Preschool (2–5 yr)*	*School Aged (6–11 yr)*	*Adolescent (12–18 yr)*
Renovascular[a]	Renal parenchymal diseases	Renal parenchymal diseases	Renal parenchymal diseases	Primary
Coarctation of the aorta	Coarctation of the aorta	Coarctation of the aorta	Renal artery stenosis	Obesity
Recessive polycystic kidney disease	Renovascular[b]	Renal artery stenosis	Obesity	Renal parenchymal diseases
Miscellaneous renal/urologic lesions	Recessive polycystic kidney disease		Primary	Renal artery stenosis
Abdominal wall defect closure	Bronchopulmonary dysplasia	Genetic disorders[c]	Genetic disorders[c]	Genetic disorders[c]
Drugs[d]	Drugs[e]	Drugs	Drugs[f]	Drugs[g]
All ages: Fluid overload; pain; endocrine disorders (excessive endogenous aldosterone; exogenous or endogenous thyroxine, corticosteroids, or catecholamines); increased intracranial pressure; drugs, corticosteroids, β_2-adrenergic agonists.				

[a]Renal artery thrombosis, renal artery hypoplasia, renal vein thrombosis.
[b]Renal artery stenosis, renal vein thrombosis.
[c]Neurofibromatosis, Williams syndrome, Turner syndrome, etc.
[d]Sympathomimetics, narcotic withdrawal (transplacental exposure).
[e]Adrenocorticotropic hormone.
[f]Decongestants, stimulants.
[g]Decongestants, stimulants, cocaine, amphetamines, anabolic steroids.

TABLE 49.4 Classification of Available Antihypertensive Agents[a]

Class	*Subclass*	*Most Frequently Used Agents*
Diuretics	Thiazides	Hydrochlorothiazide, chlorothiazide, chlorthalidone
	Thiazide-like	Indapamide
	Loop diuretics	Furosemide, bumetanide
	Potassium sparing	Spironolactone, amiloride, triamterene
Adrenergic antagonists	Selective α_1	Prazosin, doxazosin, terazosin
	Selective α_2 (central agonist)	Clonidine
	Nonselective (α_1 and α_2)	Phentolamine, phenoxybenzamine
	Selective β_1	Atenolol, bisoprolol, metoprolol, acebutolol, esmolol
	Nonselective (β_1 and β_2)	Propranolol, nadolol, pindolol, timolol
	α_1 and nonselective β	Labetalol, carvedilol
Calcium channel antagonists	Dihydropyridines	Nifedipine, amlodipine, nicardipine, felodipine, isradipine, nisoldipine
	Nondihydropyridines	Diltiazem, verapamil
Angiotensin-converting enzyme inhibitors	Sulfhydryl group	Captopril
	Dicarboxyl group	Enalapril, lisinopril, ramipril, quinapril, benazepril, moexipril, perindopril
	Phosphate group	Fosinopril
Angiotensin-II (AT-1)-receptor antagonists		Losartan, candesartan, irbesartan, olmesartan, telmisartan, valsartan
Direct vasodilators	Predominantly arterial dilation	Hydralazine, diazoxide, minoxidil
	Arterial and venous dilation	Nitroprusside
Miscellaneous	Dopamine-D1 (moderate α_2 affinity)	Fenoldopam

[a]Many older drugs (primarily centrally acting agents with significant adverse effects) that are no longer widely used in children are not listed.

ACE inhibitors, calcium channel blockers (CCBs), adrenergic inhibitors, and direct vasodilators represent the main focus of this chapter.

Although initial data concerning the pharmacokinetics, effectiveness, and safety of antihypertensives in children are becoming available, the large-scale comparative trials conducted in adults that show superiority of one drug or one therapeutic approach over another have not been conducted in children. For a variety of reasons, it is unlikely that studies similar to the widely publicized Antihypertensive and Lipid-Lowering Treatment to Prevent Heart Attack Trial (ALLHAT) (39), which compared representative drugs from four different therapeutic classes in a population of 33,357 subjects, will be conducted in children in the foreseeable future. Many similar studies are ongoing in the adult population (40). Hence, in treating children with hypertension, choices among available drug classes rely less on specific comparative data collected from pediatric patients and more on the suspected cause of the elevated BP, previous clinical experience, extrapolation from studies conducted in adults, and availability of pediatric formulations. Recommended dosing for antihypertensive agents for children and adolescents (Table 49.5) and neonates (Table 49.6) is based on currently available information and may be subject to change depending on the outcome of ongoing studies. Antihypertensive agents used in the treatment of hypertensive emergencies and urgencies are presented in Table 49.7.

ADRENERGIC AGENTS

The sympathetic division of the autonomic nervous system plays a key role in the regulation of BP. At the postganglionic synapse, norepinephrine is released from vesicles in the presynaptic membrane in response to sympathetic stimulation and binds to receptors on postganglionic effector organs. Stimulation of sympathetic nerves terminating in the adrenal medulla results in release of epinephrine and, to a lesser extent, other catecholamines into circulating blood.

The effects of the adrenergic nervous system are mediated through α and β receptors, each of which has subtypes. The α_1 adrenoceptors are located in the heart and smooth muscle in blood vessels, the intestinal tract, and the genitourinary tract. The cardiovascular effects of α_1 stimulation include vasoconstriction, increased systemic vascular resistance, and increased BP. Stimulation of α_2 receptors, which are located primarily at the postganglionic presynaptic membrane, inhibits further release of norepinephrine. Distinct subtypes of both α_1 and α_2 receptors have been identified. β_1- and β_2-adrenergic receptors are segregated based on their response to norepinephrine and epinephrine. The β_1 receptors, located primarily in the heart, adipose tissue, and juxtaglomerular cells, respond equivalently to epinephrine and norepinephrine. Stimulation of β_1 receptors results in tachycardia, increased myocardial contractility, increased conduction velocity in the atrioventricular node, and lipolysis. At β_2 receptors, response to norepinephrine is much less than that seen after stimulation with epinephrine. The β_2 receptors are found in many organs including the liver, skeletal muscle, and smooth muscle located in the vasculature and the gastrointestinal, respiratory, and genitourinary tracts. Stimulation of β_2 receptors results in smooth muscle relaxation and bronchodilation, vasodilation, and increased glucose release. As with α receptors, distinct subtypes of both β_1 and β_2 receptors have been identified.

TABLE 49.5 Drug Therapy for Children and Adolescents with Chronic Hypertension[a]

	Initial Dose	*Dosing Interval (hr)*	*Maximum Recommended dose*	*Adverse Effects*
Diuretics				
Thiazides				
Chlorothiazide	5–15 mg/kg/dose	12–24	30 mg/kg/d	Electrolyte disturbances, dehydration, hypocalciuria, nausea, vomiting, diarrhea
Chlorthalidone	0.25–0.5 mg/kg/d	24–48	1 mg/kg/d (100 mg/d)	
Hydrochlorothiazide[b]	0.25–0.5 mg/kg/d	12–24	2 mg/kg/d (100 mg/d)	
Loop diuretics				
Furosemide	0.5–1 mg/kg/dose (p.o. or i.v.)[c]	6–24	6 mg/kg/d (600 mg/d)	Electrolyte disturbances, dehydration, hypercalciuria, hyperuricemia, ototoxicity (at very high doses)
Bumetanide	0.02–0.05 mg/kg/dose (p.o. or i.v.)[c]	6–24	0.4 mg/kg/d (10 mg/d)	
Potassium-sparing agents				
Spironolactone	1 mg/kg/d	6–24	3.3 mg/kg/d (200 mg/d)	Hyperkalemia, nausea, vomiting, gynecomastia (males), breast tenderness
Adrenergic antagonists[d]				
Acebutolol[e]	Adolescents: 200 mg/d	12–24	1200 mg/d	Bradycardia, atrioventricular conduction disturbances, lethargy, vomiting, impotence
Atenolol	0.5–1.0 mg/kg/dose	24	2 mg/kg/d (200 mg/d)	
Labetalol	3–4 mg/kg/dose	8–12	10–20 mg/kg/d[f] (1,200 mg/d[f])	
Metoprolol	Adolescents: 100 mg/d	12–24	(400 mg/d)	
Propranolol	0.5–1.0 mg/kg/dose	6–12	8 mg/kg/d (640 mg/d)	
Calcium channel antagonists				
Amlodipine	0.05–0.1 mg/kg/dose	24	0.6 mg/kg/d (10 mg/d)	Hypotension, flushing, tachycardia, headache, nausea, peripheral edema
Isradipine	Adolescents: 0.15–0.2 mg/kg	12	0.8 mg/kg (20 mg/d)	
Nifedipine (sustained release)	0.25–0.5 mg/kg/dose	12–24	3 mg/kg/d	
Diltiazem (sustained release)	1.5–2.0 mg/kg/dose	24	6 mg/kg/d (360 mg/d)	
Angiotensin-converting enzyme inhibitors				
Captopril	0.3–0.5 mg/kg/dose	6–12	6 mg/kg/d (450 mg/d)	Hypotension, oliguria, acute renal failure, hyperkalemia, nonproductive cough, dizziness, neutropenia (rare), angioedema (rare)
Enalapril	0.08 mg/kg/d	12–24	0.6 mg/kg/d (40 mg/d)	
Fosinopril	0.1 mg/kg/dose	24	0.6 mg/kg (80 mg/d)	
Lisinopril	0.07 mg/kg/dose (maximum: 5 mg)	24	0.6 mg/kg/d (40 mg/d)	
Quinapril	5–10 mg/dose	24	80 mg	
Angiotensin-II-receptor antagonists				
Candesartan		24	32 mg/d	
Irbesartan	2 mg/kg/dose	24	300 mg/d	
Losartan	0.7 mg/kg/d (50 mg)	24	1.4 mg/kg/d (100 mg)	
Direct vasodilators				
Minoxidil	0.1–0.2 mg/kg/dose	12–24	1.0 mg/kg/d (50 mg/d)	Hypotension, dizziness, fluid retention, tachycardia, pericardial effusion, hypertrichosis, Stevens–Johnson syndrome (rare)

[a]Unless otherwise indicated, all doses refer to oral dosing. p.o., oral; i.v., intravenous.

[b]For treatment of chronic hypertension, the initial dose of hydrochlorothiazide is lower than the 2 mg/kg/d dosage recommended in many pediatric drug reference guides (191). Studies in adults have shown that lower doses often provided an acceptable antihypertensive effect with fewer adverse effects. Thiazides may have synergistic effects with other classes of antihypertensive agents, particularly angiotensin-converting enzyme inhibitors and angiotensin-II-receptor antagonists.

[c]Loop diuretics are useful in patients with hypertension secondary to renal diseases and volume overload but are not commonly used to treat primary hypertension. The oral bioavailability of furosemide and bumetanide is approximately 40% and 80%, respectively. This should be considered when switching between intravenous and oral dosing.

[d]The pure α-adrenergic antagonists are not widely used to treat hypertension in children, and dosing information has not been included. In adults, they have been shown to be inferior to other classes of drugs in the treatment of primary hypertension (55).

[e]Acebutolol is the only β_1-selective antagonist with intrinsic sympathomimetic activity (ISA). There are several nonselective β antagonists (carteolol, penbutolol, pindolol) with ISA, but none has been studied adequately in children.

[f]One reference suggests that children may tolerate up to 40 mg/kg/d (191). However, there are few data to support this high dose, and a more prudent maximum daily dose may be 10 to 20 mg/kg. It is not known whether the maximum daily dose (2,400 mg) in adults is appropriate for children. Adverse effects increase in frequency at daily doses exceeding 1,200 mg. Until more data are available, a maximum daily dose of 1,200 mg in children seems prudent.

TABLE 49.6 Drug Therapy for Hypertension in Neonates[a]

	Initial Dose	*Dosing Interval (hr)*	*Maximum Recommended Dose*	*Adverse Effects*
Angiotensin-converting enzyme inhibitors[b]				
Captopril	0.01 mg/kg/dose	6–12	0.5 mg/kg/dose (2 mg/kg/d)	Hypotension, oliguria, acute renal failure, hyperkalemia, seizures
Enalaprilat	5–10 μg/kg/dose (i.v.)	8–24	20 μg/kg/dose (i.v.)	
Calcium channel antagonists				
Nifedipine[c]	0.25 mg/kg/dose	6–8	3 mg/kg/d	Hypotension, flushing, tachycardia, peripheral edema
Amlodipine[c]	0.1 mg/kg/dose	24	0.6 mg/kg/d	
Adrenergic antagonists				
Propranolol	0.25–1.0 mg/kg/dose (p.o.)	6–12	5 mg/kg/d	Bradycardia, atrioventricular conduction disturbances, lethargy, vomiting
Atenolol	0.25–0.5 mg/kg/dose (p.o.)	24	2 mg/kg/d	
Labetalol	0.5–1 mg/kg/dose (p.o.), 0.25 mg/kg/dose (i.v.)[d]	8–12 (p.o.), 2–4 (i.v.)	Not known	
Diuretics				
Chlorothiazide	5–15 mg/kg/dose	12–24	30 mg/kg/d	Electrolyte disturbances, dehydration, vomiting, diarrhea
Furosemide	0.5–1 mg/kg/dose (p.o. or i.v.)[d]	12–24	4 mg/kg/d	
Bumetanide	0.05 mg/kg/dose (p.o. or i.v.)[d]	12–24	0.4 mg/kg/d	
Vasodilators				
Hydralazine[e]	0.1–0.2 mg/kg/dose (i.v.)	6–8	1 mg/kg/dose (5 mg/kg/d)	Tachycardia, emesis, diarrhea, irritability

[a]i.v., intravenous; p.o., oral.
[b]Starting doses listed are for preterm neonates and term neonates during the first few days of life. Higher initial and maximal doses may be needed in hemodynamically stable, older term neonates.
[c]Nifedipine is available only in rapid-release capsules and sustained-release tablets. The capsules contain a liquid, but the 10 mg/capsule dose is difficult to prepare for neonates. Nifedipine is no longer widely used in neonates because of difficulty preparing accurate doses, unpredictable and sometimes large decreases in blood pressure, and the availability of safer alternative drugs. An extemporaneous, orally administered suspension of amlodipine can be prepared (176).
[d]May be administered by continuous infusion.
[e]Overall use is diminishing; long-term oral administration is no longer widely used.

β-Adrenergic-receptor antagonists are distinguished by selectivity for the β_1-adrenergic receptor (Table 49.8), the presence of intrinsic sympathomimetic activity, unique pharmacologic properties (Table 49.9), and α-adrenergic blocking activity. Cardioselective drugs have greater affinity for β_1-adrenergic receptors, and nonselective agents have approximately equal affinity for both β_1- and β_2-adrenergic receptors. At higher doses, cardioselective agents may demonstrate not only β_1-antagonist activity but also some degree of β_2 antagonism. Some β-adrenergic antagonists, including acebutolol and pindolol, have small but significant β-agonist effect, known as intrinsic sympathomimetic activity. Because the agonist effect is significantly less than the antagonist effect, the antihypertensive properties of these agents are not compromised. Intrinsic sympathomimetic activity of β-adrenergic blockers helps to reduce selected adverse effects resulting from β_1 antagonism (e.g., bradycardia).

Adrenergic antagonists reversibly or irreversibly bind to α and β receptors. Receptor blockade antagonizes the effects of norepinephrine at the postganglionic synaptic membrane as well as circulating catecholamines. The resultant effects are complex and depend on the type of receptors that are blocked and the unique properties possessed by individual agents (41).

α-ADRENERGIC ANTAGONISTS

Chronic administration of peripheral α-adrenergic-receptor antagonists is uncommon in children. The prazosin arm of ALLHAT was stopped early because it was found to be inferior to other antihypertensive drugs (39). Clonidine, which stimulates central α_2 receptors, resulting in inhibition of sympathetic outflow from the vasomotor center in the brain, is occasionally used when centrally mediated hypertension is suspected or selected comorbid conditions occur. Clonidine can be administered orally or transdermally. Transdermal clonidine has been useful in patients who are not compliant with oral dosing regimens. Some patients are unable to tolerate the adverse effects frequently associated with chronic oral administration of clonidine, including somnolence and xerostomia. Clonidine should be withdrawn slowly, as rebound hypertension may occur after abrupt cessation of therapy. Other central sympatholytics are rarely used to treat hypertension in ambulatory children.

Phentolamine and phenoxybenzamine are used to treat acute, severe BP elevation, which occurs in conditions associated with excess circulating catecholamines. Phentolamine is a competitive inhibitor of α_1 and α_2 receptors useful for short-term treatment of hypertension secondary to

TABLE 49.7 Drug Therapy for Hypertensive Urgencies and Emergencies in Pediatric Patients (Excluding Neonates)

	Initial Dose	*Onset [Duration] of Action*	*Dosing Interval*	*Maximum Dose*
Hypertensive urgencies[a]				
Nifedipine	0.25 mg/kg/dose (max: 10 mg)	20–30 min [3–6 hr]	4–6 hr	0.5 mg/kg/dose 3 mg/kg/d (120 mg/d)
Captopril	0.3–0.50 mg/kg/dose (max: 50 mg)	15–30 min [dose related]	6–12 hr	2 mg/kg/dose 6 mg/kg/d (450 mg/d)
Minoxidil	0.1–0.2 mg/kg/dose (max: 5 mg)	30 min [2–5 d]	12–24 hr	0.25–1.0 mg/kg/d 1 mg/kg/d (50 mg/d)
Hypertensive urgencies or emergencies[a]				
Enalaprilat[b]	0.1 mg/kg/d (max: 1.25 mg)	5–15 min [4–24 hr]	6–24 hr	5 mg/dose (20 mg/d)
Esmolol[c]	Load: 100–500 μg/kg		Load over 1 min	500 μg/kg 1,000 μg/kg/min
	Continuous infusion: 25–250 μg/kg/min	2–10 min [10–30 min]	Titrate: 5–10 min	
Labetalol	Intermitted: 0.2–1.0 mg/kg/dose	2–5 min [2–4 hr]	10 min (as needed)	300 mg/dose
	Continuous infusion: 0.25–1.5 mg/kg/hr		Titrate: 10 min	1.5 mg/kg/hr
Nicardipine[d]	0.5–3.0 μg/kg/min (adult: 5 mg/hr)	1–2 min	Titrate: 5–15 min	Unknown (adults: 3–15 mg/hr)
Nitroprusside[e]	0.3–0.5 μg/kg/min	1–2 min [1–10 min]	Titrate: 5–10 min	8 μg/kg/min

[a]Intravenous loop diuretic therapy may be beneficial for patients with volume overload.
[b]Reduce dose of enalaprilat with concurrent diuretic therapy. Use with extreme caution in patients with bilateral renal artery stenosis.
[c]β_1 Selective at low doses, but at higher doses, β_2-antagonist activity may be observed and bronchoconstriction may occur.
[d]Avoid in patients with head trauma and space-occupying central nervous system lesions.
[e]At higher doses (>4 μg/kg/min) or in patients with renal failure, thiocyanate or cyanide concentrations should be monitored with prolonged use.

pheochromocytoma. Phenoxybenzamine irreversibly blocks α_1 and α_2 receptors but, unlike phentolamine, can be administered orally. Blockade of α receptors decreases systemic vascular resistance and lowers the BP. Hypotension may occur at higher doses.

TABLE 49.8 Classification of β-Adrenergic-Receptor Antagonists

Drug	*Intrinsic Sympathomimetic Activity*	*α-Adrenergic Activity*
β_1 Selective		
Acebutolol	Yes	No
Atenolol	No	No
Betaxolol	No	No
Bisoprolol	No	No
Esmolol	No	No
Metoprolol	No	No
Nonselective		
Carteolol	Yes	No
Penbutolol	Yes	No
Pindolol	Yes	No
Carvedilol	No	Yes
Labetalol	No	Yes
Nadolol	No	No
Propranolol	No	No
Timolol	No	No

β-ADRENERGIC ANTAGONISTS

The β-adrenergic antagonists have been used to treat hypertension in children for more than 25 years. These agents attenuate sympathetic stimulation through competitive antagonism of epinephrine and norepinephrine at β-adrenergic receptors. Reversible blockade of β-adrenergic receptors lowers the BP by several means. Depending on the underlying pathology present in individual patients and the properties of individual drugs, the initial and long-term physiologic effects may differ (41). Proposed mechanisms for the antihypertensive effect of β-adrenergic antagonism include inhibition of β_1-adrenergic receptors of juxtaglomerular cells, thus inhibiting renin release (42,43); presynaptic facilitatory β_2-adrenergic receptors at the vascular wall; norepinephrine release from sympathetic nerve endings (44); and sympathetic outflow from the central nervous system (CNS) (45). The antihypertensive effect of β-adrenergic antagonists usually results from a combination of these factors.

The immediate systemic hemodynamic effects of β-adrenergic antagonists in hypertensive subjects are reduction in myocardial contractility, cardiac output, and heart rate. In the absence of β_2-adrenergic-induced vasodilation, peripheral vascular resistance increases due to unopposed α-adrenergic activity (46,47). With long-term use of β-adrenergic antagonist therapy, heart rate and cardiac output are reduced. Unexpectedly, long-term administration of β-adrenergic antagonists has been associated with a

TABLE 49.9 Pharmacology of Adrenergic Antagonists Commonly used in Children

Drug	*First-Pass Effect*[a]	*Oral Bioavailability (%)*	T_{max} *(hr)*	*Metabolism/ Elimination*	*Elimination Half-Life (hr)*
Propranolol	Low	25–40	1–2	Hepatic	3–6
Atenolol	Low	50–60	2–4	Renal	3.5–7[b]
Bisoprolol	Moderate	80	2–4	Hepatic and renal	9–12
Acebutolol	Moderate	30–50	2–4	Hepatic and renal	3–4
Metoprolol	High	50	1–2[c]	Hepatic	3–7[d]
Labetalol	High	25	1–2[c]	Hepatic	4–8

[a]Low, <10%; moderate, 10%–30%; high, >30%.
[b]Significantly prolonged in neonates.
[c]Following oral administration.
[d]Elimination half-life in neonates is 5–10 hr.

gradual reduction in total peripheral resistance. Patients treated with β-adrenergic antagonists that possess intrinsic sympathomimetic ability are less likely to experience a drop in heart rate and cardiac output and generally manifest a lesser degree of reflex vasoconstriction (48).

β-Adrenergic antagonists generally are well absorbed after oral administration (41). Bioavailability is variable due to variation in the extent of the first-pass effect. The oral bioavailability of β-adrenergic antagonists, commonly used in children, varies widely (Table 49.9). In adults, plasma concentrations of these drugs correlate poorly with pharmacologic effects (49,50). Genetic polymorphisms for the cytochrome P450 (CYP) 2D6 isozyme may explain the exaggerated effect observed in poor metabolizers following administration of agents that are inactivated by this pathway (41).

Clinical Use in Children

The β-adrenergic antagonists have been used to treat a wide variety of conditions in children. However, few studies have focused on the use of β-adrenergic antagonists to treat pediatric hypertension (51–64). With the advent of newer and safer drugs, β-adrenergic antagonists are used less often for the treatment of hypertension in children, but still play an important role in the management of hypertension associated with several conditions and in those children who have severe hypertension requiring multiple drugs.

Propranolol was the first β-adrenergic antagonist available for the treatment of hypertension in children. Nine children with severe hypertension were treated with daily doses of 0.6 to 6.4 mg per kg of propranolol (51). Blood pressure fell in all patients. The mean reduction in systolic and diastolic BPs was 26 and 20 mmHg, respectively. There was no correlation between pretreatment plasma renin activity and the magnitude of BP reduction. In a study conducted in children with poorly controlled hypertension following renal transplantation, similar doses resulted in mean systolic and diastolic BP reduction of 12 and 15 mmHg, respectively (54). Propranolol was also shown to effectively reduce paradoxical hypertension after repair of coarctation of the aorta (55).

Despite the lack of formal efficacy data, atenolol has been widely used to treat hypertension in children. The pharmacokinetics of atenolol has been studied in children and young adults with Marfan syndrome and arrhythmias (56,57). An extemporaneous formulation has permitted use in young children where β_1 selectivity is desirable.

Metoprolol was evaluated in 16 patients, of ages 12 to 22 years, with primary or secondary hypertension (58). Nine patients were concurrently treated with diuretic therapy. The initial dose of metoprolol was 50 mg twice daily and was increased to 100 mg twice daily in nonresponders. The BP decreased to less than the 90th percentile in all subjects within 3 to 12 months. No adverse effects were reported. The mean resting heart rate fell from 87/minute to 70/minute in male patients and from 91/minute to 79/minute in female patients.

Extended-release metoprolol succinate was studied in children aged 6 to 16 years; the trial included a placebo group and three doses: 0.2 mg/kg, 1 mg/kg, and 2 mg/kg (64). All treatment groups started at the lowest dose and had weekly increases in dose until the target dose was reached. There was a dose-dependent decrease in diastolic BP decreased after 4 weeks of treatment (−7.5 mmHg for the highest dose after 2 weeks); systolic BP decreased but the group randomized to the middle dose had a greater pressure reduction compared to the highest dose (−7.7 vs. −6.3 mmHg). More than half of the participants randomized to drug treatment had reduction in BP levels below the 95th percentile compared to 26% of those randomized to placebo.

More recently, the combination of bisoprolol and hydrochlorothiazide was compared with placebo in a double-blind, randomized study conducted in children of ages 6 to 17 years (65). A dose escalation design was used to compare 2.5, 5, and 10 mg of bisoprolol combined with 6.25 mg of hydrochlorothiazide to placebo. Normalization of BP (<90th percentile) occurred in 45% of the bisoprolol/hydrochlorothiazide-treated patients and 34% of the patients who received placebo. Significant reduction in systolic and diastolic BPs was observed in children of ages 6 to 12 years but not in those of ages 13 to 17 years. To date, this is the only combination agent tested in children with hypertension (66).

Esmolol, a β_1-selective antagonist with a brief duration of action, was used to treat hypertension in the postoperative period in 20 pediatric patients, ages 1 month to 12 years, who underwent cardiac surgery (60). The BP was successfully lowered to less than the 90th percentile in all subjects. A significant reduction in heart rate was observed. The mean ± standard deviation rate of infusion was 700 ± 232 μg per kg per minute.

Adverse Effects

As a group, β-adrenergic antagonists have a relatively high therapeutic index. However, several significant adverse effects may occur during therapy. Blockade of β_2 receptors in airway smooth muscle may precipitate or exacerbate bronchospasm (61,62). Blockade of β_1-adrenergic receptors in the atria may result in bradycardia (63). Antagonism of ventricular β_1 receptors reduces cardiac output and may result in exercise intolerance, congestive heart failure, and hypotension (62). Blockade of β_1 and β_2 receptors in the gastrointestinal tract may cause constipation or dyspepsia (62). The risk of adverse effects resulting from β_2-receptor blockade may be reduced if cardioselective β-blockers are used in lower doses. However, at higher doses, β_2-antagonist activity may become evident even with β_1-selective agents.

The β-adrenergic antagonists are associated with modest changes in carbohydrate and lipid metabolism (67,68). Selective β-adrenergic antagonists, especially those with partial agonist activity or combined α and β blockade, generally have less effect on triglyceride and low-density lipoprotein and high-density lipoprotein cholesterol levels (69). Patients with diabetes mellitus have an exaggerated hypoglycemic response and in some patients, the warning signs of hypoglycemia are inhibited. For patients with labile glycemic control, β-adrenergic antagonists, including those that are cardioselective, should be avoided or used under close supervision.

Occasionally, patients treated with β-adrenergic antagonists may experience depression, fatigue, sedation, and sleep disturbances including insomnia and nightmares. The lipid solubility of β-adrenergic antagonists varies (41), and penetration of lipophilic agents into the CNS may be higher than that observed for lipophobic agents. However, the observed central adverse effects do not always correlate with higher lipid solubility.

α AND β ANTAGONISTS

Labetalol, an α_1- and nonselective β-adrenergic antagonist, has been administered intravenously to treat acute hypertensive emergencies (70,71) (Table 49.7). Both intermittent and continuous intravenous administrations have been used, but with continuous monitoring in an intensive care setting, continuous administration is often preferred. In one study of 15 subjects, infusion rates of 0.25 to 1.4 mg per kg per hour were used for several days with few adverse effects noted (70). Oral administration of labetalol to treat secondary hypertension caused by pheochromocytoma and renal or renovascular disease has been reported, but few patients and sparse data preclude any conclusions (72,73).

ANGIOTENSIN-CONVERTING ENZYME INHIBITORS

The renin–angiotensin–aldosterone system (RAAS) plays a key role in the regulation of BP. As depicted in Figure 49.1, renin catalyzes the conversion of angiotensinogen, which

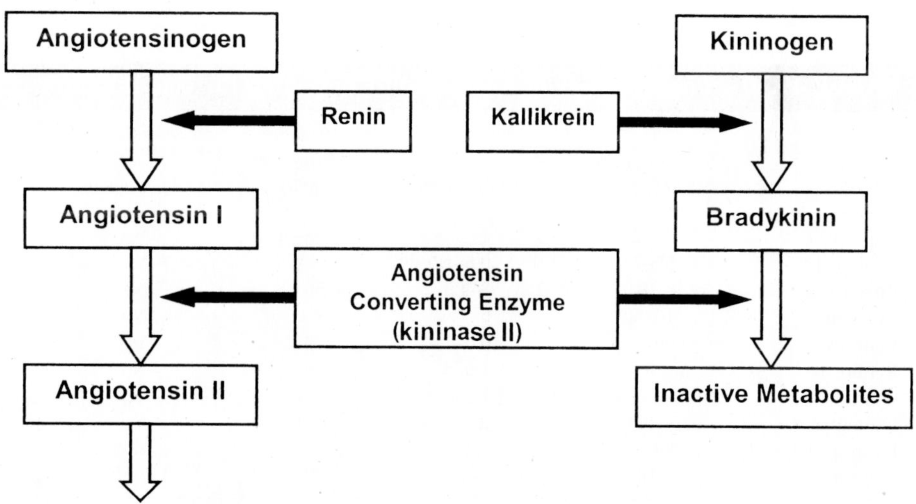

Figure 49.1. The renin–angiotensin–aldosterone system. NS, nervous system.

is synthesized primarily by the liver, to angiotensin I. In the kidney, renin is secreted by the juxtaglomerular cells located along the glomerular afferent arteriole adjacent to the macula densa. The secretion of renin is controlled by several factors, including the movement of NaCl across the macula densa, intrarenal baroreceptors, and the sympathetic nervous system. Renin release is stimulated by at least three mechanisms: decreased NaCl movement across the macula densa, reduction in hydrostatic pressure at the glomerular afferent arteriole, and stimulation of postganglionic sympathetic nerves.

Angiotensin I is a decapeptide that is rapidly cleaved by ACE to form the octapeptide angiotensin II. ACE is structurally identical to kininase II, the enzyme that converts bradykinin, a potent vasodilator, to inactive metabolites. Circulating angiotensin I is converted to angiotensin II primarily by ACE located in pulmonary epithelial cells. Angiotensin I also may be converted to angiotensin III by the combined action of ACE and aminopeptidase. The relative potencies of angiotensins I and III are less than 1% and approximately 10% to 25% of angiotensin II, respectively (74).

Angiotensin II acts to raise the BP by both rapid- and slow-onset mechanisms. A rapid increase in BP is mediated by direct vasoconstriction, stimulation of the sympathetic nervous system, and, to a lesser extent, adrenal release of catecholamines. These actions effectively raise the BP within seconds to minutes. Angiotensin II also acts directly on the proximal tubule to increase sodium reabsorption and stimulates aldosterone release from the zona glomerulosa in the adrenal cortex, resulting in increased sodium reabsorption in the distal nephron. These effects increase the BP by expanding vascular volume but require hours or days before a significant pressor response is observed.

The RAAS is also active at the tissue level in heart, brain, kidney, blood vessels, and the adrenal gland. At the local level, the RAAS plays an important role in endothelial dysfunction, vascular remodeling, ventricular hypertrophy, and stroke.

PHARMACOLOGY OF ANGIOTENSIN-CONVERTING ENZYME-INHIBITING DRUGS

ACE inhibitors have been classified into three structurally distinct groups, which have different pharmacologic profiles (see Table 49.10). Despite minor structural differences, all of these agents act to competitively inhibit binding of ACE to angiotensin I, resulting in a rapid reduction in circulating angiotensin II. Initial BP reduction primarily results from decreased sympathetic stimulation and vasodilation, leading to reduction in systemic vascular resistance. In the longer term, ACE inhibition also reduces renal NaCl reabsorption, in part because of decreased aldosterone release. Some individuals display ACE escape phenomenon or aldosterone synthesis escape, resulting in blunting of the antihypertensive response and possibly contributing to ongoing tissue injury (75). Under normal circumstances, ACE inhibitors are not associated with reflex tachycardia or reduced cardiac output (76). In children with congestive cardiomyopathy treated acutely with captopril, cardiac index increased and the BP was maintained despite a significant drop in systemic vascular resistance (77). However, in children with restrictive cardiomyopathy, cardiac index did not increase and significant hypotension ensued.

CAPTOPRIL

Captopril has been studied extensively in children with proteinuria (78), renal and renovascular hypertension, and congestive heart failure (77,79–84). Captopril effectively reduced the BP in the majority of children with severe hypertension in both the short term (79,80) and over a longer period of time (82,85).

Captopril is readily absorbed from the gastrointestinal tract, but food may reduce the extent of absorption (76). No commercially available suspension exists, but extemporaneous preparations that are stable for up to 28 days have been prepared (86). The antihypertensive effect of captopril

TABLE 49.10 Pharmacology of Angiotensin-Converting Enzyme Inhibitors

	Oral Bioavailability (%)	T_{max} *(hr)*	*Protein Binding (%)*	*Metabolism*	*Primary (Secondary) Elimination Routes*	*Elimination Half-Life (hr)*
Captopril	60–75	1	25–30	Yes	Renal (hepatic)	1–2
Enalapril	55–75	0.5–1.5	NA	Yes	Esterase (renal)	<2
Enalaprilat	<10	3–4.5	50	No	Renal	11–16
Lisinopril	10–60	6	<1	No	Renal	12
Ramipril	60	0.5–1	73	Yes[a]	Esterase (renal)	10
Ramiprilat	<10	1.5–3	56	No	Renal	10–16[b]
Quinapril	60	1	>95	Yes[c]	Esterase (renal)	1
Quinaprilat	<10	2	>95	No	Renal	2
Fosinopril	30	NA[d]	NA[d]	Yes	Esterase (renal)	<2
Fosinoprilat	<10	3–4	99	Yes[e]	Renal (hepatic)	12

[a]Two minor inactive metabolites.
[b]Extreme variability in published reports.
[c]Two inactive metabolites account for 12% of the administered dose.
[d]Not available.
[e]Metabolism becomes more important as renal function decreases.

is evident quickly, often within 15 to 30 minutes, and BP nadir is achieved in 1 to 2 hours (79,80). Maximum plasma concentrations (T_{max}) occurred between 0.5 and 2 hours in children with renal or renovascular hypertension as well as those with congestive heart failure (79–81). The BP returned to baseline after 6 to 10 hours (79). The elimination half-life of captopril in children and adolescents with normal renal function is 1 to 2 hours but increases with reduced renal function and congestive heart failure (79–80). These findings are similar to data from adult patients (76), where under normal circumstances elimination is rapid and the duration of effective BP control compared with other ACE inhibitors is brief.

Captopril has been used extensively in the neonatal population (84,87–89). Renal blood flow in the newborn, especially premature newborns, is highly dependent on an intact RAAS (90). As a result, these children often exhibit a dramatic response to ACE inhibitors. Initial attempts to use a dose similar to that for older children (0.3 to 0.5 mg per kg) resulted in profound hypotension accompanied by oliguria and renal failure in some instances (88,89). Neurologic manifestations, including seizures, were temporally related to a 40% to 72% drop in systolic BP after administration of captopril at a dose of 0.3 mg per kg (91). Subsequently, the recommended initial dose was reduced to 0.01 mg per kg and titrated upward according to response (88). No further episodes of profound hypotension were observed (88). The total dose of captopril required to control the BP was lower in neonates than that in older children (92).

ENALAPRIL AND ENALAPRILAT

Enalaprilat, the active metabolite of enalapril maleate, is poorly absorbed from the gastrointestinal tract. In adults, addition of the ester group to enalaprilat to form enalapril maleate increased oral bioavailability from less than 10% to 55% to 75% (76,93,94). Enalapril is not commercially available in a liquid preparation, but an extemporaneous suspension has been developed and tested for stability and bioequivalence (95). Instructions for preparation of the suspension are available (10).

Enalapril maleate is hydrolyzed by hepatic esterases to form enalaprilat. Peak serum concentrations of enalapril occur within 30 to 90 minutes, but enalaprilat does not peak until approximately 4 hours after administration in adults (93,96). The time to peak serum concentration (T_{max}) of enalaprilat is more variable in younger children, and the median T_{max} is 6 hours in children of ages 2 to 23 months compared with 4 hours in children of ages 12 to 16 years (10). In those patients with severe liver disease, conversion of enalapril to enalaprilat may be delayed (97). Enalaprilat is a much more potent inhibitor of ACE. The ACE-inhibiting potency of enalapril is less than 1% of that of enalaprilat (98).

Enalapril and enalaprilat are eliminated in the urine. In children of ages 2 to 16 years who received orally administered enalapril, combined urinary recovery of enalapril and enalaprilat over 24 hours was 47% to 86%, similar to that seen in adults (10). Conversion of enalapril to enalaprilat in children was approximately 65% to 70%. The mean half-life for accumulation ranged from 14.6 hours in children aged 12 to younger than 16 years to 16.3 hours in children aged 6 to younger than 12 years (10).

Enalapril and enalaprilat have been studied extensively in children with renal disease (99), congestive heart failure (100–103), and hypertension (10,104–108). In children with hypertension, enalapril effectively lowered the BP in children of ages 6 to 16 years within 2 weeks (105). The mean reductions in BP for low-, middle-, and high-dose groups are shown in Figure 49.2. The reduction in BP was significant for the middle- and high-dose groups (105). Recommended dosing for enalapril is presented in Table 49.10.

Neonates have been treated with both enalapril and enalaprilat (100,106,107). As with captopril, enalapril and enalaprilat appear to effectively reduce the BP in neonates, and dosage reductions appear to be necessary to avoid oliguria and acute renal failure (107,109). Enalaprilat has

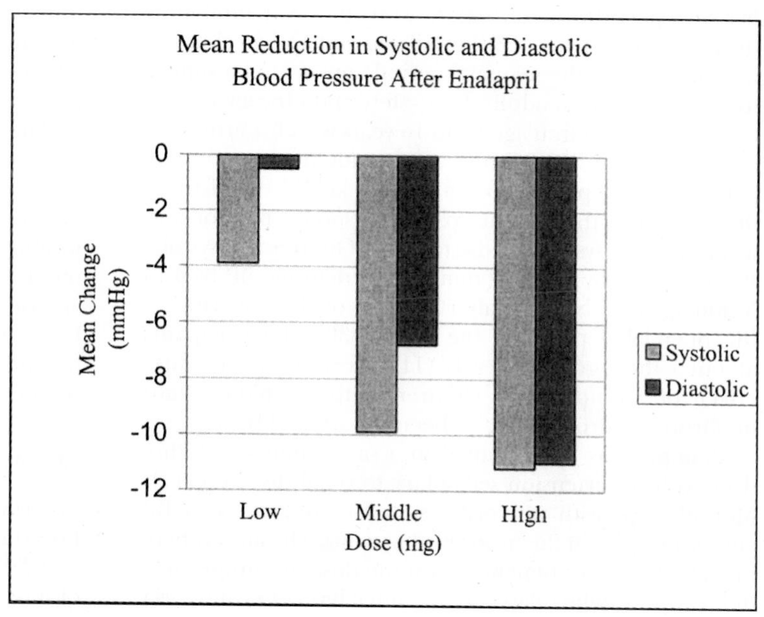

Figure 49.2. Antihypertensive effectiveness of enalapril in children of ages 6 to 16 years (n = 101). Reduction in mean systolic and diastolic blood pressure (placebo vs. enalapril). (From Wells T, Frame V, Soffer B, et al. A double-blind, placebo-controlled, dose–response study of the effectiveness and safety of enalapril for children with hypertension. *J Clin Pharmacol* 2002;42:870–880, with permission.)

been especially useful in the treatment of neonates with renovascular hypertension and in neonates who do not tolerate oral antihypertensive agents.

LISINOPRIL

Lisinopril is the lysine analogue of enalaprilat. Unlike enalapril, lisinopril does not require activation by hepatic esterases. The oral bioavailability of lisinopril in adults (110) and children (111) is 20% to 50%. A suspension is not currently marketed, but a stable extemporaneous suspension has been prepared and administered to infants and younger children (111). Median time to peak concentration after oral administration of lisinopril to children of ages 1 month to 15 years ranges from 5 to 6 hours (111). These values are similar to those historically observed in adults (110). Lisinopril is eliminated unchanged in the urine.

The effectiveness and safety of lisinopril were demonstrated in a study involving 115 children of ages 6 to 16 years (112). Lisinopril was shown to reduce both systolic and diastolic BP in a dose-dependent manner. Low doses (mean = 0.02 mg per kg) were not effective. A mean dose of 0.07 mg per kg administered once daily resulted in mean reduction in systolic and diastolic BP of 12.1 and 9.3 mmHg, respectively, over 2 weeks. Higher doses (mean = 0.61 mg per kg per dose) resulted in corresponding reductions in systolic and diastolic BP of 15.2 and 16.4 mmHg, respectively. The maximum dose of lisinopril studied was 40 mg (112).

OTHER ANGIOTENSIN-CONVERTING ENZYME INHIBITORS

Other commonly used ACE inhibitors, including quinapril, ramipril, fosinopril, benazepril, moexipril, perindopril, and trandolapril, are prodrugs that are absorbed well from the gastrointestinal tract but require bioactivation, primarily hydroxylation by hepatic esterases. As with enalapril, bioactivation delays the apparent onset of action of these agents by 30 minutes or more, making the prodrugs less suitable than captopril for use in hypertensive urgencies (76). The pharmacokinetics of fosinoprilat and quinaprilat has been published (113,114). As with other ACE inhibitors, the pharmacokinetics of fosinopril and quinapril in children who are beyond the neonatal period appears to be similar to that observed in adults. In a safety and efficacy trial of fosinopril in children aged 6 to 16 years with hypertension or high-normal BP, children were randomized to 0.1 mg per kg, 0.3 mg per kg, or 0.6 mg per kg (115). All three doses lowered the BP but no dose–response relationship was found for systolic or diastolic BP. On average, systolic BP decreased by 11 to 12 mmHg and diastolic BP by 4 to 5 mmHg from baseline after 4 weeks of therapy. During the open-label phase of the study, 83% of participants attained their goal BP levels (115). The antiproteinuric effect of fosinopril in children with steroid-resistant nephrotic syndrome has also been reported (116).

Ramipril has been studied in a small number of children with hypertension secondary to renal disease (117). Monotherapy with ramipril resulted in reduction in BP and proteinuria in the majority of patients. The antiproteinuric effect was not dependent on the dose of ramipril nor did it appear to be related to the initial level of proteinuria (117). Larger studies are needed to confirm these preliminary results.

ADVERSE EFFECTS OF ANGIOTENSIN-CONVERTING ENZYME INHIBITORS

Adverse effects related to ACE inhibitors have been well documented (82,105,112,118). In addition to hypotension, oliguria, and acute renal failure, hyperkalemia has been observed especially in children with hypertension secondary to glomerular disease. Headache and dizziness were occasionally reported. Captopril was associated with a skin rash and leukopenia in a small number of patients (82). A nonproductive cough, observed in approximately 1% to 4% of adult patients (119), has been reported in children as well (115,120,121). The cough subsides with discontinuation of ACE inhibitor therapy. Angioedema is an important but rare adverse effect of ACE inhibitors and may be fatal (121,122).

ACE inhibitors have been associated with fetal anomalies after prolonged in utero exposure during the second and third trimesters (126,127). ACE fetopathy is characterized by renal tubular dysplasia, oligohydramnios, pulmonary hypoplasia, positional deformities of the limbs and face, decreased ossification of the skull, and postnatal renal failure. ACE inhibitors should be avoided during pregnancy.

ANGIOTENSIN-II-RECEPTOR ANTAGONISTS

There are two predominant types of angiotensin-II receptors, AT-1 and AT-2 receptors. The hypertensive effects of angiotensin II appear to be mediated exclusively by the AT-1 receptors. There is some evidence that AT-1 receptors also mediate cell growth and atherosclerotic vascular changes, including proliferation of vascular smooth muscle cells and an increase in oxygen free radical generation (128). Stimulation of the AT-2 receptors appears to oppose many of the effects associated with AT-1-receptor activation, resulting in inhibition of cell growth and promotion of cell differentiation and tissue regeneration (128). An AT-4 receptor has been recently described, but its function is not completely understood (129).

The ARBs exert their effect through inhibition of the AT-1 receptor and have no apparent direct effect on AT-2 receptors. The affinity of ARBs for AT-1 is thousands of times greater than their affinity for AT-2 receptors. Unlike ACE inhibitors, angiotensin II levels increase during ARB treatment. Because the effects of RAAS are mediated through angiotensin II, the mechanism by which ARBs lower the BP is similar to that of ACE inhibitors. Pharmacokinetic parameters for ARBs commonly used in children are presented in Table 49.11.

LOSARTAN

Losartan is a competitive inhibitor of AT-1 receptors. Losartan is metabolized by CYP2C9 to form an active metabolite, E-3174, a more potent, noncompetitive inhibitor of AT-1. After an oral dose, peak serum concentrations of

TABLE 49.11 Pharmacology of Angiotensin-II-Receptor Antagonists

	Oral Bioavailability (%)	T_{max} *(hr)*	*Protein Binding (%)*	*Metabolism*	*Primary (Secondary) Elimination Routes*	*Elimination Half-Life (hr)*
Losartan	33	1	98	CYP2C9, 3A4	E-3174 (active metabolite), (renal)	1.5–2.5
E-3174	. . .	2–4	99	None	Renal, hepatic	4–9
Irbesartan	70–80	1–2	90	CYP2C9	Glucuronidation, oxidation (renal)	11–16
Valsartan	10–35	2–4	95	NA	Renal (hepatic)	6–10
Candesartan	15–25	3–4	>99	*O*-demethylation	Renal (biliary)	9

CYP, cytochrome P450; E-3174 is the pharmacologically active metabolite of losartan.

losartan and E-3174 are observed at 1 to 2 hours and 4 to 7 hours, respectively, in children of ages 1 month to 15 years (130). In children of ages 2 to 15 years, elimination of both losartan and E-3174 occurs primarily by nonrenal clearance (130). To assess the antihypertensive effect of losartan, 177 children of ages 6 to 16 years were treated with doses of losartan ranging from 2.5 to 100 mg and dose ranges were dichotomized based upon participant's weight: 20 to 49 kg and ≥50 kg (131). There was a dose–response relationship observed for diastolic BP but not for systolic BP. Diastolic BP after 3 weeks decreased by 6.0, 11.7, and 12.2 mmHg in the low-, middle-, and high-dose groups and systolic BP decreased by 4.4, 10.0, and 8.6 mmHg in the low-, middle-, and high-dose groups. An initial dose of 0.75 mg per kg once daily (maximum dose: 50 mg) lowered BP levels within 2 weeks. This study also demonstrated safety of losartan in children with chronic kidney disease whose estimated creatinine clearances were > 30 mL per minute per 1.73 m^2. Losartan has been shown to reduce proteinuria and preserve renal function in children with chronic glomerulopathies (132,133).

IRBESARTAN

Irbesartan is rapidly absorbed after oral administration in both adults and children (134). Median maximum serum concentrations are observed at 2 hours in children 6 years and older after a single dose of 2.0 mg per kg and at steady state (134). Unlike losartan, irbesartan does not have an active metabolite. Only a small fraction of an administered dose is excreted unchanged in the urine. Biliary excretion represents the major elimination pathway (135). The pharmacokinetics of irbesartan is similar in children of ages 6 and older and adults (134).

Forty-four children of ages 3.7 to 18 years were treated for 18 weeks with irbesartan (136). The initial daily dose of irbesartan ranged from 2.2 to 2.9 mg per kg and was increased in nonresponders to a maximum daily dose of 5.0 mg per kg. Mean systolic and diastolic BPs decreased by 17 and 10 mmHg, respectively, after 18 weeks of treatment. Twenty of 36 patients who had arterial hypertension at the beginning of the trial were normotensive at 18 weeks. There was no apparent relationship between dose and reduction in BP. Thirteen of the 20 patients with proteinuria experienced a 25% or greater reduction in urine protein excretion during the study (136).

VALSARTAN

Valsartan is a selective angiotensin-II-receptor blocker indicated for treatment of hypertension and heart failure in adults. As a single daily dose, it significantly lowers the BP. Two studies in children are available: a safety and efficacy trial in children 1 to 5 years of age and a pharmacokinetic study of children 1 to 16 years of age (131,137). An extemporaneous suspension of valsartan (4 mg/mL) was available to study participants. There were three treatment groups in which dosing was dichotomized based upon weight (8 up to 18 kg or ≥18 kg) to initial doses of 5, 20, and 40 mg or 10, 40, and 80 mg, respectively (138). Valsartan significantly lowered systolic and diastolic BP but not in a dose-dependent manner. Systolic BP was reduced by 8.3 to 8.6 mmHg and diastolic BP by 5.5 to 6.4 mmHg. During the open-label phase, the majority of children remained on monotherapy and attained reduction in BP to levels less than the 95th percentile based upon Task force normative thresholds. In the pharmacokinetic study valsartan was administered at a dose of 2 mg per kg of body weight with a maximum dose of 80 mg (137). The peak plasma concentration was at 2 hours, with measurable levels still present at 24 hours postdose. There were no age-related differences noted in pharmacokinetics.

CANDESARTAN

An open-label pilot study was performed in a small sample of children of ages 6 to 18 years. Candesartan was given at a starting dose of 0.05 to 0.1 mg per kg daily (11). The starting dose was stratified according to weight: 2 mg daily (20 to 39 kg), 4 mg daily (40 to 79 kg), and 8 mg daily (≥80 kg). After 2 weeks, the dose was doubled if the BP was not less than 95th percentile. Nine of 11 children required the dose increase to achieve target BP levels. This study includes ambulatory blood pressure monitoring (ABPM) in the assessment of BP response. Both clinic and ambulatory BP (ABP) were significantly reduced after treatment with candesartan. Clinic systolic and diastolic BP decreased by 10.6 and 5 mmHg, respectively, and ABP decreased by 8.1 and 8.6 mmHg, respectively.

ADVERSE EFFECTS

With the exception of cough, which is rare in patients taking ARBs, drug-related adverse effects observed during treatment with these agents are similar to those observed during treatment with ACE inhibitors. Headache, possibly related to therapy with irbesartan, has been reported in children (134). One patient experienced raised, erythematous pruritic wheals on the head and trunk within 2 hours after administration of irbesartan (136). Hyponatremia and hyperkalemia have been reported (136). As with ACE inhibitors, ARBs may cause fetal injury, particularly if administered to women during the second and third trimesters of pregnancy (139,140).

CALCIUM CHANNEL ANTAGONISTS

Calcium channel antagonists are a heterogeneous group of compounds that reduce the movement of calcium into smooth muscle cells in the heart and vasculature. These agents exert their antihypertensive effect primarily by their action on voltage-sensitive calcium channels in vascular smooth muscle cell membranes, resulting in dose-dependent inhibition of the inward flux of calcium (141). Calcium channel antagonists also have a variable effect on the sinoatrial node pacemaker and on conduction through the atrioventricular node by altering the nodal refractory period. The overall hemodynamic effect of these agents depends, in part, on their relative affinity for peripheral vascular myocytes or the myocardium. Agents with greater affinity for the heart may exhibit negative inotropic, chronotropic, and dromotropic effects (141).

On the basis of molecular structure, pharmacodynamics, and clinical indications, calcium channel antagonists can be divided into four classes: dihydropyridines, phenylalkylamines, benzothiazepines, and benzimidazolyl-substituted tetralines (143–146). All CCBs cause dilation of peripheral resistance vessels, and the net physiologic effect is a decrease in total peripheral vascular resistance. In vitro, all CCBs have negative inotropic effect, but in humans, the dihydropyridine calcium channel antagonists trigger a strong baroreflex-mediated rise in sympathetic nerve activity that blunts the negative inotropic effect (74). Because of their greater selectivity for vascular smooth muscle and minimal effect on cardiac smooth muscle, dihydropyridine calcium channel antagonists (e.g., nifedipine) are widely used to treat hypertension. Phenylalkylamines (e.g., verapamil) and benzothiazepines (e.g., diltiazem) have a depressive effect on cardiac conduction and have been used not only to lower the BP but also to control selected tachyarrhythmias. Benzimidazolyl-substituted tetralines (e.g., mibefradil) reduce the heart rate without much effect on cardiac contractility.

Administration of calcium channel antagonists initially improves glomerular filtration rate (GFR) and effective renal plasma flow (ERPF), but filtration fraction is unchanged (146–149). These changes are related to afferent arteriolar dilatation, but with improvement in hypertension, GFR and ERPF usually return to pretreatment levels within a few weeks (147), although peripheral vascular resistance remains lower. Calcium channel antagonists, particularly the dihydropyridines, acutely increase renin release, but aldosterone usually does not increase. Calcium channel antagonists may induce an acute natriuresis and diuresis (148,149), but clinically significant changes in serum electrolytes or body fluid composition are not acutely observed. With prolonged use, some dihydropyridines may cause fluid retention resulting in dependent edema.

PHARMACOLOGY

Data describing the disposition of calcium channel antagonists in children are limited. The dihydropyridine derivatives undergo a variable degree of first-pass metabolism, resulting in reduced oral bioavailability for several agents (Table 49.12). With chronic use, oral bioavailability may increase. Peak serum concentrations are attained rapidly after administration of short-acting nifedipine, but not after administration of amlodipine, felodipine, or the sustained-release preparations of nifedipine. Dihydropyridines are metabolized by CYP3A4, and the inactive metabolites are excreted in urine or the gastrointestinal tract (150). The elimination half-life for nifedipine in children of ages 5 to 68 months is 1.8 hours (151). Amlodipine is unique among calcium channel antagonists in that it has a very long elimination half-life. Verapamil and diltiazem have active metabolites (norverapamil and desacetyldiltiazem, respectively), but the potency of the metabolites appears to be less than that of the parent compounds.

CLINICAL USE IN CHILDREN

Short-acting nifedipine has been widely used to treat hypertension in children (152–155). Onset of action is apparent within 5 to 30 minutes after oral administration of nifedipine and peaks at 30 to 60 minutes (152–155). Mean reduction in systolic and diastolic BPs was 27 to 45 mmHg

TABLE 49.12 Pharmacology of Calcium Channel Antagonists

Drug	*Oral Bioavailability (%)*	*First-Pass Effect*[a]	*Protein Binding (%)*	T_{max} *(hr)*	*Metabolism*	*Elimination Half-Life (hr)*
Amlodipine	64–90	Low	93	6–12	Hepatic (CYP3A4)	30–50
Felodipine	20	High	>99	2.5–5	Hepatic/GI (CYP3A4)	11–16
Isradipine	15–24	High	95	1–2	Hepatic (CYP3A4)	8
Nicardipine	35	High	>98	1	Hepatic (CYP3A4)	8–9
Nifedipine	50–70	Moderate	96	0.5	Hepatic (CYP3A4)	2
Nifedipine GITS	50–60	Moderate	96	6	Hepatic (CYP3A4)	2

CYP, cytochrome P450; GI, gastrointestinal; GITS, gastrointestinal therapeutic system.
[a]Low, <10%; moderate, 10%–30%; high, >30%.

and 32 to 37 mmHg, respectively. The duration of effect was 4 to 6 hours after administration of nifedipine capsules, although effective antihypertensive control reportedly lasted 12 hours in a few patients (156). Mean heart rate increased significantly after acute administration of nifedipine (152,155).

Because several serious adverse effects have been reported, the use of short-acting nifedipine has become controversial (157–159). In children, adverse effects including severe hypotension and oxygen desaturation and neurologic events including stroke and deterioration in neurologic status have been reported in a retrospective review (158). Neurologic events were particularly seen in patients with acute CNS injury. In a retrospective review of 117 hypertensive patients by Blaszak et al., short-acting nifedipine was felt to be a safe antihypertensive agent in a hospital setting (160). An initial dose of less than 0.25 mg per kg is recommended in the pediatric population to avoid rapid reduction in BP. No clinically significant side effects were noted in this review despite significant reduction in systolic, diastolic, and mean arterial BP. Short-acting nifedipine may safely be used for the treatment of pediatric urgent hypertension in the hospital setting, but caution should be exercised in the home setting. Many pediatricians have abandoned the use of short-acting nifedipine.

Isradipine has also been used in children for urgent and secondary hypertension with successful reduction in both systolic and diastolic BP (161,162). A retrospective review of 72 children, of ages 1 week to 16.8 years, treated with isradipine alone or in combination with other agents demonstrated that isradipine effectively lowered the BP (161). Mean (range) daily dose was 0.36 (0.07 to 0.90) mg per kg. Isradipine was administered three times daily in 60.8% of the subjects and four times daily in 27% of the subjects. Adverse effects, including headache, flushing, dizziness, and tachycardia, were observed in 9.5% of the patients (161). Blurred vision, fatigue, and palpitations have also been reported in children who received isradipine (163).

Extended-release felodipine has been evaluated in 133 children, of ages 6 to 16 years, with essential hypertension (164). Patients were randomized to receive placebo or force titrated to one of three doses (2.5, 5, and 10 mg) administered once daily. All patients randomized to receive active drug started at 2.5 mg and were titrated at weekly intervals until maximal dose was achieved. The study duration was 3 weeks. Patients receiving 5 mg of felodipine for 2 weeks had a significant decrease in BP when compared with placebo. However, diastolic BP for subjects who received 2.5- and 10-mg doses was not different from placebo. Systolic BP was not statistically different from placebo. In a 16-week, open-label extension to the study, the 10-mg dose of felodipine failed to significantly lower the BP. Adverse effects were similar to those previously described in adults, including headache, nausea, and pedal edema.

In another study comparing extended-release nifedipine and felodipine in controlling the BP during the daytime, BP control was better in the nifedipine group (148). The pharmacokinetics of felodipine in five children with renal transplants concomitantly treated with cyclosporine has been described (165). Significant interpatient variability was observed.

Amlodipine has a long duration of action and can be dosed once daily. The availability of a stable, extemporaneous suspension that can be used in younger children offers a clear advantage over other calcium channel antagonists (166,167). Absorption of amlodipine is nearly complete and first-pass metabolism is minimal. Although the drug has an effective duration of action of more than 24 hours in adults, some children apparently require twice-daily dosing to achieve effective BP control. A randomized, double-blind, placebo-controlled trial involving 268 children of ages 6 to 16 years was conducted (168). Amlodipine, 2.5 or 5 mg, was administered for 4 weeks. Significant reductions in mean systolic and diastolic BPs were observed. In a randomized, prospective, crossover study in 11 patients with posttransplantation hypertension, amlodipine was as effective as nifedipine or felodipine (149). The adverse effects observed during treatment with amlodipine are similar to those of other calcium channel antagonists.

Nicardipine is available in oral and intravenous formulations. Intravenous nicardipine has been used to treat severe hypertension in neonates and children in an intensive care setting (169–177). The initial dosing in these reports varied from 0.2 to 5.0 μg per kg per minute, but 0.5 to 1.0 μg per kg per minute was the most commonly used initial dosing. The BP was controlled within 15 minutes in one series, but the initial rate of infusion was higher than in other studies (173). Titration of the rate of infusion occurred every 15 to 30 minutes in one report (172). The BP was controlled within hours using infusion rates from 0.3 to 5.5 μg per kg per minute, but short-term use of up to 10 μg per kg per minute has been reported (170,172–174). The heart rate increased in many patients, but because many other factors may have affected heart rate in these critically ill children, it is difficult to attribute the increase directly to nicardipine. Other reported adverse effects included clinically significant hypotension (treated with intravenous fluids and calcium), flushing, palpitations, and thrombophlebitis at the infusion site (175).

In addition to the adverse effects reported in short-term studies, calcium channel antagonists have also been associated with gingival hypertrophy, especially in transplant patients who are also receiving cyclosporine. Severe and unpredictable drop in BP is occasionally observed following oral administration of short-acting nifedipine and intravenous nicardipine (118).

DIRECT VASODILATORS

The direct vasodilators, which include hydralazine, minoxidil, diazoxide, and nitroprusside, relax vascular smooth muscle and result in vasodilation and reduced peripheral vascular resistance. Hydralazine, minoxidil, and diazoxide primarily affect arteriolar vessels. In addition to arteriolar dilation, nitroprusside also relaxes venous capacitance vessels, which results in venous pooling.

Vasodilators are seldom used as sole agents to treat hypertension over prolonged periods of time because reflex tachycardia, increased cardiac output, and sodium and water retention blunt their effectiveness. Apart from nitroprusside, which is commonly used in the management of hypertensive emergencies, vasodilators are commonly viewed as add-on therapy in children with hypertension that is difficult to control. As safe, effective alternative therapies are introduced, the use of direct vasodilators for the management of acute and chronic hypertension is decreasing.

HYDRALAZINE

Prior to the development of newer intravenous antihypertensive agents, hydralazine was often administered intravenously for hypertensive urgencies and orally to patients unresponsive to diuretics and β-blockers (2). After intravenous administration, the onset of the antihypertensive effect usually begins within 5 to 15 minutes and lasts up to 6 hours. Onset of action is delayed after oral or intramuscular administration, but the duration of action is similarly brief.

The metabolism of hydralazine is complex (176). Hydralazine is inactivated by acetylation in the gastrointestinal mucosa and liver and is subject to a significant first-pass effect (176). The slow-acetylator phenotype is associated with a significant increase in oral bioavailability compared with fast acetylators (177). However, after intravenous administration, the pharmacokinetics of hydralazine is similar in slow and fast acetylators, but the predominant metabolites are different (177).

The utility of hydralazine is limited by frequently occurring adverse effects. In addition to those common to other direct vasodilators, hydralazine has been associated with a dose-dependent, lupus-like syndrome that is possibly due to accumulation of metabolites more often found in slow acetylators (178). Acute and chronic administration of hydralazine often results in headaches, nausea, and vomiting, which can become intolerable (179). Use of hydralazine has diminished as safer alternatives have become available.

NITROPRUSSIDE

Nitroprusside is used for hypertensive emergencies and in conditions where afterload reduction is desired (Table 49.7). It is administered exclusively via the intravenous route. Nitroprusside degrades over several hours in alkaline solutions or the presence of fluorescent light. The drug must be placed in an opaque bag or syringe, and the intravenous tubing needs to be covered with aluminum foil or other opaque material to reduce decomposition.

Nitroprusside is used in the treatment of severe, symptomatic hypertension in children (180,181). The antihypertensive effect of nitroprusside is evident within 1 to 2 minutes after the infusion begins. The recommended initial rate of infusion is 0.3 to 0.5 μg per kg per minute (182). The dose can be titrated to desired effect at intervals of 5 to 10 minutes. Discontinuation of the infusion typically results in loss of effect within 3 to 5 minutes. The maximum recommended dose is 8 to 10 μg per kg per minute, but doses above 4 μg per kg per minute are not generally needed and should be used with caution, especially in patients with renal failure. In the treatment of hypertension, nitroprusside is not usually administered for more than a 2 to 3 days but has been used safely in an 11-year-old child for 28 days (183).

Twenty children, of ages 7 to 17 years, with severe arterial hypertension and encephalopathy or cardiac failure were treated with nitroprusside for 8 to 240 hours (180). All were judged to have an adequate response to therapy, and only three required nitroprusside for more than 48 hours. During treatment, infusion rates ranged from 0.5 to 3.5 μg per kg per minute. The mean (range) reductions in systolic and diastolic BPs were 47 (30 to 80) and 49 (30 to 70) mmHg, respectively. Rapid improvement in cardiac function was noted in children who presented with congestive heart failure.

Nitroprusside undergoes reduction to cyanide and nitric oxide in smooth muscle. The cyanide is converted to thiocyanate by rhodanese in the liver. Thiocyanate is excreted in the urine, but accumulation occurs in patients with renal insufficiency. Accumulation of cyanide results in inhibition of cytochrome oxidase and halts oxidative phosphorylation, resulting in shunting of pyruvate to lactate and the development of severe metabolic acidemia. Symptoms associated with thiocyanate accumulation include tachypnea, headache, nausea, vomiting, and deterioration of mental status (184). Progression to convulsions, coma, and death may occur without timely intervention.

Newer antihypertensive agents are gradually supplanting nitroprusside for the management of emergent hypertension. However, because nitroprusside decreases both capillary wedge pressure and systemic vascular resistance, it is particularly useful in treating severe hypertension associated with congestive heart failure (179).

MINOXIDIL

Minoxidil is a potent, orally administered vasodilator that is typically reserved for severe hypertension not controlled by other medications. It has also been effective when used to treat acute BP elevations in children with chronic hypertension secondary to renal disease (185).

Minoxidil is absorbed well from the gastrointestinal tract. Peak serum concentrations are observed within 20 to 60 minutes after dosing (186). Onset of action occurs within 30 minutes in most patients, but maximal effect is not observed until 2 to 4 hours after administration (185). Minoxidil undergoes both type I and type II biotransformations. It is activated in vivo by hepatic sulfotransferase. The inactive glucuronide metabolite is excreted in the urine. Because minoxidil has a relatively short elimination half-life, it is usually administered twice daily.

Several prospective studies were conducted to determine the effectiveness of minoxidil in children with uncontrolled chronic hypertension (185,187–189). Initial dosing varied from 0.05 to 0.27 mg per kg per 24 hours, but most studies used an initial dose of 0.1 to 0.2 mg per kg per 24 hours. Maximal dosing varied widely, but few children received more than 1.0 mg per kg per 24 hours. The BP was reduced effectively within 1 to 2 weeks in more than 80% of the reported patients (185,189,190). All of the patients in these studies received at least one and typically two or more antihypertensives concurrently with minoxidil.

In children with chronic hypertension treated with multiple drugs, severe, acute elevated BP can be treated successfully with minoxidil (185). Minoxidil lowered the BP to less than the 95th percentile for age in 9 of 11 children who received 0.2 mg per kg or more, but only 5 of 12 when the dose was less than 0.2 mg per kg. An antihypertensive effect was observed at 1 hour and was maximal by 2 to 4 hours.

Adverse effects related to minoxidil were frequent and included hypertrichosis, tachycardia, fluid retention, congestive heart failure, and pericardial effusion. The hypertrichosis typically is observed on the forehead, trunk, and extremities. Abnormal hair growth disappeared within 3 months after discontinuation of the drug. Administration of minoxidil during pregnancy occasionally has been associated with fetal hirsutism and other congenital anomalies (191). Minoxidil passes readily into breast milk, but adverse effects may not be discernible (192).

PRINCIPLES OF TREATMENT: RESISTANT HYPERTENSION

Hypertension that is "resistant" to drug therapy occurs frequently in children. "Resistant" hypertension is a failure to achieve expected therapeutic goals during active treatment. There are many causes for apparent resistance, including patient-related, disease-specific, and drug-related factors (Table 49.13). One of the most important tools for assessing apparent drug resistance is a thorough drug history. The drug history, coupled with scrutiny of pharmacy records and pill counts, can uncover nonadherence as well as other drug-related causes of antihypertensive "resistance." Drug-related causes of apparent resistance to therapy include drugs that interfere with the absorption of orally administered antihypertensive agents, decrease intestinal transit time, or induce drug-metabolizing hepatic enzymes. In addition, certain drugs are known to blunt the effect of selected antihypertensive agents. For example, nonsteroidal anti-inflammatory agents are known to interfere with the effectiveness of ACE inhibitors, probably by reducing the production of vasodilatory prostaglandins (193). Corticosteroids are commonly used to treat a variety of glomerular diseases in children and have been associated with the development or worsening of hypertension. Finally, the sympathomimetic agents commonly found in over-the-counter decongestants cause vasoconstriction and increased BP (194,195). Both cyclosporine and tacrolimus, which are commonly used to prevent tissue rejection in children with solid-organ transplants, to prevent graft-versus-host disease in children after bone marrow transplantation, or as second-line therapy to treat a variety of glomerular diseases in children, are known to cause hypertension (182,196). Abrupt discontinuation of clonidine has been associated with rebound hypertension, probably by increasing vasoconstriction (182). There are many other examples of drug-related hypertension, including α- and β-receptor agonists, narcotic withdrawal, methylphenidate, and amphetamines.

Medical history, physical examination, and the addition or repetition of selected diagnostic tests may uncover previously undetected secondary disease, worsening of a known relapsing and remitting diseases (e.g., vasculitis), or gastrointestinal disease that interferes with absorption of orally administered medications (e.g., gastroenteritis). Compliance with dietary salt restriction can be assessed by taking a thorough dietary history coupled with measurement of urinary sodium excretion in euvolemic patients who are not receiving diuretic therapy.

Often, a cause for resistance to antihypertensive therapy can be identified. When none of the known causes for apparent resistance is found, increasing the dose of the drug, changing to a different medication, or adding an additional antihypertensive agent may be beneficial.

TABLE 49.13 Causes of Resistance or Apparent Resistance to Antihypertensive Drug Therapy

Patient-related factors
Noncompliance
Gain in body mass
Sleep apnea
Volume overload
Excessive sodium intake
Inadequate diuretic therapy
Fluid retention secondary to vasodilator therapy
Caffeine
Disease-specific factors
Worsening of underlying disease
Missed diagnosis of secondary hypertension
Relapsing and remitting diseases
Drug-related issues
Inadequate dose or inappropriate dosing interval
Poor oral bioavailability
Rapid inactivation or elimination (e.g., nifedipine)
Hepatic induction (for drugs that undergo significant hepatic biotransformation)
Inappropriate drug combinations
Concurrent interfering drug therapy (e.g., nonsteroidal anti-inflammatory drugs, steroids, cyclosporine, sympathomimetics)

REFERENCES

1. Wells TG. Underserved therapeutic classes: examples which should not be ignored in infants and children. *Drug Inf J* 1996;30: 1179–1186.
2. Task Force on Blood Pressure Control in Children; National Heart, Lung, and Blood Institute; National Institutes of Health. Report of the Task Force on Blood Pressure Control in Children. *Pediatrics* 1977;59:797–820.
3. Task Force on Blood Pressure Control in Children; National Heart, Lung, and Blood Institute; National Institutes of Health. Report of the Second Task Force on Blood Pressure Control in Children—1987. *Pediatrics* 1987;79:1–25.
4. Food and Drug Administration, Department of Health and Human Services. Specific requirements on content and format of labeling for human prescription drugs; revision of "pediatric use" subsection in the labeling; final rule. *Fed Regist* 1994;59: 64240–64250.
5. Food and Drug Administration, Department of Health and Human Services. Regulations requiring manufacturers to assess the safety and effectiveness of new drugs and biologic products in pediatric patients; final rule. *Fed Regist* 1998;63:66631–66672.
6. Food and Drug Administration Modernization Act of 1997. Public Law 105–115, 1997.
7. Best Pharmaceuticals for Children Act. Public Law 107–001, 2002.
8. Flynn JT. Hypertension in the young: epidemiology, sequelae and therapy. *Nephrol Dial Transplant* 2009;24(2):370–375.
9. http://www.fda.gov/downloads/Drugs/DevelopmentApproval Process/DevelopmentResources/UCM049870.pdf.
10. Wells T, Rippley R, Hogg R, et al. The pharmacokinetics of enalapril in children and infants with hypertension. *J Clin Pharmacol* 2001;41(10):1064–1074.

11. Franks AM, O'Brien CE, Stowe CD, et al. Candesartan cilexetil effectively reduces blood pressure in hypertensive children. *Ann Pharmacother* 2008;42(10):1388–1395.
12. Lyszkiewicz DA, Levichek Z, Kozer E, et al. Bioavailability of a pediatric amlodipine suspension. *Pediatr Nephrol* 2003;18(7):675–678.
13. Rames LK, Clarke WR, Connor WE, et al. Normal blood pressure and the evaluation of sustained blood pressure elevation in childhood: the Muscatine study. *Pediatrics* 1978;61(2):245–251.
14. Fixler DE, Laird WP. Validity of mass blood pressure screening in children. *Pediatrics* 1983;72(4):459–463.
15. Kilcoyne MM, Richter RW, Alsup PA. Adolescent hypertension. I. Detection and prevalence. *Circulation* 1974;50(4):758–764.
16. Reichman LB, Cooper BM, Blumenthal S, et al. Hypertension testing among high school students. I. Surveillance procedures and results. *J Chronic Dis* 1975;28(3):161–171.
17. Sinaiko AR, Gomez-Marin O, Prineas RJ. "Significant" diastolic hypertension in pre-high school black and white children. The children and adolescent blood pressure program. *Am J Hypertens* 1988;1(2):178–180.
18. Update on the 1987 Task Force Report on High Blood Pressure in Children and Adolescents: a working group report from the National High Blood Pressure Education Program. National High Blood Pressure Education Program Working Group on Hypertension Control in Children and Adolescents. *Pediatrics* 1996;98(4, pt 1):649–658.
19. Din-Dzietham R, Liu Y, Bielo MV, et al. High blood pressure trends in children and adolescents in national surveys, 1963 to 2002. *Circulation* 2007;116(13):1488–1496.
20. National High Blood Pressure Education Program Working Group on High Blood Pressure in Children and Adolescents. The fourth report on the diagnosis, evaluation, and treatment of high blood pressure in children and adolescents. *Pediatrics* 2004; 114(2 Suppl, 4th Report):555–576.
21. Verdecchia P. White-coat hypertension in adults and children. *Blood Press Monit* 1999;4(3–4):175–179.
22. Sorof JM, Portman RJ. White coat hypertension in children with elevated casual blood pressure. *J Pediatr* 2000;137(4):493–497.
23. Lurbe E, Sorof JM, Daniels SR. Clinical and research aspects of ambulatory blood pressure monitoring in children. *J Pediatr* 2004; 144(1):7–16.
24. Urbina E, Alpert B, Flynn J, et al. Ambulatory blood pressure monitoring in children and adolescents: recommendations for standard assessment: a scientific statement from the American Heart Association Atherosclerosis, Hypertension, and Obesity in Youth Committee of the council on cardiovascular disease in the young and the council for high blood pressure research. *Hypertension* 2008;52(3):433–451.
25. Belsha CW, Wells TG, McNiece KL, et al. Influence of diurnal blood pressure variations on target organ abnormalities in adolescents with mild essential hypertension. *Am J Hypertens* 1998; 11(4, pt 1):410–417.
26. Daniels SR, Loggie JM, Khoury P, et al. Left ventricular geometry and severe left ventricular hypertrophy in children and adolescents with essential hypertension. *Circulation* 1998;97(19):1907–1911.
27. Hanevold C, Waller J, Daniels S, et al. The effects of obesity, gender, and ethnic group on left ventricular hypertrophy and geometry in hypertensive children: a collaborative study of the International Pediatric Hypertension Association. *Pediatrics* 2004; 113(2):328–333.
28. Lande MB, Carson NL, Roy J, et al. Effects of childhood primary hypertension on carotid intima media thickness: a matched controlled study. *Hypertension* 2006;48(1):40–44.
29. Lande MB, Kaczorowski JM, Auinger P, et al. Elevated blood pressure and decreased cognitive function among school-age children and adolescents in the United States. *J Pediatr* 2003; 143(6):720–724.
30. Sorof JM. Prevalence and consequence of systolic hypertension in children. *Am J Hypertens* 2002;15(2, pt 2):57S–60S.
31. Flynn JT. Neonatal hypertension: diagnosis and management. *Pediatr Nephrol* 2000;14(4):332–341.
32. Dillon MJ. Secondary forms of hypertension in children. In: Portman RJ, Sorof JM, Ingelfinger JR, eds. *Pediatric hypertension.* Totowa, NJ: Humana Press, 2004:159–179.
33. Mattoo TK, Gruskin AB. Essential hypertension in children. In: Portman RJ, Sorof JM, Ingelfinger JR, eds. *Pediatric hypertension.* Totowa, NJ: Humana Press, 2004:181–211.
34. de Simone G, Mureddu GF, Greco R, et al. Relations of left ventricular geometry and function to body composition in children with high casual blood pressure. *Hypertension* 1997;30(3, pt 1): 377–382.
35. Lever AF, Harrap SB. Essential hypertension: a disorder of growth with origins in childhood? *J Hypertens* 1992;10(2):101–120.
36. Okasha M, McCarron P, McEwen J, et al. Determinants of adolescent blood pressure: findings from the Glasgow University student cohort. *J Hum Hypertens* 2000;14(2):117–124.
37. Sinaiko AR, Steinberger J, Moran A, et al. Relation of insulin resistance to blood pressure in childhood. *J Hypertens* 2002;20(3): 509–517.
38. Wells T, Stowe C. An approach to the use of antihypertensive drugs in children and adolescents. *Curr Ther Res Clin Exp* 2001; 62:329–350.
39. ALLHAT Officers and Coordinators for the ALLHAT Collaborative Research Group. The Antihypertensive and Lipid-Lowering Treatment to Prevent Heart Attack Trial. Major outcomes in high-risk hypertensive patients randomized to angiotensin-converting enzyme inhibitor or calcium channel blocker vs diuretic: The Antihypertensive and Lipid-Lowering Treatment to Prevent Heart Attack Trial (ALLHAT). *JAMA* 2002;288(23):2981–2997.
40. Wang J, Staessan JA, Heagerty AM. Ongoing trials: what should we expect after ALLHAT? *Curr Hypertens Rep* 2003;5:340–345.
41. Frishman WH, Alwarshetty M. β-Adrenergic blockers in systemic hypertension. Pharmacological considerations related to the current guidelines. *Clin Pharmacokinet* 2002;41:505–516.
42. Buhler FR, Laragh JH, Baer L, et al. Propranolol inhibition of renin secretion. *N Engl J Med* 1972;287:1209–1214.
43. Keeton TK, Campbell WB. The pharmacologic alteration of renin release. *Pharmacol Rev* 1981;31:81–227.
44. Weinstock M. The presynaptic effect of beta-adrenoceptor antagonists on noradrenergic neurons. *Life Sci* 1976;19:1453–1466.
45. Garvey HL, Ram N. Centrally induced hypotensive effects of beta-adrenergic blocking agents. *Eur J Pharmacol* 1975;33:283–294.
46. Tarazi RC, Dustan HP. Beta-adrenergic blockade in hypertension. *Am J Cardiol* 1972;29:633–640.
47. Hansson L, Zweifler AJ, Julius S, et al. Hemodynamic effects of acute and prolonged beta-adrenergic blockade in essential hypertension. *Acta Med Scand* 1974;196:27–34.
48. Man in't Veld AJ. Vasodilation, not cardiodepression, underlies the antihypertensive effects of beta-adrenoceptor antagonists. *Am J Cardiol* 1971;67:13B–17B.
49. McDevitt DG, Shand DG. Plasma concentration and time course of beta blockade due to propranolol. *Clin Pharmacol Ther* 1975; 18:708–713.
50. McAreavey D, Vermeulen R, Robertson JIS. Newer beta-blockers and the treatment of hypertension. *Cardiovasc Drugs Ther* 1991; 5:577–588.
51. Griswold WR, McNeal R, Mendoza SA, et al. Propranolol as antihypertensive agent in children. *Arch Dis Child* 1978;53:594–596.
52. Bachmann H. Propranolol verses chlorthalidone—a perspective therapeutic trial in children with chronic hypertension. *Helv Paediatr Acta* 1984;39:55–61.
53. Mongeau JG, Biron P, Pichardo LM. Propranolol efficacy in adolescent essential hypertension. In: New MI, Levine LS, eds. *Juvenile hypertension.* New York: Raven Press, 1977:219–222.
54. Potter DE, Schambelan M, Salvatierra O Jr, et al. Treatment of high-renin hypertension with propranolol in children after renal transplantation. *J Pediatr* 1977;90:307–311.
55. Gidding SS, Rocchini AP, Beekman R, et al. Therapeutic effect of propranolol on paradoxical hypertension after repair of coarctation of the aorta. *N Engl J Med* 1985;312:1224–1228.
56. Phelps SJ, Alpert BS, Ward JL, et al. Absorption pharmacokinetics of atenolol in patients with Marfan syndrome. *J Clin Pharmacol* 1995; 35:268–274.
57. Buck ML, Wiest D, Gillette PC, et al. Pharmacokinetics and pharmacodynamics of atenolol in children. *Clin Pharmacol Ther* 1989;46:629–633.
58. Falkner B, Lowenthal DT, Affrime MB. The pharmacodynamic effectiveness of metoprolol in adolescent hypertension. *Pediatr Pharmacol (New York)* 1982;2:49–55.
59. Sorof JM, Cargo P, Graepel J, et al. β-Blocker/thiazide combination for treatment of hypertensive children: a randomized double-blind, placebo-controlled trial. *Pediatr Nephrol* 2002;17: 345–350.

60. Wiest DB, Garner SS, Uber WE, et al. Esmolol for the management of pediatric hypertension after cardiac operations. *J Thorac Cardiovasc Surg* 1998;115:890–897.
61. Decalmer PBS, Chatterjee SS, Cruickshank JM, et al. Beta-blockers and asthma. *Br Heart J* 1978;40:184–189.
62. Frishman W, Silverman R, Strom J, et al. Clinical pharmacology of the new beta-adrenergic blocking drugs. Part 4. Adverse effects. Choosing a beta-adrenoceptor blocker. *Am Heart J* 1979; 98:256–262.
63. Gillette P, Garson A Jr, Eterovic E, et al. Oral propranolol treatment in infants and children. *J Pediatr* 1978;92:141–144.
64. Batisky DL, Sorof JM, Sugg J, et al. Efficacy and safety of extended release metoprolol succinate in hypertensive children 6 to 16 years of age: a clinical trial experience. *J Pediatr* 2007; 150(2):134–139, 139.e1.
65. Sorof JM, Cargo P, Graepel J, et al. Beta-blocker/thiazide combination for treatment of hypertensive children: a randomized double-blind, placebo-controlled trial. *Pediatr Nephrol* 2002;17(5):345–350.
66. Flynn JT, Daniels SR. Pharmacologic treatment of hypertension in children and adolescents. *J Pediatr* 2006;149(6):746–754.
67. Artman M, Grayson R, Boerth RC. Propranolol in children: safety–toxicity. *Pediatrics* 1982;70:30–31.
68. Wells TG, Ulstrom RA, Nevins TE. Hypoglycemia in pediatric renal allograft recipients. *J Pediatr* 1988;113:1002–1007.
69. Ames RP. The effects of antihypertensive drugs on serum lipids and lipoproteins. II. Non-diuretic drugs. *Drugs* 1986;32:335–357.
70. Bunchman TE, Lynch RE, Wood EG. Intravenously administered labetalol for treatment of hypertension in children. *J Pediatr* 1992;120:140–144.
71. Mueller JB, Solhaug MJ. Labetalol in pediatric hypertensive emergencies. *Pediatr Res* 1988;23:543A.
72. Ishisaka DY, Yonan CD, Housel BF. Labetalol for treatment of hypertension in a child. *Clin Pharm* 1991;10:500–501.
73. Jureidini KF. Oral labetalol in a child with phaeochromocytoma and five children with renal hypertension. *Aust N Z J Med* 1980;10:479.
74. Hardman JG, Limbird LE, eds. *Goodman and Gilman's The pharmacological basis of therapeutics*, 10th ed. New York: McGraw-Hill, 2001.
75. Lakkis J, Lu WX, Weir MR. RAAS escape: a real clinical entity that may be important in the progression of cardiovascular and renal disease. *Curr Hypertens Rep* 2003;5(5):408–417.
76. Raia JJ Jr, Barone JA, Byerly WG, et al. Angiotensin-converting enzyme inhibitors: a comparative review. *DICP* 1990;24(5): 506–525.
77. Bengur AR, Beekman RH, Rocchini AP, et al. Acute hemodynamic effects of captopril in children with a congestive or restrictive cardiomyopathy. *Circulation* 1991;83(2):523–527.
78. Trachtman H, Gauthier B. Effect of angiotensin-converting enzyme inhibitor therapy on proteinuria in children with renal disease. *J Pediatr* 1988;112(2):295–298.
79. Sinaiko AR, Mirkin BL, Hendrick DA, et al. Antihypertensive effect and elimination kinetics of captopril in hypertensive children with renal disease. *J Pediatr* 1983;103(5):799–805.
80. Levy M, Koren G, Klein J, et al. Captopril pharmacokinetics, blood pressure response and plasma renin activity in normotensive children with renal scarring. *Dev Pharmacol Ther* 1991;16(4):185–193.
81. Pereira CM, Tam YK, Collins-Nakai RL. The pharmacokinetics of captopril in infants with congestive heart failure. *Ther Drug Monit* 1991;13(3):209–214.
82. Mirkin BL, Newman TJ. Efficacy and safety of captopril in the treatment of severe childhood hypertension: report of the International Collaborative Study Group. *Pediatrics* 1985;75(6): 1091–1100.
83. Friedman AL, Chesney RW. Effect of captopril on the renin-angiotensin system in hypertensive children. *J Pediatr* 1983; 103(5):806–810.
84. Hymes LC, Warshaw BL. Captopril. Long-term treatment of hypertension in a preterm infant and in older children. *Am J Dis Child* 1983;137(3):263–266.
85. Callis L, Vila A, Catala J, et al. Long-term treatment with captopril in pediatric patients with severe hypertension and chronic renal failure. *Clin Exp Hypertens A* 1986;8(4–5):847–851.
86. Nahata MC, Morosco RS, Hipple TF. Stability of captopril in three liquid dosage forms. *Am J Hosp Pharm* 1994;51(1):95–96.
87. Bifano E, Post EM, Springer J, et al. Treatment of neonatal hypertension with captopril. *J Pediatr* 1982;100(1):143–146.
88. O'Dea RF, Mirkin BL, Alward CT, et al. Treatment of neonatal hypertension with captopril. *J Pediatr* 1988;113(2):403–406.
89. Tack ED, Perlman JM. Renal failure in sick hypertensive premature infants receiving captopril therapy. *J Pediatr* 1988;112(5):805–810.
90. Guignard JP, Gouyon JB, John EG. Vasoactive factors in the immature kidney. *Pediatr Nephrol* 1991;5(4):443–446.
91. Perlman JM, Volpe JJ. Neurologic complications of captopril treatment of neonatal hypertension. *Pediatrics* 1989;83(1):47–52.
92. Sinaiko AR, Kashtan CE, Mirkin BL. Antihypertensive drug therapy with captopril in children and adolescents. *Clin Exp Hypertens A* 1986;8(4–5):829–839.
93. Kubo SH, Cody RJ. Clinical pharmacokinetics of the angiotensin converting enzyme inhibitors. A review. *Clin Pharmacokinet* 1985; 10(5):377–391.
94. Riley LJ Jr, Vlasses PH, Ferguson RK. Clinical pharmacology and therapeutic applications of the new oral converting enzyme inhibitor, enalapril. *Am Heart J* 1985;109(5, pt 1):1085–1089.
95. Rippley RK, Connor J, Boyle J, et al. Pharmacokinetic assessment of an oral enalapril suspension for use in children. *Biopharm Drug Dispos* 2000;21(9):339–344.
96. Ulm EH, Hichens M, Gomez HJ, et al. Enalapril maleate and a lysine analogue (MK-521): disposition in man. *Br J Clin Pharmacol* 1982;14(3):357–362.
97. Larmour I, Jackson B, Cubela R, et al. Enalapril (MK421) activation in man: importance of liver status. *Br J Clin Pharmacol* 1985; 19(5):701–704.
98. Hardman J, Limbird LE. In: Goodman and Gilman's the pharmacologic basis of therapeutics. New York: McGraw-Hill; 2001.
99. Proesmans W, Wambeke IV, Dyck MV. Long-term therapy with enalapril in patients with nephrotic-range proteinuria. *Pediatr Nephrol* 1996;10(5):587–589.
100. Nakamura H, Ishii M, Sugimura T, et al. The kinetic profiles of enalapril and enalaprilat and their possible developmental changes in pediatric patients with congestive heart failure. *Clin Pharmacol Ther* 1994;56(2):160–168.
101. Eronen M, Pesonen E, Wallgren EI, et al. Enalapril in children with congestive heart failure. *Acta Paediatr Scand* 1991;80(5):555–558.
102. Frenneaux M, Stewart RA, Newman CM, et al. Enalapril for severe heart failure in infancy. *Arch Dis Child* 1989;64(2):219–223.
103. Lloyd TR, Mahoney LT, Knoedel D, et al. Orally administered enalapril for infants with congestive heart failure: a dose-finding study. *J Pediatr* 1989;114(4, pt 1):650–654.
104. Miller K, Atkin B, Rodel PV Jr, et al. Enalapril: a well-tolerated and efficacious agent for the paediatric hypertensive patient. *J Hypertens Suppl* 1986;4(5):S413–S416.
105. Wells T, Frame V, Soffer B, et al. A double-blind, placebo-controlled, dose–response study of the effectiveness and safety of enalapril for children with hypertension. *J Clin Pharmacol* 2002; 42(8):870–880.
106. Schilder JL, Van den Anker JN. Use of enalapril in neonatal hypertension. *Acta Paediatr* 1995;84(12):1426–1428.
107. Wells TG, Bunchman TE, Kearns GL. Treatment of neonatal hypertension with enalaprilat. *J Pediatr* 1990;117(4):664–667.
108. Mason T, Polak MJ, Pyles L, et al. Treatment of neonatal renovascular hypertension with intravenous enalapril. *Am J Perinatol* 1992;9(4):254–257.
109. Dutta S, Narang A. Enalapril-induced acute renal failure in a newborn infant. *Pediatr Nephrol* 2003;18(6):570–572.
110. Lancaster SG, Todd PA. Lisinopril. A preliminary review of its pharmacodynamic and pharmacokinetic properties, and therapeutic use in hypertension and congestive heart failure. *Drugs* 1988;35(6):646–669.
111. Shaw W, Hogg R, Delucchi A, et al. Lisinopril pharmacokinetics in hypertensive children and infants. *Am J Hypertens* 2002;15: 46A.
112. Soffer B, Zhang Z, Miller K, et al. A double-blind, placebo-controlled, dose–response study of the effectiveness and safety of lisinopril for children with hypertension. *Am J Hypertens* 2003;16(10):795–800.
113. Blumer JL, Daniels SR, Dreyer WJ, et al. Pharmacokinetics of quinapril in children: assessment during substitution for chronic angiotensin-converting enzyme inhibitor treatment. *J Clin Pharmacol* 2003;43(2):128–132.
114. Wells T, Zhou SY, Hammet J, et al. Single-dose pharmacokinetics of an oral solution of fosinopril in children. *J Clin Pharmacol* 2003;43:1029.

115. Li JS, Berezny K, Kilaru R, et al. Is the extrapolated adult dose of fosinopril safe and effective in treating hypertensive children? *Hypertension* 2004;44(3):289–293.
116. Yi Z, Li Z, Wu XC, et al. Effect of fosinopril in children with steroid-resistant idiopathic nephrotic syndrome. *Pediatr Nephrol* 2006;21(7):967–972.
117. Soergel M, Verho M, Wuhl E, et al. Effect of ramipril on ambulatory blood pressure and albuminuria in renal hypertension. *Pediatr Nephrol* 2000;15(1–2):113–118.
118. Blowey DL. Safety of the newer antihypertensive agents in children. *Expert Opin Drug Saf* 2002;1(1):39–43.
119. Simon SR, Black HR, Moser M, et al. Cough and ACE inhibitors. *Arch Intern Med* 1992;152(8):1698–1700.
120. Bianchetti MG, Caflisch M, Oetliker OH. Cough and converting enzyme inhibitors. *Eur J Pediatr* 1992;151(3):225–226.
121. Donati-Genet P, Bianchetti MG. Modulators of the renin—angiotensin–aldosterone system and cough in childhood. *Pediatr Nephrol* 1996;10(4):545–546.
122. Williams GH. Converting-enzyme inhibitors in the treatment of hypertension. *N Engl J Med* 1988;319(23):1517–1525.
123. Ulmer JL, Garvey MJ. Fatal angioedema associated with lisinopril. *Ann Pharmacother* 1992;26(10):1245–1246.
124. Cooper WO, Hernandez-Diaz S, Arbogast PG, et al. Major congenital malformations after first-trimester exposure to ACE inhibitors. *N Engl J Med* 2006;354(23):2443–2451.
125. Cunniff C, Jones KL, Phillipson J, et al. Oligohydramnios sequence and renal tubular malformation associated with maternal enalapril use. *Am J Obstet Gynecol* 1990;162(1):187–189.
126. Pryde PG, Sedman AB, Nugent CE, et al. Angiotensin-converting enzyme inhibitor fetopathy. *J Am Soc Nephrol* 1993;3(9):1575–1582.
127. Sedman AB, Kershaw DB, Bunchman TE. Recognition and management of angiotensin converting enzyme inhibitor fetopathy. *Pediatr Nephrol* 1995;9(3):382–385.
128. Unger T. Blood pressure lowering and renin-angiotensin system blockade. *J Hypertens Suppl* 2003;21(6):S3–S7.
129. Ardaillou R. Angiotensin II receptors. *J Am Soc Nephrol* 1999; 10(Suppl 11):S30–S39.
130. Shaw W, Hogg R, Koch V, et al. Losartan and E-3174 pharmacokinetics in hypertensive children and infants. *J Am Soc Nephrol* 2002;13:149A.
131. Shahinfar S, Cano F, Soffer BA, et al. A double-blind, dose–response study of losartan in hypertensive children. *Am J Hypertens* 2005;18(2, pt 1):183–190.
132. Ellis D, Vats A, Moritz ML, et al. Long-term antiproteinuric and renoprotective efficacy and safety of losartan in children with proteinuria. *J Pediatr* 2003;143(1):89–97.
133. White CT, Macpherson CF, Hurley RM, et al. Antiproteinuric effects of enalapril and losartan: a pilot study. *Pediatr Nephrol* 2003; 18(10):1038–1043.
134. Sakarcan A, Tenney F, Wilson JT, et al. The pharmacokinetics of irbesartan in hypertensive children and adolescents. *J Clin Pharmacol* 2001;41:742–749.
135. Vachharajani NN, Shyu WC, Mantha S, et al. Oral bioavailability and disposition characteristics of irbesartan, an angiotensin antagonist, in healthy volunteers. *J Clin Pharmacol* 1998;38: 702–707.
136. Franscini LMD, Von Vigier RO, Pfister R, et al. Effectiveness and safety of the angiotensin II antagonist irbesartan in children with chronic kidney disease. *Am J Hypertens* 2002;15:1057–1063.
137. Flynn JT, Meyers KE, Neto JP, et al. Efficacy and safety of the angiotensin receptor blocker valsartan in children with hypertension aged 1 to 5 years. *Hypertension* 2008;52(2):222–228.
138. Blumer J, Batisky DL, Wells T, et al. Pharmacokinetics of valsartan in pediatric and adolescent subjects with hypertension. *J Clin Pharmacol* 2009;49(2):235–241.
139. Martinovic J, Benachi A, Laurent N, et al. Fetal toxic effects and angiotensin-II-receptor antagonists. *Lancet* 2001;358:241–242.
140. Magee LA. Drugs in pregnancy. Antihypertensives. *Best Pract Res Clin Obstet Gynaecol* 2001;15:827–845.
141. Janis RA, Scriabine A. Sites of action of Ca^{2+} channel inhibitor. *Biochem Pharmacol* 1983;32:3499–3507.
142. Taira N. Differences in cardiovascular profile among calcium antagonists. *Am J Cardiol* 1987;59:24B–29B.
143. Struyker-Boudier HAJ, Smits JFM, Demey JGR. The pharmacology of calcium antagonists: a review. *J Cardiovasc Pharmacol* 1990; 15(Suppl 4):S1–S10.
144. Braunwald E. Mechanism of action of calcium-channel-blocking agents. *N Engl J Med* 1982;307:1618–1627.
145. Snyder SH, Reynolds IJ. Calcium-antagonist drugs. Receptor interactions that clarify therapeutic effects. *N Engl J Med* 1985; 313:995–1002.
146. Bauer JH, Reams GP. The effects of antihypertensive therapy on renal function. In: Kaplan NM, Brenner BM, Laragh JH, eds. *Perspectives on hypertension. Vol. 3: New therapeutic strategies for hypertension.* New York: Raven Press, 1989:253–287.
147. Flynn JT. Nifedipine in the treatment of hypertension in children. *J Pediatr* 2002;140:787–788.
148. Moncica I, Oh PI, ul Qamar I, et al. A crossover comparison of extended release felodipine with prolonged action nifedipine in hypertension. *Arch Dis Child* 1995;73:154–156.
149. Rogan JW, Lyszkiewicz DA, Blowey D, et al. A randomized prospective crossover trial of amlodipine in pediatric hypertension. *Pediatr Nephrol* 2000;14:1083–1087.
150. Schran HF, Jaffe JM, Gonasun LM. Clinical pharmacokinetics of isradipine. *Am J Med* 1988;84(Suppl 3B):80–90.
151. Johnson CE, Beekman RH, Kostyshak DA, et al. Pharmacokinetics and pharmacodynamics of nifedipine in children with bronchopulmonary dysplasia and pulmonary hypertension. *Pediatr Res* 1991;29:500–503.
152. Dilmen U, Caglar MK, Senses A, et al. Nifedipine in hypertensive emergencies of children. *Am J Dis Child* 1983;137:1162–1165.
153. Lopez-Herce J, Dorao P, de la Oliva P, et al. Dosage of nifedipine in hypertensive crises of infants and children. *Eur J Pediatr* 1989; 149:136–137.
154. Lopez-Herce J, Albajara L, Cagigas P, et al. Treatment of hypertensive crisis in children with nifedipine. *Intensive Care Med* 1988; 14:519–521.
155. Siegler RL, Brewer ED. Effect of sublingual or oral nifedipine in the treatment of hypertension. *J Pediatr* 1988;112:811–813.
156. Roth B, Herkenrath P, Krebber J, et al. Nifedipine in hypertensive crises of infants and children. *Clin Exp Hypertens A* 1986;A8: 871–877.
157. Grossman E, Messerli FH, Grodzicki T, et al. Should a moratorium be placed on sublingual nifedipine capsules given for hypertensive emergencies and psuedo-emergencies? *J Am Med Assoc* 1996;276: 1328–1331.
158. Truttman AC, Zehnder-Schlapback S, Bianchetti MG. A moratorium should be placed on the use of short-acting nifedipine for hypertensive crisis. *Pediatr Nephrol* 1998;12:259–261.
159. Flynn JT. Nifedipine in the treatment of hypertension in children. *J Pediatr* 2002;140:787–788.
160. Blaszak RT, Savage JA, Ellis EN. The use of short-acting nifedipine in pediatric patients with hypertension. *J Pediatr* 2001;139: 34–37.
161. Flynn JT, Warnick SJ. Isradipine treatment of hypertension in children: a single-center experience. *Pediatr Nephrol* 2002;17: 748–753.
162. Saragoca MA, Poetela JE, Plavnick F, et al. Isradipine in the treatment of hypertensive crisis in ambulatory patients. *J Cardiovasc Pharmacol* 1992;19(Suppl 3):S76–S78.
163. Wells TG, House M, Belsha CW, et al. Treatment of pediatric hypertension with isradipine. *Clin Res* 1993;41:814A.
164. Trachtman H, Frank R, Mahan JD, et al. Clinical trial of extended-release felodipine in pediatric essential hypertension. *Pediatr Nephrol* 2003;18:548–553.
165. Blowey DL, Moncica I, Scolnik D, et al. The pharmacokinetics of extended release felodipine in children. *Eur J Clin Pharmacol* 1996;50:147–148.
166. Flynn JT, Smoyer WE, Bunchman TE. Treatment of hypertensive children with amlodipine. *Am J Hypertens* 2000;13:1061–1066.
167. Lyszkiewicz DA, Levichek Z, Kozer E, et al. Bioavailability of a pediatric amlodipine suspension. *Pediatr Nephrol* 2003;18: 675–678.
168. Flynn JT, Hogg RJ, Portman RJ, et al. Multicenter trial of amlodipine in children with hypertension. *Pediatr Res* 2002;51: 430A–431A.
169. Tobias JD. Nicardipine to control mean arterial pressure in a pediatric intensive care unit population. *Am J Anesthesiol* 1996; 23:109–112.
170. Gouyon JB, Geneste B, Semama DS, et al. Intravenous nicardipine in hypertensive preterm infants. *Arch Dis Child Fetal Neonatal Ed* 1997;76:F126–F127.

171. Michael J, Groshong T, Tobias JD. Nicardipine for hypertensive emergencies in children with renal disease. *Pediatr Nephrol* 1998;12:40–42.
172. Flynn JT, Mottes TA, Brophy PD, et al. Intravenous nicardipine for treatment of severe hypertension in children. *J Pediatr* 2001; 139:38–43.
173. Tobias JD. Nicardipine to control mean arterial pressure after cardiothoracic surgery in infants and children. *Am J Ther* 2001;8:3–6.
174. Milou C, Debuche-Benouachkou V, Semama DS, et al. Intravenous nicardipine as first-line antihypertensive drug in neonates. *Intensive Care Med* 2000;26:956–958.
175. Tenney F, Sakarcan A. Nicardipine is a safe and effective agent in pediatric hypertensive emergencies. *Am J Kidney Dis* 2000;35:E20.
176. Ludden TJ, McNay JL Jr, Shepherd AMM, et al. Clinical pharmacokinetics of hydralazine. *Clin Pharmacokinet* 1982;7:185–205.
177. Reece PA, Cozamanis I, Zacest R. Kinetics of hydralazine and its main metabolites in slow and fast acetylators. *Clin Pharmacol Ther* 1980;28:769–778.
178. Timbrell JA, Facchini V, Harland SJ, et al. Hydralazine-induced lupus: is there a toxic metabolic pathway? *Eur J Clin Pharmacol* 1984;27:555–559.
179. Chun G, Frishman WH. Rapid-acting parenteral antihypertensive agents. *J Clin Pharmacol* 1990;30:195–209.
180. Gordillo-Paniagua G, Velasquez-Jones L, Martini R, et al. Sodium nitroprusside treatment of severe arterial hypertension in children. *J Pediatr* 1975;87:799–802.
181. Benitz WE, Malachowski N, Cohen RS, et al. Use of sodium nitroprusside in neonates: efficacy and safety. *J Pediatr* 1985;106: 102–110.
182. Taketomo CK, Hodding JH, Kraus DM, eds. *Pediatric dosage handbook*, 10th ed. Hudson, OH: Lexi-Comp, 2003.
183. Luderer JR, Hayes AH, Dubynsky O, et al. Long-term administration of sodium nitroprusside in childhood. *J Pediatr* 1977;91: 490–491.
184. Linakis JG, Lacouture PG, Woolf A. Monitoring cyanide and thiocyanate concentrations during infusion of sodium nitroprusside in children. *Pediatr Cardiol* 1991;12:214–218.
185. Strife CF, Quinlan M, Waldo FB, et al. Minoxidil for control of acute blood pressure elevations in chronically hypertensive children. *Pediatrics* 1986;78:861–865.
186. Fleishaker JC, Andreadis NA, Welshman IR, et al. The pharmacokinetics of 2.5- to 10-mg oral doses of minoxidil in healthy volunteers. *J Clin Pharmacol* 1989;29:162–167.
187. Sinaiko AR, Mirkin BL. Management of severe childhood hypertension with minoxidil: a controlled clinical study. *J Pediatr* 1977;91:138–142.
188. Sinaiko AR, O'Dea RF, Mirkin BL. Clinical response of hypertensive children to long-term minoxidil therapy. *J Cardiovasc Pharmacol* 1980;2(Suppl 2):S181–S188.
189. Puri HC, Maltz HE, Kaiser BA, et al. Severe hypertension in children with renal disease: treatment with minoxidil. *Am J Kidney Dis* 1983;3:71–75.
190. Pennisi AJ, Takahashi M, Bernstein BH, et al. Minoxidil therapy in children with severe hypertension. *J Pediatr* 1977;90: 813–819.
191. Kaler SG, Patrinos ME, Lambert GH, et al. Hypertrichosis and congenital anomalies associated with maternal use of minoxidil. *Pediatrics* 1987;79:434–436.
192. Valdivieso A, Valdes G, Spiro TE, et al. Minoxidil in breast milk. *Ann Intern Med* 1985;102:135.
193. Alper AB, Calhoun DA. Contemporary management of refractory hypertension. *Curr Hypertens Rep* 1999;1:402–407.
194. Hanna JD, Chan JCM, Gill JR. Hypertension and the kidney. *J Pediatr* 1991;118:327–340.
195. Saken R, Kates GL, Miller K. Drug-induced hypertension in infancy. *J Pediatr* 1979;95:1077–1079.
196. Joss DV, Barrett AJ, Kendra JR, et al. Hypertension and convulsions in children receiving cyclosporin A. *Lancet* 1982;1:906.

CHAPTER

50

Catherine O'Brien, Jennifer Lowry, Kristine Palmer, Henry C Farrar, Gregory L Kearns, Laura P James

Gastrointestinal Drugs

INTRODUCTION

Gastrointestinal disorders are common in children and a wide variety of drugs are used to treat these conditions. The prevalence of gastroesophageal reflux disease (GERD) has been estimated to be as high as 8% in children (1,2). Although gastric and peptic ulcer diseases are responsible for significant morbidity and mortality in adults (3), these conditions are thought to be relatively infrequent in children (4). However, large-scale studies in children have yet to be performed, and the true prevalence and economic impact of pediatric ulcer disease is unknown (5). "Stress gastritis" is being increasingly recognized in children and adolescents and the most serious cases are typically secondary to *Helicobacter pylori* infection, which requires combination therapy to eradicate (6). Stress gastritis commonly occurs in critically ill hospitalized patients, including children, and many children are presumptively treated for the condition (7–9).

Children are commonly referred to as "therapeutic orphans" to reflect the relative disproportion of drug studies performed in pediatric as opposed to adult populations. Although this term was coined more than 40 years ago, it remains relevant today. Although progress has occurred in the last 15 years and an increased number of drugs have received Food and Drug Administration (FDA) approval for pediatric indications, many drugs commonly used to treat gastrointestinal conditions in children have not been thoroughly studied. This is especially true of off-patent drugs. Significant knowledge gaps remain in the pharmacology of these drugs in children, particularly for children younger than 1 year. This chapter reviews the current pediatric knowledge of drugs utilized to treat the more common pediatric gastrointestinal disorders. When available, the specific pharmacokinetics and pharmacodynamics of these drugs in children are discussed.

ANTIEMETIC AGENTS

Nausea and vomiting occur in a wide variety of diseases and clinical settings. Vomiting is controlled by the vomiting center of the medulla and has input from at least four sources, the chemoreceptor trigger zone, the cortex, the vestibular apparatus, and the gastrointestinal tract (10,11). These pathways are mediated by various neurotransmitters including serotonin (5-HT), which acts through central and peripheral 5-HT_3 receptors (12). Various clinical factors, such as the emetogenic potential of chemotherapeutic drugs or the etiology of vomiting, determine the efficacy of antiemetics. Because multiple neurotransmitters are involved in vomiting, a number of agents from various drug classes have been used to treat vomiting, including muscarinic agents, cannabinoids, steroids, and antagonists of histamine, dopamine, and serotonin receptors (10).

The dopamine antagonists (metoclopramide and the phenothiazines) and the 5-HT_3-receptor antagonists (ondansetron) are commonly used antiemetics (11,12,13). Metoclopramide blocks central dopamine receptors in the chemoreceptor trigger zone (13). Promethazine is a phenothiazine derivative with histamine H_1-receptor antagonist and anticholinergic properties. The 5-HT_3 antagonists block 5-HT_3 receptors in the enterochromaffin cells of the intestinal mucosa, thereby decreasing vagal input to the vomiting center, although these agents may also block receptors in the central nervous system (10,11,12). The high degree of receptor specificity of the 5-HT_3-receptor antagonists is associated with high efficacy and relatively fewer adverse effects of these drugs (14), compared with other agents used for this indication.

The 5-HT_3 antagonists are used for the management of anesthesia-, chemotherapy-, and radiation-related nausea and vomiting (12,15,16). Of the available drugs in this class, ondansetron has received the most study in children. The 5-HT_3 antagonists are generally viewed to be as effective as, or superior to, antidopaminergic drugs, and their efficacy is further enhanced by the adjunctive use of dexamethasone (12,15–17). Ondansetron's efficacy for the treatment of chemotherapy-related nausea and vomiting in children appears to vary by age and emetogenicity of the chemotherapeutic regimen. Younger children were shown to have better response rates in a survey study (18). In the setting of gastroenteritis, ondansetron was found to be superior to placebo or metoclopramide (19,20) or dexamethasone (21) in the management of vomiting associated with acute gastroenteritis (19–23). Ondansetron is also effective in children with gastroenteritis who fail oral rehydration therapy (22) and its use may reduce the length of stay in the emergency department (23). In addition, ondansetron given prior to ketamine for procedural sedation reduced vomiting rates in children (24). Granisetron is also approved for use in children with chemotherapy-related and postoperative nausea and vomiting (25,26).

Despite the efficacy of ondansetron in the setting of gastroenteritis, its use does not appear to be widespread. A review of antiemetic use in industrialized nations showed that up to 23% of children with gastroenteritis receive prescriptions for antiemetics. The most common drugs prescribed included promethazine, dimenhydrinate, diphenhydramine, and domperidone and prescription patterns varied by country. Promethazine was most commonly prescribed in the United States, and ondansetron compromised only 3% of prescriptions for this condition (27).

Other 5-HT_3 antagonists include dolasetron, granisetron, tropisetron, ramosetron, and palonosetron. In adults, the elimination half-lives for these compounds range from 3.9 to 10.6 hours (28). Of these compounds, palonosetron has the longest elimination rate; it has a half-life of up to 60 to 80 hours in adults, allowing for once-daily dosing and prolonged efficacy of up to 7 days (29). All drugs in this class are metabolized by CYPP450. Tropisetron and dolasetron are primarily metabolized by CYP2D6, and granisetron is primarily metabolized by CYP3A4. Ondansetron is metabolized by CYP2D6, CYP2E1, CYP3A, and CYP1A2 (28). The role of genetic variability in CYP2D6 activity has been examined as a determinant of drug efficacy (30,31). Approximately 5% to 10% of Caucasians are poor metabolizers (PMs) for CYP2D6, while 2% are considered ultrarapid metabolizers. Other ethnic populations have higher percentages of ultra rapid metabolizers. The efficacy of tropisetron and ondansetron was compared between ultra rapid and poor metabolizers for CYP2D6 in an oncology setting. Ultra rapid metabolizers were shown to have reduced control of nausea and vomiting compared with poor metabolizers following treatment with tropisetron; this effect was similar but less pronounced with ondansetron (32). These data suggest that a personalized medicine approach may be appropriate and feasible in the clinical setting of chemotherapy-induced nausea and vomiting (28).

Common adverse effects associated with ondansetron and other 5-HT_3 antagonists include anxiety, drowsiness, headache, constipation, and diarrhea (14). In addition, 5-HT_3 drugs have the potential to block either cardiac sodium or potassium channels, resulting in prolongation of the QRS or QTc intervals, respectively. Prescribing information for dolasetron and tropisetron contain warnings related to this potential cardiac toxicity (28). Granisetron altered cardiac conduction intervals in children receiving chemotherapy, but these events were asymptomatic (33). Buyukavci examined the effect of ondansetron (0.1 mg per kg infusion) versus granisetron (40 μg per kg infusion) on the electrocardiogram (ECG) and heart rate in children ($n = 22$) receiving antiemetics as prophylaxis during high-dose treatment with methotrexate (34). A decrease in heart rate at 1 and 3 hours and significant prolongation of mean QT and QTc dispersions at 1 hour after infusion were noted for granisetron. However, it should be noted that patients with these findings were asymptomatic. In contrast, no ECG or heart rate changes were noted in patients that received ondansetron. Similar findings have been reported for adults, although some case reports demonstrate increased symptomatology in select patients (35,36). It is recommended that 5-HT_3 receptor antagonists not be used in combination with drugs that have the potential to prolong QRS or QTc intervals. Concomitant use of 5-HT_3 antagonists that are highly metabolized by CYP2D6 (e.g., dolasetron, tropisetron) with drugs such as that inhibit CYP2D6 (e.g., fluoxetine, paroxetine, quinidine, or haloperidol) have the potential to cause drug interactions and possible adverse events (28). Limited pediatric data exist for the newer drugs in this class.

Pediatric dose-ranging studies of ondansetron for the management of postoperative nausea and vomiting have used doses of 0.05 to 0.2 mg per kg (37,38–45). Khalil (46) showed in a prospective, randomized, double-blind, placebo-controlled study that intravenous ondansetron (0.1 mg per kg) was safe and effective in the prevention of postoperative emesis in 1- to 24-month-old pediatric patients undergoing elective surgery under general anesthesia. In general, higher doses of ondansetron appear to have greater efficacy, although doses of 0.05 mg per kg are effective in many patients (37–39). Similar doses are frequently used to treat chemotherapy-related emesis with a titration to clinical effect (12). For treatment of vomiting-associated gastroenteritis, unit doses of 2 mg, 4 mg, and 8 mg have been used in children weighing 8 to 15 kg, 16 to 29 kg, and more than 29 kg, respectively (23). A single dose of drug is thought to be sufficient for the treatment of gastroenteritis (22). Although ondansetron is expensive, its use in this setting may avoid the need for hospitalization for intravenous hydration, especially when oral rehydration is possible.

The pharmacokinetic profile of ondansetron in children does not differ substantially from that of adults (12). The terminal elimination half-life in younger children (3 to 12 years), adolescents, and adults varies between 2.5 and 4 hours, being slightly less in younger children (12). Similarly, there are minor variations in the volume of distribution, area under the concentration versus time curve, and clearance. The 5-HT_3 antagonists are generally well absorbed (60%), although ondansetron undergoes a significant first-pass effect. Significant hepatic insufficiency may prolong the elimination of ondansetron, but toxicity has not been reported in this setting (17). Enzyme-inducing agents may enhance the elimination of ondansetron, but no toxicities secondary to drug interactions have been reported (12).

PROMETHAZINE AND METOCOPRAMIDE

Promethazine has a long history of use as an antiemetic, particularly in the management of postoperative nausea and vomiting and in the treatment of motion sickness. Side effects associated with the drug have limited its use and include sedation, extrapyramidal effects, hallucinations, seizures, tachycardia, and hypotension. Despite these concerns, it remains the most commonly prescribed antiemetic in the United States (27). In addition, metoclopramide is used as an antiemetic, but its use is associated with sedation, anticholinergic effects, and extrapyramidal symptoms (14,40). Metoclopramide is reviewed extensively in the "Prokinetic Agents" section.

ANTACIDS

Antacids are used in children for the treatment of gastritis, esophagitis, peptic ulcer disease, and GERD (41,42). In addition, they are included in combination treatment regimens for the management of *H. pylori*-related disease (42). In the past, antacids were used as prophylaxis for stress ulceration in intensive care units (8) and prior to surgical procedures. In recent years, antacids have been largely replaced by other acid-modifying drugs [e.g., H_2-receptor antagonists, proton pump inhibitors (PPIs)] due to safety and dosing concerns. Antacids are considered appropriate for use as short-term therapies (<2 weeks) for dyspepsia.

Antacids reduce and neutralize secreted gastric acid and have cytoprotective effects. Data from adult studies show that antacids at the proper doses are effective in the treatment of ulcer disease (42) and stress ulcer prophylaxis (43). Sucralfate, ranitidine, and almagate were equally effective as prophylaxis for gastrointestinal hemorrhage in critically ill children (8).

Sodium bicarbonate and calcium carbonate are the most potent antacids, followed by magnesium- and then aluminum-containing products. Sodium bicarbonate and calcium carbonate are also rapid-acting antacids. Chronic use of sodium bicarbonate is associated with fluid retention, systemic alkalosis, and the milk alkali syndrome. Calcium carbonate has a longer duration of action than sodium bicarbonate and has also been associated with hypercalcemia, hypercalciuria, renal calcium deposits, compromised renal function, and gastric acid hypersecretion (44,45). Diarrhea and hypermagnesemia are associated with the use of magnesium-containing antacids, particularly in patients with compromised renal function. Adverse events associated with the use of aluminum-containing antacids include constipation, hypophosphatemia, and hypocalcemia. Aluminum accumulation and the formation of bezoars have also been reported for aluminum-containing antacids, particularly in young infants with compromised renal function (41,47).

Concomitant use of other drugs with antacids may decrease drug absorption, and alteration of gastric pH may change the dissolution rate of drugs. Dosing of antacids 2 hours after other drugs (e.g., quinolones, H_2-receptor antagonists) may help to avoid this drug interaction (48). In general, the smallest effective dose of antacid should be utilized in children, beginning at 0.5 to 1.0 mL per kg in infants and 5 to 10 mL in children, up to a single dose of 10 to 20 mL. Administration of antacids 1 hour after meals has been shown to be effective in reducing gastric acidity in infants and to allow for reduction of the antacid dose (49). Long-term therapy (>2 to 4 weeks) with antacids in infants and children should be closely monitored for adverse effects.

PROKINETIC AGENTS

Prokinetic agents are utilized to improve gastric hypomotility, a frequent component of many pediatric gastrointestinal disorders (50). GER is the most common disorder of gastric motility in children and infants, and approximately 50% of mothers report that their infants regurgitate two or more times per day (50,51). For the majority of infants, GER is a self-limited, transient problem that resolves by 8 to 12 months of age and can be managed with nonpharmacologic therapies (51). However, pharmacotherapy may be indicated in children with pathologic GER (e.g., poor weight gain, Sandifer syndrome, esophagitis, esophageal stricture, aspiration, and airway inflammation). Surgical management is typically reserved for patients who fail therapy with acid-reducing drugs and prokinetic agents (51).

Transient relaxation of the lower esophageal sphincter is considered one of the most important factors in the pathogenesis of GER. Delayed gastric emptying is also a factor and is noted in approximately one-half of patients with GER (51). Bethanechol, metoclopramide, and erythromycin improve lower esophageal sphincter tone, and metoclopramide and erythromycin, but not bethanechol, improve gastric emptying. However, with the withdrawal of cisapride (discussed later) and the adverse effects associated with metoclopramide, other prokinetic agents, such as erythromycin, are more commonly used.

Feeding intolerance in premature newborns is another common clinical problem in pediatrics. Migrating motor complexes are responsible for phasic contractions that move distally through the intestine. These complexes appear, at least in part, to be stimulated by increased activity of the receptor for motilin, a polypeptide hormone (52,53). Infants begin to express increased numbers of motilin receptors at approximately 32 weeks of gestational age (53). Enteral feeding may result in increased release of enteric polypeptide hormones (50). Thus, prokinetic drugs that stimulate motilin receptor activity may result in improved tolerance of feeding in premature newborns. Currently, motilin receptor agonists are undergoing safety and efficacy testing in early phase clinical trials in adults with impaired gastric motor function (54–56).

BETHANECHOL

Bethanechol is an acetylcholine receptor agonist and has its greatest effect on the smooth muscle of the distal esophagus. At doses of 0.1 mg per kg, bethanechol increases the tone of the lower esophageal sphincter, whereas higher doses (0.2 mg per kg) are required to increase the amplitude and duration of esophageal peristaltic activity (57,58). These effects are absent in the upper esophagus, probably because of the predominance of striated muscle in this portion of the esophagus. Bethanechol appears to have less of an effect on gastric motility, increasing the amplitude but decreasing the frequency of antral contractions with no overall increase in gastric emptying (59). Thus, bethanechol may have a use in the treatment of GER through its effects on the lower esophageal sphincter.

Clinical studies of bethanechol in the treatment of GER have yielded mixed results. Some studies reported that bethanechol was effective in controlling clinical symptoms, improving weight gain, and reducing acid reflux by pH probe measurements; these findings have not been consistently reproduced (58,60,61). Orenstein et al. showed that children with normal lower esophageal tone by manometry actually had an increase in the number and duration of reflux episodes with bethanechol (58). Another study reported bethanechol to be comparable to liquid antacids in the treatment of GER-related symptoms (62). Although bethanechol increases lower esophageal sphincter tone, its variable effect on gastric motility likely contributes to its variable efficacy in the treatment of GER (59). The efficacy of bethanechol may also be influenced by the baseline tone of the lower esophageal sphincter (58). The optimal dose of bethanechol in children has not been clearly defined because of a lack in pharmacokinetic studies of bethanechol in children. The typical dose of bethanechol is 0.1 to 0.2 mg per kg given 30 minutes prior to feeding up to four times per day (63).

Dizziness, headache, nausea, vomiting, chest pain, bronchoconstriction, and acute dystonic reactions have been reported in association with the use of bethanechol (60,62,64). Because bethanechol is a cholinergic agonist and can precipitate bronchoconstriction, it should be avoided or used with caution in children with a history of or at risk for bronchospasm.

METOCLOPRAMIDE

Metoclopramide, 2-methoxy-5-chloro-procainamide, is a prokinetic agent commonly used to treat GER, dysmotility disorders, and feeding intolerance in infants and children. Although structurally similar to procainamide, metoclopramide is without any appreciable anesthetic or antiarrhythmic properties. Metoclopramide's mechanism of action is thought to result from a combination of central and peripheral dopamine antagonism. The drug's antiemetic effects are most likely mediated centrally at the dopamine D_2 receptor. Peripherally, the augmentation of acetylcholine release from postganglionic nerve terminals is likely responsible for the drug's effect on gastrointestinal smooth muscle (65,66). In addition, metoclopramide appears to sensitize the muscarinic receptors of gastrointestinal smooth muscle to acetylcholine (35,67). The effect of metoclopramide on cholinergic neurons is unlike that of bethanechol or other "cholinomimetic" agents, as metoclopramide does not increase gastric acid secretion, endogenous gastrin release, or salivation. The motility effects of metoclopramide appear unique to this drug class, promoting the coordination of gastric, pyloric, and duodenal motor function. This overall prokinetic effect is due to the drug's coordination of accelerated gastric emptying by increasing gastric tone, increasing the amplitude of antral contractions and relaxation of the pylorus and duodenum, while increasing the peristalsis of the jejunum, thus accelerating intestinal transit from the duodenum to the ileocecal valve (65).

Efficacy studies of metoclopramide in children have yielded variable results. Randomized, controlled studies utilizing doses of 0.1 and 0.125 mg per kg of metoclopramide every 6 hours demonstrated some improvement in reflux symptoms, with greater improvement in older children, whereas doses of 0.2 mg per kg every 6 hours significantly improved all measures of reflux disease (68,69). Improvement in GER-related symptoms have been reported in small studies of infants with GER (70,71). Hyman et al. (71) found that infants with gastroparesis following surgery demonstrated considerable improvement in gastric motility with metoclopramide, whereas infants with gastroparesis of prematurity did not have a significant change in gastric emptying. Other small studies reported improved feeding tolerance and decreased gastric residual volumes in neonates treated with metoclopramide (72,73). Metoclopramide has also been used for the treatment of chemotherapy-induced nausea and vomiting (13), postsurgical gastroparesis, and to facilitate the passage of nasoenteric feeding tubes beyond the pylorus (74,75).

A systematic review of the use of metoclopramide for the treatment of GER illustrates the contradictions in the literature for this drug. A review of 12 prospective trials (76) including 5 randomized, blinded clinical trials was conducted. Eight studies showed improvement in at least one outcome after treatment with metoclopramide; one study showed worsening of symptoms. The remaining studies showed that metoclopramide had no effect or an effect comparable to placebo. The weight of the evidence supporting the use of metoclopramide was judged to be "poor" due to the limited number of studies, small sample sizes, quality of study designs, and the lack of consistency in the literature. Given the high risk for adverse effects (detailed later), the existing evidence for its safety and efficacy was deemed "inconclusive" (76). Inconsistencies in the existing data point to the need for large clinical trials to thoroughly assess pharmacokinetics, pharmacodynamics, and safety and efficacy of metoclopramide in children.

Metoclopramide is rapidly absorbed following oral administration and substantial interindividual variation has been observed in maximal serum concentrations as well as in the drug's oral bioavailability (range, 32% to 97%) (66,77). This variation is most likely due to first-pass drug metabolism (78,79). Approximately 40% of metoclopramide is bound to plasma protein, primarily α_1-acid glycoprotein (80). The drug is readily excreted into breast milk (81). The majority of metoclopramide is metabolized in the liver by sulfation, and approximately 20% of the dose is excreted unchanged in the urine. Its elimination half-life in adults ranges from 2.5 to 5 hours (78,79).

Limited pharmacokinetic data are available to characterize the disposition of metoclopramide in children (70,78,82). One study found that children, ages 7 to 14 years, had pharmacokinetic parameters that were similar to those of adults (78). Kearns et al. (82,83) reported that the mean values for plasma clearance and volume of distribution were increased 1.4- and 2.1-fold in neonates, respectively, in comparison to values reported in adults (65). The mean value for elimination half-life in neonates was not significantly different from that in older infants, children, and adults (78,82). However, interindividual variability for elimination half-lives was large in neonates and older infants, and in several individual patients half-lives were more than 10 hours (70,82). Developmental or pharmacogenetic influences on drug metabolism, particularly in the sulfotransferase isoforms responsible for the *N*-4-sulfation of metoclopramide (78,82), may contribute to this variability. The data support a starting oral dose of metoclopramide of 0.15 mg per kg administered every 6 hours in term newborns, infants, and children (70). Lower doses (0.1 mg per kg every 6 hours) may be appropriate in the neonatal population because delayed clearance may be a concern.

Adverse reactions associated with the use of metoclopramide include drowsiness, restlessness, dry mouth, lightheadedness, and diarrhea. Overall, adverse reactions may occur in as many as 20% of patients treated with the drug and appear to be dose related. Less common adverse events include extrapyramidal effects, such as torticollis and oculogyric reactions, and are secondary to the drug's effect on dopamine and acetylcholine. Extrapyramidal effects occur in approximately 1% of patients, and young age and high dose appear to be risk factors associated with their occurrence (84,85). Avoidance of concurrent therapy with drugs with dopamine antagonist activity (e.g., phenothiazines) may help to lower the risk of extrapyramidal reactions. Rare adverse events include methemoglobinemia, seizures, elevation of serum prolactin concentrations, breast enlargement, nipple tenderness, galactorrhea, and menstrual irregularities (65,83).

Because of the effects of metoclopramide on gastric emptying and intestinal motility, it has the potential to alter the oral bioavailability and resulting serum concentration relationships (e.g., peak plasma concentration and time to peak plasma concentration) of a multitude of drugs. Studies of this potential drug interaction have yielded variable results, indicating an inconsistent effect of metoclopramide on the gastrointestinal absorption of concurrently administered drugs (77).

CISAPRIDE

Cisapride, a benzamide compound, has been shown to be effective for the treatment of GER in children (86,87). The drug enhances peripheral acetylcholine release, which subsequently increases antral motility and duodenal contractility, increases coordination of antroduodenal function, and accelerates gastric emptying (88). Cisapride has no effect on dopamine receptors (88). Cisapride also improves lower esophageal sphincter tone and esophageal contractility (67,88). In placebo-controlled studies comparing cisapride to metoclopramide, it appears to be at least as effective as, if not more effective than, metoclopramide (69,88,89). Cisapride has not been associated with the development of the extrapyramidal effects seen with other prokinetic agents.

Increased use of cisapride in the treatment of motility disorders, especially in adults, resulted in recognition of an association with electrocardiographic abnormalities, particularly the development of prolonged QTc intervals and associated ventricular arrhythmias (90). This adverse event did not appear to occur as frequently in the pediatric population (36,91). Risk factors for cardiac effects have been well described and include excessive dosing, inappropriate dosing in premature infants, treatment with drugs known to inhibit the CYP3A4 isoforms, and use in patients with existing QTc prolongation. Additional concerns include underlying cardiac disease, electrolyte disturbances, renal insufficiency, hepatic dysfunction, and concurrent therapy with medications known to alter cardiac conduction intervals (90). Because of persistent concerns over the safety, cisapride was removed from the market in the United States and Canada. The drug remains widely available throughout the rest of the world.

ERYTHROMYCIN

Erythromycin has been demonstrated to have prokinetic activity and is effective at doses less than those typically used for antimicrobial therapy (92). The drug appears to have pharmacodynamics similar to the polypeptide hormone motilin, stimulating migrating motor complexes in the gastrointestinal tract and promoting the aboral movement of nutrients (52,53). Erythromycin was found to increase the lower esophageal sphincter tone and the duration but not the amplitude of contractions of the distal esophagus in adults with GER (52). A recent review comparing erythromycin to metoclopramide supported the use of erythromycin as a prokinetic agent (93).

The optimal dose of erythromycin for improved gastrointestinal motility is 1 to 3 mg per kg. Higher doses (10 to 15 mg per kg), similar to those used in antimicrobial therapy, tend to cause continuous high-amplitude contractions or motor quiescence (94). A dose-ranging study in healthy adults noted enhanced gastric motility with increasing doses of 0.75, 1.5, and 3 mg per kg, and a 1.5 mg per kg dose of erythromycin was found to be equivalent to a standard 10-mg dose of metoclopramide (95). In a study of premature newborns, intravenous erythromycin at a dose of 0.75 mg per kg significantly increased gastric and duodenal contractions (30).

The efficacy of erythromycin in the management of feeding intolerance in premature newborns may be dependent on gestational age (92). Erythromycin did not decrease the time interval required to tolerate full feedings or decrease vomiting in two placebo-controlled clinical trials (31,96). However, in both of these studies, antimicrobial doses of erythromycin (12 to 15 mg per kg per day) were used, and the infants studied were younger than 31 of weeks of gestation. In a study evaluating age-related motilin receptor activity, infants younger than 32 weeks of gestation had no response to erythromycin, whereas 50% of children older than 32 weeks of gestation had increased motor activity with erythromycin (53). Thus, it is not clear whether lower doses may be effective in stimulating gastrointestinal motility or whether the developmental stage of migrating motor complexes is the most important limitation of erythromycin therapy.

In older children, 1 mg per kg of erythromycin was as effective as 0.15 mg per kg of metoclopramide in reducing preoperative gastric residual volumes (97). Other observational reports have described the efficacy of erythromycin in the treatment of other disorders of gastrointestinal motility (98,99). Thus, erythromycin may be useful in the treatment of gastrointestinal dysmotility in selected older children at doses of 1 to 3 mg per kg.

Ongoing studies of motilin receptor agonists, including other macrolides, will determine their safety, efficacy, and role in the pharmacologic management of impaired gastric motor function (54–56). The agonist, ABT-229, slightly, but significantly, reduced the duration of acid reflux in a dose-dependent manner in adults, although in another study this drug did not improve acid reflux-related symptoms (100,101). However, many of these studies have been unsuccessful (including ABT-229), possibly due to development of tachyphylaxis at the receptor site (102).

The inhibitory effect of erythromycin on the cytochrome P450 system, especially CYP3A4, has been well described and is a significant factor for the development of adverse drug reactions. In addition, the rapid intravenous infusion of erythromycin lactobionate has been associated with bradycardia, hypotension, prolongation of the QTc interval, and ventricular arrhythmias (103,104).

The association of erythromycin use in infants and the development of infantile hypertrophic pyloric stenosis is also of concern. After the widespread use of erythromycin for pertussis prophylaxis of newborns in a community, there was a nearly sevenfold increase in the rate of pyloric stenosis, from 4.7 to 32 cases per 1,000 livebirths, and the risk appears to increase with treatment periods of 14 days or longer (105,106). However, much of the literature on this association has been retrospective in nature and has not clearly defined a causal relationship (106). In addition, the studies that evaluated erythromycin as a prokinetic agent failed to monitor for the development of pyloric stenosis as an adverse event. Low-dose treatment with erythromycin has not been associated with the development of hypertrophic pyloric stenosis (107).

OTHER PROKINETIC AGENTS

Additional drugs that have been used as prokinetics or are under development include dopamine antagonists, serotonin agonists, and baclofen. Peripheral dopamine receptor antagonists have been used in the past for the treatment of GER. Domperidone is a D_2 antagonist that has been shown to increase motility and gastric emptying (108). However, due to its cardiovascular side effect profile including QTc prolongation, the manufacturer ceased production. Itopride is a dopamine D_2 antagonist with acetylcholinesterase inhibitory actions that is currently in clinical trials. It has compared favorably to domperidone in symptom relief, patient tolerance, safety, and efficacy (109). In a recent placebo-controlled trial, itopride was found to be superior to placebo in symptom scores of patients with functional dyspepsia (110).

Serotonin 5-HT_4 receptors are expressed on nerve terminals within the gastrointestinal tract, and binding of agonists to these receptors has been shown to enhance motility. Ongoing trials suggest that these drugs are effective in accelerating gastric and colonic emptying in adults. In addition, these drugs increase secretions, which may result in looser stools (111).

Baclofen, a derivative of γ-aminobutyric acid, has also been used extensively for the treatment of disorders involving muscular contraction. In a recent randomized, double-blind, placebo-controlled trial, baclofen was shown to reduce the incidence of transient lower esophageal sphincter relaxation and accelerated the rate of gastric emptying (112). In addition, a small study showed that baclofen reduced the number of acid reflux events from baseline measured by esophageal pH monitory. However, time of low pH and acid clearance in the esophagus was not affected (113). Although baclofen may be efficacious in some patients, its potential to cause muscle weakness may limit its widespread use, but it may be helpful in developmentally delayed children or children with spasticity who also have GERD.

H_2-RECEPTOR ANTAGONISTS

H_2-receptor antagonists are some of the most commonly used drugs in children for reflux-related symptoms, treatment of gastric or duodenal ulcers, and treatment of or prophylaxis against gastrointestinal hemorrhage (113–116). Four H_2-receptor antagonists are available for clinical use in the United States (Table 50.1). However, only ranitidine and famotidine are approved for use in both children and adolescents. Nizatidine is approved for adolescents, but not for children younger than 12 years.

The four H_2-receptor antagonists are similar to one another in efficacy but have different drug interaction and side effect profiles, based on their respective chemical structures. The original H_2-receptor antagonist, cimetidine, contains an imidazole ring. Ranitidine contains an amino methyl furan moiety, which provides greater potency and a longer duration of action. Famotidine is a thiazole ring and is 10 to 15 times more potent than ranitidine and 40 to 60 times more potent than cimetidine in inhibiting gastric acid secretion. The longer elimination half-life of famotidine may be particularly desirable for use in children by allowing for less frequent dosing (twice daily as opposed to three to four times daily for ranitidine).

The H_2-receptor antagonists reduce gastric acid secretion by acting as competitive, reversible inhibitors of histamine at the histamine H_2-receptor. The effects of histamine are mediated by binding to H_1- and H_2-receptors, and binding of histamine to H_2-receptors stimulates gastric acid secretion. H_2-receptor antagonists do not have effects on other receptors, including the H_1-receptor, or the muscarinic, nicotinic, or sympathomimetic α- or β-receptors (117). H_2-receptor antagonists also decrease the acid-secretory response of the parietal cell to stimulated acid secretion from cholinergic agents, gastrin, food, and vagal stimulation (117). However, the most prominent effects of H_2-receptor antagonists are on acid secretion and thus they are particularly effective in suppressing nocturnal acid production. Because nocturnal acid secretion is an important factor in the development of duodenal ulcers, H_2-receptor antagonists may be particularly effective for the

TABLE 50.1 Pharmacokinetics of H_2-Receptor Antagonists in Children (Mean ± SD)[a]

	Age (yr)	$t_{1/2}$ *(hr)*	V_d *(L/kg)*	*Cl*	*Ref.*
Cimetidine	9.0 (2.3)	1.4 (0.3)	1.2 (0.5)	10.4 mL/min/kg (4)	(199)
Ranitidine	12.6 (3.7)	1.8 (0.3)	2.3 (0.9)	795 mL/min/kg (334)	(129)
Famotidine	6.1 (4.9)	3.2 (3.0)	2.4 (1.7)	0.70 L/hr/kg (0.34)	(130,131)
Nizatidine	8.0 (2.4)	1.2 (0.2)	3.2 (0.6)	1.23 L/hr/kg (0.2)	(136)

[a] $t_{1/2}$, elimination half-life; V_d, volume of distribution; Cl, clearance.

management of these patients. In addition, H_2-receptor antagonists are utilized in combination with PPIs in patients who have nocturnal gastric acid breakthrough (118). Although most H_2-receptor antagonists are not thought to have direct effects on gastric motility, nizatidine has been reported to enhance gastrointestinal activity, independent of its effects on altering gastric acid secretion (119).

Several studies have evaluated the efficacy of H_2-receptor antagonists in the treatment of gastric acid-related disorders in children. Tam and Saing found that H_2-receptor antagonists were highly effective in the treatment of chronic peptic ulcer disease in children (116). High rates of ulcer healing (i.e., 91%) were observed following an 8-week course of therapy with either cimetidine or ranitidine. Only 1 treatment failure occurred among 32 patients in comparison to 16 failures in 46 children who were treated with antacids. Nagita et al. (120) found that famotidine (0.5 mg per kg twice daily, maximum 40 mg per day) was effective in healing gastroduodenal ulcers in children, and Oderda et al. found famotidine to be superior to antacids in treating children with esophagitis (121). Fewer pediatric studies have been performed with nizatidine, but a double-blind, placebo-controlled study found it to be effective in the treatment of reflux esophagitis in children (122). In an open-label, multiple-dose, randomized, multicenter trial with 210 children, Orenstein showed that nizatidine was well tolerated and effective for children aged 5 days to 18 years with GERD (123).

H_2-receptor antagonists are frequently utilized in neonatal and pediatric intensive care units as prophylaxis for gastric stress ulceration. However, their routine use in critically ill patients has been questioned due to the concern that alteration of gastric pH would allow for the overgrowth of pathogenic bacteria (115). In a neonatal study, ranitidine use, length of hospitalization, higher gastric pH, and length of antibiotic therapy were each independently associated with increased rates of bacterial colonization (124), but an increased rate of infection was not found in infants who received ranitidine. However, a more recent randomized controlled study found that GERD-affected children had an increased risk of acute gastroenteritis and community-acquired pneumonia (125). In addition, the use of H_2-blocker therapy in the very low-birth-weight infant may increase the incidence of necrotizing enterocolitis (126). A larger scale study in infants and children is needed to fully address the relationship of alkaline gastric pH and predisposition to infection.

The oral bioavailability of H_2-receptor antagonists varies depending on the specific agent, and nizatidine has the highest bioavailability (approximately 70%) of the four drugs. Antacids decrease the relative bioavailability of H_2-receptor antagonists by 12% to 25% (127). For the most part, these drugs are not highly protein bound. Between 25% and 40% of cimetidine is metabolized. Between 60% and 80% of nizatidine, ranitidine, and famotidine are eliminated by the kidneys as unchanged drugs. Dose adjustment is indicated for the H_2-receptor antagonists in children and adolescents with renal failure (128) and in infants with developmentally determined alterations in renal clearance. The H_2-receptor antagonists are not removed to any significant extent by peritoneal or hemodialysis.

The pharmacokinetics of cimetidine, ranitidine, and famotidine have been well characterized in children (129–131,132). Both glomerular filtration and tubular secretion contribute to the renal elimination of famotidine, ranitidine, and nizatidine and these processes do not reach adult maturity until 5 to 12 months of age (133,134). Consistent with the developmental profile for renal function in children during the first year of life, prolonged renal and plasma clearance for famotidine have been reported for children younger than 3 months (131,135). A report (Table 50.1) describing the disposition of nizatidine in children (mean age, 8.0 ± 2.4 years) indicates that the pharmacokinetics are very similar to that previously reported in adults (136).

The pharmacokinetics of ranitidine and famotidine have been characterized in infants (Table 50.2). Less information is available to guide the dosing of H_2-receptor antagonists in premature infants, but several pharmacodynamic studies have been performed in this population. Kuusela (137) studied 16 critically ill infants (mean gestational age, 33 weeks) and found that preterm infants required only twice-daily dosing (0.5 mg per kg per dose), whereas term infants required thrice-daily dosing (1.5 mg per kg per dose) to maintain a gastric pH of more than 4. Kelly et al. (138) found that continuous infusions of ranitidine of 0.0625 mg per kg per hour in premature infants (gestational age, 24 to 31 weeks) achieved a mean gastric pH of 4.9. Dose adjustments may be indicated in infants receiving ranitidine during extracorporeal membrane oxygenation (ECMO) (139). Wells et al. (140) reported that the elimination half-life of ranitidine was prolonged (6.6 ± 2.8 hours) in term infants receiving ECMO in comparison with data previously reported in other critically ill infants (3.5 ± 0.3 hours) (132). In this study, intragastric pH was maintained at more than 4 for 16 hours in infants who had an initial pH less than 4. On the basis of these data, intermittent dosing of every 12 hours for term infants and every 24 hours for preterm infants would appear appropriate for infants receiving ECMO. Dose titration to achieve a gastric pH of

TABLE 50.2 Pharmacokinetics of H_2-Receptor Antagonists in Infants (Mean ± SD)

	Age	*$t_{1/2}$ (hr)*	*V_d (L/kg)*	*Cl*	*Ref.*
Ranitidine	12 mo (6.9)	2.1 (1.3)	1.6 (1.0)	13.9 mL/min/kg (10.0)	(137)
Famotidine	6.6 d (4.4)	10.5 (5.4)	1.35 (0.42)	0.132 L/hr/kg (0.061)	(131)
	0–3 mo	7.6 (4.6, 12.6)[b]	1.76 (1.43, 2.18)[b]	0.2 mL/min/kg (0.14, 1.27)[b]	(135)

[a] $t_{1/2}$, elimination half-life; V_d, volume of distribution; Cl, clearance.
[b] Ninety percent confidence interval.

more than 4 may be indicated in infants and children with multiple risk factors for stress-related gastric ulceration (141).

In general, the H_2-receptor antagonists are well tolerated in children (142). Adverse reactions are more common with cimetidine than with the other drugs of this class and have been reported to be as high as 4.5% (143). Gastrointestinal symptoms, rash, and dizziness are the most common adverse effects associated with H_2-receptor antagonists (144). Central nervous system effects, including mania and seizures, have also been described with cimetidine. Elevated CNS/plasma ratios of cimetidine have been documented in adults with renal or hepatic insufficiency who experience CNS symptoms while receiving the drug (145). Adverse effects related to the endocrine system include gynecomastia, galactorrhea, impotence, and possibly a decrease in spermatogenesis (146). Elevations of serum prolactin have been associated with intravenous use of cimetidine. Thrombocytopenia and agranulocytosis are considered rare adverse effects of H_2-receptor antagonists. Bradycardia has been reported in a 4-day-old infant who received a 1 mg per kg infusion of ranitidine (147).

Drug interactions are more common with cimetidine than with the other H_2-receptor antagonist. This is secondary to the inhibitory effects of cimetidine on the cytochromes P450. Concurrent therapy of cimetidine and theophylline has resulted in the accumulation of theophylline and the development of seizures (148). Reduced drug clearance has also been reported for the coadministration of cimetidine with warfarin, phenytoin, quinidine, caffeine, metronidazole, diazepam, imipramine, lidocaine, meperidine, procainamide, propranolol, and triamterene. Although ranitidine has been reported to bind to cytochrome P450, its binding affinity is approximately 10-fold lower than that of cimetidine. Clinically significant drug interactions for ranitidine, famotidine, and nizatidine are unusual (149).

The H_2-receptor antagonists may be administered by oral, intramuscular, or intravenous routes. Oral formulations are available for all four drugs and intravenous and intramuscular formulations are available for cimetidine, ranitidine, and famotidine. Liquid pediatric formulations are available for all four H_2-receptor antagonists.

PROTON PUMP INHIBITORS

The final common pathway for acid production within the parietal cells is the H^+/K^+ adenosine triphosphatase (ATPase) enzyme transport system, commonly referred to as the proton pump. Drugs that target this pathway are a class of substituted benzimidazole compounds referred to as proton pump inhibitors (PPIs). Omeprazole, the first PPI, was approved for human use in the United States in 1988. Subsequently, four PPIs have been approved by the US FDA, including lansoprazole, pantoprazole, rabeprazole, and esomeprazole, the pure S isomer of omeprazole (150). Although only pantoprazole lacks FDA-approved product labeling in pediatric patients, none of the PPIs have approved labeling for children younger than 1 year.

PPIs are substituted 2-pyridyl methyl sulfinyl benzimidazoles (150). They are weakly basic compounds that differ from each other by molecular substituents attached to the benzimidazole and pyridine components of the molecule (Fig. 50.1). All PPIs are prodrugs, given that protonation of the nitrogen on the pyridine group produces the active form of the drug, a cyclic sulfonamide. This intermediate is trapped within the acidic environment of the parietal cell canaliculi and binds covalently to exposed cysteine thiol groups on the luminal surface of the proton pump, thus disabling it. Differences in the pK_a of the various PPIs have been shown to affect their onset of action (rapid to slower: rabeprazole > omeprazole > lansoprazole > pantoprazole) (151,152). Table 50.3 provides an overview of pharmacokinetic parameters of the currently marketed PPIs. Esomeprazole and lansoprazole are the most bioavailable of the PPIs (Table 50.3).

Considerable variability exists for the plasma concentration profiles for the PPIs due, in part, to differences in their presystemic clearance (e.g., lowest bioavailability for those drugs that are metabolized by CYP3A4) and coadministration with food (lansoprazole > omeprazole > pantoprazole) (150). Lansoprazole, pantoprazole, and rabeprazole demonstrate dose proportionality [i.e., linearity between dose and resulting area under the curve (AUC)], in contrast with omeprazole and esomeprazole, where the extent of bioavailability increases with repeated dosing (153). The PPIs are effective only if converted to their respective active moieties in the parietal cell canaliculi where active

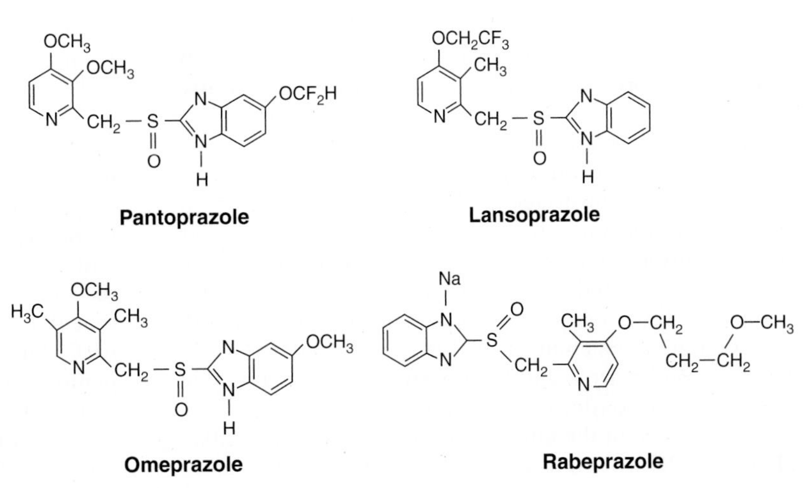

Pantoprazole

Lansoprazole

Omeprazole

Rabeprazole

Figure 50.1. Chemical structures of proton pump inhibitors.

TABLE 50.3 Comparative Average Pharmacokinetic Parameters of the Proton Pump Inhibitors in Adults[a]

Parameter	*Omeprazole 20 mg*	*Esomeprazole 40 mg*	*Pantoprazole 40 mg*	*Lansoprazole 30 mg*	*Rabeprazole 20 mg*
AUC (mg/L/hr)	0.2–1.2	12.6 (μmol/L/hr)	2–5	1.7–5	0.8
C_{max} (mg/L)	0.08–8.0	NA	1.1–3.3	0.6–1.2	0.41
T_{max} (hr)	1–3	1.6	2–4	6.3–2.2	3.1
Activation time (min)[b]	2.8/84	NA	4.6/282	2.0/90	6.3/7.2
$t_{1/2}$ (hr)	0.6–1.0	1.2–1.5	0.9–1.9	0.9–1.6	1
Cl/*F* (L/hr/kg)	0.45	NA	0.08–0.13	0.2–0.28	0.5
Bioavailability (%)	35–65	89–90	57–100	80–91	52
Protein binding (%)	95	97	98	97–99	95–98
Dose linearity	Nonlinear	Nonlinear	Linear	Linear	Linear

[a]AUC, area under the plasma concentration–time curve; Cl/*F*, apparent total plasma clearance; C_{max}, peak plasma concentration; $t_{1/2}$, elimination half-life; T_{max}, time to peak plasma concentration; NA, not available.
[b]Value independent of dose at gastric pH values of 1.2/5.1, respectively.
Source: References 128–130 and product information for respective agents.

H^+ ion secretion is taking place (150). Consequently, any condition or circumstance (e.g., administration of food, concomitant medications) that reduces H^+ ion secretion (and raises pH) by the parietal cell will prolong the time of onset of effect consequent to delayed prodrug activation (Table 50.3). Finally, examination of the average apparent oral clearance (Cl/*F*) data for the PPIs suggests possible differences among the respective drugs, with values for omeprazole and rabeprazole being generally higher than those for other compounds in the class (Table 50.3). It is important to note, however, that any apparent difference in Cl/*F* may simply reflect inter- or intrapatient differences in the extent of presystemic clearance of the drug.

In addition to tablets and capsules, several dosage forms are available that allow administration to children who cannot swallow a tablet or capsule. These include intravenous formulations, granules or powder for oral suspension, and oral disintegrating tablets (ODTs). Extemporaneous liquid formulations of these drugs have been prepared for pediatric use, although there are limited available data regarding their stability and/or bioavailability in infants and children. Given that formulation-specific differences have the potential to alter drug bioavailability in pediatric patients and therefore clinical efficacy, the impact of disrupting the integrity of a solid PPI dose form in making an extemporaneous preparation must be considered. The lansoprazole ODT is approved for use in pediatric patients (154) and affords the option of dissolution and administration via oral syringe or nasogastric tube (154,156). Although not labeled for pediatric use, omeprazole is available as single-dose powder packets for suspension. Two studies have demonstrated good stability of the prepared suspension over time when stored at 3 to 5°C. A 2 mg per mL suspension retained at least 98% of the initial concentration when stored for 45 days to 1 month (157,158). Stability at room temperature was concentration dependent, with greater stability at higher concentrations (158). Finally, esomeprazole and lansoprazole are both available as granules or powder for suspension.

As illustrated by the information contained in Table 50.3, all of the PPIs are extensively (>90%) bound to circulating plasma proteins (primarily albumin) (153). Thus, their apparent volume of distribution is limited to a physiologic space that is far less than total body water (i.e., 0.6 to 0.7 L per kg). Although drug–drug interactions between omeprazole and both phenytoin and warfarin have been reported (159), there is no evidence that these are produced as a consequence of alterations in drug–protein binding.

The PPIs are extensively metabolized by enzymatic (omeprazole, esomeprazole, lansoprazole, pantoprazole, rabeprazole) and nonenzymatic (rabeprazole) pathways (Fig. 50.2). Two cytochromes P450 are predominantly involved in catalyzing these biotransformation reactions: CYP3A4 and CYP2C19; the latter is the predominant enzyme involved in the metabolism of both omeprazole and pantoprazole. For this reason, the pharmacokinetics and pharmacodynamics of omeprazole and other PPIs have been associated with CYP2C19 activity (160). CYP2C19 is polymorphically expressed in humans (161). The poor metabolizer phenotype for CYP2C19 is produced by the inheritance of two recessive mutated alleles and is present in approximately 3% to 5% of Caucasians and African Americans and in approximately 15% to 20% of the Asian population. Although at least seven nonfunctional alleles for CYP2C19 have been identified to date (CYP2C19*2 to *8), the two most common variants, *CYP2C19*2* and **3*, previously referred to as m(1) and m(2), respectively, result from single-nucleotide substitutions that convey a dramatic reduction of enzyme activity.

The genetic polymorphism of CYP2C19 can lead to substantial differences in the disposition of a PPI. In comparison to individuals who have an extensive metabolizer (EM) phenotype for CYP2C19, poor metabolizers have a substantially higher exposure (i.e., increased plasma concentrations and AUC) from a therapeutic dose of a PPI, as reflected by recent data for omeprazole (160). Tanaka et al. (162) showed that PMs demonstrated a significantly ($p < .01$) greater AUC, longer $t_{1/2}$, and lower apparent oral clearance for pantoprazole.

In a randomized crossover study, Furuta et al. (163) assessed whether the effect of a PPI on intragastric pH correlated with CYP2C19 genotype status (i.e., a surrogate

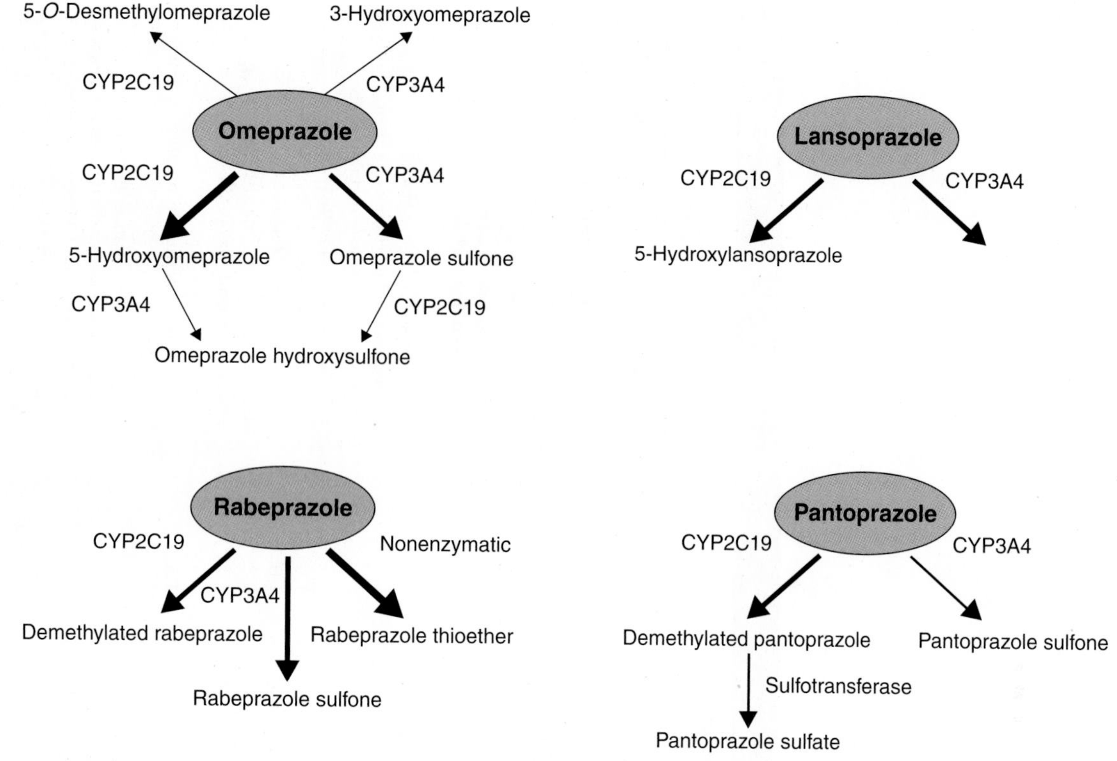

Figure 50.2. Metabolism of proton pump inhibitors. (From Ishizaki T, Horai Y. Review article: cytochrome P450 and the metabolism of proton pump inhibitors–emphasis on rabeprazole. *Aliment Pharmacol Ther* 1999;13(Suppl 3):27–36, with permission.)

measure of phenotype). The investigators demonstrated a significant ($r = .87$, $p < .0001$) correlation between mean intragastric pH and the AUC for omeprazole (ng per mL per hour). This finding indicated an association between CYP2C19 phenotype and both pharmacokinetics and pharmacodynamics as well as a possible gene–dose effect, with EMs with one functional CYP2C19 allele (i.e., the intermediate metabolizers) producing values between those from subjects who were homozygous EMs and PMs. The effect of the "intermediate metabolizer" phenotype for CYP2C19 on pantoprazole (single-dose administration) pharmacokinetics was examined by Kearns et al. (164) in a pediatric study ($n = 24$). A statistically significant difference in dose-normalized AUC (i.e., ng per mL per hour per 1 mg per kg of drug) between EMs with one versus two functional alleles was found. In addition, Furuta et al. (165) reported significant differences ($p < .001$) in cure rates for *H. pylori* infection in adults with different CYP2C19 genotypes treated with lansoprazole, clarithromycin, and amoxicillin (57.8%, 88.2%, and 92.3% for rapid, intermediate, and poor metabolizers, respectively).

Reviews examining the impact of ontogeny on drug disposition provide pharmacokinetic evidence to support reduced activity of CYP2C19 and CYP3A4 in neonates and young infants, and the potential for increased activity (relative to adults) of these enzymes in the first 4 to 5 years of life (166,167). Early data reporting the pharmacokinetics of oral omeprazole in infants and children supported a potential increase in the apparent plasma clearance in young children (168). These data prompted Hassall et al. (169) to suggest that developmental differences in omeprazole pharmacokinetics (i.e., increased clearance) were responsible for a greater dose requirement (mg per kg) of the drug in young children to ensure efficacy.

The pharmacokinetics of the PPIs has been studied in infants, children, and adolescents. A summary of the studies and pharmacokinetic parameters is provided in Table 50.4. With the exception of two studies that revealed a trend toward a more rapid clearance in infants and young children (168,170), the pharmacokinetics of omeprazole, lansoprazole, and pantoprazole do not appear to be dependent on development in infants from approximately 1 month to 16 years of age. This is not true for neonates who have lower clearance for omeprazole (171), as would be predicted by pharmacokinetic studies of other substrates for CYP2C19 (e.g., diazepam) and CYP3A4/5 (e.g., midazolam) (164). Infants and young children also appear to clear esomeprazole more rapidly than do adults and older children (112,172).

For all of the PPIs, the degree of acid suppression is well correlated with systemic drug exposure reflected by the area under the plasma concentration versus time curve (AUC) of the drug. Although omeprazole is rapidly cleared from plasma (i.e., mean elimination half-life is approximately 1 to 2 hours in CYP2C19 EMs), its pharmacologic effect can persist for 24 to 72 hours consequent to the strong binding of the active form of the drug to the receptor (160). Despite the asynchronous kinetics of elimination and response, the extent of systemic exposure to the PPIs (as determined by their pharmacokinetics) has a direct relationship with the extent and duration of drug effect (i.e., pharmacodynamics). Therefore, the selection of a PPI

TABLE 50.4 Pharmacokinetic Parameters for Infants, Children, and Adolescents[a]

Study	Drug	Patient Age	Dosing	AUC (μg/L/hr)	Clearance (L/hr/kg)	$t_{1/2}$ (hr)	Findings/Interpretations
(200)	Omeprazole i.v.	4.5–27 mo	0.56 mg/kg[b]	780[b]	0.68[b]		The AUC had positive correlation to the percentage of time pH >4 in 24 hr
			1.16 mg/kg[b]	3,950[b]	0.42[b]		
(201)	Lansoprazole p.o.	0.25–13 yr	0.73 mg/kg[b]	2,034[c]	0.76[c]	0.77[c]	AUC significantly higher in responders versus nonresponders
			1.44 mg/kg[c]	479[c]	2.94[c]	0.75[c]	
			1.36 mg/kg[c]	737[c]	2.26[c]	0.93[c]	
(202)	Lansoprazole p.o.	1–11 yr	15 mg/d	1,707[c]		0.68[c]	Lower dose with weight <30 kg; profile similar to that of adults
			30 mg/d	1,883[c]		0.71[c]	
(203)	Lansoprazole p.o.	12–17 yr	15 mg/d	1,017[c]		0.84[c]	Similar profile to adults
			30 mg/d	2,490[c]		0.95[c]	
(204)	Omeprazole i.v.	<10 d	0.4–1.2 mg/kg b.i.d.	ND	0.12–0.2	1.6–2.1	Infants <10 d of age metabolize omeprazole at a slower rate than infants (4.5–17 mo), whose metabolism is similar to that of adults
		4.5–17 mo	0.4–1.2 mg/kg b.i.d.				
(205)	Omeprazole p.o.	0–24 mo	1.0 mg/kg	658[c]		1.0[c]	Increased exposure to omeprazole in infants <5 mo of age
			1.5 mg/kg	346[c]		1.0[c]	
(168)	Omeprazole p.o.	1–6 yr	1.3 mg/kg	2,003[b]		0.85[b]	Increasing metabolism with decreasing age to second year of life
		7–12 yr	0.7 mg/kg	2,866[b]		1.74[b]	
		13–16 yr	1.1 mg/kg	3,420[b]		1.58[b]	
(170)	Lansoprazole p.o.	18 d–14 yr	17-mg single dose	3,503[c]		1.5[c]	Trend toward higher elimination rate in infants
(206)	Omeprazole p.o.	2–16 yr	0.2–0.9 mg/kg	809.5[c]	1.76[c]	0.98[c]	No apparent association between age and elimination rate constant; no difference in AUC between CYP2C19 heterozygous and homozygous extensive metabolizers
(164)	Pantoprazole p.o.	6–16 yr	20- or 40-mg single dose	4.3/45.5[d]	0.3/0.03[e]	0.6/5.8[f]	No apparent age association with oral clearance or elimination rate constant; significantly higher dose normalized AUC in CYP2C19 homozygous versus heterozygous extensive metabolizers

(207)	Pantoprazole i.v.	2–16 yr	0.8 or 1.6 mg/kg		7.6 L/hr[c]	1.1[c]	No apparent age association with clearance
(208)	Rabeprazole p.o.	12–16 yr	10-mg single dose	305[c]	0.75[c]	0.55[c]	Pharmacokinetics were similar to those observed in adults; possible accumulation with multiple doses of 20 mg
			10 mg/d	249.8[c]	0.61[c]	0.58[c]	
			20-mg single dose	557.8[c]		1.04[c]	
			20 mg/d	828.4[c]		0.97[c]	
(112)	Esomeprazole p.o.	1–24 months	0.25 mg/kg	0.65[c,g]		0.77[c]	Exposure and percentage of time pH >4 related to dosage; 0.25 mg/kg did not reduce reflux episodes
			1 mg/kg	3.51[c,g]		0.95[c]	
(172)	Esomeprazole p.o.	1–5 yr	5 mg/d	0.74[c,h]	1.01[c]	0.42[c]	Pharmacokinetics at steady state were dose and age dependent; younger children metabolized more quickly
		1–5 yr	10 mg/d	4.83[c,h]	0.39[c]	0.74[c]	
		6–11 yr	10 mg/d	3.70[c,h]	0.25[c]	0.88[c]	
		6–11 yr	20 mg/d	6.28[c,h]	0.31[c]	0.76[c]	
(209)	Esomeprazole p.o.	12–17 yr	20 mg single dose	1.58[c,h]	36.61 L/hr[c]	0.55[c]	Pharmacokinetics was dose and time dependent; similar to adults.
			20 mg/d	3.65[c,h]	15.88 L/hr[c]	0.82[c]	
			40 mg single dose	5.57[c,h]	20.78 L/hr[c]	0.86[c]	
			40 mg/d	13.86[c,h]	8.36 L/hr[c]	1.22[c]	
(210)	Lansoprazole p.o.	13–24 months	15 mg once or twice daily	1906[c,i]		0.66[c]	Results similar to older children and adults
(211)	Pantoprazole p.o.	5–16 yr	20- or 40-mg single dose	9.44 mg/L/hr[c]	0.26[c]	1.27[c]	Pharmacokinetics of p.o. and i.v. formulations were similar
	Pantoprazole i.v.	2–16 yr	0.8- or 1.6-mg/kg single dose	8.95 mg/L/hr[c]	0.20[c]	1.22[c]	

[a]AUC, area under plasma concentration–time curve; b.i.d., twice daily; i.v., intravenously; ND, no data; p.o., orally; $t_{1/2}$, elimination half-life; CYP, cytochrome P450.
[b]Median values.
[c]Mean values.
[d]Mean values normalized as mg/L/hr per 1 mg/kg for CYP2C19 extensive/poor metabolizers.
[e]Mean values as L/hr/kg for CYP2C19 extensive/poor metabolizers.
[f]Mean values for CYP2C19 extensive/poor metabolizers.
[g]AUC for the dosing interval expressed as μmol/hr/L.
[h]AUC 0–∞ expressed as μmol/hr/L.
[i]AUC 0–24 hr.

dose regimen that is associated with efficacy is predicated on providing a proper extent of systemic exposure (160).

PPIs are approved by the FDA for treatment/management of the following conditions in adults: duodenal ulcers and erosive esophagitis (treatment and maintenance), gastric ulcers, *H. pylori* infection, pathological hypersecretory conditions, and GERD. Lansoprazole and esomeprazole have been approved for the prevention of gastric ulcers associated with nonsteroidal anti-inflammatory agents; lansoprazole is also approved for the treatment of these ulcers. In recent years, all PPIs, except for pantoprazole, have received FDA approval for use in pediatric patients for the treatment of GERD. Esomeprazole and lansoprazole are also approved for the treatment of erosive esophagitis. However, PPIs still lack formal FDA approval for other pediatric conditions for which they are administered "off label," including *H. pylori* infection, adjuvant therapy in patients with cystic fibrosis, as premedication for general anesthesia, extraesophageal symptoms associated with GERD (e.g., asthma, chronic cough, sinusitis, recurrent otitis media), and apnea and/or bradycardia associated with GER and/or increased gastric residual volumes in neonates.

Of all drugs in this class, omeprazole and lansoprazole have received the most study in children. Gibbons and Gold (150) summarized data from pediatric studies of omeprazole (eight trials involving 408 children) and lansoprazole (four trials involving 184 children). The majority of subjects were older than 2 years. Collectively, these investigations demonstrated the following: a predictable time-dependent increase in gastric and esophageal pH associated with treatment, a greater than 80% symptomatic improvement while on therapy, histologic improvement/healing of gastric and esophageal lesions with maintenance therapy, an efficiency of treatment (both incidence of response and rate of onset) associated with dose escalation (e.g., omeprazole daily doses > 1.5 mg per kg and lansoprazole daily doses > 1.0 mg per kg), and a significant (>60%) relapse rate when treatment with a PPI was discontinued. More recent pediatric clinical trials of omeprazole and lansoprazole support these findings (173,174), including children 2 years of age or younger. Omeprazole has also been shown to be effective in the reduction of esophageal acid exposure in premature infants (34 to 40 weeks postmenstrual age) with symptoms of GERD (175).

Clinical trials of esomeprazole in children with GERD ranging in age from 1 month to 17 years demonstrate dose-related acid suppression, decreased esophageal acid exposure, decreased symptoms, and healing of erosive esophagitis (112,176). Pantoprazole has similarly been shown to be an effective treatment for GERD in children aged 5 to 16 years (177–179).

In addition, a few studies have examined the benefits of PPIs in children with other conditions. Esomeprazole has been demonstrated to decrease gastrointestinal symptoms in children with cysteamine-induced acid hypersecretion (180). When used with metoclopramide, esomeprazole decreased asthma exacerbations in children with asthma and concomitant GERD (181). Finally, omeprazole increased the cure rate of *H. pylori* gastritis in children aged 3 to 17 years when added to dual antibiotic therapy compared with antibiotic therapy alone (69% vs. 15%, respectively) (182).

PPIs are well tolerated in children. Headaches, nausea, and diarrhea are the most commonly reported adverse effects. A persistent, two- to fivefold rise in serum gastrin level, stimulation of enterochromaffin-like (ECL) cells (183), and histological changes in parietal cells (184) are associated with the use of PPIs. However, a review of studies reporting long-term treatment with PPIs failed to identify an association between ECL hyperplasia and progression to dysplasia and carcinoid tumors, the development of fundic cysts and polyps associated with hypertrophic parietal cells, or increased infections consequent to prolonged periods of gastric hypochlorhydria (150). Smaller studies suggested an association between PPI use and gastroenteritis or community-acquired pneumonia in children (125) as well as late onset gram-negative sepsis in very low-birth-weight infants in the neonatal intensive care unit (185). Further data is needed to confirm these findings.

The long-term safety of PPIs was examined in a cohort study of 17,489 adults that received at least one prescription for omeprazole and were followed for 4 years (186). Although all-cause mortality was increased in the first year compared with that expected for population rates, this finding was attributed to preexisting illnesses. Two studies in children have found PPIs to be safe when used for extended periods (1 to 11 years) (187,188). A recent case-control study (189) reported an association for long-term PPI use and hip fracture (adjusted odds ratio 1.44, 95% CI 1.3 to 1.59) in adults. No study has examined the association of PPI use with fractures in children.

PPIs can both inhibit and induce CYP enzymes and, as a consequence, have the potential to produce drug–drug interactions for selected pharmacologic agents (190). Omeprazole and lansoprazole have been shown to competitively inhibit CYP2C9 (K_i of 40.1 and 52.1, respectively). Both drugs noncompetitively inhibit CYP3A4, but the inhibition is weak (K_i of 84.4 and 170.4, respectively) (191). There is strong competitive inhibition of CYP2C19 by omeprazole, lansoprazole, and rabeprazole. Rabeprazole, with a K_i of 9.2, is roughly three times less potent than omeprazole or lansoprazole (K_i of 3.1 and 3.2, respectively) in inhibiting CYP2C19. Omeprazole and lansoprazole can also weakly inhibit the activity of CYP2D6 (K_i of 240.7 and 44.7, respectively). Masubuchi et al. (192) compared the induction of CYP1A2 and CYP3A4 activity in humans for three PPIs. For CYP1A2, induction potential was highest with omeprazole, followed by lansoprazole and then pantoprazole. For CYP3A4, there were no apparent differences in induction potency among the three compounds.

The potential for metabolism-based drug–drug interactions can be assessed by determining whether and how extensively a compound inhibits or induces a CYP enzyme. It is important to evaluate whether drug concentrations in the body or at the site of action are close to levels known to affect the enzyme (i.e., comparison of the K_i values for inhibition with the plasma PPI concentrations associated with therapeutic drug administration). In humans, metabolic drug–drug interactions have been reported when omeprazole is coadministered with phenytoin, diazepam, carbamazepine (191), St. John's wort (192), tacrolimus (194), saquinavir (195), nelfinavir (196), or indinavir (197). Given that the S isomer of omeprazole has less affinity for CYP2C19, the drug interaction potential of esomeprazole would be expected to be less than that of the racemic mixture (198). The absence of drug interactions reported with the other PPIs may simply reflect the larger extent to which omeprazole has been studied. Finally, evaluation of the interaction potential for the PPIs should center not only on therapeutic drugs but also on potential environmental toxicants that rely on the enzymes affected by the PPIs (e.g., heterocyclic hydrocarbons by CYP1A2) for their bioactivation.

ACKNOWLEDGMENT

This work was supported in part by grant U01 HD31324-15 (L.J.).

REFERENCES

1. Zimmermann AE, Ken Walters J, Katona BG, et al. A review of omeprazole use in the treatment of acid-related disorders in children. *Clin Ther* 2001;23(5):660–679.
2. Nelson SP, Chen EH, Syniar GM, et al. Prevalence of symptoms of gastroesophageal reflux during childhood: a pediatric practice-based survey. Pediatric Practice Research Group. *Arch Pediatr Adolesc Med* 2000;154(2):150–154.
3. Sonnenberg A, Everhart JE. The prevalence of self-reported peptic ulcer in the United States. *Am J Public Health* 1996;86(2):200–205.
4. Shoana Q, Marion R, Brendan D. Peptic ulcer disease in children. *Curr Paediatr* 2003;13(2):107–113.
5. Blecker U, Gold BD. Gastritis and peptic ulcer disease in childhood. *Eur J Pediatr* 1999;158(7):541–546.
6. Kato S, Sherman PM. What is new related to *Helicobacter pylori* infection in children and teenagers? *Arch Pediatr Adolesc Med* 2005; 159(5):415–421.
7. Cook DJ, Fuller HD, Guyatt GH, et al. Risk factors for gastrointestinal bleeding in critically ill patients. Canadian Critical Care Trials Group. *N Engl J Med* 1994;330(6):377–381.
8. Lopez-Herce J, Dorao P, Elola P, et al. Frequency and prophylaxis of upper gastrointestinal hemorrhage in critically ill children: a prospective study comparing the efficacy of almagate, ranitidine, and sucralfate. The Gastrointestinal Hemorrhage Study Group. *Crit Care Med* 1992;20(8):1082–1089.
9. Olsen KM, Bergman KL, Kaufman SS, et al. Omeprazole pharmacodynamics and gastric acid suppression in critically ill pediatric transplant patients. *Pediatr Crit Care Med* 2001;2(3):232–237.
10. Mitchelson F. Pharmacological agents affecting emesis. A review (Part I). *Drugs* 1992;43(3):295–315.
11. Milne RJ, Heel RC. Ondansetron. Therapeutic use as an antiemetic. *Drugs* 1991;41(4):574–595.
12. Culy CR, Bhana N, Plosker GL. Ondansetron: a review of its use as an antiemetic in children. *Paediatr Drugs* 2001;3(6):441–479.
13. Gralla RJ. Metoclopramide. A review of antiemetic trials. *Drugs* 1983;25(Suppl 1):63–73.
14. Goodin S, Cunningham R. 5-HT(3)-receptor antagonists for the treatment of nausea and vomiting: a reappraisal of their side-effect profile. *Oncologist* 2002;7(5):424–436.
15. Hahlen K, Quintana E, Pinkerton CR, et al. A randomized comparison of intravenously administered granisetron versus chlorpromazine plus dexamethasone in the prevention of ifosfamide-induced emesis in children. *J Pediatr* 1995;126(2):309–313.
16. Diemunsch P, Conseiller C, Clyti N, et al. Ondansetron compared with metoclopramide in the treatment of established postoperative nausea and vomiting. The French Ondansetron Study Group. *Br J Anaesth* 1997;79(3):322–326.
17. Roila F, Del Favero A. Ondansetron clinical pharmacokinetics. *Clin Pharmacokinet* 1995;29(2):95–109.
18. Holdsworth MT, Raisch DW, Frost J. Acute and delayed nausea and emesis control in pediatric oncology patients. *Cancer* 2006; 106(4):931–940.
19. Cubeddu LX, Trujillo LM, Talmaciu I, et al. Antiemetic activity of ondansetron in acute gastroenteritis. *Aliment Pharmacol Ther* 1997;11(1):185–191.
20. Reeves JJ, Shannon MW, Fleisher GR. Ondansetron decreases vomiting associated with acute gastroenteritis: a randomized, controlled trial. *Pediatrics* 2002;109(4):e62.
21. Stork CM, Brown KM, Reilly TH, et al. Emergency department treatment of viral gastritis using intravenous ondansetron or dexamethasone in children. *Acad Emerg Med* 2006;13(10): 1027–1033.
22. Leung AK, Robson WL. Acute gastroenteritis in children: role of anti-emetic medication for gastroenteritis-related vomiting. *Paediatr Drugs* 2007;9(3):175–184.
23. Freedman SB. Acute infectious pediatric gastroenteritis: beyond oral rehydration therapy. *Expert Opin Pharmacother* 2007;8(11): 1651–1665.
24. Langston WT, Wathen JE, Roback MG, et al. Effect of ondansetron on the incidence of vomiting associated with ketamine sedation in children: a double-blind, randomized, placebo-controlled trial. *Ann Emerg Med* 2008;52(1):30–34.
25. Gombar S, Kaur J, Kumar Gombar K, et al. Superior anti-emetic efficacy of granisetron-dexamethasone combination in children undergoing middle ear surgery. *Acta Anaesthesiol Scand* 2007;51(5): 621–624.
26. Berrak SG, Ozdemir N, Bakirci N, et al. A double-blind, crossover, randomized dose-comparison trial of granisetron for the prevention of acute and delayed nausea and emesis in children receiving moderately emetogenic carboplatin-based chemotherapy. *Support Care Cancer* 2007;15(10):1163–1168.
27. Pfeil N, Uhlig U, Kostev K, et al. Antiemetic medications in children with presumed infectious gastroenteritis–pharmacoepidemiology in Europe and Northern America. *J Pediatr* 2008; 153(5):659–662, 662.e1-3.
28. Kovac AL. Prophylaxis of postoperative nausea and vomiting: controversies in the use of serotonin 5-hydroxytryptamine subtype 3 receptor antagonists. *J Clin Anesth* 2006;18(4):304–318.
29. Sepúlveda-Vildósola AC, Betanzos-Cabrera Y, Lastiri GG, et al. Palonosetron hydrochloride is an effective and safe option to prevent chemotherapy-induced nausea and vomiting in children. *Arch Med Res* 2008;39(6):601–606.
30. Tomomasa T, Miyazaki M, Koizumi T, et al. Erythromycin increases gastric antral motility in human premature infants. *Biol Neonate* 1993;63(6):349–352.
31. Patole SK, Almonte R, Kadalraja R, et al. Can prophylactic oral erythromycin reduce time to full enteral feeds in preterm neonates? *Int J Clin Pract* 2000;54(8):504–508.
32. Kaiser R, Sezer O, Papies A, et al. Patient-tailored antiemetic treatment with 5-hydroxytryptamine type 3 receptor antagonists according to cytochrome P-450 2D6 genotypes. *J Clin Oncol* 2002; 20(12):2805–2811.
33. Pinarli FG, Elli M, Dagdemir A, et al. Electrocardiographic findings after 5-HT3 receptor antagonists and chemotherapy in children with cancer. *Pediatr Blood Cancer* 2006;47(5):567–571.
34. Buyukavci MMD, Olgun HMD, Ceviz NMD. The effects of ondansetron and granisetron on electrocardiography in children receiving chemotherapy for acute leukemia. *Am J Clin Oncol* 2005; 28(2):201–204.
35. Albibi R, McCallum RW. Metoclopramide: pharmacology and clinical application. *Ann Intern Med* 1983;98(1):86–95.
36. Ward RM, Lemons JA, Molteni RA. Cisapride: a survey of the frequency of use and adverse events in premature newborns. *Pediatrics* 1999;103(2):469–472.
37. Bowhay AR, May HA, Rudnicka AR, et al. A randomized controlled trial of the antiemetic effect of three doses of ondansetron after strabismus surgery in children. *Paediatr Anaesth* 2001;11(2): 215–221.
38. Lawhorn CD, Kymer PJ, Stewart FC, et al. Ondansetron dose response curve in high-risk pediatric patients. *J Clin Anesth* 1997; 9(8):637–642.
39. Splinter W, Roberts DJ. Prophylaxis for vomiting by children after tonsillectomy: dexamethasone versus perphenazine. *Anesth Analg* 1997;85(3):534–537.
40. Bartlett N, Koczwara B. Control of nausea and vomiting after chemotherapy: what is the evidence? *Intern Med J* 2002;32(8): 401–407.
41. Tsou VM, Young RM, Hart MH, et al. Elevated plasma aluminum levels in normal infants receiving antacids containing aluminum. *Pediatrics* 1991;87(2):148–151.

42. Littman A, Welch R, Fruin RC, et al. Controlled trials of aluminum hydroxide gels for peptic ulcer. *Gastroenterology* 1977;73(1):6–10.
43. Shuman RB, Schuster DP, Zuckerman GR. Prophylactic therapy for stress ulcer bleeding: a reappraisal. *Ann Intern Med* 1987; 106(4):562–567.
44. Stiel JN, Mitchell CA, Radcliff FJ, et al. Hypercalcemia in patients with peptic ulceration receiving large doses of calcium carbonate. *Gastroenterology* 1967;53(6):900–904.
45. Texter EC Jr. A critical look at the clinical use of antacids in acid-peptic disease and gastric acid rebound. *Am J Gastroenterol* 1989; 84(2):97–108.
46. Khalil SN, Roth AG, Cohen IT, et al. A double-bind comparison of intravenous ondansetron and placebo for preventing postoperative emesis in 1- to 24-month-old pediatric patients after surgery under general anesthesia. *Anesth Analg* 2005;101(2): 356–361.
47. Portuguez-Malavasi A, Aranda JV. Antacid bezoar in a newborn. *Pediatrics* 1979;63(4):679–680.
48. Flockhart DA, Desta Z, Mahal SK. Selection of drugs to treat gastro-oesophageal reflux disease: the role of drug interactions. *Clin Pharmacokinet* 2000;39(4):295–309.
49. Sutphen JL, Dillard VL, Pipan ME. Antacid and formula effects on gastric acidity in infants with gastroesophageal reflux. *Pediatrics* 1986;78(1):55–57.
50. Milla PJ. Gastrointestinal motility disorders in children. *Pediatr Clin North Am* 1988;35(2):311–330.
51. Cucchiara S, Franco MT, Terrin G, et al. Role of drug therapy in the treatment of gastro-oesophageal reflux disorder in children. *Paediatr Drugs* 2000;2(4):263–272.
52. Pennathur A, Tran A, Cioppi M, et al. Erythromycin strengthens the defective lower esophageal sphincter in patients with gastroesophageal reflux disease. *Am J Surg* 1994;167(1):169–172; discussion 72–73.
53. Jadcherla SR, Klee G, Berseth CL. Regulation of migrating motor complexes by motilin and pancreatic polypeptide in human infants. *Pediatr Res* 1997;42(3):365–369.
54. Kamerling IM, van Haarst AD, Burggraaf J, et al. Effects of a nonpeptide motilin receptor antagonist on proximal gastric motor function. *Br J Clin Pharmacol* 2004;57(4):393–401.
55. Park MI, Ferber I, Camilleri M, et al. Effect of atilmotin on gastrointestinal transit in healthy subjects: a randomized, placebo-controlled study. *Neurogastroenterol Motil* 2006;18(1):28–36.
56. McCallum RW, Cynshi O. Efficacy of mitemcinal, a motilin agonist, on gastrointestinal symptoms in patients with symptoms suggesting diabetic gastropathy: a randomized, multi-center, placebo-controlled trial. *Aliment Pharmacol Ther* 2007;26(1): 107–116.
57. Sondheimer JM, Arnold GL. Early effects of bethanechol on the esophageal motor function of infants with gastroesophageal reflux. *J Pediatr Gastroenterol Nutr* 1986;5(1):47–51.
58. Orenstein SR, Lofton SW, Orenstein DM. Bethanechol for pediatric gastroesophageal reflux: a prospective, blind, controlled study. *J Pediatr Gastroenterol Nutr* 1986;5(4):549–555.
59. Parkman HP, Trate DM, Knight LC, et al. Cholinergic effects on human gastric motility. *Gut* 1999;45(3):346–354.
60. Euler AR. Use of bethanechol for the treatment of gastroesophageal reflux. *J Pediatr* 1980;96(2):321–324.
61. Strickland AD, Chang JH. Results of treatment of gastroesophageal reflux with bethanechol. *J Pediatr* 1983;103(2): 311–315.
62. Levi P, Marmo F, Saluzzo C, et al. Bethanechol versus antiacids in the treatment of gastroesophageal reflux. *Helv Paediatr Acta* 1985;40(5):349–359.
63. Sondheimer JM, Mintz HL, Michaels M. Bethanechol treatment of gastroesophageal reflux in infants: effect on continuous esophageal pH records. *J Pediatr* 1984;104(1):128–131.
64. Shafrir Y, Levy Y, Beharab A, et al. Acute dystonic reaction to bethanechol—a direct acetylcholine receptor agonist. *Dev Med Child Neurol* 1986;28(5):646–648.
65. McCallum RW. Review of the current status of prokinetic agents in gastroenterology. *Am J Gastroenterol* 1985;80(12):1008–1016.
66. Cohen S, Morris DW, Schoen HJ, et al. The effect of oral and intravenous metoclopramide on human lower esophageal sphincter pressure. *Gastroenterology* 1976;70(4):484-487.
67. Beani L, Bianchi C, Crema C. Effects of metoclopramide on isolated guinea-pig colon. 1. Peripheral sensitization to acetylcholine. *Eur J Pharmacol* 1970;12(3):320–331.
68. Tolia V, Calhoun J, Kuhns L, et al. Randomized, prospective double-blind trial of metoclopramide and placebo for gastroesophageal reflux in infants. *J Pediatr* 1989;115(1):141–145.
69. Rode H, Stunden RJ, Millar AJ, et al. Esophageal pH assessment of gastroesophageal reflux in 18 patients and the effect of two prokinetic agents: cisapride and metoclopramide. *J Pediatr Surg* 1987;22(10):931–934.
70. Kearns GL, Butler HL, Lane JK, et al. Metoclopramide pharmacokinetics and pharmacodynamics in infants with gastroesophageal reflux. *J Pediatr Gastroenterol Nutr* 1988;7(6):823–829.
71. Hyman PE, Abrams CE, Dubois A. Gastric emptying in infants: response to metoclopramide depends on the underlying condition. *J Pediatr Gastroenterol Nutr* 1988;7(2):181–184.
72. Meadow WL, Bui KC, Strates E, et al. Metoclopramide promotes enteral feeding in preterm infants with feeding intolerance. *Dev Pharmacol Ther* 1989;13(1):38–45.
73. Sankaran K, Yeboah E, Bingham WT, et al. Use of metoclopramide in preterm infants. *Dev Pharmacol Ther* 1982;5(3–4):114–119.
74. Paz HL, Weinar M, Sherman MS. Motility agents for the placement of weighted and unweighted feeding tubes in critically ill patients. *Intensive Care Med* 1996;22(4):301–304.
75. Whatley K, Turner WW Jr, Dey M, et al. When does metoclopramide facilitate transpyloric intubation? *JPEN J Parenter Enteral Nutr* 1984;8(6):679–681.
76. Hibbs AM, Lorch SA. Metoclopramide for the treatment of gastroesophageal reflux disease in infants: a systematic review. *Pediatrics* 2006;118(2):746–752.
77. Lauritsen K, Laursen LS, Rask-Madsen J. Clinical pharmacokinetics of drugs used in the treatment of gastrointestinal diseases (Part I). *Clin Pharmacokinet* 1990;19(1):11–31.
78. Bateman DN. Clinical pharmacokinetics of metoclopramide. *Clin Pharmacokinet* 1983;8(6):523–529.
79. Ross-Lee LM, Eadie MJ, Hooper WD, et al. Single-dose pharmacokinetics of metoclopramide. *Eur J Clin Pharmacol* 1981;20(6): 465–471.
80. Webb D, Buss DC, Fifield R, et al. The plasma protein binding of metoclopramide in health and renal disease. *Br J Clin Pharmacol* 1986;21(3):334–336.
81. Kauppila A, Arvela P, Koivisto M, et al. Metoclopramide and breast feeding: transfer into milk and the newborn. *Eur J Clin Pharmacol* 1983;25(6):819–823.
82. Kearns GL, van den Anker JN, Reed MD, et al. Pharmacokinetics of metoclopramide in neonates. *J Clin Pharmacol* 1998;38(2):122–128.
83. Kearns GL, Fiser DH. Metoclopramide-induced methemoglobinemia. *Pediatrics* 1988;82(3):364–366.
84. Kris MG, Tyson LB, Gralla RJ, et al. Extrapyramidal reactions with high-dose metoclopramide. *N Engl J Med* 1983;309(7):433–434.
85. Allen JC, Gralla R, Reilly L, et al. Metoclopramide: dose-related toxicity and preliminary antiemetic studies in children receiving cancer chemotherapy. *J Clin Oncol* 1985;3(8):1136–1141.
86. Cucchiara S, Staiano A, Boccieri A, et al. Effects of cisapride on parameters of oesophageal motility and on the prolonged intraoesophageal pH test in infants with gastro-oesophageal reflux disease. *Gut* 1990;31(1):21–25.
87. Cucchiara S, Staiano A, Capozzi C, et al. Cisapride for gastro-oesophageal reflux and peptic oesophagitis. *Arch Dis Child* 1987; 62(5):454–457.
88. Barone JA, Jessen LM, Colaizzi JL, et al. Cisapride: a gastrointestinal prokinetic drug. *Ann Pharmacother* 1994;28(4):488–500.
89. Vandenplas Y, Belli DC, Benatar A, et al. The role of cisapride in the treatment of pediatric gastroesophageal reflux. The European Society of Paediatric Gastroenterology, Hepatology and Nutrition. *J Pediatr Gastroenterol Nutr* 1999;28(5):518–528.
90. Wysowski DK, Bacsanyi J. Cisapride and fatal arrhythmia. *N Engl J Med* 1996;335(4):290–291.
91. Shulman RJ, Boyle JT, Colletti RB, et al. The use of cisapride in children. The North American Society for Pediatric Gastroenterology and Nutrition. *J Pediatr Gastroenterol Nutr* 1999;28(5):529–533.
92. Curry JI, Lander TD, Stringer MD. Review article: erythromycin as a prokinetic agent in infants and children. *Aliment Pharmacol Ther* 2001;15(5):595–603.
93. Chicella MF, Batres LA, Heesters MS, et al. Prokinetic drug therapy in children: a review of current options. *Ann Pharmacother* 2005;39(4):706–711.
94. Peeters TL. Erythromycin and other macrolides as prokinetic agents. *Gastroenterology* 1993;105(6):1886–1899.

95. Boivin MA, Carey MC, Levy H. Erythromycin accelerates gastric emptying in a dose–response manner in healthy subjects. *Pharmacotherapy* 2003;23(1):5–8.
96. Stenson BJ, Middlemist L, Lyon AJ. Influence of erythromycin on establishment of feeding in preterm infants: observations from a randomised controlled trial. *Arch Dis Child Fetal Neonatal Ed* 1998;79(3):F212–F214.
97. Zatman TF, Hall JE, Harmer M. Gastric residual volume in children: a study comparing efficiency of erythromycin and metoclopramide as prokinetic agents. *Br J Anaesth* 2001;86(6):869–871.
98. Ng PC, Fok TF, Lee CH, et al. Erythromycin treatment for gastrointestinal dysmotility in preterm infants. *J Paediatr Child Health* 1997;33(2):148–150.
99. Simkiss DE, Adams IP, Myrdal U, et al. Erythromycin in neonatal postoperative intestinal dysmotility. *Arch Dis Child* 1994;71(2): F128–F129.
100. Netzer P, Schmitt B, Inauen W. Effects of ABT-229, a motilin agonist, on acid reflux, oesophageal motility and gastric emptying in patients with gastro-oesophageal reflux disease. *Aliment Pharmacol Ther* 2002;16(8):1481–1490.
101. Chen CL, Orr WC, Verlinden MH, et al. Efficacy of a motilin receptor agonist (ABT-229) for the treatment of gastro-oesophageal reflux disease. *Aliment Pharmacol Ther* 2002;16(4):749–757.
102. Thielemans L, Depoortere I, Perret J, et al. Desensitization of the human motilin receptor by motilides. *J Pharmacol Exp Ther* 2005;313(3):1397–1405.
103. Farrar HC, Walsh-Sukys MC, Kyllonen K, et al. Cardiac toxicity associated with intravenous erythromycin lactobionate: two case reports and a review of the literature. *Pediatr Infect Dis J* 1993; 12(8):688–691.
104. Fichtenbaum CJ, Babb JD, Baker DA. Erythromycin induced cardiovascular toxicity. *Conn Med* 1988;52(3):135–136.
105. Honein MA, Paulozzi LJ, Himelright IM, et al. Infantile hypertrophic pyloric stenosis after pertussis prophylaxis with erythromycin: a case review and cohort study. *Lancet* 1999;354(9196): 2101–2105.
106. Hauben M, Amsden GW. The association of erythromycin and infantile hypertrophic pyloric stenosis: causal or coincidental? *Drug Saf* 2002;25(13):929–942.
107. Maheshwai N. Are young infants treated with erythromycin at risk for developing hypertrophic pyloric stenosis? *Arch Dis Child* 2007;92(3):271–273.
108. Keady S. Update on drugs for gastro-oesophageal reflux disease. *Arch Dis Child Educ Pract Ed* 2007;92(4):ep114–ep118.
109. Sawant P, Das HS, Desai N, et al. Comparative evaluation of the efficacy and tolerability of itopride hydrochloride and domperidone in patients with non-ulcer dyspepsia. *J Assoc Physicians India* 2004;52:626–628.
110. Holtmann G, Talley NJ, Liebregts T, et al. A placebo-controlled trial of itopride in functional dyspepsia. *N Engl J Med* 2006; 354(8):832–840.
111. Camilleri M, Vazquez-Roque MI, Burton D, et al. Pharmacodynamic effects of a novel prokinetic 5-HT receptor agonist, ATI-7505, in humans. *Neurogastroenterol Motil* 2007;19(1):30–38.
112. Omari T, Davidson G, Bondarov P, et al. Pharmacokinetics and acid-suppressive effects of esomeprazole in infants 1-24 months old with symptoms of gastroesophageal reflux disease. *J Pediatr Gastroenterol Nutr* 2007;45(5):530–537.
113. Kawai M, Kawahara H, Hirayama S, et al. Effect of baclofen on emesis and 24-hour esophageal pH in neurologically impaired children with gastroesophageal reflux disease. *J Pediatr Gastroenterol Nutr* 2004;38(3):317–323.
114. Goyal A, Treem WR, Hyams JS. Severe upper gastrointestinal bleeding in healthy full-term neonates. *Am J Gastroenterol* 1994;89(4):613–616.
115. Cook DJ, Witt LG, Cook RJ, et al. Stress ulcer prophylaxis in the critically ill: a meta-analysis. *Am J Med* 1991;91(5):519–527.
116. Tam PK, Saing H. The use of H_2-receptor antagonist in the treatment of peptic ulcer disease in children. *J Pediatr Gastroenterol Nutr* 1989;8(1):41–46.
117. Wolfe MM, Soll AH. The physiology of gastric acid secretion. *N Engl J Med* 1988;319(26):1707–1715.
118. Xue S, Katz PO, Banerjee P, et al. Bedtime H2 blockers improve nocturnal gastric acid control in GERD patients on proton pump inhibitors. *Aliment Pharmacol Ther* 2001;15(9):1351–1356.
119. Sun WM, Hasler WL, Lien HC, et al. Nizatidine enhances the gastrocolonic response and the colonic peristaltic reflex in humans. *J Pharmacol Exp Ther* 2001;299(1):159–163.
120. Nagita A, Manago M, Aoki S, et al. Pharmacokinetics and pharmacodynamics of famotidine in children with gastroduodenal ulcers. *Ther Drug Monit* 1994;16(5):444–449.
121. Oderda G, Dell'Olio D, Forni M, et al. Treatment of childhood peptic oesophagitis with famotidine or alginate-antacid. *Ital J Gastroenterol* 1990;22(6):346–349.
122. Simeone D, Caria MC, Miele E, et al. Treatment of childhood peptic esophagitis: a double-blind placebo-controlled trial of nizatidine. *J Pediatr Gastroenterol Nutr* 1997;25(1):51–55.
123. Orenstein SR, Gremse DA, Pantaleon CD, et al. Nizatidine for the treatment of pediatric gastroesophageal reflux symptoms: an open-label, multiple-dose, randomized, multicenter clinical trial in 210 children. *Clin Ther* 2005;27(4):472–483.
124. Cothran DS, Borowitz SM, Sutphen JL, et al. Alteration of normal gastric flora in neonates receiving ranitidine. *J Perinatol* 1997; 17(5):383–388.
125. Canani RB, Cirillo P, Roggero P, et al. Therapy with gastric acidity inhibitors increases the risk of acute gastroenteritis and community-acquired pneumonia in children. *Pediatrics* 2006;117(5): e817–e820.
126. Guillet R, Stoll BJ, Cotten CM, et al. Association of H2-blocker therapy and higher incidence of necrotizing enterocolitis in very low birth weight infants. *Pediatrics* 2006;117(2):e137–e142.
127. Bachmann KA, Sullivan TJ, Jauregui L, et al. Drug interactions of H2-receptor antagonists. *Scand J Gastroenterol Suppl* 1994;206: 14–19.
128. Maples HD, James LP, Stowe CD, et al. Famotidine disposition in children and adolescents with chronic renal insufficiency. *J Clin Pharmacol* 2003;43(1):7–14.
129. Blumer JL, Rothstein FC, Kaplan BS, et al. Pharmacokinetic determination of ranitidine pharmacodynamics in pediatric ulcer disease. *J Pediatr* 1985;107(2):301–306.
130. James LP, Marshall JD, Heulitt MJ, et al. Pharmacokinetics and pharmacodynamics of famotidine in children. *J Clin Pharmacol* 1996;36(1):48–54.
131. James LP, Marotti T, Stowe CD, et al. Pharmacokinetics and pharmacodynamics of famotidine in infants. *J Clin Pharmacol* 1998; 38(12):1089–1095.
132. Fontana M, Massironi E, Rossi A, et al. Ranitidine pharmacokinetics in newborn infants. *Arch Dis Child* 1993;68(5 Spec No): 602–603.
133. Hook JB, Bailie MD. Perinatal renal pharmacology. *Annu Rev Pharmacol Toxicol* 1979;19:491–509.
134. Arant BS Jr. Developmental patterns of renal functional maturation compared in the human neonate. *J Pediatr* 1978;92(5): 705–712.
135. Wenning LA, Murphy MG, James LP, et al. Pharmacokinetics of famotidine in infants. *Clin Pharmacokinet* 2005;44(4):395–406.
136. Abdel-Rahman SM, Johnson FK, Manowitz N, et al. Single-dose pharmacokinetics of nizatidine (Axid) in children. *J Clin Pharmacol* 2002;42(10):1089–1096.
137. Kuusela AL. Long-term gastric pH monitoring for determining optimal dose of ranitidine for critically ill preterm and term neonates. *Arch Dis Child Fetal Neonatal Ed* 1998;78(2):F151–F153.
138. Kelly EJ, Brownlee KG, Ng PC, et al. The prophylactic use of ranitidine in babies treated with dexamethasone. *Arch Dis Child* 1992;67(4 Spec No):471.
139. Kanto WP Jr. A decade of experience with neonatal extracorporeal membrane oxygenation. *J Pediatr* 1994;124(3):335–347.
140. Wells TG, Heulitt MJ, Taylor BJ, et al. Pharmacokinetics and pharmacodynamics of ranitidine in neonates treated with extracorporeal membrane oxygenation. *J Clin Pharmacol* 1998;38(5): 402–407.
141. Marchant J, Summers K, McIsaac RL, et al. A comparison of two ranitidine intravenous infusion regimens in critically ill patients. *Aliment Pharmacol Ther* 1988;2(1):55–63.
142. Wiest DB, O'Neal W, Reigart JR, et al. Pharmacokinetics of ranitidine in critically ill infants. *Dev Pharmacol Ther* 1989;12(1):7–12.
143. Freston JW. Cimetidine: II. Adverse reactions and patterns of use. *Ann Intern Med* 1982;97(5):728–734.
144. Brogden RN, Carmine AA, Heel RC, et al. Ranitidine: a review of its pharmacology and therapeutic use in peptic ulcer disease and other allied diseases. *Drugs* 1982;24(4):267–303.

145. Schentag JJ, Cerra FB, Calleri G, et al. Pharmacokinetic and clinical studies in patients with cimetidine-associated mental confusion. *Lancet* 1979;1(8109):177–181.
146. Jensen RT, Collen MJ, Pandol SJ, et al. Cimetidine-induced impotence and breast changes in patients with gastric hypersecretory states. *N Engl J Med* 1983;308(15):883–887.
147. Nahum E, Reish O, Naor N, et al. Ranitidine-induced bradycardia in a neonate—a first report. *Eur J Pediatr* 1993;152(11):933–934.
148. Powell JR, Donn KH. Histamine H2-antagonist drug interactions in perspective: mechanistic concepts and clinical implications. *Am J Med* 1984;77(5B):57–84.
149. Smith SR, Kendall MJ. Ranitidine versus cimetidine. A comparison of their potential to cause clinically important drug interactions. *Clin Pharmacokinet* 1988;15(1):44–56.
150. Gibbons TE, Gold BD. The use of proton pump inhibitors in children: a comprehensive review. *Paediatr Drugs* 2003;5(1):25–40.
151. Kromer W, Kruger U, Huber R, et al. Differences in pH-dependent activation rates of substituted benzimidazoles and biological in vitro correlates. *Pharmacology* 1998;56(2):57–70.
152. Richardson P, Hawkey CJ, Stack WA. Proton pump inhibitors. Pharmacology and rationale for use in gastrointestinal disorders. *Drugs* 1998;56(3):307–335.
153. Stedman CA, Barclay ML. Review article: comparison of the pharmacokinetics, acid suppression and efficacy of proton pump inhibitors. *Aliment Pharmacol Ther* 2000;14(8):963–978.
154. Freston JW, Chiu YL, Mulford DJ, et al. Comparative pharmacokinetics and safety of lansoprazole oral capsules and orally disintegrating tablets in healthy subjects. *Aliment Pharmacol Ther* 2003;17(3):361–367.
155. Freston JW, Kukulka MJ, Lloyd E, et al. A novel option in proton pump inhibitor dosing: lansoprazole orally disintegrating tablet dispersed in water and administered via nasogastric tube. *Aliment Pharmacol Ther* 2004;20(4):407–411.
156. Gremse DA, Donnelly JR, Kukulka MJ, et al. A novel option for dosing of proton pump inhibitors: dispersion of lansoprazole orally disintegrating tablet in water via oral syringe. *Aliment Pharmacol Ther* 2004;19(11):1211–1215.
157. Johnson CE, Cober MP, Ludwig JL. Stability of partial doses of omeprazole-sodium bicarbonate oral suspension. *Ann Pharmacother* 2007;41(12):1954–1961.
158. Burnett JE, Balkin ER. Stability and viscosity of a flavored omeprazole oral suspension for pediatric use. *Am J Health Syst Pharm* 2006;63(22):2240–2247.
159. Prichard PJ, Walt RP, Kitchingham GK, et al. Oral phenytoin pharmacokinetics during omeprazole therapy. *Br J Clin Pharmacol* 1987;24:543–545.
160. Andersson T. Pharmacokinetics, metabolism and interactions of acid pump inhibitors. Focus on omeprazole, lansoprazole and pantoprazole. *Clin Pharmacokinet* 1996;31(1):9–28.
161. Desta Z, Zhao X, Shin JG, et al. Clinical significance of the cytochrome P450 2C19 genetic polymorphism. *Clin Pharmacokinet* 2002;41(12):913–958.
162. Tanaka M, Ohkubo T, Otani K, et al. Metabolic disposition of pantoprazole, a proton pump inhibitor, in relation to S-mephenytoin 4′-hydroxylation phenotype and genotype. *Clin Pharmacol Ther* 1997;62(6):619–628.
163. Furuta T, Ohashi K, Kosuge K, et al. CYP2C19 genotype status and effect of omeprazole on intragastric pH in humans. *Clin Pharmacol Ther* 1999;65(5):552–561.
164. Kearns G. Pantoprazole disposition in pediatrics. *Clin Pharmacol Ther* 2003;73:38.
165. Furuta T, Sagehashi Y, Shirai N, et al. Influence of CYP2C19 polymorphism and *Helicobacter pylori* genotype determined from gastric tissue samples on response to triple therapy for H pylori infection. *Clin Gastroenterol Hepatol* 2005;3(6):564–573.
166. Leeder JS, Kearns GL. Pharmacogenetics in pediatrics. Implications for practice. *Pediatr Clin North Am* 1997;44(1):55–77.
167. Alcorn J, McNamara PJ. Ontogeny of hepatic and renal systemic clearance pathways in infants: part II. *Clin Pharmacokinet* 2002;41(13):1077–1094.
168. Andersson T, Hassall E, Lundborg P, et al. Pharmacokinetics of orally administered omeprazole in children. International Pediatric Omeprazole Pharmacokinetic Group. *Am J Gastroenterol* 2000;95(11):3101–3106.
169. Hassall E, Israel D, Shepherd R, et al. Omeprazole for treatment of chronic erosive esophagitis in children: a multicenter study of efficacy, safety, tolerability and dose requirements. International Pediatric Omeprazole Study Group. *J Pediatr* 2000;137(6):800–807.
170. Tran A, Rey E, Pons G, et al. Pharmacokinetic–pharmacodynamic study of oral lansoprazole in children. *Clin Pharmacol Ther* 2002;71(5):359–367.
171. Andersson T, Borang S, Larsson M, et al. Novel candidate genes for atherosclerosis are identified by representational difference analysis-based transcript profiling of cholesterol-loaded macrophages. *Pathobiology* 2001;69(6):304–314.
172. Zhao J, Li J, Hamer-Maansson JE, et al. Pharmacokinetic properties of esomeprazole in children aged 1 to 11 years with symptoms of gastroesophageal reflux disease: a randomized, open-label study. *Clin Ther* 2006;28(11):1868–1876.
173. Khoshoo V, Dhume P. Clinical response to 2 dosing regimens of lansoprazole in infants with gastroesophageal reflux. *J Pediatr Gastroenterol Nutr* 2008;46(3):352–354.
174. Fiedorek S, Tolia V, Gold BD, et al. Efficacy and safety of lansoprazole in adolescents with symptomatic erosive and non-erosive gastroesophageal reflux disease. *J Pediatr Gastroenterol Nutr* 2005;40(3):319–327.
175. Omari TI, Haslam RR, Lundborg P, et al. Effect of omeprazole on acid gastroesophageal reflux and gastric acidity in preterm infants with pathological acid reflux. *J Pediatr Gastroenterol Nutr* 2007;44(1):41–44.
176. Croxtall JD, Perry CM, Keating GM. Esomeprazole: in gastroesophageal reflux disease in children and adolescents. *Paediatr Drugs* 2008;10(3):199–205.
177. Tsou VM, Baker R, Book L, et al. Multicenter, randomized, double-blind study comparing 20 and 40 mg of pantoprazole for symptom relief in adolescents (12 to 16 years of age) with gastroesophageal reflux disease (GERD). *Clin Pediatr (Phila)* 2006;45(8):741–749.
178. Tolia V, Bishop PR, Tsou VM, et al. Multicenter, randomized, double-blind study comparing 10, 20 and 40 mg pantoprazole in children (5-11 years) with symptomatic gastroesophageal reflux disease. *J Pediatr Gastroenterol Nutr* 2006;42(4):384–391.
179. Madrazo-de la Garza A, Dibildox M, Vargas A, et al. Efficacy and safety of oral pantoprazole 20 mg given once daily for reflux esophagitis in children. *J Pediatr Gastroenterol Nutr* 2003;36(2):261–265.
180. Dohil R, Fidler M, Barshop B, et al. Esomeprazole therapy for gastric acid hypersecretion in children with cystinosis. *Pediatr Nephrol* 2005;20(12):1786–1793.
181. Khoshoo V, Haydel R Jr. Effect of antireflux treatment on asthma exacerbations in nonatopic children. *J Pediatr Gastroenterol Nutr* 2007;44(3):331–335.
182. Cadranel S, Bontemps P, Van Biervliet S, et al. Improvement of the eradication rate of *Helicobacter pylori* gastritis in children is by adjunction of omeprazole to a dual antibiotherapy. *Acta Paediatr* 2007;96(1):82–86.
183. Gunasekaran TS, Hassall EG. Efficacy and safety of omeprazole for severe gastroesophageal reflux in children. *J Pediatr* 1993;123(1):148–154.
184. Drut R, Altamirano E, Cueto Rua E. Omeprazole-associated changes in the gastric mucosa of children. *J Clin Pathol* 2008;61(6):754–756.
185. Graham PL III, Begg MD, Larson E, et al. Risk factors for late onset gram-negative sepsis in low birth weight infants hospitalized in the neonatal intensive care unit. *Pediatr Infect Dis J* 2006;25(2):113–117.
186. Bateman DN, Colin-Jones D, Hartz S, et al. Mortality study of 18000 patients treated with omeprazole. *Gut* 2003;52(7):942–946.
187. Tolia V, Boyer K. Long-term proton pump inhibitor use in children: a retrospective review of safety. *Dig Dis Sci* 2008;53(2):385–393.
188. Hassall E, Kerr W, El-Serag HB. Characteristics of children receiving proton pump inhibitors continuously for up to 11 years duration. *J Pediatr* 2007;150(3):262–267, 267.e1.
189. Yang YX, Lewis JD, Epstein S, et al. Long-term proton pump inhibitor therapy and risk of hip fracture. *JAMA* 2006;296(24):2947–2953.
190. Kearns GL, Winter HS. Proton pump inhibitors in pediatrics: relevant pharmacokinetics and pharmacodynamics. *J Pediatr Gastroenterol Nutr* 2003;37(Suppl 1):S52–S59.
191. Ishizaki T, Horai Y. Review article: cytochrome P450 and the metabolism of proton pump inhibitors–emphasis on rabeprazole. *Aliment Pharmacol Ther* 1999;13(Suppl 3):27–36.

192. Masubuchi N, Li AP, Okazaki O. An evaluation of the cytochrome P450 induction potential of pantoprazole in primary human hepatocytes. *Chem Biol Interact* 1998;114(1–2):1–13.
193. Wang LS, Zhou G, Zhu B, et al. St John's wort induces both cytochrome P450 3A4-catalyzed sulfoxidation and 2C19-dependent hydroxylation of omeprazole. *Clin Pharmacol Ther* 2004;75(3):191–197.
194. Moreau C, Taburet AM, Furlan V, et al. Interaction between Tacrolimus and Omeprazole in a Pediatric Liver Transplant Recipient. *Transplantation* 2006;81(3):487–488.
195. Winston A, Back D, Fletcher C, et al. Effect of omeprazole on the pharmacokinetics of saquinavir-500 mg formulation with ritonavir in healthy male and female volunteers. *AIDS* 2006; 20(10):1401–1406.
196. Fang AF, Damle BD, LaBadie RR, et al. Significant decrease in nelfinavir systemic exposure after omeprazole coadministration in healthy subjects. *Pharmacotherapy* 2008;28(1):42–50.
197. Tappouni HL, Rublein JC, Donovan BJ, et al. Effect of omeprazole on the plasma concentrations of indinavir when administered alone and in combination with ritonavir. *Am J Health Syst Pharm* 2008;65(5):422–428.
198. Andersson T, Hassan-Alin M, Hasselgren G, et al. Drug interaction studies with esomeprazole, the (S)-isomer of omeprazole. *Clin Pharmacokinet* 2001;40(7):523–537.
199. Lloyd CW, Martin WJ, Taylor BD. The pharmacokinetics of cimetidine and metabolites in a neonate. *Drug Intell Clin Pharm* 1985;19(3):203–205.
200. Faure C, Michaud L, Shaghaghi EK, et al. Intravenous omeprazole in children: pharmacokinetics and effect on 24-hour intragastric pH. *J Pediatr Gastroenterol Nutr* 2001;33(2):144–148.
201. Faure C, Michaud L, Shaghaghi EK, et al. Lansoprazole in children: pharmacokinetics and efficacy in reflux oesophagitis. *Aliment Pharmacol Ther* 2001;15(9):1397–1402.
202. Gremse D, Winter H, Tolia V, et al. Pharmacokinetics and pharmacodynamics of lansoprazole in children with gastroesophageal reflux disease. *J Pediatr Gastroenterol Nutr* 2002;35(Suppl 4): S319–S326.
203. Gunasekaran T. Pharmacokinetics of lansoprazole in adolescents with GERD [Abstract]. *J Pediatr Gastroenterol Nutr* 2000;31: S97.
204. Andersson T. Pharmacokinetics of intravenous omeprazole in neonates and infants [Abstract]. *J Pediatr Gastroenterol Nutr* 2001; 33:424.
205. Andersson T. Pharmacokinetics and pharmacodynamics of oral omeprazole in infants [Abstract]. *J Pediatr Gastroenterol Nutr* 2001;33:416.
206. Kearns G. Omeprazole disposition in children following single-dose administration: relationship to CYP2C19 genotype. *J Clin Pharmacol* 2003;43(8):840–848.
207. Ferron GM. Pharmacokinetics of IV pantoprazole in pediatric patients [Abstract]. *Clin Pharmacol Ther* 2003;73:36.
208. James L, Walson P, Lomax K, et al. Pharmacokinetics and tolerability of rabeprazole sodium in subjects aged 12 to 16 years with gastroesophageal reflux disease: an open-label, single- and multiple-dose study. *Clin Ther* 2007;29(9):2082–2092.
209. Li J, Zhao J, Hamer-Maansson JE, et al. Pharmacokinetic properties of esomeprazole in adolescent patients aged 12 to 17 years with symptoms of gastroesophageal reflux disease: a randomized, open-label study. *Clin Ther* 2006;28(3):419–427.
210. Heyman MB, Zhang W, Huang B, et al. Pharmacokinetics and pharmacodynamics of lansoprazole in children 13 to 24 months old with gastroesophageal reflux disease. *J Pediatr Gastroenterol Nutr* 2007;44(1):35–40.
211. Kearns GL, Blumer J, Schexnayder S, et al. Single-dose pharmacokinetics of oral and intravenous pantoprazole in children and adolescents. *J Clin Pharmacol* 2008;48(11):1356–1365.

CHAPTER

51

Evangelia Charmandari
Tomoshige Kino
George P. Chrousos

Glucocorticoids

INTRODUCTION

Glucocorticoids regulate a broad spectrum of physiologic functions essential for life and play an important role in the maintenance of basal and stress-related homeostasis (1–3). Approximately 20% of the genes expressed in human leukocytes are regulated positively or negatively by glucocorticoids (4). Glucocorticoids are involved in almost every cellular, molecular, and physiologic network of the organism and play a pivotal role in critical biologic processes, such as growth, reproduction, intermediary metabolism, immune and inflammatory reactions, as well as central nervous system and cardiovascular functions (1–4). Physiologic amounts of glucocorticoids are also essential for normal renal tubular function and thus for water and electrolyte homeostasis. Furthermore, glucocorticoids represent one of the most widely used therapeutic compounds often employed in the treatment of inflammatory, autoimmune, and lymphoproliferative disorders (1–3).

The adrenal glands consist of the adrenal cortex and the adrenal medulla. In the fetus, the adrenal cortex is divided into two zones, the outer definitive zone and the inner fetal zone. The latter represents approximately 80% of the adrenal volume and secretes weak androgens with the delta-5 configuration (dehydroepiandrosterone, DHEA). After birth, the fetal zone regresses rapidly during the first 2 weeks and disappears almost completely by the third month of life. A few islands of cells remain which may later develop into androgen-secreting cells. During infancy and childhood, the definitive zone and perhaps remnants of the fetal zone evolve into the adult adrenal cortex, which consists of three anatomic zones: the outer *zona glomerulosa,* the intermediate *zona fasciculata,* and the inner *zona reticularis.* The *zona glomerulosa* is responsible for the production of aldosterone, the *zona fasciculata* for the production of cortisol, and the *zona reticularis* for the production of adrenal androgens. The adrenal medulla is functionally related to the sympathetic nervous system and secretes epinephrine and norepinephrine both at basal conditions and in response to stress. The adrenal cortex and medulla are embryologically and functionally interdependent, influencing each other's organogenesis, growth and function (1,2).

PATHWAYS OF STEROID BIOSYNTHESIS

The synthesis of the glucocorticoid cortisol and the mineralocorticoid aldosterone are under the control of regulatory systems that largely function independently. The major regulation of the former is by the adrenocorticotropic hormone (ACTH), while the latter is regulated primarily by the renin-angiotensin system and circulating potassium ions. All steroid hormones produced by the adrenal cortex are derived from cholesterol. Low-density lipoprotein (LDL) cholesterol is the major source of cholesterol utilized in adrenal steroidogenesis; however, the adrenal cortices can synthesize cholesterol de novo. Proteolytic and lipolytic enzymes act on LDL to release cholesterol esters for storage in lipid droplets in the adrenal steroidogenic cells (1–3).

In order for the adrenal cortex to synthesize active steroid hormones, a number of changes are required in the structure of cholesterol. Several of these reactions are catalyzed by the steroid hydroxylases, which are members of a superfamily of genes known collectively as cytochromes P450 (CYP). Adrenal steroidogenesis follows three distinct routes, which reflect the zonal differences in terms of function and regulation (Fig. 51.1).

The rate-limiting step in steroid biosynthesis is importation of cholesterol from cellular stores to the matrix side of the mitochondrial inner membrane, where the cholesterol side chain cleavage system is located. This import is controlled by the steroidogenic acute regulatory (StAR) protein, the synthesis of which is increased by trophic adrenocortical stimuli, such as ACTH (3,5,6). In addition to StAR protein, cholesterol transfer is also mediated by another protein, the peripheral benzodiazepine receptor (7) (Fig. 51.2). The first enzymatic step in steroid biosynthesis common to all steroidogenic pathways takes place in the mitochondrion and leads to the cleavage of six carbon atoms from the side chain of cholesterol, converting this C_{27} compound to the C_{21} steroid pregnenolone. This reaction is known as cholesterol side-chain cleavage and is catalyzed by the cytochrome P450 enzyme CYP11 A (P450 scc, cholesterol desmolase, side-chain cleavage enzyme), which is an integral protein of the inner mitochondrial membrane (1–3,8). Pregnenolone, the common precursor for

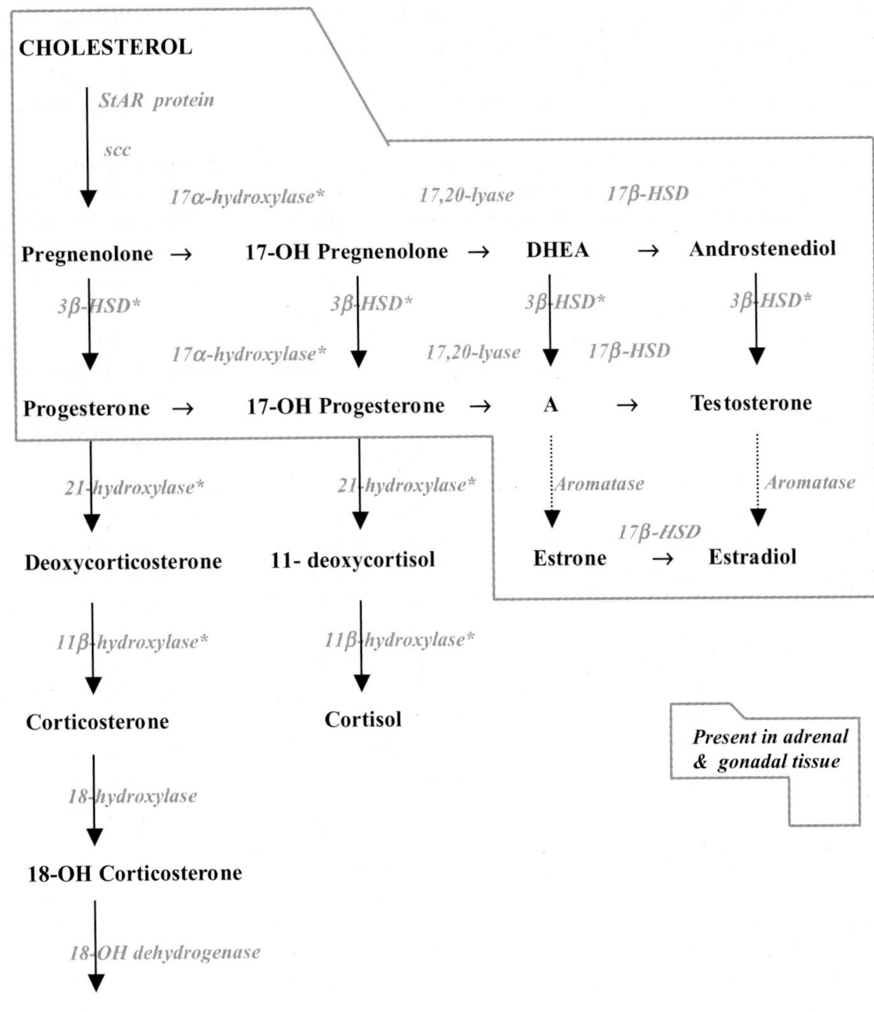

Figure 51.1. Schematic representation of adrenal steroidogenesis. Solid lines: major pathway. Dotted lines: major pathway in ovaries and testes but minor in the adrenals. *: deficient enzymatic activity results in CAH. A, androstenedione; DHEA, dehydroepiandrosterone; 3β-HSD, 3β-hydroxysteroid dehydrogenase; 17β-HSD, 17β-hydroxysteroid dehydrogenase; scc, cholesterol side-chain cleavage enzyme; StAR: steroidogenic acute regulatory protein.

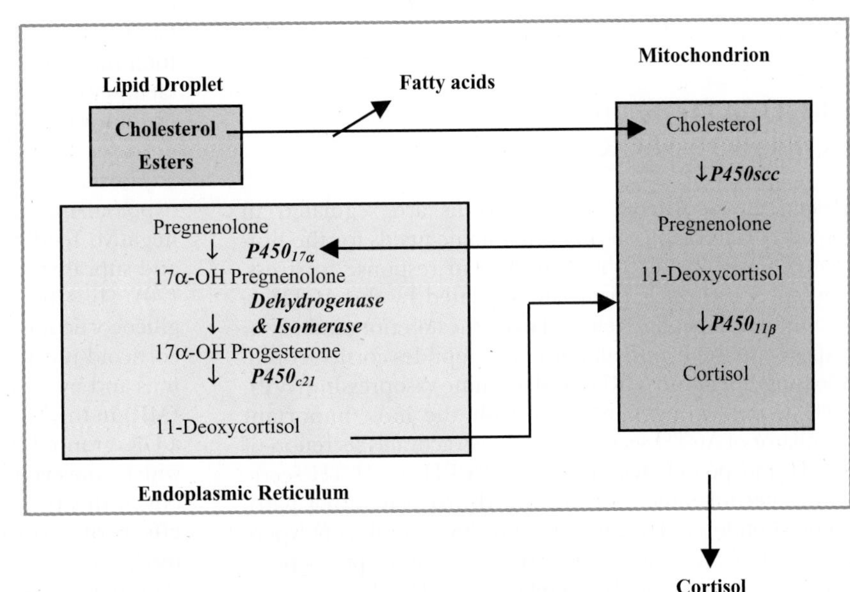

Figure 51.2. Pathway of biosynthesis of cortisol in the adrenal cortex. (Reproduced from Simpson ER, Waterman MR. Steroid biosynthesis in the adrenal cortex and its regulation by adrenocorticotropin. In: DeGroote LJ, Besser M, Burger HG, et al., eds. *Endocrinology*, Philadelphia, PA: W.B. Saunders, 1995:1630–1641.)

all steroids, then passes by diffusion from the mitochondrion to the cytoplasm where it undergoes further metabolism by several other enzymes (Fig. 51.2).

To synthesize mineralocorticoids in the *zona glomerulosa*, the microsomal 3β-hydroxysteroid dehydrogenase (3β-HSD) converts pregnenolone to progesterone (3,9). The latter is 21-hydroxylated in the cytoplasm by CYP21 (P450c21, 21-hydroxylase) to produce deoxycorticosterone (DOC). Aldosterone, the most potent 17-deoxysteroid mineralocorticoid compound, is produced by 11β-hydroxylation of DOC to corticosterone, followed by 18-hydroxylation and 18-oxidation of corticosterone (Fig. 51.1). The final three steps in aldosterone synthesis are accomplished by a single mitochondrial P450 enzyme, CYP11 B2 (P450aldo, aldosterone synthase) (10).

To produce cortisol, CYP17 (P450c17, 17α-hydroxylase/17,20-lyase) in the endoplasmic reticulum of the *zona fasciculata* and *zona reticularis* converts pregnenolone to 17α-hydroxypregnenolone (3,11). 3β-HSD in the *zona fasciculata* utilizes 17α-hydroxypregnenolone as a substrate, producing 17α-hydroxyprogesterone. The latter is 21-hydroxylated by CYP21 to form 11-deoxycortisol, which is further converted to cortisol by CYP11B1 (P450c11, 11β-hydroxylase) in the mitochondria (Fig. 51.2).

In the *zona reticularis* of the adrenal cortex and in the gonads, the 17,20-lyase activity of CYP17 converts 17α-hydroxypregnenolone to DHEA, a C_{19} steroid and sex steroid precursor. DHEA is further converted by 3β-HSD to androstenedione. In the gonads, androstenedione is reduced by 17β-hydroxysteroid dehydrogenase (12). In pubertal ovaries, aromatase (CYP19, P450c19) can convert androstenedione and testosterone to estrone and estradiol, respectively (13). Testosterone may be further metabolized to dihydrotestosterone by steroid 5α-reductase in androgen target tissues (14).

The enzymatic differences between the *zona glomerulosa* and the zona fasciculata can be summarized by stating that the *zona glomerulosa* lacks P450c17α but has the ability to catalyze the 18-oxidation of corticosterone, the precursor of aldosterone. Interestingly, this activity has been shown to be a property of the 11β-hydroxylase, which appears to be capable of 18-hydroxylation and subsequent reduction to the aldehyde aldosterone.

REGULATION OF CORTISOL SECRETION

Plasma glucocorticoid concentrations are regulated in ways that reflect the varying physiologic needs for the hormones under basal conditions and in response to stress. Cortisol secretion is primarily regulated by the ACTH, a 39-amino acid peptide released from the anterior pituitary in response to the hypothalamic neuropeptides corticotropin-releasing hormone (CRH) and arginine vasopressin (AVP). CRH is the strongest and probably the most important stimulator of ACTH secretion. AVP also activates secretion of ACTH and potentiates the effect of CRH on ACTH secretion. Catecholamines, angiotensin II, oxytocin, atrial natriuretic peptide, cholecystokinin, vasoactive intestinal polypeptide, and pituitary adenylate cyclase-activating polypeptide may also contribute to the secretion of ACTH (1–3).

ACTH is synthesized as part of a large precursor molecule of 214 amino acid, proopiomelanocortin. Depending on the cleavage enzymes, which are expressed in a tissue-specific fashion, ACTH and several other peptides, for example, NH2-terminal peptide, joining peptide, β- or γ-lipotropins, β-endorphin, α-melanocyte-stimulating hormone (αMSH), and corticotropin-like intermediate peptide, are produced. The first 18 amino acids of the *N*-terminus of ACTH are conserved through species and carry its biological activity. Thus, synthetic ACTH (1 to 24) and ACTH (1 to 18) are often used for clinical purposes instead of the full-length ACTH. The sequence of αMSH, which is contained within the ACTH molecule, stimulates the production of melanin by the melanocytes, causing skin and mucosal hyperpigmentation when secreted in excess (1–3).

ACTH is secreted in regular pulses of variable amplitude over 24 hours, with peak concentrations attained in the early morning hours (04:00 AM to 08:00 AM), thus forming the basis of the circadian pattern of ACTH and cortisol secretion (1–3,15). The acute action of ACTH is to increase the flux of cholesterol through the steroidogenic pathway, resulting in rapid production of steroids. ACTH also influences the remaining steps of steroidogenesis, as well as the uptake of cholesterol from plasma lipoproteins, thus ensuring a continuous supply of cholesterol to the mitochondria to meet the demands of activated pregnenolone biosynthesis. It also maintains the size of the adrenal glands.

CRH is the principal hypothalamic factor that stimulates the pituitary production of ACTH, while AVP plays a synergistic role (16). Both neuropeptides are produced by parvocellular neurons of the paraventricular nuclei of the hypothalamus, but are also found in other parts of the central nervous system, as well as in peripheral non-CNS locations (17). CRH and AVP are secreted in a pulsatile fashion that results in the episodic secretion of ACTH and the circadian variation of cortisol secretion. The frequency of the hypothalamic pulsations of CRH and AVP is relatively constant, while the amplitude of these secretory episodes increases in the early morning hours and during stress, resulting in major changes in the plasma concentrations of cortisol. Therefore, it is the magnitude of each pulse of CRH/AVP and consequently ACTH that determines the total daily cortisol secretion. In addition to ACTH, other factors may also play an important role in the regulation of the adrenal cortex, including neural factors, medullary peptides, and immune system products (18,19).

Cortisol is the primary negative regulator of basal hypothalamic–pituitary–adrenal (HPA) axis activity through negative feedback upon the pituitary, the hypothalamus and suprahypothalamic centers, such as the hippocampus (20). Thus, both ACTH and CRH secretion are inhibited by glucocorticoids. This effect is mediated by the classic glucocorticoid receptor α (GRα) in the pituitary and hypothalamus and by both GRα and the mineralocorticoid receptor (MR) in the hippocampus. The MR is in fact functioning as a GR, granted that the enzyme 11β-dehydrogenase type 2, which converts cortisol to the inactive cortisone, is not present in this tissue to protect it from the mineralocorticoid effects of cortisol. The concentrations of aldosterone are too low to compete with cortisol for the hippocampal MRs. Whether and to what extent direct glucocorticoid feedback on the adrenal cortex itself regulates cortisol synthesis is not clear (21).

SECRETION AND METABOLISM

In normal subjects, the secretion of glucocorticoids follows a diurnal pattern, with peak concentrations observed between 06:00 AM and 08:00 AM and lowest concentrations around midnight (22). The cortisol production rate is approximately 10 to 15 mg per m^2 per day (23). More than 90% of circulating cortisol, and to a lesser extent aldosterone, is bound tightly to corticosteroid-binding globulin (CBG) or transcortin (24). The remaining (10%) of the circulating cortisol is free or loosely bound to albumin. The free and albumin-bound fractions of cortisol represent the biologically active form of the hormone. When plasma cortisol concentrations exceed 20 μg per dL, CBG becomes fully saturated and most of the excess cortisol is biologically active. CBG is synthesized in the liver. Estrogens, thyroid hormones, pregnancy, and oral contraceptives are associated with increased CBG concentrations (24–26), whereas hypercortisolism, hepatic, or renal disease result in decreased CBG concentrations. In the presence of an intact HPA axis, alterations in CBG concentrations are likely not to affect circulating free cortisol concentrations.

The primary site of cortisol metabolism in humans is the liver, kidney, and a number of target tissues. Cytosolic and microsomal enzymes, including cytochrome P450, 5α/5β-reductase, 3α/3β-oxidoreductase, and 11β-hydroxysteroid dehydrogenase (11β-HSD), play an important role in the hepatic metabolism of cortisol (27–29). The major routes of hepatic metabolism involve A-ring and side-chain reduction followed by conjugation with glucuronic acid and sulphate (30). The inactive glucuronide and sulphate metabolites are excreted by the kidneys, whereas only less than 1% of cortisol is excreted unchanged in the urine. Therefore, the metabolic clearance of cortisol is influenced primarily by factors altering hepatic clearance and to a significant degree by renal enzymes and factors affecting renal excretion.

11β-hydroxysteroid dehydrogenase (11β-HSD) is known to modulate glucocorticoid action in tissues by altering the rate of conversion between cortisol and cortisone. There are two types of 11β-HSD: 11β-HSD type 1 (11β-HSD1) and type 2 (11β-HSD2). 11β-HSD1 acts as a reductase, catalyzing the conversion of inactive cortisone to active cortisol, and may contribute to the tissue hypersensitivity to glucocorticoids. 11β-HSD1 is widely expressed in the liver, lung, adipose tissue, vascular components, ovary, and the CNS. Increased expression of 11β-HSD1 activity in adipose tissue is associated with visceral obesity, indicating that 11β-HSD1 can enhance glucocorticoid action in local tissues (29).

In contradistinction to 11β-HSD1, the physiologic importance of the other 11β-HSD2 is well documented. Patients harboring mutations in this enzyme develop symptoms of mineralocorticoid excess, while mice bearing a deletion in this gene demonstrate glucocorticoid-dependent mineralocorticoid excess. 11β-HSD2 acts as a dehydrogenase that converts cortisol to inactive cortisone. 11β-HSD2 is expressed in classic aldosterone-sensitive tissues, such as the kidney, colon, sweat glands, and the placenta, where it protects the MR from the mineralocorticoid effects of cortisol, allowing the much lower aldosterone concentrations to exert such actions (29).

MOLECULAR MECHANISMS OF GLUCOCORTICOID ACTION

At the cellular level, the actions of glucocorticoids are mediated by an intracellular receptor protein, the GR, which functions as a hormone-activated transcription factor that regulates the expression of glucocorticoid target genes (1,31,32). The human (h) GR belongs to the superfamily of steroid/thyroid/retinoic acid receptor proteins (31). The hGR gene consists of 9 exons and is composed of a poorly conserved amino-terminal domain (NTD); a central, highly conserved DNA-binding domain (DBD); and a carboxyl-terminal, ligand-binding domain (LBD) (1,31,32). The NTD contains a major transactivation domain, termed activation function (AF)-1, which is located at amino acids 77 to 262 of the hGR. The DBD spans over amino acids 420 to 480 and contains two zinc finger motifs through which the receptor binds to specific DNA sequences in the promoter region of target genes, the glucocorticoid-response elements (GREs). The LBD contains a second transactivation domain, AF-2, as well as sequences important for interaction with heat shock proteins (HSPs), nuclear translocation, and receptor dimerization (33–35) (Fig. 51.3A, B).

Alternative slicing of the hGR gene in exon 9 generates two highly homologous receptor isoforms, termed α and β. These are identical through amino acid 727, but then diverge, with hGRα having an additional 50 amino acids and hGRβ having an additional, nonhomologous 15 amino acids (36) (Fig. 51.3A). hGRα is ubiquitously expressed in almost all human tissues and cells, resides primarily in the cytoplasm, and represents the classic GR that functions as ligand-dependent transcription factor. hGRβ is also ubiquitously expressed in tissues usually at lower concentrations than hGRα, with the exception of epithelial cells and neutrophils (36). In contradistinction to hGRα, hGRβ resides primarily in the nucleus of cells independently of the presence of ligand, does not bind glucocorticoids, and exerts a dominant negative effect upon the wild-type hGRα (32,37).

In the absence of ligand, hGRα resides primarily in the cytoplasm of cells as part of a large multiprotein complex, which consists of the receptor polypeptide, two molecules of hsp90, and several other proteins (38). The hsp90 molecules are thought to sequester hGRα in the cytoplasm of cells by maintaining the receptor in a conformation that masks or inactivates its nuclear localization signals (NLSs). Upon hormone binding, the receptor undergoes conformational changes, which result in dissociation from hsp90 and other proteins, unmasking of the NLSs and exposure of the ligand-binding pocket. In its new conformation, the activated, ligand-bound hGRα translocates into the nucleus, where it binds as homodimer to GREs located in the promoter region of target genes. hGRα then communicates with the basal transcription machinery and regulates the expression of glucocorticoid-responsive genes positively or negatively, depending on the GRE sequence and promoter context (38) (Fig. 51.4). The receptor can also modulate gene expression, as a monomer, independently of GRE binding, by physically interacting with other transcription

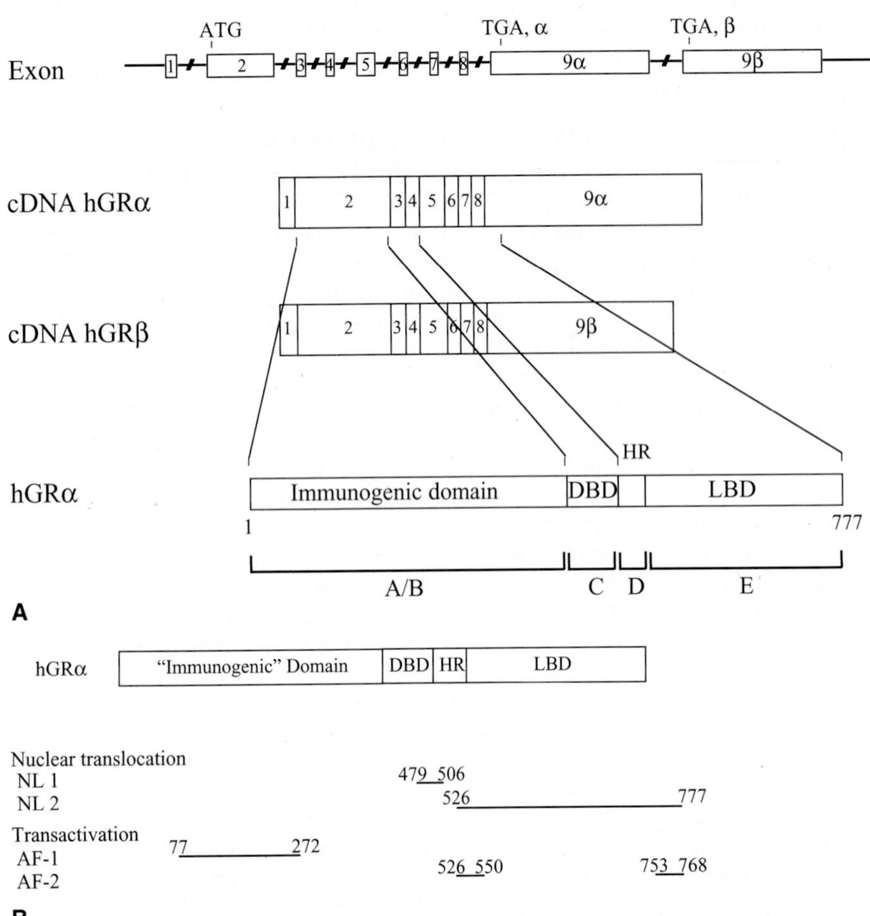

Figure 51.3. (A) Genomic and complementary DNA, and protein structures of the human glucocorticoid receptor (hGR). The hGR gene consists of 10 exons. Exon 1 is an untranslated region, exon 2 codes for the amino-terminal domain (A/B), exons 3 and 4 for the DNA-binding domain (C), and exons 5–9 for the hinge region (D), and the ligand-binding domain (E). The glucocorticoid receptor gene contains two terminal exons 9 (exon 9α and 9β) alternatively spliced to produce the classic hGRα isoform and an additional nonligand binding hGRβ isoform. (B) Functional domains of the glucocorticoid receptor. The functional domains and subdomains are indicated beneath the linearized protein structures. DBD, DNA-binding domain; LBD, ligand-binding domain; NL, nuclear localization signal; AF, activation function.

factors, such as activating protein-1, nuclear factor-κB, and signal transducers and activators of transcription (38).

Following binding to GREs, the activated hGRα enhances the expression of glucocorticoid-responsive genes by regulating the assembly of a transcriptional preinitiation complex at the promoter region of target genes. This is achieved by interaction of the liganded receptor with the basal transcription factors, a group of proteins composed of RNA polymerase II, TATA-binding protein (TBP), and a host of TBP-associated proteins (TAF_{II}s). The interaction between the activated receptor and the basal transcription factors is mediated by the coactivators, which are nucleoproteins with chromatin remodeling and other enzymatic activities (39,40) (Fig. 51.5).

The response of a single cell exposed to glucocorticoids depends on the interplay between (i) the concentration of free hormone, (ii) the relative potency of the hormone, and (iii) the ability of the cell to receive and transduce the

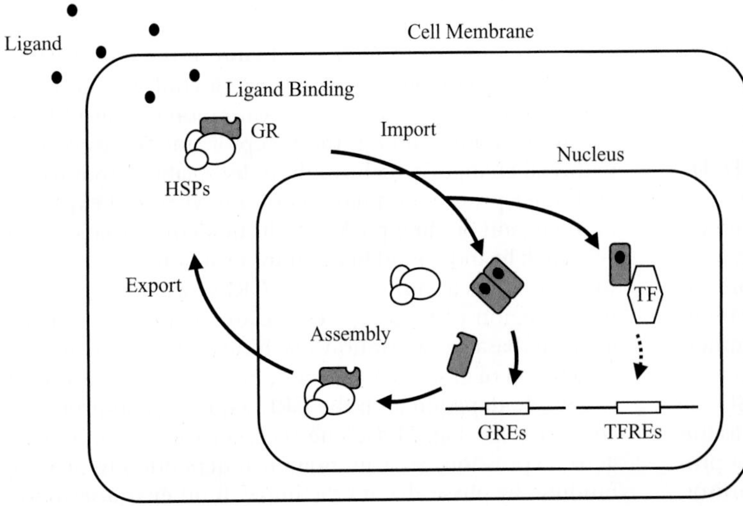

Figure 51.4. Nucleocytoplasmic shuttling of the glucocorticoid receptor. GR, glucocorticoid receptor; GRE, glucocorticoid response element; HSP, heat shock protein; TF, transcription factor; TFRE, transcription factor responsive element.

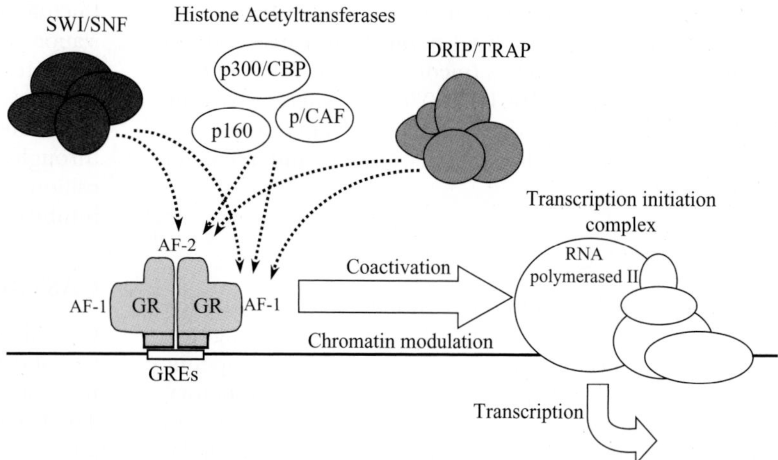

Figure 51.5. Schematic representation of the interaction of the glucocorticoid receptor with coactivators and other chromatin modulators. AF, activation function; CBP, cAMP-responsive element-binding protein (CREB)-binding protein; DRIP, vitamin D receptor-interacting protein; p/CAF, p300/CBP-associated factor; TRAP, thyroid hormone receptor-associated protein; SWI, mating-type switching; SNF, sucrose nonfermenting.

hormonal signal. The concentration of the free hormone is primarily under the control of the HPA axis but is also influenced by the plasma and tissue concentrations of CBG, whereas the relative potency of any endogenous or exogenous glucocorticoid is influenced by its bioavailability, affinity for hGR and ability to retain the hGR in the nucleus (38).

EFFECTS OF GLUCOCORTICOIDS

GROWTH AND DEVELOPMENT

Although small increases in cortisol concentrations exert a stimulatory effect on growth hormone (GH) secretion by increasing GH messenger ribonucleic acid (mRNA) levels and enhancing GH gene expression (41), significant chronic hypercortisolism results in reduced GH secretion and growth suppression (42–44), attenuation of GH response to exogenous stimuli (45,46), and inhibition of the effects of insulin-like growth factor I and other growth factors on target tissues (42,43,47). Children with Cushing syndrome have delayed or arrested growth and achieve a final adult height, which is on average 7.5 to 8.0 cm below their predicted height (42,48).

Glucocorticoids play an important role in fetal development and lung maturation by stimulating the synthesis and release of surfactant proteins (SP-A, SP-B, SP-C) (49,50). The absence of functional GR in GR −/− knockout mice leads to severe neonatal respiratory distress syndrome and death within a few hours after birth (51). Glucocorticoids also stimulate the enzyme phenylethanolamine *N*-methyltransferase, which converts norepinephrine to epinephrine in adrenal medulla and chromaffin tissue. GR −/− knockout mice do not develop an adrenal medulla.

CARBOHYDRATE AND LIPID METABOLISM

Glucocorticoids increase blood glucose concentrations through their action on glycogen, protein, and lipid metabolism. In the liver, glucocorticoids stimulate glycogen deposition, while in peripheral tissues (muscle, fat), they inhibit glucose uptake and utilization. In adipose tissue, lipolysis is activated and free fatty acids are released into the circulation (1–3). Glucocorticoids have a permissive effect on other hormones, such as catecholamines and glucagon, leading to insulin resistance and an increase in blood glucose concentrations at the expense of protein and lipid catabolism.

Glucocorticoids stimulate adipocyte differentiation and promote adipogenesis by enhancing the transcriptional activity of relevant important genes, including lipoprotein lipase, glycerol-3-phosphate dehydrogenase, and leptin (1–3). Chronic hypercortisolism leads to increased deposition of visceral or central adipose tissue. The predilection for visceral obesity may be related to the increased expression of both the GR and type-1 isozyme of 11β-hydroxysteroid dehydrogenase (11β-HSD) in omental as opposed to subcutaneous adipose tissue (52,53).

THYROID AND REPRODUCTIVE FUNCTION

Glucocorticoids suppress the thyroid axis most likely through a direct action on thyroid-stimulating hormone secretion, and they inhibit 5′ deiodinase activity, which converts thyroxin to triiodothyronine. They also act centrally to inhibit gonadotropin-releasing hormone pulsatility and release of luteinizing hormone and follicle-stimulating hormone (FSH) (1–3,48).

SKIN, MUSCLE, AND CONNECTIVE TISSUE; BONE AND CALCIUM METABOLISM

Glucocorticoids induce insulin resistance in the muscle and result in catabolic changes in muscle, skin, and connective tissue. They inhibit osteoblast function, thus explaining the osteopenia and osteoporosis associated with chronic glucocorticoid excess. Glucocorticoids also induce a negative calcium balance by inhibiting intestinal calcium absorption and increasing renal calcium excretion (1–3).

WATER AND ELECTROLYTE HOMEOSTASIS

Glucocorticoids increase blood pressure via mechanisms that involve actions on the kidney and vasculature. In vascular smooth muscle, glucocorticoids increase sensitivity to pressor agents, such as catecholamines and angiotensin II, and reduce nitric oxide-mediated endothelial dilatation.

They also increase angiotensinogen synthesis. In the kidney, cortisol acts on the distal nephron to cause sodium retention and potassium loss (mediated by the MR) depending on the activity of 11β-HSD2 (29). Elsewhere across the nephron, glucocorticoids increase glomerular filtration rate, proximal tubular epithelial sodium transport, and free water clearance (1–3).

IMMUNE FUNCTION

Glucocorticoids have profound inhibitory effects on the immune/inflammatory response (54,55). Therefore, glucocorticoids have become one of the most efficient therapeutic compounds for the management of allergic, inflammatory, and autoimmune diseases, as well as for suppressing the host immune reaction in organ transplantation. At the cellular level, the main anti-inflammatory and immunosuppressive effects of glucocorticoids include alterations in leukocyte traffic and function, decreases in production of cytokines and mediators of inflammation, and inhibition of their action on target tissues by the latter. These effects are exerted both at the resting, basal state and during inflammatory stress, when the circulating concentrations of glucocorticoids are elevated. Thus, a circadian activity of several immune factors has been demonstrated in reverse-phase synchrony with that of plasma glucocorticoid concentrations (1–3,56). Glucocorticoids increase the risk for infection, including those of bacteria, viruses, fungi, and parasites (1–3).

CENTRAL NERVOUS SYSTEM

The brain is an important target tissue for glucocorticoids. Both glucocorticoid and MRs are expressed in discrete regions of the brain, including hippocampus, hypothalamus, cerebellum, and cortex (57). Glucocorticoids cause neuronal death mostly in the hippocampus, and this effect may underlie their role in cognitive function, memory, and neurodegenerative diseases. Chronic hypercortisolism has multiple effects on CNS functions, such as cognition, mood, behavior, memory, and sleep pattern. Glucocorticoids may cause frank and Korsakoff psychosis, major depression, schizophrenia, Alzheimer disease, anorexia nervosa, and cerebrovascular brain injury, as well as cognitive disturbances, including difficulties in attention and concentration, memory disturbance, and impaired thinking. Chronic hypercortisolism may also affect the anatomy of CNS, leading to reduction of hippocampal volume, ventricular enlargement, and cortical atrophy. On the other hand, physiologic doses of glucocorticoids appear to be necessary for memory and cognitive function, as well as other important functions of the CNS (1–3).

The CNS contains two types of "glucocorticoid" receptors, which bind glucocorticoids and mediate their actions. One is the MR (type I) and the other is the classic GR (type II). The former is distributed predominantly in the limbic system, including the hippocampus, septum, septohippocampal nucleus, and amygdala, while the latter is wildly distributed in the entire CNS. Given that the CNS and in particular the hippocampus does not express 11β-HSD2, the MR may act as a high-affinity receptor for glucocorticoids in this region of the brain. It appears that the MR mediates the tonic effect of glucocorticoids on circadian fluctuations, the sensitivity of the stress response, and organization of the behavioral responses to stress, while the GR mediates the feedback inhibition of glucocorticoids on the HPA axis activity and facilitates memory storage (1–3).

In the eye, glucocorticoids raise intraocular pressure through an increase in aqueous humor production and deposition of matrix within the trabecular meshwork, which inhibits aqueous drainage (58).

GASTROINTESTINAL FUNCTION

Chronic administration of glucocorticoids increases the risk of developing peptic ulcer disease. Pancreatitis with fat necrosis is reported in patients with glucocorticoid excess. The GR is expressed throughout the gastrointestinal tract and the MR in the distal colon, and these mediate the corticosteroid control of epithelial ion transport (1–3).

TREATMENT WITH GLUCOCORTICOIDS

Natural and synthetic glucocorticoids can be used for both endocrine and nonendocrine disorders. In endocrine practice, glucocorticoids are used in establishing the diagnosis and cause of Cushing syndrome, in the hormonal replacement therapy of adrenal insufficiency and in the treatment of congenital adrenal hyperplasia, which consists of both glucocorticoid and/or mineralocorticoid substitution and suppression of excess androgen secretion. Glucocorticoids are also given in pharmacologic doses to treat patients with inflammatory, allergic, or immunologic disorders (1–3) (Table 51.1). Chronic therapy has many side effects, ranging from suppression of the HPA axis and Cushing syndrome to infections and changes in mental

TABLE 51.1 Therapeutic Indications of Corticosteroids

Disorders	*Examples*
Allergic reactions	Angioneurotic edema, asthma, urticaria
Endocrine	Replacement therapy in Addison disease, hypopituitarism, congenital adrenal hyperplasia
Gastrointestinal	Inflammatory bowel disease (ulcerative colitis, Crohn disease), chronic active hepatitis, liver transplantation/rejection
Hematologic	Leukemia, lymphoma, hemolytic anemia, idiopathic thrombocytopenic purpura
Infections	Meningococcal meningitis, septic shock
Muscular	Polymyalgia rheumatica, myasthenia gravis
Neurologic	Cerebral edema, raised intracranial pressure
Ophthalmologic	Acute uveitis, conjunctivitis, optic neuritis, choroiditis
Renal	Nephrotic syndrome, vasculitides, kidney transplantation/rejection
Respiratory	Angioedema, anaphylaxis, asthma, sarcoidosis, tuberculosis, respiratory distress syndrome
Rheumatologic	Systemic lupus erythematosus, polyarteritis nodosa, temporal arteritis, juvenile rheumatoid arthritis
Skin	Dermatitis, pemphigus, atopic dermatitis

status. Factors that influence both the therapeutic and adverse effects of glucocorticoids include the pharmacokinetic properties of the glucocorticoid, daily dosage, timing of doses during the day, individual differences in steroid metabolism, as well as the duration of treatment.

GLUCOCORTICOID REPLACEMENT THERAPY

In cortisol and aldosterone deficiency states (primary adrenal insufficiency), physiologic replacement is best achieved with a combination of hydrocortisone and the mineralocorticoid fludrocortisone; hydrocortisone alone at replacement doses does not usually provide sufficient mineralocorticoid activity for complete replacement.

In primary *Addison disease* or following bilateral adrenalectomy, hydrocortisone by mouth is usually required. This is given in two to three doses, the larger in the morning and the smaller in the evening, to mimic the normal diurnal rhythm of cortisol secretion. The optimum daily dose is determined by the clinical response. Chronic glucocorticoid therapy is supplemented by fludrocortisone. The latter is titrated clinically and on the basis of normal plasma rennin activity measurements.

In *acute adrenocortical insufficiency*, hydrocortisone is given intravenously (preferably as sodium succinate or phosphate) every 6 to 8 hours in sodium chloride intravenous infusion 0.9%.

In *hypopituitarism*, glucocorticoids should be given as in adrenocortical insufficiency, but since the production of aldosterone is regulated by the renin-angiotensin system, a mineralocorticoid is not usually required. Additional replacement therapy with levothyroxine and sex hormones should be given as indicated by the pattern of hormone deficiency. In case of thyroid and cortisol deficiency, cortisol should be given first, as hypothyroidism may mask severe cortisol deficiency, which is unleashed upon thyroid replacement.

In *congenital adrenal hyperplasia*, the anterior pituitary increases the secretion of corticotrophin to compensate for the reduced secretion of cortisol; this results in increased adrenal androgen production. Treatment is aimed at suppressing the corticotrophin secretion using hydrocortisone. Careful and continual dose titration is required to avoid growth retardation and toxicity. Salt-losing forms of congenital adrenal hyperplasia require mineralocorticoid replacement. Mineralocorticoid replacement may also be beneficial even when salt-losing symptoms are not evident (59).

GLUCOCORTICOID THERAPY

In comparing the relative potencies of corticosteroids in terms of their anti-inflammatory (glucocorticoid) effects, it should be borne in mind that high glucocorticoid activity in itself is more advantageous when it is accompanied by relatively low mineralocorticoid activity, because high doses can be given without producing salt retention as a side effect. The mineralocorticoid activity of fludrocortisone at replacement doses on the other hand is so high that its anti-inflammatory activity is of no clinical relevance. The equivalent anti-inflammatory doses of corticosteroids are shown in Table 51.2.

The relatively high mineralocorticoid activity of *hydrocortisone* and its immediate precursor *cortisone* and the resulting fluid retention make them unsuitable for disease suppression on a long-term basis. Thus, although they are preferable for adrenal replacement therapy, we recommend synthetic glucocorticoids with intermediate or long-term actions for treating diseases that require high (stress) doses of glucocorticoids. Hydrocortisone may be used on a short-term basis by intravenous injection for the emergency management of some conditions. The relatively moderate anti-inflammatory potency of hydrocortisone also makes it a useful topical corticosteroid for the management of mild inflammatory skin conditions because side effects (both topical and systemic) are less marked than those of fluorinated synthetic glucocorticoids; cortisone is not active topically.

Prednisolone has predominantly glucocorticoid activity and is the corticosteroid most commonly used by mouth for long-term disease suppression. Prednisolone or methylprednisolone can also be given parenterally. *Betamethasone* and *dexamethasone* have very high glucocorticoid activity but insignificant mineralocorticoid activity. This makes them particularly suitable for high-dose therapy in conditions where fluid retention would be a disadvantage (e.g., cerebral edema). Betamethasone and dexamethasone are fluorinated at the 9 α position and have a long duration of action. The latter, coupled with their lack of mineralocorticoid action, makes them suitable for conditions that require suppression of ACTH secretion (e.g., hard to control congenital adrenal hyperplasia). Some esters of betamethasone, beclomethasone, and dexamethasone exert a considerably marked topical effect (e.g., on the skin or the nasal or lung epithelium); use is made of this to obtain topical effects while minimizing systemic side effects (e.g., for skin applications

TABLE 51.2 Equivalent Anti-inflammatory Doses of Corticosteroids[a]

	Equivalent Dose	*Plasma Half-Life (min)*	*Biologic Half-Life (hr)*
Prednisolone	5 mg	90	18–36
≡ Betamethasone	750 μg	300	36–54
≡ Cortisone acetate	25 mg	80–118	8–12
≡ Dexamethasone	750 μg	200	36–54
≡ Hydrocortisone	20 mg	60	8–12
≡ Methylprednisolone	4 mg	180	18–36
≡ Triamcinolone	4 mg	30	18–36

[a]This table takes no account of mineralocorticoid effects, nor does it take account for variations in duration of action (59).

and inhalations). The same steroids, however, may cause skin atrophy. *Deflazacort* is derived from prednisolone and has high glucocorticoid activity (59).

Administration of Corticosteroids

Whenever possible, *local, compartmentalized treatment* with creams, intra-articular injections, inhalations, eyedrops, or enemas should be used in preference to *systemic treatment.* The suppressive action of a corticosteroid on cortisol secretion is least when it is given as a single dose in the morning. In an attempt to reduce pituitary–adrenal suppression further, the total dose for 2 days can sometimes be given as a single dose on alternate days; alternate-day administration has not been very successful in the management of asthma though. HPA axis suppression can also be reduced by means of intermittent therapy with short courses. In some conditions, it may be possible to reduce the dose of corticosteroid by adding a small dose of an immunosuppressant drug. Interestingly, when glucocorticoids are given in the context of severe stress, such as chemotherapy for leukemia, they produce very little HPA axis suppression (60).

Dosage of corticosteroids varies widely in different diseases and in different patients, and should always be individualized. If the use of a corticosteroid can save or prolong life, as in acute leukemia or acute transplant rejection, high doses may need to be given, because the complications of therapy are likely to be less serious than the effects of the disease itself.

When long-term corticosteroid therapy is used in some chronic diseases, the adverse effects of treatment may become greater than the disabilities caused by the disease. To minimize side effects, the maintenance dose should be kept as low as possible.

When potentially less harmful measures are ineffective, corticosteroids are used topically for the treatment of inflammatory conditions of the skin. Corticosteroids are used both topically (by rectum) and systemically (by mouth or intravenously) in the management of ulcerative colitis and Crohn disease. Moderate to high doses of corticosteroids are given by intravenous injection in the acute respiratory distress syndrome and in the systemic inflammatory syndrome/septic shock. Corticosteroids are recommended in meningococcal meningitis and in the recently described severe acute respiratory distress syndrome (SARS) (61,62).

Dexamethasone and betamethasone have little, if any, mineralocorticoid action and their long duration of action makes them particularly suitable for suppressing corticotropin secretion in hard to control congenital adrenal hyperplasia, where the dose should be tailored to clinical response and by measurement of adrenal androgens and 17-hydroxyprogesterone.

In acute hypersensitivity reactions, such as angioedema of the upper respiratory tract and anaphylactic shock, corticosteroids are indicated as an adjunct to emergency treatment with adrenaline (epinephrine). In such cases, hydrocortisone (as sodium succinate) by intravenous injection may be required.

Corticosteroids are preferably used by inhalation in the management of asthma, but systemic therapy in association with bronchodilators is required for the emergency treatment of severe acute asthma. Corticosteroids may also be useful in conditions such as rheumatic fever, chronic active hepatitis, and sarcoidosis; they may also lead to remissions of acquired hemolytic anemia, idiopathic nephrotic syndrome in children, and thrombocytopenic purpura. Corticosteroids can improve the prognosis of serious conditions such as systemic lupus erythematous, temporal arteritis, and polyarteritis nodosa; the effects of the disease process may be suppressed and symptoms relieved, but the underlying condition is not cured, although it may ultimately remit. It is usual to begin therapy in these conditions at fairly high doses and then to reduce the dose to the lowest dose that allows disease control (59).

SIDE EFFECTS OF CORTICOSTEROIDS

Overdosage or prolonged use may exaggerate some of the normal physiologic actions of corticosteroids leading to glucocorticoid and/or mineralocorticoid side effects.

Administration of corticosteroids may result in suppression of growth and may affect the development of puberty. It is important to use the lowest effective dose; alternate day regimens may be appropriate and limit growth reduction.

Mineralocorticoid side effects include hypertension, sodium and water retention, and potassium loss. They are most marked with fludrocortisone but are significant with cortisone, hydrocortisone, corticotropin, and tetracosactide (tetracosactrin). Mineralocorticoid actions are negligible with the high-potency long-acting glucocorticoids, betamethasone, and dexamethasone and occur only slightly with the intermediate-acting methylprednisolone, prednisolone, and triamcinolone.

Glucocorticoid side effects include obesity, especially of the centripetal type, carbohydrate intolerance and/or diabetes type 2 and osteoporosis, avascular necrosis of the femoral head, mental disturbances (insomnia, hypomania, and depression may be induced, particularly in patients with a history of mental disorder), as well as muscle wasting (proximal myopathy) (Table 51.3). Corticosteroid therapy is also weakly linked with peptic ulceration. High doses of chronically administered corticosteroids must always be gradually tapered to avoid symptoms of acute glucocorticoid deficiency. In children, administration of corticosteroids may result in suppression of growth and delay of bone age. In general, chronic use of systemic glucocorticoids in children compromises their final stature to a varying degree. Other complications include increased susceptibility to infection, poor wound healing, and activation of latent tuberculosis (59).

ADRENAL SUPPRESSION

During prolonged therapy with corticosteroids, adrenal atrophy develops and may persist for years after discontinuation of therapy. When a question about the presence of adrenal suppression is raised, a standard cortrosyn (ACTH stimulation) test may be administered. Abrupt withdrawal after a prolonged period may lead to acute adrenal insufficiency, hypotension, or death. Withdrawal may also be associated with anorexia, nausea, fever, myalgia, arthralgia, rhinitis, conjunctivitis, painful itchy skin nodules, abdominal pain, diarrhea, weight loss, and/or psychiatric manifestations.

TABLE 51.3 Effects of Chronic Pharmacologic Use of Glucocorticoids

Endocrine and metabolic
Suppression of HPA axis (adrenal suppression)
Growth failure in children
Carbohydrate intolerance
Hyperinsulinism
Insulin resistance
Abnormal glucose tolerance test
Diabetes mellitus
Cushingoid features
Moon facies, facial plethora
Generalized and truncal obesity
Supraclavicular fat collection
Posterior cervical fat deposition (buffalo hump)
Glucocorticoid-induced acne
Thin and fragile skin, violaceous striae
Impotence, menstrual disorders
Decreased TSH and T_3
Hypokalemia, metabolic alkalosis
Gastrointestinal
Gastric irritation, peptic ulcer
Acute pancreatitis (rare)
Fatty infiltration of liver (hepatomegaly) (rare)
Hemopoietic
Leukocytosis
Neutrophilia
Increased influx from bone marrow and decreased migration from blood vessels
Monocytopenia
Lymphopenia
Migration from blood vessels to lymphoid tissue
Eosinopenia
Immunologic
Suppression of delayed hypersensitivity
Inhibition of leukocyte and tissue macrophage migration
Inhibition of cytokine secretion/action
Suppression of the primary antigen response
Musculoskeletal
Osteoporosis, spontaneous fractures
Aseptic necrosis of femoral and humoral heads and other bones
Myopathy/muscle weakness
Ophthalmologic
Posterior subcapsular cataracts (more common in children)
Elevated intraocular pressure/glaucoma
Neuropsychiatric
Sleep disturbances, insomnia
Euphoria, depression, mania, psychosis
Pseudotumor cerebri (benign increase of intracranial pressure)
Cardiovascular
Hypertension
Congestive heart failure in predisposed patients

To compensate for a diminished adrenocortical response caused by prolonged corticosteroid treatment, any significant intercurrent illness, trauma, or surgical procedure requires a temporary increase in corticosteroid dose, or if already stopped, a temporary reintroduction of corticosteroid treatment. Therefore, anesthetists must know whether a patient is taking or has been taking a corticosteroid, to avoid a precipitous fall in blood pressure during anesthesia or in the immediate postoperative period.

Children on long-term corticosteroid treatment should wear an "Alert Bracelet" and carry a "Steroid Treatment Card" which gives guidance on minimizing risk and provides details of prescriber, drug, dosage, and duration of treatment, as well as an "Emergency Kit" (59).

INFECTIONS

Prolonged courses of corticosteroids increase susceptibility to infections and severity of infections; clinical presentation of infections may also be atypical. Serious infections, for example, *septicemia* and *tuberculosis*, may reach an advanced stage before being recognized, and *amebiasis* or *strongyloidiasis* may be activated or exacerbated (exclude before initiating a corticosteroid in those at risk or with suggestive symptoms). Fungal or viral *ocular infections* may also be exacerbated.

Chickenpox

Unless they have had chickenpox, patients receiving oral or parenteral corticosteroids for purposes other than replacement should be regarded as being *at risk of severe chickenpox.* Manifestations of fulminant illness include pneumonia, hepatitis, and disseminated intravascular coagulation; rash is not necessarily a prominent feature. Passive immunization with varicella-zoster immunoglobulin is needed for exposed nonimmune patients receiving systemic corticosteroids or for those who have used them within the previous 3 months; varicella-zoster immunoglobulin should preferably be given within 3 days of exposure and no later than 10 days. Confirmed chickenpox warrants specialist care and urgent treatment. Corticosteroids should not be stopped and dosage may need to be increased. Topical, inhaled, or rectal corticosteroids are less likely to be associated with an increased risk of severe chickenpox.

Measles

Patients taking corticosteroids should be advised to take particular care to avoid exposure to measles and seek immediate medical advice if exposure occurs. Prophylaxis with intramuscular normal immunoglobulin may be needed (59).

INTERACTION OF GLUCOCORTICOIDS WITH OTHER DRUGS

The interactions of corticosteroids with other drugs are listed in Table 51.4.

PREGNANCY AND BREAST-FEEDING

A review of the data on the safety of systemic corticosteroids used in pregnancy and breast-feeding has concluded the following:

- Corticosteroids vary in their ability to cross the placenta; betamethasone and dexamethasone cross the placenta readily, while most of hydrocortisone and 88% of prednisolone are inactivated by 11β-HSD2 as they cross the placenta.
- There is no convincing evidence that systemic corticosteroids increase the incidence of congenital abnormalities, such as cleft lip or palate.

TABLE 51.4 Interactions of Corticosteroids with Other Drugs[a]

ACE inhibitors	Antagonism of hypotensive effect
Acetazolamide	Increased risk of hypokalemia
Adrenergic blockers	Antagonism of hypotensive effect
α-Blockers	Antagonism of hypotensive effect
Aminoglutethimide	Metabolism of corticosteroids accelerated (reduced effect)
Amphotericin	Increased risk of hypokalemia (avoid concomitant use unless corticosteroids needed to control reactions)
Angiotensin-II-receptor antagonists	Antagonism of hypotensive effect
Antidiabetics	Antagonism of hypoglycemic effect
Aspirin (also benorilate)	Increased risk of gastrointestinal bleeding and ulceration Corticosteroids reduce plasma-salicylate concentration
Barbiturates and primidone	Metabolism of corticosteroids accelerated (reduced effect)
β-Blockers	Antagonism of hypotensive effect
Calcium-channel blockers	Antagonism of hypotensive effect
Carbamazepine	Accelerated metabolism of corticosteroids (reduced effect)
Carbenoxolone	Increased risk of hypokalemia
Cardiac glycosides	Increased risk of hypokalemia
Clonidine	Antagonism of hypotensive effect
Coumarins	Anticoagulant effect possibly altered
Diazoxide	Antagonism of hypotensive effect
Diuretics	Antagonism of diuretic effect
Diuretics, loop	Increased risk of hypokalemia
Diuretics, thiazide and related	Increased risk of hypokalemia
Erythromycin	Erythromycin possibly inhibits metabolism of corticosteroids
Estrogens	Oral contraceptives increase plasma concentration of corticosteroids
Hydralazine	Antagonism of hypotensive effect
Ketoconazole	Ketoconazole possibly inhibits metabolism of corticosteroids
Methotrexate	Increased risk of hematological toxicity
Methyldopa	Antagonism of hypotensive effect
Mifepristone	Effect of corticosteroids (including inhaled corticosteroids) may be reduced for 3–4 days after mifepristone
Minoxidil	Antagonism of hypotensive effect
Moxonidine	Antagonism of hypotensive effect
NSAIDs	Increased risk of gastrointestinal bleeding and ulceration
Nitrates	Antagonism of hypotensive effect
Nitroprusside	Antagonism of hypotensive effect
Phenytoin	Metabolism of corticosteroids accelerated (reduced effect)
Progestogens	Oral contraceptives increase plasma concentration of corticosteroids
Rifamycins	Accelerated metabolism of corticosteroids (reduced effect)
Ritonavir	Plasma concentration possibly increased by ritonavir
Somatropin	Growth-promoting effect may be inhibited
Sympathomimetics, β_2	Increased risk of hypokalemia with concomitant use of high doses
Theophylline	Increased risk of hypokalemia
Vaccines	High doses of corticosteroids impair immune response; avoid use of live vaccines
Deflazacort belongs to corticosteroids and has the following interactions information:	
Antacids	Reduced absorption of deflazacort
Dexamethasone belongs to corticosteroids and has the following interactions information:	
Ephedrine	Metabolism of dexamethasone accelerated
Indinavir	Possibly reduced plasma-indinavir concentration
Lopinavir	Possibly reduced plasma-lopinavir concentration
Ritonavir	Plasma concentration possibly increased by ritonavir
Saquinavir	Possibly reduced plasma-saquinavir concentration
Methylprednisolone belongs to corticosteroids and has the following interactions information:	
Cyclosporin	Plasma-cyclosporin concentration increased by high-dose methylprednisolone (risk of convulsions)
Erythromycin	Erythromycin inhibits metabolism of methylprednisolone
Itraconazole	Itraconazole possibly inhibits metabolism of methylprednisolone
Ketoconazole	Ketoconazole inhibits metabolism of methylprednisolone
Prednisolone belongs to corticosteroids and has the following interactions information:	
Cyclosporin	Increased plasma concentration of prednisolone
Ritonavir	Plasma concentration possibly increased by ritonavir
Beclometasone, betamethasone, budesonide, cortisone, fludrocortisone, flunisolide, fluticasone, hydrocortisone, tetracosactide, and triamcinolone belong to corticosteroids but have no additional interactions information	

[a]The above-listed interactions do not generally apply to corticosteroids used for topical action (including inhalation) (63).

- When administration is prolonged or repeated during pregnancy, systemic corticosteroids increase the risk of intrauterine growth retardation; there is no evidence of intrauterine growth retardation following short-term treatment (e.g., prophylactic treatment for neonatal respiratory distress syndrome).
- Usually, any adrenal suppression in the neonate following prenatal exposure resolves spontaneously after birth and is rarely clinically important; however, it would be safe to perform a standard cortrosyn test in the neonate to exclude adrenal suppression (Table 51.3).
- Prednisolone appears in small amounts in breast milk but doses of up to 40 mg daily are unlikely to cause systemic effects in the infant; infants should be monitored for adrenal suppression if the mothers are taking a higher dose (59).

WITHDRAWAL OF CORTICOSTEROIDS

A *gradual* withdrawal of systemic corticosteroids should be considered in those subjects whose disease is unlikely to relapse and have

- recently received repeated courses (particularly if taken for longer than 3 weeks),
- taken a short course within 1 year of stopping long-term therapy,
- other possible causes of adrenal suppression,
- received more than 40 mg daily prednisolone (or equivalent) (in adults),
- been given repeat doses in the evening, and
- received more than 3 weeks' treatment.

Systemic corticosteroids may be stopped abruptly in those whose disease is unlikely to relapse *and* who have received treatment for 2 weeks or less *and* who are not included in the patient groups described above.

During corticosteroid withdrawal, the dose may be reduced rapidly down to physiologic doses (equivalent to prednisolone 5 mg daily) and then reduced more slowly. Assessment of the disease may be needed during withdrawal to ensure that relapse does not occur.

REFERENCES

1. Stewart PM. The adrenal cortex. In: Larsen PR, Kronenberg HM, Melmed S, et al., eds. *Williams textbook of endocrinology*, 10th ed. USA: Elsevier Science, 2003:491–551.
2. Miller WL. The adrenal cortex and its disorders. In: Brook CGD, Clayton P, Brown R, eds. *Brook's clinical pediatric endocrinology*, 5th ed. UK: Blackwell Publishing Ltd., 2005:293–351.
3. Simpson ER, Waterman MR. Steroid biosynthesis in the adrenal cortex and its regulation by adrenocorticotropin. In: DeGroote LJ, Besser M, Burger HG, et al., eds. *Endocrinology*, Philadelphia, PA: W.B. Saunders, 1995:1630–1641.
4. Galon J, Franchimont D, Hiroi N, et al. Gene profiling reveals unknown enhancing and suppressive actions of glucocorticoids on immune cells. *FASEB J* 2002;16:61–71.
5. Stocco DM, Clark BJ. Regulation of the acute production of steroids in steroidogenic cells. *Endocr Rev* 1996;17:221–244.
6. Arakane F, Kallen CB, Watari H, et al. The mechanism of action of steroidogenic acute regulatory protein (StAR). StAR acts on the outside of mitochondria to stimulate steroidogenesis. *J Biol Chem* 1998;273:16339–16345.
7. Papadopoulos V. Structure and function of the peripheral-type benzodiazepine receptor in steroidogenic cells. *Proc Soc Exp Biol Med* 1998;217:130–142.
8. Nebert DW, Nelson DR, Coon MJ, et al. The P450 superfamily: update on new sequences, gene mapping, and recommended nomenclature. *DNA Cell Biol* 1991;10:1–14.
9. Cherradi N, Rossier MF, Vallotton MB, et al. Submitochondrial distribution of three key steroidogenic proteins (steroidogenic acute regulatory protein and cytochrome P450 scc and 3β-hydroxysteroid dehydrogenase isomerase enzymes) upon stimulation by intracellular calcium in adrenal glomerulosa cells. *J Biol Chem* 1997;272:7899–7909.
10. White PC, Curnow KM, Pascoe L. Disorders of steroid 11β-hydroxylase isozymes. *Endocr Rev* 1994;15:421–438.
11. Yanase T, Simpson ER, Waterman MR. 17α-hydroxylase/17,20-lyase deficiency: from clinical investigation to molecular definition. *Endocr Rev* 1991;12:91–108.
12. Penning TM. Molecular endocrinology of hydroxysteroid dehydrogenases. *Endocr Rev* 1997;18:281–305.
13. Simpson ER, Mahendroo MS, Means GD, et al. Aromatase cytochrome P450, the enzyme responsible for estrogen biosynthesis. *Endocr Rev* 1994;15:342–355.
14. Wilson JD, Griffin JE, Russell DW. Steroid 5α-reductase 2 deficiency. *Endocr Rev* 1993;14:577–593.
15. Wallace WH, Crowne EC, Shalet SM, et al. Episodic ACTH and cortisol secretion in normal children. *Clin Endocrinol (Oxf)* 1991; 34(3):215–221.
16. Itoi K, Seasholtz AF, Watson SJ. Cellular and extracellular regulatory mechanisms of hypothalamic corticotropin-releasing hormone neurons. *J Endocr* 1998;45:13–33.
17. Habib KE, Gold PW, Chrousos GP. Neuroendocrinology of stress. *Endocrinol Metab Clin North Am* 2001;30(3):695–728.
18. Ehrhart-Bornstein M, Hinson JP, Bornstein SR, et al. Intraadrenal interactions in the regulation of adrenocortical steroidogenesis. *Endocr Rev* 1998;19(2):101–143.
19. Bornstein SR, Chrousos GP. Clinical review 104: adrenocorticotropin (ACTH)- and non-ACTH-mediated regulation of the adrenal cortex: neural and immune inputs. *J Clin Endocrinol Metab* 1999; 84(5):1729–1736.
20. Keller-Wood ME, Dallman M. Corticosteroid inhibition of ACTH secretion. *Endocr Rev* 1984;5:1–24.
21. Reincke M, Beuschlein F, Menig G, et al. Localization and expression of adrenocortocotropic hormone receptor mRNA in normal and neoplastic human adrenal cortex. *J Endocrinol* 1998;156: 415–423.
22. Krieger DT, Allen W, Rizzo F, et al. Characterization of the normal temporal pattern of plasma corticosteroid levels. *J Clin Endocrinol Metab* 1971;32(2):266–284.
23. Esteban NV, Yergey AL. Cortisol production rates measured by liquid chromatography/mass spectrometry. *Steroids* 1990;55(4): 152–158.
24. Brien TG. Human corticosteroid binding globulin. *Clin Endocrinol (Oxf)* 1981;14(2):193–212.
25. Mataradze GD, Kurabekova RM, Rozen VB. The role of sex steroids in the formation of sex-differentiated concentrations of corticosteroid-binding globulin in rats. *J Endocrinol* 1992;132(2): 235–240.
26. Stolk RP, Lamberts SW, de Jong FH, et al. Gender differences in the associations between cortisol and insulin in healthy subjects. *J Endocrinol* 1996;149(2):313–318.
27. Gower DB. Steroid catabolism and urinary excretion. In: Makin HLJ, ed. *Biochemistry of steroid hormones.* Oxford, UK: Blackwell Science Ltd., 1984:349–382.
28. Iyer RB, Binstock JM, Scwartz IS, et al. Human hepatic cortisol reductase activities: enzymatic properties and substrate specificities of cytosolic cortisol Δ4–5β-reductase and dihydrocortisol-3α-oxidoreductase(s). *Steroids.* 1990;55:495–500.
29. Draper N, Stewart PM. 11beta-hydroxysteroid dehydrogenase and the pre-receptor regulation of corticosteroid hormone action. *J Endocrinol* 2005;186(2):251–271.
30. Abel SM, Maggs JL, Back DJ, et al. Cortisol metabolism by human liver *in vitro*—I. Metabolite identification and inter-individual variability. *J Steroid Biochem Mol Biol* 1992;43:713–719.
31. Carson-Jurica MA, Schrader WT, O'Malley BW. Steroid receptor family: structure and functions. *Endocr Rev* 1990;11(2):201–220.

32. Hollenberg SM, Weinberger C, Ong ES, et al. Primary structure and expression of a functional human glucocorticoid receptor cDNA. *Nature* 1985;318(6047):635–641.
33. Picard D, Yamamoto KR. Two signals mediate hormone-dependent nuclear localization of the glucocorticoid receptor. *EMBO J* 1987; 6(11):3333–3340.
34. Hollenberg SM, Evans RM. Multiple and cooperative trans-activation domains of the human glucocorticoid receptor. *Cell* 1988;55(5): 899–906.
35. Dalman FC, Scherrer LC, Taylor LP, et al. Localization of the 90-kDa heat shock protein-binding site within the hormone-binding domain of the glucocorticoid receptor by peptide competition. *J Biol Chem* 1991;266(6):3482–3490.
36. Oakley RH, Sar M, Cidlowski JA. The human glucocorticoid receptor beta isoform. Expression, biochemical properties, and putative function. *J Biol Chem* 1996;271(16):9550–9559.
37. Charmandari E, Chrousos GP, Ichijo T, et al. The human glucocorticoid receptor (hGR) beta isoform suppresses the transcriptional activity of hGRalpha by interfering with formation of active coactivator complexes. *Mol Endocrinol* 2005;19(1):52–64.
38. Bamberger CM, Schulte HM, Chrousos GP. Molecular determinants of glucocorticoid receptor function and tissue sensitivity to glucocorticoids. *Endocr Rev* 1996;17(3):245–261.
39. McKenna NJ, O'Malley BW. Combinatorial control of gene expression by nuclear receptors and coregulators. *Cell* 2002;108(4): 465–474.
40. Auboeuf D, Honig A, Berget SM, et al. Coordinate regulation of transcription and splicing by steroid receptor coregulators. *Science* 2002;298(5592):416–419.
41. Miller TL, Mayo KE. Glucocorticoids regulate pituitary growth hormone-releasing hormone receptor messenger ribonucleic acid expression. *Endocrinology* 1999;138(6):2458–2465.
42. Magiakou MA, Mastorakos G, Chrousos GP. Final stature in patients with endogenous Cushing's syndrome. *J Clin Endocrinol Metab* 1994; 79(4):1082–1085.
43. Magiakou MA, Mastorakos G, Gomez MT, et al. Suppressed spontaneous and stimulated growth hormone secretion in patients with Cushing's disease before and after surgical cure. *J Clin Endocrinol Metab* 1994;78(1):131–137.
44. Allen DB. Growth suppression by glucocorticoid therapy. *Endocrinol Metab Clin North Am* 1996;25(3):699–717.
45. Kaufmann S, Jones KL, Wehrenberg WB, et al. Inhibition by prednisone of growth hormone (GH) response to GH-releasing hormone in normal men. *J Clin Endocrinol Metab* 1988;67(6):1258–1261.
46. Miell JP, Corder R, Pralong FP, et al. Effects of dexamethasone on growth hormone (GH)-releasing hormone, arginine- and dopaminergic stimulated GH secretion, and total plasma insulin-like growth factor-I concentrations in normal male volunteers. *J Clin Endocrinol Metab* 1991;72(3):675–681.
47. Burguera B, Muruais C, Penalva A, et al. Dual and selective actions of glucocorticoids upon basal and stimulated growth hormone release in man. *Neuroendocrinology* 1990;51(1):51–58.
48. Charmandari E, Kino T, Souvatzoglou E, et al. Pediatric stress: hormonal mediators and human development. *Horm Res* 2003; 59(4):161–179.
49. Iannuzzi DM, Ertsey R, Ballard PL. Biphasic glucocorticoid regulation of pulmonary SP-A: characterization of inhibitory process. *Am J Physiol* 1993;264(3, pt 1):L236–L244.
50. Ballard PL, Ertsey R, Gonzales LW, et al. Transcriptional regulation of human pulmonary surfactant proteins SP-B and SP-C by glucocorticoids. *Am J Respir Cell Mol Biol* 1996;14(6):599–607.
51. Cole TJ, Blendy JA, Monaghan AP, et al. Targeted disruption of the glucocorticoid receptor gene blocks adrenergic chromaffin cell development and severely retards lung maturation. *Genes Dev* 1995;9(13):1608–1621.
52. Bronnegard M, Arner P, Hellstrom L, et al. Glucocorticoid receptor messenger ribonucleic acid in different regions of human adipose tissue. *Endocrinology* 1990;127(4):1689–1696.
53. Bujalska IJ, Kumar S, Stewart PM. Does central obesity reflect "Cushing's disease of the omentum"? *Lancet* 1997;349(9060): 1210–1213.
54. Chrousos GP. The hypothalamic-pituitary-adrenal axis and immune-mediated inflammation. *N Engl J Med* 1995;332(20):1351–1362.
55. Boumpas DT, Chrousos GP, Wilder RL, et al. Glucocorticoid therapy for immune-mediated diseases: basic and clinical correlates. *Ann Intern Med* 1993;119(12):1198–1208.
56. DeRijk R, Michelson D, Karp B, et al. Exercise and circadian rhythm-induced variations in plasma cortisol differentially regulate interleukin-1 beta (IL-1 beta), IL-6, and tumor necrosis factor-alpha (TNF alpha) production in humans: high sensitivity of TNF alpha and resistance of IL-6. *J Clin Endocrinol Metab* 1997; 82(7):2182–2191.
57. McEwen BS, De Kloet ER, Rostene W. Adrenal steroid receptors and actions in the nervous system. *Physiol Rev* 1986;66(4):1121–1188.
58. Wordinger RJ, Clark AF. Effects of glucocorticoids on the trabecular meshwork: towards a better understanding of glaucoma. *Prog Retin Eye Res* 1999;18(5):629–667.
59. British Medical Association & The Royal Pharmaceutical Society of Great Britain. *British National Formulary for Children.* 2006:421–430.
60. Kuperman H, Damiani D, Chrousos GP, et al. Evaluation of the hypothalamic-pituitary-adrenal axis in children with leukemia before and after 6 weeks of high-dose glucocorticoid therapy. *J Clin Endocrinol Metab* 2001;86(7):2993–2996.
61. Meduri GU, Tolley EA, Chrousos GP, et al. Prolonged methylprednisolone treatment suppresses systemic inflammation in patients with unresolving acute respiratory distress syndrome: evidence for inadequate endogenous glucocorticoid secretion and inflammation-induced immune cell resistance to glucocorticoids. *Am J Respir Crit Care Med* 2002;165(7):983–991.
62. So LK, Lau AC, Yam LY, et al. Development of a standard treatment protocol for severe acute respiratory syndrome. *Lancet* 2003; 361(9369):1615–1617.
63. British Medical Association & The Royal Pharmaceutical Society of Great Britain. *British National Formulary for Children.* 2006:767.

Tania S. Burgert
Eda Cengiz
William Tamborlane

CHAPTER 52

Insulin and Diabetes Mellitus

Prior to the advent of insulin therapy, the life expectancy of children with type-1 diabetes mellitus (T1DM) was approximately 1 year from diagnosis. Referred to as the "Pissing Evile" in 17th-century England, this disease was known for its agonizing, unremitting progression to emaciation, coma, and death (1). The revolutionary discovery of insulin changed the diagnosis of diabetes from a slowly deteriorating death sentence to a full life of near limitless possibilities. Not surprisingly, the Nobel Prize in medicine was awarded to the discoverers of insulin just 1 year after its successful extraction from beef pancreas in 1922. This insulin preparation, containing numerous impurities and varying potency, was put in use immediately for the treatment of diabetes. Since then insulin has been on the forefront of science becoming one of the best-characterized vertebrate hormones, with a wealth of data on its crystalline structure and mechanism of action at the molecular, cellular, and organ level. The gene for insulin was cloned in 1980 (2), and recombinant insulin has been available commercially since this time. Insulin therapy has recently taken a turn toward the use of insulin analogues instead of native human insulin formulations, and there are continued studies on alternative routes of delivery. Nevertheless, insulin remains one of the few drugs for which a suitable oral formulation has remained elusive.

THE DISCOVERY OF INSULIN

In 1869, a German medical student, Paul Langerhans, described a group of cells embedded within the acinar tissue of the pancreas that were dissimilar in structure to the rest of his histological preparation (1). It took another 30 years for secretory function to be ascribed to these "islets of Langerhans." Once it became apparent that the "internal secretion" of these cells had a glucose-lowering effect, the race was on for its extraction. In 1922, Banting, Best, Collip, and Macleod isolated the glucose-lowering substance from beef pancreas and attempted to treat Leonard Thompson, a severely diabetic teenager (3). After a short initial setback due to impurities of the extract, Leonard Thompson began to respond and continued to take "insulin" for the rest of his life.

TYPE-1 DIABETES MELLITUS

Type-1 diabetes mellitus (T1DM) is characterized by varying degrees of absolute (not relative) insulinopenia due to T-cell mediated autoimmune destruction of the pancreatic β cells. A decline in insulin-secreting capacity for months or years precedes the clinical manifestation of diabetes, which usually occurs once 80% of the β cells have been destroyed. It can present at any age, ranging from infancy to mid-adulthood. The incidence of T1DM has increased worldwide in all age groups (even in the very young) postulated to be due to environmental factors (4). In most countries, the highest incidence is found among children 10 to 14 years old (5) and 3 to 6 years of age. Both sexes are affected in equal parts. In the past, T1DM was thought to occur more frequently in Caucasians. However, newer reports suggest that, in certain regions in the United States, African American children may be affected as frequently as Caucasian children (6). Newly recognized cases are predominantly seen in the autumn and winter months, with many speculations as to the cause of this seasonal and long-term cyclical variation (7–9). Furthermore, the natural regional proclivity for T1DM to the northern hemisphere (such as Finland and Sweden) as opposed to the southern hemisphere (Peru and Venezuela) remains unexplained.

Common symptoms at the time of presentation include 2- to 3-week history of polyuria and polydipsia, weight loss, abdominal pain, anorexia, vomiting, and fatigue reflecting the metabolic effects of insulin deficiency. Especially in young children, a history of abdominal pain and vomiting is often misinterpreted as part of a viral syndrome. Therefore, routine urine testing of glucose and ketones are warranted in any child who presents with these complaints. Although the presence of glucosuria is a good screening tool, the following criteria have been established to confirm the diagnosis: a random serum glucose level of 200 mg per dL or more (11.1 mmol per L) must accompany symptoms suggestive of diabetes. Alternatively, a fasting serum glucose level of 126 mg per dL or more (7 mmol per L) can also establish the diagnosis. Glucosuria alone is not diagnostic of diabetes in children as it often accompanies a variety of renal tubular disorders. Glucosuria (with mild hyperglycemia) may also be stress induced during severe infection or steroid therapy. In these cases, hyperglycemia is transient and remits after convalescence. As soon as the diagnosis of diabetes is established, insulin therapy should be initiated promptly to prevent further metabolic decompensation and the development of diabetic ketoacidosis (DKA). After initiation of insulin therapy, there is a partial recovery of β-cell function. During this so-called honeymoon period, diabetes control is quite good and easy to achieve. The duration of the honeymoon period is variable, lasting from weeks up to 2 years, after which the insulin secretory capacity of the β cell declines permanently.

PHYSIOLOGIC EFFECT OF INSULIN

Although insulin has a profound effect on carbohydrates, it also exerts significant control over lipid, protein, and mineral metabolism. The most pronounced insulin effect is found at its three target tissues: liver, fat, and muscle.

The liver is a key organ in maintaining a steady state of serum glucose levels, tightly controlled by the insulin-to-glucagon ratio in the portal circulation. There is minimal direct insulin effect on the hepatocyte glucose transporter 2 (GLUT2); instead, insulin indirectly promotes glucose uptake into the liver by stimulating enzymes involved in glucose metabolism and storage. In a fasting state, low insulin levels enhance gluconeogenesis from glucose precursors, while the relative glucagon predominance stimulates glycogenolysis. Both of these processes are synergistic in achieving a steady fasting hepatic glucose production rate of 2 mg per kg per minute.

As soon as insulin levels rises postprandially, hepatic glucose production is suppressed and glycogenesis, glycolysis, and free fatty acid synthesis are enhanced. Once the liver is saturated with glycogen, any additional glucose, under the presence of insulin, is shunted to the synthesis of fatty acids. The fatty acids are esterified with α-glycerol phosphate to produce triglycerides, which are then transported as the very low-density lipoprotein (VLDL) fraction to the adipocyte.

In the adipose tissue, insulin enhances the activity of lipoprotein lipase, which is found in the capillary endothelium. Lipoprotein lipase hydrolyzes the triglycerides of the VLDL fraction to fatty acids and monoglycerides. Fatty acids are membrane permeable and can easily enter the adipocyte, where they are re-esterified to triglycerides. Insulin plays a key role in creating these fat stores by directly enhancing glucose uptake into the adipocyte through stimulating glucose transporter 4 (GLUT4), which facilitates glucose entry into the cell (see the "Insulin Receptor" section). Intracellular glucose in the adipocyte increases glycolysis, which increases the production of α-glycerol phosphate needed for fat esterification. Furthermore, insulin inhibits the breakdown of fat through inhibiting hormone-sensitive lipase, which induces lipolysis in the insulin-depleted state.

In the muscle, insulin's main function is to facilitate glucose entry into the cell by binding to the insulin receptor, which then upregulates GLUT4. Once inside the muscle, glucose is used for immediate energy expenditure and for building up muscle glycogen stores. Insulin furthermore has an anabolic effect on the muscle, promoting positive nitrogen balance by enhancing amino-acid (especially branched chain amino acids) uptake, inhibiting protein breakdown, and to a lesser extent promoting protein synthesis. During fasting (low insulin state), glucose is mainly taken up by organs that do not depend on insulin for glucose transport, such as the brain.

Insulin also activates the sodium–potassium adenosine triphosphatase (ATPase) in many cells and therefore enhances potassium flux into the cell, even in the absence of glucose movement or pH changes.

SYNTHESIS OF INSULIN

Insulin synthesis is confined to the pancreatic islet β cells. The β cells make up the bulk of the Langerhans islet and reside in the center of the islet closest to the blood supply. Glucagon-secreting α cells surround the β cells in a circular pattern. The outmost layer of the islet cell is formed by somatostatin- and gastrin-secreting δ cells. Islets containing α, β, and δ cells are mostly found in the anterior lobe, body, and tail of the pancreas. They are connected through gap junctions, a feature that has been proposed in facilitating the paracrine effect of insulin on glucagon and somatostatin. Polypeptide-producing F cells are also found in a portion of islet cells. They are restricted to those islets located in the posterior lobe of the pancreas head and are supplied by a separate vascular system. Even though the Langerhans islets are the most powerful regulators of glucose metabolism, they comprise less than 1% of the pancreatic organ mass. The average person has about 1 million islets varying in size from 50 to 300 μm in diameter.

Insulin originates in the form of a large precursor, preproinsulin, that is synthesized in the ribosome of the β cell's rough endoplasmic reticulum. This 110-amino-acid peptide is encoded by a single gene located on chromosome 11 (10). Microsomal signal peptidases rapidly excise a terminal portion of the peptide chain, leaving 86-amino-acid proinsulin to be transported to the Golgi apparatus. There it is packaged into secretory vesicles, located close to the cell membrane. The 21 amino acids adjacent to the COOH terminus of the insulin protein are referred to as the α chain. The α chain is joined via a dipeptide bond to the 31-amino-acid c (connecting) peptide. Another dipeptide link connects the c-peptide chain further to the 30 amino acids of the β chain leading up to the protein's NH_2 terminus. The tertiary structure of insulin is created by the folding and oxidation of the proinsulin in which two disulfide bridges are created between the α and β chain and another disulfide bridge within the α chain. In the secretory granules, c-peptide is split off from proinsulin, resulting in equimolar release of insulin and c-peptide. The insulin secretion process involves fusion of the cell membrane and secretory granules with subsequent exocytosis of not only insulin and c-peptide but also small amounts of proinsulin. Although c-peptide has no insulin-like effect, proinsulin has about 7% to 8% of the biological activity of insulin (11). Unlike most protein hormones, the insulin structure is highly conserved among the species. Porcine insulin differs from human insulin only by one amino acid in the β chain and bovine insulin by three amino-acid residues.

INSULIN SECRETION

Although glucose is the strongest stimulator of insulin secretion, other sugars (e.g., mannose), certain amino acids (e.g., arginine, leucine), other hormones and neurotransmitters, and vagal nerve stimulation also modulate insulin secretion, keeping glucose concentrations in a narrow range.

In the rodent, glucose is transported into the β cell by a high-capacity (GLUT2) glucose transporter (12). GLUT2 is also the predominant glucose transporter in human pancreas and liver and is capable of bidirectional transport, allowing transport in either direction depending on the glucose concentration on each side of the membrane. Other GLUT isoforms (GLUT1 or GLUT3) that are ubiquitously present in most cells may also contribute to basal transport activity into the pancreas.

After uptake into the islet cell, glucose is phosphorylated to glucose-6-phosphate by glucokinase, the rate-limiting step of glucose metabolism in the islet cell (13). Glucokinase serves as the islets' "glucose sensor" and its activity is tightly linked to glucose levels. Mutations in the glucokinase gene have been associated with defects in glucose sensing, necessitating higher glucose levels to stimulate insulin secretion. This defect is clinically referred to as MODY 2 (maturity onset diabetes of youth, form 2) leading to mild hyperglycemia (14,15).

Intracellular glucose metabolism raises ATP levels, which in turn close the potassium-dependent (K-) ATP channels in the β-cell membrane. The subsequent suppression of potassium (K) efflux leads to a progressive depolarization of the plasma membrane and the firing of action potentials. A drop in voltage follows, opening the voltage-sensitive L-type calcium channels for an influx of calcium ions (16). The rise of cytoplasmic calcium concentrations leads to a series of poorly defined reactions that culminate in the extrusion of insulin granules.

Each β cell contains thousands of K-ATP channels, which in fasting conditions are open, clamping the cell membrane potential at −70 mV. Sulphonylureas are hypoglycemic agents that are now known to modulate the K-ATP channel by attaching to a specific 145-kDa channel subunit named SUR (17). Sulphonylureas attach to the receptor and inhibit the K-ATP channel. The subsequent cascade of membrane depolarization and calcium influx then leads to an insulin secretory effect that is independent of serum glucose levels. Loss of function mutations in the gene encoding the β-cell potassium channel result in persistent hyperinsulinemic hypoglycemia of infancy (18,19). Gain of function mutations of the same gene results in certain types neonatal diabetes mellitus that can respond to sulphonylureas, and some patients can be taken off insulin (20–22).

Insulin is secreted directly into the portal vein and is immediately degraded by liver insulinases to approximately half of its original concentration. In serum, insulin levels rise to maximum levels 30 to 45 minutes after food ingestion and decline to basal levels by 2 to 3 hours postprandial. During prolonged fasting, both glucose and insulin levels will drop even further, but insulin levels will remain measurable between 2 and 5 μU per mL.

INSULIN RECEPTOR

Insulin action is mediated by the insulin receptor, a transmembrane glycoprotein present in virtually all vertebrates. Under healthy conditions, only a small proportion of the total available cell receptors are occupied to achieve maximal biological effect. High ambient insulin levels downregulate the insulin receptor by reducing the number of available insulin receptors. Furthermore, saturation of the receptor with insulin leads to "negative cooperativity," a term used for reduced affinity for insulin in the adjacent receptor. The human insulin receptor was cloned in 1985 (23), and the gene maps to the short arm of chromosome 19 (24).

The structural components of the receptor are two extracellular α subunits that are linked to each other as well as to the two β subunits by disulfide bonds, forming a heterodimer. The α subunits are external to the cell membrane and contain the hormone-binding sites. The transmembrane-spanning β subunit has three domains: extracellular, transmembrane, and cytosolic. The cytosolic domain contains tyrosine protein kinase activity. The binding of insulin at the extracellular α subunit is transduced to the intracellular β subunits, leading to rapid onset of receptor autophosphorylation (25). Among the proteins phosphorylated are the insulin receptor substrates 1–3 (IRS-1–3). IRS-1 acts as a docking protein for other proteins such as phosphatidylinositol 3 (PI3)-kinase. The cellular products created by PI3-kinase in turn appear to activate the translocation of glucose transport proteins (GLUT4) to the cell surface, facilitating glucose uptake. GLUT4 is available in the cytoplasm of all cells that have insulin-sensitive glucose transport across the cell membrane. Once insulin binds to the receptor, GLUT4 migrates to the cell surface, allowing the cell to efficiently take up glucose.

After binding to the receptor, the receptor-insulin complex is internalized and processed to release of free insulin and recycling of the receptor back to the cell membrane. Whether the internalization of insulin permits any special action of insulin at the level of the nucleus remains a speculation, and insulin action beyond receptor activation is incompletely defined.

INSULIN SIGNALING

Insulin's binding to it's receptor stimulates signal transduction pathway that culminate in GLUT4 translocation to the plasma membrane. GLUT4 is responsible for glucose uptake in all cells whose glucose transport across the cell membrane is insulin dependent. Once insulin binds to the receptor, two distinct intracellular signal transduction pathways lead to a migration of GLUT4 to the cell surface, allowing the cell to efficiently take up glucose.

The first pathway is often referred to as the IRS/phosphatidylinositol 3-kinase (PI3 K)/Akt pathway (26,27). In this pathway, IRS-1 is tyrosine phosphorylated by the insulin-stimulated tyrosine kinase activity of the insulin receptor. This allows the regulatory unit (p85) of PI3 K to dock onto the IRS-1 which in turn activates PI3 K. This leads to a generation of phosphatidylinositol 3,4,5-triphosphate (PIP3) which in turn activates the Ser/Thr kinases Akt and atypical protein kinase C (aPKC). These kinases are essential in the process of GLUT4 translocation to the cell surface, facilitating glucose uptake. The second pathway is also referred to as the Cbl–CAP pathway (28,29). Under the presence of the adapter protein CAP, the Cbl proto-oncoprotein is tyrosine phosphorylated (28). The CAP–Cbl complex then dissociates from the insulin receptor and move to a lipid raft subdomain of the plasma membrane for a second route of GLUT4 translocation (30).

INSULIN TREATMENT

Although normoglycemia is a fairly concise treatment goal in diabetes management, the clinical use of insulin is remarkably complex. With so many nutritional, hormonal, and lifestyle variables affecting glucose homeostasis, there is rarely a predictable treatment algorithm that applies to all patients, especially in children and adolescents with T1DM. Even in a single patient, treatment regiments remain under constant scrutiny warranting regular reassessments and fine-tuning. Therefore, insulin regimens are never absolute, but loose guidelines that mold with the patient throughout life.

In general, insulin requirements in a patient with newly diagnosed type-1 diabetes are calculated based on the age, pubertal status, and the presence of ketonuria. Young children (toddlers) who do not present with ketoacidosis may only require 0.3 units per kg per day. The average prepubertal child will require 0.5 to 0.75 units per kg per day, possibly more in the presence of ketosis. Pubertal children will be more insulin resistant due to their higher physiologic levels of growth hormone and usually require 1 to 1.5 units per kg per day. Within 1 to 3 weeks of commencing therapy, insulin requirements usually decrease drastically as partial remission (honeymoon period) occurs. To maximize the duration of remission, it is recommended that a twice-daily insulin regimen is maintained (even at a low dose of 0.2 units per kg per day), as long as episodes of hypoglycemia do not ensue.

ANIMAL AND HUMAN INSULIN PREPARATIONS

Today pure animal insulins are obsolete in the management of diabetes mellitus. However, the different animal preparations with their various pharmacodynamics have become the prototype after which synthetic human insulins are modeled. They are therefore of exemplifying interest.

Shortly after the discovery of insulin, pork and beef insulin products became the treatment of choice for several decades. Early on in the commercial production, trace quantities of zinc were added to produce "regular" insulin, a more stable (crystalline zinc) insulin (31). The duration of this regular insulin was on average 5 to 8 hours, often too short for overnight glucose control. Protamine, a basic fish (trout) protein, was added to slow down the absorption from the subcutis by decreasing the solubility at physiologic pH (32). Combining both zinc and protamine further extended absorption time, leading to insulin action in excess of 24 hours (33). In 1946, the Hagedorn Laboratories produced a protamine zinc insulin in which protamine was added in stoichiometric proportions to insulin, thereby reducing excess free protamine in solution. Hagedorn coined the name "isophane" (Greek: equal appearance) for the long-acting insulin, but the name did not stick and it became known as NPH (neutral protamine Hagedorn) insulin. Another method to prolongate insulin action without adding a protein was the creation of a zinc–insulin complex in the presence of large amounts of zinc and acetate buffer. Under careful pH adjustments, this insulin could be produced in a completely crystalline form (ultralente) or as an amorphous precipitate (semilente). The combination of these two zinc-acetate insulins (70% ultralente and 30% semilente) created lente insulin, with a similar duration to NPH. One of the major limitations of these animal insulins was their immunogenic potential, stemming from contamination with pancreatic extract impurities, such as animal c-peptide, proinsulin, glucagon, somatostatin, and pancreatic polypeptide (34). The foreign amino-acid sequence itself was also proposed to contribute to immunogenicity, leading to insulin resistance (35). To avoid the effect of a foreign protein sequence, a semisynthetic insulin was developed in which the human amino-acid sequence was created by switching out the differentiating amino acid in porcine insulin (36). To date, this is the only porcine-based insulin still available commercially.

With the advent of recombinant DNA technology, semisynthetic human insulins were soon joined by the production of completely synthetic human insulin in the 1980s. The initial process entailed separate production of the α and β chains from *Escherichia coli* with biochemical combination of the two chains to yield an intact molecule (37). In 1986, human insulin could be produced in its entirety from synthetic proinsulin. This method includes the insertion of a synthetic proinsulin into the genome of baker's yeast with subsequent enzymatic yield of human insulin and c-peptide. This technique allows for natural posttranslational folding of the peptide and ensures the appropriate three-dimensional structure of the molecule (38,39).

Human insulins are also marketed as regular (short acting), NPH and lente (intermediate acting), and ultralente (long acting) with identical formulations as their animal counterparts in respect to content of auxiliary substances. They have very similar biological potency to animal insulin when given intravenously (40,41). However, subcutaneous administration of intermediate- or long-acting human insulin has a shorter time-action profile than animal insulin.

INSULIN REGIMENS

The most common initial insulin regimen after diagnosis is a twice-daily injection of a mixture of human intermediate-acting (NPH) or long-acting (detemir, glargine) insulin and short-acting insulin (regular insulin) or rapid-acting insulin (insulin lispro, insulin aspart, insulin glulisine). In general, when patients are on a NPH or detemir insulin with a rapid-acting insulin regimen, two-third of the total dose is given before breakfast and one-third before dinner. The prebreakfast and predinner doses are composed of two-third intermediate-acting insulin and one-third short-acting insulin and given as a single (mixed) injection. Glargine is considered a 24-hour insulin, with some exceptions; therefore, patients receive a once a day injection of glargine with rapid-acting insulin injection for each meal.

The two-daily insulin injection regimen could be sufficient during the honeymoon period due to the fact that the endogenous insulin secretion provides much of the overnight basal insulin requirements, leading to normal fasting blood glucose values. Thus, increased and more labile prebreakfast glucose levels herald the loss of residual β-cell function often necessitating a third injection. To contain rising morning blood glucose values, the predinner dose can be separated into an injection of short-acting insulin before dinner and long-acting insulin before bedtime, thereby delaying peak action to the early morning hours. Although theoretically sound, the challenge remains to achieve normoglycemia in the morning, while avoiding nocturnal hypoglycemia during the nighttime fast. The physiologic basis for this battle with morning hyperglycemia is the dawn phenomenon, an early morning surge of counter-regulatory hormones, mainly growth hormone and cortisol. Dawn phenomenon must be differentiated from rebound hyperglycemia (Somogyi effect) that results from a counter-regulatory hormone rise in response to an untoward nocturnal hypoglycemia. Most diabetes care providers have no hesitations switching to a variety of three-injection regimens, trying to match varying peak actions with the lifestyle of the patient and his or her family. Prefilled, disposable pen devices of one type of insulin have made it easier for patients to accept split dose regimens or extra injections before lunch or before an afternoon snack. Various jet (transcutaneous pressure) injectors have also become available commercially over the last decade. Theoretically, they are indicated for children with needle phobia and are deemed to have the therapeutic advantage of increased accuracy and better subcutaneous dispersion with subsequent faster absorption. Because they are cumbersome to use and often traumatize the skin (causing greater discomfort), they have not penetrated the pediatric market very well. Disposable insulin pens with ultrafine short needles are by far the more popular alternative for a single insulin injection.

To gain better control, a third type of insulin, such as ultralente, was sometimes added to the morning or evening injection mixture to cover for waning NPH levels in the late afternoon and early morning. However, with the recent advent of the 24-hour peakless insulin glargine analogue, such regimens became a managing style of the past. Insulin glargine has a flatter and longer time-activity profile than NPH or ultralente and therefore more closely mimics the basal insulin activity of the pancreas. The only disadvantage of insulin glargine in multiple injection regimens is that it cannot be mixed with other insulins, requiring a separate injection. Unlike other long-acting insulins that are cloudy in appearance, insulin glargine is clear like the short-acting insulins. There is concern that it would be easy to confuse the two types of insulin, leading to significant dosing and administration errors. However, the fact that insulin glargine is fully suspended in solution may decrease technical errors, as it does not require resuspension prior to administration. Disposable pens with premixed-intermediate (NPH) and short-acting (insulin lispro or regular) insulin are also available, but they are rigid in their composition and allow little flexibility in fine-tuning glycemic control. They are usually used in patients whose compliance with insulin administration is at stake and the simplest dosing regimen is maintained to avoid DKA. Sometimes, these premixed preparations are indicated if it is an impossible feat for the patient or caregiver to mix insulin, resulting in major dosing errors.

When interpreting blood glucose readings, a number of factors that affect injection therapy must be considered prior to making an actual insulin dose adjustment. First and foremost, compliance and administration technique must be considered. From a psychosocial aspect, children and adolescents will often painstakingly cover up missed injections. A review of skills is equally important in uncovering technical slips, which can lead to poor glycemic control. For example, the long-acting insulins such as lente and NPH need to be resuspended prior to injection for concentration constancy between injections. Omitting this crucial step leads to great variability in glycemic control. Furthermore, the presence of hypertrophied injection sites, which results from local growth factor effect of repeated insulin injections into the same site, can slow down or decrease absorption. The site location is another factor that comes into the equation when fine-tuning insulin regimens. Insulin is absorbed most rapidly from the subcutaneous abdomen and less rapidly from the arms. Absorption is most delayed from the subcutaneous tissue in the legs. The depth of injection, the ambient temperature or the state of perfusion at the injection site can also affect absorption.

An alternative to multiple-daily injection that has revolutionized diabetes management is continuous subcutaneous insulin infusion (CSII) therapy, also referred to as insulin pump therapy. For many families, this is the preferred choice for achieving the goals of intensive therapy with increased lifestyle flexibility.

INSULIN ANALOGUES

Insulin analogues are modified human insulin molecules with altered pharmacodynamic and physicochemical properties. Using molecular technology, they were specifically designed to create a molecule to mimic endogenous insulin action. Despite the challenges with subcutaneous absorption particularly for rapid insulin analogues, both rapid- and long-acting new insulin analogues have made achieving target glycemic control with less hypoglycemia a possibility.

RAPID INSULIN ANALOGUES

New rapid insulin analogues (lispro, aspart, glulisine) reduced postprandial glucose excursions as compared to regular insulin with their earlier absorption and action profiles. The convenience of taking the injection 15 minutes before or even with the meal as opposed to 30 to 40 minutes prior to the meal also led to better compliance with therapy. Faster onset of action, earlier peak activity, and higher peak concentrations of rapid-acting analogues are particularly beneficial in overcoming problems associated with insulin resistance of puberty.

The first insulin analogue in this group did not quite make it to clinical use because of one important side effect. Asp (B10) insulin was engineered by replacing the naturally occurring histidine with aspartic acid on residue 10 of the insulin β chain and was found to be absorbed twice as fast as regular insulin (42). However, this simple amino-acid exchange altered the three-dimensional structure of insulin, leading to increased affinity of this molecule to the structurally related insulin-like growth factor (IGF)-1 receptor. Furthermore, Asp (B10) insulin demonstrated extended activation of the insulin receptor with decreased dissociation and prolonged stimulation of cellular processing (43,44). This mitogenic risk was confirmed in Sprague-Dawley rats that developed mammary tumors after supraphysiologic doses of this analogue. Further human application of this analogue has since then been halted.

In 1996, the first rapid-acting insulin analogue, insulin lispro, was FDA approved for clinical use. Insulin lispro received its name from its chemical structure in which the amino-acid lysine at position 29 of the β chain was exchanged with the position 28 proline of the same chain. This amino-acid reversal decreases the tendency to self-associate, leading to faster absorption, higher peak levels, and shorter duration of action (45). Studies comparing regular insulin and insulin lispro demonstrated no difference in affinity to the insulin receptor. There is a higher affinity to the IGF-1 receptor, but this did not cause a difference in growth-stimulating activity when compared to regular insulin (46). Clinical trials have demonstrated that insulin lispro acts within 15 minutes, peaks at approximately 1 hour, and lasts 2 to 4 hours after subcutaneous injection (45,47). Insulin lispro is stable in CSII systems and has been shown to improve postprandial glucose levels when CSII therapy was compared using regular human insulin (48–50). There is no difference in the frequency of catheter occlusion or other site-related problems with insulin lispro as compared to buffered regular insulin (49,50). However, there were recent reports of a few patients who developed marked lipoatrophy while using insulin lispro during CSII (51,52). The basis of this lipoatrophy is unclear but was resolved with use of regular human insulin. In the past, lipoatrophy was seen with the use of less purified insulins and was assumed to have an immunologic basis. Contrasting are the reports of similar immunogenicity between insulin lispro and recombinant human regular insulin (53). Also, insulin lispro has been a successful substitute for human regular insulin in several cases of presumed immunogenic insulin resistance (54,55). A concern for the use of insulin lispro (or any other rapid-acting insulin) in CSII is its short duration of action, possibly increasing the risk of DKA in cases of mechanical malfunction or catheter occlusion (56).

Another synthetic insulin analogue, insulin aspart, was approved for clinical use in the United States in June 2000. In this molecule, proline at position 28 of the β chain is substituted with negatively charged aspartic acid to reduce self-association and therefore increase rate of absorption (57). Preclinical studies have shown that the insulin aspart has the same insulin receptor and IGF-1 receptor interaction kinetics as human insulin, diminishing concerns about the mitogenic potential of insulin aspart. Similar to insulin lispro insulin, insulin aspart was conceptualized as a mealtime insulin. It is absorbed more rapidly than human regular insulin, reaches higher maximal concentrations postprandially, and has a shorter duration of action (57–59). In a multicenter study, the risk of postprandial hypoglycemia requiring third-party intervention was reduced significantly without leading to deterioration of late postprandial blood glucose levels when insulin aspart was compared to regular insulin (60).

The most recent addition to the rapid-acting insulin analogue group is insulin glulisine. It has similar pharmacokinetic, pharmacodynamic, and safety profile as compared to other rapid-acting insulin analogues. The neutral asparagine is exchanged for basic lysine at position 3 and acidic glutamic exchanged for basic lysine at position 29 as compared to human insulin β chain leading to improved solubility (61). Glulisine is formulated without the addition of zinc. It also has a different effect on activation of IRS1 and IRS2 with decreased activation of IRS1 shown by animal studies suggesting favorable effects on decreasing apoptosis (62,63). It does not appear to accumulate in patients with renal impairment (64). Insulin glulisine is comparable to other rapid-acting analogues with respect to glycemic control, and its somewhat faster absorption rate has questionable clinical significance (65). Postmeal administration of glulisine was associated with a slight reduction of weight (−0.3 kg) while premeal administration was associated with minor weight gain (+0.3 kg) (62).

After the introduction of insulin, patients experienced cutaneous reactions directly related to insulin. These immunologic reactions and skin alterations were stemming from foreign proteins from animal insulins acting as allergens. Later on, preservatives such as metacresol or agents to prolong action such as zinc protamine were reported to be the culprit of these reaction. Prevalence of hypersensitivity reactions substantially declined from 50% to 60% (66,67). Insulin therapy related lipodystrophies are still not obsolete. This group encompasses lipohypertrophy and lipoatrophy. Lipohypertrophy is a result of the insulin anabolic effect, promoting adipose tissue differentiation and growth (68). Lipoatrophy is a relatively uncommon allergic reaction mainly due to the impure insulin molecule. Fat atrophy is the result of lysosomal enzyme activity triggered by an immune-mediated inflammation (69). Lipoatrophy is not merely a cosmetic issue since the absorption of insulin from these sites is erratic (70). Local steroid injections, alternative methods of insulin delivery have been proposed for the management of lipoatrophic sites and achieved some success (71–73).

In most diabetes centers, both insulin lispro, insulin aspart, and insulin glulisine are used interchangeably when it comes to selecting a short/rapid-acting insulin for either CSII or as part of multiple-daily injection regimens. Concerns common to all new drugs hold true for these analogues as well, including lack of long-term safety profile data and the uncertainty about later in life manifestations of potential teratogenicity in humans. However, open label randomized, multicenter studies in pregnant women with T1DM found insulin lispro (74) and insulin aspart (75) to be safe for mother and offspring. Congenital abnormalities do not appear to be more frequent with either lispro or aspart use during pregnancy.

LONG-ACTING ANALOGUES

At the other end of the pharmacodynamic spectrum, insulin analogues are being developed to retard and stabilize the absorption kinetics profile to create prolonged and peakless activity. One of the first analogues developed synthetically to prolong absorption was Novosol Basal insulin. Although intraindividual variability was improved, interindividual variability remained high (76). This insulin also demonstrated poor bioavailability, necessitating very high doses. Novosol Basal was subsequently withdrawn from further studies. Ultralente and NPH fell short of the ideal basal insulin desired properties of low and constant plasma insulin levels in between meals and overnight without pronounced peak effects. This led to the investigation of new basal insulin preparations that replicate the endogenous insulin physiology.

In the spring of 2000, the FDA approved the use of insulin glargine (HOE 901), a long-acting insulin analogue for use in patients with type-1 and type-2 diabetes mellitus. The analogue resulted from the elongation of the β chain at position 30 by two arginine residues as well as by substitution of asparagine at the 21 position of the α chain with glycine. The elongation of the β chain raises the isoelectric point of the molecule from a pH of 5.4 to 6.7, increasing its solubility at acid pH and decreasing its solubility at neutral pH. Insulin glargine is therefore a stable solute in acid formulation, making it the first soluble long-acting insulin. When insulin glargine is injected into the subcutaneous tissue (neutral pH), it will precipitate, slowing and stabilizing the absorption for a peakless insulin effect (77). To enhance stabilization, the current commercial preparation of insulin glargine contains 30 mg per L of zinc, since higher concentrations of zinc did not have any added benefit (78). Insulin glargine was initially reported to have a flat profile (79); however, more recent studies demonstrate a gentle rise in effect with an unpronounced peak at 6 hours (80,81). Despite the twice-a-day use of glargine for some patients, not much of a benefit has been shown with this regimen as compared with the single day injection as basal insulin (82). Preclinical studies on insulin receptor binding and promotion of mitogenesis through "overstimulated" phosphorylation (as seen with Asp (B10) insulin) found that insulin glargine behaved like regular human insulin with respect to receptor binding, autophosphorylation, and phosphorylation of signaling elements (83). In cardiac myocytes, there was no difference in IGF-1 receptor-mediated growth-promoting activity of insulin glargine as compared with native human insulin; however, there was a higher affinity of insulin glargine to the IGF-1 receptor (84). A recent comparison of all insulin analogues confirmed a significantly greater affinity of insulin glargine for the IGF-1 receptor than human insulin (85). To date, it is unclear whether these findings carry some unrecognized safety implications. Most studies so far have not evidenced increased tumor development with insulin glargine, and its metabolic characteristics resemble human insulin more closely than the oncogenic Asp (B10) insulin (86). The major clinical benefit of a peakless basal insulin, especially for pediatric use, is the potential reduction of nocturnal hypoglycemia. In an adult study comparing nighttime hypoglycemia between NPH and insulin glargine, the frequency of hypoglycemia was reduced by 22% in the group using insulin glargine (87). A similar study comparing glycemic control between the use of insulin glargine and NPH in children and adolescents found that overall fasting blood glucose levels were significantly lower, while there was a trend toward fewer episodes of severe nocturnal hypoglycemia (88).

Newest insulin in this category, insulin detemir, was created by attaching a myristic acid to B-29 and removing threonine from B-30 of regular insulin molecule (89). This molecular change enhances albumin binding once it is injected subcutaneously leading to a slow absorption from the site and prolongation of insulin action in the circulation. Its biological duration of action is dose dependent lasting between 12 and 24 hours (81,90). It has less of a peak glucose lowering effect, which occurs later than seen in NPH insulin (91,92). It has less intrasubject insulin absorption variability, better reproducibility, and less frequent episodes of hypoglycemia as compared with NPH (93). So far, in vitro safety profiles of insulin detemir have been favorable, mostly because of its lower affinity to the IGF-1 receptor as compared with human insulin and glargine insulin (85). Furthermore, no clinically significant drug binding interference of insulin detemir albumin with other albumin binding drugs has been noted on in vitro analysis (94). Insulin detemir acts in the brain as well as in the peripheral tissue, which might lead to appetite suppression that can explain some of the reduced weight gain observed during treatment with detemir (95). A recent study comparing weight gain for patients on detemir versus glargine reported somewhat greater weight gain with the glargine group without any statistical significance (90).

The quest for new insulin analogues continues with new formulations and the methods of administration underway. VIAject is a new formulation of regular insulin with hexamers stabilized by two zinc atoms. Its absorption from the subcutaneous tissue is faster than the current rapid-acting analogues due to its favoring of the monomeric form (96). VIAject is not FDA approved yet, but phase III clinical studies showed a reduction of postprandial hyperglycemia with VIAject for patients with T1D as compared with Humulin R (96). Intradermal injection of rapid analogues by a microneedle delivery system to improve the absorption of insulin from the subcutaneous area is also being studied.

INHALED INSULIN

The concept of delivery of insulin by pulmonary route dates back to 1920s (65,97). Availability of insulin with an inhaled effective particle size of 1 to 3 μmol per L allowed it to deposit in the deep lung and be transported to the alveolar capillary (65). There are two major formulations available, aerosolized and dry powered insulin (DPI). DPI is more stable at room temperature, has less susceptibility of microbial growth, and can deliver larger doses with each inhalation (65). The bioavailability of inhaled insulin formulation is lower than that of injected forms. Thus, higher doses of inhaled insulin (approximately eight times the subcutaneous dose) are needed to achieve the same glycemic control. Inhaled insulin does not eliminate the need for basal insulin for patients with type-1 diabetes since it has a short duration of action (65).

Issues with inhaled insulin are variations in absorption, rigidity of dosing (especially for pediatric patients), effect on respiratory tract infections and smoking, long-term effects to the lungs, and possible development of anti-insulin antibodies.

There were four inhaled insulin preparations that have been developed and studied. Exubera is the only FDA-approved inhaled insulin so far; however, it was recently removed from the market due to financial issues. The development of three other inhaled insulin preparations were also halted leaving only one preparation under active investigation. This inhaled insulin formulation is a DPI entrapped with a 2 μm organic particle called Technosphere, and the manufacturing company is pursuing an FDA approval.

CONTINUOUS SUBCUTANEOUS INSULIN INFUSION

Continuous subcutaneous insulin infusion (CSII) was introduced more than 30 years ago, as a means to more closely simulate normal plasma insulin profiles than could be achieved by conventional injection regimens (98). The initial devices (insulin pumps) were cumbersome to use and there was uncertainty about the long-term benefits of intensive treatment. The results of the Diabetes Control and Complications Trial (DCCT) indicating that the long-term benefits of strict diabetes control outweigh the risks of severe hypoglycemia (99,100). As a result, intensive diabetes management has become the gold standard and insulin pump therapy is promoted by expert diabetes care providers. Meta-analysis of randomized pediatric trials comparing CSII to MDI demonstrated a significant reduction in HbA_{1c} with CSII use, but they failed to show any statistically significant difference in HbA_{1c} when compared with MDI therapy (101). There is also current data suggesting that patients with poor initial HbA_{1c} demonstrate better glycemic control when they switch from MDI to CSII therapy (102,103). The recent strides in portable computer technology have facilitated insulin pump use and increased their appeal to a wider group of patients. The vast majority of subjects enrolled in these studies chose to continue on CSII therapy even after the completion of the trials (101). Furthermore, adolescents on CSII therapy has been shown to cope better with the psychosocial aspects of having diabetes (104).

The insulin pump is composed of an insulin reservoir that is attached to a programmable beeper-like device. Since the advent of rapid-acting insulin analogues, they have become the preferred insulin used in CSII. Plastic tubing connects the insulin reservoir to a catheter that is inserted subcutaneously into either the abdomen or hip. A relatively new insulin pump, "Pod Pump," has a slightly different structure with the controlling unit similar to a palm pilot device and has direct connection to the subcutaneous tissue through a catheter without any tubing. Newer insulin pump designs such as the "Patch Pump" are also in the works and will be commercially available in the coming years.

The pump is programmed to deliver a continuous "basal rate" of rapid-acting insulin throughout the day. Basal rates can be programmed to change each hour of the day, but it is unusual to need more than six basal rates throughout the day. Variations in basal rate can be particularly beneficial overnight, since basal rates can be programmed to decrease in the early part of the night to prevent hypoglycemia and increased in the hours before dawn to keep glucose from rising. During the day, the patient "dials up" a rapid-acting insulin bolus in accordance with the carbohydrate content of the meal. This allows more flexibility with the quantity and content of food intake. The continuous basal rate eliminates the need for the use of intermediate- or long-acting insulins, and therefore meal planning does not have to center around peaking insulin action, as recommended with conventional insulin therapy.

Some of the limitations of CSII are possible encumbrance during intense exercise or contact sports. Since only rapid-acting insulin is used, any interruption in flow (catheter occlusion or disconnection) can lead to rapid deterioration of metabolic control, especially during sleeping hours. In addition, local infections at the site of catheter insertion can occur, especially if improper hygienic technique is employed or site changes are delayed. Local infection can interfere significantly with glycemic control during CSII.

New improvement in pump therapy led to advanced pump features including multiple programmable basal/bolus rates and correction factors (sensitivity factor), ability to adjust basal and bolus doses in small increments, and bolus history function to assess missing bolus doses of insulin.

Recent guidelines by Lawson Wilkins Pediatric Diabetes define clinical indications for when to consider pump therapy for children as follows: patients with recurrent severe hypoglycemia, wide fluctuations in blood glucose levels regardless of HbA_{1c}, suboptimal glycemic control with above target HbA_{1c} levels, microvascular complications and/or risk factors for macrovascular complications, or insulin regimen that compromises lifestyle despite good glycemic control (105,106). Fulfillment of one or more criteria is considered as a possible indication for initiating pump therapy provided that candidates have adequate understanding of this therapeutic tool. Same guidelines identify young children (especially infants and neonates), adolescents with eating disorders, children and adolescents with pronounced Dawn phenomenon or with needle phobia, pregnancy adolescents, ketosis-prone individuals, and competitive athletes as patient populations that might benefit from insulin pump use (105,106).

MONITORING OF GLYCEMIC CONTROL

Self-monitoring of blood glucose is central to the management of diabetes. It provides instant feedback, enabling the patient to assume immediate intervention if necessary. Furthermore, the trend analysis of daily blood glucose values over the course of a few days supplies the diabetes care provider with crucial information when readjusting insulin regiments or contemplating therapeutic strategies. The newer glucose meters are very portable and require only a tiny drop of blood. Most have computerized memories to facilitate record keeping.

Recent advances in technology introduced the possibility of monitoring glucose continuously with the availability of glucose sensors that measure interstitial glucose. Commercially available Continuous Glucose Monitor (CGM) technology emerged over the last 8 years. The first one in the market was the Medtronic Continuous Glucose Monitoring System (CGMS), which stored glucose readings every 5 minutes up to 3 days. The blood glucose values were available only after downloading the sensor without the convenience of real-time values. Guardian Medtronic CGM, as the next CGM manufactured by Medtronics, had real-time alarm for hypoglycemia without actual real-time glucose values as an added feature. GlucoWatch G2 Biographer was the first CGM with real-time glucose values. Inaccurate readings, false alarms, and local irritation on the insertion site with lack of improvement in glycemic control and hypoglycemic episodes destined GlucoWatch to become a part of CGM history rather than a popular device in use (107).

Both the new generation and old generation CGM measure interstitial fluid glucose, however, with different methods. Many of the new generation glucose sensors use needle-type catheter inserted in the subcutaneous area and has glucose oxidase at the tip. The electrochemical reaction produces an electric current directly proportional to the ambient glucose concentration that is read by the sensor and transmitted by wireless radio frequency telemetry to the receiver. Interference with glucose readings by the sensor can occur with certain substances. Glutathione, ascorbic acid, uric acid, paracetamol, isoniazid, and salicylate may become cooxidized at the sensor and lead to overestimation of glucose levels (96,108). Recent advances in the sensor technology were reported to overcome this problem (109,110).

Current CGM devices in use consist of three off-the-shelf FDA-approved brands. Minimed Paradigm and Guardian are FDA approved for children 7 to 17 years of age and adults (18 and above). They have 0.5-in., 23-gauge sensor probe with an actual sensor size of a nickel. Transmitter is $1.4 \times 1.1 \times 0.3$ in. They both display glucose values between 40 and 400 mg per dL every 5 minutes with directional trends of the last 1, 3, or 12 hours and with rate of change illustrated by arrows. Startup initialization is 2 hours. Both sensors require first calibration 2 hours after insertion and then 6 hours after the first one with consequent calibrations every 12 hours. The uniqueness of Paradigm among all other sensors is the ability to incorporate glucose data with the insulin pump (Paradigm REAL-Time 522 or 722) without the need of a separate monitor. Guardian, on the other hand, has predictive alerts that could be set to alarm 5, 10, 15, 20, 25, or 30 minutes before glucose limits have been reached or rate of change alerts when glucose levels are changing between 1.1 and 5 mg per dL per minute, in 0.1 increments. Customizable high and low alarm feature is available in both. Sensors can be worn for 3 days. Transmitter can store up to 40 minute of missed data. The sensor and pump data could be uploaded and retrospectively reviewed from a Web-based data management system.

The Dexcom STS is FDA approved for adults aged 18 years and older. It has a 13-mm, 26-gauge sensor probe and has a size of $1.5 \times 9 \times 4$ in. It displays glucose values between 40 and 400 mg per dL range every 5 minutes. Startup initialization is 2 hours and requires 2 calibrations within 30 minutes for the first calibration. Consequent calibrations are every 12 hours. It can display 1, 3, or 9 hours directional glucose trends without rate of change feature. It does not have predictive alerts but has programmable alarms for hypo- (set) and hyperglycemia (adjustable). It can be worn for 7 days. There is no transmitter memory. Downloading data from the monitor memory is possible through purchasable software to a home computer.

The Abbott Navigator is FDA approved in March 2008 for adults (18 and above). Sensor probe is 6 mm and 21 gauge. Sensor/transmitter is $2.05 \times 1.23 \times 0.43$ in. and can be worn for 5 days. The measured glucose range is between 20 and 500 mg per dL. Startup warming period is 10 hours and requires calibration at 10, 12, 24, and 72 hours after insertion without further calibration need for the final 2 days of the 5-day wear. It has a built in freestyle glucometer and displays glucose every minute with directional trends at 2, 4, 6, 12, or 24 hours and can go back to 28 days. It displays rate of change by sideway arrow (drop of glucose <1 mg per dL per minute), up arrow (raise >2 mg per dL per minute), down arrow (drop >2 mg per dL per minute), and 45° arrow (drop/raise between 1 and 2 mg per dL per minute). It allows predictive alarms 10, 20, or 30 minutes by projecting hypo- and hyperglycemia or programmable glucose levels based on trends. Data stored in the monitor could be downloaded to a Web-based data management system.

Overall percentage of error for the CGM runs around 15%. As mentioned before, accuracy depends on multiple factors such as current glucose concentration, rate of change of glucose values with poor correlation during hypoglycemia and during times of rapid change. Percentages of error for individual sensors have been reported as 17% for the Guardian RT (111), 11% to 16% for the Dexcom (62,112), and 12% to 14% for the Navigator (110,113).

The ultimate goal is to integrate the insulin pump and the glucose sensor via a control algorithm that will enable insulin delivery automatically without involving the patient. This system, the artificial pancreas, will revolutionize the diabetes management by providing a functioning bioelectronic β cell that mimics the physiologic function of pancreas. Artificial pancreas project has gained a significant momentum for the past 5 years with the advent in technology and continues to be one of the most promising areas of research in the field of diabetes management.

Another important measure of glycemic control is the percentage of glycosylated hemoglobin or hemoglobin A_{1c} (HbA_{1c}). Multiple studies have demonstrated that HbA_{1c} is a valuable prognosticator of complication risk in patients with T1DM. Glycohemoglobin is formed when glucose reacts nonenzymatically with the hemoglobin A molecule. Chromatographically, hemoglobin A can be separated into several components, expressed as HbA_{1c} fractions. The most abundant of these minor components is the HbA_{1c}, which is expressed as a percentage of total hemoglobin. A rising percentage of the glycosylated hemoglobin fraction, HbA_{1c}, indicates a higher than normal glucose exposure of the erythrocyte during its life span of 120 days. It therefore is an objective measure of glycemic control over the past 2 to 3 months. Today many pediatric diabetes centers perform a rapid HbA_{1c} analysis from capillary blood at the time of the office visit. This helps interpret the daily blood glucose log and alerts the diabetes care provider to any discrepancies. Although ambient glucose levels are the dominant influence on HbA_{1c} percentage, there are conditions that falsely lower the HbA_{1c} percentage, such as high red blood cell turnover (i.e., pregnancy or hemolysis) or the presence of a hemoglobinopathy such as sickle cell trait. If fetal hemoglobin (HbF) is elevated (such as in thalassemia, myeloproliferative disorders), the percentage of HbA_{1c} rises spuriously.

DIABETIC KETOACIDOSIS

Diabetic ketoacidosis (DKA) is a life-threatening catabolic state that occurs in the context of relative or absolute insulin deficiency. It is defined as hyperglycemia (a serum glucose of ≥300 mg per dL) and metabolic acidosis (a pH of <7.3 and a serum bicarbonate of <15 mEq per L). Around 20% to 30% of DKA episodes occur in patients who had not been diagnosed with diabetes in the past (114). In previously diagnosed children, DKA occurs with omission of insulin or under conditions that interfere with insulin action, such as the rise of counterregulatory hormones (epinephrine, norepinephrine, cortisol, growth hormone, and glucagon) and during infection, trauma, and emotional stress. Successful management of DKA requires clear comprehension of the pathophysiologic mechanisms that lead to the acid–base, fluid and electrolyte imbalance that ensues.

On a cellular level, insulinopenia creates a state of starvation, as fuel substrates cannot be taken up by the cell. Peripheral tissues are resistant to the action of insulin aggravating the insulinopenia in DKA. In muscle cells, this accelerates protein breakdown, resulting in free amino acids. In the liver, these amino acids are converted to glucose, perpetuating hyperglycemia. In light of perceived starvation, the liver further contributes to hyperglycemia by exaggerated glycogenolysis and gluconeogenesis with a rising glucagons-to-insulin ratio in the portal circulation. Hyperglycemia (above the renal threshold of 180 mg per dL) induces osmotic diuresis. Loss of water and electrolytes quickly results in hyperosmolar dehydration in these patients.

A lack of insulin in the adipose tissue activates hormone-sensitive lipoprotein lipase, releasing large amounts of fatty acids into the plasma, which are transformed to ketone bodies such as acetoacetic acid, β-hydroxybutyrate, and acetone. The rising ketonemia leads to metabolic acidosis. Ketonuria further exacerbates dehydration and loss of electrolytes.

In defense against cell shrinkage, hyperosmolarity causes the intracellular accumulation of osmoprotective molecules (myoinositol, taurine, and glutamate), which occurs most importantly in the brain cells. Although this cell preservation mechanism is beneficial during hyperosmolar dehydration, it poses a risk for the development of cerebral edema during rehydration therapy. As water freely passes through the blood–brain barrier, it is then drawn into the intracellular space by the abundance of osmols, rapidly increasing cell volume, leading to brain swelling. Other mechanisms, including increased capillary permeability, may also contribute to cerebral edema in DKA.

MANAGEMENT OF DIABETIC KETOACIDOSIS

Once the diagnosis has been established, fluid resuscitation, electrolyte management, and insulin administration are the mainstay of therapy. Key to successful recovery from DKA is frequent electrolyte monitoring, clinical evaluations, and meticulous record keeping. In the initial assessment, a complete history and physical examination should elicit any kind of precipitating infections, necessitating concomitant antibiotic therapy.

The first step in treatment of DKA is the administration of an isotonic (0.9% or normal) saline fluid bolus of 10 to 20 mL per kg of body weight (not to exceed 1 L) over 1 hour. If the patient is in shock, a 20-mL saline fluid bolus per kg body weight is rapidly administered and may be repeated to achieve hemodynamic stability. The infusion rate is then lowered to replace maintenance requirements and dehydration deficit over 36 to 48 hours. Since dehydration in DKA is intracellular, clinical measures of dehydration (such as pulse and perfusion) often underestimate the degree of deficit. A rule of thumb is to assume a 10% dehydration deficit in any child that presents in DKA. However, rehydration fluids are not to exceed 4 L per m^2 in 24 hours, as this has been associated with an increased risk of cerebral edema (115). Once the fluid bolus has been given, results of initial laboratory studies are usually available to help tailor fluid and electrolyte replacement. It is important to be aware of the frequently seen initial drop in pH after volume replacement as a result of lactic acid mobilization. Fluid administration and urine output should be carefully monitored throughout the therapy.

Sodium

At the time of presentation, patients may be hypernatremic or hyponatremic. When interpreting low-appearing sodium values from the electrolyte panel, one should be aware that they could be spuriously low due to an increase in serum glucose, lipids, and proteins. To correct for this pseudohyponatremia, 1.6 mEq per L is added to the sodium value for every 100 mg per dL of serum glucose above 100 mg per dL. This corrected sodium is then used to guide the interpretation. If corrected sodium is between 130 and 145 mEq per L, rehydration fluids can be continued with 0.45% saline (half of normal saline). Hypernatremia (>145 mEq per L) should be corrected with 0.675% saline (three-fourth of normal saline). A corrected sodium of less than 130 mEq per L requires 0.9% saline rehydration. When monitoring rehydration, the uncorrected serum sodium should always rise as the serum glucose is falling. A static uncorrected serum sodium in light of normalizing glucose levels is an ominous sign of overhydration and indicates a risk for the development of cerebral edema. When interpreting the calculated (corrected) serum sodium during fluid resuscitation, stable values are desirable but falling values should prompt an immediate decrease in the fluid rate.

Potassium

Despite total body depletion of potassium, initial potassium levels are usually normal or elevated. Insulin deficiency, acidosis, and dehydration all contribute to the relative high extracellular potassium level. Once insulin therapy is initiated, potassium is transported from the extracellular to the intracellular space, placing the patient at risk for a rapid drop in serum potassium, especially in light of total body depletion. As acidosis is corrected, each increase in serum pH by 0.1 further decreases serum potassium by 0.6 mEq per L. Therefore, close monitoring of serum potassium and administration of potassium at the time of initiation of insulin therapy will offset a precipitous drop in serum potassium. Hyperchloremic metabolic acidosis could be seen after administering potassium chloride (KCL) due to excessive chloride infusion. If the initial potassium level is more than 6.0 mEq per L, it is generally advised to hold off on adding potassium to intravenous hydration. However, once insulin infusion is started, serum potassium levels need to be monitored and potassium is added to the hydration fluid once values fall below 6.0 mEq per L. Because a precipitous drop in potassium is expected with insulin therapy, normal or low potassium levels before initiation of insulin therapy warrant higher potassium supplementation (116).

Glucose

Bedside glucose measurements are not able to accurately measure the patient's glucose level above 500 mg per dL. Blood should be sent to the laboratory for accurate assessment. The preferable collection tube is a plasma separator tube, which inhibits glucose degradation. The concentration of the intravenous insulin dose (insulin drip) is based on the age of the patient. In children aged 3 years and younger, an insulin dose of 0.05 units of short-acting insulin per kilogram per hour is cautiously administered. In all other age groups, insulin therapy is initiated at 0.1 units of short-acting insulin per kilogram per hour. In general, glucose should not be lowered faster than 100 mg per dL over an hour. When serum glucose falls below 300 mg per dL, dextrose is added to the saline solution, but the insulin drip is continued until acidosis is substantially corrected. In patients with severe hyperglycemia ($>$1,000 mg per dL), dextrose should be added earlier to avoid a precipitous drop in blood sugar that may occur with improved glomerular filtration during hydration. Once the patient is able to resume oral intake with a pH of more than 7.3 and a serum bicarbonate level of more than 15 mEq per L, the intravenous insulin can be discontinued and replaced with subcutaneous injections.

Bicarbonate and pH

In severe DKA, acidosis with a pH of less than 7.00 or a serum bicarbonate level of less than 5 mEq per L can occur. Although acidosis can be eventually corrected with insulin therapy and fluid resuscitation, bicarbonate treatment may be indicated in the ill-appearing patient, where acidosis may be impairing myocardial function. However, several caveats exist when administering bicarbonate in DKA. One of them is that the resulting rapid left shifts in the oxygen dissociation curve accelerates the entry of potassium into the cells. This could precipitate hypokalemia if potassium is not replete. It has been further stipulated that bicarbonate may worsen cerebral acidosis because it crosses the blood–brain barrier more slowly than carbon dioxide. A recent study suggests that of all the therapeutic interventions, only the administration of bicarbonate in DKA was associated with increased risk of cerebral edema (117). It is therefore not surprising that the administration of bicarbonate remains one of the most debated treatments in DKA management and if at all used, it is used sparingly (sodium bicarbonate at 1 mEq per kg given slowly over 1 to 2 hours and discontinued once pH approaches 7.1).

Calcium/Magnesium/Phosphorus

Phosphate levels are usually low and phosphate can be replaced in the form of potassium phosphate especially if PO_4 is less than 1.0 mg per dL. Since administering phosphate can lower serum calcium and magnesium, these levels should also be monitored. There are theoretical benefits to routinely using potassium phosphate instead of potassium chloride for rehydration. For example, it does not contribute to hyperchloremic metabolic acidosis and it may also help to replenish stores of 2,3-diphosphoglycerate, which are important for tissue reoxygenation. However, these effects may not outweigh the risk of hypocalcemia during phosphate administration.

Acute cerebral edema remains to be an important complication of DKA. Young children, especially younger than 3 years, with new-onset diabetes are at higher risk to develop cerebral edema. Immediate intervention is utmost important if a patient develops neurological deterioration and suggested treatment is mannitol at 1 g per kg of body weight.

OUTPATIENT MANAGEMENT

Diabetes is a demanding disease requiring a multidisciplinary team approach particularly for its outpatient management. The team ideally consists of a pediatric diabetologists, diabetes nurse specialists, social worker, dietician, and a psychologist who is experienced in the management of young patients and will focus on the needs of the patient and his/her family. The overall goal is to build a nonauthoritarian, collaborative relationship that will motivate the patients to be fully involved in their diabetes care, continue to assess the disease course, and prevent complications as much as possible.

In newly diagnosed patients, the first few weeks are critically important in the process of teaching self-management skills to the parent and child. In younger age groups, the parent is usually in daily contact with the diabetes clinical nurse specialist. Glucose levels, adjustment to diabetes, diet, and exercise are reviewed. The timing of the phone calls should be prearranged and ideally made to the same clinician. After making the insulin adjustment for the day, the rationale should be explained to the parent. Usually within 3 weeks, the parents are feeling more confidant and many are ready to attempt to make their own adjustments.

Once stabilized, regular follow-up visits on a two- to three-monthly basis are recommended for most patients. The main purpose of these visits is to ensure that the patient is achieving primary treatment goals. In addition to serial measurements of height and weight, particular attention should be paid to monitoring of blood pressure and examinations of the optic fundus, thyroid, and subcutaneous injection sites. Routine outpatient visits provide an opportunity to review glucose monitoring, to adjust the treatment regimen, and to assess child and family adjustment. Follow-up advice and support should be given by the nutritionist, diabetes nurse specialist, and psychologist or social worker. Use of the telephone, fax, or e-mail should be encouraged for adjustments in the treatment regimen between office visits.

Diet guidance for children with diabetes is best provided by a nutritionist who is an integral part of the treatment team and comfortable working with children. In addition to helping achieve optimal glucose levels and normal growth and development, nutritional management of diabetes is aimed at reducing the risk for other diseases, such as obesity, high blood cholesterol level, or high blood pressure. Underlying all of these is the establishment of sound eating patterns that include balanced, nutritious foods and consistent timing of food intake (118).

The American Diabetes Association dietary guidelines are used for dietary counseling. In addition to incorporating sound nutritional principles concerning the fat, fiber, and carbohydrate content, the importance of consistency in meal size and regularity in the timing of meals is emphasized. The prohibition of simple sugar in the diet has been de-emphasized, but it should still comprise no more than 10% of total carbohydrate intake. The success of the nutritional program may ultimately depend on the degree to which the meal planning is individualized and tailored to well-established eating patterns in the family. Moreover, flexibility can be enhanced if blood glucose–monitoring results are used to evaluate the impact of change in dietary intake.

Carbohydrate counting is an increasingly popular way to increase flexibility in food intake that is commonly used by patients using insulin pumps or multiple-daily injections. It is based on matching the amount of rapid-acting insulin that is needed for each gram or serving of carbohydrate in the meal. With instructions on how to use nutritional labels on food packages, even children can become expert at counting carbohydrates. Some foods, like pizza, that cause a prolonged increase in blood glucose levels, may require higher insulin dosing with square or dual wave bolus for insulin pump patients.

Regular exercise and active participation in organized sports have positive implications concerning the psychosocial and physical well-being of our patients. Parents and patients should be advised that different types of exercise may have different effects on blood glucose levels. For example, sports that involve short bursts of intensive exercise may increase rather than decrease blood glucose levels (119). On the other hand, long-distance running and other prolonged activities are more likely to lower blood glucose levels. Parents also need to be warned that a long bout of exercise during the day may lead to hypoglycemia while the child is sleeping during the night, which may require a reduction in the dose of intermediate-, long-acting insulin or basal rates by 20% to 50%.

Severe hypoglycemia is a common problem in patients striving for strict glycemic control with intensive treatment regimens. In the DCCT, the risk of severe hypoglycemia was threefold higher in intensively treated patients than in conventionally treated patients, and being an adolescent was an independent risk factor for a severe hypoglycemic event. The majority of severe hypoglycemic events occur overnight due, in part, to sleep-induced defects in counterregulatory hormone responses to hypoglycemia.

Monitoring glucose level is critical to detect asymptomatic hypoglycemia, especially in the young child with diabetes. The older child is usually aware of symptoms such as weakness, shakiness, hunger, or headache and is encouraged to treat these symptoms as soon as they occur. The older child who can accurately recognize symptoms is taught to immediately treat with 15 g of carbohydrate (e.g., three to four glucose tablets, 4 oz of juice, or 15 g of a glucose gel) without waiting to check a glucose level. Each episode should be assessed to make proper adjustments if a cause can be identified. Every family should have a glucagon emergency kit at home to treat severe hypoglycemia.

Children with intercurrent illnesses, such as infections or vomiting, should be closely monitored for elevations in blood glucose levels and ketonuria. On sick days, blood glucose levels should be checked every 2 hours, and the urine should be checked for ketones with every void. Supplemental doses of rapid-acting insulin (0.1 to 0.3 units per kg) should be given every 2 to 4 hours for elevations in glucose and ketones. Because of its more speedy absorption, a rapid-acting insulin analogue will lower plasma glucose faster than regular insulin. If the morning dose has not been given, and the child has a modestly elevated glucose level (150 to 250 mg per dL), small doses of NPH can be given to avoid a too rapid fall in plasma glucose levels. This works especially well in young children whose glucose levels fall quickly with rapid-acting insulin. Adequate fluid intake is essential to prevent dehydration. Fluids such as flat soda, clear soups, popsicles, and gelatin water are recommended to provide some electrolyte and carbohydrate replacement. If vomiting is persistent and ketones remain moderate or large after several supplemental insulin doses, arrangements should be made for parenteral hydration and evaluation in the emergency department.

Parents are told from the time of diagnosis that vomiting is a diabetes emergency and that they need to call for help after first checking blood glucose and urine ketone levels. This is especially true for children on pump therapy, since a catheter occlusion can throw the child into ketosis rapidly. If a pump-treated patient has elevated glucose and ketone levels, they are instructed to take a bolus injection of a rapid-acting insulin analogue by syringe. The dose of insulin varies between 0.2 and 0.4 units per kg. They are then instructed to change their infusion set and to program a temporary basal rate at twice the usual basal rate for 4 to 5 hours. Blood glucose and urine ketone levels are rechecked every hour and additional bolus doses can be given as needed. Once vomiting ceases and ketones become negative, the basal rate is returned to its usual setting. If the patient is not improving with these measures, the child should be seen.

HOW CLOSE ARE WE FOR A CURE? PANCREAS AND ISLET CELL TRANSPLANT AND IMMUNMODULATION THERAPY

Until now, transplantation of whole vascular pancreas has been reserved for patients with end-stage renal failure who are also in need of a kidney transplant. Transplant prior to renal failure has been controversial because of the considerable risks involved in the surgery itself and the lifelong immunosuppression required to prevent graft rejection. However, a recent surgical review found that, with improved operating room techniques and new immunosuppressive protocols, patient and graft survival has improved. Whole pancreas transplant may therefore be a viable option for adults with poorly controlled diabetes, before the need for kidney transplantation arises (120).

Nevertheless, the concept of whole pancreas transplant could become obsolete as protocols of islet cell transplantation are being developed. In the year 2000, the University of Alberta in Edmonton, Canada, published a minimally invasive procedure in which the portal vein is cannulated and then injected slowly with isolated islet cells. The so-called Edmonton Protocol was the first protocol to demonstrate that insulin independence could be achieved without entire pancreas transplant (121). However, subsequent multicenter trials were not this successful, with only half of the 36 subjects achieving insulin independence after 1 year (122).

The major stumbling blocks have been optimal immunosuppressive regimens. Undersuppression without corticosteroids was promoted by the Edmonton Protocol to enhance glycemic control. However, a recent study found that this might have contributed to the development of donor-specific antibodies (123). Furthermore, tacrolimus and sirolimus, the preferred immunosuppressants of the Edmonton Protocol, may have worked against success by interfering with islet cell proliferation (124). Other prohibitive factors are the need of up to four donor pancreases to harvest enough islets for transplant. As far as children are concerned, all such protocols pose an unacceptable risk of long-term immunosuppressive therapy—particularly in the area of growth and development.

The shortage of human donor pancreases has led researchers to seek out alternative ways to "grow" islet cells. Therefore, recent research has been directed toward the pluripotent stem cell of the early blastocyst, also referred to as embryonic stem cell. The first human embryonic stem cell lines were established in 1998. Although there is general consensus about the potential therapeutic benefits gained from studies with human stem cell lines, controversy still exists as to whether and how new human cell lines should be established. Embryonic stem cells have been successfully differentiated into insulin-producing cells (125) and have ameliorated hyperglycemia when transplanted into diabetic mice (126). In most studies, the insulin production and glucose responsiveness of these tissues is substantially less than those of normal β cells. A concern that often arises with embryonic stem cell therapy is their capacity to spontaneously differentiate into multiple tissues and organs. In mice, transplanted embryonic stem cells have lead to spontaneous teratoma formation (127).

Another form of stem cell being studied intently is the progenitor cell of the fetal pancreas. Although these cells are already destined to become pancreas tissue, their secretory direction has not yet been decided. The δ notch pathway is a critical factor in the decision between endocrine and exocrine function in the developing pancreas. It may be possible to modulate cell signaling in vitro so that the pancreatic duct cells (from aborted embryonic pancreas) preferentially differentiate into endocrine precursors (128). Recently, endodermal progenitor cells with multilineage potential were found in the mouse fetal liver. Dependent on the microenvironment of the host (pancreas, intestine, or liver of the mouse), these cells were able to differentiate into either pancreatic ductal/acinar cells, intestinal epithelial cells, or liver hepatocytes/cholangiocytes (129).

The third area of interest is a search for the presence of pluripotent cells in adult pancreatic tissue. It was postulated in 1993 that, after partial pancreatectomy in adult rats, proliferation and differentiation of precursor cells from the ductal epithelium can lead to the regeneration of pancreatic islets and exocrine tissue (130). In vitro studies confirmed that pancreatic ductal epithelium is composed of pluripotent cells that can be manipulated to differentiate into glucose-responsive islet tissue (131). Another location for progenitor cells has been proposed within the pancreatic islets themselves. This is a novel and distinct population of cells that expresses nestin (a neural stem cell-specific marker) but does not express insulin, glucagon, somatostatin, or pancreatic polypeptide (132). In culture, these cells rapidly proliferate and can be modulated to either demonstrate a β-cell phenotype or express exocrine pancreas markers (133).

Autoimmune origin of T1DM has been known for years and recent advances in immunomodulation therapy brought the possibility of prevention and cure of diabetes one step ahead.

Target population for the prevention studies are subjects with positive autoantibodies (IAA, GAD65, IA-2, IA-2b) and/or early β-cell dysfunction suggesting high risk of developing diabetes. Previous trials including nicotinamide (a component of vitB3), parenteral insulin use, and nasal insulin did not reveal promising results for the prevention of diabetes (134–138). However, many other prevention studies testing the effect of vitamin D3, oral insulin, docosahexaenoic acid, and delayed exposure to intact proteins are underway (http://www.jdrf.org).

Secondary intervention studies to halt β-cell destruction with chronic use of immunosuppressant were tried without much success due to serious side effects and loss of effect after sometime (139). Current immune-tolerance therapies include antigen nonspecific agents such as anti-CD3, thymoglobulin, IL-2 and sirolimus, CTLA-4Ig, and anti-CD20 are currently under research for prolongation of β-cell survival (140,141). Most recent one in the prevention trial is the GAD alum injection for new-onset T1DM patients to prolong the honeymoon phase of diabetes (142). Alternative approaches including combining immunomodulators and β-cell regenerating agents demonstrated promising results in animal studies and bring us closer to the promise the reversal of diabetes provided that clinical trials with these regimens achieve the same success. In the mean time, artificial pancreas project already utilizing off-the-shelf devices can serve as a different type of cure for children with diabetes in the near future.

REFERENCES

1. Havcock P. History of insulin therapy. In: Schade DS, Santiago JV, Skyler JS, et al., eds. *Intensive insulin therapy*, Princeton, NJ: Excerpta Medica, 1983:1–19.

2. Bell GI, Pictet RL, Rutter WJ, et al. Sequence of the human insulin gene. *Nature* 1980;284:26–32.
3. Bliss M. Banting's, Best's, and Collip's accounts of the discovery of insulin. *Bull Hist Med* 1982;56:554–568.
4. Variation and trends in incidence of childhood diabetes in Europe. EURODIAB ACE Study Group. *Lancet* 2000;355:873–876.
5. Karvonen M, Viik-Kajander M, Moltchanova E, et al. Incidence of childhood type 1 diabetes worldwide. Diabetes Mondiale (DiaMond) Project Group. *Diabetes Care* 2000;23:1516–1526.
6. Libman IM, LaPorte RE, Becker D, et al. Was there an epidemic of diabetes in nonwhite adolescents in Allegheny County, Pennsylvania? *Diabetes Care* 1998;21:1278–1281.
7. Atkinson MA. Molecular mimicry and the pathogenesis of insulin-dependent diabetes mellitus: still just an attractive hypothesis. *Ann Med* 1997;29:393–399.
8. Hiemstra HS, Schloot NC, van Veelen PA, et al. Cytomegalovirus in autoimmunity: T cell crossreactivity to viral antigen and autoantigen glutamic acid decarboxylase. *Proc Natl Acad Sci U S A* 2001;98:3988–3991.
9. Vaarala O, Hyoty H, Akerblom HK. Environmental factors in the aetiology of childhood diabetes. *Diabetes Nutr Metab* 1999;12:75–85.
10. Owerbach D, Bell GI, Rutter WJ, et al. The insulin gene is located on the short arm of chromosome 11 in humans. *Diabetes* 1981;30:267–270.
11. Porterfield S. *Endocrine physiology*. Saint Louis, MO: Mosby-Year Book, Inc., 1996.
12. Thorens B, Sarkar HK, Kaback HR, et al. Cloning and functional expression in bacteria of a novel glucose transporter present in liver, intestine, kidney, and beta-pancreatic islet cells. *Cell* 1988;55:281–290.
13. Matschinsky F, Liang Y, Kesavan P, et al. Glucokinase as pancreatic beta cell glucose sensor and diabetes gene. *J Clin Invest* 1993;92:2092–2098.
14. Froguel P, Vaxillaire M, Sun F, et al. Close linkage of glucokinase locus on chromosome 7p to early-onset non-insulin-dependent diabetes mellitus. *Nature* 1992;356:162–164.
15. Vionnet N, Stoffel M, Takeda J, et al. Nonsense mutation in the glucokinase gene causes early-onset non-insulin-dependent diabetes mellitus. *Nature* 1992;356:721–722.
16. Safayhi H, Haase H, Kramer U, et al. L-type calcium channels in insulin-secreting cells: biochemical characterization and phosphorylation in RINm5 F cells. *Mol Endocrinol* 1997;11:619–629.
17. Aguilar-Bryan L, Nichols CG, Wechsler SW, et al. Cloning of the beta cell high-affinity sulfonylurea receptor: a regulator of insulin secretion. *Science* 1995;268:423–426.
18. Thomas PM, Cote GJ, Wohllk N, et al. Mutations in the sulfonylurea receptor gene in familial persistent hyperinsulinemic hypoglycemia of infancy. *Science* 1995;268:426–429.
19. Kane C, Shepherd RM, Squires PE, et al. Loss of functional KATP channels in pancreatic beta-cells causes persistent hyperinsulinemic hypoglycemia of infancy. *Nat Med* 1996;2:1344–1347.
20. Babenko AP, Polak M, Cave H, et al. Activating mutations in the ABCC8 gene in neonatal diabetes mellitus. *N Engl J Med* 2006;355:456–466.
21. Gloyn AL, Pearson ER, Antcliff JF, et al. Activating mutations in the gene encoding the ATP-sensitive potassium-channel subunit Kir6.2 and permanent neonatal diabetes. *N Engl J Med* 2004;350:1838–1849.
22. Pearson ER, Flechtner I, Njolstad PR, et al. Switching from insulin to oral sulfonylureas in patients with diabetes due to Kir6.2 mutations. *N Engl J Med* 2006;355:467–477.
23. Ebina Y, Ellis L, Jarnagin K, et al. The human insulin receptor cDNA: the structural basis for hormone-activated transmembrane signalling. *Cell* 1985;40:747–758.
24. Seino S, Seino M, Nishi S, et al. Structure of the human insulin receptor gene and characterization of its promoter. *Proc Natl Acad Sci U S A* 1989;86:114–118.
25. Luo RZ, Beniac DR, Fernandes A, et al. Quaternary structure of the insulin–insulin receptor complex. *Science* 1999;285:1077–1080.
26. Wang Q, Somwar R, Bilan PJ, et al. Protein kinase B/Akt participates in GLUT4 translocation by insulin in L6 myoblasts. *Mol Cell Biol* 1999;19:4008–4018.
27. Bae SS, Cho H, Mu J, et al. Isoform-specific regulation of insulin-dependent glucose uptake by Akt/protein kinase B. *J Biol Chem* 2003;278:49530–49536.
28. Baumann CA, Ribon V, Kanzaki M, et al. CAP defines a second signalling pathway required for insulin-stimulated glucose transport. *Nature* 2000;407:202–207.
29. Pessin JE, Saltiel AR. Signaling pathways in insulin action: molecular targets of insulin resistance. *J Clin Invest* 2000;106:165–169.
30. Chiang SH, Baumann CA, Kanzaki M, et al. Insulin-stimulated GLUT4 translocation requires the CAP-dependent activation of TC10. *Nature* 2001;410:944–948.
31. Scott D. Crystalline insulin. *Biochem J* 1934;28:1592–1602.
32. Hagedorn H, Jensen B, Krarup N. Protamine insulinate. *J Am Med Assoc* 1936;106:177–180.
33. Scott D, Fisher A. Studies on insulin with protamine. *J Pharmacol Exp Ther* 1936;58:78–92.
34. Chance RE, Root MA, Galloway JA. The immunogenicity of insulin preparations. *Acta Endocrinol Suppl (Copenh)* 1976;205:185–198.
35. Davidson JK, DeBra DW. Immunologic insulin resistance. *Diabetes* 1978;27:307–318.
36. Morihara K, Oka T, Tsuzuki H. Semi-synthesis of human insulin by trypsin-catalysed replacement of Ala-B30 by Thr in porcine insulin. *Nature* 1979;280:412–413.
37. Goeddel DV, Kleid DG, Bolivar F, et al. Expression in *Escherichia coli* of chemically synthesized genes for human insulin. *Proc Natl Acad Sci U S A* 1979;76:106–110.
38. Thim L, Hansen MT, Norris K, et al. Secretion and processing of insulin precursors in yeast. *Proc Natl Acad Sci U S A* 1986;83:6766–6770.
39. Raskin P, Clements RS Jr. The use of human insulin derived from baker's yeast by recombinant DNA technology. *Clin Ther* 1991;13:569–578.
40. Brogden RN, Heel RC. Human insulin. A review of its biological activity, pharmacokinetics and therapeutic use. *Drugs* 1987;34:350–371.
41. Home PD, Alberti KG. Human insulin. *Clin Endocrinol Metab* 1982;11:453–483.
42. Nielsen FS, Jorgensen LN, Ipsen M, et al. Long-term comparison of human insulin analogue B10Asp and soluble human insulin in IDDM patients on a basal/bolus insulin regimen. *Diabetologia* 1995;38:592–598.
43. Bornfeldt KE, Gidlof RA, Wasteson A, et al. Binding and biological effects of insulin, insulin analogues and insulin-like growth factors in rat aortic smooth muscle cells. Comparison of maximal growth promoting activities. *Diabetologia* 1991;34:307–313.
44. Hamel FG, Siford GL, Fawcett J, et al. Differences in the cellular processing of AspB10 human insulin compared with human insulin and LysB28ProB29 human insulin. *Metabolism* 1999;48:611–617.
45. Howey DC, Bowsher RR, Brunelle RL, et al. [Lys(B28), Pro(B29)]-human insulin. A rapidly absorbed analogue of human insulin. *Diabetes* 1994;43:396–402.
46. Slieker LJ, Brooke GS, DiMarchi RD, et al. Modifications in the B10 and B26–30 regions of the B chain of human insulin alter affinity for the human IGF-I receptor more than for the insulin receptor. *Diabetologia* 1997;40(Suppl 2):S54–S61.
47. Torlone E, Fanelli C, Rambotti AM, et al. Pharmacokinetics, pharmacodynamics and glucose counterregulation following subcutaneous injection of the monomeric insulin analogue [Lys(B28), Pro(B29)] in IDDM. *Diabetologia* 1994;37:713–720.
48. Lougheed WD, Zinman B, Strack TR, et al. Stability of insulin lispro in insulin infusion systems. *Diabetes Care* 1997;20:1061–1065.
49. Zinman B, Tildesley H, Chiasson JL, et al. Insulin lispro in CSII: results of a double-blind crossover study. *Diabetes* 1997;46:440–443.
50. Renner R, Pfutzner A, Trautmann M, et al. Use of insulin lispro in continuous subcutaneous insulin infusion treatment. Results of a multicenter trial. German Humalog-CSII Study Group. *Diabetes Care* 1999;22:784–788.
51. Griffin ME, Feder A, Tamborlane WV. Lipoatrophy associated with lispro insulin in insulin pump therapy: an old complication, a new cause? *Diabetes Care* 2001;24:174.
52. Ampudia-Blasco FJ, Hasbum B, Carmena R. A new case of lipoatrophy with lispro insulin in insulin pump therapy: is there any insulin preparation free of complications? *Diabetes Care* 2003;26:953–954.
53. Fineberg NS, Fineberg SE, Anderson JH, et al. Immunologic effects of insulin lispro [Lys(B28), Pro(B29) human insulin] in

IDDM and NIDDM patients previously treated with insulin. *Diabetes* 1996;45:1750–1754.
54. Kumar D. Lispro analog for treatment of generalized allergy to human insulin. *Diabetes Care* 1997;20:1357–1359.
55. Hirsch IB, D'Alessio D, Eng L, et al. Severe insulin resistance in a patient with type 1 diabetes and stiff-man syndrome treated with insulin lispro. *Diabetes Res Clin Pract* 1998;41:197–202.
56. Attia N, Jones TW, Holcombe J, et al. Comparison of human regular and lispro insulins after interruption of continuous subcutaneous insulin infusion and in the treatment of acutely decompensated IDDM. *Diabetes Care* 1998;21:817–821.
57. Lindholm A, McEwen J, Riis AP. Improved postprandial glycemic control with insulin aspart. A randomized double-blind cross-over trial in type 1 diabetes. *Diabetes Care* 1999;22:801–805.
58. Mudaliar SR, Lindberg FA, Joyce M, et al. Insulin aspart (B28 asp-insulin): a fast-acting analog of human insulin: absorption kinetics and action profile compared with regular human insulin in healthy nondiabetic subjects. *Diabetes Care* 1999;22:1501–1506.
59. Raskin P, Guthrie RA, Leiter L, et al. Use of insulin aspart, a fast-acting insulin analog, as the mealtime insulin in the management of patients with type 1 diabetes. *Diabetes Care* 2000;23:583–588.
60. Home PD, Lindholm A, Hylleberg B, et al. Improved glycemic control with insulin aspart: a multicenter randomized double-blind crossover trial in type 1 diabetic patients. UK Insulin Aspart Study Group. *Diabetes Care* 1998;21:1904–1909.
61. Becker RH. Insulin glulisine complementing basal insulins: a review of structure and activity. *Diabetes Technol Ther* 2007;9:109–121.
62. Garg SK, Ellis SL, Ulrich H. Insulin glulisine: a new rapid-acting insulin analogue for the treatment of diabetes. *Expert Opin Pharmacother* 2005;6:643–651.
63. Garg SK. New insulin analogues. *Diabetes Technol Ther* 2005;7: 813–817.
64. Danne T, Becker RH, Heise T, et al. Pharmacokinetics, prandial glucose control, and safety of insulin glulisine in children and adolescents with type 1 diabetes. *Diabetes Care* 2005;28:2100–2105.
65. Roach P. New insulin analogues and routes of delivery: pharmacodynamic and clinical considerations. *Clin Pharmacokinet* 2008; 47:595–610.
66. Arkins JA, Engbring NH, Lennon EJ. The incidence of skin reactivity to insulin in diabetic patients. *J Allergy* 1962;33:69–72.
67. Paley R, Tunbridge R. Dermal reactions to insulin therapy. *Diabetes* 1952;1:22–27.
68. Fujikura J, Fujimoto M, Yasue S, et al. Insulin-induced lipohypertrophy: report of a case with histopathology. *Endocr J* 2005;52: 623–628.
69. Richardson T, Kerr D. Skin-related complications of insulin therapy: epidemiology and emerging management strategies. *Am J Clin Dermatol* 2003;4:661–667.
70. Young RJ, Hannan WJ, Frier BM, et al. Diabetic lipohypertrophy delays insulin absorption. *Diabetes Care* 1984;7:479–480.
71. Kumar O, Miller L, Mehtalia S. Use of dexamethasone in treatment of insulin lipoatrophy. *Diabetes* 1977;26:296–299.
72. Logwin S, Conget I, Jansa M, et al. Human insulin-induced lipoatrophy. Successful treatment using a jet-injection device. *Diabetes Care* 1996;19:255–256.
73. Whitley TH, Lawrence PA, Smith CL. Amelioration of insulin lipoatrophy by dexamethasone injection. *JAMA* 1976;235:839–840.
74. Wyatt JW, Frias JL, Hoyme HE, et al. Congenital anomaly rate in offspring of mothers with diabetes treated with insulin lispro during pregnancy. *Diabet Med* 2005;22:803–807.
75. Hod M, Damm P, Kaaja R, et al. Fetal and perinatal outcomes in type 1 diabetes pregnancy: a randomized study comparing insulin aspart with human insulin in 322 subjects. *Am J Obstet Gynecol* 2008;198:186.e1–e7.
76. Jorgensen S, Vaag A, Langkjaer L, et al. NovoSol Basal: pharmacokinetics of a novel soluble long acting insulin analogue. *BMJ* 1989;299:415–419.
77. Heinemann L, Linkeschova R, Rave K, et al. Time-action profile of the long-acting insulin analog insulin glargine (HOE901) in comparison with those of NPH insulin and placebo. *Diabetes Care* 2000;23:644–649.
78. Owens DR, Coates PA, Luzio SD, et al. Pharmacokinetics of 125I-labeled insulin glargine (HOE 901) in healthy men: comparison with NPH insulin and the influence of different subcutaneous injection sites. *Diabetes Care* 2000;23:813–819.
79. Lepore M, Pampanelli S, Fanelli C, et al. Pharmacokinetics and pharmacodynamics of subcutaneous injection of long-acting human insulin analog glargine, NPH insulin, and ultralente human insulin and continuous subcutaneous infusion of insulin lispro. *Diabetes* 2000;49:2142–2148.
80. Porcellati F, Rossetti P, Busciantella NR, et al. Comparison of pharmacokinetics and dynamics of the long-acting insulin analogs glargine and detemir at steady state in type 1 diabetes: a double-blind, randomized, crossover study. *Diabetes Care* 2007;30: 2447–2452.
81. Heise T, Nosek L, Ronn BB, et al. Lower within-subject variability of insulin detemir in comparison to NPH insulin and insulin glargine in people with type 1 diabetes. *Diabetes* 2004;53:1614–1620.
82. Porcellati F, Rossetti P, Ricci NB, et al. Pharmacokinetics and pharmacodynamics of the long-acting insulin analog glargine after 1 week of use compared with its first administration in subjects with type 1 diabetes. *Diabetes Care* 2007;30:1261–1263.
83. Berti L, Kellerer M, Bossenmaier B, et al. The long acting human insulin analog HOE 901: characteristics of insulin signalling in comparison to Asp(B10) and regular insulin. *Horm Metab Res* 1998; 30:123–129.
84. Bahr M, Kolter T, Seipke G, et al. Growth promoting and metabolic activity of the human insulin analogue [GlyA21, ArgB31, ArgB32] insulin (HOE 901) in muscle cells. *Eur J Pharmacol* 1997;320: 259–265.
85. Kurtzhals P, Schaffer L, Sorensen A, et al. Correlations of receptor binding and metabolic and mitogenic potencies of insulin analogs designed for clinical use. *Diabetes* 2000;49:999–1005.
86. Home PD, Ashwell SG. An overview of insulin glargine. *Diabetes Metab Res Rev* 2002;18(Suppl 3):S57–S63.
87. Ratner RE, Hirsch IB, Neifing JL, et al. Less hypoglycemia with insulin glargine in intensive insulin therapy for type 1 diabetes. U. S. Study Group of Insulin Glargine in Type 1 Diabetes. *Diabetes Care* 2000;23:639–643.
88. Schober E, Schoenle E, Van Dyk J, et al. Comparative trial between insulin glargine and NPH insulin in children and adolescents with type 1 diabetes. *Diabetes Care* 2001;24:2005–2006.
89. Morales J. Defining the role of insulin detemir in Basal insulin therapy. *Drugs* 2007;67:2557–2584.
90. Pieber TR, Treichel HC, Hompesch B, et al. Comparison of insulin detemir and insulin glargine in subjects with Type 1 diabetes using intensive insulin therapy. *Diabet Med* 2007;24:635–642.
91. Brunner GA, Sendhofer G, Wutte A, et al. Pharmacokinetic and pharmacodynamic properties of long-acting insulin analogue NN304 in comparison to NPH insulin in humans. *Exp Clin Endocrinol Diabetes* 2000;108:100–105.
92. Heinemann L, Sinha K, Weyer C, et al. Time-action profile of the soluble, fatty acid acylated, long-acting insulin analogue NN304. *Diabet Med* 1999;16:332–338.
93. Kurtoglu S, Atabek ME, Dizdarer C, et al. Insulin detemir improves glycemic control and reduces hypoglycemia in children with type 1 diabetes: findings from the Turkish cohort of the PREDICTIVE observational study. *Pediatr Diabetes* 2009.
94. Kurtzhals P, Havelund S, Jonassen I, et al. Effect of fatty acids and selected drugs on the albumin binding of a long-acting, acylated insulin analogue. *J Pharm Sci* 1997;86:1365–1368.
95. Hordern SV, Wright JE, Umpleby AM, et al. Comparison of the effects on glucose and lipid metabolism of equipotent doses of insulin detemir and NPH insulin with a 16-h euglycaemic clamp. *Diabetologia* 2005;48:420–426.
96. Heinemann L. Future directions for insulin therapy and diabetes treatment. *Endocrinol Metab Clin North Am* 2007;36(Suppl 2): 69–79.
97. Gaensslen M. Uber inhalation von insulin. *Klin Wochenschr* 1925;2.
98. Tamborlane WV, Sherwin RS, Genel M, et al. Reduction to normal of plasma glucose in juvenile diabetes by subcutaneous administration of insulin with a portable infusion pump. *N Engl J Med* 1979;300:573–578.
99. Group DR. The effect of intensive treatment of diabetes on the development and progression of long-term complications in insulin-dependent diabetes mellitus. The Diabetes Control and Complications Trial Research Group. *N Engl J Med* 1993;329: 977–986.
100. Group DR. Effect of intensive diabetes treatment on the development and progression of long-term complications in adolescents

with insulin-dependent diabetes mellitus: Diabetes Control and Complications Trial. Diabetes Control and Complications Trial Research Group. *J Pediatr* 1994;125:177–188.

101. Pankowska E, Blazik M, Dziechciarz P, et al. Continuous subcutaneous insulin infusion vs. multiple daily injections in children with type 1 diabetes: a systematic review and meta-analysis of randomized control trials. *Pediatr Diabetes* 2009;10:52–8.
102. Pickup JC, Kidd J, Burmiston S, et al. Determinants of glycaemic control in type 1 diabetes during intensified therapy with multiple daily insulin injections or continuous subcutaneous insulin infusion: importance of blood glucose variability. *Diabetes Metab Res Rev* 2006;22:232–237.
103. Retnakaran R, Hochman J, DeVries JH, et al. Continuous subcutaneous insulin infusion versus multiple daily injections: the impact of baseline A1c. *Diabetes Care* 2004;27:2590–2596.
104. Boland EA, Grey M, Oesterle A, et al. Continuous subcutaneous insulin infusion. A new way to lower risk of severe hypoglycemia, improve metabolic control, and enhance coping in adolescents with type 1 diabetes. *Diabetes Care* 1999;22:1779–1784.
105. Eugster EA, Francis G. Position statement: continuous subcutaneous insulin infusion in very young children with type 1 diabetes. *Pediatrics* 2006;118:e1244–e1249.
106. Ostrow D, Phillips N, Avalos A, et al. Mutational bias for body size in rhabditid nematodes. *Genetics* 2007;176:1653–61.
107. Youth and parent satisfaction with clinical use of the GlucoWatch G2 Biographer in the management of pediatric type 1 diabetes. *Diabetes Care* 2005;28:1929–1935.
108. Koschinsky T, Heinemann L. Sensors for glucose monitoring: technical and clinical aspects. *Diabetes Metab Res Rev* 2001;17:113–123.
109. Wilson DM, Beck RW, Tamborlane WV, et al. The accuracy of the FreeStyle Navigator continuous glucose monitoring system in children with type 1 diabetes. *Diabetes Care* 2007;30:59–64.
110. Weinstein RL, Schwartz SL, Brazg RL, et al. Accuracy of the 5-day FreeStyle Navigator Continuous Glucose Monitoring System: comparison with frequent laboratory reference measurements. *Diabetes Care* 2007;30:1125–1130.
111. Feldman B, Brazg R, Schwartz S, et al. A continuous glucose sensor based on wired enzyme technology—results from a 3-day trial in patients with type 1 diabetes. *Diabetes Technol Ther* 2003;5:769–779.
112. Bode B, Gross K, Rikalo N, et al. Alarms based on real-time sensor glucose values alert patients to hypo- and hyperglycemia: the guardian continuous monitoring system. *Diabetes Technol Ther* 2004;6:105–113.
113. Chase HP, Beck R, Tamborlane W, et al. A randomized multicenter trial comparing the GlucoWatch Biographer with standard glucose monitoring in children with type 1 diabetes. *Diabetes Care* 2005;28:1101–1106.
114. Falch G, Fishbein H, Ellis S. The epidemiology of diabetic ketoacidosis: a population-based study. *Am J Epidemiol* 1983;117:551.
115. Duck SC, Wyatt DT. Factors associated with brain herniation in the treatment of diabetic ketoacidosis. *J Pediatr* 1988;113:10–14.
116. Hafeez W, Vuguin P. Managing diabetic ketoacidosis—a delicate balance. *Contemp Pediatr* 2000;17:72–83.
117. Glaser N, Barnett P, McCaslin I, et al. Risk factors for cerebral edema in children with diabetic ketoacidosis. The Pediatric Emergency Medicine Collaborative Research Committee of the American Academy of Pediatrics. *N Engl J Med* 2001;344:264–269.
118. Tamborlane WV, Held N. *Diabetes.* In: Yale Guide to Children's Nutrition. New Haven, CT: Yale University Press, 1997.
119. Mitchell TH, Abraham G, Schiffrin A, et al. Hyperglycemia after intense exercise in IDDM subjects during continuous subcutaneous insulin infusion. *Diabetes Care* 1988;11:311–317.
120. Sutherland DE, Gruessner RW, Dunn DL, et al. Lessons learned from more than 1,000 pancreas transplants at a single institution. *Ann Surg* 2001;233:463–501.
121. Shapiro AM, Lakey JR, Ryan EA, et al. Islet transplantation in seven patients with type 1 diabetes mellitus using a glucocorticoid-free immunosuppressive regimen. *N Engl J Med* 2000;343:230–238.
122. Shapiro AM, Ricordi C, Hering BJ, et al. International trial of the Edmonton protocol for islet transplantation. *N Engl J Med* 2006;355:1318–1330.
123. Campbell PM, Senior PA, Salam A, et al. High risk of sensitization after failed islet transplantation. *Am J Transplant* 2007;7: 2311–2317.
124. Nir T, Melton DA, Dor Y. Recovery from diabetes in mice by beta cell regeneration. *J Clin Invest* 2007;117:2553–2561.
125. Lumelsky N, Blondel O, Laeng P, et al. Differentiation of embryonic stem cells to insulin-secreting structures similar to pancreatic islets. *Science* 2001;292:1389–1394.
126. Soria B, Roche E, Berna G, et al. Insulin-secreting cells derived from embryonic stem cells normalize glycemia in streptozotocin-induced diabetic mice. *Diabetes* 2000;49:157–162.
127. Verfaillie CM, Pera MF, Lansdorp PM. Stem cells: hype and reality. *Hematology Am Soc Hematol Educ Program* 2002:369–391.
128. Apelqvist A, Li H, Sommer L, et al. Notch signalling controls pancreatic cell differentiation. *Nature* 1999;400:877–881.
129. Suzuki A, Zheng YW, Kaneko S, et al. Clonal identification and characterization of self-renewing pluripotent stem cells in the developing liver. *J Cell Biol* 2002;156:173–184.
130. Bonner-Weir S, Baxter LA, Schuppin GT, et al. A second pathway for regeneration of adult exocrine and endocrine pancreas. A possible recapitulation of embryonic development. *Diabetes* 1993;42: 1715–1720.
131. Bonner-Weir S, Taneja M, Weir GC, et al. In vitro cultivation of human islets from expanded ductal tissue. *Proc Natl Acad Sci U S A* 2000;97:7999–8004.
132. Zulewski H, Abraham EJ, Gerlach MJ, et al. Multipotential nestin-positive stem cells isolated from adult pancreatic islets differentiate ex vivo into pancreatic endocrine, exocrine, and hepatic phenotypes. *Diabetes* 2001;50:521–533.
133. Abraham EJ, Leech CA, Lin JC, et al. Insulinotropic hormone glucagon-like peptide-1 differentiation of human pancreatic islet-derived progenitor cells into insulin-producing cells. *Endocrinology* 2002;143:3152–3161.
134. Krischer JP, Cuthbertson DD, Yu L, et al. Screening strategies for the identification of multiple antibody-positive relatives of individuals with type 1 diabetes. *J Clin Endocrinol Metab* 2003;88: 103–108.
135. Achenbach P, Warncke K, Reiter J, et al. Type 1 diabetes risk assessment: improvement by follow-up measurements in young islet autoantibody-positive relatives. *Diabetologia* 2006;49:2969–2976.
136. Gale EA, Bingley PJ, Emmett CL, et al. European Nicotinamide Diabetes Intervention Trial (ENDIT): a randomised controlled trial of intervention before the onset of type 1 diabetes. *Lancet* 2004; 363:925–931.
137. European Nicotinamide Diabetes Intervention Trial Group. Intervening before the onset of Type 1 diabetes: baseline data from the European Nicotinamide Diabetes Intervention Trial (ENDIT). *Diabetologia* 2003;46:339–346.
138. Nanto-Salonen K, Kupila A, Simell S, et al. Nasal insulin to prevent type 1 diabetes in children with HLA genotypes and autoantibodies conferring increased risk of disease: a double-blind, randomised controlled trial. *Lancet* 2008;372:1746–1755.
139. Bougneres PF, Carel JC, Castano L, et al. Factors associated with early remission of type I diabetes in children treated with cyclosporine. *N Engl J Med* 1988;318:663–670.
140. Hadjiyanni I, Baggio LL, Poussier P, et al. Exendin-4 modulates diabetes onset in nonobese diabetic mice. *Endocrinology* 2008;149: 1338–1349.
141. Bresson D, Togher L, Rodrigo E, et al. Anti-CD3 and nasal proinsulin combination therapy enhances remission from recent-onset autoimmune diabetes by inducing Tregs. *J Clin Invest* 2006;116: 1371–1381.
142. Ludvigsson J, Faresjo M, Hjorth M, et al. GAD treatment and insulin secretion in recent-onset type 1 diabetes. *N Engl J Med* 2008; 359:1909–1920.

CHAPTER

53

Delbert A. Fisher

Thyroid Hormones

Thyroid hormones are critically important to normal growth and development during infancy, childhood, and adolescence. Thyroid hormone deficiency during fetal life and infancy leads to mental retardation, and hypothyroidism during childhood and adolescence leads to growth and developmental retardation. In addition, there are significant effects of thyroid hormones on energy metabolism and on the metabolism of nutrients and inorganic ions, and these actions are important in the maintenance of normal metabolic homeostasis. In the present chapter, we review normal thyroid hormone physiology and pharmacology and the pharmacology of the drugs and chemicals used in the diagnosis and management of disorders of thyroid function.

THYROID HORMONE SYNTHESIS AND RELEASE

Thyroid hormones and analogues are tyrosine derivatives. Their structures are summarized in Figure 53.1. The only source of thyroxine (tetraiodothyronine, T_4) is the thyroid gland. The major substrates for T_4 synthesis are iodide and tyrosine (1,2). Tyrosine is not rate limiting, but iodine is a trace element, the limitation of which can severely impair thyroid hormone synthesis. The steps in thyroid hormone synthesis by the thyroid gland include iodide trapping, synthesis of thyroglobulin (Tg), organification of trapped iodide, storage of iodinated Tg in follicular colloid, endocytosis and hydrolysis of Tg to release thyroid hormones, and deiodination of monoiodotyrosine (MIT) and diiodotyrosine (DIT) with intrathyroidal recycling of the iodide (1,2) (see Fig. 53.2).

The transport of iodide across the thyroid cell membrane is the first and rate-limiting step in thyroid hormone biosynthesis. The salivary glands, gastric mucosa, uterus, mammary glands, small intestine, and placenta also are able to concentrate iodide; however, they are not capable of iodothyronine synthesis. Normally, the thyroid follicular cell generates a thyroid/serum concentration gradient of 30- to 40-fold. This gradient increases markedly when stimulated by iodine deficiency, thyroid-stimulating hormone (thyrotropin; TSH), or thyroid-stimulating immunoglobulins (TSIs), or by drugs that impair the efficiency of hormone synthesis. Several inorganic anions are capable of competitively inhibiting iodide transport; these include bromide (Br), nitrate (NO_2), thiocyanate (SCN), and perchlorate (CIO_4).

The predominant protein in thyroid colloid is Tg, a large 660-kd homodimer. The oxidation of iodide to an active intermediate is followed by iodination of Tg-bound tyrosyl residues. The thyroid gland normally contains 50 to 100 mg Tg for every 1 g of gland. The tyrosyl residues, which are the iodine acceptors of Tg, comprise about 3% of the weight of the protein, and about two-thirds of these are spatially oriented to be susceptible to iodination. Iodination of Tg tyrosyl residues forms MIT and DIT. These iodotyrosines then couple to form the iodothyronines T_3 and T_4; DIT + DIT couple to form T_4 while MIT + DIT coupling forms T_3. The relative proportions of T_3 and T_4 formed depend on the amount of available iodide. About 30% of the Tg iodoprotein is iodothyronine, with a T_4/T_3 ratio of 10:1 to 20:1.

The first step in thyroid hormone release is the endocytosis of stored colloid. The ingested colloid droplets fuse with proteolytic enzyme-containing lysosomes to form phagolysosomes in which Tg is digested to release free iodothyronines into the cytoplasm for diffusion into blood (Fig. 53.2). The MIT and DIT released during hydrolysis of Tg are largely deiodinated by a thyroidal iodotyrosine deiodinase (1,2). The free iodide enters the intracellular iodide pool and is reutilized for new hormone synthesis (Fig. 53.2). A defect in thyroidal iodotyrosine deiodinase leads to a release of iodotyrosines into the circulation and their excretion in the urine. The loss from the thyroid gland of this normally recycled iodine, amounting to 70% to 80% of the daily thyroidal iodine supply, can significantly compromise thyroid hormone synthesis.

Some Tg is released into the circulation or the perivascular compartment during the process of synthesis, and there is good evidence that Tg reaches the general circulation via thyroidal lymphatics. Circulating Tg levels are high in premature infants during the first weeks of life, and values decrease with age throughout infancy and childhood (2,3). Circulating Tg concentrations in normal children range from 2 to 70 ng per mL. Values increase after TSH administration and decrease during thyroid hormone administration.

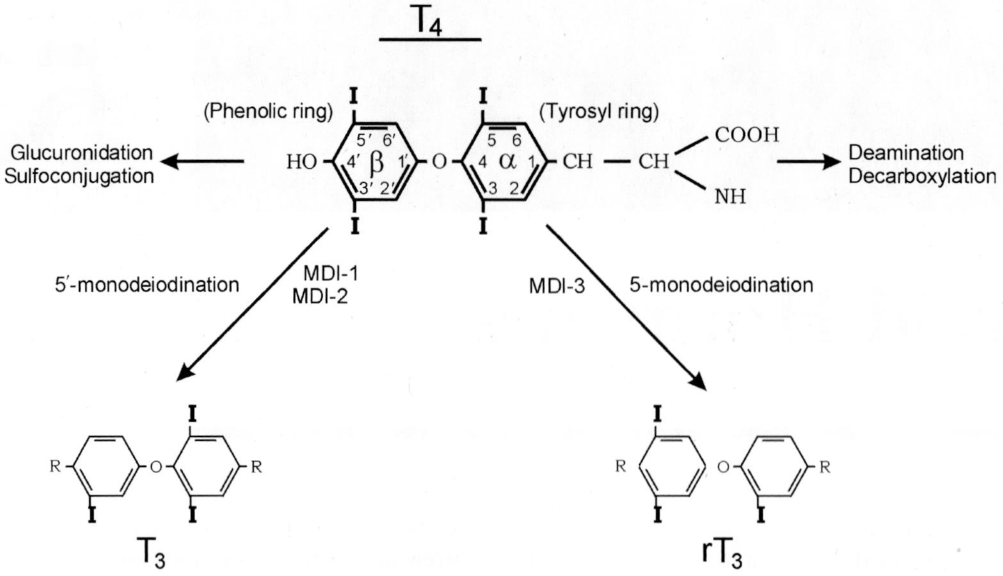

Figure 53.1. The metabolism of thyroxine (tetraiodothyronine). The major metabolic pathway is progressive monodeiodination by the three iodothyronine deiodinase enzymes, MDI-1, MDI-2, and MDI-3. Outer (phenolic) ring 5′-monodeiodination produces active 3,5,3′-triiodothyronine. Inner (tyrosyl) ring 5-monodeiodination produces inactive reverse (3,3′,5′) triiodothyronine. MDI-1 is also capable of inner ring monodeiodination. The alanine side chain of the tyrosyl ring is subject to deamination and decarboxylation. Sulfoconjugation and glucuronide conjugation reactions at the 4′-phenolic ring site occur in liver tissue.

REGULATION OF THYROID FUNCTION

Thyroid follicular cell function is regulated largely by circulating TSH and iodide levels (1,2,4). TSH stimulates production of intracellular cyclic adenosine monophosphate (cAMP), and cAMP appears to mediate most of the effects of TSH on thyroid metabolism. Pituitary TSH secretion is modulated by hypothalamic thyrotropin-releasing hormone (TRH) and negative feedback action of thyroid hormones. TRH stimulates TSH release and increases TSH synthesis as well as TSH glycosylation. Feedback control is mediated via pituitary cell T_3 nuclear receptors that modulate TSH synthesis and pituitary cell membrane TRH-receptor binding. Increased thyroid hormone levels inhibit and decreased concentrations stimulate pituitary TSH synthesis. The rate of pituitary TSH release is the net effect of the stimulation by TRH and the inhibitory effect of T_3 (see Fig. 53.3). Hypothalamic TRH production is modulated by environmental temperature via both peripheral and central (hypothalamic) thermal receptors. Decreasing environmental and body temperatures increases TRH production and increases the tonic level of TSH release. Thyroid hormones also modulate TRH synthesis within the hypothalamus.

The TRH neurons in the paraventricular hypothalamic nucleus receive input from other regions of the brain and from the circulation (4). The major afferent links to these neurons include catecholamine neurons in the brain stem and neurons from the arcuate nucleus. The former likely mediates upregulation of the TRH gene during cold exposure, while the latter mediates downregulation during starvation and illness (4). Administration of the adipocyte hormone leptin, the production of which falls during fasting, prevents the fasting-induced fall in TSH. In addition, central administration of α-melanocyte-stimulating hormone (α-MSH) prevents the fasting-induced suppression of TSH. Agouti-related peptide and neuropeptide are orexigenic peptides that are downregulated by leptin and upregulated during fasting. When administered centrally, both can suppress TRH and TSH secretion. Thus, the arcuate nucleus integrates leptin signaling and assists in the regulation of TRH gene expression as well as food intake and energy expenditure (4).

The average level of plasma iodide also is an important factor in the control of thyroid gland function (1,2). Variation in iodine intake in the physiologic range regulates thyroid membrane iodide trapping, and in pharmacologic doses iodide will block thyroid hormone synthesis. At least one important mechanism for these effects is the inhibitory action of iodide on the stimulation of cAMP by TSH.

METABOLISM OF THYROID HORMONES

The thyroid gland is the sole source of T_4, but most of the T_3 in the blood is derived from nonglandular sources via monodeiodination of T_4 in peripheral tissues (1,2) (see Fig. 53.3). Both T_3 and T_4 in the blood are associated with plasma proteins; the binding affinities of these proteins are greater for T_4 than T_3 and the concentration of T_4 in human blood is 50 to 100 times greater than that of T_3 (5). The concentrations of both are relatively constant in the

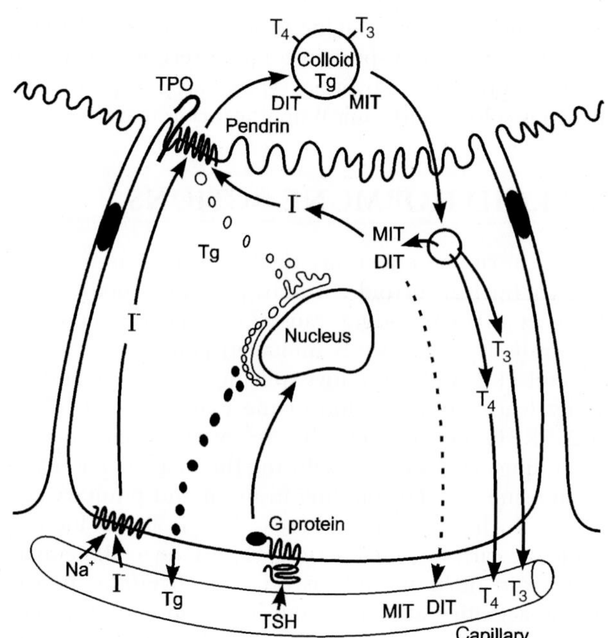

Figure 53.2. Drawing of the thyroid follicular cell illustrating thyroid hormone synthesis and secretion. TSH regulates the process through the G protein-linked plasma membrane TSH receptor. TSH binding stimulates thyroglobulin (Tg) synthesis and sodium-iodide symporter uptake of circulating iodide. Small amounts of Tg are secreted, presumably from the endoplasmic reticulum into the thyroid lymphatics. The tyrosine residues of thyroglobulin are iodinated at the apical cell membrane catalyzed by thyroid peroxidase, the organification enzyme. The pendrin protein, a chloride/iodide transporter located at the apical cell membrane, facilitates organification. The resulting monoiodotyrosine (MIT), and diiodotyrosine (DIT) moieties with appropriate spatial orientation couple to form thyroxine (T_4) and triiodothyronine (T_3) within the stored thyroglobulin molecule. TSH also stimulates endocytosis of colloid droplets and progressive thyroglobulin proteolysis within the resulting phagolysosomes. The released T_4 and T_3 are secreted into the circulation. The uncoupled MIT and DIT are deiodinated by iodotyrosine deiodinase to release iodide, which is largely recycled within the follicular cell.

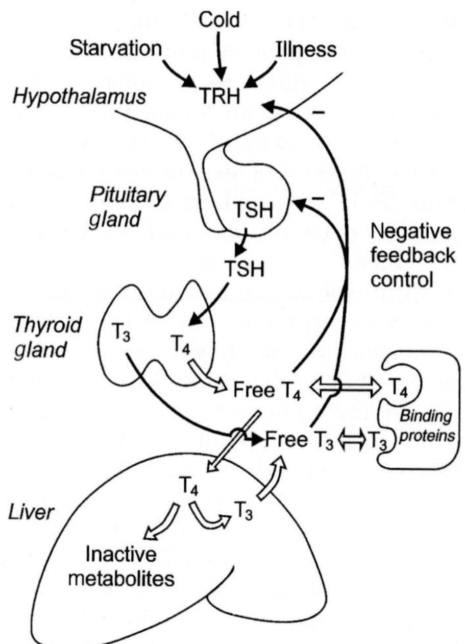

Figure 53.3. Drawing of the hypothalamic–pituitary–thyroid axis. Hypothalamic TRH stimulates pituitary TSH production, which increases thyroid follicular cell activity and thyroid hormone secretion. Most T_3 is produced in peripheral tissues (here shown as liver) from T_4 catalyzed by iodothyronine deiodinase enzymes. The deiodination process produces approximately similar amounts of T_3 and reverse (inactive) T_3 or rT_3 (see Fig. 53.1). Most circulating T_4 and T_3 are protein bound. The free fractions act via a negative feedback loop to inhibit TRH and TSH maintaining serum free hormone levels within a narrow physiologic range. TSH secretion is regulated by negative feedback of thyroid hormones on hypothalamic TRH secretion and pituitary TSH synthesis and secretion. This feedback is mediated via TRβ thyroid receptors. Cold exposure, starvation or fasting, and nonthyroidal illness also modulate TRH and TSH secretion. See text for details.

steady state. The plasma half-life of T_4 in adult humans approximates 5 days; the half-life of T_3 approximates 1 day. The circulating thyroid hormone-binding proteins include T_4-binding inter-alpha globulin (TBG), T_4-binding prealbumin (transthyretin), and albumin. TBG is the most important carrier protein for T_4; TBG and albumin seem equally important for T_3. The euthyroid steady-state concentrations of free T_4 and free T_3 approximate 0.02% and 0.20%, respectively, of the total hormone concentrations. Absolute mean free T_4 and T_3 concentrations approximate 1.5 and 0.3 ng per dL, respectively. In adolescents and adults, the plasma concentrations of the several binding proteins are 1 to 4 mg per dL for TBG, 10 to 20 mg per dL for transthyretin, and 2 to 5 g per dL for albumin. TBG levels are higher in children than in adults and decrease progressively to adult levels during adolescence.

Two major extravascular kinetic pools of T_3 and T_4 probably exist, one in which plasma–tissue interchange is rapid (chiefly liver, kidney, and lung) and one in which exchange is slow (chiefly skeletal, muscle, and skin) (6). An additional pool, chiefly in gut and bone, with an intermediate exchange rate has been suggested. Peak T_4 concentrations after single-pulse doses of labeled hormone occur in these "pools" in minutes, hours, and days, respectively. Total body T_4 distribution in adults has been estimated as follows: about 20% in plasma, 30% in fast tissues, 45% in slow tissues, and 5% in intermediate tissues.

Deiodination is the major pathway of thyroid hormone metabolism in humans. The first step in T_4 metabolism is conversion either to T_3 or to reverse T_3 (1,2,7) (Fig. 53.1). Monodeiodination of the β or outer (hydroxyl) ring produces T_3, which has three to four times the metabolic potency of T_4. Monodeiodination of the α or inner ring produces rT_3, which is metabolically inactive. Two types of outer ring iodothyronine monodeiodinase have been described (Fig. 53.1). MDI-1, predominantly expressed in liver, kidney, and thyroid, is a high Km enzyme, inhibited by propylthiouracil (PTU), and stimulated by thyroid hormone. MDI-2 also is capable of inner ring monodeiodination, particularly of T_4 sulfate (to rT_3 sulfate) and T_3 sulfate (to T_2 sulfate) (7,8). MDI-2, predominantly located in brain, pituitary, placenta, skeletal muscle, heart, thyroid, and brown adipose tissues (BATs), is a low Km enzyme insensitive to PTU and inhibited by thyroid hormone. Both MDI-1 and MDI-2 contribute to circulating T_3 production while MDI-2 acts as well to increase local tissue levels of T_3 (7,8). A third inner (tyrosyl) ring iodothyronine monodeiodinase (MDI-3) has been characterized in most tissues, including brain and placenta and more recently in uterus and fetal skin. This enzyme system catalyzes the conversion of T_4 to rT_3 and T_3 to diiodothyronine.

From 70% to 90% of circulating T_3 is derived from peripheral conversion and 10% to 25% from the thyroid gland; relative values for reverse T_3 are 96% to 98% and 2% to 4%. Progressive tissue monodeiodination reactions degrade T_3 and rT_3 to diiodo-, monoiodo-, and noniodinated thyronine. Conjugation of the phenolic ring hydroxyl group to sulfate or glucuronide produces glucuronide or sulfate analogues of the iodothyronines (7,8). These are inactivating reactions because the analogues formed do not bind to thyroid hormone receptors and are rapidly metabolized by MDI-1 or excreted in bile (7,8). The exception is T_3 sulfate which demonstrates some 20% of native T_3 bioactivity when injected into hypothyroid rats. This presumably is due to the action of tissue sulfatases or bacterial sulfatases in the intestine (8).

The alanine side chain of the inner ring of the hormones also is subject to degradative reactions, including deamination, and decarboxylation (7,8). Pyruvic acid analogues and small amounts of a lactic acid analogues have been observed in urine and bile; these have minimal biologic activity. Two enzymes, L-amino acid oxidase and thyroid hormone aminotransferase, catalyze the deamination of T_4 and T_3 to their acetic acid analogues tetrac and triac (7,8). Triac binds to the T_3 nuclear receptor with greater avidity than T_3 and demonstrates significant biologic activity when injected into animals or humans. However, relatively large doses are required because of rapid clearance and degradation via deiodination and glucuronidation (7,8). Triac has been utilized in the treatment of thyroid hormone resistance. T_4 and T_3 are potent proangiogenic agents in the chick chorioallantoic membrane model of angiogenesis and in human dermal microvascular endothelial cell assays (9). These actions are mediated via a plasma membrane hormone receptor site on integrin $\alpha_v\beta_3$. Tetrac has been shown to block this binding and to inhibit thyroid hormone action on tumor cell proliferation. Tetrac has no agonist activity at the hormone receptor site (9).

Recently, two novel thyroid hormone derivatives, 3-iodothyronamine (T1AM) and thyronamine (T0AM), products of combined thyroid hormone decarboxylation and deiodination, have been shown in mice to induce transient hypothermia, decrease aortic pressure, block carbohydrate utilization, and increase fat utilization (10,11). These molecules are present in mammalian brain, peripheral organs, thyroid gland, and blood serum. T1AM is strongly protein bound and circulating concentrations are in the microgram per deciliter range similar to T_4 (12). It has been proposed that these thionamines act via a thyronamine G-protein-coupled receptor such as the trace amine-associated receptor (TAAR1), a 7-transmembrane, G-protein-coupled receptor related to catecholamine and 5-hydroxytryptophan receptors (10). Their physiologic and clinical significance remain unclear.

THYROID HORMONE ACTIONS

Thyroid hormone effects are mediated predominantly by means of nuclear thyroid hormone protein receptors (TR), which act as DNA binding transcription factors regulating gene transcription. Two mammalian genes code for TR, Trα, and TRβ, and alternative splicing of expressed mRNA species leads to production of the major isoforms Trα1, Trα2, TRβ1, and TRβ2 (13–16). In rodent species, hepatic TR-binding activity matures during the first 3 to 5 weeks of extrauterine life. Trα binding in brain and pituitary cells appears during fetal life, whereas TRβ isoforms increase during the early neonatal period (15). In the fetal/neonatal rat, thyroid hormone effects on thermogenesis, hepatic enzyme activities, skin and brain maturation, and growth hormone (GH) metabolism mature largely during the first 4 postnatal weeks (16,17).

In the human fetus, low levels of T_4 binding have been detected in brain tissue at 10 weeks of gestational age, and hepatic, cardiac, and lung TR binding are observed at 16 to 18 weeks (16,18). Information is limited regarding the timing of appearance of thyroid hormone postreceptor effects in the human fetus. The length, weight, appearance, behavior, biochemical parameters, extrauterine adaptation, and early neonatal course of the athyroid human neonate usually are normal (16,18). Growth of the human fetus is programmed independent of thyroid hormones by a complex interplay of genetic, nutritional, hormonal, and growth factors.

Postnatal thermogenesis is mediated through BAT, prominent in subscapular and perirenal areas in the mammalian fetus and neonate. Heat production in BAT is stimulated by catecholamines by means of β-adrenergic receptors and is thyroid hormone dependent. The uncoupling protein thermogenin, or UCP-1, unique to BAT, is located on the inner mitochondrial membrane and uncouples phosphorylation by dissipating the proton gradient created by the mitochondrial respiratory chain. An iodothyronine deiodinase (MDI) in BAT mediates local T_4 to T_3 conversion. Full thermogenin expression in BAT requires both catecholamine and T_3 stimulation (19,20). UCP-2 is found in many tissues but does not appear to be regulated by β-adrenergic agonists or thyroid hormone. UCP-3 has been cloned and is expressed in muscle and white adipose tissue as well as BAT (20). Muscle UCP-3 is regulated by β_3-adrenergic stimulation and thyroid hormone and probably contributes to nonshivering thermogenesis in adult rats and presumably humans. UCP-3 mRNA levels also are regulated by dexamethasone, leptin, and starvation, but the regulation differs in BAT and muscle (20). TR-mediated thyroid hormone actions also include the synthesis of selected enzymes and proteins in liver; stimulation of myogenin, α-actin, and myosin synthesis in cardiac tissue; promotion of mammary gland development and gene expression; and stimulation of growth and development and central nervous system (CNS) maturation.

Studies in the rat model have characterized a profound effect of thyroid hormones on GH secretion and action (15,21). Hypothyroidism decreases pituitary GH content, impairs the pituitary GH response to GH-releasing hormone (GHRH), reduces basal and pulsatile GH secretion, and decreases circulating GH levels. Similar effects have been observed in hypothyroid human subjects. Hypothyroid patients show limited GH responses to insulin hypoglycemia, arginine, and GHRH, reduced nocturnal GH secretion, and reduced circulating levels of insulin-like growth factor I, (IGFI), IGF-II, IGF-binding protein-3, GH-binding protein, and bioactive IGF (22–24). There is also evidence that thyroid hormones stimulate production of other growth factors, including epidermal growth factor, nerve growth factor, and erythropoietin and have direct actions on bone, potentiating the cartilage response to IGF-I, and stimulating osteoblastic bone resorption and remodeling (25–27).

These hormonal and growth factor deficiencies contribute importantly to the disordered growth of hypothyroid infants and children, including the decreased long-bone growth, delayed bone maturation, decreased carcass growth, delayed tooth eruption, and anemia. The actions of thyroid hormones and GH are synergistic. GH administered to neonatal hypophysectomized rats increases body weight, but it has a limited effect on skeletal growth; in contrast, thyroxine accelerates skeletal growth and potentiates the GH effects. Combined treatment optimizes growth and development (21). The vast majority of infants with congenital hypothyroidism (CH) are born with normal or increased length and weight, and early adequate thyroid hormone treatment prevents development of growth retardation. There may be a transient period of growth deceleration during the early weeks of treatment (27), but even in infants with severe CH, manifested by very low serum T_4 concentrations and delayed bone maturation at birth, early, adequate treatment results in mean height and body mass index equal to or greater than values in normal children (28–31). Bone age values also are normalized by 2 to 3 years (32,33). Bone mineral density and metabolism also are normal in treated children given adequate nutrition (34).

The effects of thyroid hormones on growth and physical development extend through most of the second decade, and delayed or inadequate replacement therapy during childhood or adolescence can reduce adult height (35). Thyroxine treatment in children with growth retardation due to a prolonged period of untreated hypothyroidism usually induces marked catch-up growth, but in some instances this is inadequate to normalize adult height (35,36). Adult height is generally inversely correlated with the duration of untreated hypothyroidism prior to the advent of puberty (35). This is thought to be due to the onset of puberty, limiting the chance to achieve full growth catch-up before epiphyseal fusion. Suppression of pubertal development by administration of gonadotropin-releasing hormone plus GH was shown to improve height gain in a juvenile hypothyroid patient (35).

The critical role of thyroid hormones in CNS maturation has long been recognized. The first phase of fetal CNS maturation (neuronal multiplication, migration, and organization) occurs during the second trimester of gestation. A second phase (glial cell multiplication, migration, and myelinization) occurs during the perinatal period and extends through 3 to 4 postnatal year (16,18). Available evidence suggests that deficiency or excess of thyroid hormones alters the timing or synchronization of the CNS developmental program, presumably by altering critical homeobox gene cascades and other genetic CNS maturation events (16,18). Prior to activation of fetal thyroid function by the fetal hypothalamic–pituitary complex at midgestation, the fetus is dependent on maternal thyroid hormone which traverses the placenta in limited amounts. Several studies have shown that maternal hypothyroidism, often due to Hashimoto autoimmune thyroiditis, impairs the subsequent neuropsychological development of the offspring; even mild maternal hypothyroidism has been shown to reduce offspring IQ by 4 to 7 points (36,37).

Severe iodine deficiency with combined maternal and fetal hypothyroidism results in severe neurological impairment (cretinism), and mild endemic iodine deficiency, producing mild maternal and childhood hypothyroxinemia, has been shown to reduce the mean IQ of children (37). Sixty percent to 70% of postnatal brain growth and differentiation occurs during the first 2 years of life, and it is during this period that the CNS effects of hypothyroidism are most devastating (38). Untreated, severe CH is associated with an IQ deficit of 4 to 6 points per month during the first 5 to 7 months of postnatal life (17,37). Such infants treated promptly at birth have minimal IQ impairment, being protected in utero by the limited amounts of maternal thyroxine crossing the placenta (39–42). However, overall, a mean 6-point IQ deficit has been shown in a meta-analysis of published treatment outcome papers (40). This deficit is largely due to infants with severe disease with intrauterine hypothyroidism manifest as delayed bone maturation at birth (41,42). These data, summarized in Table 53.1, emphasize the critical role of

TABLE 53.1 Effects of Thyroid Hormone Deficiency Relative to Phase of Central Nervous System Development

Cause of Thyroid Hormone Deficiency	*Phase of CNS Development*[a]	*Severity of CNS Damage to Child*[b]
Maternal hypothyroidism	I	+
Congenital hypothyroidism		
Untreated	I + II	++++
Newborn treated	I	± to +
Combined maternal–fetal hypothyroidism (newborn treated)	I	++
Endemic iodine deficiency (no treatment)		
Mild to moderate	I + II	+ to ++
Severe	I + II	++++

[a]Phase I, neuronal multiplication, migration, and organization during second trimester of gestation; phase II, glial cell multiplication, migration, and myelinization during perinatal period and extending through 3–4 yr of age.
[b]+, 4–7 IQ points; ++++, 30–40 IQ points.

thyroid hormones in CNS development both in utero and during infancy and early childhood.

RELATIVE EFFECTS OF THYROID HORMONES VERSUS AGE

Thyroid hormone actions vary with age. Thyroid hormone deficiency during human fetal life has minimal untoward effects. Somatic growth and development and linear bone growth proceed normally in the athyroid fetus, and bone maturation is normal or minimally retarded (3 to 6 weeks) at birth (43–45). The reason(s) for the relative lack of thyroid hormone effect on fetal somatic growth is not clear. Likely explanations include low levels of active thyroid hormone in fetal serum and tissues and/or immaturity of thyroid hormone receptor responsiveness at the transcription, translation, or action levels (17,46,47).

The developmental effects of thyroid hormones, such as the CNS effects, are most obvious during infancy and early childhood. Somatic growth, bone growth and maturation, and tooth development and eruption are thyroid dependent. After 3 to 4 years of age, thyroid hormone deficiency is not associated with mental retardation, but delayed somatic and linear bone growth and delayed eruption of permanent dentition are prominent. Bone maturation, measured as bone age, also is delayed, diaphyseal bone growth is reduced, and epiphyseal growth and mineralization largely cease (2,27).

Hypothalamic and anterior pituitary function also may be abnormal in hypothyroid children. Although in most children thyroid hormone deficiency leads to a delayed sexual development, occasional children manifest precocious sexual maturation with increased levels of circulating gonadotropins (48–50). In female patients, serum prolactin levels also tend to be increased, and galactorrhea may occur if serum estrogen levels are high enough to permit breast development and milk production. These changes seem to occur in children with high serum TSH levels, and enlargement of the sella turcica has been observed. The increased serum prolactin levels are probably explained by the fact that TRH stimulates both TSH and prolactin release from the pituitary. A paracrine action of the hyperstimulated thyrotropic cells on gonadotrope cells may explain the increased gonadotropin secretion. Precocious puberty is observed only rarely, so it is possible that these patients have genetic variants of the gonadotropin receptors, which can be stimulated by the increased TSH levels (51). Similar findings have been reported for TSH and follicle-stimulating hormone (FSH) receptor variants stimulated by βHCG (51,52). When the hypothyroid state is alleviated, the manifestations of sexual precocity regress, and normal puberty ensues when the general level of maturity has progressed appropriately.

During childhood and adolescence and until epiphyseal closure, thyroid hormone deficiency leads to reduced somatic growth, reduced linear bone growth, and delayed bone maturation. In addition, epiphyseal dysgenesis is commonly observed (27,53). The effects of thyroid hormone deficiency on dental development are less profound, but delay in eruption of second dentition may occur. Abnormalities of hypothalamic–pituitary function secondary to hypothyroidism also are common in adolescence (2,27). Puberty often is delayed or incomplete. In normal women, menstrual cycles commonly are nonovulatory and bleeding may be irregular. This pattern usually is more prolonged in hypothyroid female adolescents. In addition, menorrhagia or hypomenorrhea may occur.

THYROID FUNCTION DURING INFANCY AND CHILDHOOD

IODINE METABOLISM

During prepubertal and pubertal periods of growth and development, there is a progressive growth of the thyroid gland, a progressive increase in thyroid Tg and iodothyronine stores, and a progressive increase in T_4 production rate, measured in micrograms per day (2). Measured as microgram per gram thyroid or as production relative to body mass, T_4 production decreases progressively, roughly in parallel with metabolic rate (calorie intake) (Fig. 53.4). The iodide space (on a body weight basis) in infants is relatively larger than in older children, adolescents, or adults and the thyroid iodide clearance rate is nearly three times that of adults (2). Renal iodide clearance also is high in infants and decreases progressively with age. The progressive decrease in thyroid iodide clearance may be, at least in part, secondary to the change in renal iodide clearance.

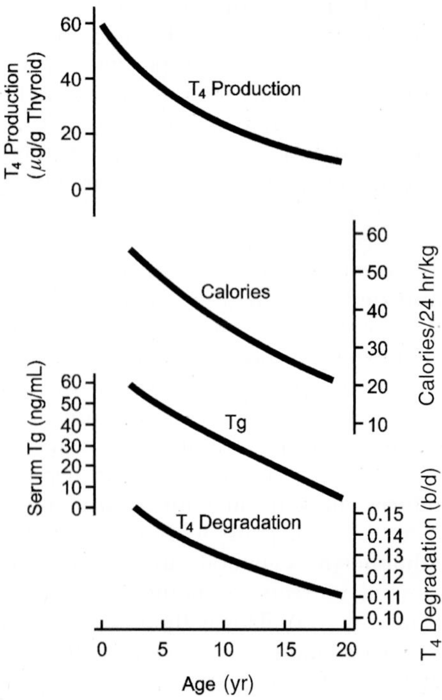

Figure 53.4. Thyroid function during childhood is characterized by a progressive increase in thyroid gland size and thyroid hormone production in μg/d. However, interpreted as μg/g thyroid gland or T_4 degradation rate (fraction of the thyroxine pool degraded daily), T_4 production decreases roughly in parallel with the decrease in metabolic rate (as calories/kg/d). The serum thyroglobulin (Tg) concentration decreases reflecting the relative decreases in T_4 secretion.

During childhood, the growth of the thyroid gland in residents of iodine-sufficient areas roughly parallels body growth. The gland volume, measured by ultrasound, increases in size from about 1.0 g at birth to a mean of about 5 g at 10 years of age. Average thyroid iodine content increases from 0.3 mg at birth to 16 mg in adolescents and adults (2,54,55). In areas of severe iodine deficiency, the thyroid weight in newborns may be 2 to 3 g, and iodine content may be as low as 40 μg. The iodide space also increases progressively in volume with age; however, the relative size (in liters per kilogram, expressed as percentage of body weight) decreases from about 50% of body weight at birth to 40% in 30-kg children (at about age 10 years) (2,56,57). These values can be compared with the 33% body weight values in 65-kg adults.

Radioiodine uptake and clearance during childhood and adolescence vary with diet and iodine intake. Values during the first 2 decades have been reported to decrease progressively or remain relatively stable (2,58). This discrepancy presumably is caused by variations in iodine intake. The data showing a decrease with age were from areas of low iodine intake in Europe and Australia. A relatively high iodine intake could tend to mask differences in uptake with age. Thyroid iodine clearance (per gram of thyroid tissue) decreases progressively with age, associated with a progressive decrease in T_4 production rate (or turnover) on a microgram per kilogram per day basis.

SERUM THYROID HORMONE CONCENTRATIONS AND T_4 PRODUCTION

Serum total free T_4 and T_3 concentrations decrease gradually with age (2). The decrease in serum total T_4 and T_3 result largely from a decrease in serum TBG concentrations that is progressive from early childhood through 15 to 16 years of age, when the mean serum TBG concentration is about the same as in adults. Reciprocal changes occur in serum transthyretin concentrations. These changes presumably reflect the effects of gonadal steroids, but other factors may be involved.

Serum free T_4 concentrations decrease slightly during childhood and adolescence (2,59,60). The percentage of iodine-131-labeled protein-bound iodine appearing in blood (percentage of dose per liter per kilogram of body weight) after labeling of the thyroid gland also decreases with age during the first 2 decades, as does T_4 turnover and production rate on a body weight basis (microgram per kilogram per day) (2,57). Estimated T_4 turnover or production rate values are 5 to 6 μg per kg per day in infants, 4 μg per kg per day in children aged 1 to 3 years, 2 to 3 μg per kg per day in children aged 3 to 9 years, and 1 μg per kg per day in adults.

The serum concentration of rT_3 remains unchanged or increases slightly during childhood and adolescence. The serum free rT_3 index (total rT_3 × fractional T_3 resin uptake) remains stable or increases slightly. Because circulating rT_3 is derived predominantly from peripheral deiodination of T_4, these observations and the fact that the mean calculated ratios of serum rT_3/serum T_4 and the free rT_3 index/free T_4 index increase progressively with age suggest that the relative rate of T_4 deiodination to rT_3 increases with age during childhood and adolescence (61). Direct measurements have not been made. The decreases with age in the ratios of serum T_3/serum rT_3 and the free T_3 index/free rT_3 index suggests a progressive decrease in the relative conversion of T_4 to T_3 with age during the first 2 decades (61).

The progressive decrease in thyroid gland T_4 production (microgram per gram), T_4 turnover, serum Tg, and thyroidal radioiodine uptake indicates a progressive relative decrease in thyroid function with age (2). The decreasing serum TSH concentration with age suggests that these decreases are mediated primarily by reduced TSH secretion. Whether this reflects decreased TRH secretion or a non-TRH mechanism is not clear. A progressive reduction in thyroid gland TSH responsiveness might also be involved.

THYROID HORMONE PREPARATIONS

The thyroid hormones as shown in Figure 53.1 are iodine-containing amino acid derivatives of thyronine (1,2). The structural requirements for bioactivity have been well defined. The two aromatic rings are essential, as is the ether linkage. The alanine side chain in position 1; halogen or methyl groups in positions 3, 5, and 3′; and the hydroxyl group in position 4 are all necessary for optimal activity. The natural hormones are levorotatory; the dextrorotatory isomers have 10% or less of the bioactivity of the L-isomers. The d-T_4 isomer had been utilized clinically in the past as a cholesterol-lowering agent but has no role in replacement therapy. Triiodothyroacetic acid (TRIAC) binds to the thyroid hormone receptor as effectively as T_3 in vitro but has a much shorter half-life in vivo. It is not available for routine clinical use but has been proposed for treatment of TSH-dependent hyperthyroidism (pituitary T_3 resistance). Tetrac and the thionamines are not available.

Several preparations of thyroid hormones are available, as summarized in Table 53.2. Na-1-thyroxine (T_4) and Na-1-triiodothyronine (T_3) are synthetic preparations of the natural hormones. These hormones also are available in combination in a 4:1 ratio of T_4 to T_3. Thyroid USP is a dried and powdered preparation of porcine or bovine thyroid gland.

Na-1-thyroxine is the drug of choice for replacement therapy. It is uniform in potency, is easily measured in serum, and it provides physiologic serum T_3 levels, since most of the circulating T_3 normally is derived from T_4 by monodeiodination in tissues. Most synthetic T_4 preparations

TABLE 53.2 Preparation and Relative Potencies of Thyroid Hormone Preparations

Preparation	*Source*	*Equivalent Dosage*
Na-1-thyroxine	Synthetic	100 μg
Na-1-triiodothyronine	Synthetic	25 μg
Na-1-thyroxine (80%) + Na-1-triiodothyronine (20%)	Synthetic	50–2.5 μg
Thyroid (USP)	Natural	60 mg

have been reformulated since 1982 to guarantee specified hormone concentrations (62). Absorption of the hormone is variable, ranging from 50% to 100%; average absorption approximates 80% (62).

There is only limited application for Na-l-triiodothyronine (T_3) in thyroid therapy. Absorption of T_3 is nearly complete after oral administration, but the serum half-life is short (1 day vs. 5 days for T_4). Blood levels are more variable and more difficult to stabilize. In adult patients with hypothyroidism, it has been suggested that partial substitution of triiodothyronine for thyroxine replacement therapy may improve mood and neuropsychological function, and it has been shown in hypothyroid adult rats that such dual treatment more reliably reproduces normal tissue levels of thyroxine and triiodothyronine (63,64). However, there is no consensus favoring combined therapy at the present time and serum and tissue levels of T_3 are normalized with T_4 therapy alone (65,66). T_3 may be useful in the early treatment of severe hypothyroidism in older children or for short-term suppression studies. It may also be useful in management of TSH-dependent hyperthyroidism.

THERAPY WITH THYROID HORMONES

CONGENITAL HYPOTHYROIDISM

Infants with congenital hypothyroidism (CH) usually have thyroid dysgenesis due to abnormal thyroid gland embryogenesis. They may have agenesis or have a residual hypoplastic gland in the normal or an ectopic location. Ten percent to 15% have an inborn abnormality in TSH secretion or response (hypothalamic–pituitary hypothyroidism) or in thyroid hormone synthesis (16,17,60). Less commonly, transient neonatal hypothyroidism can be caused by exposure to an antithyroid drug or chemical or an antithyroid antibody derived transplacentally from the mother.

In infants with CH, initial treatment with 10 to 15 μg per kg T_4 daily is desirable to consistently normalize the serum T_4 concentration (to >10 μg per dL) within 2 to 4 weeks particularly in infants with severe CH (16,17,39,67). This amounts to an initial treatment dose of 50 μg daily in most term infants. It is now clear that the major source of brain cell T_3, the receptor-active hormone, is serum T_4. Some 70% of T_3 in the cerebral cortex of neonatal rats is derived from local monodeiodination of T_4 (68–70). Thus, institution of replacement T_4 in a dose adequate to rapidly normalize the serum T_4 concentration is essential to minimize the period of CNS T_4 deficiency and help ensure optimal brain development. Replacement therapy with T_3 or mixtures of T_4 and T_3 is not recommended.

Careful monitoring of individual infants and dosage adjustment are necessary during the early weeks and months of life to guarantee adequate treatment and prevent prolonged hyperthyroxinemia. Premature synostosis with and without brain dysfunction has been reported in association with neonatal thyrotoxicosis or with excessive thyroid hormone doses in the treatment of CH (71–73). In the latter cases, the T_4 doses were in the 200 to 300 μg per day range throughout most of infancy (73). The threshold and duration of T_4 secretion or dosage required to produce premature synostosis is not clear, but the modest

TABLE 53.3 Dose of Oral Thyroxine for Replacement Therapy of Infants and Children

Age	*Daily Dose (μg/kg/d)*	*Range of Dose (μg)*
1–6 mo	7–15	30–50
6–12 mo	4–8	50–100
1–5 yr	5–6	75–150
5–10 yr	3–4	100–200
10–20 yr	1.5–3	100–250

doses recommended with careful monitoring produce little risk. It is useful to obtain serum 12 to 24 hours after the last T_4 dose to avoid the effect of transient and variable absorption. The T_4 dose can be altered so that the serum free T_4 concentration is in the upper half of the normal range.

The serum TSH concentration may be inappropriately elevated in infants with CH and may not be suppressed to normal levels with treatment (66,74,75). Adequate treatment probably should suppress serum TSH values to less than 15 mU per L by 1 to 2 months (39,67). Although the early weeks and months of treatment are critical for infants with CH, the CNS is thyroid hormone dependent for 2 to 4 years, and growth is thyroid hormone dependent during the first 2 decades of life (2,27). Thus, careful monitoring of treatment is required throughout childhood and adolescence. The total dosage of T_4 increases progressively to 200 to 250 μg daily in adolescence (Table 53.3). The dosage on a kilogram body weight basis decreases progressively to the adult value of 1.5 μg per kg per day.

Adequacy of therapy is judged by clinical evidence of normal growth and development and lack of signs and symptoms of toxicity. Growth in length and weight should be plotted monthly during the first 3 months and at 2- to 3-month intervals thereafter during the first year. Bone age should be assessed at 3 months and at 6 to 12 months of treatment. Thereafter, 12- to 24-month evaluations will suffice through 3 to 4 years. Measurements of circulating hormone concentrations are essential to assess adequacy of treatment. Measurements of T_4, TSH, and, on occasion, T_3 are helpful. Serum T_4 and free T_4 levels should be adjusted to the upper half of the normal range for age. At this time, the serum TSH level should be normal or mildly increased and the serum T_3 concentration within the normal range for age (16,17,66).

If the hypothyroidism is secondary, due to hypothalamic–pituitary dysfunction, treatment with adrenal corticosteroids and GH is necessary as deficiencies of adrenocorticotropic hormone (ACTH) and GH are documented (76). Adrenal insufficiency may be manifested as failure to thrive and/or hypoglycemia in the neonatal period. GH deficiency also may contribute to hypoglycemia and may impair growth after 3 to 6 months (76).

ACQUIRED HYPOTHYROIDISM

Acquired hypothyroidism before 5 to 6 years most commonly results from delayed failure of the thyroid remnant in infants with thyroid dysgenesis, but inborn defects in thyroid hormone synthesis, ingested goitrogens, chronic thyroiditis, or hypothalamic–pituitary disease may be involved. After 5 to 6 years of age, hypothyroidism usually is due to chronic lymphocytic (Hashimoto) thyroiditis. Surgery or radioiodine treatment also can result in hypothyroidism (2).

Irreversible brain damage is not a likely result of hypothyroidism acquired after 2 to 3 years of age. By this time, CNS growth is largely complete. Delayed growth, however, may be marked and most commonly is manifest as delayed tooth development and eruption, delayed skeletal growth and maturation, and linear growth retardation. Aberrations in pubertal development and menstrual irregularities are common (2). These manifestations are reversible with adequate replacement therapy. As in infants, the treatment of choice is oral Na-l-thyroxine. The replacement dose on a body weight basis decreases progressively with age (Table 53.3). The dosage should be adjusted at 2- to 4-month intervals to a level that maintains the serum T_4 concentration in the mid-range of normal together with normal T_3 and TSH concentrations. In contrast to adults, it is not necessary in most children with hypothyroidism to increase the dose of replacement T_4 gradually. Initial administration of the total daily estimated replacement dose will result in a gradual increase in serum T_4 concentrations over a 3- to 4-week period. If cardiac disease is suspected, more gradual replacement may be indicated.

Treatment of secondary hypothyroidism in childhood or adolescence may require simultaneous replacement with adrenal corticosteroids, GH, and gonadal steroid(s). Hashimoto thyroiditis is the most common cause of acquired hypothyroidism (2). It is an autoimmune disease associated with progressive autoimmune damage to thyroid follicular cells. The disease most frequently involves only the thyroid gland. Occasionally, however, Hashimoto thyroiditis is associated with other endocrine gland autoimmune deficiencies (77,78). These include diabetes mellitus, adrenal insufficiency, hypoparathyroidism, and, on rare occasions, hypogonadism. Autoimmune gastritis with pernicious anemia and cutaneous moniliasis are sometimes associated. Treatment of these other endocrine gland deficiencies may be necessary.

Hashimoto thyroiditis presents early as a mild-to-moderate euthyroid goiter. The disease remits spontaneously in about one-third of children (2). The remainder gradually develops hypothyroidism. There is no specific therapy, but if the goiter is large, if the serum TSH concentration is elevated, or if the patient is clinically hypothyroid, replacement therapy with Na-l-thyroxine is indicated. Some physicians favor T_4 treatment of all children with Hashimoto thyroiditis to avoid the gradual onset of mild, undiagnosed hypothyroidism.

NONTOXIC DIFFUSE GOITER

Nontoxic diffuse goiter in childhood is often referred to as simple colloid goiter (2). It is most common during adolescence in female patients, where it has been referred to as adolescent goiter. These patients are euthyroid with mild-to-moderate goiters characterized histologically by large thyroid follicles rimmed by flattened epithelial cells. The glands usually are diffusely enlarged and of nearly normal consistency, but nodularity can occur. The etiology is unclear, but some of these patients manifest multinodular goiter as adults (79,80). Systematic studies of treatment of these patients with T_4 to "suppress" the goiter have not been conducted.

THYROID NODULES

Suppressive therapy with T_4 sometimes is used to differentiate benign from malignant thyroid nodules. Diagnostic procedures usually include thyroid scanning and/or fine needle biopsy (2). In the occasional patient with an inconclusive biopsy result, a trial of suppressive T_4 therapy may be useful. In this instance, the end point is a decrease in size of the nodule or a failure of further growth over a period of 6 to 12 months. The dose of T_4 is adjusted to suppress serum TSH concentrations to the very low or undetectable level (<0.02 U per mL) using a highly sensitive TSH assay method. This may require T_4 doses 30% to 50% higher than replacement doses. T_3 is not usually used for suppression because the half-life of serum levels is relatively short (1 day vs. 5 days for T_4), and T_4 provides more reliable TSH suppression.

ANTITHYROID DRUGS

Many compounds and chemicals have been shown to inhibit the synthesis and/or metabolism of thyroid hormones. The most important of these are the thioureylenes, the iodinated organic radiographic contrast agents, iodide, and radioactive iodine.

THE THIOUREYLENES

Astwood and colleagues in the 1940s characterized a series of thioureylene drugs that inhibit thyroid hormone synthesis via a thiocarbamide group (S = C–N) (81). Several compounds have been utilized for treatment of hyperthyroidism (81). These include thiourea, thiouracil, methylthiouracil, PTU, methimazole (MMI), and carbimazole (CBI). The drugs currently used to treat hyperthyroidism include PTU, MMI, and CBI (82). CBI acts by conversion to MMI. The thioureylene drugs act by inhibiting the organification of iodine via inhibition of thyroid peroxidase activity. Inhibition of hormone synthesis results in depletion of the thyroid stores of iodinated Tg and a progressive decrease in thyroid stores of iodinated Tg and a progressive decrease in thyroid hormone secretion from the thyroid gland. In addition to blocking hormone synthesis, PTU inhibits the peripheral conversion of T_4 to T_3; MMI does not share this action (82). Effective amounts of the drugs are absorbed within 30 to 60 minutes after an oral dose. The half-life of PTU in plasma approximates 2 hours and that of MMI 6 to 13 hours. The drugs are concentrated within the thyroid, and metabolites are excreted largely in urine. They cross the placenta and appear in breast milk.

There is a significant incidence of toxic reaction to all thioureylene drugs (82,83). The incidence of major and minor toxicities is summarized in Table 53.4. The most common minor reaction is a purpuric, papular rash, which usually is mild and subsides spontaneously. Other minor reactions include nausea, headache, paresthesias,

TABLE 53.4 Characteristics of Commonly Used Thioureylene Drugs

Drug	*Blood Half-Life (hr)*	*Initial Dose (mg/kg/dose)*	*Maintenance Dose (mg/kg/d)*	*Toxic Reactions*	
				Major (%)	*Minor (%)*
Propylthiouracil	2	5–8	1–3	0.9	2.2
Methimazole	6–13	0.5–0.7	0.1–0.3	1.4	4.5
Carbimazole	. . .	0.5–0.7	0.1–0.3	0.9	2.2

hair loss, and joint pain and stiffness. Agranulocytosis, the most serious reaction, is observed in 1 in 500 to 1 in 1,000 cases. It usually develops during the first few months of treatment and may develop rapidly. Mild granulocytopenia may be due to thyrotoxicosis or may be an early sign of serious drug toxicity. Drug fever, hepatitis, nephritis, and a lupus-like reaction are rare complications. Antineutrophil cytoplasmic antibodies (ANCA) are relatively common in PTU-treated patients (4% to 46%) while the incidence of ANCA-associated vasculitis is much lower (0% to 1.4%) (83).

Should granulocytopenia be observed, frequent leukocyte counts are indicated to rule out serious drug toxicity. Routine blood counts are not helpful, since agranulocytosis can develop after several months and may appear rapidly. **The United States Food and Drug Administration reports severe liver injury and acute renal failure in children and adults treated with PTU. They recommend reserving PTU for those who cannot tolerate other treatments, including MMI, radioactive iodine, or surgery.**

SODIUM IPODATE OR IOPANOATE

These iodinated organic radiographic contrast agents have been shown to be effective antithyroid drugs (84–89). They inhibit the enzymatic monodeiodination of T_4 to T_3 and produce a rapid reduction in serum T_3 concentrations. In addition, they inhibit thyroid hormone secretion from the thyroid gland so that serum T_4 levels also fall. Chronic treatment (6 to 12 months) has been successful in 50% to more than 90% of patients with Graves disease. Sodium ipodate may be more effective than sodium iopanoic acid, but data to date are limited in this regard. Sodium ipodate has been used successfully in infants with neonatal Graves disease (88).

No serious side effects of the contrast agents have been observed to date, but experience is limited. Interestingly, in contrast to iodide, permanent blockade of thyroid function does not occur and radioiodine treatment has been applied within 2 to 4 weeks of discontinuing sodium ipodate therapy (85). These agents may be very useful for treatment of patients who develop toxicity to thioureylene drugs. They may also be useful adjuncts to other antithyroid drug regimens and may be helpful in short-term preoperative or preradioiodine treatment of severe thyrotoxicosis.

IODIDE

Iodide is the oldest antithyroid drug. In large doses (>0.1 mg per kg per day), it inhibits thyroid iodide transport, iodothyronine synthesis, and thyroid hormone release (82). As a result, there is a rapid fall in serum thyroid hormone levels that may persist several weeks. Eventually, there is an "escape" from the thyroid iodide blockade mediated in part by the inhibition of thyroid cell membrane iodide transport and a reduction in intrathyroidal iodide concentrations. Thus, iodide usually is restricted to short-term therapy (several weeks). Iodide treatment has been used in the immediate preoperative period to prepare patients for thyroidectomy and for treatment of severe thyrotoxicosis or thyroid crisis in conjunction with thioureylene drugs.

Toxic reactions to iodide are observed occasionally (82). Acute life-threatening angioedema and laryngeal edema may occur with or without a cutaneous hemorrhagic rash. Serum sickness-like manifestations also have been observed with fever, arthralgia, eosinophilia, and lymphadenopathy. Chronic intoxication (iodism) also is described, including soreness of the teeth and gums, increased salivation, nasal irritation, swelling of the eyes, headache, and chronic cough. Acneiform skin lesions, gastric irritation, and diarrhea may occur. These signs and symptoms disappear within a few days after discontinuing iodide ingestion.

Iodide preparations include strong iodine solution (Lugol's solution) for oral use and sodium iodide for intravenous use. Lugol's solution is formulated as 5% iodine and 10% potassium iodide. The iodine is reduced to iodide in the intestine before absorption. Intravenous NaI is available as a 10% solution.

RADIOACTIVE IODINE

There are several clinically useful isotopes of radioiodine (90). These include I^{131}, I^{125}, and I^{123}. The half-lives are 8 days, 60 days, and 13 hours, respectively. Gamma ray–emitting isotopes are used for scanning, whereas β radiation is desirable for tissue radiation treatment. All three isotopes are gamma emitters and are used for thyroid scanning. ^{125}I and ^{123}I are preferred because they provide lower thyroid radiation doses. I^{131} is used for treatment because of its β radiation; the average absorbed β dose per gram tissue is approximately 10 rad per day per Ci. Other isotopes of iodine are not in general clinical use.

TREATMENT OF HYPERTHYROIDISM

CHILDHOOD THYROTOXICOSIS

Hyperthyroidism in childhood usually is due to Graves disease but can be secondary to Hashimoto's thyroiditis, hyperfunctioning thyroid nodule(s), or TSH hypersecretion or an activating mutation of the TSH receptor. Treatment of Graves disease may be accomplished with antithyroid drugs, surgery, or radioiodine. Antithyroid drug treatment is still considered the initial treatment of choice by most pediatric endocrinologists (2,91). MMI is now the drug of choice.

Therapy is initiated with MMI, 0.5 to 0.6 mg per kg per day, in three divided doses at about 8-hour intervals. The dose is increased if improvement is not observed within 2 to 3 weeks. Nearly all patients will respond to MMI in doses of 1 to 1.5 mg per kg per day. However, an occasional patient may require as much as 2.3 mg per kg per day for control. MMI has a longer half-life than PTU, and some patients will maintain effective blockade of thyroid hormone synthesis with once-daily drug administration, particularly after remission has been induced. When utilized PTU dosage is 5.7 mg per kg per day.

In patients with severe disease or distressing cardiovascular symptoms, propranolol can be increased to 4 to 6 mg per kg per day.

Potassium iodide in large doses potentiates the action of thioureylene drugs. Therapeutic doses for hyperthyroidism range from 2 to 4 mg per kg per day, usually given as strong iodine solution or a saturated solution of potassium iodide. The inhibitory effect on hormone synthesis and/or release usually persists 10 to 40 days. As indicated earlier, potassium iodide is most useful for short-term treatment of severe disease and for preoperative preparation of patients for surgery.

After the patient has become euthyroid, which usually takes 30 to 90 days, the daily dose of medication can be reduced to 0.3 to 0.4 mg of MMI per kg. Treatment must be monitored with measurements of serum T_4 concentrations to ensure an adequate drug effect and avoid hypothyroidism. Measurements of serum T_3 concentration may be useful when the clinical assessment and serum T_4 measurements are in disagreement; on occasion, the antithyroid medication will be adequate to inhibit T_4 but not T_3 secretion, and the patient will appear euthyroid or even hyperthyroid, with low levels of serum T_4 and elevated serum T_3 concentrations. Measurements of thyroid-stimulating antibody levels are useful in predicting remission and are helpful in assessing drug-induced hypothyroidism (92).

Two approaches to long-term treatment have been used: (a) continue adjusting the antithyroid drug dose to maintain a euthyroid state or (b) provide a blocking dose of drugs and treat the patient with exogenous T_4. The average remission rate for Graves disease approximates 50% each 2 to 3 years. Some patients remit within 6 to 12 months, but these represent the minority. Effective drug management usually requires 2 to 5 years of continuous treatment. Markers for remission include disappearance of goiter and decreasing titers of thyroid-stimulating antibody.

If drug toxicity ensues, the drug becomes ineffective either for patient or for pharmacologic reasons, or if the goiter is large and unresponsive to a reasonable drug treatment regimen, alternative treatment may be considered. Near-total thyroidectomy for Graves disease in children is safe and effective when performed by experienced thyroid surgeons (91,93). In addition to relief of systemic symptoms, the majority of patients presenting with Graves ophthalmopathy experienced improvement of their ocular disease after operation. In 5% of patients, surgical management has allowed for detection and treatment of clinically occult thyroid malignancies. Total or near-total thyroidectomy is recommended for patients with large thyroid glands (100 g or larger) (91,93). Radioiodine is a viable alternative in the adolescent who has not gone into remission on drug therapy.

Radioiodine treatment has not been widely employed in children because of the concern about permanent hypothyroidism, radiation oncogenesis, and genetic damage (91,94). Late development of primary hypothyroidism after I^{131} therapy has occurred in every series of patients studied, regardless of the dosage of radioiodine employed. The fear of inducing leukemia and thyroid carcinoma in adult patients with radioiodine treatment has been largely alleviated. However, the thyroid glands of young animals are much more susceptible to induction of thyroid carcinoma by ionizing radiation than those of older animals, and radiation has been incriminated as an important cause of thyroid cancer in children (91,94). Currently, data are not available to assess lifetime cancer risk for children treated with I^{131} for Graves disease (91).

It has been the practice in most clinics to reserve the use of radioiodine for treatment of thyrotoxicosis in older adolescents who fail to follow a medical regimen and who cannot be adequately prepared for surgical thyroidectomy. It has been suggested that I^{131} be administered in doses delivering 300 to 400 Gy (30,000 to 40,000 cGy or rad; 360 to 480 μCi per g thyroid) to ablate the thyroid gland (91). Commonly 120 to 280 Gy (150 to 250 mCi per g thyroid) are used and may result in complete or partial thyroid gland destruction (91); 100 Gy achieves hypothyroidism in about 50% of pediatric patients, 200 Gy results in hypothyroidism in 70%, and doses of 270 Gy or larger generally assures hypothyroidism. However, results vary with thyroid gland size (91).

Adrenergic blocking drugs are useful to control the sympathetic hyperactivity. These drugs also have proven lifesaving in critically ill patients in thyroid storm, but they cannot be relied upon as the only therapy in such patients. β-Receptor blockade is potentially dangerous in patients with cardiac failure or arrhythmias.

Iodinated radiographic contrast agents (ipodate, iopanoic acid) also may be useful in the treatment of Graves hyperthyroidism (84–89). Doses of 0.01 μg per kg per day or 0.04 to 0.05 μg per kg every 3 days have been utilized successfully and have maintained remission for 6 to 8 months. There is only limited experience with their use in children.

NEONATAL THYROTOXICOSIS

Neonatal thyrotoxicosis usually is due to thyroid-stimulating antibody transferred from the mother with Graves disease. Neonatal Graves disease is rare, probably due to the low incidence of thyrotoxicosis in pregnancy (1 to 2 cases per 1,000 pregnancies) and the fact that the neonatal disease occurs in only about 1 in 70 cases of thyrotoxic pregnancy (17,95,96). In most cases, the disease is due to transplacental passage of a thyroid-stimulating antibody from a mother with active or inactive Graves disease or Hashimoto's thyroiditis (95,96). Graves disease in the newborn is manifested by irritability, flushing, tachycardia, hypertension, poor weight gain, thyroid enlargement, and exophthalmos. Thrombocytopenia, hepatosplenomegaly, jaundice, and hypoprothrombinemia have also been observed. Arrhythmias, cardiac failure, and death may occur if the thyrotoxicity is severe and the treatment is inadequate. Mortality approaches 25% in disease severe enough to be diagnosed (17,91).

The treatment of neonatal Graves disease includes sedatives and digitalization as necessary. Iodide or antithyroid drugs are administered to decrease thyroid hormone secretion (17,91,96). These drugs have additive effects with regard to inhibition of hormone synthesis; in addition, iodide will rapidly inhibit hormone release. Lugol's solution (126 mg of iodine per mL) is given in doses of one drop (about 8 mg) three times daily. MMI, CBI, or PTU is administered in doses of 0.5 to 1 mg, or 5 to 10 mg, respectively, per kilogram daily in divided doses at 8-hour intervals. A therapeutic response should be observed within 24 to 48 hours. If a satisfactory response is not observed, the dose of antithyroid drug and iodide can be increased by 50%. Adrenal corticosteroids in anti-inflammatory dosage and propranolol (1 to 2 mg per kg per day) may also be helpful. Radiographic contrast agents also may be useful in treatment (100 mg per day or 0.5 g every 3 days) either alone or more effectively in conjunction with antithyroid drug treatment (88). Rare cases of neonatal thyrotoxicosis have been reported due to an activating mutation of the TSH receptor (17,97,98). Management with iodide and/or antithyroid drugs has been successful, but the thyrotoxicosis is not transient as is the case in neonatal Graves disease. Long-term management experience is limited in such children, and surgery or radioiodine therapies must be eventually considered.

THYROTROPIN-DEPENDENT HYPERTHYROIDISM

Hyperthyroidism with diffuse goiter and elevated serum levels of TSH has been reported in some 50 patients without pituitary enlargement (2,99–101). These patients manifest a defect in the feedback control of T_3 on TSH release such that a new set point is established with hypersecretion of TSH, hypersecretion of thyroid hormone, and mild-to-moderate tissue hyperthyroidism. The rare patients with activating mutations of the TSH receptor appear clinically similar but have suppressed serum TSH concentrations. In contrast to patients with TSH-secreting tumors, the TSH-α subunit is not elevated and the TSH response to TRH is augmented.

Treatment is difficult and not generally satisfactory. Thyroid ablation by surgery or radioiodine controls the hyperthyroidism but aggravates the TSH hypersection and increases the risk of development of a pituitary adenoma. Suppression of TSH by exogenous supraphysiologic doses of thyroid hormone may aggravate the hyperthyroidism. However, this approach has been at least partially successful (99–101), and treatment with tetraiodothyroacetic acid (TETRAC) has been proposed (101). TRIAC is an experimental drug. Treatment with TRIAC has been employed in children and adults in a daily dose of 1.4 to 2.8 mg, but is not always efficacious. Dextrothyroxine, also an experimental drug, has been shown to be successful in some cases (99). When these compounds fail, the dopaminergic agent bromocriptine or somatostatin (octreotide acetate) has been employed with variable effectiveness (99,102).

SPORADIC TOXIC THYROID HYPERPLASIA

Toxic thyroid hyperplasia is a rare syndrome of childhood onset hyperthyroidism caused by activating mutations of the thyrotropin receptor (97). The mutations in the childhood onset cases produce a milder phenotype than the more severe neonatal cases and tend to be sporadic rather than familial (97,98). Diagnosis is based on elevated serum free thyroxine with suppressed TSH levels in children with diffuse goiter. Management is similar to that in children with Graves disease.

AUTONOMOUS TOXIC ADENOMAS

Autonomous functioning thyroid nodules are uncommon in childhood and adolescence. Rarely, single or multiple autonomously functioning nodules may be associated with clinical hyperthyroidism (103–107). The major causes of toxic thyroid nodules are activating mutations of the thyrotropin receptor or the intracellular linked Gsα protein (97). Such nodules are true follicular adenomas and nearly always benign; the incidence of thyroid carcinoma in functioning nodules is less than 1%. It is generally felt that function in a thyroid nodule essentially excludes a diagnosis of thyroid carcinoma. Small functional nodules usually do not produce clinical thyrotoxicosis; large nodules (>3 cm diameter) are more likely to do so. Nodular autonomy usually is discerned by thyroid radioiodine scan and confirmed if the serum TSH concentration measured by a highly sensitive TSH method is suppressed and/or is unresponsive to TRH stimulation (104,105).

The natural history of functioning thyroid nodules in the individual patient is variable. Such patients, if euthyroid, usually will remain euthyroid, but there may be a gradual increase in thyroid hormone production with development of clinical evidence of hyperthyroidism. Nodule enlargement or thyrotoxic symptoms may create the need for ablative therapy. Functioning nodules producing clinical and chemical thyrotoxicosis require surgical removal. Radioiodine treatment now tends to be reserved for older patients (>40 years of age). Antithyroid drug therapy is considered only for short-term management.

THYROID NODULES AND CANCER

THYROID NODULES

Thyroid nodules in children are significant for three reasons: they may herald underlying thyroid disease, they may be hyperfunctioning nodules and produce hyperthyroidism, or they may represent carcinoma (2,106). In the first instance, the approach is to the basic disease, often Hashimoto's thyroiditis. Functioning nodules producing clinical and chemical thyrotoxicosis require treatment, as indicated in the previous section. The likelihood of carcinoma in a cold nodule (one that does not concentrate radioiodine) in an otherwise normal thyroid gland is estimated to be 15% to 20% in children and the likelihood of carcinoma is increased if there has been exposure to external irradiation of the neck or radioactive isotopes (I^{131} or short half-life isotopes) (2,106). Most carcinomas are thyroid follicular cell neoplasms, but about 5% are medullary carcinomas secreting calcitonin and can be identified with a serum calcitonin measurement with or without stimulation testing (2,106). Fine-needle biopsy is commonly employed in differential diagnosis. The result usually is reported as malignant, suspicious, or benign. Surgery is indicated if the needle biopsy indicates a malignant lesion. Many consider that surgery also is indicated if there is a prior history of therapeutic radiation to the head or neck, if the nodule is hard, if there is evidence of tracheal invasion (dysphagia, hoarseness, or cough) or vocal cord paralysis, if adjacent lymph nodes are involved, or if there are distant metastases.

TETRAIODOTHYRONINE SUPPRESSION

If the thyroid needle biopsy result is suspicious and no thyroid malignancy criteria are present, thyroid suppression with 0.2 to 0.3 mg of Na-1-T_4 daily can be employed. If over a period of 4 to 6 months the nodule grows, or if over a period of 12 months the nodule does not decrease in size, surgery is indicated. If the nodule decreases in size, longer follow-up is in order. It is important to remember that thyroid follicular cell carcinomas in children are rather indolent neoplasms and do not require urgent treatment.

MANAGEMENT OF THYROID FOLLICULAR CANCER: USE OF RADIOIODINE

The initial approach is simple removal of the affected thyroid lobe. If frozen section reveals carcinoma, total lobectomy is indicated with as much of the contralateral lobe as possible, while attempting to preserve the parathyroid glands and recurrent laryngeal nerves. Regional lymph nodes are removed but mutilating neck dissection is contraindicated. Routine radioiodine treatment with I^{131} is of questionable benefit in children with well-differentiated thyroid carcinoma and no evidence of metastases. In patients with lymph node metastases or distant metastases to bone or lungs, postoperative I^{131} therapy is indicated (a) to ablate the residual thyroid tissue and (b) to ablate identifiable metastatic loci. A lower I^{131} dose is given to accomplish the former goal, followed by a high-dose second metastatic treatment dose. Following surgery or surgery plus radioiodine, the patient is maintained on full suppression doses of exogenous T_4 to suppress endogenous TSH. Metastatic tumor growth is assessed by serial measurements of circulating Tg. Recurrences usually are managed with repeat I^{131} treatment.

MEDULLARY CARCINOMA

Medullary thyroid carcinoma (MTC) represents neoplasia of the parafollicular "C" cells and is associated with excessive secretion of calcitonin (2,106,108). Other secretory products can include ACTH, MSH, histaminase, serotonin, prostaglandins, SRIF, and endorphin. MTC represents 4% to 10% of all malignant thyroid neoplasia: 75% of cases are sporadic and 25% familial. The prognosis is generally guarded because lymph node involvement occurs early, even when the tumor is small. Sporadic cases appear as a noniodide-concentrating (cold) thyroid nodule; the diagnosis is confirmed or suspected on the basis of needle biopsy or open biopsy. Thyroidectomy is the only current approach to treatment of medullary carcinoma, since "C" cells do not concentrate radioiodine.

Prior to 1987, the only available test for early detection of MTC in genetically at-risk patients was measurement of serum calcitonin with or without stimulation. Since then, DNA diagnosis has become the procedure of choice (2,102,108). Identification of an activating germ line mutation in the RET proto-oncogene indicates that the affected individual has a greater than 90% probability of developing MTC. The optimal treatment in children at genetic risk with RET gene mutation is early thyroidectomy before malignant transformation occurs (2,102,108). There is now a large experience correlating RET mutations with MTC aggressiveness, and high-risk mutations are ranked 1 to 3, with 3 being highest risk. It is now recommended that children with the highest risk mutations undergo prophylactic thyroidectomy before 6 months of age. Thyroidectomy before 5 years of age for level 2 risk patients and at 5 to 10 years of age for level 1 risk patients is recommended (2,108).

It is not possible to determine a priori whether an individual with apparent sporadic MTC has hereditary or sporadic disease. Available information indicates that 6% to 7% of apparent sporadic MTC patients have germ line mutations of the RET proto-oncogene. It is important to identify these individuals so that screening can be provided to other family members. For this reason, it is now recommended by the American Society of Clinical Oncology and the National Comprehensive Cancer Network that all patients with apparently sporadic MTC be tested for germ line RET gene mutations.

THYROTROPIN-RELEASING HORMONE

TRH is the first hypothalamic peptide characterized and synthesized nearly simultaneously by Guillemin and Schally (109,110). It is a tripeptide (pyroglutamyl–histidyl–proline amide) secreted by the hypothalamus into the hypothalamic–pituitary portal vascular system to stimulate TSH release from anterior pituitary thyrotroph cells. TRH acts on these cells via a specific plasma membrane receptor. TRH stimulates prolactin release and in selected circumstances can evoke GH release (111). TRH also is present in extrahypothalamic brain tissue and in extraneural tissues such as pancreas. TRH is synthesized as a 225-amino acid precursor (prepro-TRH) containing five TRH progenitor sequences (112). Processing of prepro-TRH results in cleavage of several larger peptides as well as TRH (113). The significance of these is not clear. TRH is metabolized via a pyroglutamyl amino peptidase to a cyclized metabolite, histadyl–proline diketopiperazine or cyclo (His–Pro) (111,114). Cyclo (His–Pro) also is widely distributed in brain tissue and appears to have unique bioactivities different from TRH. TRH also is deaminated and the free acid may have bioactivity (111).

The major bioactivity of TRH is the modulation, with T_3, of TSH release. TRH as the synthetic tripeptide is commercially available as a sterile, lyophilized powder (500-μg vials). The plasma half-life is very short (several minutes). The minimal intravenous dose required to evoke an increase in serum TSH is about 0.2 μg (200 ng) per kg. The TSH response increases progressively with increasing dose to plateau at 5 to 6 μg per kg. The peak rise in serum TSH is seen within 15 to 30 minutes; a secondary increase in serum T_3 levels occurs within 90 to 150 minutes (111). TRH also is active orally, but doses 20 to 40 times greater are required.

THYROTROPIN-RELEASING HORMONE TESTING

TRH is used for testing pituitary TSH reserve. An intravenous dose of TRH (7 μg per kg) is injected and measurements of serum TSH usually are conducted at 30 to 60 minutes. The TSH response, in general, is proportional to the basal TSH level. Thus, patients with primary hypothyroidism have augmented responses. Patients with hyperthyroidism have inhibited responses. The test has been utilized (a) to confirm a diagnosis of thyrotoxicosis in patients with borderline serum T_4 and T_3 concentrations (an absent TSH response to TRH supports a diagnosis of hyperthyroidism) and (b) to differentiate hypothalamic and pituitary etiologies for TSH deficiency in patients with hypothyroidism and low TSH levels (115). A normal TSH response to TRH indicates normal pituitary TSH secretory capacity and implies a hypothalamic TRH deficiency. An absent TSH response supports a diagnosis of pituitary TSH deficiency. Measurements of serum T_3 before and after 4 hours of TRH administration provide information regarding thyroid gland responsiveness. TRH has been injected intravenously in pregnant women to stimulate fetal thyroid function near term (116). A dose of 400 μg induced a marked increase in cord blood TSH within 20 minutes and evoked significant increases in cord blood T_4 and T_3 levels as well.

THYROTROPIN

Thyrotropin (TSH) is a 28- to 30-kD glycoprotein synthesized in the pituitary gland in response to TRH stimulation (117). It is a member of the glycoprotein hormone family, which includes FSH, luteinizing hormone and chorionic gonadotropin (HCG). All consist of a common α subunit and a unique β subunit. The α subunits are composed of 92 amino acids. Recombinant human TSH is now available for clinical use to stimulate thyroid cell function for diagnostic and therapeutic purposes (117,118) (Table 53.5). Recombinant human TSH (Thyrogen®, Genzyme Inc., Cambridge, MA) has replaced sterile, lyophilized TSH from animal sources for human use. It is available as a sterile, lyophilized product in kit form (two 1.1 mg vials, and two 10 mL vials of sterile water for injection). The usual dosage is 0.9 mg intramuscularly every 24 hours for two doses or every 72 hours for three doses (1.1 mg is reconstituted in 1.2 mL sterile water: 1 mL solution contains 0.9 mg TSH).

TABLE 53.5 Clinical Applications of Recombinant Human TSH

TSH stimulation test (testing thyroid reserve; confirming diagnosis of thyroid hemiagenesis; identifying "warm" thyroid nodules)
Differentiated thyroid cancer management (stimulation of thyroglobulin secretion to identify residual thyroid tissue; stimulation of radioiodine uptake in residual thyroid tissue prior to whole-body scanning)
Therapy of differentiated thyroid cancer (stimulation of thyroid tissue iodide uptake prior to therapeutic dosing with radioiodine)

REFERENCES

1. Larsen PR, Davies TF, Schlumberger MJ, et al. Thyroid physiology and diagnostic evaluation of patients with thyroid disorders. In: Larsen PR, Kronenberg HM, Melmed M, Polonsky KS, eds. *Williams textbook of endocrinology*, 11th ed. Philadelphia, PA: Saunders Elsevier, 2008:299–332.
2. Fisher DA, Grueters A. Thyroid disorders in childhood and adolescence. In: Sperling MA, ed. *Pediatric endocrinology*, 3rd ed. Philadelphia, PA: Saunders Elsevier, 2008:227–253.
3. De Nayer PH, Cornette C, Vanderschueren M, et al. Serum thyroglobulin levels in preterm neonates. *Clin Endocrinol (Oxf)* 1984; 321:148–153.
4. Hollenberg AN. Regulation of thyrotropin secretion. In: Braverman LE, Utiger RD, eds. *The thyroid, a fundamental and clinical text*, 9th ed. Philadelphia, PA: Lippincott Williams & Wilkins, 2005:197–213.
5. Benvenga S. Thyroid hormone transport proteins and the physiology of protein binding. In: Braverman LE, Utiger RD, eds. *The thyroid, a fundamental and clinical text*, 9th ed. Philadelphia, PA: Lippincott Williams & Wilkins, 2005:97–108.
6. De Stefano JJ, Fisher DA. Peripheral distribution and metabolism of the thyroid hormones: a preliminary quantitative assessment. In: Hershman JM, Bray GA, eds. *The thyroid, physiology and treatment of disease*, Oxford, UK: Pergamon Press, 1979:47–82.
7. Wu SY, Green WI, Huang WS, et al. Alternate pathways of thyroid hormone metabolism. *Thyroid* 2005;15:943–958.
8. St. Germain DL. Thyroid hormone metabolism. In: DeGroot LJ, Jameson JL, eds. *Endocrinology*, 5th ed. Philadelphia, PA: Elsevier Saunders, 2005:1861–1871.
9. Mousa SA, Bergh JJ, Dier E, et al. Tetraiodothyroacetic acid, a small molecule integrin ligand, blocks angiogenesis induced by vascular endothelial growth factor and basic fibroblast growth factor. *Angiogenesis* 2008;11:183–190.
10. Doyle KO, Suchland KL, Ciesielski TMP, et al. Novel thyroxine derivatives, thionamine and 3-iodothyronamine, induce transient hypothermia and marked neuroprotection against stroke injury. *Stroke* 2007;38:2569–2576.
11. Braulke LJ, Klingenspor M, DeBarber A, et al. 3-iodothyronamine: a novel hormone controlling the balance between glucose and lipid utilization. *J Comp Physiol B* 2008;178:167–177.
12. Geraci T, Field C, Colasurdo V, et al. 3-iodothyronamine (T1AM) levels in human serum and tissues. Program at the American Thyroid Association Meeting; October 1–5, 2008; Chicago, IL. 126.
13. Yen PM. Genomic and nongenomic actions of thyroid hormones. In: Braverman LE, Utiger RD, eds. *The thyroid, a fundamental and clinical text*, 9th ed. Philadelphia, PA: Lippincott Williams & Wilkins, 2005:135–150.
14. Munoz A, Bernal J. Biological activities of thyroid hormone receptors. *Eur J Endocrinol* 1997;137:433–445.
15. Forrest D, Golarai G, Connor J, et al. Genetic analysis of thyroid hormone receptors in development and disease. *Recent Prog Horm Res* 1996:51:1–22.
16. Brown RS, Huang SA, Fisher DA. The maturation of thyroid function in the perinatal period and during childhood. In:

Braverman LE, Utiger RD, eds. *The thyroid, a fundamental and clinical text,* 9th ed. Philadelphia, PA: Lippincott Williams & Wilkins, 2005:1013–1028.

17. Fisher DA, Grueters A. Disorders of the thyroid in the newborn and infant. In: Sperling MA, ed. *Pediatric endocrinology,* 3rd ed. Philadelphia, PA: Elsevier Saunders, 2008:198–226.
18. Bernal J. Action of thyroid hormone in brain. *J Endocrinol Invest* 2002;25:268–288.
19. Silva JE, Rabelo R. Regulation of the uncoupling gene expression. *Eur J Endocrinol* 1997;136:251–264.
20. Gong DW, He Y, Karas M, et al. Uncoupling protein-3 is a mediator of thermogenesis regulated by thyroid hormone, β3 adrenergic agonists, and leptin. *J Biol Chem* 1997;272:24129–24132.
21. Glasscock GF, Nicoll CS. Hormonal control of growth in the neonatal rat. *Endocrinology* 1981;109:176–184.
22. Snyder PJ. The pituitary in hypothyroidism. In: Braverman LE, Utiger RD, eds. *The thyroid,* Philadelphia, PA: Lippincott-Raven, 1995:836–840.
23. Meill J, Taylor A, Zini M, et al. Effects of hypothyroidism and hyperthyroidism on insulin-like growth factors (IGFs) and growth hormone and IGF binding proteins. *J Clin Endocrinol Metab* 1993; 76:950–955.
24. Chernausek SD, Turner R. Attenuation of spontaneous nocturnal growth hormone secretion in children with hypothyroidism and its correlation with plasma insulin-like growth factor-I concentrations. *J Pediatr* 1989;114:968–972.
25. Britto J, Fenton A, Holloway W, et al. Osteoblasts mediate thyroid hormone stimulation of osteoclastic bone resorption. *Endocrinology* 1994;134:169–176.
26. Huang SM, Chan SH, Wu TJ, et al. Effect of thyroid hormone on urinary excretion of epidermal growth factor. *Eur Surg Res* 1997; 29:222–228.
27. Fisher DA. Growth and development of hypothyroid infants. In: Stabler B, Bercu BB, eds. *Therapeutic outcome of endocrine disorders,* New York, NY: Springer Verlag, 2000:221–234.
28. Leger J, Czernichow P. Congenital hypothyroidism: decreased growth velocity in the first weeks of life. *Biol Neonate* 1989;55: 218–223.
29. Bucher H, Prader A, Illig R. Head circumference, height, bone age and weight in 103 children with congenital hypothyroidism before and during thyroid hormone replacement. *Helv Paediatr Acta* 1985;30:305–316.
30. Aronson R, Ehrlich RM, Bailey JD, et al. Growth in children with congenital hypothyroidism detected by neonatal screening. *J Pediatr* 1990;116:33–37.
31. Grant DB. Growth in early treated congenital hypothyroidism. *Arch Dis Child* 1994;70:464–468.
32. Chiesa A, de Papendieck LG, Keselman A, et al. Growth follow-up in 100 children with congenital hypothyroidism before and during treatment. *J Pediatr Endocrinol* 1994;7:211–217.
33. Heyerdahl S, Kase BF, Stake G. Skeletal maturation during thyroxine treatment in children with congenital hypothyroidism. *Acta Paediatr* 1994;83:618–622.
34. Leger J, Ruiz JC, Guibourdenche J, et al. Bone mineral density and metabolism in children with congenital hypothyroidism after prolonged L-thyroxine therapy. *Acta Paediatr* 1997;86:704–710.
35. Boersma B, Otten BJ, Stoelings GBA, et al. Catch-up growth after prolonged hypothyroidism. *Eur J Pediatr* 1996;155:362–367.
36. Haddow JE, Palomaki GE, Allan WC, et al. Maternal thyroid deficiency during pregnancy and subsequent neuropsychological development of the child. *N Engl J Med* 1999;341:549–555.
37. Glinoer D, Delange F. The potential repercussions of maternal, fetal, and neonatal hypothyroxinemia on the progeny. *Thyroid* 2000; 10:871–887.
38. Dobbing J. The later growth of the brain and its vulnerability. *Pediatrics* 1974;53:2–6.
39. Bongers-Schokking JJ, Koot HM, Wiersma D, et al. Influence of timing and dose of thyroid hormone replacement on development of infants with congenital hypothyroidism. *J Pediatr* 2000;136:292–297.
40. New England Congenital Hypothyroidism Collaborative. Neonatal hypothyroidism screening: status of patients at 6 years of age. *J Pediatr* 1985;107:915–919.
41. Derksen-Lubsen G, Verkerk PH. Neuropsychological development in early treated congenital hypothyroidism: analysis of literature data. *Pediatr Res* 1996;39:561–566.
42. Heyerdahl S, Oerbeck B. Congenital hypothyroidism: developmental outcome in relation to levothyroxine treatment variables. *Thyroid* 2003;13:1029–1038.
43. Letarte J, Guyda H, Dussault JH. Clinical, biochemical and radiological features of neonatal hypothyroid infants. In: Burrow GN, Dussault JH, eds. *Neonatal thyroid screening,* New York: Raven Press, 1980:225–236.
44. Price DA, Ehrlich RM, Walfish PG. Congenital hypothyroidism, clinical and laboratory characteristics of infants detected by neonatal screening. *Arch Dis Child* 1981;56:845–851.
45. Letarte J, LaFranchi S. Clinical features of congenital hypothyroidism. In: Walker P, Dussault JH, eds. *Congenital hypothyroidism,* New York: Marcel Dekker, 1983:351–383.
46. Fisher DA. The unique endocrine milieu of the fetus. *J Clin Invest* 1986;78:603–606.
47. Fisher DA, Polk DH, Wu SY. Fetal thyroid metabolism: a pluralistic system. *Thyroid* 1984;4:367–371.
48. Hemady ZS, Siler-Khodr TM, Najjar S. Precocious puberty in juvenile hypothyroidism. *Pediatrics* 1978;92:55–59.
49. Chattopadhyay A, Kumar V, Marulaiah M. Polycystic ovaries, precocious puberty and acquired hypothyroidism: the Van Wyk and Grumbach syndrome. *J Ped Surg* 2003;38:1390–1392.
50. Anasti JN, Flack MR, Frochlich J, et al. A potential novel mechanism for precocious puberty in juvenile hypothyroidism. *J Clin Endocrinol Metab* 1995;80:276–279.
51. Rodien P, Bremonte C, Sanson MLR, et al. Familial gestational hyperthyroidism caused by a mutant thyrotropin receptor hypersensitive to human chorionic gonadotropin. *N Engl J Med* 2008; 339:1823–1826.
52. Montanelli M, Delbaere A, Di Carlo C, et al. A mutation in the follicle-stimulating hormone receptor as a cause of familial spontaneous ovarian hyperstimulation syndrome. *J Clin Endocrinol Metab* 2004;89:1255–1258.
53. Reilly WA, Smyth FS. Cretinoid epiphyseal dysgenesis. *J Pediatr* 1937;11:786–796.
54. Chanoine JP, Toppet V, Lagasse R, et al. Determination of thyroid volume by ultrasound from the neonatal period to late adolescence. *Eur J Pediatr* 1991;150:395–399.
55. Delange F, Becker G, Caron P, et al. Thyroid volume and urinary iodine in European school children: standardization of values for assessment of iodine deficiency. *Eur J Endocrinol* 1997;136:180–187.
56. Ponchon G, Beckers C, DeVisscher M. Iodine kinetic studies in newborns and infants. *J Clin Endocrinol Metab* 1966;21:1392–1394.
57. Fisher DA, Oddie TH, Wait JC. Thyroid function tests: findings in Arkansas children and young adults. *Am J Dis Child* 1964;107: 282–287.
58. Beckers C, Malvaux P, De Visscher M. Quantitative aspects of the secretion and degradation of thyroid hormones during adolescence. *J Clin Endocrinol Metab* 1966;26:202–206.
59. Nelson JC, Clark SJ, Borot DL, et al. Age related changes in serum free thyroxine, during childhood and adolescence. *J Pediatr* 1993;125:899–905.
60. Delange F, Fisher DA. The thyroid gland. In: Brook CGD, ed. *Clinical paediatric endocrinology,* 3rd ed. Oxford, UK: Blackwell Science, 1995:397–433.
61. Fisher DA, Sack J, Oddie TH, et al. Serum T_4, TBG, T_3 uptake, T_3, reverse T_3 and TSH concentrations in children 1 to 15 years of age. *J Clin Endocrinol Metab* 1977;45:191–198.
62. Fish LH, Schwartz HL, Cavanaugh J, et al. Replacement dose, metabolism and availability of levothyroxine in the treatment of hypothyroidism. *N Engl J Med* 1987;316:764–770.
63. Bunevicius R, Kazanavicius G, Zalinkevicius R, et al. Effects of thyroxine as compared with thyroxine plus triiodothyronine in patients with hypothyroidism. *N Engl J Med* 1999;340:424–429.
64. Escobar-Morreale HF, del Ray FE, Obregon MJ, et al. Only the combined treatment with thyroxine and triiodothyronine ensures euthyroidism in all tissues of the thyroidectomized rat. *Endocrinology* 1996;137:2490–2502.
65. Eisenberg M, Samuels M, Distefano JJ. Extension, validation, and clinical applications of a feedback control system simulation of the hypothalamic–pituitary thyroid axis. *Thyroid* 2008;18:1071–1085.
66. Fisher DA, Schoen EJ, LaFranchi S, et al. The hypothalamic–pituitary–thyroid negative feedback control axis in children with treated congenital hypothyroidism. *J Clin Endocrinol Metab* 2000; 85:2722–2727.

67. Selva KA, Mandel SH, Rien L, et al. Initial treatment dose of L-thyroxine in congenital hypothyroidism. *J Pediatr* 2002;141:786–792.
68. Crantz FR, Silva JE, Larsen PR. An analysis of the sources and quantity of 3,5,3′ triiodothyronine specifically bound to nuclear receptors in rat cerebral cortex and cerebellum. *Endocrinology* 1982;110:367–375.
69. Silva JE, Larsen PR. Comparison of iodothyronine 5′ deiodinase and other thyroid hormone dependent enzyme activities in the cerebral cortex of hypothyroid neonatal rats. *J Clin Invest* 1982; 70:1110–1123.
70. Morreale De Escobar G, Obregon MJ, Ruiz De Ono C, et al. Transfer of thyroxine from the mother to the rat fetus near term: effects on brain 3,5,3′-triiodothyronine deficiency. *Endocrinology* 1988;122:1521–1531.
71. Daneman D, Howard NJ. Neonatal thyrotoxicosis, intellectual impairment and craniosynostosis in later years. *J Pediatr* 1980;97: 257–259.
72. Kapelman AE. Delayed cerebral development in twins with congenital hyperthyroidism. *Am J Dis Child* 1983;137:842–845.
73. Penfold JL, Simpson DA. Premature craniosynostosis, a complication of thyroid replacement therapy. *J Pediatr* 1975;86: 360–363.
74. Sato T, Suzuke Y, Taetani T, et al. Age related change in the pituitary threshold for TSH release during thyroxine replacement therapy for cretinism. *J Clin Endocrinol Metab* 1977;44: 553–559.
75. McCrossin RB, Sheffield LJ, Robertson EF. Persisting abnormality in the pituitary–thyroid axis in congenital hypothyroidism. In: Nagataki S, Stockigt JHR, eds. *Thyroid research VIII*, Canberra: Australian Academy of Sciences, 1980:37–40.
76. Van Tijn DA, de Vijlder JJM, Vulsma T. Role of corticotropin-releasing hormone testing in assessment of hypothalamic–pituitary–adrenal axis function in infants with congenital central hypothyroidism. *J Clin Endocrinol Metab* 2008;93:3794–3803.
77. Weetman AP. Autoimmune thyroid disease. In: DeGroot LJ, Jameson JL, eds. *Endocrinology*, 5th ed. Philadelphia, PA: Elsevier Saunders, 2005:1979–1993.
78. Brent GA, Larsen PR, Davies TE. Hypothyroidism and thyroiditis, In: Kronenberg HM, Melmed S, Polonsky KS, Larsen PR, eds. *Williams textbook of endocrinology*, 11th ed. Philadelphia, PA: Elsevier Saunders, 2008:377–409.
79. Derwahl M, Studer H. Multinodular goiter: much more to it than simple iodine deficiency. *Baillieres Best Pract Res Clin Endocrinol Metab* 2000;14:577–600.
80. Tajtakova M, Langer P, Gonsornikova V, et al. Recognition of a subgroup of adolescents with rapidly growing thyroids under iodine replete conditions: seven year follow-up. *Eur J Endocrinol* 1998;138:674–680.
81. Astwood EB, Bissell A, Hughes AM. Further studies on the chemical nature of compounds which inhibit the function of the thyroid gland. *Endocrinology* 1945;37:456–481.
82. Farwell AP, Braverman LE. Thyroid and antithyroid drugs. In: Hardman JG, Limberg LE, eds. *Goodman and Gilman's the pharmacological basis of therapeutics*, 10th ed. New York: McGraw Hill, 2001:1563–1596
83. Panamonta O, Sumethkul V, Radinahmed P, et al. Propylthiouracil associated antineutrophil cytoplasmic antibodies (ANCA) in patients with childhood onset Graves' disease. *J Pediatr Endocrinol Metab* 2008;21:539–543.
84. Wu SY, Chopra IJ, Solomon DH, et al. The effect of repeated administration of ipodate (Orografin) in hyperthyroidism. *J Clin Endocr Metab* 1978;47:1358–1362.
85. Shen DC, Wu SY, Chopra IJ, et al. Long term treatment of Graves' hyperthyroidism with sodium ipodate. *J Clin Endocr Metab* 1985; 61:723–727.
86. Wang YS, Tsou CT, Lin WH, et al. Long term treatment of Graves' disease with iopanoic acid (Telepaque). *J Clin Endocr Metab* 1987; 65:679–682.
87. Fontanilla JC, Schneider AB, Sarne DH. The use of oral radiographic contrast agents in the management of hyperthyroidism. *Thyroid* 2001;6:561–567.
88. Karpman BA, Rappoport B, Filetti S, et al. Treatment of neonatal hyperthyroidism due to Graves' disease with sodium ipodate. *J Clin Endocr Metab* 1987;64:119–123.
89. Laurberg P. Multi-site inhibitor by ipodate of iodothyronine secretion from perfused dog thyroid lobes. *Endocrinology* 1985;117: 1639–1644.
90. Links JM. Radiation physics. In: Braverman LE, Utiger RD, eds. *The thyroid*, 8th ed. New York: JB Lippincott, 2000:333–344.
91. Rivkees SA. Hypothyroidism and hyperthyroidism in children. In: Pescovitz OH, Eugster EA, eds. *Pediatric endocrinology*, Philadelphia, PA: Lippincott Williams & Wilkins, 2004:508–521.
92. Smith J, Brown RS. Persistence of thyrotropin (TSH) receptor antibodies in children and adolescents with Graves' disease treated using antithyroid medication. *Thyroid* 2007;17:1103–1107.
93. Sherman J, Thompson GB, Lteif A, et al. Surgical management of Graves' disease in childhood and adolescence: an institutional experience. *Surgery* 2006;140:1056–1062.
94. Maxon HR, Saenger EL. Biological effects of radioisotopes on the human thyroid gland. In: Braverman LE, Utiger RD, eds. *The thyroid*, 8th ed. New York: LB Lippincott, 2000:345–354.
95. Zakarija M, McKenzie JM, Hoffman WH. Prediction and therapy of intrauterine and late onset neonatal hyperthyroidism. *J Clin Endocr Metab* 1986;62:368–371.
96. Smallridge RC, Wartofsky L, Chopra IJ, et al. Neonatal thyrotoxicosis: alterations in serum concentrations of LATS protector, T_4, T_3, reverse T_3 and 3,3′ T_2. *J Pediatr* 1978;93:118–120.
97. Vassart G. Thyroid stimulating hormone receptor mutations. In: DeGroot LJ, Jameson JL eds. *Endocrinology*, 5th ed. Philadelphia, PA: Elsevier Saunders, 2005:2191–2199.
98. Gruters A, Schoneberg T, Biebermann H, et al. Severe congenital hyperthyroidism caused by a germ-line neo mutation in the extracellular portion of the thyrotropin receptor. *J Clin Endocrinol Metab* 1998;83:1431–1436.
99. Gurnell M, Beck-Peccoz P, Chatterjee VK. Resistance to thyroid hormone. In: DeGroot LJ, Jameson LJ, eds. *Endocrinology*, 5th ed. Philadelphia, PA: Elsevier Saunders, 2005:2227–2238.
100. Rosler A, Litvin Y, Hoge C, et al. Familial hyperthyroidism due to inappropriate thyrotropin secretion successfully treated with triiodothyronine. *J Clin Endocr Metab* 1982;54:76–82.
101. Beck-Peccoz P, Piscitelli G, Cattaneo MG, et al. Successful treatment of hyperthyroidism due to non-neoplastic pituitary TSH secretion with 3,5,3′-triiodothyroacetic acid (TRIAC). *J Endocrinol Invest* 1983;6:217–223.
102. Isales CM, Tamborlane W, Gertner JM, et al. Effect of short-term somatostatin and long-term triiodothyronine administration to a child with nontumorous inappropriate thyrotropin secretion. *Pediatrics* 1988;112:51–57.
103. Bauer AJ, Tuttle RM, Francis GL. Thyroid nodules and thyroid cancer in children and adolescents. In: Pescovitz OH, Eugster EA, eds. *Pediatric endocrinology*, Philadelphia, PA: Lippincott Williams & Wilkins, 2004:522–547.
104. Abe K, Konno M, Sato T, et al. Hyperfunctioning thyroid nodules in children. *Am J Dis Child* 1980;134:961–963.
105. Osbourne RC, Goren EN, Bybee DE, et al. Autonomous thyroid nodules in adolescents: clinical characteristics and results of TRH testing. *J Pediatr* 1982;100:383–386.
106. Pacini F, DeGroot LJ. Thyroid neoplasia. In: DeGroot LJ, Jameson JL, eds. *Endocrinology*, 5th ed. Philadelphia, PA: WB Saunders, 2005:2147–2180.
107. Schlumberger MJ, Filetti S, Hay ID. Nontoxic diffuse and nodular goiter and thyroid neoplasia. In: Kronenberg HM, Melmed S, Polonsky KS, Larsen PR, eds. *Williams textbook of endocrinology*, 11th ed. Philadelphia, PA: Elsevier Saunders, 2008:441–442.
108. Koovaraki MA, Shapiro SE, Perrier ND, et al. RET protooncogene: a review of and update of genotype–phenotype correlations in hereditary medullary thyroid cancer and associated endocrine tumors. *Thyroid* 2005;15:531–544.
109. Guillemin R. Peptides in the brain. The new endocrinology of the neuron. *Science* 1978;202:390–402.
110. Schally AV. Aspects of the hypothalamic regulation of the pituitary gland: its implication for the control of reproductive processes. *Science* 1978;202:18–28.
111. Jackson IMD. Thyrotropin releasing hormone. *N Engl J Med* 1982; 306:145–155.
112. Lechan RM, Wu P, Jackson IMD, et al. Thyrotropin releasing hormone precursor: characterization in rat brain. *Science* 1986; 231:159–161.

113. Wu P, Lechan RM, Jackson IMD. Identification and characterization of thyrotropin releasing hormone precursor peptides in rat brain. *Endocrinology* 1986;121:108–111.
114. Iruichijima T, Prasad C, Wilber JF, et al. Thyrotropin releasing hormone and cyclo (His–Pro)-like immunoreactivities in the cerebrospinal fluids of normal infants and adults and patients with various neuropsychiatric and neurologic disorders. *Life Sci* 1987;41:2419–2428.
115. Van Tijn DA, de Vijlder JJM, Vulsma T. Role of thyrotropin releasing hormone stimulation test in diagnosis of congenital central hypothyroidism in infants. *J Clin Endocrinol Metab* 2008;93:410–419.
116. Roti E, Gnudi A, Braverman LE. The placental transport, synthesis and metabolism of hormones and drugs with affect thyroid function. *Endocr Rev* 1983;4:131–149.
117. Weintraub BD, Kazlauskaite R, Grossman M, et al. Thyroid stimulating hormone and regulation of the thyroid axis. In: DeGroot LJ, Jameson JL, eds. *Endocrinology*, 4th ed. Philadelphia, PA: WB Saunders, 2001:1345–1360.
118. Torres MST, Ramirez L, Simkin PH, et al. Effect of various doses of recombinant human thyrotropin on the thyroid radioactive iodine uptake and serum levels of thyroid hormones and thyroglobulin in normal subjects. *J Clin Endocrinol Metab* 2001;86:1660–1664.

CHAPTER

54

Celia Rodd
Harvey J. Guyda

Growth Hormone

INTRODUCTION

The therapeutic use of growth hormone (GH), derived from human cadaveric pituitaries, was introduced in the late 1950s and early 1960s (1). The production of pituitary GH slowly increased over the next two decades, but supplies did not meet the treatment needs of all patients believed to have GH deficiency (GHD) due to difficulties in obtaining sufficient cadaveric pituitaries. The recognition of Creutzfeldt–Jakob disease (CJD) in recipients of pituitary-derived GH in 1985 led to its immediate discontinuation in most countries. The last two decades have seen a dramatic increase in worldwide availability of natural sequence recombinant human GH (rhGH), with improvement in treatment protocols for children with GHD. GH has been used increasingly for short children with non-GHD conditions in childhood and adolescence, including idiopathic short stature (ISS), intrauterine growth retardation (IUGR) or small for gestational age (SGA) infants, chronic renal failure (CRF), and genetic syndromes such as Turner syndrome (TS), Down syndrome (DS), and Prader–Willi syndrome (PWS). In addition, studies began in the 1990s on the adult population of childhood onset of GHD, as well as on adult-onset GHD and the elderly.

GROWTH HORMONE SECRETION

GROWTH HORMONE-RELEASING HORMONE AND SOMATOSTATIN

GH secretion is pulsatile, with diurnal variation, and varies significantly with sleep, nutrition, hormonal milieu (e.g., glucocorticoids, sex steroids), and pubertal status, with tightly controlled feedback mechanisms. GH self-entrains the ultradian rhythm of episodic GH release (2,3). The frequency of GH pulses is preserved across all species, occurring at approximately 3- to 4-hour intervals, with the largest spontaneous peaks occurring during onset of deep sleep. Somatostatin (SST) plays a critical role in the pulse frequency of GH release (4). Historically, it has been considered that only two hypothalamic hormones, growth hormone–releasing hormone (GHRH) and SST, control GH secretion: the former stimulates and the latter inhibits pituitary somatotroph release of GH (4,5). It is recognized that endogenous GHRH is required for the normal GH response to each of the following pharmacologic stimuli: L-dopa, arginine, insulin hypoglycemia, and pyridostigmine.

GROWTH HORMONE-RELEASING HORMONE RECEPTOR

GH-releasing hormone receptors (GHRHRs) are located on the pituitary somatotrophs; these receptors belong to the G protein-coupled receptor family. Homozygous or compound heterozygous inactivating mutations in the GHRHR cause complete lack of functional GHRHR protein and lack of detectable increase in serum GH to all provocative stimuli (6). These mutations cause severe familial isolated GH deficiency (IGHD type 1b), and patients have profound short stature with decreased serum levels of insulin-like growth factor-1 and -2 (IGF-1 and IGF-2) and IGF binding protein-3 (IGFBP-3). Magnetic resonance imaging (MRI) shows hypoplasia of the anterior pituitary (7). As expected, these individuals respond appropriately to exogenous GH administration.

GROWTH HORMONE SECRETAGOGUES

GH-releasing peptides (GHRPs) and nonpeptide mimetics, collectively referred to as GH secretagogues (GHSs), are a family of synthetic peptide and nonpeptide compounds that are capable of inducing GH release in all species, including humans. A novel feature is that they can stimulate GH release when given by oral, intranasal, or parenteral route (8). The coadministration of GHRP with GHRH produces a synergistic GH release. Children with classical GHD, and especially those with pituitary stalk interruption syndrome (PSIS) on MRI, have a markedly diminished GH response to GHRPs (7). This has been interpreted as a chronic absence or diminution of endogenous GHRH secretion. It should also be noted that the reliability of GH stimulation tests, with the use of GHRH or GHRPs in particular, can be improved if endogenous SST tone is modified by pretreatment with various agents, including pyridostigmine, arginine, or SST and its analogues (5,9,10).

GROWTH HORMONE SECRETAGOGUE RECEPTOR

GHS receptor (GHSR) is a G protein-coupled receptor expressed mainly in the somatotrophs of the anterior lobe of the pituitary, the hypothalamus, and the hippocampus, and on GHRH neurons. It is selective for the specific GHS peptides, such as ghrelin, which is a 28-amino acid peptide that is an endogenous ligand of GHSR. Activation of GHSR by synthetic ligands initiates and amplifies pulsatile GH release in animals, including humans, via the stimulated release of GHRH, which can be blocked by SST and GH (11). To date, four children with short stature relative to their families were found to have a shared missense mutation in the ghrelin receptor or type 1a GHSR; GH therapy has been initiated and felt to be beneficial (12).

GHRELIN

Endocrine cells in the gastric mucosa produce ghrelin, but expression in intestine, pancreas, hypothalamus, and testis has also been reported (13). Ghrelin stimulates GH secretion in vivo and from anterior pituitary cells in vitro. At least two different types of ghrelin receptors have been identified; their activation are involved in the secretion of a variety of pituitary hormones, appetite and long-term regulation of energy homeostasis (14,15).

GROWTH HORMONE GENE

The human GH gene locus is on the long arm of chromosome 17 and encodes for both pituitary GH (hGH-N), a single polypeptide chain of 191 amino acid residues that is secreted from the pituitary, as well as placental hGH (hGH-V) (16). The GH gene locus is close to the gene locus for chorionic somatotropin or human placental lactogen derived from the placenta. The primary full-length 22-kDa peptide is alternately spliced to yield a 20-kDa peptide that is cosecreted with and circulates at 5% to 10% of 22-kDa GH levels. Isolated GHD attributed to GH gene mutations may be inherited as autosomal recessive, dominant or X-linked, with the last entity being associated with hypogammaglobulinemia. Deletions of hGH-N produce very severe autosomal recessive growth failure after birth (17).

GROWTH HORMONE RECEPTOR

GH exerts many of its physiologic functions by regulating the transcription of genes of a variety of proteins, including IGF-1, transcription factors, and metabolic enzymes (18). The GH receptor was cloned in 1987 and led to the study of GH signaling at a molecular level. The cDNA for the human GH receptor encodes a 638-amino acid protein that has single extracellular, transmembrane, and cytoplasmic domains. It is a member of the cytokine/hematopoietin receptor superfamily that binds more than 25 ligands, including prolactin and leptin. In the working model of GH action, a single molecule of GH binds to two molecules of the GH receptor in a sequential fashion to form a dimer, an event that is crucial to subsequent GH-signaling events. During activation, the extracellular domain undergoes proteolytic cleavage to yield a soluble GH-binding protein in plasma or GHBP. GH binding to two receptor molecules increases the affinity of each receptor for a nonreceptor tyrosine kinase termed JAK2. Activation of JAK2 induces phosphorylation of itself and of tyrosine residues on the cytoplasmic domain of the GH receptor, initiating a cascade of signaling molecules that are beyond the purview of this chapter (18).

Inactivating mutations of the GH receptor gene or downstream signaling pathways cause the GH insensitivity syndrome (GHIS). Laron syndrome or classical GHIS is rare; its phenotype resembles that of GHD except for the presence of high serum GH concentrations and low levels of IGF-1, IFG-2, and IGFBP-3. Subcutaneous injections of recombinant IGF-1 or recombinant IGF-1–recombinant IGFBP-3 complex offer some promise of significantly improving height growth (19). A patient with a post-GH-receptor defect in conjunction with a primary immunodeficiency was described, and a mutation in the STAT5b gene has been implicated (20).

GROWTH HORMONE ACTIONS

GH is a powerful anabolic hormone, and has a broader spectrum of action than implied by its original name. The growth-promoting effects and metabolic effects of GH are mediated via interaction with the specific GH receptor and through the important intermediary IGF-1 and its receptor (18,21,22). Three general outcome measurements have been frequently assessed:

1. In childhood, auxologic measures provide parameters of linear growth response to GH: height standard deviation score (HT SDS), height velocity (HV), weight, pubertal progression, skeletal maturation, and attainment of adult final height (FH). One must distinguish between short-term changes in growth velocity and the attainment of adult FH, which may not be concordant. Thus, increased HV over intervals of less than 1 year and predictions of FH are not reliable predictors of increased adult height attainment (23–25). Age, initial HT SDS, delayed bone age, GH-secretory capacity, and GH dosage are important general predictors of a good growth response in children (24,25).
2. In both, children and adults, biochemical indices have been utilized to predict and/or monitor GH effects on cellular and tissue metabolism. GH increases protein synthesis, leading to retention of nitrogen; enhanced skeletal growth; increased sodium, phosphate, and calcium excretion; increased glucose and amino acid transport; and decreased lipogenesis. Indices of bone and mineral metabolism include calcium, phosphate, bone alkaline phosphatases, osteocalcin, propeptides of procollagen type I and type III, and bone mineral content (21). GH is the most important regulator of IGFs in all body tissues. In children and adults, there is a dose-related increase in both serum IGF-1 and IGF-II with acute GH administration (26). IGF-I increases more rapidly and to a relatively greater extent than IGF-1I. For this reason, serum IGF-I levels have become the most

commonly utilized measurement for assessing adequacy of GH secretion and monitoring the status of patients with GHD or excess.

3. Body mass index (BMI), percentage total body fat, total body or extracellular water, and bone mineral density are used most frequently to assess body composition (21). GH action on the adipocyte leads to reduction of body fat due to both decreased lipogenesis and increased lipolysis. Modest acute changes with wide variability have been observed with most of these body composition measurements.

GH dose exerts a very significant positive influence on all parameters used to assess effects on growth and metabolism. Few of the tests just described can reliably predict and/or monitor response to GH therapy. Of these, serum IGF-1 appears to offer the best indicator of the action of GH throughout all age groups. Lack of GH action is seen in children with classical GHD. In these patients, there is a decrease in serum GH, IGF-1, and IGFBP-3; decreased height SDS and growth velocity; delayed skeletal maturation; delayed pubertal onset; and increased abdominal adiposity. These are reversed with GH therapy. Excessive GH action is classically seen in patients with acromegaly, who demonstrate increased serum GH not suppressed with glucose, increased serum IGF-1 and IGFBP-3, increased BMI, and acral enlargement. With treatment of acromegaly, clinical improvement is usually best correlated with reductions in serum levels of GH and IGF-1.

THE ROLE OF THE GROWTH HORMONE–INSULIN-LIKE GROWTH FACTOR AXIS ON FETAL GROWTH REGULATION

The fetal endocrine milieu of hormones and growth factors is likely of secondary importance in the regulation of human fetal growth due to redundancy and the ability of several different systems to interact to protect fetal viability (27). In this context, GHD is relatively less important than GH insensitivity, and the paracrine/autocrine system of growth control involving local regulatory factors such as the IGFs and the IGFBPs becomes significant. IGF-1 and IGF-2 are endocrine, paracrine, and autocrine modulators of fetal growth and metabolism. In the human, circulating levels of the IGFs increase in both maternal and fetal serum during gestation, with IGF-2 present in two- to fivefold higher amount than IGF-1 (27,28). Animal gene knockout models support a predominant role for IGF-2 in fetal growth regulation (27). Therefore, IGF-2 may well be particularly important in early gestation, where it may dictate the size of the placenta and its ability to transport nutrients, both of which could profoundly affect fetal size (29).

In the human genetic model of GH insensitivity or Laron syndrome due to mutations of the GH receptor, there is a marked decrease in fetal serum IGF-1 and IGF-2, despite markedly elevated serum GH and very low serum GHBP. The neonates are small at birth (30).

THE DIAGNOSIS OF GROWTH HORMONE DEFICIENCY

The large majority of short children have nonendocrine causes for their growth failure. The variable prevalence of idiopathic GHD per million of total population from 18 to 24 per million in Europe to 287 per million in the United States is related to differences in diagnostic criteria employed (25,31). The diagnosis of GHD requires a combination of auxologic and biochemical criteria to identify the most severe or "complete" forms of GHD (32–34). Short children who are young and growing slowly are most likely to have significant GHD and to benefit most from GH treatment. A molecular genetic cause for GHD is relatively rare (35). Mutations in such genes as *Pit-1, PROP-1, HESX-1,* and *LHX3* are heritable; of note, these are usually associated with multiple hormone deficiencies as well as a positive family history (36).

The analysis of GH testing for GHD in childhood is confounded by the lack of a worldwide consensus on the definition of GHD (31–34). This difficulty largely relates to the recognition that GH secretion is a continuous spectrum with endogenous cyclicity and that children exhibit variable responses to multiple provocative stimuli. Because no one GH stimulation test has 100% sensitivity (no false negatives) and 100% specificity (no false positives), most countries have established an arbitrary cutoff to define a "normal" GH peak response to at least two provocative GH stimulation tests (31–34). However, even using these criteria, the percentage of children who retest as having "normal" GH secretion after the discontinuation of their GH treatment may be as high as 70% (31,32,37,38).

Moreover, the difficulties in assessing GH secretion in children can also be related to the lack of standardization of GH tests. A striking example was reported from France, with 6,373 GH stimulation tests from 3,233 short children with the diagnosis of GHD (39). Eleven different pharmacologic tests were used, and 62 of the possible 66 pairs were used at least once; the most frequent combination was used in only 12.7% of patients. Given the difficulty in interpretation of these findings, it is evident that only a limited number of standardized GH stimulation tests should be used. Physiologic assessment of GH secretion by frequent sampling throughout the 24-hour period is not more reliable (i.e., encompassing both sensitivity and specificity) than standard provocative GH stimulation tests, and is not used routinely for GH assessment (25,32,33).

An additional hurdle in unifying the diagnosis of GHD lies not only with nonstandardized testing protocols but the fact that GH as well as IGF-1 assays produce very disparate results on different analyzers (40). Most analyzers utilize immunochemiluminescent or immunoenzymatic GH assays, which, however, may detect different isoforms. These newer assays have led to a systematic lowering of assay results for serum GH levels. This in turn dictates that the use of arbitrary cutoff values above 8 to 10 μg per L with current assay methods should be abandoned (41). However, the cutoff level used to define GHD has not always been comparably reduced (42). To reduce such discrepancies, Japan has moved to a unified system of GH analyses, with national standardization. As a result, the diagnostic cutoff peak of GH has changed from 10 to 6 μg per L (43).

IGF-1 concentrations likewise are not standardized, similarly precluding the use of fixed reference values (44). Although subnormal serum levels of both serum IGF-1 and IGFBP-3 are believed to be highly predictive of a subnormal response to a provocative GH test in prepubertal children, two recent large retrospective studies have seriously challenged their diagnostic utility (45–47).

Once the auxological and biochemical data identify GHD, anatomic imaging by MRI is essential to allow detection of an asymptomatic CNS tumor or congenital malformations of pituitary gland. More than half of the patients with "isolated" GHD have findings of PSIS (interrupted pituitary stalk, anterior pituitary hypoplasia, and an ectopic hyperintense posterior pituitary) (48). For many of these individuals, additional anterior pituitary hormones deficiencies may be detected, either at diagnosis or later. Isolated pituitary hypoplasia has been found in about 25% of children with severe isolated GHD and surprisingly in 25% to 33% of children labeled as having ISS. This technology has not been applied in the majority of studies reported to date on FH attainment in short children treated with GH.

These issues highlight the need for clinicians to assess GH secretion only in the slowly growing short children and to be aware of the issues raised by lack of standardized GH and IGF-1 assays (32–34).

GROWTH HORMONE TREATMENT

Products and Dosage

Following the unfortunate occurrence of CJD in 1985, pituitary-derived GH was removed from production. Since then, the exclusive product has been the natural sequence recombinant GH peptide, which is distributed worldwide by several manufacturers. These products currently have a potency of 3 IU per mg and are usually administered by daily (six to seven injections per week) subcutaneous injections. These are usually given at bedtime to mimic endogenous GH secretion. The recommended doses are detailed in Table 54.1, varying from 0.18 to 0.40 mg per kg per week (0.5 to 1.2 IU per kg per week), depending on the diagnostic category. Larger GH doses are usually recommended in non-GHD children, as nonphysiologic pharmacologic doses are needed to overcome postulated "GH insensitivity."

Growth Hormone Treatment of Children with Growth Hormone Deficiency

The 40-year world experience concerning FH attainment with the use of GH to treat thousands of children with GHD has been reported (25). It is to be stressed that the criteria used for the diagnosis of GHD varied considerably, and highly variable assay methodology was used for the determination of GH values in the reported studies. In addition, the GH doses and frequency of administration were quite disparate. This makes comparisons among published studies very problematic. In addition, the vast majority of reported studies are uncontrolled, and no randomized controlled trials have been published for subjects with GHD for obvious ethical reasons.

The long-term growth response of children with GHD to pituitary GH showed an impressive mean gain of 1.9 SDS, but GHD patients still ended up near the 3rd percentile (−2.3 SDS), likely due to the late onset of less than optimal GH therapy associated with extreme short stature (−4.2 SDS) at diagnosis. GHD patients treated almost exclusively with rhGH had less height deficit at onset and achieved greater adult height than those treated with pituitary GH, with a mean additional gain of 0.9 SDS (−1.4 vs. −2.3 SDS). Although they did not achieve mean target height, the majority of GHD patients treated with rhGH achieved a normal adult height (25). This may be attributed to the fact that these patients received rhGH at larger doses, more frequently, and usually for a longer mean duration.

Final height in children with GHD arising from CNS, craniospinal, or total body irradiation may be further compromised by radiation-induced skeletal damage resulting in the inability to fully respond to GH (49). These individuals

TABLE 54.1 Cost-effectiveness of Adult Height Gain in Various Treatment Categories[a]

Study Category	*Gender*	*Untreated Adult Height (cm)*	*GH Dose (mg/kg/wk)*	*GH Treated Final Height (cm)*	*Cost/cm (1,000 USD)[b]*
Normal	M	178	...	...	...
	F	164	...	...	...
GHD	M	134–146[c]	0.18–0.35	168	10
	F	128–134[c]	0.18–0.35	155	10
PWS	M	154	0.23–0.35	+10[d]	11
	F	145–149	0.23–0.35	+10[d]	11
CRF	M	156	0.30–0.35	162–165	11–38
	F	152	0.30–0.35	151–155	11–38
ISS	M	150–170	0.20–0.40	164	22–43
	F	137–156	0.20–0.40	155	25–43
TS	F	143	0.375	146	25–28

CRF, chronic renal failure; F, female; GH, growth hormone; GHD, growth hormone deficiency; ISS, idiopathic short stature; M, male; PWS, Prader–Willi syndrome; TS, Turner syndrome.

[a]Constructed from data reported by Bryant et al. (66). Approximate mean values are expressed. For normal adult men, −2 SDS or approximate 5th percentile is 164 cm and for women, −2 SDS is 152 cm.

[b]The author converted UK estimates into US dollars (USD).

[c]Estimated from small patient numbers. Den Ouden et al. reported six adult patents with untreated multiple pituitary hormone deficiencies, who achieved heights of 148 to 193 cm (80).

[d]Data reported from only one small study with methodologic concerns.

may sustain additional deficiencies such as hypothyroidism or inability to undergo puberty, which may in turn limit height growth (49).

Patients who were younger and who had the greatest deficit in height achieved the greatest total height gain on rhGH. Delayed pubertal induction and midparental height are major factors influencing FH during rhGH treatment of children with GHD.

Growth Hormone Treatment of the Non-GH–Deficient Short Child

Despite the paucity of published controlled data that clearly indicate benefit, GH has become the most widely employed and most controversial therapeutic agent in the non-GH–deficient short child (24,25). The use of GH for the child with ISS and TS represents a significant proportion of total use, averaging from 23% to 58% in the larger series (25).

Growth Hormone Treatment in Idiopathic Short Stature

Many uncontrolled short-term studies indicate that GH administration accelerates HV in some normal short children. However, in a review of 413 short normal children treated with GH with variable doses for over 5 years, the overall mean FH gain over predicted adult height was only 2.7 cm, or +0.4 SDS (25). This resulted in a mean FH SDS of −1.7 SDS, which is nearly identical to the observed FH with spontaneous growth in 229 children with ISS (−1.5 SDS for boys and −1.6 SDS for girls) (44,45). Thus, a very significant regression toward the mean takes place, and not all short children end up being short adults.

A recent meta-analysis evaluated all randomized controlled trials assessing the impact of GH on linear growth in children with ISS; three studies included a placebo-treated control group (50). Only one trial evaluated final adult height, and another compared near final adult height in girls. Both trials had small numbers of children, many dropping out over the study interval for unspecified reasons. The first study demonstrated an apparent gain in height of 3.7 cm or 0.57 SDS (95% CI, 0.03 to 1.10) in the GH-treated group compared with controls (51). The second trial assessing final or near FH demonstrated a 6 to 7 cm gain for those treated with GH compared with controls (52). Of note, all children still ended up relatively short in both trials.

A recent publication, not included in this meta-analysis, reported on the FH outcomes of a randomized controlled study of physiologic and twice physiologic dose of GH for short non-GHD peripubertal children (53). This study was again significantly hampered because approximately 30% of those enrolled were nonadherent to the protocol, as well as the fact that the etiology was heterogeneous for the short stature and included children with SGA. If the data of all of the children were analyzed by intent to treat, then those treated with physiologic doses of GH (0.033 mg per kg per day) had similar FHs compared to the controls (−2.0 ± 0.8 FH SDS vs. −2.1 ± 0.8, $p = .053$, respectively), whereas there was a modest increase in the higher dose group versus controls (−1.5 ± 0.9 FH SDS vs. −2.1 ± 0.8, $p < .01$). The data when analyzed "per protocol" or including only those children who adhered the results would suggest modest benefit from both doses of GH; of note, many GH-treated children still ended up at less than −2 SDS (53).

In the one trial that evaluated this question, children with ISS did not have lower health-related quality of life scores than the normal population, except for social functioning (54). Treated children did not report improvements in these scores and at times had worse health-related quality of life scores than the controls (54). A reevaluation of the psychological status of both referred and population-based short children has also concluded that short stature does not appear to be associated with clinically significant psychological morbidity (54,55).

A recent statement by the Lawson Wilkins Pediatric Endocrine Society and the European Society for Paediatric Endocrinology reviewed how best to evaluate the causes of short stature, alternatives to GH therapy, many of which are not fully vetted, FH post-GH use, as well as cost/benefit analysis for this relatively expensive therapy (56).

In summary, it would thus appear from the data that the conclusion about the effect of GH and FH in children with ISS is tenuous. Prescription of GH remains a contentious issue in this otherwise healthy, well-adjusted group (57).

Growth Hormone Treatment in Turner Syndrome

Turner syndrome (TS) is not related to GHD, and the GH dose recommended, 0.375 mg per kg per week, is supraphysiologic. A recent world survey of FH in girls with TS treated with GH indicated considerable variation in the treatment protocols as to dose and age of onset of GH therapy, and in the concomitant use of estrogens or anabolic steroids (25). The mean age of onset for GH therapy varied from 10 to 15 years, with doses from 0.18 to 0.70 mg per kg per week. The mean FH of 2,211 girls with TS treated with GH was 150.0 cm, which is 5.8 cm above predicted adult height, with considerable individual variability in all studies (25). An additional report of GH treatment, at a median GH dose of 0.29 mg per kg per week, of 188 TS patients from 96 German centers from 1987 to 2000 noted a similar gain of 6.0 (−1.3 to +13) cm above the projected adult height (58). In the only randomized controlled trial of GH treatment to FH in TS reported from Canada, GH treatment significantly increased the mean FH of 69 girls: 141.4 ± 4.7 cm (mean ± 1 SD) in controls and 146.2 ± 6.5 cm in the GH group (59). It can be concluded that girls with TS *as a diagnostic group* do benefit in adult FH with GH treatment (25,58,59). However, all studies showed a poor outcome in some girls. A more efficacious intervention appears to be associated with a younger age of onset of GH treatment, larger doses of GH for longer periods, and a delay in estrogen administration until growth was nearly completed. It is critical that appropriate randomized controlled trials and meta-analyses assess which of these variables are most critical, and, more importantly, best for the patient (60,61).

Growth Hormone Treatment of Children Born with Intrauterine Growth Retardation or Small for Gestation Age

In approximately 15% to 20% of strikingly short children, postnatal growth failure is related to decreased prenatal growth velocity or intrauterine growth retardation (IUGR), resulting in infants who are small for gestation age. Most studies indicate that it is the low birth length that is most critical in the 10% to 15% of SGA infants who end up with persistent short stature during childhood and adulthood (51,52). There have been many studies assessing short-term effects of GH on children with SGA. Simon et al. reviewed the seven published trials assessing final or near-final adult height in approximately 350 children; only one was a controlled study (62). In this trial, the adolescents started with a mean height SDS of -3.2 ± 0.7; there were twice as many treated children as controls. After approximately 2.7 years, FH was obtained in all those still followed in the trial; this represented 89% of the treated and 70% of the placebo group. Both had increased their height SDS to -2.1 ± 1 versus -2.7 ± 0.9, respectively; the increases in those given GH at 0.067 mg per kg per day was significant compared with placebo ($p < .005$). Uncontrolled studies, particularly in prepubertal children often using doses of 0.067 mg per kg per day for 4 to 8 years, document more significant gains in FH SDS and without altering the age of onset of puberty; unfortunately, these were not controlled. It would appear that rhGH might normalize height if started early and using supraphysiologic doses, but additional randomized controlled studies are required for confirmation.

Growth Hormone Treatment in Children with Chronic Renal Failure

Approximately 60% of patients with chronic renal failure (CRF) have congenital disorders, and growth failure is significant from an early age (56). This is felt to be due to malnutrition, renal bone disease, acidosis, and GH insensitivity (63). The estimated mean height is −2.4 SDS from birth to 10 years, and FH is below the 3rd percentile in 33% of patients with CRF. Unlike rhGH indications for other non-GH–deficient disorders, GH is often given over shorter time intervals to increase body size pretransplant to facilitate transplantation, as well as posttransplant with the objective to improve FH. The usual rhGH dose is 0.30 to 0.35 mg per kg per week given in six to seven daily subcutaneous injections. Results from randomized controlled studies as well as NAPRTCS (North American Pediatric Renal Transplantation Cooperative Study) have demonstrated an improvement of approximately 0.5 to 1.7 SDS compared with controls, which have mean SDS of −2.9 (64,65). Posttreatment, adult height has been reported as −1.7 SDS, or 164 cm in boys and 151 to 156 cm in girls (66). Since normalization of growth and catch-up growth have also been reported with improved dialysis, the optimal approach to this multifactorial growth impairment remains to be clarified (63).

Growth Hormone Treatment in Prader–Willi Syndrome

Most patients with Prader–Willi syndrome (PWS) have deletions or an inactive portion of chromosome 15. Children with PWS have body compositions that resemble those with GHD, with mean adult height of 154 cm in men and 147 cm in women (66). The cause of the short stature is unknown, although abnormalities of the GH–IGF axis have been proposed, because reduced GH secretion has been observed. However, this interpretation is confounded by the known reduction in GH secretion seen in non-PWS obesity. Because of similarities between PWS and GHD, GH has been administered at doses of 0.20 to 0.35 mg per kg per week in the hope of increasing adult FH and improving body composition (66,67). Although increased short-term HV has been observed, reliable adult FH has not been reported. This patient population is prone to develop a number of typical adverse events with rhGH. In particular, serious concern has recently arisen because of multiple unexplained sudden deaths in PWS children early in the course of their GH treatment program (*vide infra*).

TRANSITION TO ADULT CARE

Only those children treated for GHD may be eligible to continue GH once their epiphyses have fused. One to 3 months after discontinuation of GH, they need to undergo repeat GH testing, and the cutoff to determine deficiency is more stringent (68). The GH doses typically used are about one-tenth those used in GHD children; regular IGF-1 monitoring has been advocated to maintain these concentrations in the normal range adjusted for age and sex.

GROWTH HORMONE TREATMENT RISKS

GH therapy is considered to be safe with the exception of CJD, which developed from GH and extracted from human pituitary tissue. Approximately 26 cases of this disease have been identified among the 7,700 people in the United States who received hGH from the National Hormone Pituitary Program (NHPP). An additional six overseas (National Institute of Diabetes and Digestive and Kidney Diseases, Office of Communication, March 2008) patients who received GH from US labs that produced the hormone for NHPP have also developed CJD. Unfortunately, the Web page of the European and Allied Countries Collaborative Study Group of CJD (EUROCJD; http://www.eurocjd.ed.ac.uk/) reported that as of March 2008, there have been many more cases of CJD related to GH therapy in France ($n = 100$) and in the United Kingdom ($n = 44$).

Adverse events associated with rhGH therapy include pseudotumor cerebri, slipped capital femoral epiphysis (SCFE), fluid retention, insulin resistance resulting in hyperglycemia, diabetes mellitus, and/or hyperlipidemia. Some of these issues arise more frequently in children with specific indications for rhGH therapy, see later (57).

Because GH raises serum IGF-1 concentrations, which is mitogenic, ongoing surveillance of children with GHD arising secondary to a CNS neoplasm are closely monitored for regrowth of original tumor or the diagnosis of a second neoplasm. The literature is still controversial on these points. In a recent investigation as to whether the development of a second neoplasm was more likely in childhood cancer survivors treated with rhGH versus untreated survivors, the rate ratio was 2.15 (95% CI, 1.3 to 3.5; $p < .002$) for those treated versus the untreated. Meningiomas were the most common second neoplasm diagnosed in treated group (69). Recurrence of the original tumor postinitiation of rhGH therapy is of considerable interest and the literature does not provide yet a definitive answer as to whether there is an increased risk (70).

For those children treated with supraphysiologic doses, additional scrutiny would appear to be warranted. Those treated with rhGH for ISS have few reported additional adverse events; however, this may be because relatively few children have been treated and/or the follow-up period is relatively short (49). Girls with TS treated in the National Cooperative Growth Study appear to suffer more intracranial hypertension, SCFE, scoliosis, and pancreatitis compared with children treated for other conditions (71).

Being born SGA already predisposes to insulin resistance, diabetes mellitus, the metabolic syndrome, and an apparent increased mortality attributed to coronary heart disease and stroke (72). The addition of supraphysiologic rhGH would intuitively worsen insulin sensitivity. To date, this has not been observed using our current diagnostic tools. However, the long-term risk of prolonged GH therapy has not yet been determined (73).

Pretransplant, children with CRF have increased insulin values with rhGH therapy but do not appear to have an increased risk of developing diabetes mellitus, except if the underlying diagnosis is cystinosis (74). Posttransplant, the additive use of glucocorticoids and other antirejection medications such as tacrolimus with rhGH could further predispose to glucose intolerance, and monitoring for hyperglycemia is warranted. Perhaps, more worrisome is the issue as to whether GH increases the risk of acute rejection; the literature is still unclear on this matter (65).

Since 2002, 25 GH-treated children with PWS have died, on average 4 months after GH initiation. More than two-third were due to respiratory causes, such as infections. The deaths occurred predominantly in obese males and those known to have sleep apnea (32% of deaths). Caution has been raised about prescribing GH to obese individuals with PWS, and recommendations about performing baseline and surveillance somnopolygrams have been promulgated in an attempt to reduce additional deaths (75). Of course, issues of hyperglycemia impaired insulin action, and pseudotumor cerebri with rhGH also arise in this population.

The absolute risk of each of these potential complications is likely to be very small. However, the use of increased doses of GH in children with nonendocrine short stature (>0.35 mg per kg per week or >1.0 IU per kg per week), which are twice those required to promote growth acceleration in most patients with "classical" GHD, has the potential to increase the usual risk factors. Nevertheless, when recombinant GH is administered for an approved indication at an approved dosage, it is remarkably safe (76–78).

THE USE OF GROWTH HORMONE TO INCREASE ADULT HEIGHT: HAS THE OUTCOME ACHIEVED EXPECTATIONS?

Children with short stature who begin GH treatment have the expectation of achieving not just target height but normal adult height and all the benefits that they and their families expect from this attainment. Unfortunately, this expectation has not been fulfilled for many children (25,66). Despite being treated daily with GH for many years, at considerable individual total cost, the majority of patients with classical GHD; children with ISS, SGA, CRF, or PWS; and girls with TS have not achieved "normal" adult height if the mean is used as reference (Table 54.1) (66). However, individual patients have shown dramatic responses and have surpassed target height expectations. The majority of patients with idiopathic GHD, who begin GH therapy at an earlier age, with daily administration of recombinant rather than pituitary GH at doses of 0.2 to 0.35 mg per kg per week, can be expected to achieve a FH in the normal range, with relatively normal psychosocial function.

In the last two decades, there has been expanded administration of GH to short children with normal GH secretion, to the extent that they have become the largest GH treatment category in many countries. The outcome of this increased use has been the promotion of certain legitimacy to the use of GH for the "normal short child." However, there has been inadequate debate about the reported lack of demonstrated long-term benefit in terms of either growth or psychological status and the potential for negative impact that an unfulfilled expectation may have on a short child and his or her family. The published literature on the use of GH is largely uncontrolled and does not support the view that a significant benefit will arise in the majority of idiopathic short children who have normal GH secretion by appropriate current criteria. The challenge is to develop methodology that will identify all short children, including those with genetic syndromes, who will most likely benefit from the administration of GH over a prolonged period of time. It is to be hoped that the next decade of GH research will provide additional insight to make this a truly cost-effective and globally available treatment for the majority of patients who really do require treatment with GH.

In a controversial ruling in June 2003, The US Food and Drug Administration (FDA) approved an application to begin marketing synthetic human GH for a new pediatric "indication": idiopathic short stature or ISS (79). This new indication restricts therapy to children who are more than 2.25 SD below the mean for age and sex, or the shortest 1.2% of all children. In addition, treatment is offered to boys predicted to be less than 5 ft 3.5 in. (161 cm) tall by 18 years of age and to girls likely to be shorter than 4 ft 11 in. (150 cm). The FDA approval was based on two randomized, multicenter trials that enrolled approximately 300 children with ISS, only 1 of which was controlled. There are a number of criticisms of these and other trials for ISS, which has created significant discussion amongst pediatric endocrinologists. In response to the FDA decision, the Lawson Wilkins Pediatric Endocrinology Society (LWPES) Drug and Therapeutics Committee has advised a cautionary approach (57).

REFERENCES

1. Grumbach M, Bin-Abbas B, Kaplan S. The growth hormone cascade: progress and long-term results of growth hormone treatment in growth hormone deficiency. *Horm Res* 1998;49(Suppl 2):41–57.
2. Albertsson-Wikland K, Rosberg S, Kalberg J, et al. Analysis of 24-hour growth hormone profiles in healthy boys and girls of normal stature: relation to puberty. *J Clin Endocrinol Metab* 1994;78:1195–1201.
3. Miller J, Tannenbaum G, Colle E, et al. Day-time pulsatile growth hormone secretion during childhood and adolescence. *J Clin Endocrinol Metab* 1982;55:9889–9994.

4. Tannenbaum G, Ling N. The interrelationship of growth hormone (GH)-releasing factor and somatostatin in generation of the ultradian rhythm of GH secretion. *Endocrinology* 1984;115:1952–1957.
5. Tzanella M, Guyda H, Van Vliet G, et al. Somatostatin pre-treatment enhances GH responsiveness to GHRH: a potential new diagnostic approach to GH deficiency. *J Clin Endocrinol Metab* 1996;(7):2494.
6. Salvatori R, Serpa MG, Parmigiani G, et al. GH response to hypoglycemia and clonidine in the GH-releasing hormone resistance syndrome. *J Endocrinol Invest* 2006;29(9):805–808.
7. Aguiar-Oliveira M, Gill M, de A Barretto E, et al. Effect of severe growth hormone (GH) deficiency due to a mutation in the GH-releasing hormone receptor on insulin-like growth factors (IGFs), IGF-binding proteins, and ternary complex formation throughout life. *J Clin Endocrinol Metab* 1999;84(11):4118–4126.
8. Bach M, Gormley G. Clinical use of growth hormone secretagogues. In: Smith R, Thorner M, eds. *Human growth hormone: research and clinical practice (contemporary endocrinology).* Totawa, NJ: Humana Press, 2000.
9. Cappa M, Rigamonti A, Bizzari C, et al. Somatostatin infusion withdrawal: studies in normal children and children with growth hormone deficiency. *J Clin Endocrinol Metab* 1996;84(12):4426–4430.
10. Gasperi M, Aimaretti G, Scarcello G, et al. Low dose hexarelin and growth hormone (GH)-releasing hormone as a diagnostic tool for the diagnosis of GH deficiency in adults: comparison with insulin-induced hypoglycemia test. *J Clin Endocrinol Metab* 1999;84(8):2633–2637.
11. Howard A, Feighner S, Smith R, et al. Molecular characterization of growth hormone secretagogue receptors. In: Smith R, Thorner M, et al., eds. *Human growth hormone: research and clinical practice (contemporary endocrinology).* Totawa, NJ: Humana Press, 2000.
12. Pantel J, Legendre M, Cabrol S, et al. Loss of constitutive activity of the growth hormone secretagogue receptor in familial short stature[comment]. *J Clin Invest* 2006;116(3):760–768.
13. Broglio F, Arvat E, Benso A, et al. Ghrelin: endocrine and non-endocrine actions. *J Pediatr Endocrinol Metab* 2002;15:1219–1227.
14. Muccioli G, Baragli A, Granata R, et al. Heterogeneity of ghrelin/growth hormone secretagogue receptors. *Neuroendocrinology* 2007;86:147–164.
15. Tritos N, Kokkotou M. The physiology and potential clinical applications of ghrelin, a novel peptide hormone. *Mayo Clin Proc* 2006;81(5):653–660.
16. Waxman P, Frank S. Growth hormone action. In: Conn P, Means A, eds. *Principles of molecular regulation.* Totawa, NJ: Humana Press, 2000.
17. Bona G, Paracchini R, Giordano M, et al. Genetic defects in GH synthesis and secretion. *Eur J Endocrinol* 2004;151:S3–S9.
18. Herrington J, Carter-Su C. Signaling pathway activated by GH receptor. *Trends Endocrinol Metab* 2001;12(6):252–255.
19. Savage MO, Attie KM, David A, et al. Endocrine assessment, molecular characterization and treatment of growth hormone insensitivity disorders. *Nat Clin Pract Endocrinol Metab* 2006;2(7):395–407.
20. Rosenfeld R, Kofoed E, Little B, et al. Growth hormone insensitivity resulting from post-GH receptor defects. *Growth Horm IGF Res* 2004;14:S35–S38.
21. Guyda H. How do we best measure growth hormone action? *Horm Res* 1997;48(Suppl 5):1–10.
22. Wollmann H, Ranke M. Metabolic effects of growth hormone in children. *Metabolism* 1995;44(10):97–102.
23. Allen D, Brook C, Bridges N, et al. Therapeutic controversies: growth hormone (GH) treatment of non-GH deficient subjects. *J Clin Endocrinol Metab* 1994;79:1–10.
24. Guyda H. Use of growth hormone in children with short stature and normal growth hormone release: a growing problems. *Trends Endocrinol Metab* 1994;5(8):334–340.
25. Guyda H. Four decades of GH therapy for short children: what have we achieved? *J Clin Endocrinol Metab* 1999;84(12):4307–4316.
26. Grant M, Schmetz I, Russell B, et al. Changes in IGF-I and IGF-II and their binding proteins after a single injection of growth hormone. *J Clin Endocrinol Metab* 1986;63(4):981–984.
27. Deal C, Guyda H. Regulation of fetal growth and the GH-IGF-I axis: lessons for mouse to man. *Int Growth Monit* 1994;4:2–12.
28. Gluckman P. The endocrine regulation of fetal growth in late gestation: the role of insulin-like growth factors. *J Clin Endocrinol Metab* 1995;80(4):1047–1050.
29. Roberts C, Owens J, Sferruzzi-Perri A. Distinct actions of insulin-like growth factors (IGFs) on placental development and fetal growth: lessons from mice and guinea pigs. *Placenta* 2008;29(Suppl A):S42–S47.
30. Savage M, Blum W, Ranke M, et al. Clinical features and endocrine status in patients with growth hormone insensitivity (Laron syndrome). *J Clin Endocrinol Metab* 1993;77:1465–1471.
31. Sizonenko P, Clayton P, Cohen P, et al. Diagnosis and management of growth hormone deficiency in childhood and adolescence. Part 1: Diagnosis of growth hormone deficiency. *Growth Horm IGF Res* 2001;11:137–165.
32. Guyda H. The diagnosis of growth hormone deficiency in children with short stature: is it necessary? *Hong Kong J Paediatr* 1996;1:160–168.
33. Hintz R, Lafranchi S, Lippe B, et al. The diagnosis of childhood GH deficiency revisited. *J Clin Endocrinol Metab* 1995;80(5):1532–1540.
34. Rosenfeld R, Albertsson-Wikland K, Cassorla F, et al. Diagnostic controversy: the diagnosis of childhood growth hormone deficiency revisited. *J Clin Endocrinol Metab* 1995;80:1532–1540.
35. Phillips JI, Cogan J. Molecular basis of familial human growth hormone deficiency. *J Clin Endocrinol Metab* 1994;78:11–16.
36. Force AGHT. American Association of Clinical Endocrinologists medical guidelines for clinical practice for growth hormone use in adults and children—2003 update. *Endocr Pract* 2003;9(1):65–76.
37. Ghigo E, Bellone J, Aimaretti G, et al. Reliability of provocative tests to assess growth hormone secretory status. Study in 472 normally growing children. *J Clin Endocrinol Metab* 1996;81:332–3327.
38. Longobardi S, Merole B, Pivonello R, et al. Re-evaluation of GH secretion in 69 adults diagnosed as GH-deficient patients during childhood. *J Clin Endocrinol Metab* 1996;81:1244–1247.
39. Carel J, Tresca J, Letrait M, et al. Growth hormone testing for the diagnosis of growth hormone deficiency in childhood: a population register-based study. *J Clin Endocrinol Metab* 1997;82:2117–2121.
40. Amed S, Delvin E, Hamilton J. Variation in growth hormone immunoassays in clinical practice in Canada. *Horm Res* 2008;69:290–294.
41. Celniker A, Chen A, Wert AJ, et al. Variability in the quantitation of circulating growth hormone using commercial immunoassays. *J Clin Endocrinol Metab* 1989;68:469–476.
42. Mauras N, Walton P, Nicar M, et al. Growth hormone stimulation in both short and normal statured children: use of an immunofunctional assay. *Pediatr Res* 2000;48(5):614–618.
43. Ho KK, 2007 GH Deficiency Consensus Workshop Participants. Consensus guidelines for the diagnosis and treatment of adults with GH deficiency II: a statement of the GH Research Society in association with the European Society for Pediatric Endocrinology, Lawson Wilkins Society, European Society of Endocrinology, Japan Endocrine Society, and Endocrine Society of Australia. *Eur J Endocrinol* 2007;157(6):695–700.
44. Strasburger C, Bidlingmaier M. How robust are laboratory measures of growth hormone status? *Horm Res* 2005;64(Suppl 2):1–5.
45. Tillman V, Buckler J, Kibirige M, et al. Biochemical tests in the diagnosis of childhood growth hormone deficiency. *J Clin Endocrinol Metab* 1997;82:531–535.
46. Mitchell M, Dattani M, Nanduri V, et al. Failure of IGF-I and IGBP-3 to diagnose growth hormone deficiency. *Arch Dis Child* 1999;80(5):443–447.
47. Juul A, Skakkebaek N. Prediction of the outcome of growth hormone provocative testing in short children by measurement of serum levels of IGF-I and IGFBP-3. *J Pediatr* 1997;130:197–204.
48. Nagel B, Palmbach M, Ranke M, eds. *Magnetic resonance imaging in growth hormone deficiency.* Heidelberg, Germany: Barth, 1999:65–71.
49. Hindmarsh P, Dattani M. Use of growth hormone in children. *Nat Clin Pract* 2006;2(5):260–268.
50. Bryant J, Baxter L, Cave C, et al. Recombinant growth hormone for idiopathic short stature in children and adolescents [Review]. *Cochrane Library* 2008(3):1–31.
51. Leschek E, Rose S, Yanovski J, et al. Effect of growth hormone treatment on adult height in peripubertal children with idiopathic short stature: a randomized, double-bline, placebo-controlled trial. *J Clin Endocrinol Metab* 2004;89:3140–148.
52. Cowel C. Effects of growth hormone in short, slowly growing children without growth hormone deficiency. Australian Paediatric Endocrine Group. *Acta Paediatr Scand* 1990;326(Suppl):29–30.

53. Albertsson-Wikland K, Aronson A, Gustafsson J, et al. Dose-dependent effect of growth hormone on final height in children with short stature without growth hormone deficiency. *J Clin Endocrinol Metab* 2008;93(11):4342–4350.
54. Theunissen N, Kamp G, Koopman H, et al. Quality of life and self-esteem in children treated for idiopathic short stature. *J Pediatr* 2002;140:507–515.
55. Sandberg D. Quality of life and self-esteem in children treated for idiopathic short stature. *J Pediatr* 2003;143(5):691.
56. Cohen P, Rogol A, Deal C, et al. Consensus statement on the diagnosis and treatment of children with idiopathic short stature: a summary of the Growth Hormone Society, the Lawson Wilkins Pediatric Endocrine Society, and the European Society for Paediatric Endocrinology Workshop. *J Clin Endocrinol Metab* 2008;93(11): 4210–4217.
57. Wilson TA, Rose SR, Cohen P, et al. Update of guidelines for the use of growth hormone in children: the Lawson Wilkens Pediatric Endocrinology Society Drug and Therapeutics Committee. *J Pediatr* 2003;143:415–421.
58. Ranke M, Partsch C, Lindberg A, et al. Adult height after GH therapy in 188 Ullrich–Turner syndrome patients: results of the German IGLU Follow-up Study 2001. *Eur J Endocrinol* 2002;147(5):625–633.
59. Canadian GH Advisory Committee. GH treatment to final height in Turner syndrome: a randomized controlled trial. *Horm Res* 1998; 50(Suppl 3):25.
60. Taback S, Guyda H, Van Vliet G. Pharmacological manipulation of height: qualitative review of study populations and design. *Clin Invest Med* 1999;22(2):53–59.
61. Baxter L, Bryant J, Cave C, et al. Recombinant growth hormone for children and adolescents with Turner syndrome [Review]. *Cochrane Library* 2008(3):1–28.
62. Simon D, Leger J, Carel J. Optimal use of growth hormone therapy for maximizing adult height in children born small for gestational age. *Best Pract Res Clin Endocrinol Metab* 2008;22(3): 525–537.
63. Tom A, McCauley L, Rodd C, et al. Maintenance of growth with aggressive hemodialysis therapy in children with chronic renal insufficiency. *J Pediatr* 1999;134:464–467.
64. Mehls O, Wuhl E, Tonshoff B, et al. Growth hormone treatment in short children with chronic kidney disease. *Acta Paediatr* 2008;97: 1159–1164.
65. Fine R, Stablein D. Long-term use of recombinant human growth hormone in pediatric allograft recipients: a report of the NAPRTCS Transplant Registry. *Pediatr Nephrol* 2005;20:404–408.
66. Bryant J, Care C, Mihaylova B, et al. Clinical effectiveness and cost effectiveness of growth hormone in children: as systematic review and economic evaluation. *Health Technol Assess* 2002;6(18):1–168.
67. Carrel A, Myers S, Whitman B, et al. Benefits of long-term GH therapy in Prader–Willi syndrome: a 4 year study. *J Clin Endocrinol Metab* 2002;87(4):1581–1585.
68. Molitch ME, Clemmons DR, Malozowski S, et al.; Growth Hormone Guideline Task Force. Evaluation and treatment of adult growth hormone deficiency: an Endocrine Society Clinical Practice Guideline. *J Clin Endocrinol Metab* 2006;91:1621–1634.
69. Ergun-Longmire B, Mertens A, Mitby P, et al. Growth hormone treatment and risk of second neoplasms in the Childhood Cander Survivor. *J Clin Endocrinol Metab* 2006;91:3494–498.
70. Darendeliler F, Karagiannis G, Wilton P, et al. Recurrence of brain tumours in patients treated with growth hormone: analysis of the KIGS (Pfizer International Growth Database). *Acta Paediatr* 2006;95:1284–1290.
71. Bolar K, Hoffman A, Maneatis T, et al. Long-term safety of recombinant human growth hormone in Turner syndrome. *J Clin Endocrinol Metab* 2008;93(2):344–351.
72. van Parren Y, Mulder P, Houdijk M, et al. Adult height after long-term, continuous growth hormone (GH) treatment in short children born small for gestational age: results of a randomized, double-blind, dose-response GH trial. *J Clin Endocrinol Metab* 2003;88: 3584–3590.
73. Poduval A, Saenger P. Safety and efficacy of growth hormone treatment in small for gestational age children. *Curr Opin Endocrinol Diabetes Obes* 2008;15(4):376–382.
74. Mahan J, Warady B. Assessment and treatment of short stature in pediatric patients with chronic renal disease: a consensus statement. *Pediatr Nephrol* 2006;21:917–930.
75. Tauber M, Diene G, Molinas C, et al. Review of 64 cases of death in children with Prader–Willi Syndrome (PWS). *Am J Med Genet A* 2008;146A:881–887.
76. Wilton P. Adverse events during GH treatment: 10 years' experience in KIGS, a pharmacoepidemiological survey. In: Ranke M, Wilton P, eds. *Growth hormone therapy in KIGS—10 year's experience.* Heidelberg. Germany: Barth, 1999.
77. Nishi Y, Takana T, Takano K, et al. Recent status of the occurrence of leukemia in GH-treated patients in Japan. *J Clin Endocrinol Metab* 1999;80(4):1961–1965.
78. Blethen L, Allen D, Graves D, et al. Safety of recombinant deoxyribonucleic acid-derived growth hormone. The National Cooperative Growth Study Experience. *J Clin Endocrinol Metab* 1996;81:1704–1710.
79. FDA. FDA approves Humatrope for short stature. Available at: www.accessdata.fda.gov/drugsatfda_docs/label/2008/021908s005lbl.pdf-2009-03-31.
80. Den Ouden D, Kroon M, Hoogland P, et al. A 43-year old male with untreated panhypopituitarism due to absence of pituitary stalk: from dwarf to giant. *J Clin Endocrinol Metab* 2002;87:5430–5434.

CHAPTER

55

Annie Nguyen-Vermillion
Sandra E. Juul

Hematologic Agents

INTRODUCTION

The bone marrow of a healthy growing fetus produces billions of cells each day. This challenge is greater in developing individuals than in adults because the marrow must produce enough new cells to maintain a stable cell number per body mass as the baby grows. Preterm birth or illness in the newborn period is associated with additional hematologic stressors, which can result in anemia or neutropenia. This chapter addresses multiple mechanisms of anemia and neutropenia in the newborn and reviews the use of available recombinant growth factors to treat these conditions.

ERYTHROPOIETIN

PHYSIOLOGIC AND PHARMACOLOGIC EFFECTS

Erythropoietin (Epo) is an endogenous glycoprotein that regulates erythrocyte production (1,2). Since the Food and Drug Administration (FDA) approval in 1989, many trials have been done (and reviewed) to test the safety and efficacy of recombinant human (r)Epo as an erythropoietic agent in neonates (3–5). rEpo is now widely used to treat or prevent anemia due to a variety of causes including renal failure and prematurity. Compared with adults, neonates require higher doses of rEpo per kilogram and more frequent dosing to achieve an equivalent hematopoietic response, due to their greater plasma clearance, high volume of distribution, and short fractional elimination time (6–8).

Humans have four main sites of embryonic and fetal erythropoiesis: yolk sac, ventral aspect of the aorta, liver, and bone marrow. Epo production mirrors this, beginning in the yolk sac, moving to the liver as the primary source during most of fetal life, and then switching to renal production around the time of birth. Factors regulating this switch are still not fully understood (9,10). Growth factors important for definitive erythropoiesis include Epo, stem cell factor (c-kit ligand), interleukin-3 (IL-3), IL-6, granulocyte–macrophage colony-stimulating factor (GM-CSF), and possibly insulin and insulin-like growth factor 1 (IGF-1), both of which act as nonessential survival factors for CD34+ cells (11,12). Epo maintains red cell production during fetal, neonatal, and adult life by inhibiting apoptosis of erythroid progenitors and by stimulating their proliferation and differentiation into normoblasts (13,14). Epo receptor (EpoR) density is highest in the burst-forming units erythroid and colony-forming units erythroid (Fig. 55.1). In addition to increasing and maintaining erythrocyte progenitors, Epo increases the synthesis of hemoglobin, membrane proteins, and transferrin receptors. Epo can be considered the primary growth factor in the process of erythropoiesis, as in its absence, definitive erythropoiesis does not occur: both Epo and EpoR null mutation mice die on the 13th day of intrauterine development due to absence of secondary erythropoiesis (15). Since Epo does not cross the placenta, Epo concentrations measured in the fetus reflect fetal synthesis (16).

During development, the EpoR is present on many nonhematopoietic cell types, including liver stromal cells (17), smooth muscle cells (18), myocardiocytes (19), endothelial cells (20), enterocytes (21), renal tubular cells, epithelial cells in the lung, retinal cells (22), placental tissues (23), Leydig cells (24), and cells specific to the central nervous system (25–27). The role of Epo in these tissues is under investigation.

To maintain the increase in red cell volume associated with fetal growth, it is estimated that approximately 50×10^9 erythrocytes per day must be produced. When compared with adult Epo concentrations present at the time of acute anemia, measured fetal Epo concentrations seem low in the face of such production requirements. It has, therefore, been proposed that Epo is more efficient in the stimulation of the erythropoiesis during fetal development, that it acts as a paracrine factor during hepatic hematopoiesis, and/or that other growth factors synergize with Epo. Candidate factors include hepatic growth factor, thrombopoietin, and IGF-1 (28,29). Production of Epo is stimulated by hypoxia-inducible factor 1 and 2 and is regulated by requirements for tissue oxygenation. Elevated Epo concentrations (up to 8,000 mU per mL) have been reported in pathologic states, such as fetal hypoxia, anemia, and placental insufficiency, and in infants of diabetic mothers (30,31).

In healthy term infants, serum Epo concentrations decrease following birth to reach a nadir between 4 and 6 weeks of life. By 10 to 12 weeks of life, they reach adult concentrations (approximately 15 mU per mL). In preterm

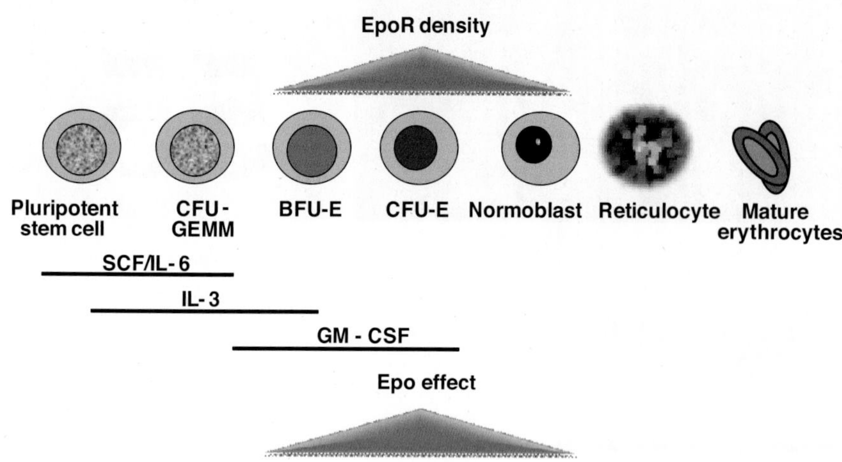

Figure 55.1. Lineage development of erythrocytes, with emphasis on growth factors and timing of erythropoietin effect. BFU-E, burst-forming unit erythroid; CFU-E, colony-forming unit erythroid; CFU-GEMM, colony-forming unit granulocyte, erythrocyte, monocyte, megakaryocyte; Epo, erythropoietin; EpoR, erythropoietin receptor; IL-6, interleukin-6; SCF, stem cell factor.

infants, the fall in Epo is more profound and persists longer, contributing to anemia of prematurity.

CLINICAL TRIALS IN NEWBORN INFANTS

Preterm infants remain among the most highly transfused patient populations despite attempts to limit phlebotomy losses, the implementation of transfusion guidelines, and the use of rEpo. Common contributors to anemia in the hospitalized preterm infant include phlebotomy loss (which may exceed the infant's circulating blood volume), short red blood cell life span (70 vs. 120 days in adults), high growth requirements, iron deficiency, inflammatory states, and anemia of prematurity. When measured, circulating Epo concentrations in this population are low relative to the degree of anemia (32). Other forms of anemia in neonates include Rh-hemolytic disease of the newborn and a variety of anemias that are associated with chronic lung disease. The role of rEpo administration has been tested in each of these conditions, and also in neonates with congenital heart disease where an elevated hematocrit is desired.

Anemia of Prematurity

The majority of erythrocyte transfusions administered to very low-birth-weight (VLBW, birth weight <1,500 g) neonates are given during the first 3 weeks of life (33). The use of rEpo to avoid excessive transfusions in preterm infants has been studied in many randomized controlled trials. Several reviews have evaluated the safety and efficacy of rEpo treatment (3,5,34). rEpo treatment used together with iron is safe, well tolerated, and decreases both the number of transfusions and the volume of blood transfused when used at doses of greater than 500 U per kg per week. However, rEpo treatment may not prevent all transfusions or even significantly decrease donor exposures. This is because clinical practice is so variable: transfusion guidelines differ in stringency, phlebotomy practices vary by institution, and the timing and dose of both rEpo and iron vary widely.

One reasonable approach to managing anemia in the extremely preterm infant is to combine the use of iron supplementation, blood transfusion, and rEpo therapy with the goal of one donor exposure per infant maximum. Optisol®-preserved blood can be stored for up to 42 days. One adult unit of blood can be divided into aliquots and assigned to one infant. The infant can be transfused with these aliquots as needed during the first 6 weeks of life (one donor exposure). Iron status should be optimized. rEpo with iron can be used to prevent further transfusions if the infant remains significantly anemic with low reticulocyte counts. Judicious phlebotomy practices should be implemented.

Hyporegenerative Anemia of Neonates with Rh-Hemolytic Disease

Infants with Rh-hemolytic disease can develop a late anemia at 1 to 3 months of life secondary to diminished erythrocyte production. The incidence of late anemia seems to be much higher in infants who receive intrauterine transfusions (35–37). In these infants, the anemia is characterized by low plasma concentrations of Epo, while erythroid progenitors remain highly responsive to rEpo in vitro (37). Studies evaluating the use of rEpo as a treatment for neonates with late hyporegenerative anemia have shown mixed results (35,38,39).

Anemia of Bronchopulmonary Dysplasia

The anemia associated with bronchopulmonary dysplasia is normocytic, normochromic, and hyporegenerative with marrow normoblast iron stains that are distinct from those observed in the anemia of chronic disorders and the anemia of prematurity (40). In a study by Ohls et al., neonates with the anemia of bronchopulmonary dysplasia received 200 U per kg of rEpo per day subcutaneously for 10 consecutive days. Infants treated with rEpo at this dose and duration had increased reticulocytes and hematocrits and required fewer transfusions than placebo recipients (41).

Neonates with Congenital Heart Disease

Infants with certain varieties of congenital heart disease often experience prolonged hospitalization, multiple invasive procedures, and significant phlebotomy losses. These neonates frequently receive multiple blood transfusions. Neonates with congenital heart disease awaiting heart transplantation who received 200 U per kg per day of rEpo had significant increase in hematocrit and a decrease in transfusions (42).

Only a limited number of studies have evaluated the role of rEpo as an alternative to transfusions in neonates awaiting cardiac surgery. In Japan, a study evaluated the effect of three doses of rEpo (300 U per kg) on transfusion requirements of infants undergoing cardiac surgery (43). A beneficial effect of rEpo has been reported among neonates who underwent open heart surgery and in those whose parents are Jehovah's Witnesses (44). Further studies evaluating the use of rEpo to reduce transfusion requirements in neonates with congenital heart disease are needed.

STRUCTURE, DOSE, ROUTES, AND REGIMENS

Recombinant human Epo is produced in Chinese hamster ovary cells by recombinant DNA technology, as a 165-amino acid glycoprotein with a molecular weight of 30.4 kDa. The human recombinant form of Epo is commercially available as epoetin alfa (rEpo) (Epogen, Amgen, Thousand Oaks, CA; Procrit, Ortho Biotech, Raritan, NJ).

A novel erythropoiesis-stimulating protein, Darbepoetin alpha (Aranesp), is a protein closely related to rEpo. It is also a 165-amino acid glycoprotein but contains five N-linked oligosaccharide chains, rather than the three contained in rEpo (45). These two additional glycosylation sites increase the molecular weight to 37.0 kDa and increase the terminal half-life threefold as determined in adult patients (46). Aranesp is available from Amgen and is formulated for intravenous and subcutaneous administration.

A wide range of dosing schedules have been used for hyporegenerative anemia in the preterm infant (50 to 700 U per kg per dose) (5,47,48). Garcia et al. showed that for every 500 U per kg per week increase in rEpo dosing, the average number of transfusions per patient decreased by three-fourth of a transfusion (5). We recommend subcutaneous administration of rEpo 400 U per kg three times per week, or daily intravenous rEpo 200 U per kg per day, for a minimum of 2 weeks (49). Alternatively, rEpo can be administered in a continuous intravenous infusion such as parenteral nutrition, using a dose of 200 U per kg per day (50). To promote effective erythropoiesis, iron must be given concomitant with rEpo. Patients on full enteral feedings who are receiving rEpo should receive 6 to 8 mg per kg per day of elemental iron. Alternatively, parenteral iron may be given at 1 mg per kg per day (49). Zinc protoporphyrin to heme ratios (ZnPP/H) may be followed weekly to assess and optimize iron status (51,52). Serum ferritin levels may also be helpful in assessing iron stores.

Aranesp has the advantage of a single once-weekly injection rather than the thrice-weekly dosing of rEpo (45). This more highly glycosylated formulation has now been well studied in adults, but there are few studies in preterm or term infants regarding the pharmacokinetics, efficacy, risks, or benefits of Aranesp in neonates (53).

PHARMACOKINETIC PROPERTIES IN NEWBORN INFANTS

rEpo can be administered by intravenous infusion or subcutaneous injection. Pharmacokinetic studies in preterm infants performed by Ohls et al. revealed that there were no differences in plasma Epo concentrations at day 3 and day 10 or in the rate of clearance between intravenously and subcutaneously administered rEpo (50). In the same study, the elimination half-life of rEpo was 17.6 ± 4.4 hours on day 3 and 11.2 ± 1.5 hours on day 10. When compared with pharmacokinetic studies performed in adults, rEpo administered to preterm infants has a three- to fourfold increase in both volume of distribution and clearance (7,50,54). The precise mechanism for Epo elimination has not been established in neonates, but it has been speculated that rEpo is eliminated by irreversible binding to its receptors on erythroid progenitor cells with subsequent internalization. Renal excretion of Epo is reported to be less than 2% of the total (nonsignificant) in adult subjects.

ADVERSE EFFECTS, TOXICITY, AND PRECAUTIONS

Known adverse effects of chronic rEpo treatment in adults include hypertension (55), thrombus formation (56), polycythemia, and red cell aplasia secondary to anti-Epo antibodies (57). Hypertensive leukoencephalopathy has also been reported in a few adult patients requiring long-term rEpo for anemia due to dialysis-dependent renal failure (58). An FDA warning was released in 2008 for patients with chronic kidney failure who receive rEpo at higher than recommended doses, as an increased risk of blood clots, strokes, heart attacks, and death have been identified. In preterm neonates, rEpo use for the treatment of anemia has been very safe with none of the adverse effects noted in adult populations (59).

One potential adverse response is unique to preterm infants. Retinopathy of prematurity (ROP) is a neonatal disease characterized by the pathophysiologic growth of immature blood vessels across the entire retina, which can trigger retinal detachment and loss of vision if unchecked (60). The disease primarily affects low-birth-weight (<1,250 g) and preterm infants born less than 31 weeks' gestation (61). Retinal vascularization occurs from 16 weeks' gestation to birth (62) and in infants born prematurely, this process can be disrupted. ROP occurs in two phases, the first involving a loss of retinal vasculature following birth and the second involving uncontrolled proliferation of retinal vessels. EpoRs are present on endothelial cells, and rEpo stimulation increases their angiogenic expression (20). Early high-dose rEpo may have a protective effect on the retina by ameliorating the first stage of ROP (63). Alternatively, the angiogenic properties of Epo may prevail, resulting in an increase in ROP, particularly if the timing of dosing coincides with second phase of ROP (63). An increased risk of ROP was identified in one meta-analysis of early use of rEpo and iron for erythropoiesis (relative risk 1.71, CI 1.15 to 2.54) (3). It is not clear whether this is an effect of rEpo or of early iron administration, since rEpo was used in conjunction with iron. Many other studies have shown no such association. No prospective randomized controlled studies have been done to study this issue.

NONHEMATOPOIETIC EFFECTS OF ERYTHROPOIETIN

Following the observations of EpoR expression in brain and other organs (22,27) and the capacity for Epo production by astrocytes (64), a broader concept of Epo as a neuroprotective molecule has emerged (65). Neuroprotection by high-dose rEpo has been demonstrated in neonatal and adult animal models of injury including hypoxia-ischemia, stroke, and hemorrhage (66–68). rEpo improves both short- and long-term outcome following unilateral neonatal brain injury in neonatal rats, decreasing structural and behavioral deficits (67,69–73). Brief courses (5 days) of high-dose rEpo have also been shown to be safe in neonatal rats with no long-term negative consequences (74). Thus, rEpo may provide an important adjunct to neuroprotective therapy in neonates. The mechanisms by which rEpo provides neuroprotection are complex and include direct neuronal effects and indirect systemic effects, as well as both early and late effects. Early effects of rEpo include antiapoptotic (75–77), anti-inflammatory (68,78), and antioxidant effects (68,76,79–82) and increased resistance to excitotoxicity (83,84). Late rEpo effects that improve brain recovery include increased neurogenesis, angiogenesis, and migration of regenerating neurons (85,86). rEpo is directly involved in prevention of oxidative stress with generation of antioxidant enzymes, inhibition of nitric oxide production, and decrease of lipid peroxidation (87). These properties of rEpo may be relevant in therapeutic prevention of injury in developing brain of premature infants, where antioxidant systems are immature. Inflammation is also an important component in the pathogenesis and progression of both preterm and term brain injury. Since rEpo has a long track record of use in preterm infants and systemic high-dose rEpo can cross the injured and intact blood–brain barrier (88,89), it has promise as a neuroprotective agent in this population.

Epo may also function as a paracrine–autocrine tissue protective hormone in other organs such as heart and kidney (90). The mechanism of rEpo action in these organ systems is thought to be similar to neuroprotective mechanisms (91,92). Clinical trials are in progress to test these hypotheses.

Clinical Studies of Neonatal Neuroprotection with Erythropoietin

Two pilot studies evaluating the safety of high-dose rEpo in preterm populations have been published (93,94). The doses included in these studies ranged from 500 to 3,000 U per kg per dose given daily for three doses. Larger randomized controlled trials to evaluate the efficacy of high-dose rEpo in preterm infants are in the planning stage, or ongoing.

Erythropoietic doses of rEpo may also be protective; however, we currently have insufficient evidence to determine this. One study reported on the long-term neurodevelopmental effects of erythropoietic doses of rEpo: VLBW infants were randomized to rEpo or control treatment from day 4 of life until 35 weeks of corrected gestational age. There were no differences in neurodevelopmental outcomes at 18 to 22 months (95). In contrast, in preterm infants weighing less than 1,000 g treated with rEpo (400 U per kg three times per week) for a similar duration, those with serum Epo concentrations greater than 500 mU per mL, had higher mental development index scores than infants with Epo concentrations of less than 500 mU per mL when tested at 18 to 22 months corrected age ($n = 6$ rEpo, $n = 6$ placebo/control) (96). This suggests that higher circulating Epo concentrations may be of benefit.

More information is needed regarding the ideal population to target for neuroprotection, the optimal rEpo dose, and duration of therapy. It is also unclear whether rEpo has a role as a prophylactic measure for at-risk extremely preterm infants, or whether it should only be used as a rescue treatment following stroke, intracranial hemorrhage, or perinatal asphyxia in term infants. Similarly, for term infants with perinatal brain injury, more data are needed. It is now possible to treat near-term brain-injured infants with hypothermia (97). The question is will additional adjunctive therapies further improve outcomes such that infants with severe hypoxic-ischemic encephalopathy also benefit? This is promising research and we anticipate that progress will be made to address these important questions in the next decade.

Potential Side Effects of High-Dose Recombinant Erythropoietin

rEpo is a potent erythropoietic growth factor. Thus, we can expect that using high doses of rEpo as neuroprotective treatment will have transient hematopoietic effects. These may include increasing erythropoiesis and possibly megakaryocytopoiesis. In the neonatal population where anemia is ubiquitous, this is unlikely to be a negative consequence but rather a beneficial side effect. It is unknown, however, how this potential increase in hematopoiesis might affect iron balance. This is important because preterm infants are at high risk for iron deficiency, since the bulk of iron transfer occurs in the third trimester. Iron is essential for normal growth and development because it is an important component of proteins and enzymes required for oxygen transport, cell division, neurotransmitter synthesis, myelination, and cellular oxidative metabolism (98). Iron deficiency can lead to adverse neurodevelopmental consequences, with deficits in executive function and memory (99). Administration of supplemental iron to preterm infants in the first 2 weeks of life is generally not advised due to the potential oxidative effects in the face of deficient antioxidative mechanisms (100). Thus, with the data available, it is not clear whether early rEpo administration for the purposes of neuroprotection should be accompanied by supplemental iron.

The role of Epo in the developing gastrointestinal tract is being defined. The EpoR is present in the developing gut, but its role is not well defined (22). Increases in villous height and crypt depth have been reported in animal models following the enteral administration of rEpo (21,22,101). Systemic absorption following enteral administration in rodents has been reported (102). Enterally administered rEpo to preterm neonates in doses up to and including 1,000 U per kg per day has resulted in no evidence of systemic absorption (103,104). The incidence of necrotizing enterocolitis seems to be lower in neonates who received rEpo (105).

The role of rEpo in a simulated amniotic fluid (SAFEstart) for enteral administration is under investigation (106–108). The sterile isotonic electrolyte solution contains rEpo and recombinant granulocyte colony-stimulating factor (rG-CSF) because both these factors are present in relatively high concentrations in second-trimester amniotic fluid, human colostrum, and human milk. SAFEstart is being evaluated as a means of reducing feeding intolerance by preventing villous atrophy among neonates who are not fed. SAFEstart is administered enterally in a volume of 20 mL per kg per day, which delivers a concentration of rEpo and rG-CSF to neonates similar to the concentration they would have received in utero had they been swallowing amniotic fluid (106–108).

Phase I studies have been conducted among neonates weighing 750 to 1,250 g who are NPO and also among neonates recovering from necrotizing enterocolitis or other surgical complications (106,107). Larger prospective, randomized, double-blinded, placebo-controlled studies are necessary to evaluate the efficacy of this solution in reducing feeding intolerance in neonates.

GRANULOCYTE COLONY-STIMULATING FACTOR

PHYSIOLOGIC AND PHARMACOLOGIC EFFECTS

Granulocyte colony-stimulating factor (G-CSF) is a physiologic regulator of neutrophil production and function (109). It is produced in vivo by multiple cell types including monocytes, macrophages, fibroblasts, and endothelial cells. G-CSF has multiple effects on white cell maturation and function, as well as other, more recently described, nonhematopoietic functions (110). These effects include clonal maturation of committed myeloid progenitors, release of neutrophils from the bone marrow to the blood, and enhancement of neutrophil functions, including chemotaxis, phagocytosis, superoxide production, and bactericidal activity (109). Administration of rG-CSF has long been used to prevent infections in patients with nonmyeloid malignancies receiving anticancer drugs and suffering febrile neutropenia. In addition, rG-CSF is used to facilitate hematopoietic recovery following bone marrow transplantation and to mobilize peripheral blood progenitor cells in healthy donors (111).

CLINICAL TRIALS IN NEWBORN INFANTS

Neonates with Bacterial Sepsis

Several small clinical trials have tested the hypothesis that rG-CSF administration to neonates with septicemia will reduce mortality, with mixed results (112–117). The benefit may depend on the patient population (preterm vs. term, proven vs. possible sepsis) and the timing and duration of drug administration. A meta-analysis of five clinical trials showed lower mortality in neonates with bacterial sepsis when rG-CSF was used (118); however, when only randomized controlled trials were considered, only a trend toward such benefit could be demonstrated. Since then, another trial has been published which also shows benefit (115). Overall, rG-CSF does appear to increase circulating neutrophil counts, but it is unclear whether this provides substantial clinical benefit. This may be due to developmental abnormalities of neonatal neutrophils (decreased adhesion, deformability, and chemotaxis) which are unchanged by rG-CSF administration. No significant adverse side effects are reported with the use of G-CSF in neonates. Adequately powered, randomized, controlled clinical trials of neutropenic infants are needed to further evaluate its efficacy as an adjunct to antibiotic therapy (119,120).

Neonates Born to Mothers with Pregnancy-Induced Hypertension

Neutropenia can be severe in neonates born to women who have pregnancy-induced hypertension (PIH) (121–123). Neutropenia associated with PIH (mediated by a circulating inhibitor to granulocytopoiesis) (121,124,125) can occur in up to 50% of exposed infants and generally resolves by 1 to 2 weeks of life. In preterm infants, neutropenia is approximately three times as common in PIH-exposed infants as compared with those unexposed and may last longer than 2 weeks (123).

Preliminary studies suggest that the use of rG-CSF (5 to 10 μg per kg per day) in neonates with neutropenia secondary to maternal PIH could be helpful (126,127). The condition is usually self-resolving; however, if the neutropenia is severe (<500 per μL) and prolonged, other diagnoses should be entertained and rG-CSF could be considered.

Neonates with Alloimmune Neutropenia

In alloimmune neutropenia, the mother becomes immunized to paternal granulocyte antigens present on fetal neutrophils (128). Maternal immunoglobulin crosses the placenta and binds to fetal neutrophils. The severity of the neutropenia is influenced by the antibody titer and the immunoglobulin G subclass involved (129). Although most neonates with alloimmune neutropenia do not require treatment, those with severe and prolonged neutropenia generally respond very well to rG-CSF therapy in doses from 5 to 10 μg per kg per day for 3 to 5 days (49). Additional doses can be given to adjust the absolute neutrophil count (ANC) so that it remains greater than 1,000 per μL. The response is clinically evident within 24 to 48 hours.

Neonates with Autoimmune Neutropenia

Autoimmune neutropenia is analogous to autoimmune hemolytic anemia and thrombocytopenia. The etiologic mechanisms remain unclear, but associations have been reported with parvovirus B 19 infection and β-lactam antibiotics (128). Neutrophil antibodies may adversely affect the function of neutrophils even in the absence of neutropenia (130). Neonates with autoimmune neutropenia respond well to rG-CSF at 10 μg per kg per day given by intravenous or subcutaneous routes. The duration of treatment is based on the resolution of the neutropenia with an ANC greater than 1,000 per μL (49).

Neonates with Chronic Idiopathic Neutropenia

Chronic idiopathic neutropenia occurs in extremely preterm infants who have no evidence of antibody-mediated neutropenia, no history of PIH, and no features that result in a specific diagnosis (123,131,132). Although these infants are generally well appearing, the ANC can be below 500 per μL for many weeks or months. This type of neutropenia can respond to rG-CSF but spontaneously remits after 3 to 6 months, so treatment may not be necessary (132,133).

The use of rG-CSF in neonates requires further studies to define the precise indications, doses, and intervals to be used.

STRUCTURE, DOSE, ROUTES, AND REGIMENS

G-CSF was first recognized and purified in the mouse and then in humans in 1986 (134). Four different commercially available forms of G-CSF exist: filgrastim (Neupogen) and filgrastim with sustained duration (Neulasta) available in the United States and Ro 25-8315 (Nartograstim) and lenograstim (Granocyte) available only in Europe (135,136).

The recommended dose of rG-CSF is 5 to 10 μg per kg per day (49). Both the intravenous and subcutaneous routes of administration are used. In general, for the treatment of neutropenia in neonates with sepsis, rG-CSF has been given once a day for 3 to 5 consecutive days (49,137). Longer dosing duration may be needed for the treatment of alloimmune and autoimmune neutropenia. In neonates with either of the latter conditions, the length of therapy should be tailored to the individual patient, as variability in antibody titers among individuals can make specific recommendations difficult.

PHARMACOKINETIC PROPERTIES IN NEWBORN INFANTS

In neonates with presumed sepsis, the half-life of filgrastim is 4.4 ± 0.4 hours, and the peak serum concentrations are dose dependent (1 μg per kg, 2,040 ± 1,340 pg per mL; 5 μg per kg, 20,000 ± 6,260 pg per mL; 10 μg per kg, 126,750 ± 22,570 pg per mL) and occur 2 hours following intravenous administration (138). Two of the subjects in this study were neutropenic, which may affect the pharmacokinetics.

In a study of 10 neutropenic neonates (5 secondary to reduced neutrophil production with PIH and intrauterine growth retardation and 5 as a result of accelerated neutrophil usage with sepsis and shock), extremely high baseline G-CSF serum and urine concentrations were measured in neutropenic patients with sepsis and shock (20,028 to 98,280 pg per mL) compared with those without (65 to 210 pg per mL) (139). This might be due to an upregulation of G-CSF production during infection or to saturation of G-CSF receptors (G-CSF-R) by endogenous G-CSF. Alternatively, expression of G-CSF-R by tumor necrosis factor α (TNF-α) or other mediators during sepsis might contribute to high circulating G-CSF concentrations (140). In vitro studies of incubations of granulocytes with TNF-α have shown a 70% reduction in the number of G-CSF-R within 10 minutes. TNF-α serum concentrations are elevated in infants with sepsis (140).

Traditional pharmacokinetic measurements can be flawed when applied to rG-CSF because of the unique manner in which G-CSF is cleared (141). Ericson et al. reported a linear relationship ($R^2 = 0.85$) between the blood neutrophil count and the rG-CSF clearance with repeated dosing (142). Kuwabara and colleagues concluded that the clearance of rG-CSF is inversely related to the dose administered and that with repeated dosing the clearance increases (143). Both postulated that rG-CSF clearance was dependent principally on saturable receptor binding, but that at very high doses, glomerular filtration and elimination in the urine become a process for nonsaturable clearance. An additional factor that complicates the analysis of rG-CSF elimination in neonates is the presence of the G-CSF-R on nonhematopoietic tissues (144).

The pegylation of filgrastim into the form known as Neulasta extends the half-life (145). When a single PEG group is attached to the N-terminal residue of rG-CSF, the circulation time increases with no effect on activity (146). Studies in animals suggest that the average elimination half-life of pegylated rG-CSF is two to four times longer than rG-CSF (147). Pegylation of filgrastim decreases its renal clearance so that clearance is almost entirely dependent on receptor-mediated elimination (148). No studies have been reported on the pharmacokinetics of Neulasta in either preterm or term neonates.

ADVERSE EFFECTS, TOXICITY, AND PRECAUTIONS

Adverse effects have rarely been described when rG-CSF is used to treat neonates with sepsis. In a 2-year follow-up of neonates who received rG-CSF for 3 days, Rosenthal et al. reported normal hematologic, immunologic, and neurologic development (149). Reductions in platelet counts have been reported after septic neonates or children were treated with rG-CSF (115,117); however, this may have been due to the underlying septic condition. Donadieu and colleagues reported thrombocytopenia after rG-CSF administration to children with chronic neutropenia in the absence of sepsis (150). Gilmore et al. noted irritability in one infant after two doses, possibly secondary to bone pain (151). No studies have evaluated the safety or efficacy of either of the pegylated forms of rG-CSF in neonates.

Concerns exist that prolonged exposure to rG-CSF might predispose neonates to myelodysplastic syndrome or to osteoporosis. Some children with Kostmann syndrome have developed leukemia while receiving rG-CSF (152). Other factors in addition to the use of rG-CSF certainly contribute to their increased risk of leukemia including structural abnormalities of the G-CSF-R (153). Neonates with Kostmann syndrome or any form of severe prolonged neutropenia who are receiving chronic rG-CSF should be monitored for the development of abnormal cytogenetics. Some children have developed osteoporosis on long-term rG-CSF therapy. However, it is unclear whether the risks of this adverse event are related to the primary disease or to the rG-CSF therapy (154,155). The administration of rG-CSF is contraindicated in any patients with known hypersensitivity to *Escherichia coli*–derived proteins or any component of the product.

NONHEMATOPOIETIC EFFECTS OF RG-CSF

As with EpoR, G-CSF-R expression is not limited to the hematopoietic system. G-CSF-R expression occurs in a variety of cell types including endothelial cells, glia, and neurons (156,157). Both G-CSF and its receptor are expressed on neuronal cells (158,159). Recent work, primarily in adult models of ischemia, has demonstrated that G-CSF has important neuroprotective properties (158,160). However, the precise mechanisms of action of C-CSF in the brain remain unclear.

rG-CSF displays anti-inflammatory properties by reducing blood–brain barrier disruption and decreasing the number of infiltrating neutrophils in the infarct penumbra (156,157). rG-CSF increases neurogenesis (158) and enhances angiogenesis following an ischemic insult (157). Whether rG-CSF can decrease neuronal injury by mobilization of hematopoietic stem cells into damaged brain areas is currently a matter of discussion (161).

Expanding evidence on the antiapoptotic effect of rG-CSF comes from several in vitro and in vivo studies. rG-CSF exerts its antiapoptotic effect by interference with various apoptotic signaling pathways such as activation of the antiapoptotic target Bcl-X_L and PI3K/phosphoinositide-dependent kinase/Akt pathway controlling neuronal survival (158).

However, data from adult studies may not be transferable to neonates. In contrast to the neuroprotective effects of G-CSF in adult models, the systemic administration of rG-CSF and stem cell factor surprisingly worsened excitotoxic brain injury in newborn mice (162).

GRANULOCYTE–MACROPHAGE COLONY-STIMULATING FACTOR

PHYSIOLOGIC AND PHARMACOLOGIC EFFECTS

Granulocyte–macrophage colony-stimulating factor (GM-CSF) acts on multiple cell lineages including macrophages, eosinophils, and, to a lesser extent, neutrophils. In animal studies, recombinant human (r)GM-CSF increases neutrophil counts and, when used prophylactically, decreases mortality due to sepsis (163).

Cairo et al. reported that rGM-CSF administration to VLBW neonates induced a significant increase in the ANC within 48 hours of administration (164,165). An increase in ANC was observed at all doses and all dosing intervals studied (5.0 μg per kg per day, 5.0 μg per kg twice daily, and 10.0 μg per kg once per day), and the increase continued for at least 24 hours after discontinuation of the rGM-CSF. At a dose of 10.0 μg per kg per day, rGM-CSF induced a significant increase in the absolute monocyte count on days 1, 4, and 6 through 9. The increase was sustained for 48 hours after the last dose. There were no significant changes in hematocrit or absolute eosinophil count at any dose level of rGM-CSF. Unfortunately, there was also no decrease in nosocomial infections (165).

CLINICAL TRIALS IN NEWBORN INFANTS

Neonatal Sepsis

The use of rGM-CSF in neonates with neutropenia and sepsis has been studied in several small clinical trials (164–167). In a prospective, randomized, controlled trial of 60 infants with neutropenia and clinical signs of sepsis, Bilgin et al. administered 5 μg per kg per day of rGM-CSF to 30 patients for 7 consecutive days (166). Twenty-five patients from the rGM-CSF group and 24 from the conventionally treated group had early-onset sepsis, and the remaining 11 patients had late-onset sepsis. Infants ranged from 28 to 41 weeks of gestational age in the rGM-CSF-treated group and from 28 to 42 weeks in the conventionally treated group. The ANC on day 7 was significantly higher in the rGM-CSF-treated group (8,088 ± 2,822 per mm^3 vs. 2,757 ± 2,822 per mm^3), and the platelet count was statistically higher on day 14 in the rGM-CSF-treated group compared with the conventionally treated group (266,867 ± 55,102 per mm^3 vs. 229,200 ± 52,317 per mm^3, $p < .01$), although this difference in platelet count probably has no clinical significance. The mortality in the rGM-CSF recipients was significantly lower than in the conventionally treated group (10% vs. 30%, respectively). A meta-analysis of both rG-CSF and rGM-CSF treatment showed no clear survival advantage for either treatment and also no harmful effects (119). There is tremendous heterogeneity in the published studies, however, both in treatment protocols and in primary endpoints. Thus, further studies are needed to clearly define the utility of such treatments.

Prophylaxis against Nosocomial Infection

Carr et al. performed the first randomized, placebo-controlled trial of rGM-CSF in 75 neonates younger than 32 weeks of gestation (168). The administration of subcutaneous rGM-CSF at 10 μg per kg per day for 5 days abolished neutropenia and sepsis-induced neutropenia in preterm neonates at high risk of sepsis.

Cairo et al. performed a randomized, placebo-controlled trial in VLBW neonates, comparing the incidence of nosocomial infections after the prophylactic use of rGM-CSF versus placebo (165). Two hundred and sixty-four VLBW neonates were randomized to receive 8 μg per kg per day of intravenous rGM-CSF or placebo over 2 hours for 7 days and then every other day for 21 days. In this study, rGM-CSF did not decrease the incidence of nosocomial infections (40% vs. 39%, rGM-CSF vs. placebo).

STRUCTURE, DOSE, ROUTES, AND REGIMENS

GM-CSF is a protein with 127 amino acids and a molecular weight of 18 to 22 kDa. rGM-CSF is marketed as Leucomax (Novartis, UK) and Leukine (Immunex, Seattle, WA). rGM-CSF is produced by many cell types and promotes the growth of precursors of several myeloid and megakaryocyte lines (169). The physiologic characteristics of rGM-CSF are somewhat similar to those of rG-CSF, but GM-CSF has a wider spectrum of action (170). As a result, monocyte, macrophage, and eosinophil counts generally increase more after rGM-CSF therapy than following rG-CSF treatment (Fig. 55.2). In addition, rGM-CSF enhances monocyte function and has a greater effect on chemotaxis and the bactericidal function of neutrophils than does G-CSF (171,172). Interactions between rG-CSF and rGM-CSF remain to be fully elucidated.

rGM-CSF has been dosed intravenously at 5 to 10 μg per kg per day in human newborn infants for prophylaxis against nosocomial infection (164). Published dosing schedules have included once a day for 7 days, twice a day for 7 days, daily for 5 days, and daily for 7 days followed by every other day for a total of 21 days (119,165–167).

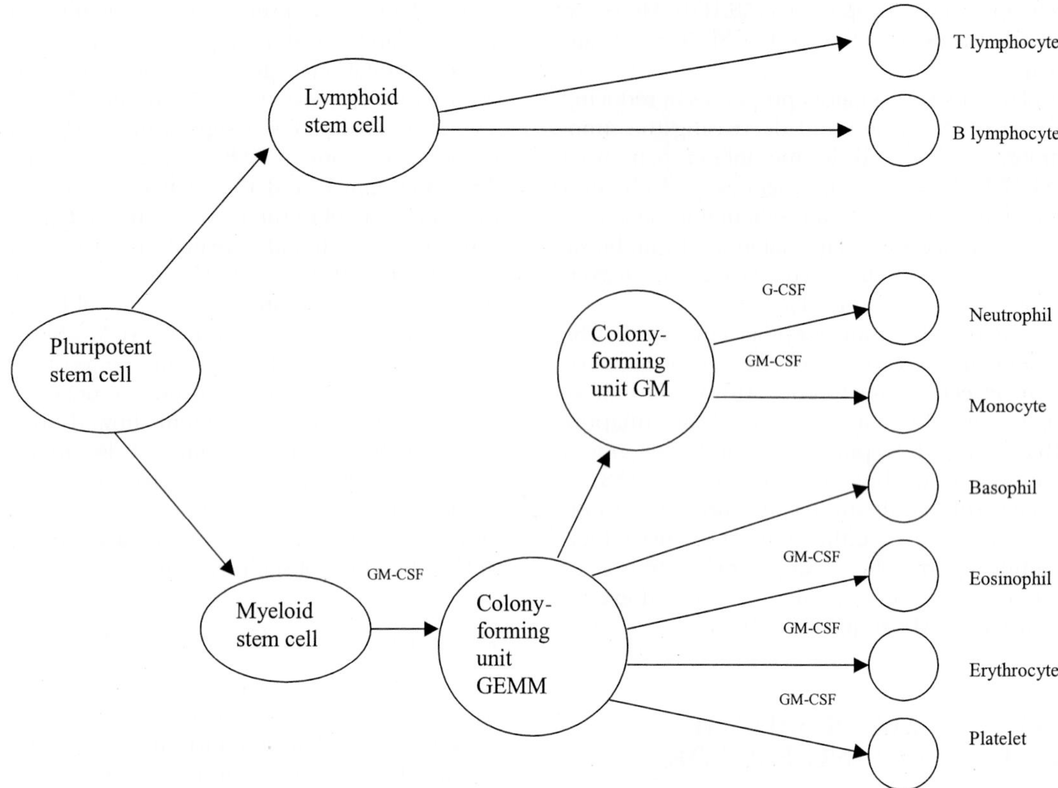

Figure 55.2. Lineage development of peripheral blood cells from pluripotent stem cell. CSF, colony-stimulating factor; GM, granulocyte–macrophage; GEMM, granulocyte, erythrocyte, monocyte, megakaryocyte. (Redrawn from Steward WP. Granulocyte and granulocyte–macrophage colony-stimulating factors. *Lancet* 1993;342:153–155, with permission.)

PHARMACOKINETIC PROPERTIES IN NEWBORN INFANTS

The distribution half-life of rGM-CSF administered intravenously is 5 to 15 minutes, and the elimination half-life is 1.4 ± 0.8 to 3.9 ± 2.8 hours (164). Peak concentrations, which occurred at the end of a 2-hour intravenous infusion, were dose dependent and were undetectable by 24 hours. After subcutaneous injection, the elimination half-life was 2.9 hours, with a peak concentration at 4 hours.

ADVERSE EFFECTS, TOXICITY, AND PRECAUTIONS

Serious adverse effects of rGM-CSF treatment of newborns have not been reported. Having said that the long-term effects of this growth factor are largely unstudied, so caution is warranted when considering its use.

REFERENCES

1. Krantz SB. Erythropoietin. *Blood* 1991;77(3):419–434.
2. Goldwasser E. Erythropoietin and the differentiation of red blood cells. *Fed Proc* 1975;34(13):2285–2292.
3. Ohlsson A, Aher SM. Early erythropoietin for preventing red blood cell transfusion in preterm and/or low birth weight infants. *Cochrane Database Syst Rev* 2006;3:CD004863.
4. Aher SM, Ohlsson A. Early versus late erythropoietin for preventing red blood cell transfusion in preterm and/or low birth weight infants. *Cochrane Database Syst Rev* 2006;3:CD004865.
5. Garcia MG, Hutson AD, Christensen RD. Effect of recombinant erythropoietin on "late" transfusions in the neonatal intensive care unit: a meta-analysis. *J Perinatol* 2002;22(2):108–111.
6. Widness JA, Veng-Pedersen P, Peters C, et al. Erythropoietin pharmacokinetics in premature infants: developmental, nonlinearity, and treatment effects. *J Appl Physiol* 1996;80(1):140–148.
7. Brown MS, Jones MA, Ohls RK, et al. Single-dose pharmacokinetics of recombinant human erythropoietin in preterm infants after intravenous and subcutaneous administration. *J Pediatr* 1993;122(4):655–657.
8. Krishnan R, Shankaran S, Krishnan M, et al. Pharmacokinetics of erythropoietin following single-dose subcutaneous administration in preterm infants. *Biol Neonate* 1996;70(3):135–140.
9. Zanjani ED. Liver to kidney switch of erythropoietin formation. *Exp Hematol* 1980;8(Suppl 8):29–40.
10. Dame C, Juul SE. The switch from fetal to adult erythropoiesis. *Clin Perinatol* 2000;27(3):507–526.
11. Muta K, Krantz SB, Bondurant MC, et al. Distinct roles of erythropoietin, insulin-like growth factor I, and stem cell factor in the development of erythroid progenitor cells. *J Clin Invest* 1994;94(1):34–43.
12. Ratajczak J, Zhang Q, Pertusini E, et al. The role of insulin (INS) and insulin-like growth factor-I (IGF-I) in regulating human erythropoiesis. Studies in vitro under serum-free conditions—comparison to other cytokines and growth factors. *Leukemia* 1998;12(3):371–381.
13. Goldwasser E. Erythropoietin and red cell differentiation. *Prog Clin Biol Res* 1981;66(pt A):487–494.
14. Koury MJ, Bondurant MC, Atkinson JB. Erythropoietin control of terminal erythroid differentiation: maintenance of cell viability, production of hemoglobin, and development of the erythrocyte membrane. *Blood Cells* 1987;13(1–2):217–226.
15. Wu H, Liu X, Jaenisch R, et al. Generation of committed erythroid BFU-E and CFU-E progenitors does not require erythropoietin or the erythropoietin receptor. *Cell* 1995;83(1):59–67.

16. Widness JA, Schmidt RL, Sawyer ST. Erythropoietin transplacental passage—review of animal studies. *J Perinat Med* 1995;23(1–2): 61–70.
17. Ohneda O, Yanai N, Obinata M. Erythropoietin as a mitogen for fetal liver stromal cells which support erythropoiesis. *Exp Cell Res* 1993;208(1):327–331.
18. Morakkabati N, Gollnick F, Meyer R, et al. Erythropoietin induces Ca2+ mobilization and contraction in rat mesangial and aortic smooth muscle cultures. *Exp Hematol* 1996;24(2):392–397.
19. Wu H, Lee SH, Gao J, et al. Inactivation of erythropoietin leads to defects in cardiac morphogenesis. *Development* 1999;126(16): 3597–3605.
20. Ribatti D, Presta M, Vacca A, et al. Human erythropoietin induces a pro-angiogenic phenotype in cultured endothelial cells and stimulates neovascularization in vivo. *Blood* 1999;93(8):2627–2636.
21. Juul SE, Joyce AE, Zhao Y, et al. Why is erythropoietin present in human milk? Studies of erythropoietin receptors on enterocytes of human and rat neonates. *Pediatr Res* 1999;46(3):263–268.
22. Juul SE, Yachnis AT, Christensen RD. Tissue distribution of erythropoietin and erythropoietin receptor in the developing human fetus. *Early Hum Dev* 1998;52(3):235–249.
23. Sawyer ST, Krantz SB, Sawada K. Receptors for erythropoietin in mouse and human erythroid cells and placenta. *Blood* 1989;74(1): 103–109.
24. Mioni R, Gottardello F, Bordon P, et al. Evidence for specific binding and stimulatory effects of recombinant human erythropoietin on isolated adult rat Leydig cells. *Acta Endocrinol (Copenh)* 1992; 127(5):459–465.
25. Konishi Y, Chui DH, Hirose H, et al. Trophic effect of erythropoietin and other hematopoietic factors on central cholinergic neurons in vitro and in vivo. *Brain Res* 1993;609(1–2):29–35.
26. Tabira T, Konishi Y, Gallyas F Jr. Neurotrophic effect of hematopoietic cytokines on cholinergic and other neurons in vitro. *Int J Dev Neurosci* 1995;13(3–4):241–252.
27. Juul SE, Yachnis AT, Rojiani AM, et al. Immunohistochemical localization of erythropoietin and its receptor in the developing human brain. *Pediatr Dev Pathol* 1999;2(2):148–158.
28. Iguchi T, Sogo S, Hisha H, et al. HGF activates signal transduction from EPO receptor on human cord blood CD34+/CD45+ cells. *Stem Cells* 1999;17(2):82–91.
29. Akahane K, Tojo A, Urabe A, et al. Pure erythropoietic colony and burst formations in serum-free culture and their enhancement by insulin-like growth factor I. *Exp Hematol* 1987;15(7):797–802.
30. Buescher U, Hertwig K, Wolf C, et al. Erythropoietin in amniotic fluid as a marker of chronic fetal hypoxia. *Int J Gynaecol Obstet* 1998; 60(3):257–263.
31. Stangenberg M, Legarth J, Cao HL, et al. Erythropoietin concentrations in amniotic fluid and umbilical venous blood from Rh-immunized pregnancies. *J Perinat Med* 1993;21(3):225–234.
32. Ohls RK, Harcum J, Li Y, et al. Serum erythropoietin concentrations fail to increase after significant phlebotomy losses in ill preterm infants. *J Perinatol* 1997;17(6):465–467.
33. Widness JA, Seward VJ, Kromer IJ, et al. Changing patterns of red blood cell transfusion in very low birth weight infants. *J Pediatr* 1996;129(5):680–687.
34. Aher S, Ohlsson A. Late erythropoietin for preventing red blood cell transfusion in preterm and/or low birth weight infants. *Cochrane Database Syst Rev* 2006;3:CD004868.
35. Dallacasa P, Ancora G, Miniero R, et al. Erythropoietin course in newborns with Rh hemolytic disease transfused and not transfused in utero. *Pediatr Res* 1996;40(2):357–360.
36. al-Alaiyan S, al Omran A. Late hyporegenerative anemia in neonates with rhesus hemolytic disease. *J Perinat Med* 1999;27(2):112–115.
37. Koenig JM, Ashton RD, De Vore GR, et al. Late hyporegenerative anemia in Rh hemolytic disease. *J Pediatr* 1989;115(2):315–318.
38. Ohls RK, Wirkus PE, Christensen RD. Recombinant erythropoietin as treatment for the late hyporegenerative anemia of Rh hemolytic disease. *Pediatrics* 1992;90(5):678–680.
39. Pessler F, Hart D. Hyporegenerative anemia associated with Rh hemolytic disease: treatment failure of recombinant erythropoietin. *J Pediatr Hematol Oncol* 2002;24(8):689–693.
40. Christensen RD, Hunter DD, Goodell H, et al. Evaluation of the mechanism causing anemia in infants with bronchopulmonary dysplasia. *J Pediatr* 1992;120(4, pt 1):593–598.
41. Ohls RK, Hunter DD, Christensen RD. A randomized, double-blind, placebo-controlled trial of recombinant erythropoietin in treatment of the anemia of bronchopulmonary dysplasia. *J Pediatr* 1993;123(6):996–1000.
42. Shaddy RE, Bullock EA, Tani LY, et al. Epoetin alfa therapy in infants awaiting heart transplantation. *Arch Pediatr Adolesc Med* 1995;149(3):322–325.
43. Ootaki Y, Yamaguchi M, Yoshimura N, et al. The efficacy of preoperative administration of a single dose of recombinant human erythropoietin in pediatric cardiac surgery. *Heart Surg Forum* 2007; 10(2):E115–E119.
44. Holt RL, Martin TD, Hess PJ, et al. Jehovah's Witnesses requiring complex urgent cardiothoracic surgery. *Ann Thorac Surg* 2004; 78(2):695–697.
45. Egrie JC, Browne JK. Development and characterization of novel erythropoiesis stimulating protein (NESP). *Nephrol Dial Transplant* 2001;16(Suppl 3):3–13.
46. Overbay DK, Manley HJ. Darbepoetin-alpha: a review of the literature. *Pharmacotherapy* 2002;22(7):889–897.
47. Maier RF, Obladen M, Scigalla P, et al. The effect of epoetin beta (recombinant human erythropoietin) on the need for transfusion in very-low-birth-weight infants. European Multicentre Erythropoietin Study Group. *N Engl J Med* 1994;330(17):1173–1178.
48. Haiden N, Klebermass K, Cardona F, et al. A randomized, controlled trial of the effects of adding vitamin B12 and folate to erythropoietin for the treatment of anemia of prematurity. *Pediatrics* 2006;118(1):180–188.
49. Calhoun DA, Christensen RD, Edstrom CS, et al. Consistent approaches to procedures and practices in neonatal hematology. *Clin Perinatol* 2000;27(3):733–753.
50. Ohls RK, Veerman MW, Christensen RD. Pharmacokinetics and effectiveness of recombinant erythropoietin administered to preterm infants by continuous infusion in total parenteral nutrition solution. *J Pediatr* 1996;128(4):518–523.
51. Juul SE, Zerzan JC, Strandjord TP, et al. Zinc protoporphyrin/heme as an indicator of iron status in NICU patients. *J Pediatr* 2003;142(3):273–278.
52. Miller SM, McPherson RJ, Juul SE. Iron sulfate supplementation decreases zinc protoporphyrin to heme ratio in premature infants. *J Pediatr* 2006;148(1):44–48.
53. Ohls RK, Dai A. Long-acting erythropoietin: clinical studies and potential uses in neonates. *Clin Perinatol* 2004;31(1):77–89.
54. Kling PJ, Widness JA, Guillery EN, et al. Pharmacokinetics and pharmacodynamics of erythropoietin during therapy in an infant with renal failure. *J Pediatr* 1992;121(5, pt 1):822–825.
55. Ismail N, Ikizler TA. Erythropoietin-induced hypertension. *J Med Liban* 1997;45(1):25–30.
56. Wolf RF, Peng J, Friese P, et al. Erythropoietin administration increases production and reactivity of platelets in dogs. *Thromb Haemost* 1997;78(6):1505–1509.
57. Casadevall N. Pure red cell aplasia and anti-erythropoietin antibodies in patients treated with epoetin. *Nephrol Dial Transplant* 2003;18(Suppl 8):viii37–viii41.
58. Delanty N, Vaughan C, Frucht S, et al. Erythropoietin-associated hypertensive posterior leukoencephalopathy. *Neurology* 1997;49(3): 686–689.
59. Ohls RK. The use of erythropoietin in neonates. *Clin Perinatol* 2000;27:681–696.
60. Tasman W, Patz A, McNamara JA, et al. Retinopathy of prematurity: the life of a lifetime disease. *Am J Ophthalmol* 2006;141(1):167–174.
61. Palmer EA, Flynn JT, Hardy RJ, et al. Incidence and early course of retinopathy of prematurity. The Cryotherapy for Retinopathy of Prematurity Cooperative Group. *Ophthalmology* 1991;98(11): 1628–1640.
62. Ashton N. Oxygen and the retinal blood vessels. *Trans Ophthalmol Soc U K* 1980;100(3):359–362.
63. Chen J, Smith LE. A double-edged sword: erythropoietin eyed in retinopathy of prematurity. *J AAPOS* 2008;12(3):221–222.
64. Masuda S, Okano M, Yamagishi K, et al. A novel site of erythropoietin production. Oxygen-dependent production in cultured rat astrocytes. *J Biol Chem* 1994;269(30):19488–19493.
65. Brines M, Cerami A. Emerging biological roles for erythropoietin in the nervous system. *Nat Rev Neurosci* 2005;6(6):484–494.
66. Brines ML, Ghezzi P, Keenan S, et al. Erythropoietin crosses the blood–brain barrier to protect against experimental brain injury. *Proc Natl Acad Sci U S A* 2000;97(19):10526–10531.
67. Demers EJ, McPherson RJ, Juul SE. Erythropoietin protects dopaminergic neurons and improves neurobehavioral outcomes

in juvenile rats after neonatal hypoxia-ischemia. *Pediatr Res* 2005; 58(2):297–301.
68. Sun Y, Calvert JW, Zhang JH. Neonatal hypoxia/ischemia is associated with decreased inflammatory mediators after erythropoietin administration. *Stroke* 2005;36(8):1672–1678.
69. Kumral A, Gonenc S, Acikgoz O, et al. Erythropoietin increases glutathione peroxidase enzyme activity and decreases lipid peroxidation levels in hypoxic-ischemic brain injury in neonatal rats. *Biol Neonate* 2005;87(1):15–18.
70. Sola A, Rogido M, Lee BH, et al. Erythropoietin after focal cerebral ischemia activates the Janus kinase-signal transducer and activator of transcription signaling pathway and improves brain injury in postnatal day 7 rats. *Pediatr Res* 2005;57(4):481–487.
71. Yatsiv I, Grigoriadis N, Simeonidou C, et al. Erythropoietin is neuroprotective, improves functional recovery, and reduces neuronal apoptosis and inflammation in a rodent model of experimental closed head injury. *Faseb J* 2005;19(12):1701–1703.
72. Liu R, Suzuki A, Guo Z, et al. Intrinsic and extrinsic erythropoietin enhances neuroprotection against ischemia and reperfusion injury in vitro. *J Neurochem* 2006;96(4):1101–1110.
73. Wen TC, Rogido M, Peng H, et al. Gender differences in long-term beneficial effects of erythropoietin given after neonatal stroke in postnatal day-7 rats. *Neuroscience* 2006;139(3):803–811.
74. McPherson RJ, Demers EJ, Juul SE. Safety of high-dose recombinant erythropoietin in a neonatal rat model. *Neonatology* 2007; 91(1):36–43.
75. Kumral A, Genc S, Ozer E, et al. Erythropoietin downregulates bax and DP5 proapoptotic gene expression in neonatal hypoxic-ischemic brain injury. *Biol Neonate* 2006;89(3):205–210.
76. Sun Y, Zhou C, Polk P, et al. Mechanisms of erythropoietin-induced brain protection in neonatal hypoxia-ischemia rat model. *J Cereb Blood Flow Metab* 2004;24(2):259–270.
77. Spandou E, Soubasi V, Papoutsopoulou S, et al. Erythropoietin prevents hypoxia/ischemia-induced DNA fragmentation in an experimental model of perinatal asphyxia. *Neurosci Lett* 2004; 366(1):24–28.
78. Villa P, Bigini P, Mennini T, et al. Erythropoietin selectively attenuates cytokine production and inflammation in cerebral ischemia by targeting neuronal apoptosis. *J Exp Med* 2003;198(6): 971–975.
79. Sakanaka M, Wen TC, Matsuda S, et al. In vivo evidence that erythropoietin protects neurons from ischemic damage. *Proc Natl Acad Sci U S A* 1998;95(8):4635–4640.
80. Bryl E, Mysliwska J, Debska-Slizien A, et al. The influence of recombinant human erythropoietin on tumor necrosis factor alpha and interleukin-10 production by whole blood cell cultures in hemodialysis patients. *Artif Organs* 1998;22(3):177–181.
81. Chattopadhyay A, Choudhury TD, Bandyopadhyay D, et al. Protective effect of erythropoietin on the oxidative damage of erythrocyte membrane by hydroxyl radical. *Biochem Pharmacol* 2000;59(4):419–425.
82. Bany-Mohammed FM, Slivka S, Hallman M. Recombinant human erythropoietin: possible role as an antioxidant in premature rabbits. *Pediatr Res* 1996;40(3):381–387.
83. Keller M, Yang J, Griesmaier E, et al. Erythropoietin is neuroprotective against NMDA-receptor-mediated excitotoxic brain injury in newborn mice. *Neurobiol Dis* 2006;24:357–366.
84. Kawakami M, Iwasaki S, Sato K, et al. Erythropoietin inhibits calcium-induced neurotransmitter release from clonal neuronal cells. *Biochem Biophys Res Commun* 2000;279(1):293–297.
85. Tsai PT, Ohab JJ, Kertesz N, et al. A critical role of erythropoietin receptor in neurogenesis and post-stroke recovery. *J Neurosci* 2006;26(4):1269–1274.
86. Wang L, Zhang Z, Wang Y, et al. Treatment of stroke with erythropoietin enhances neurogenesis and angiogenesis and improves neurological function in rats. *Stroke* 2004;35(7):1732–1737.
87. Solaroglu I, Solaroglu A, Kaptanoglu E, et al. Erythropoietin prevents ischemia-reperfusion from inducing oxidative damage in fetal rat brain. *Childs Nerv Syst* 2003;19(1):19–22.
88. Juul SE, McPherson RJ, Farrell FX, et al. Erythropoietin concentrations in cerebrospinal fluid of nonhuman primates and fetal sheep following high-dose recombinant erythropoietin. *Biol Neonate* 2004; 85(2):138–144.
89. Statler PA, McPherson RJ, Bauer LA, et al. Pharmacokinetics of high-dose recombinant erythropoietin in plasma and brain of neonatal rats. *Pediatr Res* 2007;61(6):671–675.
90. Coleman T, Brines M. Science review: recombinant human erythropoietin in critical illness: a role beyond anemia? *Crit Care* 2004;8(5):337–341.
91. Bogoyevitch MA. An update on the cardiac effects of erythropoietin cardioprotection by erythropoietin and the lessons learnt from studies in neuroprotection. *Cardiovasc Res* 2004;63(2): 208–216.
92. Fiordaliso F, Chimenti S, Staszewsky L, et al. A nonerythropoietic derivative of erythropoietin protects the myocardium from ischemia-reperfusion injury. *Proc Natl Acad Sci U S A* 2005;102(6): 2046–2051.
93. Fauchere JC, Dame C, Vonthein R, et al. An approach to using recombinant erythropoietin for neuroprotection in very preterm infants. *Pediatrics* 2008;122(2):375–382.
94. Juul SE, McPherson RJ, Bauer LA, et al. A phase I/II trial of high-dose erythropoietin in extremely low birth weight infants: pharmacokinetics and safety. *Pediatrics* 2008;122(2):383–391.
95. Ohls RK, Ehrenkranz RA, Das A, et al. Neurodevelopmental outcome and growth at 18 to 22 months' corrected age in extremely low birth weight infants treated with early erythropoietin and iron. *Pediatrics* 2004;114(5):1287–1291.
96. Bierer R, Peceny MC, Hartenberger CH, et al. Erythropoietin concentrations and neurodevelopmental outcome in preterm infants. *Pediatrics* 2006;118(3):e635–e640.
97. Higgins RD, Raju TN, Perlman J, et al. Hypothermia and perinatal asphyxia: executive summary of the National Institute of Child Health and Human Development workshop. *J Pediatr* 2006;148(2):170–175.
98. Dallman PR. Biochemical basis for the manifestations of iron deficiency. *Annu Rev Nutr* 1986;6:13–40.
99. Lozoff B, Jimenez E, Hagen J, et al. Poorer behavioral and developmental outcome more than 10 years after treatment for iron deficiency in infancy. *Pediatrics* 2000;105(4):E51.
100. Buonocore G, Perrone S, Bracci R. Free radicals and brain damage in the newborn. *Biol Neonate* 2001;79(3–4):180–186.
101. Juul SE, Ledbetter DJ, Joyce AE, et al. Erythropoietin acts as a trophic factor in neonatal rat intestine. *Gut* 2001;49(2):182–189.
102. Kling PJ, Willeitner A, Dvorak B, et al. Enteral erythropoietin and iron stimulate erythropoiesis in suckling rats. *J Pediatr Gastroenterol Nutr* 2008;46(2):202–207.
103. Juul SE. Enterally dosed recombinant human erythropoietin does not stimulate erythropoiesis in neonates. *J Pediatr* 2003; 143(3):321–326.
104. Juul SE, Christensen RD. Absorption of enteral recombinant human erythropoietin by neonates. *Ann Pharmacother* 2003;37(6): 782–786.
105. Ledbetter DJ, Juul SE. Erythropoietin and the incidence of necrotizing enterocolitis in infants with very low birth weight. *J Pediatr Surg* 2000;35(2):178–181.
106. Lima-Rogel V, Calhoun DA, Maheshwari A, et al. Tolerance of a sterile isotonic electrolyte solution containing select recombinant growth factors in neonates recovering from necrotizing enterocolitis. *J Perinatol* 2003;23(3):200–204.
107. Lima-Rogel V, Ojeda MA, Villegas C, et al. Tolerance of an enterally administered simulated amniotic fluid-like solution by neonates recovering from surgery for congenital bowel abnormalities. *J Perinatol* 2004;24(5):295–298.
108. Sullivan SE, Calhoun DA, Maheshwari A, et al. Tolerance of simulated amniotic fluid in premature neonates. *Ann Pharmacother* 2002;36(10):1518–1524.
109. Cairo MS. Neonatal neutrophil host defense. Prospects for immunologic enhancement during neonatal sepsis. *Am J Dis Child* 1989;143(1):40–46.
110. Xiao BG, Lu CZ, Link H. Cell biology and clinical promise of G-CSF: immunomodulation and neuroprotection. *J Cell Mol Med* 2007;11(6):1272–1290.
111. Bensinger W, Appelbaum F, Rowley S, et al. Factors that influence collection and engraftment of autologous peripheral-blood stem cells. *J Clin Oncol* 1995;13(10):2547–2555.
112. Kocherlakota P, La Gamma EF. Human granulocyte colony-stimulating factor may improve outcome attributable to neonatal sepsis complicated by neutropenia. *Pediatrics* 1997;100(1):E6.
113. Schibler KR, Osborne KA, Leung LY, et al. A randomized, placebo-controlled trial of granulocyte colony-stimulating factor administration to newborn infants with neutropenia and clinical signs of early-onset sepsis. *Pediatrics* 1998;102(1, pt 1):6–13.

114. Yasui K, Agematsu K, Komiyama A. Recombinant human granulocyte colony-stimulating factor therapy for sepsis in infants with neutropenia. *Pediatrics* 1999;103(6, pt 1):1310–1311.
115. Bedford Russell AR, Emmerson AJ, Wilkinson N, et al. A trial of recombinant human granulocyte colony stimulating factor for the treatment of very low birthweight infants with presumed sepsis and neutropenia. *Arch Dis Child Fetal Neonatal Ed* 2001;84(3):F172–F176.
116. Miura E, Procianoy RS, Bittar C, et al. A randomized, double-masked, placebo-controlled trial of recombinant granulocyte colony-stimulating factor administration to preterm infants with the clinical diagnosis of early-onset sepsis. *Pediatrics* 2001;107(1): 30–35.
117. Barak Y, Leibovitz E, Mogilner B, et al. The in vivo effect of recombinant human granulocyte-colony stimulating factor in neutropenic neonates with sepsis. *Eur J Pediatr* 1997;156(8):643–646.
118. Bernstein HM, Pollock BH, Calhoun DA, et al. Administration of recombinant granulocyte colony-stimulating factor to neonates with septicemia: a meta-analysis. *J Pediatr* 2001;138(6):917–920.
119. Carr R, Modi N, Dore C. G-CSF and GM-CSF for treating or preventing neonatal infections. *Cochrane Database Syst Rev* 2003(3): CD003066.
120. Carr R, Modi N. Haemopoietic growth factors for neonates: assessing risks and benefits. *Acta Paediatr Suppl* 2004;93(444):15–19.
121. Koenig JM, Christensen RD. Incidence, neutrophil kinetics, and natural history of neonatal neutropenia associated with maternal hypertension. *N Engl J Med* 1989;321(9):557–562.
122. Koenig JM, Christensen RD. The mechanism responsible for diminished neutrophil production in neonates delivered of women with pregnancy-induced hypertension. *Am J Obstet Gynecol* 1991;165(2):467–473.
123. Juul SE, Haynes JW, McPherson RJ. Evaluation of neutropenia and neutrophilia in hospitalized preterm infants. *J Perinatol* 2004; 24(3):150–157.
124. Fraser SH, Tudehope DI. Neonatal neutropenia and thrombocytopenia following maternal hypertension. *J Paediatr Child Health* 1996;32(1):31–34.
125. Brazy JE, Grimm JK, Little VA. Neonatal manifestations of severe maternal hypertension occurring before the thirty-sixth week of pregnancy. *J Pediatr* 1982;100(2):265–271.
126. Makhlouf RA, Doron MW, Bose CL, et al. Administration of granulocyte colony-stimulating factor to neutropenic low birth weight infants of mothers with preeclampsia. *J Pediatr* 1995;126(3): 454–456.
127. Kocherlakota P, La Gamma EF. Preliminary report: rhG-CSF may reduce the incidence of neonatal sepsis in prolonged preeclampsia-associated neutropenia. *Pediatrics* 1998;102(5):1107–1111.
128. Maheshwari A, Christensen RD, Calhoun DA. Immune-mediated neutropenia in the neonate. *Acta Paediatr Suppl* 2002;91(438): 98–103.
129. Maheshwari A, Christensen RD, Calhoun DA. Resistance to recombinant human granulocyte colony-stimulating factor in neonatal alloimmune neutropenia associated with anti-human neutrophil antigen-2a (NB1) antibodies. *Pediatrics* 2002;109(4):e64.
130. Lejkowski M, Maheshwari A, Calhoun DA, et al. Persistent perianal abscess in early infancy as a presentation of autoimmune neutropenia. *J Perinatol* 2003;23(5):428–430.
131. Juul S, Ledbetter D, Wight TN, et al. New insights into idiopathic infantile arterial calcinosis. Three patient reports. *Am J Dis Child* 1990;144(2):229–233.
132. Juul SE, Calhoun DA, Christensen RD. "Idiopathic neutropenia" in very low birthweight infants. *Acta Paediatr* 1998;87(9):963–968.
133. Juul SE, Christensen RD. Effect of recombinant granulocyte colony-stimulating factor on blood neutrophil concentrations among patients with "idiopathic neonatal neutropenia": a randomized, placebo-controlled trial. *J Perinatol* 2003;23(6):493–497.
134. Nagata S, Tsuchiya M, Asano S, et al. Molecular cloning and expression of cDNA for human granulocyte colony-stimulating factor. *Nature* 1986;319(6052):415–418.
135. Martin-Christin F. Granulocyte colony stimulating factors: how different are they? How to make a decision? *Anti-Cancer Drugs* 2001;12(3):185–191.
136. van der Auwera P, Platzer E, Xu ZX, et al. Pharmacodynamics and pharmacokinetics of single doses of subcutaneous pegylated human G-CSF mutant (Ro 25-8315) in healthy volunteers: comparison with single and multiple daily doses of Filgrastim. *Am J Hematol* 2001;66(4):245–251.
137. Christensen RD, Calhoun DA, Rimsza LM. A practical approach to evaluating and treating neutropenia in the neonatal intensive care unit. *Clin Perinatol* 2000;27(3):577–601.
138. Gillan ER, Christensen RD, Suen Y, et al. A randomized, placebo-controlled trial of recombinant human granulocyte colony-stimulating factor administration in newborn infants with presumed sepsis: significant induction of peripheral and bone marrow neutrophilia. *Blood* 1994;84(5):1427–1433.
139. Calhoun DA, Lunoe M, Du Y, et al. Granulocyte colony-stimulating factor serum and urine concentrations in neutropenic neonates before and after intravenous administration of recombinant granulocyte colony-stimulating factor. *Pediatrics* 2000;105(2):392–397.
140. Gessler P, Neu S, Brockmann Y, et al. Decreased mRNA expression of G-CSF receptor in cord blood neutrophils of term newborns: regulation of expression by G-CSF and TNF-alpha. *Biol Neonate* 2000;77(3):168–173.
141. Calhoun DA, Christensen RD. Human developmental biology of granulocyte colony-stimulating factor. *Clin Perinatol* 2000;27(3): 559–576, vi.
142. Ericson SG, Gao H, Gericke GH, et al. The role of polymorphonuclear neutrophils (PMNs) in clearance of granulocyte colony-stimulating factor (G-CSF) in vivo and in vitro. *Exp Hematol* 1997;25(13):1313–1325.
143. Kuwabara T, Kobayashi S, Sugiyama Y. Pharmacokinetics and pharmacodynamics of a recombinant human granulocyte colony-stimulating factor. *Drug Metab Rev* 1996;28(4):625–658.
144. Calhoun DA, Donnelly WH Jr, Du Y, et al. Distribution of granulocyte colony-stimulating factor (G-CSF) and G-CSF-receptor mRNA and protein in the human fetus. *Pediatr Res* 1999;46(3):333–338.
145. Gaertner HF, Offord RE. Site-specific attachment of functionalized poly(ethylene glycol) to the amino terminus of proteins. *Bioconjug Chem* 1996;7(1):38–44.
146. Kinstler OB, Brems DN, Lauren SL, et al. Characterization and stability of N-terminally PEGylated rhG-CSF. *Pharm Res* 1996;13(7): 996–1002.
147. Tanaka H, Satake-Ishikawa R, Ishikawa M, et al. Pharmacokinetics of recombinant human granulocyte colony-stimulating factor conjugated to polyethylene glycol in rats. *Cancer Res* 1991;51(14): 3710–3714.
148. Johnston E, Crawford J, Blackwell S, et al. Randomized, dose-escalation study of SD/01 compared with daily filgrastim in patients receiving chemotherapy. *J Clin Oncol* 2000;18(13):2522–2528.
149. Rosenthal J, Healey T, Ellis R, et al. A two-year follow-up of neonates with presumed sepsis treated with recombinant human granulocyte colony-stimulating factor during the first week of life. *J Pediatr* 1996;128(1):135–137.
150. Donadieu J, Boutard P, Bernatowska E, et al. A European phase II study of recombinant human granulocyte colony-stimulating factor (lenograstim) in the treatment of severe chronic neutropenia in children. Lenograstim Study Group. *Eur J Pediatr* 1997; 156(9):693–700.
151. Gilmore MM, Stroncek DF, Korones DN. Treatment of alloimmune neonatal neutropenia with granulocyte colony-stimulating factor. *J Pediatr* 1994;125(6, pt 1):948–951.
152. Bonilla MA, Dale D, Zeidler C, et al. Long-term safety of treatment with recombinant human granulocyte colony-stimulating factor (r-metHuG-CSF) in patients with severe congenital neutropenias. *Br J Haematol* 1994;88(4):723–730.
153. Germeshausen M, Skokowa J, Ballmaier M, et al. G-CSF receptor mutations in patients with congenital neutropenia. *Curr Opin Hematol* 2008;15(4):332–337.
154. Cottle TE, Fier CJ, Donadieu J, et al. Risk and benefit of treatment of severe chronic neutropenia with granulocyte colony-stimulating factor. *Semin Hematol* 2002;39(2):134–140.
155. Dale DC, Bolyard AA, Schwinzer BG, et al. The Severe Chronic Neutropenia International Registry: 10-Year Follow-up Report. *Support Cancer Ther* 2006;3(4):220–231.
156. Schabitz WR, Kollmar R, Schwaninger M, et al. Neuroprotective effect of granulocyte colony-stimulating factor after focal cerebral ischemia. *Stroke* 2003;34(3):745–751.
157. Lee ST, Chu K, Jung KH, et al. Granulocyte colony-stimulating factor enhances angiogenesis after focal cerebral ischemia. *Brain Res* 2005;1058(1–2):120–128.
158. Schneider A, Kuhn HG, Schabitz WR. A role for G-CSF (granulocyte-colony stimulating factor) in the central nervous system. *Cell Cycle* 2005;4(12):1753–1757.

159. Solaroglu I, Cahill J, Jadhav V, et al. A novel neuroprotectant granulocyte-colony stimulating factor. *Stroke* 2006;37(4):1123–1128.
160. Gibson CL, Jones NC, Prior MJ, et al. G-CSF suppresses edema formation and reduces interleukin-1beta expression after cerebral ischemia in mice. *J Neuropathol Exp Neurol* 2005;64(9):763–769.
161. Komine-Kobayashi M, Zhang N, Liu M, et al. Neuroprotective effect of recombinant human granulocyte colony-stimulating factor in transient focal ischemia of mice. *J Cereb Blood Flow Metab* 2006;26(3):402–413.
162. Keller M, Simbruner G, Gorna A, et al. Systemic application of granulocyte-colony stimulating factor and stem cell factor exacerbates excitotoxic brain injury in newborn mice. *Pediatr Res* 2006; 59(4, pt 1):549–553.
163. Wheeler JG, Givner LB. Therapeutic use of recombinant human granulocyte-macrophage colony-stimulating factor in neonatal rats with type III group B streptococcal sepsis. *J Infect Dis* 1992; 165(5):938–941.
164. Cairo MS, Christensen R, Sender LS, et al. Results of a phase I/II trial of recombinant human granulocyte-macrophage colony-stimulating factor in very low birthweight neonates: significant induction of circulatory neutrophils, monocytes, platelets, and bone marrow neutrophils. *Blood* 1995;86(7): 2509–2515.
165. Cairo MS, Agosti J, Ellis R, et al. A randomized, double-blind, placebo-controlled trial of prophylactic recombinant human granulocyte-macrophage colony-stimulating factor to reduce nosocomial infections in very low birth weight neonates. *J Pediatr* 1999;134(1):64–70.
166. Bilgin K, Yaramis A, Haspolat K, et al. A randomized trial of granulocyte-macrophage colony-stimulating factor in neonates with sepsis and neutropenia. *Pediatrics* 2001;107(1):36–41.
167. Venkateswaran L, Wilimas JA, Dancy R, et al. Granulocyte-macrophage colony-stimulating factor in the treatment of neonates with neutropenia and sepsis. *Pediatr Hematol Oncol* 2000;17(6): 469–473.
168. Carr R, Modi N, Dore CJ, et al. A randomized, controlled trial of prophylactic granulocyte-macrophage colony-stimulating factor in human newborns less than 32 weeks gestation. *Pediatrics* 1999;103(4, pt 1):796–802.
169. Lau AS, Lehman D, Geertsma FR, et al. Biology and therapeutic uses of myeloid hematopoietic growth factors and interferons. *Pediatr Infect Dis J* 1996;15(7):563–575.
170. Carr R, Modi N. Haemopoietic colony stimulating factors for preterm neonates. *Arch Dis Child Fetal Neonatal Ed* 1997;76(2): F128–F133.
171. Sullivan GW, Carper HT, Mandell GL. The effect of three human recombinant hematopoietic growth factors (granulocyte-macrophage colony-stimulating factor, granulocyte colony-stimulating factor, and interleukin-3) on phagocyte oxidative activity. *Blood* 1993;81(7):1863–1870.
172. Sreenan C, Osiovich H. Myeloid colony-stimulating factors: use in the newborn. *Arch Pediatr Adolesc Med* 1999;153(9):984–988.

Mary Frances Picciano
Michelle K. McGuire
Paul M. Coates

CHAPTER

56

Nutrient Supplements

INTRODUCTION

During infancy and childhood, patterns of healthy growth and development are generally predictable and orderly. Although these growth trajectories are primarily determined by genetics, environmental influences such as nutritional status can also be important. This is especially true during the most rapid periods of growth, such as those which occur in infancy and adolescence. A good example of this is protein. During early infancy, protein requirements are estimated to be 1.52 g per kg per day; this decreases gradually through childhood until it reaches 0.8 g per kg per day (1). Although obtaining adequate amounts of the essential nutrients *from foods* during periods of growth is considered most desirable, sometimes this becomes difficult, and supplementation is warranted. This is especially true for several of the micronutrients (vitamins and minerals), which are the main focus of this chapter.

Vitamins and minerals are essential for myriad functions related to growth, differentiation, and development. Vitamins can also regulate the expression of genes involved in cell proliferation and tissue specification. Minerals primarily act as enzymatic cofactors and stabilizers for enzymes and transcription factors, although some are also critical for structural purposes. Because of the far-reaching functions of vitamins and minerals, micronutrient deficiencies can have negative impacts during periods of growth and development as well as long-term effects on structural integrity. Early malnutrition may also predispose an individual to increased risk for chronic degenerative diseases (e.g., cardiovascular disease) later in life.

Because of the importance of nutritional adequacy during early life, dietary recommendations for the pediatric population are relatively well delineated, and supplementation with vitamins and minerals is sometimes used to prevent or treat nutrient inadequacies (2). The main objective of this chapter is to review a selected group of micronutrients that are most frequently provided to infants and children as dietary supplements. These include vitamin A (and the carotenoids), vitamin D, vitamin E, vitamin K, calcium, iron, zinc, iodine, and fluoride. We will also comment briefly on a group of lipids referred to as the "omega-3 fatty acids." For each of these, we will discuss their biological forms and functions, dietary sources, dietary reference intake (DRI) values, signs and symptoms of deficiencies and toxicities, and the most current recommendations for supplementation. We will also review the definition of a dietary supplement, how these products are regulated by the Food and Drug Administration, and statistics related to supplement use—especially in children.

WHAT IS A DIETARY SUPPLEMENT?

Although dietary supplements have long been available to the US consumer, they were not officially defined until 1994 when the US Congress passed the Dietary Supplement Health and Education Act (DSHEA) (3). Since that time, a "dietary supplement" has been defined as a product that meets the following requirements:

- Intended to supplement the diet or contain one or more of the following: vitamin, mineral, herb or other plant-derived substance (e.g., ginseng, garlic), amino acid, concentrate, metabolite, constituent, or extract.
- Intended for ingestion in pill, capsule, tablet, or liquid form.
- Not represented for use as a conventional food or as the sole item of a meal or diet.

DSHEA was the first legislation to clearly define dietary supplements *as foods* (as opposed to drugs) having implications for both manufacturers and consumers in terms of what was needed (or not needed) for evidence of efficacy, safety, and quality of dietary supplement products. For example, similar to how food products are handled, manufacturers are required to have evidence to support claims of efficacy and safety. However, unlike what pharmaceutical companies are required to do for drugs, food manufacturers are generally not required to seek premarket approval of their claims by the Food and Drug Administration.

DIETARY SUPPLEMENT USE IN AMERICAN CHILDREN

Use of dietary supplements in the United States is strong and growing, and it is estimated that revenue from sales of dietary supplements was more than $21 billion in 2005 (4).

Of the dietary supplements available, vitamins and minerals—as well as combinations thereof—are the most widely used types. Most (65%) of these supplements are purchased from retail establishments such as natural, health food, grocery, or drug stores; only 7% are obtained from a health practitioner.

Of special interest to this chapter is dietary supplement use among children. Ervin and colleagues compiled data from the National Health and Nutrition Examination Survey conducted between 1988 and 1994 (before the passage of DSHEA) and reported that children aged 1 to 5 years were major users of dietary supplements (5). The supplements most commonly taken by children aged 2 months to 11 years were multivitamins or combinations of multiple vitamins and minerals. Slightly less than 10% of children were taking two or more supplements.

Dietary supplement use by infants and children between 1999 and 2002 (after passage of DSHEA) has also been reported (6). In this study, the investigators used nationally representative data from the National Health and Nutrition Examination Survey, studying children (n = 10,136) from birth through 18 years. Their data indicate that 31.8% of children used dietary supplements, with the lowest use reported among infants younger than 1 year (11.9%), followed by teenagers 14 to 18 years (25.7%). Highest use was among 4- to 8-year-old children (48.5%). In an ethnic comparison, supplement consumption was found to be greatest in non-Hispanic white and Mexican American participants; lowest use was among non-Hispanic black participants. There appeared to be no difference in intake between boys and girls. These analyses suggest that the type of supplement most commonly used by children is a multivitamin/multimineral combination. Furthermore, supplement use was reported to be associated with higher income, a smoke-free environment, lower body mass index, and less daily recreational "screen time." The highest use was in children who were underweight or at risk for becoming underweight.

In summary, the use of dietary supplements and more specifically those containing vitamins and minerals is common in the pediatric American population. In the next sections, we discuss several micronutrients that are sometimes recommended as dietary supplements during infancy and childhood. We address their physiological importance, recommended intakes, signs and symptoms of deficiency and toxicity, and—when possible—recommendations for supplementation.

VITAMIN A AND THE CAROTENOIDS

The term "vitamin A" (or retinoid) refers to a group of fat-soluble compounds that all contain a complex 20-carbon structure with a methyl-substituted cyclohexenyl ring and a tetrene side chain. These compounds differ among themselves in that they can contain a hydroxyl group (retinol), aldehyde group (retinal), carboxylic acid group (retinoic acid), or ester group (retinyl ester).

The term "vitamin A" is also used to describe a series of dietary compounds (called carotenoids) that can be converted in the body to retinol, some of which are shown in Figure 56.1. These dietary substances are also called "provitamin A carotenoids" to distinguish them from other carotenoids that cannot be converted to vitamin A. Carotenoids, which usually contain 40 carbon atoms with conjugated double bonds and one or two cyclic structures, function mainly as antioxidants. Of the 600 or more carotenoids that exist in nature, β-carotene, α-carotene, and cryptoxanthin are the primary provitamin A forms. There is growing interest in both nonprovitamin A and provitamin A carotenoids, because higher dietary intakes of some forms have been associated with decreased risk for macular degeneration and cataracts, some cancers, and some cardiovascular events (7).

METABOLISM OF VITAMIN A

Regardless of whether it is consumed as preformed vitamin A or a provitamin A carotenoid, retinoids are metabolized in many organs (liver, intestine, kidney, and skin), being converted to different forms with specific functions. For example, retinal can be reversibly reduced to retinol and irreversibly oxidized to retinoic acid (8). Retinoids, bound to retinoid-binding proteins and receptors, are transported to specific sites for metabolic transformations both within the plasma and the cell.

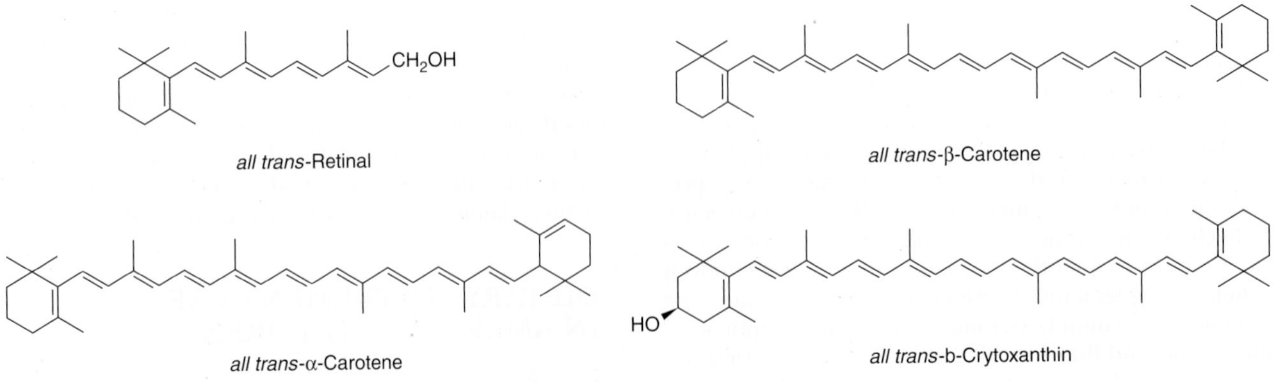

CH_2OH

all trans-Retinal

all trans-β-Carotene

all trans-α-Carotene

HO

all trans-b-Crytoxanthin

Figure 56.1. Structures of retinol and provitamin A carotenoids. (Modified from Institute of Medicine, Food and Nutrition Board. *Dietary reference intakes for vitamin C, vitamin E, selenium, and carotenoids.* Washington, DC: National Academy Press, 2000, with permission.)

PHYSIOLOGIC ROLES OF VITAMIN A

Perhaps the most thoroughly understood function of vitamin A (specifically retinal and retinoic acid) in the body is the role it plays in vision. Specifically, retinal is required for the transduction of light into neural signals necessary for vision, whereas retinoic acid is needed to maintain normal differentiation of the cornea and conjunctional membranes. However, vitamin A is also needed for a variety of other functions as well. For instance, during embryonic development, retinoic acid as well as specific retinoid receptors (retinoic acid receptor and retinoid X receptor) and retinol-binding proteins are postulated to be involved in the development of the vertebrae and spinal cord. Retinoic acid also functions in limb development and formation of the heart, eyes, and ears (8).

Retinoic acid also appears to be involved in the genesis of tissue specificity, directing undifferentiated stem cells to stop proliferating and assume a differentiated phenotype (8). In addition, retinoic acid regulates the expression of various genes that encode structural proteins involved in maintaining epithelial cell integrity (e.g., skin keratins), extracellular matrix proteins (e.g., laminin), and retinol-binding proteins and receptors. Retinoic acid is also needed to maintain adequate circulating levels of natural killer cells, increase macrophage phagocytic activity, and increase cytokines that mediate T and B lymphocyte production (9).

DIETARY SOURCES OF VITAMIN A

Preformed vitamin A is found in some animal-derived foods such as liver, dairy products, and fish. Provitamin A carotenoids tend to be plentiful in colorful fruits and vegetables, such as cantaloupe, carrots, broccoli, spinach, and some oily plants (e.g., avocado and red palm oil). The primary dietary form of provitamin A is β-carotene, which is cleaved to form free retinol in the small intestine. Note that the vitamin A content of foods or biological tissues is measured using a unit referred to as a retinol activity equivalent (RAE); 1 RAE is equivalent to 1 μg of all-trans-retinol, 2 μg of supplemental all-trans-β-carotene, 12 μg of dietary all-trans-β-carotene, or 24 μg of other dietary provitamin A carotenoids.*

DIETARY REFERENCE INTAKE VALUES FOR VITAMIN A

DRIs have been set for vitamin A during infancy. Like all of the adequate intake (AI) levels for young infants (0 to 6 months), that for vitamin A is based on the vitamin A intake of infants primarily fed human milk. The AI for this essential nutrient from 0 to 6 months is 400 μg of RAE per day; from 7 to 12 months it is 500 μg of RAE per day. Recommended dietary allowances (RDAs) for children aged 1 to 3 and 4 to 8 years are 300 and 400 μg of RAE per day, respectively, after which time they increase. Because vitamin A toxicity can occur, tolerable upper intake levels (ULs) have also been set. These values are 600 μg of RAE per day for the first 3 years of life; 900 μg of RAE per day from 4 to 8 years; 1,700 μg per day from 9 to 13 years; and 2,800 μg per day from 14 to 18 years. The AI and UL values for vitamin A (as well as the other micronutrients discussed in this chapter) during infancy are listed in Table 56.1; the AI/RDA and UL values during childhood and adolescence can be found in Table 56.2.

CONSEQUENCES OF INADEQUATE VITAMIN A INTAKE AND EFFECT OF SUPPLEMENTATION

Because human milk, bovine milk, and infant formulas are good sources of vitamin A, vitamin A deficiency in the United States is rare in infancy and childhood. However, vitamin A deficiency can occur in infants and children with fat malabsorption (2). Furthermore, vitamin A concentration in milk from mothers delivering prematurely is very low and may not provide recommended amounts (10). Thus, vitamin A nutriture may be inadequate in this subpopulation, even in developed countries.

The most common signs and symptoms of vitamin A deficiency progress from night blindness to xerosis (dryness and wrinkling of the conjunctiva) and the development of Bitot's spots, to corneal xerophthalmia, keratopathy, and finally loss of vision. In developing countries (especially Asia and Africa) vitamin A deficiency not only is the leading cause of preventable blindness but also elevates the risk of disease and death from severe infections such as diarrhea and measles (11,12). For example, children with mild xerophthalmia are at increased risk of respiratory tract infections and diarrhea, and mortality rates are up to four times greater among children with than without mild xerophthalmia. Experts estimate that between 100 and 140 million children are vitamin A deficient worldwide, 250,000 to 500,000 of whom become blind annually; half of these affected children are thought to die within 12 months of losing their sight (13). Other factors in developing countries that can influence a child's requirement for vitamin A are presence and severity of infection with parasites, inadequate iron status, low intakes of dietary fat, and protein energy malnutrition.

Fortunately, high-dose vitamin A supplementation can reduce the incidence of morbidity, including night blindness in children (13). However, vitamin A supplementation may be able to reverse the process at its early stages (14). There is also growing evidence that the risk of severe morbidity and mortality diminishes with vitamin A repletion. For example, a meta-analysis of controlled trials in several developing countries suggests a 23% to 30% reduction in mortality of young children older than 6 months after vitamin A supplementation (15). Similarly, a recent randomized trial conducted in Bangladesh showed a 15% reduction in all-causal mortality when newborns received a single, oral supplement of vitamin A (50,000 IU) at birth (16).

Vitamin A supplementation may also help prevent mortality and morbidity in very low–birth-weight (VLBW) infants. In support of this, a recent Cochrane review utilized data from eight randomized controlled trials which compared the effects of supplemental vitamin A with standard vitamin A regimes in VLBW infants (17). These authors concluded that supplementing VLBW infants with vitamin A was associated with a reduction in death or oxygen requirement at 1 month of age and oxygen requirement among survivors at 36 weeks, with the latter outcome being confined to infants with birth weight less than 1,000 g.

*Historically, vitamin A activity was described in international units (IU), with 1 μg of retinol equivalent to 3.33 IU.

TABLE 56.1 Representative Values for Nutrient Content of Mature Human Milk and Reference Intake Values for Selected Nutrients During Infancy and Childhood

Nutrient	Milk Content Per Liter[a]	Estimated Infant Intake Per Day[b]	Age (mo)	DRI[c] AI	DRI[c] UL
Retinol (μg)	300–600	200–500	0–6	400	600
			7–12	500	600
Carotenoids (mg)	0.2–0.6	0.2–0.5	–	–	–
Vitamin D (μg)[d]	0.33	0.26	0–6	5	25
			7–12	5	25
Vitamin E (mg)	3.0–8.0	2.3–6.2	0–6	4	ND
			7–12	5	ND
Vitamin K (μg)	2–3	1.6–2.3	0–6	2	ND
			7–12	2.5	ND
Calcium (mg)	200–250	156–195	0–6	210	ND
			7–12	270	ND
Iron (mg)	0.3–0.9	0.2–0.7	0–6	0.27	40
			7–12	11	40
Zinc (mg)	1.0–3.0	0.8–2.3	0–6	2	4
			7–12	3	5
Iodine (μg)	113–150	88–117	0–6	110	ND
			7–12	130	ND
Fluoride (μg)	4–15	3–12	0–6	10	700
			7–12	500	900

[a]Data from Jensen RG, ed, *Handbook of milk composition.* San Diego, CA: Academic Press, 1995; and Picciano MF. Nutrient composition of human milk. *Pediatr Clin North Am* 2001;48:53–67.
[b]Estimated intake based on milk intake of 0.78 L/d for first 6 mo of life.
[c]AI, adequate intake; DRI, dietary reference intakes; ND, no data available; UL, tolerable upper intake level. From Institute of Medicine, Food and Nutrition Board. *Dietary reference intakes for vitamin C, vitamin E, selenium, and carotenoids.* Washington, DC: National Academy Press, 2000; Institute of Medicine, Food and Nutrition Board. *Dietary reference intakes for calcium, phosphorus, magnesium, vitamin D, and fluoride.* Washington, DC: National Academy Press, 1997; Institute of Medicine, Food and Nutrition Board. *Dietary reference intakes for vitamin A, vitamin K, arsenic, boron, chromium, copper, iodine, iron, manganese, molybdenum, nickel, silicon, vanadium, and zinc.* Washington, DC: National Academy Press, 2001.
[d]The American Academy of Pediatrics recommends all breastfed infants be supplemented with 400 IU/d vitamin D beginning within the first few days of life. Formula-fed infants receiving <1 L/d vitamin D-fortified formula also need an alternative way to get 400 IU/d vitamin D, such as through vitamin supplements (2).

Improvement in vitamin A status of preterm infants is also associated with decreased incidence of and morbidity from bronchopulmonary dysplasia, indicating that vitamin A supplementation may prevent lung injury and promote healing (18). Vitamin A supplementation may be especially beneficial for extremely low–birth-weight infants. Ambalavanan and colleagues determined whether vitamin A supplementation in extremely low–birth-weight infants ($n = 807$) during the first month after birth affects survival without neurodevelopmental impairment (19). Although they found no evidence that neonatal vitamin A supplementation reduced hospitalizations or pulmonary problems after discharge, those provided with supplementation had reduced bronchopulmonary dysplasia.

Many recent studies have reported positive effects of vitamin A supplementation on overall infant and child health, especially in areas of endemic vitamin A deficiency, although others show no effect and sometimes even detrimental outcomes (20–22). An example is a randomized clinical trial of 147 severely anemic children living in Zanzibar who were being treated with the antimalarial drug sulfadoxine pyramethamine (23). The authors hypothesized that both vitamin A (100,000 or 200,000 IU depending on age) and sulfadoxine pyrimethamine treatments rapidly stimulate erythropoietin production. However, while it did reduce inflammation (as measured by C-reactive protein) and mobilized iron from stores, vitamin A supplementation decreased erythropoietin concentrations. There is also evidence of a differential response to vitamin A supplementation between boys and girls (24,25), and this interaction between vitamin A supplementation and sex on vitamin A-related outcomes warrants further study.

Because low vitamin A status has been shown to be a risk factor for maternal-to-child human immunodeficiency virus (HIV) transmission, there has also been considerable interest in whether vitamin A supplementation may be beneficial. Several intervention trials have been conducted, some of them (but not all) suggesting a positive outcome of supplementation (26). However, unease about potential negative outcomes associated with large-dose maternal or neonatal vitamin A supplementation on infant mortality in HIV-endemic areas is considerable (27). Emerging data suggest that there may exist a gene–environment interaction between having the mannose-binding lectin (MBL-2) gene

TABLE 56.2 Dietary Reference Intakes (Per Day) of Nutrients Likely to be Limiting in Diets of Children[a]

Nutrient	*Age (yr)*	*RDA/AI*[b]	*UL*	*Dietary Sources*
Retinol (μg)	1–3	**300**	600	Liver, dairy products, fish
	4–8	**400**	900	
	9–13	**600**	1,700	
	14–18	**900, 700**	2,800	
Vitamin D (μg)[c]	1–3	5	50	Fish liver oils, animal products from animals fed vitamin D, fortified milk, and cereals
	4–8	5	50	
	9–13	5	50	
	14–18	5	50	
Vitamin E (mg)	1–3	**6**	200	Vegetable oils, unprocessed cereal grains, nuts, fruits, vegetables, meats
	4–8	**7**	300	
	9–13	**11**	600	
	14–18	**15**	800	
Vitamin K (μg)	1–3	30	ND	Green vegetables, brussel sprouts, cabbage, plant oils, margarine
	4–8	55	ND	
	9–13	60	ND	
	14–18	75	ND	
Calcium (mg)	1–3	500	2,500	Dairy products, calcium-set tofu, legumes, Chinese cabbage, kale, broccoli
	4–8	800	2,500	
	9–13	1,300	2,500	
	14–18	1,300	2,500	
Iron (mg)	1–3	**7**	40	Fruits, vegetables, and fortified cereals (nonheme), meat and poultry (heme)
	4–8	**10**	40	
	9–13	**8**	40	
	14–18	**11, 15**	45	
Zinc (mg)	1–3	**3**	7	Red meats, poultry, seafoods, beans, nuts, legumes, fortified cereals
	4–8	**5**	12	
	9–13	**8**	23	
	14–18	**11, 9**	34	
Iodine (μg)	1–3	**90**	200	Sea products, processed foods, dairy products, iodized salt
	4–8	**90**	300	
	9–13	**120**	600	
	14–18	**150**	900	
Fluoride (mg)	1–3	0.7	1.3	Fluoridated water, teas, marine fish, fluoridated dental products
	4–8	1	2.2	
	9–13	2	10	
	14–18	3	10	

[a]AI, adequate intake; ND, no data available; RDA, recommended dietary allowance, in bold type; UL, tolerable upper intake level.

From Institute of Medicine, Food and Nutrition Board. *Dietary reference intakes for vitamin C, vitamin E, selenium, and carotenoids.* Washington, DC: National Academy Press, 2000; Institute of Medicine, Food and Nutrition Board. *Dietary reference intakes for calcium, phosphorus, magnesium, vitamin D, and fluoride.* Washington, DC: National Academy Press, 1997; Institute of Medicine, Food and Nutrition Board. *Dietary reference intakes for vitamin A, vitamin K, arsenic, boron, chromium, copper, iodine, iron, manganese, molybdenum, nickel, silicon, vanadium, and zinc.* Washington, DC: National Academy Press, 2001.

[b]For boys, girls.

[c]The American Academy of Pediatrics recommends that all children and teens consume 400 IU/d vitamin D from fortified foods or supplements (2).

and vitamin A intake in terms of HIV transmission during infancy (28).

CONSEQUENCES OF EXCESSIVE INTAKE OF VITAMIN A

Commonly recognized signs and symptoms of vitamin A toxicity (hypervitaminosis A) in infants and young children include skeletal abnormalities, bone tenderness and pain, increased intracranial pressure, desquamation, brittle nails, mouth fissures, alopecia, fever, headache, lethargy, irritability, weight loss, vomiting, and hepatomegaly (29). As little as 1,800 μg RAE per day can produce serious toxic effects in children. Although vitamin A toxicity is typically associated with excessive consumption of supplemental vitamin A, toxic effects have also been reported in young children fed large amounts of chicken liver daily (90 μg per g RAE) for 1 month or longer (30).

Experimental data indicate that β-carotene, even when ingested in extremely large doses, is not carcinogenic, mutagenic, embryotoxic, or teratogenic. Instead, it results in a benign disorder referred to as *hypercarotenemia*, characterized by elevated concentrations of carotenoids in serum and liver and carotenoid deposits in skin and underlying subcutaneous adipose causing the skin to become yellowish orange in color (31).

RECOMMENDATIONS FOR VITAMIN A SUPPLEMENTATION DURING INFANCY AND CHILDHOOD

The International Vitamin A Consultative Group, the World Health Organization (WHO), and the United Nations Children's Fund recommend oral doses of vitamin A for infants and young children in vitamin A-deficient populations. Specifically, the International Vitamin A Consultative Group recommends that three 50,000 IU doses of vitamin A should be given at the same time as infant vaccines during the first 6 months of life in all populations where vitamin A deficiency is an important public health problem (32). High-dose vitamin A treatment is also recommended for infants and young children with xerophthalmia, severe malnutrition, or measles. The WHO recommends broad-based prophylaxis with vitamin A in vitamin A-deficient children who suffer from xerophthalmia, measles, prolonged diarrhea, wasting malnutrition, and other acute infections. Specifically, if a child shows any ocular signs of deficiency, it is recommended that he/she receive vitamin A on days 1, 2, and 14, and then repeatedly throughout the first year of life (33). The American Academy of Pediatrics (AAP) does not make any special recommendations concerning dietary supplementation with vitamin A during infancy and childhood other than those associated with using appropriate human milk fortifiers and proprietary formulas when needed. However, there is some evidence that supplemental vitamin A may be indicated for low–birth-weight (LBW), preterm infants (10,34).

VITAMIN D

Vitamin D (technically referred to as calciferol) and its metabolites constitute a group of fat-soluble sterols that are essential for proper growth and development of the skeletal system. Vitamin D exists in two major physiologically relevant forms: vitamin D_2 (ergocalciferol) and vitamin D_3 (cholecalciferol) (Fig. 56.2). Ergosterol, the precursor to vitamin D_2, is synthesized by plants; 7-dehydrocholesterol, the precursor of vitamin D_3, is synthesized by humans and other mammals in their skin. Conversion of both precursors to active vitamin D initially requires cleavage via ultraviolet B light (UVB; 290 to 320 nm). It is because of this that vitamin D is sometimes referred to as the "sunshine vitamin" and why vitamin D deficiency is more common in areas of the world where exposure to sunlight is limited (e.g., Scandinavian countries). The availability and metabolism of vitamin D is complex, involving endogenous synthesis, sunlight exposure, dietary intake, and biotransformation to active and inactive metabolites (Fig. 56.2). Briefly, circulating vitamin D_3 is converted in the liver to 25-hydroxyvitamin D_3 and then again hydroxylated principally in the kidney to the biologically active form, 1,25-dihydroxyvitamin D_3 (calcitriol).

PHYSIOLOGIC ROLES OF VITAMIN D

Vitamin D has many roles in the body, although the most well studied relates to its importance in skeletal growth and maturation. For instance, the active metabolite (calcitriol) functions as a hormone along with parathyroid hormone (PTH) in small intestine, bone, and kidney tissues to maintain serum calcium and phosphate concentrations within physiologically optimal ranges. In addition to enhancing dietary absorption of calcium and phosphorus in the small intestine, 1,25-dihydroxy-vitamin D_3 functions with PTH to mobilize calcium from bone and increase renal resorption of calcium when blood calcium is low. Other recently recognized functions of vitamin D include immunomodulation, control of other hormone systems, inhibition of cell growth, and induction of cell differentiation (35–37).

SOURCES OF VITAMIN D AND FACTORS AFFECTING VITAMIN D STATUS

As described, the body can synthesize vitamin D given adequate precursor material and sunlight. In this way, vitamin D is often considered a conditionally essential nutrient or prohormone, instead of an essential nutrient. Nonetheless, vitamin D can be obtained from dietary sources and is therefore a nutrient. Like vitamin A, the amount of vitamin D in a food or biological material is measured by the amount of biological activity it provides. In the case of vitamin D, the IU, the biological activity of 1 μg of vitamin D is said to be 40 IU (38). One IU of vitamin D activity is equivalent to 5 ng of 25-hydroxyvitamin D_3 and 1 ng of 1,25-dihydroxyvitamin D_3.

Egg yolks, butter, whole milk, fatty fish, fish oils, and mushrooms are some of the few foods that naturally contain vitamin D, and even these foods are not especially rich sources. Therefore, obtaining an adequate intake of vitamin D solely from nonfortified foods is seldom possible (39). However, most liquid and dried milk products as well as breakfast cereals are fortified with this vitamin, and in fact most dietary vitamin D comes from these foods in the United States. Human milk is relatively low in vitamin D (0.33 μg per L IU) unless the mother is given supraphysiologic doses of the vitamin (40).

Dietary vitamin D intake can influence an individual's vitamin D status. However, perhaps more than any other nutrient, other environmental and lifestyle factors are also important. One of these factors is latitude (38). Changes in season and dark skin pigmentation also affect vitamin D status. Compared with their lighter-skin counterparts, individuals with darker skin require longer periods of sun exposure to produce similar amounts of vitamin D.

REFERENCE INTAKE VALUES FOR VITAMIN D AND RECOMMENDATIONS FOR SOLAR EXPOSURE

The AI for vitamin D during infancy, childhood, and adolescence is 5 μg per day (Tables 56.1 and 56.2). Experts

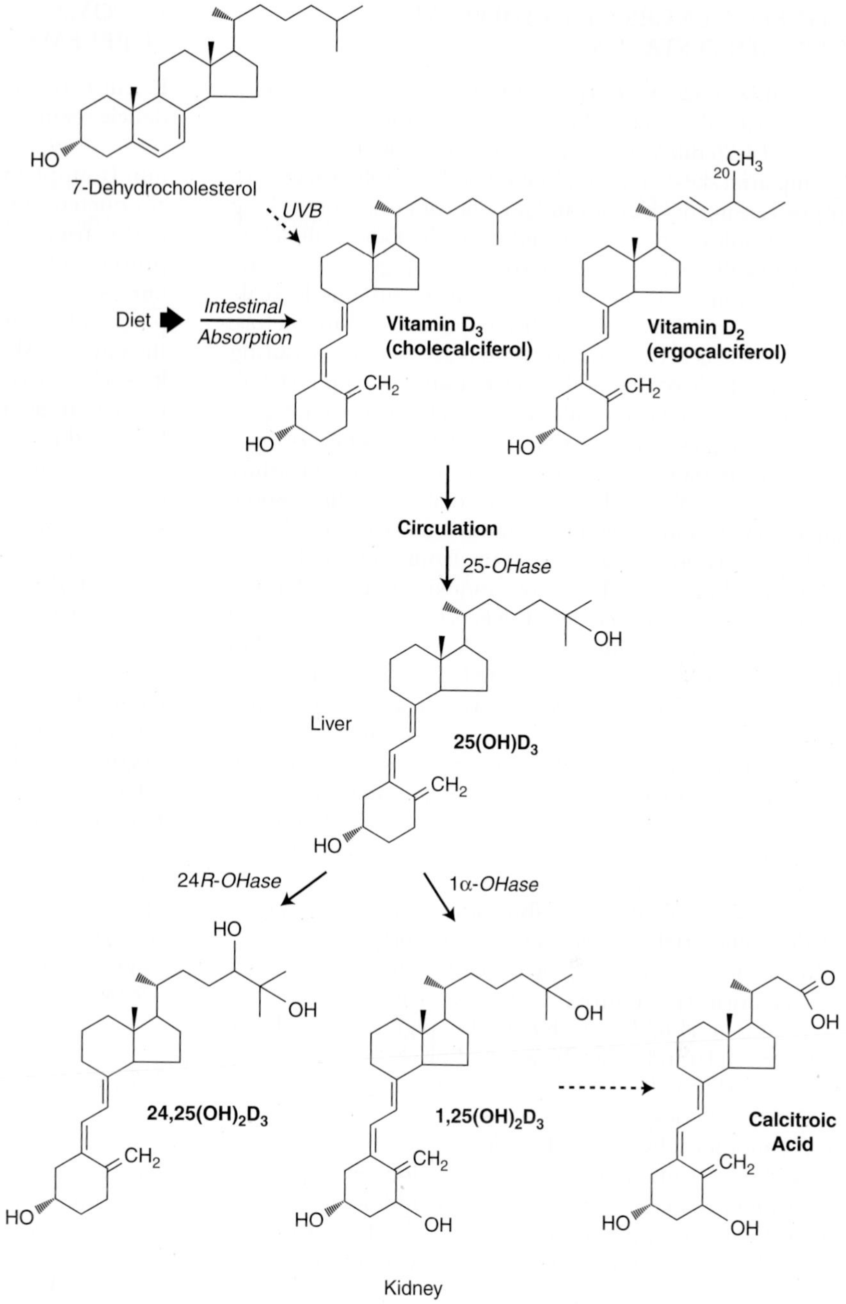

Figure 56.2. Metabolic pathways for vitamin D_3. Vitamin D_2 originates from ergosterol. Major metabolic steps in vitamin D_2 metabolism are similar to those in vitamin D_3 metabolism. 25-OHase, vitamin D 25-hydroxylase; 24R-OHase, 25(OH)D-24R-hydroxylase; 1α-OHase, 25-OH-D-1α-hydroxylase; UVB, ultraviolet B light. (Modified from Holick MF. Vitamin D. In: Olso NJA, Shike M, et al., eds. *Modern nutrition in health and disease.* Baltimore: Williams & Wilkins, 1999: 347–362, with permission.)

now agree that the dietary intake of vitamin D recommended to prevent vitamin D deficiency in normal infants cannot be met with human milk as the sole source of vitamin D. The same is likely true for dietary sources for children and adolescents. Thus, additional vitamin D must be obtained from endogenous production (via sunlight exposure) and/or supplements. Recommendations for solar exposure are discussed here, whereas recommendations for supplementation are provided in a subsequent section.

The amount of solar exposure needed to furnish adequate vitamin D is difficult to define because the amount of UVB light that penetrates skin depends on many factors such as latitude, time of day, level of air pollution, extent of skin pigmentation, sunscreen usage, and habitual dress. Nonetheless, Specker et al. suggested sun exposure of 30 minutes per week was adequate for white infants wearing only a diaper and living in Cincinnati, Ohio (USA), or 2 hours per week if they were fully clothed without a hat (41). However, dietary or supplemental sources of vitamin D become essential during the winter months at northern latitudes because intensity of and exposure to UVB radiation is insufficient to meet the needs for endogenous synthesis.

Because vitamin D toxicity can occur, ULs for this nutrient have also been set. Based on measurement of linear growth (42) and hypercalcemia (43), the UL for infants is 25 μg (1,000 IU) of vitamin D per day for the first 12 months of life; this doubles to 50 μg of vitamin D per day for children 1 to 18 years of age (38) (Tables 56.1 and 56.2).

CONSEQUENCES OF INADEQUATE VITAMIN D STATUS

Vitamin D deficiency during early life can result in a serious disease called rickets, which results from inadequate synthesis of 1,25-dihydroxyvitamin D_3. Rickets is characterized by impaired skeletal mineralization at the epiphyseal growth plates, causing deformities and poor linear growth of the long bones. Clinical signs of advanced rickets include craniotabes, frontal skull bossing, rachitic rosary (enlarged costochondral junctions), widened ribs, bowed legs, and muscle weakness. Subclinical vitamin D deficiency occurs months before signs of rickets become obvious and is assessed by measuring plasma 25-hydroxyvitamin D_3 concentration. Vitamin D deficiency later in life can result in osteomalacia, and emerging evidence suggests that low vitamin D status may be a risk factor to the development of various chronic diseases including cardiovascular disease, hypertension, diabetes mellitus, some inflammatory and autoimmune diseases, and cancer (44–46).

Until recently, rickets resulting from vitamin D deficiency was believed to be almost nonexistent in the United States. However, many cases of rickets due to low vitamin D intake and inadequate endogenous synthesis in the skin have recently been reported in the United States as well as in other Western countries such as Canada, Greece, and the United Kingdom (47–51). Vitamin D-deficiency rickets is also common in breastfed infants of Arab and south Asian countries (52). One recent estimate suggests that the annual incidence of vitamin D–deficiency rickets in developed countries ranges between 2.9 and 7.5 cases per 100,000 children (53). Other data suggest that lesser degrees of vitamin D insufficiency are also widespread (54). Vitamin D–deficiency rickets has also been reported recently in adolescence, thus making the issue of vitamin D deficiency crucial during the entire period of growth (55–57).

Infants and children with dark skin pigmentation, living at northern latitudes, or who are exclusively breastfed are at greatest risk for developing vitamin D deficiency. Vitamin D–deficiency rickets is also more common in children whose mothers observe the Islamic custom of covering their entire bodies with clothing; practice prolonged breastfeeding without vitamin supplementation or addition of vitamin D–fortified dairy products in their infants' diet; or do not themselves consume vitamin D-fortified dairy products.

CONSEQUENCES OF EXCESSIVE VITAMIN D INTAKE

Large oral doses of vitamin D lead to excessive calcium absorption by the intestine, increased bone resorption, and hypercalcemia. This condition, referred to as *hypervitaminosis D*, is characterized by elevated levels of 25-hydroxyvitamin D_3 ranging from 160 to 500 ng per mL (38). Hypercalcemia associated with hypervitaminosis D disrupts normal kidney function, resulting in polydipsia and polyuria. Anorexia, nausea, and vomiting have also been reported in individuals taking 50,000 to 200,000 IU of vitamin D per day. It is noteworthy that doses of 1,800 to 6,300 IU of vitamin D per day were reported decades ago to inhibit linear growth (38). However, that finding was not confirmed in a later study conducted over a longer period of time and with a larger number of infants (42).

RECOMMENDATIONS FOR VITAMIN D SUPPLEMENTATION

Because of growing concerns of widespread vitamin D deficiency in infants and children—especially those with dark skin—several organizations now recommend routine vitamin D supplementation in these groups. Data from studies conducted in China, the United States, and Norway show that consumption of at least 200 IU of vitamin D per day prevents clinical signs of vitamin D deficiency and maintains serum 25-hydroxyvitamin D_3 at or above 27.5 nmol per L (11 ng per mL). Indeed, this value is consistent with the current AI for vitamin D during infancy (38). However, it is clear that 25-hydroxyvitamin D_3 concentrations of more than 50 nmol per L can be maintained in exclusively breastfed infants with supplements of 400 IU of vitamin D per day, which is the amount contained in one teaspoon of cod liver oil and for which there is historic precedence of safety and prevention and treatment of rickets (58–60).

In light of the AAP recommendation that infants be kept out of direct sunlight and wear protective clothing and sunscreen when exposed to sunlight (61), it is important that special efforts be directed toward supplementing populations at increased risk of developing rickets and vitamin D deficiency. Therefore, the AAP recommends that all breastfed infants be supplemented with 400 IU of vitamin D per day beginning within the first few days of life (62). Formula-fed infants receiving less than 1 L of vitamin D–fortified formula per day also need an alternative way to get 400 IU of vitamin D per day, such as through vitamin supplements. This level of supplementation should be continued through childhood. Adolescents who do not obtain 400 IU of vitamin D per day through vitamin–D fortified milk (100 IU per 8 oz serving) and vitamin D–fortified foods should receive a vitamin D supplement of 400 IU per day.

VITAMIN E

The term "vitamin E" refers to all tocol and tocotrienol chemical derivatives that exhibit biological activity similar to that of α-tocopherol, the most abundant and active form of vitamin E. Vitamin E occurs in eight naturally occurring forms: four tocopherols and four tocotrienols (Fig. 56.3). As shown in Figure 56.3, tocopherols have similar chromanol structures, which vary only in the number and position of methyl groups on the chromanol ring: trimethyl (α), dimethyl (β or γ), and mono (δ). Tocotrienols differ from tocopherols in that they have an unsaturated side chain.

The most biologically active form of vitamin E occurs naturally in foods and thus is often referred to as "natural" α-tocopherol or more technically as RRR-α-tocopherol.[†] Synthetic vitamin E is a mixture of eight stereoisomers of α-tocopherol and is designated all-rac-α-tocopherol (often termed d,l-α-tocopherol). Compared with RRR-α-tocopherol other stereoisomers of all-rac-α-tocopherol have lower (21% to 90%) biologic activity. Absorption of α-tocopherol from natural and synthetic sources is similar. Synthetic vitamin E is preferentially degraded over the natural forms; thus, it

[†]RRR-α-tocopherol was formerly called "d-α-tocopherol."

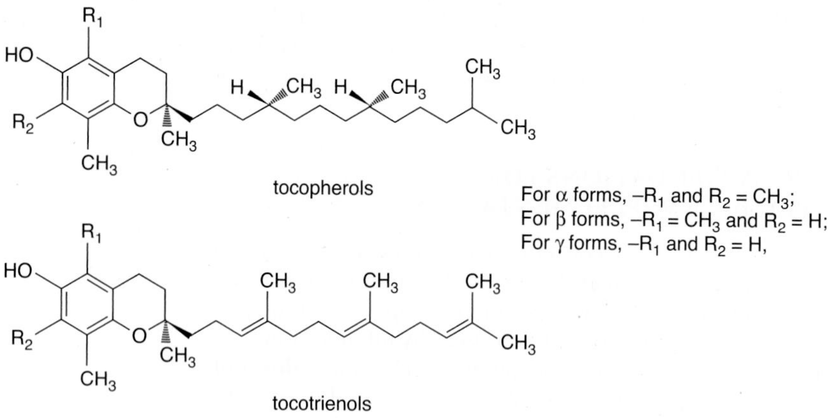

Figure 56.3. Parent forms of tocopherols and tocotrienols. (Modified from Traber MG, Sies H. Vitamin E in humans: demand and delivery. *Annual Rev Nutr* 1996;16: 321–347, with permission.)

is postulated that RRR-α-tocopherol has a specific regulatory role in a system that sorts, distributes, and degrades the different forms of vitamin E (63).

PHYSIOLOGIC ROLES OF VITAMIN E

Vitamin E has many functions in the body, the first recognized being that of reproduction. In fact, the name *tocopherol* was derived from the Greek *tokos* (childbirth) and *phero* (to bear). In general, this vitamin functions as a chain-breaking antioxidant to prevent free radical damage (64). Specifically, vitamin E typically carries out its antioxidant function within membranes. This antioxidant protection is especially important in cells that are exposed to oxygen, such as those in the lungs and red blood cells. Recent evidence also suggests a protective effect of vitamin E in the eye, such that cataract formation may be decreased with vitamin E supplementation (65).

DIETARY SOURCES OF VITAMIN E

Natural α-tocopherol is obtained largely from dietary sources such as whole grains, nuts, vegetable oils, and meats. The RRR-α-tocopherol content is especially high in wheat germ, safflower oil, and sunflower oil. Vitamin E in the diet is typically associated with polyunsaturated fatty acids (PUFAs), in particular linoleic acid. Vitamin E supplements, such as those widely consumed in the United States, are sold in the retinyl ester form and can contain natural RRR-α-tocopherol or the synthetic all-rac-α-tocopherol.

A common unit is used to express the total vitamin E activity of a food, diet, or biological sample. Traditionally, the IU for vitamin E was based on the biologic activity as determined by a rat fetal resorption assay. However, current convention is to report the vitamin E activity of a substance using units of milligrams of RRR-α-tocopherol, or RRR-α-tocopherol equivalents (αTE). For purposes of calculating vitamin E intakes in αTE, γ-tocopherol is assumed to substitute for α-tocopherol with an efficiency of 10%, β-tocopherol with an efficiency of 50%, and α-tocotrienol with an efficiency of 30%. Note that 1 mg of α-tocopherol (αTE) is equal to 1.49 IU of vitamin E.

Experts generally agree that human milk supplies an amount of vitamin E adequate to meet the requirements of term infants. Values in human milk for α-tocopherol equivalents, composed mainly of α-tocopherol, range from 3.0 to 8.0 mg per L, and the vitamin E content of milk from mothers of preterm infants is similar to that from mothers of term infants. (Table 56.1) (40). Maternal tocopherol intake via supplements does not appear to have a major influence on the vitamin E content of human milk (66).

REFERENCE INTAKE VALUES FOR VITAMIN E

The AI for vitamin E is 4 mg per day from 0 to 6 months and 5 mg per day from 7 to 12 months (Table 56.1). The RDA increases progressively to 15 mg per day during childhood and adolescence (Table 56.2). ULs for vitamin E increase from 200 to 800 during infancy, childhood, and adolescence. These values apply to any form of supplemental vitamin E, fortified foods, or a combination of the two but not vitamin E from natural forms.

CONSEQUENCES OF INADEQUATE VITAMIN E INTAKE

Vitamin E deficiency is rare in the United States but can occur in situations related to fat malabsorption. An example of rather widespread vitamin E deficiency occurred in the 1960s and the 1970s when some infant formulas contained high levels of PUFAs and low levels of vitamin E. Because PUFAs are easily damaged (oxidized) by free radicals, consumption of these formulas caused infants to have an increased need for antioxidant nutrients such as vitamin E. This event led to vitamin E fortification of infant formulas. Symptoms of vitamin E deficiency include peripheral neuropathy, hemolytic anemia, and abnormalities in platelet function.

CONSEQUENCES OF EXCESSIVE VITAMIN E INTAKE

Excessively high doses of vitamin E consumed as supplements or given as intravenous solutions have resulted in toxicity in adults and preterm infants. For instance, intravenous administration of all-rac-α-tocopherol acetate (E-Ferol; 15 to 30 mg) to VLBW preterm infants caused pulmonary deterioration, thrombocytopenia, and liver and renal failure (67). Other reports of toxicity associated with pharmacologic oral or parenteral doses of vitamin E include increased risk of necrotizing enterocolitis, sepsis, and retinal hemorrhages (64). When serum vitamin E concentrations are less than 3.5 mg per dL, adverse reactions of vitamin E supplementation are not reported in preterm infants; however, at greater concentrations adverse reactions are not uncommon (68).

RECOMMENDATIONS FOR VITAMIN E SUPPLEMENTATION

Because the vitamin E concentration in human milk is viewed to be sufficient to meet the needs of term infants, there is no evidence to support vitamin E supplementation for breastfeeding mothers and their healthy infants. However, in conditions of fat malabsorption, supplemental doses of 25 IU per kg per day of vitamin E are required to prevent deficiency. In these situations, the water-soluble form of vitamin E is preferable (2).

The usefulness of vitamin E supplementation in preterm infants is somewhat controversial (10). Some experts have suggested that LBW preterm infants receive 6 to 12 IU per kg per day of vitamin E enterally because vitamin E levels in human milk decline as lactation proceeds and because preterm infants have low stores at birth, poor absorption of fat, and increased risk of oxidative stress (66). However, the AAP does not recommend pharmacological doses of vitamin E for the prevention or treatment of retinopathy of prematurity, bronchopulmonary dysplasia, and intraventricular hemorrhage (2).

VITAMIN K

Vitamin K is a fat-soluble vitamin that functions as a coenzyme for the synthesis of biologically active proteins involved in blood coagulation and bone metabolism. For example, vitamin K-dependent carboxylase, a liver microsomal enzyme, uses vitamin K as a substrate to catalyze the posttranslational conversion of specific glutamyl residues to γ-carboxylglutamyl (Gla) residues in a number of proteins (69). Biologically activated proteins dependent on vitamin K include the clotting factors plasma prothrombin (factor II), VII, IX, and Xm as well as proteins C and S, which have anticoagulant activity. In the absence of vitamin K, hemorrhage results from the formation of biologically inactive clotting factors. Other vitamin K-dependent proteins—such as bone Gla protein (also called "osteocalcin") and matrix Gla protein—are postulated to function in the mineralization of bone, but their mechanisms of action remain unclear.

SOURCES AND FORMS OF VITAMIN K

Vitamin K found in the body is obtained from two sources—diet and synthesis by intestinal microbiota. Naturally occurring vitamin K exists in two forms: vitamin K_1 (phylloquinone), synthesized by and found in plants, and vitamin K_2 (menaquinone), synthesized by higher organisms including intestinal bacteria. A third synthetic form is called menadione (Fig. 56.4).

Most foods contain little vitamin K, and the vitamin K content of human milk is also low (2 to 3 μg per L; Table 56.1) (40). Food sources of this vitamin include green leafy vegetables (e.g., collards, spinach, salad greens), vegetable oils, and margarine (70). Although the combination of dietary vitamin K intake and intestinal synthesis in adults is typically thought to be sufficient, adequate dietary intake of vitamin K for infants aged 0 to 12 months is less likely. Aside from low levels in human milk (40), inadequate stores of vitamin K resulting from poor placental transport also contribute to the low vitamin K status in some newborn infants. In fact, serum vitamin K concentration is low or undetectable in cord blood.

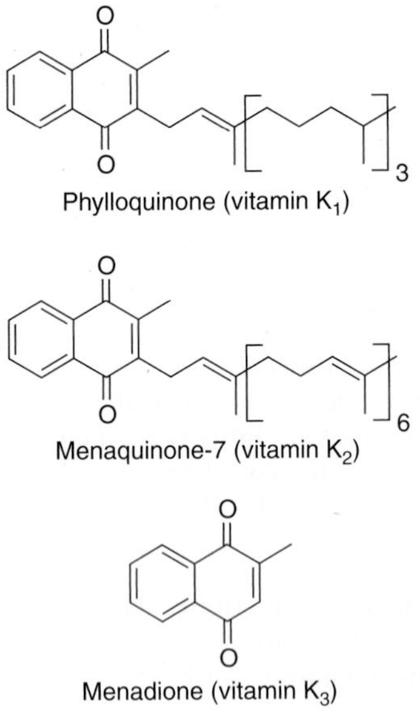

Phylloquinone (vitamin K_1)

Menaquinone-7 (vitamin K_2)

Menadione (vitamin K_3)

Figure 56.4. Biologically active forms of vitamin K. (Modified from Suttie JW. Vitamin K and human nutrition. *J Am Diet Assoc* 1992;92:585–590, with permission.)

REFERENCE INTAKE VALUES FOR VITAMIN K

Establishment of DRI values for vitamin K was challenging because the dietary requirements and metabolism of vitamin K are poorly understood. This is, in part, because of the lack of sensitive methods to assess vitamin K status (70). For example, although serum phylloquinone concentration reflects dietary intake over the previous 24 hours, it is not a good indicator of chronic vitamin K status (70).

Nonetheless, recommended intake values of this vitamin in early life have been established. The AI for infants 0 through 6 months of age was determined to be 2.0 μg of vitamin K per day and assumes that infants also receive prophylactic vitamin K at birth in amounts suggested by the American and Canadian pediatric societies (as discussed next). The AI increases to 2.5 μg per day from 7 to 12 months of life and then again to 30 and 55 μg per day at 1 and 4 years, respectively. The AI for 9- to 18-year-olds is 60 to 75 μg per day. Data on adverse effects from high vitamin K intakes are not sufficient for a quantitative risk assessment, and no adverse effects have been reported with high intakes of this vitamin. Thus, UL values have not been set.

CONSEQUENCES OF INADEQUATE VITAMIN K INTAKE

Poor vitamin K status at birth associated with bleeding during the first weeks of life is now termed *vitamin K-deficiency bleeding* (VKDB) and is categorized as early, classic, and late (71).[‡] The early form occurs in the first 24 hours of life and is characterized by cephalic hematoma and intracranial and intra-abdominal hemorrhage. Early VKDB is sometimes noted in infants born to mothers treated with anticoagulants or anticonvulsants during pregnancy. In the classic form, hemorrhage occurs between 2 and 7 days of life, with bleeding occurring from the umbilical cord stump, gastrointestinal tract, or circumcision site. Late VKDB presents between 7 days and 3 months of life, often resulting in intracranial hemorrhage and sometimes death.

VKDB occurs almost exclusively in breastfed infants who have not received vitamin K prophylaxis or have gastrointestinal disorders associated with fat malabsorption (72). Furthermore, researchers have found that most cases of late VKDB are found in infants not receiving prophylactic vitamin K treatment at birth.

CONSEQUENCES OF EXCESSIVE VITAMIN K INTAKE

Vitamin K toxicity is rare, and no adverse affects have been associated with excessive vitamin K consumption from food or supplements in recent years. An earlier report, however, of increased risk of cancer and leukemia developing during childhood raised concern about vitamin K prophylaxis (73). As a result of methodologic limitations of that study, multiple large case–cohort studies were conducted; no relationship was found between vitamin K given intramuscularly at birth and development of cancer and leukemia in children (74,75).

RECOMMENDATIONS FOR VITAMIN K SUPPLEMENTATION

The efficacy of parenteral vitamin K prophylaxis in prevention of classic VKDB is well established, and several recommendations for vitamin K supplementation and/or injection during infancy have been put forth. Both American and Canadian pediatric societies recommend that newborns receive vitamin K as phylloquinone in a single intramuscular dose of 0.5 to 1.0 mg (2,76). If this is not possible, an oral dose of 1 to 2 mg should be administered at birth, 1 to 2 weeks of age, and 4 weeks of age. Oral supplements of vitamin K are not presently licensed for newborn infants in the United States, although several researchers recommend that they be developed (77,78).

The situation for preterm infants is less well defined. Kumar et al. (71) found that premature infants given 1 mg of vitamin K intramuscularly at birth plus 60 to 130 μg per day parenterally exhibited plasma vitamin K levels directly reflective of vitamin K intakes and adequate vitamin K status. Consequently, these authors suggest that 10 μg per kg per day of vitamin K via the parenteral route of administration is more than adequate to maintain adequate vitamin K status in preterm infants. The AAP recommends that preterm infants receive 0.5 mg vitamin K as a single intramuscular dose. In conditions associated with fat malabsorption, supplemental doses of 2.5 to 5 mg two to seven times per week may be required to prevent vitamin K deficiency (2).

Maternal supplementation with vitamin K may be an alternative for parents not wishing their newborns to receive intramuscular vitamin K prophylaxis. In exclusively breastfed infants not receiving intramuscular phylloquinone at birth, vitamin K status was improved by maternal oral supplements of 5 mg per day of phylloquinone through the first 12 weeks postpartum (79).

[‡] VKDB was previously termed "hemorrhagic disease of the newborn."

CALCIUM

Calcium is the most abundant mineral in the body, being the main structural component of the skeletal system. Whereas approximately 99% of the body's calcium is in bones and teeth, the other 1% is also critical for health, being found in plasma and soft tissues where it functions in vasoconstriction, vasodilation, muscle contraction, nerve impulse transmission, and hormone secretion. Recent evidence also suggests that calcium may play a role in regulating body composition, although not all studies are in agreement (80–82). Regulation of serum calcium concentration is orchestrated by the actions of several hormones, including PTH and calcitonin.

The most commonly used index of calcium homeostasis is serum total calcium concentration, but this does not reflect dietary intake because it is tightly regulated. In fact, low serum calcium concentrations usually imply abnormal parathyroid function or kidney failure—not primary calcium deficiency. Indirect indicators of calcium adequacy, such as measurement of bone mineral content and/or density, are often used clinically to assess calcium status.

DIETARY SOURCES OF CALCIUM AND FACTORS INFLUENCING ITS BIOAVAILABILITY

Dietary calcium is found mainly in dairy products, dark-green vegetables, legumes, and fortified foods. The concentration of calcium in human milk remains relatively constant at 200 to 250 mg per L through the first 6 months postpartum and is thought to be sufficient for exclusively breastfed infants (40). Indeed, human milk satisfies infant calcium requirements, as there are no reports of calcium deficiency in vitamin D–replete, full-term infants who are exclusively breastfed (38).

Many factors influence calcium bioavailability. For example, intestinal calcium absorption depends on the availability of 1,25-dihydroxyvitamin D_3 and its intestinal receptors. The bioavailability of dietary calcium also varies approximately inversely with intake, although the absolute quantity of calcium absorbed continues to increase with intake (83). Myriad dietary constituents—in addition to vitamin D availability—also affect calcium absorption and excretion. For instance, oxalates and phytates, found mainly in vegetables and grains, inhibit absorption. Intestinal transit time and mucosal mass also affect fractional calcium absorption (84), and decreased stomach acid can reduce the solubility of insoluble calcium salts, thus decreasing absorption unless they are given with a meal. Consequently, the absorption of calcium from supplements improves when they are taken with food. Life stage also influences calcium absorption, with the highest fractional absorption seen in infancy (60%) and in early puberty (34%). Racial differences in calcium metabolism have been noted both in children and in adults. For example, African–American girls have greater absorption efficiencies than do white girls after menarche (85). Metabolic differences may contribute to the widely observed higher bone mass in African–American children, but implications for "race"-specific requirements remain unclear (38).

DIETARY REFERENCE INTAKES FOR CALCIUM

Note that because sufficient data do not exist, only AIs (not RDAs) for calcium exist. The AI for calcium is 210 mg per day from 0 to 6 months; this increases to 270 mg per day from 7 to 12 months (Table 56.1). Intake of calcium from infant formulas may need to be greater than that from human milk in order to achieve the same retention, since absolute fractional absorption of calcium from bovine milk or other formula may be lower than from human milk (86). The AI for children aged 1 to 3 years increases to 500 mg per day; for children aged 4 to 8 years is 800 mg per day; and for children aged 9 to 18 years is 1,300 mg per day (Table 56.2). These values are based on intake levels which appear to support optimal bone health, recognizing that other factors such as genetics, hormones, and physical activity all interact to affect this important outcome variable.

There is little information concerning primary calcium toxicity, and the available data on the adverse effects of excess calcium intake primarily concern calcium intake from nutrient supplements. For infants 0 through 12 months of age, further studies are needed before a UL can be established. Although the Food and Nutrition Board (FNB) recognizes that the safety of excess calcium intake in children aged 1 through 18 years has yet to be studied adequately, a UL for this age group has been established as 2,500 mg per day. This amount reflects that obtained from both diet and supplements (Table 56.2).

CONSEQUENCES OF INADEQUATE CALCIUM INTAKE

Inadequate calcium intake during infancy and childhood can have many negative effects. In LBW infants, inadequate enteral intakes of calcium result in biochemical abnormalities (e.g., hypophosphatemia), low net mineral retention, low rates of bone mineralization, and reduced linear growth (87). Low calcium intake can also contribute to the development of rickets in infants and children, especially those consuming very restrictive diets. Data also support the possibility that low bone mass may be a contributing factor to some fractures in children (88,89).

Average dietary intakes for calcium by children in the United States decline dramatically after the second year of life and are well below recommended intakes (90). In fact, only about 10% of girls and 25% of boys aged 9 to 17 years consume the AI values (91). This is important, because chronic calcium deficiency resulting from inadequate intake or poor intestinal absorption is one cause of reduced bone mass and subsequent osteoporosis. Some evidence suggests that suboptimal intakes of calcium in children and adolescents may be related to the replacement of milk intake by soft drinks and fruit juices and/or fruit drinks (92). Lactose intolerance may also impact calcium intake in some ethnic groups (2). Although there are some data to suggest that calcium supplementation may increase bone mineral content in adolescents, other data suggest that these effects are short-lived (93,94).

CONSEQUENCES OF EXCESSIVE CALCIUM INTAKE

Data on adverse effects of excess calcium intake are lacking for infants and children. In adults, however, adverse effects of excess calcium are kidney stone formation, the syndrome of hypercalcemia and renal insufficiency with and without alkalosis, and the interaction of calcium with other minerals. Hypercalcemia results in poor muscle tone; constipation; excessive urine loss; nausea; and when most severe confusion, coma and death. Although calcium can interfere with iron and zinc absorption, human studies fail to show cases in which iron and zinc depletion occurs as a result of high calcium intake. Small children may be at risk of iron and zinc deficiency when calcium intake is excessive, but no dose-response data exist.

RECOMMENDATIONS FOR CALCIUM SUPPLEMENTATION

Although human milk or infant formula provides sufficient calcium to the healthy full-term infant, premature infants have higher calcium requirements than do full-term infants. The AAP recommends that these infants' calcium requirements be met by using either human milk fortified with additional minerals or specially designed formulas for premature infants (2). Similarly, LBW infants should receive human milk fortified with additional minerals or formulas specially designed for premature infants (2).

Most experts recommend that children and teens should get as much calcium as possible *from food* because calcium-rich foods also tend to furnish other nutrients involved in calcium utilization. However, the AAP recognizes that, for children and adolescents who cannot or will not consume adequate amounts of this mineral from preferred dietary sources, the use of calcium supplements should be considered (95).

It is especially noteworthy that the AAP strongly recommends that pediatricians actively support the goal of achieving calcium intakes in children and adolescents by asking questions about dietary calcium intake and providing information about specific sources of dietary calcium that are also low in fat, such as low-fat dairy products. Establishing these healthy eating practices in childhood (as opposed to simply providing a calcium supplement) is important so that they will be followed throughout the life span.

IRON

Iron, an essential mineral, is a constituent of several classes of proteins: heme proteins (e.g., hemoglobin), iron–sulfur or other nonheme enzymes (e.g., flavoproteins), and those involved in iron storage and transport (e.g., transferrin) (96). The iron–heme complex in hemoglobin is required for the transport of oxygen from lungs to tissues, and in myoglobin it is required for the storage of oxygen for use during muscle contraction. Iron is also a cofactor in a variety of heme-containing enzymes such as cytochrome oxidase, catalase, and peroxidase. Nonheme, iron-containing enzymes such as aconitase (an iron–sulfur protein) and metalloflavoproteins such as ferredoxins are involved in oxidative metabolism. Iron also plays a role in DNA synthesis as a component of the enzyme ribonucleotide reductase.

IRON HOMEOSTASIS

Iron homeostasis is primarily maintained through the coordinated regulation of absorption and transport, and recent studies have shed considerable light on its absorption and metabolism in infancy and childhood (97). Briefly, dietary iron is solubilized in the stomach and absorbed in the duodenum in the ferrous (Fe^{2+}) form. Absorption of iron is influenced by age, iron status, state of health, form of iron ingested, gastric and luminal acidity, and several dietary components (described below). Iron uptake into the luminal surface of the mucosal epithelium is believed to be facilitated by various cell membrane proteins; however, it is unclear how such interactions determine iron bioavailability (96,98).

Iron is taken up in the small intestine by divalent metal transporter-1 and is either stored by ferritin inside the mucosal cell or transported to the systemic circulation by ferroportin, while being oxidized by hephaestin to be incorporated into transferrin (96). Hepcidin, a small peptide synthesized by the liver, can sense iron stores and regulated iron transport by inhibition of ferroportin. Note that regulation of iron transporters is immature in infants, and this may possibly explain some of the adverse effects of iron supplementation described later in this section.

Excess iron is stored intracellularly as ferritin and also hemosiderin in the reticuloendothelial system of the liver, spleen, bone marrow, and other organs. The molecular regulation of intestinal iron absorption and transport, with transcriptional, posttranscriptional, and posttranslational control mechanisms, is an ongoing area of active research. Nonetheless, it is clear that iron-regulatory proteins modulate the use of mRNA-encoding proteins that are involved in the transport, storage, and use of iron (99).

DIETARY SOURCES AND BIOAVAILABILITY OF IRON

Most dietary iron is in the plant-based nonheme form found in grains, fruits, and vegetables. This type of iron is less bioavailable than heme iron found in foods of animal origin. Dietary components known to inhibit iron absorption are calcium, phytates (such as those in legumes, rice, and grains), and polyphenols found in tea and coffee. Promoters of iron absorption include ascorbic acid (vitamin C), organic acids, and certain animal proteins.

Noteworthy is the fact that human milk is a source of highly bioavailable iron, providing 0.3 to 0.9 mg per L (40). Iron contained in cow milk and bovine-based formula is less well absorbed, and for this and other reasons is not recommended until 1 year of age (2). In addition, full-term infants are born with considerable iron stores, and these stores are mobilized during infancy. However, even these infants must eventually rely on exogenous sources because stores endowed at birth are generally depleted by 6 months.

REFERENCE INTAKES FOR IRON

Like other AIs in infancy, that for iron reflects the observed mean iron intake of infants principally fed human milk (Table 56.1); for the first 6 months of life, the AI is 0.27 mg per day. However, for reasons outlined by the FNB, there should be no expectation that an average intake of 0.27 mg per day is adequate to meet the needs of almost all individual infants (such as those fed formula), and use of the AI as an intake goal should be applied with extreme care. From 7 to 12 months, the RDA for iron increases to 11 mg per day. Recommended intakes for children then decrease to 7 mg per day at 1 year, increasing to 11 and 15 mg per day during adolescence for boys and girls, respectively (Table 56.2).

There is considerable concern about iron overload, and the UL for infants and children is 40 mg per day and is based on gastrointestinal complications of iron supplementation (Table 56.2). This value increases to 45 mg per day for adolescents. The FNB recognizes that under some circumstances individuals receiving intermittent doses of iron supplements may exceed the UL. However, the effects of intermittent dosing on gastrointestinal side effects have not been studied adequately.

CONSEQUENCES OF INADEQUATE IRON INTAKE AND EFFECT OF SUPPLEMENTATION

Iron deficiency is the most common nutritional deficiency worldwide, with the best-known consequence being anemia. It is estimated that 50% of the world's anemia burden is attributable to iron deficiency and that iron deficiency accounts for 841,000 deaths and more than 35 million disability-adjusted life years lost (100). Even otherwise healthy, full-term infants are prone to iron deficiency in the first year of life; between 3% and 30% of full-term infants develop iron deficiency during infancy, usually from 6 to 12 months of age (101). The incidence (26% and 86%) is even higher in preterm infants (102). This is partly because iron stores are especially low in preterm infants, and total body iron content has to increase at an accelerated rate postnatally. Thus, compared with term infants, preterm infants require more iron both in absolute amount and on a body weight basis.

There are many biochemical markers of mild, moderate, and severe iron deficiency. For example, chronic iron deficiency is often identified by depleted iron stores (low serum ferritin and transferrin receptor). Early functional iron deficiency can be evaluated by measuring elevated free erythrocyte protoporphyrin, decreased transferrin saturation, and/or decreased mean corpuscular volume. Iron deficiency anemia is often assessed via decreased hemoglobin and hematocrit values. Ideally, these laboratory tests should be used in combination to identify the evolution of iron deficiency through these three stages.

Diagnosis of iron deficiency during infancy is complex and lacks uniform diagnostic criteria. As in other age groups, anemia occurs after the storage and nonstorage tissue iron pools are depleted. Indicators of iron status currently most frequently used in this population are serum ferritin, transferrin receptor, percent transferrin saturation, erythrocyte protoporphyrin, mean corpuscular volume, hemoglobin concentration, and hematocrit (103). Regardless, iron supplementation during early life in otherwise healthy, breastfed infants can positively influence many of these indicators of iron status (104).

Aside from the effects of frank iron deficiency on anemia, there are also important effects of more moderate deficiency levels. For example, moderate anemia is associated with mental and motor developmental delays in children, and longitudinal studies indicate that children who were anemic in early childhood continue to have poor cognitive and motor development and depressed school achievement into middle childhood (105,106). There is also compelling evidence that iron supplementation in early life—especially in iron-deficient areas—provides benefits in terms of motor development and social–emotional behavior (107). For children older than 2 years, iron supplementation has also been associated with improvements in cognition (108). There is also some evidence that early iron supplementation may enhance physical performance in childhood and adolescence (109). However, some (but not all) studies suggest that early iron supplementation may increase the risk for infectious disease in some populations—including those at greatest risk for malaria (110,111). Furthermore, iron supplementation may have small but significant negative effects on growth in some iron-replete infants and children (112,113). Thus, there is general consensus that a single strategy for ensuring adequate iron nutrition in young children in different parts of the world is not likely satisfactory.

Another consequence of iron deficiency is enhanced heavy metal absorption and inadequate oxygen delivery. For example, clinical and epidemiologic studies have shown that absorption of lead increases with the severity of iron deficiency. Inadequate oxygen delivery during exercise and abnormal enzyme function in tissues also result from anemia. An association between iron deficiency and immune function has also been proposed (114).

CONSEQUENCES OF EXCESSIVE IRON INTAKE

Possible adverse effects of excessive dietary iron intake include promotion of cellular oxidation, impaired resistance to infection, interference with absorption or metabolism of other nutrients, and adverse reactions manifested by gastrointestinal abnormalities or behavioral disturbances. Reports of acute toxicity resulting from clinical overdoses of medicinal iron have been reported for young children (115–117), and accidental iron overdose is the most common cause of poisoning deaths in children younger than 6 years in the United States (118). And, as previously mentioned, some (but not all) studies suggest that iron supplementation may increase the disease risk in some endemic populations.

RECOMMENDATIONS FOR IRON SUPPLEMENTATION

The AAP recommends that healthy, full-term, breastfed infants receive a supplemental source of iron (approximately 1 mg per kg per day) starting at 4 to 6 months of age preferably from complementary foods (2). Iron-fortified infant cereal and/or meats are a good source of iron for initial introduction of an iron-containing food. For breastfed preterm or LBW infants, an oral iron supplement in the form of drops once a day at 2 mg per kg per day starting at 1 month should be given until 12 months of age. Note that the dose of iron (1 mg per kg) in a vitamin preparation with iron is not likely to provide sufficient iron for the preterm breastfed infant. For all infants younger than 12 months, only iron-fortified formula should be used for weaning or supplementing breast milk. Because current preterm infant and preterm discharge formulas supply only 1.8 mg per kg per day iron to the average preterm infant, formula-fed preterm infants may benefit from an additional 1 mg per kg per day iron administered as drops or in a vitamin preparation with iron. The AAP also suggests supplementation of some young children with iron during the second year, especially if the child does not have a source of meat-based iron in the diet. Common over-the-counter preparations used for iron supplementation are described in Table 56.3.

It is important to note that these recommendations may not apply to infants living in areas of endemic malaria, and the reader is urged to follow the development of recommendations for these populations as they are put forth (119). Currently, the WHO recommends that caution should be exercised in settings where the prevalence of malaria and other infectious diseases is high and that iron

TABLE 56.3 Selected Over-the-Counter Products Used for Iron Supplementation in Infants and Children

Product	*Iron Concentration (mg/mL)*	*Usual Daily Dose*
Baby vitamin drops with iron (Goldline Laboratories, Miami, FL)	10	1 mL
Ferrous sulfate drops (Fer-In-Sol, Mead Johnson, Evansville, IN, and various generic brands)	25 (125 mg/mL ferrous sulfate)	2–6 mg/kg/d
Poly-Vi-Sol with iron drops (Mead Johnson, Evansville, IN)	10	1 mL
Polyvitamin drops with iron (various brands)	10	1 mL
Tri-Vi-Sol with iron drops (Mead Johnson, Evansville, IN)	10	1 mL
Vi-Daylin ADC vitamins + iron drops (Ross Laboratories, Columbus, OH)	10	1 mL

Modified from Kleinman RE, ed. *American Academy of Pediatrics' Pediatric nutrition handbook,* 6th ed. Elk Grove Village, IL: American Academy of Pediatrics, 2008.

supplementation be targeted to those who are anemic and at risk of iron deficiency (120).

ZINC

Zinc is an essential trace mineral that has a multitude of physiologic and biochemical functions, notably in embryogenesis and growth. Zinc functions as a catalytic, structural, and/or regulatory component of nearly 300 enzymes in which it maintains structural integrity and plays a role in regulation of gene expression (121). Although the biochemical and molecular genetics of zinc function is relatively well developed, the relationships of these genetic events to zinc deficiency or toxicity and the specific functions for which zinc is particularly critical remain to be established (122). As such, explanations for depressed growth, immune dysfunction, increased diarrhea, altered cognition, host defense properties, defects in carbohydrate utilization, teratogenesis, and numerous other clinical outcomes of mild and severe zinc deficiency are not well established. This is in part due to lack of a sensitive and functional indicator of zinc nutritional status, although investigations into this are ongoing (123).

Zinc is primarily (95%) an intracellular ion, being found in all organs, tissues, fluids, and secretions of the body. Zinc concentrations are particularly high in bone, skeletal muscle, skin, liver, brain, kidney, heart, hair, and plasma. However, plasma zinc is tightly regulated and does not reflect changes in dietary intake until severe and prolonged deficiency prevails.

Homeostatic regulation of zinc metabolism is achieved principally through coordination of absorption and secretion of endogenous reserves (122). This involves adaptive mechanisms influenced by dietary zinc intake. Zinc absorption is mainly in the small intestine and is influenced by the solubility of the zinc compounds and zinc status. Zinc secretion into and excretion out of the intestine provide the major route of zinc excretion. Zinc depletion in humans is accompanied by reduced endogenous zinc losses from both pancreatic and intestinal cell secretions. Regulation of zinc absorption may provide a gross control of body zinc content, whereas endogenous zinc release provides fine control to maintain homeostasis.

DIETARY SOURCES AND BIOAVAILABILITY OF ZINC

Zinc is found primarily in foods of animal sources (e.g., oysters, red meats, poultry, and liver) but is also found in plant foods (e.g., beans, nuts, whole grains, fortified cereals, legumes) and supplements. Like iron, zinc absorption from a diet containing animal-based foods is greater than that from a purely vegetarian diet, and many dietary factors can enhance or inhibit its bioavailability. For example, large–molecular-weight compounds (e.g., phytates) and competing divalent cations (e.g., iron) inhibit zinc absorption. Conversely, low–molecular-weight ligands (e.g., cysteine) and other organic acids promote zinc absorption. Zinc depletion also increases the efficiency of intestinal absorption.

The mechanism by which zinc enters the mucosal cell is unknown. However, once inside, zinc is bound to metallothionein and is held within the cell or passes through the cell for use in zinc-dependent processes. In plasma, newly absorbed zinc circulates bound to albumin. Zinc in human milk is highly bioavailable and its concentration declines as lactation progresses (18). Like iron, the bioavailability of zinc in human milk is higher than that in bovine milk. Consequently, most formulas are supplemented with zinc to contain 5 to 7 mg per L; preterm formulas generally contain 5 to 10 mg per L.

DIETARY REFERENCE INTAKES FOR ZINC

An AI for zinc is 2.0 mg per day for infants from 0 to 6 months (Table 56.1). However, the FNB notes that the zinc bioavailability from soy formulas is significantly lower than that from milk-based formulas, and that the absorption from human milk is greater than all types of proprietary formula products. The RDA for zinc is 3 mg per day for infants and children 7 months to 3 years; 5 mg per day from 4 to 8 years; 8 mg per day from 9 to 13 years; and 9 to 11 mg per day, depending on sex, from 14 to 18 years (Table 56.2). Based on a single study by Walravens and Hambidge who fed 68 healthy, full-term infants a formula containing 5.8 mg per L zinc with no documented adverse effects, the UL for infants has been set at 4 mg per day from 0 to 6 months and 5 mg per day from 7 to 12 months (124). This value increases to 7, 12, 23, and 34 mg per day zinc at 1, 4, 9, and 14 years of age, respectively.

CONSEQUENCES OF INADEQUATE ZINC INTAKE AND EFFECT OF SUPPLEMENTATION

Zinc deficiency is difficult to detect because clinical features and laboratory indicators are not always consistent, and a reliable sensitive functional indicator of zinc is lacking. Nonetheless, in the 1970s, mild zinc deficiency was described in formula-fed infants consuming a zinc-poor formula (124). Fortification of the formula led to normal growth. Severe zinc deficiency is seen in patients with acrodermatitis enteropathica and those provided total parenteral nutrition lacking sufficient amounts of this mineral. Characteristics of severe zinc deficiency are growth retardation, alopecia, diarrhea, delayed sexual maturation and impotence, eye and skin lesions, and loss of appetite.

More recently, there has been considerable scientific attention given to the potential impact of zinc supplementation on behavior (including attention-deficit/hyperactivity disorder or ADHD) and a variety of childhood illnesses such as diarrhea and respiratory illness. However, the experimental data are conflicting and suggest a complex set of interactions that likely impact the effect of zinc nutrition on these outcomes. For instance, two separate meta-analyses have found that zinc supplementation reduced frequency and severity of diarrhea and respiratory illnesses as well as the duration of diarrheal morbidity (125,126). Another study found that zinc supplementation (70 mg per week) resulted in fewer incidents of pneumonia and decreased incidence of diarrhea; importantly, there were fewer pneumonia-related deaths in the group given zinc supplements than in the placebo group (127). However, results are not consistent across studies (128–130). This is highlighted in a study conducted in Peru in which morbidity was greater after supplementation with zinc plus multivitamins and minerals than it was after supplementation with zinc alone (131). Results of studies designed to test the effect of zinc supplementation on behavioral outcomes in children are also mixed (132,133). It is likely that other factors, such as psychosocial stimulation, interact with zinc nutrition to influence psychological outcomes (134).

CONSEQUENCES OF EXCESSIVE ZINC INTAKE

Adverse effects associated with chronic intake of excessive supplemental zinc include suppression of immune response, decreased high-density lipoprotein cholesterol, and reduced copper status. Typical signs of acute zinc toxicity include epigastric pain, diarrhea, nausea, and vomiting. In adults, acute toxicity has been associated with a dose of 225 to 450 mg of zinc as zinc sulfate (142). Chronic ingestion of zinc supplements (100 to 300 mg per day for several months) induces secondary copper deficiency caused by the competitive interaction between these elements during intestinal absorption. Zinc supplements as low as 25 mg per day have also been shown to induce copper deficiency in adults (135).

RECOMMENDATIONS FOR ZINC SUPPLEMENTATION

Because human milk may not always meet the infant's need for zinc, those fed human milk may benefit from zinc supplementation after 6 months of age, when complementary foods are introduced, particularly if such foods are low in zinc and the diet includes inhibitors of zinc absorption (136). Many premature infants fed human milk may become zinc depleted, although frank zinc deficiency may not be apparent (137).

Consequently, zinc supplements may help meet growth needs during infancy and childhood (136), particularly for infants and children at high risk of zinc deficiency (137). Addressing the apparent relationship between zinc nutrition and diarrhea, the WHO recommends zinc supplementation (10 mg per day) once a day for 10 to 14 days when an infant (<6 months old) has diarrhea; the recommended dosage increases to 20 mg per day for older infants (138). For preterm infants the AAP recommends a zinc intake of 1 to 3 mg per kg per day (2). This level of intake can be achieved through use of term or preterm formulas and human milk fortifiers. Additional supplementation is not recommended.

During the second half year of life, zinc requirements are high. Thus, zinc requirements of early childhood during the transition from milk to solid foods are also difficult to meet. Complementary foods (e.g., 50 to 70 g of lean beef per day or 40 g of dry fish per day) must provide 84% to 89% of zinc required by infants between the ages of 6 and 24 months (136). Zinc intakes by infants (137) and children in the United States and less-developed countries (139) suggest that zinc supplementation may be useful for infants and children with diets low in animal products and phytate-rich cereals and legumes. Some experts recommend that, instead of turning to supplemental forms of the mineral, parents should consider meat and/or liver instead of cereal as a "first food" for infants (140). Older infants and children who are fed a strict vegan diet may need zinc supplements because bioavailability from plants foods is low (141,142).

IODINE

Iodine is a nonmetallic trace mineral essential to humans for synthesis of the thyroid hormones thyroxine (T_4) and triiodothyronine (T_3). Thyroid hormones are necessary for regulation of human growth, development, metabolism, and reproductive function. Most iodine is concentrated in the thyroid gland; other target organs are the developing brain, muscle, heart, pituitary, and kidney. In target tissues, the physiologically active form (T_3) binds to nuclear receptors where it regulates gene expression.

Iodine is rapidly absorbed and removed from the circulation by the thyroid gland and kidneys. Iodine can also be absorbed through the skin from topical iodine applications or from iodine vapors from cleaning agents and fossil fuel combustion. The hypothalamus and pituitary are involved in the regulation of iodine metabolism. Thyrotropin-releasing hormone, a hypothalamic hormone, stimulates the release of thyroid-stimulating hormone (TSH), which in turn stimulates uptake of iodine by the thyroid gland, synthesis of thyroxine hormones, and secretion of T_3 and T_4 into the circulation. Persistently elevated levels of TSH in response to low circulating levels of T_3 and T_4 can lead to hypertrophy of the thyroid gland, and ultimately goiter formation. Excess iodine is excreted in urine, and urinary iodine is often used as an indicator of iodine status.

DIETARY SOURCES OF IODINE

The iodine content of foods depends on the iodine content of the soil and water used to grow them. Ocean fish and mollusks tend to contain high amounts of iodine because they concentrate iodine found in seawater into their tissues. However, most of the iodine in our diet comes from iodized salt, which contains about 77 μg per g of this mineral in the form of potassium iodide. Iodine concentration of human milk depends on maternal intake; typical values range from 113 to 150 μg per L (40). Nonetheless, infants fed human milk generally consume adequate quantities of this mineral. Because bovine milk is a rich source of iodine, milk-based infant formulas are also good sources.

DIETARY REFERENCE INTAKES FOR IODINE

Based on intake of iodine by exclusively breastfed infants, the AI for this mineral during the first half year of life is 110 μg per day, increasing to 130 μg per day from 7 to 12 months. The DRI committee noted, however, that there have been no studies in which the bioavailability of iodine in infant formulas and human milk has been compared. Thus, it is unknown whether this amount is actually sufficient for formula-fed infants. The RDAs for iodine are of 90 μg per day for children aged 1 to 8 years, 120 μg per day for children aged 9 to 13 years, and 120 μg per day for older children and adolescents (Table 56.2). The committee was not able to establish a UL for iodine during the first year of life, but the ULs were set at 200 μg per day for children aged 1 to 3 years; 300 μg per day from 4 to 8 years; 600 μg per day from 9 to 13 years; and 900 μg per day from 14 to 18 years.

CONSEQUENCES OF INADEQUATE IODINE INTAKE AND IODINE SUPPLEMENTATION

Although iodine intake remains a public health concern worldwide, endemic iodine deficiency was a significant problem in the United States at the beginning of the 20th century, being eliminated largely by aggressive programs encouraging the consumption of iodine-fortified salt (143). Currently, there is some controversy as to whether iodine intake is now adequate in the United States, but most data indicate that it is (144,145). Nonetheless, continued nutritional monitoring of iodine intake in the United States is warranted (146).

There is no controversy, however, that iodine deficiency remains one of the most common nutrient deficiencies worldwide (147). Manifestations of iodine deficiency take on many forms, which are collectively called *iodine deficiency disorders.* Iodine deficiency disorders include mental retardation, hypothyroidism, goiter, cretinism, and growth and developmental abnormalities. The most severe form, called cretinism, occurs when a baby is born to an iodine-deficient mother. Cretinism causes severe mental retardation, poor growth, infertility, and increased risk for mortality. When iodine deficiency occurs in childhood or later, TSH secretion greatly increases, causing the thyroid gland to grow and develop into a goiter.

Although it has long been established that iodine supplementation during pregnancy and the postnatal period could prevent cretinism and childhood goiter, more recent research suggests that it may have more far-reaching effects. Unfortunately, there are no long-term data on the effect of iodine supplementation on infant development. However, a meta-analysis of studies (n = 37; 12,291 children) conducted in China suggested that iodine supplementation (via food fortification) resulted in greater intellectual development of children who were mildly iodine deficient (148). Furthermore, data from well-controlled studies indicate that iodine repletion in moderately iodine-deficient school-aged children can improve cognitive and motor function, increase concentrations of insulin-like growth factor 1 (IGF-1) and insulin-like growth factor–binding protein 3, and improve growth (149,150).

CONSEQUENCES OF EXCESSIVE IODINE INTAKE

As mentioned, consequences of excess iodine intake for infants for the first year have not been studied sufficiently. However, to prevent high intakes of iodine, it is recommended that the only source of intake for infants in their first year of life should be food and formula (40). For older individuals, chronic excessive intakes of iodine may compromise thyroid function and also contribute to development of goiter, hypothyroidism (due to feedback inhibition of thyroid hormone synthesis), and hyperthyroidism (also called iodine-induced hyperthyroidism) (2).

RECOMMENDATIONS FOR IODINE SUPPLEMENTATION

Because human milk contains sufficient iodine as do proprietary infant formulas, the AAP does not recommend iodine supplementation during infancy (2). Furthermore, because children in the United States get an ample supply of iodine supplementation is not recommended during childhood and adolescence. However, in areas of the world where iodine is less available either naturally or because iodized salt is not routinely used, iodine supplementation may be important.

FLUORIDE

Fluoride, although not technically an essential nutrient, is a dietary mineral associated with the prevention of dental caries and more recently stimulation of new bone formation (38). Fluoride exists as the fluoride ion or as hydrofluoric acid in body fluids. Fluoride is incorporated into tooth enamel as fluorapatite during the pre-eruptive stage of enamel formation, and approximately 99% of total body fluoride is found as fluorohydroxyapatite in mineralized tissues. Present in saliva and dental plaque, fluoride helps prevent dental caries by three mechanisms: it inhibits plaque formation and decreases bacterial acid production, prevents demineralization by incorporation into tooth surface crystals, and enhances remineralization of enamel (151). At one time fluoride was thought to provide protection of pre-eruptive teeth via systemic mechanisms, but it is now generally accepted that its main effect is instead via topical use.

Fluoride is absorbed in the stomach and small intestine and excreted mainly via the kidney. For young children as much as 80% of fluoride intake can be retained by the developing skeleton and teeth (152). Body fluid and tissue concentrations of fluoride are proportional to the level of chronic intake; in other words, they are not homeostatically regulated (38).

SOURCES AND BIOAVAILABILITY OF FLUORIDE

Few foods contain fluoride naturally, with some teas and marine fish being the main exceptions. Instead, fluoride is available mainly from artificially fluoridated water supplies. Highlighting the importance of municipal water fluoridation is the fact that the Centers for Disease Control and Prevention (CDC) has named this practice one of the top 10 public health achievements in the 20th century. In the United States, communities with fluoridated water have fluoride concentrations of 0.7 to 1.11 mg per L; nonfluoridated water typically contains less than 0.4 mg per L (38). Sources of fluoride in the diet include beverages, formulas, and foods made with fluoridated water; casual ingestion of fluoride toothpaste and mouth rinses; and fluoride supplements. Fluoride has high bioavailability when sodium fluoride is ingested with water. If ingested with milk, formula, or foods that contain high concentrations of calcium or other divalent ions that form insoluble compounds, absorption may be reduced by 10% to 25%.

Fluoride intake by infants can vary widely depending on whether the infant is fed human milk or formula and whether the formula is ready-to-feed or requires reconstitution with water. Fluoride concentration of human milk typically is 4 to 15 μg per L, which results in intakes of 3 to 12 μg per day. Note that, depending on what type of water is used to reconstitute infant formula, fluoride intake by formula-fed infants can be as high as 1.0 mg per day. This is, however, highly variable. The CDC recommends that parents concerned about the effect that mixing their infant's formula with fluoridated water may have in developing enamel fluorosis can lessen this exposure by mixing formula with low-fluoride water most or all of the time (153). Bottled water known to be low in fluoride is labeled as being purified, deionized, demineralized, distilled, or prepared by reverse osmosis.

TABLE 56.4 Fluoride Supplementation Schedule[a]

	Fluoride Concentration in Local Water Supply (ppm)		
Age	*<0.3*	*0.3–0.6*	*>0.6*
Birth to 6 mo	0.00	0.00	0.00
6 mo–3 yr	0.25	0.00	0.00
3–6 yr	0.50	0.25	0.00
6 to at least 16 yr	1.00	0.50	0.00

[a]Must know the fluoride concentration in the patient's drinking water before prescribing fluoride supplements; all values are mg/d of fluoride supplement.

Modified from Kleinman RE, ed. *American Academy of Pediatrics' Pediatric nutrition handbook,* 6th ed. Elk Grove Village, IL: American Academy of Pediatrics, 2008.

DIETARY REFERENCE INTAKES FOR FLUORIDE

The AI for fluoride is 10 μg per day for infants from 0 to 6 months and 0.5 mg per day from 7 to 12 months (Table 56.1). This value increases to 0.7 mg per day from 1 to 3 years and 1 mg per day from 4 to 8 years. The UL for infants from 0 to 6 months is 0.7 mg per day and from 7 to 12 months is 0.9 mg per day. For children 1 to 3 years of age, the UL is 1.3 mg per day, and from 4 to 8 years it is 2.2 mg per day (Table 56.2).

CONSEQUENCES OF INADEQUATE FLUORIDE INTAKE AND EFFECTS OF SUPPLEMENTATION

Inadequate intake of fluoride at any age places the individual at risk for dental caries (154). As such, fluoride supplements are typically beneficial to children living in fluoride deficient areas where water fluoridation is not practiced. Furthermore, the earlier children are exposed to fluoridated water or dietary fluoride supplements, the greater the reduction in dental caries in both the primary and permanent teeth. As part of the Iowa Fluoride Study, Hamasha and colleagues documented patterns of dietary fluoride supplement use and found that 11.2% of 12-month-old infants were taking them (155). This percentage decreased to 6.3% and further to 4.7% at 12 and 96 months, respectively, and mean dosage gradually increased from 0.25 to 0.75 mg per day during this period.

CONSEQUENCES OF EXCESSIVE FLUORIDE INTAKE

Administration of supplemental fluoride must be done judiciously, because ingestion of excess fluoride can result in various degrees of fluorosis (156). Enamel fluorosis is caused by excessive fluoride intake during the pre-eruptive development of teeth. After the enamel has completed maturation, it is no longer susceptible to fluorosis. Thus, it is recommended by some that tooth brushing with fluoride-containing toothpastes should not begin until the age of 2 years and that no more than a pea-sized portion be used (157). Consequences of moderate to severe forms of fluorosis are cosmetic, being characterized by an increasing porosity, which causes the enamel to appear opaque and mottled. Mild fluorosis has no effect on tooth function and may render the enamel more resistant to caries. Clinical features include changes ranging from barely discernible to fine white lines running across the teeth and finally to entirely chalky white teeth.

RECOMMENDATIONS FOR FLUORIDE SUPPLEMENTATION

Dietary fluoride supplements in the form of tablets, lozenges, or liquids (including fluoride-vitamin preparations) have been used throughout the world since the 1940s. Most supplements contain sodium fluoride as the active ingredient. The CDC, American Dental Association, AAP, and Canadian Pediatric Society all recommend dietary fluoride supplementation aimed primarily at populations drinking suboptimally fluoridated water (2,151,158). The AAP's fluoride schedule is provided in Table 56.4. To maximize the topical effect of fluoride, tablets and lozenges are intended to be chewed or sucked for 1 to 2 minutes before being swallowed. For infants, supplements are available as a liquid and used with a dropper. Note that, to use this schedule effectively, one must know the fluoride level of the municipal water supply. This can be easily determined by contacting the local water department or visiting the CDC's Web site at http://apps.nccd.cdc.gov/MWF/Index.asp.

Because dietary fluoride supplements are intended to compensate for fluoride-deficient drinking water, the dosage schedule requires knowledge of the fluoride content of the child's primary drinking water. Consideration should also be given to other sources of water (e.g., home, child care settings, school, or bottled water) and to other sources of fluoride (e.g., toothpaste or mouth rinse), which can complicate the prescribing decision.

OMEGA-3 FATTY ACIDS

Perhaps the most recently considered dietary components in terms of supplementation during infancy and childhood are the omega-3 (ω-3 or *n*-3) fatty acids, which include the dietary essential alpha-linolenic acid (ALA; 18:3ω-3) as well as its longer-chain polyunsaturated fatty acid (LCPUFA) metabolites eicosapentaenoic acid (EPA; 20:5ω-3) and docosahexaenoic acid (DHA; 22:6ω-3). It has long been known that the omega-3 fatty acids are important in terms of visual and neurological development. More recent work, however, now suggests a host of additional physiologic roles for these compounds including being critical for optimal immune function, protecting from inflammation, and decreasing the risk for a variety of chronic degenerative diseases such as cardiovascular events. Of particular importance to pediatric nutrition is the fact that plasma and erythrocyte DHA concentrations are higher in breastfed than in formula-fed infants (159). Although this finding was initially interpreted as suggesting that infants cannot synthesize enough DHA to meet their needs, it is now clear that both term and preterm infants have this capability (160). Nonetheless, because of the importance of LCPUFA to neural development, there has been considerable interest in determining the potential importance of supplementing the infant's diet with these compounds, especially if formula feeding is practiced.

DIETARY SOURCES OF THE OMEGA-3 FATTY ACIDS

Alpha-linolenic acid is found naturally in some vegetable oils such as canola and flax seed, whereas the LCPUFAs synthesized from this essential fatty acid are found primarily in oily fish. Smaller amounts are also present in meats and eggs. Human milk contains a variety of omega-3 fatty acids, and their concentration depends greatly on the maternal diet. Because infant formulas are generally made with corn, coconut, safflower, and soy oils, unless they are fortified with LCPUFAs they contain very low levels of them. Relatively recent suggestions by some that formula-fed infants consume LCPUFA-fortified formulas, however, have resulted in these types of formulas being widely available in the United States.

DIETARY REFERENCE INTAKES FOR THE OMEGA-3 FATTY ACIDS

The AI for the omega-3 LCPUFAs during the first year of life is 0.5 g per day. After this time, the AIs refer instead to recommended intakes for ALA. Recommended intakes are 0.7 and 0.9 g per day ALA from 1 to 3 and 4 to 8 years, respectively. During the preteen years, reference intakes are slightly higher for boys than for girls (1.2 and 1.0 g per day, respectively), increasing even more during adolescence (1.6 and 1.1 g per day, respectively). There are no ULs established for this class of fatty acids.

CONSEQUENCES OF INADEQUATE OMEGA-3 FATTY ACID INTAKE AND EFFECT OF SUPPLEMENTATION

Documentation of omega-3 fatty acid deficiency in infants and children is scant. However, there is a report of a 6-year-old child who had been maintained for several weeks on a parenteral nutrition product lacking ALA (161). This resulted in numbness, weakness, blurred vision, and inability to walk, which were reversed when ALA was added to the diet. Nonetheless, because of the intense recent interest in the possibility that the omega-3 fatty acids might be conditionally essential during infancy, many studies have been conducted to investigate the effect of supplementation during early life. Specifically, most of these investigations have focused mostly on cognitive/behavioral development and visual acuity, and their results have been mixed. A meta-analysis published in 2000 that included randomized studies of term infants fed DHA-supplemented versus unsupplemented formula found an advantage of DHA consumption on behaviorally based tests of visual acuity at 2 months of age but not any other age (162). This same meta-analysis found no effect when electrophysiological methods of assessment were considered. Recent Cochrane reviews have concluded that there is likely no consistent effect of consumption of DHA-supplemented formula on visual acuity of term or preterm infants (163,164). However, other recent analyses suggest that there is "reasonably compelling" evidence of a beneficial effect in preterm, but not term infants (165). Similarly, studies designed to test the effect of long-chain omega-3 fatty acid intake during infancy on cognitive/behavioral development also provide some evidence of a potential benefit, but again the results are mixed (166,167). This area of research represents one of active scrutiny and investigation.

CONSEQUENCES OF EXCESSIVE OMEGA-3 FATTY ACID INTAKE

Although there was some concern that excessive omega-3 fatty acid intake during infancy may have detrimental effects on growth, a recent meta-analysis of 21 studies found no evidence of such an effect on term infants (168). Thus, the AAP has concluded that there is no need for concern that supplementation of the infant diet with these compounds will stunt growth (2). There is also concern that overconsumption of long-chain omega-3 fatty acids might increase the risk of conditions related to oxidative damage such as necrotizing enterocolitis and bronchopulmonary dysplasia. Presently, there are not sufficient data to support or refute these possibilities.

RECOMMENDATIONS FOR OMEGA-3 FATTY ACID SUPPLEMENTATION

The AAP has no official position on supplementation of term or preterm infant formulas with LCPUFAs in general or omega-3 LCPUFAs in particular (2). Similarly, the Life Science Research Organization Expert Panel on Nutrient Composition of Term Infant Formulas recommends neither a minimum nor maximum amount of these lipids for term infant formulas (169). The Life Science Research Organization has, however, specified a maximum (but not minimum) amount of DHA for preterm formulas (170).

SUMMARY

In summary, it is clear that supplementation of the diet with selected micronutrients and fatty acids may improve health in some infants and children. This is particularly true in the most at-risk children such as those born prematurely or of low birth weight, or those living in areas of endemic nutrient deficiencies. However, evolving data suggest complex webs of interactions more multifarious than previously recognized, and health professionals must often consider confounding factors when determining whether dietary supplementation is warranted. One of the best examples of this that has recently surfaced is that of iron supplementation which may increase morbidity and mortality in areas with endemic malaria. Thus, caution should always be used when determining whether dietary supplementation should be recommended, and altering nutrient adequacy of the diet should generally be considered carefully first. As research in this area is ongoing, remaining attentive of new recommendations from expert groups such as the AAP and WHO is critical.

REFERENCES

1. Institute of Medicine, Food and Nutrition Board. *Dietary reference intakes for energy, carbohydrate, fiber, fat, fatty acids, cholesterol, protein, and amino acids.* Washington, DC: National Academy Press, 2005.
2. Kleinman RE, ed. *American Academy of Pediatrics pediatric nutrition handbook,* 6th ed. Elk Grove Village, IL: American Academy of Pediatrics, 2008.
3. U.S. Congress. Pub L No. 103-417. Dietary Supplement Health and Education Act (DSHEA). Washington, DC: U.S. Government Printing Office, 1994.
4. Nutrition Business Journal. *NBJ's supplement business report 2006.* San Diego, CA: New Hope Natural Media, 2006.
5. Ervin RB, Wright JD, Kennedy-Stephenson J. Use of dietary supplements in the United States, 1988–94. *J Vital Health Stat* 1999; 244:1–14.
6. Picciano MF, Dwyer JT, Radimer KL, et al. Dietary supplement use among infants, children, and adolescents in the United States, 1999–2002. *Arch Pediatr Adolesc Med* 2007;161:978–985.
7. Institute of Medicine, Food and Nutrition Board. *Dietary reference intakes for vitamin C, vitamin E, selenium, and carotenoids.* Washington, DC: National Academy Press, 2000.
8. Ross AC. Vitamin A and carotenoids. In: Shils ME, Shike M, Ross AC, et al., eds. *Modern nutrition in health and disease,* 10th ed. Baltimore: Williams & Wilkins, 2005.
9. Zhao Z, Ross AC. Retinoic acid repletion restores the number of leukocytes and their subsets and stimulates natural cytotoxicity in vitamin A-deficient rats. *J Nutr* 1995;125:2064–2073.
10. Greer FR. Fat-soluble vitamin supplements for enterally fed preterm infants. *Neonatal Netw* 2001;20(5):7–11.
11. West KP Jr. Vitamin A deficiency disorders in children and women. *Food Nutr Bull* 2003;24:S78–S90.
12. World Health Organization. *Global prevalence of vitamin A deficiency,* (Micronutrient Deficiency Information System Working Paper). Geneva: 1995.
13. Katz J, West KP Jr, Khatry SK, et al. Impact of vitamin A supplementation on prevalence and incidence of xerophthalmia in Nepal. *Invest Ophthalmol Vis Sci* 1995;36:2577–2583.
14. World Health Organization. *Vitamin A supplements: a guide to their use in the treatment of vitamin A deficiency and xerophthalmia.* Geneva: 1997.
15. Fawzi WW, Chalmers TC, Herrera MG, et al. Vitamin A supplementation and child mortality. A meta-analysis. *J Am Med Assoc* 1993;269:898–903.
16. Klemm RD, Labriqu AB, Christian P, et al. Newborn vitamin A supplementation reduced infant mortality in rural Bangladesh. *Pediatrics* 2008;122:242–250.
17. Darlow BA, Graham PJ. Vitamin A supplementation to prevent mortality and short and long-term morbidity in very low birthweight infants. *Cochrane Database Syst Rev* 2007;4:CD000501.
18. Jensen RG, ed. *Handbook of milk composition.* San Diego, CA: Academic Press, 1995.
19. Ambalavanan N, Tyson JE, Kennedy KA, et al. Vitamin A supplementation for extremely low birth weight infants: outcome at 18 and 22 months. *Pediatrics* 2005;114:e249–e254.
20. Brown N, Roberts C. Vitamin A for acute respiratory infection in developing countries: a meta-analysis. *Acta Paediatr* 2004;93: 1437–1442.
21. Chen H, Zhuo Q, Yuan W, et al. Vitamin A for preventing acute lower respiratory tract infections in children up to seven years of age. *Cochrane Database Syst Rev* 2008;5:CD006090.
22. Grotto I, Mimouni M, Gdalevich M, et al. Vitamin A supplementation and childhood morbidity from diarrhea and respiratory infections: a meta-analysis. *J Pediatr* 2003;142:297–304.
23. Cusick SE, Tielsch JM, Ramsan M, et al. Short-term effects of vitamin A and antimalarial treatment on erythropoiesis in severely anemic Zanzibari preschool children. *Am J Clin Nutr* 2005;82: 406–412.
24. Diness BR, Fisker AB, Roth A, et al. Effect of high-dose vitamin A supplementation on the immune response to Bacille Calmette-Guyerin vaccine. *Am J Clin Nutr* 2007;86:1152–1159.
25. Benn CS, Martins C, Rodrigues A, et al. Randomized study of effect of different doses of vitamin A on childhood morbidity and mortality. *BMJ* 2005;331:1428–1432.
26. Wisonge CS, Shey MS, Sterne JA, et al. Vitamin A supplementation for reducing the risk of mother-to-child transmission of HIV infection. *Cochrane Database Sys Rev* 2005;4:CD003648.
27. Humphrey JH, Iliff PF, Marinda ET, et al. Effects of a single large dose of vitamin A, given during the postpartum period to HIV-positive women and their infants, on child HIV infection, HIV-free survival, and mortality. *J Infect Dis* 2006;193:860–871.
28. Kuhn L, Coutsoudis A, Trabattoni D, et al. Synergy between mannose-binding lectin gene polymorphisms and supplementation with vitamin A influences susceptibility to HIV infection in infants born to HIV-positive mothers. *Am J Clin Nutr* 2006;84:610–615.
29. American Academy of Pediatrics Committee on Infectious Diseases. Vitamin A treatment of measles. *Pediatrics* 1993;91: 1014–1015.
30. Mahoney CP, Margolis MT, Knauss TA, et al. Chronic vitamin A intoxication in infants fed chicken liver. *Pediatrics* 1980;65:893–897.
31. Underwood BA. The role of vitamin A in child growth, development and survival. *Adv Exp Med Biol* 1994;352:201–208.
32. Ross DA. Recommendations for vitamin A supplementation. *J Nutr* 2001;131:2902S–2906S.
33. World Health Organization. Treatment of associated conditions. www.searo.who.int/LinkFiles/FCH_treatment1.pdf. Accessed November 10, 2008.
34. Darlow BA, Graham PJ. Vitamin A supplementation for preventing morbidity and mortality in very low birthweight infants. *Cochrane Database Syst Rev* 2007;(4):CD000501.
35. Holick MF. Vitamin D. In: Shils ME, Shike M, Ross AC, et al., eds. *Modern nutrition in health and disease,* 10th ed. Baltimore: Williams & Wilkins, 2005.
36. Arnson Y, Amital H, Shoenfeld Y. Vitamin D and autoimmunity: new aetiological and therapeutic considerations. *Ann Rheum Dis* 2007;66:1137–1142.
37. Prentice A, Goldberg GR, Schoenmakers I. Vitamin D across the lifecycle: physiology and biomarkers. *Am J Clin Nutr* 2008;88: 500S–506S.
38. Institute of Medicine, Food and Nutrition Board. *Dietary reference intakes for calcium, phosphorus, magnesium, vitamin D, and fluoride.* Washington, DC: National Academy Press, 1999.
39. Ovesen L, Brot C, Jakobsen J. Food contents and biological activity of 25-hydroxyvitamin D: a vitamin D metabolite to be reckoned with? *Ann Nutr Metab* 2003;47:107–113.
40. Picciano MF. Nutrient composition of human milk. *Pediatr Clin North Am* 2001;48:53–67.
41. Specker BL, Valanis B, Hertzberg V, et al. Sunshine exposure and serum 25-hydroxyvitamin D concentrations in exclusively breast-fed infants. *J Pediatr* 1985;107:372–376.
42. Fomon SJ, Younoszai MK, Thomas LN. Influence of vitamin D on linear growth of normal full-term infants. *J Nutr* 1966;88:345–350.
43. Graham S. Idiopathic hypercalcemia. *Postgrad Med* 1959;25:67–72.
44. Cushman KD. Vitamin D in childhood and adolescence. *Postgrad Med J* 2007;83:230–235.
45. Harris SS. Vitamin D in type I diabetes prevention. *J Nutr* 2005; 135:323–325.
46. Holick MF. Sunlight and vitamin D for bone health and prevention of autoimmune diseases, cancers, and cardiovascular disease. *Am J Clin Nutr* 2004;80:1678S–1688S.
47. Ward LM. Vitamin D deficiency in the 21st century: a persistent problem among Canadian infants and mothers. *CMAJ* 2005;172: 769–770.

48. Kreiter SR, Schwartz RP, Kirkman HN Jr, et al. Nutritional rickets in African American breast-fed infants. *J Pediatr* 2000;137:153–157.
49. Hatun S, Ozkan B, Orbak Z, et al. Vitamin D deficiency in early infancy. *J Nutr* 2005;135:279–282.
50. Lapatsanis S, Moulas A, Cholevas V, et al. Vitamin D: a necessity for children and adolescents in Greece. *Calcif Tissue Int* 2005;77: 348–355.
51. Pal BR, Shaw NJ. Rickets resurgence in the United Kingdom: improving antenatal management in Asians. *J Pediatr* 2001;139: 337–338.
52. Dawodu A, Agarwal M, Hossain M, et al. Hypovitaminosis D and vitamin D deficiency in exclusively breast-feeding infants and their mothers in summer: a justification for vitamin D. *J Pediatr* 2003;142:169–173.
53. Kimball S, Fuleihan Gel H, Vieth R. Vitamin D: a growing perspective. *Crit Rev Clin Lab Sci* 2008;45:339–414.
54. Rovner AJ, O'Brien KO. Hypovitaminosis D among healthy children in the United States: a review of the current evidence. *Arch Pediatr Adolesc Med* 2008;162:513–519.
55. Schnadower D, Agarwal C, Oberfield SE, et al. Hypocalcemic seizures and secondary bilateral femoral fractures in an adolescent with primary vitamin D deficiency. *Pediatrics* 2006;118: 2226–2230.
56. Harkness LS, Cromer BA. Vitamin D deficiency in adolescent females. *J Adolesc Health* 2005;37:75.
57. Pettifor JM. Rickets and vitamin D deficiency in children and adolescents. *Endocrinol Metab Clin North Am* 2005;34:537–553.
58. Park EA. The therapy of rickets. *JAMA* 1940;115:370–379.
59. Mozolowski W. Jedrzej Sniadecki (1768–1883) on the cure of rickets. *Nature* 1939;143:131.
60. Rajakumar K, Thomas SB. Reemerging nutritional rickets: a historical perspective. *Arch Pediatr Adolesc Med* 2005;159:335–341.
61. American Academy of Pediatrics Committee on Environmental Health. Ultraviolet light: a hazard to children. *Pediatrics* 1999;104: 328–333.
62. Wagner CL, Greer FR; American Academy of Pediatrics Section on Breastfeeding; American Academy of Pediatrics Committee on Nutrition. Prevention of rickets and vitamin D deficiency in infants, children, and adolescents. *Pediatrics* 2008;122:1142–1152.
63. Brigelius-Flohe R, Traber MG. Vitamin E: function and metabolism. *FASEB J* 1999;13:1145–1155.
64. Traber MG, Packer L. Vitamin E: beyond antioxidant function. *Am J Clin Nutr* 1995;62:1501S–1509S.
65. Christen WG, Liu S, Glynn RJ, et al. Dietary carotenoids, vitamins C and E, and risk of cataract in women: a prospective study. *Arch Ophthalmol* 2008;126:102–109.
66. Gross SJ. Vitamin E. In: Tsang RC, Lucus A, Uauy R, et al., eds. *Nutritional needs of the preterm infant: scientific basis and practical guidelines.* Baltimore: Williams & Wilkins, 1993.
67. Arrowsmith JB, Faich GA, Tomita DK, et al. Morbidity and mortality among low birth weight infants exposed to an intravenous vitamin E product, E-Ferol. *Pediatrics* 1989;83:244–249.
68. Bell EF. Upper limit of vitamin E in infant formulas. *J Nutr* 1989; 119(Suppl 12):1829–1831.
69. Suttie JW. Vitamin K and human nutrition. *J Am Diet Assoc* 1992; 92:585–590.
70. Booth SL, Suttie JW. Dietary intake and adequacy of vitamin K1. *J Nutr* 1998;128:785–788.
71. Kumar D, Greer FR, Super DM, et al. Vitamin K status of premature infants: implications for current recommendations. *Pediatrics* 2001;108:1117–1122.
72. Greer FR. Are breast-fed infants vitamin K deficient? *Adv Exp Med Biol* 2001;501:391–395.
73. Golding J, Greenwood R, Birmingham K, et al. Childhood cancer, intramuscular vitamin K, and pethidine given during labour. *Br Med J* 1992;305:341–346.
74. McKinney PA, Juszczak E, Findlay E, et al. Case-control study of childhood leukaemia and cancer in Scotland: findings for neonatal intramuscular vitamin K. *Br Med J* 1998;316:173–177.
75. Parker L, Cole M, Craft AW, et al. Neonatal vitamin K administration and childhood cancer in the north of England: retrospective case-control study. *Br Med J* 1998;316:189–193.
76. American Academy of Pediatrics Fetus and Newborn Committee. Routine administration of vitamin K to newborns. *Pediatrics* 2003; 112:191–192.
77. American Academy of Pediatrics Vitamin K Ad Hoc Task Force. Controversies concerning vitamin K and the newborn. *Pediatrics* 1993;91:1001–1003.
78. Sutor AH. New aspects of vitamin K prophylaxis. *Semin Throm Hemost* 2003;29:373–376.
79. Greer FR, Marshall SP, Foley AL, et al. Improving the vitamin K status of breastfeeding infants with maternal vitamin K supplements. *Pediatrics* 1997;99:88–92.
80. Winzenberg T, Shaw K, Fryer J, et al. Calcium supplements in healthy children do not affect weight gain, height, or body composition. *Obesity (Silver Spring)* 2007;15:1789–1798.
81. Teegarden D. The influence of dairy product consumption on body composition. *J Nutr* 2005;135:2749–2752.
82. Lanou AJ, Barnard ND. Dairy and weight loss hypothesis: an evaluation of the clinical trials. *Nutr Rev* 2008;66:272–279.
83. Heaney RP, Weaver CM, Fitzsimmons ML. Influence of calcium load on absorption fraction. *J Bone Min Res* 1990;5:1135–1138.
84. Weaver CM, Heaney RP. Calcium. In: Shils ME, Shike M, Ross AC, et al., eds. *Modern nutrition in health and disease*, 10th ed. Baltimore: Williams & Wilkins, 2005.
85. Abrams SA, O'Brien KO, Stuff JE. Changes in calcium kinetics associated with menarche. *J Clin Endocrinol Metab* 1996;81: 2017–2020.
86. Fomon SJ, Nelson SE. Calcium, phosphorus, magnesium, and sulfur. In: Fomon SJ, ed. *Nutrition of normal infants.* St. Louis, MO: Mosby-Year Book, Inc, 1993.
87. Schanler RJ, Rifka M. Calcium, phosphorus and magnesium needs for the low-birth-weight infant. *Acta Paediatr Suppl* 1994;405: 111–116.
88. Bailey DA, Wedge JH, McCulloch RG, et al. Epidemiology of fractions of the distal end of the radius in children as associated with growth. *J Bone Joint Surg Am* 1989;71:1225–1231.
89. Parfitt AM. The two faces of growth: benefits and risks to bone integrity. *Osteoporos Int* 1994;4:382–398.
90. American Academy of Pediatrics Committee on Nutrition. Calcium requirements of infants, children, and adolescents. *Pediatrics* 1999; 104:1152–1157.
91. Cromer B, Harel Z. Adolescents: at increased risk for osteoporosis? *Clin Pediatr (Phila)* 2000;39:565–574.
92. American Academy of Pediatrics, Committee on Nutrition. The use and misuse of fruit juice in pediatrics. *Pediatrics* 2001;107; 1210–1213.
93. Wosje KS, Specker BL. Role of calcium in bone health during childhood. *Nutr Rev* 2000;58:253–268.
94. Lambert HL, Eastell R, Karnik K, et al. Calcium supplementation and bone mineral accretion in adolescent girls: an 18-mo randomized controlled trial with 2-y follow-up. *Am J Clin Nutr* 2008;87: 455–462.
95. Greer FR, Krebs NF. Optimizing bone health and calcium intakes of infants, children, and adolescents. *Pediatrics* 2006;117: 578–585.
96. Lonnerdal B, Kelleher SL. Iron metabolism in infants and children. *Food Nutr Bull* 2007;28:S491–S499.
97. Domellof M. Iron requirements, absorption and metabolism in infancy and childhood. *Curr Opin Clin Nutr Metab Care* 2007;10: 329–335.
98. Wood RJ, Ronnenberg AG. Iron. In: Shils ME, Shike M, Ross AC, et al., eds. *Modern nutrition in health and disease*, 10th ed. Baltimore: Williams & Wilkins, 2005.
99. Eisenstein RS, Ross KL. Novel roles for iron regulatory proteins in the adaptive response to iron deficiency. *J Nutr* 2003;133: 1510S–1516S.
100. Stolzfus RJ. Iron deficiency: global prevalence and consequences. *Food Nutr Bull* 2003;24:S99–S103.
101. Looker AC, Dallman PR, Carroll MD, et al. Prevalence of iron deficiency in the United States. *J Am Med Assoc* 1997;277:973–976.
102. Borigato EV, Martinez FE. Iron nutritional status is improved in Brazilian preterm infants fed food cooked in iron pots. *J Nutr* 1998;128:855–859.
103. Yip R. The changing characteristics of childhood iron nutritional status in the United States. In: Filer LJ, ed. *Dietary iron: birth to two years.* New York, NY: Raven Health Care Communications, 1989.
104. Friel JK, Aziz K, Andrews WL, et al. A double-masked, randomized control trial of iron supplementation in early infancy in healthy term breastfed infants. *J Pediatr* 2003;143:582–586.

105. Eden AN. Iron deficiency and impaired cognition in toddlers: an underestimated and undertreated problem. *Paediatr Drugs* 2005; 7:347–352.
106. Zlotkin S. Clinical nutrition: 8. The role of nutrition in the prevention of iron deficiency anemia in infants, children and adolescents. *Can Med Assoc J* 2003;168:59–63.
107. Lozoff B. Iron deficiency and child development. *Food Nutr Bull* 2007;28:S560–S571.
108. Grantham-McGregor S, Ani C. A review of studies on the effect of iron deficiency on cognitive development in children. *J Nutr* 2001;131:649S–668S.
109. Gera T, Sachdev HP, Nestel P. Effect of iron supplementation on physical performance in children and adolescents: systematic review of randomized controlled trials. *Indian Pediatr* 2007;44:15–24.
110. Lynch S, Stoltzfus R, Rawat R. Critical review of strategies to prevent and control iron deficiency in children. *Food Nutr Bull* 2007; 28:S610–S620.
111. Stolzfus RJ, Heidkamp R, Kenkel D, et al. Iron supplementation of young children: learning from the new evidence. *Food Nutr Bull* 2007;28:S572–S584.
112. Majumdar I, Paul P, Talib VH, et al. The effect of iron therapy on the growth of iron-replete and iron-deplete children. *J Trop Pediatr* 2003;49:84–88.
113. Lind T, Seswandhana R, Persson LA, et al. Iron supplementation of iron-replete Indonesian infants is associated with reduced weight-for-age. *Acta Paediatr* 2008;97:770–775.
114. Maggini S, Wintergerst ES, Beveridge S, et al. Selected vitamins and trace elements support immune function by strengthening epithelial barriers and cellular and humoral immune responses. *Br J Nutr* 2007;8:S29–S35.
115. Anderson AC. Iron poisoning in children. *Curr Opin Pediatr* 1994; 6:289–294.
116. Banner W Jr, Tong TG. Iron poisoning. *Pediatr Clin North Am* 1986; 33:393–409.
117. Vermylen C. What is new in iron overload? *Eur J Pediatr* 2008; 167:377–381.
118. Food and Drug Administration. Federal Register 62 FR 2217. http://www.fda.gov/Food/DietarySupplements/GuidanceComplianceRegulatoryInformation/ucm107366.htm. Accessed June 4, 2010.
119. Allen L, Black RE, Brandes N, et al. Conclusions and recommendations of a WHO expert consultation meeting on iron supplementation for infants and young children in malaria endemic areas. *Med Trop (Mars)* 2008;68:182–188.
120. World Health Organization. WHO statement: iron supplementation of young children in regions where malaria transmission is intense and infectious disease highly prevalent. http://www.who.int/child_adolescent_health/documents/pdfs/who_statement_iron.pdf. Accessed November 13, 2008.
121. Cousins RJ. Metal elements and gene expression. *Annu Rev Nutr* 1994;14:449–469.
122. King JC, Cousins R. Zinc. In: Shils ME, Shike M, Ross AC, et al., eds. *Modern nutrition in health and disease*, 10th. Baltimore, MD: Williams & Wilkins, 2005.
123. Fischer Walker CL, Black RE. Functional indicators for assessing zinc deficiency. *Food Nutr Bull* 2007;28:S454–S479.
124. Walravens PA, Hambidge KM. Growth of infants fed a zinc supplemented formula. *Am J Clin Nutr* 1976;29:1114–1121.
125. Aggarwal R, Sentz J, Miller MA. Role of zinc administration in prevention of childhood diarrhea and respiratory illnesses: a meta-analysis. *Pediatrics* 2007;119:1120–1130.
126. Lukacik M, Thomas RL, Aranda JV. A meta-analysis of the effects of oral zinc in the treatment of acute and persistent diarrhea. *Pediatrics* 2008;121:325–363.
127. Brooks WA, Santosham M, Naheed A, et al. Effect of weekly zinc supplements on incidence of pneumonia and diarrhoea in children younger than 2 years in an urban, low-income population in Bangladesh: randomised controlled trial. *Lancet* 2005;366: 999–1004.
128. Boron P, Tokuc G, Vagas E, et al. Impact of zinc supplementation in children with acute diarrhoea in Turkey. *Arch Dis Child* 2006;91: 296–299.
129. Sazawal S, Black RE, Ramsan M, et al. Effect of zinc supplementation on mortality in children aged 1–48 months: a community-based randomized placebo-controlled trial. *Lancet* 2007;369: 927–934.
130. Brown KH, Lopez de Romana D, Arsenault JE, et al. Comparison of the effects of zinc delivered in a fortified food or a liquid supplement on the growth, morbidity, and plasma zinc concentrations of young Peruvian children. *Am J Clin Nutr* 2007;85: 538–547.
131. Penny ME, Marin RM, Duran A, et al. Randomized controlled trial of the effect of daily supplementation with zinc or multiple micronutrients on the morbidity, growth, and micronutrient status of young Peruvian children. *Am J Clin Nutr* 2004;79:457–465.
132. Black MM. The evidence linking zinc deficiency with children's cognitive and motor functioning. *J Nutr* 2003;133:1473S–1476S.
133. Arnold LE, DiSilvestro RA. Zinc in attention-deficit/hyperactivity disorder. *J Child Adolesc Psychopharmacol* 2005;15:619–627.
134. Gardner JM, Powell CA, Baker-Henningham H, et al. Zinc supplementation and psychosocial stimulation: effects on the development of undernourished Jamaican children. *Am J Clin Nutr* 2005;82:399–405.
135. Fosmire GJ. Zinc toxicity. *Am J Clin Nutr* 1990;51:225–227.
136. Allen L. Zinc and micronutrient supplements for children. *Am J Clin Nutr* 1998;68:495S–498S.
137. Krebs NF, Westcott J. Zinc and breastfed infants: if and when is there a risk of deficiency? *Adv Exp Med Biol* 2002;503:69–75.
138. World Health Organization. Diarrhoea treatment guidelines. http://whqlibdoc.who.int/publications/2005/a85500.pdf. Published 2005. Accessed November 13, 2008.
139. Murphy SP, Calloway DH, Beaton GH. School children have similar predicted prevalences of inadequate intakes as toddlers in village populations in Egypt, Kenya, and Mexico. *Eur J Clin Nutr* 1995;49:647–657.
140. Hambidge KM, Krebs NF. Zinc deficiency: a special challenge. *J Nutr* 2007;137:1101–1105.
141. Messina V, Mangels AR. Considerations in planning vegan diets: infants. *J Am Diet Assoc* 2001;101:661–669.
142. Mangels AR, Messina V. Considerations in planning vegan diets: children. *J Am Diet Assoc* 2001;101:670–677.
143. Bleichrodt N, Shrestha RM, West CE, et al. The benefits of adequate iodine intake. *Nutr Rev* 1996;54:S72–S78.
144. Pennington JA. Intakes of minerals from diets and foods: is there a need for concern? *J Nutr* 1996;126:2304S–2308S.
145. Pearce EN. National trends in iodine nutrition: is everyone getting enough? *Thyroid* 2007;17:823–827.
146. Hollowell JG, Staehling NW, Hannon WH, et al. Iodine nutrition in the United States. Trends and public health implications: iodine excretion data from National Health and Nutrition Examination Surveys I and III (1971–1974 and 1988–1994). *J Clin Endocrinol Metab* 1998;83:3401–3408.
147. Maberly GJ, Haxton DP, van der Haar F. Iodine deficiency: consequences and progress toward elimination. *Food Nutr Bull* 2003; 24:S92–S98.
148. Qian M, Wang D, Watkins WE, et al. The effects of iodine on intelligence in children: a meta-analysis of studies conducted in China. *Asia Pac J Clin Nutr* 2005;14:32–42.
149. Zimmerman MB. The adverse effects of mild-to-moderate iodine deficiency during pregnancy and childhood: a review. *Thyroid* 2007;17:829–835.
150. Zimmermann MB, Connoly K, Bozo M, et al. Iodine supplementation improves cognition in iodine-deficient schoolchildren in Albania: a randomized, controlled, double-blind study. *Am J Clin Nutr* 2006;83:108–114.
151. Canadian Paediatric Society Nutrition Committee. The use of fluoride in infants and children. *Paediatr Child Health* 2002;7: 569–572.
152. Ekstrand J, Fomon SJ, Ziegler EE, et al. Fluoride pharmacokinetics in infancy. *Pediatr Res* 1994;35:157–163.
153. Centers for Disease Control and Prevention. Background: infant formula and the risk for enamel fluorosis. http://www.cdc.gov/FLUORIDATION/safety/infant_formula.htm. Accessed November 18, 2008.
154. Centers for Disease Control and Prevention. Recommendations for using fluoride to prevent and control dental caries in the United States. *MMWR Morb Mortal Wkly Rep* 2001;50(RR14): 1–42.

155. Hamasha AA, Levy SM, Broffitt B, et al. Patterns of dietary fluoride supplement use in children from birth to 96 months of age. *J Public Health Dent* 2005;65:1–13.
156. American Dental Association, American Academy of Pediatric Dentistry, American Academy of Pediatrics. Dosage schedule for dietary fluoride supplements. Proceedings of a workshop. Chicago, Illinois, USA. January 31–February 1, 1994. *J Public Health Dent* 1999;59:203–281.
157. Brown D, Whelton H, O'Mullane D. Fluoride metabolism and fluorosis. *J Dent* 2005;33:177–186.
158. Adair SM. Overview of the history and current status of fluoride supplementation schedules. *J Public Health Dent* 1999;59:252–258.
159. Innis SM, Akrabawi SS, Diersen-Schade DA, et al. Visual acuity and blood lipids in term infants fed human milk or formulae. *Lipids* 1997;32:63–72.
160. Uauy R, Mena P, Wegher B, et al. Long chain polyunsaturated fatty acid formation in neonates: effect of gestational age and intrauterine growth. *Pediatr Res* 2000;47:127–135.
161. Holman RT, Johnson SB, Hatch TF. A case of human linolenic acid deficiency involving neurological abnormalities. *Am J Clin Nutr* 1982;35:617–623.
162. SanGiovanni JP, Berkey CS, Dwyer JT, et al. Dietary essential fatty acids, long-chain polyunsaturated fatty acids, and visual resolution acuity in healthy full-term infants: a systematic review. *Early Hum Dev* 2000;57:165–188.
163. Simmer K, Schulzke SM, Patole S. Longchain polyunsaturated fatty acid supplementation in preterm infants. *Cochrane Database Syst Rev* 2008; (1):CD000375.
164. Simmer K, Patole SK, Rao SC. Longchain polyunsaturated fatty acid supplementation in infants born at term. *Indian Pediatr* 2009;46:783–784.
165. Gibson RA, Chen W, Makrides M. Randomized trials with polyunsaturated fatty acid interventions in preterm and term infants: functional and clinical outcomes. *Lipids* 2001;36:873–883.
166. Jensen CL, Voigt RG, Prager TC, et al. Effects of maternal docosahexaenoic acid intake on visual function and neurodevelopment in breastfed term infants. *Am J Clin Nutr* 2005;82:123–132.
167. Malcolm CA, McCulloch DL, Montgomery C, et al. Maternal docosahexaenoic acid supplementation during pregnancy and visual evoked potential development in term infants: a double blind, prospective, randomized trial. *Arch Dis Child Fetal Neonatal Ed* 2003;88:F383–F390.
168. Makrides M, Gibson RA, Udell T, et al. Supplementation of infant formula with long-chain polyunsaturated fatty acids does not influence the growth of term infants. International LCPUFA Investigators. *Am J Clin Nutr* 2005;81:1094–1101.
169. Raiten DJ, Talbot JM, Waters JH. LSRO Report: Assessment of nutrient requirements for infant formulas. *J Nutr* 1998;128:2059S–2293S.
170. Klein CJ. Nutrient requirements for preterm infant formulas. *J Nutr* 2001;132:1395S–1577S.

CHAPTER

57

Evridiki V. Fera
Paola J. Maurtua-Neumann
David W. Scheifele
Pearay L. Ogra

Childhood Vaccines

INTRODUCTION

Effective control or total elimination of many childhood infections by vaccinations is one of the most remarkable success stories of modern mankind. Immunization is also among the most cost-effective preventive measures available. Currently, about 24 bacterial and viral pathogens are the targets of immunization with specific vaccines in the United States and other parts of the world. These vaccines include replicating or nonreplicating antigens delivered via systemic intramuscular, subcutaneous, or mucosal (intranasal, oral) routes as shown in Table 57.1. To benefit fully from immunization, susceptible subjects need to receive the recommended vaccines at the recommended ages. This helps ensure protection against the peak risks of the target diseases. Of the vaccines available currently, most have been employed for Universal Childhood Vaccination Programs in different parts of the world. The recommended immunization schedules with vaccines licensed for children and adolescents in the United States for the year 2009 (1) are shown in Tables 57.2 to 57.4. This chapter provides comprehensive information about each of the available vaccines. This information is designed to meet the needs of a first-time or occasional vaccine provider. However, other health care providers who immunize very frequently may obtain additional information from other sources, such as the published statements of the Advisory Committee on Immunization Practices (ACIP) of the US Public Health Service (available online at www.cdc.gov/vaccines/), the "Red Book" from the American Academy of Pediatrics, the frequently updated Bulletins of the World Health Organization, and the *Morbidity and Mortality Weekly Report* (MMWR) from the Centers for Disease Control and Prevention (CDC), Atlanta, GA.

ANTHRAX VACCINE

The infection is caused by *Bacillus anthracis*, a spore-forming bacterium. It is a disease mainly of livestock. However, human infection may be acquired after exposure to infected animal products. The infection can be acquired through broken skin (cutaneous anthrax), by eating contaminated food (gastrointestinal anthrax), or by inhalation of anthrax spores (inhalation anthrax). Of the cases reported in the United States, 95% are cutaneous. The fatality rate for cutaneous anthrax is 5% to 20% without antibiotic treatment and less than 1% with antibiotic treatment. For those exposed through the digestive tract, the case fatality is estimated to be 25% to 60%. Before the availability of antibiotics or a vaccine, inhalation anthrax was almost always fatal. However, more recent experience suggests that early diagnosis and treatment significantly improves the prognosis and outcome.

VACCINE PREPARATIONS

Anthrax Vaccine Adsorbed (BioThrax) is a sterile, milky-white suspension (when mixed) made from cell-free filtrates of microaerophilic cultures of an avirulent, nonencapsulated strain of *B. anthracis*. The production cultures are grown in a chemically defined protein-free medium consisting of a mixture of amino acids, vitamins, inorganic salts, and sugars. The final product, prepared from the sterile filtrate culture fluid, contains proteins, including the 83 kDa protective antigen protein, released during the growth period. The final product is a nonreplicating bacterial product and is formulated to contain 1.2 mg per mL of aluminum, added as aluminum hydroxide in 0.85% sodium chloride. It also contains 25 μg per mL of benzethonium chloride and 100 μg per mL of formaldehyde, added as preservatives (1).

The current vaccine was licensed by the Food and Drug Administration (FDA) on the basis of its ability to prevent anthrax after preexposure immunization. Since anthrax immunization is considered an investigational use of an approved vaccine, informed consent is required.

VACCINE USAGE

To prevent anthrax infection before exposure, the standard schedule consists of six doses administered subcutaneously. Following the first dose, additional doses of vaccine are given at 2 and 4 weeks, followed by booster doses 6, 12, and 18 months later. Finally, an annual booster dose is recommended to maintain prolonged immunity.

In one proposed study to prevent anthrax infection among postal workers and Capitol Hill employees who

TABLE 57.1 List of Currently Available Vaccines Against Childhood Infections

	Vaccine Type		*Route of Administration*	
Vaccine	*Live (Replicating)*	*Attenuated (Nonreplicating)*	*Mucosal*	*Parenteral*
Anthrax		+		+
Diphtheria, pertussis, tetanus		+		+
Haemophilus influenzae type b		+		+
Hepatitis A		+		+
Hepatitis B		+		+
Human papilloma virus		+		+
Influenza	+	+	+	+
Japanese encephalitis		+		+
Measles, mumps, rubella	+			+
Meningococcus		+		+
Pneumococcus		+		+
Poliovirus	+	+	+	+
Rabies		+		+
Rotavirus	+		+	
Smallpox	+			+
Tuberculosis	+			+
Typhoid	+	+	+	+
Varicella-zoster	+			+
Vibrio cholera	+	+	+	+
Yellow fever	+			+

TABLE 57.2 Recommended Immunization Schedule for Persons Aged 0 Through 6 Years

	Age										
Vaccine	*Birth*	*1 mo*	*2 mo*	*4 mo*	*6 mo*	*12 mo*	*15 mo*	*18 mo*	*19–23 mos*	*2–3 yr*	*4–6 yr*
Hepatitis B	HepB	← HepB →		HepB[a]	← HepB →						
Rotavirus			RV	RV	RV						
Diphtheria, tetanus, pertussis			DTaP	DTaP	DTaP	DTaP[b]	← DTaP →				DTaP
Haemophilus influenzae type b			Hib	Hib	Hib	← Hib →					
Pneumococcal			PCV	PCV	PCV	PCV				← PPSV[1] →	
Inactivated poliovirus			IPV	IPV	← IPV →						IPV
Influenza					← Influenza (yearly) →						
Measles, mumps, rubella						← MMR →		← MMR[c] →		← MMR[1] →	
Varicella						← Varicella →		← Varicella[d] →		← Varicella[1] →	
Hepatitis A						← HepA (2 doses) →				← HepA series[1] →	
Meningococcal										← MCV[1] →	

[1]Certain high-risk groups.

[a]HepB—administration of four doses of HepB to infants is permissible when combination vaccines containing HepB are administered after the birth dose.

[b]DTaP—the fourth dose may be administered as early as age 12 months, provided at least 6 months have lapsed since the third dose.

[c]MMR—administer the second dose at age 4 through 6 years. However, the second dose may be administered before age 4, provided at least 28 days have elapsed since the first dose.

[d]Varicella—administer the second dose at age 4 through 6 years. However, the second dose may be administered before 4 years of age, provided at least 3 months have elapsed since the first dose. For children aged 12 months through 12 years, minimum interval between doses is 3 months. However, if the second dose was administered at least 28 days after the first dose, it can be accepted as valid.

DTaP, diphtheria and tetanus toxoids and acellular pertussis vaccine; HepA, hepatitis A vaccine; HepB, hepatitis B vaccine; Hib, *Haemophilus Influenzae* type b; IPV, inactivated poliovirus; MCV, meningococcal vaccine; MMR, measles, mumps, rubella; PCV, pneumococcal conjugated vaccine; PPSV, pneumococcal polysaccharide vaccine; RV, rotavirus vaccine.

TABLE 57.3 Recommended Immunization Schedule for Persons Aged 7 Through 18 Years

Vaccine	Age: 7–10 yr	11–12 yr	13–18 yr
Tetanus, diphtheria, pertussis		Tdap[a]	Tdap[2]
Human papillomavirus		HPV (three doses)[b]	HPV series[2]
Meningococcal	MCV[1]	MCV	MCV[2]
Influenza	←	Influenza (yearly)	→
Pneumococcal	←	PPSV[1]	→
Hepatitis A	←	HepA series[1]	→
Hepatitis B	←	HepB series[2]	→
Inactivated poliovirus	←	IPV series[2]	→
Measles, mumps, rubella	←	MMR series[2]	→
Varicella	←	Varicella series[2]	→

[1]Catch-up immunization.
[2]Certain high-risk groups.
HepA, hepatitis A vaccine; HepB, hepatitis B vaccine; HPV, human papillomavirus vaccine; IPV, inactivated poliovirus; MCV, meningococcal vaccine; MMR, measles, mumps, rubella; PPSV, pneumococcal polysaccharide vaccine; Tdap.
[a]Tdap—administer at age 11 or 12 years for those who have completed the recommended childhood DRP/DTaP vaccination series and have not received a tetanus and diphtheria toxoid (Td) booster dose.
[b]HPV—administer the second dose 2 months after the first dose and the third dose 6 months after the first dose (at least 24 weeks after the first dose). Tdap; tetanus toxoids, diphtheria and acellular pertussis vaccine.

may have already been exposed, recipients of the vaccine received a three-dose course with an interval of 2 weeks.

VACCINE EFFECTIVENESS

Anthrax vaccine has been found to be 92.5% effective in protecting against anthrax (both cutaneous and inhalational).

As with most vaccines, measuring anthrax antibody levels provides only an indirect measure of the vaccine's ability to prevent disease. However, 91% of adults who receive the anthrax vaccine exhibit an immune response after two or more doses, and 95% have a fourfold increase in antibodies after three doses. Higher levels of antibodies are thought to protect against anthrax, although the precise level of antibody at which protection against anthrax can be assured is not known.

The vaccine is the only aluminum-containing vaccine that is given subcutaneously. Aluminum is incorporated into many vaccines to increase their potency and produce the desired protection.

Anthrax vaccine has been recommended for use in the following groups of subjects at high risk for exposure: subjects 18 to 65 years of age who are at occupational risk of exposure to anthrax bacteria or spores; including at-risk veterinarians, livestock handlers, laboratory workers exposed to anthrax bacteria, and military personnel.

ADVERSE EFFECTS AND CONTRAINDICATION

Anthrax vaccine may cause soreness, redness, itching, swelling, and lumps at the injection site. About 30% of men and 60% of women report mild local reactions, usually lasting for only a few days. Lumps can persist for a few weeks. Between 1% and 5% of those who receive the vaccine report moderate reactions (redness, swelling) of 1 to 5 inches in diameter. Larger reactions occur in 1% of vaccine recipients.

Some vaccinees experience rashes (16%), headaches (14% to 25%), joint aches (12% to 15%), malaise (6% to 17%), muscle aches (3% to 34%), nausea (3% to 9%), chills (2% to 6%), or fever (1% to 5%) after vaccination. These symptoms usually go away after a few days. Severe allergic reactions have been reported in less than 1 out of every 100,000 doses administered (1,2).

Concerns have been raised about potential long-term effects of anthrax vaccine and the overall safety of the vaccine. A March 2000 report by the Institute of Medicine's Committee on Health Effects Associated with Exposures during the Gulf War noted that "to date, published studies have reported no significant adverse effects of the vaccine, but the literature is limited to a few short-term studies."

A review of surveillance for adverse events following anthrax vaccination found that, although there are short-term side effects—more common among women than men—"no patterns of unexpected local or systemic adverse events have been identified."

Anthrax vaccine is not recommended for postexposure protection, subjects who have recovered from an anthrax infection, and subjects who developed a serious allergic (anaphylactic) reaction to a previous dose of anthrax vaccine.

The vaccine is not indicated for preexposure protection in pregnant women, as the vaccine has not been proven to be safe in such situations, and for subjects younger than 18 years or older than 65 years, because no formal studies have been completed in these groups; subjects moderately or severely ill should consult with their physicians before receiving such vaccine.

TABLE 57.4 Catch-Up Immunization Schedule for Persons Aged 4 Months Through 18 Years

Vaccine	Minimum Age for Dose 1	Minimum Interval Between Doses: Dose 1 to Dose 2	Dose 2 to Dose 3	Dose 3 to Dose 4	Dose 4 to Dose 5
Catch-Up Schedule for Persons Aged 4 mo Through 6 yr					
Hepatitis B	**Birth**	**4 wk**	**8 wk** (and at least 16 wk after first dose)		
Rotavirus	**6 wk**	**4 wk**	**4 wk**[a]		
Diphtheria, tetanus, pertussis	**6 wk**	**4 wk**	**4 wk**	**6 mo**	**6 mo**[b]
***Haemophilus influenzae* type b**	**6 wk**	**4 wk** if first dose administered at younger than 12 mo **8 wk (as final dose)** if first dose administered at age 12–14 mo. **No further doses needed** if first dose administered at age 15 mo or older	**4 wk**[c] if current age is younger than 12 mo **8 wk (as final dose)**[c] if current age is 12 mo of older and second dose administered at younger than 15 mo. **No further doses needed** if first previous dose administered at age 15 mo or older	**8 wk (as final dose).** This dose is necessary only for children aged 12 mo through 59 mo who received three doses before age 12 mo	
Pneumococcal	**6 wk**	**4 wk** if first dose administered at younger than 12 mo **8 wk (as final dose for healthy children) children)** if first dose administered at age 12 mo or older or current age 24 through 59 mo. **No further doses needed** for healthy children if first dose administered at age 24 mo or older	**4 wk** if current age is younger than 12 mo **8 wk (as final dose for healthy children)** if current age is 12 mo or older. **No further doses needed.** For healthy children if previous dose administered at age 24 mo or older	**8 wk (as final dose).** This dose is necessary only for children aged 12 mo through 59 mo who received three doses before age of 12 mo or for high-risk children who received three doses at any age	
Inactivated poliovirus	**6 wk**	**4 wk**	**4 wk**	**4 wk**[d]	
Measles, mumps, rubella	**12 wk**	**4 wk**			
Varicella	**12 wk**	**3 mo**			
Hepatitis A	**12 wk**	**6 mo**			
Catch-Up Schedule for Persons Aged 7 Through 18 yr					
Tetanus, diphtheria/ tetanus, diphtheria, pertussis	**7 yr**[e]	**4 wk**	**4 wk** if first dose administered at younger than 12 mo **6 mo** if first dose administered at age 12 mo or older	**6 mo** if first dose administered at younger than 12 mo	
Human papillomavirus	**9 yr**	**Routine dosing intervals are recommended**			
Hepatitis A	**12 mo**	**6 mo**			
Hepatitis B	**Birth**	**4 wk**	**8 wk** (and at least 16 wk after first dose)		

(*continued*)

TABLE 57.4 Catch-Up Immunization Schedule for Persons Aged 4 Months Through 18 Years (*Continued*)

Catch-Up Schedule for Persons Aged 7 Through 18 yr (*Continued*)

Vaccine	*Minimum Age for Dose 1*	*Minimum Interval Between Doses*			
		Dose 1 to Dose 2	*Dose 2 to Dose 3*	*Dose 3 to Dose 4*	*Dose 4 to Dose 5*
Inactivated poliovirus	**6 wk**	**4 wk**	**4 wk**	**4 wk**[d]	
Measles, mumps, rubella	**12 mo**	**4 wk**			
Varicella	**12 mo**	**3 mo** if the person is younger than 13 yr **4 wk** if the person is aged 13 years or older			

[a]Rotavirus (RV)—The maximum age for the first dose is 14 weeks 6 days. Vaccination should not be initiated for infants aged 15 weeks or older (i.e., 15 weeks 0 days or older).
Administer the final dose in the series by age 8 months 0 days.
If Rotarix was administered for the first and second dose, a third dose is not necessary.
[b]Diphtheria, tetanus, pertussis (DTaP)—The fifth dose is not necessary if the fourth dose was administered at age 4 years or older.
[c]*Haemophilus influenzae* type b (Hib)—If the first two doses were PRP–OMP (Pedvax HIB or Comvax) and administered at age 11 months or younger, the third (and final) dose should be administered at age 12 through 15 months and at least 8 weeks after the second dose.
If the first dose was administered at age 7 through 11 months, administer two doses separated by 4 weeks and a final dose at age 12 through 15 months.
[d]Inactivated poliovirus (IPV)—Fourth dose is not necessary if the third dose was administered at age 4 years or older.
[e]Tetanus, diphtheria/tetanus, diphtheria, pertussis (Td/Tdap)—Tdap should be substituted for a single dose of Td in the catch-up series or as a booster for children aged 10 through 18 years: use Td for other doses.

DIPHTHERIA TOXOID

The etiologic agent of diphtheria is *Corynebacterium diphtheriae.* The most common manifestation of diphtheria is severe pharyngitis. This is caused by a toxin released by the infecting organism that damages the respiratory epithelium, causing pseudomembrane formation. Toxin dissemination can also lead to nerve and cardiac muscle damage. Without treatment mortality is high particularly as a result of airway obstruction or cardiac dysfunction. Transmission occurs from person to person by close respiratory and physical contact.

VACCINE PREPARATIONS

The vaccine (3) is based on diphtheria exotoxin, a protein that is antigenically uniform among isolates. In the manufacturing process, organisms are grown under conditions favoring toxin production. Free toxin is separated from bacteria by centrifugation and then progressively purified. Controlled exposure to formalin alters the protein structure sufficiently to abrogate toxicity while preserving antigenicity, producing a so-called toxoid. Diphtheria toxoid is usually adsorbed to an aluminum salt to enhance immunogenicity over fluid formulations. Formulations intended for young children contain more antigen (typically 6.7 to 15 Lf units per 0.5 mL dose) than formulations intended for persons older than 6 years (typically 2 Lf units per 0.5 mL dose). To make this distinction, the abbreviation D toxoid is used for pediatric formulations and the abbreviation d toxoid is used for "adult" formulations. Some products contain thimerosal preservative.

No diphtheria-only vaccine is available. Currently, the toxoid-containing vaccine includes DTaP (Diphtheria–Tetanus–acellular Pertussis) vaccine, in combination with *Haemophilus influenzae* type b (Hib) vaccine, in combination with hepatitis B and inactivated polio vaccines, in combination with Hib, hepatitis B, and inactivated polio vaccines, DT or Td (in combination with tetanus vaccine), and Tdap (Diphtheria–Tetanus–Pertussis).

Vaccines containing the whole cell pertussis component (DTP) are no longer recommended for use in the United States and are not listed here, although they are used in many other countries. Vaccines containing lower amounts of diphtheria toxoid—abbreviated with a small d—are utilized in persons aged 7 years or older. Pertussis component–containing vaccines are not available for children 7 to 9 years of age.

AVAILABLE PRODUCTS

Product Name: Diphtheria and tetanus toxoids adsorbed (DT)
Manufacturer: Sanofi Pasteur
Year Licensed: 1984

Product Name: Tetanus and diphtheria toxoids adsorbed for adult use (Td)
Manufacturers (Year Licensed): Massachusetts Public Health Biologic Laboratories (1970), Aventis Pasteur (1978)

Product Name: Tripedia (DTaP)
Manufacturer: Sanofi Pasteur
Year Licensed: 2001

Product Name: Infanrix (DTaP)
Manufacturer: GlaxoSmithKline
Year Licensed: 1997

Product Name: TriHIBit (DTaP and Hib conjugate vaccine)
Manufacturer: Sanofi Pasteur
Year Licensed: 2001

Product Name: DAPTACEL (DTaP)
Manufacturer: Sanofi Pasteur
Year Licensed: 2002

Product Name: Pediatrix (DTaP, hepatitis B, and inactivated polio vaccines)
Manufacturer: GlaxoSmithKline
Year Licensed: 2002

Product Name: DECAVAC (Tetanus and Diphtheria Toxoids Adsorbed for Adult Use—preservative free)
Manufacturer: Sanofi Pasteur
Year Licensed: 2004

Product Name: BOOSTRIX (Tetanus Toxoid, Reduced Diphtheria Toxoid and Acellular Pertussis Vaccine, Adsorbed for use in 10- to 64-year-old persons) (Tdap)
Manufacturer: GlaxoSmithKline Biologicals
Year Licensed: 2005

Product Name: ADACEL (Tetanus and Diphtheria Toxoids Adsorbed for use in 11- to 64-year-old persons)
Manufacturer: Sanofi Pasteur
Year Licensed: 2005

Product Name: Pentacel (DTaP, Hib conjugate, hepatitis B, and inactivated polio vaccines)
Manufacturer: Sanofi Pasteur
Year Licensed: 2008

All DTaP vaccines are available containing no or only trace amounts of thimerosal. Both DT and Td are available as vaccines, containing trace amounts of thimerosal, or as thimerosal-free. Tetanus toxoid (TT) is only available containing thimerosal preservative.

VACCINE USAGE

Adsorbed toxoid formulations are administered intramuscularly to minimize injection site reactions. Vaccine should be stored at 2°C to 8°C, avoiding freezing.

Diphtheria toxoid requires a series of appropriately spaced injections to reliably elicit a protective response. The number of doses needed to elicit protection varies with age. Antibody levels decline slowly and may fall below the minimum needed for protection. Periodic booster doses are recommended throughout life to maintain protection.

The recommended immunization schedule for infants and young children in the United States (3) and Canada (4) involves five doses of the pediatric (D) formulation, given at 2, 4, 6, and 15 to 18 months and 4 to 6 years. Subsequent booster doses are recommended at 14 to 16 years and every 10 years throughout adulthood, using the adult (d) formulation (see Tables 57.2 to 57.4).

VACCINE EFFECTIVENESS

Diphtheria vaccines have been routinely used since the 1930s. Clinical diphtheria is rare in well-immunized populations. Although the vaccine induces only antitoxic immune responses, prolonged use in populations has resulted in the near disappearance of circulating toxigenic organisms. In the United States, no more than five respiratory cases are reported annually, most of whom lacked adequate primary immunization. A substantial proportion of American and Canadian adults lack protective serum levels of antitoxin from not having obtained booster immunizations, but disease is rare nonetheless. Persons likely to encounter diphtheria during travel abroad or who are exposed to a case should receive a booster dose if more than 10 years has elapsed since the previous dose (and the individual had adequate primary immunization).

ADVERSE EFFECTS AND CONTRAINDICATIONS

Diphtheria toxoid vaccines are well tolerated. Occasionally, the vaccine can cause mild to moderate injection-site discomfort and low-grade fever. Booster doses may cause greater injection-site reaction with redness, swelling, and soreness. Overly frequent doses should be avoided, as they increase the risk of severe injection-site reactions. The only contraindication to its use is a history of anaphylactic reaction to a previous dose or hypersensitivity to thimerosal (thimerosal-free formulations are available) or any other vaccine component.

HAEMOPHILUS INFLUENZAE TYPE B VACCINES

Before vaccines were introduced in the late 1980s, Hib bacteria were the leading cause of purulent meningitis and epiglottis and an important cause of bacteremia, pneumonia, septic arthritis, and cellulitis in young children (5). About 1 child in 200 experienced invasive Hib infection by 5 years of age, half suffering from meningitis. The latter was the leading cause of acquired deafness and developmental delay. Hib organisms most often colonize the upper airway without causing disease and spread readily from child to child in respiratory secretions.

Immunity is associated with opsonic antibodies directed at the Hib capsular polysaccharide, polyribosyl ribose phosphate (PRP). Children do not respond to purified PRP until about 24 months of age, by which time about two-thirds of Hib cases have occurred. Response to PRP develops without T-cell help and lacks a memory component.

VACCINE PREPARATIONS

To protect the age group at greatest risk, Hib vaccines have to overcome the unresponsiveness to purified PRP characteristic of children younger than 24 months. This is achieved by chemically linking segments of PRP to the surface of carrier proteins, creating a polysaccharide–protein conjugate vaccine. Currently used carriers include tetanus toxoid (PRP-T), genetically inactivated diphtheria toxin (PRP-CRM), and outer membrane protein complex from *Neisseria meningitidis* (PRP-OMP). Uptake and processing of the linked molecules by antigen-presenting cells expose B cells responding to PRP to the cytokines released by T cells responding to carrier peptides. The T-cell help extended to B cells responding to PRP fundamentally alters the response to the polysaccharide, enabling it to develop in young infants with additional advantages of antibody avidity maturation and development of immunologic memory. The latter establishes long-term protection and the capacity for booster responses to native PRP, should individuals be colonized with Hib or cross-reacting organisms.

Current vaccines contain purified PRP conjugated to carrier proteins that vary among manufacturers. Manufacturing processes control the size and quantity of PRP molecules linked to the carrier protein, minimizing lot-to-lot variation in immunogenicity. Products are available in separate formulations or combined with other childhood vaccines.

The Hib vaccine is available as Hib (alone), Hib in combination with DTaP vaccine, and Hib in combination with recombinant hepatitis B virus (HBV) vaccine.

AVAILABLE PRODUCTS

Product: ActHIB (Hib)
Manufacturer: Aventis Pasteur
Year Licensed: 1993

Product: HibTITER (Hib)
Manufacturer: Wyeth Lederle
Year Licensed: 1990

Product: PedvaxHIB (Hib)
Manufacturer: Merck
Year Licensed: 1989

Product: Comvax (HBV-Hib)
Manufacturer: Merck
Year Licensed: 1996

VACCINE USAGE

A series of injections in the first months of life is required to elicit an antibody response. Products requiring three primary doses are given at 2, 4, and 6 months of age (see Table 57.2). Of note, PedavaxHIB by Merck requires only two primary doses, given at 2 and 4 months of age. For each product a booster dose is recommended in the second year of life. The PRP–OMP vaccine elicits the quickest response and is preferred in settings where the disease risk is high in early infancy, as in Alaskan natives (2). Fewer doses are required for children who commence immunization after 6 months of age. Booster doses later in childhood (beyond 2 years) are not required (see Tables 57.2 to 57.4).

Immunization elicits anti-PRP antibodies. The minimum protective antibody level using conjugate vaccines has not been defined, although a level of 0.15 μg per mL or more is indicative of adequate protection. The capacity for an anamnestic response upon encountering organisms may be more relevant to protection than a particular serum antibody concentration.

VACCINE EFFECTIVENESS

Virtually every healthy infant has a measurable antibody response upon completion of the recommended primary series. Antibody concentrations decline progressively thereafter but are strongly reinforced by the booster dose. With the currently used vaccines, annual Hib case totals are less than 1% of what they were before immunization became routine (6). Among the remaining cases, vaccine failures are rare; cases more often reflect incomplete immunization and parent refusal to immunize. All current products have an estimated efficacy of at least 98%.

ADVERSE REACTIONS AND CONTRAINDICATIONS

Hib conjugates cause only minor adverse effects, such as fever and injection-site morbidity, of short duration. Local reactions do not increase with successive doses. Allergy to the carrier protein and an anaphylactic reaction to a previous dose are contraindications.

HEPATITIS A VACCINE

Hepatitis A virus (HAV) causes most cases of acute hepatitis in the United States (7). Young children are often mildly ill or asymptomatic but can readily spread infection to contacts. In older children, teens, and adults, HAV infection causes substantial morbidity for 1 to 3 months (2). Infection superimposed on chronic liver disease increases the risk of fulminant hepatitis or liver failure. No chronic infection state occurs. Infection spreads through the fecal route, through direct contact with cases, or through ingestion of contaminated food or water. Recovery is associated with lifelong protection.

Vaccination programs target individuals at high risk of infection and communities with high rates or recurrent epidemics of infection (8).

VACCINE PREPARATIONS

Licensed vaccines contain inactivated HAV (9). The various vaccine strains are grown in human fibroblast cultures, purified from lysed cells, inactivated with formalin, and adsorbed to alum adjuvant. Pediatric formulations contain less antigen than do adult formulations and are intended for children older than 12 months (9). Some products may contain neomycin and other excipients.

The hepatitis A vaccine is available as HAV alone and HAV in combination with hepatitis B virus (HBV) vaccine (see Table 57.6). HAV vaccines are administered intramuscularly. They should be stored at 2°C to 8°C, avoiding freezing.

AVAILABLE PRODUCTS

Product: Havrix (HAV)
Manufacturer: GlaxoSmithKline
Year Licensed: 1995

Product: Vaqta (HAV)
Manufacturer: Merck
Year Licensed: 1996

Product: TwinRix (combined HAV, HBV)
Manufacturer: GlaxoSmithKline
Year Licensed: 2007

TABLE 57.5 Combination Vaccines

Trade Names	*Antigens*	*Antibiotics*	*Tissue Culture, Media*	*Adjuvants*	*Thimerosol*	*Formaldehyde Polysorbate 80*	*Preservatives*	*Other*	*Immunization Route*
DAPTACEL, Infanrix, Tripedia	DTaP			Aluminum	Trace (Tripedia)	Trace	None	Gelatin (Tripedia)	IM
ADACEL, Boostrix	TDap[a]			Aluminum		Trace	None	Glutaraldehyde, 2-phenoxyethanol	IM
TriHIBit[b] (Tripedia + ActHIB)	DTaP, Hib			Aluminum	Trace (Tripedia)	Trace	None	Gelatin (Tripedia)	IM
KINRIX	DTaP, IPV	Neomycin sulfate, polymyxin B	VERO, Calf serum, lactalbumin hydrolysate	Aluminum		Trace	None		IM
Pentacel[c]	DTaP, IPV, Hib	Neomycin sulfate, polymyxin B	MRC-5 cells	Aluminum		Trace	None	Glutaraldehyde bovine serum albumin, 2-phenoxyethanol	IM
Pediarix	DTaP, IPV, HepB	Neomycin sulfate, polymyxin B	VERO, Calf serum, lactalbumin hydrolysate *Saccharomyces cerevisiae*	Aluminum		Trace	None	Glutaraldehyde bovine serum albumin, 2-phenoxyethanol, ≤5% yeast protein	IM
DT	DT			Aluminum	Trace	Trace	None		IM
DECAVAC, TENIVAC, Td (generic)	Td			Aluminum	Trace (Decavac)	Trace	None	2-phenoxyethanol	IM

DTaP, diphtheria, tetanus toxoid and acellular pertussis; DT, Diphtheria and tetanus toxoids; Hib, *Haemophilus influenzae* type b; IM, intramuscular; IPV, inactivated poliovirus; Td, tetanus and diphtheria toxoids; Tdap.

[a]Vaccine is formulated with reduced quantities of diphtheria toxoid and detoxified pertussis toxoid.

[b]When Tripedia vaccine is used to reconstitute ActHIB the combination vaccine is TriHIBit.

[c]When DTaP and IPV are used to reconstitute ActHIB the combination vaccine is Pentacel.

VACCINE USAGE

Hepatitis A vaccine was introduced incrementally first in 1996 for children living in communities with the highest rates of disease and then in 1999 for children living in states/communities with consistently elevated rates of infection. The impact of immunization with hepatitis A vaccine has been a dramatic decline in the rates of disease and a sharp reduction in the groups with the highest risk of infection, Native Americans and Alaskan natives. Rates of hepatitis A infection are now similar in most areas of the United States. As a consequence, hepatitis A vaccine has now been recommended for all children in the United States 12 to 23 months of age to eliminate hepatitis A transmission nationally. A single dose elicits protective levels of antibody within 4 weeks in more than 95% of healthy recipients (10). A second dose is recommended 6 to 12 or 6 to 18 months later (depending on the product) for long-term protection. Immunity persists for at least 10 years and is expected to last much longer (11).

Universal HAV immunization of children is recommended in states or communities with higher-than-average rates of infection (10).

Individual candidates for HAV immunization include the following: children traveling to countries where HAV infection is endemic; youth at risk through use of illicit drugs in unsanitary conditions, or involvement in the sex trade or male homosexual activities, particularly involving oral–anal contact; children who have clotting factor disorders treated with clotting-factor concentrates; and children with chronic liver disease or a transplanted liver.

HAV vaccine can be given concurrently with other childhood vaccines at separate anatomic injection sites. HAV vaccine can be used to prevent infection in persons recently exposed (within 7 days) to a case and appears to be as effective as immunoglobulin.

VACCINE EFFECTIVENESS

HAV vaccines are highly effective. Universal childhood immunization programs have been shown to substantially reduce infection rates in communities across all age groups, illustrating that children are central in the transmission of this virus. Vaccination is also effective for controlling outbreaks of infection (10).

ADVERSE EFFECTS

HAV vaccines are well tolerated, with symptoms usually limited to soreness or erythema at the injection site. Rare instances of anaphylaxis have been reported. HAV vaccine should not be given to children who have had an anaphylactic reaction to a previous dose or are allergic to any constituent (e.g., neomycin). Safety of HAV administration during pregnancy has not been demonstrated.

HEPATITIS B VACCINE

The hepatitis B virus (HBV) is a DNA virus which is an important cause of liver disease that ranges in severity from a mild illness lasting a few weeks (acute) to a serious long-term illness that can lead to chronic active hepatitis or liver cancer. This virus can be transmitted through contact with infectious blood, semen, and other body fluids from having sex with an infected person, sharing contaminated needles to inject drugs, or from an infected mother to her newborn (2).

The virus contains several important antigenic components. These include hepatitis B surface antigen (HBsAg), hepatitis B core antigen (HBcAg), and hepatitis B *e* antigen (HBeAg). Humans are the only known host for HBV, although some nonhuman primates have been infected in laboratory conditions. HBV is relatively resilient and, in some instances, has been shown to remain infectious on environmental surfaces for more than 7 days at room temperature. HBV infection is an established cause of acute and chronic hepatitis and cirrhosis. It is the cause of up to 80% of hepatocellular carcinomas and is second only to tobacco among known human carcinogens (2).

VACCINE PREPARATION

Hepatitis B vaccine (Recombinant) is a noninfectious recombinant DNA hepatitis B vaccine (12). It contains purified HBsAg of the virus obtained by culturing genetically engineered *Saccharomyces cerevisiae* cells, which carry the surface antigen gene of the HBV. The surface antigen expressed in *S. cerevisiae* cells is purified by several physiochemical steps and formulated as a suspension of the antigen adsorbed on aluminum hydroxide. The preparations contain no more than 5% yeast protein. No substances of human origin are used in its manufacture.

AVAILABLE PRODUCTS

Single-antigen hepatitis B vaccines

Product: ENGERIX-B (HBV)
Manufacturer: GlaxoSmithKline
Year Licensed: 2006

Product: RECOMBIVAX-HB (HBV)
Manufacturer: Merck
Year Licensed: 2007

Combination Vaccines

- COMVAX: Combined hepatitis B-Hib conjugate vaccine. Cannot be administered before the age of 6 weeks or after the age of 71 months (see Table 57.5).
- PEDIATRIX: Combined hepatitis B, DTaP, and inactivated poliovirus (IPV) vaccine. Cannot be administered before the age of 6 weeks or after the age of 7 years (see Table 57.5).
- TWINRIX: Combined hepatitis A and hepatitis B vaccine. Recommended for persons aged 18 years or older who are at increased risk for both HAV and HBV infections (see Table 57.6) (13).

VACCINE USAGE

Each 0.5 mL dose contains 10 μg of HBsAg adsorbed on 0.25 mg aluminum as aluminum hydroxide. The pediatric formulation contains sodium chloride (9 mg per mL) and

TABLE 57.6 Combination Vaccines

Trade Names	*Antigens*	*Antibiotics*	*Tissue Culture/Media*	*Adjuvants*	*Preservatives*	*Other*	*Immunization Route*
Twinrix	HepA, HepB	Neomycin	MRC-5, *Saccharomyces cerevisiae*	Aluminium	None	Polysorbate 20, formalin, MRC-5 cellular proteins, yeast protein	IM
Comvax	Hib, HepB		*S. cerevisiae*	Aluminium	None	Sodium borate formaldehyde, ≤5% yeast protein	IM
M-M-Vax	Measles, mumps	Neomycin	Chick embryo		None	Sorbitol sodium phosphate, hydrolyzed gelatin, human albumin, fetal bovine serum	IM
M-M-R-II	Measles, mumps Rubella	Neomycin	Chick embryo, WI-38 human diploid lung fibroblasts		None	Sorbitol sodium phosphate, hydrolyzed gelatin, human albumin, fetal bovine serum	IM
Proquod	Measles, mumps Rubella, varicella	Neomycin	MRC-5, chick embryo, WI-38 human diploid lung fibroblasts		None	Hydrolyzed gelatin, monosodium L-glutamate, human albumin, sodium bicarbonate, MRC-5 cell DNA and protein, bovine calf serum	IM
Menactra	Meningococcal (groups A, C, Y and W-135) Diphtheria toxoid		*Neisseria meningitidis* A, C, Y, and W-135 strains		None	Sodium phosphate, formaldehyde	IM

HepA, hepatitis A; HepB, hepatitis B; IM, intramuscular.

phosphate buffers (disodium phosphate dehydrate, 0.98 mg per mL; sodium dihydrogen phosphate dehydrate, 0.71 mg per mL).

VACCINE EFFECTIVENESS

After three intramuscular doses of hepatitis B vaccine, more than 90% of healthy adults and more than 95% of infants, children, and adolescents (from birth to 19 years of age) develop adequate antibody responses. However, there is an age-specific decline in immunogenicity. After the age of 40 years, approximately 90% of recipients respond to a three-dose series, and by 60 years, only 75% of vaccines develop protective antibody titers.

All infants should receive the hepatitis B vaccine series as part of the recommended childhood immunization schedule. Primary vaccination consists of three or more intramuscular doses of hepatitis B vaccine. The second and third doses are administered 2 and 6 months, respectively, after the first dose (see Table 57.2). Alternate schedules have been approved for certain vaccines and/or populations (see Tables 57.2 to 57.4).

ADVERSE REACTIONS

Hypersensitivity to any component of the vaccine, including yeast, is a contraindication. This vaccine is contraindicated in patients with previous hypersensitivity to any hepatitis B–containing vaccine. As with other vaccines, vaccination of persons with moderate or severe acute illness, with or without fever, should be deferred until the acute phase of the illness is resolved. Vaccination is not contraindicated in persons with a history of multiple sclerosis, Guillain–Barré syndrome (GBS), autoimmune disease (e.g., systemic lupus erythematosus or rheumatoid arthritis), or other chronic diseases (11).

Pregnancy is not a contraindication to vaccination. Limited data indicate no apparent risk for adverse events to developing fetuses when hepatitis B vaccine is administered to pregnant women. Current vaccines contain noninfectious HBsAg and should cause no risk to the fetus (11).

Management of Infants Born to Women Who Are HBsAg Positive or Unknown

- All infants born to HBsAg-positive women should receive single-antigen hepatitis B vaccine and HBIG (0.5 mL) at 12 hours of birth or earlier, administered at different injection sites. The vaccine series should be completed according to a recommended schedule for infants born to HBsAg-positive mothers. The final dose in the vaccine series should not be administered before the age of 24 weeks (164 days).
- For preterm infants weighing less than 2,000 g, the initial vaccine dose (birth dose) should not be counted as part of the vaccine series because of the potentially reduced immunogenicity of hepatitis B vaccine in these infants; three additional doses of vaccine (for a total of four doses) should be administered beginning when the infant reaches the age of 1 month (2).
- Postvaccination testing for anti-HBs and HBsAg should be performed after completion of the vaccine series, at the age of 9 to 18 months (generally at the next well-child visit). Testing should not be performed before the age of 9 months to avoid detection of anti-HBs from HBIG administered during infancy and to maximize the likelihood of detecting late HBV infection. Anti-HBc testing of infants is not recommended because passively acquired maternal anti-HBc might be detected in infants born to HBV-infected mothers till the age of 24 months.
    1. HBsAg-negative infants with anti-HBs levels of 10 mIU per mL or more are protected and need no further medical management.
    2. HBsAg-negative infants with anti-HBs levels of less than 10 mIU per mL should be revaccinated with a second three-dose series and retested 1 to 2 months after the final dose of vaccine.
    3. Infants who are HBsAg-positive should receive appropriate follow-up.
- Infants of HBsAg-positive mothers may be breast-fed beginning immediately after birth.
- Although not indicated in the manufacturer's package labeling, HBsAg-containing combination vaccines may be used for infants aged 6 weeks or older born to HBsAg-positive mothers to complete the vaccine series after receipt of a birth dose of single-antigen hepatitis B vaccine and HBIG (2).
- Women admitted for delivery without documentation of HBsAg test results should have blood drawn and tested as soon as possible after admission.
- While test results are pending, all infants born to women without documentation of HBsAg test results should receive the first dose of single-antigen hepatitis B vaccine (without HBIG) at 12 hours of birth or earlier.
    1. If the mother is determined to be HBsAg-positive, her infant should receive HBIG as soon as possible but no later than the age of 7 days, and the vaccine series should be completed according to the recommended schedule for infants born to HBsAg-positive mothers.
    2. If the mother is determined to be HBsAg-negative, the vaccine series should be completed according to a recommended schedule for infants born to HBsAg-negative mothers.
    3. If the mother has never been tested to determine her HBsAg status, the vaccine series should be completed according to a recommended schedule for infants born to HBsAg-positive mothers. Administration of HBIG is not necessary for these infants.
- Because of the potentially decreased immunogenicity of vaccine in preterm infants weighing less than 2,000 g, these infants should receive both single-antigen hepatitis B vaccine and HBIG (0.5 mL) if the mother's HBsAg status cannot be determined at 12 hours of birth or earlier. The birth dose of vaccine should not be counted as part of the three doses required to complete the vaccine series; three additional doses of vaccine (for a total of four doses) should be administered according to a recommended schedule on the basis of the mother's HBsAg test result (2,11).

HUMAN PAPILLOMAVIRUS

Human papillomaviruses (HPVs) are a group of more than 120 different virus types. Approximately 40 HPV types are primarily sexually transmitted from person to person (e.g., genital–genital contact, oral–genital contact, and sexual intercourse), infecting the oral, anal, or genital areas of both men and women. Genital HPV infections are very common: by 50 years of age, 70% to 80% of women and a similar percentage of men will have acquired genital HPV infection. Most genital HPV infections cause no symptoms and are cleared by the immune system within a few weeks or months.

Thus, the vast majority of people recover from genital HPV infection uneventfully. However, some people develop persistent or chronic genital HPV infection, which can lead to development of genital warts and anogenital cancers, especially cervical cancer.

- Types 16 and 18 and others, known collectively as "high-risk" HPV types, may cause abnormal Pap tests and cervical cancer in women. Together types 16 and 18 cause approximately 70% of the cases of cervical cancer in the United States. Although there are a number of other risk factors for cervical cancer, being infected with a "high-risk" type HPV appears to be necessary to develop cervical cancer.
- In both men and women, "high-risk" HPV infections are also thought to cause 85% of anal cancers, 50% of other anogenital cancers, 20% of cancers of the throat and mouth, and 10% of cancers of the larynx and esophagus.
- Types 6 and 11 may cause genital warts. These two types of HPV are responsible for more than 90% of genital warts. These types may also spread from mother to infants during pregnancy or delivery and can rarely cause warts in the upper respiratory tract (throat, larynx) of the child (14,15).

VACCINE PREPARATION

Safe and effective virus-like-particle–derived recombinant vaccines have been developed against several HPV types associated with cervical cancer and genital warts. The HPV vaccine does not contain thimerosal.

AVAILABLE PRODUCTS

Product: Gardasil
Manufacturer: Merck
Year Licensed: 2006

A Quadrivalent Human Papillomavirus (Types 6, 11, 16, 18) Recombinant Vaccine was licensed by the FDA in 2006 for use in the United States.

Product: Cervarix (Types 16, 18)
Manufacturer: GlaxoSmithKline
Year Licensed in USA: 2009

Another vaccine is based on virus-like-particle of types 16 and 18 licensed by the FDA in 2009. Studies are currently in progress evaluating a vaccine consisting of large number of HPV types.

VACCINE EFFECTIVENESS

The efficacy of the HPV vaccine has been studied in women 16 to 26 years of age. In women who previously had not been exposed to the HPV types in the vaccine, the vaccine was 100% effective in preventing cervical precancers caused by the targeted HPV types and was nearly 100% effective in preventing vulvar and vaginal precancers and genital warts caused by the targeted HPV types.

If a female already has chronic infection with one of the HPV types, the vaccine will not prevent disease from that type.

Studies have shown that more than 99% of study participants developed antibodies after vaccination; antibody titers were higher for young girls than for older females participating in the efficacy trials. Routine vaccination against HPV is recommended for all girls 11 to 12 years of age. The vaccination series can be started in girls as young as 9 years of age. Catch-up vaccination is recommended for females 13 to 26 years of age who have not been vaccinated previously or who have not completed the full vaccine series, whether or not they have had sexual intercourse or previous evidence of HPV infection.

Women who are breast-feeding can receive the HPV vaccine. Moreover, immunocompromised women (from disease or medication) can receive the vaccine. However, the immune response to vaccination and vaccine effectiveness might be less than in women who are not immunocompromised.

Currently available HPV vaccine is not recommended for pregnant women since data on vaccination during pregnancy are limited. However, there is no evidence of risk to the fetus when a pregnant woman is inadvertently vaccinated; the manufacturer is maintaining a registry of pregnancy outcomes for this circumstance. Subjects with a history of immediate hypersensitivity to yeast or to any vaccine component should not receive the vaccine. Subjects with minor illnesses (e.g., diarrhea or mild upper respiratory tract infections, with or without fever) can receive the vaccine. However, those with moderate or severe acute illnesses should be deferred until after the illness improves.

VACCINE USAGE

Each dose of quadrivalent HPV vaccine is 0.5 mL, administered intramuscularly. It should be administered in a three-dose schedule (see Table 57.3). The second and third doses should be administered 2 and 6 months after the first dose. The quadrivalent HPV vaccine can be administered at the same visit when other age appropriate vaccines are provided, such as Tdap, Td, and MCV4.

ADVERSE EFFECTS

The HPV vaccine has been tested to date in more than 11,000 women (9 to 26 years of age) in many countries around the world, including the United States. These studies found that the HPV vaccine was safe and caused no serious side effects. Vaccine recipients experienced occasional pain, swelling, and redness at the injection sites.

Because these vaccines will only prevent infection with the two types of HPV that cause most cases of cervical cancer and the two types that most commonly cause genital warts, they are not expected to eliminate cancer nor genital warts related to other HPV types. Therefore, Pap screening and treatment programs for cervical cancer will still be needed. These vaccines are preventive and are expected to have no effect on preexisting infection with these HPV types. How long the vaccines will protect those who have been immunized remains to be determined (16,17).

INFLUENZA VIRUS VACCINE

Influenza virus infections affect more than 15% of children each winter, often in sharp, community-wide outbreaks. Infection causes substantial injury to the upper and lower respiratory tract, with high fever, conjunctivitis, coryza, sore throat, and prominent cough. Complications occur frequently and include otitis media, sinusitis, croup, bronchitis, and bronchopneumonia. Rarer complications include febrile convulsions, encephalopathy, and Reye syndrome. The infection spreads readily among school children and household members. Complications requiring medical care or hospitalization are more likely to occur in children younger than 2 years and in those of any age with debilitating lung or heart disease or other chronic conditions (18,19).

Immunization is recommended for children at increased risk of complications.

VACCINE PREPARATIONS

Currently licensed vaccines for children include either inactivated, nonreplicating split influenza viruses or live attenuated influenza virus vaccines. For inactivated vaccines, strains are grown in embryonated hen's eggs, then partially purified, inactivated with formalin, and disrupted with detergents. Formulations are typically trivalent, containing the three strains anticipated to spread during the following influenza season. Formulations are updated annually to match changes in circulating strains. Recent formulations have contained an influenza B strain and two influenza A strains (H_3N_2, H_1N_1). Full-dose formulations contain 15 μg of hemagglutinin antigen from each strain per 0.5-mL dose. Nonvaccine components in the vaccines may include residual egg proteins, traces of formalin, and the detergent splitting agent and thimerosal preservative, gelatin, and neomycin.

Inactivated vaccines are injected intramuscularly. They should be stored at 2°C to 8°C. A live, attenuated, trivalent vaccine (FluMist) for intranasal administration was recently licensed in the United States for use in healthy persons 2 to 49 years of age.

AVAILABLE PRODUCTS

Product: Fluarix
Manufacturer: GlaxoSmithKline
Year Licensed: 2005

Product FluMist
Manufacturer: MedImmune Vaccines
Year Licensed: 2003

Product: Fluvirin
Manufacturer: Chiron Corporation
Year Licensed: 1988

Product: Fluzone
Manufacturer: Aventis Pasteur
Year Licensed: 1978

Beginning in 2007, the FDA approved a formulation of FluMist that is stable on storage by refrigeration. FluMist and Fluarix do not contain thimerosal, and both Fluvirin and Fluzone are available with reduced thimerosal formulation. For information on the thimerosal content in these vaccines, visit the FDA Web site (www.fda.gov).

VACCINE EFFECTIVENESS

Each year, the influenza vaccine contains three virus strains, representing the influenza viruses thought to be most likely to circulate in the United States in the upcoming winter.

When the match between the virus strains in the vaccine and the circulating viruses is close, the vaccine prevents illness in up to 90% of healthy adults younger than 65 years. Among elderly people, the vaccine is about 30% to 70% effective in preventing disease, but it is 50% to 60% effective in preventing hospitalization and 80% effective in preventing influenza-related death in the elderly.

The vaccine protects between 45% and 90% of healthy children from getting influenza. Studies indicate that the older and healthier children, who have received the influenza vaccine, are more likely to be protected. Influenza vaccination has also been shown to decrease middle ear infections among young children by about 30%.

One goal for widespread influenza vaccine utilization in the United States is to decrease the transmission of influenza viruses. Epidemiologic studies have demonstrated that children have the highest rates of influenza virus infections, suggesting that universal immunization of children could result in transmission of these viruses within communities from persons providing care or who are household contacts of people who are high risk for complications form influenza (including young infants younger than 6 months for whom there is no effective vaccine and no licensed treatment), those with chronic diseases, and those who are older than 50 years (especially those who are older than 65 years) (19).

Of particular concern are health care workers who also commonly acquire influenza virus infections and who have transmitted influenza viruses in hospitals and long-term care facilities. Vaccination of health care workers has been associated with decreased deaths among nursing home residents, for example.

DOSE SCHEDULE

Trivalent inactivated vaccine (TIV) is given by the intramuscular route and live attenuated influenza vaccine (LAIV) is administered as a nasal spray (see Table 57.1). The formulations in multidose vials contain thimerosal as a preservative.

When young children (6 months until 9 years of age) are vaccinated against influenza for the first time, they should receive two doses of age-appropriate influenza vaccine given 1 month apart. Those children who received only one dose in their first year of vaccination should receive two doses in the following year. Two doses administered 4 weeks apart are also recommended for children 2 to 8 years of age who are receiving LAIV for the first time. For children 6 to 35 months of age, a half dose (0.25 mL) of TIV (injected) is recommended, in contrast with 0.5 mL which is the usual dose for everyone older than 3 years (see Tables 57.2 to 57.4) (11,19).

In the United States, Fluzone (Aventis Pasteur) may be administered to children as young as 6 months of age. Fluvirin (Novartis Corp.) should be given only to children 4 years of age and older because its efficacy in younger people has not been demonstrated. Fluarix, Flulaval, and Afluria are not licensed for use in children but are licensed for adults 18 years of age and older. LAIV (Flumist) should be given only to healthy children and adolescents, aged 2 to 17 years, and healthy adults, aged 18 to 49 years (2).

Children 9 years of age or older should receive one dose of influenza vaccine each year. Ideally, all persons in the United States should receive the influenza vaccine at the beginning of October through November each year, prior to the influenza season, which generally peaks during late December through early March. However, vaccination later in the season is considered worthwhile.

Influenza vaccine is recommended for all children older than 6 months, all adults older than 50 years, and all persons who work in the health care industry should be immunized annually. In addition, those at increased risk of developing complications from influenza should be immunized, including women who will be pregnant during the influenza season (November to April).

Influenza vaccine is recommended for all contacts of children younger than 5 years, including women who are breast-feeding. Women who are breast-feeding may receive either TIV or LAIV (unless LAIV is contraindicated because of other medical conditions). Vaccines should also be considered for those who can transmit influenza viruses to those at high risk for complications, including members of households with high-risk persons, including households that will include children younger than 6 months, persons coming in contact with children younger than 6 months, and persons who will come into contact with persons who live in nursing homes or other long-term care facilities.

In addition, influenza vaccine is recommended for children with long-term disorders of the lungs, heart, or circulation (including asthma or cystic fibrosis); metabolic diseases (including diabetes); kidney disorders; blood disorders (including anemia or sickle-cell disease); impaired immune systems (including immunosuppression caused by medications, malignancies, organ transplant, or human immunodeficiency virus [HIV] infection); and children who receive long-term aspirin therapy (and therefore have a higher chance of developing Reye syndrome if infected with influenza).

Influenza vaccine is encouraged for healthy people 6 years or older who plan to travel to foreign countries and areas where flu outbreaks may be occurring, such as the Tropics and the Southern Hemisphere from April through September; travel as part of large organized tourist groups that may include persons from areas of the world where influenza viruses are circulating; attend school or college and reside in dormitories or institutional settings; and wish to reduce their risk of becoming ill with influenza.

LAIV is not recommended for children younger than 2 years and adults older than 49 years, because safe use in these age groups has not been established; children and adolescents (2 to 17 years of age) receiving aspirin or aspirin-containing medications, because of the complications associated with aspirin and wild-type influenza virus infections in this age group; subjects with a history of asthma or other reactive airway diseases; persons with chronic underlying medical conditions that may predispose them to severe influenza infections; pregnant women; and subjects with a history of GBS.

LAIV is also not recommended for subjects who have had an anaphylactic reaction (allergic reactions that cause difficulty in breathing, which is often followed by shock) to eggs, egg products, or other components of the flu vaccine. There are antiviral agents which physicians can prescribe as an alternative for preventing influenza in such people (2,11). Children younger than 4 years should not receive Fluvirin 1 (Novartis International AG) as it has not been proven effective for this age group. LAIV should also not be given concurrently with other live-virus vaccines.

ADVERSE EFFECTS

The majority of those immunized with TIV will have no adverse reactions. Of those who do have a side effect, most will have soreness or tenderness at the injection site. Fewer than 1% of adults immunized will also experience fever, chills, or a general sense of feeling unwell that lasts for 1 to 2 days. Children are more likely to experience these symptoms.

In very rare cases (far less than 1 out of 10,000) serious reactions can occur. Subjects who have an allergy to eggs (which are used in making the vaccine) or any component of the vaccine are at greater risk for a serious allergic reaction.

Because of an increase in the frequency of GBS (a progressive disorder affecting the nervous system) associated with the 1976 swine flu vaccine, subsequent flu vaccines have been closely monitored (20). It has been estimated that about one case of GBS may occur per million persons immunized with TIV, although these cases may not be related to TIV. Persons not at high risk for developing complications from influenza, who have developed GBS within 6 weeks of a previous influenza shot, should avoid subsequent influenza shots. If the risk from influenza is high, they should be vaccinated with an age-appropriate inactivated influenza vaccine because the established benefits of the vaccine justify vaccination. LAIV should not be given to individuals who have a history of GBS because safety in those persons has not been investigated.

Influenza vaccines given as a nasal spray are being used for adults in Russia and have been under development in the United States since the 1960s. LAIV administered as a nasal spray was approved by the FDA in June of 2003. It is the first nasally administered vaccine to be marketed in the United States and the first live virus influenza vaccine approved in the United States. The possible advantages of this type of vaccine are that it is easy to administer, has the potential to induce a broad mucosal and systemic immune response, and has been shown to be approximately 87% effective in children. Although TIV and LAIV appear to have similar effectiveness and safety profiles, no study has directly compared the efficacy or effectiveness of TIV and trivalent LAIV (18).

When there is a major change in the influenza virus strain from one year to the next, epidemics or pandemics (world outbreaks) can occur. During the 20th century, there were four major pandemics; the worst caused 21 million deaths worldwide and 500,000 deaths in the United States from 1918 to 1919. Between 1957 and 1986 there were 19 different flu epidemics in the United States; several of the most recent caused more than 40,000 deaths.

JAPANESE ENCEPHALITIS VACCINE

Japanese encephalitis (JE), a mosquito-borne arboviral (Flavivirus) infection, is the leading cause of viral encephalitis in Asia (2,21). Infection leads to overt encephalitis in 1 in 20 to 1,000 infected cases. Encephalitis usually is severe, resulting in a fatal outcome in 25% of cases and residual neuropsychiatric sequelae in 50% of cases. JE acquired during the first or second trimester of pregnancy may cause intrauterine infection and miscarriage. Infections that occur during the third trimester of pregnancy have not been associated with adverse outcomes in newborns. The virus is transmitted in an enzootic cycle among mosquitoes and vertebrate amplifying hosts, chiefly domestic pigs and, in some areas, wild Ardeid (wading) birds. Viral infection rates in mosquitoes range from less than 1% to 3%. These species are prolific in rural areas where their larvae breed in ground pools and flooded rice fields.

Thus, all elements of the transmission cycle are prevalent in rural areas of Asia and human infections occur principally in this setting. Because vertebrate amplifying hosts and agricultural activities may be situated within and at the periphery of cities, human cases occasionally are reported from urban locations.

VACCINE PREPARATION

JE-VAX, Japanese Encephalitis Virus Vaccine Inactivated, is a sterile, lyophilized vaccine for subcutaneous use prepared by inoculating mice intracerebrally with JE virus, "Nakayama–NIH" strain, manufactured by The Research Foundation for Microbial Diseases of Osaka University (BIKEN). Infected brains are harvested and homogenized in phosphate buffered saline, pH 8.0. The homogenate is centrifuged and the supernatant inactivated with formaldehyde and then processed to yield a partially purified, inactivated virus suspension. This is further purified by ultracentrifugation through 40% w/v sucrose. The suspension is then lyophilized in final containers and sealed under dry nitrogen atmosphere. Thimerosal is added as a preservative to a final concentration of 0.007%. The diluent, which is sterile water, contains no preservative. Each 1.0 mL dose contains approximately 500 μg of gelatin, less than 100 μg of formaldehyde, less than 0.0007% v/v Polysorbate 80, and less than 50 ng of mouse serum protein. No myelin basic protein can be detected at the detection threshold of the assay (<2 ng per mL). Prior to reconstitution, the vaccine is a white caked powder, and after reconstitution the vaccine is a colorless transparent liquid (21).

VACCINE USAGE

JE-VAX is indicated for active immunization against JE for persons 1 year of age and older. JE-VAX should be considered for use in persons who plan to reside in or travel to areas where JE is endemic or epidemic during a transmission season. JE-VAX is NOT recommended for all persons traveling to or residing in Asia. The incidence of JE in the location of intended stay, the conditions of housing, nature of activities, duration of stay, and the possibility of unexpected travel to high-risk areas are the factors that should be considered in the decision to administer vaccine. In general, vaccination should be considered for persons spending a month or longer in epidemic or endemic areas during the transmission season, especially if travel will include rural areas. Depending on the epidemic circumstances, vaccine should be considered for persons traveling less than 30 days whose activities, such as extensive outdoor activities in rural areas, place them at particularly high risk for exposure (21).

A three-dose vaccination schedule is recommended for US travelers and military personnel on the basis of the CDC experience and a controlled immunogenicity trial performed with US military personnel. According to the CDC experience, neutralizing antibody is produced in fewer than 80% of US travelers who receive only two vaccine doses and antibody levels decline substantially in most vaccinees within 6 months. The US Army studied the immunogenicity of JE-VAX in 538 volunteers. Two three-dose regimens were evaluated (Day 0, 7, and 14 or Day 0, 7, and 30). All vaccine recipients demonstrated neutralizing antibodies at 2 months and 6 months after initiation of vaccination. The schedule of Day 0, 7, and 30 produced higher antibody responses than the Day 0, 7, and 14 schedule. Two hundred and seventy-three of the original study participants were tested at 12 months postvaccination and there was no longer a statistical difference in antibody titers between the two vaccination regimens.

The full duration of protection is unknown. Of US Army volunteers completing a three-dose regimen, 252 agreed to receive a booster dose of vaccine 1 year after the primary series. All boosted participants still had antibody 12 months after the booster. Protective levels of neutralizing antibody persisted for 24 months (2 years) in all 21 persons who had not received a booster. Definitive recommendations cannot be given on the timing of booster doses at this time (2).

VACCINE EFFECTIVENESS

The efficacy of the BIKEN Nakayama–NIH strain Japanese Encephalitis Virus Vaccine Inactivated was demonstrated in a placebo-controlled, randomized clinical trial in Thai children, sponsored by the US Army. In this trial, children between 1 and 14 years of age received BIKEN monovalent Nakayama–NIH strain (n = 21,628) or a bivalent vaccine containing the Nakayama–NIH and Beijing JE virus strains (n = 22,080) or tetanus toxoid as a placebo (n = 21,5160). Immunization consisted of two subcutaneous 1.0-mL doses of vaccine, except in children younger than 3 years who received two 0.5-mL doses (2). One case (5 cases per 100,000) of JE occurred in the monovalent vaccine group, one case (5 cases per 100,000) in the bivalent vaccine group, and 11 cases (51 cases per 100,000) in the placebo group. The observed efficacy of both monovalent and bivalent vaccines was 91% (95% confidence interval, 54% to 98%). Side effects of vaccination, including headache, sore arm, rash, and swelling, were reported at rates similar to those in the placebo group, usually less than 1%. Symptoms did not increase after the second dose. It should be noted that a schedule of two doses, separated by 7 days as employed in this trial, may be appropriate for use in residents of endemic or epidemic areas, where preexisting exposure to flaviviruses may contribute to the immune response (2).

ADVERSE REACTIONS

Adverse reactions to a prior dose of JE vaccine manifesting as generalized urticaria and angioedema are considered to be contraindications to further vaccination.

The decision to use JE-VAX should balance the risks for exposure to the virus and for developing illness, the availability and acceptability of repellents and other alternative measures, and the side effects of vaccination. Assessments should be interpreted cautiously because risk can vary within areas and from year to year and available data are incomplete. Estimates suggest that risk of JE in highly endemic areas during the transmission season can reach 1 per 5,000 per month of exposure; risk for most short-term travelers may be 1 per million or less. Although JE vaccine is reactogenic, rates of serious allergic reactions (generalized urticaria and/or angioedema) are low (approximately 1 to 104 per 10,000) (21).

Advanced age may be a risk factor for developing symptomatic illness after infection. JE acquired during pregnancy carries the potential for intrauterine infection and fetal death. These factors should be considered when advising elderly persons and pregnant women who plan visits to JE endemic areas.

There are no data on the safety and efficacy of JE vaccine in infants younger than 1 year. Whenever possible, immunization of infants should be deferred until they are 1 year of age or older (2,21).

LYME DISEASE

Lyme disease is caused by infection with *Borrelia burgdorferi*, a spiral-shaped (spirochetal) bacterium carried by deer ticks and western black-legged ticks. The ticks are often infected by feeding on the blood of the white-footed mice, white-tailed deer, or various species of birds (though these animals do not spread the disease to humans) (22).

Most (80% to 90%) of the people infected with Lyme disease develop one or more red, slowly expanding "bulls-eye" skin rashes at the tick-bite sites (erythema migrans). The rash is often accompanied by fatigue, fever, headache, stiff neck, muscle aches, and joint pain.

If diagnosed early, Lyme disease can be treated successfully with antibiotic. If the disease is left untreated, some people will develop more serious health problems such as arthritis, problems with the nervous system, pain in the large joints, and rarely, heart problems.

Lyme disease was first recognized in the United States in 1975. The number of annually reported cases of Lyme disease in the United States has increased approximately 25-fold since national surveillance began in 1982; during 1993 to 1997, a mean of 12,451 cases annually were reported by states to the CDC, and the incidence is increasing. The disease is mostly found in the northeastern, mid-Atlantic, and upper north-central regions of the United States, as well as several areas in northwestern California. Lyme disease is the most common vector-borne (spread from one host to another through a carrier such as a mosquito, fly, louse, or tick) disease in the United States (2,22).

VACCINE PREPARATIONS

In 1998, the Lyme disease vaccine, LYMErix, was approved for use in people 15 to 70 years of age. However, the vaccine was removed from the market by the manufacturer (GlaxoSmithKline) in February 2002 because of lack of demand.

KNOWN SIDE EFFECTS

The majority of those immunized (about 70% of those aged 15 to 70 years) experience no side effects. Of those who do develop side effects, most are mild and limited to the injection site, including soreness, redness, and swelling (23). Approximately 3% of those immunized experience fever, chills, or a general sense of feeling unwell that lasts for 1 to 2 days.

Although concern has been raised regarding the potential for vaccine-induced arthritis in recipients with the HLA-DR4 gene, no serious reactions have been confirmed. No vaccine is currently available for Lyme disease.

MEASLES

Measles is a serious disease caused by a highly contagious virus spread by large infectious droplets. Measles begins with fever followed by cough, runny nose, and conjunctivitis. Infections of the middle ear, pneumonia, croup, and diarrhea are common complications. Measles encephalitis occurs in 1 per 1,000 cases of natural measles, frequently resulting in significant brain damage in the survivors. Approximately 5% of children (500 out of 10,000) with measles will develop pneumonia. In addition, 1 to 3 of every 1,000 children who contract measles in the United States die from the disease. Subacute sclerosing panencephalitis (SSPE) is a rare fatal illness caused by ongoing measles virus infection of the brain. Symptoms of brain damage usually begin 7 to 10 years after infection. Death occurs 1 to 3 years after the onset of symptoms. Risk factors for developing SSPE include developing measles infection at a young age. The incidence of SSPE is estimated to be between 7 and 11 cases per 100,000 cases of measles. Measles vaccine is not associated with SSPE. Death is more common in infants, malnourished children, and among immunocompromised persons such as those with leukemia and HIV infection (24).

VACCINE PREPARATION

The first measles vaccine was licensed for use in the United States in 1963. Currently, measles vaccine is generally given in combination with mumps and rubella vaccines (MMR).

Originally, just one dose of MMR vaccine was recommended, and about 95% of children were protected. In 1989, the American Academy of Family Physicians, the American Academy of Pediatrics, and the CDC's Advisory Committee on Immunization Practices changed the recommendation to two doses so that almost all children (99.7%) would be protected. This change and a higher vaccination rate have nearly eliminated these three diseases in the United States (2,11).

AVAILABLE VACCINES

The measles vaccine is available as MMR (Measles–Mumps–Rubella), MMRV (Measles–Mumps–Rubella–Varicella Virus Vaccine Live), and Monovalent Measles (alone) (see Table 57.5).

AVAILABLE PRODUCTS

Product: ProQuad
Manufacturer: Merck
Year Licensed: 2005

Product: M-M-R II
Manufacturer: Merck
Year Licensed: 1971

Product: Attenuvax (Monovalent Measles)
Manufacturer: Merck
Year Licensed: 1963

VACCINE USAGE

Two doses of MMR vaccine are recommended for all children, including those who previously received the monovalent measles vaccine. The first dose is generally given at 12 to 15 months of age and the second dose is generally given at 4 to 6 years of age (see Tables 57.2 to 57.4). There must be a minimum of 4 weeks between doses. The second dose of MMR provides an added safeguard against all three diseases but is recommended primarily to prevent outbreaks of measles (2,11).

VACCINE EFFECTIVENESS

Ninety-five percent of those who receive the MMR or monovalent measles vaccine at 12 months of age or older are immune after the first dose. After the second dose, 99.7% of those immunized are protected. Immunity is lifelong.

Prior to licensure of the first measles vaccine in 1963, virtually every person in the United States contracted measles by the age of 20 years. Since the vaccine became available, there has been a 99% reduction in the incidence of measles. However, measles is still being "imported" from other countries. The most recent outbreaks occurred in the United States between 1989 and 1991, resulting in 755,000 cases and 123 reported deaths.

The vaccine is indicated for use in all infants 12 months of age or older. Monovalent measles vaccine is indicated for use in infants 6 to 12 months of age if there is a measles outbreak, though MMR may be used if this vaccine is unavailable; infants 6 to 11 months of age traveling to areas where measles is prevalent, though MMR may be used if this vaccine is unavailable; subjects who cannot receive one or both of the other vaccines included in MMR.

Administering the vaccine within 72 hours to people who have been exposed to measles may prevent them from developing the disease.

SIDE EFFECTS

Nearly all children who get the MMR vaccine (more than 80%) will have no side effects. Most children who develop side effects will have a mild reaction, such as soreness, redness or swelling at the site of injection, mild rash, mild to moderate fever, swelling of the lymph glands, and temporary pain, stiffness, or joint swelling.

In rare cases (far <1 child out of 10,000 given MMR), children have a serious reaction, such as lowered consciousness, coma, or hypersensitivity (anaphylaxis)—swelling inside the mouth, difficulty breathing, low blood pressure, and rarely, shock. Even more rarely, children may have developed transient thrombocytopenia. In extremely rare cases (less than 1 child out of 1,000,000 given measles vaccine) children have developed encephalitis 6 to 15 days after vaccination.

Measles and as a result MMR vaccine should not be administered to subjects with serious allergies to gelatin or any of the other components of the vaccine, women who are pregnant or trying to conceive, immunocompromised persons (with the exception of HIV-infected persons who have no symptoms of AIDS), and persons receiving chemotherapy or high doses of steroids. Subjects receiving blood products such as immune globulin should have the MMR vaccine deferred for 3 to 11 months depending on the blood product and dosage administered.

Concerns have been raised regarding the association of measles component of MMR vaccine and autism. However, the best available science indicates that the development of autism is unrelated to use of the MMR or any other vaccine. One small study seemed to postulate such a link but has subsequently been disproved by many other, larger studies. Ten of the thirteen authors of that study later retracted from their suggestion of a link between MMR vaccine and autism (2,28).

It is estimated that about 1 in every 22,000 MMR vaccinations could result in a child developing idiopathic thrombocytopenic purpura (ITP). ITP is rarely dangerous and is easily treated. ITP is generally much less serious than measles, mumps, or rubella. A recent study found that children who had ITP and later received the MMR vaccine had no vaccine-associated recurrences.

MENINGOCOCCAL VACCINE

N. meningitidis, or the meningococcus, is a bacterium that can cause a life-threatening bacteremia and or meningitis. Meningococcal disease is usually caused by groups A, B, C, Y, and W-135 of the meningococcus bacteria. Symptoms may include fever, stiff neck, sore throat, headache, muscle aches, joint pain and swelling, shock, and seizures. Complications include deafness, other neurologic impairment, and impaired circulation leading to gangrene and limb amputation. Death occurs in 10% to 14% of people with meningococcal disease and is highest in infants and adolescents (25,26).

There are approximately 2,600 cases of meningococcal meningitis in the United States each year, mostly in children younger than 5 years. Children younger than 2 years have the highest incidence, with a second peak incidence between 15 to 24 years of age. Close contacts of a person with meningococcal disease have a higher rate of infection and are at greatest risk in the first week of contact. Depending on the type of exposure some of these persons may be given antibiotics to prevent infection. Studies report that first-year college students living in dormitories have a somewhat elevated risk for meningococcal disease when compared with other undergraduate students. Large outbreaks of the disease are rare in the United States. Travelers to certain areas, particularly sub-Saharan Africa during the dry season (December through June) and travelers to Mecca during hajj may be at increased risk (26).

VACCINE PREPARATIONS

In 1978, the first meningococcal vaccines were licensed in the United States and were effective against only two of the major groups of meningococcus. Currently, licensed vaccines provide some protection against all groups except B; there is no licensed vaccine for group B in the United States

(27). In 2005, a new meningococcal diphtheria toxoid conjugated vaccine (MCV4) was licensed for subjects 11 to 55 years of age (see Table 57.6).

AVAILABLE PRODUCTS

Product: Menomune A/C/Y/W-135 (Meningococcal polysaccharide vaccine, Groups A, C, Y, and W-135 combination) (MPSV4)
Manufacturer: Aventis Pasteur
Year Licensed: 1981

Product: Menactra (Meningococcal polysaccharide [Serogroups A, C, Y, and W-135] Diphtheria Toxoid Conjugate Vaccine) (MCV4)
Manufacturer: Aventis Pasteur
Year Licensed: 2005

Menomune is available as single dose, which is thimerosal preservative-free, and 10-dose vials that contain 25 μg of thimerosal per 0.5 mL.

DOSE SCHEDULE

For children and adults 11 to 55 years of age a single vaccine dose is required. MCV4 is administered as 0.5 mL intramuscularly and MPSV4 as 0.5 mL subcutaneously (see Tables 57.2 and 57.3).

Revaccination with MCV4 should be considered for persons previously immunized with MPSV4, if they remain at increased risk for infection. If needed, children younger than 11 years may be revaccinated with MPSV4 in 2 to 3 years if they were first vaccinated before 4 years of age.

There is insufficient data available yet to guide recommendations on revaccination of persons who were previously vaccinated with MCV4.

MCV4 and MPSV4 may be administered concomitantly with other vaccines but at a different site of the body (11,26).

VACCINE EFFECTIVENESS

In older children and adults, the MPSV4 vaccine is 85% to 100% effective at preventing infection from the strains of the meningococcus used in the vaccine, and protection lasts for at least 3 years. Children younger than 2 years respond poorly to the vaccine (26).

Compared with MPSV4, MCV4 induces higher production of antibodies and protection is expected to last longer. Neither MPSV4 nor MCV4 would be expected to prevent serogroup B disease.

VACCINE USAGE

- MCV4 is the preferred vaccine and is recommended for individuals 11 to 55 years of age who are at increased risk for meningococcal disease (see Tables 57.2 and 57.3). If MCV4 is unavailable, MPSV4 is an acceptable alternative for this age group.
- MPSV4 is the only vaccine licensed for children 2 to 10 years of age.
- Currently, to more rapidly reduce disease among older adolescents, MCV4 is also recommended at high school entry (15 years of age).

The vaccine is also recommended for students living in close contact, such as in dormitories; US military recruits; subjects who might be affected during a meningococcal disease outbreak; travelers to certain parts of Africa and other locations where meningococcal disease is common; subjects with immune system disorders, terminal complement component deficiency, properdin deficiencies, or splenectomy; and laboratory personnel who are routinely exposed to the meningococcus. If at risk, MPSV4 can likely be safely given to pregnant women; however, there are no data for MCV4 given during pregnancy.

ADVERSE EFFECTS

More than half of those immunized with MPSV4 experience no adverse reactions. Mild reactions are experienced by up to 40% of those immunized and include pain and redness at the site of injection. Moreover, recipients may develop a fever after immunization. Local adverse reactions are more common among MCV4 recipients than among persons vaccinated with MPSV4 (2). In very rare cases (far less than 1 person out of 10,000), a more serious reaction to MPSV4, such as paresthesia, or an allergic response can occur (26).

The use of the vaccine is contraindicated in subjects who have had a serious reaction to previous meningococcal vaccination and in subjects who are known to be hypersensitive to any component of the vaccine or latex. MCV4 should not be given to someone known to be hypersensitive to diphtheria toxoid. It is not recommended that children younger than 11 years routinely receive the meningococcal vaccine because the infection rate among children is low, their immunity may be short-lived, and if they receive the vaccine early, subsequent doses of the vaccine may not protect them as well.

MPSV4 is to be administered subcutaneously, whereas MCV4 is to be administered intramuscularly. More than 100 persons have inadvertently received the MCV4 vaccine by the subcutaneous route, however. For a subset of these individuals, the CDC determined that—although the serologic responses were lower after MCV4 was administered subcutaneously compared to intramuscularly—the proportions of individuals who achieved antibody levels felt to be protective were similar. Therefore, the CDC did not recommend that those who had received MCV4 needed to be reimmunized (2,26).

Five cases of GBS have been reported in recipients of MCV4 (see *Morbidity and Mortality Weekly Report* (MMWR)) but it is uncertain whether they were causally related or coincidental (26).

MUMPS

Mumps is a viral infection spread from person to person by droplet. The infection begins usually with swelling and tenderness of one or more of the salivary glands. This lasts for about a week. Complications can include orchitis (20% to 50% of postpubertal males infected), brain involvement including aseptic meningitis (15% of cases), pancreatitis (2% to 5% of cases), and infection of ovaries (5% of postpubertal females). Permanent deafness may occur in about 1 per 2,000 cases.

Before widespread vaccination, there were about 200,000 cases of mumps and 20 to 30 deaths reported each year in the United States. In 1998, there were just 600 cases of mumps and no fatalities reported from the disease (2). Despite a high coverage rate with two doses of the mumps-containing vaccine, mumps outbreaks still occur. In particular, there is a group of students, roughly college-aged students, who may be less likely to have received both doses of the mumps vaccine and are incompletely vaccinated. Therefore, they are susceptible when infection is introduced and stand a higher chance of developing infections. In addition, although this is a very good vaccine, it is not perfect. About 10% of people who get both doses of the vaccine still remain susceptible to mumps.

VACCINE PREPARATIONS

The current "Jeryl Lynn" strain of mumps vaccine was developed by Dr. Maurice Hilleman, a human mumps virus isolate. This vaccine, combined with rubella or both rubella and measles vaccine (MMR), has been widely used worldwide (300 million doses given) since it was approved by the FDA in 1967 (see Table 57.6).

The mumps vaccine is available as

- MMR (Measles–Mumps–Rubella);
- MMRV (Measles–Mumps–Rubella–Varicella Virus Vaccine Live); and
- Monovalent Mumps (alone).

AVAILABLE PRODUCTS

Product: ProQuad (MMRV)
Manufacturer: Merck
Year Licensed: 2005

Product: M-M-R II
Manufacturer: Merck
Year Licensed: 1971

Product: Mumpsvax (Monovalent Mumps)
Manufacturer: Merck
Year Licensed: 1967. This vaccine is thimerosal-free.

VACCINE EFFECTIVENESS

Ninety-five percent of those who receive MMR or monovalent mumps vaccine at 1 year of age or older are immune after the first dose. Immunity is lifelong.

The use of vaccine is indicated for subjects who cannot receive one or both of the other vaccines included in MMR, and subjects who have proof of immunity to one or both of the other diseases that MMR prevents may receive the monovalent vaccine, though MMR is usually recommended (2).

DOSE SCHEDULE

The mumps vaccine is usually given with the measles and rubella vaccines in persons 12 to 15 months of age and older (see Tables 57.2 to 57.4).

Two doses of MMR vaccine administered on or after the first birthday are recommended for all children. The first dose is generally given at 4 to 6 years of age. There must be a minimum of 4 weeks between doses. The second dose of MMR provides an added safeguard against all three diseases but is recommended primarily to prevent outbreaks of measles (see Tables 57.2 to 57.4) (24).

ADVERSE EFFECTS

No serious side effects have been reported with mumps vaccine itself. However, the vaccine should not be used in subjects with serious allergies to gelatin or any of the other components of the vaccine. Women should not become pregnant within 1 month of receiving the monovalent mumps vaccine. The vaccine should not be used in immunocompromised persons (with the exception of HIV-infected persons who have no symptoms of AIDS, as noted above) and persons receiving cancer chemotherapy or high doses of steroids (2).

PERTUSSIS VACCINE

Pertussis (whooping cough) is a prolonged cough illness caused by *Bordetella pertussis* bacteria. Forceful coughing spells (paroxysms) are a distinctive feature in children, often ending with a loud intake of breath (whoop) or vomiting (30). Complications include otitis media, pneumonia, weight loss, and acute encephalopathy (rate 1 in 1,000 cases). Infants younger than 6 months may develop apnea episodes or fatal pneumonia. Infection is highly contagious during the first weeks of illness. Pertussis has been controlled by immunization since the 1950s, with recent incidence rates averaging less than 5% of rates during the preimmunization era. Nevertheless, thousands of cases are still reported annually, with albeit few fatalities. Infection is relatively common among adolescents and young adults as protection from childhood immunization wanes. These older age groups are a major reservoir of the disease and an important source of transmission to infants (30).

VACCINE PREPARATIONS

In the United States, only acellular pertussis vaccines are recommended for routine use. These vaccines contain only specific proteins purified from *B. pertussis* and adsorbed on aluminum adjuvants. These include inactivated pertussis toxin and additional proteins involved in surface attachment, such as filamentous hemagglutinin, pertactin, and fimbriae (30).

Acellular pertussis vaccine is usually combined with diphtheria and tetanus toxoids (DTaP) and may also include Hib conjugate, hepatitis B, or inactivated poliovirus vaccine (DTaP·IPV) (see Table 57.5). Products contain thimerosal or 2-phenoxyethanol preservative (see product monographs). These vaccines are administered intramuscularly in a 0.5-mL dose. They should be stored at 2°C to 8°C, avoiding freezing.

AVAILABLE VACCINES

No pertussis-only vaccine is available. The pertussis vaccine is available as (see Table 57.5)

- DTaP (Diphtheria Toxoid-Tetanus Toxoid-acellular Pertussis) vaccine;
- DTaP in combination with Hib vaccine;
- DTaP in combination with hepatitis B and inactivated polio vaccines;
- DTaP in combination with Hib, hepatitis B, and inactivated polio vaccines; and
- TdaP (Tetanus Toxoid reduced-Diphtheria-acellular Pertussis vaccine) (30,31).

Vaccines containing the whole cell pertussis component (DTP) are no longer recommended for use in the United States and are not listed here, although they are used in many other countries. Vaccines containing lower amounts of diphtheria toxoid—abbreviated with a small d—are utilized in persons 7 years of age or older. Pertussis component-containing vaccines are not available for children 7–9 years of age.

AVAILABLE PRODUCTS

Product: Tripedia (DTaP)
Manufacturer: Sanofi Pasteur
Year Licensed: 2001

Product Name: Infanrix (DTaP)
Manufacturer: GlaxoSmithKline
Year Licensed: 1997

Product: TriHIBit (DTaP and Hib conjugate vaccine)
Manufacturer: Sanofi Pasteur
Year Licensed: 2001

Product: DAPTACEL (DTaP)
Manufacturer: Sanofi Pasteur
Year Licensed: 2002

Product: Pediarix (DTaP, hepatitis B, and inactivated polio vaccines)
Manufacturer: GlaxoSmithKline
Year Licensed: 2002

Product: BOOSTRIX (Tetanus Toxoid, Reduced Diphtheria Toxoid and Acellular Pertussis Vaccine, Adsorbed for use in 10- to 18-year-old persons) (Tdap)
Manufacturer: GlaxoSmithKline
Year Licensed: 2005

Product: ADACEL (Tetanus Toxoid, Reduced Diphtheria Toxoid and Acellular Pertussis Vaccine, Adsorbed for use in 11- to 64-year-old persons) (Tdap)
Manufacturer: Sanofi Pasteur
Year Licensed: 2005

Product: Pentacel (DTap, Hib conjugate, hepatitis B, and inactivated polio vaccines)
Manufacturer: Sanofi Pasteur
Year Licensed: 2008

VACCINE USAGE

Doses are recommended to be given at 2, 4, 6, and 15 to 18 months, with a second booster dose at 4 to 6 years (see Tables 57.2 to 57.4) (33). When more rapid protection is desired, the first three doses can be given at 4-week intervals and the fourth dose given as soon as 6 months after the third dose. The dosing sequence for children not immunized in early infancy is as follows: first dose, second dose 2 months later, third dose 2 months later, fourth dose 6 to 12 months later, and final dose at 4 to 6 years, unless the fourth dose was given after 4 years of age (35) (see Table 57.3). DTaP vaccines are not recommended for children 7 years of age or older. Licensure of vaccines to boost immunity to pertussis in adolescents and adults is expected in the near future. Duration of protection has not yet been determined (2,31).

VACCINE EFFECTIVENESS

In large controlled trials, DTaP vaccination of infants reduced the risk of pertussis substantially (average reduction about 85% compared with placebo). Efficacy generally matched or exceeded that of whole-cell pertussis vaccines included in the trials. Nearly all infants have antibodies to the pertussis proteins after the third immunization, but a serologic correlate of protection has not been defined. Where acellular pertussis vaccines have been used routinely, disease control has been satisfactory in the immunized populations (33,34).

ADVERSE EFFECTS

Acellular pertussis vaccines have a substantially improved safety profile compared with previously used whole-cell pertussis vaccines. Adverse effects in young infants are infrequent and mild, consisting mainly of transient fever (in 10% to 15%) and injection-site discomfort. Booster doses are more often associated with injection-site erythema and swelling, particularly the fifth consecutive dose at 4 to 6 years. In the latter setting about 25% of children have moderate to severe redness or swelling at the injection site, but this is generally well tolerated, with minimal discomfort (30).

Use of acellular pertussis vaccines has been associated with a substantial decrease in reports of postimmunization febrile seizure or hypotonic–hyporesponsive episodes (fainting-like spells of brief duration). Anaphylactic reactions to DTaP vaccines are rare but pose a contraindication to further use. Repeat dosing after a postimmunization febrile convulsion or hypotonic–hyporesponsive episode is not contraindicated because the recurrence risk is low, whether DT or DTaP is given (30,35).

PNEUMOCOCCAL VACCINES

Streptococcus pneumoniae bacteria commonly colonize the upper airway of infants and young children, persisting for several months. Pneumococci cause opportunistic infections of the respiratory tract including purulent conjunctivitis, sinusitis, otitis media, bronchitis, and bronchopneumonia (37). Pneumococci are the leading bacterial cause of otitis media, pneumonia, and invasive bloodstream infections, including purulent meningitis. Most pneumococcal infections of children occur early in life (6 to 23 months of age) (37). The risk of infection is increased by several factors, including premature delivery, presence of chronic medical conditions, lack of breast-feeding, household crowding, and day care attendance. High rates of infection are observed in some aboriginal communities, such as Alaskan Native and Navajo communities. Children with anatomic or functional asplenia are prone to severe sepsis (37,38).

Immunity to pneumococcal infection depends mainly upon antibodies to the capsular polysaccharide of organisms, which enhance opsonization and killing by phagocytic cells. However, children younger than 2 years respond poorly to polysaccharide antigens. More than 90 distinct serotypes exist, although clinical disease is associated with fewer serotypes, which have been incorporated in different vaccine preparations.

VACCINE PREPARATIONS

Two types of pneumococcal vaccine are available, as follows:

Seven-Valent Pneumococcal Conjugate Vaccine (Prevnar)

This product contains purified capsular polysaccharide from the seven types of pneumococci that most often cause disease in young children (41–43), including types 4, 6B, 9 V, 14, 18 C, 19 F, and 23 F, covalently linked (i.e., conjugated) to CRM_{197}, a nontoxic mutant of diphtheria toxin. Each 0.5-mL dose of liquid suspension contains 16 μg of total polysaccharide and 20 μg of CRM_{197} protein, adsorbed on aluminum phosphate adjuvant, without preservative. Vaccine should be stored at 2°C to 8°C, avoiding freezing.

Twenty-Three Valent Polysaccharide Vaccine (Pneumovax, Pnu-Immune)

These products contain 25 μg of purified capsular polysaccharide (PPS) from each of 23 serotypes that commonly cause infection in children and adults. About 90% of cases of pneumococcal bacteremia and meningitis are caused by these 23 types. Dosage is 0.5 mL of the liquid suspension, injected subcutaneously or intramuscularly. Products contain thimerosal or phenol preservative (see product monographs). Products are stored at 2°C to 8°C.

AVAILABLE PRODUCTS

Product: Pneumovax 23 (PPS)
Manufacturer: Merck
Year Licensed: 1977

Product: Pnu-Immune 23 (PPS)
Manufacturer: Wyeth
Year Licensed: 1979

Product: Prevnar 7 (Conjugate)
Manufacturer: Wyeth
Year Licensed: 2000

VACCINE USAGE

Conjugate pneumococcal vaccine is recommended for routine administration to all children up to 23 months of age (see Tables 57.2 to 57.4). It is also recommended for children 24 to 59 months of age who are at increased risk of invasive pneumococcal infection. These include children with sickle-cell disease and other hemoglobin disorders, anatomic or functional asplenia, HIV infection, chronic medical conditions (e.g., functionally significant heart or lung disease, diabetes mellitus, spinal fluid leakage, and cochlear implant hearing device), and impaired immune function (including nephrotic syndrome, malignancies, long-term corticosteroid treatment, solid-organ transplants, and primary immunodeficiencies). When feasible, conjugate pneumococcal vaccine should be considered for all other children up to 59 months of age, particularly those who attend group day care facilities.

The recommended schedule for infants is four doses of conjugate vaccine, given at 2, 4, 6, and 12 to 15 months of age. The same recommendation is made for infants of low birth weight, whose first dose should be given at about 8 weeks of chronological age (see Tables 57.2 to 57.4). Children who first receive the conjugate vaccine after 6 months of age require fewer doses. After 24 months of age, one dose is sufficient for healthy children (2,11).

The dosage of conjugate vaccine is 0.5 mL, given by intramuscular injection. The conjugate vaccine can be given concurrently with other vaccines routinely administered to infants, at separate anatomic sites.

The 23-valent pneumococcal polysaccharide vaccine is used only in special circumstances in children (12). It is not recommended for use in children younger than 24 months because most fail to respond. Children 24 to 59 months of age can respond to the polysaccharide vaccine, but it is best used as a booster dose following age-appropriate immunization with conjugate vaccine in children who need broader protection because of a high risk of infection (e.g., asplenia, sickle-cell disease). Pneumococcal polysaccharide vaccine is recommended for children 6 years or older who are at high risk of infection, as it offers suitably broad protection (see Table 57.2). Polysaccharide vaccines are given by subcutaneous or intramuscular injection (see Table 57.1).

VACCINE EFFECTIVENESS

A large prelicensure controlled trial in California (42) demonstrated that pneumococcal conjugate vaccine given to infants (at 2, 4, 6, and 12 to 15 months) substantially reduced the subsequent risk of invasive pneumococcal infection (vaccine types, 97%; all types, 89%). Vaccinees also had fewer radiologically confirmed pneumonia episodes (by 21%) and otitis media episodes (by 7%) compared with control subjects. Vaccinated children are less likely to be colonized with vaccine serotypes. Routine use in infants and young children has markedly reduced the frequency of invasive infections. Routine use is expected to curb the spread of antibiotic-resistant strains, as most belong to types included in the conjugate vaccine. However, there is evidence of rising frequency of nonvaccine pneumococcal types, particularly serotype 19A.

ADVERSE EFFECTS

The conjugate vaccine is generally well tolerated (43). Minor adverse effects include fever and injection-site redness, swelling, and tenderness. Few serious adverse effects have been reported. Reactions to the polysaccharide vaccine are usually mild, consisting of redness and tenderness at the injection site. Anaphylactic reaction to a previous dose is a contraindication to further immunization. Recent observations have suggested emergence of human disease with other pneumococcal serotypes, not included in current vaccine formulation.

POLIOVIRUS VACCINES (INACTIVATED)

Poliomyelitis is a highly contagious disease caused by three distinct poliovirus, serotypes. Most infections cause asymptomatic or benign febrile illnesses, but about 1 infection in 1,000 results in paralytic disease. Destruction of anterior horn cells and motor neurons in the brain stem and/or spinal cord can compromise breathing and swallowing and cause acute flaccid limb paralysis. Three serotypes of poliovirus exist, designated types 1, 2, and 3, with type 1 most often causing paralytic disease. Infection spreads by person-to-person contact or through fecal contamination of water or food supplies. Humans are the only reservoir for poliovirus.

Paralytic poliomyelitis has been the focus of intensive, global disease eradication efforts, based on immunizing nearly all of the world's children. Polio was declared eliminated from the Western Hemisphere in 1994, but cases continue to occur in a few countries in Africa and Asia. Until global disease eradication is achieved, all children should continue to be immunized against polio. In the United States, this is accomplished most safely using IPVs, which have replaced live, oral, attenuated vaccines-oral polio vaccine (OPV) in routine use (44,45).

VACCINE PREPARATIONS

Two types of poliovaccine (OPV and IPV) were developed in the 1950s. Both were highly effective in preventing polio. Initially OPV was preferred because it helped increase community immunity to polio. However, about 1 out of 2.5 million doses of OPV distributed in the United States were associated with vaccine-associated paralytic polio. In an effort to reduce this side effect, a new polio vaccine schedule was recommended in 1997 (two doses of IPV followed by two doses of OPV). The new schedule decreased but did not guarantee elimination of vaccine-induced paralytic polio; so, effective in the year 2000, an all-IPV schedule was recommended, and OPV is no longer administered in the United States. However, OPV continues to be used in countries where wild polio infections still occur (29,45).

Inactivated poliovirus vaccines contain formalin-inactivated viruses from each of types 1 through 3 in enhanced-potency formulations. Viruses are grown in cell cultures (monkey kidney or human diploid cells, depending on the product), purified, and inactivated with formalin. Streptomycin, polymyxin B, and/or neomycin may be present in small amounts from the cell culture medium. The preservative used is 2-phenoxyethanol (not thimerosal). IPV vaccines are available alone or in combination with diphtheria and tetanus toxoids and acellular pertussis vaccines (DTaP·IPV). IPV products are injected subcutaneously in a dose of 0.5 mL. They should be stored at 2°C to 8°C.

The polio vaccine is available as Polio Vaccine Inactivated (IPV), IPV in combination with DTaP (Diphtheria–Tetanus–acellular Pertussis), and hepatitis B vaccines (see Table 57.5).

AVAILABLE PRODUCTS

Product: IPOL (Polio Vaccine Inactivated-IPV)
Manufacturer: Aventis Pasteur
Year Licensed: 1990

Product: Pediarix (IPV, DTaP, and hepatitis B vaccines)
Manufacturer: GlaxoSmithKline
Year Licensed: 2003

VACCINE USAGE

All children should receive four doses of IPV, at ages 2, 4, and 6 to 18 months and 4 to 6 years (see Tables 57.2 to 57.4) (46). The first two doses provide primary immunization, and the third and fourth doses boost protection. When combination vaccines are used, an "extra" dose is often given for convenience at 6 months of age. IPV can be given concurrently with other routinely recommended vaccines, at separate injection sites (2).

VACCINE EFFECTIVENESS

Among children given three doses of IPV (at 2, 4, and 18 months of age), 99% to 100% develop serum antibody to all three types of poliovirus. More than 90% develop antibody after two doses. Protection is expected to be long-lived. Countries that relied on IPV exclusively were able to eliminate disease.

ADVERSE EFFECTS AND CONTRAINDICATIONS

IPV is generally well tolerated, causing minimal adverse effects. IPV should not be given to children who experienced an anaphylactic reaction to a previous dose of IPV or to streptomycin, polymyxin B, or neomycin. IPV can be given during pregnancy if immediate protection is required.

IPV is the only polio vaccine recommended for children with impaired immunity and their household members. While IPV is safe for immunocompromised children, protection cannot be assured. Breast-feeding or maternal antibodies do not interfere with responses to IPV (2).

POLIOVIRUS VACCINE (LIVE-ORAL)

OPV contains live attenuated poliovirus types 1, 2, and 3 produced in monkey kidney cells or other cell cultures. Immunization with three or more doses of the vaccine induces excellent serum and secretory immune response and has been largely responsible for elimination of poliomyelitis in the United States and most other parts of the world.

Batches of polio vaccine used between 1955 and 1963 were later found to be contaminated with a virus that infects monkeys, called simian virus 40 (SV40). Studies to date have shown that those who received OPV containing SV40 are not at additional risk of complications, though scientific research is continuing. OPV produced since 1963 does not contain SV40. However, because of the fact that administration of OPV has been associated with paralytic polio due to reversion of attenuated vaccine strain to virulent phenotypes, its use has been discontinued in all countries where paralytic poliomyelitis has been eradicated. OPV is still used in a few countries where paralytic poliomyelitis continues to remain active in small endemic areas. Postvaccine experience from developed nations with OPV has shown that immunization with three doses of trivalent OPV induces protective immune response in more than 95% of children. However, when the vaccine has been administered in developing nations, the response has been significantly lower with less reliable seroconversion and antibody response especially for poliovirus type 3 serotype. The reason for the less consistent response among children in developing countries is not clear; however, most studies have concentrated on the potential role of competing enteric virus infections. Some studies have also evaluated the role of nutritional status, for example, the effect of vitamin A supplementation on the immunogenicity of OPV (29,32,47).

No OPV vaccine is currently available in the United States and other countries in the Western Hemisphere (2).

RABIES VACCINE

Rabies is an acute and almost uniformly fatal disease caused by a viral infection of the central nervous system. The rabies virus is most often spread by a bite and saliva from an infected (rabid) animal (e.g., bats, raccoons, skunks, foxes, ferrets, cats, or dogs). In the United States, rabies is most often associated with bat exposures. However, there have been rare cases in which laboratory workers and explorers in caves inhabited by millions of bats were infected by rabies virus in the air. Virtually 100% of those infected with rabies who do not receive the vaccine will die.

Although fewer than 10 human rabies fatalities occur in the United States annually, as many as 40,000 Americans receive the vaccine each year after contact with animals suspected of being rabid. An additional 18,000 people get the vaccine before exposure as a preventative measure.

Worldwide, at least 4 million subjects are vaccinated each year for rabies. The number of deaths that rabies causes each year is estimated to be at least 40,000, and as high as 70,000 if higher case estimates are used for densely populated countries in Africa and Asia where rabies is epidemic. Where data are available, there is consistent evidence that between 30% and 60% of human rabies cases occur in children younger than 15 years (48).

VACCINE PREPARATION

The first rabies vaccine was developed in early 1968; current rabies vaccine licensed for human use in the United States is derived from human diploid cell cultures or purified chick embryos.

The vaccine is available as inactivated products prepared in human diploid cell culture (HDCV), or purified chick embryo cell culture (PCEC).

AVAILABLE PRODUCTS

Product: Imovax Rabies (HDCV for pre- or postexposure)
Manufacturer: Aventis Pasteur
Year Licensed: 1980

Product: RabAvert (PCEC for pre- or postexposure)
Manufacturer: Chiron Vaccines
Year Licensed: 1997

Preexposure rabies vaccines are administered by a series of three injections:

- The first dose may be given at any time.
- The second dose should be given 7 days later.
- The third dose should be given 21 or 28 days after the first dose.
- Booster doses of vaccine are recommended every 2 years for those individuals who continue to be at increased risk of contracting rabies to maintain protective antibody levels. People who work with live rabies virus in laboratory settings should be tested every 6 months to ensure that they have adequate antibody levels and should receive boosters as necessary.

When postexposure rabies vaccines are administered:

- The number of doses required is determined by the previous immunization status of the individual.
- *Previously unvaccinated people* should receive the vaccine at 0, 3, 7, 14, and 28 days. They should also receive rabies immune globulin at the same time as the first dose of the vaccine to provide rapid protection that persists until the vaccine works.
- *Previously vaccinated people* should receive two doses of the vaccine—the first immediately, the other 3 days later. Rabies immune globulin is unnecessary and should not be given. An immunized person is anyone who has received a complete series of vaccine, or a person who has received a preexposure or postexposure series of any rabies vaccine who has an adequate rabies antibody.

VACCINE EFFECTIVENESS

All rabies vaccines licensed in the United States induce protective antibody levels after 3 doses in nearly 100% of recipients. However, previously immunized subjects must still receive 2 to 3 additional doses of the vaccine if reexposed to the virus. The vaccine is 100% effective under such circumstances as well (49).

ADVERSE REACTIONS

Mild reactions such as pain, redness, swelling, or itching at injection site are reported among 30% to 74% of those vaccinated. Headache, nausea, abdominal pain, muscle aches, and dizziness are reported in 5% to 40% of those vaccinated (49).

Serious events after current vaccine preparations are rare. However, allergic reactions including swelling and mild difficult breathing developed in 6% of patients who received booster doses of Human Diploid Cell Rabies Vaccine. In addition, three cases of neurologic illness resembling GBS, a progressive disorder affecting the nervous system, have been reported in people who receive the Human Diploid Cell Rabies Vaccine. In these cases, all patients recovered within 3 months (2,49).

Effective rabies control measures include routine immunization of dogs, cats, and ferrets, and control of stray dogs and selected wildlife. A fully vaccinated dog or cat is unlikely to become infected or to transmit rabies (2,48).

ROTAVIRUS

Rotaviruses are intestinal viruses that infect virtually all children by 3 years of age. It is the most common cause of diarrhea in children, including hospital-acquired diarrhea; childcare center outbreaks are common. The illness often also includes fever and vomiting, lasting for a week or longer and can cause persistent infection in immunocompromised people. Most rotavirus infections are mild, but about 1 in 50 cases develop severe dehydration. Each year in the United States, rotavirus infections result in the hospitalization of more than 50,000 infants younger than 2 years. In developing countries, rotavirus leads to an estimated 480,000 to 640,000 deaths each year (50).

Rotaviruses are segmented, double-stranded RNA viruses belonging to the family Reoviridae, with at least seven distinct antigenic groups (A through G). Group A viruses are the major causes of rotavirus diarrhea worldwide. Serotyping is based on the VP7 glycoprotein (G) and VP4 protease-cleaved hemagglutinin (P); G types 1 through 4 and 9 and P types 1A and 1B are most common.

VACCINE PREPARATIONS

The first rotavirus vaccine was a tetravalent, reassortant rhesus-human rotavirus vaccine licensed by the FDA in August 1998. However, in July 1999, after approximately 1 million children had been immunized with that vaccine, the CDC suspended its recommendation because of an increase in the number of children who developed "intussusceptions." Investigators calculated that the risk of intussusceptions attributable to the vaccine was about 1 per 10,000 infants vaccinated, which was about three times higher than for unvaccinated children. This vaccine was voluntarily withdrawn from the market by the manufacturer in October 1998. Those who received the vaccine in 1998 and 1999 do not have a continuing risk of developing intussusception. Subsequently, two additional vaccines were licensed in the United States; *RV5*, a pentavalent live vaccine (G 1,2,3,4, P8) contained five reassortant types developed for human and bovine parent rotavirus strains and share neutralizing epitope identity with G1, G2, G3, G4, and P8. *RV1* is also a live attenuated vaccine that contains one strain of live attenuated human rotavirus, a G1 P(8) strain. RV1 shares neutralizing epitope identity with G1, G3, G4, and G9 through the P(8) VP4 protein. RV1 does not share neutralizing identity with G2 P(4) strains (51,52).

AVAILABLE PRODUCTS

Product: RotaTeq
Manufacturer: Merck
Year Licensed: 2006

Product: RotaRix
Manufacturer: GlaxoSmithKline
Year Licensed: 2008

VACCINE USAGE

RotaTeq requires a three-dose primary series and administered at 2, 4 and 6 months of age. However, RotaRix requires only a two-dose primary series and is administered at 2 and 4 months of age. The first dose of rotavirus vaccine should be given between the ages of 6 and 14 weeks. Doses should be given at least 4 weeks apart. The final dose of rotavirus vaccine should be given before 8 months of age (see Table 57.2)(11,52).

Rotavirus vaccine may be given at the same time as other childhood vaccines.

VACCINE EFFICACY

Both RotaTeq and RotaRix have been shown to be effective against rotavirus gastroenteritis of any severity and both have high efficacy against severe rotavirus gastroenteritis. The vaccine has been recommended for use in all full-term infants who should begin the series between the ages of 6 and 14 weeks of age. Breast-fed infants can receive rotavirus vaccine.

There is limited information on the immunization of infants born at less than 37 weeks of gestation but consideration should be given for immunization of these children because they may be at increased risk for hospitalization from gastroenteritis in the first year of life.

ADVERSE REACTIONS

Children may be more likely to experience mild, temporary diarrhea or vomiting with 7 days after getting a dose of rotavirus vaccine than children who have not gotten the vaccine.

No moderate or severe reactions have been associated with these vaccines.

Rotavirus vaccines currently licensed in the United States should not be used in subjects with severe life threatening reactions to previous disease or subjects who have had life-threatening allergic reaction to latex rubber should not receive the RotaRix vaccine which is packaged in a latex applicator.

There is no safety information for administration of rotavirus vaccine to infants who are immunocompromised. However, both children and adults who are immunocompromised because of congenital immunodeficiency or following transplantation can experience severe and potentially fatal rotavirus gastroenteritis (51,52).

Infants who have received blood products should have the vaccine postponed for 6 weeks unless that delay might make the child ineligible for vaccination because of age. There is no safety information for administration of rotavirus vaccine to infants with gastroenteritis. It is recommended that rotavirus vaccine not be administered to infants with acute, moderate to severe gastroenteritis but be considered for administration to infants with mild gastroenteritis if the delay might make the child ineligible for vaccination because of age. Rotavirus vaccination series should not be initiated after 15 weeks of age.

These vaccinations should not be administered after 7 months of age because of insufficient data on vaccine safety in children who are 8 months of age and older. Vaccine should not be readministered after regurgitation or spitting out of a vaccine dose.

The risk of intussusceptions after vaccination with RotaTeq or RotaRix was evaluated in many thousands of children during the clinical trials preceding licensure. Those who received the vaccine were not at an increased risk of developing the disease than were those in the control group (51,52). However, additional postlicensure data are being collected to confirm that these vaccines are not associated with intussusceptions at a very low rate. Some cases of Kawasaki disease were identified in children younger than 1 year who had received the RotaTeq vaccine during clinical trials conducted before the vaccine was licensed. The number of Kawasaki disease reports does not exceed the number of cases expected to be seen on the basis of the usual occurrence of Kawasaki disease in children. There is no safety information related to the administration of vaccine to infants with preexisting gastrointestinal disease but vaccine might be considered for these infants if they are not receiving immunosuppressive drugs.

RUBELLA

Rubella is caused by an RNA virus that is transmitted from person to person by droplets. Rubella usually is a mild illness. Symptoms include low-grade fever and swollen lymph nodes in the back of the neck followed by a generalized rash. Complications may include joint pain, arthritis, temporary decrease in platelets, and encephalitis. Temporary arthritis may occur, particularly in adolescents and adult women. However, rubella in expectant women often leads to congenital rubella syndrome (CRS) in their fetuses. This is a disease characterized by deafness, mental retardation, cataracts and other eye defects, heart defects, and diseases of the liver and spleen that may result in thrombocytopenia. The incidence and severity of congenital defects are greater if infection occurs during the first month of gestation (2).

VACCINE PREPARATIONS

The rubella vaccine was first introduced in childhood immunizations in late 1960, with HPV-77 virus strain grown on dog kidney (HPV77/DK) or duck embryo (HPV77 DE/5) or with other live attenuated strains. These vaccines were found to be more reactogenic with high incidence of arthritis associated with vaccination especially in young children. Subsequently, Wistar strain of rubella virus RA27/3 was licensed for routine immunization in the United States and has continued to be the virus strain employed for current routine immunization with the combined mumps–measles–rubella (MMR) vaccine currently; the rubella vaccine is available as (see Table 57.6) (36,39)

- MMR (Measles–Mumps–Rubella);
- MMRV (Measles–Mumps–Rubella–Varicella Virus Vaccine Live);
- Rubella (alone).

AVAILABLE PRODUCTS

Product: ProQuad (MMRV)
Manufacturer: Merck
Year Licensed: 2005

Product: M-M-R II
Manufacturer: Merck
Year Licensed: 1971

Product: Meruvax II (Rubella)
Manufacturer: Merck
Year Licensed: 1969. This vaccine is thimerosal-free.

All MMR vaccines are available containing no thimerosal.

VACCINE USAGE

In the United States, the rubella vaccine is usually given with the measles and mumps vaccines in persons 12 to 15 months of age and older (2).

Two doses of MMR vaccine administered on or after the first birthday are recommended for all children. The first dose is generally given at 12 to 15 months of age and the second dose is generally given at 4 to 6 years of age (see Tables 57.2 to 57.4). There must be a minimum of 4 weeks between doses. The second dose of MMR provides and added safeguard against all three diseases but is recommended primarily to prevent outbreaks of measles.

Susceptible women should receive the rubella vaccine or MMR at least 28 days before getting pregnant to prevent CRS—a devastating disease that affects the babies of susceptible women exposed to rubella during their pregnancy. CRS can result in neonatal deafness, mental retardation, cataracts and other eye defects, heart defects, and hepatitis (2,53).

Because of the risk of CRS, it is particularly important that postpubertal women be immune to rubella. Routine screening of pregnant women for rubella immunity is recommended and susceptible individuals should be vaccinated when it is known that they are not pregnant. Vaccination in case of susceptible pregnant women is often given immediately after giving birth.

People susceptible to rubella working in educational institutions and childcare centers should be immunized to prevent transmission of rubella virus to pregnant women, as well as for their own protection.

Frequently, it is believed that members of the following groups should not receive the vaccine. In fact, susceptible members may still receive the vaccine: women who are breast-feeding; individuals who have HIV infection but no symptoms of AIDS; and susceptible children whose mothers or other household members are pregnant, as immunizing these contacts presents no risk to the pregnant individual.

VACCINE EFFECTIVENESS

The currently employed rubella vaccine strain (RA27/3) has been found to be highly effective in inducing a serum as well as a secretory immune response in susceptible subjects. More than 95% of subjects develop protective immunity, which is probably lifelong.

ADVERSE REACTIONS

Most subjects immunized with the live attenuated rubella vaccine alone or in combination with MMR develop no side effects or adverse reactions. Most children who have a side effect will have only a mild reaction, such as soreness, redness or swelling where the shot was given, mild rash, mild to moderate fever, swelling of the lymph glands, and temporary pain, stiffness, or temporary swelling in the joints. About 5% to 15% of children may exhibit a fever in excess of 103°F usually beginning about 7 to 12 days after the vaccine has been administered. In rare cases (about 3 children out of 10,000 given MMR, or 0.03% of recipients) a moderate reaction such as seizure related to high fever may occur. The risk of a febrile seizure after the first dose of MMRV is increased by an additional child per 1,000 (compared with children who got MMR and varicella vaccine at different sites on the same day).

Rubella vaccine in the form of MMR should not be administered to subjects who cannot receive one or both of the other vaccines included in MMR, or subjects who have proof of immunity to one or both of the diseases that MMR prevents may receive the rubella vaccine, though MMR is usually recommended.

SMALLPOX VACCINE

The global eradication of smallpox is widely considered one of the greatest achievements of modern medicine. In 1967, there were an estimated 10 million to 15 million smallpox cases in 31 countries. By 1980, there were zero cases. The eradication campaign was based on two key strategies: (a) mass vaccination and (b) the detection and containment of all cases of smallpox. This approach was possible in part because there were no animal reservoirs of smallpox. Without continuous opportunity for human-to-human spread, smallpox could not survive (54).

Currently, the only verified repositories of the virus are held in secure laboratories at the CDC in Atlanta, Georgia, and the State Research Center of Virology and Biotechnology in Koltsovo, Russia. However, it is believed that clandestine stocks of smallpox exist in 10 or more other countries (53).

Because of the events of September 11, 2001, and the subsequent spread of anthrax in October, public health officials regard the use of biological weapons by terrorists a real possibility. The United States was scheduled to destroy its remaining supply of live smallpox virus in 1996, so that no one could spread the disease accidentally or intentionally. US officials then decided to keep vials containing the virus so that scientists could use it to produce a safer smallpox vaccine, in case the virus ever escaped from the secured laboratories or was used as a bioweapon. Smallpox vaccine may also be of value in developing antiviral drugs to treat smallpox. Several deadlines for smallpox virus destruction have been set; however, officials have decided each time to keep the supply. Owing to the post-September 11 threat of terrorist attacks, the most recent destruction date, December 31, 2002, was abandoned and no new destruction date has been set.

Of all the disease-causing agents that might be used as weapons, smallpox has the potential to cause the greatest harm, since, prior to its eradication, it was considered the most devastating of all infectious diseases.

Smallpox is caused by the variola virus, a DNA virus, which can be spread from person to person via respiratory droplets produced in the nose, mouth, and throat. After a person has been exposed to the virus, there is an incubation period of between 7 and 17 days prior to the onset of symptoms, which include high fever, severe headache and backache, and often vomiting and tremors. Two to five days later, the characteristic smallpox rash develops. It beings as flat, round lesions, primarily on the face and forearms, and evolves into deep, pus-filled blisters that may cover the entire body, including the palms and soles of the feet. Some patients have a fever throughout the course of the rash (2 to 4 weeks), and often the blisters cause significant pain. In the last stage of the rash scabs form and fall off, leaving pitted scars. Some smallpox survivors are blind as a result of deep scarring in the eye area. Smallpox during pregnancy often results in miscarriage or stillbirth.

VACCINE PREPARATIONS

The only smallpox vaccine licensed in the United States is a lyophilized, live vaccinia virus prepared from the New York City Board of Health strain. The vaccine does not contain variola virus but contains a related virus called vaccinia virus, distinct from the cowpox virus initially used for immunization by Jenner. Vaccinia vaccine is highly effective in preventing smallpox, with protection waning after 5 to 10 years after one dose; protection after reimmunization has lasted longer. However, substantial protection against death from smallpox persisted in the past for more than 30 years after immunization during infancy on the basis of experience at a time of worldwide smallpox virus circulation and routine smallpox immunization practices. A smallpox immunization plan has been implemented in the United States (www.bt.cdc.gov). The plan does not include immunization of children. However, children may be at risk of vaccine complications as contacts of vaccinees. Blood donation should be deferred for 21 days after immunization or until the scab has separated. Tuberculin skin testing should be deferred for 1 month after immunization.

AVAILABLE PRODUCT

Product: ACAM2000 [Smallpox (Vaccinia) Vaccine, Live]
Manufacturer: Acambis Inc.
Year Licensed: 2007

VACCINE USAGE

Vaccine is administered using a bifurcated needle to deliver vaccine into the epidermis. Vaccine is held by capillarity between the two tines of the needle. Three skin insertions are used for primary vaccinees; 15 for repeat vaccinees.

Vaccine "take" is determined by the cutaneous reaction to the immunization: a papule should be evident at the immunization site at 3 to 5 days and should progress to a vesicle at 5 to 8 days, then a pustule reaching maximum size in 8 to 10 days. The lesion scabs and heals after 14 to 21 days, leaving a scar. There may be associated swelling, intense erythema, lymphangitis, and tenderness of regional lymph nodes. Satellite lesions at the perimeter of the immunization site may occur. People occupationally exposed to vaccinia virus (the virus in the vaccine), recombinant vaccinia viruses, or other nonvariola orthopoxviruses should be immunized every 10 years.

The smallpox vaccine is not currently recommended for or available to the general public in the United States. The smallpox vaccine is now available under limited circumstances, for example:

- Department of Defense military and civilian personnel and State Department personnel who work in high threat areas;
- Health care providers and "first responders" who volunteer for smallpox response teams;
- For laboratory workers and other at risk for exposure to the smallpox virus, or closely related viruses; and
- Participants in smallpox vaccine trials.

Recommendations for what to do in an epidemic of smallpox or a bioterrorist act with smallpox might change quickly; the most up-to-date information is provided by the CDC. In the event of exposure to smallpox virus the risk of serious complications from the vaccine among those exposed to the disease would be less than the risk of the disease, even for those listed below for whom the vaccine is generally contradicted. Vaccination within 4 days of a first exposure offers some protection against infection, and those vaccinated who do become infected are apt to have much less severe disease. The vaccine is contraindicated in the following persons in a non emergency: immunocomprimised, pregnant women or those breast feeding, children under 12 months, people with significant cardiac risk (greater than 3 risk factors) or who have a known heart conditions, as well as anyone who maybe allergic to components of the vaccine (reference: http://www.bt.cdc.gov/agent/smallpox/faq/screening.asp)

ADVERSE REACTIONS

Although the recently licensed smallpox vaccine is considered a safe vaccine, it does have potential side effects.

When the vaccine was routinely administered in the United States, the most common side effects included swollen and tender lymph nodes that lasted for 2 to 4 weeks after the vaccination site healed. Fever was common, and approximately 70% of those immunized experienced a day or more with temperatures greater than 100°F, and 15% to 20% had fevers greater than 102°F. As many as 30% of adults immunized experienced symptoms severe enough to cause them to miss at least 1 day of work. Rashes without fever can sometimes occur and generally clear without treatment.

The vaccine, in rare cases, can cause serious adverse reactions, including death. Serious reactions after the first dose of smallpox vaccine can include severe vaccinia infection in the skin of people with eczema or atopic dermatitis (<1 per 10,000 immunized). Occasionally, vaccinia necrosum, which begins with death of the tissue around the inoculation site, occurred in seriously immunocompromised people; this often-fatal reaction was rare in the past, affecting less than 1 per 10,000 immunized. Inflammation in the brain (<1 per 10,000 immunized) is another serious reaction and mainly affected children younger than 1 year when the vaccine was administered to this group. Rates of these side effects after a second dose of smallpox vaccine are lower (2).

TETANUS VACCINE

The disease is produced by *Clostridium tetani*—a hardy spore-forming organism, common in soil. It can be introduced into wounds contaminated with dirt, manure, or saliva. If the damaged tissues are lacking in oxygen, the spores can revert to active bacteria, which produce a highly potent neurotoxin, tetanospasmin (41). Dissemination of the toxin affects the central nervous system at several sites, particularly neuromuscular junctions, resulting in intense muscle contraction and involuntary spasms. The mortality is high because of prolonged problems with respiration, swallowing, nutrition, and cardiac arrhythmias. Among survivors, recovery takes several months and is not reliably associated with development of immunity.

The vaccine is prepared from altered toxin protein (toxoid).

VACCINE PREPARATIONS

The vaccine is based on tetanus toxin, a protein that is antigenically uniform among all isolates. In the manufacturing process, organisms are grown under anaerobic conditions to maximize toxin production. Free toxin is separated from bacteria by centrifugation and then progressively purified. Controlled exposure to formalin alters the protein structure sufficiently to abrogate toxicity while preserving antigenicity, producing a so-called toxoid. Tetanus toxoid is usually adsorbed to an aluminum salt to enhance immunogenicity over fluid preparations. Formulations for children younger than 7 years contain 5 to 12.5 Lf units per 0.5-mL dose, and those for older children and adults contain 5 Lf units per 0.5-mL dose. Some products contain thimerosal preservative (41).

Adsorbed toxoid formulations are administered intramuscularly to minimize injection-site reactions. Vaccine should be stored at 2°C to 8°C, avoiding freezing (55).

The tetanus vaccine is available as DTaP (Diphtheria-Tetanus-Pertussis);
DTaP in combination with Hib vaccine;
DTaP in combination with hepatitis B and inactivated polio vaccines;
DTaP in combination with Hib, hepatitis B, and inactivated polio vaccines; and
Tdap (Diphtheria–Tetanus–Pertussis), DT or Td (in combination with diphtheria vaccine), and TT (alone).

Vaccines containing the whole cell pertussis component (DTP) are no longer recommended for use in the United States and are not listed here although they are used in many other countries. Vaccines containing lower amounts of diphtheria toxoid abbreviated with a small d are utilized in persons 7 years of age and older. Pertussis component-containing vaccines are not available for children 7 to 9 years of age.

AVAILABLE PRODUCTS

Product: Tetanus toxoid (TT)
Manufacturer: Sanofi Pasteur
Year Licensed: 1978

Product: Tetanus toxoid adsorbed (TT)
Manufacturer: Sanofi Pasteur
Year Licensed: 1978

Product: Diphtheria and tetanus toxoids adsorbed (DT)
Manufacturer: Sanofi Pasteur
Year Licensed: 1984

Product: Tetanus and diphtheria toxoids adsorbed for adult use (Td)
Manufacturers (Year Licensed): Massachusetts Public Health Biologic Laboratories (1970); Aventis Pasteur (1978)

Product: Tripedia (DTaP)
Manufacturer: Sanofi Pasteur
Year Licensed: 2001

Product: Infanrix (DTaP)
Manufacturer: GlaxoSmithKline
Year Licensed: 1997

Product: TriHIBit (DTaP and Hib conjugate vaccine)
Manufacturer: Sanofi Pasteur
Year Licensed: 2001

Product: DAPTACEL (DTaP)
Manufacturer: Sanofi Pasteur
Year Licensed: 2002

Product: Pediarix (DTaP, hepatitis B, and inactivated polio vaccines)
Manufacturer: GlaxoSmithKline
Year Licensed: 2002

Product: DECAVAC (Tetanus and Diphtheria Toxoids Adsorbed for Adult use—**preservative free**)
Manufacturer: Sanofi Pasteur
Year Licensed: 2004

Product: BOOSTRIX (Tetanus toxoid, Reduced Diphtheria Toxoid and Acellular Pertussis Vaccine, Adsorbed for use in 10- to 18-year-old-persons—preservative free) (Tdap)
Manufacturer: GlaxoSmithKline
Year Licensed: 2005

Product: ADACEL (Tetanus and Diphtheria Toxoids Adsorbed for use in 11- to 64-year-old persons—preservative free) (Tdap)
Manufacturer: Sanofi Pasteur
Year Licensed: 2005

Product: Pentacel (DTap, Hib conjugate, hepatitis B, and inactivated polio vaccines)
Manufacturer: Sanofi Pasteur
Year Licensed: 2008

All DTaP vaccines are available containing no or only trace amounts of thimerosal. Both DT and Td are available as vaccines containing thimerosal preservative, containing trace amounts of thimerosal, or as thimerosal-free vaccines. TT is only available containing thimerosal preservative (2,11).

VACCINE USAGE

Tetanus toxoid vaccines require a series of appropriately spaced injections to reliably elicit a protective response. The number of primary doses needed to elicit protection varies with age (see Tables 57.2 to 57.4). Antibody levels decline slowly and may fall below the minimum protection. Periodic booster doses are recommended throughout life to maintain protection. Tetanus toxoid is usually given in combination vaccines that include diphtheria toxoid (e.g., Td) and other vaccines for children (e.g., DTaP, IPV, Hib).

The recommended immunization schedule for infants and young children in the United States involves five doses, given at 2, 4, 6, and 15 to 18 months and 4 to 6 years. Subsequent booster doses are recommended at 14 to 16 years and every 10 years throughout adulthood. In the event of a contaminated wound, a booster is recommended if 5 or more years have passed since the previous dose, provided that adequate primary immunization was given. Tetanus immune globulin can be administered for prompt passive protection of immunocompromised or inadequately primed children. In developing countries, tetanus immunization of women during pregnancy has virtually eliminated neonatal tetanus as a complication of unhygienic umbilical cord care (2,11).

VACCINE EFFECTIVENESS

Tetanus vaccines have been routinely used since the 1940s. During World War II, immunized armies were almost completely spared from tetanus. Tetanus is rare in well-immunized populations. In the United States, only 27 cases were reported in 2001, a historic low. Most cases in recent years lacked adequate primary immunization. A substantial proportion of adults lack protective serum levels of antitoxin from not having obtained booster immunizations.

Most infants and children younger than 7 years should receive DTaP beginning at 2 months of age. For children who are younger than 7 years for whom there is a reason to not give a pertussis-containing vaccine, the TD can be administered. For children 7 to 9 years of age, the Td vaccine can be administered for initial catch-up immunization. For persons 7 years of age or older, the Td vaccine should be administered every 10 years to provide continued immunity against diphtheria and tetanus and for tetanus prophylaxis for a tetanus prone injury if more than 5 years have elapsed since the last dose of a tetanus toxoid–containing vaccine.

Eleven to eighteen year olds should receive a single does of Tdap instead of a Td booster if they have completed the recommended childhood DTP/DTaP immunization series and have not received Td or Tdap. The preferred age for Tdap vaccination is 11 to 12 years (see Table 57.3). If they have already received a Td booster, it is recommended that there be an interval of at least 5 years before Tdap is administered to reduce the likelihood of local and systemic reactions. Detailed recommendations for the use of Tdap for preteens and adolescents are available from the CDC (2,11).

Adults 19 to 64 years of age should also receive a single dose of Tdap (ADACEL) to replace a single dose of Td for booster immunization if their most recent tetanus toxoid–containing vaccine was 10 or more years earlier. Tdap may be given at an interval shorter than 10 years since the last tetanus toxoid–containing vaccine to protect against pertussis, especially for the following:

- Women younger than 65 years who are planning to become pregnant.
- Adults younger than 65 years who have or anticipate having close contact with an infant younger than 12 months should receive a single dose of Tdap and trivalent inactivated influenza vaccine. Ideally, the vaccines should be given at least 2 weeks before contact.
- Health care personnel who have direct patient contact should receive a single dose of Tdap.

ADVERSE EFFECTS AND CONTRAINDICATION

Tetanus toxoid vaccines are well tolerated apart from causing mild to moderate injection site inflammation and occasional low-grade fever. Booster doses may cause greater injection-site reaction with redness, swelling, and soreness. Rare complications include brachial neuritis and GBS (55). Overly frequent doses should be avoided as they increase the risk of severe injection-site reactions. The only contraindication to its use is a history of anaphylactic reaction to a previous dose or hypersensitivity to any component of a combination vaccine.

Immunization with tetanus toxoid as a combined form with DTP should not be used in subjects:

- With a history of a serious allergic reaction (such as anaphylaxis) to any of the vaccine components.
- Subjects with a history of encephalopathy (e.g., coma or prolonged seizures) not attributable to an identifiable cause within 7 days of administration of a vaccine with pertussis components should not receive a pertussis-containing vaccine.
- Pertussis-containing vaccines (including the DTaP vaccine) are not currently recommended for children who are 7 to 9 years of age.
- Tdap is not recommended to be administered within 2 years after the most recent tetanus toxoid–containing vaccine (2,11).

TUBERCULOSIS

Tuberculosis (TB) is caused by *Mycobacterium tuberculosis.* It generally spreads through droplets from infected subjects.

Most subjects with TB show no symptoms at the time of infection. Subjects who develop symptoms usually do so within 1 to 6 months after the start of the infection. Symptoms include fever, night sweats, chills, and cough. Pneumonia, lung collapse, and enlarged lymph nodes may also occur.

The most common form of TB affects the lungs. Two forms of TB that become life-threatening are as follows:

- Miliary TB, which means the bacteria have spread throughout the lungs and into the bloodstream.
- TB meningitis (infection of the coverings of the spinal cord and/or brain by TB bacteria).

More than 25,000 new cases of TB are reported annually in the United States. People who are immunocompromised (have weakened immunity), especially those who are HIV-positive, are at increased risk of developing TB if they are exposed to the disease. Malnourished people as well as those with diabetes or kidney failure are also more likely to develop the disease if exposed (2).

VACCINE PREPARATIONS

The Bacillus Calmette-Guérin (BCG) vaccine (the human TB vaccine) is a live, attenuated bacterial vaccine made from the laboratory adapted bacterium that causes TB in cows. It was first administered to humans in 1921. It has been given to 4 billion people worldwide and has been used routinely since the 1960s in almost all the countries of the world, primarily in young infants. Changes in the TB bacteria over time have led scientists to create the different TB vaccines used throughout the world, and their effectiveness appears to be highly variable (56).

The use of available BCG vaccine is not recommended for children in the United States as it is not highly effective and may cause confusion for physicians when trying to interpret a TB skin test.

AVAILABLE PRODUCTS

Product: TICE BCG (BCG Live)
Manufacturer: Organon Teknika Corporation
Year Licensed: 1990. This vaccine is thimerosal-free.

Product: Mycobax (BCG Live)
Manufacturer: Adventis Pasteur
Year Licensed: 2000. This vaccine is thimerosal-free.

VACCINE USAGE

The vaccine is given as a single dose. Infants may receive the vaccine soon after birth, or later, but preferably before exposure to persons with active TB.

VACCINE EFFECTIVENESS

Although BCG vaccines have been administered to billions of human beings, their effectiveness in the control of active mycobacterial TB infection in humans still remains to be documented. Various well-controlled studies have drawn various and often conflicting conclusions. However, one large study found the vaccine to protect about 50% of recipients. Effectiveness rates are highest among those who get the vaccination in early childhood (57).

Those who receive the vaccine may still develop TB, but approximately 80% of recipients are protected from developing life-threatening forms of the disease, such as miliary disease and meningitis (inflammation of the brain).

Although TB vaccine is recommended by the World Health Organization, and is given in more than 100 countries, in the United States it should be considered only for infants and children who do not test positive for TB but who are:

- continually exposed to a patient with infectious TB of the lungs (and the child cannot be removed from this person) and

- exposed to a person with TB that is resistant to anti-TB drugs.

In addition, vaccination is recommended for health care workers who are employed in settings with patients who have drug-resistant TB, and where comprehensive TB infection-control precautions have been implemented but have not been successful.

ADVERSE REACTIONS

Accurate rates of adverse events due to the TB vaccine are difficult to estimate, but serious or long-term complications after TB immunization are uncommon. Frequent reactions to the TB vaccine include redness, swelling, or soreness at the injection site.

Moderate swelling of the lymph nodes in the armpits or neck, which may progress to pus-filled nodes that require drainage in some people, also occurs. In addition, swelling at the injection site may turn into a pustule and then a scar. An ulcer may develop where the shot was given in some people. These reactions occur after approximately 1% to 2% of immunizations and may last for 3 months or longer.

Because the BCG vaccine is a live vaccine, it may cause meningitis, or disseminated disease which occurs at a rate of 0.06 to 1.56 cases per 1 million vaccinated. The vaccine may also cause infection of bone growth centers, which may occur several years after the vaccine was given.

Available BCG vaccine should not be administered to HIV-infected children or children with impaired immune system and patients undergoing chemotherapy; subjects with burns or skin infections; and pregnant women (2).

TYPHOID VACCINE

Salmonella typhi is the etiological agent of typhoid fever, an acute, febrile enteric disease. Typhoid fever continues to be an important disease in many parts of the world. Travelers entering infected areas are at risk of contracting typhoid fever following the ingestion of contaminated food or water. Typhoid fever is considered to be endemic in most areas of Central and South America, the African continent, the Near East and the Middle East, Southeast Asia, and the Indian subcontinent. There are approximately 500 cases of typhoid fever per year diagnosed in the United States. In 62% of these patients the disease was acquired outside of the United States, whereas in 38% of the patients the disease was acquired within the United States. Of 340 cases acquired in the United States between 1977 and 1979, 23% of the cases were associated with typhoid carriers, 24% were due to food outbreaks, 23% were associated with the ingestion of contaminated food or water, 6% were due to household contact with an infected person, and 4% following exposure to *S. typhi* in a laboratory setting (57,58).

VACCINE PREPARATIONS

During the past 15 years, the two typhoid vaccines licensed in the United States have been widely used globally. These vaccines have largely replaced the old heat-phenol–inactivated whole-cell vaccine in many countries, including the United States. These are an oral live-attenuated strain of *S. typhi* (Vivotif Berna; Berna Biotech, SA) and a parenteral capsular polysaccharide vaccine—a piece of the bacterium that is given by injection (Typhim Vi; Aventis Pasteur).

More recently, the typhoid vaccine based on the *S. typhi* V_1 antigen has been developed and used successfully in limited field studies to control typhoid in certain endemic areas (58,59).

AVAILABLE PRODUCTS

Product: Vivotif Berna (Live attenuated Oral Vaccine)
Manufacturer: Berna Biotech, Ltd.
Year Licensed: 1994

Product: TYPHIM VI (Capsular Polysaccharide Vaccine)
Manufacturer: Berna Biotech, Ltd.
Year Licensed: 1994

VACCINE USAGE

The oral typhoid vaccine can be administered to children 6 years of age or older and adults. It is administered as a single capsule every other day for a total of four capsules. The last dose should be taken at least 1 week before travel to allow the vaccine time to work. A booster dose is needed every 5 years for people who remain at risk (59,60).

The polysaccharide typhoid vaccine can be administered to children older than 2 years. One injection is enough to provide protection. It should be given at least 1 week before travel to allow the vaccine time to work. A booster dose is needed every 2 years for people who remain at risk for exposure.

VACCINE EFFICACY

The efficacy of the two licensed vaccines ranges from 50% to 80%.

The oral vaccine has shown a protective efficacy of 62% for at least 7 years after the last dose. The inactivated vaccine for its part showed a 55% efficacy in a recent study in South Africa 3 years after immunization of children 5 to 16 years of age.

Typhoid fever is rare in the United States, so routine typhoid vaccination is not recommended. However, the following people should receive the vaccine:

- Travelers to parts of the world where typhoid fever is common. Risk is greater for travelers to the Indian subcontinent, Latin America, Asia, and Africa who may have exposure to contaminated food and drink. Since typhoid vaccine is not 100% effective, it is not a substitute for being careful about what you eat or drink.
- People in close contact with a typhoid carrier (e.g., household contacts).
- Laboratory workers who work with *S. typhi.*

Reactions to the oral typhoid vaccine include fever or headache (5%), abdominal discomfort, nausea, vomiting, or rash (rare). Reactions to the inactivated vaccine include fever (1%), headache (3%), and redness or swelling at the site of the injection (7%). Persons who have had a severe reaction to a previous dose of this vaccine should not receive another dose.

Other subjects who should not receive the live attenuated typhoid vaccine (oral) include the following:

- Persons who have had a severe reaction to a previous dose of this vaccine should not get another dose.
- Immunocompromised persons (e.g., persons with HIV/AIDS, persons receiving cancer chemotherapy, or persons receiving high doses of corticosteroids). They should get the polysaccharide typhoid vaccine instead.
- Oral typhoid vaccine should not be given within 24 hours of taking certain antibiotics.
- Children younger than 6 years (46).

VARICELLA VACCINE

Without immunization, nearly all children will experience varicella (chickenpox) infection. Children attending day care or primary school are most often affected, whereas teenagers are most severely affected. For most children, the illness is only moderately distressing, but about 5% of cases experience a complication, and as many as 1 in 200 require hospital care (61,62). Secondary bacterial infection of the skin is the most common complication, ranging from impetigo to cellulitis to necrotizing fasciitis. Other complications include otitis media, pneumonitis, hepatitis, and encephalitis/cerebellitis. Fetal injury may occur with infections during pregnancy. Reye syndrome is a risk, so use of acetylsalicylic acid should be avoided. The virus persists in nervous tissue and can cause zoster (shingles) decades after the primary infection. Immunocompromised persons may experience life-threatening disease with primary or reactivation infection.

VACCINE PREPARATIONS

The vaccine consists of lyophilized, live, attenuated varicella-zoster virus (VZV) (63). All currently licensed products are based on the Oka strain developed in Japan, but they differ slightly in potency and excipients (64). Vaccines are produced in tissue cultures, typically human diploid cells. Gelatin is added as a stabilizer. Traces of neomycin may be present. Current products are stable at 2°C to 8°C for extended periods (see product monographs for storage instructions).

Varicella vaccines are formulated as dried powders, requiring reconstitution with the supplied diluent. Reconstituted vaccine should be used promptly, according to the manufacturer's instructions. Varicella vaccines are injected subcutaneously, usually in the upper arm, in a dose of 0.5 mL.

AVAILABLE PRODUCTS

Product: ProQuad (Measles–Mumps–Rubella–Varicella Virus Vaccine Live) (MMRV)
Manufacturer: Merck
Year Licensed: 2005

Product: Varivax
Manufacturer: Merck
Year Licensed: 1995

Reconstituted MMRV must be discarded if not used within 30 minutes. The CDC recommends storage of all live vaccines in the freezer at 5°F or below. These vaccines do not contain thimerosal.

VACCINE USAGE

Children should get two doses of a varicella-containing vaccine: The first dose between 12 and 15 months of age and the second dose between 4 and 6 years of age (before entering kindergarten or first grade) (see Tables 57.2 to 57.4). People who have not been vaccinated by 13 years of age should get two doses of the vaccine, 4 to 8 weeks apart.

Note: Because varicella vaccine has been shown to be less effective when given between 1 and 29 days after MMR vaccine, it should either be given on the same day as MMR, or 30 or more days after MMR vaccine is administered.

VACCINE EFFECTIVENESS

Varicella vaccine is 85% to 90% effective for prevention of varicella and 100% effective for prevention of moderate or severe disease.

Children receiving varicella vaccine in prelicensure trials in the United States have been shown to be protected for 11 years. Studies in Japan have demonstrated protection for at least 20 years. However, breakthrough infection (i.e., cases of chickenpox after vaccination) can occur in some who have been immunized. Although breakthrough varicella usually results in mild rather than severe illness, some school outbreaks have resulted in some children with more lesions and them also being contagious. For this reason, a second dose of a varicella-containing vaccine is recommended.

The use of this live attenuated varicella vaccine is recommended for the following:

- All children aged 12 to 18 months.
- All older children and adults who have not had chickenpox and have not been vaccinated.
- If someone who has never had chickenpox disease or received the vaccine is exposed to chickenpox, giving him or her the vaccine within 72 hours will probably prevent or significantly reduce the severity of the disease. It is recommended under such circumstances.

Some children who are successfully immunized may later develop chickenpox. But it is often mild disease, although some may have more typical illness with fever and many lesions. Breakthrough varicella can be contagious. As a consequence, in June 2006, the CDC recommended a second dose of varicella-containing vaccine for all children.

ADVERSE REACTIONS

Vaccine administration induces an infection that is generally subclinical, but 15% of children experience fever and 3% to 5% develop mild skin rash when infection peaks 2 to 3 weeks later. Fever is generally mild to moderate and lasts for only

1 to 2 days but can rarely trigger a febrile convulsion. Skin rash is usually limited to a few scattered lesions, sometimes just at the injection site. Rash elements may be vesicular (in which case virus can be released and potentially communicated to contacts) or maculopapular. Transmission of vaccine virus rarely occurs and has not been documented in the absence of rash (64). Secondary vaccine virus infections in healthy persons are mild. Infrequent adverse effects include anaphylaxis, thrombocytopenia, and encephalopathy. Delayed effects include varicella zoster.

The vaccine is not recommended for children younger than 12 months because of possible interference from maternally derived antibodies. Healthy children aged 1 to 12 years require only one dose, whereas those 13 years and older require two doses, separated by at least 4 weeks. Optimal age for routine immunization is 12 to 15 months (see Tables 57.2 to 57.4) (2,11,65).

The vaccine should not be given to subjects who have had a life-threatening allergic reaction to gelatin, to the antibiotic neomycin, or (for those needing a second dose) to a previous dose of the chickenpox vaccine; those who are receiving the MMR vaccine simultaneously should not get the varicella vaccine from the same needle or in the same place on the body; and pregnant women should wait until after they give birth to receive the vaccine. Women should not become pregnant for at least 1 month after receiving the vaccine. To date, there are no reported cases of congenital varicella syndrome caused by the vaccine.

In addition, the vaccine should not be given to persons with T-lymphocyte immunodeficiency, including those with leukemia, lymphoma, other malignancies affecting the bone marrow, and congenital T-cell abnormalities. The vaccine may be given to children with acute lymphocytic leukemia under study conditions, and HIV-infected persons who are immunocompetent may be vaccinated. Susceptible family members and other contacts of HIV-infected or immunodeficient persons should receive the chickenpox vaccine, because of the risk that natural chickenpox and its complications present for these patients.

Varicella vaccine should not be given for 5 months following the receipt of antibody-containing products (e.g., blood transfusion).

VARICELLA-ZOSTER VACCINE (HERPES ZOSTER)

Herpes zoster (shingles) is a reactivation of varicella infection. The VZV—which remains in the nerve cells for life after chickenpox or after the chickenpox vaccine—may reappear as shingles in later life, particularly in the elderly and those who are immunocompromised. This is because of declining immunity to the VZV over time. Thus, anyone who has had chickenpox or the chickenpox live virus vaccine is at risk for developing shingles. Although shingles can occur at any age, the risk increases as people get older. When shingles develop, blisters appear following a dermatome distribution on the skin, generally on one side of the body. The skin blisters in shingles contain the VZV, so chickenpox-susceptible children can rarely develop chickenpox when exposed to shingles (66).

VACCINE PREPARATION

The zoster vaccine is identical to varicella vaccine but contains a higher dose of the vaccine virus. In 2006, Zostavax was licensed and recommended for routine administration to adults over the age of 60 years.

AVAILABLE PRODUCT

Product: Zostavax
Manufacturer: Merck
Year Licensed: 2006

Note: Reconstituted Zostavax must be discarded if not used within 30 minutes. The CDC recommends storage of this and all live virus vaccines in the freezer to 5°F or below. This vaccine does not contain thimerosal (2,11).

VACCINE USAGE

Zostavax should be administered immediately after it is reconstituted and is administered subcutaneously in the upper arm.

VACCINE EFFECTIVENESS

In a clinical trial of more than 38,000 individuals older than 60 years, about half of whom received the vaccine, Zostavax reduced the occurrence of shingles by about 50%. Effectiveness was greatest in the younger age groups and declined with advancing age. In those who had received the vaccine and who developed shingles, the duration (but not the severity) of postherpetic neuralgia (PHN) was reduced.

The vaccine is recommended for all individuals 60 years of age or older.

ADVERSE REACTIONS

No serious side effects have been reported to date. Duration of protection is not known at this time but appears to be more than 3 years.

Zostavax has not been studied in persons younger than 60 years.

Zostavax has not been studied among people who have already had shingles. Although recurrent cases of zoster have been described, someone who has had shingles is less likely to suffer another episode.

Currently, it is recommended that the zoster vaccine may not be administered to children as a substitute for varicella vaccine (Varivax).

It should not be administered to subjects who had had a life-threatening allergic reaction to gelatin, to the antibiotic neomycin, or to a previous dose of the chickenpox vaccine; subjects with primary or acquired immunodeficiency states, including leukemia, lymphoma of any type, other malignant neoplasm affecting the bone marrow, or lymphatic system or AIDS or other clinical manifestations of infection with HIVs; persons who are taking immunosuppressive therapy, including high-dose corticosteroids; persons with active untreated TB; and women who are or may be pregnant (2,11).

VIBRIO CHOLERAE VACCINE

Cholera is characterized by painless voluminous diarrhea without abdominal cramps or fever. Dehydration, hypokalemia, metabolic acidosis, and occasionally hypovolemic shock can occur, particularly in children. Stools are colorless, with small flecks of mucus ("rice water"), and contain high concentrations of sodium, potassium, chloride, and bicarbonate.

Vibrio cholerae is a gram-negative, curved, motile bacillus with many serogroups. Only serogroups O1, O139, and O141 cause clinical cholera associated with enterotoxin. There are three serotypes of *V. cholerae* O1: Inaba, Ogawa, and Hikojima. The two biotypes of *V. cholerae* are classical and El Tor. El Tor is more commonly observed. Since 1992, toxigenic *V. cholerae* serogroup O139 has been recognized as a cause of cholera. Nontoxigenic strains of *V. cholerae* O1 and serogroups other than O1 and O139 can cause sporadic diarrheal illness, but they do not cause epidemics (2).

During the last five decades, *V. cholerae* O1 biotype El Tor has spread from India and Southeast Asia to Africa, the Middle East, Southern Europe, and the Western Pacific Islands (Oceania). In 1991, epidemic cholera caused by toxigenic *V. cholerae* O1, serotype Inaba, biotype El Tor, appeared in Peru and spread to most countries in South and North America. In the United States, cases resulting from travel to or ingestion of contaminated food transported from Latin America or Asia have been reported. In addition, the Gulf Coast of Louisiana and Texas has an endemic focus of a unique strain of toxigenic *V. cholerae* O1. Most cases of disease from this strain have resulted from consumption of raw or undercooked shellfish (2).

Humans are the only documented natural host, but free-living *V. cholerae* organisms can exist in the aquatic environment. The usual mode of infection is ingestion of large numbers of organisms from contaminated water or food (particularly raw or undercooked shellfish, raw or partially dried fish, or moist grains or vegetables held at ambient temperature). Direct person-to-person spread has not been documented. People with low gastric acidity are at increased risk of cholera infection.

The incubation period usually is 1 to 3 days, with a range of a few hours to 5 days. Most subjects with toxigenic *V. cholerae* O1 have no symptoms, and some have only mild to moderate diarrhea lasting for 3 to 7 days; fewer than 5% have severe watery diarrhea, vomiting, and dehydration (cholera gravis) (2).

VACCINE PREPARATIONS

No cholera vaccines are available in the United States. Cholera immunization is not required for travelers entering the United States from cholera-affected areas, and the World Health Organization no longer recommends immunization for travel to or from areas with cholera infection. No country requires cholera vaccine for entry. There are currently four cholera vaccines available outside of the United States (67).

LIVE ORAL CHOLERA VACCINE

There are currently two attenuated oral cholera vaccines, CVD103-HgR (Orochol) and Peru-15 (CholeraGarde), which have been extensively tested in subjects; however, Peru-15 is still under development (68).

CVD103-HgR is normally given at a dose of 10^8 organisms per dose along with a buffer solution containing sodium bicarbonate and ascorbic acid designed to protect the live bacteria from stomach acid. This formulation was safe, immunogenic, and protective in North American volunteers. When the vaccine was given to residents in Chile and Indonesia, it was less immunogenic than expected, so the dose was increased by log 1 to improve its immunogenicity (63,69). However, even the higher dose of vaccine did not demonstrate protection in the only controlled field trial of the vaccine in Indonesia. The contrast between the high efficacy when tested in volunteers in North America and the low efficacy in Indonesia is poorly understood but may be related to preexisting natural immunity to cholera, and hence, a decreased "take" by the live vaccine. Furthermore, the rates of cholera were unusually low during the early phases of the trial, and the short-term efficacy could therefore not be determined.

KILLED ORAL CHOLERA VACCINES

There are two killed oral cholera vaccines (67,70). The killed whole cell with recombinant B subunit of the cholera toxin (WC/rCTB; Dukoral) is licensed in more than 50 countries (71), and another similar whole-cell vaccine without B subunit is licensed in Vietnam and is currently being tested in India. This vaccine has recently been licensed for use in India. The whole-cell component of the vaccine is acid stable; thus, it does not require a buffer to protect it from gastric acid. However, the B subunit is acid labile and does require a buffer. Dukoral is safe, immunogenic, and protective as documented from studies in Bangladesh, Peru, and Mozambique (70). The Bangladesh study illustrates its protective benefit in an area with high rates of malnutrition, and the study from Mozambique confirms its benefit in an area with high rates of HIV infection.

Although the vaccine was protective in these different geographic areas, the antibacterial (vibriocidal) responses were less frequent in young children (2 to 5 years) compared with older children and adults, and more doses were required to achieve a higher take rate. Similarly, the magnitude of the antitoxin responses was lower in the young age groups (2 to 5 years) than in older groups.

YELLOW FEVER

Yellow fever is an acute febrile illness associated with hepatitis, hemorrhagic fever caused by arthropod-borne viruses in many parts of the world. Epidemic yellow fever used to occur in the United States but now the disease occurs in sub-Saharan Africa and tropical South America, and parts of Asia, where it is endemic and intermittently epidemic. There are 200,000 estimated cases of yellow fever (with 30,000 deaths) per year. However, due to underreporting, only a small percentage of these cases are identified. Small numbers of imported cases also occur in countries free of yellow fever (2).

Infection causes a wide spectrum of disease. Most cases of yellow fever are mild and similar to influenza, consisting of fever, headache, nausea, muscle pain, and prominent backache. After 3 to 4 days most patients improve and their symptoms disappear. However, in about 15% of patients, fever reappears after 24 hours with severe illness, which includes hepatitis and hemorrhagic fever. Bleeding can occur from the mouth, nose, eyes, and/or stomach. Once this happens, blood appears in the vomit and feces. Kidney function also deteriorates. Half of those who develop the severe illness die within 10 to 14 days. The remainder recovers without significant organ damage (2).

VACCINE PREPARATION

Yellow fever vaccine is an attenuated, live virus vaccine that has been used since the 1930s. The isolation of the Asibi and French strains of yellow fever in 1927 enabled the development of vaccines. Scientists at the Rockefeller Foundation in New York developed a live vaccine (17D) attenuated by serial passage of the Asibi strain in embryonated chicken eggs. The 17D vaccine was first tested in 1936 in New York and in 1937 in Brazil. Although the vaccine has been available for more than 60 years, the number of people infected over the last two decades has increased and yellow fever is now a serious public health issue in a number of countries once again (72).

AVAILABLE PRODUCT

Product: YF-VAX (Live-attenuated 17D strain vaccine)
Manufacturer: Aventis Pasteur

There is no thimerosal in yellow fever vaccine.

VACCINE USAGE

The yellow fever vaccine is administered to persons of all ages as a single dose. Immunity develops by the 10th day after primary vaccination.

A booster vaccination should be administered after 10 years. Revaccination boosts antibody titer; however, evidence from several studies suggests that yellow fever vaccine immunity persists for at least 30 to 36 years and probably for life (2).

Studies have shown that the serologic response to yellow fever vaccine is not inhibited by administration of certain other vaccines concurrently at separate sites or at various intervals of a few days to 1 month. Measles and yellow fever vaccines have been administered in combination with full efficacy of each of the components; BCG and yellow fever vaccines have been administered simultaneously without interference; and typhoid, meningococcal, and yellow fever vaccines have been administered concurrently with full efficacy of each of the components.

VACCINE EFFECTIVENESS

Yellow fever vaccine is safe and highly effective. The protective effect (immunity) occurs within 1 week in 95% of people vaccinated. A single dose of vaccine provides protection for 10 years and probably for life.

Vaccination is the single most important measure for preventing yellow fever. In populations where vaccination coverage is low, vigilant surveillance is critical for prompt recognition and rapid control of outbreaks. Mosquito control measures can be used to prevent virus transmission until vaccination has taken effect (72,73).

This vaccine is recommended for use in persons 9 months of age or older, traveling to or living in areas where yellow fever infection is reported or yellow fever vaccination is required.

The vaccine is recommended for all travelers passing through or living in countries in Africa, Central America, and South America where yellow fever infection is officially reported. It is also recommended for travel outside the urban areas of countries that do not officially report yellow fever but lie in the yellow fever "endemic zones."

A vaccination certificate is required for entry to many countries, particularly for travelers arriving in Asia from Africa or South America. Fatal cases in unvaccinated tourists have been reported with an average of one a year for the past 10 years.

ADVERSE REACTIONS

Yellow fever vaccine generally has few side effects; less than 5% of vaccinees develop mild headache, muscle pain, or other minor symptoms 5 to 10 days after vaccination.

Reactions to yellow fever vaccine are generally mild. After vaccination, vaccinees have reported mild headaches, myalgia, low-grade fevers, or other minor symptoms 5 to 10 days after vaccination. In clinical trials, the incidence of mild adverse events has been approximately 25%.

Approximately 1% of vaccinees find it necessary to curtail regular activities. Immediate hypersensitivity reactions, characterized by rash, urticaria, or asthma or a combination of these, are uncommon (incidence <1 case per 131,000 vaccinees) and occur principally in persons with histories of egg allergy (73).

Rarely yellow fever vaccine can cause multiple organ system failure and encephalitis.

- Yellow fever vaccine should not be given to infants younger than 6 months because of the risk of viral encephalitis (brain inflammation) developing in the child. In most cases, vaccination should be deferred until the child is 9 to 12 months of age to minimize the risk of vaccine-associated encephalitis.
- Pregnant women should not be vaccinated because of a theoretical risk that the developing fetus may become infected from the vaccine.
- Infants 6 to 9 months of age and pregnant women should be considered for immunization only if they are traveling to high-risk areas, travel cannot be postponed, and a high level of prevention against mosquito exposure is unfeasible.
- Persons hypersensitive to eggs should not receive the vaccine because it is prepared in embryonated eggs.
- Immunocompromised persons and persons receiving cancer chemotherapy or high degrees of steroids. People with asymptomatic HIV infection may be vaccinated if exposure to yellow fever cannot be avoided (73).

REFERENCES

1. Friedlander AM, Pittman PR, Parker GW. Anthrax vaccine: evidence for safety and efficacy against inhalational anthrax. *JAMA* 1999;282:2104–2106.
2. American Academy of Pediatrics, Committee on Infectious Diseases. *Red Book: report of the committee on infectious diseases*, 27th ed. Elk Grove Village, IL, 2006.
3. Centers for Disease Control and Prevention Advisory Committee on Immunization Practices. Use of diphtheria toxoid-tetanus toxoid-acellular pertussis vaccine as a five dose series. *MMWR Recomm Rep* 2000;49(RR-13):1–16.
4. Scheifele DW, Dobson S, Kallos A, et al. Comparative safety of tetanus–diphtheria toxoids booster immunization in students in grades 6 and 9. *Pediatr Infect Dis J* 1998;17:1121–1126.
5. Cochi SL, Broome CV. Vaccine prevention of *Haemophilus influenzae* type b disease: past, present and future. *Pediatr Infect Dis J* 1986;5: 12–19.
6. Bisgard KM, Kao A, Leake J, et al. *Haemophilus influenzae* invasive disease in the United States, 1994–1995: near disappearance of a vaccine-preventable childhood disease. *Emerg Infect Dis* 1998;4: 229–237.
7. Armstrong GL, Bell BP. Hepatitis A virus infections in the United States: model-based estimates and implications for childhood immunization. *Pediatrics* 2002;109:839–845.
8. Bell BP, Shapiro CN, Alter MJ, et al. The diverse patterns of hepatitis A epidemiology in the United States—implications for vaccination strategies. *J Infect Dis* 1998;178:1579–1584.
9. Centers for Disease Control and Prevention, National Immunization Program (NIP). Hepatitis A. In: *Epidemiology and prevention of vaccine-preventable diseases ("The Pink Book")*, 8th ed. Atlanta, GA: Centers for Disease Control and Prevention, National Immunization Program (NIP), 2004:191–206.
10. Centers for Disease Control and Prevention. Prevention of hepatitis A through active and passive immunization: recommendations of the Advisory Committee on Immunization Practices (ACIP). *MMWR Recomm Rep* 1999;48(RR-12):1–37.
11. Recommended immunization schedules for persons aged 0 through 18 years—United States, 2009. *MMWR* 2009;57(51–52):Q-1–Q-4.
12. Centers for Disease Control and Prevention. Hepatitis B virus: a comprehensive strategy for eliminating transmission in the United States through universal childhood vaccination. *MMWR Recomm Rep* 1991;40(RR-13):1–17.
13. Joines RW, Blatter M, Abraham B, et al. A prospective, randomized, comparative U.S. trial of a combination hepatitis A and B vaccine (Twinrix®) with corresponding monovalent vaccines (Havrix® and Engerix-B®) in adults. *Vaccine* 2001;19:4710–4719.
14. Baseman JG, Koutsky LA. The epidemiology of human papillomavirus infections. *J Clin Virol* 2005;32(suppl 1):S16–S24.
15. Giuliano AR, Lu B, Nielson CM, et al. Age-specific prevalence, incidence, and duration of human papillomavirus infections in a cohort of 290 US men. *J Infect Dis* 2008;198:1–9.
16. Franco EL, Cuzick J. Cervical cancer screening following prophylactic human papillomavirus vaccination. *J Vaccine* 2007;26S:A16–A23.
17. Mayrand M-H, Duarte-Franco E, Coutlee F, et al. Randomized controlled trial of human papillomavirus testing versus Pap cytology in the primary screening for cervical cancer precursors: design, methods, and preliminary accrual results of the Canadian cervical cancer screening trial (CCCaST). *Int J Cancer* 2006;119:615–623.
18. Cox RJ, Brokstad KA, Ogra P. Influenza virus: immunity and vaccination strategies. Comparison of the immune responses to inactivated and live, attenuated influenza vaccines. *Scand J Immunol* 2004;59:1–15.
19. Belshe R. Current status of live attenuated influenza virus vaccine in the US. *Virus Res* 2004;103:177–185.
20. Lasky T, Terracciano GJ, Magder L, et al. The Guillain–Barre syndrome and the 1992–1993 and 1993–1994 influenza vaccines. *N Engl J Med* 1998;339:1797–1802.
21. Tsai F. Inactivated Japanese encephalitis virus vaccine: recommendations of the Advisory Committee on Immunization Practices (ACIP). *MMWR Recomm Rep* 1993;42(RR-1):1–15.
22. Evans J, Fikrig E. Lyme disease vaccine. In: Plotkin SA, Orenstein WA, eds. *Vaccines*, 3rd ed. Philadelphia, PA: WB Saunders Company, 1999:968–982.
23. Sikand VK, Halsey N, Krause PJ, et al. Safety and immunogenicity of a recombinant *Borrelia burgdorferi* outer surface protein A vaccine against Lyme disease in healthy children and adolescents: a randomized controlled trial. *Pediatrics* 2001;109:123–128.
24. Centers for Disease Control and Prevention, National Immunization Program (NIP). Measles. In: *Epidemiology and prevention of vaccine-preventable diseases ("The Pink Book")*, 6th ed. Atlanta, GA: Centers for Disease Control and Prevention, National Immunization Program (NIP), 2000:117–142.
25. Centers for Disease Control and Prevention. Prevention and control of meningococcal disease: recommendations of the Advisory Committee on Immunization Practices (ACIP). *MMWR Recomm Rep* 2000;53(RR-7):1–10.
26. Centers for Disease Control and Prevention. Meningococcal vaccine: what you need to know. (Vaccine Information Statement) (VIS). Available at: www.cdc.gov/vaccines/pubs/vis/default.htm
27. Wang VJ, Kupperman N, Malley R, et al. Meningococcal disease among children who live in a large metropolitan area, 1981–1996. *Clin Infect Dis* 2001;32:1004–1009.
28. Duclos P, Ward BJ. Measles vaccines: a review of adverse events. *Drug Saf* 1998;19:435–454.
29. Centers for Disease Control and Prevention. Poliomyelitis prevention in the United States—updated recommendations of the Advisory Committee on Immunization Practices (ACIP). *MMWR Recomm Rep* 2000;53(RR-7):1–10.
30. Cherry JD, Olin P. The science and fiction of pertussis vaccines. *Pediatrics* 1999;104:1381–1384.
31. CDC—United States, 1997–2000. *MMWR Morb Mortal Wkly Rep* 2002;51:73–76.
32. Chopra K, Kundu S, Chowdhury DS. Antibody response of infants in tropics to five doses of oral polio vaccine. *J Trop Pediatr* 1989; 35:19–23.
33. Centers for Disease Control and Prevention. Preventing tetanus, diphtheria, and pertussis among adolescents: use of tetanus toxoid, reduced diphtheria toxoid and acellular pertussis vaccines: recommendations of the Advisory Committee on Immunization Practices (ACIP). *MMWR Recomm Rep* 2006;55(RR-3):1–50.
34. Centers for Disease Control and Prevention. Preventing tetanus, diphtheria, and pertussis among adults: use of tetanus toxoid, reduced diphtheria toxoid and acellular pertussis vaccines: recommendations of the Advisory Committee on Immunization Practices (ACIP) and recommendation of ACIP, supported by the HealthCare Infection Control Practices Advisory Committee (HICPAC) for use of Tdap among health-care personnel. *MMWR Recomm Rep* 2006;55(RR-17):1–44.
35. Centers for Disease Control and Prevention. Licensure of a diphtheria and tetanus toxoids and acellular pertussis adsorbed, inactivated poliovirus, and Haemophilus b conjugate vaccine and guidance for use in infants and children. *MMWR Morb Mortal Wkly Rep* 2008;57(39):1079–1080.
36. Ogra PL, Kerr-Grant D, Umana G, et al. Antibody response in serum and nasopharynx after naturally acquired and vaccine-induced infection with rubella virus. *N Engl J Med* 1971;285:1333–1339.
37. Musher DM. Infections caused by *Streptococcus pneumoniae*: clinical spectrum, pathogenesis, immunity and treatment. *Clin Infect Dis* 1992;14:801–809.
38. Scheifele DW, Halperin S, Pelletier L, et al. Invasive pneumococcal infections in Canadian children, 1991–1998: implications for new vaccination strategies. *Clin Infect Dis* 2000;31:58–64.
39. Ogra PL, Herd JK. Arthritis associated with induced rubella infection. *J Immunol* 1971;107;810–813.
40. Fenner F, Henderson DA, Arita S, et al. *Smallpox and its eradication*. Geneva: WHO, 1998.
41. Faden H, Duffy L, Sun M, et al. Long-term immunity to poliovirus in children immunized with live attenuated or enhanced potency inactivated trivalent poliovirus vaccine. *J Infect Dis* 1993;168:452–454.
42. Black S, Shinefield H, Fireman B, et al. Efficacy, Safety and immunogenicity of heptavalent pneumococcal conjugate vaccine in children. *Pediatr Infect Dis J* 2000;19:187–195.
43. Centers for Disease Control and Prevention. Preventing pneumococcal disease among infants and young children: recommendations of the Advisory Committee on Immunization Practices (ACIP). *MMWR Recomm Rep* 2000;53(RR-7):1–10.
44. Melnick JL. Current status of poliovirus infections. *Clin Microbiol Rev* 1996;9:293–300.

45. Ogra PL, Faden HS. Poliovirus vaccines: live or dead. *J Pediatr* 1986;108:1031–1033.
46. Centers for Disease Control and Prevention. Typhoid vaccine: what you need to know. (VIS) 2004. Available at: www.cdc.gov/vaccines/pubs/vis/default.htm
47. Myaux JA, Unicomb L, Besser RE, et al. Effect of diarrhea on the humoral response to oral polio vaccination. *Pediatr Infect Dis J* 1996;15:204–209.
48. Centers for Disease Control and Prevention. Compendium of animal rabies prevention and control. *MMWR Recomm Rep* 2006;55(RR-05):1–8.
49. Moran GJ, Talan DA, Mower W, et al. Appropriateness of rabies postexposure prophylaxis treatment for animal exposure. *JAMA* 2000;284:1001–1007.
50. World Health Organization. Position paper on rotavirus. *Wkly Epidemiol Rec No. 32* 2007;82:285–296.
51. Vesikari T, Matson DO, Dennehy P, et al. Safety and efficacy of a pentavalent human-bovine (WC3) reassortant rotavirus vaccine. *N Engl J Med* 2006;354:23–33.
52. Parashar UD, Hummelman EG, Bresee JS, et al. Global illness and deaths caused by rotavirus disease in children. *Emerg Infect Dis* 2003;9:565–572.
53. Centers for Disease Control and Prevention. Rubella. In: *Epidemiology and prevention of vaccine-preventable diseases ("The Pink Book")*, 9th ed. Atlanta, Ga: CDC; 2006:155–170.
54. Henderson DA. Smallpox vaccine in vaccines. In: de Quadros CA, ed. *Preventing disease and protecting health.* Pan American Health Organization Scientific and Technical Publication No. 596 Washington DC, 2004:398.
55. Stratton KR, Howe CJ, Johnston RB. *Adverse events associated with childhood vaccines: evidence bearing on causality.* Washington, DC: National Academy Press, 1994.
56. Centers for Disease Control and Prevention. The role of BCG vaccine in the prevention and control of tuberculosis in the United States. *MMWR Recomm Rep* 1996;45(RR-4):1–18.
57. Rodrigues LC, Diwan VK, Wheeler JG. Protective effect of BCG against tuberculosis meningitis and miliary tuberculosis: a meta-analysis. *Int J Epidemiol* 1993;22:1154–1158.
58. Steinberg EB, Bishop R, Haber P, et al. Typhoid fever in travelers: who should be targeted for prevention. *Clin Infect Dis* 2004;39:186–191.
59. Murphy JR, Grez L, Schlesinger L, et al. Immunogenicity of *Salmonella typhi* Ty21a vaccine for young children. *Infect Immun* 1991;59:4291–4293.
60. Lin FY, Ho VA, Khiem HB, et al. The efficacy of a *Salmonella typhi* Vi conjugate vaccine in two-to-five year-old children. *N Engl J Med* 2001;344:1263–1269.
61. DeWals P, Blackburn M, Guay M, et al. Burden of chickenpox on families: a study in Quebec. *Can J Infect Dis* 2001;12:27–32.
62. Coplan P, Black S, Rojas C, et al. Incidence and hospitalization rates of varicella and herpes zoster before varicella vaccine introduction: a baseline assessment of the shifting epidemiology of varicella disease. *Pediatr Infect Dis J* 2001;20:641–645.
63. Simanjuntak CH, O'Hanley P, Punjabi NH, et al. Safety, immunogenicity, and transmission of a single-dose live oral cholera vaccine strain CVD 103-HgR in 24-to-59-month-old Indonesian children. *J Infect Dis* 1993;168:1169–1176.
64. Vasquez M, LaRussa PS, Gershon AA, et al. The effectiveness of the varicella vaccine in clinical practice. *N Engl J Med* 2001;344:955–960.
65. Peterson C. Varicella active surveillance and epidemiologic studies, 1995–1999. In: Guevara R, ed. *Acute communicable disease control: special studies report 1999.* Los Angeles, CA: County of Los Angeles, Department of Health Services, Acute Communicable Disease Control Unit, 2001:19–24.
66. Hope-Simpson RE. The nature of herpes zoster: a long-term study and a new hypothesis. *Proc R Soc Med* 1965;58:9–20.
67. Sack DA, Qadri F, Svennerhold A-M. Determinants of responses to oral vaccines in developing countries. *Ann Nestle* 2008;66:71–79.
68. Cooper PJ, Chico M, Sandoval C, et al. Human infection with Ascaris lumbricoides is associated with suppression of the interleukin-2 response to recombinant cholera toxin B subunit following vaccination with the live cholera vaccine CVD 103-HgR. *Infect Immun* 2001;69:1574–1580.
69. Lagos R, Avendano A, Horwitz I, et al. Tolerance and immunogenicity of an oral dose of CVD 103-HgR, a live attenuated *Vibrio cholerae* 01 strain: a double-blind study of Chilean adults. *Rev Med Chil* 1993;121:857–863.
70. Lucas MES, Deen JL, von Seidlein L, et al. Effectiveness of mass oral cholera vaccination in Beira, Mozambique. *N Engl J Med* 2005;352:757–767.
71. Clemens JD, Sack DA, Harris JR, et al. Field trial of oral cholera vaccines in Bangladesh. *Lancet* 1986;ii:124–127.
72. Monath TP. Yellow fever: an update. *Lancet Infect Dis* 2001;1:11–20.
73. Centers for Disease Control and Prevention. Adverse events associated with 17D-derived yellow fever vaccination—United States, 2001–2002. *MMWR Morb Mortal Wkly Rep* 2002;51:989–993.

CHAPTER

58

Louis Vernacchio
Allen A. Mitchell

Epidemiology of Adverse Drug Effects

INTRODUCTION

The practice of rational drug therapy requires weighing the benefits expected from the use of a given drug against its risks. Unfortunately, this ideal circumstance is rarely achieved because no matter how much we know about a drug's benefit, we often have an inadequate understanding about the frequency and severity of its adverse effects.

Historically, the lack of knowledge about adverse drug effects has been especially acute in pediatrics because of a relative scarcity of data from children. In many cases, drugs approved for adults have become widely used in children without careful consideration of potential adverse effects that may occur in the pediatric population. The growth and development that characterize children make them vulnerable to adverse outcomes unique to childhood, and often, to specific stages of childhood. The possibility of such alterations of growth, cognitive development, or specific organ development may not be appreciated in adult experience with a given drug but can have significant impact on children. Examples are numerous and include inhibition of linear growth by corticosteroids (1), tooth enamel dysplasia caused by tetracycline antibiotics (2), the association between erythromycin use and pyloric stenosis in young infants (3), and concern (still controversial) about deleterious effects of fluoroquinolones on cartilage development in prepubescent children (4). In addition to adverse outcomes that are unique to childhood, consideration must be given to the fact that children may metabolize certain drugs differently than adults, potentially leading to an increased risk of adverse effects. Chloramphenicol-induced "gray baby syndrome," in which delayed hepatic metabolism in infants leads to toxicity, is a classic example of this phenomenon (5,6).

That adverse drug reactions (ADRs) were indeed common and sometimes serious in the pediatric population was first demonstrated by systematic studies of ADRs in children that began in the 1970s (7–13). Since then, a substantial body of international literature on pediatric ADRs has confirmed and expanded these observations. In this chapter, we will focus on an epidemiologic approach to the study of adverse drug effects in children, reviewing both theoretical considerations and practical study approaches. We will attempt to emphasize aspects that are unique or especially relevant to pediatrics, using historical and current examples to illustrate the key points.

THEORETICAL CONSIDERATIONS

Whether from the clinical or epidemiologic perspective, three broad areas of information must be considered in the study of adverse drug effects: the drug of interest (the "exposure"), the adverse reaction to the drug (the "outcome"), and the nature of the patients who experience these effects (the "population").

EXPOSURE

Although the concept of exposure is straightforward, the definitions of what constitutes a drug and what constitutes an exposure are not always apparent. For example, few would quarrel with including in the definition oral and parenteral exposure to an antibiotic, but does drug exposure also include such common substances as intravenous fluids, vitamins, and oxygen? Furthermore, does the route of exposure (e.g., topical or by inhalation) affect the definition? These distinctions have important implications. As one example, because of varying definitions, three studies describing drug use in the newborn intensive care nursery (two from the same population) differed with respect to the number of drugs used in the patients, ranging from and average of 3.4 to 10.4 (13–15). Variations in the definition of what constitutes a drug exposure will clearly affect not only estimates of drug use but also the observed rates of ADRs in a given population.

Those who care for children must also consider another kind of drug exposure—the so-called inactive ingredients. These agents are included in a variety of medications to increase stability, solubility, shelf life, and the like. Although it is recognized that certain ingredients, such as sulfites and tartrazine, can produce adverse effects in sensitive individuals, observations from neonatal intensive care units have revealed that patients may suffer serious and even fatal reactions from such "inactive" ingredients as benzyl alcohol and propylene glycol (16,17). Unfortunately, agents added to active pharmaceuticals vary over time and manufacturers, and pharmacists, nurses, and physicians alike are usually unaware of the number and nature of "inactive" ingredients they are administering to patients (18). Obviously, lack of awareness about such exposures limits the likelihood of detecting their adverse effects.

A recently recognized area of concern in the pediatric population is the potential for adverse effects from "natural" products including herbs, megavitamins, and other dietary supplements. The prevalence of use of such products among children in the United States is unclear, with estimates for recent use ranging from as low as 2% to as high as 45%, depending on the population studied and the methodology used (19–24). What is not debatable is that herbal and other "natural" products have the potential for serious adverse effects in children. For example, a number of cases of sudden cardiac death and stroke have been linked to ephedra use, an herbal drug present in many diet aids, "energy" drinks, and other products specifically marketed to children (25). Less serious ADRs, such as allergic reactions and erythema nodosum linked to echinacea, have importance both because of their inherent effects and because they could be mistakenly attributed to the child's illness or to "conventional" treatments that are used concurrently (26–28).

Certainly, in terms of surveillance for potential adverse effects, a broad variety of substances and routes of administration should be considered in the definition of drug exposures. This may be of particular concern in pediatrics. The association between excessive inhaled oxygen and retinopathy in premature infants is but one dramatic example in pediatrics of the potential for a serious ADR from an intervention that, at first glance, many may not even be classified as a drug exposure (29,30).

OUTCOME

What outcomes are considered to be adverse drug effects? Much of the debate (and confusion) centers around the definition of the term "adverse drug reaction." The World Health Organization, for example, defines ADR as a response to a drug that is noxious and unintended and that occurs at doses used in humans for prophylaxis, diagnosis, or therapy (31). Although the World Health Organization definition does not exclude events that may be associated with a patient's disease state, others may exclude such events. Most definitions include noxious or pathological signs and symptoms, but do they also consider, for example, abnormalities in laboratory values in the absence of symptoms? Would asymptomatic hyperkalemia be considered an adverse reaction to potassium supplements? Many question whether certain signs and symptoms should be included as adverse reactions, particularly where they may be common, trivial, or unavoidable consequences of a drug's pharmacologic action (e.g., drowsiness with antihistamines, mild diarrhea with ampicillin, and leukopenia with cytotoxic drugs). Some would consider as ADRs only those outcomes requiring a change in drug therapy. Because few studies use a common definition of an ADR, one must be wary about making comparisons among different studies. As was the case for exposures, we prefer a broad definition of ADRs (as long as one does not give undue importance to the "total ADR rate" derived from such a definition), since it facilitates study of the broad spectrum of drug-related events.

Another source of confusion results from failure to make clear distinctions between effects of drugs that become manifest after short-term use and effects that become apparent only after long-term use. Acute effects following short-term exposure often involve allergic or hypersensitivity reactions (e.g., serum sickness with cefaclor), idiosyncratic responses (e.g., extrapyramidal signs due to phenothiazines), or extensions of a drug's known pharmacology (e.g., arrhythmias due to digitalis). Effects following long-term administration can occur in a precipitate manner (e.g., gastrointestinal bleeding from aspirin) or can have a more insidious onset (e.g., cataracts with corticosteroids); some effects may involve a latent interval, becoming apparent long after the drug exposure has ceased (e.g., adenocarcinoma of the vagina in adolescent females exposed in utero to diethylstilbestrol). A classification based on the temporal relation between duration of therapy and onset of adverse effect is particularly useful in considering various strategies for evaluating the full spectrum of ADRs.

Few ADRs represent unique clinical events. As a result, signs or symptoms that might be attributed to drug therapy by one observer might as easily be attributed to the patient's underlying disease state by another. For example, a rash occurring when amoxicillin is used to treat acute otitis media may be attributed either to the amoxicillin or to an underlying viral infection; lethargy in a patient with recurrent seizures may be attributed to the anticonvulsant used to control the seizures or to a postictal state. It is important to recognize that even healthy individuals who are receiving no medications will frequently report symptoms that are commonly considered side effects of drugs, such as fatigue, headache, and rash (32).

Reports in the mid-1970s described the difficulties inherent in attempts to establish valid and reproducible systems for implicating a particular drug in a specific adverse event (33,34). Since then, a number of researchers devised various algorithms to formally assess causality in suspected ADRs (35–37). Unfortunately, these approaches rely heavily on current information about a drug and its side effects, and they are therefore unlikely to facilitate discovery of new, previously unrecognized ADRs; in fact, by relying on current information about a drug's effects, some schemes may tend to discourage such discovery. Furthermore, effective use of the algorithms requires the availability of information (such as the results of withdrawal and rechallenge) that is often unavailable in the usual context of clinical practice. Critical assessment of specific algorithms has suggested that they have limited utility (38,39), and it is unlikely that these approaches will have major value in furthering our understanding of diverse ADRs. On the other hand, algorithms do identify the kinds of questions that must be answered to assess causality, and for this reason they can indeed prove helpful by highlighting appropriate questions in the clinician's assessment of a particular adverse event in a particular patient.

POPULATION

The third area of information needed for the study of ADRs concerns the population of patients being treated. Such information provides critical insight into both the nature of the ADRs and risk factors for their occurrence. For example, age is especially important in pediatrics as it may affect the risk of particular reactions; it is uninformative, for example, to describe the risk of sulfonamide-induced kernicterus in the entire pediatric age range, since this particular outcome is limited to newborn infants. The diseases for which patients receive drugs also affect the risk of experiencing an ADR; patients with cancer are far more likely to receive highly toxic drugs, and therefore have life-threatening adverse reactions than are other patients with less serious illnesses.

In addition to demographic factors, proper assessment of drug-effect relationships invariably requires a detailed understanding of the drug and outcome under consideration. For example, in a study of aspirin and Reye syndrome, one would be interested in whether the preceding illnesses (e.g., influenza) that prompted the aspirin use might distinguish those adversely affected by the exposure from those who were not. In a study of valproate-associated hepatotoxicity, one would wish to know whether valproate-treated epileptic patients differed from those who were treated with alternate drugs; for example, if valproate were given as a drug of "last resort," it may preferentially be administered to those who suffered ADRs on other anticonvulsants and who, therefore, may be at increased risk for ADRs on valproate.

ESTIMATING RATES OF ADVERSE DRUG REACTIONS

One of the most important aspects of ADRs is the frequency, or rate, with which they occur. In epidemiologic terms, rate refers to the number of people with the outcome of interest (the numerator) divided by the population at risk (the denominator), over a specified time. When applied to the study of ADRs, the numerator is the number of patients with reactions to a given drug, and the denominator is the number of patients exposed to that drug. The importance of the denominator is often overlooked; if penicillin-induced anaphylaxis is observed in 10 patients, the rate of this event cannot be determined unless the number of patients exposed to penicillin is also known. In statements reflecting rates of ADRs, the time reference is often implied and commonly refers to the period of drug exposure (e.g., the number of cases of anaphylaxis occurring during the course of penicillin therapy). However, for reactions that may occur after drug exposure has ceased, one must be particularly cautious that the time periods are appropriate in both the numerator and the denominator.

Finally, recall that the definition of the denominator refers to the population *at risk* for the reaction. Thus, although all penicillin-exposed patients might constitute an appropriate denominator in a consideration of anaphylaxis, since all exposed patients are at risk for anaphylaxis, the denominator for consideration of cyclophosphamide-induced azoospermia would not be all patients but only postpubescent males.

STATISTICAL CONSIDERATIONS

When a certain adverse event is observed in an at-risk population, a critical question arises as to whether that event should be attributed to the drug. In some settings, such as those involving acute events such as anaphylaxis, attribution may be straightforward. However, attribution is not straightforward for most adverse events, so the first step in answering this question is to determine the likelihood that the observed association between the drug exposure and adverse outcome is not due to chance. There are a number of statistical methods to help answer this critical question, and we will use a hypothetical example to illustrate their use.

Consider a situation in which 50 children with viral upper respiratory infections are treated with echinacea, and 15 of these patients develop a rash within days following initiation of the drug therapy. The rash rate is then 15/50, or 30%. We cannot conclude, however, that this rash rate is related to the echinacea until we compare it with the rate that would be expected among similar patients who did not receive echinacea. So, assume that among a comparable group of 50 children with viral upper respiratory infections who did not receive echinacea, 5 children developed rashes over a comparable period—a rate of 10%. The observed difference in rates (30% vs. 10%) may reflect rashes caused by the drug exposure or may merely represent a chance occurrence. Statistical testing identifies the probability of chance occurrences, and we usually state that a difference is statistically significant when the probability that the observation is due to chance is 5% or less (i.e., $p < .05$); that is, we are 95% confident that the observation is due to factors other than chance. It is important to keep in mind, however, that statistical testing is based solely on probability assessments to which we attach arbitrary cut-points; it does not provide certainty regarding the role of chance. Thus, if the echinacea–rash association is "significant" at $p = .05$, there remains a 5% probability that the observed difference in rate is due to chance. This type of error is called a "type I" or "alpha" error; it is equivalent to the "false-positive" conclusion in the evaluation of diagnostic tests. The magnitude of the alpha (false positive) error is equal to the p value that one uses to define "statistically significant" and, as noted above, is usually set at 5% (though there is no magic to that number). In our example, the likelihood that the observed difference (15/50 vs. 5/50) is due to chance is actually less than 5% (in fact, at $p = .012$, it is 1.2%). Thus, if we accept a 5% risk of making a wrong call, we can state that in this study the higher rate of rash among the echinacea-exposed children is unlikely to be due to chance (and therefore likely due to other factors, including possibly a cause–effect relationship).

Another, and often preferable, way to express the risk of an ADR in an exposed group of patients compared with an unexposed group is with the relative risk (RR) and associated confidence interval. In the context of ADRs, RR is defined as the rate of the adverse event in the exposed individuals divided by the rate in the unexposed. In the

TABLE 58.1 Number of Exposed Subjects Needed to Detect a Relative Risk of 2.0, 3.0, and 4.0 for Frequencies of Adverse Events in Unexposed Subjects of 1/50 to 1/10,000

Frequency of Adverse Event in Unexposed Subjects	*Sample Size of Exposed Subjects*		
	RR = 2.0	*RR = 3.0*	*RR = 4.0*
1/50	1,141	376	206
1/100	2,319	769	424
1/500	11,737	3,908	2,169
1/1,000	23,511	7,833	4,349
1/10,000	235,430	78,472	43,593

above example, the risk in the exposed group is 30% and that in the unexposed is 10%, yielding a RR of 3.0. In other words, rash occurred three times more commonly in the exposed individuals than in those not exposed. (If rash occurred with equal frequency in both groups, the RR would equal 1.0.) When using RR, the potential role of chance is expressed through calculation of the 95% confidence interval. In the current example, the 95% confidence interval ranges from a RR of 1.2 (the lower bound) to 7.6 (the upper bound). That the lower 95% confidence interval excludes a risk of 1.0 reflects that we are more than 95% certain that the observed association is not likely due to chance (the same information expressed by the *p* value of <.05); however, the confidence interval provides the additional information that we are 95% confident that the true RR lies between 1.2 and 7.6, and indeed is statistically more likely to be in the middle of that range and less likely to be near the extremes. Confidence intervals provide the additional benefit of statistical perspective. For a given risk estimate (e.g., RR = 3.0), *p* will be less than .05 whether the lower bound is 1.1 or 2.9, since both exclude 1.0; however, the values of the respective lower bounds should prompt the observer to recognize the more tentative nature of the former estimate.

It is useful to consider the situation in which no statistically significant difference between an exposed and unexposed group is found. Suppose our study revealed five patients with rashes among the 50 echinacea-exposed patients and five among the 50 unexposed. In this case, the RR is 1.0 and statistical testing would of course lead us to conclude that there is no evidence of a difference in rash rates between the two groups. Were these findings to be reported, it would not be unusual to see a conclusion such as the following: "Because there was no increased rate of adverse reactions among echinacea recipients, this drug appears safe." The frequency with which such statements are made reflects the failure to appreciate the very important distinction between "lack of evidence" of an association between a drug and adverse effect (i.e., no meaningful information one way or another) and "evidence of no association." In the current example, even though no association was observed, one cannot confidently rule out its existence. In fact, a study of only 50 exposed and 50 unexposed subjects would be too small to confidently rule out even fairly large increases in risk. The possibility of failing to observe an association when one actually exists is known as a "type II" or "beta" error and is comparable to the "false-negative" conclusion in the evaluation of diagnostic tests. Generally, beta is set at 0.2, meaning we are willing to accept a 20% chance of failing to detect a true association. Stated as "power" (1-beta), such a study would have an 80% chance of detecting an association where one does indeed exist.

Assuming an alpha of 0.05 and a beta of 0.2, how many exposed patients would one have to observe in order to detect various rates of ADRs? Table 58.1 presents the number of drug users needed to detect relative risks ranging from 2.0 to 4.0 for adverse events that occur among unexposed patients with varying frequencies. Thus, if the rate of a given adverse effect in the unexposed patients is 1 in 50, and if a drug is associated with a fourfold increase in risk, the increase can be detected in a sample of about 200 exposed patients. On the other hand, if the baseline rate of an adverse effect is 1 in 10,000, then nearly 44,000 exposed patients would have to be studied to detect a relative risk of the same magnitude (RR = 4.0); if the exposed patients have only a twofold increased risk of the adverse effect (RR = 2.0), its detection will require studying more than 230,000 patients exposed to the drug.

Finally, a word about relative versus absolute risk is in order. Statistical testing may reveal that an observed association between a drug exposure and given ADR is unlikely to be due to chance, and even if we assume that the observation is valid and causal (see following sections), it does not automatically follow that the increase in risk is *clinically* important. Suppose, for example, that in 100,000 children with viral upper respiratory infections treated with echinacea, a rash occurred in 100 whereas in a comparable sample of 100,000 children not treated with echinacea, a rash occurred in 25. The *relative risk* for exposed children is 4.0 with a confidence interval of 2.6 to 6.2, a highly statistically significant result. However, the *absolute risk* is only 1 per 1,000 in the exposed children compared with 0.25 per 1,000 in the unexposed, a difference in absolute risk of 0.75 per 1,000. Unless the rash in question were life-threatening, most would consider the absolute increase in risk to be clinically unimportant, regardless of the level of statistical significance.

VALIDITY

Although statistical testing is a tool that allows us to evaluate the likelihood of whether an observed association between a drug and an adverse outcome is due to chance, it in no way reflects the validity of the study that generated the data. Validity is a function of the study's design, conduct, and analysis. When it comes to drug safety, well-done randomized controlled trials provide the best assurance of validity, as it can generally be assumed that exposed and unexposed subjects are similar in terms of known and unknown factors that may affect their risks of adverse outcomes (i.e., "confounders"). In observational studies, such an assumption cannot be made. For example, if it were observed that 30% of children treated with echinacea for viral upper respiratory infection developed a rash compared with only 10% of control children, one would have to carefully assess the comparability of the two groups of children and all relevant potential confounders before concluding that the comparison was valid. If it turned out that the children treated with echinacea were more likely to have viral infections that themselves caused rashes, or were more commonly exposed to other medications that could cause rashes, one would have to question the validity of the comparison. In summary, no matter how "significant" a result is by statistical testing, such testing has relevance only if the study design is valid to answer the question of interest.

SOURCES OF ADVERSE DRUG REACTION INFORMATION

Having described the theoretical underpinnings for identifying and quantifying ADRs in children, we now focus on the sources that can provide ADR information in the pediatric population. These sources broadly fall into two categories—studies conducted prior to a drug being approved for marketing and studies conducted after a drug has come into use in children.

PREMARKETING STUDIES

In the United States, the mandate of the Food and Drug Administration (FDA) requires that the agency ensure that a drug is safe and effective before it is released to the general market. Premarketing studies are carried out according to a specified sequence: phase I studies evaluate a drug's biological effects, pharmacology, and safe dosage range in small numbers of normal human volunteers; phase II studies evaluate the drug in the treatment or prevention of a specific disease in limited numbers of patients; and in phase III studies, the drug is evaluated in selected human populations by means of clinical trials (usually randomized, double-blind studies). In phase III, the drug must be shown to be not only safe but also effective in terms of some intended use. These studies are necessarily limited in size (usually involving a total of a few hundred to a few thousand subjects).

Phase III trials are generally designed to be sufficiently large to evaluate efficacy and perhaps to evaluate expected common adverse effects; however, they are not designed to describe the full range of adverse reactions attributable to a given agent. In particular, they are unlikely to detect adverse reactions that are uncommon (occurring in as few as 1 in 100 or 1 in 1,000 drug users) and even less likely to detect reactions that occur with lower frequency (e.g., 1 in 10,000). In addition, because the duration of phase III studies tends to be quite limited, they will fail to identify those adverse effects that manifest only after long periods of use or after a latent interval from exposure. Furthermore, many types of patients who will ultimately be treated with the drug of interest are excluded from phase III studies; for example, such trials tend to exclude patients with comorbid diseases and those concurrently using other medications.

These limitations reduce the likelihood that phase III studies will detect adverse drug effects that may later be identified in various patient populations. From the pediatrician's perspective, however, premarketing studies have suffered from an additional major deficiency: historically, they have rarely evaluated drugs in children. This situation is improving with FDA efforts to encourage that children be included in clinical trials of new drugs and legislation providing for the National Institutes of Health to conduct studies of selected marketed drugs in children. However, information on many drugs currently used in children derives from drug evaluation studies that included small numbers of patients and hardly, if ever, evaluated drugs throughout the spectrum of age that concerns the pediatrician, from the premature newborn to the adolescent. As a result, most drugs in current use were released to the market without the benefit of even limited experience in pediatric age groups, and ADRs that occur uniquely or more frequently in infants and children would have necessarily gone undetected. As cited previously, examples of such reactions are numerous: sulfonamide-induced kernicterus in premature infants (40), tetracycline-induced tooth staining (2), and chloramphenicol-induced "gray baby syndrome" (5,6). Even after we have accumulated decades of experience with a given drug in the pediatric population, there is no assurance that a far more complete understanding of the drug's adverse effects will have emerged. For example, although phenytoin has been widely used as an anticonvulsant for many decades, more than 30 years of use elapsed before it was recognized that the drug may be responsible for movement disorders (41). Rash, on the other hand, has been a known adverse effect of this drug since the original studies of phenytoin were published in 1938. However, the frequency with which rash occurs is unclear; the often-quoted 5% rash rate in exposed patients can ultimately be traced to the original studies that involved a very heterogeneous and poorly described population of 200 adult and pediatric patients (42). Not only are we left with a poor understanding of the rate of rash among exposed patients, but we have virtually no understanding of factors that may make some patients more likely to develop a rash than others. Much more recent history reinforces the lack of information on risk for the most commonly used pediatric medications, as evidenced by recent findings related to over-the-counter cough and cold medications (see below).

POSTMARKETING STUDIES

Given the limitations of the premarketing drug approval process in terms of discovering certain types of adverse drug effects, postmarketing studies are critical to insuring drug safety. As mentioned previously, the premarketing approval process is particularly unlikely to identify adverse drug effects that are rare but serious, that are due to interactions with other drugs or comorbid diseases, or that result from patterns of use in the "real-world" setting of clinical medicine outside of formal trials. Various approaches to the postmarketing study of drug safety have been developed to detect and quantify these types of adverse drug effects. Each approach has its advantages and disadvantages, and a multiplicity of approaches is necessary to adequately identify and quantify adverse effects of the wide variety of drugs in clinical use. We will consider in turn the role of clinical trials and of various kinds of observational studies in the postmarketing evaluation of drug safety.

Phase IV Clinical Trials

Phase IV clinical trials are an extension of the premarketing drug approval process into the postmarketing setting. These trials are generally similar to premarketing phase III clinical trials but are conducted after the drug has been approved and is widely available for use. Phase IV trials may be designed to expand a drug's indications or may be mandated by regulatory agencies to specifically address issues raised but not resolved by the premarketing trials. In general, however, phase IV trials face the same limitations as premarketing clinical trials—they rarely focus on ADRs and, when they do, they may not account for the myriad variables that occur in routine clinical practice outside of trials such as interactions with other drugs, the effect of comorbid conditions, and patterns of use by the general public. Furthermore, their relatively small size limits their ability to identify and quantify rare but serious ADRs.

It should be noted that in some cases, very large community-based postmarketing clinical trials have been conducted specifically to detect adverse drug effects that are rare and serious or occur only in the context of typical clinical use. An example of such a study in pediatrics was a practitioner-based clinical trial conducted in the early 1990s involving more than 80,000 subjects, which demonstrated the relative safety of ibuprofen when used to treat short-term fever in children (43–45). We and others have argued that such "large simple trials" should be used more commonly in selected situations to assess the postmarketing safety of drugs, but as of yet, these types of trials remain unusual, especially in pediatrics (46,47).

Passive Surveillance/Spontaneous Reporting

Spontaneous reporting of adverse drug effects is the oldest and, to date, one of the most productive sources of information regarding ADRs. It requires three elements: one must observe an event, recognize it as a potential adverse drug effect, and report it. Such reports may be sent to drug manufacturers, to regulatory agencies, or to medical journals, where they appear as letters to the editor, case reports, or small case series.

Spontaneous reports have two major deficiencies. First, they are subject to the various biases of the observers. For example, physicians are more likely to report an adverse effect once others have; on the other hand, as the effect becomes well known, they tend to stop reporting its occurrence (this practice is encouraged by editors who view continued publication of such reports as unnecessary). Second, spontaneous reports provide no estimates of the number of patients exposed (the denominator) to the drug in question. Because spontaneous reports identify only a small fraction of all ADRs, they provide poor numerator estimates as well. As a result, estimates of the rate of adverse events usually cannot be derived and therefore cannot be compared to "baseline" rates to determine whether patients exposed to a particular drug are indeed at increased risk for an adverse effect.

Despite these deficiencies, there are situations in which adverse drug effects can be identified by spontaneous reporting; in fact, under certain circumstances, spontaneous reporting offers the most efficient mechanism for identification of new ADRs. Such discovery is most likely where the relative risk of a reaction is high, the drug is widely used, and it produces an effect that is immediate, rare, dramatic, and unrelated to the disease under treatment. For example, deafness shortly following the administration of furosemide fulfills these criteria, and such a reaction is likely to be recognized by spontaneous reports. When any one of these criteria is absent, however, discovery may be delayed substantially. Imagine a drug intended for the treatment of allergic diseases that caused urticaria in some exposed individuals; it is highly unlikely that spontaneous reporting would identify such an ADR, because most observers would likely attribute the urticaria to the patient's underlying allergic disease. The possibility of detecting an adverse effect by spontaneous reporting becomes even more remote if the effect appears long after the exposure began, and especially if it appears long after the exposure ceased. For example, the relative risk for thalidomide-induced phocomelia is extremely high, the drug was in reasonably wide use in certain countries, and the effect was very rare, dramatic, and unrelated to the disease under treatment (maternal anxiety or insomnia). However, because of the lag between exposure to the drug in early pregnancy and appearance of the malformed child at delivery, more than 6,000 babies were affected before spontaneous reporting identified the association.

Because of the theoretical usefulness and demonstrated value of spontaneous reports, it is important that practitioners remain sensitive to the possibility that an unusual event represents a previously unrecognized ADR, and that such events be reported. A number of similar independent observations, spontaneously reported by other health care professionals, will stimulate formal studies to further evaluate apparent relationships. Despite the development of sophisticated observational approaches for detecting ADRs (described below), spontaneous reports by physicians and others will continue to generate important and clinically relevant questions regarding adverse drug effects in children.

Adverse Event Registries

Adverse event registries represent attempts to centralize and formalize spontaneous reports of ADRs. Some of the first such organized registries, developed in the 1960s, were the American Medical Association's registry of blood dyscrasias which later evolved into a broad registry of ADRs and the FDA's Division of Drug Experience. Current national ADR registries include the FDA's MedWatch system (48) and Vaccine Adverse Event Reporting System (VAERS), a joint effort of the Centers for Disease Control and Prevention and the FDA (49).

The problems inherent in registries are similar to those described for spontaneous reporting—primarily, no denominators are available, so ADR rates cannot be calculated. However, like spontaneous reporting, registries have particular value in identifying strong and/or unusual associations between drugs and adverse events. For example, a small number of reports in the 1970s to the FDA registry linked central nervous system disturbances to the topical application of lindane, leading the FDA to alert practitioners to this newly discovered adverse effect (50,51). More recently, an association between the newly licensed oral rotavirus vaccine and intussusception was suggested by reports to VAERS (52).

Databases

As third parties have become more involved in the financing of medical care, record-keeping related to medical encounters has become more common. Insurance plans (e.g., Medicaid and other claims-based information sources) and health maintenance organizations, for example, have developed data files containing information on drug exposures, outcomes, and selected population variables. As a result, much attention in recent years has been devoted to utilizing such preexisting databases for the purposes of identifying and evaluating adverse drug effects. However, automated databases have limitations that are directly related to their attractiveness: they are inexpensive because they were developed for other purposes (e.g., billing), but for the same reason the information available is often inadequate to meet the needs of an epidemiologically rigorous assessment of the risks and safety of drug exposures. For example, it may be impossible or difficult to validate information on diagnosis and adverse events, and information often may not be available on critical factors, such as concurrent over-the-counter drug use (including vitamins and herbal products) or lifestyle issues such as diet and exercise. Nonetheless, there are selected situations in which automated databases can contribute useful information toward the identification and assessment of ADRs in children.

Drug Surveillance

Active approaches to the systematic discovery of ADRs vary greatly, as do the terms used to describe them. "Drug monitoring" was an early name for such activities, but it has now come to be associated with the assessment of drug levels in patients ("therapeutic drug monitoring"). More recently, the term "postmarketing surveillance" has become popular; while properly reflecting the increasing focus on the identification of ADRs once a drug has come onto the general market, this term encompasses the broad range of approaches, from spontaneous case reports, to specific studies designed to test hypotheses, to efforts designed to discover previously unrecognized ADRs. For reasons of history and personal taste, we favor "drug surveillance" as the most appropriate and established term for systematic efforts designed specifically to test and generate hypotheses regarding the effects of drugs.

The theoretical basis for drug surveillance was proposed in 1965 by Finney as "any systematic collection and analysis of information pertaining to adverse effects or other idiosyncratic phenomena associated with the normal use of drugs" (53). Beginning in the 1960s, this approach was used to study ADRs among hospitalized adults, with programs established by Cluff and colleagues (54) and Slone and colleagues [the Boston Collaborative Drug Surveillance Program (BCDSP)] (55). Information regarding drug exposure, outcome, and population characteristics was gathered by monitors employed by the programs. Cluff et al., first at Johns Hopkins and later at Gainesville, Florida, obtained information on drug exposures and selected patient characteristics from the patient record, and possible ADRs were identified by review of drug orders, patient records, and through discussions with ward physicians (56). In the BCDSP, nurses assigned to specific wards collected detailed information on variables of interest including drug exposures and potential adverse reactions. The latter came from detailed review of the patient record, attendance at ward rounds, and discussions with ward physicians. Both the Gainesville and BCDSP studies included a small number of children in their surveillance samples, but the pediatric efforts of both studies were small and short-lived (7,8,11).

In the mid-1970s, two drug surveillance efforts focused specifically on hospitalized pediatric populations. One, developed by Aranda in Montreal, was exclusively based in a newborn intensive care unit. That effort monitored 1,200 infants between 1977 and 1981 and produced useful information on the epidemiology of ADRs in this setting (57,58). The other, called the Pediatric Drug Surveillance (PeDS) program, was established in 1974 at the Children's Hospital in Boston, in collaboration with the Drug Epidemiology Unit (now the Slone Epidemiology Center) of Boston University School of Medicine. Over its 14 years, the PeDS program monitored more than 11,500 pediatric patients, from premature newborns to adolescents (13). Modeled after the BCDSP, the PeDS program provided descriptions of various aspects of drug therapy, such as rates and trends in drug exposure and clinically identified ADRs from both teaching and community hospitals (15,59,60). Known risk factors for certain reactions were also quantified (e.g., D10W-induced hyperglycemia in the newborn) (61).

A unique feature of intensive drug surveillance programs is the ability to generate hypotheses—that is, to identify previously unrecognized ADRs. For example, the PeDS program discovered sometimes serious risks associated with different medications used to sedate children for computerized tomography scans (59). The program also identified an association between intraventricular hemorrhage and low doses of heparin given to maintain the patency of infusion lines in low–birth-weight infants (62); although this procedure had been widely adopted in neonatal intensive care units, its safety had never been systematically evaluated, and it was reassuring when a randomized controlled trial, prompted by this signal, failed to show an increase in the rate of intraventricular hemorrhage among infants given heparin in this manner (63). On the other hand, we found an association between elevated levels of serum bilirubin in infants and exposure to morphine that contained the "inactive" ingredients phenol or chlorbutanol (64) and the risks of phenol and chlorbutanol in infants remain untested.

A few researchers from the United States and Europe have attempted to apply drug surveillance to the outpatient pediatric setting. Studies have reported ADR rates ranging from 1% to 6% and only rare occurrences of serious or life-threatening ADRs (65–68).

Although intensive drug surveillance has clear advantages over other approaches, it also has limitations. Programs are very expensive to develop and maintain and require multidisciplinary expertise and facilities. Because of the detailed information collected on each patient monitored in the inhospital setting, accumulation of sufficient data takes many years to accomplish. This concern is particularly problematic in pediatrics, since the marked differences in drug effects among neonates, infants, toddlers, and older children require that large numbers be monitored in each age category. Furthermore, drug surveillance programs are inefficient for the purposes of identifying relatively rare reactions, particularly if the drug involved is used infrequently.

Specific Cohort and Case-Control Studies

Cohort and case-control studies are typically employed to further investigate various hypotheses about ADRs. In cohort studies, groups of patients exposed and not exposed to a particular drug are observed for the development of adverse events that may be related to the exposure. Ampicillin was the subject of a number of such studies, leading to an understanding of the rates of rash and diarrhea attributable to this widely used agent (69–72). Cohort studies have a number of advantages, including the availability of valid information on the exposure and (usually) the outcome of interest. Because these studies identify a defined population of exposed patients, they permit one to estimate population-based rates of ADRs; however, like clinical trials, they are generally too small to efficiently detect rare events. Because cohort studies tend to involve follow-up of particular populations over some period of time, they tend to require relatively long-term involvement on the part of investigators and substantial financial support.

In case-control studies, patients with and without a given adverse event ("cases" and "controls," respectively) are identified, and the frequency of exposure to the drug in question is ascertained to determine whether exposure is more common in patients with the effect than in those without it. For example, one might identify newborn patients with cardiorespiratory collapse and patients without collapse and then ascertain exposure to benzyl alcohol-containing infusions (16). A recent example of importance to pediatrics was a case-control study, which confirmed an association between oral rotavirus vaccine and intussusception (73). Because the case-control approach begins with the outcome, that information is usually well documented and therefore valid; concern tends to focus on assuring that information on the exposure is also valid. Unlike cohort studies, which directly provide rates of adverse reactions, estimation of absolute ADR rates from case-control studies is somewhat more complicated. They are also generally inefficient for the assessment of rare exposures. On the other hand, case-control studies are useful in evaluating rare outcomes because cases can be actively sought (often across multiple centers) and then matched to controls. Whereas cohort studies tend to represent long-term efforts involving considerable cost, case-control studies are more likely to be conducted relatively quickly and inexpensively.

Although not applied frequently to pediatrics, both cohort and case-control studies can sometimes be used to generate new hypotheses regarding ADRs. In cohort studies, novel ADR hypotheses can be generated by following cohorts of individuals exposed to various drugs and monitoring for a range of adverse events. For example, the US Collaborative Perinatal Project in the 1950s and the 1960s followed drug exposures among 58,000 pregnant women and followed their offspring until age 7 years for the development of a wide range of adverse outcomes (74). In contrast, case-control studies typically focus on a particular outcome in relation to a particular exposure. However, researchers in the 1970s developed a system in which subjects with a wide variety of adverse outcomes were recruited and information on a wide range of exposures was collected. This "case-control surveillance" approach permits systematic consideration of multiple outcomes in relation to multiple exposures (75).

Proper attention to the design and conduct of a study using either the cohort or case-control approach can yield equivalently valid findings, yet some view the cohort approach as the scientifically more rigorous study design. Such a perception, we believe, reflects less the inherent qualities of the two designs and more their respective "track records." Because it is relatively easy to mount a case-control study, investigators can, without much thought to issues of design or analysis, assemble cases and controls and then seek information on exposure. By contrast, the logistics involved in most cohort studies tend to attract investigators who will commit substantial effort to the study over a relatively long time, and who can design a protocol that will pass scientific and funding reviews. It is not therefore surprising that "quick and dirty" studies are more likely to be conducted with the case-control than with the cohort approach (most often, the "dirty" reflects unrecognized or uncontrolled bias). This experience reinforces the importance of understanding that the efficiencies in time and cost inherent in the case-control approach in no way diminish the need for scientific rigor on the part of the investigators.

PEDIATRIC COUGH AND COLD MEDICATIONS—A BRIEF CASE STUDY

The recent controversy over the safety of pediatric cough and cold medications offers a case study in many of the principles governing the epidemiology of adverse drug effects in children. Cough and cold medications—which include various combinations of first-generation antihistamines, antitussives, decongestants, and expectorants—have been available over the counter and widely marketed to parents of young children for many decades. In fact, their approval predated the modern FDA system requiring rigorous premarketing evidence of safety and efficacy. Despite the absence of rigorous data, their safety in children was presumed by parents and medical professionals alike. However, throughout the 1990s and the 2000s, spontaneous case reports of serious ADRs associated with pediatric cough and cold medications were published in the medical literature (76–80). By 2007, the Centers for Disease Control and Prevention had mounted a modest drug surveillance effort and reported a significant number of serious ADRs and some deaths—largely in children younger than 2 years and largely related to the decongestant pseudoephedrine—associated with pediatric cough and cold medications (81). Following the generation of this concern, with potentially widespread and very important clinical implications, more formal studies have been conducted evaluating the prevalence of use of these medications in children (82,83) and more systematically evaluating their association with pediatric ADRs (84–86). These investigations prompted significant changes in the marketing and regulation of cough and cold medications to young children for the first time in many decades and reinforce the need for systematic assessments of the safety of the wide range of prescription and nonprescription medications [over the counter (OTC), vitamins/minerals, herbals] taken by children.

In the United States, FDA was given new authorities and mandates to require postmarketing safety studies; from the pediatric perspective, the FDA Amendments Act, as the legislation is called, gives particular prerogatives for subpopulations where premarketing safety studies were considered inadequate, and among the subpopulations it identifies are the elderly, pregnant women, and children (87). It is too soon to know whether this legislation will improve the safety of medications used in children, but the FDA Amendments Act is important for two reasons—first, it gives formal recognition to the risks resulting from lack of premarketing safety data and second, it gives those who care about the safety of pediatric therapeutics leverage to argue for the kinds of studies that, when conducted at all, have been too small, too few, and too clinically uninformative.

SUMMARY

If we are to accrue meaningful information on rates of ADRs and their associated risk factors, we need valid information on the exposure, outcome, and population under study. No single design can be expected to provide answers to all questions; rather, we need a variety of methods which, in the aggregate, will lead to critical improvements in our understanding of the nature, causes, and prevention of ADRs in children.

REFERENCES

1. Blodgett FM, Burgin L, Iezzoni D, et al. Effects of prolonged cortisone therapy on the statural growth, skeletal maturation and metabolic status of children. *N Engl J Med* 1956;254:636–641.
2. Conchie JM, Munroe JT, Anderson DO. The incidence of staining of permanent teeth by the tetracyclines. *Can Med Assoc J* 1970; 103:351.
3. Centers for Disease Control and Prevention. Hypertrophic pyloric stenosis in infants following pertussis prophylaxis with erythromycin—Knoxville, Tennessee, 1999. *MMWR Morb Mortal Wkly Rep* 1999;48:1117–1120.
4. Burkhardt JE, Walterspiel JN, Schaad UB. Quinolone arthropathy in animals versus children. *Clin Infect Dis* 1997;25:1196–1204.
5. Burns LE, Hodgman JE, Cass A. Fatal circulatory collapse in premature infants receiving chloramphenicol. *N Engl J Med* 1959;261:1318.
6. Lischner H, Seligman SJ, Krammer A, et al. An outbreak of neonatal deaths among term infants associated with administration of chloramphenicol. *J Pediatr* 1961;59:21.
7. Lawson DH, Shapiro S, Slone D, et al. Drug surveillance—problems and challenges. *Pediatr Clin North Am* 1972;19:117.
8. McKenzie MW, Stewart RB, Weiss CF, et al. A pharmacist-based study of the epidemiology of adverse drug reactions in pediatric medicine patients. *Am J Hosp Pharm* 1973;30:898–903.
9. Mullick FG, Drake RM, Irey NS. Adverse reactions to drugs: a clinicopathologic survey of 200 infants and children. *J Pediatr* 1973; 82:506–510.
10. Collins GE, Clay MM, Falletta JM. A prospective study of the epidemiology of adverse drug reactions in pediatric hematology and oncology patients. *Am J Hosp Pharm* 1974;31:968–975.
11. McKenzie MW, Marchall GL, Netzloff ML, et al. Adverse drug reactions leading to hospitalization in children. *J Pediatr* 1976;89: 487–490.
12. Whyte J, Greenan E. Drug usage and adverse drug reactions in children. *Acta Paediatr Scand* 1977;66:767–775.
13. Mitchell AA, Goldman P, Shapiro S, et al. Drug utilization and reported adverse reactions in hospitalized children. *Am J Epidemiol* 1979;110:196.
14. Aranda JV, Cohen S, Neims AH. Drug utilization in a newborn intensive care unit. *J Pediatr* 1976;89:315.
15. Lesko S, Epstein MF, Mitchell AA. Recent patterns of drug use in newborn intensive care. *J Pediatr* 1990;116:985.
16. Gershanik J, Boecler D, Ensley H, et al. The gasping syndrome and benzyl alcohol poisoning. *N Engl J Med* 1982;307:1384.
17. Glasgow AM, Boeck RL, Miller MK, et al. Hyperosmolality in small infants due to propylene glycol. *Pediatrics* 1983;72:353.
18. Hernandez-Diaz S, Mitchell AA, Kelley KE, et al. Medications as a potential source of exposure to phthalates in the U.S. population. *Environ Health Perspect* 2009;117:185–189.
19. Pitetti R, Singh S, Hornyak D, et al. Complementary and alternative medicine use in children. *Pediatr Emerg Care* 2001;17:165–169.
20. Ottolini MC, Hamburger EK, Loprieato JO, et al. Complementary and alternative medicine use among children in the Washington, DC area. *Ambul Pediatr* 2001;1:122–125.
21. Sawni-Sikand A, Schubiner H, Thomas RL. Use of complimentary/ alternative therapies among children in primary care pediatrics. *Ambul Pediatr* 2002;2:99–103.
22. Wilson KM, Klein JD. Adolescents' use of complementary and alternative medicine. *Ambul Pediatr* 2002;2:104–110.
23. Lanski SL, Greenwald M, Perkins A, et al. Herbal therapy use in a pediatric emergency department population: expect the unexpected. *Pediatrics* 2003;111:981–985.
24. Vernacchio L, Kelly JP, Kaufman DW, Mitchell AA. Medication use among children <12 years of age in the United States: results from the Slone Survey. *Pediatrics* 2009;124(2):446.
25. Haller CA, Benowitz NL. Adverse cardiovascular and central nervous system effects associated with dietary supplements containing ephedra alkaloids. *N Eng J Med* 2000;343:1833–1838.
26. Mullins RJ. Echinacea-associated anaphylaxis. *Med J Aust* 1998;168: 170–171.
27. Mullins RJ, Heddle R. Averse reactions associated with echinacea: the Australian experience. *Ann Allergy Asthma Immunol* 2002;88: 42–51.
28. Soon SL, Crawford RI. Recurrent erythema nodosum associated with *Echinacea* herbal therapy. *J Am Acad Dermatol* 2001;44: 298–299.
29. Kinsey VE, Zaharias L. Retrolental fibroplasias: incidence in different localities in recent years and a correlation of the incidence with the treatment given the infants. *JAMA* 1949;139:572–578.
30. Patz A, Hoeck LE, De La Cruz E. Studies on the effect of high oxygen administration in retrolental dysplasia. I. Nursery observations. *Am J Ophthalmol* 1952;35:1248–1253.
31. World Health Organization: International drug monitoring—the role of the hospital. *Drug Intell Clin Pharmacol* 1970;4:101.
32. Reidenberg MM, Lowenthal DT. Adverse nondrug reactions. *N Engl J Med* 1968;279:678.
33. Koch-Weser J, Sellers EM, Zacest R. The ambiguity of adverse drug reactions. *Eur J Clin Pharmacol* 1977;11(2):75–78.
34. Karch FE, Smith CL, Kerzner B, et al. Adverse drug reactions—a matter of opinion. *Clin Pharmacol Ther* 1976;19:489.
35. Karch FE, Lasagna L. Toward the operational identification of adverse drug reactions. *Clin Pharmacol Ther* 1977;21:247.

36. Naranjo CA, Busto U, Sellers EM, et al. A method for estimating the probability of adverse reactions. *Clin Pharmacol Ther* 1981;30:239.
37. Lanctot KL, Naranjo CA. Comparison of the Bayesian approach and a simple algorithm for the assessment of adverse drug events. *Clin Pharmacol Ther* 1995;58:692–698.
38. Louik C, Lacouture PG, Mitchell AA, et al. A study of adverse reaction algorithms in a drug surveillance program. *Clin Pharmacol Ther* 1985;38:183.
39. Pere JC, Begaud B, Haramburu F, et al. Computerized comparisons of six adverse drug reaction assessment procedures. *Clin Pharmacol Ther* 1986;40:451.
40. Silverman WA, Andersen D, Blanc WA, et al. A difference in mortality rate and incidence of kernicterus among premature infants allotted to two prophylactic antibacterial regimes. *Pediatrics* 1956;18:614.
41. Chalhub E, DeVivo D, Volpe JJ. Phenytoin-induced dystonia and choreoathetosis in two retarded epileptic children. *Neurology* 1976; 26:494.
42. Merritt HH, Putnam JJ. Sodium diphenylhydantoinate in the treatment of convulsive disorders. *JAMA* 1938;3:1068.
43. Lesko SM, Mitchell AA. An assessment of the safety of pediatric ibuprofen. *JAMA* 1995;273:929–933.
44. Lesko SM, Mitchell AA. Renal function after short-term ibuprofen use in infants and children. *Pediatrics* 1997;100:954–957.
45. Lesko SM, Mitchell AA. The safety of acetaminophen and ibuprofen among children younger than two years old. *Pediatrics* 1999;104:e39.
46. Mitchell AA, Lesko SM. When a randomized controlled trial is needed to assess drug safety. The case of pediatric ibuprofen. *Drug Saf* 1995;13:15–24.
47. Temple R. Meta-analysis and epidemiologic studies in drug development and postmarketing surveillance. *JAMA* 1999;281:841–844.
48. Kessler DA. Introducing MEDWatch: a new approach to reporting medication and device adverse effects and product problems. *JAMA* 1993;269:2765–2768.
49. Singleton JA, Lloyd JC, Motrey GT, et al. An overview of the vaccine adverse event reporting system (VAERS) as a surveillance system. *Vaccine* 1999;17:2908–2917.
50. Food and Drug Administration. Gamma benzene hexachloride (Kwell) and other products alert. *FDA Drug Bull* 1976;6:28.
51. Lee B, Groth P, Turner W. Suspected reactions to gamma benzene hexachloride. *JAMA* 1976;236(25):2846.
52. Centers of Disease Control and Prevention. Intussusception among recipients of rotavirus vaccine—United States, 1998–1999. *MMWR Morb Mortal Wkly Rep* 1999;48:577–581.
53. Finney DJ. The design and logic of a monitor of drug use. *J Chronic Dis* 1965;18:77.
54. Seidel LG, Thornton GF, Smith JW, et al. Studies on the epidemiology of adverse drug reactions. *Bull Johns Hopkins Hosp* 1966;119:299.
55. Slone D, Jick H, Borda I, et al. Drug surveillance utilizing nurse-monitors—an epidemiologic approach. *Lancet* 1966;ii:901.
56. Stewart RB, Cluff LE, Philip JR. *Drug monitoring: a requirement for responsible drug use.* Baltimore, MD: Williams & Wilkins, 1977.
57. Aranda JV, Portuguez-Malavasi A, Collinge JM, et al. Epidemiology of adverse drug reactions in the newborn. *Dev Pharmacol Ther* 1982; 5:173.
58. Aranda JV. Factors associated with adverse drug reactions in the newborn. *Pediatr Pharmacol* 1983;3:245.
59. Mitchell AA, Louik C, Lacouture PG, et al. Risks to children from computed tomographic scan premedication. *JAMA* 1982;247:2385.
60. Mitchell AA, Lacouture PG, Sheehan J, et al. Adverse drug reactions in children leading to hospital admission. *Pediatrics* 1988;82:24.
61. Louik C, Mitchell AA, Epstein MF, et al. Risk factors for neonatal hyperglycemia. *Am J Dis Child* 1985;139:783.
62. Lesko SM, Mitchell AA, Epstein MF, et al. Heparin use as a risk factor for intraventricular hemorrhage in low-birth-weight infants. *N Engl J Med* 1986;314:1156.
63. Chang GY, Lueder FL, DiMichele DM, et al. Heparin and the risk of intraventricular hemorrhage in premature infants. *J Pediatr* 1997; 131:362–366.
64. Lesko SM, Mitchell AA. Total bilirubin level in relation to excipients in parenteral morphine sulfate administered to seriously ill newborn infants. *Paediatr Perinat Epidemiol* 1994;8:401–410.
65. Kramer MS, Hutchinson TA, Flegel KM, et al. Adverse drug reactions in general pediatric outpatients. *J Pediatr* 1985;106:305.
66. Cirko-Begovic A, Vrhovac B, Bakran I. Intensive monitoring of adverse drug reactions in infants and preschool children. *Eur J Clin Pharmacol* 1989;36:63–65.
67. Mennitti-Ippolito F, Raschetti R, De Cas R, et al. Active monitoring of adverse drug reactions in children. *Lancet* 2000;355: 1613–1614.
68. Horen B, Montastruc J, Lapeyre-Mestre M. Adverse drug reactions and off-label drug use in paediatric outpatients. *Br J Clin Pharmacol* 2002;54:665–670.
69. Bass JW, Crowley DM, Steele RW, et al. Adverse effects of orally administered ampicillin. *J Pediatr* 1973;83:106.
70. Boston Collaborative Drug Surveillance Program. Ampicillin rashes: collaborative study. *Arch Dermatol* 1973;107(1):74.
71. Caldwell JR, Cluff LE. Adverse reactions to antimicrobial agents. *JAMA* 1974;230:77.
72. Collaborative Study Group. Prospective study of ampicillin rash. *Br Med J* 1973;1:7.
73. Murphy TV, Gargiullo PM, Massoudi MS, et al. Intussusception among infants given the oral rotavirus vaccine. *N Engl J Med* 2001; 344:564–572.
74. Heinonen OP, Slone D, Shapiro S. *Birth defects and drugs in pregnancy.* Littleton, MA: Publishing Sciences Group, 1977.
75. Slone D, Shapiro S, Miettinen OS. Case-control surveillance of serious illnesses attributable to ambulatory drug use. In: Colombo F, Shapiro S, Slone D, Tognoni G, eds. *Epidemiological evaluation of drugs.* Littleton, MA: PSG Publishing Company, 1977: 59–70.
76. Gadomski A, Horton L. The need for rational therapeutics in the use of cough and cold medicine in infants. *Pediatrics* 1992;89(4 pt 2): 774–776.
77. Gunn VL, Taha SH, Liebelt EL, et al. Toxicity of over-the-counter cough and cold medications. *Pediatrics* 2001;108(3):E52.
78. Boland DM, Rein J, Lew EO, et al. Fatal cold medication intoxication in an infant. *J Anal Toxicol* 2003;27(7):523–526.
79. Marinetti L, Lehman L, Casto B, et al. Over-the-counter cold medications-postmortem findings in infants and the relationship to cause of death. *J Anal Toxicol* 2005;29(7):738–743.
80. Wingert WE, Mundy LA, Collins GL, et al. Possible role of pseudoephedrine and other over-the-counter cold medications in the deaths of very young children. *J Forensic Sci* 2007;52(2): 487–490.
81. Centers of Disease Control and Prevention. Infant deaths associated with cough and cold medications–two states, 2005. *MMWR Morb Mortal Wkly Rep* 2007;56(1):1–4.
82. Vernacchio L, Kelly JP, Kaufman DW, et al. Cough and cold medication use by US children, 1999–2006: results from the Slone Survey. *Pediatrics* 2008;122(2):e323–e329.
83. Vernacchio L, Kelly JP, Kaufman DW, et al. Pseudoephedrine use among US children, 1999–2006: results from the Slone survey. *Pediatrics* 2008;122(6):1299–1304.
84. Watson WA, Litovitz TL, Rodgers GC Jr, et al. 2004 annual report of the American Association of Poison Control Centers Toxic Exposure Surveillance System. *Am J Emerg Med* 2005;23(5):589–666.
85. Schaefer MK, Shehab N, Cohen AL, et al. Adverse events from cough and cold medications in children. *Pediatrics* 2008;121(4): 783–787.
86. Rimsza ME, Newberry S. Unexpected infant deaths associated with use of cough and cold medications. *Pediatrics* 2008;122(2): e318–e322.
87. Food and Drug Administration Amendments Act of 2007. http://frwebgate.access.gpo.gov/cgi-bin/getdoc.cgi?dbname=110_cong_public_laws&docid=f:publ085.110. Accessed March 9, 2009.

CHAPTER

59

Michael Rieder
Bruce Carleton

Mechanisms of Adverse Drug Reactions in Children

ADVERSE DRUG REACTIONS

Children have been among the major beneficiaries of the era of Specific Therapy and the Therapeutic Revolution that started with Dömagk's description of the antimicrobial activity of Prontosil™ (1). However, as with most major advances, this has come at a price, most notably the fact that potent drugs can have potent adverse events. This was recognized very quickly, in that a number of serious adverse events associated with therapy were described in 1937, the year that sulfonamides first entered the market as antimicrobials (2). In fact, the history of drug regulation has been notable by being driven by therapeutic disasters involving children, the first of which was the Elixir of Sulfanilamide tragedy (2). Since then, it has been increasingly appreciated that adverse drug reactions (ADRs) are common and important complications of therapy that are seen with variable frequency in relation to therapy with essentially all drugs used for the care of children.

The original definition of ADRs by the World Health Organization was "any noxious, unintended, and undesired effect of a drug, which occurs at doses used in humans for prophylaxis, diagnosis, or therapy" (3). Although this is a useful definition, it is somewhat restricted in that it does not include errors in drug administration or dosing, issues that are of special relevance to children. A more useful definition is that an ADR is "an injury resulting from medical intervention related to a drug, which includes errors in administration" (4). This definition, which includes problems related to errors in drug administration, is much more useful with respect to considering ADRs that occur in children.

ADVERSE DRUG REACTIONS—THE BURDEN

ADRs are one of the most common causes of mortality and serious morbidity in developed countries (2,5,6). ADRs account for 5% of hospital admissions and complicate, at a minimal rate, 5% of the courses of most medication, with the rate climbing much higher among populations such as patients with cancer or in environments such as the critical care unit (5,6). Based on a large study of adverse events associated with therapy, it has been suggested that ADRs are the fourth most common cause of death in Canada and the United States, given that nearly 100,000 Americans a year die as a consequence of ADRs (6). The risk for children is less well defined than that for adults but does appear to be similar overall. Indeed, there may be circumstances in which the risk may be higher for children than for adults (6–9).

There are well-known risk factors for ADRs (Table 59.1) (9–11). Of note, many of the known risk factors are particularly germane for children; for example, premature neonates are at the extremes of age, often receive polypharmacy, and have developmental impairments in renal and hepatic drug clearance (12). Another underestimated factor with respect to developmental pharmacology is that the enhanced capacity of some enzymatic pathways in toddlers may also place them at increased risk for activation-induced ADRs (13). Children also cannot evaluate and express their response to medication as well as their adult counterparts.

CLASSIFICATION OF ADVERSE DRUG REACTIONS

A number of systems have been proposed to classify ADRs. At the onset, it is important to acknowledge a major nosological issue with respect to popular designation of adverse events associated with therapy. There is a common and regrettable use of the word "allergy" to apply as a blanket descriptor for all adverse events that occur in temporal relationship to drug therapy. This is both inaccurate and misleading. Although allergy in popular usage is considered to be sensitivity to a drug or chemical, in fact allergy is a very specific term, which a purist might define as an immunoglobulin E–mediated adverse event, but which is more commonly considered as an adverse reaction to a drug mediated by the immune system (14). The latter definition is much more useful, as it both speaks to mechanism and helps to guide clinical decision making as to diagnosis and therapy.

The most useful system for classifying ADRs is that described by Rawlins and Thomas, who in 1977 proposed that ADRs should be considered to be predictable or unpredictable (Table 59.2) (15). Predictable ADRs are

TABLE 59.1 Risk Factors for Adverse Drug Reactions

Extremes of age: Neonates and the elderly are at greater risk of experiencing ADRs due to hepatic enzyme immaturity and abnormality, respectively, as well as an increased chance for polypharmacy
Gender: Women experience a higher percentage of ADRs than do men
Polypharmacy: Administering multiple medications correlates with a synergistic rather than additive risk for ADRs
Disease states: Liver, kidney, and heart diseases may increase risk for ADRs, presumably by reducing the rate of drug clearance
Past history of ADR or allergy: ADRs are more frequent in patients who previously suffered an ADR or drug allergy—regardless of the class of drug to which they had experienced an adverse event to
Genetic factors: Certain genetic polymorphisms may increase risk of experiencing ADRs
Large doses: The chance of developing certain types of ADRs, notably drug hypersensitivity, appears to be greater among drugs used in higher doses

ADRs, adverse drug reactions.

TABLE 59.2 Classification of Adverse Drug Reactions

Predictable

These adverse events are predicated on the drug's known pharmacology. They are dose related and often diminish over time.

Side effects

Predictable adverse events that are consequences of the drug's pharmacology. Side effects can be troublesome but are rarely severe and often diminish over time. An example is fine hand tremor seen initially when therapy with β agonists, such as salbutamol (albuterol), is started but which often fades over time.

Secondary effects

Predictable but not inevitable adverse events that are a consequence of the drug's pharmacology. An example is pseudomembranous colitis following lincosamide therapy. A certain number of patients treated with lincosamides will have overgrowth of *Clostridium difficile*, of which a certain number will grow toxin-producing *C. difficile*, of which a certain number will develop toxin-related colitis.

Interactions

Predictable interactions occurring due to concurrent drug therapy, drug–food interactions, or drug–disease interactions. Classical examples include elevations in cyclosporine A plasma concentrations when cyclosporine A and clarithromycin are taken concurrently due to clarithromycin-inhibiting metabolism of cyclosporine A and to flushing and lightheadedness due to elevation in the plasma concentrations of nifedipine when nifedipine is taken with grapefruit juice, as grapefruit juice inhibits the intestinal metabolism of nifedipine.

Toxicity

In the case of many drugs, a high enough dose will produce toxicity, often by mechanisms different from those producing therapeutic effects. An example is aspirin, which in overdose produces toxicity by uncoupling mitochondrial oxidative phosphorylation, increasing anaerobic metabolism, and producing lactic acidosis.

Unpredictable

These adverse events are not predicated on the drug's known pharmacology and can occur via unknown or complex mechanisms. They are not typically considered as dose related, may be very severe, and may not diminish over time.

Allergic and pseudoallergic

Adverse events primarily mediated by immune-mediated or presumably immune-mediated responses. A classical example of the former is penicillin-induced anaphylaxis, a classical allergy that is still a frequent cause of mortality, while reactions to iodinated radiological contrast dyes are an example of the latter, in which case the immune system seems to be involved, but no clear mechanism has, as of yet, been delineated.

Idiosyncratic

Adverse events that are uncommon but serious consequences of therapy, which appear to occur in subsets of the population at special risk and which often appear to have complex mechanisms that can involve initial drug processing or activation followed by an immune response. Examples include clozapine-induced agranulocytosis, sulfonamide-associated toxic epidermal necrolysis or abacavir-induced Stevens–Johnson syndrome.

Intolerance

Adverse events characterized by severe side effects that occur in usual therapeutic doses when drugs are present in the blood in usual therapeutic concentrations. These adverse events appear to occur in unique subsets at special risk for reasons that remain unclear. A classical example is severe tinnitus to usual dose aspirin therapy, which can effect up to 1% of patients treated with long-term aspirin therapy.

Psychogenic

A poorly understood and difficult-to-manage type of adverse events associated with therapy, in which patients can develop disabling symptoms to a number of drugs and drug classes. The underlying mechanism(s) for these reactions is unclear, but some subsets of patients may have variant forms of panic disorder. A classical example is multiple-drug sensitivity.

ADRs, adverse drug reactions.

Determining the drug,
dose, and interval
Writing the order or
prescription

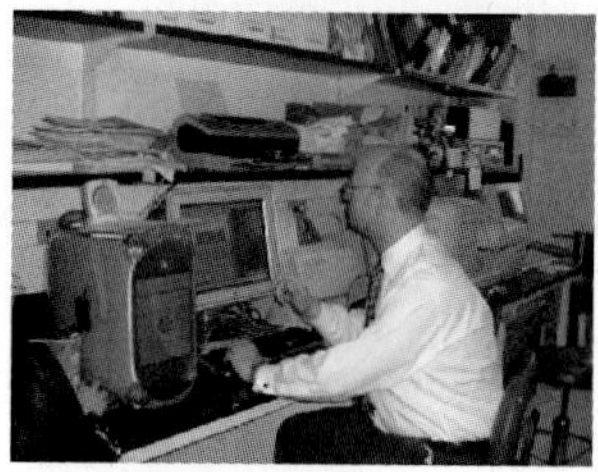

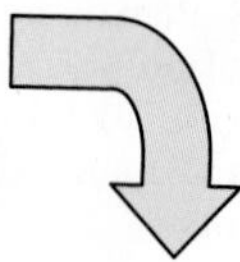

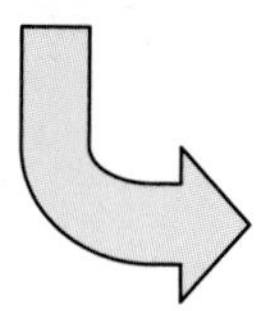

Figure 59.1. A number of factors are interrelated with respect to risk for adverse drug reactions in children, including determining the drug choice, writing the drug dose and dose interval order, dispensing and administering the drug, as well as pharmacokinetic and pharmacodynamic factors: drug absorption, distribution, metabolism, excretion, and drug action.

very common and typically not very severe. In contrast, unpredictable ADRs are much less common but often much more severe. As well, given their relatively uncommon occurrence, the vast majority of unpredictable ADRs are not described until the drug in question has gone through the development process and has been approved for general use. To illustrate, the majority of drugs are evaluated in 5,000 or fewer patients under tightly controlled circumstances prior to marketing. Many serious drug hypersensitivities occur at an incidence of 1:1,000 to 1:5,000 patients, an incidence that has potential impacts on public policy and drug regulation. However, there is essentially no chance that a hypersensitivity reaction that occurs at this rate will be detected prior to drug approval and entry into the market. This has significant implications in that serious hypersensitivity information would therefore become part of the product monograph either late or never.

MECHANISMS OF ADVERSE DRUG REACTIONS

As would be expected, the mechanisms of ADRs are dependent on the nature of the ADR, as outlined above. In the case of predictable ADRs, adverse consequences of therapy are the result of classical pharmacological determinants, and thus at different stages of development, children may be at special risk when ontologically determined alterations in pharmacokinetics or pharmacodynamics change how drugs are eliminated or how drugs act. As well, the circumstances under which drug therapy is decided upon and under which drugs are administered may predispose children at certain times in life to an increased risk for drug toxicity (Fig. 59.1). These will be considered in turn.

DEVELOPMENTAL PHARMACOLOGY

A unique issue with respect to ADRs in children, notably preterm infants, is developmental pharmacology (12). Although the admonition that "children are not small adults" is true across childhood, nowhere is this more important than in the first year of life, especially among infants born preterm. In terms of the classical pharmacological rubric of Absorption, Distribution, Metabolism, and Excretion, variations exist across all four domains, with potential impacts on the risk for ADRs.

ABSORPTION

The vast majority of drugs used in the therapy of children are given by the oral route, and there are well-described developmental differences in oral and gastrointestinal physiology between infants and older children and adults (16,17). These changes include the near-neutral pH of the newborn's stomach compared with the acidic stomach pH seen in adults and older children, delayed gastric emptying seen for the first 6 months of life, variable intestinal transit time, immature intestinal function, and altered capacity for both intestinal wall metabolism and transport. Many of these changes, notably with respect to metabolism and transporter function, remain poorly understood. The overall impact of these changes on the risk for ADRs is, for most drugs, minor. However, for some drugs, such as phenytoin, the marked differences between absorption in infants and older children place infants at an increased risk for both therapeutic failure and ADRs. Drug absorption when drugs are given via the intramuscular and pulmonary routes can vary greatly in infants, related to diminished muscular mass and muscular blood flow and to differences in pulmonary function between infants and adults (18). As well, the skin of newborns demonstrates transient, but significant, increase in percutaneous drug absorption compared with the skin of older infants, who in turn have enhanced percutaneous drug absorption compared with adults (19). This can be associated with toxicity for drugs that are not normally toxic by the cutaneous route in adults, especially if administered in large amounts (20).

DISTRIBUTION

There are substantial differences in body composition between infants and adults, with infants having 80% body water compared with 55% in adults and extracellular water of 45% in infants compared with 20% in adults (17). Also, plasma protein binding in infants is less extensive than in adults, which appears to be due to a mixture of relatively reduced binding capacity as well as relatively reduced binding affinity. As well, the blood–brain barrier of the infant is less well developed than that of adults (17). Thus, drugs that are highly protein bound may have a somewhat larger volume of distribution in infants than in adults, while drugs that normally do not cross the blood–brain barrier may be able to do so in infants. That being said, the impact of these changes on risk for ADRs is, overall, quite small.

METABOLISM

It is now well recognized that infants, notably preterm infants, have substantial differences in metabolic capacity and metabolic pathways when compared with older children and adults (12). This difference in metabolism has translated into therapeutic disaster on numerous occasions. One of the first, and among the most notable, was the chloramphenicol Grey baby syndrome (2,21,22). In the late 1950s, a syndrome characterized by cardiovascular instability with rapid progression to death was noted among infants being treated with chloramphenicol for possible sepsis (21). It has subsequently been appreciated that these infants had developmental limitations in the rate at which chloramphenicol could be metabolized via glucuronidation, with the consequence of immature glucuronidation being accumulation of chloramphenicol producing dose-dependent mitochondrial toxicity (22). This tragedy illustrated how developmental immaturity in drug metabolism capacity places neonates—especially premature neonates—at special risk (23).

It is also now appreciated that developmental expression of metabolic capacity is not uniform. Hines has described an overview that, although by his own admission somewhat simplistic, is also very useful in considering the potential impact of enzyme ontogeny on risk for ADRs (Fig. 59.2) (23). In this context, the three groups proposed are likely representative of enzymes that have substantially different biological roles. As an illustration, it is most likely that the enzymes represented in Group 1, whose peak expression occurs during the first and second trimesters of intrauterine life, have important roles in differentiation and development. The enzymes represented by Group 2 are those that appear to have relatively consistent expression, whereas the enzymes in Group 3—the largest group of enzymes—are those that have little or no function during intrauterine and early infant life, and whose expression increases over the first several years of life (Fig. 59.2). Of key relevance to risk for ADRs, the third group includes CYP2C9, CYP2D6, and CYP3A34, the major isozymes of cytochrome P450 most commonly associated with human drug oxidation, one key example being the CYP3A7 to CYP3A4 switch in which the primary isoform of CYP3A in the human fetus is 3A7 while the primary isoform in children and adults is 3A4 (23,24). Thus, infants may be at special risk when treated with drugs whose elimination is primarily dependent on these metabolic pathways. It should also be emphasized that there is considerable variation between and within enzymatic pathways as to the rate of maturation (23,25,26). Although the field of enzyme ontogeny still has many unknowns, there is now a sufficient amount of good quality data for modeling to be done to predict possible dose ranges and concentrations in infants when well-characterized drugs are used, and this modeling is becoming of increasing significance in safety pharmacology as part of drug development (27). These considerations apply to drugs given directly to the infant but also can apply to drugs delivered to the infant by breast-feeding (28). The issue of developmental alterations in drug metabolism has another side than concentration-dependent or predictable ADRs due to impaired drug clearance. There are a number of enzymes whose activity,

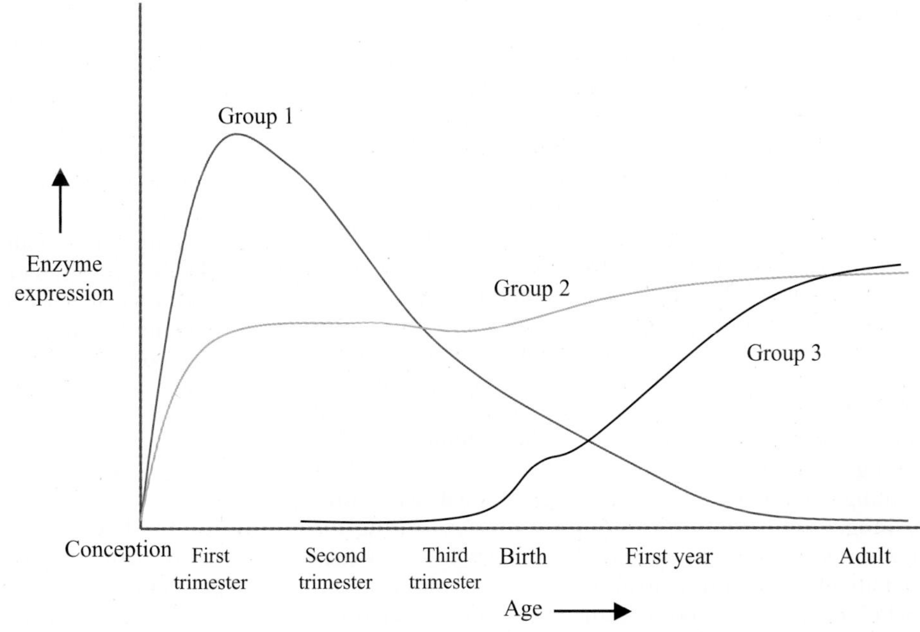

Figure 59.2. A schematic representation of the three major patterns of enzyme ontogeny (Hines RN. The ontogeny of drug metabolism enzymes and implications for adverse drug events. *Pharmacol Ther* 2008;118:250–267): with Group 1 being enzymes that are primarily expressed during the first and second trimester, Group 2 being those enzymes that are expressed relatively constantly during gestation, and Group 3 being those enzymes whose expression increases dramatically after birth. Examples of Group 1 enzymes include CYP3A7, FMO1, SULT1A3/4, and SULT1E1. Examples of Group 2 enzymes include CYP2C19, CYP3A5, and SULT1A1. Examples of Group 3 enzymes include CYP1A2, CYP2C9, CYP2D6, CYP2E1, CYP3A4, FMO3, ADH1B, ADH1C, and SULT2A1.

on a per kilogram or per metered square dose, is much more in toddlers than in adults (29). This has the potential to alter the risk for unpredictable ADRs, notably idiosyncratic ADRs such as drug hypersensitivity for which there is a reasonable body of evidence that drug bioactivation is a critical first step in initiating an immune response that ultimately determines the clinical characteristics of drug hypersensitivity (13). Thus, if a toddler had enhanced metabolic capacity, it might be possible that drugs could be activated to a greater extent than among adults, placing the toddler at unique risk for activation-induced ADRs. There is a small but compelling body of evidence supporting this; as an illustration, the risk of having a severe cutaneous reaction to lamotrigine is three times greater in children than in adults (30,31). Similarly, there is a 10-fold increase in risk for valproic acid–induced hepatotoxicity among toddlers compared with adults, while there also appears to be a 10-fold increase in the risk for cefaclor-induced serum sickness–like reactions in children compared with adults (32,33). Although the overall rate is still fairly low (1:500 for valproic acid–induced hepatotoxicity and 1:100 for cefaclor-induced serum sickness–like reactions), these represent serious and potentially life-threatening ADRs. Among children with cancer, serious ADRs are also often more common than among adults, again for reasons which currently are often not well understood (34,35). It will be important to better understand the pathophysiology of these adverse events to pursue the goal of safer drug therapy for children.

EXCRETION

As for drug metabolism, renal drug elimination also is subject to developmental expression (36). During intrauterine life, nephrons begin to form at week 5 and by week 8 become functional (37). Glomerular filtration can be appreciated early in intrauterine life and slowly increases during gestation, peaking at between 32 and 35 weeks of gestational age, while nephrogenesis ends at about 36 weeks of intrauterine life (37). At birth, glomerular filtration rate (GFR) is approximately 4 mL per minute per 1.73 m^2 body surface area; this doubles over the first several weeks of life and then rises to achieve adult values at about the end of the first year of life (36). Significantly, over the toddler years, the GFR on a relative basis is higher than in adults, resulting in enhanced clearance for drugs eliminated via the renal route compared with adults (Fig. 59.3). Thus, the developmental pharmacology of renal drug elimination is characterized by a duality, with infants—especially preterm infants—having markedly less ability to eliminate drugs via the kidney, while toddlers have an enhanced ability to do so (37).

The impact of this on drug elimination in the preterm infant has been appreciated for sometime, with the reduced ability to eliminate drugs and drug metabolites by the kidney placing newborn infants at increased risk for concentration-dependent toxicity. As an illustration, there is a substantial and robust literature on the need for altered aminoglycoside dosing—notably with respect to dosing interval—when treating newborns of different gestational ages with aminoglycoside antibiotics (38,39). Clinicians caring for newborns are typically aware of these issues and use drugs that are eliminated principally by the kidney with caution, including using, when possible, therapeutic drug monitoring to individualize therapy and reduce the risk of concentration-dependent toxicity (38,39).

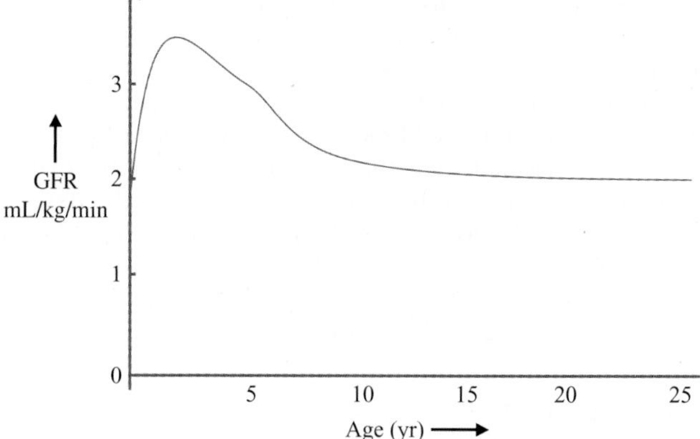

Figure 59.3. Relative glomerular filtration rate (GFR) compared to age. (Derived from Chen N, Aleksa K, Woodland C, et al. Ontogeny of drug elimination by the human kidney. *Pediatr Nephrol* 2006;21:160–168.)

It has been less well appreciated that the enhanced activity of the kidney in the toddler years may also be associated with an increased risk for other types of ADRs. One aspect of kidney function that has been somewhat underappreciated with respect to drug is renal drug metabolism (40). Although the metabolic capacity of the liver clearly overshadows that of the kidney, the kidney has substantial inherent capacity for the metabolism of many crucial molecules such as calcitriol (1,25-hydroxycholecalciferol), which is formed in kidney by the metabolism of 25-hydroxycholecalciferol. It has been appreciated for sometime that toddlers are at increased risk for nephrotoxicity from drugs such as ifosfamide, an alkylating agent widely used in the therapy of solid tumors (40). Work in our laboratory and elsewhere has suggested that this may be due to chloroacetaldehyde, which is formed in equimolar amounts to the active metabolite, ifosfamide mustard, when the parent drug ifosfamide undergoes ring hydroxylation and chloroethyl side oxidation (41). In toddlers, unbalanced production of chloroacetaldehyde versus glutathione may then lead to cellular injury and renal damage. The relevance of this hypothesis is that this offers the possibility of intervention, and pilot work has suggested that concurrent therapy with ifosfamide and the thiol donor *N*-acetylcysteine prevents the development of ifosfamide-induced nephrotoxicity in a rat model (42).

Thus, alterations in renal function in children can occur in both directions, both being associated with enhanced risk for ADRs. The strategies to reduce risk for ADRs in these cases diverge sharply, in the former case being dose monitoring and dose reduction while in the latter case it is possible that concurrent therapy models may provide an effective and alternative approach to reducing the risk of ADRs.

DRUG TRANSPORTERS

It has now been clearly demonstrated that the influx and efflux of many drugs into and out of tissues and cells are dependent on the presence of active transport systems, conventionally referred to as drug transporters (43,44).

These systems are often key determinants of the drug concentration at the target tissue, and as such of considerable importance in determining variability in drug response. Although a number of drug transporters have been found and characterized, there has been very little work on the ontogeny of drug transporters (45,46). What little work has been done suggests that there may be substantial differences in transporter expression and activity in children compared with adults; a recent animal model has demonstrated that there was very little expression of organic anion transporter 1 (OAT1), a key renal drug transporters, in fetal kidney (46). There was a sharp increase in expression of OAT1 after birth (46). The regulation of these changes, the potential impact on drug response, and the potential effect(s) on drug safety have yet to be elucidated. Given the large number and complexity of drug transporters, there is considerable research that needs to be done before we can have the same degree of confidence in appreciating impacts on drug safety as we have with the conventional pharmacokinetic concepts of absorption, distribution, metabolism, and excretion.

PHARMACODYNAMICS AND DRUG RECEPTORS

Although pharmacokinetics is an important determinant of how much drug is available to the therapeutic target, the biological response is often dictated by ligand–receptor interactions (47). The interaction between a drug and a drug receptor is the fundamental determinant of many of the effects of commonly used and therapeutically vital drugs, such as bronchodilation produced by β agonists interacting with the β receptor or analgesia produced by morphine interacting with the μ receptor, both classical cell surface G-protein–coupled receptors, to anti-inflammatory effects produced by prednisone interacting with the glucocorticoid receptor in the cytosol. As in the case of drug transporters, there has been very little work done to explore the ontogeny of drug receptors, and consequently the impact of altered receptor density or affinity on drug response in children is not well understood (48–50). This is an obvious area where clarity could provide considerable insights into variability in drug response in children. Again, much research needs to be done before we can approach our understanding of potential developmental changes in drug receptor expression or activity on the desired and adverse effects of drug therapy in children.

FORMULATION AND DOSING ISSUES

In addition to the issues with respect to the biology of drug disposition in children, there are practical issues with respect to how drugs are administered in real-world practice that can substantially alter the risk for ADRs, primarily for concentration-dependent events (Fig. 59.1). When a decision is made to prescribe therapy, the clinician must first decide upon which drug to use. The clinician must then determine a dose, dose interval, and duration of therapy. This must be communicated to the family and, in the case of prescription drugs, to the dispensing pharmacist. The drug must then be dispensed and administered to the child. Each of these events in therapy for children is fraught with the possibility of error, with the attendant risk of an ADR.

In the selection of therapy, the clinician is guided by training, experience, and the advice of experts on what constitutes the most appropriate treatment. However, in the case of children, there are many gaps both in knowledge and in knowledge translation that can result in therapeutic decisions being made on a less-than-optimal basis (51–53). In most of the developed world, the regulatory agency–approved product monograph does not contain information relevant to children's dosing or drug safety in as many as 75% of product monographs (54). As well, despite the myth that drug use in children is uncommon and then only confined to a few drug classes, it has been demonstrated that up to 20% of drug use occurs among children, and that this use crosses many therapeutic classes; a large Canadian study demonstrated that in a cohort of a million children followed for a year, there were 4.9 million prescriptions written for more than 1,200 drugs (55). Thus, without rigorous attention to drug selection, it is possible that a therapeutic decision may be made to select the wrong drug.

In terms of writing an order or prescription, drug dosing for children, especially infants, is often done on a per kilogram basis. Thus, rather than the norm in adult medicine in which there is a standard dose, the dose must often be calculated, which introduces the potential for error. It has now been clearly demonstrated that mathematical errors in writing drug doses for children is both more common than has been appreciated and also may not be an equally distributed risk; that is, there are certain groups of prescribers who are at higher risk for making errors in drug dosing (56–58). The most common extreme example of this is the 10-fold error, a phenomenon almost entirely confined to children (59). In this case, 10 times the usual dose is prescribed and given, almost always as a result of a decimal error in calculation. The fact that this error goes on to drug administration is related to a unique problem with pediatric dosage forms, in that the usual dosage and a 10-fold greater dose can often be accommodated in the same delivery vehicle, for example, the same size syringe (60). As an illustration, if an adult patient was given 10 digoxin tablets as a loading dose, this might raise a concern on the part of the pharmacist, nurse, and patient. However, the usual loading dose of digoxin for an infant and a 10-fold greater dose can be accommodated in the same syringe. There are a number of medications used in children's care for which a 5- to 10-mL dosage—easily within the range of most children's dose delivery systems—can be lethal (60). In addition, it is well known that commonly used drug dosing methods such as kitchen teaspoons can be very inaccurate, and the provision of accurate dose delivery systems for liquid medications is important in accurate dosing (61). Even when this occurs, confusion with dose delivery systems can still produce dosing errors and toxicity (62). Many of these problems can be best addressed on a system basis, that is, by the development of electronic prescribing and drug order systems that are pediatric appropriate and by the development of drug dosing systems that are child-friendly. As well, the educational and licensure systems that train and regulate child health care providers need to acknowledge, address, and evaluate strategies to improve prescribing and dispensing of medication for children.

IDENTIFICATION OF ADVERSE DRUG REACTIONS IN CHILDREN

A generic challenge in understanding ADRs is the identification of ADRs, starting with signal detection, analysis, causation evaluation, and assessment and validation. Historically, the vast majority of ADRs have not been reported to drug regulatory agencies, and underestimation of the burden of ADRs has been a systemic problem. However, there have been several developments over the past 5 years that provide hope that a new era is dawning on our understanding and approach to ADRs in children.

These developments include the creation of active surveillance networks. Although passive surveillance has been the norm, it is now clear that many common and important ADRs are not detected using the passive surveillance systems currently in place. Pioneering work using targeted active surveillance has demonstrated that this approach can not only identify serious and important ADRS at rates logarithmically greater than with passive surveillance but

TABLE 59.3 An Approach to a Suspected Adverse Drug Reaction

The first step is diagnosis: Is this an ADR or a nondrug event?

Diagnosis

History

What was the initial reason for therapy?

What was the course of events for the adverse event, notably with respect to timing and progression?

What therapy was used and in what dose?

What other therapies—current or recent—were being used?

What else is happening with the patient (including chronic health problems and food and environmental allergies)?

Physical

What are the signs of the event?

In the case of cutaneous signs, what is the distribution and nature of any cutaneous manifestations?

Differential diagnosis

The key differential is drug event versus nondrug event; that is, is the event an ADR or is it an uncommon or unexpected manifestation of the disease being treated? In many cases, this requires additional information, as there are over 2,500 drugs on the worldwide pharmaceutical market and most clinicians are familiar only with the 100-plus drugs that are used routinely in their clinical practice. In the event additional information is needed, drug information pharmacists, either in children's hospitals or as part of regional or national networks, are essential partners for the frontline clinician.

Investigation

There are relatively few confirmatory assays that can be applied to confirm a diagnosis as an ADR, and most of this small number have not been assessed in the acute state but rather have been used to confirm that a past event was an ADR. As an example, penicillin skin testing is often used to assess the possibility that urticaria accompanying penicillin therapy is due to penicillin allergy. This is almost always conducted post hoc.

Although research is ongoing on new techniques to diagnose drug allergy, the approaches being studied have not been quantified and validated sufficiently for them to be useful in a clinical context.

The next step is management: How do we deal with the consequences of the ADR?

Management

Management of an ADR is almost entirely symptomatic and supportive, with the exception of immune-mediated ADRs. In the case of serious reactions such as anaphylaxis, management should focus on supporting the airway and circulation. In the case of serious ADRs such as Stevens–Johnson syndrome or toxic epidermal necrolysis, recent evidence suggests that children who have these reactions may have a less serious course if immunomodulation in the form of intravenous immunoglobulin or adrenocorticosteroids is used. This is still controversial and the clinician caring for these patients is well advised to seek consultation with a specialist in the management of drug hypersensitivity.

During the management of the ADR, consideration must be given to the diagnosis for which therapy was given in the first circumstance; that is, has the underlying reason that the drug was administered been addressed? In the instance that it has—as an example, the otitis media for which an antibiotic was prescribed has resolved—then management can proceed directly to the ADR. In the event it has not—for example, if a child with epilepsy is still having uncontrolled seizures—then alternate therapy must be considered, bearing in mind the possibility of cross-sensitization or cross-class ADRs.

Management also includes communication. In addition to clearly communicating the fact of a diagnosed ADR plus the management plan and implications for future therapy, other health care providers involved in the circle of care for the child need to be informed so as to minimize the chance of a second ADR to the same or a similar drug. Given the complex care teams often involved in the care of children with chronic problems—who tend to be the group at highest risk for ADRs (Table 1)—this is a critical conversation.

A final consideration in management is that the fact of having had an ADR is highly likely to impact on the relationship between the clinician and the family. This may impact, as an illustration, on compliance with future therapy. In this respect, having clear communication about the fact of the ADR and the plan, both immediate and future as well as which drugs should and should not be avoided, will be much to secure a healthy clinician–patient–family relationship.

ADRs, adverse drug reactions.

Modified from Rawlins MD, Thomas SHL. Mechanisms of adverse drug reactions. In: Davis RE, Ferner RE, de Glanville H, eds. *Davies' textbook of adverse drug reactions*, 5th ed. Philadelphia, PA: Lippincott-Raven, 1998:40–64.

also that the use of active surveillance coupled with new technology can provide startling and unexpected insights into risk factors for ADRs as well as potential mechanistic insights into these adverse events (63,64). These insights in turn provide windows of opportunity for the development of strategies to identify patients at risk, including novel approaches to provide therapeutic benefit while minimizing ADR risk (34). These opportunities come with challenges that will need to be addressed if they are to achieve their full potential, including ethical, legal, economic, health care systems, and public policy issues; that being said, these novel approaches and new technologies offer the promise of an entirely new paradigm in the therapy of infants, children, and adolescents (53).

APPROACH TO ADVERSE DRUG REACTIONS IN CHILDREN

It should be emphasized that the current approach to an adverse event occurring in temporal relationship with drug therapy is almost entirely clinical. The first step is diagnosis: Is this event an ADR or not? To determine this, a stepwise approach is key in sorting out the often-complex events that happen when therapy goes wrong or is seen to go wrong (Table 59.3). It is important to keep this in mind, as a key element in the differential diagnosis—and one that is regrettably often neglected—is the consideration as to whether an undesired effect seen during therapy is due to the therapy or to the underlying disease. Once this determination has been made, the next step is management, which includes the management of both the ADR and the underlying diagnosis for which therapy was initially prescribed. The importance of clear and frequent communication with the patient, family, and other health care workers in the assessment and management of an ADR in a child cannot be overstated, given the common goal of optimal drug therapy for infants, children, and adolescents.

REFERENCES

1. Weinshilboum RM. The therapeutic revolution. *Clin Pharmacol Ther* 1987;42:481–484.
2. Choonara I, Rieder MJ. Drug toxicity and adverse drug reactions in children—a brief historical review. *Paediatr Perinat Drug Ther* 2002; 5:12–18.
3. World Health Organization Media Center. Available at: www.who.int/mediacentre/factsheets/fs293/en/index.html.
4. Bates DW, Cullen DJ, Laird N, et al. Incidence of adverse drug events and potential adverse drug events. Implications for prevention. *JAMA* 1995;274:29–34.
5. Bates DW, Spell N, Cullen DJ, et al. The costs of adverse drug events in hospitalized patients. *JAMA* 1997;277:307–311.
6. Lazarou J, Pomeranz BH, Corey PN. Incidence of adverse drug reactions in hospitalized patients: a meta-analysis of prospective studies. *JAMA* 1998;279:1200–1205.
7. Carleton BC, Smith MA, Gelin MN, et al. Paediatric adverse drug reaction reporting: understanding and future directions. *Can J Clin Pharmacol* 2007;14:e45–e57.
8. Impicciatore P, Choonara I, Clarkson A, et al. Incidence of adverse drug reactions in paediatric in/out-patients: a systematic review and meta-analysis of prospective studies. *Br J Clin Pharmacol* 2001;52: 77–83.
9. Rieder MJ. Hypersensitivity adverse drug reactions in children: pathophysiology and therapeutic implications. *Curr Ther Res Clin Exp* 2001;62:913–929.
10. Becquemont L. Pharmacogenomics of adverse drug reactions: practical applications and perspectives. *Pharmacogenomics* 2009;10: 961–969.
11. Pourpak Z, Fazlollahi MR, Fattahi F. Understanding adverse drug reactions and drug allergies: principles, diagnosis and treatment aspects. *Recent Pat Inflamm Allergy Drug Discov* 2008;2:24–46.
12. Kearns GL, Abdel-Rahman SM, Alander SW, et al. Developmental pharmacology—drug disposition, action, and therapy in infants and children. *N Engl J Med* 2003;349:1157–1167.
13. Rieder MJ. Immune mediation of hypersensitivity adverse drug reactions: implications for therapy. *Exp Opin Drug Saf* 2009;8: 331–343.
14. Assem E-SK. Drug allergy and tests for its detection. In: Davis RE, Ferner RE, de Glanville H, eds. *Davies' textbook of adverse drug reactions*, 5th ed. Philadelphia, PA: Lippincott-Raven, 1998:790–815.
15. Rawlins MD, Thomas SHL. Mechanisms of adverse drug reactions. In: Davis RE, Ferner RE, de Glanville H, eds. *Davies' textbook of adverse drug reactions*, 5th ed. Philadelphia, PA: Lippincott-Raven, 1998:40–64.
16. Strolin Benedetti M, Baltes EL. Drug metabolism and disposition in children. *Fundam Clin Pharmacol* 2003;17:281–299.
17. Bartelink IH, Rademaker MA, Schobben AF, et al. Guidelines on paediatric dosing on the basis of developmental physiology and pharmacokinetic considerations. *Clin Pharmacokinet* 2006;45: 1077–1097.
18. American Academy of Pediatrics. Committee on Drugs. Alternate routes of drug administration: advantages and disadvantages. *Pediatrics* 1997;100:143–152.
19. Ginsberg G, Hattis D, Miller M, et al. Pediatric pharmacokinetic data: implications for environmental risk assessment for children. *Pediatrics* 2004;113:973–983.
20. Rincon E, Baker RL, Iglesias AJ, et al. CNS toxicity after topical application of EMLA cream on a toddler with molluscum contagiosum. *Pediatr Emerg Care* 2000;16:252–254.
21. Sutherland JM. Fatal cardiovascular collapse in infants receiving large amounts of chloramphenicol. *AMA J Dis Child* 1959;97: 761–767.
22. de Wildt SN, Kearns GL, Leeder JS, et al. Glucuronidation in children. *Clin Pharmacokinet* 1999;36:439–452.
23. Hines RN. The ontogeny of drug metabolism enzymes and implications for adverse drug events. *Pharmacol Ther* 2008;118:250–267.
24. Leeder JS. Developmental pharmacogenetics: a general paradigm for application to neonatal pharmacology and toxicology. *Clin Pharmacol Ther* 2009;195:1–5.
25. Blake MJ, Gaedigk A, Pearce RE, et al. Ontogeny of dextromethorphan *O*- and *N*-demethylation in the first year of life. *Clin Pharmacol Ther* 2007;81:510–516.
26. Kearns GL, Robinson PK, Wilson JT, et al.; Pediatric Pharmacology Research Unit Network. Cisapride disposition in neonates and infants: in vivo reflection of cytochrome P450 3A4 ontogeny. *Clin Pharmacol Ther* 2003;74:312–325.
27. Alcorn J, McNamara PJ. Using ontogeny information to build predictive models for drug elimination. *Drug Discov Today* 2008; 13:507–512.
28. Madadi P, Koren G. Pharmacogenetic insights into codeine analgesia: implications to pediatric codeine use. *Pharmacogenomics* 2008;9: 1267–1284.
29. Strolin Benedetti M, Whomsley R, Baltes EL. Differences in absorption, distribution, metabolism and excretion of xenobiotics between the paediatric and adult populations. *Expert Opin Drug Metab Toxicol* 2005;1:447–471.
30. Hirsch LJ, Weintraub DB, Buchsbaum R, et al. Predictors of Lamotrigine-associated rash. *Epilepsia* 2006;47(2):318–322.
31. Levi N, Bastuji-Garin S, Mockenhaupt M, et al. Medications as risk factors of Stevens–Johnson syndrome and toxic epidermal necrolysis in children: a pooled analysis. *Pediatrics* 2009;123:e297–e304.
32. Anderson GD. Children versus adults: pharmacokinetic and adverse-effect differences. *Epilepsia* 2002;43(Suppl 3):53–59.
33. Kearns GL, Wheeler JG, Rieder MJ, et al. Serum sickness-like reaction to cefaclor: lack of in vitro cross-reactivity with loracarbef. *Clin Pharmacol Ther* 1998;63:686–693.
34. Ross CJ, Katzov-Eckert H, Dubé MP, et al.; the CPNDS Consortium. Genetic variants in TPMT and COMT are associated with hearing loss in children receiving cisplatin chemotherapy. *Nat Genet* 2009; 41(12):1345–1349.

35. Hausner E, Fiszman ML, Hanig J, et al. Long-term consequences of drugs on the paediatric cardiovascular system. *Drug Saf* 2008; 31:1083–1096.
36. Chen N, Aleksa K, Woodland C, et al. Ontogeny of drug elimination by the human kidney. *Pediatr Nephrol* 2006;21:160–168.
37. Solhaug MJ, Bolger JM, Jose PA. The developing kidney and environmental toxins. *Pediatrics* 2004;113:1084–1091.
38. Sherwin CM, Svahn S, Van der Linden A, et al. Individualised dosing of amikacin in neonates: a pharmacokinetic/pharmacodynamic analysis. *Eur J Clin Pharmacol* 2009;65:705–713.
39. Nielsen EI, Sandström M, Honoré PH, et al. Developmental pharmacokinetics of gentamicin in preterm and term neonates: population modelling of a prospective study. *Clin Pharmacokinet* 2009; 48:253–263.
40. Hanly L, Chen N, Rieder M, et al. Ifosfamide nephrotoxicity in children: a mechanistic base for pharmacological prevention. *Exp Opin Drug Saf* 2009;8:155–168.
41. Chen N, Aleksa K, Woodland C, et al. The effect of *N*-acetylcysteine on ifosfamide-induced nephrotoxicity: in vitro studies in renal tubular cells. *Transl Res* 2007;150:51–57.
42. Chen N, Aleksa K, Woodland C, et al. *N*-Acetylcysteine prevents ifosfamide-induced nephrotoxicity in rats. *Br J Pharmacol* 2008;153: 1364–1372.
43. Kim RB. Transporters and drug discovery: why, when, and how. *Mol Pharmacol* 2006;3:26–32.
44. Degorter MK, Kim RB. Hepatic drug transporters, old and new: pharmacogenomics, drug response, and clinical relevance. *Hepatology* 2009;50:1014–1016.
45. Johnson TN, Thomson M. Intestinal metabolism and transport of drugs in children: the effects of age and disease. *J Pediatr Gastroenterol Nutr* 2008;47:3–10.
46. Sekine T, Endou H. Children's toxicology from bench to bed—drug-induced renal injury (3): drug transporters and toxic nephropathy in childhood. *J Toxicol Sci* 2009;34(Suppl 2):SP259–SP265.
47. Maehle AH, Prull CR, Halliwell RF. The emergence of the drug receptor theory. *Nat Rev Drug Dis* 2002;1:637–641.
48. Sloboda DM, Moss TJ, Li S, et al. Expression of glucocorticoid receptor, mineralocorticoid receptor, and 11beta-hydroxysteroid dehydrogenase 1 and 2 in the fetal and postnatal ovine hippocampus: ontogeny and effects of prenatal glucocorticoid exposure. *J Endocrinol* 2008;197:213–220.
49. Subbarao P, Ratjen F. Beta2-agonists for asthma: the pediatric perspective. *Clin Rev Allergy Immunol* 2006;31:209–218.
50. Basille M, Falluel-Morel A, Vaudry D, et al. Ontogeny of PACAP receptors in the human cerebellum: perspectives of therapeutic applications. *Regul Pept* 2006;137(1–2):27–33.
51. Goodman DC. Unwarranted variation in pediatric medical care. *Pediatr Clin North Am* 2009;56:745–755.
52. Mathis L, Rodriguez W. Drug therapy in pediatrics: a developing field. *Dermatol Ther* 2009;22:257–261.
53. Leeder JS, Spielberg SP. Personalized medicine: reality and reality checks. *Ann Pharmacother* 2009;43:963–966.
54. Rieder MJ. Better drug therapy for children: time for action. *Paediatr Child Health* 2003;8:210–212.
55. Rieder MJ, Matsui DM, MacLeod S. Myths and challenges—drug utilization for Canadian children. *Paediatr Child Health* 2003; 8(Suppl A):7A.
56. Glover ML, Sussmane JB. Assessing pediatrics residents' mathematical skills for prescribing medication: a need for improved training. *Acad Med* 2002;77:1007–1010.
57. Ligi I, Arnaud F, Jouve E, et al. Iatrogenic events in admitted neonates: a prospective cohort study. *Lancet* 2008;371:404–410.
58. Kozasr E, Scolnik D, MacPherson A, et al. Variables associated with medication errors in pediatric emergency medicine. *Pediatrics* 2002;110:737–742.
59. Koren G, Barzilay Z, Greenwald M. Tenfold errors in administration of drug doses: a neglected iatrogenic disease in pediatrics. *Pediatrics* 1986;77:848–849.
60. Bar-Oz B, Levichek Z, Koren G. Medications that can be fatal for a toddler with one tablet or teaspoonful: a 2004 update. *Paediatr Drugs* 2004;6:123–126.
61. Food and Drug Administration. Guidance for Industry: Drug Delivery Devices for OTC Liquid Drug Products. US Department of Health and Human Services, Food and Drug Administration, Center for Drug Evaluation and Research, November 2009. http://www.fda.gov/ucm/groups/fdagov-public/...drugs-gen/.../ucm188992.pdf.
62. D'Alessandro LCA, Rieder MJ, Gloor J, et al. Life-threatening flecainide intoxication in a young child secondary to medication error. *Ann Pharmacother* 2009;43:1522–1527.
63. Carleton B, Poole R, Smith M, et al. Adverse drug reaction active surveillance: developing a national network in Canada's children's hospitals. *Pharmacoepidemiol Drug Saf* 2009;18:713–721.
64. Wong E, Carleton BC, Wright DF, et al. Genotypic approaches to therapy in children (GATC): using information technology to improve drug safety. *Stud Health Technol Inform* 2009;143: 209–214.

CHAPTER

60

John Chuo
George Lambert

Medication Errors

DEFINITIONS

A *medication error* is defined as the failure of a planned action to be completed as intended or the use of the wrong plan to achieve a specific aim (1). A medication error is such an error that occurs during the medication use process (2). Essentially, the right drug must be given to the right patient, in the right route, at the right dose, and at the right time (five rights) (3). Figure 60.1 illustrates the relationship among medication errors and potential, preventable, or unpreventable adverse drug events (ADEs) (4,5). ADEs are any injury due to medications (2). Preventable ADEs are medication errors that harm patients, whereas unpreventable ones are considered adverse drug reactions (ADRs) and not errors. Potential ADEs are errors that do not harm patients. A potentially harmful medication error (potential ADE) that is identified and corrected prior to drug administration is classified as a near miss, and a non-intercepted potential ADE that by chance does not result in patient injury is classified as a no-harm event. Errors can be acts of commission or omission. The authors of this chapter would like to call attention to a third error type—propagation errors—acts that permit errors committed at an earlier use process stage to pass on to the next stage or reach the patients.

INTRODUCTION

Medication errors exact a high toll on patient safety and health care costs, resulting in approximately 7,000 deaths per year (6). In the hospital setting, where most of the reports have been generated, approximately 47% of medical errors are medication related (6). Kaushal et al. reported that ADEs occur at 2.3 per pediatric admissions and approximately 19% of them are preventable (7). The 2007 Institute of Medicine (IOM) report on prevention of medication error estimates that a hospital patient may be subjected to at least one medication error per day (6). In terms of ADEs, at least 1.5 million occur each year in the United States: 380,000 to 450,000 in hospital care, 800,000 in long-term care, and 530,000 in ambulatory care. The financial burden is significant. Each medical error adds approximately 4.6 days to hospitalization and $5,857 to the patient care cost (8).

Medication errors are preventable mishaps occurring during any step of the drug use process that can lead to inappropriate drug use and patient harm (9). The opportunities for error are staggering when one considers that hundreds of medication orders are prescribed each day in larger neonatal units. Each medication use process has five steps beginning with conception to prescription, transcription dispensing, administration, and ends with effects monitoring (Fig. 60.2); each step has subprocesses that must get all five rights correct. In total, a single antibiotic order will have at least a dozen error opportunities, assuming that no process variations exist. However, medication use processes operate frequently in the midst of certain barriers that will, no doubt, produce process variation and greatly increase error opportunities. For example, distractions may cause a physician to prescribe the wrong dose; a ward clerk, nurse, or pharmacist to transcribe a written prescription incorrectly onto the pharmacy's queue; the pharmacist to make a calculation error or dispense the wrong medication; or the patient's nurse to administer the drug to the wrong patient or to the right patient at the wrong time. In the outpatient setting the patient's parent or caregiver may measure the dose incorrectly. Finally, in a patient with renal disease, the patient may start therapy with the correct drug and dose, but inadequate monitoring of serum creatinine concentrations could subsequently prevent the necessary dosage adjustment should renal function decline. Most errors fall into the commission category in which the correct medication plan is executed incorrectly. Omission errors are those in which the wrong medication plan (including no treatment) is executed. Propagation errors are "passive" in the sense that the usual safeguards (i.e., five rights checklist) are not used to stop an error committed earlier in the use process from reaching the patient. Workflows producing these errors involve complex human and environmental factors. The IOM report "To Err Is Human," attributes most patient injuries not to culpable individuals, but systemic factors such as poor communication systems, and unrealistic dependency on human memory and vigilance (1).

Prevention can happen at many levels. The IOM report summarizes patient-centered patient safety support at four levels—the federal, institution, unit, and patient. Ideally, support at each level would operationally complement one another. For example, the state of Pennsylvania mandates

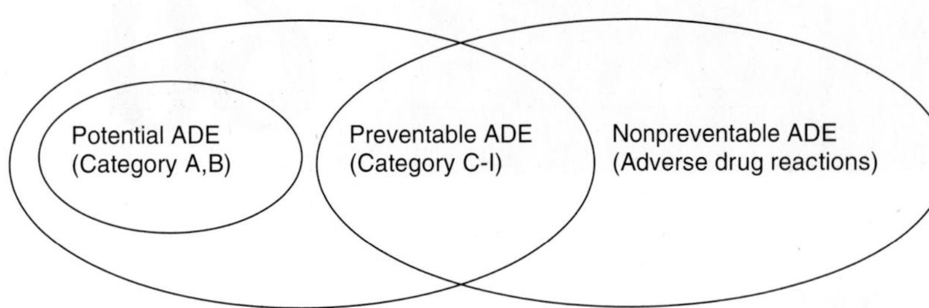

Figure 60.1. Relationship among medication errors, adverse drug events (ADE), and adverse drug reactions. [Adapted from Gandhi et al. 2000 (4) and NCC-MERP Classification for Medication Error Severity (5).]

QI reporting, the institution builds reporting infrastructure that is user-friendly and establishes a "nonblame" culture, the unit ward develops communication and educational forums that leverage the staff's expertise to identify systemic improvements (which will feedback to the institution), and the patient and family become an active part of the care team.

FREQUENCY OF MEDICATION ERRORS

Reports on medication error rates vary widely depending on the reporting mechanism (10–14). Somewhat structured written "incident reports" are most commonly used through a voluntary reporting system. Significant underreporting exists, especially for near misses. This is partly due to a hesitancy to report errors given the traditional approach to medication error management of blaming the responsible individual(s) rather than focusing on correcting a flaw in the medication delivery system that allowed the error to occur. The IOM committee, in its "Preventing Medication Errors" publication, comments that the reports of about 400,000 preventable ADE annually are likely to be underestimates. Detection methods include review of written orders, prompted reporting, chart review, electronic record extraction, and direct participation in clinical care (6). Jha et al. emphasized the complementary effect of using three methods, computerized surveillance of medical records, chart review, and voluntary reporting, together to find errors (15). Recently, trigger-based detection methods, such as the Institute for Healthcare Improvement global trigger tool, have been shown to be effective in identifying error clues in retrospective chart reviews (16). Its success has prompted adapting its use for other medical errors in clinical care.

Prescription
Handwritten or computer prescriber order typically entered by physician, nurse practitioner, or trainee.

Transcription
Critical prescription information is transferred onto the patient's medication administration record either manually or electronically.

Preparation and dispensing
Pharmacist prepares, labels, and dispenses the final drug product. Many pediatric doses require extemporaneous compounding from stock containers.

Administration
The nurse or medication technician administers the medication. In the outpatient setting, the patient or caregiver is responsible for drug administration. In either case, the five rights of medication administration should be achieved (right patient, drug, dose, time, and route)

Monitor for effects
Patients are monitored for drug reactions. Laboratory values such as plasma drug concentrations, serum creatinine concentrations, and hepatic function should be checked and drug dose or administration schedule adjusted as indicated.

Figure 60.2. Typical steps involved in the medication use process.

When studying and comparing medication error rates, it is critical to remember that the denominator may change the rate value significantly (17). For example, prescribing errors have ranged from 12.3 to 1,400 per 1,000 admissions, 0.61 to 53 per 1,000 orders, and 1.5 to 9.9 per 100 error opportunities (2,18–23). Preventable ADE rates per 1,000 admission range from 3.7 to 84.1 (24–26). Preparation and dispensing error rates are reported to be 2.6 per 1,000 admissions in general and 26% to 49% per preparation for intravenous medications (23,27,28). Errors in adults and pediatrics are approximately equal (29–34) at about 5%.

In the ambulatory setting, it is estimated that four invalid doses per 100 immunizations are given to children, or 36% of children are being immunized at least one invalid dose during childhood (35). Overimmunization happens in approximately 21% of patients (36). In two emergency room reports, 10 and 3.9 errors per 100 patients happen in the prescribing and administering phases, respectively (37). In the hospital setting, where most of the reports have been generated, approximately 47% of medication errors are medication related.

There is controversial evidence of an alarming increase in the incidence of medication errors and related mortality in the United States since the introduction of prospective pricing by Medicare in 1983 (38–42). Evaluating mortality data from the National Center for Health Statistics based on International Classification of Diseases (ICD-9) codes during the period spanning 1983 to 1998, the authors reported a 157% increase in the incidence of medication errors (38). Based on ICD-9 E850 through E858, the authors' definitions of medication errors involving the patient or medical staff included accidental drug overdoses, accidental administration of the wrong drug, and accidents involving the administration of drugs or biologic agents during medical or surgical procedures (39). The associated increase in patient mortality during this time period was 137% among hospitalized inpatients and 907% among outpatients (38). The authors mentioned that a number of potential factors contributing to the apparent increase in medication errors, including the increasing complexity of the health care system and the cost containment measures aimed at shortening the length of hospitalization, have increased the utilization of outpatient care and limited the time available for direct contact between patient and physician (38). It should be pointed out that the results of the study have been criticized for possibly mislabeling accidental poisoning deaths, a sizable proportion of which involved drugs of abuse, as medication errors (40–42). This criticism is based on the use of the term "accidental poisoning" rather than "medication error" in the *ICD-9* codes, and on the characteristics associated with the patient population. For example, of the 7,391 mortalities reported in 1993, the term "drug abuse" was used in approximately 30% of cases, whereas only 0.6% to 3.4% of cases included a description of chronic illness, such as ischemic heart disease, pulmonary disease, or cancer (42).

In summary, medication error rates are underreported. Reporting standards needs further specifications. Nevertheless, reported error rates are unacceptably high and can be used to track the effectiveness of medication error prevention programs and focus efforts.

COMMON TYPES OF MEDICATION ERRORS

It is estimated that at least 380,000 to 450,000 preventable ADEs occur in US hospitals annually (26,43). Many reported ADEs were preventable (27% to 50%) and occurred in the prescription and administration stages (39% and 38%, respectively) (44). Prescription error types were predominately wrong dose, known allergy, wrong frequency, and drug–drug interaction. In the Bates et al. study, 53% of the prescription errors were missing doses; of the remaining 250 medication errors, 31% were dose errors, 31% wrong frequency, 10% wrong route of drug administration, 6% illegible prescription handwriting, and 4% drug administration to a patient with a documented allergy to the agent, numbers that more closely resemble the percentages reported by the other studies listed in Table 60.1 (2,12,37,45,46). Leape et al. (47) analyzed 264 preventable and potential ADE events and identified the three top proximal causes of error as lack of knowledge of the drug, lack of information about the patient, and rules violations (22%, 14%, and 10%, respectively). Most errors occurred in the prescription and administration phase (39% and 38%, respectively). They found that poor access to information accounted for 78% of the errors, with the top three system failures being drug knowledge dissemination, dose and identity checking, and patient information availability (29%, 12%, and 11%, respectively). Studies also suggest that overdoses are the most common type of dosing error, with the majority of errors occurring at the drug ordering state (32,46,48). Not surprisingly the drug classes most often involved in medication errors are the ones most often prescribed to hospitalized patients (Table 60.2) (2,45,46). Antibiotics are most often associated with medication errors in the hospitalized patients, accounting for approximately 20% to 40% of all medication errors. Other drug classes commonly involved in medication errors include cardiovascular agents, gastrointestinal agents, vitamin or mineral products, electrolyte concentrates, and nonnarcotic and narcotic analgesics.

Underutilization of medications (errors of omission) deserves mention and is reported mostly by the adult literature. Most studies report a wide variation in compliance with "in time treatment" of acute myocardiac infarction, antibiotic prophylaxis, and thromboembolic prophylaxis. Depending on the exact treatment (error of omission), myocardial infarction (MI) was at 51% to 93%, surgical antibiotic prophylaxis was at 70% to 98%, and thromboembolic prophylaxis was at 5% to 90% (38–42,49–61).

TABLE 60.1 Common Types of Medication Errors, as a Percentage of Total Medication Errors Identified in Each Respective Study

Study	*Total Number of Errors (% All Orders)*	*Wrong Dose (%)*	*Wrong Schedule (%)*	*Wrong Route (%)*	*Wrong Drug or Patient (%)*	*Missing Dose*	*Known Allergy*	*Incomplete Order (%)*
Bates et al. (2)	530 (5.3)	14.5	8.1	4.9	2.1	53	2.1	. . .
Lesar et al. (45)	905 (0.31)	46.5	. . .	3.4	6.6	. . .	6.7	22.3
Lesar et al. (46)	696 (0.39)	58.3	. . .	3.3	5.4	. . .	12.9	. . .
Simborg and Derewicz (37)	105 (7.4)[a]	72.4[a]	. . .	1.9[a]	17.1[a]	. . .	. . .	. . .
	20 (1.6)[b]	35[b]		5[b]	25[b]			
Blum et al. (12)	1,012 (1.3)[c]	45[c]	27[c]	. . .	. . .	. . .	. . .	17[c]
	1,277 (2.7)[d]	58[d]	28[d]					4[d]

[a]Traditional multidose system with handwritten physician orders.
[b]Unit dose system with computerized physician order entry.
[c]Adult teaching hospital.
[d]Pediatric hospital.

TABLE 60.2 Drug Classes Most Often Involved in Medication Errors, as a Percentage of Total Medication Errors Identified in Each Respective Study

Study	*Total Number of Errors (% All Orders)*	*Antimicrobials (%)*	*Cardiovascular Agents (%)*	*Gastrointestinal Agents (%)*	*Analgesics (%)*	*Vitamins/ Electrolytes (%)*
Bates et al. (2)	530 (5.3)	19	8	. . .	7	10
Lesar et al. (45)	905 (0.31)	23.1	10.2	10.4	8.5	5.7
Lesar et al. (46)	696 (0.39)	39.7	17.5	7.3	10.2	3

MEDICATION ERRORS IN PEDIATRIC PATIENTS

Kaushal and associates investigated the frequency of medication errors, ADEs and potential ADEs in 1,120 inpatients ranging in age from neonates through adults at two teaching medical centers (29). Of 10,778 prescriptions written during the study, 616 medication errors were identified for a rate of 5.7 errors per 100 orders written. In this study, medication errors occurred at a higher rate in adult patients (8.6 errors per 100 hospital admissions) than in any other age group studied with 6.2, 4.1, 4.8, 5.8, and 6.3 medication errors per 100 admissions, respectively, in the neonatal, infant, preschool, school-aged, and adolescent cohorts ($p = .006$). In contrast, potential ADEs were identified at a significantly higher rate in neonates (2.0 potential ADEs per 100 hospital admissions) than in any other age group with 0.5, 0.8, 1.2, 1.1, and 1.4 potential ADEs per 100 admissions, respectively, in the infant, preschool, school-aged, adolescent, and adults cohorts ($p < .001$). The results of the study were also compared with those of a similar study conducted by Bates and colleagues in adult inpatients (2).

Although most studies (30–34) but not all (29) suggest that medication error rates are similar between pediatric and adult medicine, medication errors are 2½ times more likely to harm children than adults, with 30% of pediatric errors leading to disability lasting for more than 6 months and 15% leading to death (62). Several factors contribute to a higher risk of ADEs in pediatric patients when medication errors do occur (Table 60.3) (31,63–65). The Joint Commission summarized reasons for increased harm in pediatrics as (a) most medications need to be altered for pediatric use and requires pediatric-specific dosage calculations and processes that increase error opportunities, (b) many health care facilities, especially emergency rooms, lack the necessary staff orientation to pediatric care, protocols and safeguards, and reference materials, (c) children are usually less tolerant to the physiological impact of medication errors, and (d) children, especially infants, cannot communicate adverse effects effectively (66). Neonates and young infants may be less capable physiologically of coping with a medication error such as a drug overdose due to immaturity of critical body processes (29,63,64). For example, in comparison with healthy adults, the heart of newborn infants is characterized by decreased ventricular compliance, a lower ratio of contractile to noncontractile myocardial proteins, and a higher resting heart rate (67–69). Neonates therefore have a lower preload preserve and cannot tolerate volume loading as well as adults do. The higher baseline heart rate means that neonates are less capable of augmenting cardiac output by increasing heart rate without compromising diastolic filling.

It is not surprising that most harmful errors involve the wrong drug dose or happen during administration. Pharmacokinetic processes are widely variable and age specific, with highly variable age-related differences in drug absorption, distribution, metabolism, and excretion in children (70–73). The variability in pharmacokinetic processes is severalfold greater in children than in adults (70–73). Age-related differences in drug pharmacodynamics and

TABLE 60.3 Factors That Increase the Risk of Adverse Drug Reactions in Pediatric Patients (31,65)

1. Greater pharmacokinetic variability: Pharmacokinetic variables are age related and can change rapidly in young neonates, necessitating frequent drug dose and schedule adjustments; pharmacokinetic differences are magnified in preterm neonates such as in:
   a. Gastrointestinal drug absorption in neonates with increased gastric pH, delayed gastric emptying, and reduced biliary function
   b. Drug distribution in neonates with increased total body water and extracellular fluid, decreased total body fat, and decreased plasma protein binding.
   c. Drug metabolism in neonates with decreased phase I and phase II drug-metabolizing enzyme activity; both the level of activity and rate of maturation are isozyme specific
   d. Drug excretion in neonates with decreased glomerular filtration and renal tubular secretion
2. Dependence on individualized dosage calculations where calculations need to account for patient age, body weight or surface area, organ function, and disease state
3. Lack of appropriate pediatric dosage forms since younger patients often cannot or will not take oral tablets or capsules, necessitating the extemporaneous compounding of oral solutions or suspensions for many medications
4. Lack of Food and Drug Administration–approved pediatric labeling
5. Dependence on precise measurement and delivery devices: Doses of oral solutions and suspensions must be measured accurately; parenteral drug products are often delivered in smaller volumes in young neonates and infants, necessitating the use of precise infusion or syringe pumps
6. Children and infants cannot communicate adverse drug effects effectively

TABLE 60.4 Common Types of Medication Errors in Pediatric Inpatients, as a Percentage of Total Medication Errors Identified in Each Respective Study

Study	*Total Number of Errors (% All Orders)*	*Wrong Dose (%)*	*Wrong Schedule (%)*	*Wrong Route (%)*	*Wrong Drug or Patient (%)*	*Known Allergy*	*Incomplete Order (%)*
Kaushal et al. (29)	616 (5.7)	28	9.4	18	1.5	1.3	2.3
Folli et al. (31)	479 (0.47)	85	...	1.9	5.6	0.4	...
Kozer et al. (32)	271 (···)	49.1	43.2	2.6	1.8	...	...
Raju et al. (33)	315 (···)	13.7	21.6	4.1	13.3	...	...

pharmacokinetics are discussed in depth in Chapters 3 and 4. From birth to adulthood, the greatest amount of pharmacokinetic variability occurs during the neonatal period (70–73). These processes can change rapidly and dramatically during the first 4 weeks of postnatal life, as excess total body water is lost, renal and hepatic function begin to mature, and plasma protein binding begins to normalize, necessitating frequent drug dose and schedule adjustments. For example, the mean (standard deviation) total body clearance of theophylline has been shown to increase threefold between the postconceptual age of 35.5 ± 2.9 weeks and 63.2 + 14.4 weeks (21.5 + 6.9 vs. 60.7 + 14.4 mL per kg per hour, respectively) (74). This change is attributed primarily to maturation of the principal metabolic pathway in the liver, cytochrome P-450 IA2 (CYP1A2). CYP1A2 activity approaches normal by approximately 55 weeks of postconceptual age, followed by above average levels of activity during childhood and decreases to adult levels during puberty in a gender-specific fashion (75). The effect of this change in CYP1A2 activity on the elimination half-life of theophylline is dramatic, as the half-life decreases approximately 10-fold during infancy. The mean (range) half-life in premature infants (25 to 32 weeks of gestational age and 3 to 15 days of postnatal age), children (1 to 4 years of age), and adults (23 to 79 years of age) has been reported to be 30.2 (14.4 to 57.7), 3.4 (1.9 to 5.5), and 6.7 (3.6 to 12) hours, respectively (76).

Pediatric drug therapy is also frequently complicated by the wider variability in patient's body weight or body surface area and renal or hepatic function when attempting to appropriately individualize the patient's drug dose (63). This process requires accurate and current patient-specific information and accurate dosage calculation. As Table 60.4 illustrates, dosing errors are the most common type of medication errors identified in pediatric patients (29–33).

The risk of medication errors in pediatric patients can also be increased by the lack of an appropriate pediatric dose form. Solid oral dose forms are often inappropriate for younger children, yet suitable oral solutions or suspensions are not available for many drugs used to treat pediatric illnesses. As a result, pharmacists are often required to extemporaneously compound and dispense appropriate formulations for pediatric patients. Not only does this increase the risk of error by requiring additional calculations, in many instances critical information related to the stability and bioavailability of these products is not available (63).

Many drugs commonly used in pediatric medicine also continue to lack Food and Drug Administration–approved labeling (63). As a result, the optimal dose and schedule for these agents, based on the results of clinical trials, are lacking. This not only increases the risk of ADEs but also increases the likelihood of suboptimal therapy.

Pediatric patients may have higher rate of medication errors due to unique challenges with respect to drug delivery (63). Intravenous drug formulations intended for use in neonates and young infants must often be delivered in very small volumes, requiring precise, and in many instances unique, compounding procedures and specialized delivery devices such as infusion or syringe pumps. Because the drug concentration is generally higher than in the corresponding adult formulation, the risk for an ADE may be higher if a medication error is made with respect to the infusion rate. The frequent need for oral solutions or suspensions necessitates careful and precise measurement of each dose. The latter problem is complicated even further if the product is administered on an outpatient basis because the patient's parent or caregiver is generally depended on to measure and prepare for each dose (63).

IMPACT OF MEDICATION ERRORS ON PATIENT SAFETY AND TREATMENT COST

Most studies evaluating the impact of medication errors on patient safety have used ADEs or potential ADEs as the primary study outcome measure. ADEs are defined as patient injuries directly related to medication use (2). The majority of ADEs are predictable dose-related injures that are considered preventable (77–79). All preventable ADEs are therefore classified as medication errors. Nonpreventable ADEs, such as an unexpected hypersensitivity reaction to a medication, are less common and not counted as a medication error. In contrast, potential ADEs or near misses are defined as potentially harmful medication errors in which the error is either caught and corrected prior to drug administration, or cases in which the drug is given to the patient, but by chance an injury does not occur (2). An example of the latter case would be the erroneous administration of a drug to a patient with a documented allergy to the agent in which a hypersensitivity reaction does not occur. Fortunately, ADEs resulting from medication errors appear to be rare. For example, of the 530 medication errors identified by Bates and associates, only 5 (0.9%) resulted in an ADE (2). According to the results of the Harvard Medical Practice Study, 3.7% of the hospital admissions in the state of New York in 1984 were associated with an adverse event (80). Medication errors were the most common cause of these events, accounting for 19.4% of adverse events overall, meaning that approximately 0.7%

of all hospital admissions were associated with a drug-related ADE. Based on the findings of the Harvard Medical Practice Study and a similar study conducted in Colorado and Utah in 1992, the IOM's Committee on Quality of Healthcare in America estimates that 44,000 to 98,000 hospitalized patients die annually in the United States as a result of errors in medical care, the most common of which (approximately 19%) are medication errors (1,8). In other controlled studies medication errors accounted for approximately 20% to 30% of all ADEs.

Studies on the financial burden of medication errors in hospital primarily talk about cost incurred during the same hospital stay and cost of emergency room visits and hospital stays that can be attributed to earlier ADEs. In the former, a 1993 Adverse Drug Events Prevention Study reported that the additional length of hospitalization associated with the preventable ADEs was estimated at 4.6 days with an additional total cost of $5,857 (8). In a 700-bed tertiary care medical center, these results suggest an annual cost associated with preventable ADEs of $2.8 million (8). In terms of the latter, 1.4% to 28% of emergency room visits were related to ADEs, with approximately 28% to 70% of these to be preventable (15,82,83). The average cost estimates range from $1,444 to $10,375 per preventable ADE, costing hospitals as much as $1.2 million per year for all preventable ADEs in 2001 (15). In the United States, the annual additional total costs resulting from medical errors, including additional health care costs as well as disability, lost wages, and household productivity, have been estimated at $17 to $29 billion in the 1999 IOM report (1). Additional health care costs alone were estimated to account for greater than 50% of total costs.

PREVENTING MEDICATION ERRORS

The IOM report in 2007 "Preventing Medication Errors" summarized the following about medication errors—"the rates of errors and preventable harmful events are unacceptably high," the morbidity is costly, and effective error prevention strategies are available (6). Kaushal et al. report that about 20% of ADEs are preventable in pediatric hospitals (29). Preventing medication errors requires a multilevel, multidisciplinary patient-centered effort. Simultaneous engagement from all levels is critical: (a) government and state funding to help institutions implement national safe practice guidelines, (b) institutional culture transformation from one of distrust and secrecy to one of trust and teamwork, (c) self-policing individuals who hold genuine ownership and responsibility for not only the patients' clinical care but also their safe passage through the medical system, (d) focus on systemic causes of errors rather than individual blame, and (e) patients who actively participate in their medication management. At each of these levels, the focus would be at each medication management phase: prescribing, transcribing, dispensing, administering, and monitoring. Lastly, the prevention strategy requires a detailed preimplementation evaluation of the intervention's potential impact on local processes and anticipation of existing adoption barriers. According to an FMEA (Failure Mode and Effects Analysis) by Kunac and Keith looking at neonatal intensive care unit (NICU) medication safety, the top failure step was "lack of awareness of medicine safety issues." (84). The next 27 failure steps occurred in the administration stage, including environment stressors, lack of accountability, no protocols, unsafe storage of medications, dose calculation mistakes, and not checking patient identity. Similar findings were reported in another FMEA done by Williams and Tally in a US hospital, suggesting that these causes are not unique to the NICU (85). Studies also suggest that overdoses are the most common type of dosing error, with the majority of errors occurring at the drug ordering state (32,46,48).

This section discusses the advantages and drawbacks of the mechanisms used to identify and investigate medication errors. Suggestions for preventing medication errors at each stage of drug ordering and delivery process are presented.

MEDICATION ERROR IDENTIFICATION AND ANALYSIS

Accurate error identification and accounting is critical to improving processes in medication management systems in order to reduce medication errors and improve patient safety. Traditional strategies for identifying and analyzing medication errors are based primarily on incident reporting or root cause analysis (86,87). Institution-wide incident reporting systems are a requirement for all hospitals in the United States accredited by The Joint Commission on Accreditation of Healthcare Organizations (JCAHO) and include adverse events (e.g., ADEs), no-harm events, and near misses (86). Event reporting remains voluntary within hospitals. Although JCAHO does not mandate sentinel event reporting to JCAHO, it does require hospitals to perform root cause analyses and action plans for reviewable sentinel events. Some states such as Pennsylvania have established a Patient Safety Authority office that mandates the reporting of serious adverse events.

Voluntary reporting is a critical component of successful incident reporting systems. These systems were originally developed by the military to analyze military aircraft incidents and were based on the use of eyewitness accounts to identify preventable events that culminated in a "critical incident" (88). To deal with the problem of underreporting, established systems in nonmedical high-risk industries offer important incentives such as reporter confidentiality and immunity (89). These systems focus on identifying near misses and on correcting systems' flaws that allowed the events to occur rather than focusing blame on human error. However, most hospital-wide incident reporting systems are directed by the risk management department, presumably contributing to a hesitancy on the part of health care professionals to report medication errors when they occur (86). The reluctance, in part, is because "incidence reports" have traditionally been used to emphasize individual imperfections rather than solve problems within flawed systemic processes and workflows in medication management. Thus, hospital-based reporting systems tend to reflect errors more than harm (90).

Underreporting is a major drawback of many current systems, in particular the underreporting of near misses (91). For example, JCAHO has maintained since 1995 (86) a central database of "sentinel events," or events that led to serious patient injury. Voluntary reports to the database are accepted from the public, the media, the patient or patient family, and accredited hospitals. Only 1,152 events were reported between 1995 and 2001. The majority of events were self-reported by the institutions and involved serious patient injury (76% of these events were associated with patient death). In contrast, in 2001 alone a total of 192,447 medication errors were reported to MEDMARX, an Internet-accessible, anonymous database maintained by the United States Pharmacopeia since 1998 (92). Approximately 97% of the reported medication errors did not cause patient injury. Thirty-nine percent were intercepted prior to drug administration (near misses), whereas 61% were not intercepted. MEDMARX is a proprietary database, with 482 member institutions in 2002 (92). Clearly, underreporting is a major problem with most current incident-reporting systems, in part due to the lack of reporter anonymity and in many states the lack of legal immunity (86,93).

Retrospective trigger tools have emerged as a promising strategy for capturing adverse events. A pediatric-focused trigger tool to identify medication-related harm in US children's hospitals was reported by Takata et al. (94). They reviewed 960 randomly selected charts from 12 children's hospitals and found 2.49 triggers per patient, and 107 unique ADEs, yielding 11.1 events per 100 patients, 15.7 per 1,000 patient-days, and 1.23 per 1,000 medication doses. Twenty-two percent of ADEs were preventable, 17.8% identified earlier, and 16.8% mitigated. Only 3.7% of ADEs were also reported in the hospital-based occurrence reports. A NICU–focused trigger tool reported by Sharek examined 749 charts from 15 NICUs and identified 0.74 adverse events (including medication errors) per patient (95). The rate was higher for patients younger than 28 weeks' gestation and less than 1,500 g birth weight. While an overall 56% of adverse events were preventable, events that led to permanent harm were less preventable. Sixteen percent could have been identified earlier, and 6% could have been mitigated. Only 8% were also identified in existing hospital-based incident reports.

Koppel et al. reported on the identification and quantification of medication errors by evaluation of rapidly discontinued medication orders in a Computerized Physician Order Entry (CPOE) system (96). They found that of 114 rapidly discontinued orders by 75 physicians, two-thirds and 55% of orders discontinued within 45 minutes and 2 hours, respectively, were deemed inappropriate orders. This strategy presents a potentially attractive screening tool for medication errors because it can be automated with the existing CPOE system.

Root cause analysis is specifically designed to avoid many of the problems with incident-reporting systems that lead to underreporting. Although root cause analysis probably provides the most detailed and useful information regarding specific errors, it is rather resource intensive and expensive. Root cause analysis involves the formation of a multidisciplinary team that retrospectively investigates the sentinel event using chart reviews, interviews, and field observations to reconstruct the time line of events that led to the undesirable outcome and identify common underlying factors. Importantly, the focus of root cause analysis is not human error or individual blame. Rather, the emphasis is placed on correcting a flawed system by identifying "latent errors," or failures of system design, that inevitably led to the sentinel events (97). Root cause analysis is labor-intensive and cannot be applied to all medication errors. However, JCAHO requires accredited hospitals to conduct root cause analysis of all sentinel events (87). It is reasonable to assume that the quality and completeness of this extensive review process vary greatly from institution to institution. It cannot be overemphasized that critical design flaws in the health care delivery system must be effectively identified and disseminated to the health care community at large if corrective action is to be undertaken. All health care settings, whether inpatient or outpatient, must be vigilant in ensuring the quality of the root cause analysis process when investigating medication errors.

PREVENTING PRESCRIBING ERRORS

Studies in both adult and pediatric inpatients suggest that prescription errors, most commonly the wrong dose, frequency of administration, or route of administration, account for approximately 50% of all medication errors (26,29). The CPOE systems are widely proposed as a means of reducing these errors (29,98–100). Basic CPOE eliminates many of the problems associated with handwritten prescriptions, such as incomplete prescriptions or illegible handwriting, but most systems also include some form of clinical decision support software (CDSS) (98). CDSS can provide critical drug, patient, and laboratory information to the physician at the time or order entry, thereby reducing the risk of error. Critical components of an effective CPOE/CDSS system have been suggested (63). The system should generate computerized medication administration records (MARs) from a database shared by the prescriber and pharmacy, which can reduce transcription errors. The system should provide the prescriber, at the time of order entry, with patient-specific information (e.g., age, weight or body surface area, drug allergies, and pertinent laboratory variables) and a complete list of current medications. The software should be capable of not only calculating appropriate age- and weight-based doses but also incorporating important clinical data such as vital signs and laboratory values. Thus, the various patient weights entered into an electronic health information system should be standardized across vendors and clear to health care providers as to which weight is used for drug calculations. The system should have high usability scores (101), minimizing user-clicks and decision branch points to reduce potential process variations and "work-arounds." The system should provide unsolicited alerts regarding critical potential drug–drug, or drug–food interactions. Although many current vendor systems can do this, most still require extensive modifications to the architectural technical framework to optimize the efficiency of their alert capabilities. For example, if a physician interfaced with a CPOE/CDSS system to order gentamicin for a 3-month-old infant, the system could provide the patient's current weight and serum creatinine, along with the recommended weight-based dose and administration interval based on the infant's age and level of renal function. The system could also provide a complete list of the patient's positive culture and sensitivity results, along with all concomitant medications and any patient allergies. Equally important is that the system generates a standardized, complete

TABLE 60.5 Recommended Components of a Prescription (62)

1. Patient–specific information: Information should include full name, age or date of birth, current body weight, and known drug allergies
2. Drug name, strength, dose form, and number or amount to be dispensed: Generic drug names should be used exclusively and should be listed in metric units; leading zeroes should always be used for doses or less than "1" unit (e.g., 0.1 mg rather than .1 mg), whereas trailing zeroes should never be used for drug doses off whole number units (e.g., 1 mg rather than 1.0 mg)
3. Daily mg/kg drug dose: This will facilitate verification of the dose by the pharmacist and/or nurse
4. Name and contact number (pager or telephone) of prescriber
5. Complete patient instructions: Instructions should include indication for drug use, dosing instructions (dose, frequency and route of administration, and duration of therapy), and the number of authorized refills should be included; for drug products intended for outpatient use the instructions should include easily recognizable units of measure (e.g., "15 mL" should be accompanied in parenthesis by "1 tablespoonful")

prescription in a format that minimizes confusion once the prescription is reviewed by the pharmacist or nurse. For example, with respect to drug doses the use of leading zeroes should be standard for all doses less than "1" (e.g., 0.1 mg rather than .1 mg), whereas the use of trailing zeroes should be strictly prohibited for whole numbers (e.g., 1 mg rather than 1.0 mg) (102).

Kaushal and colleagues studied the rates of medication errors, potential ADEs and actual ADEs in pediatric inpatients at two teaching hospitals in which prescriptions were handwritten and concluded that 93% of potential ADEs could have been prevented by the use of CPOE (3,29). In their study, medication errors occurred at a rate of 5.7% overall, with 1.1% rate of potential ADEs, and 0.24% rate of actual ADEs. Seventy-nine percent of potential ADEs were classified as prescription errors. The authors also point out that CPOE is not a panacea, particularly in pediatric practice, where a system must have the flexibility to account for rapid and ongoing large changes in patient weight or organ function (29).

Effective physician training is also critical in eliminating prescription errors. Simulations have shown promise in effectively training residents in a safe environment to increase competence and skill (103). Studies show that medical residents are significantly more likely to commit prescription errors, particularly those involving calculation errors, than attending physicians (32,45,104). Not surprisingly, these errors are more likely to occur at the beginning of the academic year. Training should include comprehensive and repetitive written testing of dosage calculations and calculation of body surface area and conversion to metric height and weight measurements. Many institutions continue to use handwritten prescription systems, although recently great strides have been made to implement CPOE systems among academic institutions with training programs. Resident training should therefore also include repetitive testing of prescription writing, including required components of a prescription, the use of leading zeroes with decimal points and the absolute lack of a zero following a decimal point, the use of "Tall man lettering" for look-alike drug names and block lettering for units, and standardized abbreviations within and between institutions.

PREVENTING DISPENSING ERRORS

Because so many medications used in pediatric patients require extemporaneous compounding, all nonemergency medications should be prepared, labeled, and dispensed by a registered pharmacist. With traditional ward stock systems the nurse is responsible for preparing and labeling each dose using a stock drug container stored on the patient ward. Because the nurse is also responsible for drug administration, bypassing the pharmacy removes an important safety check from the drug delivery system, not to mention increasing the workload of the nursing staff. In a national survey of hospital medication–dispensing systems conducted in 1998, 50% of responding hospitals continued to use drug distribution systems that bypassed the pharmacy (105).

Pharmacists must directly verify all questionable or nonstandard drug doses or administration schedules with the prescriber prior to dispensing. In institutions utilizing handwritten prescriptions the prescriber should be careful to include all required components of the prescription (Table 60.5) and write legibly (63). Again, the pharmacist must verify any questionable information with the prescriber before dispensing the drug.

CPOE systems should be designed to share a common patient database between the prescriber and the pharmacy. The system should be capable of providing the pharmacist with current patient-specific information such as weight, serum creatinine, or liver enzyme values. The pharmacist should recalculate and verify all drug doses and verify the appropriateness of the dosing regimen based on current renal or hepatic function before dispensing.

Pharmacists are increasingly active members of the health care team, present in the patient care area and interacting with the prescriber when the prescription is written. Kaushal and colleagues concluded that the presence of a clinical pharmacist on work rounds could have prevented 94% of the potential ADEs observed in their study (29). A separate study conducted in an adult intensive care unit showed a 66% decrease in preventable ADEs with the active participation of a clinical pharmacist during rounds (106).

Automated dispensing devices are being increasingly used, particularly during hours when a pharmacist is not present. A variety of systems are available, which can be installed directly in patient care areas or at the pharmacy (107). These systems are typically stocked by the pharmacy and require the nurse to enter a password to gain access. Most systems are linked to the pharmacy computer system and are capable of automatically charging the patient as the medication is dispensed. Recommended components of these systems include a software link to the pharmacy computer system, an allowance for all new prescriptions to be reviewed by a pharmacist, stocking of all medications stored in the system by the pharmacy, verification of the placement of each medication in the unit by a registered pharmacist, and the use of unit dose medications whenever possible (63). If the nurse must prepare the dose from a stock container, another health care practitioner should verify the dose and prescription prior to drug administration.

PREVENTING ADMINISTRATION ERRORS

The nurse is generally responsible for actual medication administration in hospitalized patients, and provides the critical last check of the dose and prescription prior to drug administration (63). They have the arduous task of avoiding errors as well as preventing the propagation of errors committed earlier in the medication management from reaching the patient. Leape et al. (44) identified several systemic factors associated with medication errors, including deficient staffing and high workload. Roseman and Booker reported a positive association between medication errors and the number of patient days per month and number of shifts worked by temporary staff (108). Fewer errors occurred with increased overtime worked by permanent staff. Failure to follow policy has been cited by many authors as the number one factor associated with medication errors (109). Such failures are often due to systemic barriers, such as distractions and the lack of realistic process guidelines. A study by Pape implementing the Medication Administration Distraction Observation Sheet (MADOS) survey showed that nonmedication-related conversation is the number one distracter during medication administration. From their quasi-experimental three-group study, the authors concluded that procedural checklists are effective in reducing such distractions (110).

In hospitals where prescribers can modify medication orders easily via CPOE, nurses who rely mainly on paper MARs printed at the beginning of the shift may miss CPOE changes that happen after the start of shift. Interestingly, a recent study suggested that the use of CPOE is associated with a reduction in medication administration variance (111).

The nurse should carefully review the patient's MAR, checking the accuracy of all transcribed orders and checking for potential drug allergies or drug interactions based on concurrent medications, diet, or disease states. Any questions or discrepancies must be directly verified with the prescriber and/or pharmacist prior to drug administration. Verbal orders should be allowed only on rare emergency situations and should involve double-check safe practices. When receiving a verbal order, all information should be repeated back to the prescriber for verification, the drug name should be spelled out, and the dose should be verified. Prior to drug administration, the five rights of medication administration should be practiced: giving the right patient the right drug at the right dose, route, and time (3). The components of the medication order should be checked against the original order. The identity of the patient should be verified via two unique identifiers, and when possible, the patient or the caregiver told the name and purpose of the drug when the nurse administers the dose. This verification practice of double checks is a critical safety component when administering specific drugs known to commonly cause adverse effects, or administering drugs to patients at higher risk of medication errors and ADEs, such as intensive care unit populations.

PREVENTING OUTPATIENT AND INPATIENT MEDICATION ERRORS

Few studies have been published regarding the frequency of medication errors in the outpatient setting, although it has been estimated that 5% to 35% of outpatients experience at least one ADE annually (112,113). In pediatric outpatients, the aforementioned need with many medications to measure liquid doses from stock containers increases the potential for human error. Young children are generally not capable of acting as their own advocate. Parents or caregivers should participate as active members of the health care team, providing critical patient-specific information and monitoring throughout the therapy for the appearance of adverse effects.

The United States Pharmacopeia Center for the Advancement of Patient Safety has issued a list of recommendations for parents designed to reduce the risk of medication errors in hospitalized pediatric patients (114). On admission, parents should provide the physician with a complete list of all prescription medications, over-the-counter medications, and dietary supplements the child is currently receiving. Parents should also know their child's current height and weight and inform the physician of any drug or food allergies. If the child has potentially fatal allergy, a MedicAlert bracelet should be worn at all times while in the hospital. Because dosage calculation errors are a common cause of pediatric medication errors, parents should know their child's metric weight and verbally confirm this with physician when each prescription is written. Parents should be given both verbal and written information about each of the child's medications including possible adverse effects. To safely monitor the child's medication use, the parents should known each drug, dose and dose form, and which drug is being given, and closely monitor and report any potential adverse effect. Finally parents should be discouraged from using household measuring devices (tablespoons, etc.) when measuring doses of liquid or suspension medications. An appropriate measuring device should be supplied with the medication, and the parent instructed on the proper use of the device, including a demonstration by the parent of measuring competency. Before discharge home from the NICU with outpatient medications, the home caretakers must demonstrate to the NICU staff the caretakers' ability to obtain, dose, and administer the home medications to the patient.

SUMMARY

Medication error prevention in pediatric patients presents a formidable challenge to the health care community. Medication errors are more likely to cause ADEs in pediatric patients, particularly the youngest, sickest patients, and a variety of factors increase the risk of medication errors in this population. Effective strategies to prevent these errors must continue to focus on effective, accurate reporting and dissemination of medication errors to identify correctable deficiencies in the medication ordering and delivery system. Some ADEs cannot be prevented, but medication errors are preventable. Minimizing or eliminating medication errors can make a real difference in the quality of health care and the safety of infants and children undergoing drug treatment.

ACKNOWLEDGMENT

Many thanks to Daphne C. Papathomas for her valuable efforts in the technical preparation of this manuscript.

REFERENCES

1. Kohn LT, Corrigan JM, Donaldson MS. *To err is human: building a safer health system.* Washington, DC: National Academy Press, 1999.
2. Bates DW, Boyle DL, WanderVilet MB, et al. Relationship between medication errors and adverse drug events. *J Gen Intern Med* 1995; 10:199–205.
3. Nicholas PK, Agius CR. Towards safer IV medication administration. *Am J Nurs* 2005;105(3):25–30.
4. Gandhi TK, Seger DL, Bates DW. Identifying drug safety issues: from research to practice. *Int J Qual Health Care* 2000;12(1):69–76.
5. National Coordinating Council for Medication Error Reporting and Prevention, NCC MERP Taxonomy of Medication Errors, United States Pharmacopeia. http://www.nccmerp.org/med ErrorTaxonomy.html.
6. Philip Aspden, Julie A. Wolcott J, et al. Committee on Identifying and Preventing Medication Errors, eds. *Preventing medication errors: quality chasm series.* Institute of Medicine; National Academies Press, 2006.
7. Kaushal R, Shojania KG, Bates DW. Effects of computerized physician order entry and clinical decision support systems on medication safety: a systematic review. *Arch Intern Med* 2003;163:1409–1416.
8. Bates DW, Spell N, Cullen DJ, et al. The costs of adverse drug events in hospitalized patients. *J Am Med Assoc* 1997;277:307–311.
9. National Coordinating Council for Medication Error Reporting and Prevention. About medication errors:2002. www.nccmerp.org/ aboutmederrors.htm.
10. O'Shea E. Factors contributing to medication errors: a literature review, *J Clin Nurs* 1999;8:496–504.
11. Wears RL, Janiak B, Moorehead JC, et al. Human error in medicine; promise and pitfalls. Part I. *Ann Emerg Med* 2000;36:142–144.
12. Blum KV, Abel SR, Urbanski CJ, et al. Medication error prevention by pharmacists. *Am J Hosp Pharm* 1988;45(9):1902–1903.
13. Griffin JP, Weber JCP. Voluntary systems of adverse reaction reporting—part I. *Adverse Drug React Acute Poisoning Rev* 1985;4: 213–230.
14. Griffin JP, Weber JCP. Voluntary systems of adverse reaction reporting—part II. *Adverse Drug React Acute Poisoning Rev* 1986;5: 23–25.
15. Jha AK, Kuperman GJ, Ritternberg E, et al. Identifying hospital admissions due to adverse drug events using a computer-based monitor. *Pharmacoepidemiol Drug Saf* 2001;10(2):113–119.
16. Griffin FA, Resar RK. IHI global trigger tool for measuring adverse events. *IHI innovation series white paper.* Cambridge, MA: Institute for Healthcare Improvement, 2007.
17. Wakefield D, Wakefield B, Borders T, et al. Understanding and comparing differences in reported medication administration error rates. *Am J Med Qual* 1999;14(2):73–80.
18. Lesar TS. Prescribing errors involving medication dosage forms. *J Gen Intern Med* 2002;17(8):579–587.
19. Lapointe NM, Jollis JG. Medication errors in hospitalized cardiovascular patients. *Arch Intern Med* 2003;163(12):1461–1466.
20. Lisby M, Nielsen LP, Mainz J. Errors in the mediation process: frequency, type, and potential clinical consequences. *Int J Qual Health Care* 2005;17(1):15–22.
21. Bobb A, Gleason K, Husch M, et al. The epidemiology of prescribing errors. *Arch Intern Med* 2004;154(7):785–792.
22. Dean B, Schachter M, Vincent C, et al. Prescribing errors in hospital inpatients: their incidence and clinical significance. *Qual Saf Health Care* 2002;11(4):340–344.
23. Wintersein AG, Johns TE, Rosenberg EI, et al. Nature and causes of clinically significant medication errors in a tertiary care hospital. *Am J Health Syst Pharm* 2004;61(18):1908–1916.
24. Hardmeier B, Braunschweig S, Cavallaro M, et al. Adverse drug events caused by medication errors in medical inpatients. *Swiss Med Wkly* 2004;134(45–46):664–670.
25. Nebeker JR, Hoffman JM, Weir CR, et al. High rates of adverse drug events in a highly computerized hospital. *Arch Intern Med* 2005;165(10):1111–1116.
26. Bates DW, Cullen DJ, Laird N, et al. Incidence of adverse drug events and potential adverse drug events. Implications for prevention. *J Am Med Assoc* 1995;274:35–43.
27. Taxis K, Barber N. Ethnographic study of incidence and severity of intravenous drug errors. *Br Med J* 2003;326(7391):684.
28. Wirtz V, Taxis K, Barber ND. An observational study of intravenous medication errors in the United Kingdom and in Germany. *Pharm World Sci* 2003;25(3):104–111.
29. Kaushal R, Bates DW, Landrigan C, et al. Medication errors and adverse drug events in pediatric inpatients. *J Am Med Assoc* 2001; 285:2114–2120.
30. Fortescue EB, Kaushal R, Landigran CP, et al. Prioritizing strategies for preventing medication errors and adverse drug events in pediatric inpatients. *Pediatrics* 2003;111:722–729.
31. Folli HL, Poole RL, Benitz WE, et al. Medication error prevention by clinical pharmacists in two children's hospitals. *Pediatrics* 1987; 79:718–722.
32. Kozer E, Scolnic D, Macpherson A, et al. Variables associated with medication errors in pediatric emergency medicine. *Pediatrics* 2002;110:737–742.
33. Raju TN, Kecskes S, Thorton JP, et al. Medication errors in neonatal and paediatric intensive-care units. *Lancet* 1989;2:374–376.
34. Slonim AD, LaFleur BJ, Ahmed W, et al. Hospital-reported medical errors in children. *Pediatrics* 2003;111:617–621.
35. Butte AJ, Shaw JS, Bernstein H. Strict interpretation of vaccination guidelines with computerized algorithms and improper timing of administered doses. *Pediatr Infect Dis J* 2001;20(6):561–565.
36. Feikema SM, Klevens RM, Washington ML, et al. Extraimmunization among U.S. Children. *J Am Med Assoc* 2000;283(10):1311–1317.
37. Simborg DW, Derewicz HJ. A highly automated hospital medication system. Five years' experience and evaluation. *Ann Intern Med* 1975;83(3):342–346.
38. Bedouch P, Labarere J, Chirpaz E, et al. Compliance with guidelines on antibiotic prophylaxis in total hip replacement surgery: Results of a retrospective study of 416 patients in a teaching hospital. *Infect Control Hosp Epidemiol* 2004;25(4):302–307.
39. Quenon JL, Eveillard M, Viven A, et al. Evaluation of current practices in surgical antimicrobial prophylaxis in primary total hip prosthesis: a multicentre survey in private and public French hospitals. *J Hosp Infect* 2004;56(3):202–207.
40. Ageno W, Squizzato A, Ambrosini F, et al. Thrombosis prophylaxis in medical patients: a retrospective review of clinical practice patterns. *Haematologica* 2002;87(7):746–750.
41. Ahmad HA, Geissler A, MacLellan D. Deep venous thrombosis prophylaxis: are guidelines being followed? *ANZ J Surg* 2002;72(5): 331–334.
42. Aujesky D, Guignard E, Pannatier A, et al. Pharmacological thromboembolic prophylaxis in a medical ward: room for improvement. *J Gen Intern Med* 2002;17(10):788–791.
43. Classen DC, Pestotnik SL, Evans RS, et al. Adverse drug events in hospitalized patients. Excess length of stay, extra costs, and attributable mortality. *J Am Med Assoc* 1997;277(4):301–306.
44. Leape LL, Bates DW, Cullen DJ, et al. Systems analysis of adverse drug events. *J Am Med Assoc* 1995;274(1):35–43.
45. Lesar TS, Briceland LL, Delcoure K, et al. Medication prescribing errors in a teaching hospital. *J Am Med Assoc* 1990;263: 2329–2334.
46. Lesar TS, Briceland L, Stein DS. Factors related to errors in medication prescribing. *J Am Med Assoc* 1997;277:312–317.
47. Leape LL, Bates DW, Cullen DJ, et al. Systems analysis of adverse drug events. ADE Prevention Study Group. *JAMA* 1995;274(1): 35–43.
48. Lesar TS. Errors in the use of medication dosage equations. *Arch Pediatr Adolesc Med* 1998;152:340–344.
49. Sanborn TA, Jacobs AK, Frederick PD, et al. Comparability of quality-of-care indicators for emergency coronary angioplasty in patients with acute myocardial infarction regardless of on-site cardiac surgery (report from the National Registry of Myocardial Infarction). *Am J Cardiol* 2004;93(11):1335–1339.

50. Granger CB, Steg PG, Peterson E, et al. Medication performance measures and mortality following acute coronary syndromes. *Am J Med* 2005;118(8):858–865.
51. Roe MT, Parsons LS, Pollack CV, et al. Quality of care by classification of myocardial infarction: treatment patterns for ST-segment elevation vs. non-ST-segment elevation myocardial infarction. *Arch Intern Med* 2005;165(14):1630–1636.
52. Heineck I, Ferreira MB, Schenkel EB. Prescribing practice for antibiotic prophylaxis for 3 commonly performed surgeries in a teaching hospital in Brazil. *Am J Infect Control* 1999;27(3):296–300.
53. Vaisbrud V, Raveh D, Schlesinger Y, et al. Surveillance of antimicrobial prophylaxis for surgical procedures. *Infect Control Hosp Epidemiol* 1999;20(9):610–613.
54. Gupta N, Kaul-Gupta R, Carstens MM, et al. Analyzing prophylactic antibiotic administration in procedures lasting more than four hours: are published guidelines being followed? *Am Surg* 2003;69(8):669–673.
55. Van Kasteren ME, Kullberg BJ, de Boer AS, et al. Adherence to local hospital guidelines for surgical antimicrobial prophylaxis: a multicentre audit in Dutch hospitals. *J Antimicrob Chemother* 2003; 51(6):1389–1396.
56. Campbell SE, Walke AE, Grimshaw JM, et al. The prevalence of prophylaxis for deep vein thrombosis in acute hospital trusts. *Int J Qual Health Care* 2001;13(4):309–316.
57. Freeman C, Todd C, Camilleri-Ferrante C, et al. Quality improvement for patients with hip fracture: experience from a multi-site audit. *Qual Saf Health Care* 2002;11(3):239–245.
58. Learhinan ER, Alderman CP. Venous thromboembolism pro[phylaxis in a South Australian teaching hospital. *Ann Pharmacother* 2003;27(10):1398–1402.
59. Scott IA, Denaro CP, Flores JL, et al. Quality of care of patients hospitalized with congestive heart failure. *Intern Med J* 2003;33(4): 140–151.
60. Tan LH, Tan SC. Venous thromboembolism prophylaxis for surgical patients in an Asian hospital. *ANZ J Surg* 2004;74(6):455–459.
61. Chopard P, Dorffler-Melly J, Hess U, et al. Venous thromboembolism prophylaxis in acutely ill medical patients: definite need for improvement. *J Intern Med* 2005;257(4):353–357.
62. Fernandez CV, Gillis-Ring J. Strategies for the prevention of medical error in pediatrics. *J Pediatr* 2003;143(2):155–162.
63. Levine SR, Cohen MR, Blanchard NR, et al. Guidelines for preventing medication errors in pediatrics. *J Pediatr Pharmacol Ther* 2001;6:426–442.
64. Gupta A, Waldhauser LK. Adverse drug reactions from birth to early childhood. *Pediatr Clin North Am* 1997;44:79–92.
65. Evans RS, Pestolnik SL, Classen DC, et al. Preventing adverse drug events in hospitalized patients. *Ann Pharmacother* 1994;28:523–527.
66. The Joint Commission Preventing pediatric medication errors. http://www.jointcommission.org/sentinelevents/sentineleventalert/sea_39.htm.
67. Steinberg C, Notterman DA. Pharmacokinetics of cardiovascular drugs in children. *Clin Pharmacokinet* 1994;27:345–367.
68. Friedman WF, George BL. New concepts and drugs in the treatment of congestive heart failure. *Pediatr Clin North Am* 1984;31: 1197–1227.
69. Perloff WH. Physiology of the heart and circulation. In: Swedlow DB, Raphaely RC, eds. *Cardiovascular problems in pediatric critical care.* New York, NY: Churchill Livingstone, 1986:1–86.
70. Stewart CF, Hampton EM. Effect of maturation on drug disposition in pediatric patients. *Clin Pharm* 1987;6:548–564.
71. Morselli PL. Clinical pharmacology of the perinatal period and early infancy. *Clin Pharmacokinet* 1989;17(Suppl I):13–28.
72. Milsap RL, Jusko WJ. Pharmacokinetics in the infant. *Environ Health Perspect* 1994;102(Suppl 11):107–110.
73. Crom WR. Pharmacokinetics in the child. *Environ Health Perspect* 1994;102(Suppl 11):111–118.
74. Kraus DM, Fischer JH, Reitz SJ, et al. Alterations in theophylline metabolism during the first year of life. *Clin Pharmacol Ther* 1993;54:351–359.
75. Evans C, Lambert GH, Tucker M, et al. The effects of gender on P4501A2 activity in the human adult. *Cancer Epidemiol Biomarkers Prev* 1995;4:529–533.
76. Aranada JV, Sitar DS, Parsons WD, et al. Pharmacokinetic aspects of theophylline in premature newborns. *N Engl J Med* 1976;295: 413–416.
77. Bates DW, Leape LL, Petrycki S. Incidence and preventability of adverse drug events in hospitalized adults. *J Gen Intern Med* 1993; 8:289–294.
78. Leape LL, Brennan TA, Laird NM, et al. The nature of adverse events in hospitalized patients: results from the Harvard Medical Practice Study II. *N Engl J Med* 1991;324:377–384.
79. Melmon KL. Preventable drug reactions—causes and cures. *N Engl J Med* 1971;284:1361–1367.
80. Brennan TA, Leape LL, Laird N, et al. Incidence of adverse events and negligence in hospitalized patients: results from the Harvard Medical Practice Study 1. *N Engl J Med* 1991;324:370–376.
81. Thomas EJ, Studdert DM, Burstin HR, et al. Incidence and types of adverse events and negligent care in Utah and Colorado. *Med Care* 2000;38:261–271.
82. Dennehy CE, Kishi DT, Louie C. Drug-related illness in emergency department patients. *Am J Health Syst Pharm* 1996;53(12): 1422–1426.
83. Tafreshi MJ, Melby MJ, Kaback KR, et al. Medication-related visits to the emergency department: a prospective study. *Ann Pharmacother* 1999;33(12):1252–1257.
84. Kunac DL, Reith DM. Identification of priorities for medication safety in neonatal intensive care. *Drug Saf* 2005;28(3):251–261.
85. Williams E, Tally R. The use of failure mode effect and criticality analysis in a medication error subcommittee. *Hosp Pharm* 1994; 29:331–332,334–336,339.
86. Wald H, Shojania KG. Incident reporting. In: Shojania KG, Duncan BW, McDonals KM, et al., eds. *Making healthcare safer: a critical analysis of patient safety practices.* Rockville, MD: Agency for Healthcare Research and Quality, 2001:41–50.
87. Wald H, Shojania KG. Root cause analysis. In: Shojania KG, Duncan BW, McDonald KM, et al., eds. *Making healthcare safer: a critical analysis of patient safety practices.* Rockville, MD: Agency for Healthcare Research and Quality, 2001:51–56.
88. Flanagan J. The critical incident technique. *Psychol Bull* 1954;51: 327–358.
89. Barach P, Small S. Reporting and preventing medical mishaps: lessons from non-medical near miss reporting systems. *Br Med J* 2000;320:759–763.
90. Resar RK, Rozich JD, Simmonds T, et al. A trigger tool to identify adverse events in the intensive care unit. *Jt Comm J Qual Patient Saf* 2006;32(10):585–590.
91. Cullen DJ, Bates DW, Small SD, et al. The incident reporting system does not detect adverse drug events: a problem for quality improvement. *J Qual Improv* 1995;21:541–548.
92. Hicks RW, Cousins DD, Williams RL. *Summary of information submitted to MEDMARX, in the year 2002. The quest for quality.* Rockville, MD: USP Center for the Advancement of Patient Safety, 2003.
93. Berman S. Identifying and addressing sentinel events: an interview with Richard Croteau. *Jt Comm J Qual Improv* 1998;24:426–434.
94. Takata GS, Taketomo CK, Waite S. California Pediatric Patient safety Initiative. Characteristics of medication errors and adverse drug events in hospitals participating in the California Pediatric Patient Safety Initiative. *Am J Health Syst Pharm* 2008;65(21): 2036–2044.
95. Sharek PJ, McClead RE Jr, Taketomo C, et al. An intervention to decrease narcotic-related adverse drug events in children's hospitals. *Pediatrics* 2008;122(4):e861–e866.
96. Koppel R, Leonard CE, Localio R, et al. Identifying and quantifying medication errors: evaluation of rapidly discontinued medication orders submitted to a computerized physician order entry system. *J Am Med Inform Assoc* 2008;15(4):461–465.
97. Reason J. Human error: models and management. *Br Med J* 2000; 320:768–770.
98. Kaushal R, Bates DW. Computerized physician order entry (CPOE) with clinical decision support systems (CDSSs). In: Shojania KG, Duncan BW, McDonals KM, et al., eds. *Making healthcare safer a critical analysis of patient safety practices.* Rockville, MD: Agency for Healthcare Research and Quality, 2001:59–69.
99. Bates DW, Leape LL, Cullen DJ, et al. Effect of computerized physician order entry and a team intervention on prevention of serious medication errors. *J Am Med Inform Assoc* 1998;280: 1311–1316.
100. Bates DW, Teich J, Lee J, et al. The impact of computerized physician order entry on medication error prevention. *J Am Med Inform Assoc* 1999;6:313–321.

101. Hortman PA, Thompson CB. Evaluation of user interface satisfaction of a clinical outcomes database. *Comput Inform Nurs* 2005;23(6):301–307.
102. Lilley LL, Guanci R. Careful with the zeroes! How to minimize one of the most persistent causes of gross medication errors. *Am J Nurs* 1997;97:14.
103. Jeffrey H, Bermann M, Chen B, et al. Incorporation of a computerized human simulator in critical care training: a preliminary report. *J Trauma* 2002;53(6):1064–1067.
104. Wilson DG, McArtney RG, Newcombe RG, et al. Medication errors in paediatric practice: insights from a continuous quality improvement approach. *Eur J Pediatr* 1998;157:769–774.
105. Ringold DJ, Santell JP, Schneider PJ, et al. ASHP national survey of pharmacy practice in acute care settings: prescribing and transcribing—1998. *Am J Health Syst Pharm* 1999;56:142–157.
106. Leape LL, Cullen DJ, Clap MD, et al. Pharmacist participation on physician rounds and adverse drug events in the intensive care unit. *J Am Med Assoc* 1999;282:267–270.
107. Murray MD. Automated medication dispensing devices. In: Shojania KG, Duncan BW, McDonals KM, et al., eds. *Making healthcare safer a critical analysis of patient safety practices.* Rockville, MD: Agency for Healthcare Research and Quality, 2001: 111–116.
108. Roseman C, Booker JM. Workload and environmental factors in hospital medication errors. *Nurs Res* 1995;44(4):226–230.
109. Long G, Johnson CA. Pilot study for reducing medication errors. *Qual Rev Bull* 1981;7(4):6–9.
110. Pape T. Applying airline safety practices to medication administration. *Med Surg Nurs* 2003;12(2):77–93.
111. Taylor JA, Loan LA, Kamara J, et al. Medication administration variances before and after implementation of computerized physician order entry in a neonatal intensive care unit. *Pediatrics* 2008;121(1):123–128.
112. Hutchinson TA, Flegel KM, Kramer MS, et al. Frequency, severity and risk factors for adverse drug reactions in adult out-patients: a prospective study. *J Chronic Dis* 1986;39:533–542.
113. Hanlon JT, Schmader KE, Koronkowski MJ, et al. Adverse drug events in high risk older outpatients. *J Am Geriatr Soc* 1997;45:945–948.
114. United States Pharmacopoeia, Center for the Advancement of Patient Safety. *Tips for parents: preventing medication errors.* Rockville, MD: United States Pharmacopoeia, Center for the Advancement of Patient Safety, 2003.

CHAPTER

61

Suzanne R. White

Pediatric Poisonings and Antidotes

OVERVIEW

Poisoning is one of the most common pediatric medical emergencies. In 2006, the American Association of Poison Control Centers (AAPCC) National Poison Data System reported 1,223,815 toxic exposures in children younger than 6 years. This report included 29 fatalities and 11,062 moderate or severe complications (1). For this same age group, greater numbers were previously reported by both the National Center for Health Statistics (53 fatalities and 20,000 hospitalizations during one 12-month period) (2) and the Consumer Product Safety Commission (85,000 emergency department visits by young children annually for poisoning) (3). In 2004, the Institute of Medicine conservatively estimated the annual incidence of poisoning episodes in the United States to be 4 million cases. That year, the AAPCC captured 56% of these cases. Extrapolating the 2004 rate of reporting to AAPCC poison centers to their 2006 total volume suggests that 4,292,034 US exposures occurred (1). Although there were an estimated 30,800 fatalities in 2004, US poison centers captured only about 3.5% of these reports. These discrepant data highlight the significant underreporting of toxic exposures to poison control centers.

Overall, poisoning episodes are largely exposures and only 7.5% lead to hospitalization. Poison centers are staffed by skilled professionals whom contacted early, can treat 72.9% of children at home (1). Beyond their ability to provide immediate first aid advice and reassurance to caregivers of poisoned children, poison centers have added value. They positively affect the utilization of health care resources and they uniformly compile data that provide real-time disease surveillance and drive safety initiatives (4). They actively carry out poison prevention activities for the public and for health care professionals. Finally, recent poison center enhancements provide anxious caregivers and health care providers in all 50 United States, Puerto Rico, and the District of Columbia universal access to specially trained pharmacists, nurses, and physicians via a toll-free number. This uniform nationwide number, 1-800-222-1222, is the result of collaboration among the AAPCC, the Centers for Disease Control and Prevention, and the Health Resources and Services Administration.

The peak age for poisoning is age 1 to 3 years. The age and gender distribution of human poison exposure victims is outlined in Table 61.1. Children younger than 3 years were involved in 38.0% of exposures and 50.9% occurred in children younger than 6 years. A male predominance is found among recorded cases involving children younger than 13 years, but this gender distribution is reversed in teenagers.

The most common agents involved in toxic exposures in children younger than 6 years are listed in Table 61.2. These tend to be substances that are found in and around the home. A few studies have attempted to establish which substances are most hazardous to children younger than 6 years. The first was a large analysis of 3.8 million exposures carried out between 1985 and 1989 (5). Findings included 2,117 cases of major life-threatening toxicity and 111 fatalities. The substances with the highest hazard factors were iron, which accounted for 30% of fatalities; tricyclic antidepressants; cardiovascular agents; aspirin; hydrocarbons; and pesticides. In a summary of serious pediatric toxic exposures between 1991 and 1995 (6) (Table 61.3), the substances most commonly associated with major effects in children younger than 6 years were cleaning substances, cardiovascular agents, hydrocarbons, sedative–hypnotic agents, antidepressants, pesticides, and analgesics. The most common fatal exposures in this group were to carbon monoxide, iron, and analgesics. Adolescent fatalities were most commonly associated with exposure to hydrocarbons, antidepressants, analgesics, and cardiovascular agents.

In 2006, there were 29 fatalities reported in children younger than 6 years, similar to numbers reported over the last decade (1). The reasons for these fatal exposures are outlined in Table 61.4. Of the reported deaths in children younger than 6 years, 21 were reported as unintentional. Four deaths in children younger than 6 years were from malicious intent. Of the 21 pharmaceutical-associated fatalities, 6 involved opioids, 3 involved heparin, and 3 involved antihistamines. Of the 8 nonpharmaceutical-associated fatalities, 2 involved carbon monoxide, 2 involved hydrocarbons, and 1 each involved lead, mineral spirits, disc battery, and other foreign body. In the age range of 6 to 12 years, there were 6 reported fatalities involving 6 substances: acebutolol, antihistamine, carbon monoxide, fentanyl, mushrooms

TABLE 61.1 Age and Gender Distribution of Pediatric Exposures (1)

	Boy		*Girl*		*Unknown Gender*		*Total*		*Cumulative Total*	
Age (yr)	*Number*	*% of Age Group Total*	*Number*	*% of Age Group Total*	*Number*	*% of Age Group Total*	*Number*	*% of Age Group Total*	*Number*	*Col %*
<1	65,933	51.92	60, 616	47.74	430	0.34	126,979	5.28	126,979	5.28
1	199,553	52.03	183,399	47.82	585	0.15	383,537	15.96	510,516	21.24
2	211,865	52.64	190,006	47.21	622	0.15	402,493	16.75	913,000	37.99
3	97,530	55.31	78,418	44.48	371	0.21	176,319	7.34	1,089,328	45.32
4	46,424	56.21	335,956	43.54	204	0.25	82,584	3.44	1,171,912	48.76
5	27,321	56.77	20,615	42.84	189	0.39	48,125	2.00	1,220,037	50.76
Unk <6	1,772	46.90	1,522	40.29	484	12.81	3,778	0.16	1,223,815	50.92
6–12 (child)	87,757	57.72	63,005	41.44	1,284	0.84	152,046	6.33	1,375,861	57.24
13–19 (teenager)	78,050	46.12	90,454	53.45	733	0.43	169,237	7.04	1,545,098	64.28
Unk age child	2,704	41.54	2,424	37.24	1,381	21.22	6,509	0.27	1,551,607	64.56
Total children	**818,909**	**52.78**	**726,415**	**46.82**	**6,283**	**0.40**	**1,551,607**	**64.56**	**1,551,607**	**64.56**

cyclopeptides, and pine oil. Although children younger than 6 years were involved in the majority of exposures, they comprised just 2.4% of the verified fatalities.

Differences between pediatric and adult poisoning exist. Most toxic exposures in children younger than 6 years are accidental or unintentional. Young children often ingest or are exposed to a single substance. Furthermore, the time to discovery is brief. Most (73%) of exposures in young children are reported within 10 minutes, and children arrive to the emergency department sooner than adults. Because the child is often found with the substance, exact ingredient identification is more feasible and reliable. Generally, a smaller amount of substance is ingested by children as compared with adults. Even so, one may be seriously misguided by the universal assumption that children "only ingest small amounts of pills" or "won't ingest things that are malodorous or bad tasting."

Why does pediatric poisoning continue to occur? As just noted, most exposures in young children are accidental and unintentional. These occur as toddlers explore their environment and exhibit normal hand-to-mouth activity.

TABLE 61.2 Substances Most Frequently Involved in Pediatric (≤5 years) Exposures (1)

Substance	*Number*	*%[a]*
Cosmetics/personal care products	162,514	13.3
Cleaning substances (household)	120,250	9.8
Analgesics	103,189	8.4
Foreign bodies/toys/miscellaneous	90,906	7.4
Topical preparations	85,079	7.0
Cold and cough preparations	69,645	5.7
Vitamins	47,997	3.9
Pesticides	45,848	3.7
Plants	44,710	3.7
Antihistamines	36,591	3.0
Gastrointestinal preparations	34,099	2.8
Antimicrobials	33,832	2.8
Arts/crafts/office supplies	27,404	2.2
Hormones and hormone antagonists	23,972	2.0
Electrolytes and minerals	22,956	1.9
Cardiovascular drugs	22,868	1.9
Alcohols	21,577	1.8
Deodorizers	16,984	1.4
Food products/food poisoning	16,964	1.4
Hydrocarbons	15,989	1.3
Dietary supplements/herbals/homeopathic	15,511	1.3
Asthma therapies	15,474	1.3
Antidepressants	13,785	1.1
Sedative/hypnotics/antipsychotics	13,656	1.1
Other/unknown nondrug substances	12,504	1.0

[a]Percentages are based on the total number of exposures in children (1,223,815) rather than the total number of substances.

TABLE 61.3 Distribution of Reason for Exposure and Age for Fatalities (1)

	Age		
Reason	*≤6 yr*	*6–12 yr*	*13–19 yr*
Unintentional			
General	13	1	2
Environmental	2	1	7
Occupational	0	0	0
Therapeutic error	6	0	2
Misuse	0	0	0
Bite/sting	0	0	0
Food poisoning	0	0	0
Subtotal	21	2	11
Intentional			
Suspected suicide	0	0	26
Misuse	0	0	2
Abuse		0	16
Unknown	0	0	5
Subtotal	0	0	49
Malicious	4	2	0
Adverse reaction of drug	0	1	1
Unknown reason	4	1	1
TOTAL	**29**	**6**	**62**

TABLE 61.4 Types of Substances Responsible for Significant Pediatric Morbidity and Mortality (6)

	Age <6 yr				*Age 13–17 yr*	
	Major Effects		*Deaths*		*Deaths*	
Category	*No.*	*%*	*No.*	*%*	*No.*	*%*
Cleaning substances	277	12	7	6	1	<1
Cardiovascular agents	182	8	7	6	12	7
Hydrocarbons	168	7	5	4	56	31
Sedative–hypnotics	153	7	2	2	5	3
Antidepressants	125	6	7	6	49	27
Insecticides/pesticides	122	5	6	5	0	0
Analgesic agents	119	5	8	7	26	14
Anticonvulsants	106	5	4	3	2	1
Bites/envenomations	100	4	0	0	0	0
Stimulants/street drugs	84	4	1	<1	7	4
Iron	85	4	8	7	2	0
Carbon monoxide	42	2	18	15	5	3
Alcohols	52	2	5	4	3	2
Theophylline	38	2	3	2	3	2
Total of above substances	1,653		81		171	
Total of all substances	2,270		122		182	

Other factors include caregivers' underestimation of the developmental skills of their child, imitative behavior (watching parents take medication), "look-alike" substances or containers (similarities between the intoxicant and familiar candy or beverages), and poor packaging. Concerning packaging, the use of child-resistant containers has dramatically decreased pediatric poisoning morbidity and mortality. Nonetheless, carelessness or distraction on the part the caregiver while the product is in use limits the effectiveness of this safety feature. Illustrative of this fact is that pediatric poisoning from exposure to cleaning products in the home occurs while the product is in use in 70% of cases (7). Lack of grandparent awareness about the safe storage of their own medication is another cause for pediatric poisoning. Often, these exposures are serious because they involve highly toxic pharmaceuticals such as cardiovascular agents or antidiabetics. Grandparent's handbags, bedside stands, kitchen tables, and day-of-the-week pill dispensers are all potentially hazardous. Another important cause of poisoning, therapeutic error, constitutes 7.4% of toxic exposures and accounts for 31% of poisoning deaths in children younger than 6 years (1). Across age groups, 36% of therapeutic errors result from double dosing. This phenomenon is especially prevalent among children prescribed medication to treat attention deficit hyperactivity disorder, defining an emerging at-risk group for poisoning (8). Other therapeutic errors in children commonly result from dispensing-cup errors, 10-fold dosing errors, and drug interactions (1). Intentional poisoning may result from suicidal intent, home stressors, or substance abuse, and, unfortunately, should be considered as early as age 6 years. The most common reasons for poisoning fatality in 13- to 19-year-olds, a group with a steadily increasing fatality rate, are suicide followed by abuse.

Risk factors for pediatric poisoning have been analyzed. These include behavioral, environmental, and parental factors. Recurrent poisoning may occur in up to 30% of children with a history of previous ingestion (9). Behavioral traits in the child that predispose to accidental repeat poisoning are hyperactivity, rebelliousness, impulsivity, and pica. Environmental change or chaos, as occurs in the setting of a new home, new sibling, holiday event, or dinner preparation, presents a risk for poisoning. Parental factors include medical illness, depression, and social isolation (10,11).

APPROACH TO THE POISONED CHILD

THE ABCDs OF STABILIZATION

As with all emergencies, the initial priority in management of poisoning is stabilization. This may be accomplished by following the "ABCD" principles, or a management approach that prioritizes airway, breathing, circulation, and neurologic disability assessment. Confirmation that protective airway reflexes are intact (and if not, securement of the airway) takes precedent over all other aspects of care. The narrow-caliber pediatric airway is easily obstructed, making ingestions of corrosives, houseplants, and foreign bodies of particular concern. The airway may be further compromised or aspiration may occur during subsequent gastric decontamination procedures, such as gastric lavage or the administration of charcoal. Elective intubation in the obtunded child is always preferable to the "crash" situation. This is especially relevant when central nervous system (CNS) depressants or proconvulsants have been ingested. Next, adequate breathing must be ensured. Children more rapidly develop respiratory depression and apnea from CNS depressants than do adults. Furthermore, the classic phases seen with certain drug intoxications (respiratory alkalosis during early salicylism) may not be present, or progression to respiratory acidosis may occur more rapidly than expected. While pulse oximetry assesses oxygenation, blood gas analysis is necessary to assess adequacy of ventilation and tidal volume. Moreover, pulse oximetry will not detect carboxyhemoglobinemia and may underestimate the degree of methemoglobinemia present.

Adequacy of circulation should be clinically assessed through cardiac monitoring and blood pressure and capillary refill measurement. Intravenous access is ideally obtained quickly, while the child is well perfused, rather than after the onset of hypotension, when this becomes technically more difficult. Children are more likely to have significant volume depletion from poisoning because they are less tolerant of volume losses from sweating, diarrhea, vomiting, and cathartic use. Other "Cs" to remember include aggressive cooling in the setting of hyperthermia (as occurs with the use of anticholinergics) and complete disrobing, to reveal signs of trauma, burns, or other clues regarding the substance involved.

The "Ds" of patient stabilization include assessment of neurologic disability and decontamination. Seizures that occur as a result of poisoning should be treated with benzodiazepines or barbiturates. Phenytoin does not effectively control drug-related seizures. In patients with depressed mental status, reversible causes for coma should be sought. If CNS or respiratory depression is present, especially in the presence of miosis, naloxone, a narcotic antagonist, should be administered. The pediatric dose is 0.1 mg per kg or 2 mg intravenously. Unfortunately, narcotics are widely available in many homes and, as outlined earlier, account for a number of pediatric fatalities each year. A rapid glucose determination should be carried out. If this is not feasible, dextrose should be administered empirically as a 10% solution in neonates and 25% solution in infants at doses of 0.25 to 1.0 g per kg intravenously. Children experience glycogen depletion after only a few hours of fasting and are more prone to hypoglycemia than adults following the ingestion of agents such as ethanol. In fact, ethanol-induced hypoglycemia may occur at blood ethanol levels as low as 20 mg per dL. Flumazenil may be used to reverse the CNS-depressant effects of benzodiazepines in the setting of known single-drug benzodiazepine ingestion or conscious sedation (12). The pediatric dose is 0.01 mg per kg by slow intravenous administration. This antidote is to be avoided if the child has a history of seizures, is taking benzodiazepines therapeutically, has possibly coingested proconvulsants, or is suspected to have increased intracranial pressure. Thiamine, while typically reserved for adults with altered mental status, may be considered for lethargic children with a history of malnutrition, anorexia, on chemotherapy, or on total parenteral nutrition.

Decontamination

Dermal decontamination is carried out to decrease the level of patient exposure to the intoxicant and, in some cases, to prevent secondary spread to health care providers. Children's skin is much thinner than that of adults; therefore, both the dermal absorption of toxins and chemical burns occur more readily. Ocular chemical exposures should be of the highest priority and should be treated with immediate tepid water irrigation that begins at the scene and continues until medical evaluation is underway. The skin should be thoroughly washed with mild soap and tepid water, with attention to wounds, skin folds, hair, and nails. Close temperature monitoring is necessary in infants and young children, who may become hypothermic during the skin decontamination process.

The role of gastric emptying and other methods of gastrointestinal (GI) decontamination are areas of great controversy. Six studies have attempted to determine whether gastric emptying procedures positively affect patient outcome. One study of poisoned patients compared ipecac-induced emesis versus activated charcoal, and gastric lavage versus activated charcoal, and demonstrated benefit only in patients who were obtunded and presented within 60 minutes of ingestion. The limitations of this study are its inclusion of only five patients younger than 5 years, and the fact that some critically ill patients were excluded (13). Two additional prospective adult studies showed no difference in outcome between patients treated with gastric emptying versus those treated with charcoal alone (14,15). A small, prospective study in children treated with ipecac plus activated charcoal versus charcoal alone revealed that ipecac prolonged the time to administration of activated charcoal by an average of 100 minutes and increased the time to discharge from the emergency department by an average of 39 minutes (16). Another study compared ipecac-induced emesis followed by activated charcoal versus activated charcoal alone and found no difference in the need for hospitalization except that a higher incidence of aspiration was noted in the ipecac-treated group. On closer review, however, ipecac use in these patients was inappropriate (17). A trend toward increased referral of children to hospitals by those poison centers that used less ipecac was noted in another retrospective study (18). Demonstrating improved outcome in poisoned patients through gastric emptying procedures is difficult, given the low associated poisoning mortality. This major drawback limits the translation of the available "evidence" to strict practice guidelines, especially those that suggest complete abandonment of GI decontamination procedures. Benefit from gastric emptying may be seen in symptomatic patients presenting within the first hour after ingestion, symptomatic patients who have ingested agents that slow GI motility or are sustained-release type, and those taking massive amounts of a life-threatening substance (19). A case-by-case approach to gastric emptying decisions is warranted, and gastric decontamination methods will therefore be discussed in more detail.

Syrup of ipecac reliably produces vomiting in 85% of patients within 15 to 30 minutes of administration. The typical dose is 5 mL for children older than 6 months, 10 mL for children aged 10 to 12 months, and 15 mL for children between 1 and 12 years. The extent to which absorption of the ingested substance is prevented is dependent on the time to administration. The efficacy of ipecac dramatically declines after 30 minutes of ingestion. Overall, ipecac administration recommended by poison centers has declined significantly over the last 10 years. The use of ipecac is contraindicated in patients with depressed mental status or seizures, at high risk for aspiration, who have ingested a substance that causes altered mental status or convulsions, who have ingested a caustic or corrosive substance, who have ingested a low-viscosity petroleum distillate, or who have underlying medical conditions that may be exacerbated by vomiting, such as hypertension, bradycardia, or coagulopathy.

The risk–benefit ratio of nonprescription ipecac use and availability is being reassessed by several pediatric and toxicologic professional organizations. Pending their final recommendations, it can be stated that syrup of ipecac use in the emergency department is not appropriate (20). Furthermore, ipecac should not routinely be used in the prehospital setting but may be considered when a toxic amount of a substance has been ingested within 30 minutes. Its use may also be considered following the ingestion of toxic, large particulate matter not amenable to removal by gastric lavage (i.e., iron pills, mushrooms). A notable exception here is that ipecac should not be administered to induce emesis following button battery ingestion, as this could result in esophageal lodgment of the battery. A future alternative to syrup of ipecac, home charcoal, deserves further study but is not yet widely available in homes (21).

Gastric lavage may be considered in patients presenting within 60 minutes of the ingestion of a potentially toxic amount of a toxic substance, or for those critically ill patients for whom the time of ingestion is unknown (22). The procedure involves the orogastric placement of a 24 to 32 French Ewald tube with the patient lying in the left lateral decubitus position. Repeated instillation and removal of 50- to 100-mL aliquots of half-normal or normal saline is carried out until the lavage fluid is clear. The use of cold tap water in small children may result in hyponatremia or hypothermia. Lavage solutions employed in the past such as sodium bicarbonate or sodium phosphate are not recommended. Gastric lavage should not be performed in patients with inadequate airway protective reflexes or in those with corrosive substance ingestion. Serious potential complications from the procedure include upper airway obstruction, pulmonary aspiration, and GI tract perforation.

Activated charcoal is administered orally to most patients who have recently overdosed when contraindications do not exist. These contraindications include lack of a protected airway, potential for corrosive injury to the GI tract, and evidence of GI tract obstruction or perforation. When administered within 1 hour of ingestion, activated charcoal may reduce toxin absorption by up to 75% (23). The usual dose is 10 times that of the estimated dose of toxic substance, which is typically an unknown amount. Therefore, it generally becomes necessary to dose charcoal empirically at 0.5 to 1 g per kg of body weight. It is administered as well-mixed slurry. Most children will not voluntarily drink charcoal and may require nasogastric tube insertion. In older children, palatability may be improved through the use of a commercial cherry-flavored product, additives such as chocolate or fruit syrup, or disguising in an opaque container/opaque straw (24). Although the administration of activated charcoal has not been shown to improve patient outcome, the rationale for its administration is based on a number of theoretical benefits. These include the direct adsorption of the toxic material and the prevention of systemic absorption and the interruption of enterohepatic recirculation of specific drugs or their metabolites. In addition, based on the immense surface area of the intestinal villi, which lie in close proximity to intestinal capillaries, continuous forward movement of charcoal through the intestines may create a concentration gradient that allows systemically circulating drug to diffuse back into the gut lumen and adsorb to charcoal. This concept has been termed "gut dialysis." For some ingestions charcoal is administered in a pulse-dosed manner (as discussed later). During such practice, cathartics should be given only with the first dose of charcoal each day to prevent fluid and electrolyte imbalance. In addition, the status of intestinal activity must be monitored closely to prevent ileus-induced charcoal impaction, especially in patients with anticholinergic poisoning. Not all agents adsorb to activated charcoal. For example, metals such as iron and lithium, some pesticides, some corrosives, and some alcohols are poorly bound. Charcoal should not be given to patients who ingest corrosive agents, as it will obscure endoscopy.

Cathartics have not been shown to improve outcome following drug overdose, but they are commonly administered with the first dose of activated charcoal. They are classified as saline (magnesium citrate, magnesium sulfate) and saccharide (sorbitol). Based on their high osmolarity, they cause fluid to enter the GI tract and bowel peristalsis to increase. In addition, magnesium sulfate may stimulate the release of cholecystokinin, which increases motor and secretory action in the GI tract. Sorbitol has been demonstrated to be the most rapidly acting cathartic in terms of "time to first stool" as compared with saline cathartics. Overly aggressive use of cathartics can cause pediatric dehydration and hypermagnesemia, and they are therefore typically not used in infants. The dose in older children is 20% magnesium sulfate, 250 mg per kg; 6% magnesium citrate, 4 cc per kg; or sorbitol, 0.5 to 1 g per kg. Sorbitol is not recommended for children younger than 12 months (25).

Whole bowel irrigation is a technique increasingly employed to rid the GI tract of ingested substances that do not adsorb to charcoal, such as iron or lithium (26). Balanced polyethylene glycol solutions contain 125 mEq per L of sodium, 10 mEq per L of bicarbonate, 35 mEq per L of chloride, 80 mEq per L of sulfate, and 60 g of polyethylene glycol per L. These solutions are isoosmotic and allow for mechanical cleansing of the gut without the risk of fluid or electrolyte imbalance, even in young children. Whole bowel irrigation may also be considered in patients who are suspected to have concretions or who have ingested lead-based paint chips, massive amounts of a toxic substance, sustained-release preparations (e.g., calcium channel blockers), or drug packets. Polyethylene glycol solution is given as 20 to 40 mL per kg per hour in children. This typically requires nasogastric tube insertion, although flavored varieties may be used in the older, motivated child.

History and Physical

Once stabilization of the patient has been accomplished, a complete history should be obtained along with a complete physical examination. The history of poisoning or drug ingestion may be lacking. The clinician should always place poisoning in the differential diagnosis for children with the aforementioned risk factors for poisoning, multiple organ-system involvement, or a confusing clinical picture (27). This principle was demonstrated by a recent study that investigated poisoning as a cause of the relatively common pediatric emergency department diagnosis, "apparent life-threatening event" (ALE). In infants younger than 2 years, 18.2% of children with ALE had positive toxicology screens and 8.4% of positive screen results were considered clinically significant (i.e., identified a medication that could cause apnea or other event consistent with an ALE, even if it was a medication that the child was known to be taking). While approximately 5% of these toxicology screen results were positive for an over-the-counter cold preparation, no parent admitted to having given his or her child an over-the-counter cold preparation (28).

Vomiting is the most common presenting symptom following toxic ingestion but is a nonspecific clue. The primary goals in history acquisition are to determine the exact ingredient identification, ascertain the time of ingestion, perform dose estimation, and uncover any significant past medical history. Detailed interviews with multiple caregivers may be necessary to accomplish this. Often, it is helpful to have original household product containers and medication bottles brought to the hospital for inspection. A retrospective search of the home may be useful because children may find items that may be hidden from adult view, such as pills on the floor or discarded containers in wastebaskets. It is important to assume the worst-case scenario when calculating dose estimation. In addition, clinicians should be aware of those substances that may be potentially fatal in small or unit doses (6,29,30). Some of these substances are highlighted in Table 61.5. Fortunately, many exposures in children involve nontoxic or minimally toxic products. Substances generally considered to be minimally toxic are listed in Table 61.6. It is important to note that a nontoxic exposure may still be of concern because it could represent a suicidal gesture or a sign of caretaker distress, or indicate inadequate supervision or an unsafe environment. In addition, symptoms that occur in the setting of "nontoxic" exposure may suggest unrelated diagnoses, incorrectly identified substances, or product tampering.

Unfortunately, poisoning may be a warning sign of child abuse or neglect. Suspicions should be raised when poisoning occurs in children younger than 6 months or in those without the developmental capability to access the substance in question. Other situations suggestive of possible abuse include those in which the history provided changes or is inconsistent between caregivers. Ingestions by older children (>5 years) and ingestions of psychotropic agents, drugs of abuse, sedative–hypnotics, and ethanol are all potentially of concern. A long interval between time of ingestion and the time to presentation for medical evaluation is also suspicious. It is prudent to review previous medical records of children with poisoning; one study found that 51% had prior emergency department visits for trauma, poisoning, or failure to thrive, and 20% had evidence of abuse or neglect (31). Up to 30% of children with accidental ingestions have repeat exposures and are at risk for other injuries (32). Munchausen syndrome by proxy is an extremely rare condition that should be suspected in children with recurrent unexplained illness whose parent is a medical professional, is very willing to provide detailed data on unusual illnesses, and is overly friendly or helpful.

A meticulous physical examination should search to uncover the presence of a toxidrome. Specifically, the examination should focus on abnormalities of vital signs, mental status, pupils/fundi, mucous membrane hydration, corrosive effect on the mucous membranes and skin, bowel sounds, bladder distension, and reflexes (27). The presence of odors, bullae, cyanosis, or other skin discolorations should be noted. Miosis, bradycardia, and hypertension are unusual in pediatric patients and should point to possible drug effect (33). The clinical features of several toxidromes are outlined in Table 61.7.

TABLE 61.5 Drugs and Toxins that Can Cause Severe Toxicity to a 10-kg Child After a Small Dose

Benzocaine
Camphor
Chloroquine
Chlorpromazine
Clonidine
Codeine
Desipramine
Diphenhydramine
Diphenoxylate
Ethylene glycol
Hydroxychloroquine
Imidazolines (tetrahydrozoline, oxymetazoline, xylometazoline, naphazoline)
Imipramine
Lindane
Methanol
Methyl salicylate
Orphenadrine
Quinine
Theophylline
Thioridazine
Selenious acid (gun blueing)

TABLE 61.6 Minimally Toxic or Nontoxic Substances

Silica gel
Vitamin A and D ointment
Blackboard or sidewalk chalk
Lipsticks and noncamphor lip balms
Watercolor paints
Hand or dishwashing detergents (not dishwasher or laundry detergent or ethanol-based hand scrubs)
Calamine lotion (excluding products with antihistamines)
Clay (play)
Crayons
Diaper rash creams/ointments
Fabric softener sheets
Glow products
Glue (white arts and crafts)
Household plant food
Oral contraceptives
Pen ink
Pencils
Starch/sizing
Throat lozenges without local anesthetics
Topical antibiotics/topical steroids
Water-based paints

Laboratory

Toxicology screens are of limited value in children with the witnessed ingestion of a single substance (34,35). Such

TABLE 61.7 Toxidromes

	Opioids	*Anticholinergic*	*Cholinergic*	*Sympathomimetic*
Pulse	Decreased	Increased	Decreased	Increased
Blood pressure	Decreased	Increased	Variable	Increased
Respirations	Decreased	Variable	Variable	Increased
Temperature	Decreased	Increased	Decreased	Increased
Bowel sounds	Decreased	Decreased	Hyperactive	Normal
Skin	Sweaty	Dry, red, hot	Sweaty	Sweaty
Mental status	Depressed	Agitated delirium/seizures	Depressed/agitated	Delirium/seizures
Pupils	Miosis	Mydriasis	Miosis	Mydriasis
Other	Track marks	Urinary retention, no axillary sweat	Fasciculations Weakness, bronchospasm, bronchorrhea, ? garlic odor/pesticides	Bruxism
Examples	Codeine Other nonopiods (clonidine, γ-hydroxybutyrate)	Antihistamines	Organophosphates	Cocaine
	Heroin	Antipsychotics	Carbamates	Amphetamines
	Methadone	Scopolamine		Theophylline
	Oxycodone	Atropine		

screens may be negative even in the face of serious toxicity (36). Routine chemistries, blood gas analysis, osmolality, ketones, and lactate levels are all useful in the evaluation of metabolic acidosis, which is the most common laboratory finding. Agents that require stat analysis include iron, methanol, ethylene glycol, acetaminophen, salicylates, caffeine, carboxyhemoglobin, ethanol, digoxin, lead, lithium, methemoglobin, methotrexate, theophylline, carbamazepine, phenobarbital, valproic acid, and phenytoin. Critical early interventions may be indicated for the appropriate management of intoxication resulting from these substances, depending on specific serum or blood levels. In addition, tests in the older child or adolescent with a suspected intentional drug overdose should include routine acetaminophen and salicylate levels and consideration of a pregnancy test. Other laboratory testing should be individualized and may include a complete blood count, electrocardiogram, chest or abdominal x-ray, calcium, liver function tests, and urinalysis.

Enhanced Elimination

The elimination of absorbed, circulating toxic substances may be enhanced through a number of methods. The renal excretion of a few drugs that are weak acids can be increased by alkalinization of the urine and ion trapping the ionized form of the drug in the renal tubule. This method prevents renal tubular reabsorption of drugs such as salicylates, phenobarbital, chlorpropamide, and 2,4-dichlorphenoxyacetic acid. This technique should not be confused with the antiquated practice of forced diuresis, which employed the administration of high volumes of intravenous fluid to maintain high urinary flow rates (2 to 6 mL per kg per hour). This practice was abandoned because of serious side effects, including cerebral and pulmonary edema. The most important factor in the enhancement of renal elimination of drugs is the urinary pH and not the volume of urine output. The target urinary pH is 7.5 to 8.0 and should be monitored hourly, along with close monitoring of electrolytes and calcium. A Foley catheter is generally required (37).

Hemodialysis is another method that increases the elimination of a few specific substances. Its use was reported in children only 140 times in 2006 (1). The physical characteristics of the intoxicant determine whether it will be amenable to removal by hemodialysis. Specifically, the drug must be able to freely cross the dialysis membrane. Ideally, this necessitates a molecular weight of less than 500 daltons, high water solubility, low protein binding, and a small volume of distribution of less than 1 L per kg. Although hemodialysis has been anecdotally reported to enhance the elimination of a wide variety of intoxicants, acceptable risk-to-benefit ratios are present for only a few substances such as salicylates, phenobarbital, methanol, ethylene glycol, lithium, certain metals, and certain renally eliminated drugs in patients with renal failure. Hemodialysis is at times technically difficult in hemodynamically unstable patients and in neonates. Alternatively, exchange transfusion has been employed for the management of severe neonatal theophylline or salicylate intoxication (38–41).

The technique of hemoperfusion involves circulating blood through a cartridge filled with charcoal or resin beads that are capable of adsorbing both polar and nonpolar drugs. Hemoperfusion is typically reserved for the removal of drugs that are highly protein bound but otherwise would be amenable to hemodialysis. The technique is not limited by drug–water solubility or molecular weight. Traditionally, this modality has been employed in settings of theophylline, valproic acid, and carbamazepine poisoning. However, recent reports of high-flux hemodialysis efficiently removing these substances are emerging (42). Complications related to hemoperfusion include thrombocytopenia, leukopenia, hypoglycemia, hypocalcemia, and hemorrhage secondary to heparinization.

Multidose-activated charcoal is another method used to enhance drug elimination. Its use is warranted for the treatment of serious intoxications with phenobarbital, theophylline, carbamazepine, dapsone, and quinine (43). It may be considered for salicylate, colchicine, and amatoxin (mushroom) toxicity. Multidose charcoal is commonly recommended for the treatment of phenytoin toxicity based on volunteer data showing decreased elimination half-lives. A beneficial outcome for phenytoin-poisoned patients, however, has not been demonstrated.

TABLE 61.8 Antidotes for Poisoning

Antidote	*Toxicant*
Antivenom	Crotalids (rattlesnakes)
	North American coral snake
	Exotic snake species
	Black widow spider
	Scorpion
	Sea wasp or box jelly fish
Atropine	Organophosphates
	Carbamates
	Physostigmine
	Clitocybe, Inocybe mushrooms
Benztropine/diphenhydramine	Dystonic reaction from neuroleptic medication
Calcium	Hydrofluoric acid
	Calcium channel blocker
Chelators	
Calcium disodium ethylenediaminetetracetic acid	Lead, cadmium, copper, zinc
Deferoxamine	Iron, aluminum
Dimercaprol	Arsenic, lead, gold, inorganic mercury
D-Penicillamine	Investigational for copper, lead, mercury, arsenic, and bismuth
Dimercaptosuccinic acid (succimer)	Lead, mercury
Cyanide antidote kit	Cyanide
	Hydrogen sulfide
Digoxin-specific antibodies	Digoxin/digitoxin
	Plants such as oleander, foxglove, lily of the valley
Ethanol	Methanol
	Ethylene glycol
	Glycol ethers
4-Methylpyrazole (Antizol)	Ethylene glycol (investigational for methanol)
Flumazenil (Romazicon)	Benzodiazepines
Folic acid (leucovorin)	Methanol, methotrexate, trimethoprim
Glucagon	Beta-blockers
	Calcium channel blockers
	Insulin/oral hypoglycemic agents
Glucose	Insulin/oral hypoglycemic agents
Methylene blue	Drugs causing methemoglobinemia
Hydroxocobalamin	Cyanide
Lipid emulsion	Local anesthetics (bupivacaine)
N-Acetylcysteine	Acetaminophen, pennyroyal oil, cyclopeptide mushrooms, carbon tetrachloride
Naloxone	Opiates/narcotics
	Clonidine
	Dextromethorphan
Octreotide	Sulfonylureas
Oxygen	Carbon monoxide
Pralidoxime chloride	Organophosphates
	Carbamates
Protamine	Heparin
Pyridoxine (vitamin B_6)	Isoniazid
	Gyromitra esculenta
	Ethylene glycol
	Disulfiram
	Carbon disulfide
Thiamine	Ethanol
	Ethylene glycol
Vitamin B_{12a}	Cyanide, nitroprusside
Vitamin K_1	Coumarin
	Long-acting warfarins (rat poisons)

Antidotes

Antidote use in children, as in adults, is rarely required. Most poisonings are managed with the stabilization, decontamination, and supportive-care processes outlined earlier. When their use is necessary, however, the therapeutic indications for antidotes are generally the same as for adults. In 2006, the most commonly used antidote was a benzodiazepine, followed by naloxone and *N*-acetylcysteine (1). It should be noted that when antidote treatment is aimed at neutralizing the intoxicant, dosing may not be weight based in children. For example, if a child ingests 0.25 mg of digoxin and develops a cardiac dysrhythmia, digoxin-Fab fragments will be administered at the dose needed to neutralize the estimated amount of digoxin that is bioavailable. Another example is that the dose of antivenom administered to treat crotaline (rattlesnake) envenomation is based on the clinical severity of the envenomation and not the child's weight. Recently, Food and Drug Administration–approved antidotes such as fomepizole for the treatment of toxic alcohol exposure, crotaline Fab antivenom, and hydroxocobalamin are being used in children (44,45). Other trends in antidote use include the use of lipid emulsion to treat local anesthetic and other cardiovascular poisons and the use of octreotide following pediatric sulfonylurea poisoning. Commonly used antidotes are listed in Table 61.8.

PREVENTION

Poison prevention strategies are critical for affecting childhood safety. Examples of primary messages that clinicians should provide to caregivers are listed in Table 61.9. The most important of these is to avoid bringing toxic substances into the home. Second, all cleaning products, personal care products, and medications should be kept out of sight, on a high shelf, ideally in a locked cabinet or closet. Labeling products as hazardous with brightly colored stickers is probably not an effective deterrent (46).

Lead remains the greatest environmental hazard to US children and a key focus of poisoning prevention efforts. In 1999 to 2002, an estimated 310,000 (1.6%) US children had elevated blood lead levels (EBL defined as $\geq$10 μg per dL) and 1.4 million had blood lead levels of 5 to 9 μg per dL (almost 14%) (47). The adverse neurologic effects of lead are severe. Even low-level exposure affects intellectual development, behavior, and lifetime achievement. Since the 1980s, studies have linked blood lead levels of less than 10 μg per dL in children aged 1 to 5 years with decreased IQ and cognition, with demonstrated effects evident at about 2 μg per dL (48). No threshold for effects has been demonstrated. In 2000, the US Department of Health and Human Services adopted the goal of reducing all exposures to lead and eliminating EBLs in children by 2010. Although lead paint and dust accounts for up to 70% of EBLs in US children, the US Centers for Disease Control and Prevention estimates that 30% of current EBLs do not have an immediate lead paint source, and numerous studies indicate that lead exposures result from multiple sources. Prevention therefore requires an ongoing emphasis on controlled exposure to lead-based paint and dust and also an increased awareness of atypical sources of lead exposure. These include imported toys, jewelry, fashion accessories, folk/ethnic remedies, imported condiments, candies, pellets, bullets, and food-related items such as ceramics (49).

Another recent target of poisoning prevention efforts is the over-the-counter cough and cold product category. Serious injuries and deaths have been reported among infants and children who received over-the-counter cough and cold medicines, but most adverse events resulted from overdoses or unsupervised ingestions (50–53). To promote child safety, the Food and Drug Administration and the Centers for Disease Control and Prevention have developed materials to educate parents, health care providers, and consumers about how and when these products can be used safely. In 2008, the Consumer Healthcare Products Association announced that the leading manufacturers of pediatric over-the-counter cough and cold medicines would

TABLE 61.9 Pediatric Poisoning Prevention
Avoid bringing chemicals or medications into the home
If toxic substances must be kept in the home, keep all medications/cleaning products out of sight, on a top shelf, in a locked cabinet, or closet
Remember: out of reach ≠ out of sight
Keep regional poison control center phone sticker on each phone
Up to 30% of children who have toxic ingestions will be repeaters and are at risk for other injuries
Visitor's purses/backpacks should be kept out of reach/out of sight
Bedside stands are hazardous—do not keep mediations in this location
Do not keep medications, vitamins, or iron supplements on kitchen tables or countertops
Use only child-resistant containers
Keep syrup of ipecac in the home (1 oz per child; check expiration date)
Do not take medication in front of children
Never refer to medication as candy
Flush old medications down the toilet
Do not store cleaning products or pesticides near food or in food or beverage containers
Keep all products in their original container
Rinse out all containers thoroughly prior to disposal into the wastebasket
Double-bag (unbroken) mercury thermometers in lockable plastic baggies and take to community hazardous disposal waste site; for broken thermometers, call regional poison control center
Do not bring chemicals or products home from the workplace
Contact regional poison control center at 1-800-222-1222 for brochures on poison proofing the home and toxic plants

voluntarily modify the labels on these products to state that they should not be used in children younger than 4 years. Previous product labels stated that these medicines should not be used in children younger than 2 years. Existing products with these labels will not be removed immediately from store shelves but are expected to be replaced eventually with newly labeled products. Health care providers should be aware of the new labels and should alert parents and caregivers to this change. Additional information is available at http://www.fda.gov/bbs/topics/news/2008/new01899.html.

REFERENCES

1. Bronstein AC, Spyker DA, Cantinlena LR, et al. 2006 annual report of the American Association of Poison Control Centers' National Poison Data System (NPDS). *Clin Toxicol* 2007;45:815–917.
2. Centers for Disease Control and Prevention. Unintentional poisoning among young children—United States. *MMWR Morb Mortal Wkly Rep* 1983;32:529–531.
3. Shannon M. Ingestion of toxic substances by children. *N Engl J Med* 2000;342(3):186–191.
4. Darwin J, Seger D. Reaffirmed cost-effectiveness of poison centers. *Ann Emerg Med* 2003;41(1):159–160.
5. Litovitz T. Comparison of pediatric poisoning hazards: an analysis of 3.8 million exposure incidents. *Pediatrics* 1992;89(6):999–1006.
6. Fine JS. Pediatric principles. In: Goldrank LR, Flomenbaum NE, Lewin NA, et al., eds. *Goldrank's toxicologic emergencies*, 6th ed. New York, NY: McGraw-Hill, 1998:1687–1697.
7. Jensen G, Wilson W. Preventive implications of a study of 100 poisonings in children. *Pediatrics* 1960;65:490–496.
8. White SR, Yadao CM. Characterization of methylphenidate exposures reported to a regional poison control center. *Arch Pediatr Adolesc Med* 2000;154:1199–1203.
9. Litovitz TL, Flagler SL, Manoguerra AS, et al. Recurrent poisoning among paediatric poisoning victims. *Med Toxicol Adverse Drug Exp* 1989;4:381–386.
10. Sobel R. The psychiatric implications of accidental poisoning in childhood. *Pediatr Clin North Am* 1970;17:653–685.
11. Siebert R. Stress in families of children who have ingested poisons. *Br Med J* 1975;3:87–89.
12. Shannon M, Albers G, Burkhard K, et al. Safety and efficacy of flumazenil in the reversal of benzodiazepine-induced conscious sedation. *J Pediatr* 1997;131:582–586.
13. Kulig K, Bar-Or D, Cantrill SV, et al. Management of acutely poisoned patients without gastric emptying. *Ann Emerg Med* 1985;14: 562–567.
14. Merigian KS, Woodard M, Hedges JR, et al. Prospective evaluation of gastric emptying in the self-poisoned patient. *Am J Emerg Med* 1990;8(6):479–483.
15. Pond SM, Lewis-Driver DJ, Williams GM, et al. Gastric emptying in acute overdose: a prospective randomized controlled trial. *Med J Aust* 1995;163(7):345–349.
16. Kornberg AE, Dolgin J. Pediatric ingestions: charcoal alone versus ipecac and charcoal. *Ann Emerg Med* 1991;20(6):648–651.
17. Albertson TE, Derlet RW, Foulke GE, et al. Superiority of activated charcoal alone compared with ipecac and activated charcoal in the treatment of acute toxic ingestions. *Ann Emerg Med* 1989;18(1): 56–59.
18. Bond GR. Home use of syrup of ipecac is associated with a reduction in pediatric emergency department visits. *Ann Emerg Med* 1995; 25:338–343.
19. Bond GR. The role of activated charcoal and gastric emptying in gastrointestinal decontamination: a state-of-the-art review. *Ann Emerg Med* 2002;39:273–286.
20. American College of Emergency Physicians. Clinical policy for the initial approach to patients presenting with acute toxic ingestion or dermal or inhalation exposure. *Ann Emerg Med* 1995;25:570–585.
21. Spiller HA, Rodgers GC. Evaluation of administration of activated charcoal in the home. *Pediatrics* 2001;108(6):1–5.
22. American Academy of Clinical Toxicology, European Association of Poisons Centres and Clinical Toxicologists. Position paper: gastric lavage. *J Toxicol Clin Toxicol* 2004;42(7):933–943.
23. American Academy of Clinical Toxicology, European Association of Poisons Centres and Clinical Toxicologists. Position paper: single-dose activated charcoal. *Clin Toxicol* 2005;43:61–87.
24. Eisen TF, Grbcich PA, Lacouture PG, et al. The adsorption of salicylates by a milk chocolate–charcoal mixture. *Ann Emerg Med* 1991; 20:143–146.
25. American Academy of Clinical Toxicology, European Association of Poisons Centres and Clinical Toxicologists. Positions paper: cathartics. *Clin Toxicol* 2004;42(3):243–253.
26. American Academy of Clinical Toxicology, European Association of Poisons Centres and Clinical Toxicologists. Positions paper: whole bowel irrigation. *Clin Toxicol* 2004;42(6):843–854.
27. Henretig FM. Special considerations in the poisoned pediatric patient. *Emerg Med Clin North Am* 1994;12(2):549–567.
28. Pitetti RD, Whitman E, Zaylor A. Accidental and nonaccidental poisonings as a cause of apparent life-threatening events in infants. *Pediatrics* 2008;122(2):359–362.
29. Koren G. Medications which can kill a toddler with one tablet or teaspoonful. *Clin Toxicol* 1993;31(3):407–413.
30. Liebelt EL, Shannon MW. Small doses, big problems: a selected review of highly toxic common medications. *Pediatr Emerg Care* 1993;9(5):292–297.
31. Dine M. International poisoning of children: an overlooked category of child abuse: report of seven cases and review of the literature. *Pediatrics* 1982;70:32.
32. Baraff JL, Guterman JJ, Bayer M. The relationship of poison center contact and injury in children 2–6 years old. *Ann Emerg Med* 1992;21:153–157.
33. Bond GR. The poisoned child. *Emerg Med Clin North Am* 1995; 13(3):343–355.
34. Hepler B. Role of the toxicology testing in children. *Curr Opin Pediatr* 2001;13:183–188.
35. Hoffman RS, Nelson L. The use of toxicology testing in children. *Curr Opin Pediatr* 2001;13:183–188.
36. Wiley JF. Difficult diagnoses in toxicology. Poisons not detected by the comprehensive drug screen. *Pediatr Clin North Am* 1991; 38(3):725–735.
37. American Academy of Clinical Toxicology, European Association of Poisons Centres and Clinical Toxicologists. Positions paper: urinary alkalinization. *Clin Toxicol* 2004;42(1):1–26.
38. Shannon M, Wernovsky G, Morris C. Exchange transfusion in the treatment of severe theophylline poisoning. *Pediatrics* 1992;89: 145–147.
39. Done AK, Otterness LJ. Exchange transfusion in the treatment of oil of wintergreen poisoning. *J Pediatr* 1956;18:80–85.
40. Manikian A, Stone S, Hamilton R, et al. Exchange transfusions as an alternative to hemodialysis in severe infant salicylism [abstract]. *J Toxicol Clin Toxicol* 1996;34:585.
41. Osborn HH, Henry G, Wax P, et al. Theophylline toxicity in a premature neonate—elimination kinetics of exchange transfusion. *J Toxicol Clin Toxicol* 1993;31:639–644.
42. Dharnidharka VR, Fennell RS, Richard GA. Extracorporeal removal of toxic valproic acid levels in children. *Pediatr Nephrol* 2002;17(5): 312–315.
43. American Academy of Clinical Toxicology, European Association of Poisons Centres and Clinical Toxicologists. Position statement and practice guidelines on the use of multi-dose activated charcoal in the treatment of acute poisoning. *J Toxicol Clin Toxicol* 1999;37:731–751.
44. Osterhoudt KC. Fomepizole therapy for pediatric butoxyethanol intoxication. *J Toxicol Clin Toxicol* 2002;40(7):929–930.
45. Offerman SR, Bush SP, Moynihan JA, et al. Crotaline Fab antivenom for the treatment of children with rattlesnake envenomation. *Pediatrics* 2002;110(5):968–971.
46. Woolf AD, Lovejoy FH. Prevention of childhood poisoning. In: Haddad LM, Shannon MW, Winchester JF, eds. *Clinical management of poisoning and drug overdose*, 3rd ed. Philadelphia, PA: WB Saunders, 1998:300–306.
47. Levin R, Brown MJ, Kashtock ME, et al. Lead exposures in U.S. children, 2008: implications for prevention. *Environ Health Perspect* 2008;116(10):1285–1293.
48. Jusko TA, Henderson CR, Lanphear BP, et al. Blood lead concentrations < 10 microg/dL and child intelligence at 6 years of age. *Environ Health Perspect* 2008;116:243–248.
49. Gorospe EC, Gerstenberger SL. Atypical sources of childhood lead poisoning in the United States: a systematic review from 1966–2006. *Clin Toxicol* 2008;46(8):728–737.

50. Centers for Disease Control and Prevention. Revised product labels for pediatric over-the-counter cough and cold medicines. *MMWR Morb Mortal Wkly Rep* 2008;57(43):1180.
51. Food and Drug Administration. Cold, cough, allergy, bronchodilator, antiasthmatic drug products for over-the-counter human use. Memorandum from the Nonprescription Drug Advisory Committee meeting. http://www.fda.gov/ohrms/dockets/ac/07/briefing/2007-4323b1-02-fda.pdf. Published October 18–19, 2007.
52. Centers for Disease Control and Prevention. Infant deaths associated with cough and cold medications—two states, 2005. *MMWR Morb Mortal Wkly Rep* 2007;56:1–4.
53. Schaefer MK, Shehab N, Cohen AL, et al. Adverse events from cough and cold medications in children. *Pediatrics* 2008;121:783–787.

CHAPTER

62

Wayne R. Snodgrass
Susan C. Smolinske

Use of Herbal Products in Children: Risks and Unproven Benefits

This chapter addresses issues surrounding the use of herbal products in children. Included are descriptions of herbal products, reasons why persons use such products, the most commonly used herbals in the United States and their use during pregnancy and breast-feeding, adverse effects, drug interactions, and regulatory issues. It is clear that children are being given herbal products in the United States. It is also clear for both children and adults that too many herbal products currently do not meet Good Manufacturing Practices, that many herbal products are unpredictable in their concentrations of active ingredients, that many herbal products lack high-quality studies of efficacy, that labeling of most herbal products is not adequate, and that many herbal products pose a risk of toxicity. The benefit-to-risk ratio of most herbal products remains unknown. Because of the great demand by the public for herbal products, greater efforts and resources should be devoted to high-quality research to determine the effectiveness and the safety of herbal products.

INTRODUCTION

Use of herbal products by children is a relatively new area of interest and concern. Only very limited information regarding therapeutic efficacy and risk of adverse reactions to herbal products in adults is published in peer-reviewed medical and scientific journals. Even less is known regarding herbal products usage, efficacy, and risks in children.

OBJECTIVES

The objectives in this chapter are to describe what herbal products are, why patients and parents use them, and their adverse effects and drug interactions, and to discuss some approaches to evaluating data and clinical trials, the lack of quality control of manufacture of some herbal products, the issue of standardization of dose and active ingredients, the lack of full dose-response curve data, and the lack of high-quality clinical trials.

DEFINITION OF HERBAL PRODUCTS

Herbal products are drugs. They are complex mixtures of chemicals prepared from plants (1,2), or are parts of raw, uncooked plants. The identified or suspected active ingredients often are multichemical in nature (3). Herbal products are not required to be proven either safe or effective prior to marketing (4). The Food and Drug Administration (FDA) has minimal to no regulatory authority regarding the safety and efficacy of herbal products. The burden of proof for safety is on the FDA, not the manufacturer (5). This is the opposite situation to that of food additives and drugs. This situation likely results in an increased risk to the general public, and, unfortunately, it has been established by law. The 1994 Dietary Supplement Health and Education Act (DSHEA) categorizes herbal products as "dietary supplements." Thus, consumers have little protection against misleading or fraudulent claims made by herbal manufacturers (6,7).

Herbal products are rarely sold in child-resistant packaging (8) and are exempt from regulations that mandate imprint code identification markings. Lack of product uniformity even among batches of product from a single manufacturer has been documented. Some herbal products may contain pesticides, heavy metals, or other chemicals leached from the ambient soil media (9). There is no guarantee even on the correct identity of herbal products being sold. Herbal products may be contaminated or misidentified at any stage from harvesting through packaging (4). Some herbal products (e.g., aconite roots) may vary greatly in their alkaloid content depending on the origin, the time of harvest, and the method of processing (10). There is a lack of quality control of manufacture of many herbal products, with standards in some cases far below what is generally recognized as necessary for therapeutic drugs (11,12). Standardization of dose and active ingredients is unknown for many, and perhaps most, herbal products. For example, St. John's wort is "standardized" by its hypericin content, but hyperforin is the active ingredient. "Standardized" typically is not defined or the method stated on either the product label or a product monograph, assuming a monograph or package insert exists. Labels for dietary supplements (herbal products) may contain statements of nutrition support without preauthorization by the FDA (13,14). On June 22, 2007, the FDA passed a final rule that established a set of Good Manufacturing Practices for certain dietary supplements. Distributors have up to 3 years to comply, and bulk suppliers and some individual practitioners are exempt, thus this may not have prevented some of the large-scale contamination issues. Because most herbal products have no high-quality clinical trial studies, there is a lack of full dose-response data. Even if a dose range is recommended, typically there is no dose-response information.

Children may have a different dose response than adults, as has been well established for some therapeutic drugs. Therapeutic indices vary for herbal products and may be unpredictable, particularly in children (15). Children's doses cited by many herbal guides are strictly anecdotal (15).

About 7,000 species of plants are used in China as herbal remedies (10), and there are more than 5,000 kinds of Chinese medicinal herbs. There are more than 700 patent Chinese medicine factories, and there are more than 1,500 factories producing Chinese herbal pills and other dose forms (16). It is estimated that there are more than 20,000 herbal products on the market (17).

EPIDEMIOLOGY

An estimated 30% to 35% of adult Americans use herbal products (18). Estimates for children are based on very limited data. Approximately 11% of parents used some form of alternative medicine for their children, based on a questionnaire sent to 2,000 parents with a 96% response rate (19). It has been stated that up to 50% of children with autism in the United States probably are being given some form of complementary/alternative medicine (20). One survey of emergency department visits identified that 14.5% of women used herbal products during pregnancy and 23.5% of children younger than 16 years were given herbal preparations (21). Among teenagers who use complementary and alternative therapies, nearly 75% use herbs (6). In 142 families that brought their children to an emergency department in 2001, 45% of caregivers reported giving their children an herbal product (22).

An estimated 15% of Americans visited a provider of herbal medicine in 1998. Approximately 25% of Western drugs are isolated from plants, and another approximately 25% are modifications of substances derived from plants. Internationally, approximately 120 prescription drugs are produced directly from plant extracts. The US commercial market for herbal products was projected to be $5 billion in the year 2000 (23).

Historically, the use of plants for medicinal purposes is documented in Chinese texts of the Yellow Emperor Huang Di in 2697 B.C.E. and in the Ebers papyrus in 1550 B.C.E. (more than 800 remedies, mostly botanical). Hippocrates (466 to 377 B.C.E.) used plants in his practice of medicine.

REASONS WHY ADULTS USE HERBAL PRODUCTS

Typical adult users of herbal products are educated, middle class, white, and between the ages of 25 and 49 (24). They have a holistic belief in the integration of body, mind, and spirit. They report poorer perceived health status compared with matched nonusers of herbal products. They are not more dissatisfied with and are not more distrustful of conventional medical care. Some of these persons may be somatizers (24).

REASONS WHY CHILDREN AND ADOLESCENTS USE HERBAL PRODUCTS

One potential use of herbal products by children and adolescents is to attempt to enhance sports performance, similar to the abuse of steroids, growth hormone analogues, and so-called supplements such as creatine (25). One published source recommends, for treatment of attention deficit hyperactivity disorder in children, use of St. John's wort, kava kava, catnip, and kola nut, singly or in combination (15). A voluntary recall of ginseng products occurred after teachers reported that students were drinking ginseng extract that contained up to 24% alcohol (15). Other reports document the use of alternative medicine and/or herbal products in children for diagnoses such as juvenile arthritis, infant colic, enuresis, postoperative pain, agitation, and plantar warts (26–32).

Recently, adolescent abuse of herbal blends, purchased over the Internet, or in local alternative stores, has become epidemic. These products are distributed in Europe, and possibly manufactured in China, with common brand names of "Spice" or "Serenity". While labeled to contain a variety of herbal plants with psychoactive activity, chemical analysis has uniformly shown them to have none of the labeled content, but instead to contain "designer" drugs that act on the THC receptor, sometimes 100 times as potent. These appear to cause a higher degree of toxicity and tolerance than THC, thus posing an emerging threat (33).

High-quality clinical trials can provide valid scientific evidence of the efficacy of herbal products, both for pediatric and adult therapeutic uses. One prospective double-blind clinical trial supported the potential efficacy of one herbal tea preparation in the treatment of infant colic (34); this study is worthy of confirmation and is an example of an herbal product clinical trial that may provide useful and scientifically valid information. However, much more additional safety information is required before this product could be recommended for widespread use and incorporated into routine treatment recommendations.

UNITED STATES PHARMACOPEIA DESIGNATION

In order to obtain a United States Pharmacopeia (USP) designation and to place the letters "USP" on a label, a manufacturer must submit its product for testing by the

USP and must fulfill the standards set by the USP. Most herbal products do not have a USP designation, and it is likely that many herbal products would not meet USP standards because of factors such as batch-to-batch variability, lack of stability, and/or contaminants. A designation of NF (National Formulary) on a product without a USP designation means that the product fulfills the manufacturing quality standards set by the USP but does not have USP or FDA endorsement for the intended use (5). Most herbal products currently do not have an NF designation. The USP in the last few years has instituted a new program to certify herbal products that meet its standards, including a label designation to inform the consumer that an herbal product has met USP standards. Only a small number of herbal products have received certification by the USP.

NATIONAL CENTER FOR COMPLEMENTARY AND ALTERNATIVE MEDICINE AND OFFICE OF CANCER COMPLEMENTARY AND ALTERNATIVE MEDICINE

The National Center for Complementary and Alternative Medicine (NCCAM) is a part of the National Institutes of Health, and the Office of Cancer Complementary and Alternative Medicine (OCCAM) is at the National Cancer Institute, also part of the National Institutes of Health. These units provide information and support research involving herbal products and other types of complementary/alternative medicine (35). The Web site for NCCAM is http://www.nccam.nih.gov.

MOST COMMONLY USED HERBAL PRODUCTS IN THE UNITED STATES

The most commonly used herbal products in the United States are chamomile, echinacea, feverfew, garlic, ginger, ginkgo, ginseng, kava, saw palmetto, St. John's wort, and valerian. The commercial claims for therapeutic benefit for these herbal products typically are not substantiated by prospective, randomized, placebo-controlled, double-blind clinical trials. The claims for therapeutic use include chamomile for gastric ulcers and as a sedative, echinacea for the common cold, feverfew for migraine headache prevention, garlic for hyperlipemia and hypertension, ginger as an antemetic, ginkgo for dementia and claudication, ginseng as a "tonic," kava for anxiety, saw palmetto for prostate hypertrophy, St. John's wort for mild endogenous depression, and valerian as a sedative. There has been a surge in recent years of the use of foods, candies, or beverages promoted as energy enhancement products to adolescents. These products typically contain caffeine derived from guarana or cola nut, in doses of up to 300 mg per serving, along with other ingredients such as ginseng, vitamins, amino acids, and *Ginkgo biloba* (36).

HERBAL PRODUCTS' ADVERSE EFFECTS

A number of adverse effects of herbal products have been reported (37,38). Some of these adverse effects are severe and potentially life-threatening (39,40). Some herbal products' adverse effects have resulted in death. The World Health Organization Collaborating Center for International Drug Monitoring in Uppsala, Sweden, has had more than 5,000 reports of suspected adverse reactions that involve herbal medicines (10).

Examples of herbal products' adverse effects (some of which are based on animal or in vitro studies) include aconitum-related cardiac arrhythmias and death, aristolochia-related renal failure, chaparral-related hepatotoxicity, comfrey-related hepatotoxicity and carcinogenicity, ma huang-related hypertension and/or cerebral vascular accident (i.e., stroke) and/or cardiac arrhythmias, pokeroot-related aplastic anemia sometimes resulting in death, sassafras-related carcinogenicity, Chuen-Lin–related neonatal hyperbilirubinemia (16,41,42), and berberine-related neonatal hyperbilirubinemia (43). Other adverse effects of herbal products in children include fatal hepatic venoocclusive disease in an infant due to pyrrolizidine alkaloids in an herbal tea (44), central nervous system depression in infants due to an herbal tea (45), multiple excessive ovarian follicular development (46), aplastic anemia in a 12-year-old boy treated with an herbal product for an upper respiratory illness (47), and gynecomastia in three prepubertal boys who chronically applied topical products containing lavender or tea tree oil (48). Compared to other chemical exposures, some herbal products may be taken at doses that are relatively close to their toxic range, and they may be taken chronically (49).

Reporting of adverse effects of herbal products was formerly not mandatory for manufacturers or distributors (50). By contrast, reporting of adverse effects of therapeutic drugs is mandatory for manufacturers (3). Data from one study suggest that users of herbal products may be less likely to consult a physician for a suspected adverse reaction to an herbal product compared with a similar adverse reaction to a conventional nonprescription medicine (51). On December 22, 2006, an amendment to the FDC Act was enacted that requires a manufacturer to report a serious adverse reaction to a dietary supplement to the FDA in the same manner as that to an OTC drug and to include labeling with reporting instructions (52).

Rating of herbs by the FDA as unsafe, undefined safety, and safe is based primarily on anecdotal data and has some value as a starting point for evaluating specific herbs (53).

An indirect form of adverse effects of herbal products is the serious harm that has occurred in children with cancer when traditional chemotherapy was replaced with unproven herbal therapies (54).

HERBAL PRODUCTS–DRUG INTERACTIONS

Examples of drug interactions include aloe plus digoxin or aloe plus a diuretic resulting in hypokalemia, feverfew plus warfarin resulting in increased bleeding, garlic plus warfarin resulting in increased bleeding, ginger plus warfarin resulting in increased bleeding, gingko plus warfarin resulting in increased bleeding, ginseng plus digoxin resulting in increased plasma levels of digoxin, ginseng plus furosemide resulting in a decreased diuresis, ginseng plus warfarin resulting in a decreased international normalized ratio, kava plus sedatives resulting in central nervous system depression, ma huang plus β-blockers resulting in decreased β-blockade effect, ma huang plus monoamine oxidase inhibitors resulting in increased toxicity, ma huang plus theophylline resulting in increased toxicity, ma huang plus decongestants resulting in increased toxicity, St. John's wort plus adrenergic drugs resulting in hypertension, St. John's wort plus antidepressants resulting in serotonin syndrome, St. John's wort plus lithium resulting in increased lithium toxicity, St. John's wort plus angiotensin-converting-enzyme inhibitors resulting in hypertension, and valerian plus central nervous system depressants resulting in increased sedation.

An extremely serious drug interaction between cyclosporine and St. John's wort is important to note. Cyclosporine is metabolized by cytochrome P-450 isozyme 3A4 (CYP3A4). Because of enzyme induction of CYP3A4 by St. John's wort (twofold induction of CYP3A4 by St. John's wort; threefold induction of CYP3A4 by rifampin), acute heart rejection occurred in two heart transplant patients who started St. John's wort while receiving cyclosporine (55).

HERBAL PRODUCTS, PREGNANCY, AND BREAST-FEEDING

Approximately 26 herbs are cited for restricted use in pregnancy (56). Approximately 11 herbs are contraindicated during lactation. Most information on herbal products and breast-feeding is anecdotal and not based on scientific research (57). The herbs to avoid in pregnant women and/or women of child-bearing age include abortifacient herbs (more than 16 are known), emmenagogues (herbs that promote menstruation), nervous system stimulants, stimulant laxatives, berberine-containing herbs, pyrrolizidine alkaloid-containing herbs, and herbs with a high volatile oil content.

The herb blue cohosh is contraindicated during pregnancy. This herb has been used near the end of pregnancy to induce uterine contractions. Two newborn infants with severe toxicity due to maternal use of blue cohosh have been described. One infant was born with severe congestive heart failure, cardiogenic shock, and anterolateral myocardial infarction (58). Another infant was born with severe seizures, encephalopathy, and renal failure (59). One newborn developed extensive petechiae and purpura after exposure in utero to Evening Primrose for 1 week in an attempt to ripen the mother's cervix to ease labor (60).

Some midwives encourage the use of certain herbs as "tonics" or teas for use during pregnancy and/or lactation and also the use of some herbal products during labor and delivery (61–63). This practice has not been well studied; the risks for mother, fetus, and infant mostly are unknown. Some herbs are known animal teratogens (e.g., hellebore, hemlock, and tragacanth) (64,65). Some herbs are known human fetal toxins (e.g., blue cohosh) (64). The reported prevalence of use of Chinese herbal medicines by pregnant women in Hong Kong is 54% (42). The reasons cited for this high prevalence of use of herbal products by pregnant women included ideas such as "to ensure firm implantation of the fetus in the uterus" (42)!

The Teratology Society emphasizes the following recommendations: Dietary supplements cannot be assumed to be safe for the embryo or fetus; dietary supplements should not be labeled for use in pregnancy unless they have been shown to be safe by standard scientific methods; all dietary supplements should carry a warning that their safety in pregnancy is unknown, unless safety has been established by standard scientific means; the FDA should consider all pregnancy-related conditions to be potential "diseases" in terms of the 1994 DSHEA; and the FDA should work with the US Congress to amend the DSHEA of 1994 to ensure appropriate protection for the human embryo and fetus (64).

AN EXAMPLE: ECHINACEA

More detailed consideration of one herbal product, echinacea, will illustrate various issues regarding herbal products such as their safety versus efficacy and the lack of high-quality prospective controlled clinical trials.

Echinacea is also known as the purple coneflower, a member of the daisy family of plants, and is native to North America. It is the most popular herb in the United States. Estimated sales are $300 million annually. It is sold in various forms such as liquid extracts, tinctures, and solid dose forms. It is marketed in the United States for prevention or treatment of the common cold (coryza).

Echinacea contains a variety of different chemical compounds that have been identified as active constituents. These components include alkylamides, alkaloids, arabinogalactan, cichoric acid, flavonoids, isobutylamides, polyenes, and polysaccharides.

Echinacea has been approved only as "supportive therapy" by the Federal Health Agency in Germany for upper respiratory illnesses (URI), urogenital infections, and wounds. There are approximately 26 published controlled clinical trials regarding the efficacy of echinacea (66). None of these clinical trials are of sufficient methodologic quality to be conclusive. Deficiencies in most of these studies include treatment assignment not being randomized and treatment assignment not being blinded. One randomized, double-blind, placebo-controlled clinical trial for URI showed a statistically significant decrease in symptoms and duration of "flu-like" illness in 180 subjects (67). The effects were dose dependent and occurred at a dose of 3.6 mL per day or 180 drops per day. Another randomized, double-blind, placebo-controlled clinical trial of echinacea in recurrent URIs showed less frequent recurrences of URIs, less severe recurrences of URIs, and a 14% relative risk reduction in URIs. However, both of these two clinical trials had deficits of inadequate use or description of diagnostic criteria, randomization procedures, treatment interventions, methods for assessment of outcomes, assurance of blinding, details of results, and quality of the statistical analysis. Another randomized, double-blind, placebo-controlled clinical trial in

302 volunteers did not show a prophylactic effect for echinacea (68).

It is of note that information sources for echinacea, as well as for other herbal products, vary in the depth of analysis and evaluation. For example, echinacea is said to appear safe for use in children for colds, although there was no information on dose or duration of therapy. On the other hand, echinacea duration of use typically is restricted to 2 weeks or less. Use exceeding 8 weeks has led to immunosuppression. A warning on the bottle label that use exceeding 8 weeks may lead to immunosuppression may not be stated for many or even most products containing echinacea. This latter situation is related directly to the lack of authority for the FDA to regulate herbal products as determined by the 1994 DSHEA law passed by the US Congress.

Adverse effects of echinacea include the following: in persons with asthma, atopy, or allergic rhinitis there is increased risk of severe allergic reactions, dyspnea, and/or anaphylaxis; in persons with diabetes there may be a worsening of metabolic control. In addition, echinacea is not recommended in persons with tuberculosis, human immunodeficiency virus infection, multiple sclerosis, and autoimmune diseases.

Flavonoids in echinacea inhibit CYP3A4, an enzyme which has most of its activity in the liver, and which metabolizes approximately 40% of all drugs marketed in the United States that are cleared by the liver. Thus, it is predictable that several drug interactions with echinacea are likely to occur.

APPROACHES TO EVALUATING DATA AND CLINICAL TRIALS

Principles of rational therapy apply to herbal products just as they do to therapeutic drugs. These principles include establishing a working diagnosis, understanding the disease to be treated, choosing the best drug (considerations of benefit-to-risk ratio), individualizing treatment, choosing end points to follow to evaluate therapeutic response, and having a therapeutic contract with the patient or parent.

For a physician, evaluating therapeutic data and clinical trial data includes considerations such as the following: Was the assignment of patients to treatments really randomized? Were all clinically relevant outcomes reported? Were the study patients recognizably similar to those patients you treat? Were both statistical and clinical significance considered in the reported data? Is the therapeutic maneuver feasible in your practice? Were all patients who entered the study accounted for at its conclusion? Published checklists for evaluating clinical trial data and published studies of clinical trials may be helpful in evaluating drug therapies and herbal product therapies.

An *N* of 1 randomized clinical trial may be done in an outpatient office or clinic medical practice when the patient (parent) insists on taking (giving) a treatment that the physician thinks is useless or potentially harmful, when neither the physician nor the patient (parent) is confident of the optimal dose, and when treatment is for a chronic illness or disease.

HERBAL PRODUCTS INFORMATION SOURCES

The quality of information sources available from manufacturers for herbal products varies widely and typically is far below that available from manufacturers of marketed therapeutic drugs. In addition, lay public sources of information may be incomplete, erroneous, or even contain potentially harmful information or recommendations. For example, for herbal products containing ginger, a lay magazine article states that though ginger has not been studied in children, it is considered safe. In other words, this is simply an opinion not based on data because there are no published data on the safety of ginger in children. The same article goes on to recommend chiropractic adjustment for chronic ear infections in children, a recommendation that has no basis in biologic function or disease process (69).

The German E Commission monographs are cited widely as a reliable source of herbal information. These monographs are a compilation of the evaluations of an expert committee using the data available to them. There are few randomized, prospective, controlled clinical trial data cited or available. The German E Commission's findings are based for the most part on standardized pharmaceutical preparations found in Germany and may not necessarily be extrapolated to less-regulated products on the US market.

The Internet is a source of information on herbal products, with a wide variation in the quality of the information available. As of April 1999, there were more than 10,000 commercial Internet sites for ginkgo, 11,000 for St. John's wort, and more than 20,000 for ginseng (70).

FUTURE RESEARCH NEEDS

Future research needs related to herbal products include quantitative epidemiologic studies of the prevalence and the incidence of the use of herbal products in infants and children, the development of laboratory methods for the assay of herbal components and the synthesis of herbal ingredients, and high-quality clinical trials in children of the efficacy and the safety of very carefully selected single-chemical entities found in herbal products.

CONCLUSION

Herbal products possibly may offer some potential benefits to some children. However, insufficient quality control in manufacture despite stronger Good Manufacturing Practices (GMP) regulations and lack of consistency of many, if not most, herbal products prevent results of any high-quality clinical trial being extrapolatable to other products or possibly even to other batches of the same product from the same company. Thus, before clinical trials of herbal products are carried out, consistent quality and reproducibility of herbal products must be achieved. Then, careful selected clinical trials in adults, followed later by clinical trials in children, may be done. With this approach, the benefits of herbal products in children, if any, may be established, while the risks and adverse effects, if any, may be identified.

More immediately, epidemiologic studies of the current use of herbal products in children should be carried out; these epidemiologic studies should include collection of data regarding adverse effects of herbal products being used in children. As a first step, this would assist in identifying those herbal products posing a risk to children.

REFERENCES

1. Kemper KJ. Seven herbs every pediatrician should know. *Contemp Pediatr* 1996;13:79–93.
2. Kemper KJ. Separation or synthesis: a holistic approach to therapeutics. *Pediatr Rev* 1996;17(8):279–283.
3. Boullleta JL, Nace AM. Safety issues with herbal medicine. *Pharmacotherapy* 2000;20(3):257–269.
4. O'Hara M, Kiefer D, Farrell K, Kemper K. A review of 12 commonly used medicinal herbs. *Arch Fam Med* 1998;7:523–536.
5. Bauer BA. Herbal therapy: what a clinician needs to know to counsel patients effectively. *Mayo Clin Proc* 2000;75:835–841.
6. Gardiner P, Kemper KJ. Herbs in pediatric and adolescent medicine. *Pediatr Rev* 2000;21:44–57.
7. Zeisel SH. Regulation of "nutraceuticals." *Science* 1999;285: 1853–1854.
8. Houlder AM. Herbal medicines should be in child resistant containers. *Br Med J* 1995;310:1473.
9. Ernst E. Harmless herbs? A review of the recent literature. *Am J Med* 1998;104:170–178.
10. Chan TYK. Monitoring the safety of herbal medicines. *Drug Saf* 1997;17:209–215.
11. Liberti LE, Der Marderosian A. Evaluation of commercial ginseng products. *J Pharm Sci* 1978;67:1487–1489.
12. Heptinstall S, Awang DV, Dawson BA, Kindack D, Knight DW, May J. Parthenolide content and bioactivity of feverfew. Estimation of commercial and authenticated feverfew products. *J Pharm Pharmacol* 1992;44:391–395.
13. Anonymous. Commission on dietary supplement labels issues final report. *J Am Diet Assoc* 1998;98:270.
14. Food and Drug Administration. Current good manufacturing practice in manufacturing, packaging, labeling, or holding operations for dietary supplements; final rule. *Fed Regist* 2007;72(121): 34751–34958.
15. Turow V. Herbal therapy for children. *Pediatrics* 1998;102:1492.
16. Borins M. The dangers of using herbs. What your patients need to know. *Postgrad Med* 1998;104:91–99.
17. Buck ML, Michel RS. Talking with families about herbal therapies. *Pediatrics* 2000;136:673–678.
18. Eisenberg DM, Kessler RC, Foster C, Norlock FE, Calkins DR, Delbanco TL. Unconventional medicine in the United States: prevalence, costs, and patterns of use. *N Engl J Med* 1993;328: 246–252.
19. Spigelblatt L, Laîné-Ammara G, Pless IB, Guyver A. The use of alternative medicine by children. *Pediatrics* 1994;94:811–814.
20. AD Sandler, D Brazdziunas, WC Cooley, L Gonzalez. Counseling families who choose complementary and alternative medicine for their child with chronic illness or disability. *Pediatrics* 2001;107: 598–601.
21. Kristoffersen SS, Atkin PA, Shenfield GM. Uptake of alternative medicine. *Lancet* 1996;347:972.
22. Lanski SL, Greenwald M, Perkins A, Simon HK. Herbal therapy use in a pediatric emergency department population. *Pediatrics* 2003;111:981–985.
23. Bouldin AS, Smith MC, Garner SL. Pharmacy and herbal medicine in the U.S. *Soc Sci Med* 1999;20(3):257–269.
24. Astin JA. Why patients use alternative medicine. Results of a national study. *J Am Med Assoc* 1998;279:1548–1553.
25. Bucci LR. Selected herbals and human exercise performance. *Am J Clin Nutr* 2000;72(Suppl):624S–636S.
26. Cavalcanti FS, de Freitas GG. Alternative medicine in a patient with juvenile chronic arthritis. *J Rheumatol* 1992;19:1827–1828.
27. Southwood TR, Malleson PN, Roberts-Thomson PJ, Mahy M. Unconventional remedies used for patients with juvenile arthritis. *Pediatrics* 1990;85:150–154.
28. Klougart N, Nilsson N, Jacobsen J. Infantile colic treated by chiropractors: a prospective study of 316 cases. *J Manipulative Physiol Ther* 1989;12:281–288.
29. Leboeuf C, Brown P, Herman A, Leembruggen K, Walton D, Crisp TC. Chiropractic care of children with nocturnal enuresis: a prospective outcome study. *J Manipulative Physiol Ther* 1991;14:110–115.
30. Alibeu JP, Jobert J. Aconite in homeopathic relief of post-operative pain and agitation in children. *Pediatric* 1990;45:465–466.
31. Anonymous. Canadian Pediatric Society Statement. Megavitamin and megamineral therapy in childhood. *Can Med Assoc J* 1990;143: 1009–1013.
32. Labrecque M, Audet D, Latulippe LG, Drouin J. Homeopathic treatment of plantar warts. *Can Med Assoc J* 1992;146:1749–1753.
33. European Monitoring Centre for Drugs and Drug Addiction. Understanding the spice phenomenon. Thematic Paper; 1–37. www.emcdda.europa.eu. Published 2009.
34. Weizman Z, Alkrinawi S, Goldfarb D, Bitran C. Efficacy of herbal tea preparation in infantile colic. *J Pediatr* 1993;122:650–652.
35. Muscat M. National Cancer Institute's OCCAM partners with NCCAM to expand research on unconventional cancer treatments. *Altern Ther Health Med* 1999;5(4):26–30.
36. Clauson KA, Shields KM, McQueen CE, Persad N. Safety issues associated with commercially available energy drinks. *J Am Pharm Assoc* 2008;48(3):e55–e63.
37. Shannon M. Alternative medicines toxicology: a review of selected agents. *Clin Toxicol* 1999;37:709–713.
38. Klepser TB, Klepser ME. Unsafe and potentially safe herbal therapies. *Am J Health Syst Pharm* 1999;56:125–138.
39. Anonymous. Herbs hazardous to your health. *Am Pharm* 1984; NS24(3):20–21.
40. Furbee B, Wermuth M. Life-threatening plant poisoning. *Crit Care Clin* 1997;13:849–888.
41. Yeung CY, Lee FT, Wong HN. Effect of a popular Chinese herb on neonatal bilirubin protein building. *Biol Neonate* 1990;58:98–103.
42. Chan TYK. The prevalence, use, and harmful potential of some Chinese herbal medicines in babies and children. *Vet Hum Toxicol* 1994;36:238–240.
43. Chan E. Displacement of bilirubin from albumin by berberine. *Biol Neonate* 1993;63:201–208.
44. Roulet M, Laurini R, Rivier L, Calame A. Hepatic veno-occlusive disease in a newborn infant of a woman drinking herbal tea. *J Pediatr* 1998;112:433–436.
45. Rosti L, Nardini A, Bettinelli ME, Rosti D. Toxic effects of an herbal tea mixture in two newborns. *Acta Pediatr* 1994;83:683.
46. Cahill DJ, Fox R, Wardle PG, Harlow CR. Multiple follicular development associated with herbal medicine. *Hum Reprod* 1994; 9:1469–1470.
47. Nelson L, Shih R, Hoffman R. Aplastic anemia induced by an adulterated herbal medication. *Clin Toxicol* 1995;33:467–470.
48. Henley DV, Lipson N, Korach KS, Bloch CA. Prepubertal gynecomastia linked to lavender and tea tree oils. *N Engl J Med* 2007;356:479–485.
49. Anonymous. Herbal health. *Environ Health Perspect* 1998;106(12): A590–A592.
50. Angell M, Kassirer JP. Alternative medicine: the risks of untested and unregulated remedies. *N Engl J Med* 1998;339:839–841.
51. Barnes J, Mills SY, Abbot NC, Willoughby M, Ernst E. Different standards for reporting adverse drug reactions to herbal remedies and conventional over-the-counter medicines: face-to-face interviews with 515 users of herbal remedies. *Br J Clin Pharmacol* 1998;45:496–500.
52. Food and Drug Administration. The Dietary Supplement and Nonprescription Drug Consumer Protection Act., Public Law 109–462, Dec. 22, 2006.
53. Marderosian AD. *Natural product medicine.* Philadelphia, PA: George F. Stickley, 1988:96–104.
54. Coppes MJ, Anderson RA, Egeler RM, Wolff JE. Alternative therapies for the treatment of childhood cancer. *N Engl J Med* 1998;339:846–847.
55. Ruschitzka F, Meier PJ, Turina M, Lüscher TF, Noll G. Acute heart transplant rejection due to St. John's wort. *Lancet* 2000;355: 548–549.
56. Blumenthal M, et al. *German Commission E Monographs. Therapeutic monographs on medicinal plants for human use.* Austin, TX: American Botanical Council, 1998.

57. Kopec K. Herbal medications and breastfeeding. *J Hum Lact* 1999; 15:157–161.
58. Jones TK, Lawson BM. Profound neonatal congestive heart failure caused by maternal consumption of blue cohosh herbal medication. *J Pediatr* 1998;13:79–93.
59. Wright IMR. Neonatal effects of maternal consumption of blue cohosh. *J Pediatr* 1999;134:384–385.
60. Belew C. Herbs and the childbearing woman. Guidelines for midwives. *J Nurse Midwifery* 1999;44(3):231–252.
61. Wedig KE, Whitsett JA. Down the primrose path: petechiae in a neonate exposed to herbal remedy for parturition. *J Pediatr* 2008;152: 140–143.
62. Lee L. Introducing herbal medicine into conventional health care settings. *J Nurse Midwifery* 1999;44(3):253–266.
63. McFarlin BL, Gibson MH, O'Rear J, Harman P. A national survey of herbal preparation use by nurse-midwives for labor stimulation. Review of the literature and recommendations for practice. *J Nurse Midwifery* 1999;44:205–216.
64. Friedman JM. Teratology Society. Presentation to the FDA public meeting on safety issues associated with the use of dietary supplements during pregnancy. *Teratology* 2000;62:134–137.
65. Panter KE, Keeler RF, Buck WB. Congenital skeletal malformations induced by maternal ingestion of *Conium maculatum* in newborn pigs. *Am J Vet Res* 1985;46:2064.
66. Melchart D, Linde K, Worku F, Bauer R, Wagner H. Immunomodulation with echinacea: a systematic review of controlled trials. *Phytomedicine* 1994;1:245–254.
67. Braunig B, et al. Echinacea purpurea radix: zur starkung der korpereigenen abwehr bei grappalen infekten. *Z Phytother* 1993;13: 7–13.
68. Melchart D, Walther E, Linde K, Brandmaier R, Lersch C. Echinacea root extracts for the prevention of upper respiratory tract infections. A double-blind placebo-controlled randomized trial. *Arch Fam Med* 1998;7:541–545.
69. Zintl A. Natural cures for kids. *Ladies Home* 1998;56–62.
70. Nowak D, Zlatic T. Herbal products and the Internet: a marriage of convenience. *J Am Pharm Assoc* 1999;39:241–242.

SUGGESTED READINGS

American Academy of Pediatrics, Committee on Children with Disabilities. Counseling families who choose complementary and alternative medicine for their child with chronic illness or disability. *Pediatrics* 2001;107:598–601.

Ang-Lee MK, Moss J, Yuan CS. Herbal medicines and perioperative care. *J Am Med Assoc* 2001;286:208–216.

Anonymous. International Conference on Harmonization of Technical Requirements for Registration of Pharmaceuticals for Human Use. ICH harmonized tripartite guideline: clinical investigation of medicinal products in the pediatric population, 2002. http://www.ich.org/LOB/media/MEDIA487.pdf

Anonymous. Problems with dietary supplements. *Med Lett Drugs Ther* 2002;44:84–86.

Brue AW, Oakland TD. Alternative treatments for attention-deficit/hyperactivity disorder: does evidence support their use? *Altern Ther Health Med* 2002;8:68–74.

Cala S, Crismon ML, Baumgartner J. A survey of herbal use in children with attention-deficit-hyperactivity disorder or depression. *Pharmacotherapy* 2003;23:222–230.

Crawley FP, Kurz R, Nakamura H. Testing medications in children. *N Engl J Med* 2003;348:763–764.

Dockrell TR, Leever JS. An overview of herbal medications with implications for the school nurse. *J Sch Nurs* 2000;16:53–58.

Eisenberg DM, Davis RB, Ettner SL, et al. Trends in alternative medicine use in the United States, 1990–1997: results of a follow-up national survey. *J Am Med Assoc* 1998;280:1569–1575.

Ernst E. Serious adverse effects of unconventional therapies for children and adolescents: a systematic review of recent evidence. *Eur J Pediatr* 2003;162:72–80.

Evans WE, McLeod HL. Drug therapy: pharmacogenomics—drug disposition, drug targets, and side effects. *N Engl J Med* 2003;348:538–549.

Friedman T, Slayton WB, Allen LS, et al. Use of alternative therapies for children with cancer. *Pediatrics* 1997;100:6. www.pediatrics.org/cgi/content/full/100/6/e1.

Geissler PW, Harris SA, Prince RJ, et al. Medicinal plants used by Luo mothers and children in Bondo district, Kenya. *J Ethnopharmacol* 2002;83:39–54.

Grimm W, Müller HH. A randomized controlled trial of the effect of fluid extract of *Echinacea purpurea* on the incidence and severity of colds and respiratory infections. *Am J Med* 1999;106:138–143.

Haller CA, Benowitz NL. Adverse cardiovascular and central nervous system events associated with dietary supplements containing ephedra alkaloids. *N Engl J Med* 2000;343:1833–1838.

Heuschkel R, Afzal N, Wuerth A, et al. Complementary medicine use in children and young adults with inflammatory bowel disease. *Am J Gastroenterol* 2002;97:382–388.

Hofmann D, Hecker M, Völp A. Efficacy of dry extract of ivy leaves in children with bronchial asthma: a review of randomized controlled trials. *Phytomedicine* 2003;10:213–220.

Madsen H, Andersen S, Nielsen RG, Dolmer BS, Høst A, Damkier A. Use of complementary/alternative medicine among pediatric patients. *Eur J Pediatr* 2003;162:334–341.

Marcus DM, Grollman AP. Botanical medicines—the need for new regulations. *N Engl J Med* 2002;347:2073–2076.

Moore C, Adler R. Herbal vitamins: lead (Pb) toxicity and developmental delay. *Pediatrics* 2000;106:600–602.

Neuhouser ML, Patterson RE, Schwartz SM, Hedderson MM, Bowen DJ, Standish LJ. Use of alternative medicine by children with cancer in Washington State. *Prev Med* 2001;33:347–354.

Ottolini MC, Hamburger EK, Loprieato JO, et al. Complementary and alternative medicine use among children in the Washington, DC area. *Ambul Pediatr* 2001;1:122–125.

Pitetti R, Singh S, Hornyak D, Garcia SE, Herr S. Complementary and alternative medicine use in children. *Pediatr Emerg Care* 2001; 17:165–169.

Samenuk D, Link MS, Homoud MK, et al. Adverse cardiovascular events temporally associated with ma huang, an herbal source of ephedrine. *Mayo Clin Proc* 2002;77:12–16.

Sarrell EM, Cohen HA, Kahan E. Naturopathic treatment for ear pain in children. *Pediatrics* 2003;111:e574–e579.

Shenfield G, Lim E, Allen H. Survey of the use of complementary medicines and therapies in children with asthma. *J Paediatr Child Health* 202;38:252–257.

Sikand A, Laken M. Pediatrician's experience with and attitudes toward complementary/alternative medicine. *Arch Pediatr Adolesc Med* 1998;152:1059–1064.

Simpson N, Roman K. Complementary medicine use in children: extent and reasons. A population-based study. *Br J Gen Pract* 2001;51:914–916.

Steinbrook R. Testing medications in children. *N Engl J Med* 2002; 347:1462–1470.

Talalay P. The importance of using scientific principles in the development of medicinal agents from plants. *Acad Med* 2001;76:238–247.

Tani M, Nagase M, Nishiyama T, Yamamoto T, Matusa R. The effects of long-term herbal treatment for pediatric AIDS. *Am J Chin Med* 2002;30:51–64.

Tomassoni AJ, Simone K. Herbal medicines for children: an illusion of safety? *Curr Opin Pediatr* 2001;13:162–169.

Vessey JA, Rechkemmer A. Natural approaches to children's health: herbals and complementary and alternative medicine. *Pediatr Nurs* 2001;27: 61–67.

Webb NJ, Pitt WR. Eucalyptus oil poisoning in childhood: 41 cases in southeast Queensland. *J Paediatr Child Health* 1993;29:368–371.

Woolf AD. Herbal remedies and children: do they work? Are they harmful? *Pediatrics* 2003;112:240–246.

CHAPTER

63

Don T. Granger
Henrietta S. Bada

Pharmacologic Management of Neonatal Abstinence Syndrome

The National Survey on Drug Use and Health (NSDUH), using 2006–2007 samples, estimated that each year close to six million women of childbearing age (ages 15 and 44 years) are current users of any illicit drug (1). In addition, 5.2% of pregnant women (or an estimated 135,000) are using illicit drugs (1): this represents a 39% increase in number since the survey in 2004–2005. In the 1960s and the 1970s, heroin was the drug most commonly used by pregnant addicts, generating interests on its neonatal effects ranging from congenital malformations to normally appearing physical development with or without drug withdrawal symptomatology (2,3). This constellation of central and autonomic nervous systems signs is commonly referred to as neonatal abstinence syndrome (NAS). Because of the illicit access to heroin, the synthetic opioid methadone became a treatment of choice for opiate dependence during pregnancy; its controlled administration provided a means to achieve the goal of having improved outcomes for the exposed newborn. Methadone maintenance during pregnancy also provided the advantage of decreasing illicit drug use and improving the ability to access prenatal care (4,5), which allowed for close monitoring of maternal medical and pregnancy complications. However, it became evident that neonates show more severe signs of withdrawal manifestations including seizures with in utero methadone exposure (6–8).

In recent years as an alternative to methadone, buprenorphine is used for treatment of opiate addiction in pregnant women (9–11). Buprenorphine is a kappa receptor agonist which also exhibits μ-receptor action. Effectiveness and safety of buprenorphine are equivalent to methadone in the treatment of pregnant addicts (11) but with variable effects as to the associated prevalence and severity of NAS (12,13). Reports also show association between prenatal buprenorphine and neonatal growth parameters comparable to prenatal methadone exposure (9,12,14,15). In one study a higher birth weight was noted following buprenorphine treatment during pregnancy compared with methadone because of longer gestational age in buprenorphine exposed newborns (12).

In spite of the declining use of heroin, opioid use continues to be a public health problem. Currently, among women using illicit drugs, greater than a million and one-half are abusing or nonmedically using opioid pain relievers compared with an estimated 47,000 women who are current heroin users (1). Of those pregnant, close to 1% or an estimated 20,000 are current users of pain relievers. The commonly used painkillers are the semisynthetic opioids. They are made by simple modification of the morphine molecule with resultant phenanthrenes or alkaloids produced being codeine and thebaine. Codeine is also a semisynthetic opioid and has established clinical use as an antitussive. Having similarities to the codeine molecule and effects are the commonly abused pain relievers oxycodone (OxyContin) and hydrocodone (Lortab). Congenital malformations and neonatal withdrawal manifestations have been reported with use of codeine and opioid pain medications during pregnancy (16–19). We are now beginning to see an increased prevalence of semisynthetic opioid abuse during pregnancy with resulting increase in the number of newborns exhibiting withdrawal manifestations from these substances.

In addition to opioids, numerous other substances have reported associations with newborn drug withdrawal following in utero exposure. Examples of these substances include alcohol (20,21), barbiturates (22,23), caffeine (24), chlordiazepoxide (25), clomipramine (26), diazepam (27), ethchlorvynol (28), glutethimide (29), hydroxyzine (30), meprobamate (31), the selective serotonin reuptake inhibitors (32–34), and cocaine (35). Characteristics of withdrawal manifestations from these substances vary as to onset, severity, duration, need for treatment, and incidence (36); however, a detailed discussion on the newborn effects of prenatal use of these nonopiate drugs is beyond the scope of this chapter.

PATHOGENESIS: OPIATE EFFECTS ON THE DEVELOPING BRAIN VERSUS WITHDRAWAL

The effects of opioids or opiates on the developing brain are not limited to newborn withdrawal symptomatology. An overlap between opiate effects and withdrawal is possible based on several preclinical and human studies. Opiates act through three separate and distinct classical opioid receptor subtypes: mu, delta, and kappa (μ, δ, and κ) (37). All three receptor subtypes have been molecularly cloned and pharmacologically well characterized. These receptors have different regional central nervous system distributions and use different second messenger systems for their cellular mechanisms of action. The μ and δ receptors both inhibit adenylyl cyclase and activate outward potassium currents. The action of κ-opiate receptors is at the presynaptic terminals, through inhibition of calcium channels. The different opiates or opioids are partially selective μ-receptor agonists; differences are in pharmacokinetics and not in pharmacodynamics. Depending upon the timing of gestational exposure, the dose, kinetics, and pharmacodynamics, gross malformations may or may not be observed in the neonate. Gross abnormalities in brain development have been reported in opiate-exposed infants, for example, hydrocephaly with prenatal heroin (3) and codeine exposures (38). We recently reported on neonatal stroke following prenatal codeine prescribed as antitussive during pregnancy (19). In human neonates, prenatal opiate exposure results in a 0.5 to 2 cm decrease in head circumference (7,39–44) proportional to the decrease in body size, that is, symmetric growth restriction associated with decrease in cell number and consistent with the findings of Naeye et al. (45) in heroin exposed fetuses at 30 weeks' gestation. In animals, prenatal opioid or μ-receptor agonists' exposure results in decreased cortical density of neurons and smaller dendritic arborization and branching, therefore, affecting programming of cortical structures (46–49). The μ-receptors in developing rat brain appear early during the formation of the cortical plate (50) and μ-agonists appear to modulate cell division in the ventricular zone of late embryonic mouse cortex (51). In particular, μ-receptor agonists decrease cell division in developing cortex (51) and decrease cerebellar granule cell proliferation (52). These findings suggest a role for μ-agonists or opioids (53) in regulating neurogenesis, perhaps down regulating this critical process. Prenatal exposure to μ-agonists has been found to increase adult levels of μ-receptors in the limbic regions in the rat (54,55) but not in isocortical or striatal regions (56). Local injection of μ-agonists into the hippocampal area CA3 can impair spatial learning in rats (57) suggesting that opioids continue to play a role in the adult, different from either their developmental role in utero or their well-known role in pain modulation. Early exposure to μ-agonists therefore might lead to decrease in neurogenesis in neocortex, limbic system, and/or cerebellum, leading to decreased volumes of these brain regions and corresponding behavioral effects in overall cognition (isocortex), emotion and social interactions (limbic system), and motor learning and performance (cerebellum). These findings may explain the reported prenatal and postnatal head growth deceleration in the human newborn (7,39–44,58–61). Such findings would lend support to the role of specific biologic mechanisms for decreased brain size in infants with prenatal opiate exposure, and the associated manifestations such as hypertonicity, hyperreflexia, irritability, tremors, shrill cry, and other behavioral alterations, which are also part of the constellation of manifestations in narcotic withdrawal or NAS. No significant abnormalities on clinical magnetic resonance imaging have been noted in the immediate newborn period (62) with exposure to the opiate, buprenorphine. Findings at later ages are suggestive of decreases in brain region volumes (63) with prenatal opiate exposure, suggesting a long-lasting effect of in utero drug exposure. Of concern are the experimental studies finding effects of a high gestational dose of buprenorphine on myelination of the developing brain (64) suggested by developmental delay in myelin basic protein expression and alterations in axon–glial interactions.

PATHOGENESIS: PRENATAL OPIATE AND WITHDRAWAL MANIFESTATIONS

The central nervous and autonomic nervous systems manifestations (36) in neonates with prenatal opiate exposure comprise the neonatal narcotic withdrawal syndrome, also referred to as the "NAS." During gestation complicated by prenatal opiate exposure, the fetus receives a supply of opiate for prolonged period through the placenta and the umbilical cord. At birth the disruption of opiate supply to the fetus through the placenta is a likely explanation of the occurrence of newborn abstinence symptomatology and hence the manifestations become evident when the newly born would have metabolized and excreted the opiate from his/her system within a few days after birth.

INCIDENCE OF NAS

NAS is most common among infants born to mothers who used opiates during pregnancy. The reported incidence of NAS ranges from 21% to 93% among infants exposed to opiate in utero (14,35,36,65–67). A higher incidence is reported with in utero methadone exposure than that reported with heroin exposure (6,8). Whereas in some studies, the incidence of NAS following methadone exposure does not seem to differ significantly from the use of the newer drug, buprenorphine (13,67), other studies found a higher incidence of NAS and need for treatment in infants of mothers on methadone treatment than in infants of women treated with buprenorphine. Polydrug exposure is reported to be associated with greater severity of withdrawal manifestations (68); it also increases the odds for a neonate to develop signs of NAS; in a large cohort, a higher percentage of infants manifested the constellation of CNS/autonomic nervous system (ANS) signs consistent with withdrawal who had prenatal exposure to both opiate and cocaine than in those exposed only to either drug (35).

MONITORING OF CLINICAL MANIFESTATIONS OF NAS

Monitoring of clinical manifestations is important not only as a basis for clinical diagnosis but also in the initiation, monitoring, and discontinuation of pharmacological treatment. The CNS manifestations in NAS include a high-pitched cry, irritability, disorganized sleep pattern, hypertonia, myoclonic jerks, seizures, exaggerated Moro reflex, frequent yawning, and sneezing (35,36,69). Other signs include autonomic nervous disturbances manifested as fever, temperature instability, mottling, increased sweating, nasal stuffiness, sneezing, nasal flaring, tachypnea, and loose or watery stools (36). Additional manifestations are the gastrointestinal signs of poor feeding, uncoordinated and constant sucking, and vomiting or regurgitation, which can result in dehydration and poor weight gain (36). Onset of manifestations is noted usually within the first 72 hours of birth (2) and in some infants as late as 2 to 4 weeks of postnatal age (70). The variability of onset depends on several factors including the type of maternal drug use during pregnancy, dosage of drug of use, timing of use prior to delivery, the type of anesthesia and/or analgesia used during labor and delivery, and metabolism, accumulation, and tissue binding of the drug in the fetus, which can affect neonatal drug excretion. Duration of withdrawal manifestations is variable but signs may last for longer duration (subacute) persisting for as long as 6 months (71). Depending upon severity, NAS may require pharmacological treatment.

The severity of NAS may differ as to the gestational age of the infant at birth, the type of drug of exposure, and whether there is polydrug exposure. Less severe signs may be noted with the exposed preterm infant, which could be attributed to shorter duration of in utero opiate exposure. Caution should be taken in evaluation of symptomatology because of overlap in manifestations related to disorders of prematurity and NAS. For example, respiratory difficulty, temperature instability, and cardiovascular signs are often noted in preterm infants with respiratory distress syndrome. In late preterm and term infants, more severe symptomatology is noted with methadone exposure (72). Conflicting findings are reported from multiple studies investigating the relationship between maternal methadone dose and the severity of withdrawal manifestations and the need for pharmacologic treatment (6,73–77). In prenatal cocaine exposure, the prevalence of CNS and ANS manifestations is lower than reported with prenatal opiate exposure. Because of the persistence of neurological tone abnormalities in infants with prenatal cocaine exposure, it is in question that the CNS/ANS manifestations are due to NAS and instead are likely to be manifestations of cocaine effects (78).

Evaluation and clinical monitoring of infants with NAS are carried out using neurobehavioral assessment procedures or clinical scoring scales or tools. A commonly used scale in the clinical setting for monitoring severity and number of signs of withdrawal is the Finnegan Scoring System (79). It consists of 21 items with some being weighted according to severity (Table 63.1). Another scale for scoring narcotic withdrawal was developed by Ostrea (80), which uses ranking but with no summation scale for severity of clinical signs of withdrawal. The Finnegan Scale was later modified in the Lipsitz's tool (81) and the Neonatal Withdrawal Inventory by Zahorodny et al. (82). The Lipsitz scoring is abbreviated compared with Finnegan Scoring System and is shown in Table 63.2. Eleven items are scored, with two items (tremors and irritability) that are scored from normal (score = 0) to increasing severity with a score of 3 as worst. Five additional items are scored from 0 to 2; these are reflexes, stools, muscle tone, skin abrasions, and respiratory rate. Four items (repetitive sneezing, repetitive yawning, vomiting, and fever) are scored as not present (score = 0) or present (score = 1).

Other investigators have utilized the Neurobehavioral Assessment Scale by Brazelton (83), which has been modified to allow administration in preterm infants and those exposed to drugs in utero, through the National Institute of Child Health and Human Development Neonatal Intensive Care Unit (NICHD NICU) research network; the scale is known as the NICU Network Neurobehavioral Scale (NNNS) (84,85). In the Neurobehavioral Assessment Scale and NNNS, habituation, reflexes, tone, orientation, and state changes are assessed. The NNNS adds assessment of stress/abstinence signs and is sensitive for administration to infants of substance using mothers and those born at preterm gestation.

Some investigators utilize monitoring of physiological signals in NAS (86,87). Median activity score using a motion detector is higher in infants at pretreatment than in controls, those not requiring treatment and those stable with treatment (86). Those with NAS also demonstrate sleep deprivation, disorganization, and fragmentation; stabilization with treatment results in sleep and wakefulness similar to controls (88). Another physiological signal noted to be different in those infants exposed to opiates in utero from those nonexposed is the visual evoked potentials (89). Visual evoked potentials from those exposed are more likely to be immature or nondetectable and also smaller in amplitude than in controls. These aberrations in physiological signals may herald later problems in neurodevelopment (90).

TREATMENT OF NAS: BEHAVIORAL INTERVENTION

Recent reviews of published treatment strategies and surveys of practices among clinical centers indicate variation in approach to management of NAS. Initial management of course begins with monitoring of the exposed infants and subsequent initiation of behavioral intervention techniques when necessary. If unresponsive to these supportive measures, administration of pharmacological agents is initiated. Although these behavioral intervention modalities have been tried in nursery settings, there is no uniformity on how and when such interventions are administered to newborns with prenatal opiate exposure. The simplest and most commonly employed behavioral interventions include infant swaddling and efforts to reduce exposure to excessive light and sound in the nursery. Specifically directed interventions such as prone positioning (91) and oscillating water beds have been shown to minimize symptoms of NAS evaluated using Finnegan Scoring System (92). From a recent report, neonates born to opiate using mothers did better with rooming-in compared with historical controls not rooming-in with their mothers; those in

TABLE 63.1 Finnegan Scoring System in the Evaluation of NAS Adapted for Every 4-Hour Interval Assessment

	Signs and Symptoms	*Score*	*Hours* 12	4	8	12	4	8
Central nervous system disturbances	High-pitched cry	2						
	Continuous high-pitched cry	3						
	Sleeps <1 hr after feeding	3						
	Sleeps <2 hr after feeding	2						
	Sleeps <3 hr after feeding	1						
	Hyperactive Moro reflex	2						
	Markedly hyperactive Moro reflex	3						
	Mild tremors disturbed	1						
	Moderate–severe tremors disturbed	2						
	Mild tremors undisturbed	3						
	Moderate–severe tremors undisturbed	4						
	Increased muscle tone	2						
	Excoriation (specify area__________)	1						
	Myoclonic jerks	3						
	Generalized convulsions	3						
Metabolic vasomotor respiratory disturbances	Sweating	1						
	Fever <101°F (39.3°C)	1						
	Fever >101°F (39.3°C)	2						
	Frequent yawning (>3–4 times/interval)	1						
	Mottling	1						
	Nasal stuffiness	1						
	Sneezing (>3–4 times/interval)	1						
	Nasal flaring	2						
	Respiratory rate >60/min	1						
	Respiratory rate >60 with retractions	2						
Gastrointestinal disturbances	Excessive sucking	1						
	Poor feeding	2						
	Regurgitation	2						
	Projectile vomiting	3						
	Loose stools	2						
	Watery stools	3						
Summary	Total score							
	Scorer's initial							
	Status of therapy							

Finnegan, L.P. Neonatal abstinence syndrome: assessment and pharmacotherapy. In: Rubaltelli FF, Granti B, eds. *Neonatal therapy: an update.* Elsevier Science Publishers B. V. (Biomedical Division), 1986;122–146, with permission.

rooming-in were less likely to need pharmacotherapeutic intervention and had shorter length of hospital stay (93). These previous studies have utilized a single behavioral intervention measure and outcomes were globally measured by severity of withdrawal symptoms without systematic detailed evaluation of clusters of measures of neurobehavior such self-regulation and stress reactivity and the impact of an intervention on caretaker–child interaction. Randomized studies are lacking on the effect of a comprehensive behavioral intervention in the management of NAS. In addition, as a part of a holistic approach to behavioral intervention, providing nutritional supportive will ensure growth, while promoting self-regulation to enhance maternal–child interaction. It makes further sense that behavioral intervention in the clinical setting should continue even if the infant would require pharmacological treatment, with an approach directed to the mother–infant dyad (94).

TREATMENT OF NAS: PHARMACOLOGICAL APPROACH

Pharmacologic approaches to treating neonatal drug withdrawal vary considerably from center to center. In the 2006 US survey, only 54.5% of the responding centers had a written policy regarding management of NAS (95). Such a finding is not surprising considering the paucity of scientific data supporting the use of a specific drug therapy for NAS. It is generally agreed that an opioid is the preferred first-line drug therapy for NAS with documented maternal opiate use (96). Opioids are reported as the first-line drug in 83% of neonatal centers in the United States (95) and in 92% of the centers in the United Kingdom and Ireland (97).

Often, maternal opiate use is complicated by concurrent use of one or more substances such as benzodiazepines, barbiturates, selective serotonin reuptake inhibitors, cocaine,

TABLE 63.2 Lipsitz's Scoring System or Tool in Assessment of Narcotic Withdrawal

Signs	*Score* 0	1	2	3
Tremors (muscle activity of limbs)	Normal	Minimally when hungry or disturbed	Moderate or marked when undisturbed—subside when fed or held snugly	Marked or continuous even when undisturbed, going on to seizure-like movements
Irritability (excessive crying)	None	Slightly	Moderate to severe when disturbed or hungry	Marked even when undisturbed
Reflexes	Normal	Increased	Markedly increased	
Stools	Normal	Explosive but normal frequency	Explosive and more than 8/d	
Muscle tone	Normal	Increased	Rigidity	
Skin abrasions	No	Redness of knees and elbows	Breaking of skin	
Respiratory rate/min	<55	55–75	76–95	
Repetitive sneezing	No	Yes		
Repetitive yawning	No	Yes		
Vomiting	No	Yes		
Fever	No	yes		

Lipsitz PJ. A proposed narcotic withdrawal score for use with newborn infants. *Clin Pediatr* 1975;14(6):592–594, with permission.

marijuana, amphetamine, or methamphetamine, and legal drugs such as tobacco and alcohol. In addition, clinical management becomes difficult in many cases when historical information regarding maternal drug use is inadequate. A major component of determining the most appropriate drug therapy for neonatal withdrawal is to determine specific maternal drug use as accurately as possible.

In polydrug exposure, opioids remain as the first-line drug in 52% of US centers, followed by phenobarbital in 32% and methadone in 11% of centers (95). A second (adjunctive) therapeutic agent may be instituted if control of symptoms is not achieved with the first drug (95); adjunctive treatment may also decrease the severity of withdrawal and the infant's length of hospital stay (98,99); examples of the drugs for use in conjunction with the first-line drug are phenobarbital, clonidine, methadone, diazepam, and tincture of opium.

PHARMACOLOGIC TREATMENT OF NAS WITH OPIATE OR OPIOIDS

The terms "opiates" and "opioids" are used interchangeably to refer to naturally occurring alkaloids, including morphine and codeine. Opioid is a more general term which includes all chemicals whose mode of action is at the opioid receptors (100). For several decades, different oral opioid formulations have been used to treat NAS.

DILUTED TINCTURE OF OPIUM

Diluted tincture of opium (DTO), also known as laudanum, was used for opiate withdrawal in 20 of 47 responders in a 2006 US survey (95) but was not reportedly used in British surveys in both 1994 (101) and 2009 (97). DTO contains several narcotic alkaloids, including codeine and morphine (in a concentration of 10 mg per mL). For this reason, actual concentrations of morphine vary with each administration of the drug. For practicality of administration to neonates, DTO has typically been prepared in a 1:25 dilution, thereby creating a morphine concentration of 0.4 mg per mL. The ethanol content of DTO is diluted in this mixture from 19% to 0.7% (102). Caution is advised in the use of DTO due to fatal drug errors involving confusion between DTO and paregoric or camphorated tincture of opium.

CAMPHORATED TINCTURE OF OPIUM (PAREGORIC)

Paregoric contains morphine in a concentration of 0.4 mg per mL and is used almost exclusively for treating intractable diarrhea in adults (103). It is no longer used in the treatment of neonatal drug withdrawal because of its high ethanol content (45%). In addition, paregoric contains camphor and benzoic acid, both of which have well documented neonatal side effects (104). Deaths have been reported when patients were given tincture of opium in paregoric doses. As a result of these sentinel events, the Institute for Safe Medicine Practices recommends removing tincture of opium from hospital pharmacies and compounding aqueous oral solutions of morphine from either morphine tablets or injection (103).

MORPHINE

Morphine is the most commonly used opioid for treatment of NAS (95,97). Morphine represents the classic μ-receptor agonist and is classified as a Schedule II drug by the Drug Enforcement Agency. Morphine is derived from the poppy plant (105), which has been used for medicinal purposes for hundreds of years. Morphine was first isolated in 1804 by a German pharmacist, Friedrich Serturner (100). He named the chemical "morphium" in honor of Morpheus, the god of sleep. The use of the drug increased rapidly with the introduction of the hypodermic needle, and hundreds of thousands of soldiers during the American Civil War developed a morphine addiction (100).

The chemical structure of morphine is $C_{17}H_{19}NO_3$, consisting of a phenanthrene base with a phenolic hydroxyl group at positions 3 and an alcohol hydroxyl group at positions 6 and at the nitrogen atom (100). Morphine is readily absorbed from the gastrointestinal tract after oral administration. The molecule undergoes first-pass metabolism in the liver with subsequent bioavailability of the drug reduced to only about 25%. Upon reaching the blood–brain barrier morphine will enter the CNS a bit more slowly than other opioids as it is relatively hydrophilic with poor lipid solubility (105).

Morphine is primarily metabolized in the liver by uridine 5′-diphosphate glucuronyl transferase to morphine-3-glucuronide (M3G), with smaller amounts of morphine-6-glucuronide (M6G) produced (106). These morphine metabolites are water-soluble and undergo subsequent renal excretion (106). In spite of the polarity of these metabolites, they are able to cross the blood–brain barrier and potentiate their own clinical effects. M6G is more noted for this ability and will accumulate in patients with renal failure; consequently, it can potentiate both the degree and duration of effects of morphine in such patients. The hepatic transferase enzyme producing morphine metabolites, similar to glucuronyl transferase responsible for the conjugation of bilirubin, does not reach adult levels until 3 to 6 months of life. This maturational process also affects morphine metabolism in the first year of life (107). Although 86% of morphine elimination is in the form of M3G, elimination routes other than glucuronidation are more common in younger infants (106). Morphine can be found excreted unchanged in the urine of up to 19% of infants younger than 3 months and in 13% of older infants. Demethylation of morphine to normorphine and fecal excretion contribute very little to morphine metabolism (108).

The half-life of morphine is approximately 2 hours in adults (105) and is much longer in infants and children, 9.0 ± 3.4 hours in preterm neonates, 6.5 ± 2.8 hours in term neonates, and 2.0 ± 1.8 hours in infants and children aged 11 days to 15 years (109). Morphine clearance mirrors the maturational and postnatal increase in glomerular filtration rate, with drug clearance rising from 2.27 mL per kg per minute at 27 weeks' gestation to 7.8 mL per kg per minute at 38 weeks (110). Further increase in the clearance of morphine sulfate continues throughout the first year of life, with clearance in infants and children reaching 23.6 mL per kg per minute (106,109).

Recent data comparing use of morphine and nonopioids such as phenobarbital and chlorpromazine are very limited. One randomized controlled trial of morphine versus phenobarbital in NAS following maternal opiate use suggests that opiate therapy is superior, resulting in shorter duration of treatment (8 vs. 12 days), less likelihood of second-line treatment (47% vs. 35%), and less intensive nursing care (62% vs. 30% requiring transfer to higher newborn care) (111). A small case series reported in 2008 showed shorter duration of therapy (6 days vs. 16 days) and shorter length of stay (11 days vs. 18 days) with chlorpromazine as compared with morphine (112). Although the use of morphine seems to be the prevalent therapy, its administration (both in dosing and interval) varies considerably from center to center (97). It has been shown to be as effective as tincture of opium in the treatment of neonatal opiate withdrawal while avoiding the disadvantages of alcohol content and varying morphine doses (113).

MORPHINE DOSING IN TREATMENT OF NAS

Studies in the administration of morphine for NAS use either body weight–based dosing or symptom-based dosing, or a combination of these two regimens, that is, beginning treatment based on body weight and increasing or decreasing dosage based on severity of symptoms. Initiation of treatment and dose adjustment is based on scoring carried out every 3, 4, 6, or 8 hours. Using body weight–based dosing, the commonly used dose is between 20 and 60 μg per kg per dose (0.02 to 0.06 mg per kg per dose) given every 4 hours (range 2 to 8 hours) (8,14,69,98,111–114). If initial dosing is guided by severity of symptoms based on withdrawal scores, a high dose of 133 μg per kg per dose (0.133 mg per kg per dose every 4 hours or 0.80 mg per kg per day) may be given. Higher doses would require intensive care monitoring as well as adjunctive therapy.

Jansson et al. (104) proposes a symptom-based dosing regimen depending upon NAS scores monitored at intervals. Since most reports do not support a relationship between dose of prenatal opiate exposure and severity of manifestations of withdrawal, body weight–based dosing will not necessarily ensure that severity of withdrawal symptoms will decrease on the basis of dose per kg of body weight. Using Jansson's NAS treatment regimen, the Finnegan scores are classified into categories based on increasing severity. These categories begin from category 0 to category V. Therefore, each category is defined as follows: Category 0: scores = 0 to 8; category I: scores = 9 to 12; category II: scores = 13 to 16; category III: scores = 17 to 20; category IV: scores = 21 to 24; and category V: scores = 25 or higher. Category 0 requires no treatment and a dose of 0.04 mg of morphine is initiated when infant is assessed at category I; dose for initiation of treatment is increased by 0.04 mg with each increasing level in category upon assessment of infant with NAS. For persistence of scores within the same category, the initial dose is increased by 50% until infant has reached category 0. When scores are stable for 48 hours, the dosage is decreased by 0.02 mg every 24 hours. If reescalation of dosing is necessary, then the increase is by 25% of the initial dose. A second drug may be needed if infant is requiring greater than 0.2 mg morphine every 3 hours. Table 63.3 compares the body weight–based dosing proposed by Finnegan (115) and symptom-based approach by Jansson et al. (104), with both methods taking into consideration the severity of manifestations or increasing categories based on Finnegan scores.

METHADONE

As noted in the 2006 US survey, 20% of responders use methadone as the first-line treatment for neonatal opiate

TABLE 63.3 Comparing Body Weight–Based Dosing and Symptom-Based Dosing Using Severity of NAS as Determined from the Finnegan Scores

Body Weight–Based Dosing Finnegan and Kaltenbach (115)			*Symptom-Based Dosing Jansson et al. (104)*			
Scores	*Initial Dose of Morphine Equivalent*[a]	*Escalation Needed*	*Scores by Category*	*Initial Dose of Morphine Solution*	*Escalation as Needed*	*Reescalation if Needed (Two Scores Within Each Category)*
0–7	No treatment	. . .	Category 0: 0–8	No treatment	. . .	
8–10	0.053 mg/kg/dose q 4 hr	Increase dose by 0.02 mg (0.05 mL) with each subsequent dose	Category 1: 9–12	0.04 mg/dose	0.02 mg	0.01 mg
11–13	0.080 mg/kg/dose q 4 hr		Category II: 13–16	0.08 mg/dose	0.04 mg	0.02 mg
14–16	0.107 mg/kg/dose q 4 hr		Category III: 17–20	0.12 mg/dose	0.06 mg	0.03 mg
≥17	0.133 mg/kg/dose q 4 hr		Category IV: 21–24	0.16 mg/dose	0.08 mg	0.04 mg
If reescalation needed: resume previous dose that effected control of symptoms			Category V >25	0.20 mg/dose	0.20 mg	0.05 mg
Upon stabilization:			Upon stabilization:			
Maintain dose for 3 d			Maintain dose for 3 d			
Decrease by 10% of total daily dose every 24 hr			Decrease dose by 0.02 mg every 24 hr			
Observe at least 48 hr after drug discontinuation			Observe at least 48 hr after drug discontinuation			

[a]Paregoric (0.4 mg/mL morphine equivalent). [b]Morphine solution (0.4 mg/mL) is current formulation used by nurseries.

withdrawal (95). The methadone molecule is a synthetic μ-receptor agonist with pharmacological similarities to morphine, although longer-acting. Methadone exists in two distinct isomers, the L-isomer and the D-isomer. L-methadone is between 8 and 50 times more potent than the D-form and is responsible for virtually all of the opioid agonist effect (105). In contrast to morphine, it is absorbed well from the gastrointestinal tract and 90% becomes tightly bound to plasma proteins (105). It is basic, lipophilic, and exhibits oral bioavailability ranging from 40% to 100%. After repeated administration this lipophilic drug will gradually accumulate in fat tissue and then begins its long phase of elimination (100). The subsequent slow release of the drug from these tissue sites results in maintenance of low levels of methadone for some time even after discontinuation of the drug. Methadone is metabolized in the liver by demethylation and cyclization (cytochrome P450 system) to pyrrolidines and pyrroline (105). The metabolites are excreted almost exclusively via bile into feces, with a small portion excreted into urine (100). The drug is known to increase the QT interval and should be used with caution in cases of congenital QT prolongation, hypokalemia, or hypomagnesemia (100).

A major use of methadone is in the adult treatment of heroin addiction. Its use has recently increased, perhaps due to its cheap price and its long half-life. Unfortunately, a lack of understanding of its metabolism has contributed to a significant increase in the deaths associated with methadone use (100). The long half-life, which is reported as a mean of 19.2 hours, creates a bit of a problem in using methadone in the treatment of NAS (69,104). Because of this prolonged elimination, it is difficult to gauge clinical effectiveness of dosing changes. At the same time, some clinicians seem attracted to the longer dosing interval required for methadone as compared with morphine. Very few studies have evaluated the efficacy of methadone use in the treatment of NAS. A 2005 study comparing treatments with tincture of opium versus methadone reported similar lengths of stay (116). The Cochrane Review (2005) of opiate treatment for neonatal abstinence addressed neither the use of nor the scientific evidence supporting the effectiveness of methadone (117).

BUPRENORPHINE

Buprenorphine is a thebaine derivative, with a 25 to 40 times analgesic potency as morphine. It is a partial μ-receptor agonist, thus less likely to elicit a response similar to the full agonist morphine. It has, however, a very high binding affinity to the μ-receptor so that its effect is only partially reversed by the μ-antagonist naloxone. Maternal buprenorphine treatment clearly results in its distribution in the fetus. The exposed neonate may have serum buprenorphine concentrations that are higher than in the maternal serum (118). Cumulative or total maternal buprenorphine dose in the third trimester did not predict NAS or meconium buprenorphine and norbuprenorphine concentrations (119). Current available preparations are for intravenous and sublingual administration. Barrett and coinvestigators (120) studied the buprenorphine pharmacokinetics in newborn infants. After continuous intravenous injection and a standard infusion rate of 0.72 μg per kg per hour, mean steady-state plasma concentration was 4.3 ± 2.6 ng per mL. From a one-compartment model, the mean plasma clearance was determined to be 0.23 ± 0.07 1 per hour per kg, elimination half-life to be 20 ± 8 hours, and volume of distribution as 6.2 ± 2.11 L per kg. Therefore, clearance of buprenorphine is lower and half-life is longer compared to older children (121).

Kraft et al. performed a randomized trial on the use of buprenorphine versus neonatal opium solution in the treatment of NAS (122); the number of infants studied was small. Buprenorphine was given at a dose of 13.2 to 39.0 μg per kg per day in three divided doses by the sublingual route. Buprenorphine treatment was well tolerated with a mean length of treatment and hospital days that were 10 to 11 days shorter in the buprenorphine group compared with standard treatment (opium solution); this difference, however, was not statistically significant. The use of buprenorphine in the clinical setting is not an established practice. Randomized trials will be needed to support its use for treatment of NAS.

NONOPIATE MEDICATIONS FOR TREATMENT OF NAS

CLONIDINE

Opiate withdrawal gives rise to neuroadaptation processes which include the activation of the noradrenergic system and an associated increase in neuronal firing, glutamatergic activity and c-fos expression (123–125). Areas in the brain involved in the alterations of noradrenergic and glutaminergic activity are in the locus coeruleus and the central nucleus of the amygdala. These two regions contain colocalized opiate and noradrenergic receptors and agonists to these receptors appear to act on common effector mechanisms (126). Cessation of chronic opiate use in adults results in a constellation of manifestations, somatic and autonomic, such as shaking, tremors, anxiety, nausea, vomiting, fever sweating, insomnia, and other behavioral changes. Treatment has been directed especially in adults toward substitution of their drug of choice with decreasing dose and close monitoring during detoxification. An alternative monotherapy is the administration of an α-2-agonist. Experimental evidence suggests that both behavioral and biochemical findings support the role of noradrenergic hyperactivity in newborn opiate withdrawal (127). Therefore, the α-2-adrenergic agent, clonidine has been used in studies as a monotherapy (128) or as an adjunctive treatment of narcotic abstinence in the newborn (99).

Clonidine was first synthesized in the 1960s by Boehringer Ingelheim (129) paving the way to studies on its mechanism of action and effects on adrenergic receptors in the 1970s. The drug is primarily an antihypertensive. Clonidine stimulates the presynaptic α-2-receptors, specifically in the vasomotor center, resulting in the decrease in presynaptic calcium levels, inhibiting norepinephrine release from the sympathetic nerve endings, thereby effecting a decrease in sympathetic tone. The consequent decreases in peripheral resistance and cardiac output result in a decrease in blood pressure (130,131). Clonidine has also been found to increase antinociceptive threshold in experimental animals (132). It has been used as an adjuvant for anesthesia and for a postoperative pain relief (133). Clonidine has been suggested to be an alternative choice to benzodiazepines for premedication in infants and children since it does not have an effect on respiration (134). Its other uses include the treatment of neuropathic pain, opioid detoxification, and sleep hyperhidrosis, and as an off-label adjunctive therapy to counter the side effects of stimulant medications such as methylphenidate or amphetamine (131). In the treatment for opiate withdrawal, the centrally acting, clonidine, has more affinity to α-2 than α-1-adrenergic receptors. It inhibits firing of the noradrenergic neurons and neuronal activation in the locus coeruleus and amygdala thereby attenuating the somatic signs of opiate withdrawal (e.g., irritability, increased tendon reflexes, hypertonia, tremors) and autonomic nervous system signs of sweating, hot/cold flashes, and general restlessness (131). In neonates, manifestations of NAS have been observed to be alleviated or minimized with clonidine treatment (128,135). A recent trial involving a small number of neonates has demonstrated a potential use for clonidine as an adjunct to opiate treatment in NAS following prenatal opiate exposure (99). Clonidine has also been administered in neonates who required prolonged analgesia (136). It has been used as well with choral hydrate to treat NAS (137). Compared with morphine, treatment with the combination of clonidine and choral hydrate resulted in a significantly shorter duration of treatment, median of 14 days versus 35 days in the morphine- and phenobarbital-treated infants. Duration of hospital stay was also shorter, a median of 32 days compared with 44 days in the morphine-treated infants.

Reported dosing in the newborn infants is 3 to 5 μg per kg per day or 1 μg per kg per dose every 4 to 6 hours (128,135). Peak values occur within 3 to 5 hours of an oral dose (128). Blood levels during maintenance oral therapy are in the range of 0.1 and 0.3 ng per mL on 3 to 5 μg per kg per day dosing (128); these levels are well below those reported in case studies of accidental clonidine overdosage. A marked reduction in withdrawal manifestations is noted after clonidine administration that is maintained at a daily dose of 3 to 5 μg per kg per day for a duration of treatment ranging from 6 to 17 days with a mean 12.2 days (128). Esmaeili et al. administered clonidine as a continuous infusion at a dose of 0.5 μg per kg per hour with an increase to a maximum of 3 μg per kg per hour until relief of manifestations is observed (137). Once the maximum dose is reached, choral hydrate can be added as an adjunctive therapy at 30 to 50 mg per kg per dose and repeated as often as three times a day if needed to achieve control of symptoms.

PHENOBARBITAL

Phenobarbital with its role as a sedative has been used for several years in the treatment of NAS alone or in combination with opiate treatment. Phenobarbital is a sedative anticonvulsant which acts as an agonist to gamma aminobutyric acid (GABA) subtype A receptors, enhancing GABA–mediated action, thereby reducing neuronal excitability. Depression of neuronal excitability includes mechanisms such as suppression of glutamatergic excitatory postsynaptic potentials, voltage-dependent Ca^{2+} and Na^{+} currents, as well as activation of leak of K^{+} currents. Not all excitable tissues are affected at equivalent doses of serum concentrations. Phenobarbital is bound as 20% to 40% protein binding, but binding is less in the newborn (10% to 30% of total plasma concentration in the neonates aged 0 to 7 days). With a large percentage of the phenobarbital in plasma that is unbound, its diffusion is greater in the CNS (138,139). Brain/plasma phenobarbital concentration ratio is 0.7 similar to older children and adults (140,141). It is metabolized by the liver and excreted in the urine unchanged 25% to 50%. The elimination half-life in newborns and children ranges from 60 to 180 hours with a mean of 110 hours. Therapeutic level is between 15 to 30 μg per mL (142). Pediatric dosing for sedation is 6 mg per kg per day PO divided into three doses.

As a specific treatment of NAS, phenobarbital is reportedly used as a first-line drug in neonatal opiate withdrawal by 17% of neonatal centers in the United States. It is more commonly used as adjunctive therapy to opioid use in cases of polydrug use (32% of US centers) (95). In a randomized trial of the use of phenobarbital versus morphine in the treatment of NAS, median duration of treatment was 4 days longer when using phenobarbital (111); there was also a trend for those treated with phenobarbital to require another drug compared with those treated with morphine. As an added treatment to opiate in infants with signs of abstinence, phenobarbital administration was associated with lower maximum daily dose of opiate, less percent of time of hospitalization with Finnegan scores greater than 8, and shorter duration of hospitalization (98). These findings translate to lower average hospital cost when using phenobarbital as an adjunctive treatment to opiate than opiate alone (98). Although an anticonvulsant and a CNS depressant, phenobarbital does not necessarily prevent seizures related to withdrawal during its use as a treatment for narcotic abstinence (143). As a sedative, phenobarbital use maybe associated with less vigorous and coordinated sucking compared with opiate treatment (144).

When used for neonatal drug withdrawal, phenobarbital is given at a loading dose of 5 mg per kg IV, IM, or PO and maintained PO at a dose of 3 to 5 mg per kg divided into three doses (every 8 hours) (8). Maintenance dose may be increased by 1 mg per kg per day to a maximum of 10 mg per kg per day. Once symptomatology has decreased or infant has reached clinical stabilization (Finnegan score <8), dosage of phenobarbital is decreased by 1 mg per kg per day every other day. An alternative is a rigorous approach wherein phenobarbital is initiated at a loading dose of 20 mg per kg followed by a maintenance dose of 2 to 6 mg per kg per day, relying on optimal plasma phenobarbital concentrations (20 to 30 μg per mL) (115). If plasma level needs to be raised, then frequency of administration is changed to every 12 hours. Maximum maintenance dose may be as high as 10 mg per kg per dose every 12 hours until control of clinical manifestations, or when level of 70 μg per mL is achieved, or clinical toxicity is noted. Once control of abstinence manifestations is achieved, dosage is maintained for 72 hours and then tapering is begun by lowering the dose by 15% per day. Phenobarbital is discontinued if the serum concentration is less than 10 μg per mL and infant's abstinence scores remain less than 8.

DIAZEPAM

Diazepam, a benzodiazepine derivative, is an anxiolytic agent that reduces neuronal depolarization resulting in decreased action potentials. It enhances the action of GABA by tightly binding to A-type GABA receptors, thus opening the membrane channels and allowing the entry of chloride ions. Diazepam is metabolized primarily to *N*-desmethyl derivative, which is pharmacologically active. Other metabolites include a ring-hydroxylated derivative (methyloxazepam) and oxazepam, which is a hydroxylated and demethylated pharmacologically active metabolite of diazepam. The rate of metabolism of diazepam is lower in premature than in full-term infants, with hydroxylation and conjugation being more limited than demethylation (145).

The plasma clearance rate of diazepam in the newborn is less than that in the infant or adult. This reduced rate of plasma disappearance appears to be associated with the slower rate of metabolism of diazepam. The apparent plasma half-life of diazepam is 40 to 400 hours in the premature and 20 to 50 hours in the full-term neonates (146). For treatment of seizures, infants and children are given diazepam at a dose of 0.1 mg per kg up to a maximum of 0.3 mg per kg IV every 2 minutes; so, do not exceed a total dose of 5 mg in those aged 30 days to 5 years or a total dose of 10 mg in children aged 5 year or older. In neonatal withdrawal syndrome, diazepam is given at a dose of 0.2 to 1 mg per kg PO or slow IV infusion. It is repeated every 6 to 8 hours as required.

There are few reports on the treatment of NAS with diazepam (66,147) In the series reported by Madden et al. (66), none of the infants treated with diazepam required a second drug. However, in another series, treatment failure is lower with phenobarbital (148,149) compared with diazepam. Meta-analysis of published data indicates less treatment failure with phenobarbital compared with diazepam, whether in utero exposure involved opiate only or opiate with other drugs (150).

CHLORPROMAZINE

Chlorpromazine, a phenothiazine, is used as an adjunct premedication for anesthesia for the purpose of reducing vascular resistance. It has a sedative effect. It potentiates effects of narcotic analgesia, and it has antiemetic, antinausea, antihistaminic, hypnotic, and α-adrenergic blockade affect. Chlorpromazine is a neuroleptic agent, antagonizing the effect of dopaminergic synaptic neurotransmission. In addition to the sedative or hypnotic effect, chlorpromazine suppresses motor activity and complex behavior but intellectual functioning and response to environment remain intact. Its absorption from the gastrointestinal tract is unpredictable. When given parenterally, its bioavailability is four to ten times that of oral delivery. Chlorpromazine is lipophilic and widely distributed in the body. It is metabolized in the liver, and its metabolites are conjugated with glucuronic acid and excreted through renal processes and to a lesser extent through the liver. Elimination from plasma is variable, with an average half-life of 30 hours reported in adults. The elimination half-life in neonates following in utero exposure is 3.2 days. Minimal effective plasma levels are reported to be less than 30 ng per mL and toxic levels are at concentrations greater than 750 ng per mL. Dosage reported in newborns for sedation ranges from 0.13 to 0.88 mg per kg over an hour and maintenance dose of 0.03 to 0.21 mg per kg hour up to 47 hours (151,152). Peak plasma level for chlorpromazine is reached at 2.8 hours and half-life is reported to be 30 hours because of high protein binding of 90% or greater (112). Dosage for treatment of drug withdrawal is 0.5 to 0.7 mg per kg PO, IM, or slow IV infusion every 6 hours as required (153). Similar to other drugs for treatment of withdrawal, the effective dose is maintained for 3 to 5 days before tapering of dosage is initiated.

In the United Kingdom, chlorpromazine has been used more often than opiate for the treatment of newborn narcotic withdrawal manifestations. In 1996, a survey carried out on the management of opiate withdrawal among centers in England and Wales revealed that chlorpromazine is prescribed by 71% of those who responded and only 11% used opiates (101). In a recent report comparing the use of chlorpromazine with morphine in the treatment of NAS, duration of treatment with chlorpromazine was significantly shorter, mean of 6 days compared with a mean of 16 days with morphine treatment (112). In the same study, the duration of hospitalization was also reduced with chlorpromazine. In a more recent survey on practices regarding treatment of opiate withdrawal in the newborn, the use of chlorpromazine is actually in a decline (97) with less than 10% of those who responded are using a nonopiate drug and 92% administering opiate as the first-line drug.

SUMMARY

Clinical monitoring of infants with prenatal drug exposure for signs of NAS will allow for providing intervention. Behavioral intervention is initiated to minimize symptomatology, promote self-regulation, improve neurobehavior, support growth, and enhance dyadic interaction. However, a large percentage on infants with prenatal opiate exposure may also require pharmacological treatment. Lacking a large body of evidence in the pharmacological treatment of NAS, morphine solution is the most commonly used drug for control of newborn narcotic withdrawal manifestations. Dose of morphine may be calculated on the basis of infant's body weight or on the basis of symptoms (symptom-based). Both regimens take into consideration severity of NAS or abstinence scores. Experiences reported in the literature support drug administration at interval of 3 to 4 hours, then escalating the dosage until control of symptoms is achieved. Dosing interval of at least every 3 to 4 hours is best to avoid rebound or increase in abstinence scores that will require reescalation of dose. Once control is attained, dose is maintained for at least 48 to 72 hours, followed by decrease in dosage after 24 hours of stabilization (decrease in dose of 10% or 0.02 mg if using the symptom-based regimen). In some infants reescalation of dose may be needed during the course of weaning. Treatment maybe discontinued if infant's dose has been tapered down to at 0.02 mg per dose and the infant's Finnegan score is less than 8 for at least 24 hours duration. Increasing interval between doses as a means to wean treatment is not advisable. The Finnegan Scoring System is the commonly used tool for initiating, monitoring, and adjusting treatment. The Lipsitz's tool is an alternative scoring; scores can be summed as indicator of severity of NAS. Lastly, the long-term effects of NAS, its severity, and treatment on child development remain unclear.

REFERENCES

1. Substance Abuse and Mental Health Services Administration. Office of Applied Studies. *National household survey on drug abuse 2002, 2003, 2004, 2005, 2006, 2007,* SAMHSA, Rockville, MD; 2007.
2. Zelson C, Rubio E, Wasserman E. Neonatal narcotic addiction: 10 year observation. *Pediatrics* 1971;48:178–189.
3. Ostrea EM, Chavez CJ. Perinatal problems (excluding neonatal withdrawal) in maternal drug addiction: a study of 830 cases. *J Pediatr* 1979;94:292–295.
4. Kaltenbach K, Berghella V, Finnegan L. Opioid dependence during pregnancy. Effects and management. *Obstet Gynecol Clin North Am* 1998;25:139–151.
5. Gottheil E, Sterling RC, Weinstein SP. Diminished illicit drug use as a consequence of long-term methadone maintenance. *J Addict Dis* 1993;12:45–57.
6. Doberczak TM, Kandall SR, Friedmann P. Relationship between maternal methadone dosage, maternal-neonatal methadone levels, and neonatal withdrawal. *Obstet Gynecol* 1993;81:936–940.
7. Kaltenbach K, Finnegan LP. Perinatal and developmental outcome of infants exposed to methadone in-utero. *Neurotoxicol Teratol* 1987;9:311–313.
8. Kandall SR. *Treatment options for drug-exposed infants.* Rockville, MD: US Department of Health and Human Services, Public Health Service, National Institutes of Health, 1995.
9. Lacroix I, Berrebi A, Chaumerliac C, et al. Buprenorphine in pregnant opioid-dependent women: first results of a prospective study. *Addiction* 2004;99:209–214.
10. Johnson RE, Jones HE, Fischer G. Use of buprenorphine in pregnancy: patient management and effects on the neonate. *Drug Alcohol Depend* 2003;70:S87–S101.
11. Fischer G, Ortner R, Rohrmeister K, et al. Methadone versus buprenorphine in pregnant addicts: a double-blind, double-dummy comparison study. *Addiction* 2006;101:275–281.
12. Kakko J, Heilig M, Sarman I. Buprenorphine and methadone treatment of opiate dependence during pregnancy: comparison of fetal growth and neonatal outcomes in two consecutive case series. *Drug Alcohol Depend* 2008;96:69–78.
13. Lejeune C, Simmat-Durand L, Gourarier L, et al. Prospective multicenter observational study of 260 infants born to 259 opiate-dependent mothers on methadone or high-dose buprenorphine substitution. *Drug Alcohol Depend* 2006;82:250–257.
14. Ebner N, Rohrmeister K, Winklbaur B, et al. Management of neonatal abstinence syndrome in neonates born to opioid maintained women. *Drug Alcohol Depend* 2007;87:131–138.
15. Kahila H, Saisto T, Kivitie-Kallio S, et al. A prospective study on buprenorphine use during pregnancy: effects on maternal and neonatal outcome. *Acta Obstet Gynecol Scand* 2007;86:185–190.
16. Mangurten HH, Benawra R. Neonatal codeine withdrawal in infants of nonaddicted mothers. *Pediatrics* 1980;65:159–160.
17. Rao R, Desai NS. OxyContin and neonatal abstinence syndrome. *J Perinatol* 2002;22:324–325.
18. Van Leeuwen G, Guthrie R, Stange F. Narcotic withdrawal reaction in a newborn infant due to codeine. *Pediatrics* 1965;36:635–636.
19. Reynolds EW, Riel-Romero RM, Bada HS. Neonatal abstinence syndrome and cerebral infarction following maternal codeine use during pregnancy. *Clin Pediatr (Phila)* 2007;46:639–645.
20. Nichols MM. Acute alcohol withdrawal syndrome in a newborn. *Am J Dis Child* 1967;113:714–715.
21. Pierog S, Chandavasu O, Wexler I. Withdrawal symptoms in infants with the fetal alcohol syndrome. *J Pediatr* 1977;90:630–633.

22. Bleyer WA, Marshall RE. Barbiturate withdrawal syndrome in a passively addicted infant. *JAMA* 1972;221:185–186.
23. Desmond MM, Schwanecke RP, Wilson GS, et al. Maternal barbiturate utilization and neonatal withdrawal symptomatology. *J Pediatr* 1972;80:190–197.
24. McGowan JD, Altman RE, Kanto WP Jr. Neonatal withdrawal symptoms after chronic maternal ingestion of caffeine. *South Med J* 1988;81:1092–1094.
25. Athinarayanan P, Pierog SH, Nigam SK, et al. Chlordiazepoxide withdrawal in the neonate. *Am J Obstet Gynecol* 1976;124:212–213.
26. Musa AB, Smith CS. Neonatal effects of maternal clomipramine therapy. *Arch Dis Child* 1979;54:405.
27. Rementeria JL, Bhatt K. Withdrawal symptoms in neonates from intrauterine exposure to diazepam. *J Pediatr* 1977;90:123–126.
28. Rumack BH, Walravens PA. Neonatal withdrawal following maternal ingestion of ethchlorvynol (Placidyl). *Pediatrics* 1973; 52:714–716.
29. Reveri M, Pyati SP, Pildes RS. Neonatal withdrawal symptoms associated with glutethimide (Doriden) addiction in the mother during pregnancy. *Clin Pediatr (Phila)* 1977;16:424–425.
30. Prenner BM. Neonatal withdrawal syndrome associated with hydroxyzine hydrochloride. *Am J Dis Child* 1977;131:529–530.
31. Briggs GG, Ambrose PJ, Nageotte MP, et al. High-dose carisoprodol during pregnancy and lactation. *Ann Pharmacother* 2008; 42:898–901.
32. Austin MP. To treat or not to treat: maternal depression, SSRI use in pregnancy and adverse neonatal effects. *Psychol Med* 2006; 36:1663–1670.
33. Alwan S, Friedman JM. Safety of selective serotonin reuptake inhibitors in pregnancy. *CNS Drugs* 2009;23:493–509.
34. Thormahlen GM. Paroxetine use during pregnancy: is it safe? *Ann Pharmacother* 2006;40:1834–1837.
35. Bada HS, Bauer CR, Shankaran S, et al. Central and autonomic system signs with in utero drug exposure. *Arch Dis Child Fetal Neonatal Ed* 2002;87:F106–F112.
36. Neonatal drug withdrawal. American Academy of Pediatrics Committee on Drugs. *Pediatrics* 1998;101:1079–1088.
37. Waldhoer M, Bartlett SE, Whistler JL. Opioid receptors. *Annu Rev Biochem* 2004;73:953–990.
38. Heinonen OP, Slone D, Monson RR, et al. Cardiovascular birth defects and antenatal exposure to female sex hormones. *N Engl J Med* 1977;296:67–70.
39. Doberczak TM, Thornton JC, Bernstein J, et al. Impact of maternal drug dependency on birth weight and head circumference of offspring. *Am J Dis Child* 1987;141:1163–1167.
40. Chasnoff IJ, Hatcher R, Burns WJ. Polydrug- and methadone-addicted newborns: a continuum of impairment? *Pediatrics* 1982; 70:210–213.
41. Lifschitz MH, Wilson GS, Smith EO, et al. Factors affecting head growth and intellectual function in children of drug addicts. *Pediatrics* 1985;75:269–274.
42. Rosen TS, Johnson HL. Children of methadone-maintained mothers: follow-up to 18 months of age. *J Pediatr* 1982;101:192–196.
43. Wilson GS, Desmond MM, Verniaud WM. Early development of infants of heroin-addicted mothers. *Am J Dis Child* 1973;126:457–462.
44. Wilson GS, Desmond MM, Wait RB. Follow-up of methadone-treated and untreated narcotic-dependent women and their infants: health, developmental, and social implications. *J Pediatr* 1981;98:716–722.
45. Naeye RL, Blanc W, Leblanc W, et al. Fetal complications of maternal heroin addiction: abnormal growth, infections, and episodes of stress. *J Pediatr* 1973;83:1055–1061.
46. Zagon IS, McLaughlin PJ. Opioid antagonist-induced modulation of cerebral and hippocampal development: histological and morphometric studies. *Brain Res* 1986;393:233–246.
47. Zagon IS, McLaughlin PJ. Opioid antagonist (naltrexone) modulation of cerebellar development: histological and morphometric studies. *J Neurosci* 1986;6:1424–1432.
48. Hammer RP Jr, Ricalde AA, Seatriz JV. Effects of opiates on brain development. *Neurotoxicology* 1989;10:475–483.
49. Hauser KF, McLaughlin PJ, Zagon IS. Endogenous opioids regulate dendritic growth and spine formation in developing rat brain. *Brain Res* 1987;416:157–161.
50. Tong Y, Chabot JG, Shen SH, et al. Ontogenic profile of the expression of the mu opioid receptor gene in the rat telencephalon and diencephalon: an in situ hybridization study. *J Chem Neuroanat* 2000;18:209–222.
51. Reznikov K, Hauser KF, Nazarevskaja G, et al. Opioids modulate cell division in the germinal zone of the late embryonic neocortex. *Eur J Neurosci* 1999;11:2711–2719.
52. Hauser KF, Houdi AA, Turbek CS, et al. Opioids intrinsically inhibit the genesis of mouse cerebellar granule neuron precursors in vitro: differential impact of mu and delta receptor activation on proliferation and neurite elongation. *Eur J Neurosci* 2000; 12:1281–1293.
53. Beardsley PM, Aceto MD, Cook CD, et al. Discriminative stimulus, reinforcing, physical dependence, and antinociceptive effects of oxycodone in mice, rats, and rhesus monkeys. *Exp Clin Psychopharmacol* 2004;12:163–172.
54. Vathy I, Slamberova R, Rimanoczy A, et al. Autoradiographic evidence that prenatal morphine exposure sex-dependently alters mu-opioid receptor densities in brain regions that are involved in the control of drug abuse and other motivated behaviors. *Prog Neuropsychopharmacol Biol Psychiatry* 2003;27:381–393.
55. Schindler CJ, Slamberova R, Rimanoczy A, et al. Field-specific changes in hippocampal opioid mRNA, peptides, and receptors due to prenatal morphine exposure in adult male rats. *Neuroscience* 2004;126:355–364.
56. Slamberova R, Rimanoczy A, Schindler CJ, et al. Cortical and striatal mu-opioid receptors are altered by gonadal hormone treatment but not by prenatal morphine exposure in adult male and female rats. *Brain Res Bull* 2003;62:47–53.
57. Meilandt WJ, Barea-Rodriguez E, Harvey SA, et al. Role of hippocampal CA3 mu-opioid receptors in spatial learning and memory. *J Neurosci* 2004;24:2953–2962.
58. Wilson GS, McCreary R, Kean J, et al. The development of preschool children of heroin-addicted mothers: a controlled study. *Pediatrics* 1979;63:135–141.
59. Rosen TS, Johnson HL. Long-term effects of prenatal methadone maintenance. *NIDA Res Monogr* 1985;59:73–83.
60. Hans SL. Developmental consequences of prenatal exposure to methadone. *Ann N Y Acad Sci* 1989;562:195–207.
61. Johnson H, Diano A, Rosen T. 24-month neurobehavioral follow up of methadone-maintained mothers. *Inf Behav Dev* 1984;7: 115–123.
62. Kahila H, Kivitie-Kallio S, Halmesmaki E, et al. Brain magnetic resonance imaging of infants exposed prenatally to buprenorphine. *Acta Radiol* 2007;48:228–231.
63. Walhovd KB, Moe V, Slinning K, et al. Volumetric cerebral characteristics of children exposed to opiates and other substances in utero. *Neuroimage* 2007;36:1331–1344.
64. Sanchez ES, Bigbee JW, Fobbs W, et al. Opioid addiction and pregnancy: perinatal exposure to buprenorphine affects myelination in the developing brain. *Glia* 2008;56:1017–1027.
65. Fricker HS, Segal S. Narcotic addiction, pregnancy, and the newborn. *Am J Dis Child* 1978;132:360–366.
66. Madden JD, Chappel JN, Zuspan F, et al. Observation and treatment of neonatal narcotic withdrawal. *Am J Obstet Gynecol* 1977; 127:199–201.
67. Jones HE, Johnson RE, Jasinski DR, et al. Buprenorphine versus methadone in the treatment of pregnant opioid-dependent patients: effects on the neonatal abstinence syndrome. *Drug Alcohol Depend* 2005;79:1–10.
68. Fulroth R, Phillips B, Durand DJ. Perinatal outcome of infants exposed to cocaine and/or heroin in utero. *Am J Dis Child* 1989; 143:905–910.
69. Oei J, Lui K. Management of the newborn infant affected by maternal opiates and other drugs of dependency. *J Paediatr Child Health* 2007;43:9–18.
70. Kandall SR, Gartner LM. Late presentation of drug withdrawal symptoms in newborns. *Am J Dis Child* 1974;127:58–61.
71. Desmond MM, Wilson GS. Neonatal abstinence syndrome: recognition and diagnosis. *Addict Dis* 1975;2:113–121.
72. Zelson C, Lee SJ, Casalino M. Neonatal narcotic addiction. Comparative effects of maternal intake of heroin and methadone. *N Engl J Med* 1973;289:1216–1220.
73. Dashe JS, Sheffield JS, Olscher DA, et al. Relationship between maternal methadone dosage and neonatal withdrawal. *Obstet Gynecol* 2002;100:1244–1249.

74. Kuschel CA, Austerberry L, Cornwell M, et al. Can methadone concentrations predict the severity of withdrawal in infants at risk of neonatal abstinence syndrome? *Arch Dis Child Fetal Neonatal Ed* 2004;89:F390–F393.
75. Ostrea EM, Chavez CJ, Strauss ME. A study of factors that influence the severity of neonatal narcotic withdrawal. *J Pediatr* 1976; 88:642–645.
76. McCarthy JJ, Leamon MH, Parr MS, et al. High-dose methadone maintenance in pregnancy: maternal and neonatal outcomes. *Am J Obstet Gynecol* 2005;193:606–610.
77. Berghella V, Lim PJ, Hill MK, et al. Maternal methadone dose and neonatal withdrawal. *Am J Obstet Gynecol* 2003;189:312–317.
78. Chiriboga CA, Kuhn L, Wasserman GA. Prenatal cocaine exposures and dose-related cocaine effects on infant tone and behavior. *Neurotoxicol Teratol* 2007;29:323–330.
79. Finnegan LP. Neonatal abstinence syndrome: assessment and pharmacotherapy. In: Rubaltelli FF, Granati B, eds. *Neonatal therapy: an Update.* Amsterdam, NY-Oxford: Elsevier Science Publishers B.V. (Biomedical Division) 1986:122–146.
80. Ostrea EM, ed. *Infants of drug dependent mothers.* Philadelphia, PA: WB Saunders, 1993.
81. Lipsitz PJ. A proposed narcotic withdrawal score for use with newborn infants. A pragmatic evaluation of its efficacy. *Clin Pediatr (Phila)* 1975;14:592–594.
82. Zahorodny W, Rom C, Whitney W, et al. The neonatal withdrawal inventory: a simplified score of newborn withdrawal. *J Dev Behav Pediatr* 1998;19:89–93.
83. Brazelton T. *Neonatal Behavioral Assessment Scale.* Philadelphia, PA: JB Lippincott, 1984.
84. Lester BM, Tronick EZ, Brazelton TB. The Neonatal Intensive Care Unit Network Neurobehavioral Scale procedures. *Pediatrics* 2004;113:641–667.
85. Lester BM, Tronick EZ, LaGasse L, et al. Summary statistics of Neonatal Intensive Care Unit Network Neurobehavioral Scale scores from the maternal lifestyle study: a quasinormative sample. *Pediatrics* 2004;113:668–675.
86. O'Brien C, Hunt R, Jeffery HE. Measurement of movement is an objective method to assist in assessment of opiate withdrawal in newborns. *Arch Dis Child Fetal Neonatal Ed* 2004;89:F305–F309.
87. Lodge A, Marcus MM, Ramer CM. Part II. Behavioral and electrophysiological characteristics of the addicted neonate. *Addict Dis* 1975;2:235–255.
88. O'Brien CM, Jeffery HE. Sleep deprivation, disorganization and fragmentation during opiate withdrawal in newborns. *J Paediatr Child Health* 2002;38:66–71.
89. McGlone L, Mactier H, Hamilton R, et al. Visual evoked potentials in infants exposed to methadone in utero. *Arch Dis Child* 2008;93:784–786.
90. McGlone L, Mactier H, Weaver LT. Drug misuse in pregnancy: losing sight of the baby? *Arch Dis Child* 2009;94:708–712.
91. Maichuk GT, Zahorodny W, Marshall R. Use of positioning to reduce the severity of neonatal narcotic withdrawal syndrome. *J Perinatol* 1999;19:510–513.
92. Oro AS, Dixon SD. Waterbed care of narcotic-exposed neonates. A useful adjunct to supportive care. *Am J Dis Child* 1988;142:186–188.
93. Abrahams RR, Kelly SA, Payne S, et al. Rooming-in compared with standard care for newborns of mothers using methadone or heroin. *Can Fam Physician* 2007;53:1722–1730.
94. Velez ML, Jansson LM, Schroeder J, et al. Prenatal methadone exposure and neonatal neurobehavioral functioning. *Pediatr Res* 2009;66(6):704–709.
95. Sarkar S, Donn SM. Management of neonatal abstinence syndrome in neonatal intensive care units: a national survey. *J Perinatol* 2006;26:15–17.
96. Johnson K, Gerada C, Greenough A. Treatment of neonatal abstinence syndrome. *Arch Dis Child Fetal Neonatal Ed* 2003;88: F2–F5.
97. O'Grady MJ, Hopewell J, White MJ. Management of neonatal abstinence syndrome: a national survey and review of practice. *Arch Dis Child Fetal Neonatal Ed* 2009;94:F249–F252.
98. Coyle MG, Ferguson A, Lagasse L, et al. Diluted tincture of opium (DTO) and phenobarbital versus DTO alone for neonatal opiate withdrawal in term infants. *J Pediatr* 2002;140:561–564.
99. Agthe AG, Kim GR, Mathias KB, et al. Clonidine as an adjunct therapy to opioids for neonatal abstinence syndrome: a randomized, controlled trial. *Pediatrics* 2009;123:e849–e856.
100. Trescot AM, Datta S, Lee M, et al. Opioid pharmacology. *Pain Physician* 2008;11:S133–S153.
101. Morrison CL, Siney C. A survey of the management of neonatal opiate withdrawal in England and Wales. *Eur J Pediatr* 1996;155: 323–326.
102. Levy M, Spino M. Neonatal withdrawal syndrome: associated drugs and pharmacologic management. *Pharmacotherapy* 1993; 13:202–211.
103. Institute for Safe Medication Practices. Confusion between opium tinctures marks need for community high alert list. http://www.ismp.org/Newsletters/ambulatory/archives/ 200605_1.asp. Published 2006.
104. Jansson LM, Velez M, Harrow C. The opioid-exposed newborn: assessment and pharmacologic management. *J Opioid Manag* 2009;5:47–55.
105. Gutstein HB, Akil H. Opioid analgesics. In: Brunton LL, Lazo JS, Parker KL, eds. *Goodman and Gilman's the pharmacological basis of therapeutics,* 11th ed. Hightstown, NJ: Mc Graw-Hill Companies, 2006:547–590.
106. Bouwmeester NJ, Anderson BJ, Tibboel D, et al. Developmental pharmacokinetics of morphine and its metabolites in neonates, infants and young children. *Br J Anaesth* 2004;92:208–217.
107. Onishi S, Kawade N, Itoh S, et al. Postnatal development of uridine diphosphate glucuronyltransferase activity towards bilirubin and 2-aminophenol in human liver. *Biochem J* 1979;184: 705–707.
108. McRorie TI, Lynn AM, Nespeca MK, et al. The maturation of morphine clearance and metabolism. *Am J Dis Child* 1992;146: 972–976.
109. Kart T, Christrup LL, Rasmussen M. Recommended use of morphine in neonates, infants and children based on a literature review: part 1—pharmacokinetics. *Paediatr Anaesth* 1997;7:5–11.
110. Scott CS, Riggs KW, Ling EW, et al. Morphine pharmacokinetics and pain assessment in premature newborns. *J Pediatr* 1999;135: 423–429.
111. Jackson L, Ting A, McKay S, et al. A randomised controlled trial of morphine versus phenobarbitone for neonatal abstinence syndrome. *Arch Dis Child Fetal Neonatal Ed* 2004;89:F300–F304.
112. Mazurier E, Cambonie G, Barbotte E, et al. Comparison of chlorpromazine versus morphine hydrochloride for treatment of neonatal abstinence syndrome. *Acta Paediatr* 2008;97:1358–1361.
113. Langenfeld S, Birkenfeld L, Herkenrath P, et al. Therapy of the neonatal abstinence syndrome with tincture of opium or morphine drops. *Drug Alcohol Depend* 2005;77:31–36.
114. Improving treatment for drug-exposed infants: the recommendations of a consensus panel. In: U.S. Department of Health and Human Services, ed. *Treatment Improvement Protocol (TIP).* Washington DC: Center for Substance Abuse Treatment, 1993.
115. Finnegan LP, Kaltenbach K. Neonatal abstinence syndrome. In: Hoekelman RA, Friedman SB, Nelson N, Seidel HM, eds. *Primary pediatric care,* 2nd ed. St. Louis: C.V. Mosby, 1992:1367–1378.
116. Lainwala S, Brown ER, Weinschenk NP, et al. A retrospective study of length of hospital stay in infants treated for neonatal abstinence syndrome with methadone versus oral morphine preparations. *Adv Neonatal Care* 2005;5:265–272.
117. Osborn DA, Jeffery HE, Cole M. Opiate treatment for opiate withdrawal in newborn infants. *Cochrane Database Syst Rev* 2005; 20(3):CD002059.
118. Marquet P, Chevrel J, Lavignasse P, et al. Buprenorphine withdrawal syndrome in a newborn. *Clin Pharmacol Ther* 1997;62: 569–571.
119. Kacinko SL, Jones HE, Johnson RE, et al. Correlations of maternal buprenorphine dose, buprenorphine, and metabolite concentrations in meconium with neonatal outcomes. *Clin Pharmacol Ther* 2008;84:604–612.
120. Barrett DA, Simpson J, Rutter N, et al. The pharmacokinetics and physiological effects of buprenorphine infusion in premature neonates. *Br J Clin Pharmacol* 1993;36:215–219.
121. Olkkola KT, Maunuksela EL, Korpela R. Pharmacokinetics of intravenous buprenorphine in children. *Br J Clin Pharmacol* 1989; 28:202–204.
122. Kraft WK, Gibson E, Dysart K, et al. Sublingual buprenorphine for treatment of neonatal abstinence syndrome: a randomized trial. *Pediatrics* 2008;122:e601–e607.

123. Maldonado R. Participation of noradrenergic pathways in the expression of opiate withdrawal: biochemical and pharmacological evidence. *Neurosci Biobehav Rev* 1997;21:91–104.
124. Rasmussen K. The role of the locus coeruleus and N-methyl-D-aspartic acid (NMDA) and AMPA receptors in opiate withdrawal. *Neuropsychopharmacology* 1995;13:295–300.
125. Rasmussen K, Brodsky M, Inturrisi CE. NMDA antagonists and clonidine block c-fos expression during morphine withdrawal. *Synapse* 1995;20:68–74.
126. Freedman JE, Aghajanian GK. Opiate and alpha 2-adrenoceptor responses of rat amygdaloid neurons: co-localization and interactions during withdrawal. *J Neurosci* 1985;5:3016–3024.
127. Little PJ, Price RR, Hinton RK, et al. Role of noradrenergic hyperactivity in neonatal opiate abstinence. *Drug Alcohol Depend* 1996;41:47–54.
128. Hoder EL, Leckman JF, Poulsen J, et al. Clonidine treatment of neonatal narcotic abstinence syndrome. *Psychiatry Res* 1984;13: 243–251.
129. Stahle H. Clonidine. In: Bindra JS, Lednicer D, eds. *Chronicles of drug discovery*. New York, NY: John Wiley & Sons, 1982:87–111.
130. Houston MC. Clonidine hydrochloride. *South Med J* 1982;75: 713–719.
131. Crassous PA, Denis C, Paris H, et al. Interest of alpha 2-adrenergic agonists and antagonists in clinical practice: background, facts and perspectives. *Curr Top Med Chem* 2007;7:187–194.
132. Paalzow G, Paalzow L. Clonidine antinociceptive activity: effects of drugs influencing central monoaminergic and cholinergic mechanisms in the rat. *Naunyn Schmiedebergs Arch Pharmacol* 1976; 292:119–126.
133. Ghignone M, Quintin L, Duke PC, et al. Effects of clonidine on narcotic requirements and hemodynamic response during induction of fentanyl anesthesia and endotracheal intubation. *Anesthesiology* 1986;64:36–42.
134. Bergendahl H, Lonnqvist PA, Eksborg S. Clonidine in paediatric anaesthesia: review of the literature and comparison with benzodiazepines for premedication. *Acta Anaesthesiol Scand* 2006;50: 135–143.
135. Hoder EL, Leckman JF, Ehrenkranz R, et al. Clonidine in neonatal narcotic-abstinence syndrome. *N Engl J Med* 1981;305: 1284.
136. Leikin JB, Mackendrick WP, Maloney GE, et al. Use of clonidine in the prevention and management of neonatal abstinence syndrome. *Clin Toxicol (Phila)* 2009;47:551–555.
137. Esmaeili A, Keinhorst A, Schuster T, et al. Treatment of neonatal abstinence syndrome with clonidine and chloral hydrate [published online ahead on print October 19, 2009]. *Acta Paediatr* 2010;99:209–214.
138. Lous P. Blood serum and cerebrospinal fluid levels and renal clearance of phenemal in treated epileptics. *Acta Pharmacol Toxicol (Copenh)* 1954;10:166–177.
139. Waddell WJ, Butler TC. The distribution and excretion of phenobarbital. *J Clin Invest* 1957;36:1217–1226.
140. Jalling B. Plasma concentrations of phenobarbital in the treatment of seizures in newborns. *Acta Paediatr Scand* 1975;64: 514–524.
141. Vajda F, Williams FM, Davidson S, et al. Human brain, cerebrospinal fluid, and plasma concentrations of diphenylhydantoin and phenobarbital. *Clin Pharmacol Ther* 1974;15:597–603.
142. Gal P, Toback J, Boer HR, et al. Efficacy of phenobarbital monotherapy in treatment of neonatal seizures—relationship to blood levels. *Neurology* 1982;32:1401–1404.
143. Kandall SR, Doberczak TM, Mauer KR, et al. Opiate v CNS depressant therapy in neonatal drug abstinence syndrome. *Am J Dis Child* 1983;137:378–382.
144. Kron RE, Litt M, Eng D, et al. Neonatal narcotic abstinence: effects of pharmacotherapeutic agents and maternal drug usage on nutritive sucking behavior. *J Pediatr* 1976;88:637–641.
145. Mandelli M, Tognoni G, Garattini S. Clinical pharmacokinetics of diazepam. *Clin Pharmacokinet* 1978;3:72–91.
146. Morselli PL, Franco-Morselli R, Bossi L. Clinical pharmacokinetics in newborns and infants. Age-related differences and therapeutic implications. *Clin Pharmacokinet* 1980;5:485–527.
147. Nathenson G, Golden GS, Litt IF. Diazepam in the management of the neonatal narcotic withdrawal syndrome. *Pediatrics* 1971; 48:523–527.
148. Finnegan LP, Michael H, Leifer B, et al. An evaluation of neonatal abstinence treatment modalities. *NIDA Res Monogr* 1984;49: 282–288.
149. Kaltenbach K, Finnegan LP. Neonatal abstinence syndrome, pharmacotherapy and developmental outcome. *Neurobehav Toxicol Teratol* 1986;8:353–355.
150. Osborn DA, Jeffery HE, Cole MJ. Sedatives for opiate withdrawal in newborn infants. *Cochrane Database Syst Rev* 2005;20(3): CD002053.
151. Root B, Loveland JP. Premedication of children with promethazine, propiomazine, and mepazine: comparison of oral and intramuscular routes. *J Clin Pharmacol J New Drugs* 1970;10: 182–193.
152. Larsson LE, Ekstrom-Jodal B, Hjalmarson O. The effect of chlorpromazine in severe hypoxia in newborn infants. *Acta Paediatr Scand* 1982;71:399–402.
153. Kahn EJ, Neumann LL, Polk GA. The course of the heroin withdrawal syndrome in newborn infants treated with phenobarbital or chlorpromazine. *J Pediatr* 1969;75:495–500.

CHAPTER

64

Kelly P. Shaw
Shannon Manzi

Drug Interactions in Newborns and Children

INTRODUCTION

The administration of multiple drugs to one patient is a common occurrence, in particular when the patient is a critically, or chronically, ill newborn or child. The risk of drug interactions increases in relation to the number of medications being administered. In addition to drug–drug interactions, more is being learned about drug–herb, drug-dietary supplement, and drug–food interactions. These interactions can range in severity from theoretical to clinically significant, including prolonged morbidity and even mortality. This chapter reviews the principal information concerning the properties and mechanisms of drug–drug interactions.

ABSORPTION/ADMINISTRATION

Simultaneous administration of orally administered drugs sets the stage for potentially clinically significant drug–drug interactions. Absorption of drugs from the gastrointestinal (GI) tract is complex and may be impacted in a variety of ways. Numerous factors are accountable in determining the amount of drug that is absorbed by the body, including age, hydrochloric acid secretion, gastric emptying time, intestinal motility, and bile acid secretion. The primary mechanism of absorption is passive diffusion of nonionized drug molecules via the lipophilic GI mucosa. Subsequently, drugs that change the pH, gastric emptying time, or GI motility will interact with the absorption of other medications. Drug interactions related to GI absorption generally fall into one of eight categories: adsorption, complexation or chelation, resin binding, increased GI motility, decreased GI motility, increased gastric pH, decreased intestinal flora, and the modification of metabolism within the GI wall.

Interactions of adsorption are best described with activated charcoal. The large surface area of activated charcoal allows for adsorption of other drugs and this feature is utilized advantageously in the treatment of toxic exposures and overdose.

It is well documented that some antibiotics such as fluoroquinolones and tetracycline will bind to iron, calcium, calcium-fortified foods, and antacids if given concomitantly (1,2). This insoluble complex puts the patient at risk for potential of treatment failure based on little or no systemic absorption and may lead to the development of resistant organisms. Phenytoin is another example wherein orally administered drug may also bind to heavy metals, as well as enteral tube feedings (3,4). When these interactions go unrecognized, subtherapeutic phenytoin levels and a subsequent loss of seizure control may result. To best avoid these interactions, the iron, calcium, and antacids must be given either 2 hours before or 2 hours after the dose of the object drug. It is also suggested that continuous enteral feeding be halted for 2 hours before and after phenytoin administration.

Cholestyramine and sucralfate will physically bind other medications such as fluoroquinolones, ketoconazole, phenytoin, warfarin, valproic acid, and digoxin. In some circumstances, administering the drug 2 hours before cholestyramine or sucralfate and monitoring for effects will be adequate. In other cases, the combination may be best avoided entirely, such as with cholestyramine and warfarin.

Erythromycin, a macrolide antibiotic, is known to increase gut motility and, in recent years, has been exploited for this property as an alternative to cisapride. Cisapride was removed from the market secondary to life-threatening arrhythmias and torsades de pointes that occurred when combined with other drugs that inhibited the cytochrome P3A4 isoenzyme, depleted electrolytes, or prolonged QT interval. Historically there was concern in regard to the impact of increasing gut motility being tied to a potential decrease in the extent of drug absorption—for example, it was reported that the bioavailability of a digoxin tablet formulation (not *Lanoxin*) was reduced when taken concomitantly with metoclopramide therapy (5). More recently, however, reports of the opposite effect have surfaced where tacrolimus toxicity was associated with concomitant metoclopramide therapy (6). This drug–drug interaction is likely the result of enhanced absorption of tacrolimus secondary to metoclopramide, whereby coadministration of the metoclopramide substantially improves gastric motility and promotes delivery of tacrolimus to the absorption sites in the small intestine. Drugs that delay gastric emptying will usually slow the transition of a drug into the small intestine, thus delaying and possibly decreasing absorption.

Other interactions can be exploited to enhance absorption of a drug. Didanosine liquid is prepared with antacid suspension to ensure adequate pH for optimal stability. The role of pH in the absorption of ketoconazole is well described, an acidic medium being required for dissolution and subsequent absorption. Administration of ketoconazole in the presence of proton-pump inhibitors, H_2-blockers, or antacids severely hinders ketoconazole bioavailability. Ferrous sulfate is converted to the more absorbable ferric state in the presence of vitamin C. Many medications should be taken with food to enhance absorption, whereas some drugs should be given on an empty stomach. Often, the presence of food will delay the absorption but not impact the overall bioavailability of the drug. Consistency, either with or without food, should be the aim for patients taking medications with the potential for fluctuations in serum levels and resultant toxicities such as phenytoin, propranolol, and warfarin.

Intestinal flora plays an important role in body homeostasis. These bacteria, present widely in the large intestine, may have a role in drug interactions for medications that are recirculated back into the intestine after initial absorption, as in the case of oral contraceptives. It is understood that oral contraceptives are absorbed undergoing a significant first-pass effect, are conjugated in the liver, and are subsequently eliminated via the bile. Intestinal flora hydrolyzes the eliminated drug, yielding free estrogen that can then be reabsorbed. The presence of the intestinal flora is essential to maintain adequate serum concentrations of estrogen to prevent pregnancy. Although there is some controversy regarding this interaction, when a woman taking oral contraceptives is also subject to antibiotic treatment, if intestinal flora is compromised, the estrogen level may drop putting her at risk for unintended pregnancy (7).

In addition, P-glycoprotein, a genetically encoded and widely distributed drug efflux pump, has been described in significant drug interactions. P-glycoprotein is highly expressed in normal tissues, including the columnar epithelial cells in the intestine (8). Induction and inhibition of intestinal P-glycoprotein is reported to play a role in several drug interactions (8). The specific roles of P-glycoprotein in interactions are complex and are still being elucidated. For example, paclitaxel bioavailability rises in the presence of ciclosporin, a potent inhibitor or P-glycoprotein, suggesting that P-glycoprotein serves as an intestinal barrier preventing paclitaxel absorption. Likewise, P-glycoprotein inhibition by verapamil has been associated with improved digoxin absorption and elevated digoxin levels (8).

Drug interactions occurring during the administration phase are not only limited to the oral route. Intravenous aminoglycoside antibiotics can be inactivated if given within 30 minutes of a penicillin derivative. Postexposure prophylaxis that requires both passive immune globulin and active vaccine immunization should be given at distinct injection sites on different extremities to avoid diminishing the immune response to the vaccine.

Similar to taking advantage of enteral drug interactions to enhance a drug effect, injectable drug interactions can at times be useful. Epinephrine, a potent vasoconstrictor will decrease blood flow to an area. When added to a local anesthetic during laceration treatment, the epinephrine creates a more visible working environment. The lack of blood flow also enhances the efficacy by decreasing the absorption of the local anesthetic.

DISTRIBUTION

Distribution of medications is dependent upon total body water, extracellular fluid, percentage of adipose tissue, and the capacity to bind to plasma proteins. Albumin and α-1 glycoprotein are the primary circulating plasma proteins to which drugs bind. Albumin is the predominant plasma protein and binds in particular to acidic and neutral drugs, whereas α-1 glycoprotein preferentially binds basic drugs (9). Variations in plasma protein concentration are seen secondary to certain disease states and can influence free drug concentration. Drug interactions occur because of competition for binding sites on these proteins. In effect, one drug displaces the other off the binding site, or alternatively, occupies the site, not allowing the other drug to bind.

An interaction will not be clinically significant unless the involved drugs are highly protein bound (>95%) or have very narrow therapeutic indices. A classic example is phenytoin, which not only is involved in physical binding interactions discussed previously, as well as cytochrome P450 interactions to be discussed later, but also is generally between 89% to 93% protein bound with a very narrow therapeutic window. When phenytoin is given in conjunction with salicylates or valproic acid, the free fraction of phenytoin increases because of competition for the same plasma protein binding sites. Should the free fraction of phenytoin rise above 2 μg per dL, toxicity is generally seen consisting of ataxia, nystagmus, increased seizure activity, and if high enough, coma.

METABOLISM

The liver is the most important organ involved in drug metabolism, although metabolism also takes place to a degree in the blood, GI tract, kidney, lung, skin, and placenta. Drug metabolism is divided into two categories, phase I (oxidation, reduction, hydrolysis) and phase II (conjugation) reactions. Phase I reactions generally result in a compound that is less toxic and more hydrophilic, allowing for efficient excretion. At times, phase I reactions lead to the metabolism of a parent compound or prodrug into the active metabolite (e.g., acetaminophen, methanol, enalapril). Mixed function oxidases, or the cytochrome P450 (CYP450) system of enzymes, are responsible for the bulk of Phase I reactions. Phase II reactions generally terminate the biologic activity of the drug and prepare it for elimination through conjugation with glucuronide, sulfate, or glycine; although the compounds have a larger molecular weight, they are more water-soluble.

The CYP450 enzymes are unique isoenzymes found primarily in the liver and are responsible for the metabolism of many drugs and toxins. (Table 64.1) The enzymes are so named because of the absorption of light at a wavelength of 450 nm and are grouped into families 1, 2, and 3 and then divided into subfamilies A to E. The individual member enzymes are then further designated by a number (e.g., 3A4, 2D6). These enzymes are genetically encoded and therefore are associated with interpatient variability; this variability makes it difficult to predict who will experience an adverse reaction or exaggerated drug interaction. Age-related development of CYP450 enzymes matures and even surpasses adult capacity during the first year of life (10).

Inducers are drugs that are capable of increasing CYP450 enzyme activity by increasing enzyme synthesis. These drugs will enhance the enzyme's metabolizing capacity, speeding up substrate drug metabolism, and decreasing the object drug effect. The time onset of enzyme induction is dependent upon the half-life of the inducing drug. An inducer such as phenobarbital, with a long half-life can take up to a week to have an impact. In contrast, a decrease in the concentration of a drug metabolized by CYP2C9 can occur within 24 hours after the initiation of rifampin, a rapid and potent inducer (11).

The inhibition of CYP450 enzymes may occur secondary to competitive binding between two drugs or to permanent inactivation (12). Generally, inhibition begins after the first dose of the inhibitor and the duration of inhibition correlates with the half-life of the drug. Most commonly these interactions result in the slow down of substrate drug metabolism, yielding increased plasma concentrations, increased drug effect, and thereby increased risk of adverse events. Drugs have been intentionally combined to exploit CYP450 inhibition; the protease inhibitor ritonavir, a potent CYP3A4 inhibitor, is added to lopinavir and elvitegravir to boost serum levels in patients with human immunodeficiency virus (13,14).

CYTOCHROME P1A2

Nearly 15% of medications used today are metabolized by cytochrome P1A2 (CYP1A2), most notably caffeine, theophylline lidocaine, tricyclic antidepressants, and warfarin. The activity of CYP1A2 can be induced by cigarette smoke, charbroiled foods, and cruciferous vegetables (e.g., cabbage, broccoli). Several medications can also affect CYP1A2 activity. Phenobarbital, carbamazepine, and rifampin induce CYP1A2 as well as several other enzymes, leading to clinically relevant drug interactions. Inhibitors of CYP1A2 include cimetidine, ciprofloxacin, erythromycin, fluvoxamine, and grapefruit juice. Omeprazole and ritonavir simultaneously induce CYP1A2 and inhibit one or more other enzymes.

CYTOCHROME 2B6

The significance of cytochrome 2B6 (CYP2B6) in drug metabolism has only recently become apparent. CYP2B6 is genetically polymorphic and is implicated in the metabolism of a growing number of clinically important drugs. It is estimated that nearly 8% of drugs on the market are metabolized via CYP2B6 (15). Clinically used drugs that are known to be metabolized by CYP2B6 include chemotherapeutics such as cyclophosphamide, ifosfamide, the antiestrogen tamoxifen, as well as efavirenz, ketamine, propofol, and diazepam (16,17). Ritonavir, a protease inhibitor, is known to be a CYP2B6 inducer, which may explain the increased elimination of several drugs as demonstrated with bupropion (18). Genetic polymorphisms occur in approximately 3% of whites and up to 20% of blacks, being poor metabolizers, this seems to predict a more complicated clinical course and greater risk of toxicity-driven drug discontinuation (15).

CYTOCHROME 2C8

Cytochrome 2C8 (CYP2C8) has been studied to a lesser extent than its familial counterparts. Comprising approximately 7% of total microsomal CYP content in the liver, it caries out oxidative metabolism in nearly 5% of drugs cleared via phase I processes (19). Therapeutic agents metabolized by CYP2C8 include paclitaxel, amiodarone, rosiglitazone, cerivastatin, and fluvastatin. Known inhibitors of CYP2C8 consist of trimethoprim, gemfibrozil, montelukast, and ketoconazole, as well as several known CYP3A4 substrates—amitriptyline, terfenadine, and triazolam—causing up to 50% inhibition of CYP2C8 activity (19). Several genetic polymorphisms have been identified with CYP2C8, the most common of which is seen in roughly 18% of blacks and rarely in whites.

CYTOCHROME P2C9

Cytochrome P2C9 (CYP2C9) is responsible for the metabolism of several common medications including ibuprofen, carvedilol, celecoxib, losartan, phenytoin, glyburide, and warfarin (11). Rifampin and rifabutin are powerful inducers of CYP2C9 activity and will therefore decrease serum concentrations of the above substrates. Other inducers include carbamazepine, ethanol, and phenobarbital. Warfarin is produced as a racemic mixture of R-warfarin and S-warfarin, with the S-enantiomer being responsible for the predominance of pharmacologic activity. S-warfarin is principally metabolized via CYP2C9; inhibition of this enzyme pathway results in clinically significant drug–drug interactions, such that the Food and Drug Administration approved updated labeling for warfarin in 2007 remarking on this pharmacogenetic issue (20). Known inhibitors of CYP2C9 include fluconazole, ketoconazole, metronidazole, amiodarone, lovastatin, and even a number of flavonoids, secondary metabolites of many plants consumed by humans in a typical diet (21). Genetic polymorphisms occur in up to one-third of whites, contributing to abnormally decreased enzyme activity in these individuals (22).

CYTOCHROME P2C19

Like several other monoamine oxidases, cytochrome P2C19 (CYP2C19) has been shown to exhibit a genetic polymorphism; 3% to 6% of Caucasians, 15% to 20% of Japanese,

TABLE 64.1 Cytochrome P450 Substrates, Inhibitors, and Inducers

1A2	*2B6*	*2C8*	*2C9*	*2C19*	*2D6*	*2E1*	*3A3/4*	
				Substrates				
Acetaminophen	Bupropion	Amiodarone	Amitriptyline	Amitriptyline	Amitriptyline	Acetaminophen	Alfentanil	Lidocaine
Amitriptyline	Cyclophosphamide	Amodiaquine	Celecoxib	Carisoprodol	Amphetamine	Benzene	Alprazolam	Loratadine
Caffeine	Diazepam	Carbamazepine	Diclofenac	Citalopram	Atomoxetine	Caffeine	Amiodarone	Lovastatin
Clomipramine	Efavirenz	Cerivastatin	Fluoxetine	Clomipramine	Carvedilol	Chlorzoxazone	Amitriptyline	(not pravastatin)
Clozapine	Ifosfamide	Chloroquine	Flurbifrofen	Cyclophosphamide	Chlorpheniramine	Dapsone	Amlodipine	Methadone
Cyclobenzaprine	Ketamine	Cyclophosphamide	Fluvastatin	Diazepam	Chlorpromazine	Dextromethorphan	Atorvastatin	Midazolam
Estradiol	Propofol	Dapsone	Glipizide	Fluoxetine	Clomipramine	Ethanol	Bromocriptine	Nefazodone
Fluvoxamine	Tamoxifen	Diclofenac	Glyburide	Imipramine	Clozapine	Enflurane	Budesonide	Nicardipine
Haloperidol		Fluvastatin	Ibuprofen	Indomethacin	Codeine	Halothane	Bupropion	Nifedipine
Imipramine		Ibuprofen	Irbesartan	Lansoprazole	Desipramine	Isoflurane	Buspirone	Nimodipine
Mexiletine		Ifosfamide	Losartan	Nelfinavir	Dextromethorphan	Isoniazid	Caffeine	Omeprazole
Naproxen		Methadone	Naproxen	Omeprazole	Encainide	Sevoflurane	Calcium channel blockers	Ondansetron
Olanzapine		Morphine	Phenytoin	Pantoprazole	Flecainide	Theophylline	Carbamazepine	Paclitaxel
Ondansetron		Paclitaxel	Piroxicam	Phenytoin	Fluoxetine	Venlafaxine	Cisapride	Paroxetine
Pentazocine		Repaglinide	Rosiglitazone	Primidone	Fluvoxamine		Clomipramine	Pimozide
Propranolol		Rosiglitazone	Sulfamethoxazole	Progesterone	Haloperidol		Clonazepam	Progesterone
Ropivacaine		Troglitazone	Tamoxifen	Proguanil	Imipramine		Cocaine	Protease inhibitors
Tacrine		Torsemide	Torsemide	Propranolol	Lidocaine		Codeine	Quetiapine
Theophylline		Verapamil	Tolbutamide	Teniposide	Methadone		Cyclosporine	Quinidine
TCAs		Zopiclone	*S*-Warfarin	TCAs	Metoclopramide		Dapsone	Quinine
Verapamil				*R*-Warfarin	Metoprolol		Dexamethasone	Rifabutin
R-Warfarin					Mexiletine		Dextromethorphan	Rifampin
Zileuton					Nortriptyline		Diazepam	Ritonavir
Zolmitriptan					Olanzapine		Diltiazem	Salmeterol
					Ondansetron		Disopyramide	Saquinavir
					Oxycodone		Doxycycline	Sertraline
					Paroxetine		Ergotamine	Sildenafil
					Perphenazine		Erythromycin	Simvastatin
					Propafenone		Ethinyl estradiol	Tacrolimus
					Propranolol		Ethosuximide	Tamoxifen
					Risperidone		Etoposide	Theophylline

(*continued*)

TABLE 64.1 Cytochrome P450 Substrates, Inhibitors, and Inducers (*Continued*)

1A2	*2B6*	*2C8*	*2C9*	*2C19*	*2D6*	*2E1*	*3A3/4*	
					Sertraline		Fentanyl	Trazodone
					Tamoxifen		Finasteride	Triazolam
					Thioridazine		Fluconazole	TCAs
					Timolol		Fluoxetine	Venlafaxine
					Tramadol		Haloperidol	Verapamil
					Trazodone		Ifosfamide	Vinca alkaloids
					TCAs		Imipramine	Warfarin
					Venlafaxine		Indinavir	Zolpidem
							Isradipine	
							Itraconazole	
							Ketoconazole	
							Lansoprazole	
				Inhibitors				
Amiodarone	Clopidogrel	Amitriptyline	Amiodarone	Cimetidine	Amiodarone	Disulfiram	Amiodarone	
Cimetidine	Thiotepa	Gemfibrozil	Cimetidine	Felbamate	Bupropion	Methylpyrazole	Cimetidine	
Ciprofloxacin	Ticlopidine	Ketoconazole	Clopidogrel	Fluoxetine	Celecoxib		Ciprofloxacin	
Clarithromycin		Montelukast	Fluconazole	Fluvoxamine	Chloroquine		Clarithromycin	
Erythromycin		Terfenadine	Fluoxetine	Indomethacin	Chlorpheniramine		Diltiazem	
Fluoxetine		Triazolam	Fluvastatin	Ketoconazole	Chlorpromazine		Erythromycin	
Fluvoxamine		Trimethoprim	Fluvoxamine	Lansoprazole	Cimetidine		Fluconazole	
Gatifloxacin			Isoniazid	Omeprazole	Citalopram		Fluoxetine	
Grapefruit juice			Lovastatin	Paroxetine	Clemastine		Fluvoxamine	
Interferon			Metronidazole	Ritonavir	Clomipramine		Grapefruit juice	
Levofloxacin			Paroxetine	Ticlopidine	Cocaine		Itraconazole	
Mexiletine			Phenylbutazone	Topiramate	Diphenhydramine		Ketoconazole	
Ofloxacin			Probenecid		Doxorubicin		Nefazodone	
Nefazodone			Ritonavir		Escitalopram		Nifedipine	
Ticlopidine			Sertraline		Fluoxetine		Omeprazole	
			Sulfamethoxazole-trimethoprim		Haloperidol		Propoxyphene	

			Teniposide		Hydroxyzine		Protease inhibitors
			Zafirlukast		Indinavir		Verapamil
					Methadone		
					Metoclopramide		
					Paroxetine		
					Perphenazine		
					Propoxyphene		
					Quinidine		
					Ranitidine		
					Ritonavir		
					Sertraline		
					Terbinafine		
					Thioridazine		
					Ticlopidine		
				Inducers			
Broccoli	Ritonavir	Cortisol	Carbamazepine	Carbamazepine	Pregnancy	Chronic ethanol	Carbamazepine
Brussels sprouts		Dexamethasone	Ethanol	Norethindrone		Isoniazid	Dexamethasone
Carbamazepine		Phenobarbital	Phenobarbital	Prednisone		Ritonavir	Efavirenz
Charbroiled food		Rifampin	Phenytoin	Rifampin		Tobacco	Griseofulvin
Cigarette smoke			Primidone				Nevirapine
Modafinil			Rifabutin				Phenobarbital
Nafcillin			Rifampin				Phenytoin
Omeprazole			Secobarbital				Prednisone
Phenobarbital							Rifabutin
Phenytoin							Rifampin
Rifampin							Ritonavir
Ritonavir							St John's wort
Tobacco							Sulfinpyrazone
							Troglitazone

Data from http//medicine.uipui.edu/flockhart/table.htm; Shannon M. Drug–drug interactions and the cytochrome P450 system: an update. *Pediatr Emerg Care* 1997;13(5):350–353; Totah RA, Terrie AE. Cytochrome P450 2C8: substrates, inhibitors, pharmacogenetics, and clinical relevance. *Clin Pharm Ther* 2005;77:341–352; Taketomo CK, Hodding JH, Kraus DM. *Pediatric dosage handbook*, 10th ed. Cleveland: Lexicomp Inc, 2003–2004; and Flockhart DA. Drug Interactions: Cytochrome P450 Drug Interaction Table. Indiana University School of Medicine (2007). http://medicine.iupui.edu/clinpharm/ddis/table.asp. Accessed February 28, 2009.

and 10% to 20% of African Americans are poor metabolizers (23,24). Medications metabolized by CYP2C19 include several benzodiazepines, citalopram, tricyclic antidepressants, omeprazole, and warfarin, as well as the antiepileptics phenytoin, phenobarbital, and valproic acid (25,26). The isoenzyme is of major relevance to anticancer drug and antiepileptic drug interactions. Induction or inhibition of CYP2C19 can cause a decrease in anticancer drug concentrations. Similarly, enzyme inhibition or induction by anticancer drugs may lead to toxicity or loss of seizure control. This complex relationship is important particularly in the treatment of patients with brain cancer (22). Known inducers of CYP2C19 include carbamazepine, phenytoin, rifampin, and phenobarbital, whereas inhibitors consist of fluoxetine, sertraline, fluvoxamine, omeprazole, ritonavir, and isoniazid.

CYTOCHROME P2D6

Cytochrome P2D6 (CYP2D6) is an extensively studied polymorphic drug-metabolizing enzyme. Although it comprises a relatively small percentage (2% to 6%) of the total CYP450 in the liver, it is involved in the metabolism of many drugs, up to 25% of all drugs (27). Greater than 50 medications rely on CYP2D6 for metabolism, including β-blockers, analgesics, antidepressants, and antiemetics. Approximately 7% to 10% of whites are poor metabolizers of medications utilizing CYP2D6; these patients are then at risk for drug accumulation and toxicity from substrates of this enzyme, such as amitriptyline, metoprolol, paroxetine, and risperidone (11). The conversion of codeine to the active form, morphine, is catalyzed by CYP2D6; therefore, patients with low-enzyme activity demonstrate a poor analgesic response. The predictability of this response has prompted discussion in favor of genotype-influenced rational prescribing (28). Currently, there is a US Food and Drug Administration–approved, commercially available test (Amplichip) for determining CYP2D6 genotype.

Unlike other CYP450 enzymes, there are no known inducers of this activity except pregnancy. Several medications inhibit CYP2D6, the most potent include cimetidine, diphenhydramine, fluoxetine, haloperidol, paroxetine, and codeine.

CYTOCHROME P2E1

Although cytochrome P2E1 (CYP2E1) metabolizes a relatively small fraction, approximately 1.5% metabolic activity in the liver, this enzyme plays a significant role in the activation and inactivation of toxins (24). Cytochrome P2E1 metabolizes primarily small organic molecules (e.g., ethanol, carbon tetrachloride) as well as acetaminophen and dapsone. The product of acetaminophen's CYP2E1 metabolism is a highly reactive intermediate, *N*-acetyl-*p*-benzoquinoneimine (NAPQI), a hepatotoxin that must be detoxified by conjugation with glutathione. Chronic ethanol use, as seen in patients with alcohol dependence, results in increased risk for hepatotoxicity secondary to acetaminophen due to the ethanol induction of CYP2E1 as well as a secondary depletion of glutathione stores (29). Induction of CYP2E1 leads to a greater percentage of acetaminophen being metabolized to NAPQI. Research continues to explore the benefits of using inhibitors such as disulfiram to prevent the toxicity associated with some CYP2E1 metabolites (29).

CYTOCHROME P3A3/4

Cytochrome P3A (CYP3A) is both the most abundant and clinically significant family of CYP450 enzymes, metabolizing virtually 50% of marketed drugs. The CYP3A family comprises four major enzymes: CYP3A3, CYP3A4, CYP3A5, and CYP3A7. Cytochrome P3A4 is the most common and is implicated in the most drug interactions. Because these enzymes are so closely related (most are 97% similar), they are often referred to as the subfamily name, CYP3A. Close to 60% of the liver's total CYP450 is CYP3A, and the presence of CYP3A in the small intestine results in decreased bioavailability of many drugs (30). Among the many significant CYP3A inhibitors are grapefruit juice, the macrolides erythromycin and clarithromycin, the antifungals ketoconazole and itraconazole, the antidepressants fluoxetine and fluvoxamine, the anti-HIV agent ritonavir, and calcium channel blockers such as verapamil.

Clopidogrel, an oral antiplatelet medication, is metabolized to an active thiol metabolite by the CYP3A4 enzyme. Variability in patient response has led to investigation of the mechanism, which has been at least partly attributed to drug–drug interactions in some patients (31). Intake of calcium channel blockers, known to inhibit CYP3A, has been associated with a reduced efficacy of clopidogrel to inhibit platelet aggregation. It is, however, this same interaction, inhibition of CYP3A that permits the use of ritonavir as a boosting agent for other protease inhibitors (32,33).

Cytochrome P3A inducers include the dexamethasone, rifampin, carbamazepine, phenobarbital, and phenytoin. Following the resurgence of tuberculosis (TB) in the United States in the late 1980s through early 1990s, the annual rate of TB has declined steadily. Unfortunately, however, that decrease has now slowed, and the proportion of multidrug resistant TB cases contributed by foreign-born persons continues to rise (34). Given these data it is not surprising that rifampin, an inducer of the CYP3A subfamily, continues to play a role in clinically relevant drug interactions. Of particular clinical significance is the potential reduction of oral contraceptive efficacy by rifampin, since estradiol levels can be reduced by rifampin-mediated CYP3A induction (23).

N-ACETYLTRANSFERASE

Acetylation is a unique, non-CYP pathway of drug metabolism. Dapsone, hydralazine, isoniazid, procainamide, and sulfonamides are examples of drugs metabolized via acetylation. Acetylation polymorphisms, being discovered nearly 50 years ago, are well described (35). Variants in the alleles coding for the conjugating *N*-acetyltransferase enzymes occur in nearly half of Americans, white and black, resulting in slow acetylators. Slow acetylator phenotypes occur in 60% to 70% of Northern Europeans and 5% to 10% of Asians (36). These slow acetylators demonstrate enhanced toxicity but longer drug effectiveness. The fast acetylator phenotypes may not demonstrate the desired therapeutic response to treatment.

HUMAN ETHER-A-GO-GO–RELATED GENE

The human ether-a-go-go–related gene (hERG) is responsible for the potassium channels mediating ventricular repolarization. Drug-induced cardiac arrhythmias, specifically *torsades de pointes* (TdP), are of considerable concern, in particular in patients genetically predisposed to long QT syndrome. Genetic abnormalities predispose patients to either long QT syndrome or short QT syndrome, both of which could result in fatal cardiac arrhythmia (37). The potassium channel is also sensitive to drug binding, as well as changes in extracellular potassium levels, both of which may give rise to decreased channel function and subsequent acquired long QT syndrome. Drugs that can cause QT prolongation include antiarrhythmics (especially Class 1A and Class III), antipsychotics, quinolones, and macrolide antibiotics. The administration of drugs metabolized by CYP3A4 oxidases such as terfenadine, cisapride, pimozide, and astemizole are particularly vulnerable when coadministered with agents that inhibit CYP3A4 such as ketoconazole, erythromycin, and clarithromycin.

ELIMINATION/EXCRETION

Elimination and excretion of drugs occur primarily via the kidneys. Biliary secretion, plasma esterases, and other minor pathways are important routes, albeit less common than renal elimination. Renal elimination is dependent upon multiple factors such as glomerular filtration rate, tubular secretion, and tubular reabsorption.

Glomerular filtration hinges upon the protein-binding characteristics of the drug and the glomerular filtration rate. Changes in glomerular filtration rate are often the result of changes in blood pressure or glomerular hydrostatic pressure—both of which can be the result of drug therapy. Drug interactions occurring under these circumstances are considered indirect interactions, as it is the nephrotoxicity induced by one drug that causes the adverse effects of the object drug. For example, excessive antihypertensive therapy may result in diminished renal blood flow. In such a case, drugs primarily eliminated via glomerular filtration will accumulate and have the potential to cause toxicity (38).

Urinary alkalinization and acidification by some medications can cause others to be more (or less) readily excreted. Other agents can inhibit renal tubular secretion and assist in maintaining higher serum concentrations than the body would otherwise allow. A classic example is the use of probenecid and penicillin, secondary to probenecid blocking the tubular secretion of β-lactams. More recently, probenecid has been studied for use with the antiviral oseltamivir for treatment and prophylaxis in the event of an influenza pandemic (39). Oseltamivir is administered as a prodrug, which is rapidly hydrolyzed to its active metabolite, which is then subject to excretion via glomerular filtration and renal tubular secretion. Administration of probenecid results in marked reductions in renal clearance and subsequent elevations in plasma area-under-the-curve. Researchers are hopeful that this interaction can be exploited to allow for considerable dose saving (11). In contrast, probenecid has also become an integral part of the regimen for decreasing the nephrotoxic effects of cidofovir by limiting the exposure of renal proximal tubular cells to the drug (40). Finally, probenecid should not be used with sulfonamides, ketorolac, or methotrexate because of increased serum concentrations and half-life, resulting in increased toxicity (41).

An additional interaction involving renal tubular secretion that can be potentially detrimental is that of methotrexate and the proton-pump inhibitor omeprazole. By inhibiting hydrogen ions (protons) in the renal tubules, omeprazole may also inhibit methotrexate elimination as it is actively secreted in the distal tubules with hydrogen ions via the H^+/K^+-ATPase pump (42). A more recent trial supports this interaction via another mechanism: here four proton-pump inhibitors were analyzed and demonstrated a significant inhibition of breast cancer resistance protein–mediated transport of methotrexate for elimination (43). These interactions can result in prolonged elevated serum concentrations, particularly concerning after treatment with a high-dose regimen for cancer therapy.

Interactions involving the use of potassium-sparing diuretics such as spironolactone with drugs or herbal supplements that can increase serum potassium levels are also concerning. Here serum potassium escalates secondary to a drug-induced impairment of the renin-angiotensin-aldosterone system that regulates potassium excretion. Following publication of the findings that mortality was significantly lowered in patients on spironolactone in the Randomized Aldosterone Evaluation Study (RALES), reports of hyperkalemia climbed (44,45). Impaired renal function and the addition of several other medications are thought to compound the retention of potassium. For this reason, when combined with spironolactone, the following agents can increase potassium, possibly leading to hyperkalemia and cardiac arrest if not intercepted: nonsteroidal anti-inflammatory drugs, COX-2 inhibitors, angiotensin-converting enzyme inhibitors, angiotensin II receptor antagonists, β-blockers, cyclosporine, tacrolimus, heparin, ketoconazole, trimethoprim, and pentamidine (46–48). Patients receiving these medications with spironolactone warrant intensive monitoring of renal function and potassium levels.

SUMMARY

The mechanisms of drug interactions are varied, typically including object and subject drugs though may include herbal supplements and foods. As the knowledge of drug interactions increases, it is important to have on-hand drug interaction resources available to ensure patient safety. Being informed about the potential for drug interactions is the best way to prevent them from occurring. Moreover, understanding the mechanisms of drug interactions will assist all clinicians in avoiding these serious, often, preventable events (Table 64.2). It is important to bear in mind that although interactions follow a predictable pattern, there is often interpatient variability. Any potential interaction must be evaluated using patient-specific data to best determine the most beneficial course of action.

TABLE 64.2 Questions to Help the Clinician Detect Drug Interactions

1. Identification of the nature of the interaction
   - Is there a potential interaction between a drug and another drug, disease, food, nutrition, or combination of any of these factors?
2. Understanding the mode of action of the interaction
   - Can the pharmacokinetic interaction be explained in terms of absorption, distribution, metabolism, or elimination of the drug?
   - Is the interaction pharmacodynamic?
   - What is the time course of the interaction? Several factors will affect the time course of the interaction, such as the mechanism of the interaction, the pharmacokinetics of the object drug, the nature of the interacting drug (inhibitor, inductor, substrate), the sequence of prescription, and the baseline concentration of the target drug.[a]
   - Is this interaction well documented in published work, or are there strong suspicions (theoretical or clinical) to expect that an adverse drug interaction might take place?
   - Would the potential interaction appear when a drug is added or discontinued?
3. Identification of potential or real clinical outcomes for the patient
   - What are the short- and long-term clinical outcomes for the patient?
   - Is the patient having new problems (e.g., falls and gait difficulties, bleeding, blood pressure changes, confusion) that can be explained by a drug interaction?
   - Does the patient have risk factors that might increase the likelihood of an adverse outcome (e.g., with regard to comorbidities, other drugs taken, dose and duration of treatment, pharmacogenetics)?[b]
4. Monitoring and follow-up for potential drug interactions
   - Is an appropriate monitoring plan in place—for example, INR, serum drug concentration, electrolytes, blood pressure, glucose concentration, and who is responsible for follow-up to promote continuity of care? Does this plan account for the estimated time course of the interaction?[c]
   - Are caregivers vigilant to monitor for the appearance of new symptoms after any changes to drug treatment?
   - Has the drug interaction been documented in the patient's medical record?

[a]For example, a patient on chronic treatment with a drug that induces CYP3A4, (e.g., rifampicin) who is then given a CYP3A4 substrate will experience little or no effect from the CYP3A4 substrate, starting with the very first dose of the substrate. If, however, the same two drugs are given but the inducer is added to the substrate, the interaction will take much longer to develop. Another example would be a patient who is just on the verge of toxic effects from drug A when an inhibitor of drug A's metabolism is added (drug B). Drug A might normally take days to achieve a new steady-state serum concentration when drug B (inhibitor of drug A) is added. In most people, the interaction would be delayed. However, if the patient was only a few drug molecules away from toxicity, he may develop toxic effects in less than 24 hours.
[b]For example, a patient on warfarin who is started on thyroid supplement for hypothyroid is at greater risk of overanticoagulation and bleeding than a patient on chronic thyroid supplement treatment who is started on warfarin.
[c]For example, it can take 7–10 days for the international normalized ratio (INR) to stabilize after a patient on warfarin starts taking a CYP2C9 inhibitor.
Reproduced from Mallet L. The challenge of managing drug interactions in elderly people. *Lancet* 2007;370:185–191, with permission.

REFERENCES

1. Wallace AW, Victory JM, Amsden GW. Lack of bioequivalence when levofloxacin and calcium-fortified orange juice are coadministered to healthy volunteers. *J Clin Pharmacol* 2003;43(5):539–544.
2. Neuhofel AL, Wilton JH, Victory JM, et al. Lack of bioequivalence of ciprofloxacin when administered with calcium-fortified orange juice: a new twist on an old interaction. *J Clin Pharmacol* 2002;42(4):461–466.
3. Au Yeung SC, Ensom MH. Phenytoin and enteral feedings: does evidence support an interaction? *Ann Pharmacother* 2000;34(7–8):896–905.
4. Faraji B, Yu PP. Serum phenytoin levels of patients on gastrostomy tube feeding. *J Neurosci Nurs* 1998;30:55–59.
5. Manninen V, Melin J, Apajalahti A, et al. Altered absorption of digoxin in patients given propantheline and metoclopramide. *Lancet* 1973;301:398–400.
6. Prescott WA Jr, Callahan BL, Park JM. Tacrolimus toxicity associated with concomitant metoclopramide therapy. *Pharmacotherapy* 2004;24(4):532–537.
7. Summers A. Interaction of antibiotics and oral contraceptives. *Emerg Nurs* 2008;16(6):20–21.
8. Lin JH, Yamazaki M. Role of P-glycoprotein in pharmacokinetics. *Clin Pharmacokinet* 2003;42(1):59–98.
9. Kremer JMH, Wilting JAAP, Janssen LHM. Drug binding to human alpha-1-acid glycoprotein in health and disease. *Pharmacol Rev* 1988;40(1):1–47.
10. Kearns GL, Abdel-Rahman SM, Alander SW, et al. Developmental pharmacology—drug disposition, action, and therapy in infants and children. *N Engl J Med* 2003;349:1157–1167.
11. Lynch T, Price A. The effect of cytochrome P450 metabolism on drug response, interactions, and adverse effects. *Am Fam Physician* 2007;76:391–396.
12. Shannon M. Drug–drug interactions and the cytochrome P450 system: an update. *Pediatr Emerg Care* 1997;13(5):350–353.
13. Molto J, Barbanoh MJ, Miranda C, et al. Simultaneous population pharmacokinetic model for lopinavir and ritonavir in HIV-infected adults. *Clin Pharmacokinet* 2008;47(10):681–692.
14. Mathias AA, West S, Hui J, et al. Dose-response of ritonavir on hepatic CYP3A activity and elvitegravir oral exposure. *Clin Pharm Ther* 2009;85(1):64–70.
15. Nolan D, Phillips E, Mallal S. Efavirenz and CYP2B6 polymorphism: implications for drug toxicity and resistance. *Clin Infect Dis* 2006;42:408–410.
16. Turpeinen M, Raunio H, Pelkonen O. The functional role of CYP2B6 in human drug metabolism: substrates and inhibitors in vitro, in vivo and in silico. *Curr Drug Metab* 2006;7(7):705–714.
17. Hodgson E, Rose RL. The importance of cytochrome P450 2B6 in the human metabolism of environmental chemicals. *Pharmacol Ther* 2007;113:420–428.
18. Kharasch ED, Mitchell D, Coles R, et al. Rapid clinical induction of hepatic cytochrome P450B6 activity by ritonavir. *Antimicrob Agents Chemother* 2008;52(5):1663–1669.
19. Totah RA, Terrie AE. Cytochrome P450 2C8: substrates, inhibitors, pharmacogenetics, and clinical relevance. *Clin Pharm Ther* 2005;77:341–352.
20. Huang S-M, Temple R. Is this drug or dose for you?: impact and consideration of ethnic factors in global drug development, regulatory review, and clinical practice. *Clin Pharm Ther* 2008;84(3):287–294.
21. Si D, Wang Y, Guo Y, et al. Mechanism of CYP2C9 inhibition by flavones and flavonols. *Drug Metab Dispos* 2009;37:629–634.

22. Lee C, Goldstein JA, Pieper JA. Cytochrome P450 2C9 polymorphisms: a comprehensive review of the in-vitro human data. *Pharacogenetics* 2002;12:251–263.
23. Cupp MJ, Tracy TS. Cytochrome P450: new nomenclature and clinical implications. *Am Fam Physician* 1998;57(1):107–116.
24. Wijnen PAHM, Buijshc OD, Drent M, et al. Review article: the prevalence and clinical relevance of cytochrome P450 polymorphisms. *Aliment Pharmacol Ther* 2007;26(Suppl 2):211–219.
25. Yap KY, Chui WK, Chan A. Drug interactions between chemotherapeutic regimens and antiepileptics. *Clin Ther* 2008;30(8):1385–1407.
26. Uno T, Sugimoto K, Sugawara K, et al. The effect of CYP2C19 genotypes on the pharmacokinetics of warfarin enantiomers. *J Clin Pharm Ther* 2008;33:67–73.
27. Goetz MP, Kamal A, Ames MM. Tamoxifen pharmacogenomics: the role of CYP2D6 as a predictor of drug response. *Clin Pharmacol Ther* 2008;83(1):160–166.
28. Lanfear DE, McLeod HL. Pharmacogenetics: using DNA to optimize drug therapy. *Am Fam Physician* 2007;76:1179–1182.
29. Lin JH. CYP induction-mediated drug interactions: in vitro assessment and clinical implications. *Pharm Res* 2006;23(6):1089–1116.
30. Manzi SF, Shannon M. Drug interactions—a review. *Clin Pediatr Emerg Med* 2005;6:93–102.
31. Siller-Matula JM, Lang I, Christ G, et al. Calcium-channel blockers reduce the antiplatelet effect of clopidogrel. *J Am Coll Cardiol* 2008;52:1557–1563.
32. Zhou SF, Xue CC, Yu XQ, et al. Clinically important drug interactions potentially involving mechanism-based inhibition of cytochrome P450 3A4 and the role of therapeutic drug monitoring. *Ther Drug Monit* 2007;29(6):687–710.
33. Mathias AA, West S, Hui J, et al. Dose-response of ritonavir on hepatic CYP3A activity and elvitegravir oral exposure. *Clin Pharmacol Ther* 2009;85(1):64–70.
34. Pratt R, Robinson V, Navin T, et al. Trends in tuberculosis—United States, 2007. *MMWR Morb Mortal Wkly Rep* 2008;57(11):281–285.
35. Spielberg SP. N-acetyltransferases: pharmacogenetics and clinical consequences of polymorphic drug metabolism. *J Pharmacokinet Biopharm* 1996;24(5):509–519.
36. Wilkinson G. Pharmacokinetics. In: Hardman JG, Limbird LE, Gillman AG, eds. *Goodman & Gilman's the pharmacologic basis of therapeutics*, 10th ed. New York, NY: McGraw-Hill, 2001.
37. Hancox JC, McPate MJ, Harchi AE, et al. The hERG potassium channel and hERG screening for drug induced torsades de pointes. *Pharmacol Ther* 2008;119:118–132.
38. Hansten PD, Horn JR. *Drug interactions analysis and management 2008.* St. Louis, MO: Wolters Kluwer Health, 2008.
39. Wattanagoon Y, Stepniewska K, Lindegardh N, et al. Pharmacokinetics of high dose oseltamivir in healthy volunteers. *Antimicrob Agents Chemother* 2009;53:945–952.
40. Cundy KC. Clinical pharmacokinetics of the antiviral nucleotide analogues cidofovir and adefovir. *Clin Pharmacokinet* 1999;36(2):127–143.
41. Watson Laboratories I. Probenecid [package insert]. 2003.
42. Beorlegui B, Aldaz A, Ortega A, et al. Potential interaction between methotrexate and omeprazole. *Ann Pharmacother* 2000;34:1024–1027.
43. Suzuki K, Doki K, Homma M, et al. Co-administration of proton pump inhibitors delays elimination of plasma methotrexate in high-dose methotrexate therapy. *Br J Clin Pharmacol* 2009;67(1):44–49.
44. Hauben M, Reich L, Gerrits CM, et al. Detection of spironolactone-associated hyperkalemia following the Randomized Aldactone Evaluation Study (RALES). *Drug Saf* 2007;30(12):1143–1149.
45. Juurlink DN, Mamdani MM, Lee DS, et al. Rates of hyperkalemia after publication of the Randomized Aldactone Evaluation Study. *N Engl J Med* 2004;351:543–551.
46. Saklayen MG, Gyebi LK, Tasosa J, et al. Effects of additive therapy with spironolactone on proteinuria in diabetic patients already on ACE inhibitor or ARB therapy: results of a randomized, placebo-controlled, double-blind, crossover trial. *J Investig Med* 2008;56(4):714–719.
47. Svensson M, Gustafsson F, Glatius S, et al. Hyperkalemia and impaired renal function in patients taking spironolactone for congestive heart failure: retrospective study. *BMJ* 2003;327:1141–1142.
48. Palmer BF. Managing hyperkalemia caused by inhibitors of the renin-angiotensin-aldosterone system. *N Engl J Med* 2004;351:585–592.

APPENDIX

A1

Mirjana Lulic-Botica
J. V. Aranda

Drug Formulary for the Newborn

TABLE A1.1 Commonly Used Medications in a Newborn Intensive Care Unit

Medication	*Dosage*	*Comments*
Acetaminophen (Tylenol)	10–15 mg/kg/dose q6–8 hr p.o/p.r., max 90 mg/kg/day (term neonate) 60 mg/kg/day (preterm neonate)	• Contraindicated in G6PD deficiencies • Caution in liver failure
Acetaminophen w/codeine elixir (Tylenol w/codeine)	0.5–1 mg codeine/kg/dose p.o. q4–6 hr	• Contains 12 mg codeine + 120 mg acetaminophen per 5 mL. • Elixir contains sodium benzoate as preservative • Contraindicated in G6PD deficiency
Acyclovir (Zovirax)	20 mg/kg/dose i.v. q8 hr (neonatal HSV)	• Infuse over 1 hr: monitor BUN, SCr, liver enzymes, CBC • For 14–21 day in HSV infection • Dose adjust with elevated serum creatinine levels

Serum Creatinine Level (mg/dL)	*Dose (mg/kg/dose)*	*Interval (hr)*
0.8–1.1	20	q12
1.2–1.5	20	q24
>1.5	10	q24

Medication	*Dosage*	*Comments*
Adenosine (Adenocard)	50 mCg/kg rapid i.v.p. over 1–2 seconds Increase dose by 50 mCg/kg increments q2 min until return of sinus rhythm; max 250 mCg/kg	• Flush with saline immediately post dose • Adenosine 6 mg/2 mL vial size: Dilute 2 mL adenosine vial with 18 mL of normal saline for final concentration of 300 mCg/mL • After converting SVT to normal sinus rhythm give digoxin or propranolol • Decreased effect when theophylline/caffeine on-board due to competitive antagonism
Albumin 5%/25%	0.5–1 g/kg/dose i.v. over 30–120 min	• Administer through 5-μm filter • Isotonic crystalloid solutions should be used first line (*Neonatal Resuscitation guidelines 2005* state that an isotonic crystalloid rather than albumin is the solution of choice for volume expansion in the delivery room (Class IIb; LOE 7). • May be placed in TPN when treating fluid overload due to third spacing • Too rapid of infusion may result in vascular overload • 25% concentration should be avoided secondary to possible risk of hemolysis and IVH in preterm neonates

(*continued*)

TABLE A1.1 Commonly Used Medications in a Newborn Intensive Care Unit (*Continued*)

Medication	*Dosage*	*Comments*
		• If 25% concentration required secondary to renal failure and fluid restriction, it must be Y-in to main i.v. or TPN so that final concentration is ≤5% • Albumin infusions should be administered within 6 hr of preparation
Alteplase (TPA) (Activase)	**For catheter occlusion**: 0.5–1 mg via catheter; dwell time 2 hr Aspirate out of catheter. DO NOT INFUSE. May repeat in 1 hr for one more dose **Thrombolytic therapy:** **Dose:** 0.1–0.6 mg/kg/hr for 6 hr	• Please note: syringes are frozen, so allow for thaw time • Contraindicated: bleeding • **Chest 2008 guidelines regarding thrombolytic therapy in neonates**: "We recommend against thrombolytic therapy for neonatal VTE unless major vessel occlusion is causing critical compromise of organs or limbs (Grade 1B)"
Amikacin	0–4 wk <1,200 g: 7.5 mg/kg/dose i.v. q18–24 hr Postnatal age: <7 day, 1,200–2,000 g: 7.5 mg/kg/dose i.v. q12 hr >7 day, 1,200–2,000 g: 7.5–10 mg/kg/dose i.v. q8–12 hr >7 day, 1,200–2,000 g: 10 mg/kg/dose i.v. q8 hr	• Reserved for tobramycin-resistant gram-negative pathogens • **Therapeutic levels**: peak 20–30 mCg/mL, trough <4 mCg/mL • Monitor BUN, SCr, urine output
Aminophylline	Loading dose: 5 mg/kg/dose i.v. over 30 min Maintenance dose: 1.5–3 mg/kg/dose i.v. q8–12 hr Aminophylline drip—start at 0.2 mg/kg/hr i.v. 6 wk–6 mo: 0.5 mg/kg/hr 6 mo–1 yr: 0.6–0.7 mg/kg/hr	• Apnea level 7–12 mCg/mL • BPD level: 10–15 mCg/mL • Half-life is variable per age: Premature 20–30 hr Term 10–25 hr <6 mo 14 hr >6 mo 5 hr • Serum levels reduced in neonates because of decreased binding of theophylline to fetal albumin, resulting in greater free drug. • Draw theophylline level 3 days after therapy initiated or changed • Adjust frequency of theophylline dosing in anticipation of change of half-life • Toxic levels can result in tachycardia, PVC, seizures • Increases theophylline level: erythromycin, furosemide, hypothyroid • Decreases theophylline level: phenobarbital, phenytoin, rifampin, high protein diet • In preterm infants approximately 30% of aminophylline or theophylline is converted to caffeine
Amiodarone (Cordarone)	Loading dose: 5 mg/kg slow i.v.p. over 5 min Maintenance dose: 5–15 mCg/kg/min Max: 15 mCg/kg/min	• Standard continuous concentrations: 1 mg/mL, 2 mg/mL, 4 mg/mL • Limited data available in neonates; safety and efficacy not established • Class II antiarrhythmic which inhibits adrenergic stimulation and decreases A-V conduction • Contains benzyl alcohol • NOT compatible with heparin, sodium bicarbonate • Monitor for signs of hypo/hyperthyroidism (contains 37% iodine by weight) • Inhibits cytochrome P-450 isoenzyme: Increases plasma levels of digoxin, theophylline, and phenytoin

(*continued*)

TABLE A1.1 Commonly Used Medications in a Newborn Intensive Care Unit (*Continued*)

Medication	*Dosage*	*Comments*
Amoxicillin (Amoxil)	20–30 mg/kg/day p.o. div q12 hr 10–20 mg/kg p.o. qday for prophylaxis due to hydronephrosis	• Prophylaxis to continue until VCUG (voiding cystourethrography) completed • Powder for oral suspension is stable for 14 days under refrigeration after reconstitution
Amoxicillin/ clavulanic acid (Augmentin)	30 mg/kg/day p.o. div q12 hr	• Clavulanic acid binds and inhibits β-lactamases which inactivate amoxicillin • Administer with feeds to decrease GI side effects
Amphotericin B (conventional)	Dose: 1 mg/kg i.v. over 2–3 hr Bladder irrigation: 5–15 mg/100 cc. Instill 10 cc/kg via catheter; clamp for 60–120 min; perform irrigation 3–4 times/day for 2–4 days	• Total cumulative dose 15 mg/kg • Total cumulative dose 20–25 mg/kg for persistent fungemia or CNS involvement • Binds to ergosterol altering cell membrane permeability causing leaking of cell components • Monitor BUN, SCr, liver enzymes, electrolytes (hypokalemia, hypomagnesemia) and CBC • DO NOT FLUSH WITH ANY SOLUTIONS CONTAINING SALINE • Final concentration 0.1 mg/mL • Fluid restricted patients may concentrate up to 0.5 mg/mL in D5W/D10W through a central venous catheter • Poor CSF penetration
Amphotericin B lipid complex (Abelcet)	5 mg/kg/dose i.v. q24 hr infuse over 2 hours (may be dosed up to 7.5–10 mg/kg in refractory cases per infectious disease recommendation)	• Restricted criteria at most institutions and may require approval by infectious disease specialist • Exhibits nonlinear kinetics with high tissue concentration in liver, spleen, and lung. • First-line antifungal agent at Hutzel Women's Hospital for treatment of suspected fungal infection. • Empirical antifungal therapy for suspected candidiasis has been shown to improve mortality and morbidity • DO NOT use lipid complex Amphotericin B (ABLC) for *Candida lusitaniae and Candida guilliermondii* • Compatible in D5W/D10W • DO NOT ADD HEPARIN • Monitor renal, hepatic, electrolyte, and hematological status • Final concentration: 1 mg/mL • Maximum concentration of 2 mg/mL may be used in fluid-restricted patients • No guidelines regarding dose adjustment requirement in renal failure
Ampicillin	Postnatal <7 days <2 kg: 25 mg/kg/dose i.v./i.m. q12 hr; 50 mg/kg/dose i.v./i.m. q12 hr (suspected meningitis) >2 kg: 25 mg/kg/dose i.v./i.m. q8 hr; 50 mg/kg/dose i.v./i.m. q8 hr (suspected meningitis) GBS meningitis 200 mg/kg/day i.v. div q8 hr Postnatal >7 days <1,200 g: 25 mg/kg/dose i.v./i.m. q12 hr 1,200–2,000 g: 25 mg/kg/dose i.v./i.m. q8 hr >2,000 g: 25 mg/kg/dose i.v./i.m. q6 hr	• Incompatible with TPN
Ampicillin/sulbactam (Unasyn)	>1 mo old: 100–150 mg ampicillin/kg/day div q6 hr Meningitis: 200–400 mg ampicillin/kg/day div q6 hr	• Reserved for infants >1 mo old secondary to sulbactam component • Sulbactam is a β-lactamase inhibitor

(*continued*)

TABLE A1.1 Commonly Used Medications in a Newborn Intensive Care Unit (*Continued*)

Medication	*Dosage*	*Comments*
Atenolol (Tenormin)	0.8–1 mg/kg/dose p.o. qday MAX: 2 mg/kg/day	• Selective β1 blocker • 2 mg/mL oral solution compounded from tablets • Monitor blood pressure, heart rate, and respiratory rate
Atropine	Bradycardia: 0.02 mg/kg/dose i.v./i.m./s.c./e.t. May repeat q5 min up to 1 mg total dose	• Treatment of sinus bradycardia • 0.25 mg/5 mL (0.05 mg/mL)
Azithromycin (Zithromax)	<6 mo: 10 mg/kg/dose i.v. qday for 5 days (pertussis)	• No dosing guidelines for treatment of ureaplasma infections
Aztreonam (Azactam)	< or = 2 kg 60 mg/kg/day i.v. div q12 hr >2 kg 90 mg/kg/day i.v. div q8 hr	• Treatment for multidrug resistant aerobic gram-negative infections
Beractant (Survanta)	4 mL/kg intratracheal q6 hr for up to four doses if required	• Criteria: $FiO_2 > 0.3$ and MAP >7 • 25 mg/mL (4 mL, 8 mL)
Sodium citrate/citric acid (Bicitra)	2–3 mEq/kg/day div q6–8 hr p.o.	• Each mL contains 1 mEq of bicarbonate and 1mEq sodium • Monitor serum Na, K, $HCO3^-$, urine pH • Conversion to bicarbonate may be impaired with hepatic failure • Polycitra contains 2 mEq/mL bicarbonate, 1 mEq/mL potassium, and 1 mEq/mL sodium • Polycitra K contains 2 mEq/mL bicarbonate and 2 mEq/mL potassium
Bumetanide (Bumex)	0.01–0.05 mg/kg/dose p.o./i.v. q24–48 hr	• Monitor serum electrolytes, renal function, urine output
Calcitriol (Rocaltrol)	Hypoparathyroidism: 0.04–0.08 mCg/kg p.o. qday Hypocalcemia (premature infants): 1 mCg p.o. qday for 5 days	• Oral solution 1 mCg/mL
CALCIUM SALTS	Hypocalcemia: 50–150 mg/kg/day div q4–6 hr (expressed as elemental calcium)	
Calcium glubionate	Hypocalcemia: 50–150 mg/kg/day div q4–6 hr (Dose expressed in mg of elemental calcium)	• 6.5% syrup contains 115 mg elemental calcium per 5 mL = 1.2 mEq calcium/mL
Calcium gluconate	Symptomatic hypocalcemia: 100–200 mg/kg/dose i.v. q6 hr	• 10% gluconate contains 9 mg/mL elemental calcium • Order 2–4 doses for symptomatic hypocalcemia • Avoid giving via UAC (umbilical artery catheter) • Not recommended for infusion with TPN due to Ca-PO4 ratio limitations • Ionized calcium is preferred measurement due to poor correlation between serum ionized calcium (free) and total serum calcium especially with low albumin states and acid/base imbalances • Initiate as bolus for true hypocalcemia only • Normal calcium levels: • Preterm <1 wk 6–10 mg/dL • Term <1 wk 7–12 mg/dL • Total corrected calcium in low albumin states: Total corrected Ca: = Total serum Ca + 0.8 (4 − measured serum albumin) • Calcium corrections based on the above calculations may be inaccurate in the neonatal population • Ionized calcium level should be obtained if hypocalcemia is considered to be clinically significant.

(continued)

TABLE A1.1 Commonly Used Medications in a Newborn Intensive Care Unit (*Continued*)

Medication	*Dosage*	*Comments*
Caffeine citrate (Cafcit) (Specify caffeine citrate on order)	Loading dose: 20 mg/kg i.v./p.o. Maintenance dose: 5 mg/kg/day i.v./p.o.	• Trough level: 5–25 mCg/mL • Consider switching to p.o. as soon as possible due to cost • Caffeine citrate is ½ caffeine base • Order dose as caffeine citrate • May require larger maintenance dose for preterm infants • i.v. 60 mg/3 mL = $31, p.o. 20 mg/mL $0.50
Captopril (Capoten)	Premature neonates: 0.01 mg/kg/dose p.o. q8–12 hr Term neonates: 0.05–0.1 mg/kg/dose p.o. q8–24 hr; titrate up to 2 mg/kg/day	• Administer 1 hr before feeding • Management of CHF, HTN • ACE inhibitor which decreases angiotensin II, which increases plasma renin activity and decreases aldosterone secretion • Monitor blood pressure, serum creatinine, CBC, serum potassium
Carbamazepine (Tegretol)	10–20 mg/kg/day p.o. div b.i.d.–t.i.d. Maximum 35 mg/kg/day	• Therapeutic range: 4–12 mCg/mL • Adjust dose to clinical response and levels • Adjuvant agent in neonates not responding to conventional therapy • Cytochrome P450 isoenzyme: may induce metabolism of midazolam, phenytoin, theophylline, valproic acid, and topiramate
Carnitine	20 mg/L standard in TPN for all neonates less than or equal to 5 kg Dose of 10–20 mg/kg/day have been used in preterm infants whose triglyceride levels remain high	• Prevention and treatment of carnitine deficiency • Facilitates transport of long chain fatty acids into mitochondria
Caspofungin (Cancidas)	1 mg /kg i.v. over 2 hr	• Safety and efficacy not established in children • Reserved for last-line therapy secondary to refractory fungemia • Infectious disease approval only • FDA approved for aspergillosis, invasive refractory candidiasis, esophageal candidiasis • Noncompetitive inhibitor of beta- (1,3)-glucan synthase in the echinocandin class • Dilute to final concentration of 0.2 mg/mL • Monitor for increase in liver enzymes, infusion-related reactions (thrombophlebitis) • DO NOT USE DILUENTS/FLUSHES CONTAINING DEXTROSE • Restricted criteria at most institutions and may require approval by infectious disease specialist
Cefazolin (Ancef)	<7 days: 20 mg/kg/dose i.v. q12 hr >7 days <2 kg: 20 mg/kg/dose i.v. q12 hr >2 kg: 20 mg/kg/dose i.v. q8 hr	• Infuse over 30 min
Cefdinir (Omnicef)	>6 mo–1 yr: 7 mg/kg/dose p.o. q12 hr for 10 day	• Third-generation oral cephalosporin
Cefepime (Maxipime)	50 mg/kg/dose i.v. q12 hr Febrile neutropenia: 50 mg/kg/dose i.v. q8 hr	• Reserve for ceftazidime-resistant gram-negative pathogens • Monitor closely for increases in bilirubin especially in preterm infants • Fourth-generation cephalosporin • No data for infants less than 2 mo • Dose adjust in renal impairment
Cefpodoxime (Vantin)	>6 mo: 5 mg/kg/dose p.o. q12 hr	• Third-generation oral cephalosporin • Monitor CBC, liver enzymes

(*continued*)

TABLE A1.1 Commonly Used Medications in a Newborn Intensive Care Unit (*Continued*)

Medication	*Dosage*	*Comments*
Cefotaxime (Claforan)	0–4 wk <1200 g: 50 mg/kg/dose i.v./i.m. q12 hr >1200 g and >7 days: 50 mg/kg/dose q8 hr	• Compatible with TPN • Third-generation cephalosporin • Used for empiric coverage of late-onset sepsis with Vancomycin
Ceftazidime (Fortaz)	50 mg/kg/dose i.v. q12 hr >1200 g and >7 days: 50 mg/kg/dose i.v. q8 hr	• Compatible with TPN • Third-generation cephalosporin
Ceftriaxone (Rocephin)	Gonococcal prophylaxis: 25–50 mg/kg i.m./i.v. × one dose (NOT to exceed 125 mg)	• Third-generation cephalosporin • Good penetration into CSF (meningitis) • Generally not used in the neonatal population for indications other than gonococcal prophylaxis secondary to potential bilirubin displacement • NOT compatible with calcium or calcium containing solutions (TPN). Immediate precipitation will result
Cephalexin (Keflex)	25–50 mg/kg/day p.o. div q6–8 hr Severe infections: 50–100 mg/kg/day p.o. div q6–8 hr Otitis media: 75–100 mg/kg/day p.o. div q6 hr	• 250 mg/5 mL oral suspension
Cholestyramine 5%	5% cream: apply three to four times a day to diaper rash area	• Reserved for severe diaper rash • Compounded by pharmacy
Chloral hydrate (Noctec)	Sedative: 25 mg /kg/dose p.o. prior to procedure Hypnotic: 50–75 mg/kg/dose p.o./p.r.	• Avoid in hepatic/renal failure • Use caution in neonates especially in preterm neonates with repeated doses due to accumulation of active metabolite TCE (trichloroethanol) • Prolonged use is associated with a direct hyperbilirubinemia • Contains sodium benzoate (preservative) which is associated with gasping syndrome in large doses in neonates
Chlorothiazide (Diuril)	10–30 mg/kg/day p.o. div q8–12 hr 2–6 mg/kg/day i.v. div q12 hr	• Monitor electrolytes at initiation of therapy • May require sodium supplementation for diuretic-induced hyponatremia • Generally initiated for babies >1 mo
Ciprofloxacin (Cipro)	Reported: 7–40 mg/kg/day div q12 hr	• Ciprofloxacin is not considered a first-line agent in the neonatal population secondary to reported adverse events related to joints and or surrounding tissues (cartilage in animals) • Reserved for documented multi-resistant aerobic gram-negative bacilli
Clindamycin (Cleocin)	<7 day and <2000 g: 5 mg/kg/dose i.v. q12 hr >2000g: 5 mg/kg/dose i.v. q8 hr >7 day: <1,200 g: 5 mg/kg/dose i.v. q12 hr 1200–2000 g: 5 mg/kg/dose i.v. q8 hr >2000g: 20–30 mg/kg/day i.v. div q6–8 hr	• Compatible with TPN • Infuse slowly over 30 min • Contains benzyl alcohol • Preferred agent for *mycoplasma hominis* cultured from endotracheal tube
Cloxacillin (Tegopen)	>1 month: 50–100 mg/kg/day p.o. div q6	• Use with MSSA (methicillin-sensitive staphylococcus aureus) • Oral antistaphylococcal penicillin
Colistimethate (Colistin)	2.5–5 mg/kg/day i.v. div q6–12 hr	• Restricted criteria at most institutions and may require approval by infectious disease specialist • Safety and efficacy in neonates has not been established. • Should be reserved for use for life-threatening infections caused by organisms resistant to traditional antimicrobials

(*continued*)

TABLE A1.1 Commonly Used Medications in a Newborn Intensive Care Unit (*Continued*)

Medication	*Dosage*	*Comments*
		• Adjust dose in renal impairment • Does NOT penetrate CSF • Monitor for nephrotoxicity and neurotoxicity
Cosyntropin (Cortrosyn)	0.015 mg/kg/dose i.v./i.m.	• Diagnostic agent for adrenocortical insufficiency • i.m. concentration 0.25 mg/mL • i.v.p.: administer in 2–5 mL of normal saline over 2 min
Cyclopentolate 1% (Cyclogyl Tropicamide)	ROP (retinopathy of prematurity examination): one drop into each eye 10–30 min prior to examination May repeat × one dose in 5 min	• Used in diagnostic procedures requiring mydriasis and cycloplegia • Monitor blood pressure and heart rate
Cysteine	40 mg cysteine per gram of amino acids (Trophamine) 3 g/kg/day of amino acids provide 120 mg/kg/day of cysteine	• Supplement to Trophamine amino acid solution • Monitor BUN, SCr, acid–base balance • MAX 120 mg/kg/day • Addition of cysteine to TPN solutions enhances the solubility of calcium and phosphate but can increase the need for acetate in the TPN
Desmopressin (DDAVP)	0.1 mg p.o. qday (range 0.1–0.5 mg p.o. qday per endocrinology) 5 mCg/day intranasally div one to two times/day (range 5–30 mCg/day)	• Treatment for diabetes insipidus • Crush tablet in Ora-sweet to make 0.1 mg/mL
Dexamethasone (Decadron)	Airway edema/extubation: 0.5–2 mg/kg/day i.v. div q6 for 4 doses (begin 24 hr prior to extubation) CLD (chronic lung disease): 0.5 mg/kg/day i.v. div q12 hr × 5 day Taper 0.3 mg/kg/day div q12 hr × 3 day 0.15 mg/kg/day div q12 hr × 3 day 0.07 mg/kg/day div q12 hr × 3 day	• Monitor BP, glucose metabolism, GI bleed, weight loss • Consider concomitant ranitidine therapy (total daily dose of ranitidine may be placed in TPN) • Use of dexamethasone is controversial in CLD and the AAP statement in Pediatrics February 2002 states "the routine use of systemic dexamethasone for the prevention or treatment of CLD in infants with VLBW is not recommended" and "current use of dexamethasone should be limited to infants on maximal ventilator and oxygen support" • Before treatment, the parents should be informed of the potential lifesaving benefit and the uncertain additional risk of neurological injury, and informed consent should be obtained

Glucocorticoid	*Approximate Equivalent Dose (mg)*
Short acting	
Hydrocortisone	20
Intermediate acting	
Methylprednisolone	4
Prednisolone	5
Prednisone	5
Long acting	
Dexamethasone	0.75

Medication	*Dosage*	*Comments*
Diazoxide (Proglycem)	10–15 mg/kg/day p.o. div q8–12 hr	• Inhibits pancreatic insulin release • For hypoglycemia due to hyperinsulinemia • Peak hyperglycemic effect within 1 hr
Dicloxacillin	25–50 mg/kg/day p.o. div q6 hr	• Monitor for elevated liver enzymes, thrombocytopenia, and eosinophilia
Osteomyelitis	50–100 mg/kg/day div q6 hr	• Food decreases rate and extent of absorption
Digoxin (Lanoxin)	(see table below)	• Give ½ TDD as initial dose, then ¼ TDD for two doses q6–12 hr • Adjust dose for renal impairment • Therapeutic range 0.8–2 ng/mL • Draw trough level just prior to next dose • Half-life: Preterm 61–70 hr Term 35–45 hr

	TDD (mCg/kg)		*Main Dose (mCg/kg)*	
	p.o.	*i.v.*	*p.o.*	*i.v.*
Preterm	20–30	15–25	5–7.5	4–6
Full-term	25–35	20–30	6–10	5–8

TDD, Total digitalizing dose

(*continued*)

TABLE A1.1 Commonly Used Medications in a Newborn Intensive Care Unit (*Continued*)

Medication	*Dosage*	*Comments*
Diltiazem (Cardizem)	1.5–2 mg/kg/day p.o. div t.i.d.–q.i.d.	• Management of paroxysmal supraventricular tachycardias (PSVT), atrial fibrillation, atrial flutter • i.v. form reserved as antiarrhythmic • Cytochrome P450 isoenzyme • Diltiazem may increase serum concentrations of carbamazepine, digoxin, and midazolam, and increase effect of fentanyl and rifampin.
Diphenhydramine (Benadryl)	5 mg/kg/day p.o./i.v. div q6–8 hr	• Additive sedative when given concomitantly with other CNS depressants
Dobutamine	2–20 mCg/kg/min i.v. continuous titrate to response	• Std continuous concentrations: 0.8 mg/mL, 1.6 mg/mL, 3.2 mg/mL • Compatible with TPN • Half-life = 2 minutes • DO NOT infuse through UAC • Stimulates β1 adrenergic receptors and increases heart rate, increases contractility • Little effect on β2 or alpha receptors • Treat extravasations with phentolamine • Consider double-concentrating infusion drip especially in the ELBW neonate to minimize volume occupied by continuous drip infusions

Desired dose (mCg/kg/min)	*Rate (mL/hour) = Factor × Weight (kg) Concentration*		
	0.8 mg/mL	*1.6 mg/mL*	*3.2 mg/mL*
2	0.15	0.075	0.037
3	0.225	0.112	0.056
4	0.3	0.15	0.075
5	0.375	0.187	0.093
6	0.45	0.225	0.112
7	0.525	0.262	0.131
8	0.6	0.3	0.15
9	0.675	0.337	0.169
10	0.75	0.375	0.188
11	0.825	0.412	0.206
12	0.9	0.45	0.225
13	0.975	0.487	0.243
14	1.05	0.525	0.262
15	1.125	0.562	0.281
16	1.2	0.6	0.3
17	1.275	0.637	0.319
18	1.35	0.675	0.338
19	1.425	0.712	0.356
20	1.5	0.75	0.375

Medication	*Dosage*	*Comments*
Dopamine	5–20 mCg/kg/min i.v. continuous Titrate to response	• Standard2 continuous concentrations: 0.8 mg/mL, 1.6 mg/mL, 3.2 mg/mL • SEE above table for quick rate calculation • Half-life = 2 minutes • DO NOT infuse through UAC • Treat extravasation with phentolamine • LOW DOSE: Stimulates dopaminergic receptors—renal and mesenteric vasodilatation • INTERMEDIATE DOSE: Stimulates both dopaminergic and β1 adrenergic ↑HR/Clearance • HIGH DOSE: Stimulates α-adrenergic receptors; ↑BP and vasoconstriction
Enalapril (Vasotec)	0.1 mg/kg/day p.o. q24 hr 5–10 mCg/kg/dose i.v. q8–24 hr	• Injection contains benzyl alcohol as preservative • Use with caution in preterm neonates • Adjust dose in renal impairment • Indicated for mild–severe hypertension, CHF, and asymptomatic left ventricular dysfunction

(*continued*)

TABLE A1.1 Commonly Used Medications in a Newborn Intensive Care Unit (*Continued*)

<table>
<tr><th>Medication</th><th>Dosage</th><th>Comments</th></tr>
<tr><td>Enoxaparin (Lovenox)</td><td>Prophylaxis: 0.75 mg/kg/dose s.c. q12 hr
Treatment: 1.5 mg/kg/dose s.c. q12 hr</td><td>
<ul>
<li>Treatment or prophylaxis of thromboembolic disorders</li>
<li>Potentiates the action of antithrombin III and inactivates coagulation factor Xa.</li>
<li>Monitor: CBC, platelets, stool occult tests, and other signs of excessive bleeding or bruising</li>
<li>Closely monitor platelet decreases of <100,000 or >50% from baseline</li>
<li>Required therapeutic doses as high as 2.5 mg/kg/dose s.c. q12 reported in literature for preterm neonates</li>
<li>Can be reversed with protamine but not completely; only 60%–75% of aXa activity can be reversed</li>
<li>Monitor antifactor Xa levels:</li>
</ul>
<table>
<tr><th>aXa Level</th><th>Level Interpretation</th><th>When to Repeat Levels</th></tr>
<tr><td><0.35 units/mL</td><td>↑ dose by 25%</td><td>4 hr after next dose</td></tr>
<tr><td>0.35–0.49 units/mL</td><td>↑ dose by 10%</td><td>4 hr after next dose</td></tr>
<tr><td>0.5–1 units/mL</td><td>Continue same dose</td><td>Next day, repeat in 1 wk, and then every month</td></tr>
<tr><td>1.1–1.5 units/mL</td><td>↓ dose by 20%</td><td>Before next dose</td></tr>
<tr><td>1.6–2 units/mL</td><td>Hold dose for 3 hr and then ↓ dose by 30%</td><td>Before next dose, then 4 hr after next dose</td></tr>
<tr><td>>2 units/mL</td><td>Hold doses until aXa level is ≤0.5 units/mL and then decrease dose by 40%</td><td>Before next dose and every 12 hr until level <0.5 units/mL</td></tr>
</table>
Adapted from Mongale Chalmers E, Chan A, DeVeber G, Kirkham F, Massicotte P, Michelson AD. Antithrombotic therapy in neonates and children: American College of Chest Physicians Evidence-Based Clinical Practice Guidelines (8th Edition). Chest 2008;133:887S–968S.
</td></tr>
<tr><td>Epinephrine</td><td>Bradycardia:
0.01 mg/kg/dose i.v. 0.03 mg/kg/dose intratracheal
(0.1–0.3 mL/kg/dose using 1:10,000 concentration)
May repeat every 3–5 min as needed.
Hypotension (inotrope):
0.05–1 mCg/kg/min. Titrate dose to desired effect</td><td>
<ul>
<li>Std continuous concentrations: 1 mg/100 mL, 5 mg/100 mL</li>
<li>Half-life = 2 minutes</li>
<li>DO NOT infuse through UAC</li>
<li>Treat extravasation with phentolamine</li>
</ul>
</td></tr>
</table>

(*continued*)

TABLE A1.1 Commonly Used Medications in a Newborn Intensive Care Unit (*Continued*)

Medication	*Dosage*	*Comments*
	(see rate table below)	
Erythromycin	10 mg/kg/dose i.v./p.o. q6 hr Ethylsuccinate: for chlamydial conjunctivitis and pneumonia: 12.5 mg/kg/dose p.o. q6 hr × 14 day	• Compatible with TPN • Reduces theophylline clearance; monitor levels
Erythropoietin (Epogen)	50–200 units/kg/dose s.c. q. MWF Or 100 units/kg/dose s.c. 5 times/wk Or 200 units/kg/dose s.c. every other day for 10 doses i.v. route requires an increase of 30%–50% of dose	• Supplement with iron concurrently to provide for increased requirements during expansion of red cell mass
Esmolol (Brevibloc)	SVT Loading dose: 100–500 mCg/kg over 1 min Maintenance dose: 200 mCg/kg/min Titrate 50–100 mCg/kg/min q5–10 min (range: 300–1,000 mCg/kg/min)	• Standard continuous concentrations: 5 mg/mL, 10 mg/mL, 20 mg/mL • Class II antiarrhythmic for SVT • Blocks response to β1-adrenergic stimulation • Use in extreme caution in patients with hyperreactive airway disease • DO NOT administer through UAC line
Fentanyl (Sublimaze)	Sedation/analgesia: 1–4 mCg/kg/dose q2–4 hr Continuous: 0.5–2 mCg/kg bolus, then 0.5–1 mCg/kg/hr	• Standard continuous concentrations 5 mCg/mL, 10 mCg/mL, 40 mCg/mL • Compatible with TPN • Adjust dose in renal failure • Reverse with naloxone • Slow i.v.p. over 3–5 min to prevent chest wall rigidity • Less histamine effect (more suitable in CLD with less airway narrowing • Less GI motility impairment, less urinary retention Decreases peripheral vascular resistance which is potentially useful in PPHN

Rate (mL/hour) = Factor × Weight (kg)

Desired dose (mCg/kg/min)	Concentration 0.01 mg/mL	0.05 mg/mL
0.05	0.3	0.06
0.1	0.6	0.12
0.15	0.9	0.18
0.2	1.2	0.24
0.25	1.5	0.3
0.3	1.8	0.36
0.35	2.1	0.42
0.4	2.4	0.48
0.45	2.7	0.54
0.5	3	0.6
0.55	3.3	0.66
0.6	3.6	0.72
0.65	3.9	0.78
0.7	4.2	0.84
0.75	4.5	0.9
0.8	4.8	0.96
0.85	5.1	1.02
0.9	5.4	1.08
0.95	5.7	1.14
1	6	1.2

Fentanyl: Rate (mL/hr) Factor × Weight (kg)

Dose desired (mCg/kg/hour)	Concentration 5 mCg/mL	10 mCg/mL
0.5	0.1	0.05
1	0.2	0.1
2	0.4	0.2
3	0.6	0.3
4	0.8	0.4
5	1	0.5

(*continued*)

TABLE A1.1 Commonly Used Medications in a Newborn Intensive Care Unit (*Continued*)

<table>
<tr><th>Medication</th><th>Dosage</th><th>Comments</th></tr>
<tr><td>Ferrous Sulfate (Fer-in-sol)</td><td>2–4 mg elemental iron/kg/day div q12–24 hr
Max 15 mg/day = 0.6 mL/day</td><td>• Fer-in-sol contains 25 mg elemental iron/mL
• Delaying initiating iron supplementation for infant until 1 mo of age since oral iron may reduce vitamin E absorption
• Iron fortified formulas contain 12-mg iron/L providing approximately 2 mg/kg/day</td></tr>
<tr><td>Filgrastim (Neupogen)</td><td>5–10 mCg/kg/day i.v./s.c. once daily for 3–5 days</td><td>• For neutropenic neonates with sepsis
• Discontinue filgrastim when ANC >1,000/mm^3 for 3 day
• ANC = (neutrophils + bands) (WBC × 10)</td></tr>
<tr><td>Fluconazole (Diflucan)</td><td>Systemic fungal infection:
10 mg/kg/dose i.v./p.o. qday (higher dose up to 12 mg/kg/day for Candida parapsilosis or with CNS involvement)
Prophylaxis regimen at Hutzel Women's Hospital:
3 mg/kg/dose i.v./p.o.
<table>
<tr><th>Postmenstrual Age (wk)</th><th>Postnatal Age (d)</th><th>Dosing Interval (hr)</th></tr>
<tr><td>≤29</td><td>0–14</td><td>72</td></tr>
<tr><td></td><td>>14</td><td>48</td></tr>
<tr><td>30–36</td><td>0–14</td><td>48</td></tr>
<tr><td></td><td>>14</td><td>24</td></tr>
<tr><td>37–44</td><td>0–7</td><td>48</td></tr>
<tr><td></td><td>>7</td><td>24</td></tr>
<tr><td>≥45</td><td>>0</td><td>24</td></tr>
</table></td><td>• Second-line agent at our institution for infections with Candida species after persistent positive blood culture taken at 48–72 hr while on lipid complex amphotericin b (ABLC)
• DO NOT use fluconazole for Candida krusei
• Monitor liver enzymes
• Adjust for renal failure
• Oral bioavailability >90%
• Prophylaxis regimen provides targeted short-term fluconazole prophylaxis for VLBW infants at greatest risk for invasive fungal infections (IFI) during periods of broadspectrum antibiotic administration
• Criteria for prophylaxis: <1,500 g, <6 wk postnatal AND with one of the following:
central venous access
parenteral nutrition
endotracheal intubation
history of necrotizing enterocolitis</td></tr>
<tr><td>Flucytosine Ancobon</td><td>25–100 mg/kg/day div q12–24 hr</td><td>• Therapeutic level: 25–100 mCg/mL
• Draw level 2 hr postdose on or after day 4
• Good CNS penetration
• Not to be used as monotherapy
• Monitor liver enzymes, bone marrow suppression, BUN, SCr, and crystalluria</td></tr>
<tr><td>Flumazenil (Romazicon)</td><td>0.01 mg/kg i.v. over 15 s; repeat every minute for cumulative dose of 0.05 mg/kg or total of 1 mg whichever is lower</td><td>• Treatment of benzodiazepine overdose
• Onset of action within 1–3 min</td></tr>
<tr><td>Fosphenytoin (Cerebyx)</td><td>Loading dose for status epilepticus:
15–20 mg PE/kg i.v. over 10 min
Maintenance dose:
4–6 mg PE/kg/day i.v.</td><td>• DOSE expressed as phenytoin sodium equivalents (PE)
• Phenytoin 1 mg = fosphenytoin 1 mg PE
• MAX 3 mg/PE/kg/min
• Monitor phenytoin serum concentrations</td></tr>
<tr><td>Furosemide (Lasix)</td><td>1–2 mg/kg/dose q12–24 hr i.v./p.o./i.m.</td><td>• Monitor electrolytes
• Poor oral bioavailability
• Compatible with TPN</td></tr>
<tr><td>Ganciclovir (Cytovene)</td><td>Congenital CMV infections:
6 mg/kg/day i.v. q12 hr for 6 wk</td><td>• Congenital CMV infections as recommended by infectious disease specialist and manifests with hearing loss and learning disabilities
• CMV IgM (+) indicates current/recent exposure
• Adjust dose in renal failure
• Monitor CBC, platelets, urine output, SCr, and liver enzymes
• Handle and dispose of as chemotherapeutic agent</td></tr>
</table>

(*continued*)

TABLE A1.1 Commonly Used Medications in a Newborn Intensive Care Unit (*Continued*)

Medication	*Dosage*	*Comments*
Gentamicin	Hutzel women's hospital regimen for early onset sepsis (<7 days) <1200 g: 3 mg/kg/dose i.v. q36 hr 1,200–2,000 g: 3 mg/kg/dose i.v. q24 hr >2,000 g: 3.5 mg/kg/dose i.v. q24 hr Postnatal age >7–10 days <1200 g: 3–4 mg/kg/dose i.v. q24 hr 1,200–2,000 4 mg/kg./dose i.v. q24 hr >2,000 g: 4–5 mg/kg/dose i.v. q24 hr	• Therapeutic level • Peak 6–12 mCg/mL • Trough 0.5–1.2 mCg/mL • Concentration dependent killing • Desired peak level = Eight times MIC • Target synergy dose is 1.5 mg/kg/dose • Target synergy peak level is 3–4 mCg/mL
Glucagon	Hypoglycemia: 0.02–0.03 mg/kg i.v./i.m. × one dose. May repeat × one dose in 20 min if needed	• Dilute with manufacturer-provided diluent to final concentration of 1 mg/mL
Glycopyrrolate (Robinul)	p.o. 40–100 mCg/kg/dose 3–4 times a day i.m./i.v. 4–10 mCg/kg/dose q3–4 hr	• Decreases oral secretions • Oral absorption is poor • Contains benzyl alcohol as preservative and should therefore be used with caution in neonates when given parenterally
Heparin flush	10 Units q24 hr as heparin flush for CVC (Broviac) catheter	• See attached guideline on use of heparin to maintain line patency in the neonatal intensive care unit
Heparin	Loading dose 75 units/kg over 10 minutes Maintenance Dose 28 units/kg/hr Adjust to APTT of 60–85 seconds (see APTT adjustment table below)	• Standard continuous concentrations: 10 units/mL, 50 units/mL, 100 unit/mL • Treatment of thrombosis • Obtain APTT 4 hr after initiation of infusion and every 4 hr after infusion rate change • Monitor for signs of bleeding • Contraindicated in IVH, GI bleed, platelets <50,000 • Adapted from Mongale Chalmers E, Chan A, DeVeber G, Kirkham F, Massicotte P, Michelson AD. Antithrombotic therapy in neonates and children: American College of Chest Physicians Evidence-Based Clinical Practice Guidelines (8th Edition). *Chest* 2008;133:887S–968S

APTT (seconds)	*Dose Adjustment*	*Time to Repeat APTT*
<50	50 units/kg bolus, increase infusion rate by 10%	4 hr after infusion change
50–59	Increase infusion rate 10%	4 hr after infusion change
60–85	Continue same rate	4 hr after infusion change
86–95	Decrease infusion rate 10%	4 hr after infusion change
96–120	Hold infusion 30 min; then ↓ infusion rate by 10%	4 hr after infusion change
>120	Hold infusion 60 min; then ↓ infusion rate by 15%	4 hr after infusion change

Medication	*Dosage*	*Comments*
Homatropine (Ispoto-Homatropine) 2%	Uveitis: One drop two to three times a day into affected eye(s)	• Anticholinergic agent producing cycloplegia and mydriasis
Hyaluronidase (Amphadase)	Inject 150 units (1 mL) divided as five separate 0.2 mL subcutaneous/intradermal injections around the periphery of the extravasation site at the leading edge	• See attached guideline on the management of neonatal extravasations • Initiate immediately and ideally within 1 hr of extravasation • Initiate for Stage III/IV infiltrate • Do not inject intravenously
Hydralazine (Apresoline)	0.1–0.2 mg/kg/dose i.v. q6–8 hr Maximum 3.5 mg/kg/day i.v. 0.25–1 mg/kg/dose p.o. q6–8 hr Maximum 5 mg/kg/day p.o.	• Low bioavailability when given orally

(*continued*)

TABLE A1.1 Commonly Used Medications in a Newborn Intensive Care Unit (*Continued*)

Medication	*Dosage*	*Comments*
Hydrocortisone (Solu-cortef)	Hypotension: 2 mg/kg i.v. × 1 dose then 1 mg/kg/dose i.v. q6 hr Anti-inflammatory or immunosuppressive: 1–5 mg/kg/day i.v. Chronic lung disease (CLD): 0.5 mg/kg/dose i.v. q6 hr × 3 days, then 0.5 mg/kg/dose i.v. q8 hr × 3 days, then 0.5 mg/kg/dose i.v. q12 hr × 3 days, then 0.5 mg/kg/dose i.v. q24 hr × 1 day (total cumulative dose: 14 mg/kg over 10 days) OR 0.5 mg/kg/dose i.v. q12 hr for 12 days, then 0.25 mg/kg/dose i.v. q12 hr for 3 days (total cumulative dose: 13.5 mg/kg over 15 days)	• Third-line agent for treatment of hypotension in neonates not responding to inotropes for a short-course therapy (up to 5 days) • Studies have shown that preterm neonates with critical cardiovascular compromise will respond to hydrocortisone treatment; evidence that VLBW neonates have impaired cortisol production in response to stress or endogenous or exogenous corticotropin • Extended therapy will require slow tapering • Monitor for edema, hypokalemia, hyperglycemia, growth suppression, suppression of HPA function • Physiologic replacement doses of hydrocortisone are approximately 14 mg/m^2/days in the neonate • Corticosteroids may facilitate extubation in ventilator-dependent neonates with established or evolving BPD • Early, low-dose hydrocortisone treatment does not appear to be associated with increased cerebral palsy. • Before treatment, the parents should be informed of the potential life-saving benefit and the uncertain additional risk of neurological injury, and informed consent should be obtained
Ibuprofen (Motrin, Advil)	Analgesic: 4–10 mg/kg/dose p.o. q6– 8 hr MAX 40 mg/kg/day Intravenous (For PDA treatment): Neonates 500–1500 g and ≤32 wk gestational age Initial dose of 10 mg/kg/dose i.v. × one dose followed by 5 mg/kg/dose i.v. q24 hr × 2 doses (three-dose course)	• Analgesic/antipyretic • Use with caution with impaired renal or hepatic function • Criteria for initiation of treatment in patent ductus arteriosus (PDA): Echo confirmation of PDA with left-to-right shunting, check IVH status, check urine output and serum creatinine, check platelet count • Hold subsequent intravenous dose if urine output decreases to less than 0.6 mL/kg/hr • A second course of treatment may be given if the ductus arteriosus fails to close or reopens • Infuse through dedicated line over 15 min • Monitor BUN, SCr, platelets, urine output • Contraindications: active bleeding, significant thrombocytopenia (platelets <60K), BUN > 30, SCr >1.4, urine output < 1 mL/kg/hour coagulation defects, necrotizing enterocolitis
Imipenem/cilastatin (Primaxin)	0–4 wk, <1200 g : 20 mg/kg/dose i.v. q18–24 hr </= to 7 days: 1200–1500 g: 20 mg/kg/dose iv q12 hr </= to 7 days: >1500 g: 25 mg/kg/dose iv q12 hr >7 day 1,200–1,500 g: 20 mg/kg/dose i.v. q12 hr >1,500 g: 25 mg/kg/dose i.v. q8 hr 1–3 months: 25 mg/kg/dose iv q6 hrs	• Restricted criteria at most institutions and may require approval by a infectious disease specialist • Reserved for more serious or refractory gram-negative infections with documented resistance to all other β-lactams • Monitor for seizures • Dose adjust in renal impairment
i.v. immune globulin (IVIG)	500–1000 mg/kg/dose i.v. for one dose over 2–6 hr	• Infuse via dedicated line • Restricted criteria at most institutions: Neonatal platelet alloimmunization May require approval by hematology disease specialist

(*continued*)

TABLE A1.1 Commonly Used Medications in a Newborn Intensive Care Unit (*Continued*)

Medication	*Dosage*	*Comments*
Indomethacin (Indocin)	Treatment of PDA: (i.v.): *Age at First Dose* / *Dose #1* / *Dose #2* / *Dose #3* <48 hr: 0.2 mg/kg, 0.1 mg/kg, 0.1 mg/kg 2–7 day: 0.2 mg/kg, 0.2 mg/kg, 0.2 mg/kg >7 day: 0.2 mg/kg, 0.25 mg/kg, 0.25 mg/kg Dosing regimen q12 hr. Consider q24 regimen in the ELBW neonate or with urine output < 1 mL/kg/hr.	• Change to q24 in the ELBW neonate or if urine output <1 mL/kg/hr • Decreases renal and GI blood flow • Hold dose with oliguria UO <0.6 mL/kg/hr • Monitor BUN, SCr, platelets, urine output • Incompatible with TPN and lipids • Use immediately after reconstitution • Indomethacin is tightly bound to albumin and may displace bilirubin • Contraindicated: active bleeding, significant thrombocytopenia (platelets <60K), BUN > 30 SCr >1.6 (as high as 1.8 reported), coagulation defects, NEC • Do not administer via UAC.
Insulin (Insulin R)	0.05–0.2 units/kg/hr continuous intravenous infusions 0.05–0.2 units/kg subcutaneously q6–12 hr	• Standard continuous concentrations: 0.5 units/mL, or 1 unit/mL • Use for persistent glucose intolerance in ELBW • Compatible with or in TPN • Preterm infants are insulin resistant • Treatment for hyperkalemia requires glucose load of 5 mg/kg/min • Flush approximately 10 mL through tubing to saturate binding sites of tubing • Will require multiple dilutions for dose preparation in the ELBW neonate
Insulin, aspart (Novolog)	0.05–0.2 units/kg subcutaneously q6–12 hr	• High-alert medication • Rapid acting insulin • Will require multiple dilutions for dose preparation in the ELBW neonate
Iron dextran	Anemia of prematurity: 0.4–1 mg/kg/day i.v. continuous infusion (in total parenteral nutrition) With (concomitant) erythropoietin therapy: 20 mg/kg/wk i.v.	• Can be added to TPN • Will discolor TPN (rust color) • Monitor for rust color precipitates
Isoniazid	Treatment: 10–15 mg/kg/days p.o. daily or divided q12 hr Prophylaxis: 10 mg/kg/day p.o. once a day	• Monitor liver enzymes • Cytochrome P450 inhibitor—may increase concentrations of phenytoin, carbamazepine, and diazepam
Isoproterenol	0.05–2 mCg/kg/min	• Standard continuous concentrations: 20 mCg/mL, 40 mCg/mL • Do not administer through UAC • Indicated for ventricular arrhythmia secondary to AV nodal block
Lansoprazole (Prevacid)	0.7–1.66 mg/kg/dose p.o. once daily	• Incompatible with TPN
Levothyroxine (Synthroid)	10–15 mCg/kg/day p.o. 5–8 mCg/kg/day i.v.	• Administer i.v. dose immediately after reconstitution • Give oral dose on empty stomach • IV dose = 50–75% of oral dose
Lidocaine 1%	2–5 mg/kg subcutaneously 0.5–1 mg/kg endotracheally	• Use subcutaneously for ring or nerve blocks • Consider adding sodium bicarbonate to buffer lidocaine to decrease pain • Lidocaine also available as topical spray
Lidocaine/prilocaine (EMLA)	Topical agent: 0.5–2 g under occlusive dressing 1 hr prior to procedure (1 g = 1 mL)	• Apply 2 g = 2 mL for term infants and 0.5 g = 0.5 mL for preterm infants • Appears safe in preterm infants when applied in small amounts once daily

(*continued*)

TABLE A1.1 Commonly Used Medications in a Newborn Intensive Care Unit (*Continued*)

Medication	*Dosage*	*Comments*
Linezolid (Zyvox)	10 mg/kg/dose i.v./po q8 hr (Use q12 hr in neonates <1,200 g and <7 days)	• Restricted criteria at most institutions and may require approval by an infectious disease specialist • Reserved for documented vancomycin-resistant *enterococcus* (VRE) or documented infection with vancomycin-resistant *Staph aureus* or vancomycin-resistant *coagulase-negative staph* • Monitor CBC/platelets for pancytopenia; ALT, optic neuropathy (long-term treatment), renal function • Enhanced vasopressor effects (dopamine, epinephrine) when given concomitantly with linezolid • Oral bioavailability 100%
Loperamide Imodium	0.08–0.24 mg/kg/day p.o. div b.i.d.–t.i.d. MAX 2 mg/dose	• Acts directly on intestinal muscles to inhibit peristalsis and prolong transit time • Used in neonates with high output stoma post small bowel resections • May increase risk of bacterial overgrowth • Use caution in hepatic dysfunction
Lorazepam (Ativan)	Status Epilepticus: 0.05 mg/kg i.v. over 2–5 min May repeat in 10–15 min Anxiety/sedation 0.05–0.1 mg/kg/dose i.v.p. q4–8 hr	• Preparation contains benzyl alcohol and therefore use with caution especially in preterm infants due to neurotoxicity and myoclonus • Dilute with sterile water 1:1 prior to infusion • Should be infused in a dedicated line (drug compatibility issues) • Incompatible with TPN • Slow i.v.p. over 2 min
Magnesium sulfate	Hypomagnesemia: 25–50 mg/kg/dose **magnesium sulfate i.v.** q8–12 hr for 2–3 doses Infuse slowly over 2–4 hr	• 25–50 mg/kg/dose magnesium sulfate = 0.2–0.4 mEq magnesium/kg/dose • 1 g of magnesium sulfate = 98.6 mg **elemental** magnesium = 8.12 mEq magnesium • Do not exceed 1 mEq/kg/hr
Medium-chain triglyceride (MCT oil)	Supplement with feeding to add an additional 10 kcal/kg/day Preterm Neonates: 0.2–0.3 mL per feed (every 3 hr)	• Medium chain triglycerides are composed of fatty acids with chain length varying from 6–12 carbon atoms • 1 mL = 7.7 calories • DOES NOT provide any essential fatty acids since it contains ONLY saturated fats
Meropenem (Meropenem)	Postnatal 0–7 days: 20 mg/kg/dose i.v. q12 hr Postnatal >7 days: 1,200–2,000 g: 20 mg/kg/dose i.v. q12 hr >2,000 g: 20 mg/kg/dose i.v. q8 hr	• Restricted criteria at most institutions and may require approval by an infectious disease specialist • Treatment of multidrug–resistant gram-negative and gram-positive aerobic and anaerobic pathogens • Safety and efficacy in children <3 mo of age have not been established • Adjust dose in renal impairment
Methadone	Neonatal abstinence syndrome: 0.05–0.2 mg/kg/dose i.v./p.o. q12–24 hr Taper dose by 10%–20%/wk	• Extended elimination half-life and therefore difficult to taper doses. Consider alternative agents • Cytochrome P-450 isoenzyme substrate • Carbamazepine, phenytoin, nevirapine, nelfinavir, and rifampin may increase the metabolism of methadone and precipitate withdrawal • Methadone may increase zidovudine serum concentrations

(*continued*)

TABLE A1.1 Commonly Used Medications in a Newborn Intensive Care Unit (*Continued*)

Medication	*Dosage*	*Comments*
Methylprednisolone (Solu-medrol)	Status asthmaticus: 2 mg/kg i.v. × one loading dose, then 1 mg/kg/dose i.v. q6 hr	• ONLY sodium succinate salt can be given intravenously (i.v.) • Short-course burst in preterm neonates for 5 days to assist in weaning off the ventilator when settings are no longer weanable and oxygenation not maintained
Metoclopramide (Reglan)	0.1–0.2 mg/kg/dose i.v./p.o. q6 hr	• Monitor for extrapyramidal reactions: tardive dyskinesia, dystonia • Potent dopamine receptor antagonist • Increases gastric emptying time
Metronidazole (Flagyl)	0–4 wk, <1,200 g: 7.5 mg/kg/dose i.v. q48 hr <7 days, <2 kg 7.5 mg/kg i.v. q24 hr <7 days, >2 kg 7.5 mg/kg i.v. q12 hr >7 days, <2 kg 7.5 mg/kg i.v. q12 hr >7 days, >2 kg 15 mg/kg i.v. q12 hr	• Do not refrigerate since precipitation may occur • Use with caution in patients with liver impairment
Micafungin (Mycamine)	10 mg/kg/dose i.v. qd (based on preliminary pharmacokinetic data)	• Restricted criteria at most institutions and may require approval by an infectious disease specialist • At Hutzel women's hospital: Add a third agent (echinocandin) for infections with all *Candida* species if: persistent fungemia, repeat blood culture taken at 48–72 hr remain positive despite combination therapy with ampho B lipid complex (ABLC) and fluconazole • Appears that neonates have increased clearance requiring a higher dose • Monitor CBC, platelets, liver enzymes, and bilirubin levels • No adjustment required in renal impairment
Midazolam (Versed)	0.05–0.15 mg/kg slow i.v.p. q2–4 hr 0.1–0.3 mg/kg/dose intranasal 0.15–0.45 mg/kg/dose ORALLY Continuous infusion: Initial 0.03–0.06 mg/kg/hr = 0.5–1 mCg/kg/min).	• Standard continuous concentrations: 0.5 mg/mL, 1 mg/mL, and 5 mg/mL • Sedative/hypnotic • NO analgesic properties • Use preservative free vials
Milrinone (Primacor)	Loading dose: 50 mCg/kg i.v. over 15 min Maintenance dose: 0.5 mCg/kg/min (reported range: 0.25–1 mCg/kg/min)	• Standard continuous concentrations: 0.1 mg/mL, 0.2 mg/mL • Inhibits PDE III which increase cAMP • Short-term treatment of acute decompensated heart failure. • Incompatible with furosemide • Use caution in renal dysfunction
Morphine sulfate	0.05–0.2 mg/kg/dose i.v.p./s.c./i.m. q4 hr p.r.n. 0.15–0.6 mg/kg p.o. q4 hr p.r.n. 0.03–0.1 mg/kg/dose p.o. q3–4 hr Continuous infusion: 0.01–0.03 mg/kg/hr = 10–30 mCg/kg/hr Neonatal abstinence syndrome: 0.04 mg/kg = 0.1 mL/kg p.o. q3–4 hr (reported range 0.03–0.1 mg/kg/dose) Increase dose by 0.02 mg/kg = 0.05 mL/kg per dose as needed until desired response is achieved Taper 10%–20% per day as tolerated	• Standard continuous concentrations: 0.2 mg/mL, 0.5 mg/mL • Monitor for respiratory depression, O_2 saturation, urinary retention, decreased bowel sounds • Continuous infusion for greater than 5 day will likely develop withdrawal with an abrupt discontinuation • Use preservative-free product • Rate of morphine elimination is much slower in the neonate due to decrease in clearance rates resulting in higher serum concentrations

(*continued*)

TABLE A1.1 Commonly Used Medications in a Newborn Intensive Care Unit (*Continued*)

Medication	*Dosage*	*Comments*
Multivitamin (Poly-Vi-Sol) (AquaADEK)	Term infant: 1 mL/day Preterm infant: 1 mL/day div q6–12 hr	• AquaDEKs multivitamin drops differ from Poly-Vi-Sol in terms of a higher concentration of vitamin A, C, E, B_6, B_{12}, and vitamin C. ADEK also contain 400 mCg vitamin K, 15 mCg biotin, 5 mg zinc, 3 mg β-carotene, niacin, pantothenic acid, selenium, β-carotene, and coenzyme Q10.
Nafcillin	0–4 wk, <1,200 g: 25–50 mg/kg/dose q8–12 hr </= 7 days, 1200–2000 g: 25 mg/kg/dose iv q12 hrs </= 7 days, >2000 g: 25 mg/kg/dose iv q8 hrs > 7 days, 1200–2000 g: 25 mg/kg/dose iv q8 hrs > 7 days, >2000 g: 25 mg/kg/dose iv q6 hrs	• Use for methicillin sensitive *staphylococcus aureus* (MSSA). Use caution in severe hepatic impairment
Naloxone (Narcan)	0.1 mg/kg i.v./i.m./s.c. Repeat every 2–3 min as needed for recurrent apnea and hypoventilation	• Management of neonatal opioid-induced depression • Should be avoided in babies whose mothers are suspected of having had long-term exposure to opioids (Class indeterminate)
Nevirapine (Viramune)	Prevention of maternal-fetal HIV transmission: 2 mg/kg p.o. × one dose as a single dose at 2–3 days of age if mother received intrapartum single-dose of nevirapine or at birth if mother did NOT receive intrapartum single-dose of nevirapine	• 2007 Perinatal HIV Guideline Working Group • Nonnucleoside reverse transcriptase inhibitor • Use with 6-wk zidovudine prophylaxis to infant • Bioavailability >90% • 50 mg/5 mL oral suspension • Cytochrome P-450 isoenzyme substrate inducer and inhibitor • Look-alike, sound-alike medication: May be confused with nelfinavir (Viracept)
Nystatin	Oral candidiasis: 100,000 units p.o. q.i.d. (50,000 units to each side of cheek)	• Shake suspension well before use • Concentration: 100,000 units/mL
Octreotide (Sandostatin)	Persistent hyperinsulinemic hypoglycemia: 2–10 mCg/kg/day i.v. div q12 hr Increase dose per patient response MAX 40 mCg/kg/day Chylothorax: 0.5 – 4 mCg/kg/hr continuous infusion for 1–2 wk. Titrate to response Reported range: 0.3–4 mCg/kg/hr	• Only Sandostatin injection may be intravenously, intramuscularly, and subcutaneously • Dilute continuous infusion in 50–200 mL of dextrose 5% or normal saline
Omeprazole (Prilosec)	1 mg/kg/day once or twice daily p.o.	• Proton-pump inhibitor which decreases the acid produced in the stomach • Used in neonates for severe reflux
Opium tincture, diluted (Laudanum)	0.08–0.2 mg/dose p.o. q3–4 hr p.r.n. DO NOT CONFUSE WITH CAMPHORATED TINCTURE OF OPIUM (PAREGORIC)	• Treatment of neonatal narcotic abstinence • Initiate dose at 0.08 mg for term infants every 3 hr ATC; may be titrated to response slowly wean as tolerated • Monitor respiratory and cardiac status, abdominal distension and loss of bowel sounds, and decreased urine output
Oxacillin	0–4 wk, <1,200 g: 25 mg/kg/dose i.v. q12 hr <7 day: 1,200–2,000 g: 25–50 mg/kg/dose i.v. q12 hr > 2 kg: 25–50 mg/kg/dose i.v. q8 hr > 7 day: 1,200–2,000 g: 25–50 mg/kg/dose i.v. q8 hr >2,000 g: 25–50 mg/kg/dose i.v. q6 hr	• Monitor liver enzymes, bilirubin, CBC, BUN, SCr

(*continued*)

TABLE A1.1 Commonly Used Medications in a Newborn Intensive Care Unit (*Continued*)

Medication	*Dosage*	*Comments*
Pancuronium (Pavulon)	0.1 mg/kg i.v.p. q1 hr p.r.n. 0.02 – 0.04 mg/kg/hr (0.4–0.6 mCg/kg/min) continuous i.v. infusion	• Standard continuous concentrations: 0.1 mg/mL, 0.5 mg/mL • Monitor BP; infant must be intubated and sedated • Adjust in renal impairment • Continuous infusions are used rarely in the neonatal population when adequate and appropriate sedation is provided • Consider use of muscle relaxant to facilitate acute respiratory failure or hyperventilation ventilator management (PPHN) • Prolonged skeletal muscle paralysis in the preterm neonate is not advised
Penicillin G, aqueous	Proven or highly probably congenital syphilis: 50,000 Units/kg/dose i.v. q12 hr × 7 day, then 50,000 units/kg/dose i.v. q8 hr thereafter for a total of 10 days	• Compatible with TPN and lipid • 10-day treatment for congenital syphilis
Penicillin G benzathine	50,000 units/kg × one dose i.m.	• One dose i.m. only for asymptomatic congenital syphilis in neonates >1,200 g
Penicillin G procaine	50,000 units/kg/day i.m. q24 h × 10 days	• i.m. only • Use with caution in neonates due to procaine toxicity and sterile abscesses
Phenobarbital	Loading dose: 15–20 mg/kg/dose i.v./p.o. Maintenance dose: 5 mg/kg/day i.v./p.o. div q12 hr	• Therapeutic level: 15–40 mCg/mL • Half-life in neonates 45–200 hr • Obtain trough level just before next dose • May give additional 5 mg/kg boluses q15 min until seizure controlled. MAX 40 mg/kg
Phentolamine (Regitine)	Dilute 5 mg vial with 10 mL normal saline preservative free Administer 0.1 mL injections subcutaneously around the periphery of the extravasation site at the leading edge Do not exceed a maximum dose of 0.1 mg/kg or 2.5 mg total	• Use for extravasations with alpha-adrenergic drugs
Phenylephrine 2.5%	One drop 15–30 min prior to retinopathy of prematurity examination	• Use only the 2.5% ophthalmic solution in neonates • Apply pressure to the lacrimal sac postadministration to minimize systemic absorption

Phenytoin (Dilantin)	Loading dose:
	15–20 mg/kg i.v./p.o. × one dose
	Maintenance dose:
	5 mg/kg/day maintenance dose div q12 hr (reported range: 5–8 mg/kg/day)
		• Maximum infusion rate 0.5–1 mg/kg/min
		• Initiate maintenance dose 12 hr after loading dose
		• Therapeutic range: 8–15 mCg/mL
		• Therapeutic free (unbound) range: 1.5–2.5 mCg/mL (up to 20% free)
		• Oral loading doses should be divided in 2–3 doses q2 hr to ensure complete oral absorption
		• Monitor free and total serum concentrations in patients with hyperbilirubinemia, hypoalbuminemia, renal dysfunction, and uremia
		• Neonates have increased free fraction due to decreased protein binding
		• Follows dose-dependent Michaelis–Menten pharmacokinetics
		• Draw trough level just before next dose
		• Postload/peak: 1 hr after end of infusion
		• Give oral dose 2 hr before feeds if possible
		• Drug interactions:
		  • Phenytoin can decrease serum concentrations of theophylline, dopamine
		  • Phenytoin serum concentrations can be decreased by zidovudine, continuous nasogastric feeds

(*continued*)

TABLE A1.1 Commonly Used Medications in a Newborn Intensive Care Unit (*Continued*)

Medication	*Dosage*	*Comments*
Phosphate, Na/K	Low dose: 0.08 mmol/kg Intermediate dose: 0.16–0.24 mmol/kg For serum level 0.5–1 mg/dL High dose: 0.36 mmol/kg For serum level <0.5 mg/dL	• Infuse slowly over 1–2 hr (max: 0.06 mmol/kg/hr) • Peripheral line max concentration: 0.05 mmol/mL • Central line max concentration: 0.12 mmol/mL • Neonates are in positive phosphate balance and only 60% of phosphate absorbed from diet is excreted in the urine • High serum phosphate level in neonates is NOT a manifestation of a lower GFR rate but of a higher proximal tubular reabsorption capacity • Normal serum phosphate levels in a neonate are 4.8–8.2 mg/dL
Phytonadione (Vitamin K)	Hemorrhagic disease of newborn: 0.5 mg s.c./i.m., birth weight <1,500 g 1 mg s.c./i.m., birth weight >1,500 g	• Subcutaneous is the preferred route • Vitamin K deficiency due to malabsorption, decreased synthesis of vitamin K, and drug interactions
Piperacillin	≤7 days: 50 mg/kg/dose i.v. q8 hr > 7 days: 50 mg/kg/dose i.v. q6 hr	• Synergy with aminoglycosides • Adjust with renal dysfunction
Piperacillin/tazobactam (Zosyn)	150–300 mg/kg/day of piperacillin component i.v. div q6–8 hr	• Restricted criteria at most institutions and may require approval by an infectious disease specialist • Adjust dose for renal dysfunction • Tazobactam prevents degradation of piperacillin by binding to β-lactamases • Tazobactam component does not provide any additional coverage for *Pseudomonas aeruginosa*
Plasma protein fraction (Plasmanate)	10 mL/kg i.v. over 30–60 min. May repeat dose if needed	• Isotonic crystalloid solutions should be used first line (Neonatal Resuscitation guidelines 2005 states that an isotonic crystalloid rather than albumin is the solution of choice for volume expansion in the delivery room (Class IIb; LOE 7). • Avoid 25% concentration in preterm neonates because of increased risk for IVH
Poractant alfa (Curosurf)	Intratracheal: Initial dose: 2.5 mL/kg/dose (200 mg/kg/dose), then 1.25 mL/kg/dose (100 mg/kg/dose) q12 hr for up to two additional doses MAX 5 mL/kg	• Treatment of respiratory distress syndrome (RDS) in premature infants • Criteria: FiO2 >0.3 and MAP >7 • Unused AND unopened vials warmed to room temperature may be returned to refrigerator within 24 hr (warming: ONCE ONLY). • 80 mg/mL (1.5 mL, 3 mL)
Potassium supplements	0.5–1 mEq/kg/dose slow i.v. (Max 1 mEq/kg/hr) Hypokalemia secondary to diuretics: 1–2 mEq/kg/day p.o. daily or divided q12 hrs	• Infuse 0.3–0.5mEq/kg/hr (Max rate: 1 mEq/kg/hr) • MUST be diluted prior to i.v. administration • Peripheral line concentration: 0.08 mEq/mL • Central-line concentration 0.15 mEq/mL • p.o. formulation should also be diluted prior to administration • Normal daily requirement 2–6 mEq/kg/day

(*continued*)

TABLE A1.1 Commonly Used Medications in a Newborn Intensive Care Unit (*Continued*)

Medication	*Dosage*	*Comments*
Prednisolone	Asthma exacerbations: 1–2 mg/kg/day div b.i.d.	• Look-alike sound-alike medication; may be confused with PredniSONE
Prednisone	Asthma exacerbations 1–2 mg/kg/day div b.i.d.	• Look-alike sound-alike medication; may be confused with PrednisoLONE
Propranolol (Inderal)	0.25 mg/kg/dose p.o. q6–8 hr up to maximum of 5 mg/kg/day 0.01 mg/kg slow i.v.p. over 10 min. Repeat every 6–8 hr up to maximum of 0.15 mg/kg/dose i.v. q6–8 hr	• Do not abruptly discontinue therapy. Taper over 2 wk • Cytochrome P-450 isoenzyme and substrate
Prostaglandin E1 (Alprostadil) (Prostin VR)	0.05–0.1 mCg/kg/min (up to 0.4 mCg/kg/min has been reported) *Final Concentration* — *Rate Calculation [Multiply Factor × Wt (kg)]* 5 mCg/mL — 0.6–1.2 mL/kg/hr 10 mCg/mL — 0.3–0.6 mL/kg/hr	• Maximum 0.4 mCg/kg/min • Std continuous concentrations: 5 mCg/mL, 10 mCg/mL • Monitor for apnea, hypocalcemia, hypoglycemia, and hypokalemia • Infuse through UVC at ductal opening • Therapeutic response indicated with increase in pH and increase with systemic blood pressure. Once stable the rate may be decreased by 50% • Long-term use of prostaglandin E1 can lead to gastric outlet obstructions, cortical hyperostosis • Observe closely for extravasations secondary to high osmolarity
Pyridoxine (vitamin B_6)	Pyridoxine-depended seizures: 10–100 mg p.o./i.m./i.v.	• Prevention and treatment of pyridoxine-dependent seizures in infants
Ranitidine (Zantac)	< 2 wk: 1 mg/kg/dose i.v./p.o. q12 hr >1 mo: 2–4 mg/kg/day i.v. div q6–8 hr 2–4 mg/kg/day p.o. div q12 hr Continuous: 0.0625 mg/kg/hr (range 0.04–0.1 mg/kg/hr)	• Compatible with TPN and lipids • Safety and effectiveness of use in neonates less than 1 month has not been established • Use with caution when thrombocytopenia present • H2 blocker use as been associated with late onset sepsis and NEC. It should be discontinued as soon as possible • There is wide variability among institutions in patterns of use of ranitidine and other similar medications. Randomized-controlled trials are needed to develop a consistent evidence-based approach • Dose adjust in renal impairment
Rifampin (Rifadin)	10–20 mg/kg/day p.o./i.v. div q12 hr	• Causes red/orange discoloration of body secretions • Used with vancomycin for synergy for *staphylococcal* infections • Slow i.v. over 30 min • May need to increase dose of theophylline, digoxin if given concomitantly • Monitor liver enzymes, CBC, bilirubin, platelets
Sildenafil (Revatio)	Pulmonary hypertension: 0.25–1 mg/kg/dose p.o. q6–12 hr (Wide range of doses has been reported. Further studies are needed to determine optimal dose in the neonatal population)	• Phosphodiesterase Type-5 (PDE5) inhibitor • Monitor blood pressure closely due to vasodilator effects • Monitor platelets, ROP (retinopathy of prematurity), loss of hearing • Cytochrome P450 isoenzyme and substrate
Silver sulfadiazine (Silvadene)	Apply once or twice daily	• Acts on bacterial cell wall and cell membrane

(*continued*)

TABLE A1.1 Commonly Used Medications in a Newborn Intensive Care Unit (*Continued*)

Medication	*Dosage*	*Comments*
Sodium bicarbonate	HCO_3 needed (mEq) = Base deficit (mEq/L) × 0.3 × Wt (kg)	• Maximum concentration 0.5 mEq/mL • Infuse through dedicated line and monitor closely for extravasation • Tissue necrosis can occur due to the hyperosmolarity of sodium bicarbonate. (4.2% = 0.5 mEq/mL = 900 mOsm/L) • Not compatible with calcium or any calcium-containing solution. Immediate precipitation will result • Not compatible with TPN • Administer slowly at max rate of 10 mEq/min or 1 mEq/kg/hr
Sodium chloride	Correction of hyponatremia: mEq sodium needed = [desired sodium (mEq/L) − actual sodium (mEq/L)] × 0.6 × Wt (kg)	• Maintenance requirements: Preterm: 2–8 mEq/kg day Term: 1–4 mEq/kg day • Serum/plasma levels: Preterm: 132–140 mEq/L Term: 133–142 mEq/L >2 months: 135–145 mEq/L
Sodium polystyrene sulfonate (Kayexalate)	1 g/kg/day p.o./PR q6 hr	• 1 g of resin binds approximately 1mEq potassium • Use with caution in neonates especially in preterm neonates with rectal route secondary to reported perforations • Does NOT rapidly reverse hyperkalemia • Sodium content approximately 100 mg/g
Spironolactone (Aldactone)	1–3 mg/kg/dose p.o. divided q8–24 hr	• Monitor electrolytes, BUN, SCr
Sulfacetamide (Bleph-10)	1–2 drops q1–3 hr × 7–10 day (during daytime) Ointment: 1–4 times per day and at bedtime	• Treatment and prophylaxis of conjunctivitis
Sulfamethoxazole/ trimethoprim (Bactrim)	> 2 mo: Mild–moderate infections: 6–12 mg TMP/kg/day i.v. div q12 hr	• Cytochrome P450 inhibitor • Bioavailability 90%–100% • Dose recommendations are based on the trimethoprim (TMP) component • Dose adjust in renal impairment
Theophylline	See aminophylline	
Ticarcillin/clavulanate (Timentin)	200–300 mg ticarcillin component/kg/day div i.v. q6–8 hr	• Restricted criteria at most institutions and may require approval by an infectious disease specialist • Antibacterial activity is synergistic when given concomitantly with aminoglycosides • Adjust dose in renal dysfunction • Monitor BUN, SCr, liver enzymes, CBC
Tobramycin (Tobrex)	Preterm <1000 g: 3.5 mg/kg/dose i.v. q24 hr 0–4 wk, <1,200 g 2.5 mg/kg/dose q18 hr >7 day, <2 kg 2.5 mg/kg/dose q8–12 hr >7 day >2 kg 2.5 mg/kg/dose q8 hr	• Therapeutic levels: • Peak 4–12 mCg/mL • Trough 0.5–1.2 mCg/mL • Reserved for gentamicin-resistant gram-negative pathogens • Concentration-dependent killing • Peak level desired is eight times the MIC
Topiramate (Topamax)	1–3 mg/kg/dose p.o. daily (max 25 mg) Increase weekly by 1–3 mg/kg/day divided p.o. b.i.d. (Maintenance dose: 5–9 mg/kg/day p.o. div b.i.d.)	• Cytochrome P450 inhibitor • Topiramate may increase phenytoin levels and phenytoin and carbamazepine may decrease topiramate levels

(*continued*)

TABLE A1.1 Commonly Used Medications in a Newborn Intensive Care Unit (*Continued*)

Medication	*Dosage*	*Comments*
Trace metals (PTE-5)	Product that is used in TPN: 0.2 mL/kg/day of PTE-5 Contents per mL of PTE-5 *Cr* | *Cu* | *I* | *Mn* | *Se* | *Zn* 1 mCg | 0.1 mg | ··· | 25 mCg | 15 mCg | 1 mg	• Metals may accumulate in conditions of renal failure or biliary obstruction • Must be diluted prior to use • Remove copper and manganese for biliary obstruction with marked increase in liver enzymes
Tromethamine (THAM)	Neonates: 1 mL/kg for each pH unit below 7.4 Empiric dose based upon base deficit: Dose = Wt (kg) × base deficit (mEq/L) × 1.1 Maximum 500 mg/kg/dose = 13.9 mL/kg/dose of a 0.3M solution	• Infuse slowly over 1 hr • Do not infuse through a UAC line • Indicated in severe metabolic acidosis in patients where sodium or CO_2 elimination is restricted and received maximum dose of sodium bicarbonate (8–10 mEq/kg/24 hr) • 1 mM = 120 mg = 3.3 mL = 1mEq of THAM • Avoid use in renal dysfunction
Tropicamide 1% (Mydriacyl)	Cycloplegia: 1–2 drops (1%) May repeat in 5 min	• Eye examination must be performed within 30 min • Apply pressure to lacrimal sac postadministration to minimize systemic absorption
Ursodiol (Actigall) (UDCA)	Biliary atresia: 10–15 mg/kg/day once daily TPN-induced cholestasis 10 mg/kg/dose p.o. t.i.d.	• Treatment of cholestasis associated with total parenteral nutrition, biliary atresia, and cystic fibrosis • Monitor direct biliary levels • Hydrophobic bile acid that decreases both secretion of cholesterol from liver and its intestinal absorption
Valproic acid (Depakene, Depakote)	i.v.: 10–15 mg/kg/day div q6 hr Increase by 5–10 mg/kg/day weekly until therapeutic level obtained p.o.: 10–15 mg/kg/day div q.d.–t.i.d. Increase by 5–10 mg/kg/day weekly until therapeutic level obtained Rectal: Loading dose: 17–20 mg/kg Maintenance dose: 10–15 mg/kg/dose q8 hr	• Monitor trough concentrations closely • Therapeutic range: (increased free fraction in neonates) Total: 40–80 mCg/mL Free: <15–20 mCg/mL • Neonates will have an increased free fraction due to decreased protein binding • Monitor liver enzymes, bilirubin, CBC, platelets, serum ammonia • Monitor above closely secondary to reports of hepatic failure, pancreatitis, and hyperammonemic encephalopathy. Contraindicated in severe hepatic dysfunction • VPA is a CYP2D6 isoenzyme inhibitor: will increase levels of phenobarbital can displace phenytoin from protein binding sites • Reserved agent as recommended by neurology for refractory uncontrolled seizures in neonates not responding to more standard treatment modalities

(*continued*)

TABLE A1.1 Commonly Used Medications in a Newborn Intensive Care Unit (*Continued*)

Medication	*Dosage*	*Comments*

Vancomycin	<7 day <1,200 g 15 mg/kg i.v. q24 hr
	1,200–2,000 g 10–15 mg/kg i.v. q12–18 hr
	>2,000 g 10–15 mg/kg i.v. q8–12 hr
	>7 day < 2,000 g 10–15 mg/kg i.v. q8–12 hr
	>7 day > 2,000 g 15–20 mg/kg i.v. q8 hr
		• Therapeutic levels:
		  • Peak: 25–40 mCg/mL
		  • Trough 5–15 mCg/mL
		• More aggressive target peak and trough serum concentrations for vancomycin may be required in certain disease states such as endocarditis, meningitis, and osteomyelitis
		• Neonates: Postnatal age >14 days and less than 1,200 g may eliminate vancomycin at a quicker rate at this later postnatal age requiring a shorter frequency dosing regimen. Consider q12–18 hr dosing interval
		• Desired trough level should be 4× MIC
		• Obtain levels if course >3 days and every 7 days as therapy continues
		• Monitor BUN, SCr 2–3 times a week
		• Incompatible with heparin >1:1
		• Time-dependent killing T > MIC

Vitamin A (Aquasol A)	5,000 international units i.m. every Monday, Wednesday, and Friday	• 12 doses total or up to postnatal age of 28 days • Protect from light • Studies have shown a decrease in chronic lung disease among ELBW infants, decrease in sepsis, and increase overall survival (NNT = 13)
Vitamin D (Ergocalciferol)	400–1,200 International Units p.o. once a day	• Monitor alkaline phosphatase levels • 8,000 IU/mL
Vitamin E	25–50 International Units PO once a day	• Routine administration for ROP or BPD secondary to O_2 therapy is not recommended by AAP

Zidovudine (Retrovir)	1.5 mg/kg/dose i.v. q6 hr
	2 mg/kg/dose p.o. q6 hr
	Premature neonates < 35 wks gestational age at birth:
	  2 mg/kg/dose p.o. q12 hr
	  1.5 mg/kg/dose i.v. q12 hr
	Increase to 2 mg/kg/dose p.o. q8 hrs at 2 weeks of age if >/= 30 weeks at birth
	Increase to 2 mg/kg/dose p.o. q8 hrs at 4 weeks of age if < 30 weeks at birth
		• Length of therapy: 6 wk
		• Monitor CBC
		• Formerly known as AZT

AAP, American Academy of Pediatrics; ABLC, amphotericin b lipid complex; ACE, angiotensin converting enzyme; ANC, absolute neutrophil count; APTT, activated partial thromboplastin time; ATC, around the clock; AV, atrioventricular; BP, blood pressure; BPD, bronchopulmonary dysplasia; BUN, blood urea nitrogen; CBC, complete blood count; CHF, chronic heart failure; CI, cardiac index; CLD, chronic lung disease; CMV, cytomegalovirus; CNS, central nervous system; CSF, cerebral spinal fluid; CVC, central venous catheter; div, divided; D5W, dextrose 5% in water; D10W, dextrose 10% in water; ELBW, extremely low birth weight; FDA, Food and Drug Administration; GA, gestational age; GBS, group B streptococcus; GI, gastrointestinal; G6PD, glucose 6 phosphate dehydrogenase deficiency; HPA, hypopituitary axis; HSV, herpes simplex virus; HTN, hypertension; i.m., intramuscular; IU, international units; IVH, intraventricular hemorrhage; i.v.p., intravenous push; MAP, mean arterial pressure; MIC, minimum inhibitory concentration; MWF, Monday, Wednesday, Friday; NEC, necrotizing enterocolitis; NNT, number needed to treat; NS, normal saline; PDA, patent ductus arteriosus; PDE, phosphodiesterase; plat, platelets, PPHN, persistent pulmonary hypertension in newborns; PK, pharmacokinetics; p.o. oral; p.r., rectal; PVC, premature ventricular contractions; ROP, retinopathy of prematurity; s.c., subcutaneous; SCr, serum creatinine; SVT, supraventricular tachycardia; TDD, total digitalizing dose; TPA, tissue plasminogen activator; TPN, total parenteral nutrition; UAC, umbilical artery catheter; UO; urinary output; UVC, umbilical venous catheter; VLBW, very low birth weight; VPA, valproic acid; VTE, venous thromboembolism.

TABLE A1.2 Recommended Childhood Immunization (0–6 yr) Schedule for United States 2009[a]

	Birth	*2 mo*	*4 mo*	*6 mo*	*6–12 mo*	*12–15 mo*	*15–18 mo*	*19–23 mo*	*2–3 yr*	*4–6 yr*
Diphtheria, tetanus, acellular pertussis		X	X	X			X			X
Haemophilus influenzae type B		X	X	X		X				
Hepatitis A							(Two doses)			
Hepatitis B	X	X			X					
Influenza					GIVE YEARLY INFLUENZA VACCINE					
Meningococcal									MCV	
MMR						X				X
Pneumococcal –conjugated 7		X	X	X		X				
Polio virus -inactivated		X	X		X				X	
Rotavirus		X	X	X						
varicella						X				X

MCV, meningococcal conjugated vaccine; MMR, measles, mumps, rubella.
Use of combination vaccine products is encouraged at initiation of 2-month vaccine administration to decrease number of required injections. See table below for combination products available.

TABLE A1.3 Hepatitis-B Surface Antigen Status (HepBsAg)

Mother's Hepatitis-B Surface Antigen Status (HepBsAg)	*Hepatitis-B Vaccine Schedule*	*Hepatitis-B Immune Globulin Schedule (HBIG)*
Positive	Dose #1 @ birth (≤12 hr) Dose #2 @ 1–2 mo Dose #3 @ 6 mo	Hepatitis-B immune globulin Dose @ birth (≤12 hr)
Negative	Dose #1 @ birth (before discharge)[a] Dose #2 @ 1–2 mo Dose #3 @ 6–18 mo	Not required
Unknown	Dose #1 @ birth (≤12 hr) Dose #2 @ 1–2 mo Dose #3 @ 6 mo	Determine the mother's HepBsAg status as soon as possible postdelivery. Preterm neonates (<2 kg): Dose @ birth (≤12 hr) Mother's HepBsAg status must be determined within 12 hr postdelivery for the preterm infant. If not determined within 12 hr the HBIG must be given due to less reliable immune response Term neonates Administer HBIG within 7 days if mother tests HepBsAg positive

[a]The first dose of hepatitis B vaccine should be administered at the time of birth for term infants. Preterm infants should receive the first dose of hepatitis B vaccine at the time of discharge or by 1 month chronological age regardless of weight. This initial vaccine, however, should not be counted in the required three doses to complete the immunization series.

TABLE A1.4 Vaccines[a]

Vaccines	*Dosage*	*Notes*
Diphtheria, tetanus, and acellular pertussis (DTaP) (Infanrix, Tripedia)	0.5 mL i.m.	• The fourth dose may be administered as early as 12 months as long as 6 months has elapsed since the third dose • Administer final dose in the series at 4–6 yr
DTaP/HIB (TriHiBit)	0.5 mL i.m.	• Do NOT use at 2,4, and 6 months • Can be used as final dose in infants >12 months
DTaP/IPV/HIB (Pentacel)	0.5 mL i.m.	• The vaccine is approved for use in infants and children ages 6 wk through 4 yr • Four doses given at 2, 4, 6, and 15–18 months of age
Haemophilus B conjugate vaccine PedvaxHIB (Act-HIB)	0.5 mL i.m.	• Minimum age of 6 wk • The conjugate HIB vaccines licensed for use in infants are interchangeable • Act-HIB: Previously unvaccinated infants aged 2 through 6 months should receive three doses of vaccine administered 2 months apart, followed by a booster dose at age 12–15 months • PedvaxHIB: Unvaccinated children aged 2 through 11 months should receive two doses of vaccine 2 months apart, followed by a booster dose at 12–15 months of age
Hepatitis A (Havrix) (Vaqta)	0.5 mL i.m. administered as two injections 6–12 mo apart	• Minimum age of 12 months for first dose
Hepatitis B vaccine (Recombivax HB, Engerix-B)	0.5 mL i.m. Strength for each brand is different: 10 mCg = 0.5 mL = Engerix-B 5 mCg = 0.5 mL = Recombivax-HB	• Administer the first dose of monovalent hepatitis B vaccine to ALL newborns before hospital discharge or by 1-months chronological age • Mothers HepBsAg unknown should receive the vaccine within 12 hr of birth. Preterm infants should receive HBIG as well if status is not determined within 12 hr • Thimerosal-free vaccine • Four doses of Hep B to infants are permissible when combination vaccines are administered after the birth dose • Premature infants <2 kg should receive four total doses
Hepatitis B vaccine/ DTaP/IPOL Combination vaccine (Pediarix)	0.5 mL i.m.	• This combination vaccine should not be used in infants younger than 6 wk. Therefore, it should be initiated at 2-months immunization schedule • Use of this combination vaccine at each routine immunization schedule will result in administration of a fourth dose of hepatitis B vaccine (accepted on routine schedule)
Hepatitis B vaccine/ haemophilus B conjugate Combination vaccine (Comvax)	0.5 mL i.m.	• This combination vaccine should not be used in infants younger than 6 wk. Therefore, it should be initiated at 2 months immunization schedule
Influenza vaccine (inactivated) (Fluzone)	TIV: 6–35 mo: 0.25 mL i.m. >3 yr old: 0.5 mL i.m.	• Minimum age of 6 months (trivalent inactivated influenza vaccine (TIV)) • Minimum age of 2 yr for live, attenuated influenza vaccine (LAIV) • Administer annually to children 6 months to 18 yr • Administer two doses at least 4 wk apart in children <9 yr old who have received the influenza vaccine for the first time
Measles/mumps/rubella (MMR)	0.5 mL i.m.	• Minimum age of 12 months
Pneumococcal, conjugated 13-valent (Prevnar)	0.5 mL i.m.	• Minimum age of 6 wk for pneumococcal conjugate vaccine (PCV) and minimum of 2 yr for pneumococcal polysaccharide vaccine (PPSV)
Polio vaccine, enhanced inactivated (IPOL)	0.5 mL i.m./s.c.	• This vaccine contains all three serotypes of polio vaccine virus
Rotavirus live (pentavalent) (Rotateq) (Rotarix)	2 mL p.o.	• ORAL vaccine • Administer the first dose before 15 wk and final dose by 8 months • Fecal shedding of vaccine virus was evaluated in a subset of persons enrolled in the phase III trials. Vaccine virus was shed by 9% of 360 infants after dose 1, but none of 249 and 385 infants after doses 2 and 3, respectively • Fecal shedding of rotavirus antigen was evaluated in all or a subset of infants from seven studies in various countries. After dose 1, rotavirus antigen shedding was detected by ELISA in 50% to 80% (depending on the study) of infants at approximately day 7 and 0% to 24% at approximately day 30. After dose 2, rotavirus antigen shedding was detected in 4% to 18% of infants at approximately day 7, and 0% to 1.2% at approximately day 30. The potential for transmission of vaccine virus to others was not assessed • Administer to hospitalized infants AT THE TIME OF DISCHARGE due to fecal shedding of vaccine virus (up to 15 days)
Varicella live (Varivax)	0.5 mL i.m.	• Minimum age of 12 months • Avoid use of salicylates for 6 wk following vaccination due to potential increase risk of Reye's syndrome

i.m., Intramuscular; p.o., oral; s.c., subcutaneous.

[a]Report all serious adverse reactions to the US Department of Health and Human Services (DHHS) Vaccine Adverse Event Reporting System (VAERS): 1-800-822-7967.

TABLE A1.5 Immune Globulins

Immune Globulins	*Dosage*	*Notes*
Hepatitis B immune globulin (HBIG)	0.5 mL i.m.	• HepBsAg–positive mothers: Administer within 12 hr of birth • Efficacy decreases significantly if treatment is delayed > 48 hr • HepBsAg unknown mothers: Administer HBIG and hepatitis B vaccine to preterm infants within 12 hr of life. Administer hepatitis B vaccine to term infants within 12 hr of life and HBIG within 7 day of life.
Palivizumab (Synagis)	15 mg/kg i.m.	• Give monthly throughout RSV season (November–March) for Midwest • Eligibility criteria: Infant with chronic lung disease of prematurity Infants born before 32 wk of gestation Infants born at 32–35 wk of gestation with at least two risk factors • The updated recommendations of palivizumab administration and major policy changes include: Modification of recommendations for initiation and cessation of RSV prophylaxis based on current CDC descriptions of seasonality (geographical regions in United States) Maximum of five doses in all geographic areas Modification of risk factors for severe disease in infants born between 32 and 35 wk of gestation For infants 32 through 35 wk of gestation who qualify for prophylaxis based on presence of risk factors, prophylaxis is recommended until 90 day of age (maximum of 3 doses)
Varicella immune globulin (VariZIG)	<10 kg 125 units i.m.	• Administer to infants whose mothers have an onset of varicella 5 days or less prior to delivery or in the first 48 hr after delivery • Or if < 32 wk of gestation and exposed to varicella • Most effective if given within 48–96 hr of exposure • VZIG has been discontinued by the manufacturer; VariZIG is an investigational product available by IND application.

CDC, Centers for Disease Control and Prevention; HepBsAg, hepatitis B surface antigen; i.m., intramuscular; IND, investigational new drug; RSV, respiratory syncytial virus.

TABLE A1.6 Respiratory Medications

Respiratory Medication	*Dosage*	*Notes*
Acetylcysteine (Mucomyst)	0.5 mL of 20% t.i.d./q.i.d. nebulized	• Use for patients with abnormal or viscous mucous secretions • Exerts mucolytic action through its free sulfhydryl group which opens up the disulfide bonds in mucoproteins and ↓ viscosity
Albuterol (Ventolin)	0.5–1 mg inh in 2 mL 0.9% sodium chloride q4–6 hr 0.1–0.45 mg/kg/hr continuous nebulization	• Monitor for tachycardia, CNS, hypokalemia, tremor • May administer more often in severe cases • Continuous infusion: nebulized at constant rate of 2 mL/hr in the newborn • Dose calculated/100 mL = dose(mg/kg/hr) × Wt (kg) × 50 • Tachyphylaxis with prolonged use
Budesonide (Pulmicort)	0.25 mg inh daily b.i.d.	• Used on a limited basis in neonatal population for infants who have developed chronic lung disease and remain on respiratory support • Does not work immediately. Allow for minimum of 2–3 wk of therapy to determine any potential benefits in terms of decreasing respiratory support • Up to 39% of oral inhalation is systemically absorbed • Monitor for growth suppression, adrenal suppression, hypokalemia, growth of *Candida* in mouth/nares
Cromolyn (Intal)	>2 yr old: 20 mg inh four times a day	• Generally not recommended for neonates and preterm infants • Prevents mast cell release of histamine, leukotrienes • Monitor for wheezing, congestion, and lacrimation • Does not work immediately—need to be on consistent regimen for 2–4 wk
Ipratropium (Atrovent)	Neonates: 25 mCg/kg/dose inh three times a day Infants: 125–250 mCg inh three times a day	• Blocks the action of acetylcholine at parasympathetic sites in bronchial smooth muscle causing bronchodilation • Additive effects with anticholinergics
Vaponephrine (Racepinephrine)	0.25–0.5 mL of 2.25% racemic epinephrine in 2 mL 0.9% sodium chloride nebulized q6 hr	• For stridor (short-term treatment)

b.i.d., Twice daily; inh, inhaled; q, every; q.d., daily; q.i.d., four times; t.i.d. thrice daily.

TABLE A1.7 Infusion of Medications Through the Umbilical Artery Catheter (UAC)

Drugs that should not be routinely administered through the UAC include any agents that are
- Hyperosmolar agents (osmolality > serum 281–289 mOsmol/L)
- Vasoconstrictor agents
- Irritants
- Alkalinic agents

Complications (rates reported: 1.5% to 23%)
- Vascular: thrombus, emboli, vasospasms, and hypertension
- Infections: colonizations of 39% reported after 6 days of UAC placement, systemic infections
- Perforation
- Miscellaneous

Placement:
- HIGH: catheter tip high in the aorta at T4–T11 level
- LOW: catheter tip at L4

Medications that CAN be infused through the UAC:
Medications and flushes should be infused slowly over 20–30 min, be dilute and isotonic as possible
- Albumin
- Aminophylline
- Ampicillin
- Blood products
- Cefotaxime (Cephalosporins)
- Dexamethasone
- Dextrose (maximum 15%)
- Digoxin
- Furosemide
- Gentamicin
- Heparin
- Hydrocortisone
- Maintenance i.v.s with dextrose
- Electrolytes
- Pancuronium
- Penicillin G
- Phentolamine
- Sodium bicarbonate—consider diluting
- Total parenteral nutrition (TPN)

Medications that CANNOT be infused through the UAC
- Acyclovir
- Alprostadil
- Amphotericin B
- Caffeine
- Calcium gluconate (or any salt)
- Diazepam
- Dobutamine
- Dopamine
- Epinephrine
- Fat emulsion
- Immune globulin
- Indomethacin
- Isoproterenol
- Lorazepam
- Metoclopramide
- Norepinephrine
- [a]Phenobarbital
- Phenytoin
- Potassium boluses
- Propranolol
- Tromethamine (THAM)
- [a]Vancomycin

[a]Relative contraindication with reported vasospasm and skin blanching.

REFERENCES

1. Bryant BG. Drug, fluid, and blood products administered through the umbilical artery catheter: complications experiences from one NICU. *Neonatal Netw* 1990;9(1):27–46.
2. Green C, Yohanna MD. Umbilical arterial and venous catheters: placement, use and complications. *Neonatal Netw* 1998;17(6):23–27.
3. Hodding JH. Medication administration via the umbilical arterial catheter: a survey of standard practices and review of the literature. *Am J Perinatol* 1990;7(4):329–332.
4. Ankola PA, Atakent YS. Effect of adding heparin in very low concentration to the infusate to prolong the patency of umbilical artery catheters. *Am J Perinatol.* 1993;10(3):229–232.
5. Fletcher MA, Brown DR, Landers S, Seguin J. Umbilical arterial catheter use: report of an audit conducted by the study group for complication of perinatal care. *Am J Perinatal* 1994;11(2):94–99.
6. Smith L, Dills R. Survey of medication administration through umbilical arterial and venous catheters. *Am J Health Syst Pharm* 2003;60:1569–1572.
7. Stocker M, Berger TM. Arterial and central venous catheters in neonates and infants. *Anaesthesist* 2006;55(8):873–882.
8. Butler-O'Hara M, Buzzard CJ, Reubens L, McDermott MP, DiGrazio W, D'Angio CT. A randomized trial comparing long-term and short-term use of umbilical venous catheters in premature infants with birth weights of less than 1251 grams [published online ahead of print June 19, 2006]. *Pediatrics* 2006;118(1):e25–e35.
9. Furdon SA, Horgan MJ, Bradshaw WT, Clark DA. Nurses' guide to early detection of umbilical arterial catheter complications in infants. *Adv Neonatal Care* 2006;6(5):242–256; quiz 257–260.
10. Havranek T, Johanboeke P, Madramootoo C, Carver JD. Umbilical artery catheters do not affect intestinal blood flow responses to minimal enteral feedings [published online ahead of print March 29, 2007]. *J Perinatol* 2007;27(6): 375–379.

TABLE A1.8 Neonatal Intravenous Push Medications

Medication	*Dose*	*Comments*
Adenosine (Adenocard)	50–100 mCg/kg rapid i.v.p. over 1–2 s Increase dose by 50–100 mCg/kg increments q1–2 min until return of normal sinus rhythm MAX 300 mCg/kg or until termination of PSVT	• Flush with saline immediately post each dose administration • Adenosine 6 mg/2 mL vial: Take 1 mL of adenosine and dilute with 0.9% NS 9 mL for a final concentration of 300 mCg/mL • Half-life: <10 seconds
Albumin 5% (Buminate)	0.5–1 g/kg/dose i.v. (5–10 mL/kg/dose) i.v.p. over 10 min MAX 2–4 mL/min	• Administer through 5 micron filter • Consider normal saline as colloid. (Neonatal Resuscitation guidelines 2005: An isotonic crystalloid rather than albumin is the solution of choice for volume expansion in the delivery room (Class IIb; LOE 7) (1–3).
Atropine	0.01–0.03 mg/kg/dose over 1 min	
Calcium gluconate	100–200 mg/kg/dose i.v.p. over 10–30 min	• Do NOT administer through UAC line
Dextrose	1–2 mL/kg of D10W i.v.p. over 1 min	
Digoxin (Lanoxin)	Preterm neonate: Loading dose: 15–25 mCg/kg/dose slow i.v.p. over 5–10 min Maintenance dose: 4–6 mCg/kg/dose slow i.v.p. over 5 min Term neonate: Loading dose: 20–30 mCg/kg/dose slow i.v.p. over 5–10 min Maintenance dose: 5–8 mCg/kg/dose slow i.v.p. over 5 min	• Therapeutic range 0.8–2 ng/mL • Half life varies: • Preterm neonate 61–70 hr • Term neonate 35–45 hr
Epinephrine (1:10,000)	0.01–0.03 mg/kg/dose rapid i.v.p. (0.1–0.3 mL/kg of 1:10,000 solution) 0.3–1 mL/kg/dose endotracheally (ET)	• Repeat every 3–5 min as needed • Do NOT administer through UAC line
Fentanyl (Sublimaze)	1–4 mCg/kg/dose i.v.p. slowly over 3–5 min	• Slow i.v.p. over 3–5 min to prevent chest wall rigidity • Reverse with naloxone • Less histamine release (more suitable in CLD due to less airway narrowing) • Less GI motility impairment, less urinary retention • Decreases peripheral vascular resistance which is potentially useful in PPHN
Furosemide (Lasix)	1–2 mg/kg/dose i.v.p. over 2–4 min	• Monitor electrolytes
Hydralazine (Apresoline)	0.1–0.2 mg/kg/dose q4–6 hr p.r.n.	• Max 3.5 mg/kg/day divided q4–6 hr • Administer i.v.p. over 1 min • (Max 0.2 mg/kg/min)
Lorazepam	0.05–0.1 mg/kg/dose i.v.p. over 2–5 min May repeat subsequent doses in 10–15 min	• Preparation contains benzyl alcohol and therefore should be used with caution in the preterm infant due to potential neurotoxicity, myoclonus and "gasping syndrome" • Dilute with sterile water or normal saline 1:1 prior to administration • Infuse through dedicated line.
Midazolam (Versed)	0.05–0.15 mg/kg/dose i.v.p. over 5 min	• No analgesic properties • CNS side effects include paradoxical excitement, rhythmic myoclonic jerking (in preterm infants approximately 8% incidence), tonic-clonic movements
Morphine sulfate	0.05–0.2 mg/kg/dose i.v.p. over 5 min	• Monitor for respiratory depression, O_2 saturation, urinary retention, decreased bowel sounds
Naloxone	0.1 mg/kg/dose rapid i.v.p. Repeat every 2–3 min as needed	• Use with caution in infants of opioid-dependent mothers
Pancuronium (Pavulon)	0.1 mg/kg/dose i.v.p. over 1 min	• Monitor BP; neonate must be intubated and sedated • Adjust dose in renal impairment
Phenobarbital	Loading dose: 20 mg/kg/dose i.v.p. over 20 min Additional 5–10 mg/kg bolus doses may be required until seizure controlled maximum of 40 mg/kg total Maximum infusion rate of 1 mg/kg/min	• Therapeutic level: 15–40 mCg/mL • Half-life in neonates: 45–200 hr • Do NOT administer through UAC line

(*continued*)

TABLE A1.8 Neonatal Intravenous Push Medications (*Continued*)

Medication	*Dose*	*Comments*
Phenytoin (Dilantin)	Loading dose 20 mg/kg/dose i.v.p. over 20 min Maximum infusion rate 0.5–1 mg/kg/min	• Do NOT administer through UAC line
Plasma protein fraction (Plasmanate)	10–15 mL/kg/dose i.v.p. over 10 min	• Use 0.9% normal saline when possible: 0.9% NS 500 mL $ <1 Plasmanate/albumin 50 mL $ 62 • Isotonic crystalloid solutions should be used first line for acute volume expansion (Neonatal Resuscitation guidelines 2005 states that albumin-containing solutions are not the fluid of choice for initial volume expansion secondary to increased risk of infections and associated increased mortality. (Class IIb, LOE 7)
Sodium bicarbonate	1–2 mEq/kg/dose i.v. over at least 30 min. Maximum 1 mEq/kg/hr	• Infuse through dedicated line and monitor closely for extravasation. Tissue necrosis can occur because of the hyperosmolarity of sodium bicarbonate. (4.2% = 0.5 mEq/mL = 900 mOsm/L) • Not compatible with calcium or any calcium-containing solution. Immediate precipitation will result • Sodium bicarbonate is not a recommended therapy in the neonatal resuscitation guidelines and therefore rapid i.v. infusions are **not** administered
Tromethamine (THAM)	1–2 mmol/kg/dose slow i.v.p. Maximum rate of 1 mL/min (1 mmol = 3.3 mL of 0.3M solution = 120 mg = 1 mEq of THAM)	• Do NOT infuse through a UAC line • Indicated in severe metabolic acidosis in patients where sodium is elevated or bicarbonate elimination is restricted or patient received maximum dose of sodium bicarbonate (8–10 mEq/kg/day)

CLD, Chronic lung disease; GI, gastrointestinal; i.v.p., intravenous push; PPHN, persistent pulmonary hypertension in newborns; PSVT, paroxysmal supraventricular tachycardia; UAC, umbilical artery catheter.

REFERENCES

1. So KW, Fok TF, Ng PC, Wong WW, Cheung KL. Randomized controlled trial of colloid or crystalloid in hypotensive preterm infants. *Arch Dis Child Fetal Neonatal Ed* 1997;76:F43–F46.2.
2. Emery EF, Fok TF, Ng PC, Wong WW, Cheung KL. Randomized controlled trial of colloid infusions in hypotensive preterm infants. *Arch Dis Child* 1992;67:1185–1188.
3. Oca MJ, Nelson M, Donn SM. Randomized trial of normal saline versus 5% albumin for the treatment of neonatal hypotension. *J Perinatol* 2003; 23:473–476.
4. Jacob M, Chappell D, Conzen P, Chappell D, Conzen P, Wilkes MM, Becker BF, Rehm M. Small-volume resuscitation with hyperoncotic albumin: a systematic review of randomized clinical trials. *Crit Care* 2008;12(2):R34.
5. Taketomo CK, Jodding JH, Kraus DM. *Lexicomp-pediatric dosage handbook*, 15th ed. Lexi-Comp. 2008.
6. Young TE, Mangum B. Neofax 2009. 22nd Edition. Offered by Thomson Reuters.
7. Communication directly with manufacturer or package insert.

TABLE A1.9 Therapeutic Drug Monitoring (TDM) and Drug Sampling Times

Drug	Infusion Time	Therapeutic Range	When to Draw Levels	Comments
Amikacin	0.5 hr	Peak: 20–30 mCg/mL Trough: <4 mCg/mL	Trough: ½ hr prior to dose Peak: ½ hr after end of infusion	Reserved for tobramycin-resistant gram-negative bacteria Dose 7.5 mg/kg/dose i.v. × 1 in renal failure patients—draw random level in 24 hr and redose when level is <4 mCg/mL
Caffeine (Cafcit)	0.5 hr	5–25 mCg/mL	Draw trough level just prior to next dose	Long half-life: 45–100 hr. Draw trough level at steady state after day 5 of therapy
Carbamazepine (Tegretol)	N/A	4–12 mCg/mL	Just prior to next dose	ORAL form only Carbamazepine may be administered rectally if required: Give same total daily dose but give in small diluted multiple doses (dilute with water)
Digoxin (Lanoxin)	Slowly over 5–10 min	0.8–2 ng/mL	Draw trough level just prior to next dose or at least 6 hr after dose given	Give ½ TDD as initial dose then 1/4 TDD times two doses q6–12 hr apart Half-life: Preterm 61–70 hr Term 35–45 hr
Enoxaparin (Lovenox)	N/A	Antifactor Xa level: 0.5–1 unit/mL is therapeutic	4 hr postdose	Initiate dose at 1.5 mCg/kg/dose s.c. q12 and titrate per aXa levels Monitor for signs of bleeding Repeat level if extremely low or high prior to dose change
Flucytosine (Ancoban)	N/A	25–100 mCg/mL	L2 hr postdose after at least 4 day of therapy	ORAL form only Good CNS penetration Not to be used as monotherapy
Gentamicin	0.5 hr	Peak: 3–10 mCg/mL Trough: <1.2 mCg/mL	Trough: ½ hr prior to dose Peak: ½ hr after end of infusion	Gent levels for synergy: Peak 3–4 mCg/mL Trough <1 mCg/mL Levels not routinely done Dosing in renal failure patients 2 mg/kg/dose i.v. × 1—draw random in 24 hr and redose when level is ≤1.2 mCg/mL
Heparin	Continuous infusion	APTT 60–85 seconds	Obtain APTT 4 hr after initiation of continuous infusion and every 4 hr after infusion rate change	Loading dose: 75 units/kg, then maintenance dose: 28 units/kg/hr
Levetiracetam (Keppra)	0.5 hr	Trough: 5–30 mCg/mL	Trough: just before dose	Exact dosing in neonates not established. Second- or third-line agent used in refractory seizures. Loading dose: 10–20 mg/kg/dose, then 5–10 mg/kg/day divided in two to three doses. May increase by 10 mg/kg/day if tolerated to maximum of 60 mg/kg/day
Phenobarbital	Slow i.v.p. over 20 min Maximum infusion rate 1 mg/kg/min	15–40 mCg/mL	Draw trough level just prior to next dose Postload/peak: 1 hr after end of infusion	Initiate maintenance dose 12 hr after loading dose
Phenytoin (Dilantin)	Slow i.v.p. over 20 min Maximum infusion rate of 0.5–1 mg/kg/min	Total: 8–15 mCg/mL Free: 1.5–2.5 mCg/mL	Draw trough level just prior to next dose Postload/peak: 1 hr after end of infusion	Initiate maintenance dose 12 hr after loading dose Oral loading dose should be administered in 2–3 doses q2 hr to ensure complete oral absorption

(continued)

TABLE A1.9 Therapeutic Drug Monitoring (TDM) and Drug Sampling Times (*Continued*)

Drug	*Infusion Time*	*Therapeutic Range*	*When to Draw Levels*	*Comments*
Theophylline (Aminophylline is an i.v. product)	Aminophylline 0.5 hr	AOP: 7–12 mCg/mL BPD: 10–15 mCg/mL	Draw trough level just prior to next dose Peak: 1 hr postdose Cont infusion: 16–24 hr after initiation of infusion	Apnea 7–12 mCg/mL BPD 10–15 mCg/mL $t_{1/2}$ variable by age: Premature 20–30 hr Term 10–25 hr <6 mo 14 hr >6 mo 5 hr Draw level 3 days after therapy initiated or changed Adjust frequency and dosing in anticipation of change of half-life
Tobramycin	0.5 hr	Peak: 3–10 mCg/mL Trough: <1.2 mCg/mL	Trough: ½ hr prior to dose Peak: ½ hr after end of infusion	Reserve for documented *Pseudomonas aeruginosa* or other gram-negative pathogen resistant to gentamicin Dosing in renal failure patients 2 mg/kg/dose i.v. i.v. × 1—draw random in 24 hr and redose when level is ≤1 mCg/mL
Valproic acid (Depacon)	1 hr	Total: 40–80 mCg/mL Free: <15 mCg/mL	Draw trough level just before next dose	Increase in free fraction in neonates Consult neurology prior to initiation Side effects: Hyperammonemic encephalopathy, pancreatitis, thrombocytopenia, ↑ liver enzymes, and liver failure
Vancomycin	1 hr	Peak: 25–40 mCg/mL Trough: 5–20 mCg/mL	Trough: ½ hr prior to dose Peak: 1 hr after infusion	No need for levels for empiric 3 days rule outs Desired trough level should be 4× MIC Target higher trough levels with MIC >1 as tolerated More aggressive target trough concentrations are required in disease states such as meningitis, endocarditis, pneumonia, and osteomyelitis Obtain levels if course of therapy >3 days and every 7 days as therapy continues

AOP, Apnea of prematurity; BPD, bronchopulmonary dysplasia; CNS, central nervous system; i.v., intravenous; i.v.p., intravenous push; MIC, minimum inhibitory concentration; $t^{1/2}$: half-life; TDD, total digitalizing dose.

TABLE A1.10 Drug Compatibility with Neonatal TPN and Fat Emulsion at Y-Site (Terminal Injection Site)

Medication	*Compatibility with TPN*	*Compatibility with Lipids*	*Comments*
Acyclovir	N	N	
Albumin	Y	Y	
Alprostadil	N	NI	
Amikacin	Y	N	Incompatible with heparin at concentrations >1 unit/mL
Aminophylline	Y	Y	1 mg/mL concentration ONLY compatible. 5 mg/mL is incompatible with Trophamine
Amphotericin B	N	N	
Amphotericin B lipid complex	N	N	
Ampicillin	N	Y	More stable in NS/SW than dextrose
Ampicillin/sulbactam (Unasyn)	N	NI	
Amiodarone (Cordarone)	N	NI	
Atropine	Y	NI	
Azithromycin	NI	NI	
Bumetanide	N	Y	
Caffeine	Y	Y	
Calcitriol	NI	NI	
Calcium Gluconate	[a]	Y	[a]Potential for precipitation based on specific TPN and the Ca-PO4 ratio. Infuse bolus doses over 30 min NOT with TPN when possible so as to avoid precipitation and decrease osmolality.
Caspofungin	N	N	
Cefazolin	Y	Y	
Cefepime	Y	NI	
Cefotaxime	Y	Y	
Cefoxitin	Y	Y	
Ceftazidime	Y	Y	
Ceftriaxone	Y	Y	
Chlorothiazide	N	NI	
Clindamycin	Y	Y	
Colistimethate (Colistin)	NI	NI	
Dexamethasone	Y	Y	
Digoxin	Y	Y	
Dobutamine	Y	Y	
Dopamine	Y	Y	
Enalapril	N	Y	
Epinephrine	Y	N	
Erythromycin	Y	Y	
Esmolol	N	NI	
Fentanyl	Y	Y	
Fluconazole	Y	Y	
Furosemide	Y[a]	Y	[a]Furosemide must be administered IV push; Dex/AA will degrade furosemide when mixed together for several hours
Ganciclovir	Y	N	
Gentamicin	Y	Y	Incompatible with heparin at concentrations >1 unit/mL
Glucagon	NI	NI	
Glycopyrrolate	N	NI	
Heparin	Y	Y[a]	[a]Not compatible at concentrations >100 units/mL
Hydralazine	Y	N	
Hydrocortisone	Y	Y	
Ibuprofen	NI	NI	
Imipenem–cilastatin	Y	Y	
Indomethacin	N	NI	
Insulin, regular	Y	Y	
Iron dextran	Y	N	Usually placed in TPN. Mix only in Dex/AA solutions containing at least 2% amino acids
Isoproterenol	Y	Y	
Levetiracetam	NI	NI	

(*continued*)

TABLE A1.10 Drug Compatibility with Neonatal TPN and Fat Emulsion at Y-Site (Terminal Injection Site) (*Continued*)

Medication	*Compatibility with TPN*	*Compatibility with Lipids*	*Comments*
Levothyroxine	N	N	
Lidocaine	Y	Y	
Linezolid	Y	NI	
Lorazepam	N	N	
Magnesium sulfate	Y	N	
Meropenem	Y	Y	
Methicillin	Y	NI	
Methylprednisolone	Y	Y	
Metoclopramide	Y	Y	
Metronidazole	Y	Y	
Micafungin	NI	NI	
Midazolam	N	N	Damage to emulsion integrity
Milrinone	Y	NI	
Morphine	Y	Y	
Nafcillin	Y	Y	
Oxacillin	Y	Y	
Pancuronium	Y	NI	
Penicillin G	Y	Y	
Phenobarbital	N	N	
Phenytoin	N	N	Incompatible with heparin at concentrations >1 unit/mL
Phosphates	N	N	
Phytonadione	Y	NI	
Piperacillin	Y	Y	
Piperacillin/tazobactam	Y	Y	
Potassium salts	Y	Y	
Propranolol	NI	NI	
Pyridoxine	NI	Y	
Ranitidine	Y	Y	
Rifampin	NI	NI	
Sodium Bicarbonate	N	Y	
Ticarcillin	Y	Y	
Ticarcillin–clavulanate	Y	Y	(Timentin)
Tobramycin	Y	Y	Incompatible with heparin at concentrations >1 unit/mL
Trimethoprim/sulfamethoxazole	N	Y	(Bactrim, Septra)
Tromethamine (THAM)	N	N	
Valproic acid	N	N	
Vancomycin	Y	Y	Incompatible with heparin at concentrations >1 unit/mL
Zidovudine	Y	Y	

N, no; NI, no information; NS, normal saline; SW, sterile water; Y, Yes.
NI should be treated as incompatible.

REFERENCES

1. King Guide to Parenteral Admixtures.
2. Lexi-Comp, Pediatric Dosage Handbook, 16th Ed. Lexi-Comp. 2009–2010.
3. Micomedex- IV compatibility online.
4. Phelps SJ, Hak EB, Crill C. *Guidelines for administration of intravenous medications to pediatric patients.* 9th ed.
5. Trissel LA. *Handbook on injectable drugs*, 15th ed.
6. Veltri M. Y-site Compatibility of IV drugs with Trophamine PN Solutions.
7. Young TE, Mangum B. *Neofax 2008.* edn.
8. Zenk K, Sills JH, Keopprel RM. *Neonatal medications and nutrition*, 3rd ed.

GUIDELINES FOR HEPARIN USE TO MAINTAIN LINE PATENCY IN THE NEONATAL INTENSIVE CARE UNIT

ISSUE

The overuse of heparin is a risk factor to the neonate. Heparin is a risk factor for neonatal candidiasis. Other risk factors for neonatal candidiasis include extremely low gestational age, thrombocytopenia, use of skin emollients, intralipids, enclosed humid environment, lack of breast milk feeds, lack of enteral feeds, hyperglycemia-insulin

Type of Line	*Can the IV Site be Locked?*	*Recommendations for Flush When Locking the IV Site*	*Should Heparin be Added to IV Fluids?*	*Recommendation for the Addition of Heparin to IV Fluids*	*Recommended Minimum Volume to be Infused in Line*
Peripheral	Yes	0.5 mL preservative free normal saline (0.9% sodium chloride) every 8 hr	No	None	1 mL/hr
PICC (any gauge)	No	None	Yes	Heparin 0.5 units/mL for rates: <2 mL/hr May exclude the ELBW critically ill neonate	1 mL/hr
Hickman–Broviac, CVC	Yes	Heparin 10 units daily	No	None	2 mL/hr
UAC	No	None	Yes	Heparin 0.5 units/mL	0.5 mL/hr
UVC	No	None	No	None	1 mL/hr
Secondary UVC (Double lumen)	Yes	Heparin 10 units daily	No	None	No minimum
Femoral	Yes	Heparin 10 units daily	No	None	No minimum

CVC, central venous catheter; ELBW, extremely low birth weight; IV, intravenous; PICC, peripherally inserted central catheter; UAC, umbilical artery catheter; UVC, umbilical venous catheter.

therapy, use of cephalosporins, hydrocortisone, and heparin.

Other risk factors related to heparin include increased risk of heparin induced thrombocytopenia (HIT), bleeding, and long-term effects on bones.

RECOMMENDATIONS FOR USE OF HEPARIN

1. The use of heparin will be reserved on the basis of the above guidelines. Normal saline locks will be flushed with 0.9% sodium chloride.
2. If the total intravenous infusion rate is less than 2 mL/hr for PICC line, add heparin 0.5 units/mL to TPN or maintenance intravenous fluid.
   a. The ELBW neonate may be excluded in the first few days of life since the initial total fluid goals are low and concomitant continuous infusions may be infusing. The addition of heparin based on rate is under the assumption that the neonate has adequate oral intake with heparin added to maintain patency of line for a short duration until that oral fluid goal is achieved.
3. It is not necessary to add heparin to every intravenous fluid that is being coinfused with TPN or the main IV fluid.
4. UAC minimum infusion rates of 0.5 mL/hr should be reserved for the ELBW infant.

INFILTRATE MANAGEMENT FOR THE NEONATE

BACKGROUND

Neonates are more prone to extravasations secondary to smaller veins, more reactive veins which vasoconstrict more readily, and immature skin structure.

PURPOSE

To provide prompt, appropriate management of extravasation from agents that may cause severe tissue damage when infiltrated (outside the blood vessel).

DEFINITIONS

Extravasation: Discharge or escape of drug from a blood vessel into the tissue which can cause pain, burning, inflammation, necrosis, sloughing, or ulceration of the tissue.

CLASSES OF AGENTS WHICH MAY CAUSE EXTRAVASATION

A) Vesicant—an agent that produces blistering or tissue damage (necrosis) on exposure
   a. Chemotherapeutic agents
B) Hyperosmolar—an agent which alters cellular fluid balance and may lead to cell damage or death
   a. Acyclovir, alprostadil (Prostaglandin E1), aminophylline, calcium chloride, calcium gluconate, contrast media, dextrose >10% concentration, diazepam, indomethacin, ibuprofen, lorazepam, phenytoin, potassium chloride, sodium bicarbonate, sodium chloride 0.9%, thiopental, total parenteral nutrition (TPN)/lipid emulsion.
C) Vasoconstrictor—an agent that restricts local blood flow and may lead to ischemic necrosis
   a. dobutamine, dopamine, epinephrine, norepinephrine, phenylephrine, vasopressin

SIGNS AND SYMPTOMS OF EXTRAVASATION

Swelling
Pain
Erythema

POTENTIAL EXTRAVASATION OUTCOMES

Vessel damage
Necrosis
Skin sloughing
Discoloration
Gangrene
Surgical repair/amputation
Scarring

ASSESSMENT: STAGING OF EXTRAVASATION

STAGING OF IV INFILTRATES

Stage	*Characteristics of Infiltrate*
Stage I	Painful IV site, NO erythema, NO swelling, NO drainage. Flushes with ease
Stage II	Painful IV site, slight swelling (0%–20%), redness, NO blanching, good pulse below site, 1–2 seconds capillary refill below site
Stage III	Painful IV site, marked swelling (30%–50%), blanching, skin cool to touch, good pulse below infiltration site, 1–2 seconds capillary refill below infiltration site
Stage IV	Painful IV site, severe swelling (>50%), blanching, skin cool to touch, decreased or absent pulse[a], capillary refill greater than 4 seconds[a], skin breakdown or necrosis[a].

[a]The presence of any one of these characteristics constitutes a Stage IV infiltrate.
Adapted from Flemmer and Chan 1993; Millam 1988; Winskunas 1990. *Pediatr Nurs* 1993;19(4):355–359 and *Pediat Nurs* 1999;25(2): 167–180.

EXTRAVASATION TREATMENT

TREATMENT FOR EXTRAVASATION OF HYPEROSMOLAR AGENTS

1. Minimize tissue exposure
   a. Discontinue administration of medication immediately
   b. Remove catheter
   c. Notify physician or Neonatal Nurse Practitioner (NNP)
   d. Determine stage of infiltrate
   e. Stage III and IV infiltrates require antidote treatment
2. Minimize inflammation, swelling, and discomfort
   a. Avoid applying pressure to site
   b. DO NOT apply warm or cold compresses
   c. Elevate extremity if possible and if tolerated
   d. Observe site for pain, erythema, swelling, induration, progression of lesion size, signs of skin breakdown every 30 min for 1 hr and then every hour for 4 hr.
3. Administer antidote—hyaluronidase (Amphadase)
   a. Hyaluronidase is a mucolytic enzyme which modifies the normal intercellular tissue barrier/permeability through hydrolysis of hyaluronic acid. This allows for the rapid dispersion of extravasated fluid through tissues
   b. Initiate immediately and ideally within 1 hr of extravasation
   c. Initiate for Stage III/IV infiltrate
   d. Inject 150 units (1 mL) as five separate 0.2 mL subcutaneous/intradermal injections around the periphery of the extravasation site at the leading edge
   e. Use 26-gauge needle and change needle after each injection

TREATMENT OF EXTRAVASATION OF VASOCONSTRICTOR AGENTS

1. Minimize tissue exposure:
   a. Discontinue administration of medication immediately
   b. Assess and document pulse and circulation distal to the extravasated area
   c. Notify physician
   d. Determine stage of infiltrate
      i. Stage III and IV infiltrates require antidote treatment
2. Minimize inflammation, swelling, and discomfort
   a. Elevate extremity as patient tolerates if possible
   b. DO NOT apply warm or cold compresses
   c. Observe site for pain, erythema, swelling, induration, progression of lesion size, signs of skin breakdown every 30 min for 1 hr and then every hour for 4 hr
3. Administer antidote-phentolamine (Regitine)
   a. Phentolamine is an α-adrenergic blocking agent that produces peripheral vasodilation. Phentolamine reverses dermal necrosis produced by vasopressor (α-adrenergic) infiltration
   b. Prepare diluted phentolamine with final concentration of 0.5 mg/mL. (Dilute 5 mg in 10 mL preservative free 0.9% NaCl)
   c. Administer 0.1 mL injections subcutaneously around the periphery of the extravasation site at the leading edge
   d. Use 26-gauge needle and change needle after each injection site
   e. Do not exceed a maximum dose of 0.1 mg/kg or 2.5 mg
   f. Generally only 2–3 injections required
   g. Monitor vital signs every 15 min for 2 hr and watch for complications of hypotension and tachycardia

TABLE A1.11 Intravenous Extravasation Medications

Extravasated Drug	*Antidote*	*Dilution*	*Intervention*
Hyperosmolar agents: Acyclovir Alprostadil—(Prostaglandin E1) Aminophylline Calcium chloride Calcium gluconate Contrast media Dextrose >10% Diazepam Indomethacin Ibuprofen Lorazepam Phenytoin Potassium chloride Sodium bicarbonate Sodium chloride greater than 0.9% Thiopental TPN and lipids	Hyaluronidase (Amphadase)	Draw up 150 units (1 mL) into syringe	1. Notify physician or NP 2. Determine stage of infiltrate. Stage III or IV extravasations meet criteria for hyaluronidase administration 3. Physician/NP to inject 150 units (1 mL) as five separate 0.2 mL subcutaneous injections around the periphery of the extravasation site at the leading edge 4. Use 26-gauge needle and change needle after each injection site 5. Physician or NP to document description of wound and procedure in the progress note section of infant's medical record 6. Document medication administration
Vasoconstrictor agents: Dobutamine Dopamine Epinephrine Norepinephrine Phenylephrine Vasopressin	Phentolamine (Regitine)	Dilute phentolamine to final concentration of 0.5 mg/mL. (Dilute 5 mg in 10 mL preservative free 0.9% NaCl.)	1. Notify physician or NP 2. Determine stage of infiltrate. Stage III or IV extravasation meets criteria for phentolamine administration 3. Physician/NP to administer 0.1 mL injections subcutaneously around the periphery of the extravasation site at the leading edge 4. Use 26-gauge needle and change needle after each injection site 5. Do not exceed a maximum dose of 0.1 mg/kg or 2.5 mg 6. Generally, only two to three injections required 7. Monitor for signs of hypotension and tachycardia

NP, Nurse practitioner; TPN, total parenteral nutrition.

POSTEXTRAVASATION WOUND HEALING—USE OF HYDROGELS

1. Initiate therapy upon collaboration with the physician.
2. Draw up 10 mL of preservative free normal saline into a 10 mL (cc)syringe. In another 10-mL syringe squeeze the contents of the hydrogel tube. Place both syringes in the isolette to warm their contents. Warming may take 15–20 min.
3. Measure the size of the wound, that is, length and width, and record findings.
4. Put on sterile gloves. Irrigate the affected area with the warmed preservative free normal saline. Do not touch the wound with the syringe tip.
5. Place the affected limb into a sterile polyethylene bag forming a "glove" or "boot." A sterile urine collection bags may be used. The mouth of the bag may need to be cut to allow for placement over the extremity. Leave a small opening where the syringe filled with the hydrogel will be injected. Make sure that glove/boot is large enough to allow for full extension of the affected extremity.
6. Squirt hydrogel into the bag to completely cover the wound forming a thin layer between bag and wound. Use 5–10 mL from the syringe containing the hydrogel, depending on the size of the extravasation.
7. Ensure that wound is covered at all times and that the bag does not come in contact with the wound surface.
8. The neck of the bag is closed using surgical tape.
9. An additional bag may be placed over the polyethylene bag to minimize disruption of applied thick layer of gel. Secure the bag with surgical tape, taking care to avoid making the tape too tight around the extremity.
10. A splint may be applied to the extremity to support the weight of the gel.
11. Dressing may be left on for 3 day.
12. Monitor for signs of infection with each dressing change.
13. Do dressing changes every 3 day. Slide bag off limb and irrigate with normal saline. No contact as rubbing or patting of the wound site is required.
14. Monitor for signs of infection.
15. During healing, a pale yellow, semisolid fibrinous layer may develop but this does not affect the healing process. Do not disturb this layer.
16. Healing process is dramatic but slow and may require five to seven dressing changes.
17. Document interventions and neonate's responses each shift with the nursing assessment.

NICU IV ELECTROLYTE SUPPLEMENTATION GUIDELINES

BACKGROUND

Blood/serum osmolarity 300–310 mOsm/L
Isotonic solution 280–310 mOsm/L

The tonicity of a solution dictates whether it should be infused peripherally or centrally. When solutions with extremes of tonicity are infused, fluids shift into or out of cells. This resulting change in cell size of the vein wall will cause the inflammatory and clotting process to occur which can lead to phlebitis and thrombophlebitis.

PERIPHERAL IV MAXIMUM OSMOLARITY: 900 MOSM/L FOR NON-TPN SOLUTIONS

Ability of peripheral veins to dilute parenteral infusions is compromised when osmolarity is greater than 900 mOsm/L.

Hypotonic solutions such as 0.2% normal saline (1/4 NS) can cause the red blood cell to swell and burst and can result in hemolytic anemia.

DEFINITIONS

1. **Osmolarity**
   The concentration of the solute in a solution per unit of solvent, usually mmol solute per liter.
2. **Tonicity**
   Frequently used in place of osmotic pressure or tension is related to the number of particles found in solution. Osmolarity is most often used when referring to blood and tonicity is most often used when referring to intravenous fluid, but the terms may be used interchangeably.
3. **Isotonic**
   Of equal tension. Denoting a solution having the same tonicity as another solution with which it is compared.
4. **Hypertonic**
   Having a higher concentration of solute particles per unit volume than a comparison solution, regardless of kinds of particles. A solution in which cells shrink due to efflux of water.
5. **Hypotonic**
   Having a lower concentration of solute particles per unit volume than a comparison solution, regardless of kinds of particles. A solution in which cells expand because of influx of water.

TABLE A1.12 Osmolarity of Common Intravenous Admixture Fluids in NICU

Solution Type	*Osmolarity (mOsm/L)*
0.2% normal saline	77
0.45% normal saline	154
0.9% normal saline	308
Dextrose 5% in water	252
Dextrose 10% in water	505
D5W/0.2% NS	321
D5W/0.45% NS	406
D5W/0.9% NS	560
D10W/0.2% NS	573
D10W/0.45% NS	661
D10W/0.9% NS	817
D5W/0.2% NS/20KCl/L	360
D10W/0.2% NS/20KCl/L	613
D5W/0.2% NS/20KCl/L/Calcium 560 mg/L elemental	401
D10W/0.2% NS/20KCl/L/Calcium 560 mg/L elemental	654
D5W/0.9% NS/20KCl/L	604
D10W/0.9% NS/20KCl/L	857
D5W/0.9% NS/20KCl/L/calcium 560 mg/L elemental	645
D10W/0.9% NS/20KCl/L/calcium 560 mg/L elemental	898

NS, normal saline.

TABLE A1.13 Osmolarity of Common Electrolyte Additives

Electrolyte	*Strength*	*Osmolarity Per mL*
NaCl	2.5 mEq/mL	5 mOsm/mL
Na Acetate	2 mEq/mL	5 mOsm/mL
Potassium chloride/acetate	2 mEq/mL	4 mOsm/mL
Magnesium sulfate	125 mg/mL	4.06 mOsm/mL
Calcium gluconate	100 mg/mL	0.308 mOsm/mL
Phosphate—as potassium	3 mmol/mL	7.4 mOsm/mL
Phosphate—as sodium	4 mEq/mL	12 mOsm/mL

POTASSIUM REPLACEMENT GUIDELINES

INDICATION

Serum potassium <3 mEq/L
Incorporate into maintenance intravenous solution for serum levels ≥3 mg/dL; intermittent intravenous potassium administration should be reserved for severe depletion.

DOSE

0.5–1 mEq/kg/dose potassium chloride **intravenous slowly** over 1–2 hr × one dose

PREPARATION

Peripheral 0.08 mEq/mL final concentration
Central 0.15 mEq/mL final concentration

POTASSIUM MUST ALWAYS BE DILUTED

DAILY REQUIREMENTS:

Term infant: 1–2 mEq/kg/day
Preterm infant: 2–6 mEq/kg/day

REFERENCE RANGE

3.4–5 mEq/L

(Please note that electrolytes obtained by heel stick in this population will often be hemolyzed and result in an artificially high potassium level. A suspected true elevation of the potassium level may result in electrocardiographic changes and will require confirmation with a repeat level obtained arterially.)

CONCOMITANT DRUG THERAPIES WHICH MAY REQUIRE LARGER MAINTENANCE POTASSIUM

Continuous albuterol respiratory treatment; amphotericin B, diuretics, and caspofungin

NOTES

Infuse slowly over 1–2 hr. Continuous cardiac monitoring (may cause cardiac arrhythmias) is required during infusion.

Monitor site closely during infusion since infiltrations can cause severe tissue damage.

MAGNESIUM REPLACEMENT GUIDELINES

INDICATION

Serum magnesium <1.5 mEq/L

DOSE

Magnesium sulfate 25–50 mg/kg/dose **IV** q8–12 hr for 2–3 doses

Infuse slowly over 2–4 hr

PREPARATION

125 mg/mL

DAILY REQUIREMENTS

Term infant: 0.125–0.25 mEq/kg/day (1.6–3.1 mg/kg/day)

Preterm infant: 0.25–0.5 mEq/kg/day (3.1–6.3 mg/kg/day)

REFERENCE RANGE

1.5–2.3 mEq/L

CONCOMITANT DRUG THERAPIES WHICH MAY REQUIRE LARGER MAINTENANCE MAGNESIUM

Amphotericin B

NOTES

Infuse slowly over 2–4 hr. Hypotension may result with rapid intravenous administration. Monitor blood pressure and monitor for cardiac arrhythmia and respiratory and central nervous system depression.

Overdoses may be treated with calcium gluconate.

PHOSPHATE REPLACEMENT GUIDELINES

INDICATION

Exact treatment in terms of dosing of severe hypophosphatemia may be difficult since the extent of total body deficits and response to therapy may be difficult to predict. Aggressive doses of phosphate may result in a transient serum elevation followed by redistribution into intracellular compartments or bone tissue.

Intestinal absorption by the oral route is unreliable and large doses of phosphate may cause diarrhea.

Low dose	When losses are recent and uncomplicated
Intermediate dose	Serum phosphate 0.5–1 mg/dL
High dose	Serum phosphate <0.5 mg/dL

(Note: These guidelines for dose replacement are based on adult serum phosphate levels. The renal handling of phosphate by the neonatal kidney is different than the adult. Adults maintain a neutral phosphate balance by excreting the same amount of phosphate as they absorb by the gastrointestinal tract. Neonates are in positive phosphate balance and only 60% of phosphate absorbed from diet is excreted in the urine. This high serum phosphate level in neonates is NOT a manifestation of a lower glomerular filtration rate but of a higher proximal tubular reabsorption capacity. Normal serum phosphate levels in a neonate are 4.8–7.2 mg/dL and in an adult are 2.3–5 mg/dL)

DOSE

Replacement

Low dose	0.08 mmol/kg sodium phosphate **IV** × 1 dose Infuse slowly over 2–4 hr
Intermediate dose	0.16–0.24 mmol/kg sodium phosphate **IV** × 1 dose Infuse slowly over 2–4 hr
High dose	0.36 mmol/kg sodium phosphate **IV** × 1 dose Infuse slowly over 2–4 hr

PREPARATION

Central: 0.05 mmol/mL
Peripheral: 0.12 mmol/mL

DAILY REQUIREMENTS

Term: 25–40 mg/kg/day
Preterm: 60–140 mg/kg/day

REFERENCE RANGE

Newborn: 4.2–9 mg/dL (Note that range is higher for infants than for adults)

6 wk–18 months: 3.8–6.7 mg/dL

NOTES

Non–total parenteral nutrition (TPN) maintenance intravenous solutions containing phosphate CANNOT contain calcium. These solutions in the absence of buffering agents such as amino acids and cysteine placed in TPN are NOT COMPATIBLE.

Infuse slowly over 2–4 hr. Monitor for hypocalcemia and hypotension.

CALCIUM REPLACEMENT GUIDELINES

INDICATION

Serum calcium (<7 mg/dL)

Note that the direct correlation between serum ionized calcium and total serum calcium is poor especially in states of low albumin or acid/base imbalances. Direct measurement of ionized calcium is recommended.

Total corrected calcium (with low albumin) = Total serum calcium + 0.8 (4 − measured serum albumin)

DOSE

Replacement

200–800 mg/kg/day IV divided q6 hr as calcium gluconate

MAINTENANCE

Intravenous solutions containing calcium that wish to match the current TPN concentration are expressed as "elemental calcium of 560 mg/L as calcium gluconate" which is then 3,000 mg/L.

Please note that calcium and phosphorus content will be halved if amino acid concentration is <15 g/L or if neonate is >2 kg with a total fluid goal of >120 mL/kg/day.

PREPARATION

50 mg/mL for doses less than 150 mg
100 mg/mL (straight drug)

DAILY REQUIREMENTS

Term: 0.5–2.5 mEq/kg/day
Preterm: 4–5 mEq/kg/day

REFERENCE RANGE

Newborns 7–12 mg/dL

NOTES

Non-TPN maintenance intravenous solutions containing calcium CANNOT contain phosphate. These solutions in the absence of buffering agents such as amino acids and cysteine placed in TPN are NOT COMPATIBLE.

Monitor intravenous sites closely for infiltration. Rapid intravenous administration can cause bradycardia and arrhythmias.

SODIUM REPLACEMENT GUIDELINES

INDICATION

Serum sodium <130 mEq/L

DOSE

Correction of hyponatremia:

mEq sodium needed = Desired sodium (mEq/L) − actual sodium (mEq/L) × 0.6 × Wt (kg)

Replace sodium gradually. Replace half the calculated amount over 12–24 hr.

MAINTENANCE

Standard TPN solution contains 26 mEq/L Na

IV maintenance solutions wishing to match the TPN concentration should contain 0.3% normal saline = 26 mEq/L

PREPARATION

1/2 normal saline (0.45%) = 77 mEq/L
Normal saline (0.9%) = 154 mEq/L

Hypertonic saline (3%) = 513 mEq/L (Reserved for only acute life-threatening symptomatic hyponatremia.)

DAILY REQUIREMENTS

Premature neonates: 2–8 mEq/kg/day
Term neonates 1–4 mEq/kg/day

REFERENCE RANGE

Premature neonates: 132–140 mEq/L
Term neonates 133–142 mEq/L
Infants >2 months 135–145 mEq/L

NOTES

Hypertonic 3% saline should be reserved in life-threatening emergencies (1,025 mOsm/L) and can cause phlebitis (administer via central line only).

Excessive dosage or too rapid administration rate can cause pulmonary edema and lead to sudden increases in serum osmolality that may result in central nervous system hemorrhage.

DISCLAIMER/NOTICE

This version of Hutzel Women's Hospital formulary has been edited for content and length. Drug information is constantly evolving because of ongoing research, clinical experience and government regulations. It is often subject to interpretation and evaluation of the clinician. Although great care has been taken to ensure the accuracy of the information presented, the reader is advised that the authors, editors, reviewers, contributors, and Hutzel Women's Hospital cannot be held responsible for the continued currency of the information or for any errors, omissions, or applications of this information, or for any consequences arising subsequently. The decisions regarding drug therapy must be based on the independent judgment of the clinician, changing information about a drug (e.g., as reflected in the literature, the manufacturer's most current product information), and changing medical practices. This appendix is intended for use in conjunction with other necessary information and is not intended to be solely relied upon by any user.

Shannon F. Manzi
Alana Arnold
Al Patterson

APPENDIX

A2

Pediatric Drug Formulary

DISCLAIMER

This version of the Children's Hospital of Boston formulary supported by Lexicomp platform has been edited for content and length. The nature of drug information is constantly evolving because of ongoing research and clinical experience and is often subject to interpretation. Although great care has been taken to ensure the accuracy of the information presented, the reader is advised that the authors, editors, reviewers, contributors, and Children's Hospital of Boston cannot be held responsible for the continued currency of the information or for any errors, omissions, or applications of this information, or for any consequences arising subsequently.

Because of the dynamic nature of drug information, readers are advised that decisions regarding drug therapy must be based on the independent judgment of the clinician, changing information about a drug (e.g., as reflected in the literature and the manufacturer's most current product information), and changing medical practices. Therefore, these data are intended to be used in conjunction with other necessary information and are not intended to be solely relied upon by any user.

TABLE A2.1 Pediatric Drug Formulary[a,b,c,d]		
Medication	*Dosage*	*Comments*
Abacavir (Ziagen)	8 mg/kg/dose p.o. b.i.d.; max dose: 300 mg b.i.d.	• Hypersensitivity in 5%—DO NOT rechallenges
Acetaminophen Tylenol)	Pre-op loading dose: 30 mg/kg/dose p.r. for 1 dose Emergency department: high dose (may only be prescribed by attending or fellow) 40 mg/kg/dose p.r. for 1 dose 10–15 mg/kg/dose p.o./p.r. q4 hr p.r.n. Not to exceed max of 4 g/day or 75 mg/kg/day, whichever is less	• All acetaminophen orders will be automatically discontinued after 72 hr; infants and children with continued fever, viral illness, dehydration, nausea, and vomiting may be at a higher risk for hepatic injury; consider using ibuprofen or morphine if round-the-clock doses are needed
AcetaZOLamide (Diamox)	20 mg/kg/day i.v./p.o. div q6 hr; increase by 25 mg/kg/day; a maximum dose of 100 mg/kg/day has been used	• Adjust dosing interval in renal impairment
Acetylcysteine (Mucomyst) ☹	Acetaminophen poisoning: • Oral: 140 mg/kg, followed by 17 doses of 70 mg/kg q4 hr; repeat dose if emesis occurs within 1 hr of administration • Intravenous: If approved by toxicology, 150 mg/kg i.v. over 60 min followed by 50 mg/kg i.v. over 4 hr then 100 mg/kg over 16 hrs. Secretion management, inhalation: • Infants: 1–2 mL of 20% solution or 2–4 mL of 10% solution via nebulizer t.i.d.–q.i.d. • Children: 3–5 mL of 20% solution or 6–10 mL of 10% solution via nebulizer t.i.d.–q.i.d. • Adolescents: 5–10 mL of 10%–20% solution via nebulizer t.i.d.–q.i.d. Renal protection for radiographic contrast agent-induced reductions in renal function: oral, 10 mg/kg/dose up to 600 mg p.o. b.i.d. on day prior to and day of procedure Meconium ileus equivalent: oral, rectal irrigation, 5–30 mL of 10%–20% solution 3–6 times/day for at least 24 hr and symptom improvement	• Injection: restricted to toxicology • Treatment should still be considered in patients presenting late; minimize free water in pediatric patients, dilute to no less than 30 mg/mL in D5W • Patients should receive an aerosolized bronchodilator 10–15 min prior to inhaled acetylcysteine
Acyclovir (Zovirax)	Herpes simplex virus encephalitis: 60 mg/kg/day i.v. div q8 hr Varicella zoster virus and herpes simplex virus: 30 mg/kg/day i.v. div q8 hr 80 mg/kg/day p.o. div 3–5 times/day Oral max: 3,200 mg/day	• Adequate hydration required to prevent nephrotoxicity: 1.5 times maintenance IVF per day recommended, or 2 times maintenance 1 hr before and during, and 1 hr after, acyclovir infusion; carefully monitor urine output (must be ≥1.5 mL/kg/hr) • Dose for obese patients should be based on ideal body weight
Adenosine (Adenocard)	Children <50 kg: • Neonates: 0.05 mg/kg i.v. × 1 dose; if not effective within 2 min, increase dose by 0.05-mg/kg increments q2 min to a maximum dose of 0.25 mg/kg or until termination of PSVT • Infants and children: PALS dose for treatment of SVT 0.1 mg/kg (max: 6 mg); if not effective, give 0.2 mg/kg (max: 12 mg) • Children and adolescents weighing ≥50 kg and adults: 6 mg; if not effective within 1–2 min, 12 mg may be given; may repeat 12 mg × 1	• May need to use higher dose for refractory SVT • Administer simultaneously with NS flush, may use three-way stopcock
Albuterol (Proventil, Ventolin)	0.5% inhalation solution INH q1–6 hr p.r.n.: • <10 kg: 0.25 mL/dose • 10–30 kg: 0.5 mL/dose • >30 kg: 1 mL/dose Inhalation: MDI: 90 mcg/actuation • Children <12 yr: 1–2 inhalations 4 times/day • Children ≥12 yr to adults: 2–4 inhalations q4–6 hr Maximum 12 inhalations/day during maintenance therapy Intensive care patients: continuous nebulized albuterol at 0.5 mg/kg/hr	• Aerosolized: dilute 0.5% solution with 1–2 mL of NS and administer with appropriate small-volume nebulizer • Suggested β_2-agonist total max: 20 mg/hr

(*continued*)

TABLE A2.1 Pediatric Drug Formulary[a,b,c,d] (*Continued*)

Medication	*Dosage*	*Comments*
Allopurinol (Aloprim)	Prevention of acute uric acid nephropathy in myeloproliferative neoplastic disorders: Children ≤10 yr: • Intravenous: 100 mg/m^2/dose i.v. q8 hr; max dose: 600 mg/day • Oral: <6 yr: 50 mg p.o. t.i.d.; 6–10 yr: 100 mg p.o. t.i.d. Children >10 yr and adults: • Intravenous: 200–400 mg/m^2/day i.v. in 1–3 div doses; max: 600 mg/day • Oral: 600–800 mg/day p.o. in 2–3 div doses	• Begin 1–2 day before chemotherapy • Adjust dose in renal impairment • Daily doses >300 mg should be administered in divided doses
Alprazolam (Xanax)	Children <18 yr: initial doses of 0.005 mg/kg or 0.125 mg p.o., increase by increments of 0.125–0.25 mg/dose; maximum of 0.02 mg/kg/dose or 0.06 mg/kg/day Adults: 0.25–0.5 mg p.o. 2–3 times/day, titrate dose upward; max dose: 10 mg/day	• Adequate studies in children have not been completed
Alprostadil (Prostin)	Neonates and infants: 0.05–0.1 mcg/kg/min; maintenance 0.01–0.4 mcg/kg/min	• With therapeutic response, rate is reduced to lowest effective dosage
Alteplase (tPA) (Activase)	Catheter clearance, volume of catheter + 10%: max of 2 mg/2 mL in clogged port for 20 min–2 hr, then withdraw Systemic thrombolytic therapy: 0.1–0.6 mg/kg/hr i.v. × 6 hr	• Central venous catheter occlusion: dose listed is per lumen; for multilumen catheters, treat one lumen at a time • Consult hematology service for all continuous infusions
Amikacin (Amikin)	15–22.5 mg/kg/day i.v. div q8 hr	• Restricted to ID service • Check trough level prior to third dose; check peak level after third dose • Goal: pre, <10 mcg/mL; post, 15–30 mcg/mL
Aminocaproic acid (Amicar)	Load: 50–100 mg/kg i.v. × 1 Maintenance: continuous infusion of 30 mg/kg/hr i.v. OR 100 mg/kg/dose i.v./p.o. q6 hr Max dose: 30 g/day	

Aminophylline	All doses based on aminophylline
	Apnea of prematurity:
	• Loading dose: 5 mg/kg p.o./i.v. × 1
	• Maintenance: initial: 5 mg/kg/day p.o. div q12 hr; increased doses may be indicated as liver metabolism matures (usually >30 day of life)
	Treatment of acute bronchospasm:
	• Loading dose (in patients not currently receiving aminophylline or theophylline): 6 mg/kg (based on aminophylline) given i.v. over 20–30 min
	• Approximate i.v. maintenance dosages are based on continuous infusions; intermittent dosing (often used in children <6 mo of age) may be determined by multiplying the hourly infusion rate by 24 hr and dividing by the desired number of doses/day (usually in 3–4 doses/day):
	  • 6 wk–6 mo: 0.5 mg/kg/hr
	  • 6 mo–1 yr: 0.6–0.7 mg/kg/hr
	  • 1–9 yr: 1–1.2 mg/kg/hr
	  • 9–12 yr and young adult smokers: 0.9 mg/kg/hr
	  • 12–16 yr: 0.7 mg/kg/hr
		• Monitor serum levels to determine appropriate doses
		• Theophylline levels should be initially drawn after 3 day of therapy; repeat levels are indicated 3 day after each increase in dose or weekly if on a stabilized dose

Amiodarone (Cordarone)	VF/VT arrest: 5 mg/kg i.v./i.o. rapid push Dysrhythmia (unstable): 5 mg/kg i.v./i.o. over 20–60 min Max: 300 mg/dose	• Dilute in D5W only • Glass container only for large-volume parenteral
Amoxicillin (Amoxil) ☺	40–120 mg/kg/day p.o. div q8 hr; max: 3 g/day	• Usual 80 mg/kg/day
Amoxicillin/clavulanic acid (Augmentin) ☺	Augmentin tablets: 40 mg/kg/day p.o. div q8 hr Augmentin ES-600 liquid: 40–90 mg/kg/day p.o. div q8 hr Max: 3 g as amoxicillin/day	• Dosed as amoxicillin • Diarrhea associated w/higher doses of clavulanic acid
Amphotericin B (Fungizone)	0.5–1 mg/kg/dose i.v. q. day, max: 1.5 mg/kg/day Cystic fibrosis: 15 mg INH b.i.d.	• Max concentration for fluid-restricted patients 0.2 mg/mL via central line

(*continued*)

TABLE A2.1 Pediatric Drug Formulary[a,b,c,d] (*Continued*)

Medication	*Dosage*	*Comments*
Amphotericin B liposomal (Ambisome)	3 mg/kg/day i.v. q. day, max: 5 mg/kg/day	• ID approval required
Ampicillin	200–400 mg/kg/day i.v. div q6 hr; max: 12 g/day	
Ampicillin/sulbactam (Unasyn)	200 mg/kg/day i.v. div q6 hr Max: 8 g/day as ampicillin May add extra ampicillin for total 12 g/day	• Dose based on ampicillin component
Amprenavir (Agenerase) ☹	Oral solution: 22.5 mg/kg/dose p.o. b.i.d. Capsule: 20 mg/kg/dose p.o. b.i.d. Max doses: • Solution: 2,800 mg/day • Capsules: 2,400 mg/day	• Avoid high-fat meals • Solution and capsules not equivalent on a mg-per-mg basis
Aspirin	10–15 mg/kg/dose p.o. q4–6 hr p.r.n. Acute myocardial infarction: 325 mg p.o. (chewed) × 1 dose Kawasaki disease: 80–100 mg/kg/day p.o. div q6 hr until fever resolves, then 3–5 mg/kg/day p.o. q. day	
Atenolol (Tenormin)	Initial: 0.8–1 mg/kg/dose p.o. q. day Range: 0.8–1.5 mg/kg/dose p.o. q. day Max: 2 mg/kg/dose p.o. q. day	
Atovaquone (Mepron)	Treatment: 40 mg/kg/day p.o. div q12 hr; max: 1,500 mg/day Prophylaxis: 30–45 mg/kg/day p.o. q. day	
Atropine	Premedication for rapid-sequence intubation (<7 yr): 0.02 mg/kg/dose i.v./i.o. Bradycardia: 0.02 mg/kg/dose i.v./i.o.; repeat × 1 p.r.n. min 0.1 mg/dose, max: 1 mg/dose	• If giving via endotracheal tube, dose is 2–10 × i.v. dose • Dilute ETT dose in 3–5 mL of NS and follow with several positive-pressure breaths
Azathioprine (Imuran)	Initial: 2–5 mg/kg/dose p.o./i.v. q. day Maintenance: 1–3 mg/kg/dose p.o./i.v. q. day	
Azithromycin (Zithromax) ☺	Otitis media: 30 mg/kg (max: 1,500 mg/dose) p.o. × 1 dose GABHS pharyngitis: 12 mg/kg/day q. day × 5 day OR 10 mg/kg/dose p.o. q. day × 1 day, then 5 mg/kg/dose p.o. q. day × 4 day Community-acquired pneumonia: 10 mg/kg/dose i.v./p.o. q. day × 1 day (max: 500 mg/dose), followed by 5 mg/kg/dose p.o./i.v. q. day (max: 250 mg/dose) × 4 day *Chlamydia* prophylaxis postsexual assault: 1,000 mg p.o. × 1 dose	
Aztreonam (Azactam)	90–120 mg/kg/day i.v. div q6–8 hr; max: 8 g/day	
Baclofen (Lioresal)	Oral: • 2–7 yr: initial 10–15 mg/day div q8 hr; max: 40 mg/day • >8 yr: titrate dosage as above, max: 60 mg/day • Adults: 5 mg 3 times/day, max: 80 mg/day Intrathecal: Screening dosage: 50 mcg for 1 dose and observe for 4–8 hr; very small children may receive 25 mcg; if ineffective, a repeat dose increased by 50% (e.g., 75 mcg) may be repeated in 24 hr; if still suboptimal, a third dose increased by 33% (e.g., 100 mcg) may be repeated in 24 hr; patients who do not respond to 100 mcg intrathecally should not be considered for continuous chronic administration via an implantable pump Maintenance intrathecal dose: continuous infusion Initial: depends on the screening dosage and its duration: • If the screening dose duration >8 hr: daily dose = effective screening dose • If the screening dose duration <8 hr: daily dose = twice effective screening dose Continuous intrathecal infusion dose mcg/hr = daily dose div by 24 hr	• Titrate dose q3 day in increments of 5–15 mg/day • Further adjustments in infusion rate may be done q24 hr p.r.n.; for spinal cord–related spasticity, increase in 10%–30% increments/24 hr; for spasticity of cerebral origin, increase in 5%–10% increments/24 hr

(*continued*)

TABLE A2.1 Pediatric Drug Formulary[a,b,c,d] (*Continued*)

Medication	*Dosage*	*Comments*
	Average daily intrathecal dose: • Children ≤12 yr: 100–300 mcg/day (4.2–12.5 mcg/hr); doses as high as 1,000 mcg/day have been used • Children >12 yr and adults: 300–800 mcg/day (12.5–33 mcg/hr); doses as high as 2,000 mcg/day have been used	
Basiliximab (Simulect)	Children <35 kg: renal transplantation: 10 mg i.v. within 2 hr prior to transplant surgery, followed by a second 10-mg dose i.v. 4 day after transplantation Children ≥35 kg and adults: renal transplantation: 20 mg i.v. within 2 hr prior to transplant surgery, followed by a second, 20-mg i.v. dose 4 day after transplantation	• The second dose should be withheld if complications occur (including severe hypersensitivity reactions or graft loss)
Benztropine (Cogentin)	Drug-induced extrapyramidal reaction: • >3 yr: 0.02–0.05 mg/kg/dose p.o./i.m./i.v. q. day–b.i.d. • Adults: 1–4 mg/dose p.o./i.m./i.v. q. day–b.i.d. Parkinsonism: 0.5–6 mg/day p.o. in 1–2 div doses; begin with 0.5 mg/day; increase in 0.5-mg increments at 5- to 6-d intervals to achieve the desired effect	• Use in children <3 yr should be reserved for life-threatening emergencies
Beractant (Survanta)	Prophylactic treatment: give 4 mL/kg as soon as possible; as many as 4 doses may be administered during the first 48 hr of life, no more frequently than 6 hr apart Rescue treatment: give 4 mL/kg as soon as the diagnosis of RDS is made; may repeat if needed, no more frequently than q6 hr to a maximum of 4 doses	• The need for additional doses is determined by evidence of continuing respiratory distress or if the infant is still intubated and requiring at least 30% inspired oxygen to maintain a PaO_2 ≤80 torr
Bisacodyl (Dulcolax)	Oral: • 3–12 yr: 5–10 mg or 0.3 mg/kg/day p.o. q. day • ≥12 yr and adults: 5–15 mg/day p.o. q. day Rectal: • 2–11 yr: 5–10 mg/day p.r. q. day • ≥12 yr and adults: 10 mg/day p.r. q. day	• <2 yr: 5 mg/day p.r. q. day
Botulinum toxin type A (Botox)	Strabismus: Children 2 mo–12 yr: • Horizontal or vertical deviations <20 prism diopters: 1.25 units into any one muscle • Horizontal or vertical deviations 20–25 prism diopters: 1–2.5 units into any one muscle • Persistent VI nerve palsy of ≥1 mo duration: 1–1.25 units into the medial rectus muscle Children ≥12 yr and adults: • Horizontal or vertical deviations <20 prism diopters: 1.25–2.5 units into any one muscle • Horizontal or vertical deviations 20–50 prism diopters: 2.5–5 units into any one muscle • Persistent VI nerve palsy of ≥1 mo duration: 1.25–2.5 units into the medial rectus muscle Spasticity associated with cerebral palsy, children >18 mo to adolescents: small muscle, 1–2 units/kg; large muscle, 3–6 units/kg; maximum dose per injection site 50 units; maximum dose for any one visit 12 units/kg, up to 400 units; no more than 400 units should be administered during a 3-mo period	• For strabismus, reexamine patient 7–14 day after each injection to assess effects; dose may be increased up to twofold of the previously administered dose; do not exceed 25 units as a single injection for any one muscle
Budesonide (Pulmicort Turbuhaler, Pulmicort Respules)	Intranasal: children ≥6 yr and adults, Rhinocort: initial, 8 sprays (4 sprays/nostril) per day (256 mcg/day); after symptoms decrease (usually by 3–7 day), reduce dose slowly q2–4 wk to the smallest effective dose Nebulization: children 12 mo–8 yr, Pulmicort Respules: • Previously treated with bronchodilators alone: initial, 0.25 mg b.i.d. or 0.5 mg once daily; max dose: 0.5 mg/day • Previously treated with inhaled corticosteroids: initial, 0.25 mg b.i.d. or 0.5 mg once daily; max dose: 1 mg/day • Previously treated with oral corticosteroids: initial, 0.5 mg b.i.d. or 1 mg once daily; max dose: 1 mg/day	• Administer via a Nebulizer Medication System with filter; requires no further dilution

(*continued*)

TABLE A2.1 Pediatric Drug Formulary[a,b,c,d] (*Continued*)

Medication	*Dosage*	*Comments*
	Oral inhalation, children ≥6 yr: • Previously treated with bronchodilators alone or with inhaled corticosteroids: initial, 200 mcg (1 puff) b.i.d.; max dose: 400 mcg (2 puffs) b.i.d. • Treated with oral corticosteroids: initial, 400 mcg (2 puffs) b.i.d. (maximum dose)	
Bumetanide (Bumex)	Neonates: 0.01–0.05 mg/kg/dose i.v./i.m./p.o. q24–48 hr Infants and children: 0.015–0.1 mg/kg/dose i.v./i.m./p.o. q6–24 hr (max dose: 10 mg/day)	
Bupropion (Wellbutrin)	Children and adolescents: 1.4–6 mg/kg/day p.o. q. day	
Caffeine citrate	Apnea of prematurity: oral: • Loading dose: 10–20 mg/kg as caffeine citrate (5–10 mg/kg as caffeine base) • Maintenance dose: 5–10 mg/kg/day as caffeine citrate (2.5–5 mg/kg/day as caffeine base) once daily starting 24 hr after the loading dose	• If theophylline has been administered to the patient within the previous 5 day, a full or modified loading dose (50%–75% of a loading dose) may be given at the discretion of the physician • Maintenance dose is adjusted based on patient's response (efficacy and adverse effects) and serum caffeine concentrations
Calcitriol (Rocaltrol)	Management of hypocalcemia in patients with chronic renal failure: Hemodialysis patients: Intravenous: • Children: 0.01–0.05 mcg/kg i.v. 3 times/wk • Adults: 0.5 mcg (0.01 mcg/kg) i.v. 3 times/wk; may increase dose by 0.25- to 0.5-mcg increments at 2- to 4-wk intervals until an optimal response is achieved; range 0.5–3 mcg (0.01–0.05 mcg/kg) Oral: • Children: 0.25–2 mcg/day p.o. q. day • Adults: 0.25 mcg p.o. q. day; may increase in 0.25-mcg increments at 4- to 8-wk intervals; range 0.5–1 mcg/day Nonhemodialysis patients: moderate-to-severe renal failure (CrCl 15–55 mL/min; corrected for surface area in children): oral: • Children <3 yr: 0.01–0.015 mcg/kg p.o. once daily • Children ≥3 yr and adults: 0.25 mcg/day p.o. q. day (max dose: 0.5 mcg/day) Hypoparathyroidism/pseudohypoparathyroidism: oral (evaluate dose at 2- to 4-wk intervals): • Children <1 yr: 0.04–0.08 mcg/kg p.o. q. day • Children 1–5 yr: 0.25–0.75 mcg p.o. q. day • Children >6 yr and adults: 0.5–2 mcg p.o. q. day Vitamin D-dependent rickets: children and adults, oral: 1 mcg p.o. once daily Vitamin D-resistant rickets (familial hypophosphatemia): children and adults, oral: • Initial: 0.015–0.02 mcg/kg p.o. once daily • Maintenance: 0.03–0.06 mcg/kg p.o. once daily • Max dose: 2 mcg p.o. once daily Hypocalcemia in premature infants: oral, 1 mcg p.o. once daily for 5 day Hypocalcemic tetany in premature infants: i.v., 0.05 mcg/kg i.v. once daily for 5–12 day	• Maintain calcium levels of 9–10 mg/dL
Calcium carbonate	Recommended daily allowance (dose is in terms of elemental calcium): • <6 mo: 400 mg/day • 6–12 mo: 600 mg/day • 1–10 yr: 800 mg/day • 11–24 yr: 1,200 mg/day • Adults >24 yr: 800 mg/day	

(*continued*)

TABLE A2.1 Pediatric Drug Formulary[a,b,c,d] (*Continued*)

Medication	*Dosage*	*Comments*
	Hypocalcemia (dose depends on clinical condition and serum calcium level): oral (dose expressed in mg of elemental calcium): • Neonates: 50–150 mg/kg/day p.o. in 4–6 div doses; not to exceed 1 g/day • Children: 45–65 mg/kg/day p.o. in 4 div doses • Adults: 1–2 g or more per day p.o. in 3–4 div doses	
Calcium CHLORIDE	10–20 mg/kg/dose central i.v./i.o., slowly	• 10% solution = 100 mg/mL • Must further dilute prior to administration
Calcium GLUCONATE	100–200 mg/kg/dose central i.v./i.o., slowly Max: 3 g/dose	• 10% solution = 100 mg/mL
Captopril (Capoten)	Neonates: 0.05–0.1 mg/kg/dose p.o. t.i.d. Children: 0.3–0.5 mg/kg/dose p.o. t.i.d. Adults: 6.25–25 mg/dose p.o. t.i.d.	
Carbamazepine (Tegretol, Carbatrol)	10–35 mg/kg/day p.o. div b.i.d.–t.i.d.	• Dose individualized based on levels • Suppositories made by pharmacy
Carnitine (Carnitor)	Primary carnitine deficiency: oral: • Children: 50–100 mg/kg/day p.o. div b.i.d.–t.i.d., max: 3 g/day • Adults: 330–990 mg/dose p.o. b.i.d.–t.i.d. Valproic acid toxicity: prophylaxis: 50–100 mg/kg/day p.o. div b.i.d.–t.i.d. Active hepatotoxicity/overdose: • Oral: 150–500 mg/kg/day p.o. div b.i.d.–t.i.d., max: 3 g/day • Intravenous: 50 mg/kg i.v. load, followed (in severe cases) by 50 mg/kg/day infusion; maintenance: 50 mg/kg/day i.v. div q4–6 hr, increase as needed to a maximum of 300 mg/kg/day ESRD patients on hemodialysis: • Intravenous: adults, predialysis carnitine levels below normal (30–60 μmol): 10–20 mg/kg i.v. after each dialysis session; maintenance doses as low as 5 mg/kg may be used after 3–4 wk of therapy depending on response (carnitine level) Supplement to parenteral nutrition: neonates, 10–20 mg/kg/day in parenteral nutrition solution	• Dosage must be individualized based on patient response; higher doses have been used
Caspofungin (Cancidas)	For patients weighing <15 kg: • Loading dose: 1.5 mg/kg i.v. × 1 (max: 70 mg) • Daily dose: 1 mg/kg/day i.v. q. day (max: 50 mg) For patients weighing >15 kg: • Loading dose: 70 mg/m^2 i.v. × 1 (max: 70 mg) • Daily dose: 50 mg/m^2/day i.v. q. day (max: 50 mg)	• Adjust dose in hepatic dysfunction
Cefazolin (Kefzol, Ancef)	50–150 mg/kg/day i.v. div q8 hr Max: 12 g/day	• Usual adult 2 g/dose
Cefdinir (Omnicef)☺	Infants and children (≥6 mo–12 yr): • Otitis media or pharyngitis/tonsillitis: 14 mg/kg/day p.o. div q12 hr for 5–10 day or 14 mg/kg/day p.o. q. day for 10 day • Skin and soft tissue infection: 14 mg/kg/day p.o. div b.i.d. for 10 day • Acute maxillary sinusitis: 14 mg/kg/day p.o. div q12 hr for 10 day or 14 mg/kg/day p.o. q. day for 10 day Children >12 yr and adults: • Acute exacerbations of chronic bronchitis or pharyngitis/tonsillitis: 600 mg p.o. q. day for 10 day or 300 mg p.o. q12 hr for 5–10 day • Skin and soft tissue infection or community-acquired pneumonia: 300 mg p.o. q12 hr for 10 day • Acute maxillary sinusitis: 600 mg p.o. q. day for 10 day or 300 mg p.o. q12 hr for 10 day	• Max: 600 mg/day • Adjust dose in renal impairment

(*continued*)

TABLE A2.1 Pediatric Drug Formulary[a,b,c,d] (*Continued*)

Medication	*Dosage*	*Comments*
Cefepime (Maxipime)	150–200 mg/kg/day i.v. div q8 hr; max: 6 g/day	• Adjust dose in renal impairment
Cefotaxime (Claforan)	150–300 mg/kg/day i.v. div q6–8 hr; max: 12 g/day	• Adjust dose in renal impairment
Cefoxitin (Mefoxin)	80–160 mg/kg/day i.v. div q6–8 hr; max: 12 g/day	• Adjust dose in renal impairment
Ceftazidime (Fortaz)	150 mg/kg/day i.v. div q8 hr, max: 6 g/day Cystic fibrosis: 150–200 mg/kg/day i.v. div q8 hr (max: 6 g/day)	• Adjust dose in renal impairment
Ceftriaxone (Rocephin)	50–100 mg/kg/day i.v./i.m. q12–24 hr, max: 4 g/day Postsexual assault (gonorrhea prophylaxis): 125 mg i.m. × 1	• Do not use in infants <14 day or in those with hyperbilirubinemia
Celecoxib (Celebrex)	Adolescents: oral, initial dose 400 mg, followed by an additional 200 mg if needed on day 1; maintenance dose 200 mg twice daily p.r.n.	
Cephalexin (Keflex) ☺	25–100 mg/kg/day p.o. div q.i.d.; max: 4 g/day	
Cetirizine (Zyrtec)	2–5 yr: 2.5–5 mg/day p.o. div q. day–b.i.d. ≥6 yr: 5–10 mg/day p.o. div q. day–b.i.d.	
Charcoal, activated	1 g/kg/dose p.o./n.g. × 1 dose; max: 60 g/dose	• Do not use sorbitol-containing product for repetitive dosing • May repeat dose as necessary (q4–6 hr) for agents with enterohepatic recirculation or bezoar formation • Single dose: 1 g absorbs 100–1,000 mg of poison
Chloral hydrate	Procedural sedation: 50–100 mg/kg/dose p.o./p.r. × 1; may repeat in 30 min with 25–75 mg/kg p.o./p.r. × 1	• Max total dose: 100 mg/kg or 1 g for infants <1 yr, 2 g for children; whichever is less
Chlorothiazide (Diuril)	20–40 mg/kg/day i.v./p.o. div q12 hr	
Ciprofloxacin (Cipro) ☺	20–30 mg/kg/day i.v. div q12 hr; max: 800 mg/day Severe *Pseudomonas aeruginosa*: 30 mg/kg/day i.v. div q12 hr; max: 1.2 g/day 20–30 mg/kg/day p.o. div q12 hr; max: 1.5 g/day Cystic fibrosis: 40 mg/kg/day p.o. div q12 hr; max: 2 g/day	
Cisatracurium (Nimbex)	Children 2–12 yr: initial 0.2 mg/kg i.v., followed by maintenance dose of 0.03 mg/kg i.v. p.r.n. Children >12 yr to adults: initial 0.15–0.2 mg/kg i.v., followed by maintenance dose of 0.03 mg/kg i.v. q40–60 min p.r.n. Continuous infusion 0.1–0.2 mg/kg/hr i.v.	• Reserved for patients with renal dysfunction
Citalopram (Celexa)	Children and adolescents: obsessive compulsive disorder (unlabeled use): 10–40 mg/day p.o.	
Clarithromycin (Biaxin) ☺	15 mg/kg/day p.o. div b.i.d.; max: 1 g/day	
Clindamycin (Cleocin) ☺	25–40 mg/kg/day i.v. div q8 hr, max: 4.8 g/day; 10–30 mg/kg/day p.o. div q8 hr, max: 1.8 g/day	
Clonazepam (Klonopin)	Infants and children <10 yr or 30 kg: • Initial: 0.01–0.03 mg/kg/day (max: 0.05 mg/kg/day) p.o. div b.i.d.–t.i.d.; increase by no more than 0.5 mg every third day until seizures are controlled or adverse effects seen • Maintenance: 0.1–0.2 mg/kg/day p.o. div t.i.d.; not to exceed 0.2 mg/kg/day Children ≥10 yr (>30 kg) and adults: • Initial daily dose not to exceed 1.5 mg p.o. div t.i.d.; may increase by 0.5–1 mg every third day until seizures are controlled or adverse effects seen • Maintenance: 0.05–0.2 mg/kg/day p.o. div t.i.d.; do not exceed 20 mg/day	• Note this is frequently confused with clonidine. Please use caution.

(*continued*)

TABLE A2.1 Pediatric Drug Formulary[a,b,c,d] (*Continued*)

Medication	*Dosage*	*Comments*
Clonidine (Catapres, Duraclon)	Hypertension: oral, initial 5–10 mcg/kg/day p.o. div q8–12 hr; increase gradually, if needed, to 5–25 mcg/kg/day in div doses q6 hr; max dose: 0.9 mg/day ADHD: oral, initial: 0.05 mg/day p.o. q. day, increase q3–7 day by 0.05 mg/day to 3–5 mcg/kg/day p.o. div t.i.d.–q.i.d.; usual max dose: 0.3–0.4 mg/day Clonidine tolerance test (test of growth hormone release from the pituitary): oral, 0.15 mg/m^2 or 4 mcg/kg p.o. as a single dose Analgesia: epidural (continuous infusion), reserved for cancer patients with severe intractable pain, unresponsive to other analgesics or epidural or spinal opiates; initial, 0.5 mcg/kg/hr; adjust with caution, based on clinical effect; do not exceed adult doses Transdermal: children may be switched to the transdermal delivery system after oral therapy is titrated to an optimal and stable dose; a transdermal dose approximately equivalent to the total oral daily dose may be used	• Clonidine patches may be cut if necessary to provide appropriate dose • 8 mcg/kg/day has been used for ADHD • Note this has been confused with clonazepam (Klonopin). Please use caution.
Codeine	0.5–1 mg/kg/dose p.o. q3–4 hr p.r.n.	• Usual adult 30–60 mg/dose
Colistimethate (Coly-Mycin)	Children and adults: 2.5–5 mg/kg/day i.v./i.m. div b.i.d.–q.i.d. Inhalation: 75 mg + 3 mL NS (4 mL total) via nebulizer b.i.d.	• Adjust intravenous dose in renal dysfunction
Corticotropin (Acthar-HP)	Infantile spasms: • 150 units/m^2 i.m. q. day × 2 wk • 30 units/m^2 i.m. q. day × 3 day • 15 units/m^2 i.m. q. day × 3 day • 10 units/m^2 i.m. q. day × 3 day • 10 units/m^2 i.m. q.o.d. × 6 day	• Monitor blood pressure, electrolytes
Cromolyn (Intal)	Nebulization solution: children >2 yr and adults, initial 20 mg q.i.d.; usual dose 20 mg 3–4 times/day Metered spray: • Children 5–12 yr: initial 2 inhalations q.i.d.; usual dose 1–2 inhalations 3–4 times/day • Children ≥12 yr and adults: initial 2 inhalations q.i.d.; usual dose 2–4 inhalations 3–4 times/day Prevention of allergen- or exercise-induced bronchospasm: administer 10–15 min prior to exercise or allergen exposure but no longer than 1 hr before: • Nebulization solution: children >2 yr and adults, single dose of 20 mg • Metered spray: children >5 yr and adults: single dose of 2 inhalations	
Cyclosporine (Neoral, Gengraf, Sandimmune)	Intravenous: • Initial: 5–6 mg/kg/dose i.v. administered 4–12 hr prior to organ transplantation • Maintenance: 2–10 mg/kg/day i.v. in div doses q8–24 hr; patients should be switched to oral cyclosporine as soon as possible Oral: solution or soft gelatin capsule (Sandimmune): • Initial: 14–18 mg/kg/dose p.o. administered 4–12 hr prior to organ transplantation • Maintenance, postoperative: 5–15 mg/kg/day p.o. div q12–24 hr; maintenance dose is usually tapered to 3–10 mg/kg/day Oral: solution or soft gelatin capsule in a microemulsion (Gengraf, Neoral): based on the organ transplant population • Initial: same as the initial dose for solution or soft gelatin capsule	• Brands NOT interchangeable, order must specify brand name • Cyclosporine doses should be adjusted to maintain whole-blood HPLC trough concentrations in the reference range • A 1:1 ratio conversion from Sandimmune to Neoral or Gengraf has been recommended initially; however, lower doses of Neoral or Gengraf may be required after conversion to prevent overdose

(*continued*)

TABLE A2.1 Pediatric Drug Formulary[a,b,c,d] (*Continued*)

Medication	*Dosage*	*Comments*
	OR • Renal: 9 mg/kg/day (range 6–12 mg/kg/day) • Liver: 8 mg/kg/day (range 4–12 mg/kg/day) • Heart: 7 mg/kg/day (range 4–10 mg/kg/day)	
Cyproheptadine Periactin)	Allergic conditions: • Children: 0.25 mg/kg/day or 8 mg/m^2/day p.o. in 2–3 div doses OR • 2–6 yr: 2 mg q8–12 hr (not to exceed 12 mg/day) • 7–14 yr: 4 mg q8–12 hr (not to exceed 16 mg/day) • Adults: 4–20 mg/day div q8 hr (not to exceed 0.5 mg/kg/day) Appetite stimulation (anorexia nervosa): >13 yr, 2 mg p.o. q.i.d.; may be increased gradually over a 3-wk period to 8 mg p.o. q.i.d. Migraine headaches: • Children: 4 mg p.o. b.i.d.–t.i.d. • Adults: 4–8 mg p.o. t.i.d. Spasticity associated with spinal cord damage: ≥12 yr, 4 mg p.o. q.h.s.; increase by 4 mg/dose q3–4 day; average daily dose 16 mg in div doses; not to exceed 36 mg/day	• Reduce dose in patients with significant hepatic dysfunction
Dapsone	Prophylaxis for first episode of opportunistic infection: *Toxoplasma gondii*: children ≥1 mo of age, 2 mg/kg or 15 mg/m^2 (max dose: 25 mg) p.o. once daily in combination with pyrimethamine 1 mg/kg p.o. once daily and leucovorin 5 mg p.o. q3 day Primary and secondary PCP prophylaxis: 2 mg/kg/day p.o. once daily, max dose: 100 mg/day, or 4 mg/kg/dose p.o. once weekly, max dose: 200 mg/dose Leprosy: 1–2 mg/kg/day p.o. given once daily in combination therapy; max dose: 100 mg/day	• Do not use in patients with G6PD deficiency
Desmopressin (DDAVP)	Diabetes insipidus: • Oral: 0.05 mg p.o. b.i.d.; titrate to desired response; range 0.1–1.2 mg p.o. div 2–3 times/day • Intranasal: children 3 mo to ≥12 yr, initial (using 100 mcg/ mL nasal solution) 5 mcg/day (0.05 mL/day) div 1–2 times/day, range 5–30 mcg/day (0.05–0.3 mL/day); children >12 yr and adults, initial (using 100-mcg/mL nasal solution) 5–40 mcg (0.05–0.4 mL) div 1–3 times/day • Intravenous, subcutaneous: children >12 yr and adults, 2–4 mcg/day in 2 div doses or 1/10 of the maintenance intranasal dose Hemophilia: • Intravenous, subcutaneous: children ≥3 mo and adults, 0.3 mcg/kg beginning 30 min before procedure; may repeat dose if needed • Intranasal: children >12 yr and adults, using high-concentration Stimate nasal spray: ≤50 kg: 150 mcg (1 spray) >50 kg: 300 mcg (1 spray each nostril) Nocturnal enuresis: • Intranasal: children ≥6 yr (using 100-mcg/mL nasal solution), initial 20 mcg (0.2 mL) at bedtime, range 10–40 mcg; it is recommended that 1/2 of the dose be given in each nostril • Oral: children >12 yr, 0.2–0.4 mg p.o. once before bedtime	• Adjust morning and evening doses separately for an adequate diurnal rhythm of water turnover • The nasal spray pump delivers doses of 10 mcg (0.1 mL) or multiples thereof; other doses must be given via the rhinal tube • Repeat use of the nasal spray in hemophilia is determined by the patient's clinical condition and laboratory work; if using preoperatively, administer 2 hr before surgery
Dexamethasone (Decadron)	Croup: 0.6 mg/kg/dose i.m./p.o. × 1, max: 10 mg/dose Inflammation: 0.5–2 mg/kg/day i.v./p.o. div q6–8 hr	• Dexamethasone 1 mg = methylprednisolone 5 mg

(*continued*)

TABLE A2.1 Pediatric Drug Formulary[a,b,c,d] (*Continued*)

Medication	*Dosage*	*Comments*
Dextroamphetamine Dexedrine)	ADHD: • <3 yr: not recommended • 3–5 yr: initial, 2.5 mg/day p.o. given every morning; increase by 2.5 mg/day at weekly intervals until optimal response is obtained, usual range is 0.1–0.5 mg/kg/dose every morning with maximum of 40 mg/day given in 1–3 div doses per day • 6 yr: 5 mg p.o. once or b.i.d.; increase in increments of 5 mg/day at weekly intervals until optimal response is reached, usual range is 0.1–0.5 mg/kg/dose every morning (5–20 mg/day) with maximum of 40 mg/day given in 1–3 div doses per day Narcolepsy: • Children 6–12 yr: initial 5 mg/day, may increase at 5-mg increments at weekly intervals until optimal response is obtained; max dose: 60 mg/day • Children >12 yr and adults: initial 10 mg/day, may increase at 10-mg increments at weekly intervals until optimal response is obtained; max dose: 60 mg/day Exogenous obesity: >12 yr and adults, 5–30 mg/day p.o. in div doses of 5–10 mg given 30–60 min before meals	
Dextrose	0.5–1 g/kg i.v./i.o.	• D25W 2–4 mL/kg • D10W 5–10 mL/kg
Diazepam (Valium, Diastat)	Rectal: • Gel, <5 yr: 0.5 mg/kg/dose p.r. q2 hr p.r.n. • Gel, 6–11 yr: 0.3 mg/kg/dose p.r. q2 hr p.r.n. • Gel, ≥12 yr: 0.2 mg/kg/dose p.r. q2 hr p.r.n. • Injection given p.r. 0.5 mg/kg p.r. × 1 Intravenous: 0.05–0.2 mg/kg/dose i.v. q2–4 hr p.r.n., max: 10 mg/dose Oral: 0.1–0.8 mg/kg/day p.o. div q6–8 hr, max: 10 mg/dose	• May use undiluted injectable preparation rectally • Max i.v. 0.6 mg/kg per 8-hr period
Didanosine (Videx)	90–120 mg/m^2/dose p.o. b.i.d.; max: 200 mg/dose	
Digoxin (Lanoxin)	Loading (see note for frequency): Oral: • Neonates: 20–35 mcg/kg p.o. • 1 mo–2 yr: 35–60 mcg/kg p.o. • 2 yr–5 yr: 30–40 mcg/kg p.o. • 5–10 yr: 20–30 mcg/kg p.o. • >10 yr: 10–15 mcg/kg p.o. • Adult: 0.75–1 mg p.o. Intravenous: • Neonates: 15–30 mcg/kg i.v. • 1 mo–2 yr: 30–50 mcg/kg i.v. • 2–5 yr: 25–35 mcg/kg i.v. • 5–10 yr: 15–30 mcg/kg i.v. • >10 yr: 8–12 mcg/kg i.v. • Adult: 0.5–1 mg i.v. Maintenance: Oral: • Neonates: 2.5–5 mcg/kg/dose p.o. b.i.d. • 1 mo–2 yr: 5 mcg/kg/dose p.o. b.i.d. • 2–10 yr: 2.5–5 mcg/kg/dose p.o. b.i.d. • >10 yr: 2.5–5 mcg/kg/dose p.o. q. day • Adult: 0.125–0.25 mg p.o. q. day, max: 0.5 mg/day Intravenous: • Neonates: 2–4 mcg/kg/dose i.v. q12 hr • 1 mo–2 yr: 3.5–6 mcg/kg/dose i.v. q12 hr • 2–10 yr: 3–4 mcg/kg/dose i.v. q12 hr • >10 yr: 2–3 mcg/kg/dose i.v. q24 hr • Adult: 0.1–0.4 mg i.v. q24 hr	• Loading dose should be divided to provide ½ the total dose at initial dose, then give ¼ of the dose at 6- to 12-hr intervals × 2 doses • Adjust dose in renal dysfunction • Dose on lean body weight

(*continued*)

TABLE A2.1 Pediatric Drug Formulary[a,b,c,d] (*Continued*)

Medication	*Dosage*	*Comments*
Diphenhydramine (Benadryl)	1 mg/kg/dose i.v./p.o. q6 hr p.r.n.	• Usual adult 25–50 mg/dose
DoBUTamine	2.5–20 mcg/kg/min i.v.	• Central line preferred
Docusate (Colace) ⊗	5 mg/kg/day p.o. in 1–4 div doses OR • <3 yr: 10–40 mg/day p.o. in 1–4 div doses • 3–6 yr: 20–60 mg/day p.o. in 1–4 div doses • 6–12 yr: 40–150 mg/day p.o. in 1–4 div doses • Adolescents and adults: 50–400 mg/day p.o. in 1–4 div doses	• May use several drops of the liquid in ear canal to remove cerumen buildup
DoPamine	2.5–20 mcg/kg/min i.v.	• If starting in shock state, begin at 10 mcg/kg/min • Central line preferred
Dornase alfa (Pulmozyme)	>5 yr: 2.5 mg/day inhaled q. day–b.i.d.	• Select nebulizers in conjunction with a Pulmo-Aide or a Pari-Proneb compressor • b.i.d. dosing may be beneficial in some patients, especially older than 21 yr or with forced vital capacity >85%
Dronabinol (Marinol)	Antiemetic: 5 mg/m^2/dose p.o. 1–3 hr before chemotherapy, then give 5 mg/m^2/dose p.o. q2–4 hr after chemotherapy for a total of 4–6 doses/day; dose may be increased up to a maximum of 15 mg/m^2 per dose if needed	• Dose may be increased in 2.5 mg/m^2 increments
Doxycycline	2–4 mg/kg/day p.o./i.v. div q12–24 hr; max: 200 mg/day	• Use in patients >8 yr; only exception is treatment of Rocky Mountain spotted fever, pneumonic plague
Efavirenz (Sustiva)	• 10–15 kg: 200 mg p.o. q. day • 15–20 kg: 250 mg p.o. q. day • 20–25 kg: 300 mg p.o. q. day • 25–32.5 kg: 350 mg p.o. q. day • 32.5–40 kg: 400 mg p.o. q. day • 40 kg: 600 mg p.o. q. day Max: 600 mg/day	• Take at bedtime to improve tolerability of CNS side effects
Enalapril (Vasotec)	Initial: 0.1 mg/kg/day p.o. div q. day–b.i.d., titrate up to max 0.5 mg/kg/day Usual adult: 10–40 mg/day p.o. div q. day–b.i.d. Max: 40 mg/day	• Adjust dose in renal dysfunction
Enalaprilat (Vasotec i.v.)	5–10 mcg/kg/dose i.v. q8–12 hr Usual adult: 0.625–1.25 mg i.v. q6 hr Max: 5 mg i.v. q6 hr	• Adjust dose in renal dysfunction • Use caution, note dosing difference from oral preparation.
Enoxaparin (Lovenox)	DVT treatment: • <2 mo = 1.5 mg/kg/dose s.c. q12 hr • ≥2 mo = 1 mg/kg/dose s.c. q12 hr DVT prophylaxis: • <2 mo = 0.75 mg/kg/dose s.c. q12 hr • ≥2 mo = 0.5 mg/kg/dose s.c. q12 hr	• For treatment, check LMWH level 4 hr after dose • Goal, antifactor Xa 0.4–0.6 units/mL
Epinephrine	Intramuscular (1:1,000): 0.01 mL/kg/dose (0.01 mg/kg) s.c./i.m.; max: 0.5 mL/dose Intravenous (1:10,000): 0.1 mL/kg/dose (0.01 mg/kg) i.v./i.o. q3 min Continuous infusion: 0.05–2 mcg/kg/min i.v. Endotracheal tube (1:1,000): 0.1 mL/kg/dose (0.1 mg/kg) ETT q3 min	• Dilute ETT dose in 3–5 mL of NS and follow with several positive-pressure breaths • Central line preferred for continuous infusion
Erythromycin	15–50 mg/kg/day i.v. div q6 hr; max: 4 g/day 30–50 mg/kg/day p.o. div q6 hr; max: 3.2 g/day Prokinetic: • Children: initial 3 mg/kg/dose i.v. infused over 60 min followed by 20 mg/kg/day p.o. in 3–4 div doses before meals, or before meals and at bedtime • Adults: initial 200 mg i.v. followed by 250 mg p.o. t.i.d. 30 min before meals	

(*continued*)

TABLE A2.1 Pediatric Drug Formulary[a,b,c,d] (*Continued*)

Medication	*Dosage*	*Comments*
Erythropoietin alfa (Epogen)	Anemia of prematurity: 25–100 units/kg/dose i.v./s.c. 3 times/wk or 100 units/kg/dose i.v./s.c. 5 times/wk or 200 units/kg/dose q.o.d. for 10 doses Anemia in cancer patients: 150 units/kg/dose i.v./s.c. 3 times/wk; max: 1,200 units/kg/wk Anemia in chronic renal failure: 50–150 units/kg/dose i.v./s.c. 3 times/wk	
Esmolol (Brevibloc)	500 mcg/kg i.v. × 1 over 1 min; then continuous infusion 50 mcg/kg/min i.v. If no response in 4 min, repeat 500 mcg/kg i.v. × 1 over 1 min, then continuous infusion 100 mcg/kg/min i.v. Max: 200 mcg/kg/min	• Some cardiology centers use lower initial doseing (50 mcg/kg/dose x 1)
Ethambutol (Myambutol)	Tuberculosis: 15–25 mg/kg/day p.o. once daily OR 50 mg/kg/dose p.o. twice weekly, not to exceed 2.5 g/dose Nontuberculous mycobacterial infection: 15 mg/kg/day p.o. q. day, not to exceed 1 g/day	
Ethosuximide (Zarontin)	<6 yr: initial 15 mg/kg/dose p.o. div b.i.d., max: 250 mg/dose; titrate q4–7 day; usual maintenance 15–40 mg/kg/day, max: 1.5 g/day >6 yr: initial 250 mg/dose p.o. b.i.d., increase by 250 mg per dose q4-7 day, up to 1.5 g/day	• Give with food • Goal: trough 40–100 mcg/mL
Etomidate (Amidate)	Rapid sequence intubation: 0.3 mg/kg/dose i.v. × 1 dose	• One dose only; not for continuous infusion
Fentanyl (Sublimaze)	1–2 mcg/kg/dose i.v. q1 hr p.r.n. Procedural sedation: 1–2 mcg/kg/dose i.v. × 1 (max: 100 mcg/dose); repeat dose 1 mcg/kg/dose (max: 50 mcg/dose) q3 min p.r.n. sedation; total max 5 mcg/kg	• Usual adult 100 mcg/dose • Adjust dose in renal dysfunction
Ferrous sulfate ☹	Severe iron-deficiency anemia: 4–6 mg elemental iron/kg/day p.o. in 3 div doses Mild-to-moderate iron-deficiency anemia: 3 mg elemental iron/kg/day p.o. in 1–2 div doses Prophylaxis: 1–2 mg elemental iron/kg/day p.o.	• Dose expressed in terms of elemental iron
Filgrastim (Neupogen)	Neonates: 5–10 mcg/kg/day s.c./i.v. once daily for 3–5 day has been administered to neutropenic neonates with sepsis Children and adults: 5–10 mcg/kg/day s.c./i.v. (~150–300 mcg/m^2/day) once daily for up to 14 day until ANC = 10,000/mm^3 Cancer patients receiving bone marrow transplant: 5–10 mcg/kg/day s.c./i.v. administered ≥24 hr after cytotoxic chemotherapy and ≥24 hr after bone marrow infusion	• Dose escalations of 5 mcg/kg/day may be required in some individuals when response at 5 mcg/kg/day is not adequate • If administering i.v., add albumin 2 mg/mL to D5W prior to adding filgrastim
Fluconazole (Diflucan) ☺	Load: 6–12 mg/kg i.v./p.o. × 1 dose Maintenance: 3–12 mg/kg/dose i.v./p.o. q. day Max: 800 mg/day	
Flucytosine (Ancobon)	100–150 mg/kg/day p.o. div q6 hr	• Monitor levels: pre >25 mcg/mL; post 40–60 mcg/mL
Flumazenil (Romazicon)	Benzodiazepine reversal: 0.01 mg/kg/dose i.v., max: 0.2 mg/dose; may repeat p.r.n. to 0.05 mg/kg or 1 mg total, whichever is less	
Fluoxetine (Prozac)	Children 5–18 yr: initial doses of 5–10 mg/day (or 10 mg given 3 times a week) may result in less adverse effects; dose is titrated upward as needed; usual dose 20 mg/day	• Some studies have reported 20–40 mg/day in older children with OCD and Tourette syndrome • Use caution in children, increased risk of suicidal ideation

(*continued*)

TABLE A2.1 Pediatric Drug Formulary[a,b,c,d] (*Continued*)

Medication	*Dosage*	*Comments*
Fluticasone (Flovent, Flonase)	Asthma: Inhalation: • Children ≥4–11 yr: dosing based on previous therapy: Flovent, Diskus, and Rotadisk; bronchodilator alone: recommended starting dose 50 mcg b.i.d.; highest recommended dose 100 mcg b.i.d. Inhaled corticosteroids: recommended starting dose 50 mcg b.i.d.; highest recommended dose: 100 mcg b.i.d.; a higher starting dose may be considered in patients previously requiring higher doses of inhaled corticosteroids • Children 11 yr: dosing based on previous therapy: Flovent, Diskus, and Rotadisk; bronchodilator alone: recommended starting dose 100 mcg b.i.d.; highest recommended dose 500 mcg b.i.d. Inhaled corticosteroids: recommended starting dose 100–250 mcg b.i.d.; highest recommended dose 500 mcg b.i.d.; a higher starting dose may be considered in patients previously requiring higher doses of inhaled corticosteroids Flovent MDI: dosing based on previous therapy Bronchodilator alone: recommended starting dose 88 mcg b.i.d.; highest recommended dose: 440 mcg b.i.d. Inhaled corticosteroids: recommended starting dose 88–220 mcg b.i.d.; highest recommended dose 440 mcg b.i.d.; a higher starting dose may be considered in patients previously requiring higher doses of inhaled corticosteroids Oral corticosteroids: recommended starting dose 880 mcg b.i.d.; highest recommended dose 880 mcg b.i.d.; starting dose is patient dependent; in patients on chronic oral corticosteroids therapy, reduce prednisone dose no faster than 2.5 mg/day on a weekly basis; begin taper after ≥1 wk of fluticasone therapy Rhinitis: intranasal, children ≥4 yr and adolescents: initial 1 spray (50 mcg/spray) per nostril once daily; patients not adequately responding or patients with more severe symptoms may use 2 sprays (100 mcg) per nostril; depending on response, dosage may be reduced to 100 mcg daily; total daily dose should not exceed 2 sprays in each nostril (200 mcg/day); dosing should be at regular intervals	• Titrate to the lowest effective dose once asthma stability is achieved; children previously maintained on Flovent Rotadisk may require dosage adjustments when transferred to Flovent Diskus
Fluticasone/salmeterol (Advair)	Children ≥12 and adults: oral inhalation, one inhalation b.i.d., morning and evening, 12 hr apart Max dose: fluticasone 500 mcg/salmeterol 50 mcg, one inhalation b.i.d.. See package insert for detailed information on transitioning patients from fluticasone or budesonide	• Dosing for <12 yr not approved, although single inhaler products of fluticasone and salmeterol have been used • Advair Diskus is available in 3 strengths, initial dose prescribed should be based on previous asthma therapy • Dose should be increased after 2 wk if adequate response is not achieved
Folic acid	Deficiency: • Infants: 15 mcg/kg/dose i.v./i.m./s.c./p.o. q. day, max: 50 mcg/day • 1–10 yr: 1 mg/day i.v./i.m./s.c./p.o. initial, then 0.1–0.4 mg/day • >11 yr: 1 mg/day i.v./i.m./s.c./p.o. initial, then 0.5 mg/day	• Normal total folate 5–15 ng/mL
Fomepizole (Antizol)	Methanol, ethylene glycol, propylene glycol toxicity: 15 mg/kg i.v. loading dose × 1, then 10 mg/kg/dose i.v. q12 hr; at 48 hr, increase dose to 15 mg/kg/dose i.v. q12 hr; if on hemodialysis, interval should be changed to q6 hr	• Also referred to as 4-MP
Fosphenytoin (Cerebyx)	20 mg PE/kg i.v. load; in status epilepticus run at 3 mg PE/kg/min, max: 150 mg PE/min; then 5–8 mg PE/kg/d i.v./i.m. div q12 hr	• PE = phenytoin equivalents • Hypotension may occur during bolus infusion, slow rate • Trough level: total = 10–20 mcg/mL, free = 0.4–1.4 mcg/mL

(*continued*)

TABLE A2.1 Pediatric Drug Formulary[a,b,c,d] (*Continued*)

Medication	*Dosage*	*Comments*
Furosemide (Lasix)	1 mg/kg/dose i.v./p.o. q6 hr Continuous infusion 0.05–0.1 mg/kg/hr	• Suggested max: 6 mg/kg/day
Gabapentin (Neurontin) ☺	Initial dose 5 mg/kg/day p.o. q. day, usual dose 8–35 mg/kg/day p.o. div t.i.d., max dose up to 90 mg/kg/day (or 3,600 mg/day) has been reported Adult: initial dose 300 mg p.o. q. day, increase by 300 mg each day; usual dose 900–1,800 mg/day p.o. div t.i.d., max dose of 3,600 mg/day has been well tolerated	• Liquid must be refrigerated
Ganciclovir (Cytovene)	10 mg/kg/day i.v. div q12 hr, then may switch to oral: • Children: maintenance dose, prophylaxis of CMV disease in solid-organ transplant patients: oral, 500 mg/m²/dose p.o. q8 hr OR 30 mg/kg/dose q8 hr with food, max: 1,000 mg/dose • Adults: maintenance 1,000 mg p.o. t.i.d. or 500 mg p.o. 6 times/day q3 hr during waking hours	• Follow chemotherapy precautions • Dose adjustment required in renal dysfunction
Gentamicin	• <35 wk GA: <30 day old: 3 mg/kg i.v. q24 hr • ≥35 wk GA: <30 day old: 4 mg/kg i.v. q24 hr • >1 mo–10 yr: 7.5 mg/kg i.v. q24 hr or div q8 hr • >10 yr: 6 mg/kg i.v. q24 hr or div q8 hr	• Check peak/trough with third dose • Exclusions from extended interval program include CrCl <60 mL/min/1.73 m²; febrile neutropenia; cystic fibrosis; endocarditis; patients with rapid fluid shifts • Dose in obese patients based on adjusted body weight: AdjBW = 0.4 × (ABW − IBW) + IBW, where ABW is actual body weight, IBW is ideal body weight
Glycopyrrolate (Robinul)	Secretory control: • Oral: 40–100 mcg/kg/dose p.o. t.i.d.–q.i.d. • Intravenous: 4–10 mcg/kg/dose i.v. t.i.d.–q.i.d.	• May use injectable product orally
Haloperidol (Haldol)	0.025–0.075 mg/kg/dose i.v./i.m. q6 hr; followed by ½ initial dose q2 hr p.r.n.; max: 10 mg/dose	
Heparin	75 units/kg i.v. × 1, then continuous infusion as follows: • <1 yr: 28 units/kg/hr i.v. • ≥1 yr: 20 units/kg/hr i.v.	• Adjust based on heparin levels
Hydralazine (Apresoline)	0.1–0.5 mg/kg/dose i.v. q4–6 hr p.r.n.	• Usual adult 20 mg/dose
Hydrocortisone (Solu-Cortef)	Emergent: 1–2 mg/kg i.v. × 1 Stress dose: 50 mg/m² i.v. × 1, then 50 mg/m²/day i.v. div q6–8 hr Maintenance dose: 10–20 mg/m²/day i.v./p.o. div q6–8 hr	
Hydromorphone (Dilaudid)	Acute pain (moderate to severe): • Children ≥6 mo and <50 kg: Oral: 0.03–0.08 mg/kg/dose p.o. q3–4 hr p.r.n. Intravenous: 0.015 mg/kg/dose i.v. q3–6 hr p.r.n. • Children >50 kg and adults: opiate-naive, 1–2 mg p.o./s.c./i.v. q3–4 hr p.r.n.; usual adult 2 mg, some adults may require 4 mg; patients with prior opiate exposure may require higher initial doses	• Use caution in opiate naïve patients. Use lowest dose possible.
Hydroxyzine (Atarax, Vistaril)	Oral: 2 mg/kg/day p.o. div q6–8 hr p.r.n. Intramuscular: 0.5–1 mg/kg/dose i.m. q4–6 hr p.r.n.	• Has been used intravenously with caution
Hypertonic saline 3%	4 mL/kg i.v. over 20 min if seizing secondary to hyponatremia; continuous infusion 1–2 mL/kg/hr i.v.	• Must be obtained from pharmacy • Ensure gradual correction if nonacute hyponatremia
Ibuprofen (Motrin)	10 mg/kg/dose p.o. q6 hr p.r.n.	• Usual adult 600–800 mg/dose
Imipenem/cilastatin (Primaxin)	• <3 mo: 100 mg/kg/day i.v. div q6 hr • >3 mo: 60–100 mg/kg/day i.v. div q6 hr Max: 4 g/day	
Infliximab (Remicade)	Crohn disease: moderately to severely active: 5 mg/kg i.v. as a single infusion over a minimum of 2 hr Fistulizing: 5 mg/kg i.v. as an infusion over a minimum of 2 hr; dose repeated at 2 and 6 wk after the initial infusion	• Dosing has ranged from 3 to 10 mg/kg i.v. infusion repeated at 4- or 8-wk intervals • Infusion reactions common, may need to premedicate

(*continued*)

TABLE A2.1 Pediatric Drug Formulary[a,b,c,d] (*Continued*)

Medication	*Dosage*	*Comments*
	Rheumatoid arthritis (in combination with methotrexate therapy): 3 mg/kg i.v. followed by an additional 3 mg/kg at 2 and 6 wk after the first dose; then repeat q8 wk thereafter	
Indinavir (Crixivan)	350–500 mg/m^2/dose p.o. t.i.d.; alternatively, adults 800 mg p.o. b.i.d. plus ritonavir booster; max: 800 mg p.o. t.i.d.	• Administer on empty stomach • Adjust dose in hepatic dysfunction
Insulin (regular) (Humulin R)	Acute symptomatic hyperkalemia: 0.1 units/kg i.v./s.c. × 1; DKA: continuous infusion 0.1 units/kg/hr i.v.	• Prime tubing 15 min prior to infusion to ensure adequate dosing • Do not use bolus dosing for DKA
Ipratropium (Atrovent)	Nebulization: • <10 kg: 0.25 mg INH q20 min × 3 doses with albuterol • >10 kg: 0.5 mg INH q20 min × 3 doses with albuterol MDI: • 3–12 yr: 1–2 puffs t.i.d., max: 6 puffs/24 hr • >12 yr: 2 puffs q.i.d., max: 12 puffs/24 hr	• No benefit seen in acute asthma with continuing treatment after initial emergency room doses
Isoniazid	10–20 mg/kg/day p.o. q. day; max: 300 mg/day	• Consider prophylactic pyridoxine therapy
Ketamine (Ketalar)	Procedural sedation: 1–2 mg/kg/dose i.v. × 1 (max: 100 mg/dose), repeat dose 0.5 mg/kg/dose i.v. (max: 50 mg/dose) q2–5 min p.r.n. sedation, max: 5 mg/kg or 500 mg; OR 4–5 mg/kg/dose i.m. with atropine 0.02 mg/kg/dose (min 0.1 mg, max: 0.5 mg) × 1, may repeat ketamine 2 mg/kg i.m. × 1 if inadequate sedation in 10 min Rapid sequence intubation: 0.5–2 mg/kg/dose i.v.; OR 3–7 mg/kg/dose i.m. × 1	• Drug of choice for RSI in status asthmaticus
Ketorolac (Toradol)	• 8–12.5 kg: 4 mg i.v. q6 hr × 24–72 hr • 12.5–25 kg: 7.5 mg i.v. q6 hr × 24–72 hr • >25–50 kg: 15 mg i.v. q6 hr × 24–72 hr • >50 kg: 30 mg i.v. q6 hr × 24–72 hr	• Absolute maximum: 5 day of therapy • p.r.n. orders are not accepted
Labetalol (Normodyne, Trandate)	0.25–1 mg/kg/dose i.v. q4–6 hr, max: 20 mg/dose Continuous infusion 0.25–1 mg/kg/hr, max: 3 mg/kg/hr	
Lactulose	Constipation: • Children: 7.5–15 mL/day p.o. div q. day–b.i.d. • Adults: 15–30 mL/day p.o. div q. day–b.i.d. Max: 60 mL/day	
Lamivudine (Epivir)	4 mg/kg/dose p.o. b.i.d.; max: 150 mg b.i.d.	• Also referred to as 3TC • May be administered with food • Do not use with zidovudine • Adjust dose in renal dysfunction
Lamotrigine (Lamictal)	Not recommended for children <17 kg Regimens containing valproic acid: • Weeks 1 and 2: 0.15 mg/kg/day p.o. in 1–2 doses, round down to nearest 5 mg • Weeks 3 and 4: 0.3 mg/kg/day p.o. in 1–2 doses, round down to nearest 5 mg • After week 4, titrate to effect, increase q1–2 wk by 0.3 mg/kg/day, rounded down to nearest 5-mg dose; usual maintenance 1–5 mg/kg/day in 1–2 doses (max: 200 mg/day) Regimens containing enzyme-inducing AEDs without valproic acid: • Weeks 1 and 2: 0.6 mg/kg/day p.o. div b.i.d., rounded down to nearest 5 mg • Weeks 3 and 4: 1.2 mg/kg/day p.o. div b.i.d., rounded down to nearest 5 mg • After week 4, titrate to effect, increase q1–2 wk by 1.2 mg/kg/day, rounded down to nearest 5 mg; usual maintenance 5–15 mg/kg/day p.o. div b.i.d. (max: 400 mg/day) Dosage, adult and children >12 yr: Regimens containing valproic acid • Weeks 1 and 2: 25 mg p.o. q.o.d. • Weeks 3 and 4: 25 mg p.o. q. day	• Titrate slowly • Educate patients to report appearance of rash immediately

(*continued*)

TABLE A2.1 Pediatric Drug Formulary[a,b,c,d] (*Continued*)

Medication	*Dosage*	*Comments*
	• After week 4, titrate to effect, increase q1–2 wk by 25–50 mg/day; usual maintenance 100–400 mg/day p.o. div b.i.d.; usual dose 100–200 mg/day if on valproic acid ONLY Regimens containing enzyme-inducing AEDs without valproic acid: • Weeks 1 and 2: 50 mg p.o. q. day • Weeks 3 and 4: 100 mg/day p.o. div b.i.d. • After week 4, titrate to effect, increase q1–2 wk by 100 mg/day; usual maintenance 300–500 mg/day p.o. div b.i.d.	
Lansoprazole (Prevacid)	0.5–1.6 mg/kg p.o. q. day GERD, erosive esophagitis: children 1–11 yr: • ≤30 kg: 15 mg p.o. q. day • >30 kg: 30 mg p.o. q. day Duodenal ulcer: children ≥12 yr and adults, 15 mg p.o. q. day for 4 wk; maintenance therapy 15 mg p.o. q. day Primary gastric ulcer (and also associated with NSAID use): children ≥12 yr and adults, 30 mg p.o. q. day for up to 8 wk Pathological hypersecretory conditions: children ≥12 yr and adults, initial 60 mg p.o. q. day; adjust dose based on patient response; doses of 90 mg p.o. b.i.d. have been used; administer doses >120 mg/day in div doses Reflux esophagitis: children ≥12 yr and adults, 30–60 mg p.o. q. day for 8 wk *Helicobacter pylori*-associated antral gastritis: 30 mg p.o. b.i.d. for 2 wk (in combination with 1 g amoxicillin and 500 mg clarithromycin given b.i.d. for 14 day)	• Limited data in children
Levetiracetam (Keppra)	13–30 mg/kg/day p.o. div q. day–b.i.d.; max: 4 g/day 30 mg/kg/dose IV × 1 over 15 min, 10–100 mg/kg/day	• Doses over 300 mg/kg/day have been used
Levonorgesterol (Plan B)	1.5 mg p.o. × 1	• Package includes both tablets and patient instructions
Levothyroxine (Levoxyl, Synthroid)	Oral: • 0–6 mo: 8–10 mcg/kg or 25–50 mcg p.o. q. day • 6–12 mo: 6–8 mcg/kg or 50–75 mcg p.o. q. day • 1–5 yr: 5–6 mcg/kg or 75–100 mcg p.o. q. day • 6–12 yr: 4–5 mcg/kg or 100–150 mcg p.o. q. day • >12 yr: 2–3 mcg/kg or ≥150 mcg p.o. q. day • Growth and puberty complete: 1.6 mcg/kg p.o. q. day	• Conversion to i.v. or i.m.: use 50%–75% of the oral dose
Lidocaine	1-2 mg/kg i.v./i.o. × 1; continuous infusion 20–50 mcg/kg/min i.v./i.o. Prevention of ICP spikes during suctioning: 1 mg/kg via ETT × 1 prior to suctioning	• If giving via endotracheal tube, dose is 2–4 × i.v. dose • Dilute ETT dose in 3–5 mL of NS and follow with several positive-pressure breaths
Linezolid (Zyvox)	• <12 yr: 30 mg/kg/day i.v./p.o. div q8 hr (max: 1.8 g) • >12 yr: 20 mg/kg/day i.v./p.o. div q12 hr (max: 1.2 g)	• Acts as weak MAOi—watch for potential drug–drug and drug–food interactions
Lithium (Eskalith, Lithobid)	15–60 mg/kg/day p.o. div t.i.d.–q.i.d., max: 2.4 g/day If using sustained-release preparation, give total daily dose in two divided doses	• Adjust dose in renal dysfunction • Avoid NSAIDs and thiazide diuretics
Loperamide (Immodium)	Acute diarrhea: Initial doses (in first 24 hr): • 2–5 yr: 1 mg 3 times/day • 6–8 yr: 2 mg b.i.d. • 8–12 yr: 2 mg 3 times/day After initial dosing, 0.1 mg/kg doses after each loose stool, but not exceeding initial dose Chronic diarrhea: 0.08–0.24 mg/kg/day div 2–3 times/day, max: 2 mg/dose Traveler's diarrhea: treat for no more than 2 day: • 6–8 yr: 1 mg after first loose stool followed by 1 mg after each subsequent stool; max: 4 mg/day	

(*continued*)

TABLE A2.1 Pediatric Drug Formulary[a,b,c,d] (*Continued*)

Medication	*Dosage*	*Comments*
	• 9–11 yr: 2 mg after first loose stool followed by 1 mg after each subsequent stool; max: 6 mg/day • 12 yr to adults: 4 mg after first loose stool followed by 2 mg after each subsequent stool; max: 8 mg/day	
Lopinavir/ritonavir (Kaletra)	• 7–15 kg: 12 mg lopinavir/3 mg ritonavir/kg/dose p.o. b.i.d. • 15–40 kg: 10 mg lopinavir/2.5 mg ritonavir/kg/dose p.o. b.i.d. • >40 kg: 400 mg lopinavir/100 mg ritonavir p.o. b.i.d.	• Administer with food • Refrigerate capsules and oral solution
Loratadine (Claritin)	• 2–5 yr: 5 mg p.o. q. day • ≥6 yr: 10 mg p.o. q. day	
Lorazepam (Ativan)	0.05–0.1 mg/kg/dose i.v./p.o. q4–8 hr p.r.n., max: 4 mg/dose Continuous infusion 0.05–0.1 mg/kg/hr i.v. Status epilepticus: 0.1 mg/kg/dose i.v./i.m. q5–15 min × 2–3 doses	• Use caution with continuous infusion and subsequent propylene glycol toxicity
Magnesium sulfate	Asthma: 40 mg/kg i.v. slow over 20 min Torsades de pointes: 25–50 mg/kg/dose i.v. slow Max: 2 g/dose	
Mannitol 20%	0.5–1 g/kg/dose i.v. over 20 min for increased ICP/cerebral edema, then 0.25–1 g/kg/dose i.v. q4–6 hr p.r.n.	• Use filter during administration • Never give as continuous infusion
Megestrol (Megace)	Cachexia: 4–8 mg/kg/day p.o. in 2–4 div doses	• Restricted to infectious disease service
Meropenem (Merrem)	60–120 mg/kg/day i.v. div q8 hr	• Usual course of therapy is 3–6 wk
Mesalamine (Asacol)	Capsules 50 mg/kg/day p.o. div q6–12 hr; tablets 50 mg/kg/day p.o. div q8–12 hr	• Oral products are formulated to slowly release therapeutic quantities of drug throughout the GI tract
Methadone	0.025–0.1 mg/kg/dose i.v. q4–12 hr p.r.n.	• Increase dosing interval after 2–3 doses to prevent accumulation
Methylphenidate (Ritalin, Ritalin XR, Metadate, Concerta)	≥6 yr: 0.3 mg/kg/dose p.o. before breakfast and lunch, max: 5 mg/dose, increase by 0.1 mg/kg/dose every week p.r.n.; usual dose: 0.3–1 mg/kg/day, max: 2 mg/kg/day or 60 mg/day, whichever is less	• Some patients may require t.i.d. dosing • If using sustained-release products, titrate with regular product and convert based on 8-hr increments
Methylprednisolone (SoluMedrol)	Asthma, anti-inflammatory: 2 mg/kg × 1 dose load, then 1 mg/kg/dose i.v. q6–12 hr Pulse therapy: 30 mg/kg/day i.v. for 1–5 day, max 1.5 g/day	• Administer doses >1 g over at least 1 hr
Metoclopramide (Reglan)	0.1–0.2 mg/kg/dose i.v./p.o. q6 hr p.r.n., max: 10 mg/dose High-dose regimen: 1 mg/kg/dose (max: 50 mg/dose) i.v./p.o. q6 hr p.r.n. nausea with acetaminophen overdose or chemotherapy	• If using high-dose regimen, consider adding diphenhydramine
Metolazone (Zaroxolyn)	0.2–0.4 mg/kg/day p.o. div q12–24 hr	
Metronidazole (Flagyl) ☹	30 mg/kg/day i.v./p.o. div q6 hr, max: 4 g/day Postsexual assault: 2 g p.o. × 1 dose	
Midazolam (Versed)	0.05–0.1 mg/kg/dose i.v./i.m. q1–2 hr p.r.n., max: 10 mg/dose Continuous infusion 0.05–0.1 mg/kg/hr i.v. Procedural sedation: • Intravenous: 0.05–0.1 mg/kg/dose i.v. × 1 (max: 2 mg/dose), may repeat q3 min at 0.05 mg/kg (total max: 0.3 mg/kg or 10 mg, whichever is less) • Oral: 0.25–0.75 mg/kg/dose p.o., max: 12 mg/dose • Intranasal: 0.2 mg/kg/dose	
Milrinone (Primacor)	50 mcg/kg i.v. × 1, then 0.25–1 mcg/kg/min i.v.	
Minocycline (Minocin)	>8 yr: 4 mg/kg p.o./i.v. followed by 2 mg/kg/dose p.o./i.v. q12 hr	• Use only in patients >8 yr old
Montelukast (Singulair)	• 2–5 yr: 4 mg/day • 6–14 yr: 5 mg/day • >14 yr: 10 mg/day	

(*continued*)

TABLE A2.1 Pediatric Drug Formulary[a,b,c,d] (*Continued*)

Medication	*Dosage*	*Comments*
Morphine	• <6 mo: 0.05 mg/kg/dose i.v. q2–4 hr p.r.n. • >6 mo: 0.05–0.1 mg/kg/dose i.v. q2 hr p.r.n. Continuous infusion: 0.05–0.1 mg/kg/hr i.v.	• Usual adult 10 mg/dose i.v.
Nalbuphine (Nubain)	Opiate-induced pruritus: 10–20 mcg/kg/dose i.v. q3–6 hr p.r.n. Pain: 0.1–0.15 mg/kg/dose i.v. q3–6 hr p.r.n.	
Nalmefene (Revex)	Opioid reversal: 0.25 mcg/kg/dose i.v. q2 min (max: 40 mcg/dose) to a max of 1 mcg/kg	• Total max dose: 0.5 mg
Naloxone (Narcan)	Opioid reversal: • Full reversal: 0.1 mg/kg/dose i.v./i.m./ETT • Graded reversal: 1–10 mcg/kg/dose i.v./i.m. Max: 2 mg/dose • Continuous infusion for pruritus: 0.25 mcg/kg/hr	If giving via endotracheal tube, dose is 2–10 × i.v. dose • Dilute ETT dose in 3–5 mL of NS and follow with several positive-pressure breaths • Note that higher doses must be used in Suboxone overdoses
Nelfinavir (Viracept)	55 mg/kg/dose p.o. b.i.d.; max: 1,250 mg p.o. b.i.d.	• Administer with food • Powder may be mixed with water, milk, pudding, or formula
Neostigmine (Prostigmin)	Nondepolarizing paralytic reversal: 0.07 mg/kg i.v. × 1; max: 5 mg total	• Premed first with glycopyrrolate 5–15 mcg/kg/ dose i.v.
Nevirapine (Viramune)	Initial: 120 mg/m^2/dose p.o. q. day, then increase to 120 mg/m^2/dose p.o. b.i.d. at 14 day	
Nifedipine (Procardia)	0.25–0.5 mg/kg/dose p.o. q6 hr; max: 10 mg/dose	• Must withdraw liquid from capsule for doses <10 mg
Nitazoxanide	Diarrhea: • 12–47 mo: 100 mg p.o. q12 hr for 3 day • 4–11 yr: 200 mg p.o. q12 hr for 3 day	
Nitrofurantoin (Macrodantin)	5–7 mg/kg/day p.o. div q6 hr; max: 400 mg/day UTI prophylaxis: 1–2 mg/kg/day p.o. q. day, max: 100 mg/day	
Nitroglycerin	0.5–5 mcg/kg/min i.v.	• Check cyanide and thiocyanate levels, especially if dose >4 mcg/kg/min or if used for >3 day
Nitroprusside	0.5–10 mcg/kg/min i.v.	
Norepinephrine (Levophed)	0.05–1 mcg/kg/min i.v.	• Central line preferred
Nortriptyline (Pamelor)	Depression: 1–3 mg/kg/day p.o. div t.i.d.–q.i.d., max: 150 mg/day Nocturnal enuresis: • 20–25 kg: 10 mg p.o. q.h.s. • 25–35 kg: 10–20 mg p.o. q.h.s. • 35–54 kg: 25–35 mg p.o. q.h.s.	• Give 30 min prior to bedtime for nocturnal enuresis • Adjust dose in hepatic insufficiency
Octreotide (Sandostatin)	Bolus: 1–2 mcg/kg i.v./s.c., max: 50 mcg/dose Continuous infusion: 1–2 mcg/kg/hr i.v., max: 50 mcg/hr	
Omeprazole (Prilosec)	1 mg/kg p.o. q. day, may increase to b.i.d.; usual adult 20 mg/day; max: 3.3 mg/kg/day	
Ondansetron (Zofran)	Nononcology nausea and vomiting: • <5 kg: 0.5 mg i.v./p.o. q8 hr p.r.n. • 5–30 kg: 1 mg i.v./p.o. q8 hr p.r.n. • ≥30 kg: 2 mg i.v./p.o. q8 hr p.r.n. Chemotherapy-associated nausea and vomiting: 0.45 mg/kg/day i.v./p.o. q24 hr or div q8 hr	
Oseltamivir (Tamiflu)	Treatment: • <15 kg: 30 mg p.o. b.i.d. • 15–23 kg: 45 mg p.o. b.i.d. • >23–40 kg: 60 mg p.o. b.i.d. • >40 kg: 75 mg p.o. b.i.d.	
Prophylaxis	• <15 kg: 30 mg p.o. q. day • 15–23 kg: 45 mg p.o. q. day • >23–40 kg: 60 mg p.o. q. day • >40 kg: 75 mg p.o. q. day	

(*continued*)

TABLE A2.1 Pediatric Drug Formulary[a,b,c,d] (*Continued*)

Medication	*Dosage*	*Comments*
Oxacillin	150–200 mg/kg/day i.v. div q4–6 hr; max: 12 g/day	• Adjust dose in renal dysfunction
Oxcarbazepine (Trileptal)	20–75 mg/kg/day p.o. div b.i.d.–q.i.d.; max: 5.4 g/day	
Oxybutynin (Ditropan)	0.1–0.2 mg/kg/dose p.o. q6–12 hr; max: 5 mg/dose	
Oxycodone	Immediate release 0.05–0.15 mg/kg/dose p.o. q4–6 hr p.r.n.; usual max: 10 mg/dose	• If using sustained-release OxyContin, divide total daily dose b.i.d.–t.i.d.
Palivizumab (Synagis)	15 mg/kg/dose i.m. every month during RSV season in high-risk patients	• Approval form must be submitted
Pamidronate (Aredia)	0.5–1 mg/kg i.v. q. day for 3 day, may repeat in 4–6- mo intervals	
Pancuronium (Pavulon)	0.1 mg/kg/dose i.v. q1–2 hr p.r.n.; continuous infusion: 0.1 mg/kg/hr i.v.	
Pantoprazole (Protonix)	0.5–1 mg/kg/day i.v./p.o. div q. day–b.i.d.; adult 40 mg i.v. q. day	• Use within 2 hr of reconstitution
Penicillin G (aqueous)	100,000–400,000 unit/kg/day i.v. div q4–6 hr; max: 24 million unit/day	
Penicillin G Benzathine	50,000 unit/kg i.m. × 1; max: 1.2 million unit/dose	• i.m. only
Penicillin VK ⊗	25–50 mg/kg/day p.o. div q6–8 hr; max: 2 g/day	
Pentamidine (Pentam 300)	Treatment of *Pneumocystis carinii* pneumonia: 4 mg/kg/day i.v./i.m. (i.v. preferred) once daily for 14–21 day Prophylaxis for *P. carinii* pneumonia: load 4 mg/kg/dose i.v. daily for 3 day then 4 mg/kg/dose i.v./i.m. q2–4 wk OR Inhalation every month via Respirgard II nebulizer: • Infants <1 yr: 2.27 mg/kg × nebulizer output (L/min) × weight (kg) divided by alveolar ventilation (L/min) • Children <5 yr: some institutions have used a dose of 8 mg/kg INH every month • Children ≥5 yr: 300 mg/dose INH every month Treatment of trypanosomiasis: 4 mg/kg/day i.m. once daily for 10 day Treatment of visceral leishmaniasis: 2–4 mg/kg/day i.m. once daily or q2 day for up to 15 doses	• Aerosolized pentamidine is administered at doses adjusted for min ventilation and weight
Pentobarbital (Nembutal)	Procedural sedation: • Intravenous: 1–2 mg/kg/dose (max: 100 mg/dose) i.v. q5 min until asleep (total max: 6 mg/kg or 300 mg, whichever is less) • Oral: 2–6 mg/kg/dose p.o. × 1	
Phenazopyridine (Pyridium)	12 mg/kg/day p.o. div t.i.d. for 2 day; max: 200 mg/dose	
Phenobarbital	20 mg/kg i.v. load, then 5 mg/kg/day i.v./p.o. div q12–24 hr	• Trough level 15–40 mcg/mL
Phentolamine (Regitine)	Treatment of pressor extravasation: dilute 2.5–5 mg phentolamine in 5–10 mL NS, infiltrate area with approx 1 mL within 12 hr of extravasation, max: 0.1 mg/kg or 2.5 mg, whichever is less Diagnosis of pheochromocytoma: 0.05–0.1 mg/kg/dose i.v. × 1 dose, max: 5 mg/dose	
Phenylephrine (Neosynephrine)	0.1–0.5 mcg/kg/min i.v.	• Central line preferred
Phenytoin (Dilantin)	5–8 mg/kg/day p.o. div q. day–t.i.d.	• Dose individualized based on levels
Phytonadione (vitamin K_1)	1–5 mg/dose s.c. q24 hr × 3 day 2.5–5 mg/dose p.o. q24 hr; may also be given three times per week	• Must be given SLOWLY if using i.v. route
Piperacillin/tazobactam (Zosyn)	200–300 mg/kg/day i.v. div q6 hr Cystic fibrosis: 300–500 mg/kg/day i.v. div q6 hr Max: 18 g as piperacillin/day	• Dosed as piperacillin

(*continued*)

TABLE A2.1 Pediatric Drug Formulary[a,b,c,d] (*Continued*)

Medication	*Dosage*	*Comments*
Potassium chloride	Intravenous: 0.25–1 mEq/kg/dose i.v. over at least 1 hr Oral: 2–5 mEq/kg/day p.o. div b.i.d.–q.i.d.	• PIV max: 80 mEq/L • CVL max: 200 mEq/L • Patient must be placed on CV monitor if >0.25 mEq/kg/hr • Patient must be in intensive care unit if >0.5 mEq/kg/hr • Dilute oral solution prior to administration
Prednisone/ prednisOLone (Deltasone, Prelone, Orapred) ☹	Asthma: 2 mg/kg p.o. × 1, then 2 mg/kg/day p.o. div q12 hr Anti-inflammatory: 0.5–2 mg/kg/day div q. day–q.i.d. Max: 80 mg/dose	• Patients may prefer taste of Orapred, keep refrigerated
Primidone (Mysoline)	10–25 mg/kg/day p.o. div b.i.d.–q.i.d.; max: 2 g/day	• Therapeutic range 5–12 mcg/mL
Procainamide (Procan)	• <1 yr: load 3–7 mg/kg i.v. over 30 min; then 20–80 mcg/kg/min • >1 yr: load 5–15 mg/kg i.v. over 30 min; then 20–80 mcg/kg/min	• Final concentration for maintenance infusion 2–8 mg/mL
Prochlorperazine (Compazine)	0.4 mg/kg/day p.o./p.r. div q6 hr p.r.n., 0.13 mg/kg/dose i.m. q6 hr p.r.n.; max: 10 mg/dose	• Use i.v. with caution
Promethazine (Phenergan)	Antiemetic: 0.25–1 mg/kg p.o./p.r./i.m. q4–6 hr p.r.n.; max: 25 mg/dose	• Use i.v. with caution
Propranolol (Inderal)	Hypertension/arrhythmias: Oral: • Neonates: 0.25 mg/kg/dose p.o. q6–8 hr • Children: initial: 0.5–1 mg/kg/day p.o. div q6–8 hr; maintenance 1–5 mg/kg/day p.o. div q6–8 hr Intravenous: • Neonates: 0.01 mg/kg/dose i.v. q6–8 hr p.r.n. (max: 1 mg/dose) • Children: 0.01–0.1 mg/kg/dose i.v. q6–8 hr p.r.n. (max: 3 mg/dose) Migraine headache prophylaxis: 0.6–1.5 mg/kg/day p.o. div q8 hr, max: 4 mg/kg/day	
Pseudoephedrine (Sudafed)	• <2 yr: 1 mg/kg/dose p.o. q6 hr p.r.n. • 2–5 yr: 15 mg p.o. q6 hr p.r.n. • 6–12 yr: 30 mg p.o. q6 hr p.r.n. • >12 yr: 60 mg p.o. q6 hr p.r.n.	
Pyrazinamide	20–30 mg/kg/day p.o. q. day; max: 2 g/day	
Racemic epinephrine (Vaponefrin)	2.25% inhalation solution: 0.25 mL (<5 kg), 0.5 mL (>5 kg) INH q1 hr p.r.n.	• May use epinephrine injection equivalent dose: racemic epinephrine 10 mg = L-epinephrine 5 mg
Ranitidine (Zantac) ☹	3 mg/kg/day i.v. div q8 hr, max 180 mg/day; 4–6 mg/kg/day p.o. div q12 hr, max 300 mg/day; continuous infusion 0.15 mg/kg/hr i.v.	
Rifabutin (Mycobutin)	*Mycobacterium avium* complex (MAC): 5–6 mg/kg/day p.o. q. day (max: 75 mg/day) Prophylaxis for first episode of MAC in human immunodeficiency virus (HIV)-infected patients: • Children <6 yr: 5 mg/kg once daily • Children ≥6 yr: 300 mg once daily Prophylaxis for recurrence of MAC in HIV-infected patients: 5 mg/kg p.o. once daily (max: 300 mg/day) in combination with clarithromycin	• Limited studies in children • In patients who experience GI upset, rifabutin can be administered 150 mg b.i.d. with food
Rifampin (Rifadin)	10–20 mg/kg/day p.o. div q. day–b.i.d.; max: 1.2 g/day	
Risperidone (Risperdal)	Pervasive developmental disorder (unlabeled use): initial 0.25 mg b.i.d.; titrate up to 0.25 mg/day q5–7 day; optimal dose range 0.75–3 mg/day Autism (unlabeled use): initial 0.25 mg q.h.s.; titrate to 1 mg/day (0.1 mg/kg/day) Schizophrenia: initial 0.5 mg b.i.d.; titrate as necessary up to 2–6 mg/day	

(*continued*)

TABLE A2.1 Pediatric Drug Formulary[a,b,c,d] (*Continued*)

Medication	*Dosage*	*Comments*
	Bipolar disorder (unlabeled use): initial 0.5 mg; titrate to 0.5–3 mg/day Tourette disorder (unlabeled use): initial 0.5 mg; titrate to 2–4 mg/day	
Ritonavir (Norvir) ☹	350–450 mg/m^2/dose p.o. b.i.d.; booster dose 100–200 mg/ m^2/dose p.o. b.i.d.; max: 600 mg/dose b.i.d.	• Administer with food • Oral solution may be mixed with milk, pudding, or formula
Rocuronium (Zemuron)	Rapid sequence intubation: 0.6–1.2 mg/kg/dose i.v./i.m. × 1 dose	• Use higher end of dosing range if giving i.m.
Salmeterol (Serevent)	• >4 yr: MDI 42 mcg (2 puffs) inhaled q12 hr • >4 yr: Diskus 50 mcg (1 puff) inhaled q12 hr	• NOT for rescue therapy
Saquinavir (Fortovase)	50 mg/kg/dose p.o. t.i.d. If in combination with nelfinavir: 33 mg/kg/dose p.o. t.i.d. Max: 1,200 mg/dose t.i.d.	• Administer with food • Sun exposure may cause photosensitivity reactions
Sertraline (Zoloft)	• 6–12 yr: initial 25 mg/day p.o. q. day, titrate at weekly intervals until effect, max: 200 mg/day • >12 yr: initial 50 mg/day p.o. q. day, titrate at weekly intervals until effect, max: 200 mg/day	• Use caution in children, increased risk of suicidal ideation
Sirolimus	• ≥13 yr, <40 kg: loading dose 3 mg/m^2 (day 1), followed by a maintenance of 1 mg/m^2/day • Adults ≥40 kg: loading dose: for de novo transplant recipients, a loading dose of 3 times the daily maintenance dose should be administered on day 1 of dosing; maintenance dose 2 mg/day; doses should be taken 4 hr after cyclosporine, and should be taken consistently either with or without food	• Adjust dose in hepatic impairment
Sodium bicarbonate	1 mEq/kg = 1 mL/kg i.v./i.o. slow Tumor lysis syndrome: D5W with 75 mEq/L sodium bicarbonate at 125 mL/m^2/hr to maintain urine pH 7–8 and SG ≤ 1.010	• Use 0.5 mEq/mL concentration for neonates
Sodium chloride	Maintenance: • Premature neonates: 2–8 mEq/kg/day p.o./i.v. div q. day–t.i.d. • Term neonates: 1–4 mEq/kg/day p.o./i.v. div q. day–t.i.d. • Children: 3–4 mEq/kg/day p.o./i.v. div q. day–t.i.d. Severe hyponatremia: see hypertonic saline	
Sodium polystyrene (Kayexalate)	1 g/kg/dose (max: 15 g/dose) p.o. q6 hr OR 1 g/kg/dose (max: 50 g/dose) p.r. q2–6 hr	Avoid sorbitol containing preparations for the PR route
Spironolactone (Aldactone)	1–3 mg/kg/day p.o. div q12–24 hr	
Stavudine (Zerit)	• <30 kg: 1 mg/kg/dose p.o. b.i.d. • 30–59 kg: 30 mg p.o. b.i.d. • >60 kg: 40 mg p.o. b.i.d. Max: 40 mg b.i.d.	• May be administered with food
Succinylcholine (Quelicin)	Rapid-sequence intubation: 1–2 mg/kg/dose i.v. × 1 dose; 3–4 mg/kg/dose i.m. × 1 dose; max: 150 mg/dose	• Premed with atropine <7 yr • Use 2 mg/kg/dose i.v. if <1 yr • Contraindicated in hyperkalemia, myopathies, "old" trauma
Sucralfate (Carafate)	40–80 mg/kg/day p.o. div q6 hr; max: 1 g/dose	• Dose based on trimethoprim (TMP) component
Sulfamethoxazole/ trimethoprim (Bactrim)	8–20 mg TMP/kg/day i.v./p.o. div q6–12 hr Treatment of *P. carinii* pneumonia: 20 mg TMP/kg/day i.v. div q6 hr	
Tacrolimus (Prograf, Protopic)	Oral: 0.15–0.3 mg/kg/day p.o. div q12 hr Intravenous: 0.05–0.15 mg/kg/day i.v. continuous infusion Topical: 0.03% ointment applied b.i.d.	• Oral dose conversion is 4–5 times the i.v. dose • Titrate to levels of 5–10 ng/mL in stem cell transplant • Children require higher doses than adults

(*continued*)

TABLE A2.1 Pediatric Drug Formulary[a,b,c,d] (Continued)

Medication	*Dosage*	*Comments*
Tenofovir (Viread)	• 10–20 kg: 75 mg p.o. q. day • 21–35 kg: 150 mg p.o. q. day • 36–50 kg: 225 mg p.o. q. day • >50 kg: 300 mg p.o. q. day	• Take with meals • Give 1 hr prior to or 2 hr after didanosine
Terbutaline (Brethine)	10 mcg/kg i.v./s.c. × 1, then 0.4–6 mcg/kg/min i.v.	• Suggested max total β_2-agonist dose = 20 mg/hr
Tetracycline	>8 yr: 25–50 mg/kg/day p.o. div q6 hr; max: 3 g/day	• For patients >8-yr-old
Thiamine (vitamin B_1)	Neonatal seizures: 100 mg i.v. × 1 dose Mitochondrial defect: 100–200 mg p.o. q. day	
Thiopental (Pentothal)	Rapid-sequence intubation: 4–6 mg/kg/dose i.v. × 1 dose	• Hypotension common, do not use in hypovolemic/hypotensive patients
Tiagabine (Gabatril)	Initial dose 0.1 mg/kg/day p.o. (max: 4 mg/dose) q. day for 1 wk; then increase by 0.1 mg/kg/day (max: 4 mg) for wk 2, then by 0.1–0.2 mg/kg/day (max 8 mg) weekly thereafter; titrate to effect Usual dose is 0.3–1.25 mg/kg/day p.o. div t.i.d.; max dose: 32 mg/day Adult: initial dose 4 mg/day p.o. q. day for 1 wk; then increase by 4–8 mg/day each week div b.i.d.–q.i.d., titrate to response; max dose: 56 mg/day	• t.i.d. dosing may be better tolerated
Tobramycin (Nebcin)	See gentamicin TOBI nebs: 300 mg INH b.i.d. Cystic fibrosis: 10–12 mg/kg/day i.v. div q8–12 hr	• Cystic fibrosis patients require higher dosing • Individualize dose based on levels and MIC of organism
Topiramate (Topamax)	Initial dose 0.5–1 mg/kg/day p.o. div b.i.d. for 1 wk; then increase by 0.5–1 mg/kg/day each week; titrate to effect Adult: initial dose 50 mg/day p.o. q. day for 1 wk; then 100 mg/day p.o. div b.i.d. for 1 wk, increase by 50 mg/day each week, titrate to response Usual dose 200 mg p.o. b.i.d.; max dose: 1,600 mg/day	Usual minimally effective dose is 6 mg/kg/day div b.i.d.; doses as high as 50 mg/kg/day have been used in children receiving other enzyme-inducing AEDs
Ursodiol (Actigall)	Biliary atresia: 10–15 mg/kg/day p.o. q. day TPN-induced cholestasis: 30 mg/kg/day p.o. div t.i.d. Cystic fibrosis: 30 mg/kg/day p.o. div q. day–t.i.d. Max: 300 mg/dose	• Use oral suspension formulation without sorbitol to avoid diarrhea
Valacyclovir (Valtrex)	Treatment (not prophylaxis): 45–50 mg/kg/day p.o. div t.i.d.; max: 3 g/day	
Valganciclovir (Valcyte)	• <15 kg: induction 15 mg/kg/dose p.o. b.i.d. for approximately 14 day; maintenance 15 mg/kg/dose p.o. q. day • >15 kg: induction: 500 mg/m^2/dose p.o. b.i.d. for approximately 14 day; maintenance 500 mg/m^2/dose p.o. q. day	
Valproic acid (Depacon, Depakote, Depakene)	20 mg/kg i.v./p.o. load × 1 dose Initial: 15 mg/kg/day i.v. div q6 hr; 15 mg/kg/day p.o. div q8 hr Usual range: 20–100 mg/kg/day in div doses	• In status epilepticus, administer at 5 mg/kg/min • Routine i.v. doses, administer over 1 hr • May require up to 100 mg/kg/day if on enzyme-inducing AEDs • Desired trough 50–100 mcg/mL • May add carnitine for liver protection with high doses
Vancomycin ⊗	40–60 mg/kg/day i.v. div q6–8 hr Use 60 mg/kg/day i.v. div q6 hr for CNS infection Antibiotic-associated pseudomembranous colitis: • Children: 40 mg/kg/day p.o. in div doses q6 hr for 7–10 day; not to exceed 2 g/day • Adults: 0.5–2 g/day p.o. in div doses q6–8 hr	• Usual adult dose 2 g/day i.v. div q12 hr • Check trough with third dose, trough 5–15 mcg/mL • Adjust dose in renal dysfunction

(*continued*)

TABLE A2.1 Pediatric Drug Formulary[a,b,c,d] (*Continued*)

Medication	*Dosage*	*Comments*
Vasopressin (Pitressin)	Diabetes insipidus: 0.5 milliunit/kg/hr i.v., double dose q30 min p.r.n. to effect (UO < 2 mL/kg/hr) to max 10 milliunit/kg/hr GI bleed: 2–5 milliunit/kg/min i.v., titrate as needed; once no bleeding × 12 hr taper off over 24–48 hr	
Vecuronium (Norcuron)	0.1 mg/kg/dose i.v. q1 hr p.r.n. Continuous infusion 0.05–0.07 mg/kg/hr i.v. Rapid-sequence intubation 0.3 mg/kg i.v. × 1 dose× 1 dose	• Not routinely used for RSI due to long duration of effect
Voriconazole (Vfend)	Loading dose 12 mg/kg/day p.o./i.v. div q12 hr for 1 day, then 6–8 mg/kg/day p.o./i.v. div q12 hr; max: 600 mg/day	• Do not use i.v. formulation in patients with CrCl <50 mL/min/1.73 m^2
Warfarin (Coumadin)	Load on day 1: 0.2 mg/kg p.o. × 1 (max: 10 mg); further loading and maintenance dosing based on INR; usual maintenance 0.1 mg/kg/day with great variation	• Counsel patients on drug–food interactions
Zalcitabine (Hivid)	0.005–0.02 mg/kg/dose p.o. t.i.d.; max: 0.75 mg t.i.d.	• Also referred to as dDC • Administer on empty stomach • Adjust dose in renal dysfunction
Zidovudine (Retrovir)	Neonates: 2 mg/kg/dose p.o. q.i.d. OR 1.5 mg/kg/dose i.v. q6 hr Children: 160 mg/m^2/dose p.o. t.i.d. OR 120 mg/m^2/dose i.v. q6 hr Max: oral 200 mg/dose t.i.d. Continuous infusion 20 mg/m^2/hr i.v.	• Also referred to as AZT • May be administered with food • Adjust dose in severe renal and hepatic dysfunction
Zonisamide (Zonegran)	Initial 2–4 mg/kg/day p.o. div q. day–t.i.d.; usual 4–8 mg/kg/day p.o. div q. day–t.i.d. recommended max is 12 mg/kg/day Adult: initial 100–200 mg/day p.o. div q. day–t.i.d. (titrate to 200–400 mg/day over 2 wk) Max dose: 600 mg/day	• Studies have used up to 20 mg/kg/day for infantile spasms

[a]☹, poor palatability; ☺, excellent palatability.
[b]i.o., intraosseous; i.m., intramuscular; i.v., intravenous; n.g., nasogastric; p.o., oral; p.r., rectal: s.c., subcutaneous.
[c]b.i.d., twice daily; div, divided; p.r.n., as needed; q, every; q. day, daily; q.h.s., at bedtime; q.i.d., four times a day; q.o.d., every other day; t.i.d., thrice daily.
[d]ADHD, attention deficit and hyperactivity disorder; AED, antiepileptic drug; ANC, absolute neutrophil count; CMV, cytomegalovirus; CNS, central nervous system; CrCl, creatinine clearance; CV, cardiovascular; CVL, central venous line; DVT, deep vein thrombosis; D5W, dextrose 5% in water; D10W, dextrose 10% in water; D25W, dextrose 25% in water; ESRD, end-stage renal disease; ETT, endotracheal tube; GA, gestational age; GABHS, group A beta-hemolytic streptococcus; GERD, gastroesophageal reflux disease; GI, gastrointestinal; HPLC, high powered liquid chromatography; ICP, intracranial pressure; ID, infectious disease; INH, inhaled; INR, international normalized ratio; IVF, intravenous fluid; LMWH, low-molecular-weight heparin; MAOi, monoamine oxidase inhibitor; MDI, metered dose inhaler; MIC, minimum inhibitory concentration; NS, normal saline; NSAIDs, nonsteroidal anti-inflammatory drugs; OCD, obsessive compulsive disorder; PaO_2, partial pressure of oxygen in arterial blood; PALS, pediatric advanced life support; PCP, *Pneumocystis Carinii* pneumonia; PIV, peripheral intravenous (line, catheter); PSVT, paroxysmal supraventricular tachycardia; RDS, respiratory distress syndrome; RSI, rapid sequence intubation; RSV, respiratory syncytial virus; SCI, spinal cord injury; SG, specific gravity; SVT, supraventricular tachycardia; TMP, trimethoprim; TPN, total parenteral nutrition; UO, urine output; UTI, urinary tract infection; VF/VT, ventricular fibrillation/ventricular tachycardia.

Index

Index

Note: Page numbers followed by f indicate figure; those followed by t indicate table.

D

I

J

K

L